AF710863

SURGICAL INFECTIOUS DISEASES

— *Third Edition* —

Richard J. Howard, MD
Professor
Department of Surgery
University of Florida
Gainesville, Florida

Richard L. Simmons, MD
Chairman
Department of Surgery
University of Pittsburgh
Pittsburgh, Pennsylvania

APPLETON & LANGE
Norwalk, Connecticut

Notice: The authors and the publisher of this volume have taken care to make certain that the doses of drugs and schedules of treatment are correct and compatible with the standards generally accepted at the time of publication. Nevertheless, as new information becomes available, changes in treatment and in the use of drugs become necessary. The reader is advised to carefully consult the instruction and information material included in the package insert of each drug or therapeutic agent before administration. This advice is especially important when using new and infrequently used drugs. The publisher disclaims any liability, loss, injury, or damage incurred as a consequence, directly or indirectly, of the use and application of any of the contents of this volume.

Copyright © 1995 by Appleton & Lange
A Simon & Schuster Company
Copyright © 1988 by Appleton & Lange
Copyright © 1982 by Appleton-Century-Crofts

All rights reserved. This book, or any parts thereof, may not be used or reproduced in any manner without written permission. For information, address Appleton & Lange, 25 Van Zant Street, East Norwalk, Connecticut 06855.

95 96 97 98 99 / 10 9 8 7 6 5 4 3 2 1

Prentice Hall International (UK) Limited, *London*
Prentice Hall of Australia Pty. Limited, *Sydney*
Prentice Hall Canada, Inc., *Toronto*
Prentice Hall Hispanoamericana, S.A., *Mexico*
Prentice Hall of India Private Limited, *New Delhi*
Prentice Hall of Japan, Inc., *Tokyo*
Simon and Schuster Asia Pte. Ltd., *Singapore*
Editora Prentice Hall do Brasil Ltda., *Rio de Janeiro*
Prentice Hall, *Englewood Cliffs, New Jersey*

Library of Congress Cataloging-in-Publication Data

Surgical infectious diseases / [edited by] Richard J. Howard, Richard L. Simmons. — 3rd ed.
p. cm.
Includes bibliographical references and index.
ISBN 0-8385-8754-2
1. Surgical wound infections. I. Howard, Richard J.
II. Simmons, Richard L., 1934–
[DNLM: 1. Surgical Wound Infection. WO 185 S9617 1994]
RD98.3.S953 1994
617′.01—dc20
DNLM/DLC 94-20995
for Library of Congress CIP

Production Editor: Elizabeth C. Ryan
Production Service: Spectrum Publisher Services
Designer: Penny Kindzierski
Cover: Mary Skudlarek

ISBN 0-8385-8754-2

PRINTED IN THE UNITED STATES OF AMERICA

Contents

Contributors

George L. Adams, MD
Professor and Head
Department Otolaryngology
University of Minnesota
Minneapolis, Minnesota

Augusto Aguirre, MD
Senior Attending Pathology Staff
Riverside Methodist Hospitals
Clinical Assistant Professor of Pathology
College of Medicine, Ohio State University
Columbus, Ohio

David H. Ahrenholz, MD
Associate Director, The Burn Center
Ramsey Medical Center
St. Paul, Minnesota
Assistant Professor
Department of Surgery
University of Minnesota
St. Paul, Minnesota

Daniel B. Allen, MD
Senior Resident in General Surgery
University of California Davis–East Bay
Research Fellow, Department of Surgery
University of California–San Francisco
San Francisco, California

Raymond A. Amoury, MD
Surgeon-in-Chief, The Children's Mercy Hospital
Kansas City, Missouri
Katharine Berry Richardson Professor of Pediatric Surgery
University of Missouri
Kansas City School of Medicine
Clinical Professor of Surgery
Creighton University School of Medicine
Omaha, Nebraska
Consultant in Surgery
Truman Medical Center and St. Luke's Hospital
Kansas City, Missouri

Louis H. Aulick, PhD
Professor, Department of Physiology
Marshall University School of Medicine
Huntington, West Virginia

Henry H. Balfour, Jr., M.D.
Professor of Laboratory Medicine, Pathology and Pediatrics
University of Minnesota Medical Sciences Center
Minneapolis, Minnesota

Perry Black, MD
Hahnemann University Hospital
Professor and Chairman, Department of Neurosurgery
Hahnemann University
Philadelphia, Pennsylvania

Itzhak Brook, MD, MSc
Consultant, Infectious Diseases
Naval Hospital
Bethesda, Maryland
Consultant, Infectious Diseases
Hospital for Sick Children
Georgetown University Medical Center
Washington, DC
Professor of Pediatrics
Georgetown University School of Medicine
Washington, DC

Steve E. Calvano, PhD
Associate Professor of Surgery
Cornell University Medical College
New York, New York

Michael E. Carey, MD
Professor of Neurosurgery
Louisiana State Medical School
New Orleans, Louisiana

Frank B. Cerra, MD
Director, Critical Care and Clinical Nutrition
University Hospital
Professor of Surgery
University of Minnesota
Minneapolis, Minnesota

Robert E. Condon, MD
Chairman, Department of Surgery
Medical College of Wisconsin/Froedtert Memorial Lutheran Hospital/Milwaukee County Medical Complex
Ausman Foundation Professor
Medical College of Wisconsin
Milwaukee, Wisconsin

Timothy P. Connall
Surgical Research Fellow
Department of Surgery
University of California, Irvine Medical Center
Orange, California

A. Benedict Cosimi, MD
Chief, Transplantation Unit
Massachusetts General Hospital
Claude E. Welch Professor of Surgery
Harvard Medical School
Boston, Massachusetts

Scott F. Davies, MD
Director, Pulmonary and Critical Care Medicine
Hennepin County Medical Center
Associate Professor
University of Minnesota School of Medicine
Minneapolis, Minnesota

Steve H. Dougherty, MD
Director, Surgical Infectious Diseases
R. E. Thomason Hospital
Associate Professor of Surgery and Microbiology
Texas Tech University, Regional Academic Health Center at El Paso
El Paso, Texas

David L. Dunn, MD, PhD
Head, Surgical Infectious Diseases
University of Minnesota Hospital and Clinic
Professor of Surgery
University of Minnesota
Minneapolis, Minnesota

Richard F. Edlich, MD, PhD
Distinguished Professor of Plastic Surgery and Biomedical Engineering
University of Virginia School of Medicine
Charlottesville, Virginia

Thomas J. Enright, MD
Assistant Consulting Professor of Surgery
Duke University Medical Center
Consultant Veterans Affairs Medical Center
Asheville, North Carolina

Sydney M. Finegold, MD
Staff Physician, Medical Service
VA Medical Center West Los Angeles
Professor of Medicine
Professor of Microbiology and Immunology
UCLA School of Medicine
Los Angeles, California

Mitchell P. Fink, MD
Chief, Division of Trauma and Critical Care
Beth Israel Hospital
Associate Professor of Surgery
Harvard Medical School
Boston, Massachusetts

Robert H. Fitzgerald, Jr., MD
Professor and Chairman
Department of Orthopedic Surgery
Wayne State University School of Medicine
Detroit, Michigan

Wesley Furste, MD
Honorary Surgical Staff
Riverside Methodist Hospitals
Grant Medical Center
Clinical Professor of Surgery, Emeritus
College of Medicine, Ohio State University
Columbus, Ohio

Julio Garcia-Aguilar, MD
Resident
Division of Colon and Rectal Surgery
Clinical Resident, Department of Surgery
University of Minnesota
St. Paul, Minnesota

Hugh A. Gelabert, MD
Assistant Professor of Surgery
UCLA School of Medicine
Los Angeles, California

Dale N. Gerding, MD
Chief, Medical Service
VA Lakeside Medical Center
Professor and Associate Chairman, Department of Medicine
Northwestern University
Chicago, Illinois

Gary W. Gibbons, MD
Clinical Chief, Division of Vascular Surgery
New England Deaconess Hospital
Associate Clinical Professor of Surgery
Harvard Medical School
Boston, Massachusetts

Toni Hau, MD, PhD
Chief of General Surgery
Nordwest-Krankenhaus Sanderbusch
Privat-Dozent
Medizinische Hochschule Hannover
Sande, Germany

David N. Herndon, MD
Chief of Staff
Shriners Burns Institute
Jesse H. Jones Distinguished Professor of Burn Surgery
University of Texas Medical Branch
Galveston, Texas

Monto Ho, MD
Director, Clinical Microbiology
University of Pittsburgh Medical Center
Professor of Medicine, Microbiology, and Pathology
University of Pittsburgh
Pittsburgh, Pennsylvania

Richard J. Howard, MD
Professor
Department of Surgery
University of Florida
Gainesville, Florida

Thomas K. Hunt, MD
Director, Wound Healing Laboratory
University of California San Francisco Medical Center
Professor
University of California–San Francisco
San Francisco, California

Sandra S. Kaplan, MD
Medical Director, Hematology Laboratory
Presbyterian University Hospital
Professor of Pathology
University of Pittsburgh School of Medicine
Pittsburgh, Pennsylvania

Patrick J. Kelly, MD
Orthopedic Surgeon, Emeritus
Mayo Clinic
Professor of Orthopaedic Surgery, Retired
Mayo Clinic and Mayo Medical School
Rochester, Minnesota

Ernst Klar, MD
Assistant Professor of Surgery
University of Heidelberg
Heidelberg, Germany

David R. Knighton, MD
Medical Director
Institute for Reparative Medicine
Clinical Associate Professor
University of Minnesota
St. Louis Park, Minnesota

Daniel V. Landers, MD
Associate Professor Obstetrics, Gynecology, and Reproductive Science
San Francisco General Hospital
San Francisco, California

James T. Lee, Jr., MD, PhD, FACS
Associate Professor of Surgery
University of Minnesota
Associate Chief of Surgery
VA Medical Center
Minneapolis, Minnesota

William Lineaweaver, MD
Associate Professor
Division of Plastic Surgery and Division of Hand Surgery
Stanford University Medical Center
Stanford, California

Pamela A. Lipsett, MD
Assistant Professor
Department of Surgery
Johns Hopkins Medical Institutions
Baltimore, Maryland

Michael T. Lotze, MD
Chief, Section of Surgical Oncology
University of Pittsburgh Medical Center
Professor of Surgery, Molecular Genetics, and Biochemistry
University of Pittsburgh
Pittsburgh, Pennsylvania

Stephen F. Lowry, MD
Attending Surgeon
New York Hospital
Professor of Surgery
Cornell University Medical Center
New York, New York

Mark A. Malangoni, MD
Chairperson
Department of Surgery, MetroHealth Campus
MetroHealth Medical Center
Professor and Vice Chairman
Department of Surgery
Case Western Reserve University School of Medicine
Cleveland, Ohio

William J. Martin, PhD
Director of Microbiology, Immunology, and Virology
Associated Clinical Laboratories
Clinical Pathology Institute
Erie, Pennsylvania

Susan A. McCarthy, PhD
Assistant Professor
Departments of Surgery and Molecular Genetics and Biochemistry
University of Pittsburgh School of Medicine
Pittsburgh, Pennsylvania

Thomas M. McCormack, MD
Senior Instructor
Division of Neurosurgery
Hahnemann University
Philadelphia, Pennsylvania

Jonathan L. Meakins, MD
Chief of Surgery
Royal Victoria Hospital
Edward W. Archibald Professor of Surgery
McGill University
Montreal, Quebec
Canada

Lee S. Monroe, MD
Senior Consultant in Gastroenterology
Scripps Clinic and Research Foundation
Clinical Professor of Medicine
University of California
San Diego, California

Wesley S. Moore, MD
Professor of Surgery
Chief, Section of Vascular Surgery
UCLA School of Medicine
Los Angeles, California

A. B. Nathens, MD
Resident, General Surgeon
Department of Surgery
University of Toronto
Toronto, Ontario
Canada

Thuan T. Nguyen, MD
Clinical Burn Fellow
Shriners Burns Institute
Galveston, Texas

Phillip K. Peterson, MD
Professor of Medicine
University of Minnesota Medical School
Director, Infectious Diseases
Hennepin County Medical Center
Minneapolis, Minnesota

Henry A. Pitt, MD
Professor of Surgery
The Johns Hopkins Hospital
Baltimore, Maryland

Reuben Ramphal, MD
Associate Professor
Division of Infectious Diseases
Department of Medicine
Gainesville, Florida

Kenneth H. Rand, MD
Associate Professor of Pathology and Medicine
University of Florida
Gainesville, Florida

James A. Roberts, MD
Head, Department of Urology
Tulane Regional Primate Research Center
Professor and Associate Chairman (Research)
Tulane University School of Medicine
Covington, Louisiana

George T. Rodeheaver
R. F. Edlich Research Professor of Plastic Surgery
University of Virginia School of Medicine
Charlottesville, Virginia

David A. Rothenberger, MD, FACS
Chief, Division of Colon and Rectal Surgery
Clinical Professor
Department of Surgery
University of Minnesota
St. Paul, Minnesota

Ori Rotstein, MD
Associate Professor of Surgery
Toronto General Hospital
Toronto, Ontario
Canada

Robert H. Rubin, MD
Chief of Transplant Infectious Disease
Massachusetts General Hospital
Director, Center for Experimental Pharmacology and Therapeutics
Harvard–M.I.T. Division of Health Sciences and Technology
Associate Professor of Medicine
Harvard Medical School
Boston, Massachusetts

Randi L. Rutan, RN, BSN
Research Nurse/Clinical Data Coordinator
Shriners Burns Institute
Galveston, Texas

George A. Sarosi, MD
Professor and Vice-Chairman
Department of Internal Medicine
Director, Division of General Medicine
University of Texas Health Sciences Center
Houston, Texas

Gordon Francis Schwartz, MD
Attending Surgeon
Thomas Jefferson University Hospital
Consultant in Surgery—Pennsylvania Hospital and Chestnut Hill Hospital (Philadelphia), and The Bryn Mawr Hospital (Bryn Mawr)
Professor of Surgery
Jefferson Medical College
Philadelphia, Pennsylvania

Stewart M. Scott, MD
Chief of Surgery
VA Medical Center
Asheville, North Carolina
Consulting Professor of Surgery
Duke University Medical Center
Durham, North Carolina

Gulshan K. Sethi, MD
Professor of Surgery
Medical Director Circulatory Sciences Program
University of Arizona
Tucson, Arizona

Richard L. Simmons, MD
Chairman
Department of Surgery
University of Pittsburgh
Pittsburgh, Pennsylvania

Joseph S. Solomkin, MD
Director, Surgical Infectious Diseases Division
University Hospital
Associate Professor of Surgery
University of Cincinnati College of Medicine
Cincinnati, Ohio

Wiley W. Souba, MD, ScD
Chief, Division of Surgical Oncology
Massachusetts General Hospital
Professor of Surgery
Harvard Medical School
Boston, Massachusetts

Harvey J. Sugerman, MD
David Hume Professor of Surgery
Vice-Chairman for Research and Education
Medical College of Virginia
Richmond, Virginia

Richard L. Sweet, MD
Chairman
Department of Obstetrics, Gynecology, and Reproductive Sciences
University of Pittsburgh School of Medicine
Pittsburgh, Pennsylvania

Timothy Takaro, MD
Consulting Professor of Surgery
Duke University Medical Center
Consultant, VA Medical Center
Asheville, North Carolina

John G. Thacker, MD
Professor of Mechanical and Aerospace Engineering
University of Virginia
Charlottesville, Virginia

Alonzo P. Walker, MD
Associate Professor of Surgery
Department of Surgery
Medical College of Wisconsin
Milwaukee, Wisconsin

Andrew L. Warshaw, MD
Chief of General Surgery and Associate Chief of the Surgical Services
Massachusetts General Hospital
Harold and Ellen Danser Professor of Surgery
Harvard Medical School
Boston, Massachusetts

Carol L. Wells, PhD
Associate Professor
Departments of Laboratory Medicine & Pathology and Surgery
University of Minnesota
Minneapolis, Minnesota

Russell A. Williams, MD
Vice Chairman
Department of Surgery
University of California
Irvine Medical Center
Professor of Surgery
University of California, Irvine College of Medicine
Orange, California

Douglas W. Wilmore, MD
Director, Laboratory for Surgical Metabolism and Nutrition
Brigham and Women's Hospital
Frank Sawyer Professor of Surgery
Harvard Medical School
Boston, Massachusetts

Samuel E. Wilson, MD
Chairman
Department of Surgery
University of California
Irvine Medical Center
Professor of Surgery
University of California, Irvine College of Medicine
Orange, California

Alastair C. J. Windsor, MB, BS, FRCS
Surgical Research Fellow
Medical College of Virginia
Richmond, Virginia

Marcos A. Wolff, MD
Fellow, Division of Adult Infectious Diseases
Shands Hospital
Fellow
University of Florida
Gainesville, Florida

Lowell S. Young, MD
Chief, Division of Infectious Diseases
California Pacific Medical Center
Clinical Professor of Medicine
University of California–San Francisco
San Francisco, California

Preface

Surgical infections—infections that require operative intervention or that result as a complication of surgery—will always be with us. Our understanding of the mechanisms of infection, the responses to infection, and of the mediators of those responses has advanced substantially since the second edition of *Surgical Infectious Diseases* was published in 1989. These new developments are covered in the first three parts of the third edition. Also, a new chapter on mediators of immunity and infection has been added to this edition.

Currently, biologic agents that affect the activities of these mediators are being tested. Although none have yet been proven effective, they hold great promise as an entirely new area of attack on the effects of infection. In the meantime antimicrobials directed at the infecting agent, operative treatment of the infection, and general support of the patient remain the mainstays of treating surgical infections. We have prepared the third edition of *Surgical Infectious Diseases* primarily to cover recent important advances in these areas.

Future changes in the structure and financing of health care will emphasize both cost and quality. Preventing postoperative surgical site infections and other nosocomial infections will be even more important because hospitals with low nosocomial infection rates will have lower costs and rank higher on quality measures, thereby attracting managed-care contracts. Nosocomial infections and their prevention are discussed in the sections on wound infection and infections arising in the hospital.

We appreciate all those persons whose patience and assistance have made this book possible. The chapter authors took time from their busy schedules to add their expertise to this book, Ms. Thelma Lewis retyped many manuscripts, and Ms. Rebecca Pfeifer provided valuable editorial assistance.

SURGICAL MICROBIOLOGY

PART I

Overview of Etiologic Agents of Surgical Infections

CHAPTER 1

Carol L. Wells, Richard J. Howard

A myriad of microorganisms inhabit the human body, but only a small fraction characteristically cause disease. Only a fraction of the organisms associated with disease typically cause surgical infections, that is, infections that appear to be a consequence of operative or other trauma or infections for which surgical therapy may be required.

TYPES OF MICROORGANISMS

The classification of microorganisms is based on their structural properties (Table 1–1). Microorganisms can be placed into groups based on the increasing complexity of their structure: (1) viruses; (2) prokaryotes, which lack a true nucleus and include bacteria, rickettsiae, chlamydiae, and mycoplasmas; and (3) eukaryotes, which have a nucleus bounded by a nuclear membrane and include protozoa and fungi.

Multicellular eukaryotic parasites, such as nematodes (roundworms), cestodes (tapeworms), and trematodes (flukes) are not microorganisms but can cause infection.

Viruses

Viruses are among the smallest (20 to 300 nm diameter) infectious agents and have the simplest structure (Fig. 1–1). They are obligate intracellular parasites, which originally were distinguished by their small size (*filterable viruses*). However, some small prokaryotes (chlamydiae, rickettsiae, and mycoplasmas) also share these properties, so that the only unique features of viruses are their simple structures and modes of replication. Whereas bacteria and higher organisms reproduce by binary cell division, viral multiplication occurs by synthesis of the individual components within the host cell, followed by assembly into complete virus particles. Viruses differ from each other in size and shape, in chemical composition of the genome, and in types of cells they can infect.

A complete virus particle, a *virion,* has a central core of genetic material surrounded by a protein coat, which protects the nucleic acid from the nucleases in the environment and serves as a vehicle for transmission from one host to another. The nucleic acid accounts for only a small part of the total mass of the virion—approximately 1 percent in the case of the influenza virus. All viruses have a central core containing either RNA or DNA, but not both. The nucleic acid can be either single- or double-stranded. Most DNA viruses of clinical importance have double-stranded DNA, whereas medically important RNA viruses have either single- or double-stranded RNA. Viruses have relatively lim-

TABLE 1–1. CLASSIFICATION OF MICROORGANISMS

Microorganism	Mean Diameter (μm)	Mass (daltons)	Number of Genes
Viruses			
Poliovirus	0.02–0.03	2.5×10^6	7–8
Herpesviruses	0.10–0.20	6×10^7	150
Vaccina	0.20–0.30	1.6×10^8	4×10^2
Prokaryotes			
Bacteria			
Escherichia coli	$0.6 \times 1–3$	3.9	6×10^3
Bacillus anthracis	1.3×10		
Spirochetes	$0.10 \times 5–20$		
Chlamydiae	0.20–0.30	4×10^8	10^3
Mycoplasma	0.20–0.30	5×10^8	10^3
Rickettsiae	0.30–0.60	10^9	2×10^3
Eukaryotes			
Fungi	2–4		
Protozoans			
Entamoeba histolytica	40		
Human cells	8–50	1.6×10^{12}	3×10^6

ited genetic capacity (see Table 1–1). For instance, the genome of poliovirus codes for only seven or eight polypeptides, whereas herpesviruses have sufficient genetic information to code for 150 polypeptides.

The nucleic acid is surrounded by a protein coat, the *capsid*. The capsid is composed of individual polypeptide units, capsomeres (see Fig. 1–1). Some of the factors used in classification of viruses include the number of capsomeres and the configuration or symmetry of the nucleocapsid (helical, icosahedral, complex). The capsid protects the nucleic acid from physical and chemical inactivation and may also play a role in viral attachment to sites on susceptible cells.

Some viruses have a second coat, the *envelope*. The envelopes of viruses consist of lipids and proteins (often linked to carbohydrates). The proteins of the envelope are determined by the viral genome, but the lipid and carbohydrate come from the host cell. Viruses that assemble in the cell nucleus (eg, herpes simplex virus, cytomegalovirus) acquire much of their lipid from nuclear membrane as they "bud" from the nucleus—a process similar to reverse pinocytosis. Enveloped RNA viruses (eg, the influenza virus), which assemble in the cytoplasm, bud from the plasma membrane and acquire their envelope lipids and carbohydrates from the cytoplasmic membrane. The presence of lipid in the envelope prevents formation of a rigid structure, and the outer surface of enveloped viruses makes the virus sensitive to organic solvents, such as ether. This lipoprotein envelope is an integral part of the virion and aids in attachment and penetration of the virus into cellular hosts.

All viruses are obligate intracellular parasites because they are entirely dependent on host cells for energy generation and for biosynthesis. Many viruses are not completely devoid of enzymes: they may contain enzymes important in the replication of their nucleic acid such as reverse transcriptase, found in the retroviruses.

Two virus-related particles differ from complete viruses in that they contain nucleic acid or protein, but not both. *Viroids,* the etiologic agents of serious diseases of many plants, have no capsid and consist of nothing but RNA. *Prions,* by contrast, consist solely of protein and may be the transmissible agents of slowly evolving diseases, such as Kuru and Creutzfeldt–Jakob disease, once thought to be transmitted by "slow viruses."

Prokaryotes

Bacteria. Bacteria are the smallest organisms that contain all the biosynthetic machinery and energy-generating mechanisms required for an inde-

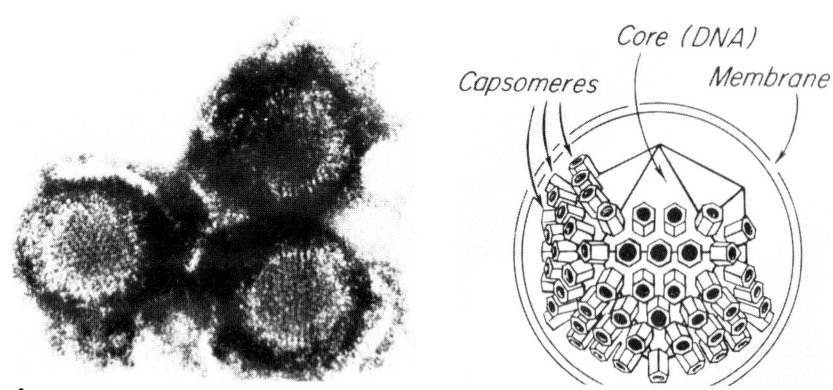

A B

Figure 1–1. A. Cytomegalovirus negatively stained with uranyl acetate. The capsomeres and irregularly shaped surrounding envelope are readily seen. *(From Lee FK, Nahmias AJ, Stagno S:* N Engl J Med *229:1266, 1978.)* **B.** Schema of a typical herpesvirus. The central core contains DNA. The core is surrounded by a layer of protein called the capsid, which is composed of individual units termed capsomeres. The capsid of herpesviruses is an icosahedron that has 162 capsomeres. Herpesviruses acquire a membrane coat (envelope) when they bud from the nuclear membrane of the host cell.

pendent existence and for self-replication. Bacteria are prokaryotic organisms because they lack a true nucleus surrounded by a nuclear membrane, chromosomes, and a mitotic apparatus (Fig. 1–2). The most obvious differences between bacterial and animal cells are size and simplicity of structure (see Table 1–1). Bacteria have three general shapes: rods (eg, *Escherichia coli, Bacteroides fragilis*), spheres (eg, *Staphylococcus aureus, Streptococcus pyogenes*), and spirals (eg, *Treponema pallidum*).

Bacterial Structure

NUCLEAR BODY. Although bacteria lack a true nucleus, a nuclear region consisting of DNA fibrils can be seen in electron micrographs (see Fig. 1–2). Furthermore, these concentrations of DNA have also been recognized as discrete nuclear bodies under light microscopy using DNA-specific stains. Bacterial DNA exists as a single circular molecule, and bacteria are thus considered to have a single chromosome. The DNA of a typical bacterium (*E. coli*) weighs 3×10^9 daltons, compared with 2.5×10^6 daltons for poliovirus and 1.6×10^{12} daltons for a human somatic cell (see Table 1–1). When unfolded, the DNA is approximately 1000 times as long as the bacterium.

Outside the large circular chromosome (nuclear body), some bacteria contain small autonomously replicating DNA strands called *plasmids*. Plasmids contain a variety of genes, some of which may code for antibiotic resistance. Because plasmids can be transferred between bacteria by conjugation, they have been called resistance transfer factors, or R factors. Plasmids are common in enteric bacteria such as *E. coli, Salmonella* species, and *Shigella* species. In 1959, strains of *Shigella* suddenly appeared that were resistant to four widely used antibiotics: sulfonamides, chloramphenicol, streptomycin, and tetracycline. A plasmid that had genes for resistance to each of the four antibiotics had been introduced into these *Shigella*.

CYTOPLASMIC CONTENTS. Bacterial cytoplasm is densely populated with ribosomes. Bacteria have 70S ribosomes composed of 50S and 30S subunits. Animal cells have larger 80S ribosomes. Ribosomes are the sites where synthesis of polypeptides from amino acids occurs. Many bacteria also have granular inclusions that contain cellular storage materials, such as glycogen and lipid. Bacteria do not have mitochondria, but enzymes and cytochromes involved in electron transport and oxidative phosphorylation are located on the plasma membrane.

PLASMA MEMBRANE. The cytoplasmic membrane is a typical lipid bilayer that appears as a dark-light-dark band using transmission electron microscopy

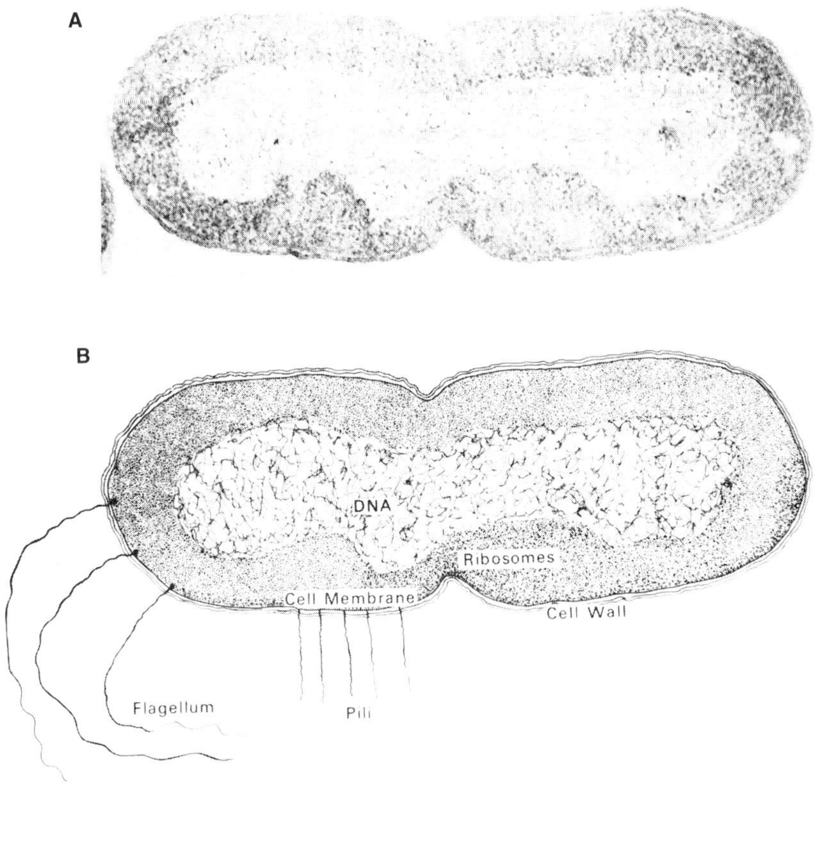

Figure 1–2. A. Transmission electron micrograph showing *Escherichia coli* with central nucleoid containing DNA fibers coagulated by the fixative osmium tetraoxide. There is no distinct nuclear membrane, a feature that differentiates prokaryotic cells from eukaryotic cells. A central constriction in the membrane can be seen indicating that cell division has begun. The dark area surrounding the nucleoid is filled with ribosomes. No flagella or fimbriae can be seen in this photograph. *(From Woldringh CL, de Jong MA, van den Berg W, Koppes L: J Bacteriol 131:270, 1977).* **B.** Schema of *E. coli* cell showing essential structural features of a typical bacterium. Flagella and fimbriae can be located over the entire cell surface.

(see Fig. 1–2). The plasma membrane's major functions are to provide: (1) selective permeability and transport of solutes into the cell, (2) electron transport and oxidative phosphorylation, (3) excretion of exoenzymes, and (4) a repository for enzymes responsible for synthesis of DNA, cell wall polymers, and membrane lipids.

Mesosomes are convoluted invaginations of the cytoplasmic membrane. Septal mesosomes serve as the attachment sites of the bacterial chromosome to the cytoplasmic membrane. They are also involved in cell division. The extra membrane of the mesosome may facilitate separation of the segregating chromosomes and the initiation of a membrane bridge between two newly formed cells. Lateral mesosomes, attached to nonseptal regions of the bacterium, are involved in protein secretion.

CELL WALL. Gram-positive bacteria have a rigid, relatively thick (15 to 80 nm) electron-dense cell wall, external to the plasma membrane. The cell wall gives shape to the bacterium and enables the plasma membrane to resist bursting as a result of the high intracellular osmotic pressure (5 atmospheres for gram-negative bacteria and up to 20 atmospheres for gram-positive bacteria). In gram-negative bacteria, this electron-dense layer is only 2 to 3 nm thick. Gram-negative bacteria have an additional trilaminar outer membrane layer 6 to 18 nm thick (Figs. 1–3 and 1–4). Differences in cell wall structure determine whether bacteria are gram-positive or gram-negative.

The walls of gram-positive bacteria have a basic structure of peptidoglycan, consisting of polysaccharide chains (the backbone) of alternating residues of N-acetylglucosamine and N-acetylmuramic acid. These polysaccharide chains are cross-linked by polypeptide chains (nine amino acids long in the case of *S. aureus*). Gram-positive bacteria may also have teichoic acids covalently bound to some N-acetylmuramic acid residues. Teichoic acids are polymers of either ribitol or glycerol residues that protrude from the cell and provide much of the antigenic specificity.

The cell walls of gram-negative bacteria also contain peptidoglycan, but there is much less of it than in gram-positive bacteria, and there is no teichoic acid. The outer membrane of a gram-negative bacterium is a lipid bilayer that resembles the plasma membrane (see Fig. 1–3). This outer membrane contains lipopolysaccharide and is also known as endotoxin because it is toxic and is firmly bound to the bacterial cell. Lipopolysaccharide is described as having three layers: lipid A (the innermost layer), followed by a core polysaccharide, and then an outermost polysaccharide containing specific O antigens. The innermost areas are the most conserved among gram-negative bacteria; the outer O antigens vary widely among different species/strains, contributing to the antigenic diversity of enteric bacteria. This tremendous antigenic diversity has made it extremely difficult for research scientists to design a single antiendotoxin antibody that is broadly cross-reactive among different species/strains of gram-negative bacteria.

CAPSULE. Capsules are loose, gel-like structures composed of polysaccharides, polypeptides, or both. In some bacterial species (eg, *Haemophilus influenzae*), capsular polysaccharide has immunologi-

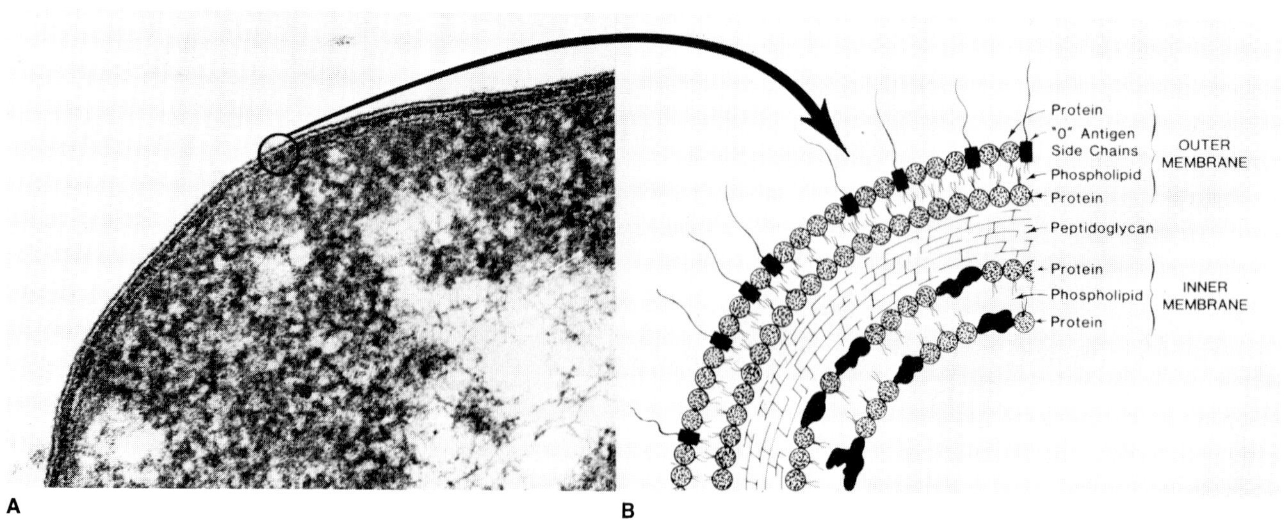

Figure 1–3. A. *Escherichia coli* cell wall (×200,000). *(Courtesy of RGE Murray.)* **B.** Schema of *E. coli* cell envelope.

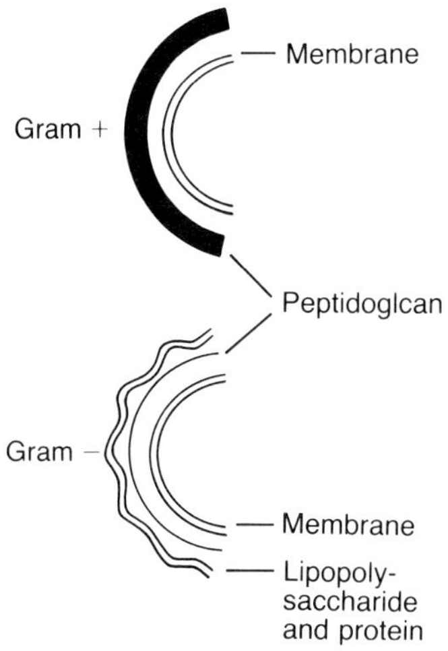

Figure 1–4. Comparison of cell wall of gram-positive and gram-negative bacteria. *(From Brock TD, Smith DW, Madigan MT: Biology of Microorganisms, 4th ed. Englewood Cliffs, NJ, Prentice Hall, 1984.)*

cal specificity that can be used to identify different bacterial strains or bacterial types within a given species. Capsules are visualized most easily by negative staining with India ink, where the capsule appears as a clear layer (or halo) between the black ink particles and the dark bacterial cell. Capsules also impart a glistening, mucoid appearance to colonies on agar medium. Capsules protect bacteria from phagocytosis, and their presence is usually correlated with virulence. Capsule formation is determined in part by the environment of the bacterium. Bacteria tend to form capsules in host tissues. When grown in vitro, however, bacteria tend not to make capsules unless specific nutrients are provided.

FLAGELLA, FIMBRIAE, AND FIBRILS. Flagella, fimbriae, and fibrils are hair-like appendages on the surfaces of some bacteria (Fig. 1–5). Flagella are relatively long structures (3 to 20 μm by 10 to 25 nm), while fimbriae are shorter and thinner than flagella, and fibrils are shorter than fimbriae. Flagella and fimbriae are composed of repeating protein units (flagellin and pilin, respectively) and can be found on some gram-negative and some gram-positive bacteria. In contrast, fibrils are only found on some gram-positive bacteria and are described as a fuzzy surface layer composed of protein or polysaccharide. Flagella and fimbriae often confer serologic specificity. There is evidence that flagella, fimbriae, and fibrils may play important roles in bacterial attachment to mucosal surfaces and therefore function as adhesins (Fig. 1–6). Adhesins are often considered to be virulence factors.

The ability of flagella to function as adhesins is a relatively new concept. Historically, flagella have been recognized solely as the primary mechanism of bacterial locomotion. Flagella are classified as polar (at one or both poles of the bacterium) or peritrichous (distributed over the entire bacterial surface). The number of flagella is generally correlated with motility of the organism. Hence some species in the genus *Proteus* have numerous peritrichous flagella and "swarm" (form a thin spreading film) on the surface of an agar plate.

Although the ability of flagella to function as adhesins is a relatively new concept, fimbrial adhesins have been studied for years. Experimental antifimbrial vaccines have been used both therapeutically and prophylactically to help prevent and/or treat infections that involve bacterial attachment to a mucosal surface, such as *E. coli* urinary tract infections and *Neisseria gonorrhoeae* genital infections. The term pili has often been used interchangeably with the term fimbriae; in precise usage, however, pili should be reserved for the specialized fimbriae that function in bacterial conjugation and mediate transfer of chromosomal elements in conjugating gram-negative bacteria.

SPORES. Spores provide a vehicle to survive adverse conditions and are formed by some gram-positive bacteria, including *Bacillus* species and *Clostridium* species. Spores are much more resistant to the lethal effects of heat, drying, freezing, radiation, and toxic chemicals than are vegetative bacterial cells. The spore wall and cortex contain protein and peptidoglycan. The central core contains the complete genome of the vegetative cell. A variety of catabolic and biosynthetic enzymes is also present. Bacterial spores have no metabolic activity but can recover from this dormant state when exposed to the appropriate environmental conditions.

Rickettsiae. The rickettsiae are nonmotile, small bacteria that appear as spherical forms (0.3 μm in diameter) or as short rods (0.3 × 1.0 μm). Clinically important rickettsiae are obligate intracellular parasites that multiply within host cells. Because of their small size and because they are obligate intracellular organisms, rickettsiae were at one time thought to constitute a separate phylum between viruses and bacteria. However, rickettsiae are true bacteria: (1) they multiply by binary fission; (2) they contain both DNA and RNA; (3) they contain enzymes of the Krebs cycle and of electron transport; (4) at least one species contains muramic acid, a constituent found only in bacterial cell walls; and (5) their growth is inhibited by antibacterial agents.

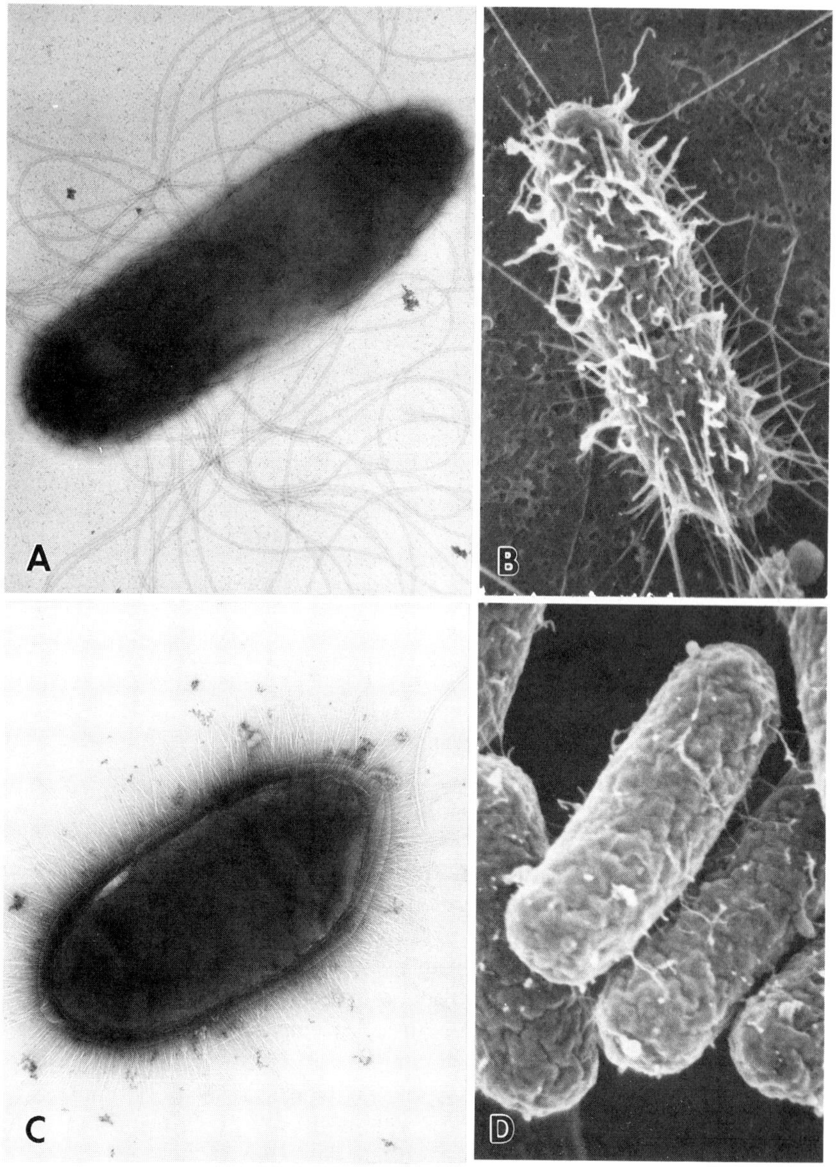

Figure 1–5. **A.** Negatively stained image of *Proteus mirabilis* showing numerous peritrichous flagella. **B.** Scanning electron micrograph of another strain of *P. mirabilis* that is both fimbriated (relatively short, straight appendages) and peritrichously flagellated. **C.** Negatively stained image of a fimbriated strain of *Escherichia coli* showing numerous fimbriae distributed around the entire surface of the bacterium. **D.** Scanning electron micrograph showing *E. coli* fimbriae mediating contact between adjacent bacterial cells.

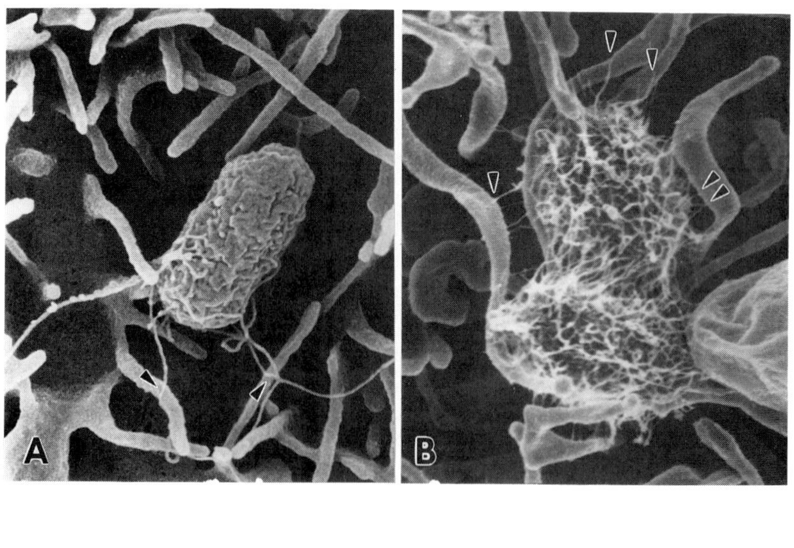

Figure 1–6. Scanning electron micrographs showing adherence of enteric bacteria to the apical microvilli of cultured intestinal epithelial cells (ie, Caco-2 cells). **A.** *Escherichia coli* with several elongated flagella mediating adherence to individual microvilli (arrowheads). **B.** Two heavily fimbriated, rod-shaped *Proteus mirabilis* with numerous fimbriae mediating adherence to microvilli, and with some of the points of contact highlighted with arrowheads.

The survival of most rickettsiae requires that they be transmitted from one host to another in a manner that minimizes their exposure to the extracellular environment. Most rickettsiae therefore have an arthropod vector. Rickettsial diseases are characterized by fever, headache, myalgia, and an exanthematous rash and include louse-borne typhus fever, murine typhus, Q fever, Rocky Mountain spotted fever, and scrub typhus.

Chlamydiae. Chlamydiae are small (0.2 to 0.3 μm in diameter) obligate intracellular bacteria. Their ribosomes are similar to those of other bacteria, and, like other bacteria, they contain both DNA and RNA, multiply by binary fission, contain peptidoglycan in their cell walls, and are susceptible to antibiotics. Isolated chlamydiae lack the ability to synthesize their own proteins, DNA, and RNA, but they can do so within host cells. Chlamydiae lack energy-producing enzyme systems and cannot synthesize adenosine triphosphate; so that they depend on host cells for generating metabolic energy. They produce typical cytoplasmic inclusions (termed inclusion bodies) in infected cells, which are pathognomonic. *Chlamydia psittaci* is the etiologic agent of psittacosis in birds and of respiratory disease in humans; indeed, the prevalence of psittacosis in birds prohibits their use as pets in nursing homes or in homes for the elderly. *Chlamydia trachomatis* is associated not only with trachoma but also with inclusion conjunctivitis, lymphogranuloma venereum, pneumonitis, and a variety of sexually transmitted diseases including nongonococcal urethritis, pelvic inflammatory disease in females, and gay bowel syndrome in homosexual men.

Mycoplasmas. Mycoplasmas are the smallest (150 to 300 nm in diameter) cells capable of independent extracellular existence (Fig. 1–7). Because they lack cell walls, mycoplasmas do not stain well with Gram stain and are typically resistant to antimicrobials, such as penicillin, that inhibit cell wall synthesis. Mycoplasmas require sterols for growth. *Mycoplasma pneumoniae* causes primary atypical pneumonia, a disease most often seen in young adults. Other mycoplasmas, such as *M. hominis* and *M. salivarium,* rarely cause disease but are normal flora of the oral cavity and are common laboratory contaminants of tissue culture cell lines.

Ureaplasma urealyticum is closely related to the mycoplasmas and requires urea for growth. The organism is normal flora of the respiratory and urogenital tracts and has also been associated with nongonococcal urethritis acquired through sexual contact.

Eukaryotes

Fungi. Fungi are eukaryotic cells (Figs. 1–8 to 1–10). Their DNA is separated into chromosomes during cell division, and the nuclei are separated from the cytoplasm by a nuclear membrane. Their nuclei also contain nucleoli and histones, features lacking in bacteria. Unlike prokaryotic cells, the cytoplasm of fungi contains organelles such as mitochondria and endoplasmic reticulum. The plasma membrane of fungi contains sterols, a component absent from the plasma membranes of bacteria.

Fungi have a rigid cell wall, external to the plasma membrane, that serves to protect the cell from osmotic disruption. Fungi grow as either yeasts (single-celled organisms that reproduce by budding) or molds (multicellular, filamentous colonies). The cell wall of fungi does not contain peptidoglycan but is composed almost entirely of polysaccharide. Molds have tubular branching hyphae (see Fig. 1–10) that are either septate (individual cells separated by cross walls) or aseptate (with sparse cross walls). In many fungi, the principal structural material is chitin, a polymer of N-acetylglucosamine residues. Some yeasts also have a polysaccharide capsule surrounding the cell wall that, like bacterial capsules, inhibits phagocytosis (see Fig. 1–8).

Specialized reproductive cells that are capable of developing into mature fungi are called spores in clinical medicine (see Fig. 1–10). [However, fungal taxonomists use the term conidia (singular, conidium) to more correctly refer to the majority of spores seen in the clinical microbiology laboratory.] Of the estimated 80,000 species of fungi, only about 100 cause disease (mycoses) in humans. Of all the species of fungi in the world, a single species (*Candida albicans*) accounts for approximately 60 percent of all fungal isolates in a typical clinical mycology laboratory. Fungal diseases are classified as systemic, subcutaneous, cutaneous, and superficial mycoses.

Systemic (deep) mucoses affect internal organs, such as the liver, lung, or brain, and often produce a granulomatous reaction in the host. Fungi capable of causing systemic disease include *Histoplasma capsulatum, Blastomyces dermatitides, Cryptococcus neoformans,* and *Coccidiodes immitis.* Other fungi, such as *C. albicans, Aspergillus* species, and *Mucor* species, are opportunists and usually cause systemic disease only in hosts with compromised immune systems. Subcutaneous mycoses are characterized by lesions in the deeper layers of the skin (below the epidermis) and follow traumatic implantation of the fungus. The most prevalent subcutane-

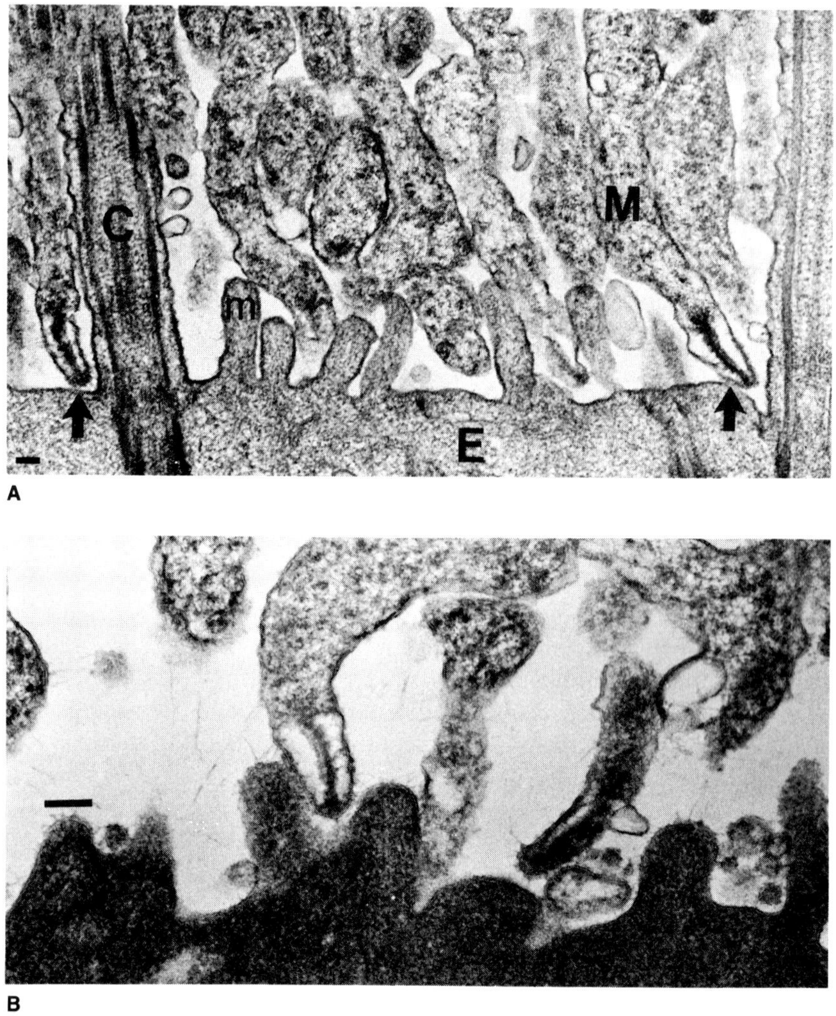

Figure 1–7. A. *Mycoplasma pneumoniae* in tracheal ring organ culture for 72 hours. There is heavy parasitemia of the cell with specialized tips for attachment to tracheal cells (arrows) closely apposed to the bases of the cilia and microvilli. Scale bar = 0.1 μm. C, cilium; M, mycoplasma; m, microvillus; E, epithelium. **B.** *Mycoplasma pneumoniae* in infected tracheal ring showing classical filamentous structure of the organism, its tip touching a nonciliated cell. The encircling unit membrane, the body containing ribosomes, and fibrils of nuclear material are all present. Scale bar = 0.1 μm. *(From Wilson MH, Collier AM: J Bacteriol 125:332, 1976.)*

ous mycosis in the United States is sporotrichosis caused by *Sporothrix shenkii,* a soil organism. Sporotrichosis is seen with some frequency in persons who tend roses and acquire a skin wound from a rose thorn contaminated with the fungus. Cutaneous mycoses (dermatomycoses) are relatively superficial infections of keratin-rich structures such as hair, nails, and epidermis. Dermatophytic infec-

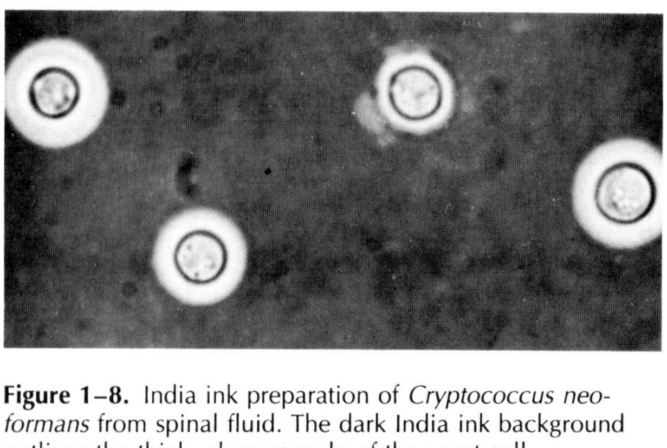

Figure 1–8. India ink preparation of *Cryptococcus neoformans* from spinal fluid. The dark India ink background outlines the thick, clear capsule of the yeast cell.

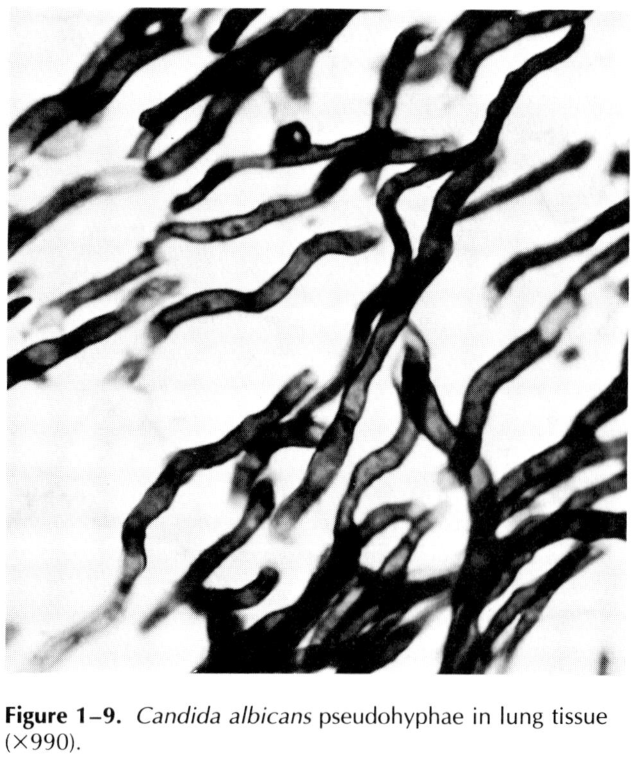

Figure 1–9. *Candida albicans* pseudohyphae in lung tissue (×990).

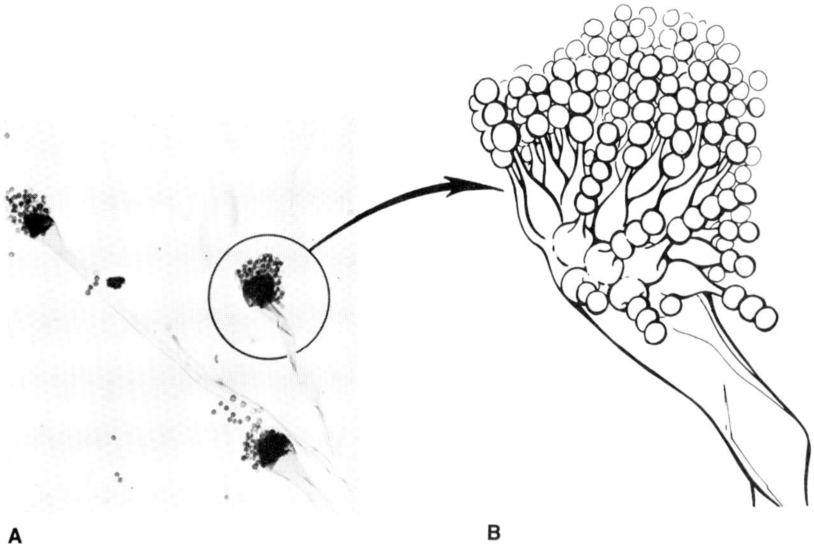

Figure 1–10. *Aspergillus fumigatus.* **A.** Long conidiophores (structures bearing conidia) have vesicle-like tips. **B.** The tip of the vesicle is covered with flask-shaped phialides to which chains of conidia are attached.

tions are caused by fungi belonging to the genera *Trichophyton, Epidermophyton,* and *Microsporum.* Superficial mycoses involve only the most superficial layers of the epidermis or the hair shaft, and living tissue is not affected. There is no pain, and the patient typically sees a physician for cosmetic reasons. For example, *Malassezia furfur* is a lipophilic yeast that infects the stratum corneum causing discolored or depigmented areas of skin. (*Malassezia furfur* has also been isolated from the blood of hospitalized infants fed liquid diet containing a high lipid concentration.)

Protozoa. Protozoa are unicellular, eukaryotic microorganisms. Their cellular structure has many characteristics in common with human cells. Like all eukaryotic cells, protozoa have a true nucleus with a nuclear membrane, mitotic structure, histones, chromosomes, and a nucleolus. Their cytoplasm contains well-defined organelles such as mitochondria and endoplasmic reticulum. The plasma membrane is stabilized with sterols. Unlike fungi, however, there is no cell wall. Small protozoa, such as *Leishmania,* measure 2 × 4 μm, whereas the giant ameba, with a diameter of approximately 1 mm, is visible to the naked eye.

HOST-MICROBE RELATIONSHIPS

Humans are normally colonized with a wide variety of microorganisms (see Chap. 3). Bacteria are extremely prevalent on the human body and outnumber all eukaryotic cells by 10:1. It is estimated that 10^{14} bacteria live on the skin and mucous membranes, including the oral, respiratory, gastrointestinal, and genitourinary surfaces. Each site provides numerous ecological niches suitable for different types of bacteria. Although much less studied than the bacterial flora, a variety of viruses (approximately 150), fungi, and protozoa are also members of the normal microbial flora of humans.

The normal microflora are extremely beneficial to the host. For example, certain species of intestinal bacteria synthesize vitamin K, which is required by the host for normal hemostasis. Dense populations of bacteria in the mouth, intestinal tract, and vagina help exclude potential pathogens by competing for attachment sites and available nutrients. In one widespread outbreak of salmonellosis attributed to contaminated milk, persons most likely to become infected were those taking broad spectrum antibiotics that altered the composition of their normal intestinal microflora.

The human body has a number of natural barriers to prevent colonization of potentially pathogenic microbes. Skin cannot be penetrated by bacteria unless there is a break in the integrity of the epithelium. Skin also provides a hostile environment to many microbes: it is dry and mildly acidic (due to the breakdown of lipids into fatty acids), contains a normal microbial flora to compete for ecological niches, and undergoes desquamation. In the respiratory tract, bronchial and tracheal cilia keep the mucous layer moving upward toward the pharynx. Intestinal mucus and intestinal peristalsis, as well as the flow of urine, tears, and saliva, help prevent invading microbes from adhering to epithelial surfaces. The human body produces several potent antibacterial chemicals, such as gastric acid, spermine, and lysozyme.

Disease results from the interplay of the infectious dose of a microbe coupled with the host's state of immunity. A frank pathogen is one that typically causes disease in a normal host, for example, *Yersinia pestis,* the etiologic agent of the plague of the Middle Ages. An opportunistic pathogen is one that causes disease in a compromised host, such as those persons who are very young, very old, alcoholic, diabetic, or nutritionally deficient. Other compromised hosts include trauma patients, postsurgical patients, cancer patients, and organ transplant recipients. The number of microbes necessary to cause disease in the majority of normal adults is termed the infectious dose, which varies with the microbial species. For example, the infectious dose for a healthy adult is approximately 10^7 *Salmonella* organisms, 200 *Shigella* organisms, and 1 *Mycobacterium tuberculosis.*

MICROBIAL PATHOGENICITY

Microbial pathogens have some unique characteristics that facilitate the production of disease. These characteristics are often called virulence factors, among which are toxins that alter normal physiology, enzymes that destroy host tissue, and capsules that inhibit phagocytosis. Such disease-producing abilities characterize the pathogen in contrast with the commensal or saprophytic microbe. We simply do not understand how most pathogens cause disease, especially microbes of low pathogenicity. However, some of the primary ways by which microbes can avoid host defenses and cause clinical disease are discussed as follows.

Microbial Adherence and Internalization at Epithelial Surfaces

Because many infections originate in the respiratory, gastrointestinal, or genitourinary tract, an important initial step is often the ability of a microbe to adhere to an epithelial surface. There are two potential outcomes of bacterial adherence to epithelial cells: colonization and internalization. For pathogens that are internalized, it is generally accepted that attachment is an initial step.

Viruses appear to attach to epithelial cells via pairs of complementary receptors on the microbe and the cell. The influenza virus attaches to respiratory epithelial cells because the viral hemagglutinin reacts with neuraminic acid receptors on the epithelial cell. Other viruses (eg, poliovirus, adenovirus) attach to susceptible cells because there are specific receptors on these cells for viral capsid protein. The flagellated protozoan, *Giardia lamblia,* appears to use its ventral sucking disk to adhere to the microvillous border of the small intestine; there is no evidence of parasite invasion or toxin production, but the parasitized epithelial cells do not secrete and absorb macromolecules in a normal manner.

Bacterial adherence and internalization by epithelial surfaces are currently an active area of research, and our knowledge in this area is rapidly expanding. There is recent evidence that bacteria can bind either directly or indirectly to epithelial cells, facilitating bacterial colonization and possibly internalization. As an example of direct binding, *Yersinia enterocolitica* has been shown to bind to certain receptors on eukaryotic cells called integrins, which often function to bind the cell to its own cellular matrix proteins. These integrin receptors colocalize with a variety of actin-associated proteins in the host cell, triggering the "zipper mechanism" of bacterial internalization where the mammalian cell surface wraps completely around the bacterium using a series of advancing receptor-ligand interactions. It should be emphasized that integrins may not be the only receptors capable of coupling the process of bacterial adherence and mobilization of the host cell cytoskeleton.

If a bacterium binds indirectly to the host cell, certain polysaccharides and/or proteins secreted by the host cell mediate contact between the bacterium and the eukaryotic cell. The proteins most involved in mediating indirect binding include proteins of the extracellular matrix such as fibronectin, laminin, collagen, and vitronectin. Examples of bacteria that bind indirectly include *S. pyogenes* and *S. aureus.* It has been postulated that binding via extracellular matrix proteins is of low affinity and does not result in bacterial internalization.

Bacterial fimbriae have widely been studied as structures that mediate bacterial adherence to mucosal surfaces (see Fig. 1–6B). Fimbriae are composed of protein and have lectin-like activity. (*Lectins* are defined as proteins or glycoproteins of nonimmune origin that agglutinate cells or precipitate complex carbohydrates.) Fimbriae mediate bacterial binding to a variety of glycoconjugates, many of which are linked to host membrane lipids. For example, many strains of *E. coli* possess type 1 fimbriae, which bind to mannose receptor sites on epithelial cells. Recent evidence suggests that fimbrial binding facilitates colonization, but not bacterial internalization, possibly due to low binding affinity and/or low number of receptor-ligand contacts.

Mechanisms Whereby Microbes Resist Phagocytosis

The directed movement of phagocytes toward a target is called chemotaxis. Bacteria produce a number of chemical signals (chemoattractants) that attract phagocytic leukocytes. (Bacteria also stimulate the host to produce chemoattractants.) Some bacterial products can also stimulate macrophages to secrete cytokines that increase the adhesiveness of endothelial cells for neutrophils and monocytes. For example, bacterial endotoxin stimulates macrophages to secrete factors that induce a class of surface receptors called endothelial-leukocyte adhesion molecules (ELAMs). ELAMs facilitate the endothelial adhesion and subsequent diapedesis of phagocytes from the circulation to infected sites.

One way for a microbe to avoid phagocytosis is to interfere with chemotaxis. Some streptococci secrete a streptolysin that inhibits polymorphonuclear neutrophil (PMN) chemotaxis. The same streptolysin is also lethal for phagocytes. Many bacteria (eg, *Streptococcus pneumoniae, Hemophilus influenzae, Klebsiella pneumoniae, Salmonella typhi*) and fungi (eg, *Histoplasma capsulatum, Cryptococcus neoformans*) possess antiphagocytic capsules. Unless antibodies specific for the capsular polysaccharide are present, phagocytosis is impossible. Capsules are strongly correlated with virulence. For instance, as few as ten encapsulated *S. pneumoniae* can kill a mouse when it is inoculated intraperitoneally, whereas 10,000 bacteria are required if the bacteria have had their capsules removed by hyaluronidase. If the mouse is rendered incapable of forming antibodies (opsonins) against the capsule, a single bacterium is sufficient to cause death. Thus, the pneumococcus is a potent pathogen indeed in the young who have not been immunized by prior exposure in the splenectomized patient who is deficient in producing antibody, and in the elderly who have lost prior immunity.

Another mechanism that bacteria use to resist phagocytosis is exhibited by *S. aureus*. A component of the cell wall, protein A, inhibits the phagocytosis even of opsonized bacteria. Protein A acts by blocking the Fc portion of IgG antibody, preventing binding of the Fc portion to the PMN receptors. Protein A is found only on highly pathogenic staphylococci and may thus be an important virulence factor. *Staphylococcus aureus* also produces catalase, an enzyme that enables it to degrade hydrogen peroxide, a potent bactericidal component of the PMN myeloperoxidase-hydrogen peroxide-halide system. Group A streptococci have at least two antiphagocytic components: an outer hyaluronate capsule and an M protein (associated with fimbrial appendages).

Intracellular and Extracellular Survival of Microbes

The majority of microbes that cause disease are quickly killed by phagocytic leukocytes, for example, *S. pyogenes* and *S. aureus*. By contrast, facultative intracellular pathogens are those that are not only capable of extracellular growth but that can also survive (and possibly replicate) intracellularly in host cells; classical examples include *Listeria monocytogenes, S. typhi,* and *M. tuberculosis*. Obligate intracellular pathogens are those microbes that are capable of growth only within host cells and include viruses, rickettsiae, chlamydiae, and some protozoa.

In recent years, the concept of a phagocytic cell has evolved to include a distinction between professional and nonprofessional phagocytes. Professional phagocytes are those cells that ingest microbes as a primary function, that is, polymorphonuclear leukocytes and mononuclear phagocytes (circulating monocytes and tissue macrophages) (Fig. 1–11). Nonprofessional phagocytes are other cells that have also been shown to internalize microbes and include some endothelial cells, some epithelial cells (some enterocytes and some pigment epithelial cells in the neural retina), some neurons, and some fibroblasts. Even hepatocytes are hosts for intracellular pathogens like *Plasmodium* organisms (malaria) and *Listeria*. It is not clear how the organisms become internalized, however.

The mechanisms responsible for intracellular survival vary among microbial species and are often

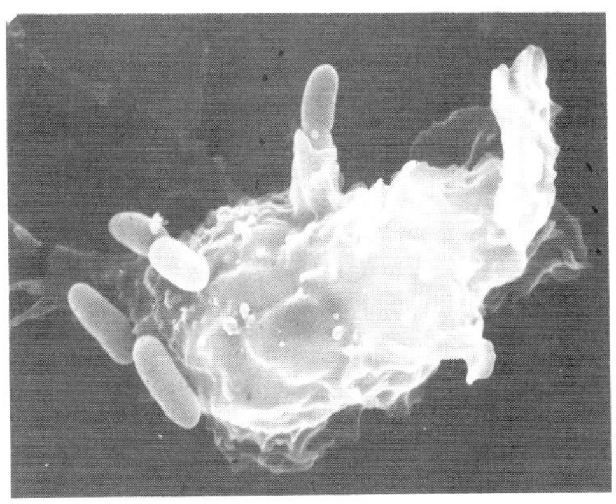

Figure 1–11. Scanning electron micrograph of a mouse peritoneal macrophage with four adherent, rod-shaped *Escherichia coli* (left edge of phagocyte), and other *E. coli* (top, middle of photograph) partially engulfed by a pseudopod formed during phagocytosis.

not well understood. In professional phagocytes, microbes are typically internalized into a phagocytic vacuole, which subsequently fuses with cytoplasmic lysosomes, releasing lysosomal granules into the vacuole, facilitating microbial degradation.

Some microbes have elaborate mechanisms to avoid intracellular killing within the vacuole. Intracellular survival of the protozoan *Toxoplasma gondii* appears to be dependent on the absence of specific antibody. In the absence of antibody, *T. gondii* enters into a phagosome that fails to be acidified or to fuse with lysosomes; that is, the phagosomal-lysosomal membrane is stabilized. Conversely, if *T. gondii* is nonviable or opsonized with IgG, the phagocytic vacuole fuses with lysosomes and become acidified. The Fc receptor appears to play a critical role in this latter process, because if the receptor is modified (truncated) experimentally, the *T. gondii*-containing vacuole does not fuse with the lysosomes. Thus, in this instance, the fate of the internalized microbe depends on the nature of the cellular receptor mediating microbial internalization.

Some bacteria, such as *S. typhimurium* and *M. tuberculosis,* also survive intracellularly by preventing fusion of the phagosome-lysosome membrane. Microbial growth within the vacuole is typically not possible due to an acidic pH, the presence of lysosomal enzymes, and a limited availability of nutrients such as iron. Some microbes can prevent acidification of the vacuole, although at least one microbe has been shown to require an acidified phagolysosome for growth. Microbes that escape the vacuole are more likely to survive intracellularly; for example, one virulence factor of *L. monocytogenes* is the production of an extracellular hemolysin (listeriolysin) that facilitates escape from the membrane-bound vacuole into the more friendly environment of the host cell cytoplasm. *Listeria monocytogenes* has also been observed to spread from cell to cell by polymerization of host cell actin filaments that form a growing "tail" at one end of the vacuole and appear to propel the *Listeria*-containing vacuole through the plasma membrane of one epithelial cell and into the plasma membrane of an adjacent cell.

Microbial Toxins

Microbial toxins are substances that either damage host cells or interfere with host defense mechanisms. Toxins may act locally or at sites distal to the organism producing the toxin. Toxins can be classified either by target site in the host or by site of association with the microbe. Thus neurotoxins affect the nervous system, enterotoxins affect the gastrointestinal tract, leukotoxins affect leukocytes, and cytotoxins affect host cells in general. The term exotoxin refers to a toxin released into the surrounding environment. Endotoxin refers to a toxin that is intimately associated with the microbe. An intracellular toxin is one that is released during microbial lysis.

The remainder of this discussion deals with bacterial toxins because much more is known about bacterial toxins compared to the toxins of other microbes. This approach is not meant to imply that other microbes do not synthesize toxins. For example, some fungi manufacture very potent toxins that have been used in germ warfare, and some toxigenic mushrooms can be lethal within hours of ingestion by the host (Table 1–2).

Bacterial Toxins. Some bacteria manufacture a single toxin that is implicated in pathogenesis, while others manufacture a host of toxic components that may have undefined roles in pathogenicity. Bacterial toxins are often coded in plasmids or in temperate bacteriophages, and nontoxigenic strains exist for many toxigenic species. Thus, in any given clinical specimen, the mere isolation of microbial species known to produce a toxin does not confirm the presence of the corresponding toxin in that patient.

Bacterial Exotoxins. Exotoxins are secreted by a variety of bacterial species including *Clostridium bot-*

TABLE 1–2. TOXICITY OF WELL-KNOWN POISONS AND BACTERIAL TOXINS

Poison or Toxin	Toxicity for Humans (mg)[a]
Strychnine	100
Arsenic	100
Cyanide	50
Cobra venom	25
Endotoxin	100
Clostridium botulinum	
Botulinum toxin type A	0.00009
Botulinum toxin type D	0.00003
Clostridium tetani toxin	0.0001
Clostridium welchii toxin	0.28
Clostridium novyi toxin	0.001
Shigella dysenteriae neurotoxin	0.00006
Corynebacterium diphtheriae toxin	0.02

[a] The numbers given here are approximations from animal data. Because animal species may vary in susceptibility to toxins, the figures will vary according to the species on which the toxicity is based. Therefore, these numbers must be regarded as rough approximations for a 70-kg human.

ulinum, C. tetani, C. difficile, C. perfringens, Vibrio cholera, E. coli, Shigella species, *Salmonella* species, *Aeromonas* species, *Staphylococcus* species, *Pseudomonas* species, and *Corynebacterium diphtheriae.* Almost all exotoxins are proteins and are readily inactivated by heat, formaldehyde, and other chemical treatments. These inactivated toxoids often retain their antigenic determinants and are suitable for active immunization against the toxin.

In some instances, a bacterial exotoxin has a clearly defined role in pathogenicity. For example, *C. diphtheriae* colonizes the oropharynx of the host and secretes a potent exotoxin with systemic activity. The molecular mechanism involved in this toxemia has carefully been elucidated (Table 1–3). The genes for toxin production are coded on a bacteriophage. Nontoxigenic strains are rarely associated with clinical disease but can be converted to virulent strains following insertion of the appropriate bacteriophage. The pathogenesis of *C. tetani* is similar to that of *C. diphtheria* in that *C. tetani* remains localized (in a wound), while it secretes a spasmogenic exotoxin (a neurotoxin) that has systemic effects. Diphtheria and tetanus are rare diseases in the United States due to widespread active immunization with the corresponding toxoid.

While some diseases are caused by toxigenic bacteria that replicate within the human body, other diseases are caused by ingestion of preformed toxin(s) in contaminated food (intoxications). The most common etiology of food poisoning in the United States is ingestion of food contaminated with enterotoxins of *S. aureus.* A rarc cause of food poisoning in the United States is ingestion of the botulinum toxin in food contaminated with *C. botulinum.* The rarity of this event is fortunate because botulinum toxin is among the most potent poisons known; it has been speculated that the amount of toxin that can be contained on the head of a pin would kill forty adults. Because *C. botulinum* can be found worldwide in the soil, it is likely that humans occasionally ingest this organism without ill effects, highlighting the protective effect of the normal intestinal flora that function to exclude pathogenic microbes. Another form of botulism (ie, infant botulism) occurs following ingestion of *C. botulinum* into the intestinal tract of an infant with an underdeveloped intestinal flora; here the organism replicates and secretes its potent exotoxin, resulting in a disease that ranges from "failure to thrive" to sudden infant death. Because *C. botulinum* is so ubiquitous, and because it can cause paralysis of the respiratory tree, it has even been speculated to be an unstudied and undocumented cause of failure to wean an ICU patient from a respirator. As a result of its paralytic effects, botulinum toxin is being tested as a therapeutic agent for the treatment of some hyperactive muscle disorders such as strabismus, hemifacial spasm, and blepharospasm.

Clostridium perfringens is an example of an organism that secretes numerous exotoxins, some of which have a clearly defined role in pathogenicity while others have only a speculated role. Some of these toxins are enzymes and include hyaluronidase, collagenase, proteinase, and deoxyribonuclease. These enzymes have various roles in microbial virulence (Table 1–4). Eleven or more toxins are produced, in various patterns, by five different types of *C. perfringens.* Alpha-toxin (lecithinase) is the principal determinant of pathogenicity in gas gangrene. This toxin is lethal and necrotizing and likely acts on lecithin-containing lipoproteins in cell membranes. This toxin can have widespread effects

TABLE 1–3. MODE OF ACTION EXOTOXINS SECRETED BY SOME OF THE MORE PROMINENT TOXIGENIC BACTERIA

Exotoxin	Mode of Action on Host Target Cells
Diphtheria toxin	Single polypeptide chain with a B fragment that binds to eukaryotic cells and an A fragment that is transported across the cell membrane and catalyzes the transfer of ADP-ribose from NAD to elongation factor 2, thereby interfering with protein synthesis
Pseudomonas toxins	Similar to the action of diphtheria toxin
Cholera toxin	B component attaches to ganglioside receptors on the surface of a susceptible cell, and an A component activates adenyl cyclase, causing outpouring of fluids and massive diarrhea
E. coli heat-labile enterotoxin	Similar to cholera toxin (nucleotide sequence 80% homologous) but causes milder disease called "traveler's diarrhea"
Botulinum toxin	Binds to neuromuscular junctions of parasympathetic nerves and blocks acetylcholine release, causing muscle paralysis
Tetanus toxin	Spasmogenic toxin fixes to neural gangliosides and blocks glycine release, permitting contraction of antagonistic muscles

TABLE 1–4. EXAMPLES OF EXTRACELLULAR ENZYMES ASSOCIATED WITH MICROBIAL VIRULENCE

Enzyme	Mode of Action
Hyaluronidase	"Spreading factor"; promotes diffusion through connective tissue by depolymerizing hyaluronic acid; may facilitate microbial invasion
Coagulase	Causes plasma to clot; may contribute to production of fibrin barrier around certain lesions (converts fibrinogen to fibrin)
Staphylokinase	Causes lysis of fibrin; produced by staphylococci
Streptokinase	Causes lysis of fibrin; may contribute to spreading of streptococcal lesions
Streptodornase	Degrades nucleic acids; may contribute to infection spread
Streptolysin O	Binds to cholesterol-containing membranes, generating slits and pores
Collagenase	Breaks down muscle collagen
Erythrogenic toxin	Responsible for the rash of scarlet fever
Hemolysins	May act as leukocidins; role not clearly defined
Alpha-toxin	Forms pores in cell membranes; cytolysin

due to the presence of lecithin in the membranes of a wide variety of cell types. Alpha-toxin may also cause platelet aggregation and thrombosis. Theta-toxin binds to cholesterol on cell membranes and may initiate the hemolysis seen in gas gangrene. *Clostridium perfringens* is also a common cause of food poisoning, attributable to an enterotoxin that is synthesized during sporulation of the organism.

Staphylococcus aureus produces both a cell-bound and an extracellular coagulase that causes clotting of plasma in vitro. Although the ability to produce coagulase is correlated with virulence of *S. aureus,* there is no evidence that the coagulase itself is responsible for this virulence. It has been hypothesized that by converting fibrinogen to fibrin, coagulase contributes to pathogenicity by entrapping the bacteria in the clot, thus protecting them from phagocytes. Pathogenic strains of *S. aureus* that do not elaborate coagulase, however, produce similar tissue lesions and are no more readily phagocytosed. When grown in broth, *S. aureus* also elaborates a necrotizing toxin that can cause necrosis of cells. Its role in actual infections is not known.

Clostridium difficile is a toxigenic species frequently seen in the hospital setting. This organism produces an enterotoxin (toxin A) and a cytotoxin (toxin B). It was originally thought that isolation of *C. difficile* from the stool of a patient was always indicative of active disease. However, epidemiological data indicate that *C. difficile* is carried in the normal flora of healthy adults and that its prevalence increases with the use of broad spectrum antibiotics. The isolation of the organism and/or its toxin is not conclusive evidence of active disease. In addition, the physician should be cautioned that some of the laboratory techniques currently used for isolation of *C. difficile* do not distinguish between toxigenic and nontoxigenic strains.

Bacterial Endotoxins. Endotoxins form the outer layer of the cell wall of gram-negative bacteria and can also be found in a cell-free form following degradation of the cell wall. Unlike most exotoxins, endotoxins are heat stable and cannot be converted to toxoids. Endotoxins are macromolecular complexes of phospholipids, polysaccharide, and protein. Their toxic biologic properties are associated with the lipid A portion of the lipopolysaccharide (LPS) moiety.

Bacterial endotoxin is involved in the pathogenesis of a variety of clinical disorders, including various liver diseases, acute renal failure, glomerulonephritis, inflammatory bowel disease, adult respiratory distress syndrome, and toxic shock syndrome. However, bacterial endotoxin is most prominently involved in septic shock. The mortality associated with gram-negative bacteremia remains high (20 to 50 percent), in spite of adequate antimicrobial therapy. The most important negative prognostic indicator of gram-negative bacteremia is the development of septic shock, a syndrome mediated by bacterial endotoxin. Septic shock often precedes multiple organ failure and is characterized by hypotension, oliguria, hypoxia, acidosis, microvascular alterations, and disseminated intravascular coagulation. It has been estimated that the mortality associated with septic shock is 75 percent. Implicated pathogens include enteric gram-negative bacteria, as well as other nonenteric gram-negative bacteria, including *Haemophilus influenzae, Neisseria meningitidis, N. gonorrhoeae,* and *Bordetella pertussis.* In addition to endotoxin, substances associated with other microbes may also mediate septic shock;

a variety of microbes have been implicated in this scenario including spirochetes, rickettsiae, mycoplasmas, parasites, viruses, and fungi. It is also possible that some microbial components greatly augment the host's susceptibility to an otherwise harmless concentration of endotoxin. For example, the toxic shock toxin (TSST-1) produced by some strains of *S. aureus* (which has no known endotoxin) markedly augments the lethality of otherwise innocuous quantities of *E. coli* endotoxin.

The molecular structure of lipopolysaccharide consists of three regions: an O-specific side chain, a "core" polysaccharide, and inner lipid A region (Fig. 1–12). Most of the pathophysiological and immunological activities of LPS are attributed to the lipid A region. The O region is the most immunogenic, and specific anti-O antibodies are highly protective in animal models. Unfortunately, the structure of the O antigen is extremely diverse among gram-negative species/strains. There have been many attempts to design an antiendotoxin vaccine to be used for passive protection in high-risk patients. This has proved to be a formidable task. The innermost portions of LPS molecule contain the conserved regions that should be most suitable for a broadly cross-reactive vaccine. Attempts have been made to use "rough mutants" (lacking the O region and part of the core polysaccharide) to raise a suitably cross-reactive antiendotoxin vaccine. However, the innermost portions of the LPS molecule are not highly immunogenic, and antisera raised against these regions often do not react with many of the clinically relevant varieties of LPS molecules.

The biological effects of endotoxin are legion. It is virtually impossible to construct an exhaustive list of these effects, although some attempt has been made in Table 1–5. Much, if not all, endotoxin toxicity is attributed to a variety of mediators made by the host in response to LPS, rather than to endotoxin itself. Some of these mediators include arachidonic acid derivatives, reactive oxygen intermediates, endorphins, coagulation factors, and platelet-activating factor. Other molecules associated with disseminated intravascular coagulation are tissue factor and intercellular adhesion molecule 1 (ICAM-1).

Many recent studies involving the activity of endotoxin have centered on the role of various host cytokines in mediating septic shock, that is, tumor necrosis factor α (TNF-α), interferon α/β (INF-α/β), and interleukins 1, 2, and 6 (IL-1, IL-2, IL-6). Of these latter mediators, TNF has received the most attention. Macrophages are the primary source of many mediators of endotoxin shock, including TNF (originally called cachectin). TNF is pyrogenic and induces septic shock following injection into experimental animals. Passive immunization with TNF protects laboratory animals from the lethal effects of endotoxin. High levels of circulating TNF have been associated with a poor prognosis in septic patients. However, it should be stressed that other experiments have demonstrated that TNF is not the sole mediator of septic shock. It is likely that septic shock results from a complex interplay of a variety of cytokine and noncytokine mediators that have overlapping and/or synergistic effects. To add to the confusion, it has even been proposed that lipid A analogs of low toxicity (and with antiendotoxin effects) be used therapeutically as endotoxin antagonists in gram-negative septicemia and septic shock.

Because endotoxin has been associated with septic shock, several attempts have been made to correlate levels of circulating endotoxin with the severity of shock or with prognosis. These attempts have led to considerable confusion because the results have been extremely variable. This variation is most likely due to the fact that the levels of circulating endotoxin appear to be transient, and it is difficult to use one time point, or even several time

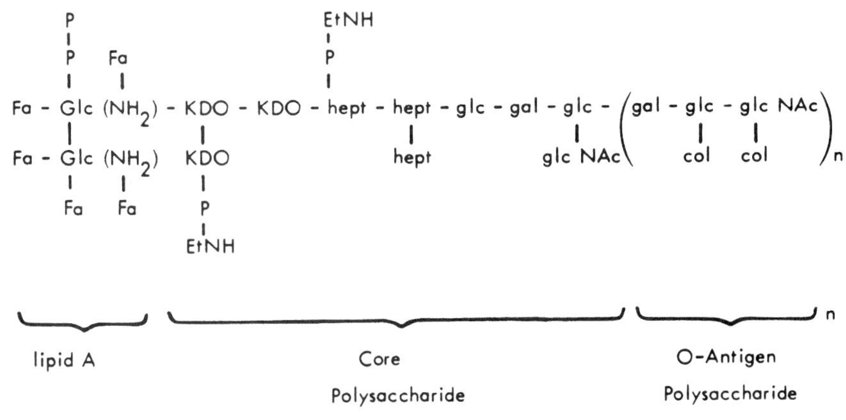

Figure 1–12. Chemical structure of *Escherichia coli* lipopolysaccharide (endotoxin). Fa, fatty acid; P, phosphate; Glc (NH_2), glycosamine; KDO, 2-keto 2-deoxyoctulosonate; EtNH, ethanolamine; hept, L-galactose; glcNAc, N-acetylglucosamine; col, colitose. *(From Morrison DC, Ulevitch RJ: Am J Pathol 93:525, 1978.)*

TABLE 1–5. SOME OF THE VARIED BIOLOGIC ACTIVITIES OF ENDOTOXIN

Releases pyrogens from neutrophils	Decreased liver glycogen
Affects thermoregulatory center in hypothalamus	Hyperlipidemia
Shifts erythropoiesis from bone marrow to spleen	Increases liver protein synthesis
Bone marrow necrosis	Decreases serum iron/iron-binding capacity
Leukopenia followed by leukocytosis	Decreases thirst, appetite, gastric emptying
Thrombocytopenia	Induces diarrhea
Platelet aggregation and activation	Increases antigen processing
Release of platelet constituents	Stimulates reticuloendothelial system
Disseminated intravascular coagulation	Enhances blood clearance of colloidal carbon
Activates complement by alternative pathway	Increases nonspecific resistance to bacteria, fungi, viruses
Decreases systemic pressure	B cell mitogen; adjuvant for variety of antigens
Decreases cardiac output	Releases mediators from macrophages
Decreases venous return	Increases phagocytosis and bacterial killing in vitro
Increases peripheral resistance	Activates macrophages
Pooling of blood	Induces various prostaglandins and cytokines
Releases/activates histamine, serotonin, kinins	Localized and generalized Shwartzman's reaction
Release of ACTH and growth hormone	Hyperglycemia followed by hypoglycemia
Stimulates antiendotoxin antibodies	Antitumor activity
Increases plasma cortisol	Binds to hydrophobic antibiotics (eg, polymyxin B)

points, to monitor the endotoxin concentration in a given patient.

Despite the hundreds of articles dealing with the chemistry and biologic effects of endotoxin, its role in the initiation of clinical infection is not clear. However, much circumstantial evidence supports its pivotal role in the pathogenesis of overwhelming gram-negative sepsis and possibly multiple organ failure.

Superantigens

There is recent evidence that proteins (toxins) made by certain bacteria can serve as *superantigens* that trigger massive cytokine release. Such microbial superantigens may plan an important role in the pathogenesis of a variety of acute and chronic disease in humans. Normally, a typical protein antigen is initially processed by the immune system in the following manner: the antigen is internalized by an antigen-presenting cell (eg, macrophage), then degraded into antigenic peptides by intracellular proteases, which subsequently bind to the major histocompatibility complex (MHC). The peptide-MHC complex is then expressed on the surface of the antigen-presenting cell and is recognized by a clone of T cells specific for the antigenic epitope. The specific T cell clone is then activated to release cytokines that "help" expand the clone and recruit B cells and cytotoxic T cells to mediate the various immune responses.

The reaction is specific to the congenitally committed clone for that epitope and is thereby a contained specific response. Superantigens differ from other antigens in that they do not require immunological processing by an antigen-presenting cell. Rather, superantigens interact directly with class II MHC molecules on macrophages, and this complex interacts directly with the T cell receptor—but not with the part that normally accepts the antigenic epitope. Instead, the superantigen binds with a portion of the T cell receptor (TcR)—that is, the variable of the beta chain (V_{β}). Thus, many clones of T cells are stimulated regardless of the antigenic specificity of the TcR. The end result is a massive release of lymphokines and monokines. Of special importance is the release of INF-γ and IL-2 by the T cell and of IL-1 and TNF by the macrophage. Both IL-1 and TNF are strongly implicated in the pathogenesis of fever and shock; INF-γ is a major cytokine that upregulates TNF and IL-1 production by the macrophages.

To date, the recognized superantigens include antigens associated with human immunodeficiency virus (HIV), various pyrogenic toxins of streptococci and staphylococci (some scarlet fever toxins, some staphylococcal enterotoxins, some toxins of *Strepto-*

coccus sanguis and groups B, C, F, and G streptococci, as well as toxic shock syndrome toxin 1), streptococcal M protein, and staphylococcal exfoliative toxin. Superantigens have been implicated in a variety of diseases, many of which were once thought to be allergic and autoimmune reactions. These diseases include rheumatic fever, guttate psoriasis, Kawasaki syndrome, arthritis, and atopic dermatitis. Because superantigens are associated with the induction of shock-like syndromes, it has been speculated that superantigens may play a role in the pathogenesis of septic shock.

INFECTIOUS DISEASE AS A RESULT OF HOST RESPONSE TO INFECTION

If no toxic agent is implicated in microbial pathogenesis, disease is often produced as a result of the host response to the microbe. The immune response to infections may have evolved as protective devices, but these devices can themselves produce inflammation, cell infiltration, and tissue destruction and may even ultimately lead to death. For example, pneumococcal pneumonia is characterized by lung consolidation mediated by a massive leukocytic infiltrate. The lesions seen in tuberculosis (granulomas and caseous necrosis) are associated with cell-mediated immune response and activated macrophages.

Perhaps the best known disease caused by the host immune response is rheumatic fever, which follows group A streptococcal infections. Streptococci have antigens that cross-react with heart muscle; therefore, antibodies against these streptococcal antigens can react with heart muscle and valve tissue. The resulting antigen-antibody complexes can activate both the complement cascade and inflammatory changes, which lead to myocarditis and endocarditis. Because many strains of streptococci have these antigens, recurrent attacks of rheumatic fever can occur.

Antibodies to other microbes also form during the course of infection, and antigen-antibody complexes can themselves lead to disease. For example, immune complexes can become deposited on the basement membranes of the renal glomerulus and blood vessels. In these sites, immune complexes activate the complement system and produce inflammation and immune injury. This injury causes acute glomerulonephritis and vasculitis. Kidney deposits of immune complexes have been found in people with hepatitis B infection, infection with *S. pyogenes,* and malaria. These glomerulonephritides are usually acute. The antigen responsible for chronic glomerulonephritis has not been identified.

Delayed-type hypersensitivity reactions to microbial antigens are responsible for some of the most prominent clinical manifestations of microbial disease. For example, dermatophytes grow in the stratum corneum of the skin. These fungi do not seem to produce any irritant or toxins that directly damage the skin; however, after 2 to 3 weeks, the advancing border of the infection may become inflamed. This inflammation stems from the host immunity to the dermatophyte. This immunity then produces most of the pathology observed in clinical dermatophytoses, including erythema and edema. The cell-mediated immune damage has some benefit to the host, because it prevents the spread or the lateral migration of the fungus within the skin. If cell-mediated immunity does not develop, the skin does not become inflamed but the infection is not eradicated. Consequently, in patients without the ability to express cell-mediated immunity, the infected skin is only minimally inflamed, but the fungus infection persists to produce scaling erythema, pruritus, fissures, and cracks. The acute inflammatory type of skin infection usually heals spontaneously or responds well to treatment. The chronic or noninflammatory type of infection, however, associated with failure to express cell-mediated immunity to the fungus, is relapsing and responds poorly to treatment.

Another example of the immune response contributing to disease is experimental lymphocytic choriomeningitis virus in mice. Infection of healthy, adult animals with this virus produces choroiditis and meningitis. A persistent carrier state ensues, however, if lymphocytic choriomeningitis is inoculated into immunologically incompetent neonatal mice within 24 hours of birth, or into adult mice that have been immunosuppressed and are unable to mount an immune response against the virus. Both inoculated neonatal mice and adult immunosuppressed mice persistently carry the virus but do not develop meningitis or choroiditis. Histologically, lymphocytic infiltrates can be seen in the choroid plexus and meninges of animals that develop choriomeningitis. Thus, in these animals, the immune response to the virus is responsible for the cerebral injury and subsequent death. Lymphocytic choriomeningitis virus can be detected by immunofluorescence in the cerebrum and cerebellum, liver, and other organs of mice inoculated at birth, despite lack of cellular destruction or pathologic or functional changes. If, however, immune lymphocytes are passively transferred to these animals, these mice rapidly die of diffuse tissue damage caused by a vigorous inflammatory infiltrate.

PATTERNS OF INFECTION

Organotrophism

For reasons that are not clearly understood, some bacteria are highly selective in the surfaces or tissues they infect or invade. For example, *S. pneumoniae* and *M. tuberculosis* have a predilection for the lung; *S. pyogenes* and *C. diphtheriae* infect the oropharynx; *Salmonella* species and *C. difficile* infect the intestinal tract; *S. pneumoniae* and *N. meningitidis* are frequent etiologic agents of meningitis; and *E. coli* is the primary cause of urinary tract infections. Clearly, some of these patterns reflect the preferred ecological niches of the organisms (eg, *S. pneumoniae* colonizes the pharynx) and some represent known and unknown receptor–ligand interactions (eg, *E. coli* bind to urothelium), but their pathogenetic factors remain to be elucidated.

Time Course of Infection

Microorganisms can cause infections that have different time courses: acute, chronic, persistent (latent), and slow. These divisions are for convenience, because microbes can cause more than one pattern of infection. Furthermore, acute infections can become chronic, or latent, or can develop into slow infections, and latent infections can become acute infections.

Acute infections have an abrupt onset and last for several days or several weeks. Most acute surgical infections are localized to one organ or body region, as occurs in pneumonia, cellulitis, carbuncle, abscess, pyelonephritis, peritonitis, or infection of an artificial valve or aortic graft.

Disseminated infections involve multiple tissues or organs and are spread via the bloodstream. Disseminated infections are rare in surgical patients, but, when they do occur, they are frequently fatal. In addition, surgical patients with compromised host defenses are susceptible to opportunistic disseminated bacterial, fungal, and viral diseases.

Inapparent infections occur when the host has evidence of infection but there are no clinical manifestations and no disease occurs. Most infections with poliovirus and mumps virus are inapparent; patients manifest serum antibody to the virus but have never had clinical disease. Inapparent infection also occurs with *H. capsulatum, M. tuberculosis, C. immitis, T. pallidum, S. pyogenes* (streptococcus carrier), *S. typhi,* and others.

Chronic infections last from weeks to months and years and are particularly common with facultative intracellular pathogens. Most surgical infections do not fall into this category, but the surgeon can encounter leprosy, syphilis, tuberculosis, anthrax, and osteomyelitis.

Persistent (latent) infections occur when the microbial parasite and host have reached an equilibrium so that the microbe does not cause disease but remains in the host—unaffected by host defenses. Viruses, especially members of the herpesvirus family, are the best examples of persistent infections. Herpes zoster virus can persist in the dorsal root ganglia for years without causing disease, only to appear as an acute case of zoster when the appropriate stimulus reactivates it. Herpes simplex virus, the etiologic agent of fever blister, is also a latent virus that can be reactivated by stress, heat, actinic radiation, and illness. Most adults have been infected by another herpesvirus, cytomegalovirus (an inapparent infection). It can remain latent until reactivated by pregnancy, immunosuppression, or cancer chemotherapy. All latent herpesviruses can be reactivated by operation, immunosuppressive drugs, or cancer chemotherapy. Syphilis, tuberculosis, and other bacteria may exist as latent infection, and their reactivation may present with local (and therefore surgical) manifestations.

Slow viral infections refer to viral infections that may require several years to become clinically manifest. Virus replication is not slow, but the disease occurs over a prolonged period. Almost all slow virus disease primarily affects the central nervous system. Subacute sclerosing panencephalitis is caused by measles viruses. Other slow virus infections are Kuru and Creutzfeldt-Jakob disease, which may actually be due to a new type of infectious agent, a prion, which contains protein but no detectable RNA or DNA.

Synergistic Infections

According to Koch's postulates, an infectious agent is documented if it can be isolated from an infected site, inoculated into a healthy host, and reproduce the pathogenesis of the disease. If all diseases had a single etiologic agent, antimicrobial therapy could be more easily targeted at the offending agent. However, some diseases are clearly the result of a complex interplay of several etiologic agents. Peritonitis, caused by bowel spillage, typically results in the isolation of 5 to 13 different bacteria that are a mixture of strictly anaerobic and facultative species. Gas gangrene, actinomycosis, Vincent's angina, and Meleney's synergistic gangrene of the abdominal wall are other examples of synergistic infections that challenge the physician's ability to target therapy toward a specific etiologic agent.

SUMMARY

The etiologic agents of surgical infections are legion and include viruses, bacteria, fungi, and protozoa. A broad-based knowledge of the patterns of pathogenicity exhibited by these microbes should aid the physician in the diagnosis and treatment of the majority of infectious diseases associated with surgical patients.

BIBLIOGRAPHY

Baron S: Medical Microbiology, 3rd ed. New York, Churchill Livingstone, 1991.

Bayston KF, Cohen J: Bacterial endotoxin and current concepts in the diagnosis and treatment of endotoxemia. J Med Microbiol 31:73, 1990.

Davis BD, Dulbecco R, Eisen HN, Ginsberg HS: Microbiology, 4th ed. Philadelphia, Lippincott, 1990.

Falkow S, Isberg RR, Portnoy DA: The interaction of bacteria with mammalian cells. Annu Rev Cell Biol 8:333, 1992.

Gorbach SL, Bartlett JG, Blacklow NR (eds): Infectious Diseases, Philadelphia, Saunders, 1992.

Joklik WK, Willett HP, Amos DB, Wilfert CM: Zinsser Microbiology, 19th ed. Norwalk, CT, Appleton & Lange, 1988.

Morrison DC, Ryan JL: Bacterial Endotoxic Lipopolysaccharides. Ann Arbor, MI, CRC Press, 1992.

Schlievert PM: Role of superantigens in human disease. J Infect Dis 167:997, 1993.

Laboratory Diagnosis of Infections

CHAPTER 2

Kenneth H. Rand, Henry H. Balfour, Jr.

A microbiology laboratory is essential for establishing the cause of infectious diseases. The clinical picture is often sufficient to narrow the differential diagnostic possibilities to several microorganisms, but it is unwise to rely solely on clinical data to diagnose and treat surgical infections. Knowledge of how to use the diagnostic microbiology laboratory is vital for the surgeon. This chapter will not make the reader a microbiologist, but sufficient detail is given so that the surgeon can correctly interpret the results received from the diagnostic microbiology laboratory. In addition, a working knowledge of the techniques for each type of culture provides insight into the limitations of the diagnostic procedures.

COLLECTION OF SPECIMENS

Specimen collection and transport are the foundation for reliable microbiologic diagnosis. A culture report is only as good as the specimen cultured. If specimens are inappropriately collected and transported, the causative agent can be lost, and other organisms that are actually contaminants may be erroneously considered as pathogens.

General Principles

Knowledge of normal flora is important for developing a rational approach to the collection of specimens and interpretation of the results. The skin, upper respiratory tract, intestinal tract, female genital area, and open wounds all have or develop normal microbial flora. The presence of normal flora is a problem that may be circumvented or minimized in one of the following ways.

1. Look only for organisms that may be pathogenic, such as group A beta-hemolytic streptococci or *Corynebacterium diphtheriae* in the throat. Indicate this to the microbiology laboratory when sending the specimen for culture.
2. Cleanse the area with an appropriate disinfectant to eliminate surface flora or contaminants. This is especially important when obtaining material from wounds.
3. Completely bypass areas of normal flora to reach tissue or body cavities not normally colonized with microbial agents; for example, aspirate the bladder to obtain a urine sample for culture.
4. Use quantitation as a means of determining

probable disease association, such as quantitative clean-catch urine specimens or bacterial counts from Gram stains of tissues.

Adequate equipment and materials are important in the collection and transport process, and new equipment and transport systems are being devised constantly (Fig. 2–1). Some prove to be valuable, but their adoption by a hospital requires actual clinical trial within the immediate environment.

Another important part of the collection process is the use of an appropriate requisition form. A completed requisition slip should accompany each specimen. The laboratory personnel can do a much better job with a specimen if they know the suspected organism (if possible), the clinical diagnosis, and recent antibiotic therapy.

Collection of Specimens for Bacterial, Fungal, and Parasitic Examination

Abscesses. If possible, prepare the abscess surface with povidone-iodine solution and let it dry. Aspirate 1 to 5 ml of purulent material with a sterile syringe and needle. Expel air from the syringe and inject the sample into an anaerobic transport media, which can also be used for aerobic and fungal cultures. Swabs should not be used because: (1) the amount of material collected is too small; (2) swabs provide an inadequate sample of the total specimen; (3) contamination with surface flora is common; and (4) exposure to air, which is unsatisfactory for anaerobic cultures, is unavoidable.

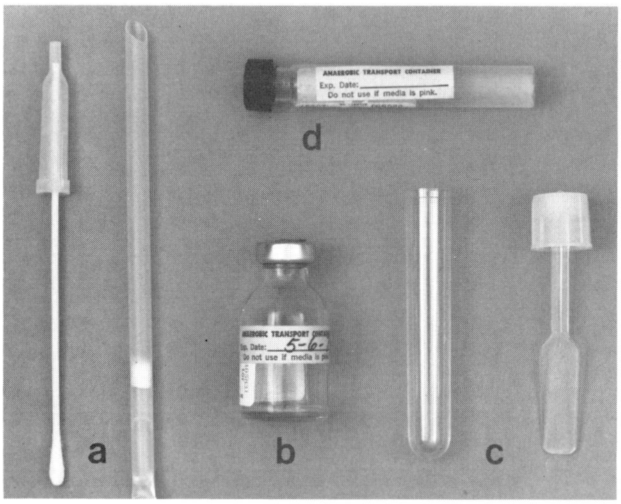

Figure 2–1. Devices useful for collection and transport of specimens. **a.** Culturette swab and tube (Marion Scientific, Kansas City, MO). **b.** Anaerobic transport vial (Gibco Diagnostics, Madison, WI). **c.** Swube paddle and tube (Becton, Dickinson & Co., Oxnard, CA). **d.** Anaerobic transport tube (Gibco Diagnostics, Madison, WI).

Actinomyces. See next section on anaerobic cultures.

Anaerobic Cultures. Collect specimens in special anaerobic containers as supplied by the laboratory. Routinely culture all abscesses and body fluids for anaerobes, except cerebrospinal and joint fluids, which rarely are infected with anaerobes. If anaerobes are specifically suspected, also culture wounds, drainage, endometrium, tissue, cerebrospinal fluid, and joint fluid. If urine is to be cultured for anaerobes, it must be obtained by suprapubic aspiration.

Whenever possible, aspirate material for culture. Expel air from the syringe and inject the specimen into an anaerobic vial. Put tissue samples into an anaerobic tube specifically designed for this purpose and follow the instructions for use of the particular tube. Specimens obtained for anaerobic culture may also be used for routine and fungal cultures.

Routine specimens from the following areas *should not be* cultured for anaerobes because they contain anaerobes as normal flora: mouth, throat, bronchus (unless washings are collected by a covered brush system), skin, cervix, urethra, and vagina. In addition, sputum and stool should not be cultured for anaerobes.

Blood Cultures. Proper preparation of the skin is critical before performing a venipuncture. The following procedure is recommended. Scrub the venipuncture site for 2 minutes with povidone-iodine or chlorhexidine surgical scrub, dry it with sterile gauze, and then cover the site with povidone-iodine or chlorhexidine solution and allow it to dry. Do not touch the venipuncture site after cleansing unless your finger has been similarly cleaned or you are wearing sterile gloves. Follow the directions established for the blood culture collecting device in use; this should include both an aerobic and an anaerobic bottle.

Laboratory personnel are frequently asked how many blood samples should be drawn. If acute sepsis, acute untreated bacterial pneumonia, meningitis, or acute bacterial endocarditis is suspected, two sets of samples (20 ml per set for adults) should be obtained from separate sites (left and right arms) before empirical therapy is begun. For patients with fever of unknown origin or suspected subacute bacterial endocarditis, three sets of blood samples should be obtained on the first day. Draw the samples at least 60 minutes apart. If the culture results are negative after 24 hours, draw two or three more samples. If five or six blood-culture results are negative, special culture techniques may be needed. If the patient has received antibiotics, inoculation of at least one hypertonic blood culture bottle or one resin-containing bottle should be done to remove the antibiotics. Data indicate that patients with suspected acute infections rarely have positive blood culture results after five or six cultures have been negative. Although previous antimicrobial therapy may delay the growth of organisms, culturing more than five or six samples does not increase the yield of positive results. There are no specific guidelines to follow in cases of suspected infection after various types of operations. One must assume in these cases that cultures of blood will be valuable any time conditions change.

Body Fluid Culture, Except Urine and Cerebrospinal Fluid. For percutaneous collection, prepare the skin as for samples for blood culture. Aspirate the fluid with a sterile syringe and needle. Expel air from the syringe, and inject the sample into the anaerobic transport media provided by the hospital or clinic. Do not collect the specimen on swabs, and do not use blood culture systems for these samples.

Bronchoscopic Washing. Collect the washings using a covered brush system, and place it in an anaerobic tube or other anaerobic collection vial. More recently, bronchoalveolar lavage has proved to be an excellent method for obtaining appropriate material for culture. It provides excellent material not only for routine bacteria but also for unconventional agents such as mycoplasmas, *Chlamydia,* and viruses, and for agents that cannot be grown but only stained, such as *Pneumocystis carinii.*

Bullous Lesions, Cellulitis, Petechiae, or Vesicles. Cleanse the skin as for blood culture sampling. The lesion must not be ruptured during preparation. Aspirate sample material with a sterile syringe and needle; do not use swabs. Transport to laboratory in anaerobic transport media as described above. If no aspirate is available, sterile normal saline for injection (without preservative) may be injected and aspirated at the lesion edges.

Petechiae present special collection problems. After the skin is cleansed, the lesion is excoriated with a needle. This material can be used to inoculate a chocolate agar plate or to prepare a smear for Gram stain directly at the bedside. Swabs are not acceptable because of possible contamination with surface flora.

Catheters. To culture venous or arterial catheters, disinfect the entry site, remove the catheter, clip off the tip, and drop it aseptically into a sterile container. Do not culture Foley catheters, because a positive result does not correlate with urinary tract infection. If infection is suspected, culture the urine.

Cerebrospinal Fluid. Gloves, gown, and mask must be worn to avoid contamination of the cerebrospinal fluid (CSF). They also protect the operator from transmissible pathogens.

Prepare the skin as for blood culture sampling, drape the surrounding skin with sterile linen, and collect 2 to 5 ml of CSF in a sterile, screw-capped (leakproof) tube. Ideally, separate specimens should be collected for culture, cell counts, and chemical determinations.

Cervix. Use a speculum lubricated with water, not a petroleum-based product, to examine the cervix os and collect a culture sample. Insert a swab into the distal portion of the cervical os, rotate gently, and allow it to remain for 10 to 30 seconds so that it is saturated. For gonococcal cultures, immediately inoculate a warm (room temperature) Thayer-Martin agar plate at one edge. Send the plate to the laboratory immediately. For nongonococcal cultures, place the specimen in a Culturette tube (Marion Scientific Corporation, Kansas City, MO) or other satisfactory transport system.

The workup for sexually transmitted diseases must also include *Chlamydia.* Several excellent methods exist including direct detection by fluorescent antibody, by ELISA, and, in the very near future, by polymerase chain reaction (PCR) as well as culture. Although these are excellent diagnostic methods, in cases of suspected rape or child abuse, courts generally have accepted only the results of *Chlamydia* culture.

Endometrium. Insert a speculum to examine the cervical os. Remove the mucous plug, wipe the cervical os with povidone-iodine solution, and aspirate material by needle and syringe or by a double-lumen catheter. The catheter technique involves first making a slight cut in the end of a No. 16 straight rubber catheter. Insert the catheter through the cervical os, pass a No. 8 infant feeding tube or intravenous catheter through the lumen of the rubber catheter to avoid contamination by normal flora, and aspirate the material. If an anaerobic culture is desired, expel air from the syringe and inject the material into an anaerobic vial. If the specimen is to be cultured only for aerobic and facultative organisms, place the aspirate in a sterile tube. Do not collect the specimen on swabs because it will be contaminated with normal cervical and vaginal flora.

Eye. Collect culture samples from the eye by retracting the lower lid and blotting the conjunctiva or pus with a swab. Avoid the lid margins and eyelashes, or the sample may be contaminated. Place the swab into a Culturette tube or other suitable transport system. Special transport media should be used for *Chlamydia* culture in infants.

Fungal Cultures. For culture of blood see the previous section on blood cultures.

Systemic Fungi. When systemic fungi such as *Histoplasma, Blastomyces,* or yeast are suspected, collect the specimen as described for bacterial culture from appropriate sites. If coccidioidomycosis is suspected, the mycology laboratory must be notified so that the culture plates are not inadvertently opened, exposing the laboratory workers.

For the culture of dermatophytes from skin, cleanse the area with 70 percent alcohol, scrape off some skin at the active border of the lesion (including some healthy skin), and place the scrapings in a dry, sterile container. The same procedure should be used for nails, except that the initial portions of the nails should be discarded and deeper scrapings sent for culture.

Gonococcal Cultures. In females, collect cervical specimens using the method previously described. In addition, if there is purulent material in the urethra, swab it and inoculate it directly onto a warm Thayer-Martin agar plate. If no purulent material is seen in the urethra, collect an anal sample by inserting a swab approximately 3 cm into the anal canal. Move the swab from side to side to sample the crypts and leave it for 10 to 30 seconds to allow for absorption of organisms. Inoculate it directly onto a warm Thayer-Martin plate. Do not make a smear, because gonococcal infection cannot be confirmed or ruled out by Gram staining material from this source. Send the culture to the laboratory immediately.

In males, collect a sample of the urethral exudate with a swab. If no exudate is present, use a sterile bacteriologic loop and gently scrape the mucosa of the anterior urethra. Alternately, a flexible wire swab may be inserted into the urethra. Inoculate the specimen directly onto a warm Thayer-Martin plate and also prepare a smear. An anal culture should also be collected. If intracellular gram-negative diplococci are seen in the Gram-stained smear of a urethral exudate from a male, it is essentially diagnostic of gonococcal infection; the Gram stain will be positive in 95 percent of cases of male gonococcal urethritis.

Malarial and Other Blood Parasites. Blood collected from the finger or earlobe should be used to prepare both thick and thin films when plasmodia or other parasites are suspected. The thick films need to dry at room temperature for 8 to 12 hours before staining is done. Collect two sets of specimens approximately 8 hours apart each day for 3 days.

Mycobacterium Cultures

SPUTUM. Do not submit a 24-hour specimen of sputum for mycobacteria cultures. Collect the first morning sputum on three separate days, and send each separately (see section on sputum collection that follows). Refrigerate specimens until they are sent to the laboratory. If the patient is not producing sputum, induce its production by having the patient inhale a warm aerosol of sterile 1 percent aqueous sodium chloride. The best time for this procedure is in the morning before breakfast. Induced sputum is superior to a gastric specimen, but a combination of both will give more positive culture results than either will alone.

GASTRIC WASHINGS. The specimen should be collected through a nasogastric tube 30 minutes after induction of sputum. If the specimen is not sent to the laboratory within 1 day, the acid should be neutralized by adding about 100 mg of powdered sodium carbonate.

URINE. A 24-hour specimen of urine should not be used for culture. Collect the first morning midstream urine on three separate days, and send each as a separate specimen (see section on urine collection). The specimens should be refrigerated if there is delay in sending them to the laboratory.

Nasopharynx. Cultures of the nasopharynx are indicated only for diagnosis of streptococcal disease in infants, for *Bordetella pertussis* (whooping cough), and to detect carriers of *Neisseria meningitidis.* The patient should be comfortably seated, with the head tilted back. A flexible wire swab is inserted through a nasal speculum into the posterior nasopharyngeal area. The swab is gently rotated and allowed to remain in place for 20 to 30 seconds. The swab is placed in a Culturette tube or other satisfactory transport system. If *B. pertussis* is suspected, immediately inoculate fresh Bordet-Gengou plates previously ordered from the microbiology laboratory. If the culture is being used to detect *N. meningitidis* carriers, be sure to indicate this on the request slip.

Nocardia. See section on fungi.

Nose. Samples from the nose are taken by swabbing the anterior nares with a sterile swab and placing it in a Culturette tube or other satisfactory transport system.

Peritoneal Fluid. See body fluid section.

Pinworm Ova. Use a Swube paddle (Falcon, Division of Becton, Dickinson & Co., Oxnard, CA) to collect a pinworm ova specimen in the morning before the patient has bathed or defecated (see Fig. 2–1). Hold the paddle by its cap and remove it from the tube. Separate the buttocks and press the tacky surface against several areas of the perianal region. Replace the paddle in the tube and send it to the laboratory. Three consecutive morning specimens should be collected to ensure detection of pinworm infection.

Pleural Fluid. See body fluid section.

Skin. See bullous lesions, cellulitis, petechiae, or vesicles.

Sputum. Interpretation of the sputum Gram stain and culture can be extremely difficult because: (1) it is almost always contaminated with upper airway normal flora, and (2) there is a high incidence of upper respiratory tract colonization with potentially pathogenic gram-negative rods, such as *Klebsiella* and *Pseudomonas.* Simply recovering one of these potential pathogens from a sputum culture does not mean the patient has pneumonia caused by that organism. Nonetheless, certain findings are helpful. If the Gram-stained sputum contains more than 25 polymorphonuclear leukocytes per low-power field, and fewer than ten epithelial cells per low-power field, it may be considered a valid specimen. Under these conditions, if literally sheets of gram-negative rods are seen, it is extremely likely the patient has a gram-negative pneumonia. A heavy predominance of lancet-shaped diplococci is suggestive of pneumonia caused by *Streptococcus pneumoniae;* large numbers of tiny, pleomorphic gram-negative rods are suggestive of *Haemophilus.* If such a specimen contains predominantly gram-negative diplococci, including intracellular bacteria within polymorphonuclear leukocytes, strong consideration must be given to *Branhamella catarrhalis.* The microbiology laboratory should be alerted to look for this organism, since it is often resistant to the penicillins. Interpreting sputum cultures from intubated patients requires some experience, but, in general, in the presence of many polymorphonuclear leukocytes, a culture growing 3+ or 4+ gram-negative rods must be taken very seriously, particularly if the Gram stain shows large numbers of gram-negative rods as well.

A sputum culture is distinctly valuable if a pathogen that rarely contaminates the mouth or pharynx is isolated, such as *Cryptococcus* or *M. tuberculosis.*

Stool

Stool Bacterial Culture. Stool cultures are useful for isolation of *Salmonella, Shigella,* and *Campylobacter* species routinely. In special cases culture for *Yersinia, Vibrio,* or *Clostridium difficile* may be indicated. A test for *C. difficile* toxin may also be indicated for diagnosis of antibiotic-associated colitis. Acute typhoid fever is best diagnosed from blood cultures because the bacteria are rarely found in the stool during the acute phase of the illness. Diarrhea caused by enterotoxigenic *Escherichia coli* can now be diagnosed by stool culture, but the laboratory must be alerted so that special media can be used. *Staphylococcus aureus* and *Candida albicans* must be present in large numbers in Gram stain of the feces to justify a diagnosis of staphylococcal or candidal enteritis; isolation of either organism alone is not sufficient—they are part of the normal fecal flora.

The specimen should be collected in a sterile bedpan or on newspaper over the toilet seat. Place a portion in a sterile nonpaper container with a lid. Send the specimen to the laboratory immediately. If a rectal swab must be used instead of a stool specimen, insert the swab 3 cm into the anal canal and leave it in for 20 to 30 seconds. Place the swab in a Culturette tube or other transport system. One specimen should be tested during the acute illness.

Request a smear for fecal leukocytes; their presence will differentiate bacterial gastroenteritis from nonspecific, toxic, or viral diarrhea. In the absence of fecal leukocytes, more than one stool culture cannot be justified.

Stool for Ova and Parasites. Stool samples to test for ova and parasites should be collected in the same manner as for bacterial culture. Specimens should not be mixed with urine or toilet bowl water because this destroys the protozoan trophozoites. The parasites are not passed consistently. A maximum of three normally passed specimens should be collected on three alternate days or, more cost effectively, daily for 3 days. If no parasites are found after three tests, one saline-purged stool may be obtained, or rectal biopsy material can be submitted. If all four specimens reveal no ova and parasites, the patient probably does not have an intestinal parasitic infection. Stools from patients receiving antidiarrheal compounds, antibiotics, antacids, oils, bismuth, or barium are unsuitable for examination. Wait at least 7 days after barium or bismuth administration before collecting a specimen suspected of containing parasites. Never transport stools in an incubator, because it enhances the disintegration of trophozoites. Liquid or soft stools should be brought to the laboratory immediately, whereas formed stools can be refrigerated.

It is important to tell the laboratory which organisms are suspected (eg, *Schistosoma, Giardia*). The patient's travel history will assist the laboratory personnel to perform optimal examinations of each specimen.

Throat. Because of the presence of the normal upper-airway bacterial flora, throat cultures should be done only to look for specific pathogens of therapeutic importance (eg, group A *Streptococcus pyogenes*). Because up to 10 to 20 percent of the normal population may be colonized with *S. pneumoniae* or *N. meningitidis,* recovery of these potential pathogens must be interpreted on clinical grounds.

Culture samples from the throat can be taken with the help of a tongue blade and bright light. Swab both tonsillar areas, posterior pharynx, and areas of inflammation, ulceration, or exudation. Place the swab in a Culturette tube or other transport device. If *C. diphtheriae* is suspected, the swab should be rubbed firmly over the lesion or, if possible, inserted beneath the tonsillar membrane. If *B. pertussis* is suspected, a posterior nasopharyngeal swab should be obtained. Consult the microbiology laboratory for the appropriate medium to be inoculated at the bedside. Send the culture to the laboratory immediately.

Urethra. See gonococcal cultures.

Urine. Because overnight incubation in the bladder yields the highest bacterial counts, the first morning urine sample is the best specimen to culture.

For clean-catch or midstream specimens, either assist the patient or give both verbal and written instructions, which include the following for females. Have the patient remove her undergarments and wash her hands with soap and water and dry them with a disposable paper towel. With one hand, the patient or nurse should spread the labia and keep them apart for the rest of the procedure. Using a fresh povidone-iodine swab for each motion, wipe the inner labial tissues down one side from front to back; then wipe the other side from front to back. With another fresh swab, wipe the center from front to back. Repeat until thoroughly clean, and finally dry the area with sterile gauze. Have the patient void a small amount of urine into the toilet or a bedpan. The flow is stopped briefly and then is continued into a sterile specimen container. A few drops are adequate for culture, but 5 to 10 ml are ideal. Be careful not to touch the inner part of the container or lid while the container is being capped.

In males, have the patient wash his hands with soap and water and dry them with a disposable paper towel. Retract the foreskin, if necessary. Using a povidone-iodine swab, clean the glans and meatus thoroughly and wipe with sterile gauze. Ask the patient to void a small amount into the toilet or a bedpan. The flow should be stopped briefly, then another 5 to 10 ml are voided into a sterile specimen container.

In infants or small children, after cleaning the periurethral tissues, place a sterile urine bag over the labia or penis to collect urine. If no urine is present after 30 minutes, reclean the patient and attach a new bag. If it is impossible to obtain urine or if the culture yields a mixture of organisms, a suprapubic aspiration is recommended.

The suprapubic tap is the most desirable technique for infants and small children. The suprapubic area should be scrubbed with povidone-iodine surgical scrub. Paint the area with povidone-iodine solution and allow it to dry. Using a sterile syringe and needle, aspirate a few milliliters of urine from the bladder. Inject the urine into a sterile container. If an anaerobic culture is desired, expel the air and inject the sample into an anaerobic vial.

All specimens should be refrigerated if there is to be a delay in transport to the laboratory. Urine for culture should never be taken from a bedpan or urinal, nor should a specimen be brought from home because any contaminants will have multiplied, and false-positive results are common.

Venereal Disease. If *Chlamydia* or *Gonococcus* is suspected, the appropriate sections in this chapter should be consulted.

HAEMOPHILUS DUCREYI. Special chocolate agar (with and without vancomycin) should be ordered from the laboratory before collection and should be present at the patient's bedside for immediate incubation. The ulcer base should be cleansed thoroughly with a sterile gauze pad moistened in sterile saline. A sterile swab moistened in sterile saline should then be applied to the cleansed ulcer base and immediately rolled at the edge of the chocolate plate. Only then should it be rolled at the edge of the plate with vancomycin. The plates should be taken to the laboratory immediately. A direct smear must be interpreted with caution because other gram-negative bacteria (eg, *Bacteroides fragilis*) have morphology similar to *H. ducreyi.*

SYPHILIS. Serologic tests are best for the diagnosis of syphilis. Many laboratories do not perform dark-field examinations for syphilis because substantial expertise is required to differentiate *Treponema pallidum* from saprophytic treponemes.

When obtaining specimens from open lesions, always wear rubber gloves. First remove surface crusts or scabs, cleanse several times with a saline-soaked gauze sponge. Dry the surface and abrade it until it bleeds. Remove the blood by gentle sponging, and when a serum exudate appears touch it with a No. 1 coverslip. Invert the coverslip on a slide, and seal the edges with Vaseline or other suitable sealing material. Immediately send the specimen for dark-field examination. Delay will result in loss of motility of the spirochetes.

Wounds. To collect culture samples from closed wounds, use the technique described in the section in bullous lesions.

For open wounds, clean the sinus tract opening or wound surface with a sterile, water-soaked sponge. Be careful not to use bacteriostatic saline. Scrapings of the wound are best because the contribution of the surface flora is minimized. Alternatively, aspirate the material with a sterile syringe and needle or catheter. Do not use swabs. If little fluid is present, inject a small amount of sterile water and aspirate. Place any material into a sterile container. If an anaerobic culture is desired, expel any air bubble from the syringe and inject the sample into an anaerobic vial or place curettings into an anaerobic tube. Send the specimen to the laboratory immediately, and indicate the site of the wound on the request slip.

Viruses. We recommend collecting viral specimens from all patients in whom viral infections are clinically suspected (Table 2–1). Collect the specimens as outlined in Table 2–2. When submitting specimens for viral culture, always send an additional serum sample for acute viral antibody titers. If no virus is isolated, submit a second sample 2 to 6 weeks later. The diagnosis can then be made by finding an antibody titer rise, as described later in this chapter.

TRANSPORTATION OF SPECIMENS

Although some specific directions for specimen transport were already included, they are worth repeating. Even when the sample is obtained by the best technique available, organisms can be altered or lost if inappropriate storage and transportation

TABLE 2–1. WHICH PATIENTS TO STUDY FOR VIRAL INFECTIONS AND WHAT TO COLLECT

General Disease Category	Specimens Recommended for Viral Cultures
Neonatal	Throat swab, fresh morning urine; vesicular fluid or swabs if rash is present
Respiratory (index or lower respiratory tract involvement)	Throat swab
Central nervous system	Throat swab; stool or rectal swab (stool is preferable); urine, CSF, biopsy material; vesicular fluid if available
Gastrointestinal	Throat swab, stool or rectal swab
Exanthems	Throat swab; stool or rectal swab; vesicular fluid if present
Fever of unknown origin	Throat swab; urine, stool, heparinized blood
Infections in immunocompromised patients	Throat swab; urine, heparinized blood, bronchoalveolar lavage

TABLE 2–2. COLLECTION OF SPECIMENS FOR VIRAL DIAGNOSIS

Specimen	Method
Throat swab	Swab posterior pharynx briskly with two sterile, dry, cotton-tipped applicators. (If respiratory syncytial virus is suspected, it may be preferable to insert one swab into the nasopharynx and use the other to swab the posterior pharynx. They can be sent to the laboratory as one specimen.) Insert the tips of the applicators into a sterile tube containing medium suitable for bacteriologic cultures such as trypticase soy or Hank's balanced salt solution. Culturette tubes are acceptable.
Rectal swab	Insert two cotton-tipped applicators at least 3 cm into the rectum. The swab should be stained with stool. Transport as a throat swab.
Vesicular lesions	If vesicles are intact, aspirate at least six lesions with a 25-gauge needle attached to a tuberculin syringe. Replace the hub on the needle. Label the syringe appropriately and send to the laboratory.
Urine, stool, cerebrospinal fluid, biopsy, or autopsy	Collect in sterile containers. At least 1 g of tissue or stool, 2 ml of spinal fluid, and 20 ml of urine are adequate.
Heparinized blood (for viral isolation)	Draw at least 10 ml of blood and place in a heparinized tube at once; shake gently to ensure anticoagulation.
Serum (for antibody tests)	Two specimens are preferred; the first should be collected as soon after onset of acute illness as possible, and the second 2 to 6 weeks later. Collect 7 ml of blood, if possible, in a plain (not anticoagulated) tube. Avoid hemolysis and do not freeze.

methods are used. Some organisms, including enteric gram-negative rods, anaerobes, myxoviruses, and herpesviruses, do not survive outside the body for long and are particularly susceptible to drying. Culterette tubes contain a small amount of Stuart's medium in a capsule, which is broken after the swab has been inserted in the tube, to provide enough liquid medium to keep the specimen moist.

When the specimen collected is a body fluid, many organisms will proliferate in the fluid at room temperature. If a urine specimen cannot be delivered to the laboratory within 20 minutes after collection for bacterial culture or within 4 hours for viral isolation, the sample should be held in a refrigerator (4C). Refrigerator temperatures, however, are deleterious to the types of fastidious bacteria that may be found in body fluids, and specimens containing these must be delivered to the laboratory immediately. Specimens should not be frozen for storage.

Serum samples for antibody titers may be shipped, if necessary, at room temperature if the sera have been separated from the clot. Most serologic tests measure IgG antibody, which is extremely stable unless the specimen is grossly contaminated with bacteria. Even IgM can usually survive shipment at room temperature. Sera may also be stored or shipped frozen, but whole blood should never be frozen because hemolysis renders most serologic tests impossible.

For anaerobic cultures, particularly those placed in tubes, rapid transportation is essential because the anaerobic atmosphere can become aerobic and the fastidious anaerobes will be lost (see Fig. 2–1).

A good clinical microbiology laboratory will have arranged for messenger services and timed specimen pickup; these are critically important. It is an excellent idea to monitor the time from collection of specimens to the time the laboratory has logged them in.

BEST METHODS OF LABORATORY DIAGNOSIS

The best laboratory procedures for making an accurate identification of each microbial agent are summarized in Table 2–3.

Direct Microscopic Examination

Direct Gram stains of certain clinical specimens are extremely valuable (Fig. 2–2). One of the most useful is Gram staining the spinal fluid sediment, which can give a presumptive diagnosis of *Haemophilus influenzae, N. meningitidis,* or *S. pneumoniae* meningitis. It is also very useful to perform Gram stains on purulent exudates to determine immediately the types of organisms involved and their relative numbers. The Gram stain is especially useful when anaerobes are suspected. A satisfactory method is given in Table 2–4.

A Gram stain can give not only rapid information as to the class and general morphology of the organism but also important quantitative information. For example, in mixed infections, the most prevalent organism cannot always be gleaned from a culture because the rates of growth differ. If a

TABLE 2–3. CLINICAL MICROBIOLOGY LABORATORY ISOLATION AND IDENTIFICATION

Agent	Best Method for Diagnosis[a]
Bacteria	Isolation of organisms on agar or in both media; direct Gram stains of certain specimens valuable
Chlamydiae	Inoculation into cell culture and identification of inclusion bodies in infected cells
Fungi	Isolation of organisms on selective media, such as Saboraud's; detection of antigen by latex agglutination useful for *Cryptococcus;* India ink preparation of cerebrospinal fluid; KOH preparation of direct specimens
Mycobacteria	Culture definitive but slow; acid-fast stains of sputum or lymph nodes valuable
Mycoplasma pneumoniae	Serology; fourfold or greater rise in complement-fixing titers or elevated cold agglutinins
Parasites	
Helminths	Identification of ova or larvae in stool preparations
Protozoa	Direct microscopic identification of organisms in stool, tissue, or blood specimens; specific stains sometimes useful
Rickettsiae	Serology; fourfold rise in complement-fixing tests or elevated *Proteus* agglutinins
Viruses	Isolation in cell cultures or fourfold rise in serum antibody titers

[a] Molecular diagnostic techniques may replace many of these methods.

TABLE 2–4. METHOD OF GRAM STAINING

Procedure: Prepare smear and fix with heat.

1. Flood slide with crystal violet (solution A). Add about 3 drops solution B. Wash with tap water.
2. Flood slide with iodine. Wash with tap water.
3. Decolorize with acetone-alcohol until no more purple is seen in the washings (about 10 seconds, depending on thickness of smear). Wash with tap water.
4. Flood slide with safranin. Wash with tap water. Blot dry with clean blotter, bibulous paper, or paper towel.

Reagents

Solution A—crystal violet	
Crystal violet, Cl 42555	20 g
Distilled water	2000 ml
Solution B—sodium bicarbonate	
$NaHCO_3$	100 g
Distilled water	2000 ml
Iodine (dilute 1:10 for working solution)	
Iodine crystals	100 g
Potassium iodide (KI)	5 g
Sodium hydroxide pellets	20 g
Distilled water	500 ml
Add sodium hydroxide pellets slowly to 50 ml water. After pellets have dissolved, add iodine and potassium iodide. Add 300–400 ml water and mix until iodine goes into solution. Dilute to total of 500 ml. Dilute 1:10 before using.	
Acetone alcohol	
Acetone	1000 ml
Alcohol (95% ethyl)	1000 ml
Safranin	
Safranin O, Cl 50240	40 g
Distilled water	2000 ml

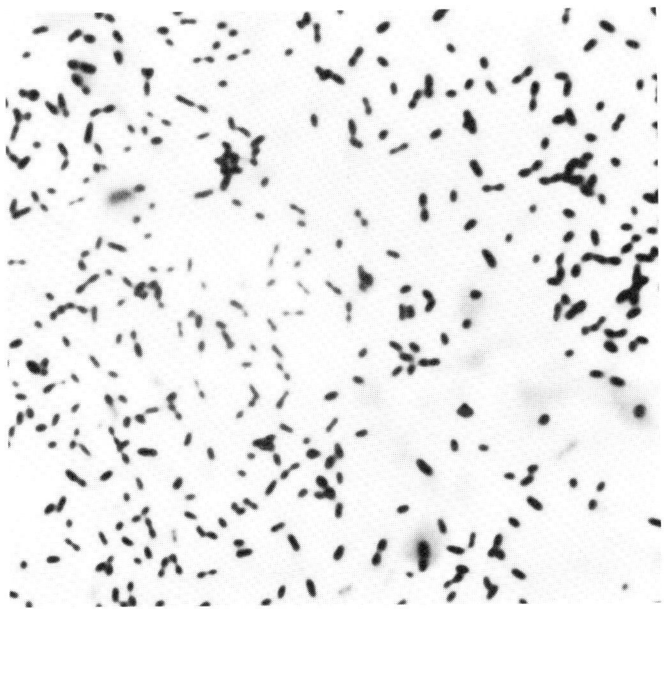

Figure 2–2. Gram stain of cerebrospinal fluid showing typical gram-positive diplococci, indicating the presence of *Streptococcus pneumoniae. (Courtesy of Louise Hofherr, University of Minnesota, Minneapolis.)*

large number of a slow-growing organism were present in the wound, only a few organisms may become apparent on the culture plate. A smaller number of a fast-growing organism may proliferate and appear to be more important on culture. The truly predominant organism may be identifiable on initial smear and Gram stain.

Direct examination of the specimen in actinomycosis, for example, may demonstrate the presence of the diagnostic sulfur granules. If these are seen, an acid-fast stain should also be performed. *Actinomyces* are not acid fast, and this distinguishes them from *Nocardia,* which are acid fast and may produce a similar granule.

Direct examination of all specimens sent for fungal cultures should be performed. This is best done by suspending a portion of the specimen in a potassium hydroxide solution. The potassium hydroxide dissolves the tissue elements and reveals the fungal hyphae or mycelium. Although a specific identification of the fungus cannot always be made, its presence in the tissue indicates a fungal infection and thus helps to determine that any fungus subsequently isolated is not a contaminant.

Bacterial Identification

For bacteria, microbiology laboratories use various media and atmospheres for isolation of organisms. The media most commonly employed include 5 percent sheep blood agar for growth of most organisms, MacConkey agar or eosin methylene blue for gram-negative rods, and trypticase soy or thioglycollate broth for more fastidious organisms or those present in smaller numbers. Many laboratories also include media such as colistin-nalidixic acid agar or phenylethyl alcohol agar for isolation of gram-positive organisms. The majority of bacterial species will grow in the media mentioned. Some, such as *H. influenzae,* require special growth factors that are present in chocolate agar. *Neisseria gonorrhoeae* and *N. meningitidis* are particularly fastidious and require either chocolate or Thayer-Martin agar and incubation in carbon dioxide. This emphasizes again the need to specify, on the requisition slip, the clinical diagnosis and what organisms are suspected. Culture techniques for anaerobic bacteria are discussed in Chapter 6.

After isolation, organisms are identified on the basis of colonial morphology, Gram stain, and biochemical and serologic tests. Isolation and identification of commonly isolated bacteria is relatively rapid, within 24 to 48 hours. Some particularly fastidious anaerobes may require several weeks before a definitive identification can be made.

If one suspects the presence of a certain organism and the laboratory does not report it, consultation with the laboratory personnel is recommended. If a fastidious organism was suspected and not indicated on the requisition slip, the proper medium may not have been inoculated, or the specimen collection and transport may have been imperfect. It is tremendously useful to the laboratory to obtain feedback on patients who appear to have classic diseases but in whom the causative organism was not found (eg, a patient with scarlet fever from whom group A beta-hemolytic streptococci were not isolated). Only through a continual feedback between the clinician and the laboratory can optimal service for the patient be provided.

Quantitative cultures are occasionally of great value. The best example is urine, in which a properly collected specimen containing 100,000 colonies or more of a single gram-negative rod is statistically linked to urinary tract infection, whereas a culture with colony counts lower than that or a culture containing mixed organisms is usually not indicative of a bona fide infection. Here again, not only the quantity of organisms present but also the method of specimen collection is critical. For example, culturing any quantity of bacteria in a suprapubic tap would be significant, whereas greater than 100,000 colonies of mixed skin flora such as alpha streptococci or *Corynebacterium* species in a clean-catch sample from a woman would probably be insignificant.

Quantitative cultures of tissue in burns and other wounds have been used to determine when to graft or otherwise secondarily close open wounds. For accuracy, the tissue submitted to the laboratory should weigh at least 0.5 g, which would be a piece measuring about 2 × 1 × 0.5 cm. Punch biopsies are also widely used. The tissue is weighed on an analytic balance and the bacterial count determined by direct culture after homogenization. A semiquantitative technique has also been devised, which involves the examination of Gram-stained material under an oil immersion lens.

Legionella pneumophila (legionnaires' disease bacillus) may be isolated using special media. However, lung biopsy or pleural fluid has the best yield for culture. Sputum and bronchial washings must be cultured in selective media to suppress the normal respiratory flora that will overgrow the slower-growing *L. pneumophila.* For detection of the organism in these latter specimens, the direct fluorescent antibody technique can also be used. Antiserum for this test is available commercially. Yet, it is critical to have experienced personnel examine these specimens. In addition to culture and immunofluorescence tests, serologic detection of antibody production may be used to diagnose legionnaries' disease.

In the last few years, latex agglutination tests have become widely available for the direct detection of bacterial antigens in body fluids, particularly CSF. Antibodies specific for bacterial antigens are coated on latex beads. When mixed with body fluids containing the specific organisms, an agglutination reaction takes place. Reagents are now commercially available for the direct and rapid detection of *H. influenzae, S. pneumoniae, N. meningitidis,* and group B *Streptococcus.* These tests may be carried out on CSF, serum, pleural fluid, and urine; however, many body fluids such as serum and urine may give nonspecific agglutination reactions since these fluids must be highly concentrated for the test. In general, these tests are from 80 to 95 percent as sensitive as culture. In no case can they substitute for clinical judgment.

When several organisms have been isolated, interpretation of culture results is difficult. An example is a culture of peritoneal fluid. Often the specimen will contain many fecal organisms, especially when the infection has just begun. In these cases it should suffice for the laboratory to report the culture as "mixed fecal flora" (Fig. 2–3). Isolation and identification of all the anaerobic organisms are tedious, time consuming, and expensive. It is impossible to be certain which organisms are the initial pathogens in mixed infections because relatively avirulent organisms can act synergistically. Selection of appropriate antimicrobial therapy is therefore complex. If fecal-like flora are present, the clinician can assume the presence of *B. fragilis,* the most antibiotic-resistant of the anaerobes, and treatment should include an appropriate antibiotic such as metronidazole, imipenem, amoxacillin/sulbactam, or ticarcillin/clavulanate.

Isolation and identification of facultative organisms, such as *E. coli,* from peritoneal fluid is simpler than is identification of anaerobes, but the interpretation of the importance of each in a mixed infection is still difficult. Predominance does not necessarily equate with clinical significance.

Wound cultures also present problems of interpretation when several organisms are isolated. However, if the specimen has been collected to eliminate any contaminating surface flora, the isolated organisms will be more significant. We again emphasize the importance of proper collection of specimens to obtain worthwhile results.

Chlamydia ***Identification.*** To diagnose nongonococcal urethritis in males, insert a swab of 2 to 5 cm into the urethra. In females, swab the cervix. Place the specimen *immediately* into the transport medium appropriate for *Chlamydia* supplied by the laboratory and send it directly to the laboratory. Lung tissue obtained by biopsy or autopsy should be treated in the same way.

These intracellular organisms grow only in living cells and are transmitted by direct contact. There are now three clinically important species of *Chlamydia: C. trachomatis,* which consists of 15 serotypes; *C. psittaci,* which produces the zoonosis psittacosis; and *C. pneumoniae* (TWAR), which also produces pneumonia in adolescents and adults. These organisms can be isolated in embryonated eggs, but certain cell cultures, such as McCoy, are ideal. The presence of *Chlamydia* is detected approximately 2 days after inoculation by finding typical cytoplasmic inclusion bodies after the cell cul-

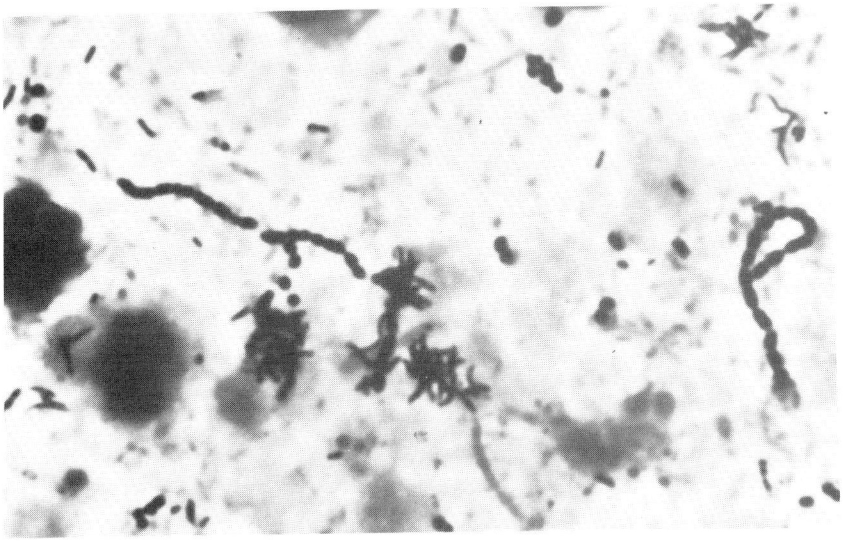

Figure 2–3. Gram stain of peritoneal fluid showing various rods, pleomorphic rods, and cocci typical of fecal flora. *(Courtesy of Louise Hofherr, University of Minnesota, Minneapolis.)*

tures have been stained with iodine. In the case of conjunctivitis, typical cytoplasmic inclusion bodies may be seen in Giemsa-stained conjunctival scrapings. Because of the technical difficulty and cost, most clinical laboratories do not offer cultures for *Chlamydia.* Recently, however, monoclonal antibodies specific for *Chlamydia* have become commercially available, and there are now readily available reagents for the direct detection of *Chlamydia* in air-dried smears from infected tissues. In preparing smears for fluorescent antibody staining for *Chlamydia,* it is critical that the actual mucosal epithelial cells be scraped and smeared; the urethral exudate is of no value.

Mycobacterium *Identification.* The most important mycobacterial agent is *M. tuberculosis,* but the so-called atypical organisms also cause disease. The definitive method of diagnosis is culture, which by classic methods may require 6 to 8 weeks for culture and identification. A radiometric method (Bactec) has become available in which radioactive substrates are incorporated into the medium. Mycobacteria (or other contaminating bacteria) metabolize these substrates to radioactive carbon dioxide, which can be detected by sampling the gas in the bottle. *Mycobacterium tuberculosis* can be detected in 1 to 3 weeks routinely by this method. With the use of DNA probes, *M. tuberculosis* complex and *M. avium-intracellulare* may now be definitively identified within days of growth in liquid medium. Other atypical mycobacteria still require biochemical tests and growth on solid media for definitive identification. Recently, the incidence of *M. tuberculosis* has increased because of the increasing number of AIDS cases, and multiply resistant strains have emerged. Therefore, antibiotic susceptibility testing has assumed new importance. Patients with positive AFB smears must remain in respiratory isolation for at least 2 weeks of treatment *and* must have responded clinically before isolation can be discontinued. Selective stains, including modifications of the Ziehl-Nielson acid-fast procedure and fluorescent staining of the organisms, have achieved importance. Neither of these stains differentiates between *M. tuberculosis* and the atypical mycobacteria.

Mycoplasma *Identification.* *Mycoplasma pneumoniae* can be grown on a cell-free medium (eg, Hayflick), but growth of these organisms is relatively slow, and definitive identification takes approximately 3 weeks. For this reason, routine cultures for *Mycoplasma* are rarely done, and serologic techniques are used to make the diagnosis. A four-fold or greater rise in *M. pneumoniae* complement-fixing titers is diagnostic. A nonspecific test, the cold-agglutinin titer, is readily available in most laboratories, and if titers are elevated or rising a presumptive diagnosis of *M. pneumoniae* infection can be made. Some children will not develop elevated cold agglutinins in the presence of mycoplasmal infection. Conversely, adults may have positive cold agglutinins associated with *Chlamydia* or non-mycoplasmal infections.

Unlike *M. pneumoniae,* the genital mycoplasmas, *Mycoplasma hominis* and *Ureaplasma urealyticum,* can readily be cultured. When they are recovered from genital cultures, however, their significance is difficult to assess because from 30 to 40 percent of sexually active women carry these organisms without symptoms. Nevertheless, they have been associated with postpartum fever, infections following urogenital surgery, and neonatal pneumonia. If recovered from an abscess, blood, or a normally sterile body fluid or tissue, they may be presumed to be pathogenic.

Parasitic Identification

Helminth infections are best identified by a parasitologist skilled in microscopic morphologic identification of characteristic ova or larvae. These are found in stool preparations that have been collected as outlined in the preceding section.

Protozoa are identified directly by microscopic examination of the specimen and are rarely cultured. Stools are best examined fresh (preferably liquid since the yield from formed stools is quite low). Stools may also be preserved with polyvinyl alcohol (PVA) and stained with trichrome (Wheatley) stain. Several direct antigen tests are now available for such organisms as *Giardia* end cryptosporidia.

In an immunocompromised patient in whom *Pneumocystis carinii* infection is suspected, the bronchoalveolar lavage sediment should be examined with methenamine silver or Giemsa stain. *Pneumocystis* can be confirmed using a specific fluorescent antibody.

Malarial and other blood parasites are identified by microscopic examination of the blood by an experienced parasitology technologist. Periodic specimens are needed to ensure detection of the organisms in all stages of the life cycle.

Rickettsial Identification

Rickettsiae can be grown in embryonated eggs and some tissue cultures, but for practical purposes, serologic techniques are used for diagnosis. Nonspecific tests, such as *Proteus* agglutinins, are sometimes helpful, but the definitive method is to document a fourfold or greater rise in complement-fixing antibody to the specific organisms in question. These latter tests are usually available only at the Centers for Disease Control and Prevention. The most important organism in the United States is *Rickettsia rickettsiae,* the cause of Rocky Mountain spotted fever. The rash of this infection is characteristic, being maculopapular, purpuric, sometimes bullous, and frequently involving the palms and the soles. Because the illness progresses fairly rapidly, antimicrobial therapy with tetracycline or chloramphenicol is usually begun before serologic confirmation of the diagnosis is made.

Fungal Identification

The diagnosis of fungal diseases frequently requires histopathologic, serologic, morphologic, and culture techniques. Fungi are usually isolated on selective media designed to suppress more rapidly growing bacteria so that the fungi can have an opportunity to multiply and be identified. Fungi grow more slowly than bacteria, and cultural isolation may require 4 to 6 weeks.

For *Cryptococcus neoformans* it may be possible to demonstrate the presence of encapsulated yeast in spinal fluid sediment by the use of India ink. Although other yeasts may produce capsules, these are not found in spinal fluid; therefore a positive India ink test is virtually diagnostic of *C. neoformans* meningitis. Organisms are not always demonstrable in spinal fluid, however, and serologic techniques have been developed. Currently, the cryptococcal latex agglutination test is about 95 percent as sensitive as culture and can be performed within hours. Furthermore, as the disease is treated, test results will remain positive for months to years, even though the cultures have become negative. Generally, however, the titer falls progressively in successfully treated patients.

Viral Identification

Viral Isolation Techniques. Most clinical virology laboratories rely on cell cultures to isolate viruses. Confluent monolayers of cells are prepared in tubes or plates. As soon as the specimen is received in the laboratory, antibiotics are added (usually a combination of penicillin, gentamicin, and amphotericin B) to prevent bacterial and yeast overgrowth. A small portion of each specimen, approximately 0.2 ml, is inoculated at least two tubes or two wells of the appropriate cell lines. Because no single line will support the growth of all human viruses, a combination of cell lines (typically three) is used: (1) cynomolgus monkey kidney, which best supports the growth of myxoviruses and enteroviruses; (2) a continuous line of human epithelial cells (HEp-2), which are ideal for isolation of respiratory syncytial and adenoviruses; and (3) a diploid fibroblast cell line (human foreskin cells or MRC-5), which best supports the growth of human cytomegalovirus. The inoculated cells are examined microscopically at least every other day for the presence of cytopathic effect produced by virus. If cytopathic effect is observed, the technologist can frequently recognize it as typical of a particular virus. For example, the cytopathic effect produced by cytomegalovirus is distinctive. The type of cytopathic effect and ability to grow in certain cell lines often suggest the presumptive virologic diagnosis. As soon as cytopathic effect is detected, the physician can be informed that the virus has been isolated. This can usually be accomplished within a week except for cytomegalovirus, which is relatively slow growing and may require 4 weeks of observation before cytopathic effect is seen.

Newer methods combine cell culture with enzyme-linked or fluorescent antibody staining. From 24 to 48 hours after inoculation, cultures for herpes simplex virus type 1 or 2 or cytomegalovirus may be fixed and stained by either direct or indirect fluorescent antibody or ELISA methods. Commercially available methods using this shell vial technique are currently available for CMV and the respiratory viruses (influenza A and B; parainfluenza 1, 2, and 3; respiratory syncytial virus; and adenovirus).

Direct Detection Methods. Reliable reagents are commercially available for the direct detection of several viral antigens. Air-dried smears of vesical scrapings for herpes simplex type 1 or 2 or for varicella-zoster can be specifically stained with monoclonal antibodies to the appropriate agent, followed by fluorescein-conjugated antibody to the murine monoclonal antibody. Direct detection of adenovirus influenza A and respiratory syncytial virus in nasopharyngeal swabs is also possible by similar methods with commercially available reagents.

Viral Serologic Tests. The measurement of serum antibodies has two major clinical applications: (1) diagnosis of acute viral illness when virus cannot be recovered from clinical specimens or is present only in the stool, and (2) determination of immune status. Because rubella may be teratogenic, assessment of rubella immunity is necessary for unvaccinated women of childbearing age. In the future it may be necessary to check the immune status in women who have received rubella vaccine and possibly in recipients of measles and mumps vaccine as well. In these instances the diagnostic virology laboratory can assist in deciding which patients need to be reimmunized.

Six serologic procedures are commonly used to measure viral antibodies.

1. Complement fixation (CF) is still used by a number of viral diagnostic laboratories. Although not as sensitive as most of the other methods, it has the advantage of measuring antibodies to groups rather than single types of viruses. For example, CF tests can be done for adenovirus and in most instances will detect infection with any of the more than 30 adenovirus serotypes.
2. Hemagglutination-inhibition (HI) testing is sensitive and relatively specific. Rubella and measles antibodies are most commonly measured by the HI method. Since HI antibodies persist for life, the HI test is useful for determination of immune status. CF antibodies often decline to undetectable levels several years after infection, and hence the CF test is not as useful as the HI procedure for the determination of immune status.
3. Immunofluorescence is quite sensitive if done by experienced technologists. For antibody determinations, indirect immunofluorescence is the technique most often employed.
4. Neutralizing antibodies are usually measured by incubating serial dilutions of the patient's serum with virus and then inoculating the virus-serum mixtures into cell cultures. If the antibody is not present, the virus produces cytopathic changes in the cells. The antibody titer is usually expressed as the highest dilution of serum that prevents the development of cytopathic effect in 50 percent of the inoculated cell cultures. This method is sensitive and very specific.
5. Precipitin testing can be done by simple diffusion or counterimmunoelectrophoresis. It is specific but relatively insensitive.
6. Radioimmunoassay can be used to identify viral antigens or antibodies. This technique is probably the most sensitive method available for detection of viral antibodies and antigens, but it requires expensive equipment and carries a small risk of exposure to radioactivity. It is rarely used now.
7. Enzyme-linked immunosorbent assay (ELISA), first developed in the mid-1970s is more sensitive than any of the other serologic methods except radioimmunoassay, and it is equally specific. Viral antigen(s) and appropriate control antigen(s) are allowed to bind to plastic microtiter wells. After incubation with sera, binding is detected by a second antibody, which has been chemically linked to an enzyme such as alkaline phosphatase or horseradish peroxidase. When the enzyme substrate is added, color develops, which is read spectrophotometrically. The method readily lends itself to semiautomation; and with commercial reagents now available for nearly every medically important virus, ELISA is likely to be the state-of-the-art serologic method for years to come.

Interpretation of Virology Results. The significance of viral isolation varies according to the source of the specimen (Table 2–5). Isolation of virus from any of the sites in the first group listed is diagnostic of a viral infection in that area. For example, isolation of herpes simplex from corneal scrapings is diagnostic of herpes keratitis. Because viruses can be found in stool specimens of asymptomatic persons, especially children, isolation of virus from stool alone is not diagnostic.

Viral Antibody Titers. A fourfold rise or decline in serum antibody titer is considered diagnostic of a recent infection. Although paired specimens are preferred, a single titer can sometimes be useful. A high titer suggests a recent infection, whereas a negative titer during convalescence excludes that particular virus. The presence of serum antibody usually connotes immunity. For example, it is ex-

TABLE 2–5. SIGNIFICANCE OF VIRAL ISOLATION

Source of Positive Culture	Interpretation
Autopsy Blood Biopsy tissue Cerebrospinal fluid Exudates and transudates Eye Cervix Skin lesions	Virtually diagnostic of infection in the site cultured
Throat[a] Urine[a]	Virus isolated is probably associated with clinical illness
Stool[a]	Virus isolated is possibly associated with clinical illness

[a] Isolation of virus from these specimens would be diagnostic if accompanied by serologic evidence of homologous virus infection.

tremely rare for individuals with detectable rubella hemagglutination-inhibition antibodies to subsequently develop clinical rubella.

Tests for IgM antibodies are now widely available commercially, both by the indirect fluorescent antibody method and by ELISA. Because a positive test result is presumptive evidence for recent or current viral infection, the tests are very attractive. Unfortunately, they are fraught with false-positive results, most often the presence of IgG antibodies to the same agent together with detectable or even undetectable levels of rheumatoid factor. The IgM rheumatoid factor binds to the IgG antibodies bound to the virus, resulting in a false-positive result when the anti-IgM conjugate is applied. The only way this pitfall can be avoided is to remove the IgG prior to testing, which can be done by first putting the sera through a Sephadex column and then testing it, or by using only those ELISA kits that incorporate this feature.

NEWER METHODS IN MICROBIOLOGY

DNA Hybridization

Tests that use direct hybridization of DNA probes are now available for the detection of *Mycoplasma pneumoniae, Legionella pneumophila, Neisseria gonorrheae,* and *Chlamydia trachomatis.* The advantage of these methods for the first two organisms is their rapidity, since both are relatively difficult organisms to grow. In the case of the latter, the advantages are speed and convenience. Because direct probes generally require more than 10^3 organisms for a positive test, they are slightly less sensitive than culture methods. However, because they take only a few hours to perform and organisms need not be viable, they can be very useful.

Polymerase Chain Reaction

Recently, an entirely new approach based on amplification of DNA has been developed. Known as PCR (for polymerase chain reaction), this method uses two oligonucleotide primers (usually 20 to 30 bp in length) that specifically bind to the target DNA on opposite strands at a distance of 100 to 1000 bp apart (Figure 2–4). In the presence of these primers and a very heat-stable DNA polymerase (called Taq), the target DNA is heated to 95C to separate the DNA strands. The temperature is then lowered to 55C to 60C, so that the primers can specifically anneal to the sequence that matches and then raised to 72C for the Taq polymerase to extend the primer, copying the original sequence. Repeated cycles of heating, annealing, and extension then yield amplification of the DNA product, whose size is equal to the length of DNA between the primers. The PCR product may be detected by agarose gel electrophoresis and staining with ethidium bromide. Although 30 to 40 cycles are ample when there is a high starting concentration of the target sequences, that number is insufficient for the maximum sensitivity needed for the detection of pathogens in patient specimens. In general, the PCR product is either detected by hybridization with a specific labeled probe or by a second round of PCR using specific primers, internal to the first set. In theory, PCR can detect as few as 1 to 10 DNA copies per reaction mixture.

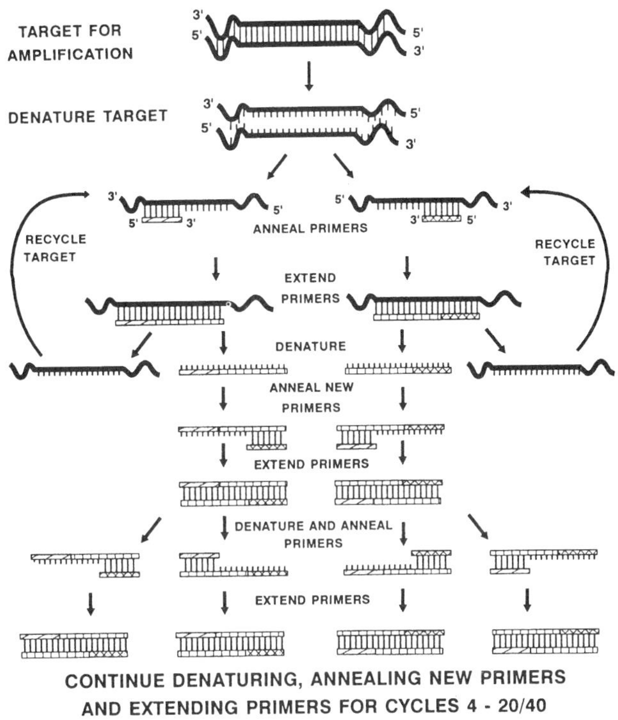

Figure 2–4. Basic steps in PCR amplification involve alternating a denaturing step, a reannealing or hybridization step, and an enzymatic step. In the first step, DNA is denatured and allowed to reanneal so that most single strands of DNA hybridize to a primer sequence of nucleotides. The primer serves as the start point for the enzymatic addition or extension of nucleotides with the original DNA strand serving as the model or template for the synthesis of more DNA fragments. The reaction is thermally cyclic and normally consists of 20 to 40 cycles. Different cycling times and temperatures can optimize the process, but most cycles are in the range of minutes so that a complete amplification of a sequence can be completed in a few hours. (*From Wolcott M: DNA-based rapid methods for the detection of food borne pathogens. J Food Protection 54:387, 1991.*)

At the present writing, PCR is only available in research laboratories and a few specialized commercial laboratories for detection of human immunodeficiency virus (HIV-1 and -2), cytomegalovirus (CMV), herpes simplex virus (HSV), parvovirus, human T lymphotrophic virus I (HTLV-1), hepatitis B, and hepatitis C. A commercial kit for detection of *Chlamydia trachomatis* is expected to be widely available in hospital laboratories soon, followed by kits for *Mycobacterium tuberculosis, Neisseria gonorrheae,* Lyme disease, and many others. The role of PCR in the diagnosis of infectious diseases is likely to increase and change in the future as more clinical correlation is obtained. At the moment, PCR for HSV can be done on spinal fluid in cases of suspected HSV encephalitis, providing rapid, noninvasive, laboratory confirmation on which treatment can be based. However, because of the cost of the test, there would be no reason to use it for the diagnosis of a cold sore or a recurrent genital lesion. In the case of HIV, PCR is primarily used to determine whether infants born to HIV seropositive mothers are infected. The published data appear to show that PCR for *Chlamydia* is equivalent to or more sensitive than culture. If cost is equivalent, PCR could well replace it. In the case of tuberculosis, PCR is likely to have equivalent sensitivity to culture but can have results in 1 to 2 days. However, culture will still be needed to determine antibiotic resistance. Because of high cost and relative complexity, PCR is unlikely to replace culture entirely, but rather PCR will supplement it in areas where cultures are too slow or insensitive.

BIBLIOGRAPHY

Balows A, Hausler WJ, Shadomy HJ: Manual of Clinical Microbiology, 5th ed. Washington, DC, American Society for Microbiology, 1991.

Baron EJ, Finegold SM: Bailey and Scott's Diagnostic Microbiology, 8th ed. St. Louis, Mosby, 1990.

Koneman EW, Allen SD: Color Atlas and Textbook of Diagnostic Microbiology, 4th ed. Philadelphia, Lippincott, 1992.

Lennette EH: Laboratory Diagnosis of Viral Infections. New York, Marcel Dekker, 1992.

Indigenous Microbial Flora of Humans

CHAPTER 3

Itzhak Brook

Most of the human body mucosal and epithelial surfaces are covered with aerobic and anaerobic microorganisms that are referred to as the normal or indigenous flora.[1] The surfaces of the body that are inhabited by normal flora are the skin, conjunctiva, mouth, nose, throat, lower intestinal tract, vagina, and urethra. The organisms that reside at these sites are predominantly anaerobic and are actively multiplying. The trachea, bronchi, esophagus, stomach, and upper urinary tract are not normally colonized by indigenous flora. However, a limited number of transient organisms may be present at these sites from time to time. Such changing patterns of colonization are dependent on differences in the environment, such as oxygen tension and pH, and availability of nutritional factors, plus variations in the ability of bacteria to adhere to these surfaces. Microflora also vary within different microenvironmental niches on a given surface. In the oral cavity, for example, the microorganisms present in the buccal folds differ in strain type and concentration from those isolated from the tongue or gingival sulci. Nevertheless, the organisms that prevail in one body system predictably belong to certain major bacterial species. These sets of bacterial flora, with their predictable pattern, remain stable through life, despite perturbing factors. The relative and total colony counts, however, can be affected by various factors, such as age, diet, anatomic variations, illness, hospitalization, and antimicrobial therapy.

Anaerobes outnumber aerobic bacteria on all mucosal surfaces, and certain organisms predominate at the difference sites (Table 3–1). The predominance of anaerobic bacteria in the intestinal and genitourinary tracts and their scarcity at other sites are partially due to the differences in oxygen tension at these locations. The number of anaerobes at a site is generally inversely related to the oxygen tension. Their predominance in the skin, mouth, nose, and throat, which are exposed to oxygen, is explained by the anaerobic microenvironment generated by the coexistent facultative bacteria that consume oxygen.

Knowledge of the composition of the flora at certain sites is useful for predicting which organisms may be involved in an infection adjacent to that site. This is helpful in the selection of logical empiric antimicrobial therapy before the precise microbial etiology of the infection is known. Furthermore, it can also be helpful in determining the source and significance of microorganisms recovered from unrelated sites of the body. For example, bacterial endocarditis caused by *Enterococcus faecalis* is more often associated with urinary tract infection, while alpha-hemolytic streptococcus endocarditis is more often seen in patients with poor dental hygiene and tooth extraction.

TABLE 3–1. NORMAL AEROBIC AND ANAEROBIC MICROBIAL FLORA[a]

Area	Aerobes	Anaerobes
Oral cavity	10^8–10^9	10^9–10^{11}
Upper gastrointestinal tract	10^2–10^5	10^3–10^7
Lower gastrointestinal tract	10^5–10^9	10^{10}–10^{12}
Vagina	10^8	10^8

[a] Number of organisms per gram of secretion or contents.

A knowledge of the indigenous microbiota is also helpful in determining the consequence of overgrowth of one microorganism by another. For example, the overgrowth of *Candida* within the gastrointestinal tract is frequent in patients given neomycin because it inhibits the bacteria of the family Enterobacteriaceae but has little effect on *Candida*. Clindamycin and other antimicrobial agents that suppress the intestinal anaerobic bacteria are select for the growth of *Clostridium difficile*. Uncontrolled proliferation of *C. difficile* can result in the elaboration of a potent enterotoxin that may cause pseudomembranous enterocolitis.

Recognition of the normal flora can also help the clinical microbiology laboratory in choosing proper culture media that will inhibit certain organisms regarded as contaminants. Proper media can be used to enhance the growth of expected pathogens that reside as part of the indigenous flora in proximity to the infected site. The usefulness of such information is apparent during investigation of bacteremia of unknown origin, for which the presence of certain organisms can suggest a possible port of entry (ie, *Clostridium* and *Bacteroides fragilis* usually originate from the gastrointestinal tract).[2]

The normal flora are not just a potential hazard for the host but also a beneficial partner. An example for such synergy is the development of vitamin K deficiency following antimicrobial therapy, which suppresses the gut flora that produces this vitamin. Normal body flora also serve as protectors from colonization or subsequent invasion by potentially virulent bacteria. In instances where the host defenses are impaired or breach occurs in the mucous membranes or skin, however, the members of the normal flora can cause infections.

SKIN

The most common members of the cutaneous microflora belong to the bacterial genera *Staphylococcus, Micrococcus, Corynebacterium, Propionibacterium, Brevibacterium,* and *Acinetobacter* and the yeast *Pityrosporum* (Table 3–2). The indigenous microbiota of the skin will vary greatly depending on the sites of the body and the characteristics of the skin at these sites. The anaerobic propionibacteria, for example, live preferentially in the lipid-secreting glands of the dermis. Most other species are found only on desquamating epithelial cells of the stratum corneum. Organisms, such as viruses, that require living cells for hosts must invade cells of the basal epithelial layers, where there is active cellular metabolism.

Some important pathogens commonly found in skin are only transient residents that contaminate the area around orifices. The oral region or sites that can be in contact with the oropharyngeal flora (ie, nipples, fingers, genitalia) can become colonized with aerobic and anaerobic organisms that originate from the oral flora.[3] These organisms include *Haemophilus* species, *Staphylococcus aureus, Peptostreptococcus* species, *Fusobacterium* species, and pigmented *Prevotella* and *Porphyromonas* species. Similarly, the rectal and vulvovaginal areas and lower extremities can become colonized with organisms that originate from the colon and vaginal flora. These include *Escherichia coli, Enterococcus* species, *B. fragilis* groups, *Clostridium* species (in the rectal area) or *Neisseria gonorrhea,* group B *Streptococcus,* and *Prevotella* species (vaginal origin). Because of this spread, these organisms can cause local infections (wounds, abrasions, infected burns, or decubitus ulcers) or serve as a source of systemic spread or bacteremia.[2]

The anaerobic microflora of the skin and the external auditory canal usually are made up of the genus *Propionibacterium.*[4–6] The majority of the isolates of the genus *Propionibacterium* are *P. acnes,* while *P. granulosum* and *P. avidum* can be recovered less frequently. One finds *P. acnes* and *P. granulosum* on skin with a high sebum content, while *P. acnes* is found essentially in all postpubertal individuals. *Propionibacterium granulosum* is found regularly in 10 to 20 percent of individuals in numbers about 10- to 100-fold fewer than *P. acnes.* The third species, *P. avidum,* is present in the axilla and requires an environment that has a high availability of water rather than abundant lipids. Species of *Eubacterium* and *Peptostreptococcus* may also be encountered. These organisms grow within the openings of the sebaceous glands. Consequently, their distribution is proportional to the number of glands, the amount of sebum produced, and the composition of skin surface lipids.[5]

Propionibacterium species are capable of producing free fatty acids from triglycerides by generating lipase.[7] The degree of hydrolysis of sebum triglycerides varies but is the most effective by

TABLE 3–2. PREDOMINANT HUMAN MICROBIAL FLORA

Type of Bacteria	Body Site: Skin	Conjunctiva	Nasopharynx	Oral Cavity	Lower Gastrointestinal Tract	Genitourinary Tract
Aerobic and facultative						
Staphylococcus species	+	+	+			
Streptococcus species	+	+	+	+	+[a]	+
Haemophilus species				+		
Moraxella catarrhalis				+		
Enterobacteriaceae					+	+
Anaerobic						
Veillonella species				+	+	+
Peptostreptococcus species	+	+	+	+	+	+
Actinomyces species				+		+
Bifidobacterium species				+	+	+
Eubacterium species				+	+	+
Lactobacillus species					+	+
Propionibacterium species	+	+	+		+	+
Clostridium species					+	
Fusobacterium species				+		
Bacteroides species				+	+	+
Prevotella species				+[b]		+[c]
Porphyromonas species				+[b]		

[a] *Enterococcus* species.
[b] Pigmented species.
[c] *Prevotella bivia* and *Prevotella disiens*.

P. acnes and *P. granulosum*.[8] These fatty acids have strong antibacterial and antifungal activity and can interfere with the growth of nonindigenous microorganisms on skin surfaces. *Staphylococcus* species, *Streptococcus pyogenes*, and aerobic gram-negative bacilli are sensitive to these fatty acids. The fatty acids generated by *Propionibacterium* species may therefore play a role in excluding more virulent organisms from the skin surfaces, thus maintaining the stability of the cutaneous flora. However, the fatty acids produced by *Propionibacterium* species may play a deleterious role in the development of acne. These acids generated in the hair follicles and sebaceous gland ducts can cause an inflammatory response, resulting in the production of acne lesions.[9]

CONJUNCTIVA

The normal conjunctival flora contain *Staphylococcus epidermidis* (in approximately 40 to 50 percent of conjunctivae), *Corynebacterium* species (in 20 to 25 percent, and alpha-hemolytic streptococci (in 10 to 15 percent) (see Table 3–2).

Anaerobic bacteria were recovered from up to 20 percent of the conjunctival cultures obtained from normal individuals.[10–12] The predominant isolates in descending order of frequency were *P. acnes, P. avidum, P. granulosum, Peptostreptococcus* species, and *Eubacterium* species. These organisms were also recovered from parts adjacent to the conjunctiva such as the eyelids and lacrimal sac. *Propionibacterium acnes* was isolated from normal noninflamed conjunctiva of 18.5 percent of the children studied,[12] as compared to 46.0 percent of adults.[11]

NOSE AND NASOPHARYNX

The bacterial flora of the nose are similar to that of the skin (see Table 3–2). *Staphylococcus aureus, S. epidermidis,* alpha-hemolytic streptococci, diphtheroids, *P. acnes,* and anaerobic and microaerophilic streptococci compose the largest number of bacteria in the nasal passages.[13]

Patients and hospital staff often carry *S. aureus* that is frequently resistant to antimicrobials. Colonization with these organisms has been incriminated in the spread of these bacteria within the hospital and they present an epidemiological and therapeutic dilemma.[14]

Potentially virulent organisms such as *Streptococcus pneumoniae, Neisseria meningitidis,* and *Haemophilus influenzae* may be isolated in some individuals' nasopharynges. Their exact significance in these settings is unclear, since they generally lack virulence factors such as specific polysaccharide complexes.

OROPHARYNX

The microflora of the oral cavity are complex and contain many kinds of aerobic and facultative and obligate anaerobes. The establishment of the normal oral flora is initiated at birth. Certain organisms such as lactobacilli and anaerobic streptococci, which establish themselves at an early date, reach high numbers within a few days. *Actinomyces, Fusobacterium,* and *Nocardia* are acquired by the age of 6 months. Following that time, *Prevotella, Porphyromonas, Bacteroides, Leptotrichia, Propionibacterium,* and *Candida* also are established as part of the oral flora.[15] *Fusobacterium* populations reach high numbers after dentition and attain maximal numbers at the age of 1 year. The most predominant group of facultative microorganisms native to the oropharynx are the alpha-hemolytic streptococci (or the viridans group of streptococci), which include the species *Streptococcus mitis, S. milleri, S. sanguis, S. intermedius, S. salivarius,* and several others.[15,16] Other groups of organisms native to the oropharynx are *Moraxella catarrhalis* and *H. influenzae,* which are capable of producing beta-lactamase and may spread to adajcent sites causing otitis, sinusitis, or bronchitis. Encapsulated *H. influenzae* organisms also induce serious infections such as meningitis and bacteremia. The oropharynx also contains *S. aureus* and *S. epidermidis* that can also produce beta-lactamase and take part in chronic infections.

The normal oropharynx is seldom colonized by gram-negative Enterobacteriaceae. In contrast, hospitalized patients are generally heavily colonized with these organisms. The reasons for this change in microflora are not known but may be related to changes in the glycocalyx of the pharyngeal epithelial cells or due to selection processes that occur following the administration of antimicrobial therapy.[17,18] The shift from predominantly gram-positive to gram-negative bacteria is thought to contribute to the high incidence of pneumonia caused by gram-negative bacteria in patients with severe illness.

Oropharyngeal selective decontamination using topical application of polymyxin B, neomycin, and vancomycin was successful in reducing tracheobronchial colonization with *S. aureus* and gram-negative bacteria, as well as the occurrence of pneumonia caused by these organisms.[19] The efficacy of these agents may be due to their antibacterial activity against potential aerobic pathogens and lack of activity against anaerobic bacteria.

Anaerobic bacteria are present in large numbers in both the mouth and the oropharynx, particularly in patients with poor dental hygiene, caries, or periodontal disease. Anaerobic bacteria outnumber the aerobic counterpart in a ratio of 10:1 to 100:1. The predominant anaerobes are anaerobic streptococci, *Veillonella* species, *Bacteroides* species, pigmented *Prevotella* and *Porphyromonas* species (previously called *Bacteroides melaninogenicus* group), and *Fusobacterium* species.[1] These organisms are a potential source of a variety of chronic infections such as otitis, sinusitis, aspiration pneumonia, and lung abscesses and abscesses of the oropharynx and teeth. Up to 50 percent of the pigmented *Prevotella, Porphyromonas,* and *Fusobacterium* species can produce beta-lactamase.[20]

Anaerobic bacteria can adhere to tooth surfaces and contribute, through the elaboration of metabolic products, to the production of both caries and periodontal disease that can range from gingivitis to periodontitis.[15]

The recovery rate of aerobic and anaerobic beta-lactamase-producing bacteria (BLPB) in the oropharynx has increased in recent years, and these organisms were isolated in more than one-half of the patients with head and neck infections.[20] BLPB can be involved directly in the infection and protecting not only themselves from the activity of penicillins but also penicillin-susceptible organisms. This can occur when the enzyme beta-lactamase is secreted into the infected tissue or abscess fluid in sufficient quantities to break the penicillin's beta-lactam ring before it can kill the susceptible bacteria.[21]

The high incidence of recovery of BLPB in upper respiratory tract infections may be due to the selection of these organisms following antimicrobial therapy with penicillins. Emergence of penicillin-resistant flora can occur following only a short course of penicillin.[22,23]

The distribution of organisms within the oral cavity seems to be a function of their ability to adhere to the oral mucous membrane surfaces. The differences in numbers of the anaerobic microflora probably occur because of a considerable variation in the oxygen concentration in parts of the oral cavity.

The periodontal pockets are the most anaerobic area in the oral cavity. The maxillary and mandibular buccal folds contain less oxygen (less than 0.4 percent) than the tongue surfaces (more than 12.4 percent). The buccal folds are more anaerobic than the gingival sulcus.

The ratio of anaerobic bacteria to aerobic bacteria in saliva is approximately 10:1. The total count of anaerobic bacteria is 1.1×10^8/ml (Fig. 3–1). The gram-negative anaerobic species found in the oral cavity include *Fusobacterium* species (especially *Fusobacterium nucleatum*), pigmented *Prevotella* and *Porphyromonas, Bacteroides* species, *Porphyro-*

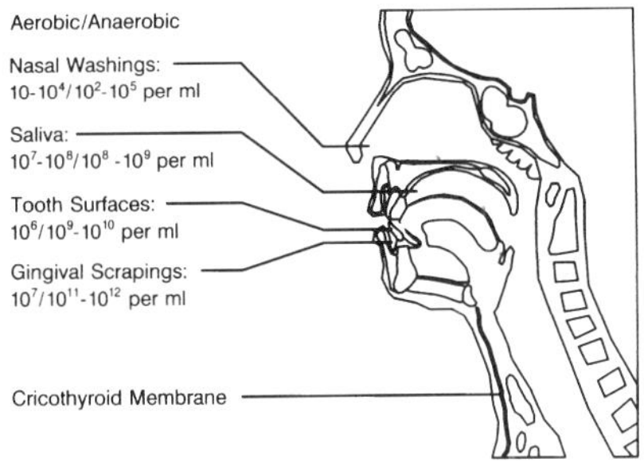

Figure 3–1. Concentrations of the microflora of the oral cavity.

monas gingivalis, Prevotella oralis, Prevotella oris, Prevotella buccae, Prevotella disiens, and *Bacteroides ureolyticus.*

The number of anaerobic strains varies between locations in the oropharynx. Loesche et al[24] found the prevalence of *Clostridium* to be 10 percent of the flora of periodontal pockets, 38 percent in normal gingival crevices, and 44 percent in carious teeth. Pigmental *Prevotella* and *Porphyromonas* represent less than 1 percent of the coronal tooth surface but constitute 4 to 8 percent of gingival crevice flora. *Veillonella* represents 1 to 3 percent of the coronal tooth surface, 5 to 15 percent of the gingival crevice flora, and 10 to 15 percent of the tongue flora. Microaerophilic streptococci predominate in all areas of the oral cavity and reach high numbers in the tongue and cheek.[25] Other anaerobes prevalent in the mouth are *Actinomyces,* anaerobic cocci, treponemas, *Leptotrichia buccalis, Bifidobacterium, Eubacterium,* and *Propionibacterium* (see Table 3–2).[26,27]

GASTROINTESTINAL TRACT

The alimentary tract of the newborn is generally sterile. Within hours after delivery it becomes colonized with organisms that are acquired from the mother during delivery when the newborn aspirates material from the cervical canal.[28] Early gut colonization with *Bacteroides* species, *Clostridium* species, and group B streptococci has been noted more often in infants delivered vaginally than in those delivered by cesarean section.[29]

Streptococci, enterococci, and staphylococci usually are present in the first days of life. Even the meconium, the first stool passed, contains bacteria.[30] At the end of the first week of life the fecal flora are predominantly anaerobic and contain *Bifidobacterium* species and *Clostridium* species. The most common facultative fecal flora are *Escherichia coli* and *Streptococcus faecalis,* which reach 10^8 to 10^{10} organisms/g of feces.[29]

There also are differences in bacterial flora of breast-fed and formula-fed infants. In breast-fed infants, *Bifidobacterium* becomes the predominant anaerobe.[31] In full-term infants delivered vaginally, *B. fragilis* is established by the first week in 22 percent of breast-fed infants as compared to 61 percent of formula-fed infants.[32] As breast-fed children grow and are weaned, the numbers of *Bifidobacterium* decrease, while the numbers of *Bacteroides* increase until they outnumber *Bifidobacterium* by a ratio of 3:1.

The type of delivery, the dietary constituents, and the gestational age all influence the colonization pattern of anaerobic bacteria.[32] By 4 to 6 days virtually all full-term, formula-fed, vaginally delivered infants are colonized by anaerobic bacteria, 61 percent of the infants harboring *B. fragilis.* In contrast, anaerobes are found altogether in only 59 percent and *B. fragilis* in 9 percent of infants delivered by cesarean section, confirming that significant contamination occurred during passage through the birth canal. *Veillonella* organisms are more commonly found in infants delivered by cesarean section. Both premature births and breast feeding are less frequently associated with anaerobe colonization in general, and *B. fragilis* is less likely to be found in breast-fed infants than in their formula-fed counterparts. Studies of newborn infants with congenital small bowel obstruction establish that colonization of the small bowel occurs through the oral route. In infants with obstruction distal to the ligament of Trietz, fecal-type flora are found immediately proximal to the site of obstruction, and the distal bowel remains sterile.[33]

The fate of swallowed bacteria and their ability to colonize the gut depend on a number of factors: ability to adhere to mucosa, environmental factors of diet, nutrient availability, chemical and pH conditions, secretory immunoglobulins, intestinal motility, and interference by other bacteria.[30,34–36]

The gastrointestinal flora are dynamic and vary at different locations. The changes in the flora can be unique to each patient and depend on factors such as anatomic changes, diet, state of health, and ingestion of medication that may alter the acidity of the stomach. Factors that interfere with colonization are active peristalsis, gastric acidity, and relatively high oxidation-reduction potential.

The upper regions of the normal gastrointestinal tract are sparsely populated with microorganisms while the lower region is heavily colonized. The changes in the gastrointestinal flora between the upper and lower regions are gradual and are both quantitative and qualitative. The esophagus, stomach, duodenum, jejunum, and proximal ileum normally contain relatively few bacteria. However, the flora become more complex and the number of different bacterial species increases in the distal portion of the gastrointestinal tract.[36]

The stomach is seeded constantly with bacteria from the drainage of nasopharyngeal and salivary secretions and usually contains fewer than 1000 organisms/ml. Only a few of these organisms are anaerobic.[35] The low pH and the high oxygen tension in the stomach are responsible for the small number of organisms that survive in the stomach. However, patients who receive antacids or H_2 blockers or have gastric bleeding have a higher pH, which can lead to an increase in the bacterial contents of the stomach, and subsequently of the upper gastrointestinal tract.[37]

The bacterial counts in the small intestine are relatively low, with total counts of 10^2 to 10^5 organisms/ml. The predominant bacteria above the ileocecal valve are gram-positive facultative, while below the valve *Bacteroides* (mostly the *B. fragilis* group), *Bifidobacterium, Lactobacillus,* and coliform are the major isolates.[30]

The colon contains the largest numbers of microorganisms of any inhabited region of the human body (see Table 3–1). The mean number of bacteria in the colon is approximately 10^{12} bacteria/g fecal material. Approximately 99.9 percent of these bacteria are anaerobic (the ratio of aerobes to anaerobes is 1:1,000 to 1:10,000), and the colon contains 300 to 400 different species or types of bacteria.

Bacteroides is the predominant bacterial genus in the intestine, present at approximately 10^{11} organisms/g dry weight.[35] The two species most frequently isolated are *B. vulgatus* and *B. thetaiotaomicron,* although *B. distasonis, B. fragilis,* and *B. ovatus* are also common. Among the gram-positive rods, *Bifidobacterium adolescentis, Eubacterium aerofaciens, Eubacterium lentum,* and *Clostridium ramosum* predominate.[38]

The *B. fragilis* group of organisms undergoes important morphological changes as the organism transforms itself from a member of the normal gut flora to a pathogen causing abscesses and bacteremia. The frequency of encapsulated and piliated *Bacteroides* species was determined among isolates from normal flora and abscesses.[39] Most of these isolates were members of the *B. fragilis* group. Of the strains of *Bacteroides* species isolated, 45 of 54 (83 percent) recovered from blood and 31 of 40 (78 percent) found in abscesses were encapsulated. In contrast, only 7 of 71 (10 percent) similar strains isolated from the feces or pharynx of healthy persons were encapsulated ($P < 0.001$) (see the distribution only in *B. fragilis* group in Fig. 3–2). Pili were observed in 3 of 54 (6 percent) strains isolated from blood, 30 of 40 (75 percent) of those recovered from abscesses ($P < 0.001$), and 49 of 71 (69 percent) of those found in normal flora ($P < 0.001$).

The findings in this study suggest that *Bacteroides* species express different morphological features at different sites. Such changes may enable these organisms to adjust to varying environmental conditions, some bacterial structures being accordingly advantageous or detrimental.[39]

Pili enable *Bacteroides* species that colonize mucous membranes to adhere to these membranes.[40] However, because they are not exposed to macrophages during colonization, capsules do not provide them with any advantage.[41] In abscesses, capsules provide protection from macrophages, and pili enable the organisms to attach to their surroundings. In contrast, the presence of pili may interfere with systemic spread, since piliated organisms may be more easily phagocytosed.[42] In a manner similar to that of *E. coli*[43] and *H. influenzae,*[44] *Bacteroides* species may be able to modulate pilus formation in relation to environmental conditions. The gastrointestinal tract contains numerous members of the *B. fragilis* group but apparently only those that can adapt to the changing environment can cause illness and are therefore more pathogenic.

Anatomic and physiologic derangement of the gastrointestinal tract can lead to bacterial overgrowth in the upper small bowel.[36] Proliferation of a colonic-type flora in the small intestine may be accompanied by a variety of metabolic disturbances

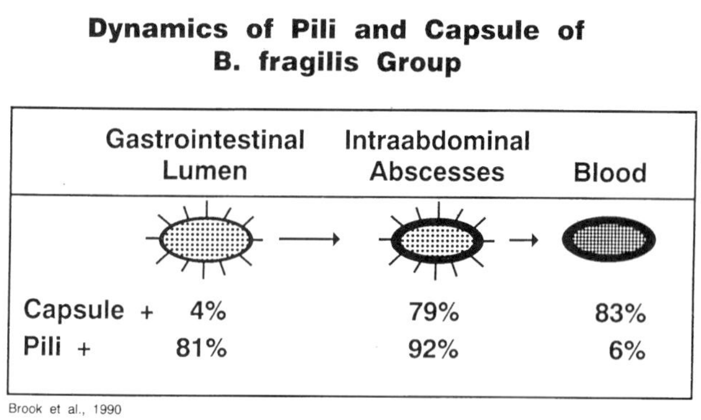

Figure 3–2. Pili and capsule development in *Bacteroides fragilis* group in intra-abdominal infection. (*From Brook I, Myhal LA, Dorsey CH: Encapsulation and pilus formation of Bacteroides spp. in normal flora abscesses and blood. J Infect 25:251, 1991.*)

including steatorrhea, vitamin deficiencies, and carbohydrate malabsorption. A significant increase in the bacterial population in the small bowel can be demonstrated in patients with hypochlorydia whether due to atrophic gastritis, intake of antacids or cimetidine, or a surgical procedure.[34,36,37] This increase in intestinal bacteria has also been observed in patients with ineffective peristalsis, multiple diverticula, cirrhosis, chronic malnutrition, excessive small bowel resection, and abdominal irradiation. Malabsorption of fat is the most common clinical manifestation of bacterial overgrowth and results in steatorrhea and vitamin B_{12} deficiency.[36,45] The role of the intestinal flora in the induction of systemic or gastrointestinal malignancy has been investigated. However, no clear-cut association has thus far been found.[36]

Acute diarrheal illness produces profound alterations in the bacterial populations of the gastrointestinal tract. Under certain conditions, the resident microflora are eclipsed by an identifiable pathogen.[35] The rapid transit of diarrheal stool results in a marked reduction in the anaerobic population of the large bowel. In patients with cholera, the concentration of *Bacteroides* in the feces decreases to 10^5 organisms/ml, a reduction by a factor of 10^5 to 10^6.[36] Apparently, these changes are secondary to the underlying acute process because resolution of diarrhea is accompanied by rapid restitution of the normal flora.

The normal colonic microflora tend to be relatively constant in an individual and constitute an important defense mechanism against infection.[36] Organisms belonging to thc normal flora, such as *B. fragilis,* are capable of protecting against infection by *Salmonella* and *Pseudomonas aeruginosa.*[36] Suppression of the anaerobic normal flora by antimicrobials effective against most anaerobic bacteria except *C. difficile* has been incriminated in the etiology of pseudomembranous enterocolitis.[46]

Animal studies have provided evidence that colonic microflora interfere with the establishment of nonindigenous, potentially virulent, organisms in the intestinal tract. Anaerobic bacteria appear to be actively involved in this process. The exclusion of invaders by the indigenous flora was termed *colonization resistance* by van der Waaij et al.[47]

The potential importance of preserving the normal anaerobic flora of the gut was illustrated in several studies that demonstrated the adverse effects of antimicrobials on the flora.[48,49] Berg[48] demonstrated that treatment of mice with oral antibiotics (penicillin, clindamycin, and metronidazole) that suppress the multiplication of anaerobes increased the gut population of Enterobacteriaceae and was associated with increased translocation of these organisms to mesenteric lymph nodes. Van der Waaij et al[49] described a decreased resistance to colonization with gram-negative bacteria during treatment of mice with broad spectrum antibiotics.

Selective decontamination of the gut as an attempt to eradicate only the aerobic gram-negative bacilli by using antimicrobial agents effective against them only has gained increased interest in clinical studies.[50–52] The subjects of these studies were generally immunosuppressed individuals and those prone to infections. The antimicrobials used were either nonabsorbable agents such as polymyxin, neomycin, and bacitracin or absorbable agents such as trimethoprim/sulfamethoxazole and the quinolones.[52] However, in contrast to selective decontamination of the oropharynx flora,[19] there is no consensus yet regarding the practical implications of using selective decontamination of the gut flora. This topic deserves further study.

GENITOURINARY TRACT

The kidneys, ureters, and bladder do not usually contain indigenous microbiota. The most distal portions of both the male and female urethra, however, are colonized with small numbers of bacteria (10^2 to 10^4 organisms/ml urine). The microorganisms that may colonize the outermost portion of the urethra can be aerobic (eg, staphylococci, nonhemolytic streptococci, diphtheroids, and enteric rods) and anaerobic organisms (eg, *Bacteroides, Prevotella, Fusobacterium, Peptostreptococcus, Eubacterium, Clostridium.*[53,54]

The vagina contains a complex microbial flora.[55–57] Lactobacilli colonize the vagina shortly after birth, because of the mother's hormonal stimulation. As this effect wanes, lactobacilli are replaced with gram-positive cocci. At puberty the cyclic hormonal stimulation ensues and the glycogen content of squamous epithelium increases again and this is correlated with the return of lactobacilli. Lactobacilli metabolize glycogen, thus producing lactic acid, which contributes to a low vaginal pH (4.5 to 5.5) in adults.[55–57] The low pH selects for certain microorganisms, such as *Candida albicans* and anaerobic bacteria, but inhibits the growth of more fastidious bacteria including certain Enterobacteriaceae.

The normal vaginal flora are fairly homogeneous. The mean number of bacteria in the vagina and cervix is approximately 10^8 organisms/ml of secretion (range 10^5 to 10^{11}). Cervical canal flora are composed of mixed aerobic and anaerobic flora.[55–59]

The aerobic components consist of lactobacilli, group B and group D streptococci, *S. epidermidis, S. aureus,* and gram-negative enteric rods such as *E. coli.*[60]

The anaerobic component consists predominantly of *Lactobacillus, Peptostreptococcus* species, *P. bivia, P. disiens,* and *Bacteroides* species.[55–59] *Clostridium perfringens* and other clostridia can also be found. A variety of anaerobic strains can be recovered from various individuals.[55–59] For example, peptostreptococci are reported in 7 to 57 percent of women. Gram-negative anaerobic rods are recovered from 57 to 65 percent of women. The predominant gram-negative anaerobic strains are *P. disiens, P. bivia,* pigmented *Prevotella* and *Porphyromonas, B. fragilis* group, and *P. oralis.*[58] *Veillonella* organisms can be recovered from 27 percent, *Bifidobacterium* species from 10 to 72 percent, and *Eubacterium* species from 15 percent. *Clostridium* species are recovered from 17 percent, and these are isolates of *Clostridium bifermentans, C. perfringens, C. ramosum,* and *C. difficile.*

Variations in cervical and vaginal flora are affected by age, pregnancy, and the menstrual cycle. The microflora in females before puberty, during childbearing years, pregnancy, and after menopause are not uniform. Colonization with lactobacilli is low in children and in postmenopausal women, while it is high in pregnant women and those in their reproductive years. Although differences in colonization between age groups occur in organisms other than *Lactobacillus,* the vaginal flora of children contain many of the aerobic strains recovered from adult women.

The influence of pregnancy on the vaginal flora is of particular interest because the newborn is exposed to that flora during passage through the birth canal or through exposure to infected amniotic fluid.[28] Most reports[28,60–62] indicate that the bacterial component of the vaginal flora during pregnancy generally is identical to that found prior to pregnancy; the major change is an increase in the colonization by lactobacilli. This increase in the number of the avirulent lactobacilli at the expense of the more virulent groups of microorganisms may serve to protect the fetus, so that the infant is exposed to benign organisms while passing through the heavily colonized birth canal.

Data collected from animals[63,64] indicate that estrogen can increase the bacterial population of the female genital tract, while progesterone decreases it. The influence of these hormonal changes on the quantitative isolation of microorganisms in the menstrual cycle is yet to be studied.

REFERENCES

1. Socransky SS, Manganiello SD: The oral microflora of man from birth to senility. J Periodontol 42:485, 1971.
2. Brook I: Anaerobic bacteremia: 12 years experience in two military hospitals. J Infect Dis 160:1071, 1989.
3. Brook I, Finegold SM: Aerobic and anaerobic microbiology of cutaneous abscesses in children. Pediatrics 67:891, 1981.
4. Marples RR, McGinley KJ: *Corynebacterium acnes* and other anaerobic diphtheroids from human skin. J Med Microbiol 7:349, 1974.
5. McGinley KJ, Webster GF, Leyden JJ: Regional variations of cutaneous propionibacteria. Appl Environ Microbiol 35:62, 1978.
6. Brook I: Microbiological studies of the bacterial flora of the external auditory canal in children. Acta Otolaryngol 91:285, 1981.
7. Weaber K, Freedman R, Eudy WW: Tetracycline inhibition of a lipase from *Corynebacterium acnes.* Appl Microbiol 21:639, 1971.
8. Puhvel SM, Reisner RM, Sokamoto M: Analysis of lipid composition of isolated human sebaceous gland homogenates after incubation with cutaneous bacteria. Thin layer chromatography. J Invest Dermatol 64:406, 1975.
9. Strauss JS, Kligman AM: The pathologic dynamics of acne vulgaris. Arch Dermatol 82:779, 1960.
10. Perkins RE, Kundsin RB, Pratt MV, et al: Bacteriology of normal and infected conjunctiva. J Clin Microbiol 1:147, 1975.
11. Brook I, Petit TH, Martin WJ, et al: Anaerobic and aerobic bacteriology of acute conjunctivitis. Ann Ophthalmol 11:389, 1979.
12. Brook I: Anaerobic and aerobic bacterial flora of acute conjunctivitis in children. Arch Ophthalmol 98:833, 1980.
13. Brook I: Aerobic and anaerobic bacteriology of purulent nasopharyngitis in children. J Clin Microbiol 26:592, 1988.
14. Boyce JM: Methicillin-resistant *Staphylococcus aureus.* Detection epidemiology and control measures. Infect Dis Clin North Am 3:901, 1989.
15. Marsh PD: Microbiology of dental plaque in health and disease. In Ivanyi L (ed): Immunological Aspects of Oral Diseases. Lancester, MTP Press, 1986, p 13.
16. Bowden GHW, Ellwood DC, Hamilton IR: Microbial ecology of the oral cavity. Adv Microb Ecol 3:135, 19XX.
17. Valenti WM, Trudell RG, Bentley DW: Factors predisposing to oropharyngeal colonization with gram-negative bacilli in the aged. N Engl J Med 298:1108, 1978.
18. Johanson WG Jr, Woods DE, Chauduri T: Association of respiratory tract colonization with adherence of gram-negative bacilli to epithelial cells. J Infect Dis 139:667, 1979.

19. Pugin J, Auckenthaler R, Lew DP, et al: Oropharyngeal decontamination decreases incidence of ventilator-associated pneumonia: a randomized, placebo-controlled, double-blind clinical trial. JAMA 265: 2704, 1991.
20. Brook I: Beta-lactamase–producing bacteria in head and neck infection. Laryngoscope 98:428, 1988.
21. Brook I: The role of beta-lactamase–producing bacteria in the persistence of streptococcal tonsillar infection. Rev Infect Dis 6:601, 1984.
22. Brook I, Gober AE: Emergence of beta-lactamase-–producing aerobic and anaerobic bacteria in the oropharynx of children following penicillin chemotherapy. Clin Pediatr (Phila) 23:338, 1984.
23. Tuner K, Nord CE: Emergence of beta-lactamase–producing microorganisms in the tonsils during penicillin treatment. Eur J Clin Microbiol 5:399, 1986.
24. Loesche WJ, Hockett RN, Syed SA: The predominant cultivable flora of tooth surface plaque removed from institutionalized subjects. Arch Oral Biol 17:1311, 1972.
25. Gibbons RJ: Aspects of the pathogenicity and ecology of the indigenous oral flora of man. In Ballows A, Dedaan RM, Dowell VR Jr, et al (eds): Anaerobic Bacteria, Role in Disease. Springfield, IL, Charles C Thomas, 1974, p 267.
26. Loesche WJ: The role of spirochetes in periodontal disease. Portside Symp Adv Dent Res 2:275, 1988.
27. Moore WEC: Microbiology of periodontal disease. J Periodont Res 22:335, 1987.
28. Brook I, Barrett CT, Brinkman CR, et al: Aerobic and anaerobic bacterial flora of the maternal cervix and newborn gastric fluid and conjunctiva: a prospective study. Pediatrics 63:451, 1979.
29. Rotimi VO, Olowe SA, Ahmed I: The development of bacterial flora of premature neonates. J Hyg (Lond) 94:309, 1985.
30. Gorbach SL, Nahas L, Lerner PI, et al: Studies of intestinal microflora. I. Effects of diet, age, and periodic sampling on numbers of fecal microorganisms in man. Gastroenterology 53:845, 1967.
31. Mata LJ, Urrutia JJ: Intestinal colonization of breast-fed children in an area of low social-economic level. Ann NY Acad Sci 176:93, 1971.
32. Long SS, Swenson RM: Development of anaerobic fecal flora in healthy newborn infants. J Pediatr 91:298, 1977.
33. Bishop RF, Anderson CM: The bacterial flora of the stomach and small intestine in children with intestinal obstruction. Arch Dis Child 35:487, 1960.
34. Snepar R, Poporad GA, Romano JM, et al: Effect of cimetidine and antacid on gastric microbial flora. Infect Immun 36:518, 1982.
35. Finegold SM, Sutter VL, Mathisen GE: Normal indigenous intestinal flora. In Hentges DJ (ed): Human Intestinal Microflora in Health and Disease. New York, Academic Press, 1983, p 3.
36. Simon GL, Gorbach SL: Intestinal flora in health and disease. Gastroenterology 86:177, 1987.
37. Howden CW, Hunt RH: Relationship between gastric secretion and infection. Gut 28:96, 1987.
38. Finegold SM, Sutter VL, Sugihara PT, et al: Fecal microbial flora in Seventh Day Adventist populations and control subject. Am J Clin Nutr 30:1781, 1977.
39. Brook I, Myhal LA, Dorsey CH: Encapsulation and pilus formation of *Bacteroides* spp. in normal flora abscesses and blood. J Infect 25:251, 1992.
40. Okuda K, Slots J, Genco RJ: *Bacteroides gingivalis, Bacteroides asaccharolyticus,* and *Bacteroides melaninogenicus* subspecies: cell surface morphology and adherence to erythrocytes and human buccal epithelial cells. Curr Microbiol 6:7, 1981.
41. Simon GL, Klempner MS, Kasper DL, et al: Alterations in opsonophagocytic killing by neutrophils of *Bacteroides fragilis* associated with animal and laboratory passage: effective capsular polysaccharide. J Infect Dis 145:72, 1982.
42. Beachey EH: Bacterial adherence: adhesion receptor interactions mediating the attachment of bacteria to mucosal surfaces. J Infect Dis 143:325, 1981.
43. Eisenstein BI: Phase variation of type I fimbriae in *Escherichia coli* is under transcriptional control. Science 214:337, 1980.
44. Sterk LMT, Van-Alphen L, Geelen-van Den Broek L, et al: Different binding of *Haemophilus influenzae* to human tissue by fimbriae. J Med Microbiol 35:129, 1991.
45. Wolin MJ: Metabolic interactions between intestinal microorganisms. Am J Clin Nutr 27:1320, 1974.
46. Bartlett JG: Antibiotic-associated pseudomembranous colitis. Rev Infect Dis 1:530, 1979.
47. Van der Waaij D, Berghuis de Vries JM, Lekkerkerk van der Wees JEC: Colonization resistance of the digestive tract in conventional and antibiotic-treated mice. J Hyg 69:405, 1971.
48. Berg RD: Promotion of the translocation of enteric bacteria from the gastrointestinal tracts of mice by oral treatment with penicillin, clindamycin, or metronidazole. Infect Immun 33:854, 1981.
49. Van der Waaij O, Hofstra IT, Wiegersma N: Effects of beta-lactam antibiotics on the resistance of the digestive tract of mice to colonization. J Infect Dis 146:417, 1982.
50. Rozenberg-Arska M, Dekker AW, Verhoef J: Ciprofloxacin for selective decontamination of the alimentary tract in patients with acute leukemia during remission induction treatment: the effect on fecal flora. J Infect Dis 142:104, 1985.
51. Tetteroo GWM, Wagenvoort JHT, Bruning HA: Role of selective decontamination in surgery. Br J Surg 79:300, 1992.
52. Klastersky J: A review of chemoprophylaxis and therapy of bacterial infection in neutropenic patients. Diagn Microbiol Infect Dis 12:201s, 1989.
53. Bran JL, Levison ME, Kaye D: Entrance of bacteria into the female urinary bladder. N Engl J Med 286:626, 1972.
54. Marrie TJ, Harding GKM, Ronald AR: Anaerobic and

aerobic urethral flora in healthy females. J Clin Microbiol 8:67, 1978.
55. Bartlett JG, Onderdonk AB, Drude E, et al: Quantitative bacteriology of the vaginal flora. J Infect Dis 136:271, 1977.
56. Onderdonk AB, Polk BF, Moon NE, et al: Methods for quantitative vaginal flora studies. Am J Obstet Gynecol 128:777, 1977.
57. Sautter RL, Brown WJ: Sequential vaginal cultures from normal young women. J Clin Microbiol 11:479, 1980.
58. Ohm MJ, Galask RP: Bacterial flora of the cervix from 100 prehysterectomy patients. Am J Obstet Gynecol 12:683, 1975.
59. Larsen B, Galask RP: Vaginal microbial flora and theoretic relevance. Obstet Gynecol 55(Suppl):1005, 1980.
60. Holdeman LV, Johnson JL: *Bacteroides disiens* sp. nov. and *Bacteroides bivius* sp. nov. from human clinical infections. Int J Syst Bacteriol 27:337, 1977.
61. Goplerud CP, Ohm MJ, Galask RP: Aerobic and anaerobic flora of the cervix during pregnancy and the puerperium. Am J Obstet Gynecol 126:858, 1976.
62. Tashjian JH, Coulan CB, Washington JA: II. Vaginal flora in asymptomatic women. Mayo Clin Proc 51:557, 1976.
63. Larsen B, Markovetz AJ, Galask RP: The role of estrogen in controlling the genital microflora of female rats. Appl Environ Microbiol 34:534, 1977.
64. Larsen B, Markovetz AJ, Galask RP: The bacterial flora of the female rat genital tract. Proc Soc Exp Biol Med 151:571, 1976.

BIBLIOGRAPHY

Gayah H, Verhoef J: Current topic: colonization resistance. Eur J Clin Microbiol 7:91, 1988.

Hentges DJ (ed): Human Intestinal Microflora in Health and Disease. New York, Academic Press, 1983.

Hill GB: Anaerobic flora of the female genital tract. In Lambe OW, Genec KJ, Mayberry-Carson S (eds): Anaerobic Bacteria: Selected Topics. New York, Plenum Publishing, 1980, p 39.

Simon GL, Gorbach SL: Intestinal microflora. Med Clin North Am 66:557, 1982.

The Pyogenic Cocci

CHAPTER 4

Marcos A. Wolff, Reuben Ramphal, Phillip K. Peterson

The occurrence of infections caused by pyogenic cocci appears to be a cyclical phenomenon. Staphylococci and streptococci accounted for the majority of wound infections in the preantibiotic era. However, the number of infections declined sharply after the introduction of penicillin. Infections caused by *Staphylococcus aureus* reached epidemic proportions in the 1950s, then declined gradually following the introduction of methicillin. Methicillin-resistant strains of staphylococci appeared in the 1960s and have subsequently become a worldwide clinical problem. In recent years there has been an overall increase in the incidence of staphylococcal infections, the reasons for which are not clear. Severe toxigenic streptococcal infections have also reemerged in the past few years and enterococci have now become important nosocomial pathogens. Currently, *Staphylococcus aureus* and *Staphylococcus epidermidis* show a significant level of resistance to β-lactams; gonococci and pneumococci have developed penicillin resistance; and enterococci are beginning to show ampicillin and vancomycin resistance. Thus the role of the pyogenic cocci as pathogens is in a state of flux, requiring constant evaluation. The same can be said of therapy for these organisms.

The purpose of this chapter is to outline what is known at the cellular and molecular levels about the pathogenesis of staphylococcal, streptococcal, and neisserial infections.

STAPHYLOCOCCI

Identification and Classification

The genus *Staphylococcus* is comprised of facultatively anaerobic gram-positive cocci, which ferment glucose, produce catalase, and tend to form irregular grape-like clusters. Staphylococci are members of the family Micrococcaceae, the other genus of this family being *Micrococcus*. Unlike staphylococci, micrococci are usually strict aerobes and do not ferment glucose. A variety of biochemical tests can be used to identify a number of staphylococcal species.[1] The most widely recognized staphylococcal species are *S. aureus, S. epidermidis,* and *S. saprophyticus. Staphylococcus aureus* is the best characterized and also clearly the most pathogenic of these species.

Staphylococcus aureus strains usually produce golden or pale yellow colonies on solid media, hence the name of the species and its distinction from the white colonies of *S. epidermidis*. Pigment production is an unstable characteristic; some *S. aureus* strains produce only white colonies. *Staphylococcus aureus* is more consistently, and most practically, identified by its production of coagulase.[2] Many laboratories define *S. aureus* as a coagulase-positive staphylococcus, whereas coagulase-negative staphylococci are referred to as *S. epidermidis*. However, there are rare strains of *S. aureus* that are coagulase negative, and some laboratories define *S. aureus* as staphylococci that produce deoxyribonuclease (DNase), a characteristic that also correlates highly with this species. Unfortunately, a number of coagulase-negative, DNase-positive staphylococci belong to species other than *S. aureus*.[3]

Pathogenesis

Source of Infection. The natural habitat of staphylococci is the body surface of many species of mammals and birds. Staphylococci are also found in the air and dust of occupied buildings and in milk, food, and sewage.[2] *Staphylococcus aureus* is a commensal bacterium found on moist areas of skin and in the anterior nares of up to 40 percent of healthy persons.[4] *Staphylococcus epidermidis* is an ubiquitous member of the flora of the skin and mucous membranes. Carriers of *S. aureus* can serve as reservoirs of this microorganism, and the skin often provides a vehicle for spread of staphylococci from person to person. The hospital environment is particularly favorable for transmission of *S. aureus.* Organisms can be transferred from patient to patient by the hands of attendants, and airborne transmission of staphylococci can be facilitated by improper room ventilation, as well as by the clothing of nurses and physicians.[5]

Staphylococcus aureus remains the most common pathogen isolated from operative wound infections, having been reported to be responsible for 17 percent of postoperative wound infections in a recent survey.[6] Such patients are a serious source of nosocomial staphylococcal infection, and some means of isolation should be practiced. Another source of infection, particularly for methicillin-resistant *S. aureus* (MRSA), is through the hospital admission of an infected or colonized patient from a chronic care facility.[7]

Staphylococcus epidermidis infection is largely a product of modern medical and surgical technology. Although this staphylococcal species is not as pathogenic as *S. aureus,* it is particularly well suited for a tenacious existence in the presence of foreign bodies such as prosthetic heart valves and joints, ventricular shunts, and plastic catheters.

Bacterial Factors. Although *S. aureus* is one of the principal bacterial pathogens that causes human infections, experimental infections can be produced only when high numbers of bacteria are used, and low numbers of bacteria can actually accelerate wound healing.[8] In a series of classic experiments, Elek[9] and Elek and Conen[10] demonstrated that it required a minimum of 7.5×10^6 cocci to produce a pustule when bacteria were injected intradermally, subcutaneously, or in full thickness wounds of volunteers. No differences were found in the virulence of strains obtained from clinical lesions, from healthy carriers, and from epidemic sources. When organisms were introduced by skin sutures left in situ, 500 times fewer bacteria produced severe local abscesses. In one volunteer a suture containing only 100 cocci caused suppuration. To date the mechanisms by which foreign bodies enhance pathogenicity remain largely unexplained. However, recent studies suggest that organisms growing on such surfaces are protected by a surrounding biofilm or exopolysaccharide "slime."[11] Another important aspect of the pathogenesis of S. aureus infection is the role of trauma. Whereas large inocula are required to produce infection in intact skin, the mere shaving of skin with a razor significantly reduces the inoculum required to cause infection.[12]

A variety of virulence factors have been described for *S. aureus.* However, it has also become clear that there is no known single important staphylococcal virulence factor, but rather that there is an array of mechanisms by which these bacteria can both evade host defenses and injure the host. Virulence factors of *S. aureus* can be divided into two general categories: (1) bacterial cell surface components, and (2) extracellular products (Fig. 4–1).

Bacterial Cell Surface Components. The cell wall of most *S. aureus* strains is composed of three major constituents—peptidoglycan, teichoic acid, and protein A. The peptidoglycan (mucopeptide) is a polysaccharide with extensively cross-linked peptide side chains. Attached to the carboxyl group of each N-acetylmuramic acid molecule is a short peptide, which is usually cross-linked by a pentaglycine bridge to a neighboring peptide unit. About 50 percent of the weight of the cell wall is contributed by peptidoglycan, which provides rigidity.[13] Cell wall teichoic acids, comprising about 40 percent of cell wall weight, are charged polymers of ribitol-phosphate with N-acetyl-D-glucosamine and D-alanine substituents. Protein A, contributing about 5 percent of the cell wall weight, is covalently linked to the peptidoglycan component.

Many strains of *S. aureus* possess a cell wall peptidoglycan that has been associated with pathogenicity.[14] When injected intradermally in animals, this cell wall "aggressin" inhibits edema production and migration of leukocytes, thus allowing bacteria to multiply and to produce necropurulent lesions. *Staphylococcus aureus* peptidoglycan also possesses endotoxin-like properties[15] and can activate both the classic and alternative pathways of the serum complement system and elicit a cell-mediated immune response (Fig. 4–2).

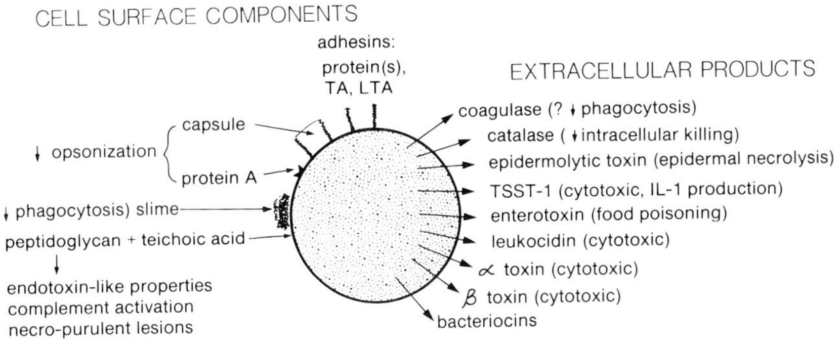

Figure 4–1. Virulence factors of *Staphylococcus aureus* and their proposed biologic effects.

A role in the pathogenesis of *S. aureus* infections has not been defined for teichoic acid, although it appears that this cell wall component may contribute to complement activation.[16] Therefore, along with protein A and peptidoglycan, teichoic acid may contribute to the formation of pus, which is a major manifestation of staphylococcal infection. The teichoic acids are largely responsible for the serologic specificity of staphylococci, and high titers of antibodies have been found in patients with serious or deep-seated staphylococcal infections.[17] Testing for the development of teichoic acid antibodies may be of diagnostic value in certain clinical settings.

Other cell wall components of *S. aureus* play different roles in pathogenesis, e.g. proteinaceous adhesins which bind to fibronectin, laminin and collagen are thought to play a role in colonization and localization of this organism in tissue.[18,19,20]

Some *S. aureus* strains also possess capsules. The capsule is believed to be antiphagocytic[21] and hence serve as a virulence factor in the same way as it is seen in classically encapsulated organisms, such as pneumococcus. Finally the ability of some strains to produce a more loosely surface-associated exopolysaccharide, or glycocalyx (slime), has been identified as a potential virulence factor in the pathogenesis of *S. aureus* osteomyelitis.[22]

Extracellular Products. Many *S. aureus* strains produce a large number of extracellular, enzymatically active factors that are believed to be important in

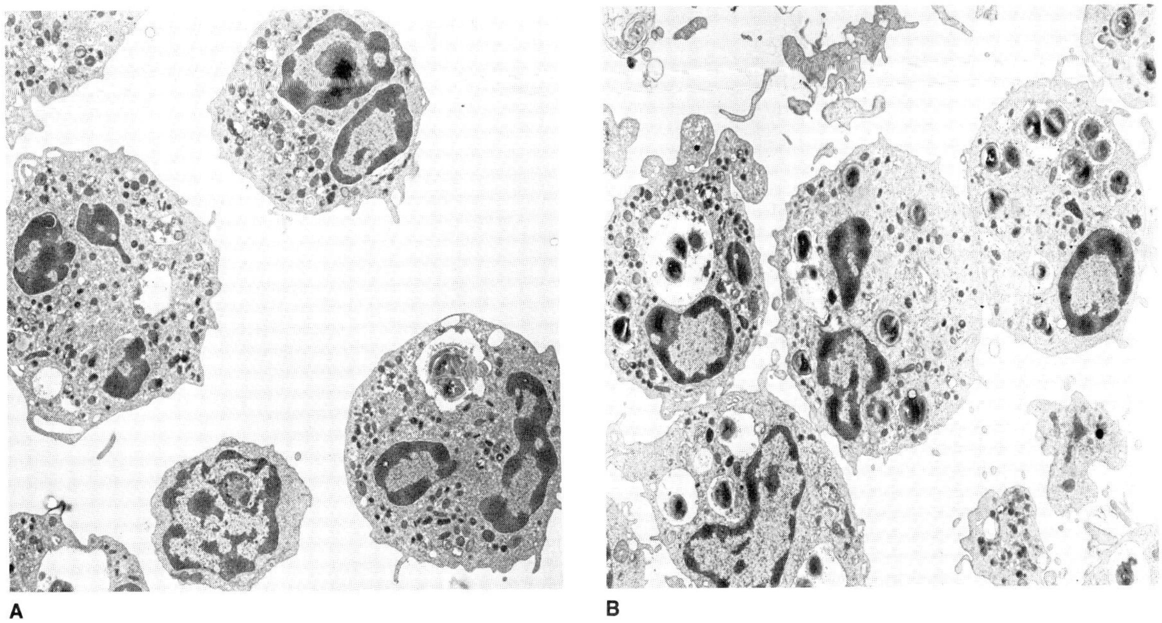

Figure 4–2. Electron micrograph of human polymorphonuclear leukocytes incubated with equal concentrations of **A,** an encapsulated *Staphylococcus aureus* strain, and **B,** an unencapsulated variant. Bacteria were incubated in normal human serum before being added to the leukocytes. Note the paucity of ingested encapsulated bacteria in comparison to the unencapsulated organisms.

the pathogenesis of staphylococcal disease. The enzyme coagulase is used to differentiate the more pathogenic coagulase-positive staphylococcal species. Although early investigators suggested that coagulase protected staphylococci from phagocytosis, this concept has been disputed.[23] Studies have shown that coagulase-negative, DNase-positive variants of *S. aureus* are significantly less virulent than are related coagulase-positive, DNase-negative variants,[24] suggesting that coagulase plays a role in virulence.

Catalase, another staphylococcal enzyme, may protect bacteria from the lethal effects of hydrogen peroxide produced by phagocytic cells and thereby function as a virulence factor.[25] This observation may in part explain the previously recognized ability of some staphylococci to survive within phagocytic cells.

About one-third of the clinical isolates of *S. aureus* produce a toxin capable of causing staphylococcal food poisoning,[26] which is characterized by vomiting and diarrhea 1 to 6 hours after ingestion of this enterotoxin. It is believed that enterotoxins enter the circulation in an unchanged state via the digestive tract and that their activity is mediated via the central nervous system.

Epidermolytic toxin can cause a variety of skin lesions, the most characteristic of which are the diffuse exfoliative bullae seen in children with staphylococcal scalded skin syndrome. Only certain staphylococcal strains (phage group II) are capable of producing this toxin.

The toxic shock syndrome (TSS) was first described in children in 1978,[27] then in menstruating women who were using tampons,[28] and more recently in association with postoperative wound infections, localized abscesses, and even staphylococcal colonization.[29] This syndrome is caused by at least three staphylococcal toxins (TSST-1, enterotoxins B and C).[30] Menstrual cases are caused primarily by strains secreting TSST-1, whereas nonmenstrual cases are caused primarily by strains producing enterotoxins B and C.[31] These toxins are believed to act on blood vessels as well as on the immune system, leading to the release of cytokines, which are responsible for the clinical manifestations of shock, rash, and fever. Although the number of menstrual TSS cases has decreased markedly in recent years, less severe forms of the illness are now well recognized, and the disease has been observed in patients of both sexes with otherwise benign wound infections.[33] It is likely that TSST-1 acts as a "superantigen"—that is, a molecule that binds the V_β chain of the T cell receptor to the major histocompatibility molecule on the macrophage. This triggers a massive cytokine cascade from both T lymphocytes and macrophages that results in a shock-like picture. Other superantigens are toxic products of other gram-positive organisms.

Host Factors. In many microbial infections, disease is in part produced by the host's inflammatory response to the invading microorganisms. Staphylococcal disease is no exception. The intense suppurative host response provoked by this pathogen is responsible for many of the localized manifestations of staphylococcal disease.

The invaded host's major means of defense against staphylococci is provided by phagocytic cells. Patients with quantitative or qualitative defects of these cells are predisposed to recurrent and severe staphylococcal diseases (see Chapter 13).

Clinical Manifestations and Therapeutic Considerations

As discussed, the clinical manifestations of staphylococcal disease are largely the combined result of bacterial toxicity and host response to this organism. Because specific disease entities involving staphylococci and their treatment are dealt with in subsequent chapters, selected clinical problems will be mentioned here briefly. A review of staphylococcal diseases has been provided by Musher and McKenzie[32,34] and Sheagren.[35,36]

As soon as *S. aureus* gains access to the circulation, the potential for serious disease is present, even in the host with normal immune defense mechanisms. *Staphylococcus aureus* bacteremia is therefore regarded as a serious clinical problem because of its well-recognized pathogenicity, as witnessed by its ability to establish infection on normal heart valves and to localize in other deeper foci, including bone, kidney, and brain. The management of staphylococcal bacteremia is problematic. There is evidence that the presence of a removable focus of infection, such as an infected intravenous line, allows short-term therapy (not less than 10 days).[37,38] However, a number of these cases will result in complications or relapse. Thus many authorities continue to recommend 4 to 6 weeks of parenteral antistaphylococcal therapy for all cases of *S. aureus* bacteremia. The treatment of each case of *S. aureus* bacteremia should be individualized and patients should be monitored with repeat blood cultures and serum erythrocyte sedimentation rate measurements at the end of treatment if short-course therapy is instituted. Monitoring a patient for the development of antistaphylococcal antibodies may help predict which patients are more likely to have deep-seated infection and would therefore benefit from long-term therapy.[39,40]

In contrast to the case with *S. aureus,* the isolation of coagulase-negative staphylococci from a blood culture usually signifies contamination of the culture from the skin. When multiple blood cultures are positive, however, infective endocarditis or an infected foreign body must be considered. These organisms can also cause suppurative[41] and lower urinary tract infections. In recent years coagulase-negative staphylococci have been assuming an increasingly important status as nosocomial pathogens.[42]

An important aspect of the management of most staphylococcal abscesses is incision and drainage. For some infections, such as cutaneous abscesses or wound infections that are not recurrent or severe or associated with systemic symptoms, incision and drainage are sufficient treatment, and antibiotic therapy is not required. Abscesses that involve internal organs generally necessitate operative drainage, although occasionally antibiotic therapy alone can be curative. Foreign bodies or necrotic tissue must generally be removed or debrided for effective eradication of infection. Generally, because of the widespread emergence of penicillin resistance among staphylococci, a penicillinase-resistant antibiotic must be used. When parenteral therapy is indicated, drugs such as nafcillin or oxacillin can be used. The dosage and duration of therapy, neither of which has clearly been established for any of the staphylococcal diseases, are generally decided by considerations related to the nature and severity of the disease being treated. A first-generation cephalosporin can be used in the penicillin-allergic patient who does not have a history of an immediate or accelerated type of hypersensitivity. Vancomycin is the drug of choice for infections caused by coagulase-negative and methicillin-resistant strains.[43,44] Although there are in vitro and animal studies that indicate that aminoglycosides or rifampin may provide a synergistic effect when used in combination with penicillinase-resistant penicillins, the benefit of combination therapy has not been established with certainty in humans. Quinolones, while showing in vitro activity against *S. aureus,* have been associated with the emergence of resistant strains and therapeutic failures.[45]

STREPTOCOCCI

Identification and Classification

Bacteria belonging to the genus *Streptococcus* are gram-positive, ovoid or spherical cells arranged in chains or pairs. Streptococci are nonsporing, usually nonmotile, and fail to reduce nitrate. They ferment carbohydrates with the production of acid, but never gas. Unlike staphylococci, streptococci are catalase negative. Streptococci are similar to staphylococci in that they are facultatively anaerobic. The strictly anaerobic chain-forming cocci (anaerobic streptococci) differ so greatly from the streptococci in their metabolic characteristics that they are excluded from the genus *Streptococcus* and therefore will not be discussed in this chapter. Although not of major surgical significance, the pneumococci are recognized as a separate and well-defined streptococcal species.

Three major characteristics are used for the classification of the streptococci: (1) changes induced by colonies of bacteria grown on sheep blood agar (beta-hemolysis, ie, complete destruction of erythrocytes; alpha-hemolysis, ie, zones of greenish discoloration containing intact red cells; gamma-hemolysis, no hemolysis in the surrounding culture medium); (2) serologic reactions (Lancefield classification); and (3) biochemical and physiologic characteristics such as the production of specific enzymes and the ability to grow in the presence of various chemical substances. On the basis of these characteristics many of the streptococci can be identified at a species level (Table 4–1). Although this method of classification is somewhat cumbersome, it is clinically relevant. When provided such information about a streptococcal isolate, the clinician: (1) may have a better appreciation of the most likely source of infection; (2) may anticipate specific complications (eg, endocarditis, rheumatic fever, suppurative foci); and (3) may make significant therapeutic decisions regarding choice of antibiotic and operative intervention. Some of the tests used to identify the streptococcal species that are the most pathogenic in humans are listed in Table 4–1.

In 1933 Lancefield described a method for classifying beta-hemolytic streptococci. She used a precipitin reaction and antigens extracted from these bacteria. Originally, five antigenic groups were identified (A, B, C, D, and E). There are now 20 groups (A through H and K through V). The Lancefield serologic classification is based on a heat- and acid-stable carbohydrate antigen located in the cell walls of organisms of all groups except groups D and N (which are identified on the basis of a lipoteichoic acid moiety). Although a number of clinical isolates are nongroupable,[46] serologic classification remains a valuable method.

Group A streptococci, the most common streptococcal pathogens of humans, constitute a single species (*S. pyogenes*). Almost all group A strepto-

TABLE 4–1. GENERAL CHARACTERISTICS OF *STREPTOCOCCUS* AND *ENTEROCOCCUS* SPECIES COMMONLY PATHOGENIC FOR HUMANS

Species	Serologic Group	Hemolysis	Identifying Features	Common Infections	MICs of Benzyl Penicillin (μg/ml)[a]
S. pyogenes	A	β^b	Bacitracin susceptibility[b]	Skin, wound, respiratory tract (nonsuppurative complications)	0.005
S. agalactiae	B	β^b	Hippurate hydrolysis, CAMP test	Neonatal meningitis, bacteremia, genitourinary tract	0.05
Enterococci *E. faecalis* *E. faecium* *E. durans*	D	α,β,γ	Bile-esculin hydrolysis, salt tolerant	Endocarditis, intra-abdominal and intrapelvic, urinary tract	2
Nonenterococci S. bovis S. equinus	D	α,β,γ	Bile-esculin hydrolysis, not salt tolerant	Endocarditis	0.06
Viridans streptococci *S. mutans* *S. mitis* *S. salivarius* *S. sanguis* *S. milleri group*		α,γ		Endocarditis Abscesses	0.012
S. pneumoniae		α^b	Bile solubility, optochin susceptibility	Pneumonia, otitis media, meningitis	0.01

[a] Concentrations given are approximate estimates of mean minimal inhibitory concentrations (MICs) taken from many sources.
[b] An occasional exception.

cocci are beta-hemolytic and are extremely susceptible to bacitracin—two features that are commonly used in the presumptive identification of this species. Group A streptococci can be subclassified according to their cell wall protein antigens (M and T). More than 80 M types are recognized.

Group B streptococci also comprise only one species, *S. agalactiae.* Group B streptococci are almost always beta-hemolytic, and virtually all produce hippuricase, an enzyme that hydrolyzes hippuric acid. Most of the other beta-hemolytic streptococci do not produce this enzyme; however, some strains of enterococci hydrolyze hippuric acid.

There are five organisms of clinical importance within group D. They belong to two genera: *Enterococcus* and *Streptococcus.* The three enterococcal species—*E. faecalis, E. faecium,* and *E. durans,* are collectively referred to as enterococci. The two nonenterococcal species—*S. bovis* and *S. equinus*—share the group D antigen and, also like the enterococci, give a positive bile-esculin reaction. Tolerance to 6.5 percent NaCl broth is a major characteristic of the enterococci, a feature used in distinguishing them from the nonenterococcal species. The separation of these two groups is of major clinical significance, as the enterococci are much less susceptible to penicillin, and important therapeutic considerations are based on the identification of this group when endocarditis is diagnosed.

The viridans streptococci are comprised of at least 13 species, of which five are commonly encountered (see Table 4–1). All species are non-beta-hemolytic and also by definition are not non-beta-hemolytic members of group A, B, D, and N. Although many viridans streptococci cannot be grouped by the Lancefield classification, there are strains that do react with antisera to groups H, K, and O. These species of streptococci do not grow in broth containing 6.5 percent NaCl and do not give a positive bile-esculin reaction.

Streptococcus pneumoniae is an easily distinguishable alpha-hemolytic streptococcal species that shares a number of immunologic cross-reactions with the viridans group.[47] Pneumococci have a characteristic lanceolate morphology and are arranged in pairs or chains. Solubility in bile and susceptibility to optochin are two tests commonly used in the clinical laboratory to distinguish this species (see Table 4–1). The pneumococci possess one of a series of antigenically specific capsular polysaccharides. By using antisera to these polysaccharides, 84 pneumococcal types can be identified; however, 23 types cause about 90 percent of all serious infections.[48] Polysaccharides from these 23 types are included as antigens in the current pneumococcal vaccine. When pneumococci react with homologous anticapsular serum, a capsular precipitin reaction (quellung reaction) occurs, and the capsule appears refractile under the microscope. An omniserum containing antibodies to all 84 pneumococcal types can be used in identifying pneumococci.

Pathogenesis

Source of Infection. Group A streptococci that cause soft tissue infections are spread by direct contact of an injured area with the organisms in the environment; pharyngitis is spread by large airborne droplets. The spread of group A streptococci that causes pyoderma and impetigo is enhanced by crowding and poor hygiene. Several outbreaks of group A streptococcal wound infections have been linked to airborne transmission in the operating room.[49–51] Skin or wound infections and the respiratory tract are the most frequent sources for group A streptococcal bacteremia.[46]

The epidemiology of group B streptococcal infections indicates that the female genital tract is the primary reservoir of these organisms; the frequency of carriage has been variously reported from less than 5 to 25 percent.[52] The acquisition rate of group B streptococci is high in infants born of colonized mothers, but the risk of clinical disease is low. The portal of entry of group B streptococci that causes neonatal meningitis or bacteremia, respiratory distress, and pneumonia probably involves multiple body orifices. Group B streptococci can also be isolated from rectal swabs and from urethral cultures of asymptomatic males and females—these sites also may be important reservoirs.

Enterococci and *S. bovis* are normal residents of the bowel and vagina. Endogenous infection from one of these sites appears to be the major source of a diverse group of clinical diseases, including nosocomial enterococcal urinary tract infection, intra-abdominal or intrapelvic infection, bacteremia, and endocarditis. In surgical practice they are most often found in mixed infections in wounds or in intraperitoneal sepsis. Recent studies have shown that colonized hospital personnel are probably the primary disseminators of nosocomial enterococcal infections.[53]

The viridans streptococci are found as part of the normal flora of many of the body's surfaces, including the mouth and bowel. They are the most prominent inhabitants of the oral cavity, an important portal of entry for infections such as endocarditis and brain abscess. The bowel may be an important source of *S. milleri,* occasionally found in intra-abdominal abscesses.[54]

Pneumococci colonize the respiratory tract of from 30 to 60 percent of "healthy people." Epidemiologic evidence indicates that person-to-person spread of these organisms may be facilitated by viral infection of the upper respiratory tract. The portal of entry for many pneumococcal infections is presumably this site. Overwhelming pneumococcal infection is the principal late septic complication after splenectomy and is the principal cause of primary peritonitis in children.

Bacterial Factors of Group A Streptococci. Group A streptococci are the most pathogenic and most thoroughly studied of the streptococcal groups. This is the only streptococcal species associated with suppurative and nonsuppurative complications, that is, acute rheumatic fever and poststreptococcal glomerulonephritis. As was pointed out for *S. aureus,* both bacterial cell surface components and extracellular products play a role in pathogenesis (Table 4–2). Wannamaker[55] has reviewed these bacterial factors in detail.

Bacterial Cell Surface Components of Group A Streptococci. The cell surface of the group A streptococcus is currently regarded as a mosaic network comprised of four major constituents—hyaluronic acid, Lancefield group-specific carbohydrate, peptidoglycan, and surface proteins (M, T, and R antigens). Although there is evidence that the hyaluronic acid capsule is antiphagocytic, its role in pathogenicity in human infections is not established. The group-specific carbohydrate is a polysaccharide polymer of

TABLE 4–2. VIRULENCE FACTORS OF GROUP A STREPTOCOCCI

Bacterial Factors	Biologic Effects
Cell surface components	
M protein	Antiphagocytic (decreased opsonization)
Hyaluronic capsule	Antiphagocytic
Peptidoglycan	Endotoxin-like properties, necropurulent lesions
Lipoteichoic acid	Attachment to epithelial cells
Extracellular products	
Streptolysins O and S	Cytotoxic
Proteinase	Cytotoxic
Hyaluronidase, streptokinase	Promote spread of infection
Pyrogenic exotoxins	Rash, shock

N-acetyl-D-glucosamine and L-rhamnose. This polymer has antigenic components that cross-react with glycoprotein from human cardiac valves, but its role in the pathogenesis of rheumatic carditis is unknown.

The M protein of group A streptococci, which is located in hair-like structures of fimbriae on the cell surface (Fig. 4–3), is a major virulence factor for this group of organisms.[56] Group A variant strains lacking M protein rarely cause human disease because they are readily phagocytized by human leukocytes. The exact mechanism by which M protein interferes with phagocytosis is unclear. There is evidence, however, that it may do so by inhibiting bacterial opsonization by masking the cell surface components that are responsible for activation of the alternative complement pathway.[57] Alternatively, the binding of fibrinogen to M protein may block bacterial recognition of the organisms by opsonic complement molecules.[58] Type-specific, anti-M protein antibodies are essential for promoting efficient phagocytosis of M protein-positive strains. The T and R proteins are not important for virulence and do not stimulate protective antibodies.

The peptidoglycan component of the streptococcal cell wall has a structure and significance similar to that of the staphylococcal peptidoglycan. It gives the cells its shape and rigidity, and it shares antigens. Such sharing may be involved in natural immunity to gram-positive bacteria. Streptococcal peptidoglycan, like staphylococcal peptidoglycan, produces fever and local Shwartzman's reaction in rabbits. Peptidoglycan also produces dermal necrosis with infiltration of polymorphonuclear leukocytes and can activate the alternative pathway of complement.[59] Thus this cell wall constituent shares a number of characteristics of the endotoxins of gram-negative bacteria.

The initiation of infection in the upper respiratory tract requires that group A streptococci possess a mechanism for adhering to mucosal cells of the pharynx and tonsils. Adherence to epithelial cells appears to be a property of lipoteichoic acid, which is located in the surface fimbriae of group A streptococci along with M proteins. Fibronectin on the surface of host cells appears to be the attachment site for the lipoteichoic acid adhesive of group A streptococci.[58,60]

Extracellular Products of Group A Streptococci. Group A streptococci release a large array of toxins and enzymes, some of which have been implicated in pathogenesis. Two distinct hemolysins, O and S, are produced by group A streptococci. Streptolysin S is responsible for the beta-hemolysis that surrounds colonies on the surface of blood agar; subsurface hemolysis is caused by oxygen-labile, streptolysin O. Streptolysin O, a potent cardiotoxin,[61] can act on any sterol-containing membrane, including the cell membranes of polymorphonuclear leukocytes and platelets and of mammalian mitochondria. Measurement of antibodies to this hemolysin has been useful as a diagnostic test in recent group A streptococcal infection. Because streptolysin S, which also has leukotoxic properties, is nonantigenic, it has been suggested that it might be active during repeated streptococcal infections and in recurrences of rheumatic fever.[62] Streptococcal proteinase may be responsible for tissue invasion or tissue damage. DNases, hyaluronidase,

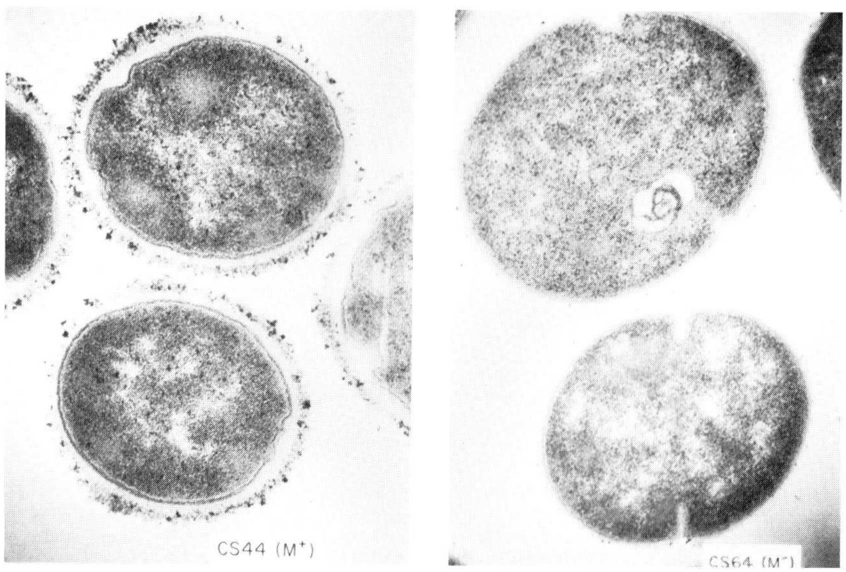

Figure 4–3. Electron micrographs of an M protein-positive, group A streptococcal strain, CS44 (M^+), and an M protein-negative variant of this strain, CS64 (M^-). The hair-like structures seen on the surface of CS44 contain M protein, a major streptococcal virulence factor. *(Photomicrographs courtesy of PP Cleary.)*

and streptokinase may all promote spread of infection.

Although the pathogenesis of group A streptococcal infections is multifactorial, it has become clear that a specific syndrome, the *streptococcal toxic shock syndrome,* is the product of a single toxin, pyrogenic toxin A, which is structurally related to the staphylococcal toxin causing the same syndrome.[63] It probably acts by virtue of its "superantigen" character, which permits the triggering of release of both T cell and macrophage cytokines. The cytokine cascade leads to a shock-like state.

Bacterial Factors in Other Streptococci. Bacterial factors involved in the pathogenicity of streptococcal infections caused by species other than group A are not as clearly understood. Although the factors responsible for virulence in group B streptococci are largely unknown, immunologic studies suggest that virulence may be related to the capsular antigen. Sialic acid, a major constituent of the polysaccharide capsules of group B streptococci, has been considered a possible virulence factor for invasion of neonatal meninges. The presence of sialic acid in all serotypes, however, does not explain the propensity of type III organisms for invasion of this site.[64] Sialic acid residues, present in the type-specific capsule of all five group B streptococcal serotypes, are antiopsonic, and this may play a major role in virulence.[65] The function of extracellular products of group B streptococci in pathogenesis is obscure.[54]

The major virulence factor of *S. pneumoniae* appears to be its capsular polysaccharide. The antiphagocytic property of this cell surface component may be similar to that of the capsular polysaccharide found in some staphylococcal strains. This polysaccharide appears to mask cell wall peptidoglycan from the opsonic activity of certain serum factors, in particular, the complement system.[66] Type-specific anticapsular antibodies promote phagocytosis of these organisms and are, in general, protective against serious infection—hence the renewed interest in capsular antigen vaccines for susceptible individuals.

Adherence is a major factor involved in the pathogenesis of endocarditis caused by both the group D organisms and by the viridans streptococci. These organisms have the potential to adhere to damaged or abnormal heart valves. It is possible that glucan, a dextran frequently produced by endocarditis-associated species of streptococci, may contribute to the stickiness of these bacteria and may thus play a role in the initiation of this infection.[67,68] Exopolysaccharide production within cardiac vegetations may permit the sustained survival of viridans streptococci at this body site.[69] The ecologic or pathogenetic role of these organisms in mixed infections is unknown.

Host Factors. Mechanisms of host response to, and defense against, streptococci are in many respects similar to those seen with staphylococci. An intact integument and mucous membrane barrier are of primary importance in defense against streptococci. Breaks in these barriers are essential for tissue invasion and the bacteremia seen with many of the streptococcal species. Purulent infections of the tonsils and pharynx by group A streptococci can occur without local trauma.

Many streptococci have a predilection for certain hosts.[55] The majority of group B streptococcal infections occur in neonates or mothers in the postpartum period. In other adults, group B infections appear to be largely opportunistic, occurring with a high frequency in diabetics, patients with chronic liver disease, or people with underlying malignancy.[70] Another example of special host requirements for some streptococcal infections is the finding that the pharyngeal cells of patients with rheumatic heart disease have an increased avidity for adherence of rheumatic fever-associated group A streptococci, a phenomenon that may be important in the pathogenesis of rheumatic fever.[71] In burn patients who have received skin grafts, infections with group A streptococci can lead to graft rejection. An important host factor to consider when one is dealing with bacteremia or endocarditis caused by *S. bovis* is the association of these prob lems with occult carcinoma of the colon[72] or chronic liver disease.[73] Host defenses are discussed in Chapter 13.

Clinical Manifestations and Therapeutic Considerations

Streptococcus pyogenes (group A streptococci) remain the most common cause of human streptococcal infections. These organisms can cause infections of almost any organ system, although the skin, subcutaneous tissues, and pharynx are by far the most frequently affected sites.[74] The pyogenic potential of these organisms is perhaps best demonstrated by the striking propensity for empyema formation after *S. pyogenes* pneumonia. There has been a resurgence of nonsuppurative complications of *S. pyogenes* infection, namely, acute rheumatic fever, which has been caused by type M-18 strains.[75] The streptococcal toxic shock syndrome has been increasingly reported. In a recent review, necrotizing fascitis, with or without myositis, was the most common soft tissue infection associated[76] with a toxic shock picture and required extensive surgical debridement for treatment. This syndrome may also be a potential postoperative complication of routine surgical procedures, presenting with shock and multiorgan failure, in some patients with no site of infection being apparent at presentation.[77,78] The most benign-appearing as well as the most extensive soft tissue infections can produce the shock-like picture caused by toxins that behave as superantigens.

Group B streptococci are an important cause of infection in neonates, primarily meningitis and bacteremia; however, a significant number of bacteremic infections also occur in adults. Bacteremia in adult patients is often a hospital-acquired infection and is associated with a high mortality rate, especially in the elderly.[79] Serious infections caused by other streptococcal serogroups have been described[80–82] and cellulitis developing in limbs of coronary bypass patients after saphenous phlebectomy is a well-recognized manifestation of non-group A beta-hemolytic streptococci.[83]

Infections caused by group D streptococci are particularly important in hospitalized patients, a fact that is partially related to their existence as part of the normal flora of the genitourinary and gastrointestinal tracts. The insertion of instruments in the genitourinary tract can lead to urinary tract infection, bacteremia, and endocarditis. Perforation of the gastrointestinal tract or infection of the pelvic organs is a common association with the development of intra-abdominal or intrapelvic infection caused by a mixed bacterial flora, including group D enterococci. Operative intervention is usually mandatory. As has already been pointed out, the distinction between enterococcal and nonenterococcal group D species is important in guiding antibiotic therapy. Of all the streptococcal species the enterococci are routinely resistant to penicillin (see Table 4–1), so ampicillin is generally substituted. When enterococci are the cause of endocarditis, gentamicin should be added to the regimen because of its therapeutic synergy. Vancomycin should be used in the penicillin-allergic patient. None of the currently available cephalosporin or cefamycin antibiotics are active against enterococci. Increasing resistance among enterococci, particularly among isolates that cause nosocomial infections, requires that careful susceptibility testing be performed on isolates causing serious infections so that optimal antibiotic therapy can be selected.

The viridans streptococci remain the most common cause of infective endocarditis. Although not generally pyogenic, one species, *S. milleri,* is highly pyogenic, being found in abscesses in many sites such as the liver and brain.[54] The isolation of *S. milleri* from a blood culture should alert the physician to look for such a complication. This is one reason for the proposal that clinical microbiology laboratories should routinely speciate the viridans streptococci.

Penicillin is still the best drug for group A streptococcal infections. Fortunately, resistance to penicillin has not appeared among group A streptococci, although resistance to erythromycin may be increasing. Cephalosporins can be used as an alternative in patients with a history of penicillin allergy that is not of the immediate type. Although penicillin is also the best drug for pneumococcal infections, the recent emergence of resistant strains is a cause of concern.[84,85] Pneumococci isolated from blood or cerebrospinal fluid (CSF) should be tested for resistance to penicillin using a 1 μg oxacillin disk, which distinguishes strains that are susceptible from those that are relatively resistant (MIC = 0.12 to 1.0 μg/ml) and fully resistant (MIC > 1.0 μg/ml) to penicillin.[86] Penicillin, or an appropriate alternative drug, should also be used prophylactically in patients at high risk for rheumatic fever recurrences, infective endocarditis (congenital heart disease, valvular heart disease, and prosthetic grafts and valves), and overwhelming pneumococcal infection (anytime after splenectomy). Immunization with the 23-valent pneumococcal vaccine appears to be warranted in all patients who are functionally asplenic or who have undergone splenectomy.[87] Ideally, pneumococcal vaccine should be given 10 to 14 days before an elective splenectomy because of the importance of the spleen in processing antigen. Even vaccination will not prevent all pneumococcal sepsis in asplenic patients, and long-term chemoprophylaxis may be necessary.

NEISSERIAE

Identification and Classification

Although other members of this group of microorganisms can cause human disease, *Neisseria gonorrhoeae* and *N. meningitidis* are clearly the most pathogenic species for humans. These bacteria are gram-negative, spherical or ovoid cocci found in pairs with flattened adjacent sides. They do not produce spores, are nonmotile, and are strict aerobes. Neisseriae produce indophenol oxidase, and a positive oxidase reaction, although not specific for this group, is used in the process of identification. Gonococci and meningococci are relatively fragile organisms with fastidious nutritional and growth requirements. This characteristic necessitates special care in the transport of clinical specimens, special culture media (chocolate agar or Thayer-Martin medium), and the presence of carbon dioxide and humidity to assure growth. Differentiation between gonococci and meningococci is often based on their different means of breakdown of specific sugars with concomitant production of acid (gonococci degrade only glucose, meningococci degrade maltose and glucose, and neither species can degrade sucrose or lactose).

Immunofluorescence tests can be used to distinguish gonococci from other neisseriae and for the subtyping of gonococci. Different gonococcal strains can also be identified by specific growth requirements (*auxotyping*) and by various outer membrane antigens.[89] The serogroups of meningococci (A, B, C, D, X, Y, and Z) are differentiated on the basis of specific polysaccharides found on the bacterial surface, all of which, except for serogroups B and D, are clearly capsular in nature.

Pathogenesis

Source of Infection. *Neisseria gonorrhoeae* and *N. meningitidis* are both specifically human pathogens. Gonococci can infect epithelial cells of the urethra, endocervix and canal, pharynx, and conjunctiva. Gonococcal infection is transmitted from person to person by the apposition of these mucosal surfaces, usually during sexual contact. Infection is not necessarily accompanied by symptoms, and asymptomatic carriers are the primary reservoir for gonococcal infection. Contiguous spread of bacteria from the endocervix can result in endometritis, salpingitis, tubo-ovarian abscess, and peritonitis. Invasion from any infected mucosal surface into the bloodstream can result in the clinical syndrome of disseminated gonococcal infection.

Neisseria meningitidis can be found as a member of the normal flora of the pharynx (the carrier rate has been variously reported from 2 to 38 percent). Although the attack rate clearly increases with crowding (eg, among military recruits) and with exposure to patients with active infection, the relationship between colonization and the development of overt disease is not entirely clear. In the case of meningococcal meningitis, for example, the portal of entry is often covert. Surgically treatable metastatic abscesses are rare complications of meningococcemia.

Bacterial Factors. The cell surface of gonococci has several functions in pathogenesis (Table 4–3). The outer membrane of the gonococcal cell envelope contains several constituents that are important in this regard—outer membrane protein, lipopolysaccharide, and pili (hair-like structures traversing the cell wall). Endotoxin is one part of the lipopolysaccharide component. Pili appear to be important for the initial attachment to epithelial cells and may also inhibit phagocytosis and bacterial killing.[90] Resistance to phagocytosis may also be correlated with the protein components of the outer layer of the cell surface.[91] Outer membrane protein II plays a role in the attachment of gonococci to epithelial cells.[92] The mechanisms of attachment to and penetration of epithelial cells by meningococci bear close similarities to those of gonococci.[93] The surface of some gonococci may be encapsulated, and encapsulated strains are resistant to non–antibody-mediated phagocytosis. Most meningococcal strains are encapsulated, and the capsule is presumably an important bacterial defense factor.

The ability of some microorganisms to acquire iron within a host is an important determinant both of virulence and of the nature of the engendered infection.[94] Strains of *N. gonorrhoeae* isolated from patients with disseminated gonococcal infection have an enhanced ability to acquire iron in an experimental host, when compared to urogenital isolates from patients with uncomplicated infection. *Neisseria meningitidis,* which can produce septicemia and disseminated infection, is also unaffected by reduced iron concentrations.[94]

IgA protease is an extracellular enzyme produced by both gonococci and meningococci. The only known substrate for this enzyme is human immunoglobulin of the IgA1 subclass, which is important

TABLE 4–3. VIRULENCE FACTORS OF *N. GONORRHOEAE*

Bacterial Factors	Biologic Effects
Cell surface components	
Lipopolysaccharide (endotoxin)	Cytotoxic, pyrogenic
Pili	Attachment to epithelial cells, inhibits phagocytosis, killing
Outer membrane proteins	Inhibits phagocytosis, attachment to epithelial cells
Capsule	Inhibits phagocytosis
Iron-binding ability	Promotes survival, dissemination
IgA protease	Degrades local IgA

in local mucosal immune defense. Mulks and Plaut[95] have shown that all clinical isolates of *N. gonorrhoeae* and *N. meningitidis* tested were IgA protease positive, in contrast to eight species of nonpathogenic neisseriae that commonly colonize the normal human nasopharynx.

Host Factors. Inhibition of attachment of *N. gonorrhoeae* to epithelial cells is, at least in part, associated with the local production of antibody. Tramont[95] has shown that antibodies of the classes IgG and IgA (primarily secretory IgA) are capable of inhibiting such attachment. Other humoral factors and polymorphonuclear leukocytes appear to have a major role in the killing of gonococci and in preventing invasion and spread of infection.

Whereas serum by itself does not possess significant bactericidal activity for staphylococci or streptococci, serum is clearly bactericidal for a number of gonococcal strains. Both antibodies and the complement system are involved in the bactericidal action. Patients with deficiencies of the terminal, lytic, components of the complement cascade are especially prone to recurrent episodes of disseminated gonococcal and meningococcal disease.

Host factors that may promote the spread of gonococcal infections into the endometrial cavity and the fallopian tubes include menstruation and the implantation of an intrauterine device. Host defenses are more thoroughly discussed in Chapter 13.

Clinical Manifestations and Therapeutic Considerations

Gonococcal infection remains an extremely important social problem.[97] Gynecologists, urologists, orthopedic surgeons, and even general surgeons will encounter this disease in its local and systemic manifestations (eg, skin lesions, tenosynovitis, acute septic arthritis, pelvic peritonitis).[98] In contrast, most patients with meningococcal disease (ie, patients with meningitis, meningococcemia, or pneumonitis) will not be seen in surgical consultation.

About 10 to 20 percent of the exposed females who become infected with gonococci develop acute salpingitis (acute pelvic inflammatory disease). When pelvic inflammatory disease is complicated by the development of tubo-ovarian abscess, surgical intervention is generally warranted. Anorectal infection, seen primarily in females, neonates, and homosexual males, usually involves rectal bleeding. Anorectal infection can be complicated by pararectal abscess formation or fistula in ano. Spread of gonococci into the upper abdomen can result in gonococcal perihepatitis (Fitz-Hugh-Curtis syndrome). Patients with this disease have right upper quadrant or bilateral upper abdominal pain and tenderness. The clinical findings, plus mild liver function test abnormalities and associated nonvisualization of the gallbladder on oral cholecystography, can mimic acute cholecystitis. Epididymitis and prostatitis are seldom caused by gonococci, presumably because of early antibiotic therapy.

Penicillin remains an excellent drug for meningococcal infection, but the rapid spread of plasmid-mediated, penicillinase-producing strains of gonococci, first recognized in 1975,[99] has made this agent inadequate as first line treatment for gonococcal infections. Ceftriaxone is the currently recommended antibiotic of choice for treating gonococcal infections, with quinolones as alternative.[100] Because a percentage of patients with gonorrhea are also infected with chlamydia, a drug active against this organism should be given concomitantly.

REFERENCES

Staphylococci

1. Kloos WE, Lamber DW Jr: Staphylococci. In: *Manual of Microbiology,* 5th ed. Washington, DC, American Society for Microbiology, 1991, p 223.
2. Wilson GS, Miles A: Virology and immunity. In Topley WWC, Wilson GS: Principles of Bacteriology, Vol 1, 6th ed. Baltimore, Williams & Wilkins, 1975, p 764.
3. Gramoli JL, Wilkinson BJ: Characterization and identification of coagulase-negative, heat-stable deoxyribonuclease-positive staphylococci. J Gen Microbiol 105:275, 1978.
4. Williams REO, Blowers R, Garrod LP, Shooter RA: Hospital Infections, 2nd ed. London, Lloyd-Luke, 1966.
5. Lidwell OM, Brock B, Shooter RA, et al: Airborne infection in a fully air-conditioned hospital. IV. Airborne dispersal of *Staphylococcus aureus* and its nasal acquisition by patients. J Hygiene 75:445, 1975.
6. Anonymous: Nosocomial infection rates for interhospital comparison: limitations and possible solutions. Infect Control Hosp Epidemiol 12:609, 1991.
7. Muder RR, Brennen C, Wagener M, et al: Methicillin-resistant staphylococcal colonization and infection in a long-term care facility. Ann Intern Med 114:107, 1991.
8. Levenson SM, Kan-Gruber D, Gruber C, et al: Wound healing accelerated by *Staphylococcus aureus.* Arch Surg 118:310, 1983.
9. Elek SD: Experimental staphylococcal infections in the skin of man. Ann NY Acad Sci 65:85, 1956.
10. Elek SD, Conen PE: The virulence of *Staphylococcus pyogenes* for man: A study of wound infection. Br J Exp Pathol 38:573, 1957.

11. Costerton JW: The etiology and persistence of cryptic bacterial infections: A hypothesis. Rev Infect Dis 6(Suppl):608, 1984.
12. Morse SI. Studies on the chemistry and immunochemistry of *Staphylococcus aureus.* J Exp Med 115:295, 1962.
13. Ghuysen JM, Strominger JL, Tipper DJ: Bacterial cell walls. Compr Biochem 26:53, 1968.
14. Van der Vijver JCM, Van Es-Boon MM, Michel MF: A study of virulence factors with induced mutants of *Staphylococcus aureus.* J Med Microbiol 8:279, 1975.
15. Rotta J: Endotoxin-like properties of the peptidoglycan. Z Immunitaetsforsch 149:230, 1975.
16. Wilkinson BJ, Kim Y, Peterson, PK, et al: Activation of complement by cell surface components of *Staphylococcus aureus.* Infect Immun 20:338, 1978.
17. Crowder JG, White A: Teichoic acid antibodies in staphylococcal and nonstaphylococcal endocarditis. Ann Intern Med 77:87, 1972.
18. Kuusela P: Fibronectin binds to *Staphylococcus aureus.* Nature 276:718, 1973.
19. Lopes JD, dos Reis M, Brentani RR: Presence of laminin receptors in *Staphylococcus aureus.* Science 229:275, 1985.
20. Vercellotti GM, McCarthy JB, Lindholm P, et al: Extracellular matrix proteins (fibronectin, laminin, and type IV collagen) bind and aggregate bacteria. Am J Pathol 120:13, 1985.
21. Peterson PK, Wilkinson BJ, Kim Y, et al: Influence of encapsulation on staphylococcal opsonization and phagocytosis by human polymorphonuclear leukocytes. Infect Immun 19:943, 1978.
22. Gristina AG, Oga M, Webb LX, Hobgood CD: Adherent bacterial colonization in the pathogenesis of osteomylitis. Science 228:990, 1985.
23. Cawdery M, Foster WD, Hawgood BC, Taylor C: The role of coagulase in the defense of *Staphylococcus aureus* against phagocytosis. Br J Exp Pathol 50:408, 1969.
24. Hasegawa N, San Clemente CL: Virulence and immunity of *Staphylococcus aureus* BB and certain deficient mutants. Infect Immun 22:473, 1978.
25. Mandell GL: Catalase, superoxide dismutase, and virulence of *Staphylococcus aureus.* In vitro and in vivo studies with emphasis on staphylococcal-leukocyte interaction. J Clin Invest 55:561, 1975.
26. Casman EP: Staphylococcal enterotoxin. Ann NY Acad Sci 128:124, 1965.
27. Todd J, Fishaut M: Toxic-shock syndrome associated with phage-group-I staphylococci. Lancet 2:1116, 1978.
28. Shands KN, Schmid GP, Dan BB, et al: Toxic-shock syndrome in menstruating women: association with tampon use and *Staphylococcus aureus* and clinical features in 52 cases. N Engl J Med 303:1436, 1980.
29. Chesney PJ: Clinical aspects and spectrum of illness of toxic shock syndrome: overview. Rev Infect Dis 11:S1, 1989.
30. Schlievert PM: Staphylococcal enterotoxin B and toxic-staphylococcal shock toxin-1 are significantly associated with nonmenstrual toxic shock syndrome. Lancet 1:1149, 1986.
31. Kain KC, Schulzer M, Chow AW: Clinical spectrum of nonmenstrual toxic shock syndrome (TSS): comparison with menstrual TSS by multivariate discriminant analyses. Clin Infect Dis 16:100, 1993.
32. Musher DM, McKenzie SO: Infections due to *Staphylococcus aureus.* Medicine (Baltimore) 56:383, 1977.
33. Bartlett P, Reingold AL, Graham DR, et al: Toxic shock syndrome associated with surgical wound infections. JAMA 247:1448, 1982.
34. Musher DM, McKenzie SO: Infections due to *Staphylococcus aureus.* Medicine (Baltimore) 56:383, 1977.
35. Sheagren JN: *Staphylococcus aureus:* the persistent pathogen, I. N Engl J Med 310:1368, 1984.
36. Sheagren JN: *Staphylococcus aureus:* the persistent pathogen, II. N Engl J Med 310:1437, 1984.
37. Iannini PB, Crossley K: Therapy of *Staphylococcus aureus* bacteremia associated with a removable focus of infection. Ann Intern Med 84:558, 1976.
38. Raad II, Sabbagh MF. Optimal duration of therapy for catheter-related *Staphylococcus aureus* bacteremia: a study of 55 cases and review. Clin Infect Dis 14(1):75, 1992.
39. Tuazon CU, Sheagren JN, Choa MS, et al: *Staphylococcus aureus* bacteremia: relationship between formation of antibodies to teichoic acid and development of metastatic abscesses. J Infect Dis 137:57, 1978.
40. Verbrugh HA, Nelson RD, Peterson PK, Thompson RL: Serology of *Staphylococcus aureus* infections using multiple antigens and serum samples. J Infect Dis 148:608, 1983.
41. Polaczek-Kornecka B, Dziadur-Goldsztajn Z, Komorowski A: Coagulase-negative staphylococci in clinical surgery. In Jeljaszewicz J (ed): Staphylococci and Staphylococcal Diseases, published as supplement 5 to Zentralblatt für Bakteriologie, Parasitenkunde, Intfektionskrankheiten und Hygiene. New York, Fischer Verlag, 1976, p 145.
42. Lowy FD, Hammer SM: *Staphylococcus epidermidis* infections. Ann Intern Med 99:834, 1983.
43. Hackbarth CJ, Chambers HF: Methicillin-resistant staphylococci: detection methods and treatment of infections. Antimicrob Agents Chemother 33:995, 1989.
44. Wadsworth SJ, Ki-Ho K, Satishchandran V, et al: Development of new antibiotic resistance in methicillin-resistant but not methicillin-susceptible *Staphylococcus aureus.* J Antimicrob Chemother 30:821, 1992.
45. Trucksis M, Hooper DC, Wolfson JS: Emerging resistance to fluoroquinolones in staphylococci: an alert. Ann Intern Med 114(5):424, 1991.

Streptococci

46. Duma RJ, Weinberg AN, Medrek TF, Kunz LJ: Streptococcal infections: A bacteriologic and clinical study of streptococcal bacteremia. Medicine (Baltimore) 48:87, 1969.

47. Wannamaker LW, Matsen JM (eds): Streptococci and Streptococcal Diseases: Recognition, Understanding and Management. New York, Academic Press, 1972, p 355.
48. Bolan G, Broome CV, Facklam RR, et al: Pneumococcal pneumonia efficacy in selected populations in the U.S. Ann Intern Med 104:1, 1986.
49. Gryska PF, O'Dea AE: Postoperative streptococcal wound infection. The anatomy of an epidemic. JAMA 213:1189, 1970.
50. Berkelman RL, Martin D, Graham DR, et al: Streptococcal wound infections caused by a vaginal carrier. JAMA 247:2680, 1982.
51. Paul SM, Genese C, Spitalny K: Postoperative group A B-hemolytic *Streptococcus* outbreak with the pathogen traced to a member of a healthcare worker's household. Infect Control Hosp Epidemiol 11:643, 1990.
52. Facklam RR: A review of the microbiological techniques for the isolation and identification of streptococci. CRC Crit Rev Clin Lab Sci 6:287, 1976.
53. Moellering RC Jr: Emergence of enterococcus as a significant pathogen. Clin Infect Dis 14:1173, 1992.
54. Parker MT, Ball LC: *Streptococcus milleri* as a pathogen for man. In Parker MT (ed): The Pathogenic Streptococci: Streptococcal Disease in Man and Animals. Chertsey, Surrey, Reedbooks, 1980.
55. Wannamaker LW: Immunology of streptococci. In Nahmias AJ, O'Reilly R (eds): Immunology of Human Infections. New York, Plenum, 1980.
56. Fox EN: M proteins of group A streptococci. Bacteriol Rev 38:57, 1974.
57. Peterson PK, Schmeling D, Cleary PP, et al: Inhibition of alternative complement pathway opsonization by group A streptococcal M protein. J Infect Dis 139:575, 1979.
58. Beachey EH, Simpson WA, Ofek I, et al: Attachment of *Streptococcus pyogenes* to mammalian cells. Rev Infect Dis 5(Suppl):670, 1983.
59. Greenblatt J, Boackle RJ, Schwab JH: Activation of the alternative complement pathway by peptidoglycan from streptococcal cell wall. Infect Immun 19:296, 1978.
60. Stanislawski L, Simpson WA, Hasty D, et al: Role of fibronectin in attachment of *Streptococcus pyogenes* and *Escherichia coli* to human cell lines and isolated oral epithelial cells. Infect Immun 48:257, 1985.
61. Halbert SP: Streptolysin O. In Ajl SJ, Kadis S, Montie TC (eds): Microbial Toxins, Vol III. New York, Academic Press, 1970, p 69.
62. MacLeod CM: Hypersensitivity and disease. In Lawrence HS (ed): Cellular and Humoral Aspects of the Hypersensitive States, New York, PB Hoeber, 1959, p 615.
63. Stevens DL, Tanner MH, Einship J, et al: Severe group A streptococcal infections associated with a toxic shock-like syndrome and scarlet fever toxin A. N Engl J Med 321:1, 1989.
64. Patterson JH, Hafeez AEB: Group B streptococci in human disease. Bacteriol Rev 40:744, 1976.
65. Shigeoka AO, Rote NS, Santos JI, Hill HR: Assessment of the virulence factors of group B streptococci: correlation with sialic acid content. J Infect Dis 147:857, 1983.
66. Wilkinson BJ, Peterson PK, Quie PG: Cryptic peptidoglycan and the antiphagocytic effect of the *Staphylococcus aureus* capsule: model for the antiphagocytic effect of bacterial cell surface polymers. Infect Immun 23:502, 1979.
67. Parker MT, Ball LC: Streptococci and aerococci associated with systemic infection in man. J Med Microbiol 9:275, 1976.
68. Ramirez-Ronda CH: Adherence of glucan-positive and glucan-negative streptococcal strains to normal and damaged heart valves. J Clin Invest 62:805, 1978.
69. Mills J, Pulliam L, Dall L, et al: Exopolysaccharide production by viridans streptococci in experimental endocarditis. Infect Immun 43:359, 1984.
70. Lerner PI, Gopalakrishna KV, Wolinsky E, et al: Group B streptococcus (*S. agalactiae*) bacteremia in adults: analysis of 32 cases and review of the literature. Medicine (Baltimore) 56:457, 1977.
71. Selinger DS, Julie N, Reed WP, Williams RC Jr: Adherence of group A streptococci to pharyngeal cells: a role in the pathogenesis of rheumatic fever. Science 201:455, 1978.
72. Murray HW, Roberts RB: *Streptococcus bovis* bacteremia and underlying gastrointestinal disease. Arch Intern Med 138:1097, 1978.
73. Zarkin BA, Lillemoe KD, Cameron JL, et al: The triad of *Streptococcus bovis* bacteremia, colonic pathology and liver disease. Ann Surg 211(6):786, 1990.
74. Peter G, Smith AL: Group A streptococcal infections of the skin and pharynx, I and II. N Engl J Med 297:311, 365, 1977.
75. Veasy LG, Wiedmeier SE, Orsmond GS, et al: Resurgence of acute rheumatic fever in the intermountain area of the United States. N Engl J Med 361:421, 1987.
76. Wood TF, Potter MA, Jonasson O: Streptococcal toxic shock-like syndrome. The importance of surgical intervention. Ann Surg 217(2):109, 1993.
77. Barter T, Dascal A, Carroll K, Curley FJ: Toxic strep syndrome. Arch Intern Med 148:1421, 1988.
78. Hoge CW, Schwartz B, Talkington DF, et al: The changing epidemiology of invasive group A streptococcal infections and the emergence of streptococcal toxic shock-like syndrome: a retrospective population-based study. JAMA 269:384, 1993.
79. Gallagher PG, Watanakunakorn C: Group B streptococcal bacteremia in a community teaching hospital. Am J Med 78:795, 1985.
80. Auckenthaler R, Hermans PE, Washington JA II: Group G streptococcal bacteremia: clinical study and review of the literature. Rev Infect Dis 5:196, 1983.

81. Lam K, Bayer AS: Serious infections due to group G streptococci: report of 15 cases with in-vitro-in-vivo correlations. Am J Med 75:561, 1983.
82. Libertin CR, Hermans PE, Washington JA: Beta-hemolytic group F streptococcal bacteremia: a study and review of the literature. Rev Infect Dis 7:498, 1985.
83. Baddour LM, Bisno AL: Non-group A beta-hemolytic streptococcal cellulitis: association with venous and lymphatic compromise. Am J Med 79:155, 1985.

Pneumococci

84. Feldman C, Kallenbach JM, Miller SD, et al: Community-acquired pneumonia due to penicillin-resistant pneumococci. N Engl J Med 313:615, 1985.
85. Isolation of multiple antibiotic-resistant pneumococci—New York. MMWR 34:545, 1985.
86. Klugman KP, Koornhof HJ: Drug resistance patterns and serogroups or serotypes of pneumococcal isolates from cerebrospinal fluid or blood, 1979–1986. J Infect Dis 158:956, 1988.
87. Austrian R: The assessment of pneumococcal vaccine. N Engl J Med 303:578, 1980.
88. Musher DM: Infections caused by *Streptococcus pneumoniae:* clinical spectrum, pathogenesis, immunity and treatment. Clin Infect Dis 14:801, 1992.

Gonococci

89. Johnston KH, Holmes KK, Gotschlich EC: The serological classification of *Neisseria gonorrhoeae,* I. Isolation of the outer membrane complex responsible for serotype specificity. J Exp Med 143:741, 1976.
90. Ofek I, Beachey EH, Bisno AL: Resistance of *Neisseria gonorrhoeae* to phagocytosis: relationship to colonial morphology and surface pili. J Infect Dis 129:310, 1974.
91. King GJ, Swanson J: Studies on gonococcus infections, XV. Identification of surface proteins of *Neisseria gonorrhoeae* correlated with leukocyte association. Infect Immun 21:575, 1978.
92. Swanson J: Gonococcal adherence: Selected topics. Rev Infect Dis 5(Suppl):678, 1983.
93. McGee ZA, Stephens DS, Hoffman LH, et al: Mechanisms of mucosal invasion by pathogenic *Neisseria.* Rev Infect Dis 5(Suppl):708, 1983.
94. Payne SM, Finkelstein RA: The critical role of iron in host-bacterial interactions. J Clin Invest 61:1428, 1978.
95. Mulks MH, Plaut AG: IgA protease production as a characteristic distinguishing pathogenic from harmless Neisseriaceae. N Engl J Med 299:973, 1978.
96. Tramont EC: Inhibition of adherence of *Neisseria gonorrhoeae* by human genital secretions. J Clin Invest 59:117, 1977.
97. Hook EW III, Holmes KK: Gonococcal infections. Ann Intern Med 102:229, 1985.
98. O'Brien JP, Goldenberg DL, Rice PA: Disseminated gonococcal infection: a prospective analysis of 49 patients and a review of pathophysiology and immune mechanisms. Medicine (Baltimore) 62:395, 1983.
99. Sparling PF, Holmes KK, Wiesner PJ, Puziss M: Summary of the conference of the problem of penicillin-resistant gonococci. J Infect Dis 135:865, 1977.
100. Guidelines for treatment of sexually transmitted diseases. MMWR 38(S8):1, 1989.

BIBLIOGRAPHY

Brittigan BE, Cohen MS, Sparling PF: Gonococcal infection: a model of molecular pathogenesis. N Engl J Med 312:1683, 1985.

Feldman HA: Meningococcal infections. Adv Intern Med 18:177, 1972.

Jeljaszewicz J (ed): Proceedings of the 3rd International Symposium on Staphylococci and Staphylococcal Infections. New York, Springer-Verlag, 1976.

Kreig NK, Holt JG (eds): Bergey's Manual of Determinative Bacteriology. Baltimore, Williams & Wilkins, 1984.

Manjo G: The Healing Hand: Man and Wound in the Ancient World. Cambridge, MA, Harvard University Press, 1975.

Parker MT (ed): The Pathogenic Streptococci. Chertsey, Surrey, Reedbooks, 1980.

Patterson MJ, Hafeez A: Group B streptococci in human disease. Bacteriol Rev 40:774, 1976.

Sparling PF, Lee TJ: Gonorrhea: new insights and problems. In Weinstein L, Field BN (eds): Seminars in Infectious Disease, Vol 1. New York, Stratton Intercontinental Medical Book Corporation, 1978, p 34.

Enteric Gram-Negative Bacteria and Pseudomonads

CHAPTER 5

William J. Martin, Lowell S. Young

Once considered saprophytes of limited virulence, the gram-negative bacilli along with the staphylococci and the enterococci now comprise the single greatest infection hazard in hospitalized patients.[1–3] The principal reason for this shift has been the fact that debilitated individuals, who in another era would have been considered unacceptable for surgery, now qualify for a variety of surgical procedures. Gram-negative bacilli are true pathogens in such hosts.

Although the gram-negative bacilli have frequently been viewed as a single group of potential pathogens, important taxonomic differences do exist, even among members of the family Enterobacteriaceae. The microorganisms described in this chapter are currently included in two large families of gram-negative bacilli: Enterobacteriaceae and Pseudomonadaceae. However, because of the frequent appearance of *Pseudomonas* and a variety of nonenteric bacilli in surgical infections and because of their presence in "mixed infections" including enteric gram-negative organisms, it seems appropriate to discuss the bacteriology and basic clinical syndromes associated with these organisms. The Enterobacteriaceae account for approximately 80 percent and the nonfermenters, which includes the pseudomonads, account for an additional 12 percent of the aerobic or facultative gram-negative bacilli isolated in all clinical specimens.[4]

Table 5–1 is an attempt to group aerobic or facultative gram-negative bacilli by their order of clinical importance. Some of these organisms of lesser surgical significance are discussed in Chapter 9.

MICROBIOLOGIC ASPECTS OF GRAM-NEGATIVE BACILLI

Basic Structure of the Gram-Negative Bacillary Organisms

Aerobic gram-negative bacilli of clinical importance are non–spore-forming organisms that fail to take the Gram stain, may or may not be motile, and have certain structural or cell wall constituents that underlie this tinctorial property. Bacterial nomenclature is a constantly changing field (see Table 5–1), and recognition that organisms previously grouped on the basis of biochemical and antigenic properties may in fact not be closely related. In recent years, however, nucleic acid hybridization techniques have provided a powerful tool that better defines the evolutionary relationships of all organisms.[5] Indeed, it is the application of this technology along with the author's knowledge of how it is to be used that forms the current nomenclature and classification system employed by the Centers for Disease Control and Prevention (CDC) and used in this chapter.

TABLE 5–1. AEROBIC AND FACULTATIVE GRAM-NEGATIVE BACTERIA OF SURGICAL SIGNIFICANCE

Important	Occasionally Important	Rarely Significant
Enterobacteriaceae	Enterobacteriaceae	
Escherichia coli	*Citrobacter*	*Achromobacter*
Enterobacter	*Edwardsiella*	*Alcaligenes*
Klebsiella	*Providencia*	*Flavobacterium*
Proteus	*Salmonella*	*Moraxella*
Serratia	*Shigella*	*Eikenella*
	Yersinia	*Kingella*
	Acinetobacter calcoaceticus	
Pseudomonas aeruginosa	*Acinetobacter lwoffi*	
	Aeromonas	
	Legionella	
	Pasteurella	
	Pseudomonas, not *aeruginosa*	
	Vibrio	
	Xanthomonas maltophilia	

The basic cell wall structure of clinically significant gram-negative bacilli includes most of the components that are illustrated in Figure 5–1. Many organisms, such as *Klebsiella pneumoniae* and *Escherichia coli,* are encapsulated with a polysaccharide-containing material. Designation for this encapsulated material is K, or capsular antigen, but other synonymous terms have been the Vi antigen of *Salmonella typhi* and the serotype antigen of *K. pneumoniae.* The acidic, negatively charged, structural capsule may allow the organisms to resist phagocytosis and can be an important virulence factor. Penetrating through the outer capsule of motile organisms is a relatively large proteinaceous whip-like structure called flagellum (flagella, plural), which carries the H antigen. Motility may be an important microbial factor involved in pathogenesis of infections such as occur in the urinary tract, which are usually ascending infections. Localized surface structures called pili or fimbriae that protrude from the capsule or outer cell wall facilitate attachment of infecting microbes to the mucosa of alimentary, respiratory, or genitourinary tracts. Pili-mediated ability to attach to surfaces is probably important in the initial interaction between parasite and host.

Much attention has been focused on the somatic heat-stable cell wall antigens, the so-called O antigens of gram-negative bacilli. Other synonyms for these structures are lipopolysaccharide or endotoxin. Most gram-negative bacilli contain endotoxins, the material left (both structurally and in terms of biologic activity) after cell wall structures are boiled for 30 to 60 minutes. When these endotoxins are injected, they elicit fever, leukopenia followed by leukocytosis, and, if given in sufficient quantities, hemodynamic instability leading to shock and death.

The structure of bacterial endotoxins has been elucidated in the past 15 years. Lipopolysaccharide

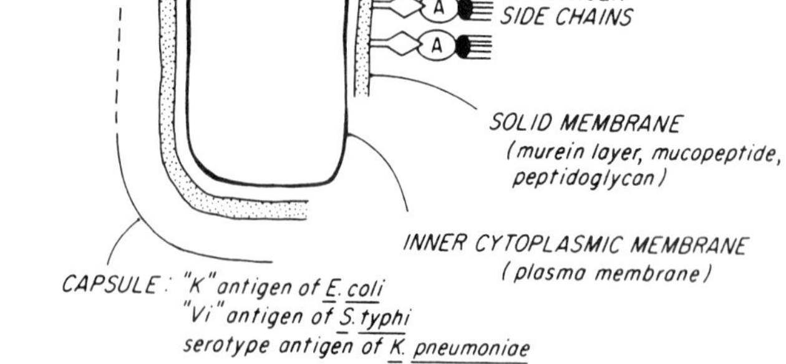

Figure 5–1. The major cell wall antigens of the gram-negative bacillus. Some are flagellated (H antigen) and may have capsules (K antigen). The O, or heat-stable, somatic antigen is part of the outer of three membranes and contains lipid A, which is responsible for endotoxicity. *(From Young LS, Martin WJ, Meyer RD, et al: Ann Intern Med 86:456, 1977, with permission of the publishers.)*

derived from strains of organisms that are usually isolated from urinary tract infections or bloodstream invasion has three regions or layers:

1. The *outer membrane* contains O-specific lipopolysaccharides, that is, repetitive units of specific sugars that convey the serologic specificity of an organism. Thus the familiar O agglutination pattern reported from *Salmonella* and *E. coli* reflects the ability of specific antiserum to agglutinate these organisms in high dilution. The O-specific lipopolysaccharide in turn is linked to a core region, which consists of common repetitive sugars linked to an inner core comprised of ketodeoxyoctonate linked to lipid A. Lipid A appears to be a "toxic" component of the lipopolysaccharide structure.[6] Minute quantities of endotoxin cause gelation in vitro of an extract from the horseshoe crab, *Limulus polyphemus.* However, the limulus assay has not proved to be a clinically useful bioassay for detecting circulating endotoxemia.[7] The structure of the core glycolipid is widely shared among gram-negative bacteria; antibodies to it are broadly cross-reactive. Since the lipid A appears to be responsible for all the toxic biologic properties of lipopolysaccharide, it is possible that vaccines or antisera could be developed to protect against many types of gram-negative bacillary infections (see "Immunity Against Gram-Negative Bacilli," p. 68). One reservation about this approach, however, is that other determinants more peripheral to the cell wall membrane may obscure or protect the core, so that antibodies directed against core regions may not have direct access to neutralize the toxic effects of lipopolysaccharides.

   O-antigenic structures and capsular antigens may further enhance resistance to phagocytosis as well as to the bactericidal activity of serum complement plus circulating antibodies. The so-called outer membrane portion of the gram-negative bacillary wall thus contains capsules (for encapsulated organisms), lipopolysaccharide, and protein constituents.
2. The *intermediate layer* is composed of murein or mucopeptide, and it is at this structure that beta-lactam agents (penicillins, cephalosporins) exert their effect in disrupting cell wall synthesis.
3. The inner cell wall membrane, or *cytoplasmic membrane,* is the truly limiting structure in the presence of beta-lactam antibiotics; organisms exposed to penicillin-type agents tend to swell up and form spheroplasts that are osmotically fragile.

Cell wall structures of gram-negative bacilli appear to be related to some properties of invasiveness, but extra-cellular products such as tissue-destroying proteolytic enzymes and exoenzymes can also function as virulence factors.

For example, exotoxins from enteropathogenic *E. coli* are most responsible for the production of diarrhea in a manner analogous to cholera toxin. Most clinical isolates of *P. aeruginosa* produce both proteolytic enzymes and at least one exotoxin. Exotoxin A, the best characterized of these *Pseudomonas* toxins, is a potent inhibitor of protein synthesis, similar to diphtheria toxin. Just as antibodies directed against capsular and outer membrane components (O-specific lipopolysaccharide, core glycolipid) can protect against the sequelae of shock and death complicating bacteremic infections,[8–10] antibodies directed against toxins such as exotoxin A are also protective.[11]

Taxonomy and Nomenclature

Family Enterobacteriaceae. The best known and most easily recognized of the gram-negative facultative bacilli (ie, bacilli that grow aerobically and under conditions of increased CO_2) are the bacteria that currently make up the family Enterobacteriaceae. In 1972 there were 11 genera and 26 species in the family Enterobacteriaceae,[12] whereas in 1984 there were 22 genera, 69 species, and 29 biogroups or enteric groups.[13] Members of this family are usually motile, although the *Shigella* and *Klebsiella* are nonmotile. The motile species possess peritrichous flagella, differing from members of the family Pseudomonadaceae, which have polar flagella. Several strains of *Salmonella, Shigella, Escherichia, Klebsiella, Enterobacter,* and *Proteus* possess fimbriae or pili.

All species of enteric bacilli ferment D-glucose. Aerogenic (ie, gas-producing) and anaerogenic forms are found. The absence of gas in the fermentation of carbohydrates is characteristic of some genera. Nitrates are reduced to nitrites and are catalase positive. Indophenol-oxidase is not produced.

The family is composed of a large and diverse group of organisms varying in antigenic structure and biochemical properties. The genera within the

TABLE 5–2. CURRENT CDC CLASSIFICATION OF THE ENTEROBACTERIACEAE

Budvicia aquatica[a]
Buttiauxella agretis
Cedecea davisae[a]
- *C. lapagei*[a]
- *C. neteri*[a]
- *Cedecea* species 3[a]
- *Cedecea* species 5[a]

Citrobacter freundii[a]
- *C. diversus*[a]
- *C. amalonaticus*[a]
- *C. amalonaticus* biogroup 1[a]

Edwardsiella tarda[a]
- *E. tarda* biogroup 1[a]
- *E. hoshinae*[a]
- *E. iotaluri*

Enterobacter aerogenes[a]
- *E. cloacae*[a]
- *E. agglomerans*[a]
- *E. gergoviae*[a]
- *E. sakazakii*[a]
- *E. taylorae*[a]
- *E. amnigenus* biogroup 1[a]
- *E. amnigenus* biogroup 2
- *E. intermedium*
- *E. asburiae*[a]
- *E. cancerogenous*
- *E. dissolvens*
- *E. nimipressuralis*

Obesumbacterium proteus biogroup 2
Pragia fontium
Proteus mirabilis[a]
- *P. vulgaris*[a]
- *P. penneri*[a]
- *P. myxofaciens*

Providencia rettgeri[a]
- *P. stuartii*[a]
- *P. acalifaciens*[a]
- *P. rustigianii*[a]
- *P. heimbachae*

Rahnella aquatilis[a]
Salmonella
- Subgroup 1 strains
  - Most serotypes[a]
  - *S. typhi*[a]
  - *S. choleraesuis*[a]
  - *S. paratyphi* A[a]
  - *S. gallinarum*[a]
  - *S. pulloram*[a]
- Subgroup 2 strains[a]
- Subgroup 3a strains (arizona)[a]
- Subgroup 4 strains[a]
- Subgroup 5 strains[a]
- Subgroup 6 strains[a]

Serratia marcescens[a]
- *S. marcescens biogroup 1*[a]
- *S. liquefaciens* group[a]

family have been established mainly on the basis of biochemical characteristics. Original species designations are still widely used and were established by both biochemical and ecologic criteria. The antigenic complexity of these bacteria has led to the development of antigenic schemes, patterned after the Kauffmann-White scheme for *Salmonella,* in which numerous serotypes based on O and H antigen typing were derived. Many of these serotypes are biochemically similar and can be distinguished only by serologic procedures.[12]

Although the classification system of Edwards and Ewing[12] has had the greatest impact on clinical microbiologists and infectious disease physicians in this hemisphere, the most recent classification and nomenclature of these organisms are shown in Table 5–2. These changes are currently being used by the CDC[14] and consist of 26 genera, 93 species, and 19 biogroups or enteric groups. A variety of taxonomic criteria were used and included the use of antibiotic susceptibility patterns, species- or gene-specific bacteriophages, computer analyses, sophisticated biochemical and immunochemical patterns, and, most importantly, nucleic acid hybridization techniques.[5] The reader should understand that the dynamics of any classification system is undergoing constant change and, although confusing to some, an attempt should be made to try to define all microorganisms so that they have the same meaning for all.

Family Pseudomonadaceae. The family Pseudomonadaceae currently consists of four genera: *Pseudomonas, Xanthomonas, Frateuria,* and *Zoogloea.*[15] The genus *Pseudomonas* is widely distributed in nature. Some species are pathogenic for humans, others for animals or plants; gram negative and rarely nonmotile, they are motile by one or more polar flagella. The type species *P. aeruginosa* is a polar monotrichous, gram-negative rod occurring singly, in pairs, or in short chains. On blood agar the organism grows as a large, flat colony with a ground-glass appearance and produces a zone of hemolysis. In patients with cystic fibrosis, mucoid strains are frequently isolated from the sputum. The colonies tend to spread and give off a character-

TABLE 5–2. (continued)

Escherichia-Shigella	*S. oderifera* biogroup 1[a]
E. coli[a]	*S. odifera* biogroup 2[a]
E. coli inactive[a]	*S. plymuthica*[a]
Shigella, O groups A, B, C[a]	*S. ficaria*[a]
S. sonnei[a]	*S. entomophila*
Escherichia fergusonii[a]	*"Serratia" fonticola*[a]
E. hermannii[a]	*Tatumella ptyseos*[a]
E. vulnaeris[a]	*Yersinia enterocolitica*[a]
E. blattae	*Y. frederiksenii*[a]
Ewingella americana[a]	*Y. intermedia*[a]
Hafnia alvei[a]	*Y. kristensenii*[a]
H. alvei biogroup 1	*Y. rohdei*[a]
Klebsiella pneumoniae[a]	*Y. pestis*[a]
K. oxytoca[a]	*Y. pseudotuberculosis*[a]
K. ornithinolytica[a]	*Y. aldovae*
K. planticola[a]	*Y. bercoveiri*[a]
K. ozaenae[a]	*Y. mollaretii*[a]
K. rhinoscleromatis[a]	*"Yersinia" ruckeri*[a]
K. terrigena	*Xenorhabdus luminescens* (25C)
Kluyvera ascorbata[a]	*X. luminescens* DNA group 5[a]
K. cryocrescens[a]	*X. nematophilus* (25C)
Koserella trabulsii[a]	Enteric group 58[a]
Leclercia adecarboxylata[a]	Enteric group 59[a]
Leminorella grimontii[a]	Enteric group 60[a]
L. richardii[a]	Enteric group 63
Moellerella wisconsensis[a]	Enteric group 64
Morganella morganii[a]	Enteric group 68[a]
M. morganii biogroup 1[a]	Enteric group 69
S. rubidaea[a]	Enteric group 90

[a] Occurs in clinical specimens.

Adapted from Farmer JJ III, Kelly MT: Enterobacteriaceae. In Balows A, Hausler WT Jr, Herrmann KL, et al (eds): Manual of Clinical Microbiology, 5th ed. Washington, DC, ASM, 1991, p 360.

istic grape-like odor. Most strains excrete pyocyanin and fluorescein (pyoverdin), giving the colony a characteristic blue-green color; approximately 4 percent are apyocyanogenic.

Identification

Lactose-Fermenting Members of Enterobacteriaceae. A large number of organisms within the family Enterobacteriaceae ferment lactose and can tentatively be identified by the reactions shown in Figure 5–2 and in triple sugar iron (TSI) agar as seen in Table 5–3. Some lactose-positive species exhibit a delayed reaction, and the vast majority of the clinically important isolates fall into one of these categories. The lactose reaction can provide important information in the bacteriologic evaluation of a gram-negative rod. For example, clinicians should know that the lactose-positive organisms—*E. coli* and *Klebsiella*—tend to be more susceptible to antimicrobial agents like one of the cephalosporins and chloramphenicol, whereas organisms that do not or slowly ferment lactose—*Pseudomonas, Serratia, Enterobacter,* indole-positive *Proteus*—often require therapy with potentially toxic agents like aminoglycosides.

The classic IMViC [indole, methyl red, Voges-Proskauer, and citrate (the "i" is inserted for euphony)] reaction is used primarily to distinguish between the coliform bacteria but may also be applied advantageously to other organisms in the family. Again, final identification must depend on an extended profile of biochemical tests.

A large number of rapid methods using a battery of test substrates designed to reduce the amount of time for identifying members of the En-

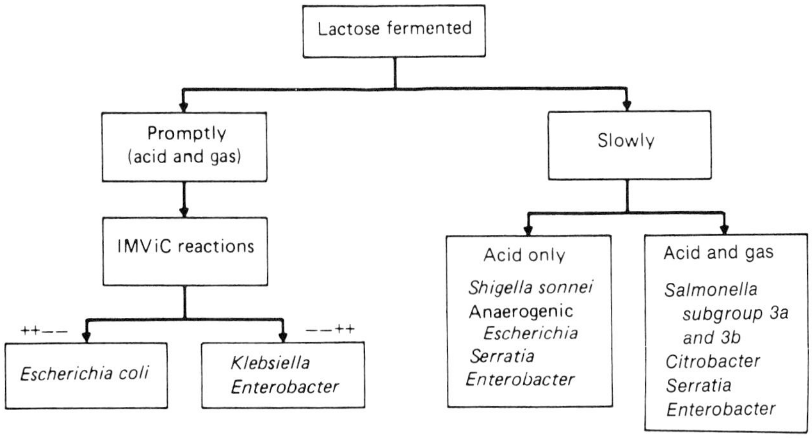

Figure 5–2. Immediate screening and tentative identification of Enterobacteriaceae by lactose, IMViC, and triple sugar iron (TSI) reactions.

terobacteriaceae as well as other gram-negative bacilli have been developed commercially. Many of these systems have been rated as good, with an accuracy correlation ranging from 87 to 96 percent or higher depending on the number and variety of cultures tested. A large number of these rapid test systems are in common use today in most laboratories.

IMMUNITY AGAINST GRAM-NEGATIVE BACILLI

Host defenses against infection are extensively covered in Chapter 12 and in other reviews.[9,16,17] Only a brief summary will be made of the mechanisms that appear to prevent normal individuals from developing systemic enterobacillary infection.

Many individuals have circulating antibodies against disease-causing organisms without history of disease.[18] Natural antibodies probably result from gastrointestinal colonization or inapparent infection. Another possibility is that these antibodies developed after exposure to avirulent organisms that share antigens with disease-causing microbes. Cross-reactions between cell wall components of pneumococci and gram-negative organisms like *E. coli* and *Klebsiella* have been described.[19]

The obvious risk of gram-negative bacillary infection, particularly *P. aeruginosa* infection in the neutropenic patient, attests to the critical role of neutrophils in the defense against systemic invasion by gram-negative rods; monocytes appear to be less active and efficient phagocytes for encapsulated bacteria. For neutrophils to function optimally, opsonic support through the complement and antibody systems is required.[17,20] The antibodies are of the IgG and IgM class and are heat stable, but IgM requires complement in order to act as an opsonin. IgA is the primary antibody of the mucosal surfaces, and both IgA and IgG have been implicated in blocking the attachment of microbes to mucosal surfaces. Diseases such as acquired or native hypogammaglobulinemia are clearly associated with increased susceptibility to infection, and the prospect for survival from bacteremic gram-negative bacillary infections even in patients with normal levels of phagocytic cells but decreased antibody levels has been shown to be poor.[10] Thus neither an adequate antibody level nor an adequate number of circulating phagocytes (usually a neutrophil count in excess of 1000) by itself is sufficient for adequate defenses against disease-causing pyogenic organisms.

From a therapeutic standpoint granulocyte transfusions have given way to use of colony-stimulating factors to raise the peripheral neutrophil count in neutropenic patients.[22] Use of antisera, either in the form of pooled human gamma globulin

TABLE 5–3. REACTIONS OBSERVED IN TSI AGAR

Reactions	Explanation	Examples
Acid butt (yellow), alkaline slant (red)	Glucose fermented	*Shigella*
Acid throughout medium, butt and slant yellow	Lactose or sucrose or both fermented	*Escherichia coli*
Gas bubbles in butt, medium sometimes split	Aerogenic culture	*Enterobacter* species
Blackening in the butt	Hydrogen sulfide produced	Most *Salmonella* species
Alkaline slant and butt (medium entirely red)	None of the three sugars fermented	*Pseudomonas*

(IgG)[23,24] or monoclonal antibodies (IgM), that react with lipid A is more controversial. Despite some encouraging clinical trials,[25,26] reservations about the clinical benefits of such immunotherapy have been raised.[27] Additional supportive human clinical trials of immunotherapy will be necessary before endotoxin-reactive monoclonal antibodies are licensed and available for general use.

Cell-mediated immunity does not appear to have a major role in defenses against gram-negative bacillary organisms, although some diseases characterized by depressed cell-mediated immunity have been associated with parallel deficiencies in humoral defenses and phagocytic cell function.

IMPORTANT ENTEROBACTERIACEAE

The epidemiology of infections with these organisms is of the utmost importance in current hospital practice.[28,29] Chapter 26 is devoted to nosocomial problems.

Escherichia Coli

Escherichia coli is a motile, flagellated, usually piliated bacillus, whose biochemical characteristics have been well described.[4,6] It is the most common facultative aerobic gram-negative bacillus in the gastrointestinal tract and in biliary and mixed intra-abdominal infections associated with perforations of the gastrointestinal tract. The ascending course of these organisms from feces to urethra, ureter, kidney, and ultimately to blood is thought to account for their predominance as a cause of both urinary tract infections and bacteremia.

These organisms can also be an important cause of gram-negative pneumonia.[30,31] Wound infections, osteomyelitis, and meningitis appear to develop either as a result of direct extension of infection from a primarily infected site or on a bacteremic basis. *Escherichia coli* is also an important cause of diarrhea.

Diarrhea-producing strains of *E. coli* attach more readily (adhere) to gastrointestinal mucosal surfaces through their piliated surface structures. Once they are adherent, there appear to be four mechanisms for the pathogenesis of diarrhea: (1) enteroinvasive or local invasion (mucosal penetration) in a manner akin to invasiveness of *Shigella* species; (2) enterotoxigenic strains that trigger intestinal secretions by one of several heat-labile or heat-stable extracellular toxins in a manner analogous to cholera (the diarrhea-producing characteristics seem linked to a plasmid that contains chromosomal material coding for the production of the exotoxin); (3) enteropathic *E. coli* consisting of specific serotypes that historically have been associated with outbreaks of infantile diarrhea but possess pathogenic mechanisms not related to any of these; and (4) strains associated with hemorrhagic colitis (enterohemorrhagic), namely, *E. coli* 0157:H7, that produce one or more serotoxins and have been detected in most outbreaks of infection linked to consumption of undercooked beef.[32]

Several methods are now available for epidemiologic studies of *E. coli* infections. These include tracing of biologic properties of the organism (enzyme production and utilization of certain substrates are the basis for so-called biotyping schema) and the more classic identification of cell wall surface structures by agglutination reactions using O, K, and H antigens. Techniques such as electrophoresis, agglutination, and immunodiffusion have been used.[33] The ability to type *E. coli* by agglutination reactions or related methods may be of value in certain epidemiologic situations, such as an outbreak of nosocomial infections or the identification of the cause of infectious diarrhea.

Fortunately, *E. coli* are usually sensitive to a wide variety of antimicrobial agents including the tetracyclines, chloramphenicol, the broad spectrum penicillins, cephalosporins, the aminoglycosides, and trimethoprim-sulfamethoxazole. For uncomplicated urinary tract infections, sulfonamides will suffice, and the efficacy of bacteriostatic agents like tetracyclines and chloramphenicol is as good as with bactericidal agents if the organisms are susceptible in vitro. Chloramphenicol's superior distribution into fatty tissues and into the central nervous system places it at a singular advantage in infections occurring in the central nervous system and possibly in the lung. The latter infections, however, should be severe before this agent is used. For neutropenic patients the use of bactericidal agents is to be preferred, particularly the pairing of one of the beta-lactam (ampicillin or cephalosporin) agents with an aminoglycoside to achieve a bactericidal and possibly synergistic effect.[34]

Klebsiella, Enterobacter, Serratia

Organisms belonging to this group of enteric organisms are important causes of surgical infections associated with the biliary tree and the perforations of the gastrointestinal tract. Originally, the serotypes described by Friedlander, *K. pneumoniae* A through F (now redesignated 1 through 6), were recognized as the etiologic agents of a life-threatening, gram-negative pneumonia afflicting alcoholics. Today we realize that this particular type of pneumonitis is not unique to the lower-numbered serotypes of *Klebsiella*. In fact, *Klebsiella, Enterobacter,* and *Serratia* can all be important causes of pneumonia as well as urinary tract infections.

Klebsiella *Species*. Within the genus *Klebsiella,* seven species have been recognized and include *K. pneumoniae, K. ozaenae, K. rhinoscleromatis, K. oxytoca, K. planticola, K. ornithinolytica,* and *K. terrigena* (see Table 5–2). Approximately 95 percent of the clinical isolates encountered in the laboratory are *K. pneumoniae.* The indole-positive species *K. oxytoca* makes up the majority of the remaining 5 percent. These organisms are usually encapsulated and often produce large mucoid colonies on agar. Of the *Klebsiella* types, approximately 80 have been identified by their specific agglutination patterns. Strains of *K. ozaenae* usually belong to type 4, 5, or 6, and strains of *K. rhinoscleromatis* to type 3. Clinical isolates of *K. planticola, K. terrigena,* and *K. ornithinolytica* are extremely uncommon.[14]

Patients who develop community-acquired (ie, nonnosocomial) *Klebsiella* pneumonia are often afflicted with a disease such as alcoholism. In the classic radiologic description this infection was found to involve the upper lobes. Sputum has been described as both bloody and mucoid, and the consolidated parenchyma of the involved lobe may be "bowed" or bulging as the fissure is demarcated by x-ray. Nonetheless, these features are not a reliable basis for distinguishing *K. pneumoniae* infection from other bacterial or even fungal pneumonias. Histopathologically, *Klebsiella* pneumonitis is a necrotizing process characterized by destruction of alveolar septate linings and occasional cavitation.

Klebsiella pneumoniae accounts for up to 10 percent of all hospital-acquired infections. Urinary tract infections are most common, followed by lower respiratory tract and wound infections. Increased risk of infection has been associated with Foley catheterization and endotracheal intubation. Multi drug-resistant strains of *Klebsiella* have become endemic in a number of institutions.

Klebsiella rhinoscleromatis is a cause of scleroma, a chronic granulomatous process of the nasal mucosa, paranasal sinuses, pharynx, larynx, middle ear, and the respiratory epithelium down to the bronchi.[35] Histologically, there is evidence of necrosis and fibrosis. Large foamy cells containing rod-shaped, gram-negative organisms (Mikulicz cells) can be seen. This invasive growth, which can invade bone and result in the destruction of respiratory passages, has been mistaken for a neoplastic process or a mycobacterial disease. The disease is endemic in Eastern Europe (Slavic leprosy), but the organism is actually of low infectivity and appears to spread by close and prolonged exposure between afflicted persons. Antimicrobial treatment of scleroma must be combined with surgical excision for optimum benefit.

Klebsiella ozaenae has been isolated from patients with a chronic atrophic rhinitis called ozaena. Histopathologically, there is loss of mucosal architecture; clinically, there is a chronic production of a foul-smelling discharge. In contrast to scleroma, ozaena is not believed to be a primary bacterial process and may have multiple causes, with other gram-negative organisms acting as copathogens. This organism could also be an opportunistic secondary invader of damaged nasal mucosa. Many patients in technologically advanced societies have the isolates recovered from sputum or bronchoalveolar lavage. This organism is generally not a pathogen but can cause pneumonia or other deep-seated infection.

As a group, organisms belonging to the genus *Klebsiella* are susceptible to cephalosporins, chloramphenicol, tetracyclines, the aminoglycosides, polymyxins, and trimethoprim-sulfamethoxazole. Also it has been recognized by some investigators that *K. oxytoca* is somewhat more susceptible to many of these agents than is *K. pneumoniae.* The important factor is that except for *K. ozaenae, Klebsiella* species are usually resistant to ampicillin, carbenicillin, and ticarcillin; when these drugs are used in systemic therapy for *Pseudomonas* and *Serratia, Klebsiella* species, which may coexist, are not likely to be eradicated.

Enterobacter *Species*. The genus *Enterobacter* currently includes 13 species, of which *E. aerogenes, E. cloacae,* and, to a lesser extent, *E. agglomerans* are perhaps the most important. In contrast to *Klebsiella, Enterobacter* species rarely cause primary infection alone but are often isolated in combination with *E. coli* or *Klebsiella* from biliary or intraperitoneal infections and from the sputum, urine, or wound drainage from hospitalized patients. In intensive care units, *Enterobacter* and *Serratia* species have been a particularly vexing cause of cross-infection in patients who have indwelling urethral catheters, endotracheal tubes, or tracheostomies. Outbreaks of septicemia have also been implicated with contaminated parenteral fluids or with indwelling venous catheters.[29]

Serratia *Species*. Members of the genus *Serratia* have been recognized as significant human pathogens only within the last 25 years and currently include nine species and one biogroup.[14,36] Of these lactose-negative, gram-negative organisms, *S. marcescens, S. liquefaciens,* and *S. rubidaea* are considered the most important clinically. *Serratia marcescens* has been particularly implicated in the following types of nosocomial infections: (1) bacteremia linked to indwelling intravenous or intraperitoneal catheters or to instrumentation of the genitourinary tract and (2) pneumonia associated with contaminated inhalation therapy equipment. Both *S. marcescens* (mainly) and *Pseudomonas aeruginosa* are often superinfecting pathogens that affect patients initially receiving such broad spectrum antimicrobials as the cephalosporins, ampicillin, and the tetracyclines. Septic arthritis caused by *Serratia* organisms occasionally occurs and may be introduced into joints after aspiration or injection of medication or as a result of bacteremia. *Serratia marcescens* may be a common infecting organism in heroin addicts. Of the newly described species, *S. entomophila* has not been isolated from human specimen material.[14]

Serratia organisms tend to be highly resistant to penicillin G, ampicillin, and polymyxins. The agents of choice are aminoglycosides (gentamicin or amikacin), high concentrations of the extended spectrum penicillins like carbenicillin or ticarcillin, and the combination of trimethoprim and sulfamethoxazole. New cephalosporins (eg, "third generation" compounds) are generally quite active in vitro, but quite rapid emergence of resistance may be observed in a clinical setting. This phenomenon of resistance is probably related to inducible beta-lactamases, which may also be detected in strains of *Enterobacter, Citrobacter,* and *Pseudomonas* species.[37] Chloramphenicol may be active but should probably be considered after the other agents have failed.

Proteus, Providencia, Morganella

Four species are currently assigned to the genus *Proteus—vulgaris, mirabilis, penneri,* and *myxofaciens*—and five species to the genus *Providencia* as well—*alcalifaciens, rettgeri, stuartii, rustigianii,* and *heimbachae.* Both of these genera and *Morganella morganii* are gram-negative, motile, pleomorphic rods. Typically, they are lactose negative and are distinguished from other enteric bacilli by having the enzyme phenylalanine deaminase. One of the most typical microbiologic properties of *P. mirabilis* and *P. vulgaris* is their ability to swarm on moist agar media. Discrete colonies are surrounded by a thin bluish-gray, confluent surface growth that occurs over a wide temperature range and complicates the isolation of other organisms present in mixed culture.

These organisms are generally not carried in the stools of healthy individuals but can be found in patients receiving oral antimicrobial therapy. The most common site of infections with many of these organisms is the urinary tract, but it is a frequent isolate in mixed infections related to gastrointestinal perforations and has been implicated in bacteremic infections, wound infections, pulmonary infections, and brain abscesses.

Proteus mirabilis is the most common strain encountered clinically and may cause 10 percent of all urinary tract infections. It often represents an even larger proportion of organisms causing hospital-acquired urinary tract infections. Several properties appear to underlie the pathogenicity of these genera for the urinary tract. Because many strains are urease producers, these organisms are able to split urea and form ammonium hydroxide. The shift in urinary pH to a markedly alkaline range potentiates the formation of stones. Stones may account for the chronicity or recurrence of urinary tract infections as a result of one or more species of these bacteria because they act as a foreign body, and organisms remaining viable in the stony matrix could be protected from the effects of antimicrobial therapy. Another factor that contributes to the uropathogenicity of these strains is that many, if not all, of these organisms are piliated and can attach to urothelium.[38]

One of the most noteworthy clinical microbiologic aspects of infections due to this group of bacteria is the differing antimicrobial susceptibility of the indole-positive versus indole-negative strains. *Proteus mirabilis,* the indole-negative species and also the best known species, is usually susceptible to high concentrations of penicillin G, although most clinicians tend to use ampicillin, amoxacillin, or a cephalosporin. This species is usually susceptible to other agents as well, including tetracyclines, chloramphenicol, and the aminoglycosides. On the other hand, the indole-positive and less common strains—*P. vulgaris, P. rettgeri, P. stuartii,* and *M. morganii*—can be quite antibiotic resistant and are best treated with the aminoglycosides, trimethoprim-sulfamethoxazole, and third-generation cephalosporins. Some of the most resistant gram-negative organisms now encountered in the hospital, and of particular concern because some are aminoglycoside resistant, belong to *P. rettgeri* and *P. vulgaris* species.

Proteus stuartii has been implicated as a serious cause of complicated nosocomial urinary tract infections and in life-threatening infections occurring in burn units. *Proteus stuartii* is highly resistant to a number of conventionally used antimicrobial agents such as ampicillin, cephalosporins, and chloramphenicol, and it usually requires aminoglycoside therapy. However, even in this group a number of organisms are gentamicin resistant and may require therapy with amikacin.

OCCASIONALLY IMPORTANT ENTERIC ORGANISMS

Salmonella and *Shigella*

Salmonella and *Shigella* are the classic gram-negative enteric pathogens associated with abdominal pain and diarrheal syndromes. Both groups of organisms contain many important species and serotypes, and the clinical manifestations can be protean. Perhaps the greatest concern to practicing surgeons is the likelihood that acute salmonellosis or shigellosis can mimic an acute surgical abdomen. Table 5–4 is an attempt to summarize some of the bacterial pathogens, including *Salmonella* and *Shigella,* which might cause a clinical picture leading to surgical intervention. It is not clear whether surgical intervention should be discouraged (see discussion on yersiniosis); in fact it might be encouraged even if the infection turns out to be amenable to antibiotic treatment alone.

Diarrhea is not a necessary clinical manifestation of either disease. In the early stages of classic typhoid, for instance, constipation or even intestinal obstruction may be the major clinical finding. This paradoxical observation has often been a stumbling block to the correct perception of the underlying diagnosis. Furthermore, *S. typhi* is classically associated with biliary tract disease and can on occasion mimic acute cholecystitis; chronic carriage of typhoid bacilli is more commonly associated with biliary stones, and cure of typhoid carriers may require cholecystectomy.

TABLE 5–4. GRAM-NEGATIVE BACILLARY INFECTIONS WITH SYMPTOMS THAT CAN BE CONFUSED WITH ACUTE SURGICAL ABDOMEN

Enterobacteriaceae
- *Salmonella* species
- *Shigella* species
- *E. coli* (enteropathogenic, enterohemorrhagic, enteroinvasive, enterotoxigenic)
- *Yersinia* species

Campylobacter
Vibrio cholerae
Vibrio parahaemolyticus
Vibrio vulnificus
Rarely: *Citrobacter, Edwardsiella, P. aeruginosa, Klebsiella, Aeromonas*

Shigella. Shigellosis appears to cause a diarrheal syndrome either on the basis of local invasion of the gastrointestinal mucosa or the elaboration of a diarrhea-producing exotoxin. Its hallmark is a fairly short incubation period (average 2 days), fever, crampy abdominal pain, and a diarrheal product characterized by both blood and mucus. Abdominal tenderness is usually general, and the abdominal wall is not rigid. Sigmoidoscopy can reveal hyperemia, small bleeding sites, and purulent mucus secretions, and Gram stain or methylene blue stain of feces reveals myriad fecal leukocytes (the latter being a helpful sign of intestinal shigellosis as opposed to other diarrheal entities).

Salmonella. Salmonellosis has innumerable animal reservoirs, and most people acquire the infection from environmental or food-borne sources. The mechanism of the diarrhea is unknown, and the disease is usually self-limited and requires only symptomatic treatment. Acute food poisoning (ie, *Salmonella* enterocolitis) is characterized by short incubation periods (18 to 72 hours), nausea, vomiting, colicky abdominal pain, and rapid onset of diarrhea. The finding of mucus and blood in the stool is less common than it is in shigellosis. Occasionally, severe abdominal tenderness even with rebound occurs, which can be confused with acute appendicitis or acute cholecystitis. Usually, however, the disease subsides within 5 days.

Of particular interest are the extraintestinal manifestations of salmonellosis. Although relatively few individuals are found to be bacteremic, organisms may cause arthritis, acute pericarditis, and appendicitis and have been found to colonize aortic aneurysms, causing primary peritonitis, pyelonephritis, and osteomyelitis. An increased susceptibility to *Salmonella* infections has been classically associated with asplenia such as occurs during the natural history of sickle cell anemia. There is a striking tendency of *Salmonella* species to be localized at sites of preexisting vascular disease (eg, aneurysms, vascular grafts).

Recognition of salmonellosis in patients with acquired immune deficiency syndrome (AIDS) has been described by several investigators.[39–41] There appears to be a high propensity of *Salmonella typhimurium* to invade the bloodstreams of these patients, which suggests that in the appropriate clinical settings the organism may be considered as an opportunistic pathogen.[39,40] Unlike other infections in patients with AIDS, this infection can be treated.[40]

Typhoid fever is on the decline in areas of improved sanitation. Immunization has had a questionable impact on its incidence. The overall mortality may reach 10 percent in certain series, with dangerous complications being intestinal hemorrhage and perforation of the bowel. The distinction between typhoid and other *Salmonella* enteric fevers (eg, paratyphoid) is difficult to make on clinical grounds alone.

Treatment. Although shigellosis should be treated with antimicrobial drugs, uncomplicated *Salmonella* diarrhea should not be treated. Good studies have shown that antibiotic treatment actually prolongs gastrointestinal carriage and selects for resistant fecal organisms. On the other hand, there is not much dispute about treating extraintestinal salmonellosis.

In many parts of the world, *Salmonella* and *Shigella* are often quite resistant to antimicrobials such as tetracyclines, ampicillin, and sulfonamides. Chloramphenicol is the best agent for typhoid, though ampicillin is quite effective if given in adequate parenteral dose for susceptible organisms. Trimethoprim-sulfamethoxazole appears to be effective for both gastrointestinal and systemic *Salmonella* and *Shigella* infections.

Yersinia

These organisms are gram-negative coccobacillary forms of which three species are recognized as important pathogens for humans: (1) *Y. pestis,* the agent of bubonic plague or the "black death"; (2) *Y. pseudotuberculosis,* an occasional human pathogen known to cause tuberculous-like lesions in animals; and (3) *Y. enterocolitica,* by far the most important species because it is now recognized as an important cause of diarrhea and abdominal symptoms.

Yersinia enterocolitica. Appreciation of the importance of *Y. enterocolitica* in human disease stems from investigations of both sporadic and epidemic cases of enterocolitis, often accompanying abdominal symptoms in a manner that has mimicked acute appendicitis. Usually this organism produces a relatively mild and self-limited disease, which requires no treatment, but sometimes septicemias can occur. Severe diarrhea, often bloody, and temperatures in excess of 38C (102F) mimic disease caused by other intestinal pathogens such as *Shigella, Salmonella,* and enteropathogenic *E. coli.* Furthermore, mesenteric lymphadenitis due to *Y. enterocolitica* may occur with or without gastrointestinal symptoms and cause a syndrome indistinguishable from acute appendicitis. The appendix may be normal, but one study has demonstrated that approximately 5 percent of appendectomies will yield positive cultures of *Y. enterocolitica.*[42] For this reason, inflamed mesenteric nodes should be cultured when a normal appendix is discovered during operations for acute appendicitis. Recovery of *Y. enterocolitica* could alert the community to the possibility of an epidemic of pseudoappendicitis. Such epidemics have occasionally been traced to a common source such as contaminated food or water.[43]

Although the true incidence of yersinosis is not well defined, the infection is most prevalent in the cooler regions of North America and Europe. In many parts of the world, *Y. enterocolitica* exceeds *Shigella* and is equal to *Salmonella* as a cause of acute gastroenteritis. Different serotypes are associated with human infections in different regions of the world. For example, sporadic infections caused by serovar 0:3 and, to a lesser extent, serovar 0:9 are predominant in Europe, Canada, and Japan, whereas in the United States most reported outbreaks have been caused by serovar 0:8.[44]

The only definitive means for diagnosing *Y. enterocolitica* infection is culture of stool or mesenteric nodes and, in recent years, improvements have been made in the development of selective plating media for isolation of this organism.[45] Bacteremia is uncommon. Unfortunately, cultural recovery even with the best available techniques, including the use of cold enrichment (when feces are incubated at cold temperatures, this organism grows, whereas the growth of other bacteria is inhibited), is slow, and appendectomy should not be deferred awaiting laboratory confirmation.

Most cases of mesenteric adenitis resolve spontaneously, but there may be late complications of disease (such as infectious arthritis possibly as a result of an autoimmune mechanism). Symptomatic treatment with fluids and bed rest is indicated in the milder cases, and there is no evidence that antimicrobial therapy shortens the course of the disease. Serious infections, on the other hand, particularly in the immunocompromised patient, require aggressive antimicrobial therapy with chloramphenicol, the aminoglycosides, or trimethoprim-sulfamethoxazole.

Yersinia pestis. *Yersinia pestis* is the cause of all the clinical forms of plague. It is not an enteric organism.[46] The epidemiology of plague is complex, and foci occur throughout the world wherever wild rodents with fleas interact with people. It is endemic in the Rocky Mountain region of the United States. Rat-borne plague is a far less serious problem in urban areas than previously, and now wild mammal transmission in the rural areas predominates (ie, ground squirrels, prairie dogs, chipmunks). Human plague may result from pneumonic spread, human flea transmission, or contact with infected exudates.

Yersinia pestis in fleas develops into masses of organisms, which block the upper gut. Attempts to swallow blood lead to regurgitation of the organisms into the site of the bite. The human is an accidental victim of a bite by a rat flea or by contact with infected tissue in carnivores or other wild rodents. The local tissues in the regional nodes become necrotic, infarcted, inflamed, hemorrhagic, and edematous, and progressive toxemia leads to death. The usual incubation period of bubonic plague is 2 to 6 days, and the severity at onset is variable. Initially, malaise, fever, pain, and tenderness occur in the area of the regional lymph nodes. Bubos (enlarged fluctuant nodes) most often appear in the inguinal or axillary regions, but any subcutaneous site is susceptible. Intermittent bacteremia is common. The progression of infection in bacteremia can be extremely rapid, and in some patients the onset of clinical toxicity is sudden and bubo formation can be delayed, making the diagnosis difficult.

The diagnosis depends on suspecting the disease, aspirating a bubo, and culturing the blood. A rapid tentative diagnosis can be made on smear if Giemsa or Wayson stains are used. Gram stain preparations do not show the characteristic bipolarity. Fluorescent antibody tests on aspirated material will confirm the diagnosis. Bubos should not be excised or incised and drained for diagnostic purposes. Tularemia is a common incorrect diagnosis, and cultures of aspirates that are negative at 24 hours should increase the suspicion of plague or tularemia. Acute and convalescent sera are useful in epidemics.

Therapy should be started immediately. Streptomycin is the best drug, but other effective drugs include kanamycin, chloramphenicol, tetracyclines, and sulfadiazine. Quarantine of all patients and patient contacts should be carried out, and prophylactic chemotherapy should be instituted for contacts. Shock may require steroid administration.

A heat-killed vaccine is available that is reasonably effective in preventing disease. Booster injections are recommended every 6 months, but the principal protective method is environmental sanitation.

Citrobacter

Organisms belonging to the genus *Citrobacter* are closely related to the *Salmonella*. There are extensive cross-reactions between these organisms and other members of the family Enterobacteriaceae. Currently consisting of three species and a biogroup, *Citrobacter* organisms are occasionally isolated from a variety of clinical sources and are most commonly implicated in urinary and respiratory tract infections.[47] *Citrobacter diversus* is an important cause of central nervous system infection in neonates. Cerebral abscesses, endocarditis, and sepsis secondary to contaminating intravenous fluids have been reported. The two most commonly encountered species of *Citrobacter* are *C. diversus* and *C. freundii*. *Citrobacter diversus* are found to be resistant to ampicillin and carbenicillin but susceptible to cephalothin, whereas strains of *C. freundii* are variably sensitive to all of these agents. *Citrobacter amalonaticus* is isolated from feces on occasion and rarely from extraintestinal sources.[14]

Hafnia Alvei

These organisms are more closely related to the genus *Enterobacter*. Clinical isolates have been mainly nosocomial in origin, and the types of infection include pneumonia, urinary tract infection, and surgical wounds. Most aminoglycosides, chloramphenicol, tetracyclines, and carbenicillin are active against this agent, but *Hafnia* species are resistant to ampicillin and cephalosporins.

Edwardsiella Tarda

This group of organisms is similar to *Salmonella* in terms of the clinical disease produced, but the two genera are not closely related. The species name *tarda* refers to the relative slowness of this organism in fermenting various biochemical substrates. Rarely isolated, most human strains have been obtained from cases of acute gastroenteritis.[48] The syndrome involves intermittent watery diarrhea that persists for a few days but may last up to 2 weeks. Occasionally, low-grade fever and vomiting are present. Although the organism has been recovered from the stools of entirely asymptomatic individuals, *E. tarda* has been implicated as the source of bloodstream infection, liver abscess, meningitis, and soft tissue infection. Most cases of gastroenteritis associated with this organism resolve without treatment. As with the management of *Salmonella* gastroenteritis, normal individuals probably should not receive antimicrobial therapy. For systemic infections the organism is sensitive to a variety of common antimicrobials including ampicillin, cephalosporins, chloramphenicol, tetracyclines, and aminoglycosides.

Only described recently, the other two species and biogroup are extremely rare.[14]

OTHER GENERA AND SPECIES

There are several genera (and species) of Enterobacteriaceae that are now being recognized more often in the clinical microbiology laboratory (see Table 5–2). However, very little is known about their cause and effect other than they are infrequently isolated and little is known of their clinical significance. When isolated, many of the different genera have been recovered from blood cultures, suggesting that at least for now they are rare opportunistic pathogens.[14]

FAMILY PSEUDOMONADACEAE

Pseudomonas Aeruginosa

As mentioned earlier in this chapter, *Pseudomonas aeruginosa* (*Bacillus pyocyaneus*) is an organism that technically does not belong within the family Enterobacteriaceae but is properly categorized within the family Pseudomonadaceae. In clinical practice, *P. aeruginosa* is probably the most important of the gram-negative rods referred to as nonfermenters.[49] This term encompasses a taxonomically heterogeneous group of bacilli that have two important characteristics: they fail to ferment carbohydrates, and they are obligate aerobes. These two features are highly important in selection of laboratory techniques for the detection and identification of these microorganisms.

Because *P. aeruginosa* infections commonly occur in association with gastrointestinal disease, respiratory failure, urinary tract abnormalities, burns, or other situations in which gram-negative enteric bacilli are often encountered, it is proper to consider *P. aeruginosa* when evaluating the enteric bacteria. The experience of many medical centers is that among the systemic and pulmonic gram-negative bacillary infections, those caused by *P. aeruginosa* rank highest in mortality.[9,49] This high mortality appears to be a reflection of the predilection of this organism for neutropenic subjects, subjects with thermal injury, and recipients of organ transplants.[49,50]

There is no consensus about the basis for the human virulence of *P. aeruginosa*. A number of interesting studies have investigated the ability of the organism to elaborate extracellular virulence factors such as exoenzymes and toxins,[11,51] the heat-stable cell wall structures that appear to convey resistance to phagocytosis,[20] and the physical properties of the microbe that allow it to survive in adverse environmental conditions.[49] Indeed, one of the most simplistic explanations for the opportunistic nature of *P. aeruginosa* is its saprophytic qualities, that is, it has minimal nutritional requirements, and limited carbon sources will permit luxuriant growth. It survives readily in water, soil, and food products and is so hardy that commonly used detergents and disinfectants have little effect on its viability. Because pseudomonads will survive in any moist environment, medical equipment using water is commonly contaminated.

Epidemiology. Attempts to colonize normal volunteers with *P. aeruginosa* have been unsuccessful unless concomitant antimicrobial agents like ampicillin have been given,[52] and this organism is not likely to be found in the gastrointestinal tract of normal individuals. Furthermore, leukocytes and sera from normal individuals show an excellent ability to phagocytose and kill strains of *P. aeruginosa* from a wide variety of sources.[20] The incidence of gastrointestinal carriage in hospitalized or clinically ill patients receiving special diets or antibiotics, however, many approach 50 percent. It seems, then, that the host is continually assaulted with strains of *P. aeruginosa* that abound in the environment and in ingested materials. Colonization occurs only with some debility of the host, and colonization usually precedes bacteremia, particularly in the neutropenic patient.[53]

A number of serologic typing systems have been used to study the epidemiology of *P. aeruginosa*,[54] and a number of cross-reactions have been noted. Agglutination tests have identified 10 to 17 O-antigenic serotypes, but Fisher et al[55] have seven antisera that can adequately identify approximately 90 percent of clinically important strains. Other methods for epidemiologic study include phage typing and pyocin typing. All these techniques have been extremely useful in determining which nosocomial outbreaks of *P. aeruginosa* have a common source or an epidemic strain as opposed to multiple sources of infection.

Virulence Factors. The principal surface antigen implicated in resistance to phagocytosis is lipopolysaccharide or endotoxins.[56] Besides surface antigens, which are identified by agglutination reactions, the extracellular products of *P. aeruginosa* may be important virulence factors. Exotoxin A (of several exotoxins) is a potent inhibitor of protein synthesis, somewhat analogous to activity of diphtheria toxin.[11,51] Furthermore, most disease-causing *P. aeruginosa* elaborate potent proteolytic enzymes such as elastase and lecithinase.[51,57] At present it is not possible to conclude which if any of these factors is most critical in the pathogenesis of *P. aeruginosa* infection.

Clinical Manifestations. Clinically, the onset of *Pseudomonas* bacteremia may be fulminant with a rapid progression to hypotension and shock. In a small percent of patients, bacteremia is accompanied by a striking necrotizing vasculitis.[58] The name *ecthyma gangrenosum* is the classic term for these lesions. Initially, the first indication of vasculitis is a vesicle or bulla surrounded by a slightly raised halo of erythema. Within a matter of hours the central vesicle or bulla progresses to frank ulceration. The halo of erythema may become darkly ecchymotic (and might be mistaken for just subcutaneous bleeding in thrombocytopenic patients). Histopathologically, organisms are found invading the venular side of the vascular bed and appear to trigger thrombosis and infarction.[59] Some ecthyma gangrenosum skin lesions may be singular, while other patients may have showers of them. They appear on any surface of the body including the trunk, back, and extremities, but the area that should be carefully examined is the perirectal area. Although some lesions have been attributed to a hypersensitivity phenomenon, the recovery of the organisms by aspiration or biopsy is readily achieved if the patient is not receiving systemic antimicrobial drugs. Thus the finding of these lesions is prima facie evidence of bacteremia, and the patient should be treated.

The proclivity of *P. aeruginosa* to cause necrotizing vasculitis is one of the striking features of bacteremic disease syndromes, and these may also involve the gastrointestinal tract and the lungs. Indeed, the so-called shock lung syndrome may reflect the activation of complement, coagulation, and kinin systems, with the lung serving as one of several target organs. The rapid development of pulmonary infiltrates with evidence for increased alveolar capillary-arterial oxygen gradient may be a reflection of a diffuse intrapulmonary capillary leak triggered by bacterial products such as *Pseudomonas* endotoxins. The mortality in this complication is high, and aggressive antimicrobial therapy and maintenance of ventilatory function are imperative.

Pseudomonas aeruginosa infections can involve all major organs and soft tissue sites. The organism can cause central nervous system infections, particularly meningitis and brain abscess, in patients with immunodeficiency or in individuals who have intracerebral catheters or shunts in place. External ear infections due to *P. aeruginosa* are quite common but may not necessarily call for the use of systemic antimicrobial therapy. Bone infections frequently represent a superinfection, that is, the onset of a *Pseudomonas* infection following an initial process caused by staphylococci. Caution must be exercised in interpreting the results of sinus tract cultures in diagnosing osteomyelitis. Biopsy of infected bone should be undertaken before committing the patient to a prolonged course of potentially toxic antipseudomonal therapy.

Pulmonary infections caused by *P. aeruginosa* are among the greatest therapeutic challenges that clinicians now face. Highly mucoid strains of *Pseudomonas* have caused life-threatening disease in children with cystic fibrosis. Mucoid strains of *P. aeruginosa* are rarely encountered in other types of *Pseudomonas* infection, but the nonmucoid strains are a particular problem in hospital-acquired aspiration pneumonia. These pneumonias tend to occur in intensive care units or burn units and in critically ill patients receiving assisted ventilation.

Intra-abdominal and urinary infections often present as superinfections after antimicrobial therapy for another infection has been initiated. Foreign bodies such as Foley catheters, intra-arterial and intravenular catheters, peritoneal lavage devices, and prostheses serve as the nidus of persistent infection. *Pseudomonas* arthritis and osteomyelitis develop on a bacteremic basis in heroin addicts, who also are prone to *Pseudomonas* endocarditis, a lethal complication that may require excision of infected cardiac valves.[60]

Treatment. Four groups of antimicrobial drugs that are widely available can be used for *P. aeruginosa* infection: the aminoglycosides (gentamicin, tobramycin, amikacin, netilmicin), the antipseudomonal penicillins (carbenicillin, ticarcillin, mezlocillin, azlocillin, piperacillin), and the polymyxins (polymyxin B, colistin) (Table 5–5). Historically, polymyxins were relatively ineffective, supposedly because of nephrotoxicity.

During the last half of the decade two most important advances in the antimicrobial chemotherapy of *P. aeruginosa* infections have occurred with the appearance of compounds of the cephalosporin and quinolone classes that have potent antipseudomonal activity. The earlier, prototype agents of each class—cephalothin of the cephalosporins and nalidixic acid of the quinolones—lacked antipseu-

TABLE 5–5. ANTIMICROBIAL SUSCEPTIBILITY OF *PSEUDOMONAS* SPECIES

Species	Aminoglycosides[a]	Carbenicillin[b]	Polymyxins[c]	Tetracyclines	Chloramphenicol	Sulfa
P. aeruginosa	+	+	+	0	0	0
P. cepacia	0	±	0	0	±	+[d]
P. fluorescens	+	0	+	+	±	
X. maltophilia	0	±	+	±	±	±[d]
P. stutzeri	+	+	+	+	±	
P. pseudomallei	±	+	0	+	+	+
P. putida	+	0	+	±	0	

+, usually susceptible; ±, variable; 0, resistant.
[a] Amikacin, gentamicin, tobramycin.
[b] Or ticarcillin.
[c] Polymixin B or colistin.
[d] Trimethoprim-sulfamethoxazole preferred.

domonal activity. Molecular modifications have endowed newer agents of each class with variable in vitro effects against *P. aeruginosa*. Compounds such as cefotaxime, ceftizoxime, and ceftriaxone have modest antipseudomonal activity and should not be used as monotherapy for systemic infection. Cefoperazone, cefsulodin, and ceftazidime are more potent antipseudomonal cephoalosporins but are still recommended for use in combinations with aminoglycosides for therapy of severely immunocompromised hosts. New beta-lactam agents that are not cephalosporins (eg, aztreonam, imipenem) are quite active in vitro against *P. aeruginosa* in a manner similar to or better than the three aforementioned cephalosporins.

The quinolones (examples of which are norfloxacin and ciprofloxacin, still experimental in the United States but not elsewhere) are attractive. Norfloxacin is the first orally absorbed agent to be active against *P. aeruginosa* since carbenicillin indanyl. Still, caution must be exercised in employing oral therapy for systemic infection. It seems likely that the new quinolones will have a major role for therapy of pseudomonal urinary tract infections and may be used as follow-up therapy after parenteral antibiotics are used to treat the acute stages of systemic infections.

Prevention. Prevention of *Pseudomonas* infections may be possible through the use of immunoprophylactic measures such as the administration of a vaccine or immunoglobulin, approaches that have been successfully demonstrated experimentally and in some clinical trials.[21,23,61] The use of granulocyte transfusions may be of benefit in neutropenic patients. Because the transfused white cells are short-lived, multiple daily transfusions are needed until the patients' own leukocytes return in sufficient numbers.[22]

Nonaeruginosa *Pseudomonas* Species

Table 5–6 is a summary of nonaeruginosa pseudomonads of occasional medical and surgical importance. The three most important species listed are *P. cepacia, Xanthomonas maltophilia,* and *P. pseudomallei.* All are found in soil and water and cause illnesses similar to those caused by *P. aeruginosa.* Unfortunately, their antibiotic sensitivity patterns are different.

Pseudomonas cepacia is a recent appellation for organisms previously designated as *P. multivorans* or *K. kingae.* The organism has occasionally been encountered in wound and genitourinary tract infections. It colonizes foot ulcers or traumatized skin, leading to the peculiar syndrome known as

TABLE 5–6. NONAERUGINOSA *PSEUDOMONAS* SPECIES OF OCCASIONAL MEDICAL AND SURGICAL IMPORTANCE

Species	Reference	Clinical Associations
P. cepacia	62	Septicemia, "foot rot," endocarditis, wound infections, GU infections
P. fluorescens	66	Wounds, respiratory infections, catheter-associated bacteremia
X. maltophilia[a]	64	Respiratory infections, ulcers, abscesses, wound infections, granulomas
P. stutzeri	65	Wounds, osteomyelitis, otitis
P. pseudomallei	63	Necrotizing pneumonia and metastatic disease
P. putida	66	Wounds, GU infections, catheter associated bacteremia
P. putrefaciens	65	Wounds, abscesses, bacteremia

[a] Also called *P. multivorans* or *X. kingae.*

foot rot.[62] The most serious infections with *P. cepacia* are endocarditis (as in abusers of intravenous drugs), septicemia, and meningitis. *Pseudomonas cepacia* appears to be a nosocomial pathogen of increasing importance that, like strains of *P. aeruginosa,* contaminates inhalation therapy equipment, water baths, and sinks. Also, it has been isolated from outbreaks associated with contaminated blood products or infusion fluids.

Pseudomonas pseudomallei is found in Southeast Asia. The syndrome of necrotizing pneumonia with occasional septicemia and metastatic spread of disease was recognized in U.S. troops in Vietnam.[63]

Xanthomonas maltophilia can occasionally cause nosocomial respiratory infections, wound infections, and granulomatous infections.[64,65]

Depending on the clinical circumstances, presumed infection by these organisms should be approached either cautiously or aggressively. Recovery of nonaeruginosa pseudomonads from skin or the oropharynx may represent new colonization. These organisms tend to overgrow during the selection pressure of antimicrobial therapy. On the other hand, the isolation of the organism in pure culture from a transtracheal aspirate, bone aspirate, carefully collected urine, or from blood unquestionably indicates infection that requires urgent treatment.

REFERENCES

1. Young LS, Martin WJ, Meyer RD, et al: Gram-negative rod bacteremia: microbiologic, immunologic, and therapeutic considerations. Ann Intern Med 86:456, 1977.
2. Bennett JV: Incidence and nature of endemic and epidemic nosocomial infections. In Bennett JV, Brachman PS (eds): Hospital Infections. Boston, Little, Brown, 1979, p 233.
3. Musher DM: Cutaneous and soft-tissue manifestations of sepsis due to gram-negative enteric bacilli. J Infect Dis 2:854, 1980.
4. Finegold SM, Martin WJ: Bailey and Scott's Diagnostic Microbiology, 6th ed. St. Louis, Mosby, 1982.
5. Brenner DJ: Taxonomy, classification, and nomenclature of bacteria. In Balows A, Hausler WJ Jr, Herrmann KL, et al (eds): Manual of Clinical Microbiology, 5th ed. Washington, DC, American Society of Microbiology, 1991, p 209.
6. Rietschel ET, Wollenwelser HW, Russa R, et al: Concepts of the chemical structure of lipid A. Rev Infect Dis 6:432, 1984.
7. Young LS: Opsonizing antibodies, host factors, and the limulus assay for endotoxin. Infect Immun 12:88, 1985.
8. McCabe WR, Kreger BE, John M: Type-specific and cross-reactive antibodies in gram-negative bacteremia. N Engl J Med 287:261, 1972.
9. Young LS, Mandell GL, Douglas RG, Bennett JE: Principles and Practice of Infectious Diseases. New York, Wiley, 1990, p 617.
10. Zinner SH, McCabe WR: Effects of IgM and IgG antibody in patients with bacteremia due to gram-negative bacilli. J Infect Dis 133:35, 1976.
11. Pollack M, Young LS: Protective activity of antibodies to exotoxin A and lipopolysaccharide at the onset of *Pseudomonas aeruginosa* septicemia in man. J Clin Invest 63:276, 1979.
12. Edwards PR, Ewing WH: Identification of Enterobacteriaceae, 3rd ed. Minneapolis, Burgess, 1972.
13. Farmer JJ III, Davis BR, Hickman-Brenner FW, et al: Biochemical identification of new species and biogroups of *Enterobactericeae* isolated from clinical specimens. J Clin Microbiol 21:46, 1985.
14. Farmer JJ III, Kelly MT: Enterobacteriaceae. In Balows A, Hausler WJ Jr, Herrmann KL, et al (eds): Manual of Clinical Microbiology, 5th ed. Washington, DC, American Society of Microbiology, 1991, p 360.
15. Krieg NR, Holt JG (eds): Bergey Manual of Systematic Bacteriology, Vol 1. Baltimore, Williams & Wilkins, 1984.
16. Stossel TP: Phagocytosis. N Engl J Med 290:717, 1974 (Part I); 290:774, 1974 (Part II); 290:833, 1974 (Part III).
17. Müller-Eberhard HJ: Complement. Ann Rev Biochem 44:697, 1975.
18. Young LS, Stevens P: Cross-protective immunity to gram-negative bacilli: studies with core glycolipid of *Salmonella minnesota* and antigens to *Streptococcus pneumoniae.* J Infect Dis 136(Suppl):S174, 1977.
19. Robbins JB, Myerowitz RL, Whisnant JK, et al: Enteric bacteria cross-reactive with *Neisseria meningitidis* groups A and C and *Diplococcus pneumoniae* types I and III. Infect Immun 6:651, 1972.
20. Young LS, Armstrong D: Human immunity to *Pseudomonas aeruginosa,* I. In vitro-interaction of bacteria, polymorphonuclear leukocytes, and serum factors. J Infect Dis 126:257, 1972.
21. Young LS, Meyer RD, Armstrong D: *Pseudomonas aeruginosa* vaccine in cancer patients. Ann Intern Med 79:518, 1973.
22. Lieschke GJ, Burgess AW: Drug therapy: granulocyte colony-stimulating factor and granulocyte macrophage colony-stimulating factor. N Engl J Med 327:28, 99, 1992.
23. The Intravenous Immunoglobulin Collaborative Study Group: Prophylactic intravenous administration of standard immune globulin as compared with core-lipopolysaccharide immune globulin in patients at high risk of postsurgical infection. N Engl J Med 4:234, 1992.
24. Siber GR: Immune globulin to prevent nosocomial infections. N Engl J Med 4:269, 1992.
25. Ziegler EJ, Fisher CJ Jr, Sprung CL, et al: Treatment of gram-negative bacteremia and septic shock

with HA-1A human monoclonal antibody against endotoxin—a randomized double-blind, placebo controlled trial. N Engl J Med 324:429, 1991.
26. Greenman RL, Schein RMH, Martin MA, et al: A controlled clinical trial of E5 murine monoclonal IgM antibody to endotoxin in the treatment of gram-negative sepsis. JAMA 266:1097, 1991.
27. Wenzel RP. Anti-endotoxin monoclonal antibodies—a second look. N Engl J Med 326:1151, 1992.
28. Brachman PS: Epidemiology of nosocomial infections. In Bennett JV, Brachman PS (eds): Hospital Infections. Boston, Little, Brown, 1979, p 9.
29. Goldmann DA, Maki DG, Bennett JV: Intravenous infusion-associated infections. In Bennett JV, Brachman PS (eds): Hospital Infections. Boston, Little, Brown, 1979, p 443.

Enterobacteriaceae

30. Lorber B, Swenson RM: Bacteriology of aspiration pneumonia. A prospective study of community- and hospital-acquired cases. Ann Intern Med 81:329, 1974.
31. Tillotson JR, Lerner AM: Characteristics of pneumonias caused by *Escherichia coli.* N Engl J Med 277:115, 1967.
32. Doyle MP: Pathogenic *Escherichia coli, Yersinia enterocolitica,* and *Vibrio parahaemolyticus.* Lancet 336:1111, 1990.
33. Orskov I, Orskov F, Jann B, Jann K: Serology, chemistry and genetics of O and K antigens of *Escherichia coli.* Bact Rev 41:667, 1977.
34. Anderson ET, Young LS, Hewitt WL: Antimicrobial synergism in the therapy of gram-negative rod bacteremia. Chemotherapy 24:45, 1978.
35. Reyes E: Rhinoscleroma. Observations based on a study of two hundred cases. Arch Dermatol 54:531, 1946.
36. Wilfert JN, Barrett FF, Kass EH: Bacteremia due to *Serratia marcescens.* N Engl J Med 279:286, 1968.
37. Sanders CC, Sanders WE: Emergence of resistance during therapy with newer beta lactam antibiotics: role of inducible beta lactamases and implications for the future. Rev Infect Dis 5:639, 1983.
38. Silverblatt FJ: Host parasite interactions in the rat renal pelvis. A possible role for pili in the pathogenesis of pyelonephritis. J Exp Med 140:1696, 1974.
39. Bottone EJ, Wormser GP, Duncanson FP: Nontyphoidal salmonella bacteremia as an early infection in the acquired immunodeficiency syndrome. Diag Microbiol Infect Dis 2:247, 1984.
40. Glaser JB, Morton-Kute L, Berger SR, et al: Recurrent *Salmonella typhimurium* bacteremia with the acquired immuno-deficiency syndrome. Ann Intern Med 102:189, 1985.
41. Profeta S, Forrester C, Eng RHK, et al: Salmonella infections in patients with acquired immunodeficiency syndrome. Arch Intern Med 145:670, 1985.
42. Bottone EJ: *Yersinia enterocolitica:* a panoramic view of charismatic microorganism. CRC Crit Rev Microbiol 5:211, 1977.
43. Black RE, Jackson RJ, Tsai T, et al: Epidemic *Yersinia enterocolitica* infection due to contaminated chocolate milk. N Engl J Med 298:76, 1978.
44. Cover TL, Aber RC: *Yersinia enterocolitica.* N Engl J Med 321:16, 1989.
45. Head CB, Whitly DA, Ratman S: Comparative study of selective media for recovery of *Yersinia enterocolitica.* J Clin Microbiol 16:615, 1982.
46. Poland JD: Plague. In Hoeprich PD (ed): Infectious Diseases: A Modern Treatise of Infectious Processes. Hagerstown, MD, Harper & Row, 1977, p 1050.
47. Lipsky BA, Hook EW III, Smith AA, Plorde JJ: Citrobacter infections in humans: experience at the Seattle Veterans Administration Medical Center and a review of the literature. Rev Infect Dis 2:746, 1980.
48. Jordan GW, Hadley WK: Human infection with *Edwardsiella tarda.* Ann Intern Med 70:283, 1969.
49. Young LS, Armstrong D: *Pseudomonas aeruginosa* infections. CRC Crit Rev Clin Lab Sci 3:291, 1972.
50. Lau WK, Young LS, Black RE, et al: Comparative efficacy and toxicity of amikacin/carbenicillin versus gentamicin/carbenicillin in leukopenic patients: A randomized prospective trial. Am J Med 62:959, 1977.

Pseudomonads

51. Young LS: The role of exotoxins in the pathogenesis of *Pseudomonas aeruginosa* infections. J Infect Dis 142:626, 1980.
52. Buck AC, Cooke EM: The fate of ingested *Pseudomonas aeruginosa* in normal persons. J Med Microbiol 2:521, 1969.
53. Moody MR: Effect of acquisition on the incidence of *Pseudomonas aeruginosa* in hospitalized patients. In Young VM (ed): *Pseudomonas aeruginosa:* Ecological Aspects and Patient Colonization. New York, Raven, 1977, p. 111.
54. Farmer JJ III, Herman LG: Epidemiological fingerprinting of *Pseudomonas aeruginosa* by the production of and sensitivity of pyocin and bacteriophage. Appl Microbiol 18:760, 1969.
55. Fisher MW, Devlin HB, Gnabasik FJ: New immunotype schema for *Pseudomonas aeruginosa* based on protective antigens. J Bacteriol 98:835, 1969.
56. Cruz SJ Jr, Pitt TL, Furer E, Germamier R: Role of lipopolysaccharide in virulence of *Pseudomonas aeruginosa.* Infect Immun 44:508, 1984.
57. Wretlind B, Mollby R, Wadstrom T: Separation of two hemolysins from *Aeromonas hydrophila* by isoelectric focusing. Infect Immun 4:503, 1971.
58. Forkner CE, Frei E III, Edgcomb JH, Utz JP: *Pseudomonas* septicemia. Observations on twenty-three cases. Am J Med 25:877, 1958.
59. Dorff GJ, Geimer NJ, Rosenthal DR, Rytel MW: *Pseudomonas* septicemia. Illustrated evolution of its skin lesion. Arch Intern Med 128:591, 1971.

60. Reyes MP, Palutke WA, Wylin RF, Lerner AM: *Pseudomonas* endocarditis in the Detroit Medical Center. Medicine (Baltimore) 52:173, 1973.
61. Alexander JW, Fisher MW, MacMillan BG: Immunological control of *Pseudomonas* infection in burn patients: a clinical evaluation. Arch Surg 102:31, 1971.
62. Taplin D, Bassett DCJ, Mertz PM: Foot lesions associated with *Pseudomonas cepacia.* Lancet 2:568, 1971.
63. Spotnitz M, Rudnitzky J, Rambaud JJ: Melioidosis pneumonitis. Analysis of nine cases of a beginning form of melioidosis. JAMA 202:950, 1967.
64. Gilardi GL: *Pseudomonas maltophilia* infections in man. Am J Clin Pathol 51:58, 1969.
65. Gilardi GL: Infrequently encountered *Pseudomonas* species causing infection in humans. Ann Intern Med 77:211, 1972.
66. von Graevenitz A, Weinstein J: Pathogenic significance of *Pseudomonas fluorescens* and *Pseudomonas putida.* Yale J Biol Med 44:265, 1971.

Anaerobic Bacteria

CHAPTER 6

Sydney M. Finegold

There is considerable disagreement as to how to define an anaerobe. A practical operational definition is that an anaerobe is a bacterium that requires reduced oxygen tension for growth; it cannot grow on the surface of solid media in 10 percent carbon dioxide in air (18 percent oxygen). Facultative organisms can grow in either the presence or the absence of air. The term microaerophilic is commonly used for organisms that grow poorly or not at all in air but that will grow distinctly better under 10 percent carbon dioxide in air (reduced oxygen content) or anaerobically. Aerotolerant organisms are anaerobes that tolerate oxygen well enough to grow to some extent on the surface of freshly prepared solid media.

CLASSIFICATION

Anaerobic bacteria are represented by all morphologic types. The most commonly encountered are the gram-negative anaerobic bacilli, which are seen in at least one-third of clinically significant anaerobic infections. Although there are a large number of gram-negative anaerobic cocci, the gram-positive anaerobic cocci are clearly more important. The gram-positive spore-forming anaerobic rods are next to last in frequency of isolation from clinical infections, but they are important as potent toxin producers and can produce devastating disease. Finally, there are gram-positive, non–spore-forming anaerobic bacilli, but only *Actinomyces,* certain *Propionibacterium* species, and *Bifidobacterium dentium* are of much clinical significance.

Table 6–1 is a simplified classification of the anaerobes of greatest clinical importance. Five organisms or groups taken together account for two-thirds of all clinically significant anaerobic infections. Included are the *Bacteroides fragilis* group, the anaerobic cocci, the pigmented anaerobic gram-negative rods (*Porphyromonas* and certain *Prevotella* species), and *Clostridium perfringens.* A table is included on the common anaerobic pathogens in each of the chapters on regional infections.

Gram-Negative Bacilli

Bacteroides, Prevotella, Porphyromonas, Bilophila, and *Fusobacterium* are the pathogenic organisms of the gram-negative non-spore-forming rods. The others are of much less clinical significance. Because of their fastidious requirements for growth and their inability to form spores, the anaerobic gram-negative rods are apparently commensal with people. They dominate the normal flora of the mouth, the intestines, and the female genital tract numerically and, as strict anaerobes, can produce foul odor and gas. Many grow slowly, taking a week or longer for identification (largely because of the presence of multiple organisms in mixed culture), which neces-

TABLE 6–1. MAJOR ANAEROBES ENCOUNTERED CLINICALLY

- Gram-negative bacilli
  - *Bacteroides fragilis* group
    - Especially *B. fragilis, B. thetaiotaomicron, B. distasonis, B. ovatus, B. vulgatus*
  - Other *Bacteroides*
    - *B. gracilis*
    - *B. ureolyticus*
  - *Porphyromonas* species
    - Especially *P. asaccharolytica*
  - Pigmented *Prevotella* species (*P. corporis, P. denticola, P. intermedia, P. loescheii, P. melaninogenica, P. nigrescens*)
  - Other *Prevotella* species
    - *P. oris*
    - *P. buccae*
    - *P. oralis* group
    - *P. bivia*
    - *P. disiens*
  - *Fusobacterium* species
    - *F. nucleatum*
    - *F. necrophorum*
    - *F. mortiferum*
    - *F. varium*
  - *Bilophila wadsworthia*
- Gram-positive cocci
  - *Peptostreptococcus*
    - Especially *P. anaerobius, P. intermedius,*[a] *P. micros, P. magnus, P. asaccharolytica, P. prevotii*
  - Microaerophilic streptococci[a]
- Gram-positive spore-forming bacilli
  - *Clostridium perfringens*
  - *C. ramosum*
  - *C. septicum*
  - *C. novyi*
  - *C. histolyticum*
  - *C. sporogenes*
  - *C. sordellii*
  - *C. bifermentans*
  - *C. fallax*
  - *C. difficile*
  - *C. innocuum*
  - *C. botulinum*
  - *C. tetani*
- Gram-positive non–spore-forming bacilli
  - *Actinomyces* (*israelii, meyerii, naeslundii, odontolyticus, viscosus*)
  - *Propionibacterium propionicum*
  - *Propionibacterium acnes*
  - *Bifidobacterium dentium*

[a] Not true anaerobes.

sitates the use of empiric drug therapy for the patient. Certain anaerobes, such as *Bacteroides gracilis* and *Bilophila,* may actually take a week to grow.

Although most anaerobic gram-negative rods are pleomorphic, *Bacteroides fragilis* is a relatively nonpleomorphic organism, sometimes difficult to distinguish from *Escherichia coli,* although *B. fragilis* typically shows pale, irregular staining. It is frequently associated with *E. coli. Bacteroides fragilis* is the most clinically significant of these bacilli. It is the most common anaerobic organism in clinical infections, including septicemia.

Pigmented anaerobic gram-negative rods are usually found mixed with other *Prevotella* and with *Bacteroides.* Although they may be difficult to maintain in pure culture, they grow well when mixed with other anaerobes. These organisms are active in establishing synergistic infections.

Fusobacterium, Bacteroides, and *Prevotella* have been implicated in many localized infections. The ear, nose, and throat regions were common sites of infection by anaerobes before the widespread use of penicillin and other antibiotics for the treatment of undiagnosed acute pharyngitis. Other infections attributed to the gram-negative anaerobic organisms are peritonitis and abscesses of the abdominal cavity and pelvis; acute appendicitis (*Bilophila* is quite common here, along with the *Bacteroides fragilis* group and other anaerobes); pneumonia, lung, liver, and brain abscesses; infections of the gallbladder; perirectal infections; and pilonidal and sebaceous cyst infections. *Bacteroides* and *Fusobacterium* infections often cause thrombophlebitis and secondary septic embolization to the liver, lungs, peritoneum, and joints. *Bacteroides* bacteremias are less frequently recognized now; most cases originate from the gastrointestinal tract. Most of the *Fusobacterium* and *Prevotella* bacteremias originate from upper respiratory sites.

Gram-Positive Cocci

Peptococcus *and* Peptostreptococcus. *Peptostreptococcus* is the more significant pathogen and has been associated with anaerobic myositis, joint infection, breast abscess, septic abortion, liver abscesses, and empyema, as well as with gram-negative anaerobic rods and *Bacteroides* in a variety of mixed infections. With the exception of *Peptococcus niger,* all pathogenic species formerly in the genus *Peptococcus* have been transferred to the genus *Peptostreptococcus.* Both *Peptococcus* and *Peptostreptococcus* can produce a foul odor and gas. *Peptostreptococcus* organisms occur normally in the vagina, mouth, and feces.

Gram-Positive Spore-Forming Bacilli

Clostridium. The characteristics, classification, and pathogenic properties of the clostridia are the best understood of all the anaerobic bacilli. They are the only spore-forming anaerobic organisms, and their identification depends on the demonstration of spores, which can be difficult in the case of *C. perfringens* and *C. ramosum*. *Clostridium perfringens,* the most common pathogenic species, does not produce spores in tissues. Although most of the clostridia are obligate anaerobes, two species, *C. tertium* and *C. histolyticum,* can grow aerobically, and *C. perfringens* is quite aerotolerant. Only a dozen or so of the more than 100 species of clostridia are associated with human disease. Tetanus produced by *C. tetani* and botulism caused by *C. botulinum* are more properly described as intoxications rather than infections (see Chap. 50). In addition to *C. perfringens,* the less common *C. novyi* and *C. septicum* and the still rarer *C. histolyticum, C. bifermentans,* and *C. fallax* are all capable of causing myonecrosis (gas gangrene), anaerobic cellulitis, septic abortions, and operative wound infections. *Clostridium difficile* causes pseudomembranous colitis. Clostridia are found as part of the normal bowel flora, in the soil, and irregularly in the mouth and the female genital tract.

Gram-Positive Non–Spore-Forming Bacilli

Actinomyces. *Actinomyces israelii, A. naeslundii,* and other *Actinomyces* (and *Propionibacterium propionicum*) have been identified as a part of the normal flora of the mouth and the female genital tract. *Actinomyces israelii* also occurs in the intestines of humans but never exists as a saprophyte outside the body. Most strains of *A. israelii* are obligate anaerobes and will not grow on Sabouraud medium, which typically supports fungal growth. Other *Actinomyces,* however, are aerobic or aerotolerant. Clinical infections by *Actinomyces* or *P. propionicum* are always endogenous, complex, and are often accompanied by anaerobic cocci, pigmented anaerobic gram-negative bacilli, *Actinobacillus actinomycetemcomitans,* and staphylococci. These concomitant organisms lower the oxidation-reduction potential and secrete enzymes that facilitate tissue invasion by disrupting the mechanical structure of the tissues. Sulfur granules can usually be detected in the purulent material obtained from *Actinomyces* infections. The gram-positive rods result from fragmentation of the short branching filaments and can often be confused with those of *Propionibacterium acnes,* but the catalase-positive activity of the latter will distinguish the two organisms. *Actinomyces viscosus,* however, is also catalase-positive.

Propionibacterium. The anaerobic diphtheroid *Corynebacterium acnes* has been reclassified as *Propionibacterium acnes.* This organism is significant because it is probably the most prominent bacterium of the normal skin flora and is often a contaminant in mixed cultures. It also occurs in the mouth and in the intestinal tract. *Propionibacterium acnes* can be confused with *A. israelii.* On occasion, *P. acnes* has been implicated as a primary pathogen in cases of sinusitis, infected prosthetic devices, and endocarditis either with or without rheumatic heart disease.

Other gram-negative non–spore-forming rods (*Eubacterium, Bifidobacterium,* and *Lactobacillus*) have seldom been associated with clinical infections, except for *B. dentium,* which has been recovered occasionally from serious pulmonary infection.

Eubacterium. *Eubacterium nodatum,* in particular, may be found in women with intrauterine contraceptive devices and a clinical picture like actinomycosis. *Eubacterium lentum* is also recovered from various infections on occasion.

Gram-Negative Cocci

Veillonella. *Veillonella* is the most common gram-negative anaerobic coccus found in humans. This strict anaerobe is found normally in the mouth, upper respiratory tract, vagina, and intestinal tract. Strains of *Veillonella* have been identified from abscesses, cysts, pleural fluid, bone and joint infection, and other infections, usually in combination with other anaerobic or aerobic bacteria.

GROWTH CHARACTERISTICS

Certain characteristics of anaerobes present problems in clinical identification.[1,2] For example, gram-positive anaerobic bacteria commonly destain and may therefore appear gram-negative. Occasionally, young gram-negative forms appear to be gram-positive or contain gram-positive granules. Certain short bacilli, the pigmented anaerobic gram-negative rods, commonly look like cocci. On occasion, cocci may be pleomorphic enough to appear to be short rods. Spores are often difficult to detect. This is especially true in the cases of *C. perfringens* and *C. ramosum.* Finally, some of the anaerobic organisms, particularly a number of clostridia, are aerotolerant and will grow to some extent on the surface of culture media. Thus it can be difficult to decide whether a given organism is anaerobic, although experienced bacteriologists usually do not find these characteristics to be major problems. Table 6–2 lists certain microscopic characteristics and the morphologic features of colonies of the more common anaerobic bacteria.

The simplest and most practical way to cultivate clinically significant anaerobic bacteria is in a GasPak (BBL) or similar jar. After appropriate plates are inoculated and placed into this jar, the anaerobic atmosphere is created by adding 10 ml of water to a commercially available gas-generating packet and then placing the lid on the jar. Hydrogen and carbon dioxide are liberated, and the hydrogen combines with oxygen in the jar in the presence of catalysts incorporated in a basket on the underside of the jar lid. This produces water and makes conditions within the jar anaerobic. The procedure is so simple that house staff members, if provided with the jars and appropriate plate media, can set up the cultures themselves if necessary. Fresh media or prereduced anaerobically sterilized (PRAS) media (commercially available) should be used. However, specialized techniques are required (1) to ensure that anaerobes growing on the plates do not die, (2) to determine that a given colony represents a true anaerobe and not a facultative organism, and (3) to identify the organisms accurately. Jars should not be opened until after 48 hours of incubation. The jars should only be opened by experienced bacteriologists to examine plates and to subculture. When results are needed as soon as possible, duplicate samples can be taken so that one jar can be opened early.

TABLE 6–2. MICROSCOPIC CHARACTERISTICS AND MORPHOLOGY OF COLONIES OF COMMONLY ENCOUNTERED ANAEROBES

Anaerobes	Microscopic Morphology	Morphology of Colonies on Blood Agar
Bacteroides fragilis group	Gram-negative bacilli with rounded ends, pleomorphic, may be coccobacillary, may show vacuolation and bipolar staining	Convex, entire, white-gray, semitranslucent, may be mucoid, shiny
Pigmented *Prevotella* and *Porphyromonas*	Gram-negative short bacilli with rounded ends, often coccobacillary	Convex, entire edge, glistening or dull, yellow-beige-brown to black depending on length of incubation, medium, etc
Fusobacterium nucleatum	Gram-negative bacilli, slender, spindle-shaped with tapered ends, sometimes in pairs end to end	Convex, glistening with internal iridescent flecking or raised opaque "bread crumb" colonies; greening of medium
Fusobacterium necrophorum, F. mortiferum, F. varium	Very pleomorphic, filamentous, irregularly staining, gram-negative bacilli; swellings along filaments; large, free round bodies	Often "fried egg" colonies; raised center; flat, irregular periphery; center opaque, edge translucent
Peptostreptococcus	Gram-positive spherical or elongated cocci, occurring singly, in pairs, or in chains	Convex, gray to white, opaque, shiny or dull, entire edge; small
Clostridium perfringens	Gram-positive bacilli, broad, relatively short, with blunt ends; spores rare	Low convex, semiopaque, shiny, entire, with double zone of hemolysis: narrow zone of complete hemolysis surrounded by a larger zone of incomplete hemolysis
Other clostridia	Thin to broad gram-positive bacilli; may or may not show spores	
Gram-positive non–spore-forming bacilli		
Bifidobacterium	Pleomorphic; often have bifurcated ends but may be club-shaped or coccobacillary	Convex, white, smooth
Propionibacterium propionicum	Thin, filamentous, long, branching; may be club-shaped	Convex to low convex
Propionibacterium, other	Regular or club-shaped, palisading or "Chinese-letter" arrangement may be seen	Convex, white to pink, entire edge
Actinomyces	Thin, filamentous, long, branching	Smooth to rough "molar tooth" colonies

ANAEROBES AS NORMAL FLORA

Anaerobes are prevalent as normal flora throughout the body, and most surgical anaerobic infections arise from indigenous organisms that gain entrance to deeper or devitalized tissues[3,4] (see Chap. 3). If an infection occurs in relation to a given mucosal surface, the normal flora at that site can provide a guide to the specific organisms that should be encountered (Fig. 6–1). It is also important to recognize that since anaerobes are prevalent as normal flora, specimens for culture must be obtained in such a way as to preclude mixing in normal flora with organisms causing the infection.

Table 6–3 lists the incidence of normal anaerobic flora at various sites throughout the body. All mucosal surfaces are heavily populated with anaerobic as well as aerobic bacteria. Anaerobes always outnumber aerobic or facultative bacteria. In the mouth and upper respiratory tract, anaerobes outnumber aerobes 10 : 1. In the colon, anaerobes outnumber aerobes 1000 : 1. Thus *E. coli* makes up only one-tenth of 1 percent of the total colonic flora, and the *B. fragilis* group is numerically dominant. In addition to mucosal surfaces, the skin has an indigenous flora, which includes certain anaerobes, particularly *P. acnes* and anaerobic cocci.

The normal anaerobic flora can be modified by disease, impaired drainage, and antimicrobial therapy. Normally the stomach contains less than 10^3 organisms per milliliter (usually transient oral flora), and obligate anaerobes are absent. The small bowel flora is also relatively simple, with total counts of 10^4 to 10^5/ml, or less, except for the distal ileum, where counts range from 10^6/ml to somewhat higher levels. High in the small bowel the

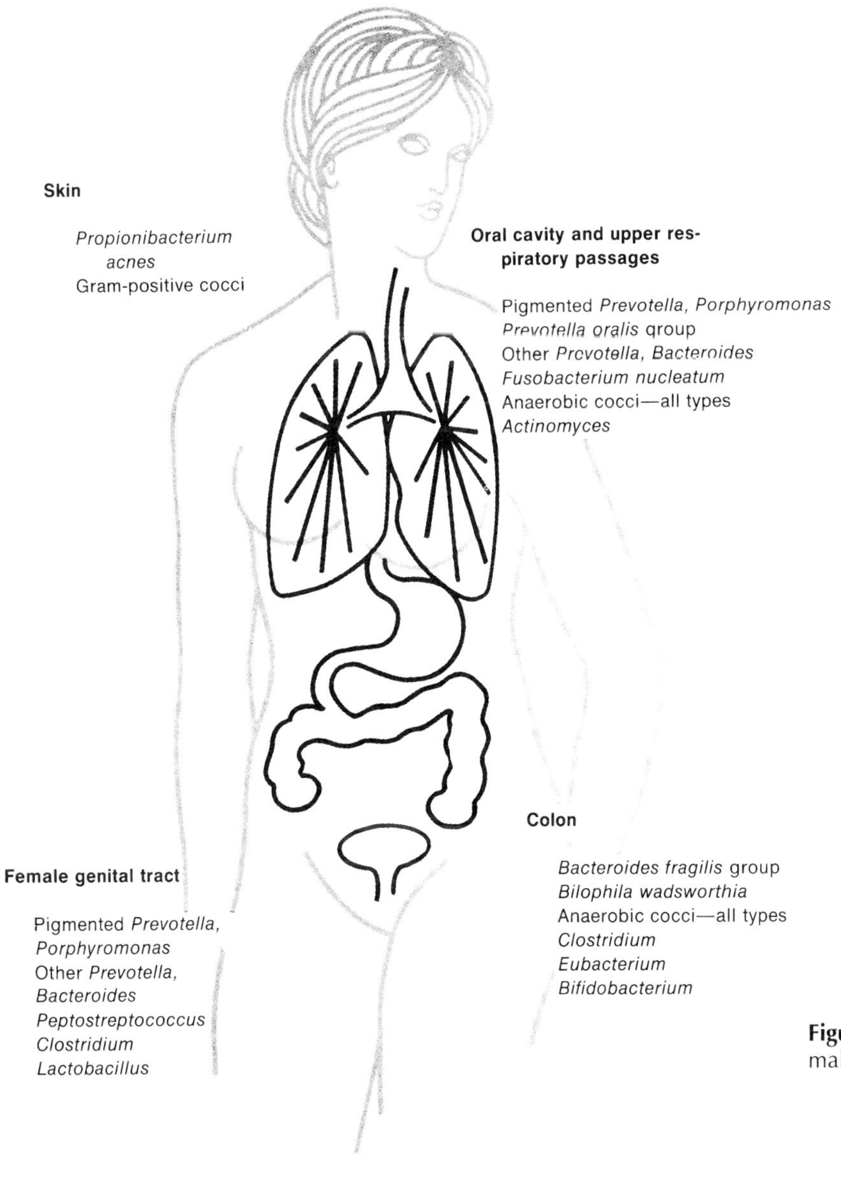

Figure 6–1. Predominant anaerobes of the normal flora.

TABLE 6–3. INCIDENCE OF VARIOUS ANAEROBES AS INDIGENOUS FLORA IN HUMANS

	Gram-Positive							Gram-Negative			
	Clostridium	*Actinomyces*	*Bifidobacterium*	*Eubacterium*	*Lactobacillus*[a]	*Propionibacterium*	Cocci	*B. fragilis* group	*Fusobacterium*	Other GNR	Cocci
Skin	0	0	0	+/−	0	2	1	0	0	0	0
Upper respiratory tract[b]	0	1	0	+/−	0	1	1	0	1	2	1
Mouth	+/−	1	1	1	1	+/−	2	0	2	2	2
Intestine	2	+/−	2	2	1–2	+/−	2	2	1	2	1
External genitalia	0	0	0	U	0	U	1	+/−	+/−	1	0
Urethra	+/−	0	0	U	+/−	0	+/−	+/−	+/−	1	U
Vagina	+/−	+/−	+/−	+/−	2	+/−	2	+/−	+/−	1	+/−
Endocervix	+/−	0	0	+/−	1	+/−	2	+/−	+/−	1	+/−

U, unknown; Ø, not found or rare; +/−, irregular; 1, usually present; 2, usually present in large numbers.
[a] Includes anaerobic, microaerobic, and facultative strains.
[b] Includes nasal passages, nasopharynx, oropharynx, and tonsils.
From Summanen P, Baron EJ, Citron DM, et al: Wadsworth Anaerobic Bacteriology Manual, 5th ed. Belmont, CA, Star Publishing, 1993.

flora consists entirely of gram-positive facultative forms—streptococci, lactobacilli, and yeasts. The farther one goes distally in the small bowel, the more the flora varies. In the terminal ileum there are equal numbers of aerobes and anaerobes. The major anaerobes encountered are *Bacteroides, Prevotella,* and *Bifidobacterium,* the latter usually nonpathogenic. In the presence of bleeding or obstructing duodenal ulcer or with gastric ulcer or carcinoma, the flora of the stomach and upper small bowel is usually more profuse and may include anaerobes, coliforms, and other organisms found in fecal flora. The impact of antimicrobial therapy will of course depend on levels of drug achieved and the susceptibility of the normal flora. Thus a knowledge of the pharmacology and antibacterial spectrum of various antimicrobial drugs will permit one to anticipate which elements of the normal flora will be suppressed, and to what extent, and also to predict which resistant organisms are likely to colonize that area. Because the normal flora of the body constitutes one of the most important defense mechanisms, antimicrobial agents should be used only when specifically indicated.

INCIDENCE AND TYPES OF ANAEROBIC INFECTIONS

Anaerobic bacteria may participate in any type of infection caused by any type of bacterium.[5–25] No organ or tissue is immune. Well-documented data on the impressive incidence of anaerobic bacteria in major infections involving the lung and pleural space, intra-abdominal sites, and the female genital tract have been available for some time. Additional data continually accumulate to indicate that anaerobes are important in many other categories of infection throughout the body. Table 6–4 shows a number of types of surgical infections in which anaerobes are common. Table 6–5 correlates the specific anaerobic bacteria recovered with the type of infection.

SURGICAL EPIDEMIOLOGY

Almost all anaerobic infections are endogenous. In the case of *Clostridium,* an organism widely distributed in soil and nature, there may be occasional exogenous infections, particularly relating to trauma. Nevertheless, most cases of clostridial myonecrosis that follow war injury are of endogenous origin and are primarily related to difficulties in maintaining good personal hygiene under battle conditions. Also, clostridial myonecrosis after operation is probably caused by a patient's own fecal flora rather than by spores of clostridia in the operating suite (even though the latter have been found).

Anaerobic infection may be facilitated by diagnostic and therapeutic modalities used in the hospital that lead to impaired blood supply, tissue necrosis, and breakdown of mucosal barriers, which create ideal conditions for invasion and multiplication of anaerobes from the normal flora. Radiation, cytotoxic drugs, and corticosteroids generally predispose to infection, anaerobic or otherwise. Antimicrobial therapy may select out resistant anaerobes, such as *B. fragilis,* which may then cause infection under appropriate conditions. Transmission of infection caused by anaerobes from animal to human has rarely been documented. Human-to-human transmission is even more rare, with the exception of certain venereal diseases. Infection following animal or human bites frequently involves anaerobic organisms, however. Administration of anesthetics or drugs that compromise consciousness, of course, may predispose to aspiration and subsequent pulmonary infection.

PATHOGENESIS OF ANAEROBIC INFECTIONS

Predisposing Conditions

Essentially all anaerobic infections arise endogenously. Under certain circumstances, anaerobes of the indigenous flora have an opportunity to penetrate tissues and cause infection. Poor vascular supply and necrosis of tissue lower the oxidation-reduction potential, favoring their growth. The oxidation-reduction potential of the intestinal tract, necrotic tissue, and abscess cavities ranges from −150 to −250 mV. Accordingly, factors that predispose to anaerobic infection include vascular disease, epinephrine injection, cold, shock, edema, trauma, operation, foreign bodies, malignancy, and gas production by microorganisms. Prior infection with aerobic or facultative bacteria also makes conditions more favorable for anaerobic growth by lowering the oxidation-reduction potential. Under certain circumstances, such as aspiration pneumonia, the normal flora may be carried into another area normally free of bacteria and set up an infection.

As with infection involving aerobic or facultative bacteria, conditions that impair host defense mechanisms and prior antimicrobial therapy to which the infecting organisms are resistant (ie, aminoglycosides, trimethoprim/sulfamethoxazole, and most quinolones in the case of most anaerobes) may pave the way for anaerobic infection.

Aerotolerance

Certain elements of the normal flora that are sensitive to oxygen appear to be unable to participate in infections. In general, the pathogenic anaerobes are more aerotolerant—some surprisingly so. This feature, of course, permits these organisms to survive after the normally protective mucosal barrier is broken, until conditions are satisfactory for their multiplication and further invasion. After the process has started, anaerobes can multiply rapidly and maintain their own reduced environment by virtue of excretion of end products of fermentative metabolism, including short-chain fatty acids, organic acids, and alcohols.

Mixed Infections

At least two-thirds of the infections in which anaerobes participate are mixed, with both anaerobes and facultative or occasionally aerobic bacteria participating together.[5] Participation of the anaerobes in these mixed infections is often facilitated by the nonanaerobes. Lowering of the oxidation-reduction potential by growth of the nonanaerobes has already been mentioned. Other bacteria may also supply anaerobes with necessary growth factors. This has been demonstrated in mixed infections involving pigmented anaerobic gram-negative rods, which often require vitamin K or analogs and whose growth may be stimulated by hemin and other, unknown, factors. In some cases the mucosal barrier may have been penetrated early in the course of an infection by only facultative bacteria. Thus acute otitis media and acute sinusitis frequently involve only facultative bacteria, but chronic otitis media and chronic sinusitis often involve anaerobes or are mixed. There are examples of specific synergy, such as postoperative bacterial synergistic gangrene, which requires the combination of a microaerophilic (or sometimes anaerobic) streptococcus and *Staphylococcus aureus* (or sometimes a gram-negative facultative bacillus) (see Chap. 7).

Involvement of anaerobes in infections may depend on resistance of certain of these organisms to normal defense mechanisms. This may include resistance to normal bactericidal activity of serum and to phagocytosis. This will be discussed further.

Enzymes

Superoxide dismutase has been found in a number of anaerobes, including members of the *B. fragilis* group. In general, there is a good correlation between superoxide dismutase activity and oxygen tolerance. Although catalase is found in some anaerobes, such as some members of the *B. fragilis* group, there is no relationship between catalase activity and oxygen tolerance. A number of anaerobes produce beta-lactamases, which accounts for their resistance to certain cephalosporins and penicillins.

TABLE 6–4. SURGICAL INFECTIONS COMMONLY INVOLVING ANAEROBES

Infection	Percentage of All Cultures Yielding Anaerobes	Proportion of Cultures Positive for Anaerobes Yielding Only Anaerobes
Bacteremia	10	4/5
Ocular infections	38	10/43
Corneal ulcers	7	9/11
Central nervous system		
Brain abscess	89	1/2–2/3
Subdural empyema	29 (84 cases)	
Epidural abscess	39 (41 cases)	
Head and neck		
Chronic sinusitis	52	4/5[a]
Chronic otitis media	56	1/10
	59	11/115
	33	0
Cholesteatoma	92	1/11
Neck space infections	100	3/4
Wound infection following head and neck surgery	95	0
Peritonsillar abscess	94	6/32
	76	6/28
Dental, oral, facial		
Orofacial, of dental origin	94	4/10
Dental abscess, endodontic origin	100	8/12
Thoracic		
Aspiration pneumonia	93	1/2[b]
	62	1/3
	100	1/3
Lung abscess	93	1/2–2/3
	85	3/4
Bronchiectasis	56	0/5
	27	
	17 (18 cases)	3/3
Empyema (nonsurgical)	76	29/63
Abdominal		
Intra-abdominal infection (general)	86	1/10
	90	1/3
	81	1/3
	94	1/7
Appendicitis with peritonitis	92	8/71
Liver abscess	52	1/3
Other intra-abdominal infection (postsurgery)	93	1/6
Wound infection following bowel surgery	60 (33 cases)	5/20
Biliary tract	45	0
	41	2/117
Obstetric-gynecologic		
Miscellaneous types	100	1/3
	74	1/3
	72	
Pelvic abscess	88	1/2
Vulvovaginal abscess	75	1/4
Vaginal cuff abscess	98	1/30
Septic abortion, sepsis	69	18/20
	67	
	63	
Pelvic inflammatory disease	25	1/14
	48	1/7
Soft tissue and miscellaneous		
Nonclostridial crepitant cellulitis	75	1/12
Pilonidal abscess	88 (41 cases)	

TABLE 6–4. (continued)

Infection	Percentage of All Cultures Yielding Anaerobes	Proportion of Cultures Positive for Anaerobes Yielding Only Anaerobes
Bite wound infections		
Dog bites	30–41	
Human bites	50–56[c]	
Diabetic foot ulcers	95	1/20
Infected diabetic gangrene (deep tissue culture)	85	1/11
Soft tissue abscesses	60	1/4
Cutaneous abscesses	62	1/5
Decubitus ulcers with bacteremia	63	10/12
Osteomyelitis	40	1/10
Gas gangrene (clostridial myonecrosis)	100	
Breast abscess (nonpuerperal)	53	5/8
	83	18/34
	79	5/41
Perirectal abscess	77 (74 cases)	

[a] Twenty-three of twenty-eight cultures (82%) yielding heavy growth of one or more organisms had only anaerobes present.
[b] Aspiration pneumonia occurring in the community rather than in the hospital involves anaerobes to the exclusion of aerobic or facultative forms two-thirds of the time.
[c] Includes clenched fist injuries.
Adapted from Summanen P, Baron EJ, Citron DM, et al: Wadsworth Anaerobic Bacteriology Manual, 5th ed. Belmont, CA, Star Publishing, 1993.

Plasmids and chromosomal elements that code for resistance to several antimicrobial agents and for transferable resistance have been found in *Bacteroides* and in *Clostridium.* These points will be discussed in the treatment section.

Exotoxins

In the case of clostridia, the most virulent of all anaerobes, various exotoxins produced by these organisms are responsible for the nature of the local lesions and the systemic manifestations.[26–31] However, the modes of action of the toxins and the individual importance of each are complex and unclear. Lecithinases, such as those produced by *C. perfringens* (alpha-toxin) and *C. novyi* (gamma-toxin), can damage or destroy cell membranes. Capillaries are made freely permeable to fluid and protein, and the resulting extravasation of fluid can cause increased anoxia in tissues. Lysis of red blood cells by alpha-toxin of *C. perfringens* is almost certainly the cause of the hemolytic anemia and hemoglobinuria seen in sepsis with this organism. The collagenases of *C. perfringens* and *C. histolyticum* destroy collagen barriers in the tissues and thus prevent localization of the infection. Destruction of reticulin around capillaries and procoagulant activity lead to hemorrhage and thrombosis, with further decrease in the oxidation-reduction potential. Proteolysis provides additional amino acids and peptides for bacterial growth. The hyaluronidase of *C. perfringens* greatly facilitates spread of the organism through the tissues. Other factors produced by pathogenic clostridia presumably are important in pathogenesis as well, but it is difficult to prove. Included would be deoxyribonucleases (*C. perfringens* and *C. septicum*), lipases (*C. novyi*), proteinases (*C. histolyticum*), and fibrinolysins. Other toxins produced by clostridia include hemolysins, neuraminidase, phospholipase, lysolecithinase, elastase, and leukocidin. *Clostridium perfringens* and *C. difficile* both produce an enterotoxin. *Clostridium difficile,* the cause of most cases of pseudomembranous colitis related to antimicrobial therapy, also produces other toxins, including one that has a cytopathic effect on almost all tissue culture cell lines and an enterotoxin.

The gram-negative anaerobic rods also produce certain exotoxins.[28] Pigmented anaerobic gram-negative rods may produce collagenase. Certain *Bacteroides* produce neuraminidase. *Bacteroides fragilis* produces a heparinase that may contribute to intravascular clotting, and so an increased dosage of heparin is required in treating the septic thrombophlebitis that may be seen during the course of infection due to this organism. The lipopolysaccharides of *B. fragilis, B. vulgatus,* and *F. mortiferum* activate the Hageman factor and thereby initiate coagulation. *Porphyromonas asaccharolytica* has ex-

TABLE 6–5. INCIDENCE OF SPECIFIC ANAEROBES IN VARIOUS INFECTIONS (WADSWORTH VA MEDICAL CENTER EXPERIENCE 1984–1990)

Parameter	Blood	CNS[a]	Head and Neck Infections	Dental	Human Bites	Animal Bites	TTA[b] and Pleural	Lung	Appendiceal Tissue or Abscess
Number of specimens	161	50	60	12	7	21	90	32	70
Number of specimens yielding anaerobes	147	19	37	11	3	10	38	11	66
Bacteroides fragilis	41	2	5	3	0	0	2	0	35
B. thetaiotaomicron	7	0	3	0	0	0	1	0	25
Other *B. fragilis* group	14	0	7	0	0	1	4	1	60
Bilophila wadsworthia	0	0	0	0	0	0	1	0	29
Prevotella melaninogenica group	0	3	10	5	0	0	18	5	3
P. intermedia-corporis	3	2	4	10	1	0	9	2	7
Other pigmented *Prevotella*	1	3	8	8	0	0	11	0	3
Porphyromonas asaccharolytica	1	0	0	0	0	0	0	0	2
Porphyromonas species	1	2	4	2	0	1	0	1	6
B. gracilis	1	1	2	0	0	0	1	1	6
Other *B. ureolyticus* group	2	0	6	6	0	1	4	1	3
P. oralis group	0	2	8	8	0	0	13	1	0
Other *Bacteroides/Prevotella* species	3	0	5	0	1	0	10	0	29
Fusobacterium nucleatum	4	3	3	5	1	1	8	2	10
F. necrophorum	1	0	0	0	0	0	0	0	2
F. mortiferum/varium	0	0	0	0	0	0	0	0	3
Other *Fusobacterium* species	4	3	5	5	1	2	0	0	3
Other gram-negative bacilli	2	2	2	3	0	1	5	1	8
Peptostreptococcus species	16	8	20	5	2	3	16	2	34
Anaerobic *Streptococcus* species	3	2	3	6	2	0	7	0	11
Veillonella species	4	0	4	5	0	1	10	1	1
Other gram-negative cocci	2	0	0	3	1	0	4	0	1
Clostridium perfringens	32	1	0	0	0	2	1	0	1
Other *Clostridium* species	21	0	0	1	0	1	2	0	19
Actinomyces species	0	7	9	7	1	1	4	0	5
Bifidobacterium species	1	1	0	5	0	0	0	0	0
Eubacterium species	3	2	8	10	1	2	10	0	21
Lactobacillus species	1	1	4	9	0	1	11	6	15
Propionibacterium acnes	7	11	10	1	1	4	5	3	5
Propionibacterium species	1	1	2	3	0	4	1	1	0
Other gram-positive bacilli	1	0	1	6	1	1	2	2	12
Staphylococcus saccharolyticus	1	0	2	0	0	1	1	1	1

[a] Central nervous system.
[b] Transtracheal aspiration.
[c] Mostly from appendiceal infections.
[d] Designations stated on culture requisition.
From Summanen P, Baron EJ, Citron DM, et al: Wadsworth Anaerobic Bacteriology Manual, 5th ed. Belmont, CA, Star Publishing, 1993.

tensive proteolytic activities, rendering it capable of hydrolyzing gelatin, casein, coagulated protein, plasma protein, and azacol, as well as collagen. *Fusobacterium necrophorum* produces leukocidin and hemolysin. Most strains of *P. intermedia* produce a lipase. All species of the *B. fragilis* group, except for *B. vulgatus,* produce extracellular hyaluronidase and chondroitin sulfatase. Elastase is rarely found in *Bacteroides*. Other enzymes produced by certain members of the genus *Bacteroides* include fibrinolysin, lysozyme, lecithinase, deoxyoxyribonuclease, phosphatase, protease, and lipase.

							Miscellaneous Soft Tissue Infections	
Peritoneal Fluid[c]	Gallbladder	Abdominal, Other	Osteomyelitis[d]	Foot Ulcer[d]	Decubitus Ulcer	Perirectal Abscess	*Below the Waist*	*Above the Waist*
126	20	15	72	278	15	15	80	33
74	17	5	20	148	8	12	32	9
37	3	3	2	17	2	8	9	0
34	0	2	2	1	0	1	4	0
93	3	8	4	15	7	10	19	0
30	0	0	0	0	0	0	0	1
3	0	1	1	15	0	0	3	2
16	0	1	2	6	0	1	4	1
5	1	1	3	15	2	3	11	0
1	0	0	0	3	0	0	8	0
3	0	0	3	5	0	2	3	0
9	0	0	1	1	0	2	0	1
3	0	0	4	10	0	3	8	0
7	0	0	0	10	0	1	1	0
24	1	2	5	22	1	4	15	3
14	0	0	0	9	0	1	1	1
2	0	0	0	1	0	0	0	0
2	0	0	0	0	0	0	0	0
7	0	0	1	5	0	2	1	0
12	0	0	0	3	0	1	7	0
41	0	3	34	225	11	10	64	9
13	1	0	3	14	2	0	4	1
3	0	0	1	9	0	1	3	0
1	0	0	0	2	1	1	2	1
1	0	3	0	4	0	0	0	0
28	3	6	0	1	1	1	3	0
6	0	0	4	7	1	1	7	1
0	0	0	0	0	0	0	1	0
29	0	2	3	19	1	4	7	3
15	0	0	0	12	1	1	3	0
3	0	1	1	14	0	1	1	4
2	0	0	0	5	1	0	0	3
15	0	1	2	4	0	0	1	0
0	0	0	0	0	0	0	1	0

Endotoxins

There have been a number of studies of the endotoxin of various gram-negative anaerobic rods.[31] In the case of the *B. fragilis* group, the endotoxin does not contain lipid A, 2-ketodeoxyoctanate, or heptose. It also lacks beta-hydroxymyristic acid. This endotoxin exhibits poor biologic activity in various test systems. *Porphyromonas asaccharolytica* also does not have any beta-hydroxymyristic acid; its endotoxin is biologically impotent. The endotoxin of other pigmented anaerobic gram-negative rods and *P. oralis* show weak biologic activity. The endotoxins of *F. necrophorum* and *F. nucleatum* vary to some extent from strain to strain in terms of content of 2-ketodeoxyoctanate and sugars and in biologic activity, but many or most strains show strong biologic activity, comparable to that of *Salmonella enteritidis*.

HOST DEFENSE MECHANISMS AND IMMUNITY

The oxidation-reduction potential of healthy tissues is well above levels necessary for anaerobic growth. Thus anaerobes cannot multiply in normal tissues. Atraumatic inoculation of guinea pigs with toxin-free spores of *Clostridium tetani* does not cause tetanus. Wounds, however, are by their very nature traumatic, and it is trauma that both initiates colonization by anaerobes and provides the atmosphere for their multiplication. Vascular damage or vascular insufficiency is probably the most important predisposing factor for anaerobic infection. Tissue damage results in a fall in both Eh and pH, and these changes, together with the breakdown of protein to produce amino acids, lead to conditions highly favorable for the growth of anaerobic bacteria. Postoperative gas gangrene following clean operations is most often encountered in patients with arterial insufficiency—patients with diabetes mellitus, atherosclerosis, and frostbite. Operations that require the use of tourniquets or bloodless field techniques favor growth of anaerobes that may be introduced into the operative site. The same is true for procedures in which there is imperfect hemostasis, excessive heat coagulation of tissues, or prolonged and traumatic use of retractors. War wounds are the classic examples of wounds that contain large amounts of necrotic tissue, providing suitable conditions for anaerobic bacterial invasion. In addition, neither cellular nor humoral components of the host defense systems[32–34] can reach the bacteria in an avascular microenvironment.

Both cell-mediated and humoral immunity may be important in protection against anaerobic infections. Certain anaerobes, such as pigmented anaerobic gram-negative rods, may inhibit phagocytosis and the killing of other organisms that may be found together with them in mixed infection. The capsules of certain organisms, such as *B. fragilis, P. asaccharolytica,* and *C. perfringens,* may be important factors in determining anaerobic infection. The mechanism by which the capsule facilitates infection with these organisms remains to be determined. There is no definitive evidence that the capsule interferes with phagocytosis, but it is a possibility. It is interesting that *B. fragilis* strains adhere to rat peritoneal mesothelium better than do unencapsulated species of *Bacteroides*.

Polymorphonuclear leukocytes have both oxygen-dependent and oxygen-independent microbicidal systems. Components of both of these systems might be important in phagocytic killing of anaerobes under conditions of varying oxygen tension. Studies performed to date have not provided a clear-cut picture of the situation. One study indicated normal killing of *B. fragilis* within polymorphonuclear leukocytes under anaerobic conditions, and another study noted normal killing of this organism under aerobic conditions. Neither random migration of polymorphonuclear leukocytes nor chemotaxis in response to factors generated by immune complexes in plasma differed significantly under aerobic or anaerobic conditions. However, chemotaxis in response to factors generated by bacteria in plasma was depressed under anaerobic conditions; one of the organisms used in this study was *B. fragilis*.

Bacteroides fragilis is more resistant to the normal bactericidal activity of serum than are other members of the *B. fragilis* group. *Fusobacterium mortiferum* is killed by serum alone or serum plus white blood cells under both aerobic and anaerobic conditions. Under anaerobic conditions, *B. thetaiotaomicron* and *B. fragilis* are phagocytosed and killed intracellularly by human polymorphonuclear leukocytes in the presence of normal serum, but not by either leukocytes or serum alone. In an aerobic environment, similar results are obtained except that *B. fragilis* is phagocytosed and killed intracellularly to some extent in the absence of serum.

Immunoglobulin and components of the alternate complement pathway participate in opsonization of *B. fragilis* and *B. thetaiotaomicron.* Antibody to the capsular polysaccharide of *B. fragilis* can be induced in animals by infection with encapsulated strains or by implantation of the capsular material itself (along with outer membrane components that stimulate antibody response). This type of immunization confers significant protection in animals against subsequent abscess development caused by *B. fragilis.* Furthermore, a study of women with acute pelvic inflammatory disease demonstrated antibody to the capsular antigen of *B. fragilis* in those in whom *B. fragilis* was part of the infecting flora.[35]

Various techniques have been used to demonstrate antibodies in animals experimentally infected and in people undergoing natural infection. With some of the gram-negative anaerobic bacilli, there may be significant cross-reactions between species. Normal subjects can also show antibody to various gram-negative anaerobic bacilli.

Endotoxins of gram-negative anaerobic bacilli have been studied for their influence on blastic transformation of lymphocytes and on polymorphonuclear leukocyte migration. The reactions are proportionate to the potency of the endotoxin and therefore more impressive in the case of *Fusobacterium* than with *Bacteroides*.

It is clear that *B. fragilis* is involved in infection more commonly than other members of the *B. fragilis* group (such as *B. vulgatus* or *B. ovatus*), despite the fact that *B. fragilis* may be outnumbered by these other members in the normal colonic flora. This may be due to encapsulation of *B. fragilis* in contrast to the usual lack of a capsule in other members of the *B. fragilis* group. As suggested earlier, the capsule may interfere with host defense mechanisms. The same may apply to *P. asaccharolytica,* which appears to be more important in infection than other pigmented anaerobic gram-negative rods that are not encapsulated.

DIAGNOSTIC CONSIDERATIONS

A list of clues suggesting that a patient may have an anaerobic infection is given in Table 6–6. The only specific clue to anaerobic infection is foul or putrid odor to secretions. Only anaerobic infection produces this type of odor, although the absence of a foul odor does not exclude the possibility of anaerobes being involved in infection. Certain anaerobes, particularly some of the cocci, do not produce the end products of metabolism that have this characteristic odor. In other cases, there will not be communication between the infected site and the examiner's nose. The remainder of the clues are not specific but nonetheless are helpful, particularly when two or more are present together. Location of infection in proximity to a mucosal surface is a clue because this is a major location for indigenous anaerobic flora. Tissue necrosis and gas in tissues or discharges are nonspecific, but they are commonly encountered with anaerobic infections. They can also occur in other types of infection and in the absence of infection, but they should make one suspect an anaerobic infection. Three types of malignancy have a special association with anaerobic infections—bronchogenic carcinoma, carcinoma of the colon, and uterine cancer.

TABLE 6–6. CLUES TO ANAEROBIC INFECTION

1. Foul odor to specimen
2. Location of infection in proximity to a mucosal surface
3. Infections secondary to human or animal bite
4. Gas in specimen
5. Previous therapy with aminoglycoside antibiotics (such as neomycin, gentamicin, and amikacin), trimethoprim/sulfamethoxazole, and most quinolones
6. Black discoloration of blood-containing exudates; these exudates may fluoresce red under ultraviolet light (pigmented *Prevotella* or *Porphyromonas* infections)
7. Presence of "sulfur granules" in discharges (actinomycosis)
8. Unique morphology on Gram stain
9. Failure to grow, aerobically, organisms seen on Gram stain of original exudate
10. Growth in anaerobic zone of fluid media or of agar deeps
11. Growth anaerobically on media containing 75 to 100 μg/ml of kanamycin, neomycin, or paromomycin (or medium also containing 7.5 μg/ml of vancomycin, in the case of gram-negative anaerobic bacilli)
12. Characteristic colonies on agar plates anaerobically (eg, *F. nucleatum* and *C. perfringens*)
13. Young colonies of pigmented anaerobic gram-negative rods may fluoresce red under ultraviolet light (blood agar plate)

Clinical Specimen Collection

Specimen collection and transport are important considerations if the surgeon wishes to document the role of anaerobes in an infection.[2] The best anaerobic bacteriology laboratory is necessarily limited by the nature of the specimen submitted and the care that was taken in transporting it. Table 6–7 lists the recommended methods of specimen collection for a variety of anaerobic infections.

Ideally, all types of specimens should be cultured for anaerobes for these simple reasons: (1) anaerobes are commonly involved in a variety of infections; (2) any type of infection may involve these organisms; and (3) many nonanaerobic organisms (especially streptococci) will grow better under anaerobic conditions than aerobically. There are practical limitations, however. Anaerobes are so prevalent as normal flora that no specimen likely to be contaminated with normal flora should be cultured for anaerobic organisms. This only imposes an unnecessary chore on the bacteriology laboratory and provides data that can be seriously misleading. The following types of specimens should *not* routinely be set up for anaerobic culture: gingival or oral swabs, gastric contents, small bowel contents, feces, expectorated sputum, voided urine, vaginal or endometrial swabs, and bronchoscopically obtained specimens when specially protected brushes or bronchoalveolar lavage are not used. In certain instances, exceptions will have to be made. For example, in suspected "blind loop syndrome" quantitation of the aerobic or facultative and anaerobic flora of the small bowel or afferent gastric loop contents may be important in diagnosis and in guiding therapy.

TABLE 6–7. SPECIMEN COLLECTION FOR ANAEROBIC CULTURE

Site of Infectious Process	Appropriate Specimen[a]	Collection Method[a]
Head and neck	Aspirate	Percutaneous needle aspiration
	Tissue biopsy	Surgically obtained
Periodontal	Gingival pocket debris	Sterile paper points into anaerobic transport broth
	Aspirate	Scaler or needle aspiration
Pulmonary	Lung aspirate	Percutaneous needle aspiration of lung
	Tissue biopsy	Surgically obtained tissue biopsy
	Deep bronchial secretions	Transtracheal aspirate, protected, bronchial brush, or bronchoalveolar lavage
Joint	Joint fluid	Percutaneous needle aspiration
Abdominal	Peritoneal fluid	Percutaneous needle aspiration
	Abscess contents	Aspirate obtained at surgery or under CT or ultrasound guidance (avoiding contamination with bowel contents)
	Bile	Bile obtained at surgery
	Tissue biopsy	Surgically obtained
Female genital tract	Peritoneal fluid	Culdocentesis
	Endometrial material	Endometrial suction or protected collector
	Tissue biopsy (others)	Surgically obtained
Bone	Biopsy	Curettings or scrapings obtained surgically
	Aspirate	Aspirate of deep tissue via uninvolved skin surface
Other soft tissue	Tissue biopsy	Surgically obtained
	Aspirate	Percutaneous needle aspiration
	Tissue	Curettings
Urine	Bladder urine	Suprapubic aspirate

[a] Aspirates should be performed after decontamination of intact skin surface with alcohol followed by povidone-iodine.

From Summanen P, Baron EJ, Citron DM, et al: Wadsworth Anaerobic Bacteriology Manual, 5th ed.

The most important consideration is to protect the organisms in the specimen from exposure to oxygen. Details of specimen transport, Gram staining, examination, and culture are presented in Chapter 2.

Special Collection Problems

Aspiration Pneumonia. Obtaining a proper specimen when aspiration pneumonia is suspected is a major problem. If there is a complicating empyema, the empyema fluid will ordinarily reflect the bacterial flora of the parenchymal disease, and information obtained from blood cultures may be useful if bacteremia is present. However, most cases of aspiration pneumonia or other anaerobic pulmonary infection are not complicated by bacteremia. Even when bacteremia occurs, only one or two of the many organisms present are cultured. Thus, at least in patients who are seriously ill, it is often desirable to do percutaneous transtracheal aspiration to bypass normal upper respiratory tract flora and to obtain the true infecting flora. Patients with severe hypoxia, hemorrhagic diathesis, or severe intractable cough should not be subjected to this procedure. If bronchoscopy is indicated to remove aspirated particulate matter, a double-sheathed bronchial brush may permit the retrieval of a reliable specimen for anaerobic and aerobic culture. (The effectiveness of this procedure depends on quantitative culture.) Without meticulous care and the use of such a double-protected brush, however, normal and transient oral flora, which may or may not actually be involved in the aspiration pneumonia, will be inadvertently cultured. It is also likely that bronchoalveolar lavage can provide reliable bacteriologic information if quantitative culture is performed.

Female Genital Infection. In the case of female genital tract infections with cul de sac abscess, culdocentesis after decontamination of the vaginal wall with povidone-iodine should yield the causative agents. Some claim that a few drops of material obtained by culdocentesis, without a cul de sac collection, will accurately reflect the bacteriology of the deeper infection. Double-protected biopsy devices (eg, Pipelle®) may be used to obtain material from the endometrial cavity in the case of endometritis. This may not be reliable in postpartum endometritis, since there is significant contamination of the endometrial cavity with vaginal flora after delivery.

Special Diagnostic Tests

Direct gas-liquid chromatography of clinical specimens may occasionally provide important clues to the presence of certain gram-negative anaerobic bacilli.[2] Presence of large amounts of butyric acid in the absence of isobutyric or isovaleric acid is indicative of the presence of *Fusobacterium* species. The presence of succinic acid in a specimen that shows only gram-negative bacilli on Gram stain is indicative of *Bacteroides.* The presence of both succinic and isobutyric acids in a specimen indicates that *Bacteroides* is present. Fluorescent antibody procedures have been developed for identification of *Actinomyces* and of certain gram-negative anaerobic bacilli in clinical material. The reagents for *Actinomyces* are not generally available.

Serologic tests are not yet practical diagnostic aids. Commercially available *C. difficile* antitoxins will neutralize the toxins produced by *C. difficile,* the principal cause of pseudomembranous colitis related to antimicrobial therapy. Thus the use of such antibody to block the cytopathic effect of *C. difficile* toxin in tissue culture constitutes a diagnostic test. Both the organism and its toxin may be present in the absence of pseudomembranous colitis on occasion, particularly in patients treated with certain cephalosporins; therefore it is necessary to demonstrate the presence of the typical plaques or pseudomembrane in addition to the toxin for definitive diagnosis.

Molecular techniques such as DNA probes are coming into use, primarily for identification of isolated organisms, but few are available commercially so far.

PROTOTYPIC INFECTIONS

In general, anaerobic infections are characterized by abscess formation and tissue destruction. Some prototypic infections will be discussed here, and some are covered in greater detail in other chapters.

Brain Abscess

Brain abscess begins as an acute suppurative encephalitis and eventually becomes localized and encapsulated; the vast majority of brain abscesses yield anaerobic bacteria. The most important underlying condition is chronic otitis media, with or without mastoiditis. Infection of the lung or pleural space is the second most common underlying condition for anaerobic brain abscess, and chronic sinusitis is third. Other underlying conditions include dental or oral infection, infection in the tonsillar or pharyngeal area, congenital heart disease, and trauma. Gram-negative anaerobic bacilli and anaerobic and microaerophilic streptococci are the most common causative agents; however, anaerobes of all other types occasionally may be found (see Chap. 34).

Aspiration Pneumonia

Aspiration pneumonia, a common postoperative complication, involves oral anaerobic bacteria in almost all cases. The three major anaerobes found are the pigmented anaerobic gram-negative rods group, *Fusobacterium nucleatum,* and anaerobic cocci, but there are a number of others such as the *P. oralis* group, *P. oris, P. buccae, B. gracilis, P. bivia,* and *B. fragilis.*

There is a distinct difference, however, between aspiration pneumonia occurring in the community and that occurring within the hospital. Community-acquired aspiration pneumonia (ie, an individual aspirating after a cerebrovascular accident at home) involves primarily anaerobic bacteria and viridans streptococci from the oral flora. *Bacteroides fragilis* or other beta-lactamase-producing anaerobes may be recovered from 30 percent of the cases. Because of the resistance problem the addition of metronidazole or clindamycin to penicillin G (or use of another appropriate regimen) is recommended in seriously ill patients.

Aspiration within the hospital frequently involves, in addition to indigenous oral flora, potential nosocomial pathogens that have colonized the upper respiratory tract. Therapy for this type of aspiration pneumonia is much more difficult. In addition to coverage for anaerobes, one must often cover nonanaerobic gram-negative bacilli (including *Pseudomonas aeruginosa* at times) and *S. aureus.* The earliest manifestation of the disease is pneumonitis alone. Without effective therapy, necrotizing pneumonia or lung abscess, either of which may be complicated by empyema, can occur.

Intra-Abdominal Infection

Intra-abdominal infection, particularly peritonitis and intra-abdominal abscess, is discussed in Chapter 38. Anaerobes can be recovered from the majority of such infections but are seldom recovered in pure culture.[11–13] Most infections are mixed, containing both anaerobes and facultative or aerobic bacteria. In most of these infections, the source of the organism is the bowel flora, particularly the flora of the colon. Accordingly, the *B. fragilis* group, and *B. fragilis* and *B. thetaiotaomicron* in particular, is recovered regularly. Other gram-negative anaerobic rods may also be found. Anaerobic cocci are commonly found, as are clostridia, especially *C. perfringens* and *C. ramosum*.

Postabortal Sepsis

Anaerobes are important in postabortal sepsis. Although clostridia account for only a small percentage of these infections, they often cause the most severe and dramatic illnesses. Clostridial infection of the uterus starts as a localized chorioamnionitis with invasion in the placenta of a dead fetus. This process, known as fetal emphysema, is relatively benign, but the gaseous vaginal discharge, crepitus of the uterine wall, and striking radiographic findings may make it difficult to distinguish from more serious infections. The next stage is a low-grade endometritis with vaginal discharge and uterine tenderness, with or without gas formation. The most severe form of this process extends beyond the endometrium to the uterine muscle and results in necrosis, which may be accompanied by perforation, peritonitis, and bacteremia. The patient is toxic, exhibits tachycardia out of proportion to the fever, and has uterine and abdominal pain and foul gaseous vaginal discharge that reveals numerous clostridia on direct Gram stain. A unique and dramatic clinical picture accompanies severe clostridial sepsis—hemolytic anemia, hemoglobinemia, hemoglobinuria, disseminated intravascular coagulation, bleeding tendency, bronze-colored skin, hyperbilirubinemia, shock, and anuria. *Clostridium perfringens* is the key pathogen in patients with sepsis and hemolytic anemia. It may also be important in less severe cases of postabortal sepsis, along with anaerobic streptococci, gram-negative anaerobic bacilli (including, at times, *B. fragilis*), other clostridia, aerobic streptococci (most often group A), and coliforms.

Gas Gangrene

A classic but fortunately uncommon variety of anaerobic infection is clostridial myonecrosis, or gas gangrene.[29] The term gas gangrene should be limited to those infections that invade muscle and produce massive necrosis of tissue. It is a clinical syndrome, and clostridial species other than *C. perfringens* may be involved. Gas gangrene usually manifests itself with a sudden appearance of pain and heaviness in the region of an injury. The onset may be so sudden that it suggests a vascular accident. The pain steadily increases in severity but remains localized, spreading as the infection itself spreads. Soon local edema and a thin hemorrhagic exudate can be noted. The tachycardia is out of proportion to the slight elevation of temperature. The skin is tense, white, often marbled, colder than normal, and very tender. Bronze discoloration increases with time. Local swelling and toxemia increase gradually, and the serous discharge becomes more profuse. Bullae filled with dark red or purplish fluid appear, and gas becomes manifest, although usually in relatively small amounts. A peculiar sweet smell may be present. The patient may remain clear mentally with a profound terror of impending death; a toxic delirium is also characteristic. Later, there may be overwhelming prostration and toxemia. As time goes on there may be a drop in blood pressure. The patient has a peculiar gray pallor, weakness, and profuse sweating.

The evidence of the disease at the skin surface and the clinically demonstrable gas are relatively minor compared to the extensive involvement of underlying muscle, which can be seen only at operation. At first the muscle is pale and edematous, but later the color changes, the blood supply is lost, contractility disappears, and gas may be seen. As the disease progresses, the muscle becomes red with mottled purple and the consistency becomes pasty or mucoid. Finally, the muscle is diffusely gangrenous, dark greenish purple or black, friable, and even liquefied.

Clostridium perfringens is present in 80 percent of cases, *C. novyi* in 40 percent, *C. septicum* in 20 percent, and *C. bifermentans* in a few cases. *Clostridium histolyticum* and *C. fallax* are uncommon. The diagnosis of clostridial myonecrosis is made clinically. When material can be obtained for Gram stain, the characteristic large, relatively broad, gram-positive (or gram-variable) bacilli may be an important clue, as is disruption of white blood cells caused by the action of the toxin. Definitive identification of clostridia in the wound is not of great value, however, because many wounds, particularly traumatic wounds, may be colonized with these organisms without evidence of infection. It is crucial to keep in mind that the infection may spread rapidly and irreversible tissue changes may develop in a matter of hours. Accordingly, immediate operative exploration is indicated when suspicion exists. It is important to recognize also that gas gangrene may occur after elective surgery, especially operations on the lower limbs, bowel, and gallbladder. A common error is to leave casts, splints, or dressings undisturbed. At the slightest suspicion of infection, they must be removed and the wound thoroughly inspected.

Pseudomembranous Colitis

The primary cause of antimicrobial agent-induced pseudomembranous colitis is now known to be the toxins of *C. difficile.*[23] Whether the postoperative pseudomembranous colitis sometimes seen prior to the antimicrobial era was also due to this organism is unknown. Similarly, it is not known whether ischemic colitis may involve this organism and its toxins, although there is some evidence that they may be involved. Essentially all antimicrobial agents with the exception of vancomycin are capable of inducing this complication, but it is seen most often after clindamycin, lincomycin, ampicillin, and the cephalosporins. The entire spectrum of clinical colitis can be seen ranging from a relatively mild diarrhea to severe intractable diarrhea, toxic megacolon, perforation of the colon, shock, and sometimes death. The sine qua non of antibiotic-associated pseudomembranous colitis is the presence of the distinctive elevated yellowish plaques on the colonic mucosa, or frank pseudomembrane. Recovery of *C. difficile,* even in high numbers, and demonstration of the cytotoxin of this organism, even in high titer, do not necessarily establish the diagnosis, because these may be seen on occasion in the course of antimicrobial therapy without any evidence of colon pathology. Colonoscopic or proctoscopic examination is the best way to establish the diagnosis. It must be kept in mind that some lesions, particularly early in the course of the illness, may be found only on the right side of the colon.

Intestinal Overgrowth Syndromes

Bowel bacterial overgrowth syndromes (blind loop syndrome) may result from prior operations, such as production of an afferent loop or ileal bypass for obesity, and operation may be required to correct the cause of bacterial overgrowth in the bowel. The steatorrhea and macrocytic anemia, which are important findings in this process, are a result of deconjugation of bile acids and adsorption of vitamin B_{12}, usually high in the small bowel. Various anaerobes, notably members of the *B. fragilis* group, are important in this regard, along with other types of organisms (see Chap. 42).

Infection in Malignancy

The strong association between *C. septicum* infection and malignancy should be mentioned. Carcinoma of the colon and cecal pathology of other types should be suspected in patients who have infection with *C. septicum.*

Actinomycosis

Actinomycosis is frequently grouped with fungal infections because of its clinical resemblance. *Actino-*

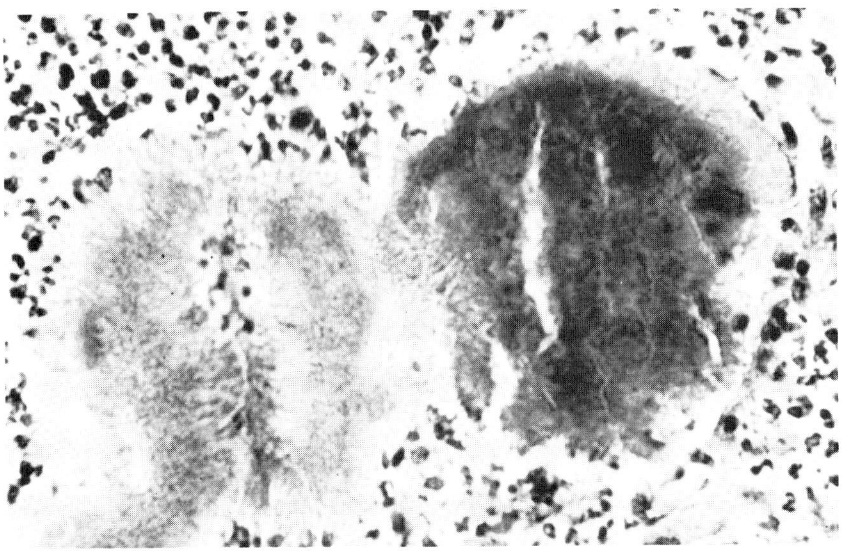

Figure 6–2. Abdominal actinomycosis. "Sulfur granule" expressed from purulent material draining from fistula. Note the fine filaments of the organisms at the periphery (×472).

TABLE 6–8. SUSCEPTIBILITY OF ANAEROBES TO ANTIMICROBIAL AGENTS[a]

Percentage of Strains Susceptible at Breakpoint	*B. fragilis* Species	*B. fragilis* Group (Excluding *B. fragilis*)	*B. gracilis*[b]	Other *Bacteroides*	*Fusobacterium*
Greater than 95%	Ampicillin+Sulbactam Piperacillin+Tazobactam Ticarcillin+Clavulanate Cefoperazone+Sulbactam Imipenem Chloramphenicol Metronidazole	Ampicillin+Sulbactam Piperacillin+Tazobactam Ticarcillin+Clavulanate Cefoperazone+Sulbactam Imipenem Chloramphenicol Metronidazole	Imipenem Chloramphenicol	Piperacillin Ampicillin+Sulbactam Ticarcillin+Clavulanate Cefoperazone Cefotaxime Cefoxitin Cefoperazone+Sulbactam Ceftizoxime Imipenem Chloramphenicol Clindamycin	Penicillin G Piperacillin Ampicillin+Sulbactam Piperacillin+Tazobactam Ceftizoxime Imipenem Chloramphenicol Clindamycin Metronidazole
85–95%	Cefotetan Cefoxitin Clindamycin Piperacillin	Piperacillin	Metronidazole	Cefotetan Ceftazidime Ceftriaxone	Ticarcillin+Clavulanate Cefoperazone Cefotaxime Cefotetan Cefoxitin Ceftriaxone Cefoperazone+Sulbactam
70–84%	Ceftizoxime Moxalactam	Cefoxitin Clindamycin	Piperacillin Ampicillin+Sulbactam Moxalactam Cefoperazone+Sulbactam	Penicillin G Moxalactam	Ceftazidime Moxalactam
50–69%	Cefoperazone Cefotaxime Ceftazidime Ceftriaxone	Cefoperazone Cefotetan Ceftizoxime Moxalactam	Penicillin G Ticarcillin+Clavulanate Cefoperazone Cefotaxime Cefotetan Cefoxitin Ceftizoxime Clindamycin		
Less than 50%	Penicillin G	Penicillin G Cefotaxime Ceftazidime Ceftriaxone	Ceftazidime		

Percentage of Strains Susceptible at Breakpoint	*Bilophila*	*Peptostreptococcus*	*Clostridium perfringens*	Other *Clostridium* Species	Non–spore-forming Gram-Positive Rods
Greater than 95%	Chloramphenicol Metronidazole Imipenem Ticarcillin Ticarcillin+Clavulanate Cefoxitin	Penicillin Piperacillin Ampicillin+Sulbactam Ticarcillin+Clavulanate Cefoperazone Cefotetan Ceftazidime Ceftriaxone Moxalactam Cefoperazone+Sulbactam Imipenem Chloramphenicol	All drugs are active at ≥95% level	Amoxicillin Ampicillin Carbenicillin Penicillin G Piperacillin Ticarcillin Ampicillin+Sulbactam Imipenem Chloramphenicol Metronidazole	Penicillin G Piperacillin Ampicillin+Sulbactam Ticarcillin+Clavulanate Cefotaxime Ceftizoxime Imipenem Chloramphenicol
85–95%	Clindamycin	Metronidazole			Cefotetan Cefoxitin Ceftazidime Ceftriaxone Cefoperazone+Sulbactam Clindamycin
70–84%	Cefotaxime Cefotetan	Clindamycin		Cefoxitin Moxalactam Clindamycin	Cefoperazone Moxalactam
50–69%				Cefoperazone Cefotaxime Ceftizoxime Ceftriaxone	Metronidazole
Less than 50%	Penicillin G Ceftizoxime			Ceftazidime	

[a] These data represent a compilation of studies from the Wadsworth Anaerobe Laboratory. The ranking within a group does not reflect degree of activity; drugs are arranged by classes.
[b] Strains that were previously identified as *B. gracilis* will probably be split into several different taxa. Also, if one uses formate/fumarate (a growth supplement for *B. gracilis*) in the test medium, many strains will have considerably lower MICs with certain antibiotics. The susceptibility patterns will also vary among the new taxa.
Adapted from Finegold SM, Baron EJ, and Wexler H. A Clinical Guide to Anaerobic Infections. Belmont, CA: Princeton Scientific Productions/Star Publishing, 1992.

myces israelii is actually an anaerobic bacterium that is part of the normal flora and is the usual cause of actinomycosis in people, although *A. naeslundii* or other members of the genus, as well as *Propionibacterium propionicum,* have been implicated in human disease. *Actinomyces bovis* is primarily a pathogen of swine and cattle. The bacterium is an anaerobic gram-positive rod that grows in thin filamentous strands at 37C. Tangled masses of organisms form macroscopic specks known as sulfur granules, which are the hallmark of the infection.

Actinomycosis is a chronic suppurative infection producing abscess cavities, separated by bands of fibrosis and interconnected by fistulous tracts. At the periphery of the lesion, granulomas consisting of large, lipid-laden macrophages can sometimes be found imparting a yellow color to the tissue. Spread may be hematogenous but is usually by direct extension.

Three main types of infection are recognized—cervicofacial, thoracic, and abdominal.[15,16] Cervicofacial disease usually begins in the mouth or oropharynx, commonly the result of a break in the normal protective barriers (eg, gingivitis). The infection extends into adjacent bone and burrows through soft tissues, producing multiple abscesses with interconnecting fistulas and sinus tracts that drain to the skin surface. Pus expressed from the sinus tracts frequently contains the sulfur granules, the matted masses of organisms that are characteristic of actinomycosis. There is little pain until the infection is far advanced.

Pulmonary actinomycosis is a chronic fibrosing and abscess-forming infection, which frequently resembles tuberculosis or malignancy. As in any aspiration pneumonia, the abscesses may also contain multiple organisms from the mouth. Direct involvement of the pleura and adjacent ribs is common, but free pleural effusions are rare.

Abdominal actinomycosis frequently is first manifested as a fistula in the abdominal wall. The organism gains access to the peritoneal cavity either by hematogenous spread from the oral pharynx or by direct penetration of the bowel mucosa (from within by a sharp object such as a fishbone or from without by a penetrating wound). Appendicitis may be a primary source of abdominal actinomycosis.

There have been many reports of chronic endometrial actinomycosis, most frequently related to intrauterine devices used for contraception. The infection may spread to the adjacent fallopian tubes.

Osteomyelitis caused by actinomycosis is indistinguishable from hematogenous osteomyelitis caused by other bacteria and can be found in any bone in the body.

Examination of fresh pus from draining sinuses frequently shows the characteristic sulfur granules. They are easiest to find on gauze dressings used to cover sinuses, and they appear as small 1- to 2-mm yellow granules. Crushed granules stained with Gram stain show gram-positive branching filamentous organisms (Fig. 6–2).

Direct anaerobic culture of pus of resected tissue will frequently yield the organism, although *Actinomyces* is quite fastidious. Small, white colonies appear in 2 to 5 days and can be subcultured under strict anaerobic conditions.

Skin tests and serology ordinarily play no role in the diagnosis.

The best treatment is prolonged use of penicillin. High dose intravenous therapy is given for 2 to 3 weeks, followed by oral penicillin for 6 to 12 months. Incision and drainage of abscesses should be done only after institution of penicillin coverage. Clindamycin, and sometimes a tetracycline or erythromycin, can be used in penicillin-sensitive patients. The nature of accompanying flora may influence the choice of therapy.

TREATMENT OF ANAEROBIC INFECTIONS

There are three principles of treatment of anaerobic infections: (1) make the tissue environment hostile for anaerobic proliferation; (2) check the spread of anaerobic bacteria to healthy tissues; and (3) neutralize the toxins.

To control the local environment, a variety of surgical measures includes debridement of dead tissue, removal of foreign bodies, drainage of pus, excision of malignancies, improvement of circulation to the part, and improved oxygenation of tissues. The surgeon must also obtain material for diagnosis by biopsy or aspiration.

Antimicrobial therapy is also important to prevent the spread of infection. In vitro susceptibility tests, properly performed, serve as a guide to drug therapy for anaerobic infections. In view of the increasing resistance of many anaerobes to antimicrobial agents, it is desirable for hospitals to do periodic surveys of susceptibility and to do susceptibility studies on individual isolates from seriously ill patients or patients not responding to empiric therapy. Patterns of susceptibility are most useful for initiating therapy in an empiric manner. Table 6–8 lists the most common anaerobic bacteria and their susceptibility to various agents. In serious anaerobic infections, antimicrobial therapy must be intensive and prolonged, because these infections have a tendency to relapse if therapy is discontinued too soon. In the case of anaerobic pulmonary infections, therapy is usually required for several weeks. Liver abscess and other intra-abdominal infections may require even more prolonged therapy.

Bacteroides fragilis is a particular problem; it is both the most commonly encountered of all anaerobes and the most resistant to antimicrobial agents. The beta-lactamase produced by the *B. fragilis* group is one of the major means by which this organism manifests resistance to certain antimicrobial agents. The beta-lactamases produced are primarily cephalosporinases but also account for significant destruction of penicillins. Other anaerobic bacteria also produce beta-lactamases, most of which are primarily penicillinases.

The nature of the various organisms in mixed infections will influence the choice of drugs. Drugs active against anaerobic bacteria in vitro may be quite inactive against accompanying aerobic or facultative organisms, and vice versa. Other factors that influence choice of drugs include the toxicity of the various agents, whether or not the patient is allergic to given agents, the lack of penetration of the central nervous system of certain drugs (eg, by clindamycin), the excellent bactericidal activity of metronidazole, and the renal and hepatic functional status of the patient. Patients who are very ill with suspected anaerobic pulmonary infection, in whom the bacteriology is not yet worked out, should receive therapy adequate to cover the most resistant organisms. In the case of hospital-acquired aspiration pneumonia, additional therapy may be required for the nonanaerobic bacteria present.

In patients with antimicrobial agent-associated pseudomembranous colitis caused by *C. difficile,* discontinuation of the offending antimicrobial agent is the first step. In patients who are relatively sick, oral vancomycin (125 to 500 mg given at 6-hour intervals) should be given for 10 days to 2 weeks. The smaller dose is usually effective. Oral metronidazole, 500 mg q6h, is as effective and much cheaper. Patients should be observed carefully for at least 4 to 6 weeks after discontinuation of therapy, because relapse occurs in about 30% of patients.

REFERENCES

1. Holdeman LV, Cato EP, Moore WEC (eds): Anaerobe Laboratory Manual, 4th ed. Blacksburg, VA, Virginia Polytechnic Institute and State University, 1977, pp 1–156.
2. Summanen P, Baron EJ, Citron DM, et al: Wadsworth Anaerobic Bacteriology Manual, 5th ed. Belmont, CA, Star Publishing, 1993, pp 1–230.
3. Hentges DJ (ed): Human Intestinal Microflora in Health and Disease. New York, Academic Press, 1983.
4. Rosebury T: Microorganisms Indigenous to Man. New York, McGraw-Hill, 1962.
5. Finegold SM: Anaerobic Bacteria in Human Disease. New York, Academic Press, 1977, pp 1–710.
6. Finegold SM, George WL: Anaerobic Infections in Humans. San Diego, CA, Academic Press, 1989, pp 1–851.
7. Finegold SM, Goldstein EJC (eds): Proceedings of the First North American Congress on Anaerobic Bacteria and Anaerobic Infections. Clin Infect Dis 16 (Suppl. 4):5159–5457, 1993.
8. Styrt B, Gorbach SL: Recent developments in the understanding of the pathogenesis and treatment of anaerobic infections. N Engl J Med 321:240, 298, 1989.
9. Anderson CB, Marr JJ, Ballinger WF: Anaerobic infections in surgery: clinical review. Surgery 79:313, 1976.
10. Sim FH: Anaerobic infections. Orthop Clin North Am 6:1049, 1975.
11. Bennion RS, Baron EJ, Thompson JE Jr, et al: The bacteriology of gangrenous and perforated appendicitis—revisited. Ann Surg 211:165, 1990.
12. Bennion RS, Thompson JE, Baron EJ, Finegold SM: Gangrenous and perforated appendicitis with peritonitis—treatment and bacteriology. Clin Ther 12:31, 1990.
13. Finegold SM, Bennion RS, Thompson JE, et al: Gangrenous and/or perforated appendix: clinical outcome and in vitro susceptibility testing. Hosp Pract 25:3, 1990.
14. Willis AT: Clostridia of Wound Infection. London, Butterworths, 1969, pp 1–470.
15. Wohlgemuth SD, Gaddy MC: Surgical implications of actinomycosis. South Med J 79:1574, 1986.
16. Dove J. Actinomycosis in surgical biopsies. J R Soc Med 72:106, 1979.
17. Bohnen JMA, Solomkin JS, Dellinger EP, et al: Guidelines for clinical care: anti-infective agents for intra-abdominal infection: a Surgical Infection Society policy statement. Arch Surg 127:83, 1992.
18. Nichols RL, Condon RE: Role of the endogenous gastrointestinal microflora in postoperative wound sepsis. Surg Annu 7:279, 1975.
19. Walker AP, Edmiston CE Jr, Krepel CJ, Condon RE: A prospective study of the microflora of nonpuerperal breast abscess. Arch Surg 123:908, 1988.
20. Wittmann DH, Bergstein JM, Frantzides C: Calculated empiric antimicrobial therapy for mixed surgical infections. Infection 19(Suppl 6):S345, 1991.
21. Nichols RL: Surgical wound infection. Am J Med 91(Suppl 3B):54S, 1991.
22. Finegold SM, Baron EJ, Wexler H: A Clinical Guide to Anaerobic Infections. Belmont, CA, Star Publishing, 1992.

23. Rolfe RD, Finegold SM (eds): *Clostridium difficile:* Its Role in Intestinal Disease. Orlando, FL, Academic Press, 1988, pp 1–408.
24. Krohn MA, Hillier SL, Lee ML, et al: Vaginal *Bacteroides* species are associated with an increased rate of preterm delivery among women in preterm labor. J Infect Dis 164:88, 1991.
25. Hillier SL, Krohn MA, Kiviat NB, et al: Microbiologic causes and neonatal outcomes associated with chorioamnion infection. J Infect Dis 165:955, 1991.
26. Stevens DL, Mitten J, Henry C: Effects of alpha and theta toxins from *Clostridium perfringens* on human polymorphonuclear leukocytes. J Infect Dis 156:324, 1987.
27. Stevens DL, Troyer BE, Merrick DT, et al: Lethal effects and cardiovascular effects of purified alpha- and theta-toxins from *Clostridium perfringens.* J Infect Dis 157:272, 1988.
28. Kasper DL, Finegold SM (eds): Virulence factors of anaerobic bacteria (symposium). Rev Infect Dis 1:245, 1979.
29. MacLennan JD: The histotoxic clostridial infections of man. Bacteriol Rev 26:177, 1962.
30. Hofstad T: Virulence factors in anaerobic bacteria. Eur J Clin Microbiol Infect Dis 11:1044, 1992.
31. Zaleznik DF, Kasper DL: Role of bacterial virulence factors in pathogenesis of anaerobic infections. In Finegold SM, George WL (eds): Anaerobic Infections in Humans. San Diego, Academic Press, 1989, pp 81–95.
32. Crabb JH, Finberg R, Onderdonk AB, Kasper DL: T cell regulation of *Bacteroides fragilis*—induced intraabdominal abscesses. Rev Infect Dis 12(Suppl. 2):S178, 1990.
33. Hofstad T: Immune responses to anaerobic gram-negative bacteria in health and disease. Nahrung 28:717, 1984.
34. Kasper DL, Finberg RF, Crabb J, Onderdonk AB: Immune mechanisms in the prevention of intra-abdominal abscess formation. Scand J Infect Dis Suppl 62:29, 1989.
35. Paavonen J, Valtonen VV, Kasper DL, et al: Serological evidence for the role of *Bacteroides fragilis* and *Enterobacteriaceae* in the pathogenesis of acute pelvic inflammatory disease. Lancet 1:293, 1981.

BIBLIOGRAPHY

Finegold SM: Anaerobic Bacteria in Human Disease, New York, Academic Press, 1977.

Finegold SM, George WL: Anaerobic Infections in Humans. San Diego, Academic Press, 1989.

Finegold SM, Goldstein EJC (eds): Proceedings of the First North American Congress on Anaerobic Bacteria and Anaerobic Infections. Clin Infect Dis 16(Suppl. 4): 5159–5457, 1993.

Styrt B, Gorbach SL: Recent developments in the understanding of the pathogenesis and treatment of anaerobic infections. N Engl J Med 321:240, 298, 1989.

Willis AT: Clostridia of Wound Infection. London, Butterworths, 1969.

CHAPTER 7

Mixed and Synergistic Infections

David H. Ahrenholz, Richard L. Simmons

Since the era of Pasteur and Koch, emphasis in the discipline of infectious diseases has been on the study of diseases caused by individual pathogenic organisms. Koch's postulates are easily fulfilled only if a single species can be grown in pure culture and reinoculated to produce a specific disease. Thus, traditional textbooks of infectious disease are organized according to the individual causative agents and their microbiologic characteristics. Similarly, surgeons frequently refer to the infections they treat as being caused by individual bacterial species.

It is increasingly apparent, however, that many infections treated by surgeons are caused by combinations of organisms rather than single pathogens. Three trends have directed attention to this fact: (1) the discovery of antibiotic therapy effective against pyogenic cocci, so that life-threatening diseases caused by other pathogens now predominate; (2) the increased frequency of opportunistic infections; and (3) the recognition of the role of anaerobic bacteria as copathogens.

The majority of surgical infections result from breaks in the normal cutaneous or mucosal barriers that permit the endogenous mixed flora on these surfaces to penetrate and infect the surrounding tissue. There is little understanding of how the individual microbial components of such complex mixtures interact with each other or with the tissue defenses, but a profound simplification of the normal cutaneous and mucosal flora occurs after inoculation into tissues, and certain bacteria frequently emerge as principal copathogens.

Mixed and synergistic surgical infections usually contain anaerobic bacteria for two reasons: (1) the inocula contain mixed anaerobes; and (2) surgical infections take place in anaerobic environments, where blood supply is deficient and necrotic debris is plentiful. Even if aerobes are present in the initial inoculum, they soon deplete the available local oxygen. At that point, facultative organisms can switch to anaerobic metabolism, while the strict aerobes cannot survive. Finally, anaerobic fermentative metabolic pathways release a variety of complex organic compounds used as substrates by other anaerobic bacteria.

MIXED BACTERIAL COLONIZATION OF BODY SURFACES

Most body tissues are isolated from contact with bacteria, and the presence of bacteria in these areas is pathognomonic of infection. Exceptions are the skin and mucous membrane surfaces of the respiratory, alimentary, and external genital tracts. These surfaces represent two distinct physical barriers to bacterial invasion, the cornified skin and the mucosa-lined surface. The skin is specifically adapted to resist water loss and withstand abrasion. It loses most of its resistance to bacterial invasion if subjected to prolonged contact with moisture. The mucosa-lined tracts retain their effectiveness as microbial barriers under wet conditions, but this ability is rapidly lost if they are allowed to dry completely.

The microbial ecology of the skin and the mucosa-lined tracts is only partially understood. Many resident and transient microbial species coexist on the skin, and mechanisms exist for reestablishing a fairly stable population of mixed microbes whenever the balance has been temporarily disturbed (see Chap. 3). Only *Staphylococcus epidermidis* and diphtheroids survive as residents on the rather dry, lipid-rich, mildly acidic, nutritionally deprived surfaces of normal glabrous skin (see Chaps. 3 and 31). Fecal gram-negative bacilli and oral streptococci, which frequently contaminate normal skin, survive only transiently unless moisture is constantly provided. Even then, colonization is impossible unless the normal flora are displaced or eradicated. For example, the vaginal organisms deposited on the skin of the neonate during delivery are rapidly replaced by the normal cutaneous flora from the environment.[1]

The mucosa-lined surfaces possess a more complex ecosystem. The oral cavity becomes inoculated with bacteria within hours of birth by nursing or contact with environmental surfaces.[1] The ability of bacteria to adhere to surfaces is a prerequisite to survival within the mouth, since the oral cavity is constantly washed by saliva and intermittently exposed to the abrasive effects of eating, toothbrushing, and dental flossing. Different types of bacteria preferentially adhere to each type of surface.[2] *Streptococcus sanguis* organisms have such a high affinity for dental enamel that chewing only temporarily displaces them. *Streptococcus salivarius* has a similar affinity for the tongue and oral mucosa. Some other bacterial genera attach specifically to plaque streptococci and not to teeth enamel.[3] Even *Streptococcus mutans,* the organism most frequently associated with dental caries, has surprisingly little intrinsic affinity for dental enamel, and its survival as a pathogen depends on a complex set of interactions with other flora. Dental plaque begins as a storage form of glucose for *S. sanguis,* within the confines of which huge numbers of aerobic and anaerobic bacteria can grow. *Streptococcus mutans* releases acids during growth that remain in contact with dental enamel under a blanket of plaque and etch it away, exposing dentin. Numerous aerobic and anaerobic bacteria then invade and destroy the exposed dentin, resulting in dental caries.[4]

Anaerobic organisms flourish in the oral cavity, not only on exposed plaque-covered surfaces but especially within the gingival cleft, where the oxygen tension is very low.[5] The fermentative metabolic pathways used release a variety of complex organic compounds that function as substrates for other bacteria. The majority of oral organisms require extremely low oxygen environments and complex organic substrates for growth. Most of these organisms have not yet been grown in vitro.

The remainder of the gastrointestinal tract is also sterile at birth but becomes contaminated almost synchronously with the oral cavity. The empty stomach represents an effective acidic deterrent to the development of a resident gastric population of bacteria. With each food bolus, the pH temporarily rises, and oral bacteria traverse the stomach to the small bowel.

Bacteria resident in the small bowel must adhere to bowel mucosa or be washed away by the fecal stream. Because of the rapid transit time of intestinal contents, bacterial populations remain low and are supplemented by the intermittent influx of oral microorganisms. A few specifically adherent bacteria have been identified: for example, travelers' diarrhea is caused by an adherent, enterotoxigenic strain of *Escherichia coli*. The ability to adhere to small bowel mucosa is associated with cell surface antigens, and diarrhea is produced by an enterotoxin, each property being coded separately by the bacterial genome. If the organism has only the surface antigen or only the ability to produce the toxin, disease does not result.[6] Travelers' diarrhea can be prevented if purified cell surface antigen is ingested before the pathogenic *E. coli.*

In the colon, bacterial adherence to the mucosa is less critical because the flow of the fecal stream is intermittent. Here, aerobic bacteria rapidly remove available oxygen, and multiple species of anaerobes flourish, out-numbering aerobes 1000 to 1 (see Chap. 3). Bacteria in stool number $10^{11.5}$ per gram of feces, representing hundreds of species.[7] Bacteria comprise half the total weight of feces.

The significance of the normal colonic microbial interactions in humans is poorly understood. Clearly, the normal gastrointestinal flora inhibit the colonization by pathogenic bacteria (eg, *Salmonella, Shigella, Pseudomonas*).[7,8] No detectable nutritional effects other than excessive water and electrolyte loss are noted in patients who have undergone colectomy. In ruminant animals, such as cattle, however, anaerobic bacteria in the foregut break down cellulose into fatty acids and alcohols, which are directly absorbed into the bloodstream. The bacteria are then digested in the hindgut and serve as a significant source of nutrients. There is little evidence for such beneficial interactions between humans and their colonic flora. Bacterial growth is probably a secondary phenomenon as the colon absorbs water and stores feces before evacuation.

The male genital tract, except for the distal urethra, remains sterile throughout life in the absence of infection. The female tract, however, becomes colonized by fecal organisms early in life. During the childbearing years, lactobacilli come to predominate. Their presence usually inhibits the growth of other organisms, but during pregnancy, the vaginal secretions change, and overgrowth by *Candida albicans* or other organisms frequently results. Vaginal secretions represent too little flow to physically remove bacteria, and bacterial adherence to the vaginal mucosa is not essential to colonization. Virulent strains of the gonococcus, however, have surface pili and a high affinity for urethral mesothelium. Nonpiliated strains of gonococcus have a much lower affinity for genitourinary epithelium and are much less virulent.[9]

Bacterial Competition

The microbial world is generally characterized by a fierce competition for available nutrients, especially under aerobic conditions. Any aerobic organism that gains a temporary advantage will multiply and displace other organisms by sheer weight of numbers. Not every species, however, can metabolize every available energy source. If oxygen and sufficient glucose are available in a given microenvironment, inoculation of aerobic organisms will result in a bacterial population explosion, as glucose is actively transported across the bacterial cell wall and used as a rich energy source. Use of all other energy sources is repressed by specific genetic control mechanisms. As the glucose is depleted, enzymes for transport and use of other substrates are derepressed or induced by specific organic compounds. The first bacterial species to produce the enzymatic machinery to utilize a secondary energy source will proliferate. This sequence may be repeated endlessly. One of the reasons *Pseudomonas* species are so ubiquitous in nature is that they carry the genetic information to use over 100 organic substrates for energy.

Aerobic organisms in the presence of oxygen preferentially oxidize organic substrates to carbon dioxide and water. This results in the highest energy yield and permits exponential growth. Under anaerobic conditions, fermentative processes must be used, typically producing less than 5 percent of the energy available by oxidative metabolism. Thus obligate anaerobes rarely show the explosive growth potential of aerobes even under ideal conditions and may require days or weeks for culture in vitro.

Anaerobic metabolism also produces many complex organic end products, most of which can be used as energy sources by another microorganism. Complex bacterial interactions are thus characteristic of anaerobic environments. Surgical infections, which occur under conditions of injury and tissue death, frequently provide a relatively anaerobic environment. Since polymicrobial contamination is inevitable whenever the mechanical barriers of skin or mucosa are breached, many surgical infections initially contain multiple organisms. The mixture tends to persist when anaerobic metabolism fosters complex substrate production.

Most bacteria have but one response to the presence of nutrients—rapid growth and reproduction. Those that reproduce most rapidly are most successful. Some bacteria, however, have other competitive mechanisms for survival in mixed colonies. Some secrete antibiotics: the bacteriocins of *Bacillus* species, for example, are locally bacteriostatic or bactericidal. In fact, all naturally occurring antibiotics are microbial products and facilitate survival of the organism.

Other bacteria rely on their ability to rapidly alter the available nutrients into forms unusable by their competitors. For example, lactobacilli, which are very acid tolerant, rapidly convert glucose to lactic acid. This process has a low energy yield but has two advantages: it removes glucose available for the growth of other bacteria and produces an acidic environment that is inhibitory to most other bacterial species. Similarly, *S. mutans* in the mouth rapidly converts ingested sucrose to dextran polymer, which is unsuitable as an energy source to most other bacteria. The dextran in this case acts as a surface to which a variety of bacteria can adhere secondarily, but only those that produce dextranase can use the material for growth.[10]

If a bacterial species can occupy all the available binding sites on a surface, it can successfully dominate the microenvironments. *Streptococcus sanguis* has a high affinity for tooth enamel and can prevent colonization of the teeth by introduced *S. mutans*. If *S. sanguis* is removed by toothbrushing, *S. mutans* will adhere readily to the teeth. However, once *S. mutans* becomes established, the dextran it elaborates creates a new area for bacterial adherence.[11]

The preceding examples of bacterial competition illustrate the general principle of *amensalism,* in which interacting bacteria derive no benefit from the interaction. Examples of true *parasitism,* in which the parasite derives benefit at the expense of the host, are rare in bacterial interactions. A few intracellular parasites of bacteria are known, such as *Bdellovibrio,* which attacks *E. coli.* However, bacterial interactions become remarkedly altered when one organism produces an end product that another organism can use as a substrate for growth. This is an example of *commensalism*—mutual association with benefit to one partner without adverse effects on either. Often the bacteria are found in association because the substrate that the dependent partner consumes is unavailable elsewhere. The association can become *symbiotic* when both partners benefit from the association, a common occurrence. Many bacteria are rapidly inhibited by the accumulation of their metabolic end products. A second organism that removes these end products allows the continued growth of the first organism.[12]

Microbial Synergism

A useful term in describing microbial infections is *synergism,* an effect on the host found in the presence of two or more organisms not seen with either organism alone. Many bacteria involved in synergistic infections are not considered typical pathogens, that is, organisms capable in pure culture of invading a normal host. Opportunistic organisms are those that can establish an infection only in a host with impaired defense mechanisms. Trauma, especially extensive burns, neoplastic disease, collagen-vascular disease, and chemotherapy, can all alter the host defense mechanisms and allow the establishment of opportunists. The term *opportunistic synergism* probably best describes the sequence of events in which a pathogenic organism invades a host, establishes a disease, and suppresses local or systemic host defenses to the extent that an opportunistic organism can become established. These synergistic effects have been reviewed by Mackowiak.[13] Virtually any opportunistic organism can produce disease if host defenses are sufficiently impaired. By extension of this concept, the organisms need not even be synchronously present. For example, rheumatic fever after group A streptococcal infection resulting in valvular heart damage can predispose to bacterial endocarditis years later. In this chapter, we will emphasize synergistic infections, where two bacteria synchronously produce an effect not seen with either alone. As noted above, not all bacterial synergistic actions produce disease.

Mechanisms of Microbial Synergism. Mackowiak[13] identifies four principal mechanisms of microbial interactions that are synergistic:

1. One organism may facilitate transmission to or colonization of the host by a second organism.
2. The organism may lower local or systemic host resistance, allowing invasion by a second organism.
3. One organism may provide growth factors for another organism.
4. One organism may increase the virulence of another.

Increased Transmission. Synergistic mechanisms may have only an indirect effect on the host. In the broadest sense, some microbial interactions merely increase the transmission of a virulent organism. For example, *Treponema pallidum* is a virulent organism capable of penetrating intact skin, but it is extremely sensitive to oxygen and dies rapidly on exposed surfaces. Nevertheless, the open chancre of primary syphilis has a redox potential of −180 to −250 mV and is teeming with the spirochetes, which are readily transmitted by direct contact. Apparently *Fusobacteria, Bacteroides,* and anaerobic streptococci, which are regularly isolated from these lesions, serve to maintain the low redox potential necessary for survival and transmission of the spirochete.

In humans, influenza virus produces changes that increase the susceptibility of patients to secondary pyogenic pneumonia. Initially, this was thought to be due to edema and cellular debris producing suitable culture material for the secondary bacterial pathogens. There is now increasing evidence that primary viral infections produce anatomic alterations in the tracheal epithelium, allowing adherence of bacterial pathogens. Fainstein et al[14] found an increased adherence of *Staphylococcus aureus, Haemophilus influenzae,* and *Streptococcus pneumoniae* to tracheal epithelium both in naturally acquired acute respiratory illness and in volunteers inoculated with influenza virus vaccine. To produce clinical influenza in swine, a virus and *H. influenzae* must be inoculated intranasally.[15]

Eichenwald et al[16] found that simultaneous infection with a respiratory virus and a bacterial pathogen in the nasopharynx of infants results in a much greater spread to the surrounding environment of both organisms. These organisms may then infect other children nearby. Children with a marked rhinorrhea exhibit a stuffy-nose syndrome, with frequent sneezing, snorting, and coughing. Asymptomatic children may also disseminate bacteria and have been called "cloud babies." In both groups, the ability to spread organisms is correlated with the presence of both a respiratory virus and a bacterial pathogen. In the first group, it is possible that the severe rhinorrhea found when both organisms are present results in increased coughing, which spreads the organism as an aerosol. In asymptomatic infants, the presence of a virus allows persistence of pathogenic bacteria that would otherwise be readily eliminated. These increased numbers of pathogens are spread to the local environment, and the incidence of infection increases.

Lowered Host Resistance

BREAKDOWN IN LOCAL DEFENSE. There is a time-dependent factor in many synergistic interactions. Commonly, the presence of one organism alters the local conditions so that a second organism can become established. The first organism is then no longer required to maintain the disease. If the order of introduction of these organisms is reversed, the disease does not result.

Certainly the most common form of bacterial interaction occurs when a pathogenic organism causes a break in anatomic defenses, which subsequently allows one of a variety of opportunistic organisms to invade the host. This anatomic deformity can be either chronic scarring or an acute open lesion. Acute rheumatic fever that follows a streptococcal infection can produce chronic changes in the heart valves that predispose to late bacterial endocarditis. Because the events in this chain of action are widely separated in time, they do not fit the definition of true synergistic infection. A similar example is the damage to fallopian tubes caused by gonorrhea that predisposes women to recurrent salpingitis. The scarring is a permanent anatomic change. The salpingitis in the scarred tubes is usually a mixed bacterial infection with organisms less virulent than the gonococcus.

Any pathogen that produces an open lesion of a cutaneous or mucosal surface can permit secondary invasion by other organisms. Classic veterinary examples include foot rot in sheep,[17] liver granulomas of turkeys,[18] and liver abscesses of cattle,[14] which all produce huge economic losses for farmers.

In humans, the nematode *Strongyloides* can carry enteric bacteria from the intestine to various internal organs during its migration from the bowel. Polymicrobial septicemia is said to be suggestive of *Strongyloides* enteric infection.[15] *Trichinella spiralis* and *Nematospiroides dubius* possibly transmit *Salmonella typhimurium*.

LoVerde et al[19] have found an association between *Schistosoma* species and *Salmonella*. Pili on *Salmonella* specifically adhere to the tegument of the male schistosomes, producing persistent *Salmonella* infections in humans. The mucosal lesions produced by the worms may contribute to the disease as well. Many more prosaic examples can be cited. Typhoid perforations of the distal ileum, perforated amebic ulcers, and actinomycotic abscesses all lead to polymicrobial intra-abdominal infections.

These examples represent a breach of the local physical barriers to microbial invasion. Many infections seen in clinical surgical practice result when earlier tissue damage so impairs local host defenses or so alters the tissue microenvironment that superinfection results. The classic example is the indolent diabetic foot ulcer produced by trauma to a relatively ischemic and neuropathic area. Colonization of the lesion with mixed flora may be stable for prolonged periods until a predominant set of pathogens emerges.

Secondary infections of chronic visceral abscesses and necrotic granulomas are more exotic examples of breakdown in local defense. Secondary bacterial infection of an amebic liver abscess, an aspergilloma in an old tuberculous cavity, or invasive pulmonary aspergillosis emerging from a resolving pyogenic lung abscess in a transplant recipient are sometimes seen.

BREAKDOWN OF SYSTEMIC DEFENSES. A variety of pathogens (eg, measles virus, Epstein-Barr virus, cytomegalovirus, *Mycobacterium tuberculosis,* and *H. capsulatum*) are capable of suppressing cell-mediated immunity (Table 7–1).[13] Cytomegalovirus infections increase the lethality of *Pseudomonas, Staphylococcus,* and *Candida* infections in mice, and bacterial superinfection of cytomegalovirus-infected patients is a common lethal syndrome in recipients of organ transplants.[20] Other infections (eg, influenza, measles, mumps, and herpesvirus) can produce a nonspecific suppression of fixed and circulating phagocytic cells. Malaria and influenza have been implicated in the suppression of humoral immunity, but exact mechanisms are unclear.

Temporary depression of cell-mediated immunity occurs in a variety of infections,[13] although there is little direct evidence that this increases the risk of secondary infections. An exception is the increased incidence of tuberculosis during epidemics

TABLE 7–1. STUDIES DEMONSTRATING SUPPRESSION OF CELL-MEDIATED IMMUNITY DURING INFECTIONS

Infection	Animal Studied	In Vitro Studies[a]	In Vivo Studies[a]	Immunogen[b]
Influenza	Human		+	T, H, C, Cx, Tr
Parainfluenza	Mouse		+	*Listeria monocytogenes*
Measles	Human		+	T
Infectious mononucleosis	Human	+	+	C, SK, SD
Herpes simplex	Human	+		HSV-1
Cytomegalovirus	Human	+	+	M, P, PM
Tuberculosis	Human		+	T, H, C, M
Histoplasmosis	Human	+		H
Leprosy	Human	+	+	L, T, C, Tr, P
Syphilis	Human	+		P
Pertussis	Human		+	T
Streptococcus	Human		+	T
Trypanosomiasis	Rabbit	+	+	T
Toxoplasmosis	Mouse		+	*Schistosoma mansoni*
Live virus vaccines[c]	Human	+	+	H, C, P, PM

[a] + denotes type of study.
[b] C, *Candida*; Cx, coccidioidin; H, histoplasmin; HSV-1, herpes simplex virus type 1; L, lepromin; M, mumps; P, phytohemagglutinin; PM, pokeweed mitogen; SD, streptodornase; SK, streptokinase; T, tuberculin; Tr, trichophyton.
[c] Rubeola, rubella, mumps, and attenuated influenza virus vaccines.
From Mackowiak PA: N Engl J Med 298:21, 1978.

of measles. Measles in malnourished infants in some tropical countries is associated with herpetic ulcerations of the mouth, which in turn become infected by mixed oral flora, leading to the gangrenous infection known as "noma" (chancrum orum).[21] Adenoviral infections are more frequent after smallpox and typhoid vaccination. The commonly observed activation of herpes labialis during pyogenic infections suggests that this is a result of a temporary depression of cell-mediated immunity. Conversely, resistance to experimental herpes infections is increased by BCG or *Corynebacterium parvum* inoculation, both documented stimulators of cell-mediated immunity.[13]

Because the AIDS virus selectively destroys CD4+ lymphocytes, subsequent infection with other organisms such as *M. tuberculosis, M. avium-intracellulare,* pneumocystis, toxoplasmosis, cryptococcus, CMV, or herpes virus is virtually inevitable. AIDS is fatal not as a primary infection but because of the opportunistic infections that it permits.[22] (See Chap. 11.)

Many microorganisms, especially viruses, nonspecifically impair the reticuloendothelial system, which may allow secondary invasion by opportunistic organisms (Table 7–2).[13] Suppression of phagocytosis is transient and species specific and may be directly related to the quantity of virus present. Viruses apparently can produce a metabolic block of the glycolytic pathway in the phagocytic cell to prevent phagocytosis.[13]

There are experimental studies to show that infection by a phagocytosis-suppressing virus followed by bacterial infection produces a higher mortality rate than is found with the individual organisms alone. This occurs only when the viral infection precedes the bacterial infection. Organisms that produce a chronic hemolytic state, such as *Plasmodium* and *Bartonella,* may also impair phagocytosis by iron overload of the reticuloendothelial system.[13]

In addition, the capsule from many types of bacteria is capable of blocking phagocytosis.[23] The presence of encapsulated organisms, such as *Bacteroides fragilis* or *Prevotella melaninogenica,* may therefore prevent phagocytosis of other organisms present within a mixed inoculum.[24] A few bacteria secrete substances (leukocidins) that are directly cytocidal to phagocytic cells—*S. aureus, F. necrophorum,* and group A *Streptococcus pyogenes.*[25]

Microorganisms can alter the humoral immune system as well. Antibody production may be inhibited or enhanced, or the complex interactions of immunoregulation may be disturbed. The agents

TABLE 7–2. STUDIES DEMONSTRATING SUPPRESSION OF THE RETICULOENDOTHELIAL SYSTEM DURING VIRAL INFECTIONS

Infection	Animals Studied	In Vitro Studies[a]	In Vivo Studies[a]	Phagocyte Challenge
Influenza	Mouse, guinea pig	+	+	*Haemophilus influenzae Bacillus anthracis,* Baker's yeast, *S. aureus, S. pneumoniae, Staphylococcus epidermidis*
Parainfluenza	Mouse	+		*H. influenzae, S. aureus*
Adenovirus	Human	+		*Neisseria meningitidis*
Sandfly fever	Human	+		*S. aureus,* aggregated albumin
Mumps	Guinea pig	+		*Bacillus anthracis*
Reovirus	Mouse		+	*S. aureus*
Herpes simplex	Human	+		Endotoxin
Measles	Human	+		Endotoxin

[a] + denotes type of study.
From Mackowiak PA: N Engl J Med 298:21, 1978.

known to be associated with inhibition of antibody production are listed in Table 7–3. The mechanisms of suppression are unknown, but hypotheses include: (1) an infection of the B lymphocytes themselves, (2) competitive inhibition of noncommitted antibody-producing cells, and (3) neoplastic transformation by viruses.[13] In addition, interferon induced by viral infection may suppress antibody synthesis.

Malaria in the experimental animal impairs humoral immunity by an unknown mechanism, resulting in protection from spontaneous autoimmune

TABLE 7–3. STUDIES DEMONSTRATING SUPPRESSION OF THE HUMORAL IMMUNE SYSTEM BY AGENTS OR MEDIATORS INVOLVED IN HUMAN INFECTIONS

Agent or Mediator	Animal Studied	In Vitro Studies[a]	In Vivo Studies[a]	Immunogen
Influenza virus	Mouse		+	*S. pneumoniae*
Lymphocytic choriomeningitis virus	Mouse		+	Ovalbumin, human serum albumin, sheep erythrocytes
Junin virus	Guinea pig		+	Human erythrocytes
Newcastle disease virus	Rabbit	+		Egg albumin, bovine serum, albumin
Malaria	Human, mouse		+	Tetanus toxoid, sheep erythrocytes, *Salmonella typhi* (O antigen)
Trypanosoma brucei	Mouse		+	Sheep erythrocytes
Toxoplasma gondii	Mouse		+	Sheep erythrocytes
Trichinella spiralis	Mouse		+	Sheep erythrocytes
Endotoxin	Rabbit, mouse		+	*Neisseria meningitidis,* actinophage, sheep erythrocytes
Interferon	Mouse	+	+	Sheep erythrocytes, concanavalin A, phytohemagglutinin, lipopolysaccharide

[a] + denotes type of study.
From Mackowiak PA: N Engl J Med 298:21, 1978.

disease. Malaria also enhances the oncogenic potential of certain viruses, for example, induction of lymphomas in mice is enhanced by *Plasmodium berghei* infection. Dengue is normally a mild febrile illness but becomes hemorrhagic fever if the patient has circulating heterologous dengue antibodies.[26] This may occur by passive transfer of antibodies from mother to child or by earlier infection with a heterologous strain. Similarly, unusually severe respiratory syncytial viral infections can occur in those persons previously inoculated with an attenuated vaccine.[27]

Certain microorganisms may stimulate IgA blocking antibodies that protect secondary pathogens from circulating IgM. The secondary invaders are coated with IgA, thereby blocking IgM attachment, which normally would result in death of the cells by phagocytosis or complement activation. Within dental plaque, secretory IgA, as well as IgG, IgM, and lactoferrin, are extensively degraded by resident bacteria, especially *Streptococcus, Bacteroides,* and *Capnocytophagia* species.[28]

Nutritional Synergism. The third mechanism by which microbes interact occurs when one organism provides a growth factor for another organism. For example, tetanus spores inoculated into normal viable tissue will not germinate unless other facultative bacteria are present to provide the proper oxidation-reduction potential. It has been assumed that this is the major mechanism by which aerobic and anaerobic bacteria interact in mixed surgical infections. Most species of anaerobic bacteria are so sensitive to oxygen that even a few minutes exposure to room air is lethal. Even *B. fragilis,* the most common anaerobic pathogen in humans, is unable to grow in such conditions, although it can survive for extended periods of time in contact with oxygen.

Infections involving *Toxoplasma gondii* and cytomegalovirus are common in patients with disseminated cancer. In these infections, both organisms occupy the same cells, and the *Toxoplasma* rosettes tend to form around the cytomegalovirus inclusion bodies. There is speculation that *Toxoplasma* derives nutrients in this way.[29]

Several other well-documented examples are known. In the synergistic gangrene of Meleney, the microaerophilic, nonhemolytic *Streptococcus* thrives only if hyaluronidase and a heat-labile growth factor usually provided by *S. aureus* are present.[17] *Prevotella melaninogenica* has a requirement for vitamin K, which facultative diphtheroids apparently provide in many mixed infections.[30] Additional synergistic interactions also have been identified between *Streptococcus pyogenes* and *Staphylococcus aureus,* which cause a rather severe form of necrotizing fasciitis.[31]

In fusospirochetal gingivitis, four types of organism are typically isolated. These include *Treponema microdentium,* a small *Fusobacterium,* an anaerobic hemolytic *Streptococcus,* and an anaerobic *Vibrio.* Combinations of three or fewer of these organisms usually fail to produce characteristic necrotic lesions. Socransky et al[32,33] showed that *T. microdentium* requires isobutyrate, polyamines, and a low redox potential for growth. The organism could be grown in the presence of a facultative diphtheroid accompanied by either a *Fusobacterium* or a motile, gram-negative, anaerobic rod (*Prevotella*).

Brook has studied the relative growth rates of both aerobes and anaerobes in murine subcutaneous abscesses. The addition of *Bacteroides* species markedly increased the rate of growth for most facultative organisms.[34] *Candida albicans* also stimulates the growth of *Staphylococcus aureus* intraperitoneally in mice.[35] Nutritional factors may be responsible, but blockade of phagocytosis is a more likely mechanism.

Conferred Virulence. The fourth mechanism of microbial synergism occurs when one organism confers increased virulence onto another microorganism. *Entamoeba histolytica* usually exists as a commensal organism in the large intestine, feeding on bacteria and superficial mucosal cells. It can become highly invasive in laboratory animals only if allowed to associate for 6 to 12 hours with certain bacteria before inoculation. This suggests that some virulence factors are derived from the intestinal bacteria.[12]

The best example, however, is the transmission of antibiotic resistance factors between organisms. This is especially common among the Enterobacteriaceae but has also been demonstrated from *E. coli* to *B. fragilis*. Transmissible drug resistance was discovered in Japan in 1959, when a strain of *Shigella* resistant to chloramphenicol, tetracycline, streptomycin, and sulfonamides was isolated from a patient with dysentery.[36] Since that time, resistant strains to most of the commercially available antibiotics have been found throughout the world. Strains resistant to ampicillin, kanamycin, neomycin, chloramphenicol, streptomycin, tetracycline, sulfonamides, and penicillin are especially common. Multiple antibiotic resistance is usually transmitted to an extrachromosomal plasmid consisting of two parts. The first part is an r-determinant, which codes for resistance to one or more antibiotics. The resistance transfer factor (RTF) is an independent sex factor responsible for the formation of sex pili.

Pili-bearing bacteria attach to nonpili-bearing cells and transfer the resistance plasmid by conjugation. The recipient cell now becomes fertile and, after forming its own sex pili, can further transmit the resistance factor.

Transmission of drug resistance is different from selection of drug-resistant organisms, in that multiple drug resistance is usually transmitted. This is especially important in diseases being treated with multiple antibiotics because emergence of resistant strains requires multiple sequential mutations, whereas antibiotic resistance can be transmitted in one step during conjugation.[36]

Gram-positive organisms are also capable of transmitting a plasmid for the enzyme beta-lactamase. This splits the lactam ring of penicillin, conferring penicillin resistance. Gram-positive cells do not undergo conjugal transfer but rely on transduction by a viral vector. As viral phage particles are formed in a bacterial cell, they sometimes incorporate parts of the bacterial genome, including plasmids keying for beta-lactamase. These phage particles can then specifically attach to phage-susceptible strains of bacteria. After attachment, the genetic contents are injected into the cell, which can now elaborate beta-lactamase. The cell is not always killed after injection of the viral genome if the viral genome is incomplete or if the cell undergoes lysogeny in which a specific repressor for expression of the viral genome is elaborated, preventing cell lysis. The virally injected DNA can then undergo recombination with the bacterial genome to allow replication and expression of the antibiotic resistance plasmid. These resistance mechanisms are described in greater detail by Joklik and Willett.[36]

Even in the absence of direct transmission from one organism to another, bacteria producing penicillinase, cephalosporinase, or other extracellular enzymes that inactivate antibiotics can protect otherwise sensitive copathogens from these antibiotics. The best examples are penicillin-resistant mixed infections with *S. aureus,* where the extracellular penicillinase protects the penicillin-sensitive copathogens.[37] This also probably occurs with *Bacteroides* infections, since virulent *B. fragilis* strains elaborate many enzymes, including a penicillinase and cephalosporinase.[38]

DIAGNOSTIC CLUES TO MIXED BACTERIAL INFECTIONS

The mixed infections of greatest importance to surgeons contain bacteria or fungi, and anaerobes are usually present. The findings suggestive of anaerobic infection are also associated with many mixed infections. The clinical clues to anaerobic infections provided by Finegold are equally applicable to mixed infections (Table 7–4).[39] Especially suggestive are a foul odor, extensive tissue necrosis, gas in the tissue, or discharge.

Infections of tissue in proximity to a mucosal surface characteristically contain mixed flora. These include dental infections, aspiration pneumonia, lung abscess, bronchiectasis, peritonitis, intra-abdominal abscess, wound infection following bowel surgery or trauma, perirectal or ischial rectal abscess, gas-forming or necrotizing soft tissue infections, infections following human bites, and many gynecologic infections. Although most cutaneous infections are caused by *S. aureus,* mixed infections are becoming more common (see Chap. 31).

When the Gram stain shows a mixture of morphologic types of bacteria, failure to isolate more than one organism is usually due to inadequate anaerobic technique. But it is useless to culture for mixed organisms when specimens are contaminated with normal flora, such as throat cultures, gingival or vaginal swabs, expectorated sputum, gastric contents, small bowel contents, or feces. These specimens will be incorrectly reported as mixed infections. Culture results of tissue biopsy specimens are more reliable. The collection and transport of specimens for anaerobic cultures have been described (see Chap. 2). The pathogenic aerobes are relatively easy to culture and identify, and the clinician is aware of their presence early. The surgeon depends on the Gram stain to indicate a

TABLE 7–4. CLINICAL CLUES TO POSSIBLE MIXED BACTERIAL INFECTION

I. Clinical setting suggestive of infection due to colonization by bacteria normally resident on mucosal or skin surfaces
   A. Soft tissue infection due to acute or chronic skin breaks, especially of perineal region and feet
   B. Intra-abdominal infection due to a perforated viscus
   C. Gynecologic infections after instrumentation or operation
   D. Soft tissue infections of head and neck due to mucosal trauma or disease
   E. Infection after human or animal bite
II. Infection associated with malignancy or other process resulting in tissue destruction
III. Necrotic tissue, skin necrosis, pseudomembrane formation
IV. Gas in tissues or discharges
V. Foul-smelling discharge

Adapted from Finegold SM: Anaerobic Bacteria in Human Disease, Orlando, Academic Press, 1977, p 41.

mixed infection until the anaerobic cultures are examined and reported (usually 48 hours).

In many mixed infections, the limitations of the laboratory will prevent the identification of some of the organisms present. Not every organism is virulent, however, and, with time, only a few species persist. Sequential culturing of mixed infections will identify the microflora that emerge in the face of surgical or antimicrobial therapy.

PRINCIPLES OF TREATMENT OF MIXED BACTERIAL INFECTIONS

The surgical management of mixed soft tissue infections is largely determined by the level of tissue invaded and presence or absence of pus or necrotic tissue (Table 7–5).[40–44] Infections of skin (level 1) rarely require surgery and respond to local care, elevation, and antibiotics. In subcutaneous tissue (level 2), incision and drainage of purulent abscess material are often curative, even without antibiotics. Infections of the fascial planes or muscle (levels 3 and 4) are major infections requiring surgical debridement to remove necrotic tissue and obtain adequate cultures (see Chap. 31).

Localized purulent fluid collections usually respond to aspiration but mixed infections of body cavities, such as acute peritonitis, mandate exploratory surgery to control the source of contamination, irrigate the body cavity, drain loculated pockets of pus, and aspirate fluid for cultures (see Chap. 38). Antibiotic choice is often guided by the Gram stain of recovered fluid.

Pathogens in Mixed Bacterial Infections

Not all organisms are major pathogens in mixed infections.[43,44] The virulence of the pyogenic cocci, the enteric gram-negative facultative organisms, pseudomonads, and mycobacteria is well established. The pathogenic role of other bacteria is variable (see Chap. 9).

The role of some anaerobic bacteria found in mixed infections is uncertain. A bacterial species is a pathogen requiring treatment if: (1) there is repeated isolation of the same organism from a patient over a period of time, (2) the organism is grown in pure culture, or (3) if the Gram stain or quantitative culture shows that one organism predominates.[39] These criteria define certain anaerobic organisms that are pathogens, and infections with such organisms should be treated (see Tables 7–1 and 7–6).

Bacteroides fragilis is the most commonly pathogenic anaerobe in clinical infections and is most resistant to antimicrobial agents.[39] It is isolated in pure culture more often than any other anaerobic organism. Other *Bacteroides* species, such as *B. thetaiotaomicron,* appear virulent, whereas *B. ovatus* and *B. ruminocoli* are less often associated with infection. *Prevotella melaninogenica,* which is commonly found in mixed bacterial infections, is so dependent on other organisms to supply growth factors that, alone, it is rarely capable of causing disease.[39]

Of the anaerobic gram-positive cocci, *Fusobacterium nucleatum, F. necrophorum,* and *F. varium* are commonly found as part of the mixed flora and are capable of causing infections in pure culture.

TABLE 7–5. INFECTIONS ASSOCIATED WITH MIXED BACTERIA

Soft tissue	
Skin (level 1)	Human bite cellulitis
Subdermis (level 2)	Perineal or pilonidal abscess, diabetic foot ulcer, Meleney ulcer, postoperative wound infection
Fascia (level 3)	Necrotizing fasciitis
Muscle (level 4)	Nonclostridial myonecrosis
Body cavities	
Abdomen	Peritonitis
Thorax	Empyema
Sinuses	Sinusitis, mastoiditis
Middle ear	Bacterial otitis media
Oropharynx	Vincent's disease, peritonsillar abscess
Organs	
Lung	Aspiration pneumonia, lung abscess
Breast	Breast abscess
Liver, spleen, brain	Visceral abscess
Uterus	Postpartum endometritis, septic abortion
Fallopian tubes	Salpingitis

Adapted from Bartlett JG: Anaerobic bacteria: general concepts. In Mandel GL, Douglas RG, Bennett JE (eds): Principles and Practice of Infectious Diseases, New York, Churchill Livingstone, 1990, p 1834.

TABLE 7–6. MAJOR ANAEROBIC COPATHOGENS ASSOCIATED WITH MIXED BACTERIAL INFECTIONS

Gram-negative bacilli
- *Bacteroides fragilis*[a]
- *Prevotella melaninogenica*[a]
- *Fusobacterium nucleatum*[a]
- *F. necrophorum*
- *F. varium*
- *F. mortiferum*

Gram-positive cocci[a]
- *Peptococcus* (especially *P. magnus, P. asaccharolyticus, P. prevotii*)
- *Peptostreptococcus* (especially *P. anaerobius, P. intermedius,*[b] *P. micros*)
- *Microaerophilic cocci* and *streptococci*

Gram-positive spore-forming bacilli
- *Clostridium perfringens*[a]
- *C. ramosum*
- *C. septicum*
- *C. novyi*
- *C. histolyticum*
- *C. sporogenes*
- *C. sordellii*

Gram-positive non–spore-forming bacilli
- *Actinomyces*
- *Arachnia*
- *Eubacterium* (especially *E. lentum, E. limosum, E. alactolyticum*)
- *Bifidobacterium eriksonii*

[a] These five organisms or groups of organisms account for two-thirds of all clinically signifcant anaerobic isolates.
[b] *P. intermedius* is actually microaerophilic and belongs in the genus *Streptococcus*.
From Finegold SM: Anaerobic Bacteria in Human Disease, Orlando, Academic Press, 1977, p. 68.

The microaerophilic streptococcus can also cause infection, although the viridans group of streptococci is less pathogenic.[39]

Most clostridial species, including *Clostridium perfringens* and *C. septicum,* clearly can cause serious infections, as can *Actinomyces* species, *Arachnia,* and *Bifidobacterium eriksonii*.[43,44]

Many bacteria are benign and not capable of causing infection by themselves, including most species of *Bifidobacterium, Propionibacterium,* and *Eubacterium,* most anaerobic lactobacilli (with the exception of *Lactobacillus catenaforme*), and most spirochetes, except *T. pallidum*. None of these require treatment in immunocompetent hosts.[39]

Antibiotic Choice in the Treatment of Mixed Infections

The debate over the optimal antibiotic treatment of mixed bacterial infections will not be resolved in this brief chapter (see Chap. 29). In relatively healthy persons undergoing early operative treatment of localized infections, eradication of one synergistic group (facultative organisms or anaerobes) may be sufficient for cure.[45–47] But several investigators have reported bacteremia and death caused by the untreated group of organisms, especially in elderly or immunocompromised patients.[48,49] Therefore most clinicians begin empirical treatment with antibiotics effective against both facultative gram-negative organisms and anaerobes when their presence is suspected in clinical infection.

Cephalosporins such as cefoxitin, cefotetan, and cefotaxime and semisynthetic penicillins are relatively nontoxic and have antibacterial activity against facultative and anaerobic organisms. A number of beta-lactam antibiotics are effective for primary treatment in otherwise healthy individuals or for prophylaxis after abdominal trauma.[50,51]

Imipenim/cilastatin has been used for more severe, deep-seated infections in frail or elderly patients. Semisynthetic penicillins (ticarcillin/clauvulanate) and ampicillin/sulbactam use a beta-lactamase inhibitor for increased efficacy.[52] Chloramphenicol is an older and more toxic drug that is often overlooked but remains a useful agent in highly selected, seriously ill patients. Single agents can safely be used in primary treatment of mixed infections.[53]

Infections caused by mixed gram-positive organisms usually respond to cephalosporins or clindamycin. Vancomycin is effective for severe infections caused by mixed staphylococci and streptococci, despite recent reports of vancomycin resistance.[54,55] Gentamicin has a marked synergistic action with vancomycin against staphylococci and streptococci.[56]

Many surgeons prefer a combination of two or more antibiotics for treatment of mixed infections. An aminoglycoside is often combined with clindamycin, metronidazole, or a semisynthetic penicillin.[57–59] Pharmacokinetic studies prevent excessive or inadequate serum levels and minimize toxic side effects.[60] Aztreonam can be substituted for the aminoglycoside in patients with renal failure. No single antibiotic or combination of agents has demonstrated superior efficacy in a randomized, stratified clinical trial for treatment of mixed infections.[52,53,61–64]

The culture reports should be examined to confirm the presence of mixed organisms and assure the antibiotics are appropriate. *Enterococcus* occasionally emerges as a predominant organism after treatment and usually responds to ampicillin.[51,65] But strains resistant to even vancomycin and gentamicin are increasingly prevalent.[55] If *Candida* superinfection occurs, modest doses of amphotericin (0.5 mg/kg/day) are very effective.[66] Fluconazole may be less satisfactory as an alternative agent.[67]

In addition, preliminary reports indicate hyperbaric oxygen, combined with appropriate antibiotics and extensive surgical debridement, decreases the morbidity and mortality of severe mixed soft tissue infections,[68] although no randomized clinical or experimental trials have been performed.[69,70]

HUMAN MIXED INFECTIONS

Mixed infections in humans are usually the result of inoculation of soft tissue or a body cavity by oral flora, enteric flora, or the synergistic combination of *Staphylococcus aureus* and streptococci. Abscesses of solid organs such as liver, spleen, or brain are more rarely encountered (see Table 7–5).

Mixed Infections with Oral Flora

The oral flora contain large numbers of the viridans group of streptococci, including *S. sanguis, S. salivarius,* and *S. mutans,* which have little ability to invade tissues.[71] In a gingival crevice, anaerobes such as *Prevotella melaninogenica, Viellonella, Actinomyces,* and the spirochetes, including *Spirillum* and *Treponema* species, proliferate. Most of these organisms are of low virulence alone but, as a mixture, are responsible for such destructive lesions as necrotizing gingivitis, noma, and tropical ulcer.[72] They also have been isolated from peritonsillar, pharyngeal space, and otogenic cerebral abscesses.[73–75]

Much of the evidence for the synergistic interactions of oral microorganisms is summarized in Table 7–7.[32,33,76–82] Fusiform and spirochetal organisms predominate in these infections. In necrotizing gingivitis, for example, four zones of tissue destruction are found.[80] In the deepest zone, spirilliform organisms invade healthy tissue. Next is a necrotic area and then a zone infiltrated by leukocytes. At the surface is a confluent bacterial mat. The invading spirochetes produce the necrosis supported by the other synergistic bacteria.

Most oral spirochete species have not been cultured because their nutritional requirements are so complex. For example, *Treponema microdentium* requires isobutyrate, polyamines, and an anaerobic environment for growth.[32] Diphtheroids and fusobacteria may supply these factors in clinical infections.

Fusobacterium necrophorum is a virulent organism even in pure culture. It produces a potent leukocidal exotoxin.[78,79] Other products include a hemolysin, a cytoplasmic toxin, and cell wall proteolytic enzymes.[77]

Corynebacterium pyogenes, a facultative diphtheroid, lowers the redox potential in mixed infections, allowing the growth of anaerobes. It secretes a growth factor for *F. necrophorum* and vitamin K required by *P. melaninogenica*.[78,79]

Prevotella melaninogenica is associated with many oral flora infections.[43,44] It elaborates a capsule that blocks phagocytosis of nearby organisms[33]

TABLE 7–7. MECHANISMS OF BACTERIAL SYNERGISM IN FUSOSPIROCHETAL INFECTIONS

Interacting Organisms	Mechanisms	References
Organisms usually present: a spirochete (*Treponema* or *Spirillum* species), a diphtheroid (*Corynebacterium* species), a fusiform rod (*Fusobacterium*), a gram-negative anaerobic rod (*Prevotella*)		
Fusobacterium necrophorum	Destroys leukocytes (leukocidin)	78,79
	Also produces a hemolysin and cytoplasmic toxin	77
	Produces cell wall-bound proteolytic enzymes	77
	Produces viable L-form after penicillin therapy	77
Corynebacterium pyogenes	Lowers pH for anaerobes	78,79
	Growth factor for *F. necrophorum*	78,79
	Provides vitamin K for *P. melaninogenica*	80
Diphtheroids with either *Fusobacterium* or gram-negative anaerobic rod (*Prevotella*)	*T. microdentium* requires isobutyrate, polyamines, and lowered Eh for growth	32
Treponema microdentium	Invades surrounding tissue, allowing other bacteria to proliferate	80
Prevotella melaninogenica or *B. fragilis*	Encapsulated forms produce an antiphagocytic capsule	33
P. melaninogenica required for experimental fusospirochetal infection in guinea pigs	Unknown	33
F. necrophorum liver abscesses are potentiated by *P. melaninogenica, B. fragilis,* or *F. nucleatum*	Unknown	81

and requires hemin and vitamin K for growth. Fusiform bacteria and spirochetes isolated from human dental infections are insufficient to produce necrotizing infections in guinea pigs in the absence of *P. melaninogenica.* The most severe infections occur when spirochetes, diphtheroids, fusiform rods, and gram-negative anaerobic rods are combined (see Table 7–7).[33] One or more of these organisms may be omitted if the local conditions already facilitate the growth of the other bacteria.

Necrotizing Gingivostomatitis (Trench Mouth). Necrotizing gingivostomatitis characteristically occurs in young adults under conditions of stress, poor nutrition, and poor oral hygiene. It is extremely painful, with rapid invasion of the gingiva around the teeth producing pockets of necrosis. Ultimately, there is a breakdown of the dental ligament and surrounding bone, with loss of the teeth. The disease is prevented by good nutrition combined with daily plaque removal. For acute infection, warm water lavage with gum debridement and scaling of the teeth provides symptomatic relief and rapid healing. In patients with fever, lymphadenopathy, or septicemia, penicillin or erythromycin is given orally. These agents are of little benefit without effective local care.

Vincent's Disease. A similar disease, also called Vincent's angina or Vincent's stomatitis, causes a pseudomembranous ulceration of tonsils, pharynx, tongue, or oral mucosa. The onset is usually sudden with mild fever accompanied by pain, lymphadenopathy, difficulty in eating, and foul breath. These pharyngeal diseases may resemble diphtheria. Direct wet smear examination under dark-field microscopy reveals the spirochetal flora.

Peritonsillar Abscess. Peritonsillar and deep pharyngeal space abscesses caused by mixed oral flora produce intense local pain, swelling, and systemic toxicity. These lesions dissect through adjacent tissue planes and may cause septicemia or airway obstruction. The agents include streptococci, anaerobic bacteria, or mixed aerobic and anaerobic organisms. Therapy is high-dose penicillin and surgical drainage with daily debridement (see Chap. 33).

Tropical Ulcer, Noma. Tropical ulcer is a fusospirochetal infection with oral flora but typically occurs on the ankle following injury or abrasion. A similar lesion of the face is called noma. Malnutrition and skin maceration are common predisposing factors. Pain, fever, toxemia, and marked disability are characteristic. The ulcer rapidly enlarges and may extend deeply, with destruction of underlying muscle, tendon, or bone. Treatment requires large doses of parenteral penicillin and local debridement. Oral tetracycline or metronidazole have proved effective. After control of the infection, a large granulating tissue defect remains that often requires skin grafting (see Chap. 31).

Human Bite Infections. Human bite infections result from the inoculation of mixed oral flora into tissue planes. These most frequently occur on the hand, especially after fist fights, or in the relatively avascular cartilage of the ear. There is usually a delay of hours or days before the patient seeks medical attention for marked swelling and erythema spreading from the laceration or puncture wound.

Immediate elevation and treatment with parenteral penicillin or a cephalosporin is indicated. Most are mixed oral flora infections, which may include *Eikenella corrodens.*[83] This organism responds to penicillin but is resistant to semisynthetic penicillins, clindamycin, and metronidazole. Inability to flex or extend a finger usually indicates a tendon sheath abscess that requires urgent surgical drainage. Soft tissue loss may cause permanent disability (see Chap. 47).

Mixed Infections with Enteric Flora

Relatively few of the hundreds of bacteria that inhabit the gastrointestinal tract are especially virulent (see Chap. 3). Meleney et al.[84] and later Altemeier[85] observed that combinations of enteric flora produced an increased mortality when injected intraperitoneally in dogs.

A series of experiments in rats have confirmed the synergistic nature of intraperitoneal infections.[86–91] Feces from grain-fed rats inoculated intraperitoneally consistently failed to produce intraperitoneal infection. The colonic flora of animals fed meat, however, became very similar to that of the human, and 27 species could be isolated from rat feces. Intraperitoneal implantation of feces[87,88] in a double-gelatin capsule containing barium sulfate and anaerobic growth media resulted in a two-stage intraperitoneal infection. The first stage consisted of free peritonitis characterized by *E. coli* septicemia and large numbers of *E. coli* in the peritoneal fluid. Lesser numbers of *B. fragilis, F. necrophorum,* and enterococci were isolated. Other isolates of the original 27 species were rare. Surviving animals formed intraperitoneal abscesses consisting of larger numbers of *B. fragilis* and lesser numbers of *E. coli, F. necrophorum,* and enterococci.[86–88]

In a subsequent study, the facultative aerobes *E. coli* and enterococcus and the obligate anaerobes *B. fragilis* and *F. necrophorum* were mixed in various combinations before intraperitoneal implantation.[88] During the free peritonitis stage, bacteremia with *E. coli* produced the highest mortality. Survivors developed abscesses only if the intraperitoneal inoculum contained a facultative and an anaerobic species. Mixed anaerobes or mixed facultative organisms did not produce abscesses.

Next, animals were given various antibiotics, alone or in combination. Antibiotics effective against *E. coli* prevented lethal septicemia but had no effect on the incidence of abscesses. Antibiotics effective against anaerobes had no effect on *E. coli* septicemia but virtually eliminated subsequent abscesses. Combinations of antibiotics effective against both classes of organisms resulted in the lowest mortality and the lowest residual infection rate.[61,92] Clearly, the pattern of infection of the mixture depended on both aerobic and anaerobic organisms.

The mechanisms of interaction in mixed enteric infections are listed in Table 7–8. Facultative organisms, such as *E. coli* and *Enterococcus,* can consume local oxygen and lower the redox potential. In addition, pathogenic anaerobes, such as *B. fragilis,* have an inducible superoxide dismutase system, which may protect anaerobes in nonreduced environments.

Bacteroides species have a number of virulence factors that make them good synergistic partners.[93] They secrete extracellular enzymes, including pronases, penicillinases, lipases, and heparinases. Extracellular beta-lactamases protect both the *Bacteroides* organisms and any other bacteria from the effects of penicillin or cephalosporin antibiotics.[94] The digestive enzymes elaborated by *Bacteroides* species break down tissue, producing a good culture medium for other organisms in a mixed infection. In addition, *Bacteroides* heparinase may stabilize local fibrin deposits, preventing influx of antibiotics, antibodies, and complement and allowing abscess formation.[95] *Bacteroides fragilis* has a capsule that protects aerobic bacteria from local phagocytosis.[23,24] Tofte et al[96] have reported that *Bacteroides* when incubated in normal serum with *E. coli,* can bind opsonins and thereby reduce phagocytosis of *E. coli*. Even after *B. fragilis* has been phagocytosed by neutrophils, it produces succinate, which inhibits its intracellular killing by leukocytes.[97]

TABLE 7–8. MECHANISMS OF BACTERIAL SYNERGISM AMONG MIXED ENTERIC ORGANISMS

Organisms	Mechanisms
Organisms usually present: facultative gram-negative rod (*E. coli, Klebsiella*), anaerobic gram-negative rod (*B. fragilis*), facultative gram-positive cocci (*Enterococcus*), anaerobic gram-positive rods or cocci (*Peptostreptococcus* or *Peptococcus*)	
Facultative organisms, such as *E. coli* or *Enterococcus*	Lowers redox potential Secretes growth factors, possibly vitamin K, especially for *Bacteroides* species May release catalase to protect *Bacteroides* species
B. fragilis, P. melaninogenica[a]	Produces an antiphagocytic capsule Elaborates penicillinases or cephalosporinases Elaborates other digestive enzymes Produces heparinase to stabilize fibrin deposits and decrease influx of antibiotics, antibodies, and complement

Intra-Abdominal Infections. Mixed enteric infections usually originate from a break in the bowel mucosa, releasing the organisms into the surrounding tissue and producing peritonitis or soft tissue abscesses. The symptoms manifested are determined by the duration and intensity of inflammation before the release of bacteria, the quantity of inoculum released, and the source of the inoculum, because the distal gastrointestinal tract contains far more virulent mixtures of bacteria than do gastric or duodenal contents (see Chap. 31).

Necrotizing Soft Tissue Infections. Necrotizing fasciitis can be produced by mixed enteric organisms. This severe soft tissue infection spreads along the fascial cleft between superficial and deep fascia, leaving the overlying skin intact. During the Civil War, this disease was called "hospital gangrene." Meleney and others cultured group A beta-hemolytic streptococci alone or in combination with *S. aureus,*[98] but this disease is most commonly caused by mixed facultative and enteric flora.[99,100]

This is a virulent infection in diabetics and others with compromised immune defenses. The immunodepressed patient presents with minimal constitutional symptoms. The physician finds a draining wound, which may have surrounding anesthetic skin, or only an area of spreading redness and swelling resembling severe cellulitis. The patient becomes rapidly toxemic and ultimately hypotensive. Opening the wound shows extensive subcutaneous necrosis beneath relatively intact skin. Fluid resuscitation, broad spectrum antibiotics, and surgical debridement of all necrotic tissue are lifesaving[101] (see Chap. 31).

Mixed Infections with *Staphylococcus Aureus* and Streptococci

Because *Staphylococcus aureus* and many streptococci are such virulent organisms alone, this combination of bacteria has received little attention as a synergistic cause of surgical infection, despite Meleney's work in the 1930s.[102] But their consistent association in such diverse disease states as impetigo, progressive cutaneous ulcers, and necrotizing fasciitis should not be overlooked.[42]

Gram-Positive Necrotizing Fasciitis. Meleney initially cultured group A beta-hemolytic streptococci from a severe form of necrotizing fasciitis.[98] *Staphylococcus aureus* was frequently present but not considered a causative organism. But Giuliano et al[99] in 1977 recognized necrotizing fasciitis could result from either mixed enteric organisms or combined *Staphylococcus aureus* and streptococci, including enterococci. Subsequently, Seal and Kingston[31] have confirmed that these bacteria interact synergistically to produce necrotizing fasciitis in animals.

The clinical picture is indistinguishable from fascial infections caused by enteric organisms. But antibiotics effective against enterococcus and penicillinase-producing staphylococci should be used when wound fluid shows only gram-positive cocci. Surgical debridement is always indicated after fluid resuscitation.[101]

Meleney Ulcer. This disease has a variety of names, including progressive synergistic gangrene and Meleney synergistic gangrene, and is functionally equivalent to tropical ulcer or noma caused by oral organisms. Brewer and Meleney,[103] in 1926, first described this unusual chronic progressive cutaneous infection following drainage of an appendiceal abscess and reviewed 18 cases in the literature. The infection is characterized by a painful, tender area of erythema and swelling, with a central purplish zone that expands slowly with central gangrene. It was inexorably progressive until wide total excision was performed. This progressive ulcerating infection was, for surgeons, the prototype of synergistic soft tissue infections—even though it is now so rare that few surgeons have seen a case, and its character may have changed in the antibiotic era.

Meleney's cultures showed a synergistic infection with a microaerophilic streptococcus (originally *Streptococcus evolutus* and now probably *Streptococcus intermedius*) and *S. aureus* from these lesions.[98] In the original study, coliforms were isolated but were not felt to be pathogenic organisms. Both the streptococcus and staphylococcus could be recovered from the central necrotic area, but the reddened edge contained only the streptococcus. Meleney found subsequently that the infection could be reproduced in dogs only by the synchronous injection of both organisms.

Treatment with penicillin or cephalosporins is usually effective when combined with debridement of all necrotic tissue. Today, this disease is also produced by mixed enteric organisms including *Enterobacter aerogines, Proteus* species, and anaerobes, especially in areas of ischemia. Debridement and revascularization procedures are adjuncts to antibiotic treatment.

REFERENCES

1. Drasar BS, Hill MJ: Human Intestinal Flora. London, Academic Press, 1974.
2. Mergenhagen SE, Rosan B (eds): Molecular basis of oral microbial adhesion. Washington, DC, American Society of Microbiology, 1985.
3. Kolenbrander PE, Andersen RN, Holdeman LV: Coaggregation of oral *Bacteroides* species with other bacteria: central role in coaggregation bridges and competitions. Infect Immun 48:741, 1985.
4. MacDonald J, Socransky S, Gibbons R: Aspects of the pathogenesis of mixed anaerobic infections of mucous membranes. J Dent Res 42:529, 1963.
5. Moore WEC, Holdeman LV, Smibert RM, et al: Bacteriology of severe peridonitis in young adult humans. Infect Immun 38:1137, 1982.
6. Evans DG, Satterwhite TK, Evans DJ Jr, Dupont HL: Differences in serological responses and excretion patterns of volunteers challenged with enterotoxigenic *Escherichia coli* with and without the colonization factor antigen. Infect Immun 19:883, 1978.
7. Hentges DJ: Role of intestinal microflora in host defense against infection. In Hentges DJ (ed): Human Intestinal Microflora in Health and Disease. New York, Academic Press, 1983, p 311.
8. Kennedy MJ, Volz PA: Ecology of *Candida albicans* gut colonization: inhibition of *Candida* adhesion, colonization, and dissemination from the gastrointestinal tract by bacterial antagonism. Infect Immun 49:654, 1985.
9. Tramont EC, Hodge WC, Gilbreath MJ, Ciak J: Differences in attachment antigens of gonococci in reinfection. J Lab Clin Med 93:730, 1979.

10. Gibbons RJ: Ecology and cariogenic potential of oral streptococci. In Wannamaker LW, and Matsen JM (eds): Streptococci and Streptococcal Diseases, Recognition, Understanding and Management. New York, Academic Press, 1972, p 355.
11. Shulman JA: Streptococci of the viridans group. In Mandell GL, Douglas RG, Bennett JE (eds): Principles and Practices of Infectious Diseases, Vol 2. New York, Wiley, 1979, p 1612.
12. Williams REO: Benefit and mischief from commensal bacteria. J Clin Pathol 26:811, 1973.
13. Mackowiak PA: Microbial synergism in human infections [2nd of 2 parts]. N Engl J Med 298:83, 1978.
14. Fainstein V, Musher DM, Cate TR: Bacterial adherence to pharyngeal cells during viral infection. J Infect Dis 141:172, 1980.
15. Easterday BC: Animal influenza. In Kilbourne ED (ed): The Influenza Viruses and Influenza. New York, Academic Press, 1975, p 449.
16. Eichenwald HF, Kotsevalov O, Fasso LA: Some effects of viral infection on aerial dissemination of staphylococci and on susceptibility to bacterial colonization. Bacteriol Rev 25:274, 1961.
17. Roberts DS: Synergistic mechanisms in certain mixed infections. J Infect Dis 120:720, 1969.
18. Walker-Smith JA, McMillan B, Middleton AW, et al: Strongyloidiasis causing small bowel obstruction in an aboriginal infant. Med J Aust 2:1263, 1969.
19. LoVerde PT, Amento C, Higashi GI: Parasite-parasite interaction of *Salmonella typhimurium* and *Schistosoma*. J Infect Dis 141:177, 1980.
20. Simmons RL, Matas AJ, Rattazzi LC, et al: Clinical characteristics of lethal cytomegalovirus infection following renal transplantation. Surgery 82:537, 1977.
21. Whittle HC, Smith JS, Kogbe GI, et al: Severe ulcerative herpes of mouth and eye following measles. Trans R Soc Trop Med Hyg 73:66, 1979.
22. Selik RM, Chu SY, Buehler JW: HIV infection as leading cause of death among young adults in US cities and states. JAMA 269:2991, 1993.
23. Wade BN, Kaspar DL, Mandell GL: Interactions of *Bacteroides fragilis* and phagocytes: studies with pure organisms, purified capsular polysaccharide and clindamycin-treated bacteria. J Antimicrob Chemother 17(suppl C):51, 1983.
24. Jones GR, Gemmel CG: Impairment by *Bacteroides* species of opsonization and phagocytosis of enterobacteria. J Med Microbiol 15:351, 1982.
25. Fales WH, Warner JF, Teresa GW: Effects of *Fusobacterium necrophorum* leukotoxin on rabbit peritoneal macrophages in vitro. Am J Vet Res 38:491, 1977.
26. Monath TP: Flavovirus (St. Louis encephalitis and dengue). In Mandell GL, Douglas RG, Bennett JE (eds): Principles and Practices of Infectious Diseases, Vol 2. New York, Wiley, 1979, p 1248.
27. Kim HW, Canchola JG, Brandt CD, et al: Respiratory syncytial virus disease in infants despite prior administration of antigenic inactivated vaccine. Am J Epidemiol 89:422, 1969.
28. Hsu SD, Cole MF: Structural integrity of host defense factors in dental plaque. Infect Immun 50:398, 1985.
29. Gelderman AH, Grimley PM, Lunde MN, Rabson AS: *Toxoplasma gondii* and cytomegalovirus: mixed infection by a parasite and a virus. Science 160: 1130, 1968.
30. Gibbons RJ, MacDonald JB: Hemin and vitamin K compounds as required factors for the cultivation of certain strains of *Bacteroides melaninogenicus*. J Bacteriol 80:164, 1960.
31. Seal DV, Kingston D: Streptococcal necrotizing fasciitis: development of an animal model to study its pathogenesis. Br J Exp Pathol 56:813, 1988.
32. Socransky SS, Loesche WJ, Hubersak C, MacDonald JB: Dependency of *Treponema microdentium* on other oral organisms for isobutyrate, polyamines, and a controlled oxidation-reaction potential. J Bacteriol 88:200, 1964.
33. Socransky SS, Gibbons RJ: Required role of *Bacteroides melaninogenicus* in mixed anaerobic infection. J Infect Dis 115:247, 1965.
34. Brook I: Enhancement of growth of aerobic and facultative bacteria in mixed infections with *Bacteroides* species. Infect Immun 50:929, 1985.
35. Carlson E, Johnson G: Protection by *Candida albicans* of *Staphylococcus aureus* in the establishment of dual infection in mice. Infect Immun 50:655, 1985.
36. Joklik WK, Willett HP (eds): Zinsser Microbiology, 18th ed. Norwalk, CT, Appleton-Century-Crofts, 1984.
37. Fong IW, Engelking ER, Kirby WMM: Relative inactivation by *Staphylococcus aureus* of eight cephalosporin antibiotics. Antimicrob Agents Chemother 9:939, 1976.
38. Rudek W, Haque R: Extracellular enzymes of the genus *Bacteroides*. J Clin Microbiol 4:458, 1976.
39. Finegold SM: Anaerobic Bacteria in Human Disease. New York, Academic Press, 1977.
40. Kolbacha ME, Stankiewicz JA, Clift SE: Severe soft tissue infection of the face and neck: a classification. Laryngoscope 92:1135, 1982.
41. Ahrenholz DH: Necrotizing soft tissue infections. Surg Clin North Am 68(1):199, 1988.
42. Ahrenholz DH: Necrotizing fasciitis and other infections. In Rippe JM, Irwin RS, Alpert JS, Fink MP (eds): Intensive Care Medicine, 2nd edition. Boston, Little, Brown, 1991, p 1334.
43. Bartlett JG: Anaerobic bacteria: general concepts. In Mandel GL, Douglas RG, Bennett JE (eds): Principles and Practice of Infectious Diseases, 3rd edition. New York, Churchill Livingstone, 1990, p 1828.
44. Finegold SM: General aspects of anaerobic infection In Finegold SM, George WL (eds): Anaerobic Infections in Humans. San Diego, Academic Press, 1989, p 137.
45. Thadepalli H, Gorbach SL, Broido PW, et al: Abdominal trauma, anaerobes, and antibiotics. Surg Gynecol Obstet 137:270, 1973.

46. Leigh DA: *Bacteroides* infections. Lancet 2:1081, 1973.
47. Gorbach SL, Bartlett JG: Anaerobic infections. N Engl J Med 290:1177, 1237, 1289, 1974.
48. Fry DE, Garrison RN, Polk HC Jr: Clinical implications in bacteroides bacteremia. Surg Gynecol Obstet 149:189, 1979.
49. Solomkin JS, Flohr AB, Quie PG, Simmons RL: The role of *Candida* in intraperitoneal infections. Surgery 88:524, 1980.
50. File TM, Tan JS: Treatment of bacterial skin and soft tissue infections. Surg Gynecol Obstet 172(Suppl): 17, 1991.
51. Feliciano DV, Gentry LO, Bitondo CG, et al: Single agent cephalosporin prophylaxis for penetrating abdominal trauma. Results and comment on emergence of the enterococcus. Am J Surg 152:674, 1986.
52. Karam GH, Sanders CV, Aldridge KE: Role of newer antimicrobial agents in treatment of mixed aerobic and anaerobic infection. Surg Gynecol Obstet 172(Suppl):17, 1991.
53. Saunders CV, Aldridge KE: Current antimicrobial therapy of anaerobic infections. Eur J Clin Microbiol Infect Dis 11:999, 1992.
54. Walsh CT: Vancomycin resistance: decoding the molecular logic. Science 261:308, 1993.
55. Spera RV Jr, Farber BF: Multiply-resistant *Enterococcus faecium.* The nosocomial pathogen of the 1990s. JAMA 268:2563, 1992.
56. Wilhelm MP: Vancomycin. Mayo Clin Proc 66:1165, 1991.
57. Thadepalli H, Gorbach SL, Broido P, Norsen J: A prospective study of infections in penetrating abdominal trauma. Am J Clin Nutr 25:1405, 1972.
58. Stone HH, Fabian TC: Clinical comparison of antibiotic combinations in the treatment of peritonitis and related mixed aerobic-anaerobic surgical sepsis. World J Surg 4:415, 1980.
59. Sen P, Apuzzio J, Reyelt C, et al: Prospective evaluation of combinations of antimicrobial agents for endometritis after cesarean section. Surg Gynecol Obstet 151:89, 1980.
60. Bakker-Woudenber IA, Roosendaal R: Impact of dosage schedule of antibiotics on the treatment of serious infections. Intensive Care Med 16:S229, 1990.
61. Weinstein W, Onderdonk A, Bartlett J, et al: Antimicrobial therapy of intraabdominal sepsis. J Infect Dis 132:282, 1975.
62. Solomkin JS, Meakins JL, Allo MD, et al: Antibiotic trials in intra-abdominal infections. Ann Surg 200:29, 1984.
63. Dellinger EP: Design and evaluation of clinical trials of antimicrobial agents in surgery. Surg Gynecol Obstet 172(Suppl):17, 1991.
64. Christou NV, Barie PS, Dellinger EP, et al: Surgical Infection Society intra-abdominal infection study. Prospective evaluation of management techniques and outcome. Arch Surg 128:193, 1993.
65. Dougherty SH: Role of enterococcus in intraabdominal sepsis. Am J Surg 148:308, 1984.
66. Solomkin JS, Simmons RL: *Candida* infections in surgical patients. World J Surg 4:381, 1980.
67. Graninger W, Presteril E, Schneeweiss B, et al: Treatment of *Candida albicans* fungaemia with fluconazole. J Infect 26:133, 1993.
68. Riseman JA, Zamboni WA, Curtis A, et al: Hyperbaric oxygen therapy for necrotizing fasciitis reduces mortality and the need for debridements. Surgery 108:847, 1990.
69. Stevens DL, Bryant AE, Adams K, et al: Evaluation of therapy with hyperbaric oxygen in clostridial myonecrosis. Clin Infect Dis 17:231, 1993.
70. Heimbach D: Editorial response: use of hyperbaric oxygen. Clin Infect Dis 17:239, 1993.
71. Bowden GHW, Ellwood DC, Hamilton IR: Microbial ecology of the oral cavity. Adv Microbial Ecol 3:135, 1979.
72. Slots J: Subgingival microflora and periodontal disease. J Clin Periodontol 6:351, 1979.
73. Labrolia JD, Mascare J, Alpert B: The microbiologic flora of orofacial abscesses. J Oral Maxillofac Surg 41:711, 1983.
74. Ferreira MC, Araujo WC, Otto SS, Uzeda M: Anaerobic and facultative microbial organisms in chronic tonsillitis. Ear Nose Throat J 58:35, 1979.
75. Ingham HR, Selkon JB, Roxby CM: Bacteriological study of otogenic cerebral abscesses: chemotherapeutic role of metronidazole. Br Med J 2:991, 1977.
76. Brook I, Hunter V, Walker RI: Synergistic effect of *Bacteroides, Clostridium, Fusobacterium,* anaerobic cocci and aerobic cocci on mortality and induction of subcutaneous abscesses in mice. J Infect Dis 149:924, 1984.
77. Langworth BF: *Fusobacterium necrophorum:* its characteristics and role as an animal pathogen. Bacteriol Rev 41:373, 1977.
78. Roberts DS: The pathogenic synergy of *Fusiformis necrophorus* and *Corynebacterium pyogenes.* I. Influence of the leucocidal exotoxin of *F. necrophorus.* Br J Exp Pathol 48:665, 1967.
79. Roberts DS: The pathogenic synergy of *Fusiformis necrophorus* and *Corynebacterium pyogenes.* II. The response of *F. necrophorus* to a filterable product of *C. pyogenes.* Br J Exp Pathol 48:674, 1967.
80. MacDonald JB, Socransky SS, Gibbons RJ: Aspects of the pathogenesis of mixed anaerobic infections of mucous membranes. J Dent Res 42:529, 1963.
81. Hill G, Osterhout S, Pratt P: Liver abscess production by non-spore-forming anaerobic bacteria in a mouse model. Infect Immun 9:599, 1974.
82. Smith DT: Fusospirochetal disease of the lungs produced with cultures from Vincent's angina. J Infect Dis 46:303, 1930.
83. Goldstein EJC, Barone M, Miller TA: *Eikenella corrodens* in hand infections. J Hand Surg 8:563, 1983.
84. Meleney F, Olpp J, Harvey H, Zaytseff-Jern H: Peritonitis: II. Synergism of bacteria commonly found in peritoneal exudates. Arch Surg 25:709, 1932.
85. Altemeier W: The pathogenicity of the bacteria of ap-

pendicitis peritonitis. An experimental study. Surgery 11:374, 1942.
86. Weinstein WM, Onderdonk AB, Bartlett JG, Gorbach SL: Experimental intra-abdominal abscesses in rats: development of an experimental model. Infect Immun 10:1250, 1974.
87. Onderdonk AB, Weinstein WM, Sullivan NM, et al: Experimental intra-abdominal abscesses in rats: quantitative bacteriology of infected animals. Infect Immun 10:1256, 1974.
88. Onderdonk AB, Bartlett JG, Louie T, et al: Microbial synergy in experimental intra-abdominal abscess. Infect Immun 13:22, 1976.
89. Kelly MJ: The quantitative and histologic demonstration of pathogenic synergy between *Escherichia coli* and *Bacteroides fragilis* in guinea pig wounds. J Med Microbiol 11:513, 1978.
90. Dunn DL, Rotstein OD, Simmons RL: Fibrin in peritonitis: IV. Synergistic intraperitoneal infection due to *Escherichia coli* and *Bacteroides fragilis* within fibrin clots. Arch Surg 119:139, 1984.
91. Rotstein OD, Pruett TL, Simmons RL: Lethal microbial synergism in intra-abdominal infections. Arch Surg 120:146, 1985.
92. Nichols RL, Smith JW, Fossedal EN, Condon RE: Efficacy of parenteral antibiotics in the treatment of experimentally induced intraabdominal sepsis. Rev Infect Dis 1:302, 1979.
93. Rotstein OD, Pruett TL, Simmons RL: Mechanisms of microbial synergy in polymicrobial surgical infections. Rev Infect Dis 7:151, 1985.
94. O'Keefe JP, Tally FP, Barza M, Gorbach SL: Inactivation of penicillin G during experimental infection with *Bacteroides fragilis*. J Infect Dis 137:437, 1978.
95. Gesner BM, Jenkin CR: Production of heparinase by *Bacteroides*. J Bacteriol 81:595, 1961.
96. Tofte RW, Peterson PK, Schmeling D, et al: Opsonization of four *Bacteroides* species: role of the classical complement pathway and immunoglobulin. Infect Immun 27:784, 1980.
97. Rotstein OD, Nasmith PE, Grinstein S: The *Bacteroides* by-product succinic acid inhibits neutrophil respiratory burst by reducing intracellular pH. Infect Immun 55:864, 1987.
98. Meleney FL: Hemolytic streptococcus gangrene. Arch Surg 9:317, 1924.
99. Giuliano A, Lewis F Jr, Hadley K, Blaisdell FW: Bacteriology of necrotizing fasciitis. Am J Surg 134:52, 1977.
100. Stone HH, Martin JD Jr: Synergistic necrotizing cellulitis. Ann Surg 175:702, 1972.
101. Pessa ME, Howard RJ: Necrotizing fasciitis. Surg Gynecol Obstet 161:357, 1985.
102. Meleney F: Bacterial synergism in disease processes with confirmation of synergistic bacterial etiology of certain type of progressive gangrene of abdominal wall. Ann Surg 94:961, 1931.
103. Brewer GE, Meleney FL: Progressive gangrenous infection of the skin and subcutaneous tissues, following operation for acute perforative appendicitis. A study in symbiosis. Ann Surg 84:438, 1926.

BIBLIOGRAPHY

Finegold SM, George LW: Infections in Human Diseases. New York, Academic Press, 1989.

Surgical Parasitology

CHAPTER 8

Lee S. Monroe

Not infrequently, a surgeon will be faced with problems produced by parasitism. Modern travel has become important in introducing exotic infections into the United States. To cope with this problem a new specialty of travel medicine called *emporiatics* is emerging. Many of the diseases addressed by this subspecialty are caused by parasites, so it is important for the clinician to be aware of certain problems not indigenous to North America. A summary of the life cycle and methods of diagnosis for selected parasites will be included. Opportunistic infections, such as pneumocystosis cryptosporidiosis toxoplasmosis, or strongyloidiasis, which may become rampant in the immunosuppressed or deficient patient, are discussed in Chapter 51.

PROTOZOA

Entamoeba histolytica. Amebiasis has a worldwide distribution and is the most important of the parasitic problems regularly encountered by the surgeon in the United States.

Life Cycle, Pathogenesis, and Pathology. Infection with *E. histolytica* is acquired by the ingestion of food or water contaminated with mature cysts. The vegetative form, the trophozoite, is destroyed by hydrochloric acid, whereas cysts survive gastric transit. Upon exposure to the alkaline milieu of the small bowel, excystation and division occur with the formation of eight metacystic trophozoites, which become lodged within the crypts of the cecum. In this locale the trophozoites develop, feed, grow, and multiply, usually as commensals. As fecal material solidifies, encystation of the ameba takes place. Cysts of *E. histolytica* in cool moist surroundings may remain viable for a month and are resistant to the common germicides as well as chlorinated water. Fortunately, they are destroyed by heat over 50C.[1] Potentially contaminated water should be boiled.

Most trophozoites inhabit the colonic mucosa as commensals, but active tissue invasion will occur under certain conditions. Factors such as the strain or virulence of the organism and host resistance are commonly cited[2] as influencing the ability of the trophozoite to invade. Malnutrition, avitaminosis, dietary factors (a fish or wheat diet), or steroid administration may predispose to infection.[3–5] Bacteria of the gut play a permissive role in the development of invasive amebiasis. Phillips et al[6,7] found that infection did not occur in the germ-free guinea pig until the intestinal tract was contaminated with bacteria (eg, *Clostridium perfringens* or *Bacillus subtilis*).

Although similar by light microscopy, the trophozoites of *E. histolytica* apparently vary considerably in their invasive capability and this is thought to be related to the electrophoretic patterns of the isoenzymes (zymodemes) found in culture extracts. By electron microscopy, trophozoites with invasive properties are thought by some to have a "fuzzy" surface comprised of complex membranous dendritic extensions, which contain lytic enzymes.[8] On contact, surface-active lysosomes are probably released, destroying tissue cells and defensive macrophages or lympocytes. In addition, *E. histolytica* produces proteases, which are markers of pathogenicity and contribute to the degredation of collagen.[9]

Probably as a combination of these factors, *E. histolytica* penetrates the depths of the colonic crypts at separate localities. The initial invasion is usually unaccompanied by inflammatory reaction, and with progressive involvement the muscularis mucosa is penetrated, and lateral spread begins. Overlying surface epithelium is then breached, and typical circumscribed flask-shaped ulcers are formed (Fig. 8–1). Ulcers may eventually involve the muscularis and become confluent. At this time, bacterial invasion with inflammatory cell reaction is the rule. Although amebic ulcers can be disseminated, they are usually limited to the cecum. Less commonly, there is involvement of the rectosigmoid and other parts of the colon; rarely, the ulcerations may appear in the ileum near the ileocecal junction.[10] On occasion, tissue reaction includes an exuberant fibroblastic, eosinophilic, and lymphocytic response. Such lesions (amebomas) occur in 1 to 5 percent of cases of amebic colitis and may mimic adenocarcinoma or inflammatory bowel disease (Fig. 8–2).[10,11]

With the invasion of trophozoites, mesenteric

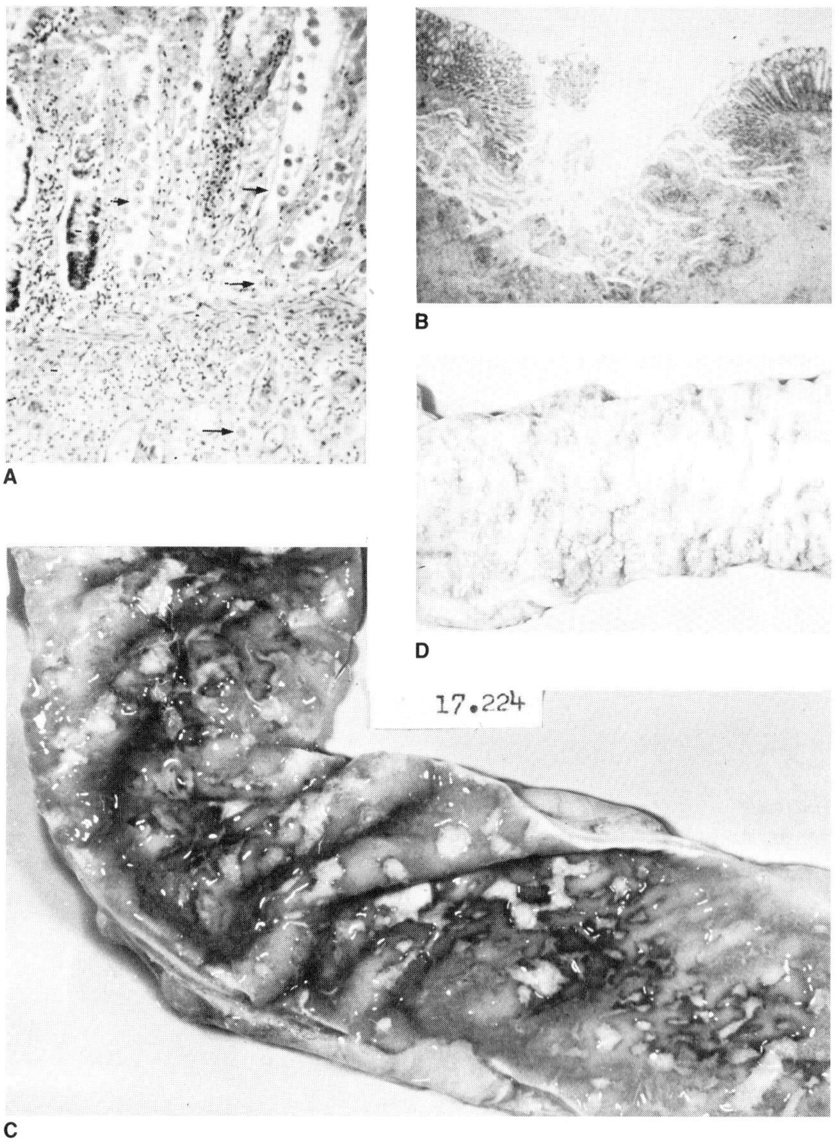

Figure 8–1. Amebic colitis. **A.** Histologic section of a colon showing trophozoites of *Entamoeba histolytica* within the crypts, lamina propria, and submucosa; little inflammatory response is present. **B.** Typical flask-shaped ulcer. **C.** Gross appearance of ulcers in amebic colitis (chronic phase) with normal mucosa between areas of ulceration. **D.** Secondarily infected amebic colitis grossly resembling chronic ulcerative colitis. *(From Monroe LS: Amebiasis. In Berk JE, Haubrich WS, Kalser MH, et al (eds): Bockus Gastroenterology, Vol. 7, 4th ed. Philadelphia, Saunders, 1985, p 4259.)*

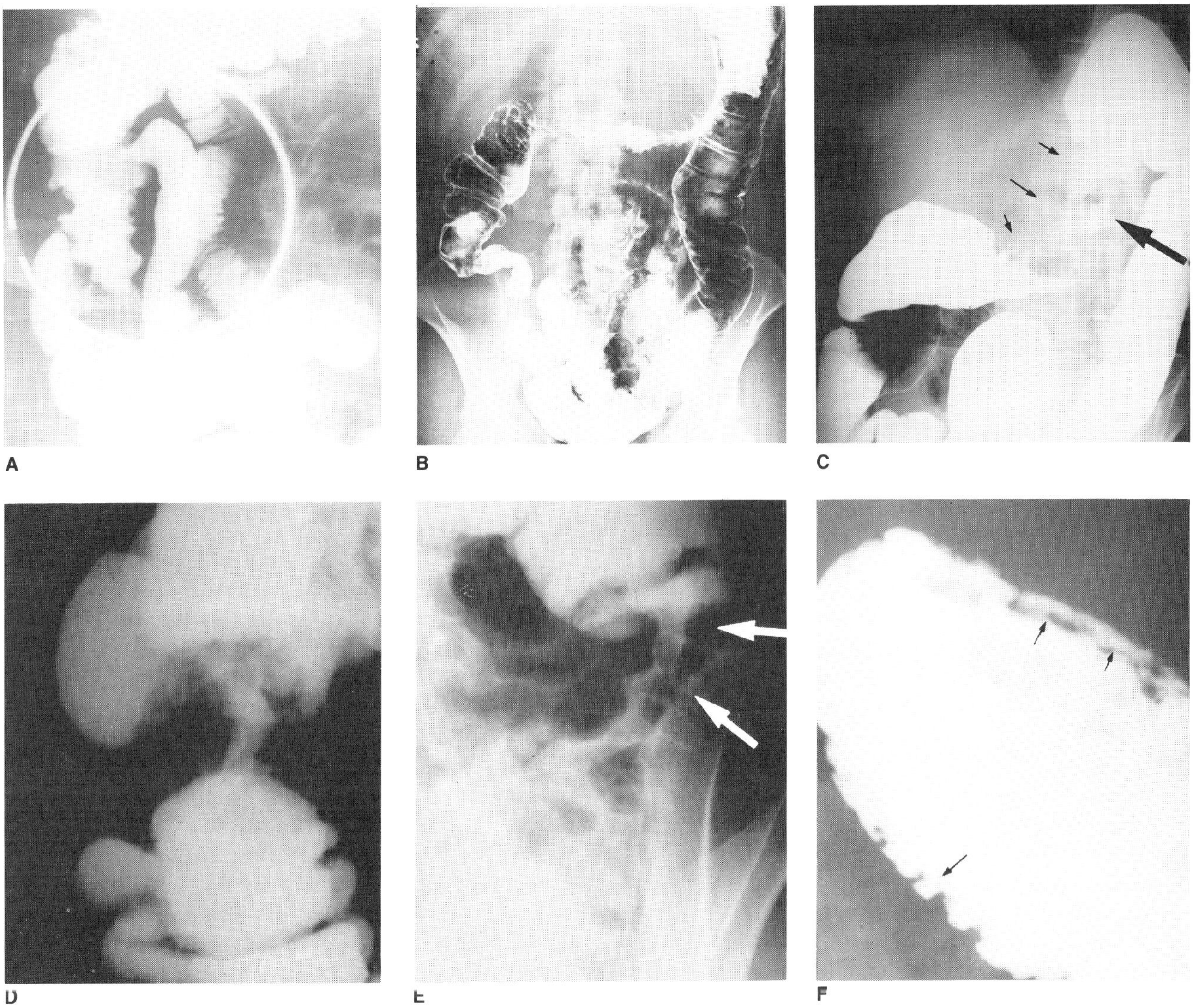

Figure 8–2. Radiographic appearance of amebic colitis and amebic granuloma. **A.** Conical cecum of amebic cecitis. **B,C.** Segmental involvement of the transverse colon. Note similarity to granulomatous colitis. **D.** Amebic granuloma (ameboma) of ascending colon, which simulates carcinoma. **E.** Amebic granuloma, descending colon. **F.** Collar-button and undetermined amebic abscesses. *(**A** to **D** courtesy of Jorge Lega-Siccar; **E** and **F** courtesy of Robert Berk.)*

venules may be entered and the amebae swept into the portal circulation to reach the liver. There most trophozoites are eradicated, but when circumstances are favorable, tiny colonies coalesce to form an abscess. Portal hemodynamics favor involvement of the right lobe. Within the abscess, trophozoites accumulate at the periphery while at the central portion variable amounts of blood, necrotic hepatic cellular debris, and leukocytes accumulate. The physical appearance of the fluid from an amebic hepatic abscess depends on the age of the lesion. With lesions of short duration, 3 weeks or less, the aspirate is thick, usually dark red, and most often bacteriologically sterile. When abscesses are older, the contents are often pale yellow, of thinner consistency, and may have a marbled appearance (caused by blood streaking). The aspirate of such amebic hepatic abscesses, unless secondarily infected, is odorless (in contrast to abscesses produced by anaerobes), a finding that is important to the surgeon who is attempting to determine the cause of a lesion at the operating table. Amebic abscesses are multiple in 30 percent of the cases, and the majority of single lesions usually arise from a coalition of smaller lesions. Trophozoites of *E. histolytica* collect on the periphery of an abscess and therefore are best demonstrated in the last material to be aspirated.

An enlarging amebic hepatic abscess may rupture into surrounding structures, to produce such complications as bronchohepatic fistula, empyema, pericarditis, or peritonitis (see Chap. 38). As a secondary, rare complication of such abscess, metastatic involvement (via the bloodstream) can occur in nearly any part of the body, particularly the lungs, brain, spleen, and kidneys.

Clinical Manifestations. The identification of amebic forms in stool (cysts or trophozoites) does not necessarily indicate infection. In fact, the majority of *E. histolytica* exist as commensals within the gut and are not responsible for any pathologic change. On the other hand, when invasion of the intestine occurs, the resulting symptoms are widely variable. Indeed, some patients without intestinal complaints can harbor invasive trophozoites, which produce symptoms only after invading the liver. Mild diarrhea is the most common manifestation of intestinal involvement. The onset after exposure averages 7 days, and stools are usually watery or poorly formed. As a rule, the initial accompanying systemic manifestations are not prominent, as with the bacillary dysenteries. Acute cecal involvement can produce right lower quadrant pain and localized tenderness, which simulates acute appendicitis. In certain parts of the world, particularly in tropical zones, acute dysentery with bloody diarrhea, dehydration, and electrolyte losses may occur. Such a fulminant process is more common in the malnourished, elderly, or immunosuppressed patient.[12]

Complications of intestinal amebiasis include perforation, hemorrhage (rare), stenosis, granuloma, and hepatic abscess formation. Chapter 40 contains a detailed description of the clinical manifestations and treatment of amebic liver abscesses (Fig. 8–3). Only a few additional points are discussed here. Secondary infection is reported in 10 to 30 percent of cases.[13] It is probable that modern bacteriologic methods will find coliforms and anaerobes to be the most common offenders; however, staphylococci and streptococci are the most frequently reported organisms. Such secondary infection should be suspected when the patient is in an unusually toxic condition and does not respond to antiamebal drugs and when the liver aspirate is malodorous. Any region of the body can be involved by metastatic amebiasis, and this event is rather uniformly antedated by an amebic hepatic abscess. Brain, lung, and kidney are among the rare sites of such secondary involvement.

Diagnosis. The clinician must be aware of the possibility of amebiasis among the jungle of conditions that produce symptoms such as diarrhea, hepatomegaly, right upper quadrant pain, or right basilar pulmonary lesions. The requisite diagnostic maneuvers are relatively simple. The most precise diagnosis requires the demonstration of some form of *E. histolytica*, and fortunately coprology or examination of an aspirate is a rapid method. It is important, however, to remember that the majority of persons who harbor *E. histolytica* in the gut have no significant pathology that can be attributable to the organism; also, the demonstration of an amebic form (particularly cysts) does not necessarily indicate that the symptoms are related. In the stool, amebae may appear intermittently, influenced adversely by medications (mineral oil, kaolin, bismuth, antibiotics) or hypertonic enemas. At the time of sigmoidoscopy, the examining physician should obtain multiple specimens by scraping or aspiration from a suspicious lesion, and such material should be prepared in a saline mount for prompt examination. While microscopy is pending, an electric heating pad, turned to low setting, makes an

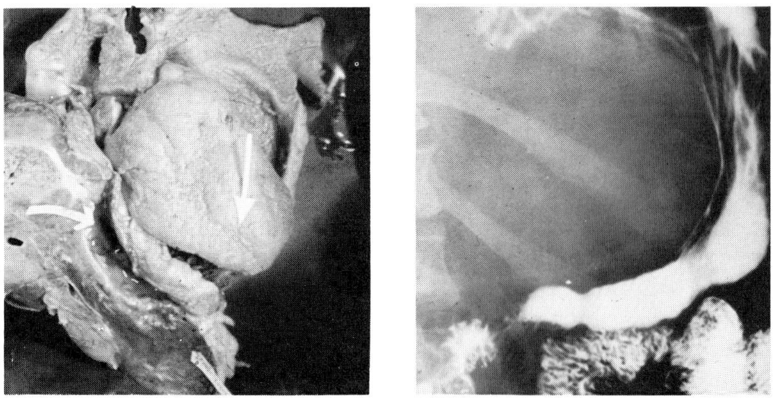

A B

Figure 8–3. **A.** Section through the liver showing abscess of the left lobe with perforation into the pericardium and secondary pericarditis. **B.** Radiograph showing lateral displacement of the stomach by a large left lobe abscess.

ideal slide storage area; the warmth helps preserve the motility of trophozoites. To obtain specimens from an ulcerating lesion of the bowel or skin, the clinician should scrape or aspirate the overhanging margins, the site of the greatest concentrations of amebae.

Inasmuch as the motile, blood-containing trophozoite is important in the diagnosis of amebic dysentery, laboratory attention should be focused on the demonstration of this form. The ideal material for this purpose is obtained either at sigmoidoscopy or from warm liquid stools after a saline cathartic (sodium sulfate or buffered phosphosoda). Alicna and Fadell[14] have demonstrated that the examination of three specimens on successive days will greatly increase the accuracy of coprology. Trophozoites will be scarce in solid stools, but cyst recovery can be enhanced by using a concentration technique (formalin ether or zinc sulfate). Whenever possible, a positive specimen should be preserved by a permanent staining technique (trichrome or iron hematoxylin). Remember that coprology is a poor method for confirming the presence of an amebic hepatic abscess (less than 50 percent of stools are positive); for this purpose, scanning techniques and serology are valuable (see Chap. 40).

Spurred by the development of axenic antigen, which has greatly improved specificity, serologic study has become increasingly important for diagnosis. The tests available from the parasitology division of the Centers for Disease Control include indirect hemagglutination and enzyme immunoassay (Table 8–1). Usually, however, the results must be obtained within a short period, so it is important to have serologic testing available to every hospital laboratory. The precipitin test (agar gel diffusion) and the latex agglutination test are optimal and avoid the technical difficulties of the other procedures and can be done in the average hospital laboratory.[15] In symptomatic intestinal amebiasis, 70 to 90 percent of serologic tests are positive. In the commensal state a lower percentage of serologic tests are positive. Electrophoretic studies of the isoenzymes found in the extracts of *E. histolytica* have been shown to differentiate pathogenic from nonpathogenic strains.[16–18] Eighteen zymodemes have been identified, of which types II and XI are associated with intestinal and liver involvement, respectively. Commensal strains have other types of zymodemes. As this technique requires culture, it has epidemiologic rather than clinical usage.

Circulating antibodies may persist for years; therefore in endemic areas a positive result is not necessarily an indication of a currently active infection. In the United States, however, where the background of infection is extremely low, a positive test is most often accompanied by invasive amebiasis.

TABLE 8–1. SEROLOGIC TESTS FOR HELMINTHIC AND PROTOZOAL INFECTIONS

Parasitic Infection	Tests Available[a]
Protozoa	
Amebiasis	IHA,[b] EIA[c]
American trypanosomiasis (Chagas' disease)	IIF,[b] CF[b]
Nematodes	
Trichinosis	BF[b]
Cestodes	
Cysticercosis	IB[b]
Echinococcosis	
(*E. granulosis*)	EIA,[c] IHA,[b] IB[b]
(*E. multilocularis*)	IHA[b]
Trematodes	
Schistosomiasis	EIA,[b] IB[b]
Paragonimiasis	IB[b]

[a] IHA, indirect hemagglutination; EIA, enzyme immunoassay; IIF, indirect immunofluorescence; CF, complement fixation; BF, Bentonite flocculation; IB, immunoblot.
[b] Serologic assays performed by the Immunodiagnostic Reference Laboratory, Parasitic Disease Branch, CDC, tel: (404) 488-4311.
[c] Commercial kits available through LMD Laboratories, Carlsbad, CA 92008.

Scanning (ultrasound, isotopic, and computerized axial tomography) techniques have been improved to vastly simplify the diagnosis of amebic hepatic abscess (see Chap. 40). X-ray study of the colon gives important clues (see Fig. 8–2). Amebic typhlitis is characterized by a conical, stiff-appearing cecum, which is unassociated with involvement of the ileum. It is also important to recognize that an ameboma can manifest a configuration identical to carcinoma or the segmental involvement of Crohn's disease.

On rare occasions, colonoscopy is useful to differentiate ameboma, carcinoma, or inflammatory bowel disease. The ulcers of amebic colitis can be biopsied for identification of trophozoites.

A therapeutic trial was formerly an important step in the diagnosis of liver abscess. With current scanning and serologic techniques, it is seldom necessary today. Furthermore, if metronidazole were to be used in such a regimen, the clinician should be alert to the fact that this drug is effective in certain anaerobic infections[19] so that a clinical response would not necessarily indicate *E. histolytica* as the culprit.

Treatment. The drugs used in the medical treatment of amebiasis are outlined in Table 8–2.[20–22]

TABLE 8–2. DRUG THERAPY OF *ENTAMOEBA HISTOLYTICA*

Drug	Average Adult Dose	Duration (days)	Clinical Indications	Adverse Effects
Iodoquinol[a] (di-iodohydroxyquin, USP)	650 mg tid	20	Commensal state	Diarrhea, mild iodism, interference with thyroid function tests, occasional subacute myeloptic atrophy—rare
Diloxanide furoate[b]	500 mg/kg/d in 3 doses	10	Commensal state	Occasional mild gastrointestinal upset
Paromomycin[b]	25–30 mg tid	7	Commensal state	Gastrointestinal disturbances, VIII nerve, renal damage—rare
Metronidazole[a] plus iodoquinol	750 mg tid	10	Symptomatic intestinal or hepatic abscess	Diarrhea, vomiting, dizziness, depression, fall in blood pressure with alcohol; leukopenia
Tinidazole[a] plus iodoquinol	600–800 mg tid	5	Symptomatic intestinal or hepatic abscess	Nausea, vomiting, metallic taste
Dehydroemetine[a] plus iodoquinol	1–1.5 mg/kg/d (max 90 mg/d)	5	Symptomatic intestinal or hepatic abscess	Diarrhea, painful injection site, neuropathy; potentially toxic to heart, liver, and kidneys
Chloroquine phosphate[a] plus iodoquinol	600 mg base qd/2d; then 300 mg base for 2–3 weeks	14–21	Symptomatic intestinal or hepatic abscess	Nausea, vomiting, diarrhea, skin eruptions, blood dyscrasias—rare; corneal opacity, retinal injury—rare

[a] Drug of choice.
[b] Alternatives.
Adapted from Medical Letter on Drugs and Therapeutics.[20]

Most drugs that eliminate cysts or trophozoites from the gut do not destroy tissue-invading trophozoites. For example, using di-iodohydroxyquin (iodoquinol) because cysts were found in the stool does not guarantee that amebic liver involvement will not develop. Thus it is good practice to always include a direct-acting luminal amebicide (ie, di-iodohydroxyquin) with a drug active against trophozoites within tissue (metronidazole, tinidazole, dehydroemetine or chloroquine).

The surgeon is cautioned to rule out amebiasis before initiating treatment for a complication of inflammatory bowel disease, inasmuch as corticosteroids can greatly predispose to metastatic amebiasis. For example, if a perforation of the colon (particularly the cecum) is encountered, diagnostic testing (serologic and coprologic) should be an urgent requirement. If such studies are not available on a timely basis, drug treatment with a tissue-active drug should be started (see Table 8–2).

The treatment of amebic hepatic abscess should be varied depending on the particular situation. Although aspiration of an abscess is a routine procedure in certain parts of the world, local experience with the morbidity and mortality of secondarily infected abscesses has led to a selective approach. Aspiration is undertaken (1) when there are manifestations of impending performation, (2) when the response to appropriate antiamebics is unsatisfactory in 72 hours, and (3) in left lobe abscess unless response to medical treatment is prompt and dramatic. In such a case, open drainage is the safest procedure. The techniques of aspiration and open drainage are described in Chapter 40. The abscess should be evacuated as completely as possible, and the last bit of aspirate, which contains the highest concentration of trophozoites, should immediately be submitted for microscopy. Systemic tissue-active amebicides are always indicated in liver abscess and usually have been given before aspiration is undertaken. Bacterial cultures should always be carried out to detect superinfections.

Abscesses that metastasize to distant organs (ie, brain, lung, kidney) carry a high mortality. The treatment, in addition to tissue-active antiamebicides, usually requires surgical drainage of the lesion.

Balantidium coli. Balantidiasis is caused by a ciliated protozoan, *B. coli*, that commonly infects primates, rats, and swine and has a worldwide distribution. Humans, on occasion, can acquire the infection and sometimes develop perforation of the colon or appendix.

Morphology, Life Cycle, and Pathology. The trophozoites of *B. coli* are large, measuring 50 to 200 μm in their long axis, and as a result can be seen with the naked eye in fresh saline mounts. Configuration of the motile form is slightly lemon shaped with a prominent cytostome visible at the narrow end. The prominent macronucleus and micronucleus are distinctive features in stained specimens.[1] Furthermore, in fresh preparations, activity of the cilia produces prominent eddy currents about the living organism.

The life cycle of *B. coli* is generally similar to that of *E. histolytica*, except that many areas of the colon are commonly involved. Protein starvation, vitamin deficiency, and alcoholism may play a permissive role in the establishment of infection. More than 50 percent of infected humans have lived near swine.[23]

Within the colon, *B. coli* most often exists as a harmless commensal; however, when invasion of the epithelium occurs, sloughing ulcers are formed. These do not acquire the overhanging edge often produced by amebic ulceration and in addition are accompanied by a marked degree of vascular thrombosis and bleeding. In histologic sections, trophozoites may be seen teeming in the exudate and penetrating below the submucosa of an ulcer. Some investigators have reported a hyaluronidase-like substance secreted from the trophozoite and have suggested that this may facilitate tissue invasion. On rare occasions, ulcers of the cecum or appendix may deepen with perforation and the development of peritonitis. Distant metastasis of the parasite is reported, but it is rare.[24]

Clinical Manifestations. Balantidiasis must be considered in any acute diarrheal condition, but especially when the following clinical features are found: (1) close contact with pigs, (2) residence in a tropical area (although the condition has been reported in the United States and Canada), (3) malnutrition, and (4) acute diarrhea with a prominent amount of blood and mucus in the stool. Perforation of a balantidial abscess is often heralded by abdominal pain, rigidity, and diminished bowel sounds. Before the use of tetracyclines for such an acute abdomen, mortality was in the neighborhood of 30 percent.

Diagnosis. Unless the patient has received earlier antibiotic treatment, the diagnosis is easily made by examination of material aspirated from ulcerating lesions at the time of proctosigmoidoscopy. Balantidiasis should be considered whenever discrete ulcers with intervening normal mucosa are observed. It should enter into the differential diagnosis of granulomatous colitis and amebiasis. Fortunately, in the usual dysenteric case the wet preparation teems with organisms, and trophozoites can be identified with the naked eye. The diarrheal stool produced by *B. coli* often has a diffusely bloody or blood-streaked appearance. When stools are solid or semiformed, cysts are found on examination of the stool. As with amebiasis, eosinophilia is not a feature of the infection.[25]

Treatment. For the carrier state or invasive balantidial colitis the primary treatment is tetracycline (average adult dose of 0.5 g four times a day for 10 days), and alternate drugs are di-iodohydroxyquin (0.650 g tid for 20 days, and metronidazole (750 mg, tid for 5 days). As in any acute diarrheal condition, fluid and electrolyte replacement is equal in importance to drug therapy. If the clinical signs of perforation appear during the course of an acute balantidial colitis, prompt laparotomy is indicated. Rapid preliminary restoration of fluid and electrolyte balance may be life saving, because many of these patients are nearly moribund at the time of intestinal perforation.

Trypanosoma cruzi. Infection with *T. cruzi* may result in gastrointestinal or urinary tract hypomotility that requires operative intervention. American trypanosomiasis (Chagas' disease) afflicts approximately 17 to 24 million people in the Western Hemisphere, with South America and particularly Brazil harboring the majority of cases. Chagas' disease extends northward through Central America to Mexico and is occasionally documented in the southern and southwestern United States.[26,27]

Morphology and Life Cycle. Trypanosoma cruzi is the only trypanosome to exhibit both leishmanial and trypanosomal stages in humans. In the Wright-stained blood smear the trypanosome assumes a U or C shape, and the organism approximates 15 to 20 μm in length.

The vertebrate hosts of *T. cruzi* include humans and various wild and domestic animals, and at least 40 species of triatomids (reduviid bugs) transmit the infection (Fig. 8–4).[28] Infection with Chagas' disease is favored by unsanitary rural living conditions, in particular, primitive habitations containing chinks and cracks that provide hiding for the triatomids. These biting insects emerge at

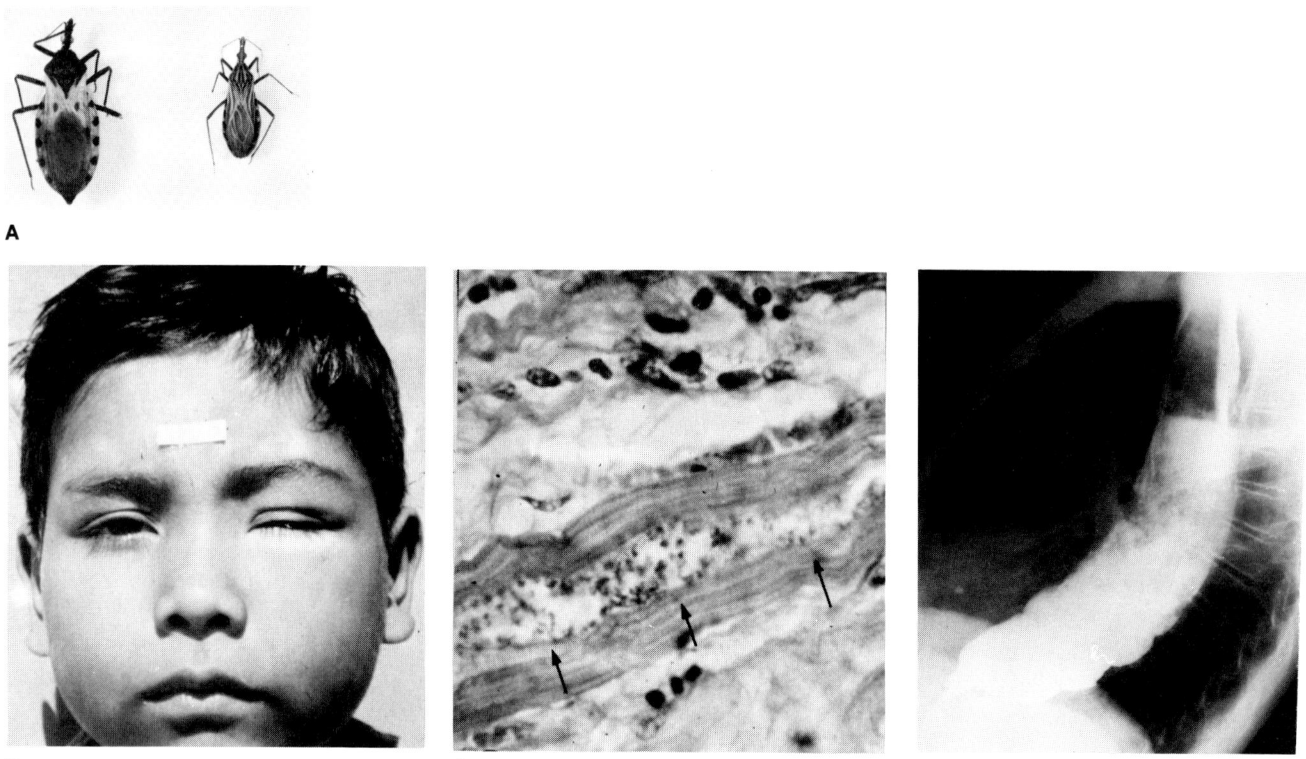

A B C D

Figure 8–4. **A.** Adult and nymph of triatoma, *Rhodnius prolixus.* **B.** Unilateral facial cellulitis, Romaña's sign. **C.** Pseudocyst (leishmanial forms) in the myocardium. **D.** Megaesophagus caused by Chagas' disease. *(From Monroe LS: The gastrointestinal parasites of man. In Berk JE, Haubrich WS, Kalser MH, et al (eds): Bockus Gastroenterology, Vol 7, 4th ed. Philadelphia, Saunders, 1985, p 4285.)*

night to seek a blood meal. While feeding, the triatomid defecates, and if the feces contain infective metacyclic forms, the protozoa enter the subcutaneous tissues through the punctured skin. Infection can also be introduced through abraded skin, the conjunctiva, by blood transfusion, or, rarely, congenitally via the placenta. Once within the host, the trypanosomes enter macrophages and transform to leishmanias. In turn, the leishmanias spread to local nodes where the parasites multiply by binary fission. From these sites, intermediate forms (crithidial and leptomonas) are carried by the blood and lymph to distant sites throughout the body.

Pathology and Clinical Manifestations. Immunosuppression of both cellular and humoral systems by *T. cruzi* may facilitate spread of the organism.[29] At the original site of infection an inflammatory reaction characterized by lymphocytes, plasma cells, reticulum cells, and fibroblasts arises. This locus appears as an erythematous nodular (or ulcerated) lesion called a chagoma and is associated with enlargement of regional lymph nodes. An even more common initial lesion is a unilateral facial and orbital edema associated with conjunctivitis (Romaña's sign) (see Fig. 8–4). Although the associated fever may continue, the local lesions usually subside within 30 days. In approximately 25 percent of cases, local signs are lacking, and the signs of invasion are easily confused with a variety of febrile disease states.[30] During the acute invasive phase the patient may remain febrile from 4 to 5 weeks, and hepatosplenomegaly may persist for months. In the acute phase, myocarditis may develop with cardiac enlargement, congestive heart failure, the appearance of first-degree heart block, and T-wave inversion.

Patients recovering from acute Chagas' disease (some are asymptomatic) have a positive complement-fixation test (Machado-Guerreiro reaction). Months to years later the subacute or chronic manifestations may appear with the development of electrocardiographic conduction defects and arrhythmias. Congestive heart failure may result.

The inflammatory reaction that attends leishmanial invasion produces degeneration of ganglion cells—a late feature of visceral Chagas' disease. The symptoms resulting from such loss of ganglion cells are variable. In mild cases, patients may be asymptomatic. Gastrointestinal symptoms develop late and may not appear until 2 to 20 years after the acute infection has subsided. "Megas" of various organs develop, especially the colon and esophagus. Stomach, small bowel, ureters, and bladder are afflicted less often.

With the development of megacolon the patient develops a slowly progressing constipation. Esophageal stasis may not produce symptoms but often gives rise to dysphagia and regurgitation similar to that found in achalasia. As in the latter condition, secondary complications of aspiration pneumonitis, abscess, and carcinoma may arise.

Diagnosis. The appearance of a lesion suggesting a chagoma or Romaña's sign should, in an endemic area, immediately raise suspicion. Within the first 6 weeks (during the febrile period) the demonstration of trypanosomes in the blood smear or lymph node aspirate is confirmatory. Also during this acute period, xenodiagnosis* is positive in upward of 80 percent of cases.

In the subacute and chronic stages of the disease the indirect immunofluorescence and complement-fixation tests are the most frequently used. Within the first 2 months the indirect immunofluorescence test is most often positive; later the complement-fixation is positive in over 90 percent of those originally infected (see Table 8–1).

In the late stages the x-ray appearance of the megaesophagus is indistinguishable from that of achalasia (see Fig. 8–4), and the manometric profile is similar. The x-ray configuration of Chagas' megacolon is one of uniform dilatation and atony, resembling secondary megacolon rather than Hirschsprung's disease, which is accompanied by narrow bowel segments.

Treatment. Although patients with acute Chagas' disease can be treated with such antitrypanosomal drugs as nitrofurans (Nifurtimox) or Benznidazole, there is no currently satisfactory medical treatment.[28] Nifurtimox is available from the Parasitology Division, Centers for Disease Control.[20] With the development of megaesophagus the patient should be treated as for achalasia. This includes elevation of the head of the bed to prevent nocturnal regurgitation and the institution of bag or balloon dilation (bougienage is not satisfactory, as the lower sphincter will not be sufficiently weakened by this procedure). It is doubtful that surgery is often warranted in view of the generally satisfactory results reported from dilation—45 percent cured, 51 percent improved. When surgery is undertaken, a Heller procedure or subtotal esophagectomy has been advocated.[31] Ferreira-Santos[31] reports carcinoma in 10 percent of 75 cases of esophageal surgery for Chagas' disease.

Softeners (such as dioctyl sulfosuccinate) and enemas have value to prevent impaction. Particularly in children, such enemas should be of physiologic saline to avoid water intoxication. Rarely, hemorrhage from a stercoraceous ulcer, obstruction, or perforation will mandate surgery. Patients who are completely obstipated are usually poor risks and may require proximal colostomy for decompression and the removal of impacted stool. Resection of the rectosigmoid is a more definitive procedure when the patient's condition permits.

* An uninfected triatomid is allowed to bite and consume blood from a suspected case. The feces of the insect are then examined for metacyclic trypanosomes at biweekly intervals for a period of 2 months before the test is declared negative.

HELMINTHS

Nematodes

Anisakis marina. Fully developed (third stage) ascaris-type larvae of the genus *Anisakis* are capable of producing an ulcerative and granulomatous lesion of both the upper and lower gastrointestinal tracts (anisakiasis). Originally described as *herring-worm disease*, it is contracted by the indigestion of raw or partially cooked marine fish.[32] Although the majority of cases have been reported from the Netherlands and Japan, the infection may be considered in any maritime area where raw fish is consumed (ie, Mexico and California).

Morphology and Life Cycle. The adult *A. marina* is a nematode inhabiting the intestinal tracts of whales, porpoises, seals, and sea lions. Although the details of the life cycle are largely unknown, the immature eggs are probably discharged with the feces into the sea, where larvae develop within plankton, which are eaten by fish and squid. The marine mammal acquires the infection through its diet (Fig. 8–5).[33] The apparent recent increase in reported cases may have been due to the changes in the methods of fish preparation, for example, no longer filleting fish immediately after a catch. The refrigeration of whole fish allows larvae to migrate from the gut into the musculature.

Pathology and Clinical Features. After infected raw fish has been eaten, the larvae from the fish burrow

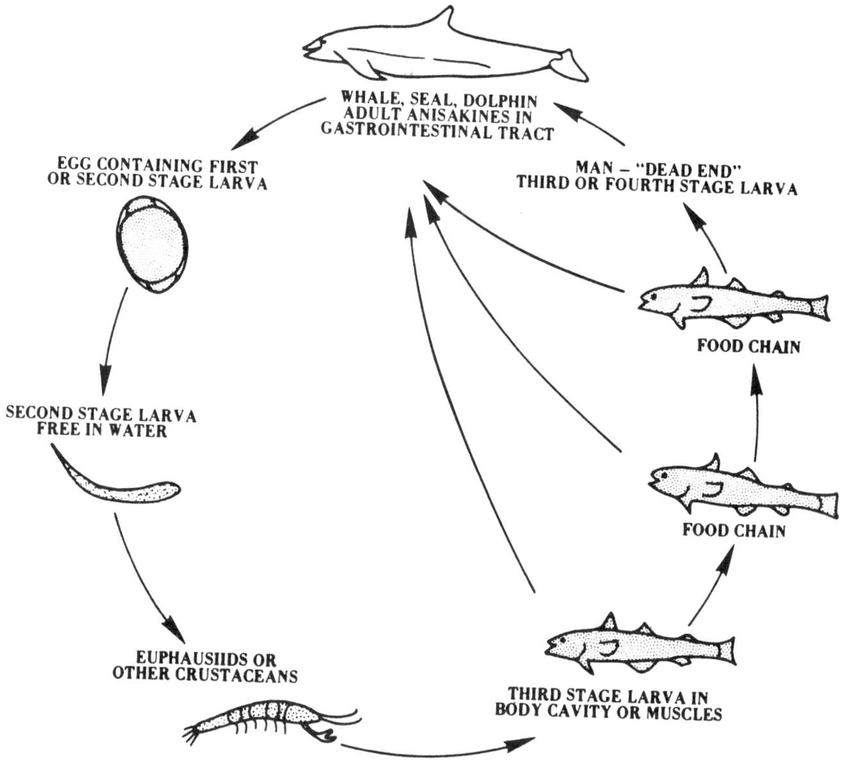

Figure 8–5. Suspected life cycle of anisakine larvae. *(Courtesy of Armed Forces Institute of Pathology 76-6006.)*

into the human gut mucosa, where an ulcerative and granulomatous lesion is formed. The stomach is involved more than the small bowel and colon are. Perforation is rare but may occur at any site from the stomach to the colon. Repeated invasion with subsequent sensitization may help enhance tissue reactivity. Histologically, the lesion appears as an eosinophilic granuloma, and occasionally the etiology is recognized when the larva is identified within the reactive tissue.

Crampy abdominal pain and fever are primary manifestations and may persist for months. Perforation is accompanied by signs of peritonitis.

Diagnosis. Although the endoscopist can rarely identify a larvae, it is unusual for the diagnosis to be made before laparotomy. Anisakiasis should be considered whenever a patient who eats raw fish develops acute and chronic abdominal symptoms.[34] In chronic infection, x-ray study may reveal stenotic lesions of the bowel simulating Crohn's disease. Ishimura et al[35] in a review of presumed regional enteritis in Japan, found 13 of 50 cases to have been caused by *A. marina*. Other than the identification of the larva within the lesion, there is no reliable way to diagnose the infection.[36] Eosinophilia is inconstant, varying from 3 to 34 percent.

Treatment. Under circumstances in which the clinician is highly suspicious of anisakiasis, a medical trial with thiabendazole (25 mg/kg, bid, for 3 days) might prove worthwhile. Most patients undergo resection of the afflicted portion of the intestinal tract without a preoperative diagnosis. Operation carries a high mortality, and staphylococcal enteritis is a common complication. Removal of the larvae with biopsy forceps at the time of endoscopy has produced symptomatic relief.

Angiostrongylus costaricensis. In Central America an occasional eosinophilic granuloma in the terminal ileum, appendix, or cecum is caused by this nematode. In 1971, Morera and Cespedes described *A. costaricensis* (a metastrongylid), defined its life cycle, and located the adults in the mesentery of the small bowel.[37,38]

Morphology and Life Cycle. The adult male and female *A. costaricensis* range from 20 to 33 mm in length and have a cephalic extremity that lacks a buccal capsule. The morphologic details of the adults and larvae forms are best described by Morera.[39]

The adult worms inhabit the mesenteric arterioles of various species of rats. Embryonated eggs enter the bowel and exit with the feces. The intermediate larval stages develop within the common garden slug, and the infective third-stage larvae are extruded with the slime as the mollusk travels. Rats and people acquire the infection through the ingestion of contaminated vegetables. From the gut the larvae pass through the local lymphatics and penetrate the lumen of the mesenteric arteries, where maturation occurs.

Pathology and Clinical Features. A granulomatous response develops with abundant eosinophils and plasma cells in the tissues of the mesentery, bowel wall, and lymphatics. Although the condition has been recognized from the terminal ileum to the ascending colon, the appendix and cecum are most commonly invaded. The adults reside in the vessels at a distance from the bowel wall and thus will not be included in the usual surgical specimen.

Abdominal pain and fever are the earliest symptoms. A mass in the right lower quadrant suggests an appendiceal abscess or tumor. Leukocytosis is variable, sometimes reaching 50,000 white blood cells per cubic millimeter. X-ray examination may reveal a stenotic lesion of the bowel. Eosinophilia is usually a prominent feature and may give a clue to diagnosis.

Diagnosis and Treatment. Because the eggs and larvae of *A. costaricensis* are not recognized in the stool, most cases are diagnosed preoperatively as a bowel lesion. A precipitin reaction has been developed for the diagnosis; however, a clinical correlation is lacking.[40] When a partial obstruction of the ileum or a mass that resembles an appendiceal abscess is associated with an eosinophilia and occurs within an endemic area (Central America), this diagnosis should be considered. Most of these patients do well after resection of the inflammatory mass and the involved mesentery. Thiabendazole has been suggested[20] as treatment but data are lacking.

Ascaris lumbricoides. The large nematode *A. lumbricoides* is the most prevalent helminth infection. In certain parts of the world, more than 90 percent of the population harbor the parasite. The condition is ubiquitous but is more common in humid tropical areas, particularly when night soil is used as a fertilizer. Accumulations of these worms produce intestinal obstruction. The helminth has a propensity for entering small orifices—a habit that frequently produces a biliary tract or a pancreatic manifestation.

Morphology and Life Cycle. The adult male *A. lumbricoides* resembles a large, pale earthworm, measuring 15 to 31 cm in length and 2 to 4 mm in diameter, and is easily identified by a sharp central curve to the tail and the presence of a pair of copulatory spicules.[1] The female is somewhat larger, and a single fertile female can extrude an average of 200,000 eggs per day, so the concentration of eggs in the feces is enormous.

Fertilized eggs pass via the feces, are extremely resistant to the usual methods of water purification, and may retain their infectious potential for up to 6 years.[41] When ingested, the larvae erupt and penetrate the small intestine wall to reach the mesenteric lymphatics or portal venules. They proceed to the lungs and, after a few days, rupture into the alveolar spaces. The larvae then migrate up the bronchial tree, are swallowed, and reach the small intestine, where maturation occurs in about 70 days.

Clinical Manifestations and Diagnosis. Maximal larval migration through pulmonary arteries occurs 5 to 6 days after infection and is often accompanied by symptoms. Patients develop chills, fever, cough, dyspnea, and asthmatic attacks. Examination reveals corresponding bronchial rales, and x-ray examination may demonstrate the changes of a bronchopneumonia or findings suggestive of miliary tuberculosis. After about 10 days the symptoms begin to subside and completely disappear within 3 weeks. The degree of symptomatology is related to previous exposure, which produces sensitization, and the size of the original larval inoculum.

By far the most troublesome complication of ascariasis is the development of intestinal obstruction (Fig. 8–6). Ascarids have a tendency to intertwine themselves. In infants, as few as ten worms can occlude the ileum, the most vulnerable site in all age groups. Abdominal scout films can be helpful, and stool studies (if stool can be obtained from the rectal ampulla by digital examination) should reveal *Ascaris* eggs. A soft periumbilical mass is sometimes noted. Intestinal obstruction can be associated with intussusception or volvulus. Perforation of the bowel, secondary to ascarid obstruction, may occur at any level. For example, an ascarid intruding into the lumen of the appendix may produce an abscess with perforation. *Ascaris lumbricoides* also has a propensity to invade the site of a recent intestinal anastomosis, with resultant perforation. When the helminth enters the peritoneal cavity, localized or generalized peritonitis may occur.

On occasion, although ascarids may enter the peritoneum without inducing pain, they may produce a syndrome characterized by an abdominal mass, leukocytosis, and fever. Such entry occasionally occurs without a demonstrable site of gut perforation.

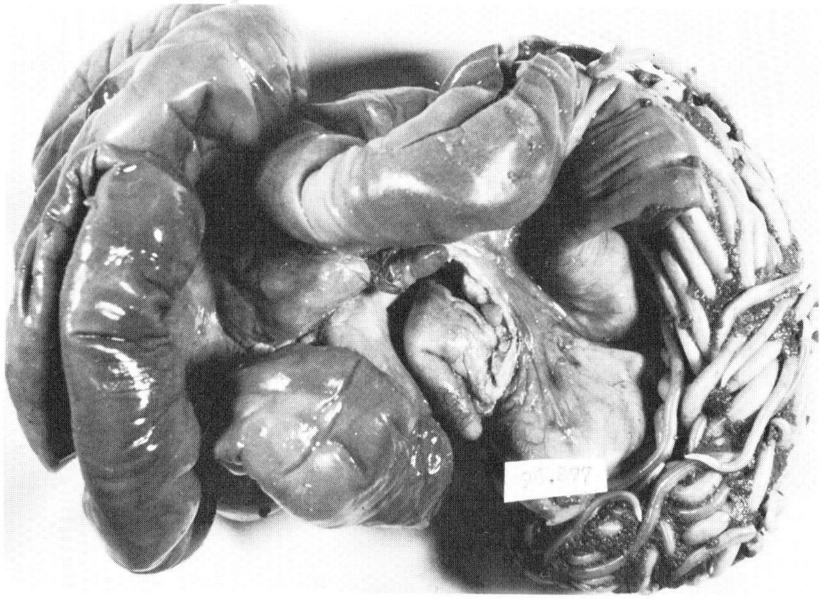

Figure 8–6. Autopsy specimen of ascarids producing intestinal obstruction and bowel necrosis. *(Courtesy of Rudolfo Céspedes.)*

Ascarids may migrate into the biliary and pancreatic tree, causing cholangitis and pancreatitis. In localities such as the Far East where patients with enormous worm burdens are encountered, hepatic abscess secondary to migrating ascarids is called *Hong Kong liver*. In addition, the irritant effects of eggs produces granulomatous lesions and an exuberant cholangitis with pylephlebitis. Such involvement of the biliary system is usually accompanied by hepatomegaly and liver tenderness. Leukocystosis varies from 12,000 to 20,000 white blood cells per cubic millimeter, and eosinophilia is usually mild. Rarely, ascarids reach an arterial lumen, pulmonary parenchyma, eustachian tube, or larynx.

Treatment. Uncomplicated intestinal ascariasis requires only the administration of an appropriate drug (mebendazole, pyrantel pamoate, and albendazole are currently preferred) (Table 8–3). Such drug therapy is 77 to 100 percent effective, and the side effects are minimal. If complications that require operations occur, medical therapy should be instituted after recovery.

Intestinal obstruction produced by ascariasis is an emergency. If it is recognized, nonoperative therapy is sometimes effective. This consists of (1) fluid and electrolyte replacement, (2) nasogastric suction for the relief of distension and vomiting, and (3) enemas with physiologic saline to remove ascarids that clog the colon. If vomiting subsides within 4 to 6 hours, suction is discontinued, and one of the drugs (see Table 8–3) is instilled via a nasogastric tube. On the other hand, if obstruction is not relieved within 24 hours, an operation should be undertaken. The simplest procedures is to milk the worm bolus from the ileum into the large bowel. Enemas can complete the evacuation most easily if the bolus of worms is small. When the obstruction in the ileum cannot be dislodged, resection with end-to-end anastomosis is recommended. A simple enterotomy to extract the ascarids frequently leads to infection and disruption of suture lines.

If biliary or pancreatic ascariasis is suspected and eggs are in the stool, primary drug treatment should be initiated. When symptoms do not abate after 3 weeks, an exploration or endoscopic lavage is in order. Removal of helminths from the biliary or pancreatic systems may be instrumental in relieving the manifestations of acute cholangitis or pancreatitis. Surgical cholangiography and pancreatography are important to rule out the presence of residual helminths. Other than the use of appropriate drugs and operative or endoscopic cleansing of the ductal system, little can be done following the development of ascaris liver abscess.

Helminths in ectopic locations will seldom be diagnosed preoperatively. When they are encountered, simple removal and a search for residual infecting worms usually suffices.

Dirofilaria *Species.* Infection with *Dirofilaria* species (heartworm) is cosmopolitan in certain carnivores, including dogs and cats. In people this parasitosis may appear as a subcutaneous swelling, a coin lesion of the lung, or rarely as an adult parasite within the cardiovascular system. More than 70 cases of human dirofilariasis have been recognized.[42]

TABLE 8–3. DRUG THERAPY OF COMMON HELMINTH INFECTIONS OF SURGICAL INTEREST

Organism	Drug	Average Adult Dose	Duration	Adverse Reactions and Comments
Nematodes				
Ascaris lumbricoides	Mebendazole (Vermox)	100 mg bid	3 d	Occasional: diarrhea and abdominal discomfort
	Albendazole (Zentel)	400 mg	1 d	Occasional: diarrhea, abdominal pain. Rare: leukopenia, alopecia, elevated transaminase
	Pyrantel pamoate (Antiminth)	11 mg/kg (max 1 g)	1 d	Occasional: nausea, vomiting, rash, fever, headache
Enterobius vermicularis	Mebendazole[a]	100 mg; repeat in 2 weeks	1 d	See above
	Pyrantel pamoate	11 mg/kg (max 1 g); repeat in 2 wk	1 d	See above
	Albendazole	400 mg repeat in 2 wk	1 d	See above
Trichuris trichiura	Mebendazole[a]	100 mg bid	3 d	See above
	Albendazole	400 mg	1 d	See above
Cestodes				
Taenia solium	Praziquantel (Biltricide)	5–10 mg/kg	1 d	Common: headache, drowsiness, GI disturbances, eosinophilia. Rare: Pruritis, rash
	Niclosamide (Yomesan)	2 g	1 d	Occasional: nausea, abdominal discomfort
Cysticercosis	Praziquantel	50 mg/kg/d in 3 doses	15 d	See above
	Albendazole	15 mg/kg/d in 3 doses; may repeat	28 d	See above
Echinococcus granulosus hydatidosis	Albendazole	400 mg bid; may repeat	28 d	See above
Echinococcus multilocularis	Albendazole of possible benefit			See above
Trematodes				
Clonorchis sinensis	Praziquantel	25 mg/kg tid	1 d	Common: drowsiness, GI disturbances, fever, eosinophilia. Uncommon: headache, dizziness
Fasciola hepatica	Bithionol (Bitin)	30–50 mg/kg on alternate days	10–15 doses	See above Photosensitivity, diarrhea, vomiting
Paragonimus westermani	Praziquantel	25 mg/kg tid	2 d	See above
Schistosoma mansoni, haematobium, japonicum	See Table 8–4			

[a] Probable drug of choice.
Adapted from Medical Letter on Drugs and Therapeutics.[20]

Life Cycle and Pathology. The adult worm is most often found within the right heart and pulmonary artery of a dog, where microfilariae are released into the bloodstream. Mosquitoes are intermediate hosts to the microfilariae and transmit the infection to definitive hosts, including humans. Because humans are poor hosts, it is unusual to have adult parasites develop within the pulmonary artery or right heart, and, as a rule, involvement is not associated with symptoms. Microfilaremia does not occur within humans, and the parasite typically produces a pulmonary infarct[42,43] or subcutaneous mass.[44,45]

Dirofilaria tenuis produces a subcutaneous inflammatory swelling in the raccoon and is believed by some to be the chief cause of cutaneous masses caused by dirofilariasis in people. *Dirofilaria conjunctivae*, a related species, relies on the raccoon as a host and can produce an inflammatory mass in the eye of humans. The intermediate host of *D. conjunctivae* is the flea.[46] In humans, *D. immitis* microfilariae produce an infarct within the small branches of the pulmonary artery. The resultant x-ray picture may appear as a coin lesion, which simulates early cancer.

Clinical Features and Diagnosis. Heartworms in the dog can produce cor pulmonale or pulmonary disease. In humans, fewer than six cases of right heart involvement have been reported. The infection is usually asymptomatic but may cause subcutaneous masses or pulmonary coin lesions. Other than the identification of a helminth within infected tissue, there is no reliable diagnostic tool.

Treatment. Although drugs are used to treat canine heartworm, the disease in humans does not require treatment except to exclude cancer or explain subcutaneous masses.

Dracunculus medinensis. Infection with the nematode *D. medinensis* occasionally produces an erythematous, serpiginous tract in the subcutaneous tissue. Blisters usually develop in the skin of the lower extremities, where the gravid female discharges larvae. Dracunculiasis occurs predominantly in Africa and Asia, although cases have been reported from the West Indies to South America.[47]

The adult females are extremely long, 70 to 120 cm, in contrast to the tiny male, which averages 12 to 29 mm.[47] The larvae, discharged from the gravid female, enter a freshwater cyclops. Humans are infected by drinking water containing such parasitized copepods. Within the gut the larvae penetrate the intestinal wall to enter the retroperitoneal tissues, where maturation and fertilization occur. After about 12 months the females migrate to the subcutaneous tissues and subsequently penetrate the skin to discharge their larvae. Infection is usually recognized by the appearance of either a long subcutaneous tract or cutaneous blister (Fig. 8–7). At times a portion of the nematode may protrude from the skin.

Treatment consists of dissection and removal of the worm. The classic maneuver of winding the protruding nematode on a stick is not recommended, because the worm can rupture, with a resultant violent tissue reaction (see Fig. 8–7B). Thiabendozole and metronidazole may be effective in killing the worm but should not be substituted for surgery.

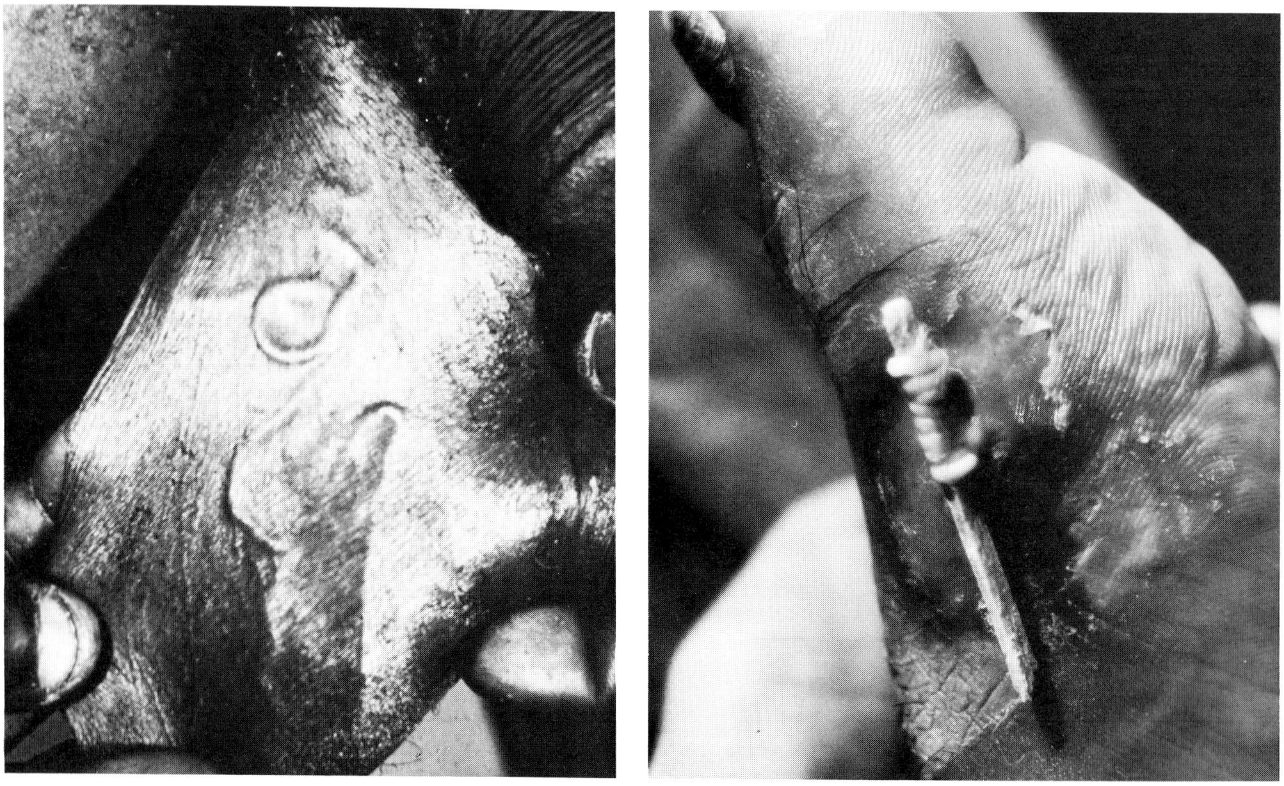

A B

Figure 8–7. *Dracunculus medinensis.* **A.** The tortuous tract of the female is evident in the subcutaneous tissue of the scrotum. *(Courtesy of Armed Forces Institute of Pathology, 67-1563-6; contributed by Dr. Everett L. Schiller.)* **B.** The folk remedy of winding the protruding *D. medinensis* on a stick—not recommended.

Enterobius Vermicularis

A plague to nervous parents, the ubiquitous pinworm is rarely the cause of any concern to the surgeon. The importance of *E. vermicularis* lies in the fact that the helminth can be incidentally found in surgical specimens, particularly the appendix or fallopian tubes. In addition, it should be considered as a rare cause of inflammatory reactions in these areas.

The adults inhabit the right colon (cecum and appendix) and the adjacent small bowel. The gravid females migrate to the rectum and during the night pass through the sphincter to deposit their eggs on the perineal surfaces. Eggs are relatively resistant to drying and disinfectants and when ingested complete the simple oral-anal cycle. The symptoms of infection are usually exceedingly mild and are limited to a pruritus produced by the ovipositing female. The role of enterobiasis in the production of acute appendicitis is probably minimal, but convincing cases are reported.[48] Migrating gravid females may pass through the vagina and produce an endometritis, salpingitis, or granulomatous nodules within the peritoneal cavity.[49] The diagnosis of enterobiasis is based on the recovery of typical eggs. Stool specimens or fingernail dirt are good sources. In addition, eggs may be recovered from the perianal area by the cellophane tape technique (clear adhesive tape is placed sticky side down on the uncleansed perineum and then transferred to a slide for microscopic examination). Drug treatment is outlined in Table 8–3, and one of those listed should be given to all members of a family.

Onchocerca volvulus. Infection with the filarial nematode *O. volvulus* is an important parasitic infection in Africa and in Central America. It produces subcutaneous nodules and microfilariae, which give rise to important cutaneous and ocular lesions. It has been estimated that 50 million persons are infected in Equatorial Africa and 200,000 in Central and South America.[50]

Morphology, Life Cycle, and Pathology. The adults of *O. vulvulus* are long (to 50 cm), slender nematodes that form masses to form nodules within the subcutaneous tissue. These onchocercomas release microfilariae, which can either infect the flies of the Simuliidae family or cause ocular and cutaneous reactions within the host. Although these lesions are usually located in the subcutaneous tissue above the waist, they may also be found adherent to periosteum and in bone. Microfilariae produce ocular lesions, which are characterized pathologically as limbitis, uveitis, and optic atrophy. Furthermore, microfilariae produce edema and lichenification of the skin.

Diagnosis. The demonstration of microfilariae from skin snips, involved skin, or aspiration from subcutaneous nodules confirms the diagnosis. An eosinophilia in the range of 35 percent is usually present. When a patient resides in an endemic zone, the appearance of subcutaneous nodules should raise clinical suspicion. Frequent cross-reactions limit serologic diagnostic methods.

Treatment. Chemotherapy with drugs such as ivermectin 150 mg/kg once and repeated every 6 to 12 months has proved of great value. Nevertheless, the chief method is surgical removal of the subcutaneous onchocercomas. This measure reduces the number of microfilariae and diminishes the danger of ocular damage. The removal of onchocercomas can easily be accomplished with the use of local anesthesia. The lesions are enclosed in a fibrous layer that usually offers a cleavage plane.

Toxocara canis *and* T. cati. The ascarids *T. canis* and *T. cati* commonly infect domestic dogs and cats, as well as related wild species. Accidental ingestion of eggs gives rise to the syndrome of visceral larva migrans and can on rare occasion be produced by a variety of spirurid, filarial, strongyloid nematodes. Children playing in contaminated areas may become infected by the ingestion of eggs. The life cycle is abortive in humans, and larvae do not mature into adult helminths. The larvae penetrate the intestinal wall and produce eosinophilic granulomas and abscesses of the liver. Less commonly, larvae may reach the central nervous system or lung, and rarely the eye. At this latter site the larvae may produce a severe chorioretinitis or endophthalmitis, which ends in blindness. Such lesions are usually unilateral, and enucleation is sometimes carried out with the presumptive diagnosis of retinoblastoma or other malignancy.[51]

The diagnosis of toxocariasis should be suspected when a child develops cough, hepatomegaly, lymphadenopathy, and lung infiltrates, and on laboratory examination a hypergammaglobulinemia and persistent eosinophilia are documented. Suspicion is further heightened if household pets can be shown to harbor *Toxocara* species and if the child is known to eat dirt. Stool examination is, of course, worthless, as the larvae do not develop into adults. Liver biopsy may be diagnostic, and such material should be serially sectioned. Because the lesions are unevenly distributed, failure to find the larvae or granuloma does not rule out the diagnosis. With ocular involvement the larvae can occasionally be seen by slit-lamp examination. Eye lesions are unilateral, and the absence of calcifications favors a parasitic rather than a neoplastic etiology.

Currently at the Centers for Disease Control and Prevention (CDC), enzyme immunoassay (EIA) using toxocaral larval antigen has a specificity of 78 to 92 percent.[52] Because of cross-reactivity, positive results are not absolute proof of infection.

Primary treatment of toxocariasis consists of preventing reinfections, that is, separation of the patient from infected pets and the prevention of dirt eating. If additional infection can be prevented, most patients begin to improve within weeks. Treatment with thiabendazole, diethylcarbamazine, and mebendazole has been suggested; however, the latter two are deemed investigational by the FDA.[20] Additional rapid clinical improvement following the use of corticosteroids has been suggested.[53] If a larva can be identified by slit-lamp examination, thiabendazole has been used, with probable benefit.

Trichuris trichiura. Infection with whipworm, *T. trichiura*, a cosmopolitan nematode, is commonly asymptomatic. Occasionally, however, particularly in children, the infection may be fulminant and lead to colonic ulceration and rectal prolapse.

Morphology and Life Cycle. Averaging 30 to 50 mm in length, the adult worms (Fig. 8–8) are narrowed in their anterior portion. The male is characterized by its coiled posterior end with a projecting spicule.[54] The eggs are a deep brown and are distinguished by bipolar plugs and an ovoidal shape. The life cycle is simple and parallels that of *Enterobius vermicularis*. Excreted in the feces, the eggs maturate, and, when they are ingested, larvae erupt and begin their development within the villi of the small intestine. Within 30 days the parasites migrate to the proximal colon, where they reside with their slender esophagi burrowed beneath the mucosa. These helminths may survive as long as 3 years.[55]

Clinical Manifestations. Trichuriasis is seldom accompanied by symptoms. Severe infection can initiate diarrhea, debility, and blood loss. When more than 300 helminths are present, iron deficiency can be expected. In children infection of the rectosigmoid may precipitate diarrhea, tenesmus, and rectal prolapse. Rarely, ulcerations produced by infection will lead to perforation with the signs of peritonitis.

Diagnosis. The eggs of *T. trichiura* are easily recognized. Adults rarely may be identified in the mucosa of a rectal prolapse or during colonoscopic examination (see Fig. 8–8).

Treatment. Mebendazole is a well-tolerated anthelminic; 100 mg twice a day for 3 days will cure 90 percent of adults (see Table 8–3). Albendazole 400 mg in a single dose is an alternative drug.

The surgeon may be called for advice regarding a patient (usually a child) with rectal prolapse. The etiology can often be established with identification of adult whipworms residing within the prolapsed mucosa. The first maneuver is gentle digital replacement of the prolapsed segment. Next, oral drugs are used to prevent tenesmus and treat the infection. If a patient with severe trichuriasis and

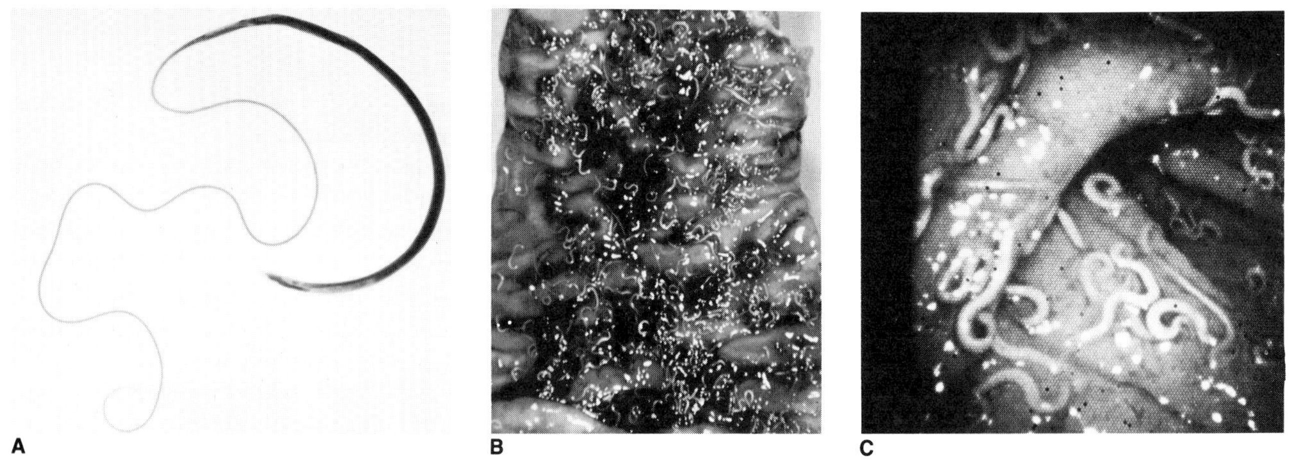

Figure 8–8. A. Adult *Trichuris trichiura* (length 50 mm). **B.** An autopsy specimen of colon heavily infected with *T. trichiura. (Courtesy of Rudolfo Céspedes.)* **C.** Colonoscopic view of *T. trichiura* in situ in cecum. *(From McCaffery TD: Gastrointest Endosc 21:172, 1975.)*

diarrhea develops signs of intestinal perforation, laparotomy should be undertaken. Unfortunately, trichuriasis is seldom a pure infection, and the clinician should always be alert to the necessity of treatment for an additional pathogen such as hookworm or *Ascaris*. Drug therapy should follow any operation to eradicate residual helminths.

Cestodes

Echinococcus granulosa. Cystic hydatid disease (CHD) or echinococcosis is an important parasitic infection of humans and other animals (dogs, wolves, and cats). Humans usually become infected by the ingestion of viable eggs that originate in dog feces. The larvae produce cystic lesions, 75 percent of which arise in the liver (see Chap. 31); however, nearly every organ in the body can be invaded.

The condition is cosmopolitan but is particularly prevalent where sheep are raised as in South America, South Africa, and Central Europe. Sixty-nine cases have been reported in the United States.[56]

Morphology and Life Cycle. The adult *E. granulosus* is a small tapeworm, measuring 3 to 6 mm in length with three proglottids. The rostellum has a double crown of hooks, and the scolex has four suckers. The eggs cannot be distinguished from other *Taenia* species.[57]

Eggs or sloughed proglottids are passed in the feces of the definitive host, and when the eggs are ingested by an intermediate host (usually sheep), including humans, the larvae usually pass to the liver but also to the lung, spleen, central nervous system, and bone. In the liver the cysts grow slowly, averaging 2 to 3 cm a year, until they reach a huge size and contain several liters of fluid. The fully developed cyst (Fig. 8–9) contains a peripheral zone of fibrous tissue that may calcify, an intermediate chitinous layer, and an inner germinal layer, which produces brood capsules and proscolices. When such scolices break loose into the hydatid fluid, they, along with free daughter cysts, are termed *hydatid sand* (see Fig. 8–9).

Clinical Aspects and Diagnosis. When cystic lesions of subcutaneous tissue, liver, lung, bone, spleen, or brain are encountered, CHD should be ruled out. A mature cyst has a thin, dense radiopaque wall and such a finding usually indicates a dormant state. Computed tomography (CT) can aid in determining progression. In approximately 80 percent of the cases the cysts involve the right lobe of the liver and are multiple 25 percent of the time. The pressure of cyst fluid is high (averaging 40 to 80 cm of water, and the pressure on the biliary tree produces jaundice in approximately one-third of the patients. After many asymptomatic years, a patient may be found to have an abnormal mass during a routine physical examination. Vilardel[58] described pain resembling that of biliary colic on one-half of 98 patients with hydatid liver cysts. Other manifestations included eosinophilia in 55 percent, palpable mass in 53 percent, fever in 27 percent, and pruritus in 24 percent. The hydatid cysts appear as a smooth rounded mass, which may be tender but is not characteristically hard. Uncommonly, vascular compression may produce a Budd-Chiari syndrome or splenomegaly. A hydatid liver cyst will perforate into the biliary tree approximately 25 percent of the time. Uncommonly, rupture can occur into the gastrointestinal tract or pleural or peritoneal space (see Chap. 31).

Serologic testing using enzyme immunoassay (EIA) or indirect hemagglutination (IHA) are of value in confirming the diagnosis of CHD (see Table 8–1). Further confirmation of a positive test can be obtained by the immunoblot assay and is performed at the CDC.[52] The intradermal Casoni test and IHA together give a positive reaction in 92 percent of known cases.[59] The Casoni test is false positive, however, in about 18 percent of cases.[58] Unfortunately, serologic procedures, while important diagnostically, do not indicate whether a cyst is enlarging. This distinction must be made using clinical evidence (observed enlargement, tenderness). Radiographically, the presence of a densely calcified cyst is an important clue to a dormant cyst.

Treatment. A densely calcified hydatid cyst that is not producing symptoms can be observed and operation deferred. In the majority of cases, however, an operation is recommended because of the danger of rupture of the cyst and progressive destruction of the liver. A variety of solutions (2 percent formalin cetrimide, povidone-iodine, 30 percent saline) have been instilled in cysts to sterilize their contents; however, the effectiveness is uncertain and complications may arise (ie, sclerosing cholangitis or local perotonitis). The benzimidazoles have an important role in the management of CHD. The first drug shown to have a therapeutic effect was mebendazole; however, high doses (50 mg/kg) for long periods up to 3 months were necessary. Albendazole (400 mg bid for 28 days, repeated as necessary) is the current treatment of choice, although some patients will require excision of the cyst. Praziquantel may be useful preoperatively in the event of a spill

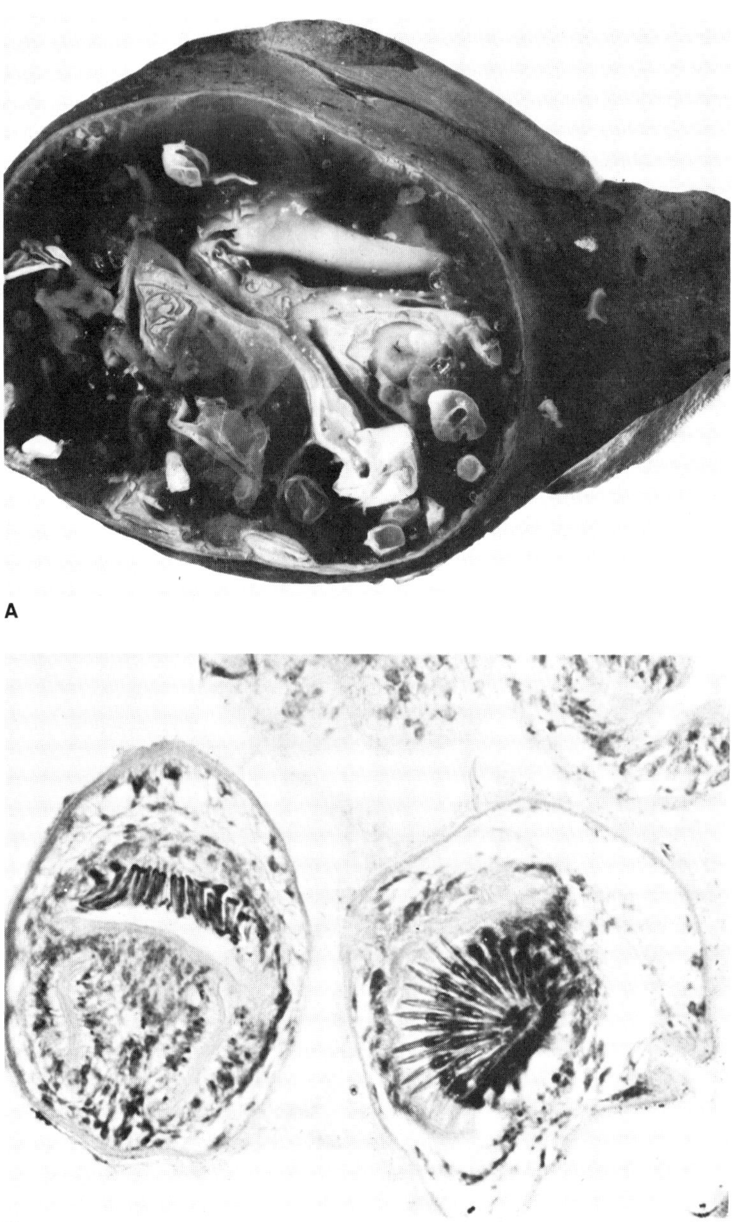

A

B

Figure 8–9. A. Large unilocular hydatid cyst of the liver, with free daughter cysts in fluid. B. Scolices and *E. granulosus* in the blood capsule. *(Courtesy of Armed Forces Institute of Pathology N-31977 and 70-8831.)*

of cystic fluid.[20] Details of treatment are given in Chapter 31.

Echinococcus multilocularis. An unusual but deadly variant caused by *E. multilocularis* produces alveolar hydatid disease (AHD). AHD is found in southern Germany, Austria, Switzerland, and Russia near the Bering Sea. The adult *E. multilocularis* is smaller than *E. granulosus*. The larvae of *E. multilocularis* cannot produce a confined colony of organism as does *E. granulosus*. The alveolar hydatid proliferates by exuberant budding—a feature that makes this infection behave as if it were a malignancy.

The intermediate hosts of *E. multilocularis* are small rodents, and the definitive hosts are usually foxes and other members of the dog family. Humans usually become the accidental intermediate hosts by eating vegetable material contaminated by egg-containing feces.

In more than 90 percent of patients the liver is involved and is gradually destroyed by invasive cystic masses. Diagnostic measures as for *E. granulosus* are of value. Needle biopsy should not be done because of the danger of spread of infection. Surgical resection of the infected portion of the liver, combined with medical therapy, is the chief hope for cure (see Chap. 31). Albendazole (400 mg bid for

2 to 3 months) may be of value; however, data are scarce.[60]

Taenia solium *and* Cysticercus cellulosae. Wherever undercooked pork is consumed, infection with *T. solium* will be encountered. When humans become the intermediate host, the larval form of the parasite *C. cellulosae* may produce an important cause of space-occupying intracranial lesion.[61]

Morphology and Life Cycle. The adult *T. solium* is characterized by a scolex having four suckers and a rostellum encircled by a double row of hooklets.[62] The gravid proglottid is distinguished by having fewer lateral uterine branches (7 to 13) than does the corresponding proglottid of *T. saginata*. The adult *T. solium* resides in the upper gut of humans, the only known definitive host. When passed in the feces, living proglottids may be ingested by a variety of mammalian intermediate hosts. Within the gut of the intermediate host the eggs hatch, penetrate the wall, and migrate throughout the body to develop in 60 to 90 days as infective bladder worms.

When eggs are accidentally ingested, humans become the intermediate hosts, with the development of cysticerci within tissues. As a rule, however, humans acquire the adult *T. solium* through the ingestion of *C. cellulosae* present in raw or undercooked meat, especially in countries where the quality of meat inspection is uncertain, for example, Mexico.

Clinical Features. People are seldom aware that they are harboring an adult *T. solium*. Mild aberrations of appetite, abdominal discomfort, and diarrhea are reported. Cysticercosis may produce symptoms referable to the site—brain, heart, lungs, muscles, liver, and eye. No tissue is immune to invasion. When nonvital structures, such as the subcutaneous tissue, are involved, the patient may be completely unaware of infection. The most serious complication of cysticercosis is the development of a cerebral lesion with the resultant edema and gliosis. Such diverse conditions as brain tumor, pseudotumor, syphilitic meningitis, or the cerebral atrophies may be mimicked. On the other hand, silent cerebral cysticercosis can develop, the diagnosis being made by the x-ray visualization of end-stage intracranial calcifications.

Diagnosis. As the eggs of various *Taenia* species are indistinguishable, the recognition of *T. solium* infection rests with the identification of the typical scolex or gravid proglottid. The definitive histologic diagnosis of cysticercosis depends on the demonstration of an invaginated scolex with four suckers and two rows of hooklets.

The sudden appearance of subcutaneous nodules associated with acute central nervous system complaints (particularly jacksonian convulsions) should suggest cysticercosis. Computerized axial tomography (CAT) is often a diagnostic aid. In the eye, examination may reveal a cysticercus within the vitreous. With end-stage lesions, calcifications may be seen scattered throughout skeletal muscle or within the brain (Fig. 8–10). It should be remembered that such calcified lesions are rarely, if ever, symptom producing and that active *C. cellulosae* are not radiopaque. Eosinophilia is variable and is rarely helpful. The CDC provide an immunoblot test for cysticercosis. The test has a high sensitivity and specificity.

Treatment. The medical therapy for intestinal *T. solium* and for cysticercosis is outlined in Table 10–3. Praziquantel, a chemotherapeutic agent originally developed to treat schistosomiasis, is a major breakthrough in the therapy of cysticercosis, and clinical improvement occurs in the majority of cases.[63,64] Albendazole is an effective alternative drug. When larval *T. solium* infections are so treated, an inflammatory reaction produced by the death of cysts may cause additional damage in ocular, cerebral, or spinal lesions. Çorticosteroids should be given for 2 to 3 days before and during treatment but may not completely suppress complications. The appearance of ring enhancement (caused by an inflammatory response) can be docu-

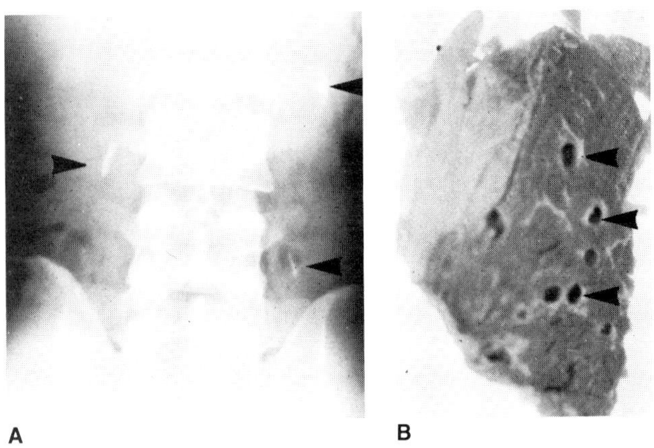

Figure 8–10. A. X-ray showing "rice grain" calcifications in skeletal muscles, produced by larvae of *Taenia solium*. **B.** Skeletal muscle of a hog infected with cysticerci of *T. solium* (measly pork). *(From Monroe LS: The gastrointestinal parasites of man. In Berk JE, Haubrich WS, Kalser MH, et al (eds): Bockus Gastroenterology, Vol 7, 4th ed. Philadelphia, Saunders, 1985, p 4310.)*

mented by CAT scanning. In unresponsive cases or in those in which the lesion is life threatening, surgery should be undertaken. Removal of the cyst and decompression of hydrocephalus are the most common procedures involving the central nervous system. Calcified cysticerci are not in themselves a surgical indication because the *C. cellulosae* are dead. In such a case with a neurologic disorder a different cause should be sought.

Trematodes

Clonorchis sinensis. Infection with the Chinese liver fluke *C. (Opisthorchis) sinensis* is common in the areas of Asia bounded by the China Sea. An autopsy series from Hong Kong found evidence of clonorchiasis in 65 percent of deaths. Inasmuch as the adult flukes may survive in biliary passages for more than 20 years, the condition is frequently detected in Asiatics who have moved long ago from areas where it is endemic.

Morphology and Life Cycle. The average adult *C. sinensis* ranges from 10 to 25 mm in length and has an anterior and ventral sucker. The eggs are small, averaging 27 to 35 μm, and have a prominent "shoulder" adjacent to the operculum.[65]

Cats, pigs, camels, rats, and dogs are important reservoir hosts of *C. sinensis*. On reaching water with the feces, the eggs are ingested by snails and undergo metamorphosis. After 4 to 5 weeks, cercariae emerge and penetrate freshwater fish where metacercariae encyst in the flesh. People (and other flesh eaters) acquire the infection from undercooked fish. The metacercariae are released and penetrate the duodenal mucosa to migrate to the biliary tree, seeking as a rule the smaller branches of the left lobe of the liver where maturation occurs (see Fig. 8–11).

Pathology and Clinical Manifestations. Although mild asymptomatic infections are common, the presence of *C. sinensis* in the biliary passages provokes a marked inflammatory reaction called *pipestem fibrosis*. A portal-type cirrhosis with its complications, ascites and varices, may follow. More frequently, complications of clonorchiasis include the development of biliary calculi centering about eggs or adults and the occurrence of acute suppurative cholangitis. The latter condition, cholangiohepatitis, can be acute or chronic and is associated with intrahepatic stones, abscesses, and ductal strictures. The incidence of cholangioma is reported by Hou[66] to be increased in clonorchiasis; in fact, 15

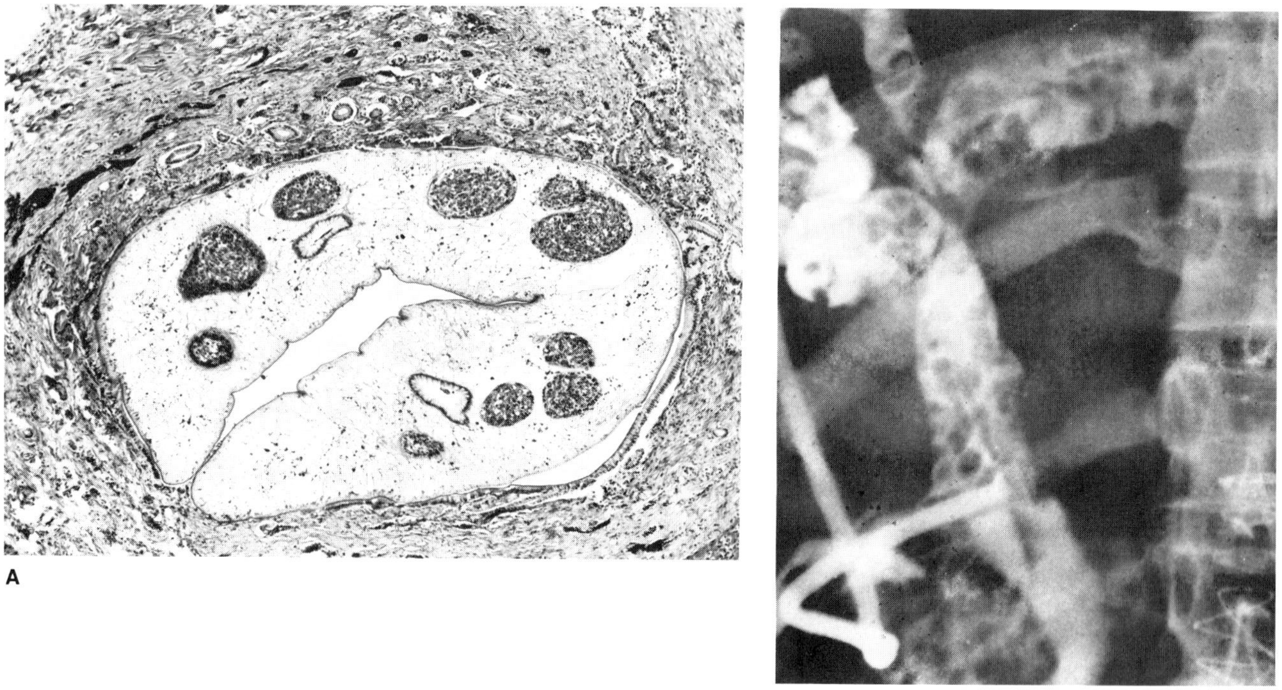

A

B

Figure 8–11. A. Section through posterior portion of *Clonorchis sinensis* in a bile duct, showing testis and cecae (×31.5) **B.** T-tube cholangiogram showing ductular dilatation and numerous parasites. *(Courtesy of Armed Forces Institute of Pathology 74-11157 and 69-5522-3.)*

percent of primary carcinoma of the liver in Hong Kong may be induced by this infection. The presence of *C. sinensis* within the pancreatic ductal system has been found in as many as 37 percent of autopsy reports of clonorchiasis; however, the associated pancreatitis is usually mild.

There is no characteristic pattern of the infection produced by *C. sinensis*, and symptoms may occur before eggs are detectable in the stool. Many light infections are asymptomatic. A tender, enlarged liver accompanied by chills, fever, and malaise are frequent early signs in heavy infections. Fluctuating jaundice is usually obstructive in character, and eosinophilia to 40 percent may accompany the illness. Colicky right upper quadrant and epigastric pain may simulate or be caused by associated cholelithiasis and choledocholithiasis. Late rare manifestations of advanced disease are those that accompany decompensated cirrhosis.

Diagnosis. Clonorchiasis should be suspected when a patient develops signs of hepatic, biliary, or pancreatic disease and has eaten raw freshwater fish from an endemic area. Eosinophilia indicates a possible parasitic cause. The final diagnosis depends on finding the tiny operculated egg in the stool. A concentration technique (such as the formalin-ether method) will facilitate recovery of the eggs. Serologic tests have been described but are not available clinically. Retrograde endoscopic cholangiography should prove to be a useful tool in delineating the strictures and stones associated with cholangiohepatitis.

Treatment. There is no completely satisfactory drug treatment for clonorchiasis. Praziquantel (25 mg/kg tid, for 1 day) has been tried with some success (see Table 8–3).

Exploration of the common bile duct with removal of flukes, detritus, and associated stones has been of value in advanced cases of cholangiohepatitis. Symptomatic cholelithiasis, developing in a parasitic locus, would require cholecystectomy. Operative cholangiography, common duct exploration, and lavage should probably be carried out whenever cholecystectomy is performed. ERCP with removal of flukes and ductal lavage can also be of value.

Fasciola hepatica. Human infection with *F. hepatica* (fascioliasis) occurs wherever sheep are raised. Forty-nine cases reported from England in 1968 illustrate the problem produced by the ingestion of parasitized water plants (particularly watercress).[1,67–69] Because humans are poor hosts for the parasite, the flukes frequently localize ectopically in subcutaneous tissue, lung parenchyma, peritoneum, brain, and stomach rather than the usual site—the biliary tree.

Morphology, Life Cycle, and Diagnosis. The adult *F. hepatica* has a broadly ovoidal shape with a distinctive cephalic cone. The average length (30 mm) and the branching intestinal cecae are distinguishing features. The eggs of *F. hepatica* are operculated, large, and easily confused with those of other trematodes. The animal hosts of *E. hepatica* include sheep, goats, cattle, and a variety of wild herbivores. Eggs are passed with the feces. When they reach water, the eggs mature to develop miracidiae, which penetrate snails and eventually acquire the cercarial form. Such cercariae leave the snail and encyst on aquatic plants, which are food for grazing animals. When consumed by the definitive host, including humans, the larvae hatch, move through the intestinal tract, traverse peritoneal surfaces, enter the liver, and finally arrive in the biliary tree. Ectopic migration can occur to any organ but is particularly frequent in subcutaneous tissues. In herbivores, the flukes within the biliary tree evoke an intense inflammatory reaction with a predominant eosinophilic component. Local abscesses are common, and the term *sheep liver rot* describes the infected organ.

In humans, the larval migration is accompanied by eosinophilia, which subsides as the fluke matures. The ingestion of contaminated water plants (particularly watercress) is followed within 7 to 14 days by a febrile illness and an eosinophilia. The appearance of a coin lesion in the lung or a mass in the subcutaneous tissues should further increase suspicion. Mature eggs are rarely seen in the stool, and coprology is of little value. The ultimate diagnosis is usually made by recovery of the adult trematode at the time of biliary exploration. The larvae can occasionally be identified when removed from their aberrant site.

Treatment. Whenever fascioliasis is diagnosed, medical treatment should be instituted with bithionol (30 to 50 mg/kg for 1 day and then on alternate days or 10 to 15 doses) (see Table 8–3). The surgeon may encounter flukes at the time of cholecystectomy. In such a case ERCP or operative cholangiography and common duct exploration should be undertaken for the removal of residual helminths.

Paragonimus westermani. Infection with the lung fluke *P. westermani* and closely related species is widely distributed in areas of the Far East. Humans acquire the disease after eating freshwater crustaceans or their juice. Lesions may develop in the lungs, subcutaneous tissue, spinal canal, brain, liver, pancreas, and peritoneal surfaces. Some manifestations may require surgical intervention.

Morphology, Life Cycle, and Pathology. The adult *P. westermani* resides in humans and a variety of domesticated and wild animals. The adult flukes average 7.5 to 20 mm in length and have an elongated oval shape.[70] There are anterior and ventral suckers. The adults, which reside in pulmonary cysts, pass eggs that exit the body via sputum or feces. On reaching water the miracidia hatch to enter snails, the usual pattern for trematodes. After further development, cercariae emerge from the snails and encyst as metacercariae in the gills and muscles of crustaceans. When ingested by an appropriate definitive host, the metacercariae penetrate the upper small intestine and enter the abdominal cavity; from there they may penetrate the diaphragm, enter the pleural cavity, and invade the lungs. It requires about 70 days for the flukes to mature and produce eggs. After such an odyssey it is not surprising that larval forms may reach widespread ectopic areas in the body, that is, liver, bone, pancreas, and subcutaneous tissue.

The oval pulmonary parasitic cysts, averaging 0.6 to 3.3 cm in greatest dimension, are thin-walled and usually discernible as firm masses at or near the pleural surface. On section, one and occasionally more flukes may be seen. The lung parenchyma surrounding the cysts is hemorrhagic. The inflammatory reaction shows varying numbers of neutrophils and mononuclear cells with eosinophils predominating. Charcot-Leyden crystals may be present in the necrotic center of such a cyst. Inflammatory changes peripheral to the cyst may lead to bronchitis, peribronchitis, and bronchopneumonia. The contents of a ruptured cyst enter the bronchi and produce a cough and many times bronchopneumonia. The foreign protein may stimulate a granulomatous reaction with giant cells of the Langhans type, and, as a late event, ossification of the granuloma and cysts can occur.

Although no region escapes infection, cutaneous paragonomiasis has a predilection for the subcutaneous tissue of the trunk. A typical cyst would appear in the abdominal wall and measure 2 to 3 cm in diameter. Histologically, the parasite and eggs can be identified in about 50 percent of cases. Granulomas with foreign body giant cells and eosinophilia dominate the tissue response.

Clinical Manifestations. With pulmonary involvement, cough with the production of blood-tinged sputum is common. The condition is often chronic, extending over years; however, aside from periodic bouts of pleuritic pain, patients as a rule show relative well-being. Examination of the sputum should be done repeatedly by concentration techniques and direct smear when the patient is from an endemic area.

On x-ray examination the peripheral circumscribed pulmonary lesions of paragonimiasis are often coin lesions, and the differential diagnosis includes the infectious granulomas, tumor, and other parasites. In at least 40 percent of the cases the x-ray picture is indistinguishable from tuberculosis. Examination of sputum and stool for typical eggs is an important diagnostic measure when an Asiatic with such an x-ray picture is being evaluated.

Cerebral paragonimiasis may initiate with progressive neurologic symptoms and signs of a space-occupying intracranial lesion. The most common first sign is a jacksonian or grand mal seizure. Headache, hemiplegia, and nuchal rigidity occur to a lesser degree.

Diagnosis. The diagnosis may be confirmed by the identification of large operculated eggs in the sputum or spinal fluid; however, the passage of eggs from pulmonary lesions may be sporadic and serodiagnosis may be necessary. The Centers for Disease Control offer an immunoblot assay that has a high specificity and was positive in 96 percent of patients with parasitologically confirmed *P. westermani* infections.[52]

Treatment. Praziquantel (25 mg/kg tid for 1 to 2 days) or bithionol (30 to 50 mg/kg on alternate days for 10 to 15 doses) should be given as soon as the diagnosis is made (see Table 10–3). Data on cure rates are sparse, but they probably exceed 90 percent. An operation is still indicated for a localized, space-occupying, intracranial or spinal lesion.

Schistosoma mansoni. Schistosomiasis is the most important parasitic infection of people.[71,72] It has been estimated that there are 29 million cases of *S. mansoni*, 39 million *S. haematobium*, and 46 million *S. japonicum* infections in the world. *Schistosoma mansoni*, along with *S. haematobium*, is found in the Nile Basin and other parts of Africa. Foci of *S. mansoni* also exist in Central and South America (particularly Puerto Rico). Although the vectors are present, the condition is not acquired within the continental United States.

Morphology and Life Cycle. *Schistosoma mansoni* is a trematode. The adults reside within the venous radicles of the hemorrhoidal plexus.[73] The paired worms are usually located in the vasculature near the rectum and sigmoid. Eggs with a subterminal spine are deposited in the immediate submucosal area. On transiting the mucosa, the eggs mix with the stool, reach water, and the miracidium develops to enter a snail.[74] Within the snail, division and metamorphosis occur, with the release of a forked-tailed cercaria. These motile cercariae penetrate the exposed skin or when swallowed transit the gut to enter local lymphatics, from whence they migrate to the lungs. From this latter site the schistosomes reach the liver, probably via the bloodstream. Maturation continues, and the developing adults migrate against the blood current to their final habitat. The time from cutaneous penetration to final maturation and egg deposition is approximately 40 to 50 days.

Pathology and Clinical Features. Within minutes to hours after entry of cercariae into the skin a urticarial rash may develop; the eruption can last for several days. Systemic symptoms are usually absent during the stage of larval migration to early oviposition.[73] Beginning with the onset of sustained oviposition, however, the acute stage commences, with fever, abdominal pain, and diarrhea. Fever is usually remittent, with afternoon elevations, and continues for approximately 2 weeks. During this period, physical findings may include a generalized lymphadenopathy and a mild hepatomegaly. Periorbital edema and transitory urticarial rashes may also be present during this stage. A leukocytosis in the range of 20,000 white blood cells per cubic millimeter is accompanied by an eosinophilia with values averaging 30 to 75 percent.[73] In the chronic stage, tissue alterations caused by *S. mansoni* can be attributed to the adult worms, their eggs, toxic products, and the host's reaction to the parasitism. Probably the most significant pathology is produced by the eggs, which induce granulomas or pseudotubercules with phlebitis in the liver, intestine, lungs, bladder, heart, and other organs.[75] Within the colon this process leads to a progressive fibrosis with mucosal ulceration and occasionally the production of inflammatory polyps and papillomas. Eggs that circulate into the liver induce phlebitis and allergic hyperreactive proliferation within the portal tracts. A concentric fibrosis occurs about the portal tracts, and, in association, reticulin fibers proliferate in an "onion skin" configuration. A Symmers' fibrosis can be produced, with the liver appearing "as if a number of clay pipestems had been thrust at various angles through the organ" (Fig. 8–12). Portal hypertension with congestive splenomegaly, hypersplenism with anemia, leukopenia, and thrombocytopenia may ensue. This cirrhosis is presinusoidal, so that the measurement of wedged hepatic vein pressure does not reflect the elevated portal vein pressure. In the severe case, garden variety portal or postnecrotic cirrhosis develops. The adult worms inhibit chiefly the hemorrhoidal plexus, so in contrast to the eggs they contribute little to the hepatic pathology.

In advanced cases, bleeding from esophageal varices occurs. Inasmuch as parenchymal function remains good because of adequate perfusion of the lobula, these bleeding episodes are usually well tolerated by the patient. In fact, liver function study results are only mildly disturbed in most cases.[73]

Cardiopulmonary schistosomiasis produces a spectrum of pathologic changes including the development of diffuse minute arteriovenous fistulas with subsequent deficient oxygenation.[73]

The appearance of the rectosigmoid mucosa is variable, and many mild cases may appear normal even though superficial ulcerations and progressive thickening of the mucosa may mimic granulomatous colitis, inflammatory stricture, or carcinoma.[74] Hyperplastic (inflammatory) polyps of the colon can develop under the stimulus of eggs within the mucosa and simulate the pseudopolyps of chronic ulcerative colitis. Such polyps can disappear with medical treatment.

Diagnosis. The diagnosis of *S. mansoni* is most easily made by biopsy of the rectal mucosa. Multiple specimens are best taken from an upper rectal valve. Observation of the flickering flame cell or motility of the miracidium gives a clue to egg viability. It should be noted that after treatment the exterior shell may remain intact for months to years, although the egg is nonviable. This differentiation is important because the mere presence of eggs does not indicate the need for treatment. Coprology is much less successful, so it should not be used in lieu of biopsy to help identify eggs.

Serologic studies can be useful in those cases when eggs cannot be demonstrated. At the Centers for Disease Control specimens are tested (EIA) using adult *S. mansoni* antigen and a positive reaction indicates infection with *Schistosoma* species.[52] A more specific diagnosis utilizing immunoblots based on travel history then aids in species identification (see Table 8–1).

Treatment. Drugs used in the treatment of schistosomiasis are outlined in Table 8–4. Fortunately,

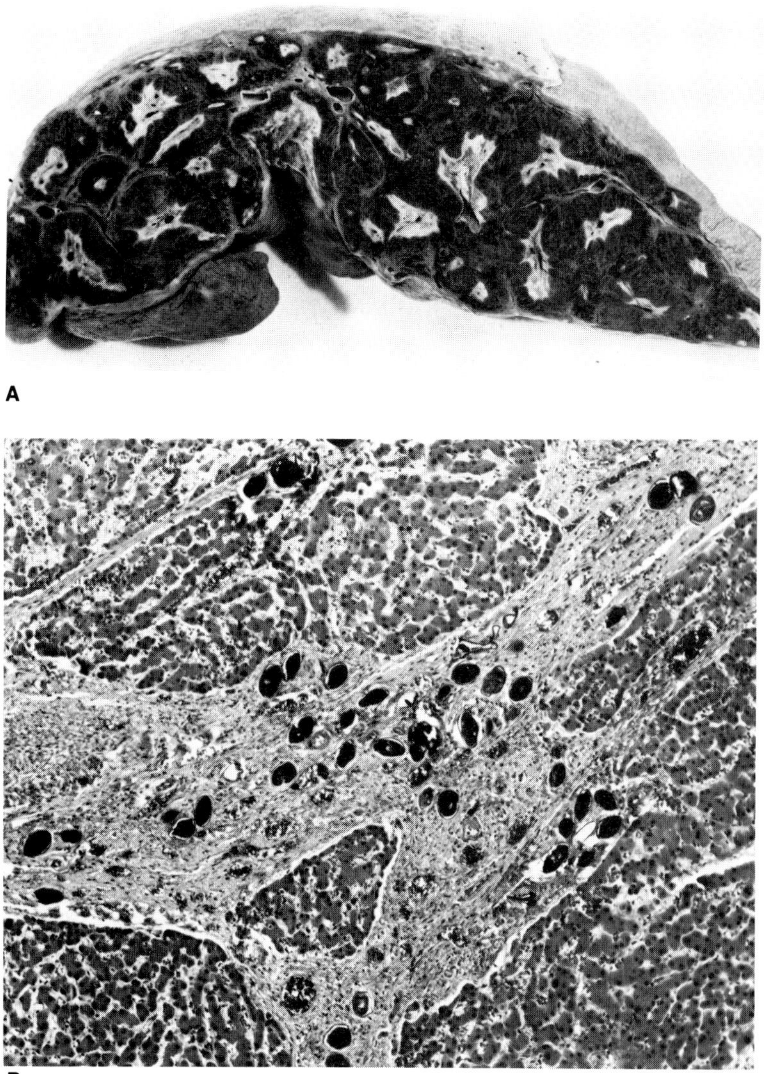

Figure 8–12. A. A liver showing classic Symmers' pipestem fibrosis. The lobular architecture is preserved, while the parenchyma may be distorted by bands of fibrous tissue in the smaller portal areas. B. Eggs in a bland area of mature fibrosis (×58.75). *(Courtesy of Armed Forces Institute of Pathology 83437 and 749593.)*

within recent years a number of potent and less toxic drugs have been developed and have replaced older medications. Praziquantel (Biltricide), a heterocyclic pyrazinoesoquinolone, is a broad spectrum agent effective against all types of human schistosomiasis. No major toxicity has been reported, and praziquantel also represents an advance in therapy of fluke infections (including clonorchiasis, paragonimiasis). Oxaminiquine (Vansil), a tetrahydroquinole, is an alternative drug for treatment of *S. mansoni*. Adverse reactions are more common than for praziquantel. With currently available less toxic drugs, medical treatment is being increasingly stressed in the poor risk patient and as an adjunct to surgery.

Bleeding esophageal and gastric varices, secondary to portal hypertension, are common complications of hepatosplenic schistosomiasis. As a rule these patients tolerate hemorrhage better than do patients with portal hypertension from portal cirrhosis, and encephalopathy and functional renal failure rarely ensue. Such hemorrhages usually respond to blood replacement, pitressin, and esophageal tamponade. When bleeding episodes become frequent, a variety of surgical procedures have been proposed. Portal caval shunt has been widely used. In endemic areas, splenectomy is favored. Prata[75] lists the following advantages of splenectomy: (1) elimination of the discomfort of a large abdominal swelling, (2) immediate correction of hypersplenism, (3) cure of infantilism, (4) improvement in the general state of the patient, and (5) reduction in portal pressure by about 40 percent. Ligation of esophageal varices has been proposed but is seldom indicated because the bleeding usually arrests with conservative measures.

Inflammatory and granulomatous lesions may produce obstructive or compressive lesions of the

TABLE 8–4. DRUGS USED IN THE TREATMENT OF SCHISTOSOMIASIS

Drug	Adult Dose	Days	Adverse Effects
Schistosoma mansoni			
Praziquantel	40 mg/kg (in 2 doses)	1	Occasional: headache, abdominal discomfort, nausea, dizziness, eosinophilia
Oxamniquine	15 mg/kg (single dose)	1	Occasional: headache, fever, diarrhea, rash, ECG and EEG changes, transaminase elevations
Schistosoma japonicum			
Praziquantel	60 mg/kg (in 3 doses)	1	Occasional: headache, abdominal discomfort, nausea, dizziness, eosinophilia
Schistosoma haematobium			
Praziquantel	40 mg/kg (in 2 doses)	1	Occasional: headache, abdominal discomfort, nausea, dizziness, eosinophilia
Schistosoma mekongi			
Praziquantel	60 mg/kg/d (in 3 doses)	1	See above

Adapted from Medical Letter on Drugs and Therapeutics.[20]

bowel or peritoneum. These masses, which resemble tumors, may become large and require resection for relief.

Schistosoma haematobium. Infection with *S. haematobium* is common in the Nile Valley and in many areas of Africa, the Middle East, and southwestern India. The life cycle of the parasite is similar to that of *S. mansoni* and *S. japonicum*. The adult worms lodge in the vascular plexus of the pelvis and bladder. *Schistosoma haematobium* is the chief cause of urogenital schistosomiasis with its exudative and granulomatous involvement of the bladder and ureters. Obstructive uropathy with hydroureter and hydronephrosis may ensue, but in the young it is reversible with medical treatment. Masses of eggs with surrounding connective tissue frequently produce a bilharzioma, which may simulate an exophytic tumor.[73,77]

Radiography can demonstrate calcified eggs in the bladder wall. Ulceration of the bladder often produces hematuria, and inflammatory polyps may simulate carcinoma. To complicate the matter, there is a high incidence of malignancy associated with schistosomal bladder disease; of these, 50 percent are squamous cell, 40 percent transitional cell, and 10 percent adenocarcinoma.[77] *Schistosoma haematobium* rarely causes cirrhosis but along with the other species can involve the central nervous system to produce jacksonian epilepsy or the manifestations of transverse myelitis. The diagnosis of *S. haematobium* is made by identifying typical eggs in rectal biopsy, in a centrifuged urine specimen, or in histologic sections and occasionally serology may be helpful; see under *S. mansoni*. In addition to medical treatment (see Table 8–4), an operation to relieve chronic obstructive uropathy or associated neoplasm is often life-saving.

Schistosoma japonicum. The Oriental blood fluke *S. japonicum* is encountered in the Far East. The basic life cycle is that common to all the schistosomes. The adults reside in the tributaries of the inferior mesenteric veins. As with *S. mansoni*, the liver and intestinal tract are chiefly involved, although infection of the central nervous system can be severe. Diagnosis is best made via rectal biopsy with recovery of eggs or serology; see under *S. mansoni*. The often-described tiny lateral spine is not seen in most specimens. Currently, praziquantel (20 mg/kg tid for 1 day) is the drug of choice (see Table 8–4).

Schistosoma mekongi. There are other schistosomes of lesser medical importance that rarely infect humans. *Schistosoma mekongi*, a parasite of dogs, seen in Thailand, Laos, and Cambodia, is similar in morphology and pathogenicity to *S. japonicum*; however, the eggs are distinguished by their smaller size. Praziquantel is the treatment of choice (see Table 8–4).

Subcutaneous Helminths

The surgeon is often called upon to excise a subcutaneous nodule or to biopsy an inflammatory serpiginous cutaneous lesion. As these may be parasitic in origin, it is important to understand the diverse causes. Table 8–5 outlines the most im-

TABLE 8–5. HELMINTHIC INFECTIONS PRODUCING CUTANEOUS LARVAE MIGRANS AND SUBCUTANEOUS LESIONS IN HUMANS

Organism	Characteristic Skin Lesion
Nematodes	
Dirofilaria immitis, D. tenuis (nonhuman)	Subcutaneous mass
Dracunculus medinensis	Subcutaneous, migrating tunnel
Human hookworm	
Ancylostoma duodenale	Ground itch (purplish macules, pruritic, urticaria)
Necator americanus	
Nonhuman hookworm	
A. braziliense	Creeping eruption (pruritic, migrating, inflammatory tunnel)
A. caninum	
Gnathostoma spinigerum (nonhuman)	Migrating subcutaneous masses, intermittent urticaria, creeping eruption (rare)
Onchocerca volvulus	Subcutaneous masses (nonmigrant)
Cestodes	
Taenia solium (cysticercosis)	Subcutaneous masses
Sparganosis (nonhuman)	Subcutaneous masses
Trematodes	
Fasciola hepatica	Subcutaneous masses
Paragonimus westermani	Subcutaneous masses
Schistosoma (human) *mansoni, haematobium, japonicum*	Urticarial, patchy
Avian *schistosomes* (nonhuman)	Swimmer's itch (urticarial)
Freshwater and salt water	

portant of the helminths that produce skin lesions. Some of these are discussed in Chapter 31. For lesions produced by arthropods a parasitology text should be consulted.[1]

In making a diagnosis of a cutaneous or subcutaneous parasitic infection, it is important to take a careful medical history: that is, the ingestion of undercooked chicken or fish for gnathostomiasis; the exposure to stagnant water in association with avian schistosomiasis, and the geographical location of the patient. Furthermore, the physical characteristics of the lesion—subcutaneous nodule, creeping eruption, or patchy edema—may indicate its cause. For example, the most common cause of creeping eruption is exposure of the skin to the infective larvae of hookworms that infect animals, that is, *Ancylostoma braziliense* and *A. caninum*. In the biopsy of all migrating lesions (including the deep subcutaneous lesions produced by gnathostomiasis), it should be remembered that the larvae are usually ahead of the advancing inflammatory tract they produce and that tissue excised for biopsy must include this region. Unfortunately, it is seldom possible to make species identification from biopsy material, and the pathologist must usually be content with recognition of the family or genus. Several subcutaneous parasitic diseases have already been discussed. (See sections on *Dirofilaria immitis* and *D. tenuis Dracunculus medinensis; Onchocerca volvulus*; as well as sparganosis and cysticercosis, caused by cestodes; and the trematodes, *F. hepatica, P. westermani, S. mansoni, S. japonicum*, and *S. haematobium*.)

Ancylostoma duodenale *and* Necator americanus *(Human Hookworm).* The skin of the lower extremity is usually involved when the filariform larvae of hookworms gain entrance to the body. The lesion is a tiny purplish pruritic macule that persists for several days. Histologically, edema with a neutrophilic and inflammatory infiltrate is present. Secondary infection produces a condition known as ground itch.[78,79]

Ancylostoma braziliense *and* A. caninum *(Nonhuman Hookworm).* Infection with the larvae of the dog and cat hookworm produces a cutaneous lesion, which is indistinguishable from infection with the human species.[80] Involvement often occurs on the trunk, since many persons acquire the infection while sunbathing on a beach contaminated with animal feces. The lesion is more chronic than those produced by human hookworms, and a pruritic inflammatory migrating tunnel is frequently observed. Albendazole and mebendazole (see under *Trichuris trichiura*, Table 8–3) are usually effective in treatment, as is local freezing.

Strongyloides stercoralis. Penetration of the skin by infective filariform larvae can produce lesions identical to those of hookworms. Such lesions usually occur on the lower extremities but may occur in the perianal area when hemorrhoidal tags or redundant mucosa promote the collection of stool.

Gnathostoma spinigerum. Infection with this nematode is an unusual cause of larva migrans in humans and is endemic in Southeast Asia, India, and China.[81] The adult nematodes inhabit the gastric wall of wild and domestic members of the dog and cat family. The life cycle requires the passage of larvae through a cyclops and a wide variety of secondary intermediate hosts (freshwater fish and other animals, particularly chickens, that consume fish). Within 48 hours of the ingestion of infected foods (undercooked fish or chicken), allergic and abdominal symptoms ensue, and cutaneous manifestations begin in approximately 1 month. The typical lesion is subcutaneous rather than cutaneous, as with hookworms, and appears as a rounded, erythematous bulging that is intensely pruritic. The appearance of lesions is episodic. Usually the larvae will migrate rapidly for 1 week and then become dormant for 2 to 6 weeks. The lesion can advance at the rate of 1 cm per hour. The central nervous system is rarely involved by this parasite.[82]

Schistosoma, *Avian*. Dermatitis produced by invasion with the cercariae of nonhuman schistosomes is characterized by intense pruritus and the appearance of patchy urticarial macules and papules. The lesions disappear after 7 to 10 days, leaving residual pigmented spots. The condition should be suspected when a rash appears after the patient has been swimming in fresh, salt, or brackish water. Treatment consists of systemic antihistamines, local antipruritic medications (calamine lotion), and topical corticosteroids.[83]

Acknowledgment. Grateful acknowledgment for aid in the preparation of this chapter is extended to G. E. Cosgrove (deceased) and A. C. Olson, Jr., of the Parasitology Study Group of the San Diego Zoo Hospital.

REFERENCES

Protozoa

1. Faust EC, Russel PF, Jung RC: Craig and Faust's Clinical Parasitology, 8th ed. Philadelphia, Lea & Febiger, 1970.
2. Neal RA: Pathogenesis of amebiasis. In Cahill KM (ed): Clinical Tropical Medicine, Vol II. Baltimore, University Park Press, 1972, p 134.
3. Elsdon-Dew R: Factors influencing the pathogenecity of *Entamoeba histolytica*. Proceedings of the World Congress of Gastroenterology. Baltimore, Williams & Wilkins, 1959, p 770.
4. Villarejos VM: Studies on the pathogenicity of *Entamoeba histolytica* and other ameba species. PhD dissertation, Tulane University, New Orleans, 1961.
5. Teodorovic S, Ingals JW, Greenbergh L: Effects of corticosteroids on experimental amoebiasis. Nature (London) 197:86, 1963.
6. Phillips BP, Gorstein F: Effects of different species of bacteria on the pathology of enteric amebiasis in monocontaminated guinea pigs. Am J Trop Med 15:863, 1966.
7. Phillips BP, Wolfe PA, Bartgis IL: Studies on the ameba-bacteria relationship in amebiasis. Am J Trop Med 7:392, 1958.
8. El-Hashimi W, Pittman F: Ultrastructure of *Entamoeba histolytica* trophozoites obtained from the colon and from in vitro cultures. Am J Trop Med 19:215, 1970.
9. McKerrow JH. The Role of Proteinases in the Pathogenesis of Parasitic Diseases. In Leech JH, Sande MA, Root RK (eds). Parasitic Infections. New York, Churchill Livingstone, 1988, p 51.
10. Connor DH, Neafie RC, Meyers WM: Amebiasis. In Binford CH, Connor DH (eds): Pathology of Tropical and Extraordinary Diseases, Vol 1. Washington, DC, AFIP, 1976, p 308.
11. Tucker PC, Webster PD, Kilpatrick ZM: Amebic colitis mistaken for inflammatory bowel disease. Arch Intern Med 135:681, 1975.
12. Juniper K: Amoebiasis. Clin Gastroenterol 7:3, 1978.
13. Lamont NH, Pooler NR: Hepatic amoebiasis: a study of 250 cases. Q J Med 27:389, 1958.
14. Alicna AD, Fadell BJ: Advantage of purgation in recovery of intestinal parasites and their eggs. Am J Clin Pathol 31:139, 1959.
15. Monroe LS, Korn ER, Fitzwilliam SJ: A comparative study of the latex agglutination and the gel diffusion precipitin tests in the diagnosis of amebic liver abscess. Am J Gastroenterol 58:52, 1972.
16. Sargeaunt PG: Biochemical Homogeneity of *Entamoeba histolytica* Isolates, Especially Those from Liver Abscess. London School of Hygiene and Tropical Medicine, Keppel Service, London WCIE 7HTT.
17. Sargeaunt PG, Williams JE, Grene JD. The differentiation of invasive and non-invasive *Entamoeba histolytica* by isoenzyme electrophoresis. Trans R Soc Trop Med Hyg 72:519, 1978.
18. Sargeaunt PG, Williams JE: Electrophoretic isoenzyme patterns of the pathogenic and non-pathogenic intestinal amoebae of man. Trans R Soc Trop Med Hyg 73:225, 1979.
19. Galgiani JN: Metronidazole for anaerobic bacterial infections. Drug Ther P 155, Nov 1978.
20. Drugs for parasitic infections. Med Lett Drug Ther 35 (911): 111–122, 1993.
21. Monroe LS: Amebiasis. In Berk JE, Haubrich WS,

Kalser MH, et al (eds): *Bockus Gastroenterology*, Vol 7, 4th ed. Philadelphia, Saunders, 1985, p. 4250.
22. Krogstad DJ, Spencer HC, Healy GR: Current concepts in parasitology: Amebiasis. N Engl J Med 298:262, 1978.
23. Baskerville L, Yusufuddin A, Ramchand S: *Balantidium* colitis. Report of a case. Am J Dig Dis 15:727, 1970.
24. Cespedes R, Rodriguez O, Valverde O, et al: Estudio de un caso anatomoclinico masivo con lesiones y presencia del parasito en el intestino delgado y pleura. Acta Med Cost 10:135, 1967.
25. Neafie RC: Balantidiasis. In Binford CH, Conner DH (eds): Pathology of Tropical and Extraordinary Diseases, Vol 1. Washington, DC, AFIP, 1976, p 325.
26. Woody NC, Woody HB: American trypanosomiasis. In clinical and epidemiologic background of Chagas' disease in the United States. J Pediatr 58:568, 1961.
27. WHO: Chagas' disease: Report of a study group. WHO Tech Rep Ser No 202, 1960.
28. Edgcomb JH, Johnson CM: American trypanosomiasis (Chagas' disease). In Binford CH, Connor DH (eds): Pathology of Tropical and Extraordinary Diseases, Vol 1. Washington, DC, AFIP, 1976, p 244.
29. Kierszenbaum F, Sztein MB. Mechanisms underlying immunosuppression induced by *Trypanosoma cruzi*. Parasitol Today 6:261, 1990.
30. Andrade ZA, Andrade SC: Chagas' disease (American trypanosomiasis). In Marcial-Rojas RA (ed): Pathology of Protozoal and Helminthic Diseases. Baltimore, Williams & Wilkins, 1971, p 69.
31. Ferreira-Santos R: Tratamento cirurgico do megaesofago. In Cancado JR (ed): Doenca del Chagas. Belo Horizonte, Minas Gerais, 1968, p 592.

Anisakids

32. Van Thiel PH, Kuipers FC, Roskam RT: A nematode parasitic to herring, causing acute abdominal syndromes in man. Trop Geogr Med 12:97, 1960.
33. Yokogawa M, Yoshimura H: Clinicopathologic studies on larval anisakiasis in Japan. Am J Trop Med 16:723, 1967.
34. Yoshimura H: Parasitic granuloma with special reference to clinical pathology of anisakis-like larva infection in the digestive apparatus of man. Jpn J Parasitol 15:32, 1966.
35. Ishimura H, Hawasaka H, Kikuchi Y: Acute regional ileitis in Hokkaido with special reference to intestinal anisakiasis. Sapporo Med J 32:183, 1967.
36. Arean VM: Anisakiasis. In Marcial-Rojas RA (ed): Pathology of Protozoal and Helminthic Disease. Baltimore, Williams & Wilkins, 1971, p 846.

Angiostrongylus Costaricensis

37. Morera P, Cespedes R: *Angiostrongylus costaricensis n. sp.* (Nematoda: Metastrongylidae) a new lungworm occurring in man in Costa Rica. Rev Biol Trop 18:173, 1971.
38. Morera P, Cespedes R: *Angiostrongilosis abdominal.* Acta Med Cost 14:159, 1971.
39. Morera P: Life history and redescription of *Angiostrongylus costaricensis.* Morera and Cespedes, 1971. Am J Trop Med Hyg 22:613, 1973.
40. Sauerbrey M: A precipitin test for the diagnosis of human abdominal angiostrongyliasis. Am J Trop Med Hyg 26:1156, 1977.

Ascaris

41. Pawlowski ZS: Ascariasis. Clin Gastroenterol 7:157, 1978.

Dirofilaria

42. Tuazon RA, Firestone F, Blaustein AU: Human pulmonary dirofilariasis manifesting as a "coin" lesion. A case report. JAMA 199:45, 1967.
43. Gershwin LJ, Gershwin ME, Kritzman J: Human pulmonary dirofilariasis. Chest 66:92, 1974.
44. Blecka LJ, Miller A, Craf EC: Human subcutaneous dirofilariasis in Illinois. JAMA 240:245, 1978.
45. Beaver PC, Samuel WN: Dirofilariasis in Canada. Am J Trop Med Hyg 26:329, 1977.
46. Harrison EG, Thompson JH: Dirofilariasis. In Marcial-Rojas RA (ed): Pathology of Protozoal and Helminthic Diseases. Baltimore, Williams & Wilkins, 1971, p 903.

Dracunculus Medinensis

47. Neafie RC, Connor DH, Meyers WM: Dracunculiasis. In Binford CH, Connor DH (eds): Pathology of Tropical and Extraordinary Diseases, Vol 2. Washington, DC, AFIP, 1976, p 397.

Enterobius Vermicularis

48. Duran-Jorda F: Appendicitis and enterobiasis in children: a histological study of 691 appendices. Arch Dis Child 32:208, 1957.
49. Moreno E: Enterobiasis (oxyuriasis, pinworm infection). In Marcial-Rojas RA (ed): Pathology of Protozoal and Helminthic Diseases. Baltimore, Williams & Wilkins, 1971, p 760.

Onchocerea Volvulus

50. Connor DH, Heafie RC: Onchocerciasis. In Binford CH, Connor DH (eds): Pathology of Tropical and Extraordinary Diseases, Vol II. Washington, DC, AFIP, 1976, p 360.

Toxocara Canis and *T. Cati*

51. Arean VM, Crandall CA: Toxocariasis. In Marcial-Rojas RA (ed): Pathology of Protozoal and Helminthic Diseases. Baltimore, Williams & Wilkins, 1971, p 808.
52. Wilson M, Schantz P: Nonmorphologic diagnosis of parasitic infections. In Balows A, Hausler WJ, Hermann KL, et al (eds): Manual of Clinical Microbiology, 5th ed. Washington, DC, American Society of Microbiology, 1991, p 717.

53. Krupp IM: A pet disease: visceral larva migrans. Drug Ther p 143, May 1978.

Trichuris Trichiura

54. Ramirez-Weiser RR: Trichuriasis. In Marcial-Rojas RA (ed): Pathology of Protozoal and Helminthic Diseases. Baltimore, Williams & Wilkins, 1971, p 658.
55. Neafie RC, Connor DH: Trichuriasis. In Binford CH, Connor DH (eds): Pathology of Tropical and Extraordinary Diseases, Vol II. Washington, DC, AFIP, 1976, p 415.

Echinococcus Granulosus and *E. Multilocularis*

56. Miller CW, Ruppanner R, Schwabe CW: Hydatid diseases in California: study of hospital records, 1960 through 1969. Am J Trop Med Hyg 20:904, 1971.
57. Sparks AK, Connor DH, Neafie RC: Echinococcosis. In Binford CH, Connor DH (eds): Pathology of Tropical and Extraordinary Diseases, Vol II. Washington, DC, AFIP, 1976, p 530.
58. Vilardel F: *Echinococcus* (hydatid) cysts of the liver. In Bockus HL (ed): Gastroenterology, Vol III. Philadelphia, Saunders, 1976, p 570.
59. Poole JB, Marcial-Rojas RA: Echinococcosis. In Marcial-Rojas RA (ed): Pathology of Protozoal and Helminthic Diseases. Baltimore, Williams & Wilkins, 1971, p 635.
60. Wilson JF, Rauch RL, Malon BJ, et al: Albendazole in alveolar hydatid disease. Am J Trop Med Hyg 37(1):162, 1987.
61. Marquez-Monter H: Cysticercosis. In Marcial-Rojas RA (ed): Pathology of Protozoal and Helminthic Diseases. Baltimore, Williams & Wilkins, 1971, p 592.
62. Sparks AK, Neafie RC, Connor DH: Cysticercosis. In Binford CH, Connor DH (eds): Pathology of Tropical and Extraordinary Diseases, Vol II. Washington, DC, AFIP, 1976, p 539.
63. Botero D, Castano S: Treatment of cysticercosis with praziquantel in Colombia. Am J Trop Med Hyg 31:811, 1982.
64. Praziquantel—a new antiparasitic drug. Med Lett Drug Ther 34(865):17, 1992.

Clonorchis Sinensis

65. Dooley JR, Neafie RC: Clonorchiasis and opisthorchiasis. In Binford CH, Connor DH (eds): Pathology of Tropical and Extraordinary Diseases, Vol II. Washington, DC, AFIP, 1976, p 509.
66. Hou PC: The relationship between primary carcinoma of the liver and infestation with *Clonorchis sinensis*. J Pathol Bacteriol 72:239, 1956.

Fasciola Hepatica

67. Norton RA, Monroe LS: Infection by *Fasciola hepatica* acquired in California. Gastroenterology 41:46, 1961.
68. Ashton WLG, Boardman PL, Everall PH, Houghton AWJ: Human fascioliasis in Shropshire. Br Med J 3:500, 1970.
69. Hardman EW, Jones RLH, Davies AH: Fascioliasis—a large outbreak. Br Med J 3:502, 1970.

Paragonimus Westermani

70. Meyers WM, Neafie RN: Paragonimiasis. In Binford CH, Connor DH (eds): Pathology of Tropical and Extraordinary Diseases, Vol II. Washington, DC, AFIP, 1976, p 517.

Schistosomes

71. Stoll NR: This wormy world. J Parasitol 33:1, 1947.
72. Warren KS: The relevance of schistosomiasis. N Engl J Med 303:203, 1980.
73. Marcial-Rojas RA: *Schistosoma mansoni*. In Marcial-Rojas RA (ed): Pathology of Protozoal and Helminthic Diseases. Baltimore, Williams & Wilkins, 1971, p 373.
74. Mendes TE: The schistosomiases. In Bockus HL (ed): Gastroenterology, Vol 4. Philadelphia, Saunders, 1976, p 220.
75. Prata A: *Schistosoma mansoni*. Clin Gastroenterol 7:49, 1978.
76. Nebel OT, el Masry NA, Castell DO, et al: Schistosomal disease of the colon: a reversible form of polyposis. Gastroenterology 67:939, 1974.
77. McCully RM, Barron CN, Cheever AW: Schistosomiasis (bilharziasis). In Binford CH, Connor DH (eds): Pathology of Tropical and Extraordinary Diseases, Vol II. Washington, DC, AFIP, 1976, p 482.

Subcutaneous Helminths

78. Meyers WM, Neafie RC, Connor DH: Ancylostomiasis. In Binford CH, Connor DH (eds): Pathology of Tropical and Extraordinary Diseases, Vol II. Washington, DC, AFIP, 1976, p 421.
79. DeLeon E, Maldonado JF: Uncinariasis (ancylostomiasis). In Marcial-Rojas RA (ed): Pathology of Protozoal and Helminthic Diseases. Baltimore, Williams & Wilkins, 1971, p 734.
80. Meyers WM, Neafie RC: Creeping eruption. In Binford CH, Connor DH (eds): Pathology of Protozoal and Extraordinary Diseases, Vol. II. Washington, DC, AFIP, 1976, p 437.

Gnathostomes

81. Swanson VL: Gnathostomiasis. In Marcial-Rojas RA (ed): Pathology of Protozoal and Helminthic Diseases. Baltimore, Williams & Wilkins, 1971, p 871.
82. Swanson VL: Gnathostomiasis. In Binford CH, Connor DH (eds): Pathology of Tropical and Extraordinary Diseases, Vol II. Washington, DC, AFIP, 1976, p 471.
83. Hunter GW: Schistosome cercarial dermatitis and other rare schistosomes that may infect man. In Marcial-Rojas RA (ed): Pathology of Protozoal and Helminthic Diseases. Baltimore, Williams & Wilkins, 1971, p 450.

BIBLIOGRAPHY

Ash LR, Orihel TC: Atlas of Human Parasitology, 2nd ed. Chicago, American Society of Clinical Pathology Press, 1984.

Binford CH, Connor DH (eds): Pathology of Tropical and Extraordinary Diseases, Vols. 1, 2. Washington, DC, AFIP, 1976.

Hunter GW, Swartzwelder JC, Clyde DF: Tropical Medicine. Philadelphia, Saunders, 1976.

Mandell GL, Douglas RG Jr, Bennett JE (eds): Protozoal Diseases, Section C (Part III). In: Principles and Practice of Infectious Diseases, Vol II. New York, Wiley, 1979.

Mandell GL, Douglas RG Jr, Bennett JE (eds): Diseases Due to Helminths, Section H (Part III). In: Principles and Practice of Infectious Diseases, Vol II. New York, Wiley, 1979.

Marcial-Rojas RA (ed): Pathology of Protozoal and Helminthic Diseases. Baltimore, Williams & Wilkins, 1971.

Opportunistic Bacteria

CHAPTER 9

Dale N. Gerding

This chapter is a potpourri of microorganisms rarely encountered by most surgeons and not comprehensively discussed elsewhere in this text. The organisms range from conventional gram-negative and gram-positive bacteria to mycobacteria, nocardiae, spirochetes, rickettsiae, chlamydiae, and mycoplasmas. Some cause infections that are specifically related to surgical procedures, particularly in immunosuppressed patients, and many are likely to require surgical consultation for diagnosis or treatment. The discussion of each organism is designed to provide the essentials of identification, pathogenesis, clinical illness, diagnosis, and treatment. Special emphasis has been placed on the clinical features that are of surgical interest and importance. In this third edition, previously discussed organisms have been updated and newer references have been added. New organisms include *Borrelia burgdorferi, Legionella* species, *Branhamella* (*Moraxella*) *catarrhalis, Capnocytophaga* species, and *Chlamydia pneumoniae*.

The number of microorganisms known to cause disease in humans continues to expand, as does knowledge of the type of infection caused by previously known pathogens. These newer aspects of infectious disease have been emphasized, particularly as they apply to the immunocompromised patient. Because of the large number of pathogenic organisms, however, it is not possible to discuss them all. The selection is somewhat arbitrary, but it is designed to include the organisms that surgeons in the Western world will encounter. Discussions of taxonomy have been minimized because of controversy in this area. Newer nomenclature has been used, but older names and synonyms are included to reduce confusion.

GRAM-POSITIVE BACTERIA

Genus *Bacillus*

Bacillus organisms are aerobic, spore-forming bacilli, which are usually gram positive but may be gram variable. The majority are nonpathogenic for humans, with the notable exception of *B. anthracis,* and are commonly found in soil, water, dust, animal feces, and animal products. *Bacillus* species have been recognized recently as causative agents of infection, particularly in immunosuppressed patients.

Bacillus anthracis

Morphology and Identification. *Bacillus anthracis* is the cause of human and animal anthrax. It is a rod-shaped, gram-positive bacillus 1 μm × 3 to 10 μm. Although it grows best under aerobic conditions, it can also grow anaerobically, potentially causing confusion with clostridial organisms. The organism grows well on ordinary culture media at 37C. *Bacil-*

lus anthracis is nonmotile and forms capsules in sodium bicarbonate agar under incubation with 5 percent CO_2. Both a gamma phage test and fluorescent-antibody stain are available from the Centers for Disease Control for rapid identification. Good bacteriologic safety techniques are essential in handling suspected anthrax specimens, especially avoidance of aerosol production when working with material containing spores.

Epidemiology and Pathogenesis. Approximately 20,000 to 100,000 cases of anthrax occur annually in the world; less than ten occur in the United States each year. Most cases result from contact with animal products, especially goat and sheep hides, hair, wool, and meat. Most recent American cases have been acquired by handlers of imported wool and yarns. Anthrax is acquired by the deposition of *B. anthracis* spores directly into the skin, by inhalation of spores, and, rarely, by consumption of contaminated meat. Infection may be confined to local skin lesions or extend to regional lymph nodes in the lung or gastrointestinal tract with production of toxin and resultant necrosis, hemorrhage, and edema.

Clinical Manifestations. The majority of infections are acquired by the cutaneous route and usually remain localized. After a 1- to 7-day incubation, typical skin lesions evolve through an initial papule, which progresses to a vesicle or ring of vesicles, followed by development of a depressed ulcer covered by black eschar. Most lesions occur on the hands, arms, or head, and they heal with the formation of a scar. The respiratory syndrome usually begins as a mild, nonspecific, flu-like illness with a nonproductive cough. It progresses to development of severe respiratory distress with fever, rales, and occasionally pleural effusion and subcutaneous edema of the upper torso. Meningitis can also develop. Gastrointestinal anthrax may be of importance to surgical consultants because its symptoms resemble an acute surgical abdomen with elevated leukocyte count, nausea, vomiting, fever, abdominal pain, and occasionally bloody diarrhea. An oropharyngeal form of anthrax associated with the ingestion of uncooked or undercooked beef and buffalo has recently been described in Thailand. Patients presented with pharyngeal ulceration, edema, cervical lymphadenopathy, and occasionally pharyngeal pseudomembranes.[1]

Diagnosis. A history of animal or animal product contact, particularly in a geographic area endemic for anthrax, should arouse suspicion. Diagnosis is dependent on isolation of *B. anthracis* from clinical material. Moistened swabs should be used to obtain material from vesicular skin lesions and from under the edge of eschars. The diagnosis of anthrax may also be established by a fourfold rise in indirect hemagglutination titer in paired sera.

Treatment and Prognosis. Penicillin, administered orally for mild cases but intravenously or intramuscularly in severe cases, is the best drug for the treatment of anthrax. Local excision of cutaneous lesions can lead to spread of infection. Topical antibiotics should also be avoided. The expected survival in treated cutaneous anthrax is over 99 percent. In contrast, pulmonary anthrax is almost always fatal, despite antibiotic therapy, and gastrointestinal anthrax is fatal 25 to 50 percent of the time. Three of twenty-four patients with oropharyngeal anthrax died.[1]

Bacillus *Species*

Morphology and Identification. Bacillus species other than anthrax are responsible for a small but increasing number of human infections. These organisms are indistinguishable on Gram stain from the anthrax bacillus, and differentiation requires detailed biochemical testing. *Bacillus subtilis* and *B. cereus* are most frequently associated with human disease.[2,3]

Epidemiology and Pathogenesis. Human infection caused by these organisms is extremely rare and except for eye infections occurs almost exclusively in intravenous drug abusers or immunosuppressed hosts.[3,4] The exception to this rule is food poisoning caused by *B. cereus,* which is due to an enterotoxin.[5]

Clinical Manifestations and Diagnosis. A variety of systemic infections with *Bacillus* species has been reported, including endocarditis, pneumonia, bacteremia, eye infections, wound infections, and urinary tract infections.[2,4] There are two types of *B. cereus* food poisoning—an acute upper gastrointestinal syndrome that resembles staphylococcal food poisoning and an acute diarrheal illness similar to *Clostridium perfringens* food poisoning. Fried rice is often implicated. Diagnosis is made by isolation of the organism from suspect foods or the stool; however, *B. cereus* organisms may be normal inhabitants of the stool.[5] Diagnosis of systemic illness is based on the isolation of *Bacillus* species from blood or body fluids. Trauma surgeons should be aware of *Bacillus* species infections following motor vehicle accidents.[6]

Treatment and Prognosis. Antibiotic therapy is indicated only for systemic infection. Unlike the anthrax bacillus, many *Bacillus* species are resistant to penicillins and cephalosporins, and in vitro studies have demonstrated that tetracyclines, gentamicin, kanamycin, chloramphenicol, and vancomycin have been most effective against a variety of strains. In general, *B. subtilis* tends to be penicillin and cephalosporin sensitive, whereas most *B. cereus* are resistant to these drugs. *B. cereus* food poisoning is self-limited and does not require antibiotic therapy.[5]

Genus *Corynebacterium*

Organisms of the genus *Corynebacterium,* with the exception of the diphtheria bacillus, are seldom pathogenic for humans. These organisms are gram-positive, non-spore-forming, non-acid-fast, nonencapsulated rods. They are aerobic or microaerophilic and, when grown on nutritionally deficient media, exhibit terminal clubbing, from which the group derives its name.

Corynebacterium diphtheriae

Morphology and Identification. Corynebacterium diphtheriae are gram-positive, irregularly staining rods that are 0.3 to 0.8 μm × 1 to 8 μm. Confirmation of *C. diphtheriae* requires isolation in pure culture and biochemical and toxigenicity testing. Presumptive identification can be made when L- and V-shaped organisms (Chinese characters) and granules that appear as polar bodies are seen on Loeffler alkaline methylene blue stain.

The presence of diphtheria toxin can be tested for by an in vivo guinea pig inoculation test or by an in vitro gel-diffusion test. A positive toxigenicity test is essentially proof that the organism is *C. diphtheriae,* because only *C. ulcerans* can also produce a toxin that is neutralized by diphtheria antitoxin.

Epidemiology and Pathogenesis. Diphtheria is a worldwide disease, but in the late 1980s and early 1990s fewer than ten cases per year occurred in the United States. Inadequately immunized persons are most often affected, especially children who have not been immunized and older adults whose immunity has waned. The disease occurs most often in the colder months of the year, and it is thought to be spread by droplets and close personal contact. Convalescent or healthy carriers are the presumed reservoir of disease between epidemics. The most frequent site of illness is the upper respiratory tract, although skin infections occur.

The lethal nature of the disease is primarily related to the production of an exotoxin, an acidic globular protein (molecular weight about 62,000) that acts by interfering with polypeptide synthesis in the cell.[7] The production of toxin is mediated by parasitization of the diphtheria organisms by a specific bacteriophage.[8] Local invasiveness of the organism is probably necessary for clinical illness.

Clinical Manifestations. Most patients exhibit upper respiratory symptoms of sore throat, nonproductive cough, low-grade fever, and malaise. In severe cases, cervical adenopathy may be prominent with additional soft tissue swelling. Most characteristic is a thick, adherent membrane in the pharynx with severe local inflammation and edema. The membrane may appear gray, green, or black and consists primarily of fibrin, necrotic epithelium, lymphocytes, and polymorphonuclear leukocytes. Local concomitant infection with group A streptococci is frequent. Pharyngeal edema and membrane formation may be sufficiently severe to cause respiratory obstruction. Occasionally the ear, eye, and genitalia are infected. Also, infection of preexisting skin lesions such as stasis ulcers or burns can occur in temperate climates, although it is more common in the tropics.

Myocarditis and polyneuritis, manifestations of diphtheria toxemia, appear 1 or more weeks after the onset of clinical illness. Congestive heart failure, heart block, or other cardiac arrhythmias may be evident. Polyneuritis is most frequent in the cranial nerves, and patients exhibit difficulty in swallowing and have a nasal voice.

Diagnosis. The diagnosis is established by isolation of *C. diphtheriae* and proof of toxin production. Pharyngeal swabs, or preferably portions of pharyngeal membranes, should be submitted to the laboratory for culture. Clinical diagnosis of the disease is particularly difficult in mild cases when a pharyngeal membrane is not present. In patients who have the late manifestations, such as congestive heart failure, heart block, or polyneuritis, it may be impossible to prove the cause. A history of pharyngeal infection will help establish the diagnosis.

Treatment and Prognosis. Specific therapy is directed at neutralizing toxin by the use of a horse antitoxin; 30,000 to 40,000 units of antitoxin are injected intramuscularly in moderately severe cases. Severely ill patients can be treated with up to 80,000 units. Because approximately 10 percent of patients will develop allergic reactions to horse serum, a careful history of allergy should be taken, and tests for hypersensitivity to horse serum should be done before administration. Antibiotic treatment is an adjunct to antitoxin and is used to eliminate the organism from the pharynx and prevent spread to other persons. Penicillin or erythromycin is preferred and can be used to treat asymptomatic carriers.

Although immunization has reduced the frequency of diphtheria, the mortality remains between 5 and 10 percent. Most deaths are the result of either respiratory obstruction by the pharyngeal lesion or subsequent myocarditis.

Prevention. Diphtheria is usually prevented by immunization with diphtheria toxoid, a formalin-detoxified preparation commonly administered in childhood. Immunity, however, is not lifelong and requires repeated boosters in later life.

Corynebacterium *Species*

Morphology and Identification. Corynebacteria other than *C. diphtheriae* are usually saprophytic or weakly pathogenic for humans. They are frequently reported from pharyngeal, conjunctival, or skin isolates as "diphtheroids." They can be distinguished from *C. diphtheriae* on the basis of morphology, biochemical reactions, failure to produce an exotoxin, and hemolysis.

Epidemiology and Pathogenesis. Members of the genus *Corynebacterium* are normal inhabitants of the pharynx, skin, and conjunctivae. With a few exceptions they are pathogenic only in immunologically compromised patients. A localized skin eruption, characterized by mild inflammation, scaling, and weeping in body folds or intertriginous areas and termed *erythrasma* has been attributed to *C. minutissimum*. *Corynebacterium* species are often isolated from polymicrobial skin infections, particularly from foot infections in diabetic patients, and should not be ignored as contaminants.[9] *Corynebacterium (Rhodococcus) equi* is known to cause pneumonia in immunosuppressed patients, particularly renal transplant recipients.[10] Bacteremia with corynebacteria organisms of the JK group (*C. jeikeium*) has been described in immunosuppressed patients or those with intravenous or prosthetic devices.[11,12] Prosthetic heart valve infection by "diphtheroids" is frequently due to *C. jeikeium*.

Treatment and Prognosis. Erythrasma is usually treated with topical antibacterial soaps, but erythromycin may be required in severe cases. Unlike *C. diphtheriae,* most *Corynebacterium* species have exhibited resistance to commonly used antibiotics such as penicillin G,[11] and susceptibility testing is essential. Most successful treatments of diphtheroid infections, however, have included penicillin G with the addition of an aminoglycoside. *Corynebacterium jeikeium* bacteremias and prosthetic device infections should be treated with vancomycin until susceptibilities are available as these strains are widely antibiotic resistant.[12]

Listeria and *Erysipelothrix*

Although *Listeria* and *Erysipelothrix* differ in their pathogenicity and the type of disease they cause, they will be discussed together because of their similar morphologic and cultural appearances and because both are associated with disease in animals as well as people.

Listeria monocytogenes

Morphology and Identification. The genus *Listeria* is of uncertain affiliation. These small, gram-positive coccobacillary organisms frequently appear in pairs and chains and may be confused with diplococci. They are not encapsulated, they lack spores and are motile when grown at 18C to 20C. They can be grown on ordinary laboratory media, usually aerobically, but they are also facultatively anaerobic.

Epidemiology and Pathogenesis. Listeria monocytogenes is a ubiquitous organism that causes disease in both animals and people.[13] It has been isolated from animals, birds, water, sewage, and soil and is carried in the stool in a small proportion of patients; the carriage rate is increased among close contacts of patients with listeriosis. Milk, cheese, and raw vegetables have been implicated in spread of the disease.[13] Normal people may be infected with *Listeria*, but most cases are associated with immunologic compromise or advanced age. *Listeria monocytogenes* can also cause abortion or perinatal infection in both mother and child. Infection in the mother is usually benign and nonspecific, whereas the newborn has signs of meningitis or pneumonia and frequently hepatosplenomegaly and a rash. The importance of underlying malignant disease, particularly lymphoma and leukemia, as an associated factor in *Listeria* infection has been emphasized. Listerial meningitis and bacteremia without meningitis have been reported in kidney transplant recipients.[14]

Clinical Manifestations and Diagnosis. Both normal and immunosuppressed patients will have typical symptoms of septicemia or meningitis. Diagnosis is based almost entirely on the isolation and identification of *L. monocytogenes* from infected tissues or body fluids. Occasionally the organism may be isolated from skin lesions in the newborn. Serologic tests are not clinically useful. Physicians should always be alert to the possibility of *Listeria* when diphtheroids are reported from Gram smears or cultures of spinal fluid.

Treatment and Prognosis. Death from *Listeria* infection is most common in the neonatal period, particularly if the infection is contracted transplacentally. Listeriosis in some immunosuppressed patients, particularly kidney transplant recipients, has been associated with a remarkably low mortality (5 to 10 percent).[14] This may be related to the higher frequency of *Listeria* bacteremia without meningitis in this group of patients. The organism is sensitive to a large number of antibiotics including ampicillin, penicillin, erythromycin, tetracycline, and gentamicin. The addition of an aminoglycoside to penicillin or ampicillin demonstrates synergistic killing in vitro, but the clinical benefit is unclear. Rifampin also exhibits in vitro synergy with penicillin or ampicillin, and trimethoprim-sulfamethoxazole exhibits good activity in vitro. Penicillin G or ampicillin in high intravenous doses is still the best treatment for *Listeria* infections. If combination penicillin-aminoglycoside treatment is elected, the aminoglycoside should be administered intrathecally or intraventricularly to assure adequate concentrations in the cerebrospinal fluid in meningitis. Renal transplant recipients should be treated for at least 3 weeks; there is a relapse rate of 35 percent when shorter periods are used.[15]

Erysipelothrix rhusiopathiae

Morphology and Identification. Erysipelothrix rhusiopathiae, formerly designated *E. insidiosa,* is the only member of the genus *Erysipelothrix*. The organism is a slender, gram-positive rod 0.2 to 0.4 μm $\times$ 0.5 to 2.5 μm. The organism can be grown on ordinary bacteriologic media. It develops circular transparent colonies, which may produce a green appearance around the margin when grown on blood agar.

Epidemiology and Pathogenesis. Erysipelothrix rhusiopathiae is common in nature and is the cause of swine erysipelas. In humans, erysipeloid is the most common form of infection. This inflammatory eruption usually occurs on the hands as a purplish erythema, with sharply demarcated margins that are irregular and slightly raised. Histologic examination reveals inflammation of the dermis with gram-positive bacilli identifiable on Gram stain. Fish handlers, butchers, veterinarians, fishermen, abattoir workers, and cooks are most susceptible to infection because of their contact with potentially contaminated fish and animal products. Local infection is thought to occur by primary inoculation through skin injury. A more severe form of disease with fever, systemic illness and septicemia, and occasionally endocarditis, arthritis, and meningitis is also described. The systemic form may occur with or without the presence of skin lesions.[16]

Clinical Manifestations. The majority of patients have the previously described lesions of the hands; edema may be severe enough to restrict finger motion. Lymphangitis and lymphadenitis or other systemic signs of illness are ordinarily absent. Itching, burning, and tenderness are typical. Signs and symptoms of systemic illness and endocarditis cannot be distinguished from those caused by other organisms. Both normal and abnormal cardiac valves can be involved in endocarditis.

The diagnosis of cutaneous infection can readily be made by the typical appearance of the skin lesions and can be confirmed from biopsy specimens taken from the advancing margin of a lesion. The biopsy sample should be submitted for both histologic examination and culture in glucose infusion broth. Diagnosis can also be made by injection and aspiration of normal saline at the margin of the lesion. The organism is readily grown from ordinary blood culture media in cases of septicemia or endocarditis.

Treatment and Prognosis. Erysipelothrix rhusiopathiae is typically sensitive to penicillin, cephalosporins, erythromycin, and clindamycin but not to vancomycin or the aminoglycosides. Localized skin lesions can be treated with a single intramuscular injection of long-acting benzathine penicillin or with oral erythromycin. Penicillin G is the best treatment for endocarditis and should be administered in high doses for 4 to 6 weeks.

GRAM-NEGATIVE BACTERIA

Francisella tularensis

Morphology and Identification. Francisella tularensis is a genus of uncertain affiliation. It is also known as *Brucella tularensis* or *Pasteurella tular-*

ensis. These non-spore-forming organisms are small, coccobacillary, gram negative, nonmotile, unencapsulated, and 0.2 μm × 0.2 to 0.7 μm.

Epidemiology and Pathogenesis. Francisella tularensis is the cause of tularemia. The organism is a parasite of numerous mammals (cottontail rabbits, beaver, muskrats, moles, squirrels, rats, mice). The most frequent arthropod vectors are the tick and the deerfly.[17,18] Most infections are thought to be caused by passage of the organism through the skin, either via scratches or breaks in the skin during the handling of contaminated animal products or by entry at the time of a vector bite. A pneumonic form of the disease may be acquired by inhalation of the organism.

Clinical Manifestations. Four types of tularemia are traditionally described. The most common, the ulceroglandular forms, appears 80 to 90 percent of the time, followed by the nonspecific "typhoidal" form of tularemia.[18] Oculoglandular tularemia is the most rare, occurring in less than 1 percent of cases. The fourth type, pneumonic tularemia, may occur as an isolated event or in association with any of the other three forms.

Ulceroglandular disease is characterized by a cutaneous ulcer at the site of inoculation and local lymphadenopathy. Oculoglandular tularemia is associated with conjunctivitis with local lymphadenopathy; the typhoidal form of the disease exhibits only nonspecific febrile symptoms that occasionally are accompanied by nonproductive cough. Patients experience a high fever, 40C to 41C, and abrupt onset. Severe headache is not unusual, and hepatomegaly and splenomegaly are usually present.

Diagnosis. Because of the difficulty of isolating the tularemia organism, the diagnosis frequently hinges on a high index of clinical suspicion. A history of animal contact, particularly with rabbits or tick or insect bites, is particularly important, as is examination for the presence of tender lymphadenopathy and skin ulceration. Culture of sputum on special media will occasionally yield the organism. Gram stain is usually not helpful.

In the majority of patients the diagnosis is reached retrospectively by use of a serum agglutination test. Titers become positive after 10 to 14 days with peak titers of 1:1280 at 4 to 8 weeks of illness. A serial rise in agglutinin titers at 1- to 2-week intervals is diagnostic. The differential diagnosis is difficult because it includes all the rare ulceroglandular diseases (eg, cat-scratch fever, *Yersinia pseudotuberculosis, Pasteurella multocida* bite infection, plague, chancroid, melioidosis, sporotrichosis).

Treatment and Prognosis. The mortality rate with untreated tularemia pneumonia may be as high as 30 percent; the mortality with untreated ulceroglandular disease is only about 5 percent. Streptomycin, the most effective antibiotic, is usually administered for at least 1 week. Other aminoglycosides should also be effective, but clinical experience is limited.

Pasteurella multocida

Morphology and Identification. Pasteurella multocida, also known as *P. septica,* is a non-spore-forming gram-negative bacillus 1 to 1.8 μm × 0.3 to 0.5 μm, which is nonmotile and bipolar staining. It is a facultative anaerobe that grows on ordinary media and is oxidase and catalase positive and citrate negative, does not liquefy gelatin, and reduces methylene blue.

Epidemiology and Pathogenesis. Pasteurella multocida is a normal inhabitant of the upper respiratory and digestive tracts of healthy animals and birds. It is the cause of cholera in fowl and hemorrhagic septicemia in cattle and other animals.[19] Human infection is associated with close contact with animals, particularly bites from cats and dogs (cat-bite fever).[20] Rare cases of pneumonia, brain abscess, meningitis, peritonitis, and septicemia have been reported.[21] In patients with respiratory infection the organism is usually associated with bronchiectasis, chronic bronchitis, and bronchogenic carcinoma. On pathologic examination, specimens exhibit evidence of acute inflammation that is indistinguishable from that caused by other pyogenic organisms.

Clinical Manifestations and Diagnosis. The majority of patients have acute cellulitis with purulent drainage, lymphangitis, and regional adenopathy, associated with a recent animal bite or scratch, particularly when caused by a cat. Occasionally, acute and chronic cough develop with or without evidence of pulmonary infiltration and consolidation. Severe septicemia can also develop, particularly in patients who are immunosuppressed. In addition, alcoholics can develop spontaneous bacterial peritonitis. Physicians should be suspicious of *P. multocida* when Gram stain of an infected animal bite or scratch shows gram-negative coccobacillary organisms. Routine culture techniques will identify the organism.

Treatment and Prognosis. *Pasteurella multocida* is susceptible to penicillin G, ampicillin, chloramphenicol, parenteral cephalosporins, and the tetracyclines but is usually resistant to erythromycin, clindamycin, vancomycin, and the aminoglycosides.[21] Local infections should be drained and penicillin administered. The use of penicillin for the empiric treatment of patients with animal bites is an unsettled issue, but selective use has been recommended for deep bites that involve tendon or bone. Others recommend the uniform use of systemic antibiotics for any animal wound that requires suturing.[20] The prognosis is excellent in localized infections, and death is rare except in immunocompromised patients.

Streptobacillus moniliformis and *Spirillum minor*

These two gram-negative organisms will be discussed together because of their similar propensity to cause rat-bite fever. *Streptobacillus moniliformis* and *Spirillum minor* belong to different bacterial genera, and each causes a somewhat different clinical illness.

Morphology and Identification. *Streptobacillus moniliformis* is a gram-negative, 1 μm × 1 to 5 μm pleomorphic bacillus that often forms long filaments. It is aerobic or facultatively anaerobic. *Spirillum minor* is also a gram-negative bacillus, 2 to 5 μm in length with two to six spirals and bipolar tufts of flagella. The organism has not been cultivated in vitro. Identification is dependent upon its appearance on wet mounts examined with a dark-field microscope, or on blood films stained with Giemsa or Wright stains.

Epidemiology and Pathogenesis. Disease caused by *S. moniliformis* (streptobacillary fever) is rare but is still the most common type of rat-bite fever in the United States. Most illness is associated with a rodent bite or the bite of an animal (weasel, cat) that has fed on infected rodents. This organism is also thought to have been the cause of a large milk-borne epidemic of streptobacillary fever in Haverhill, Massachusetts.[22] Many reported cases in the United States derive from bites of experimental rats in the laboratory.[23] *Spirillum minor,* the causative organism of spirillary fever (Sodoku), was first described in Japan but is also sporadically reported from the United States, Asia, and Europe. It too is contracted from rat bites.

Both organisms are thought to disseminate through the blood-stream, although *S. moniliformis* infection may be restricted to the site of the bite and local lymph nodes. Examination of infected tissue reveals only a nonspecific chronic inflammatory response, with microorganisms visible. In fatal cases the organism has disseminated to various organs.

Clinical Manifestations. Clinical symptoms after a streptobacillary infection tend to occur earlier than in the spirillary form of the disease. Chills, fever, malaise, headache, and rash occur within 10 days of the rat bite. About one-fourth of the patients with streptobacillary fever have local lymphangitis and lymphadenitis. The original site of the bite is usually healed but may still be quite tender. Migratory polyarthritis is present in half the patients with streptobacillary fever but is unusual in spirillary fever. Patients with spirillary fever usually have no symptoms until at least 7 days after being bitten. The rash in spirillary fever is usually purplish red and macular and occurs with approximately the same frequency (75 percent) as in streptobacillary fever. False-positive serologic test results occur for syphilis in approximately 25 percent of streptobacillary fevers and 50 percent of spirillary fevers.

Diagnosis. Definitive diagnosis in streptobacillary fever depends on the isolation of *S. moniliformis* from blood, the site of the bite, skin pustules, or joint fluid. If there is no recent rodent bite, the differential diagnosis must include Rocky Mountain spotted fever, rickettsial-pox, meningococcemia, syphilis, and the viral exanthems. A serum agglutination test for *S. moniliformis* may be useful if cultures are negative; titers of 1:80 are diagnostic. The diagnosis of spirillary fever requires a demonstration of *S. minor* in a dark-field preparation of infected exudate or blood. Blood films stained with Giemsa or Wright stains may also reveal the organism. If these initial examinations fail to demonstrate the organism, the only diagnostic recourse is to inoculate mice and guinea pigs.

Treatment and Prognosis. Mortality in untreated streptobacillary fever may exceed 10 percent, while mortality in spirillary fever is approximately one-half of that. Penicillin is the best treatment for both infections. Streptomycin, tetracycline, and chlortetracycline have been effective alternatives; however, the choice should be based on susceptibility testing of *S. moniliformis.* The use of penicillin prophylactically at the time of a rat bite has been recommended, but its ability to prevent rat bite fever is unproven.

Eikenella corrodens

Morphology and Identification. Eikenella corrodens is a pathogen of humans that is facultatively anaerobic and grows best under increased carbon dioxide tension. In the past this organism has been termed HB-1 and *Bacteroides corrodens*. More recently the strictly anaerobic *B. corrodens* has been separated from the microaerophilic *E. corrodens. Eikenella corrodens* is a nonmotile, small, gram-negative bacillus that grows slowly on sheep blood agar plates. Colonies are small (0.5 mm) at 24 hours and typically do not reveal pitting or corroding of the surface until at least 48 hours of incubation. The organisms are oxidase positive and urease negative.

Epidemiology and Pathogenesis. Eikenella corrodens is a member of the normal oral flora of humans and may also be a normal resident of the fecal flora. Most clinical infections have implicated oral or gastrointestinal secretions as the source of the infective organism. Breaks in normal mucosal integrity, for example, lacerations of the oral mucosa, periodontal infection, bites, and abdominal operations, permit invasion of tissue. In addition, there seems to be a unique relationship among *E. corrodens,* cutaneous abscesses, and the practice of subcutaneous or intravenous injection of methylphenidate. The majority of infections are indolent abscesses, which frequently reveal multiple organisms, particularly anaerobic bacteria and streptococci, in addition to *Eikenella.*

Clinical Manifestations and Diagnosis. Most patients will have abscesses of the head and neck, particularly the mouth, and dental abscesses. Other sites of infection include abdominal abscesses, endocarditis, meningitis, and osteomyelitis.[24,25] Pneumonia, lung abscess, and empyema usually involve *E. corrodens* in mixed culture. Cutaneous abscesses are frequently associated with drug abuse or with trauma to the hands from human teeth. Diagnosis is based on Gram stain and culture of abscesses. Patients typically have a rather quiescent, indolent history of abscess formation after trauma or injury, particularly to the head, neck, and hands. Abscess material may be particularly foul smelling, which suggests that the infection is anaerobic in origin. Because of this the patient may be empirically treated with clindamycin for a presumptive diagnosis of anaerobic abscess and fail to respond because of the resistance of *E. corrodens* to clindamycin and lincomycin.

Treatment and Prognosis. Surgical drainage combined with appropriate antimicrobial treatment, usually with ampicillin or penicillin, results in rapid cure of abscesses. Alternate antibiotics are tetracycline and possibly erythromycin or chloramphenicol; however, some strains can be resistant to the latter two drugs. Organisms typically exhibit high resistance to methicillin, clindamycin, lincomycin, and metronidazole.[24,25] Cephalosporins are generally not as active as penicillin G, but cefoxitin and several of the third-generation cephalosporins appear to be active in vitro.[26] In vitro susceptibility tests should be performed to determine optimal antibiotic therapy for endocarditis in the penicillin-allergic patient.

Bordetella pertussis

Morphology and Identification. Bordetella pertussis is a minute coccobacillus, 0.2 to 0.3 μm $\times$ 0.5 to 1.0 μm. It is nonmotile and produces smooth, pearly, glistening, small colonies on Bordet-Gengou medium. Along with *B. parapertussis* and *B. bronchiseptica, B. pertussis* is the cause of whooping cough. In addition to culture techniques, immunologic diagnosis can be made using a fluorescent-antibody staining technique either on direct nasopharyngeal smears or on specimens obtained from culture media.

Epidemiology and Pathogenesis. Whooping cough is largely a disease of unimmunized young children. The disease is acquired by droplet spread from clinical cases or even adult carriers.[27] The frequency of pertussis has decreased since the advent of widespread immunization in childhood. Immunity is not lifelong, however, and side effects of the vaccine prohibit its use in older children and adults, which leads to susceptibility with increasing age. Infection appears to be limited primarily to the upper respiratory tract and bronchi, where large numbers of organisms are found enmeshed in a mucosal exudate. Bronchopneumonia is unusual.

Clinical Manifestations. Whooping cough has been divided into three phases, which follow an incubation period of approximately 1 to 3 weeks. The initial or catarrhal phase of the illness also lasts 1 to 3 weeks and is characterized by rhinorrhea, conjunctivitis, and generalized upper respiratory symptoms. Next the paroxysmal stage begins and lasts an additional 2 to 6 weeks with severe episodic coughing. The disease acquires its name from the characteristic crowing (whooping) sound made during inspiration after coughing spells. A child may appear remarkably well between the sieges of coughing, but vomiting or cyanosis during paroxysms suggests the diagnosis.[28] A third phase of convalescence lasts an additional 2 to 3 weeks.

Diagnosis. Culture for *B. pertussis* should be performed by using long, thin, nasopharyngeal swabs, which should be plated on Bordet-Gengou medium at the bedside or taken immediately to the laboratory. Growth is slow and usually does not occur for 48 to 96 hours. Fluorescent antibody studies may be performed immediately on direct swabs.

Treatment and Prognosis. Treatment of the infected patient is designed primarily to assure adequate oxygenation and nutrition. Antibiotics do not alter the clinical course of the illness, and certain antibiotics do not even eliminate the organism.[28,29] Erythromycin for 10 to 14 days is recommended to reduce spread of infection to other susceptible persons. Tetracycline and chloramphenicol are effective but potentially more toxic, and ampicillin is ineffective.[29] The fatality rate is approximately 5 per 1000. The ultimate treatment is prevention by means of adequate immunization of children. Chemoprophylaxis with erythromycin has been recommended, especially for those with inadequate immunization as children. The efficacy of this practice has not been unequivocally documented.

Haemophilus influenzae

Morphology and Identification. Haemophilus influenzae are minute gram-negative rods 0.2 to 0.3 μm × 0.5 to 2.0 μm and coccobacillary in appearance. They are notoriously difficult to recognize on Gram stains of clinical material and may appear to be gram positive. Both encapsulated and unencapsulated types have been described in clinical illness, but of the six capsular types, type b is by far the most frequent pathogen. The organism grows aerobically, does not produce spores, and produces acid from glucose and sucrose.

Epidemiology and Pathogenesis. Haemophilus influenzae is a normal inhabitant of the upper respiratory tract, particularly in young children. The organism usually causes upper respiratory infection from the age of 6 months to about 3 years. Typical infections include epiglottitis, otitis media, tracheobronchitis, laryngitis, and pneumonia, but cellulitis, arthritis, pericarditis, osteomyelitis, and meningitis also occur frequently.[30] Bacteremia may accompany any of these infections. Among adults, pneumonia due to *H. influenzae* has become increasingly frequent. The virulence of the organism is thought to be associated with the capsule; however, the precise mechanism by which a normal respiratory inhabitant becomes pathogenic is not known. Immunity is related to the develoment of specific antibodies to the capsule, which are lacking in young children but are present in most adults and older children.

Clinical Manifestations. Most patients are young children whose symptoms begin with nonspecific upper respiratory symptoms, cough, hoarseness, fever, and occasionally stridor. Acute epiglottitis has a rapid onset. The pharynx becomes beefy red, and the epiglottis is swollen and may completely close, necessitating tracheostomy. Signs and symptoms in meningitis cannot be distinguished from illness caused by other pyogenic organisms.

Diagnosis. Diagnosis is dependent on the isolation and identification of the organism from infected exudates or body fluids such as sputum, throat swabs, and cerebrospinal fluid. Caution must be exercised in the interpretation of Gram smears because the organism may appear gram-positive and may resemble diplococci. For spinal fluid specimens, rapid detection of *H. influenzae* may be accomplished by the use of counterimmunoelectrophoresis.

Treatment and Prognosis. During the 1970s, *H. influenzae* resistant to ampicillin became sufficiently prevalent to contraindicate the empiric use of ampicillin for serious infections.[31] Effective alternative antibiotics include chloramphenicol for treatment of meningitis and the newer cephalosporins, cefotaxime, ceftizoxime, ceftriaxone, and cefuroxime.[32–35] Rifampin has been used successfully for the eradication of the pharyngeal carriage state. Vaccines that are effective against *H. influenzae* have been developed and are in widespread use with a resultant decline in serious *H. influenzae* infections in children.

Other *Haemophilus* Species

Other species of the genus *Haemophilus* that are known or suspected to cause disease in people include *H. parainfluenzae, H. haemolyticus, H. parahaemolyticus, H. aphrophilus, H. aegyptius,* and *H. ducreyi.*

Haemophilus ducreyi. Chancroid, a soft, painful, venereal ulcer, is caused by *H. ducreyi*. Lesions are more frequent in the male and usually occur under the foreskin or around the corona of the glans penis and occasionally on the penile shaft. Inguinal adenopathy may or may not be present. Special techniques using media containing blood or serum are required to culture *H. ducreyi.* Demonstration of small, gram-negative coccobacilli on direct Gram smear of the lesion may be used as presumptive diagnosis of chancroid if a dark-field examination for syphilis is negative. Gram stains of aspirates of inguinal nodes may also be used to establish the diagnosis. *Haemophilus ducreyi* is frequently resistant to traditional therapeutic agents such as sulfonamides, tetracycline, and ampicillin. Most patients with chancroid are best treated with either erythromycin or trimethoprim-sulfamethoxazole (TMP-SMX), including a single-dose regimen that has proven clinically effective.[36–38] Needle aspiration or drainage of inguinal abscesses or buboes is usually necessary only if fluctuance is present.[36,37]

Haemophilus aphrophilus. *Haemophilus aphrophilus* can be found among the normal oral and pharyngeal flora and is occasionally the cause of endocarditis, brain abscess, bacteremia, meningitis, pneumonia, or soft tissue abscesses. It may be difficult to distinguish from *Actinobacillus actinomycetemcomitans,* which can cause similar clinical illness. Patients with *H. aphrophilus* infection have a high frequency of trauma, oropharyngeal infection, and underlying malignancies or are undergoing chemotherapy for cancer.[39] Endocarditis is the most frequently reported infection due to *H. aphrophilus,* followed by brain abscess.[39,40] Results of in vitro antimicrobial susceptibility testing of *H. aphrophilus* suggest that chloramphenicol, tetracycline, streptomycin, and gentamicin may be effective drugs. Susceptibility to penicillin G and ampicillin is variable, and the preferred treatment, particularly for endocarditis, remains unsettled, but susceptibility to newer parenteral cephalosporins should be obtained.

Haemophilus parainfluenzae. A prominent feature of recently recognized acute and subacute bacterial endocarditis caused by *H. parainfluenzae* is the high incidence of major arterial occlusion secondary to emboli. This organism can be regularly isolated from the upper respiratory tract of healthy persons and only rarely causes human disease. Combination treatment with a penicillin (ampicillin) and an aminoglycoside appears to be most effective.

Haemophilus aegyptius. *Haemophilus aegyptius* has been the cause of acute conjunctivitis.

Calymmatobacterium granulomatis

Morphology and Identification. This small, pleomorphic, gram-negative rod, formerly known as *Donovania granulomatis,* causes granuloma inguinale. It is extremely difficult to culture this organism, which requires either inoculation of egg yolks or egg yolk slants. On Wright stain the organisms appear blue and exhibit bipolar staining (Donovan bodies), frequently within the vacuoles of large phagocytic cells.

Epidemiology and Pathogenesis. Fewer than 100 cases of granuloma inguinale are reported in the United States per year, mostly in the southeastern states. Over 90 percent of the time the disease is localized to the genital and groin area and traditionally has been thought to be disseminated by sexual contact; however, the rate of transmission appears to be quite low. The organism has been isolated from stools, raising the possibility of acquisition from the patient's own flora. The ulcer base is infiltrated with mononuclear cells, particularly large macrophages filled with organisms. Lesions begin as papules, which slowly ulcerate. Infection may extend from the genital area with development of large inguinal nodes. Occasionally, lesions have been noted in bone, joints, and liver.

Clinical Manifestations and Diagnosis. Patients are rarely seen during the acute stage of the illness, which is characterized by papules and small ulcers on the vulva, perineum, groin, glans penis, or penile shaft. Later lesions are hypertrophic and may resemble carcinoma. Lesions are typically long-standing, destructive, and painless but not insensitive.[41] Diagnosis is accomplished by microscopic examination of Wright- or Giemsa-stained smears of scrapings or biopsies at the advancing margin of ulcerative lesions. Dark-field examination should be performed to rule out syphilis. Although complement-fixation serologic tests are available, they lack specificity and cross-react with other venereal diseases. Granuloma inguinale is considered a probable premalignant lesion, and carcinoma must always be suspected in hypertrophic lesions.[42]

Treatment and Prognosis. A number of antibiotic regimens have been successful, including tetracycline, chloramphenicol, erythromycin, streptomycin, and gentamicin. Oral treatment with tetracycline is usually continued for 10 to 20 days. The disease may reappear years later, despite adequate treatment. Treatment of late lesions may result in stricture of the urethra, vagina, or anus.

Brucella Species

Brucellae are the causative organisms of brucellosis (formerly undulant fever) in humans. They primarily infect the genitourinary tract of a variety of animals and are associated with abortion. Species pathogenic for humans and their usual animal hosts are *B. abortus* (cattle), *B. suis* (swine), and *B. melitensis* (sheep and goats); however, there is a wide overlap in the susceptibility of various animals to *Brucella* species. More recently, *B. canis* (dogs) has also been associated with disease in humans.[43]

Morphology and Identification. The organisms are short, coccobacillary, gram-negative rods. They are nonmotile, strict aerobes, some of which require the addition of CO_2 for growth. Growth of *Brucella* organisms on ordinary media is slow. Cultures of body fluids should be held for 21 days before being reported as negative.

Epidemiology and Pathogenesis. Human brucellosis is acquired by contact with infected animals or animal products. Most cases in the United States occur in Texas and the southwestern states bordering on Mexico. The majority of cases in the United States have occurred in adult men who work in meat-packing plants. Other sources of brucellosis include ingestion of unpasteurized dairy products and consumption of foreign cheese, particularly goat cheese from Mexico. From 1967 to 1977, 17 cases in the United States were attributed to *B. canis* acquired through contact with dogs. The organism probably causes infection by entering the body through breaks in the skin or by ingestion or inhalation. Organisms spread rapidly, are phagocytosed by macrophages and polymorphonuclear leukocytes, and multiply within phagocytic vacuoles.[44]

Clinical Manifestations. The diagnosis is particularly difficult if a history of animal contact has not been obtained because the symptoms are nonspecific—fever, chills, sweats, malaise, weakness, body aches, anorexia, and weight loss. Headache is reported in about half the patients. Lymphadenopathy, splenomegaly, and hepatomegaly can be evident in up to 25 percent of patients, but the results of physical examination are usually normal. Occasionally, patients will exhibit symptoms of dysuria, testicular pain, arthralgias, respiratory symptoms, visual disturbances, tinnitus, loss of balance, and mental depression. Because of the nonspecificity of acute symptoms the differential diagnosis in acute brucellosis includes a variety of bacterial, parasitic, viral, and fungal diseases.

Diagnosis. The majority of brucellosis infections are diagnosed by demonstration of a serologic rise in agglutinating antibody to *B. abortus* antigen. Agglutinating titers almost always exceed 1:160 within 2 to 3 weeks of acute illness. Titers may remain elevated for years, and their significance in chronic brucellosis can be difficult to interpret. Blood is the most frequent source of the organism during the acute phase, while aspirates of bone, joint fluid, or soft tissue abscess may reveal the organism in chronic brucellosis.

Treatment and Prognosis. Mortality is low with antimicrobial therapy in brucellosis, and even without treatment most patients recover spontaneously. Most of the deaths are associated with infective endocarditis. If acute brucellosis is diagnosed or suspected, antimicrobial therapy should be instituted. In vitro susceptibility testing suggests that the tetracycline antibiotics, as well as erythromycin, gentamicin, kanamycin, streptomycin, and rifampin, are quite active against *Brucella* organisms.[45] Patients are usually treated with a tetracycline for 3 to 4 weeks; however, relapses may be forestalled when combination therapy with tetracycline (or doxycycline) and streptomycin is used. Trimethoprim-sulfamethoxazole has also proved effective, but the failure rate is 5.7 percent and the relapse rate is 12 percent or more. The most popular current regimen is doxycycline plus rifampin for 45 days.[45]

Vibrio Species

Organisms of the genus *Vibrio* are currently divided into at least three categories: (1) *V. cholerae*; (2) the so-called nonagglutinable (NAG) or noncholera (NCV) vibrios or non-O1 *V. cholerae,* which produce primarily diarrheal illness; and (3) the halophilic vibrios, which include *V. parahaemolyticus, V. alginolyticus, V. vulnificus,* and *V. fluvialis.*

Vibrio cholerae *and Non-O1* V. cholerae *(Noncholera Vibrios)*

Morphology and Identification. The *V. cholerae* organism is a short, slightly curved, 0.5 μm × 1.5 to 3.0 μm gram-negative, motile rod, which is facultatively anaerobic and oxidase positive. Both nonselective and selective media should be used for the initial isolation of the organism from stool. Direct fluorescence microscopy on stool specimens using fluorescein-labeled, type-specific antibody can also be used for rapid presumptive diagnosis. Non-O1 *V. cholerae* are indistinguishable morphologically or biochemically from *V. cholerae* but fail to agglutinate with *V. cholerae* antiserum.[46]

Epidemiology and Pathogenesis. Humans are the only known hosts of *V. cholerae,* and the disease is endemic to portions of India and Bangladesh. Periodic pandemics have swept the world since 1800. Cases have been sporadic in western Europe and the United States since 1960 with 65 cases reported in the United States from the Gulf of Mexico.[47] In 1991 an epidemic of cholera struck Peru, the first time in this century that cholera was reported in South America.[47] The major mode of transmission appears to be infected water. Asymptomatic cases usually outnumber clinical cases, so that control is difficult. A gallbladder-carrier state may develop, but its importance in promulgation of the disease is unknown. The pathogenesis of clinical cholera is one of the best known of all infectious diseases. Illness results from the action of a protein enterotoxin that binds to small-bowel epithelial cells and stimulates production of adenylcyclase, leading to increased concentrations of intracellular cyclic AMP and secretion of electrolytes into the small bowel. Non-O1 *V. cholerae* is usually acquired by ingestion of seafood, particularly raw oysters, but has also occurred among travelers.[47]

Clinical Manifestations and Diagnosis. The patient with cholera typically has no fever or abdominal pain but has abrupt, watery diarrhea without blood or mucus, with initial signs of fluid depletion, including poor skin turgor, thready pulse, low blood pressure, tachycardia, and tachypnea. Most adults remain alert, but children may exhibit stupor and convulsions in severe cases. Although many patients have mild illness with relatively small amounts of fluid loss, up to 1 liter per hour may be lost from the gastrointestinal tract. Diarrhea may continue for as long as 7 days. Where the disease is endemic, a presumptive diagnosis can be made on the basis of the clinical evidence. Ultimate diagnosis is established by culture of the organism from stool and identification with specific agglutinating antisera.

Treatment and Prognosis. The mainstay of cholera treatment is fluid and electrolyte replacement. For severely ill patients and those unable to take oral fluids, intravenous replacement is necessary, but oral therapy has become an accepted treatment for those less seriously ill.[48] The failure rate of oral therapy (15 to 20 percent) is highest in those patients with the greatest amount of diarrhea (greater than 20 ml/kg/h). For oral replacement, either glucose (20 g/liter) or sucrose (40 g/liter) is required to facilitate the uptake of sodium by the intestinal epithelium. The duration and volume of diarrhea can be reduced by the use of antibiotics. Tetracycline is usually used, but organisms are also susceptible to ampicillin, chloramphenicol, and sulfonamides. The mortality rate in treated cholera should be under 1 percent as demonstrated in the Peruvian outbreak in 1991.[48]

Halophilic Vibrios

Morphology and Identification. The most important organism among the halophilic vibrios is *V. parahaemolyticus,* which is one cause of acute diarrhea associated with seafood consumption. In addition, *V. alginolyticus* has been found in bacteremias and wound infections associated with a marine environment. More recently, *V. vulnificus* has been implicated as the cause of bacteremia and wound infections in people exposed to seawater.[49,50] The organisms are gram-negative, facultative anaerobes that require 1 to 3 percent sodium chloride in media for growth, hence the "halophilic" grouping.

Epidemiology. Infection with all these organisms is associated either with exposure to seawater or ingestion of seafoods. Gastroenteritis caused by *V. parahaemolyticus* is the most common cause of food poisoning in Japan. In the United States all cases have been reported from Eastern or Gulf Coast states. Most Japanese infections are associated with eating raw seafood, but in the United States infections have been associated with cooked crab, shrimp, lobster, or oysters.[49] Most patients exhibit cramping diarrhea, which begins 6 to 36 hours after ingestion of the suspect food. About one-half of the patients have vomiting, and one-fourth have fever. Symptoms usually subside spontaneously after 24 to 48 hours. Both *V. alginolyticus* and *V. vulnificus* have been isolated from infected wounds of persons working in or near seawater and have also been isolated from seawater, particularly in warm weather months when the frequency of gastroenteritis peaks.

Pathogenesis. The pathogenesis of *V. parahaemolyticus* infection is not clearly understood. Pathogenicity is linked to a hemolysin. A dysentery-like illness in a minority of patients suggests that the organism can invade the intestinal mucosa at times. *Vibrio vulnificus* causes wound infections by direct inoculation from shellfish or seawater. It also appears to cause bacteremia in patients with liver disease after oral ingestion of seafoods such as raw oysters.[50]

Clinical Manifestations. Patients with *V. parahaemolyticus* infection present with cramping and watery diarrhea with occasional vomiting and nausea. Blood and mucus may be found in the stool. *Vibrio vulnificus* also can cause a gastroenteritis.[49] Patients do not have bacteremia and usually have a history of recent seafood ingestion. Patients with skin or wound infections exhibit an intense cellulitis at the site of entry of the organism. Patients with *V. vulnificus* wound infections may also exhibit signs of systemic infection, including fever and chills, and have positive blood cultures. Patients with *V. vulnificus* bacteremia not associated with wound infection may exhibit erythematous or ecchymotic areas on the extremities, which form bullae or vesicles and then become necrotic ulcers. On biopsy these lesions reveal a vasculitis in the skin and subcutaneous tissues.[46] *Vibrio alginolyticus* produces wound and ear infections.[46]

Diagnosis. Diagnosis of *V. parahaemolyticus* gastroenteritis can be made by isolation of the organism from stool and from suspect seafoods. Patients with *V. parahaemolyticus* gastroenteritis may have red cells and leukocytes in stool on microscopic examination. Diagnosis of *V. vulnificus* infection is made from blood, stool, or wound cultures. *Vibrio alginolyticus* is usually found in wounds.

Treatment and Prognosis. *Vibrio parahaemolyticus* food poisoning or gastroenteritis is a self-limited disease in the majority of patients and does not require treatment; the efficacy of antibiotics in severe cases is unknown. Antibiotics are strongly recommended for treatment of *V. vulnificus* infections, but the optimal regimen is not known. The halophilic vibrios are susceptible to broad-spectrum antibiotics including ampicillin, cephalosporins, gentamicin, tetracycline, and chloramphenicol. Tetracycline is probably the preferred agent. Prognosis in *V. parahaemolyticus* gastroenteritis is excellent. In contrast, the mortality rate with *V. vulnificus* infection approaches 50 percent in bacteremic patients.[49,50]

Campylobacter Species

Morphology and Identification. *Campylobacter* species (formerly called *Vibrio fetus*) are non-spore-forming, microaerophilic, spirally curved, gram-negative rods that are motile by means of a single polar flagellum. There are now at least six species of *Campylobacter* known, but two, *C. jejuni* and *C. fetus,* cause the majority of human disease. It tolerates anaerobic conditions but fails to grow under atmospheric conditions. Recovery of the organism from stool in outbreaks of diarrhea has been facilitated by selective media containing vancomycin, polymyxin B, and trimethoprim.

Epidemiology and Pathogenesis. *Campylobacter fetus* is a well-known pathogen of animals, causing abortion in cattle and sheep and enteritis in calves and pigs. Although some cases in humans may be related to animal contact, the majority are due to ingestion of contaminated food such as unpasteurized milk, undercooked meats, or contaminated surface water. Cases of bacteremia are more frequent with *C. fetus* and are presumed to be acquired by the gastrointestinal route. Household contacts, particularly children, have acquired the disease. The exact pathogenic mechanism of the disease remains unexplained, as there is evidence of both enterotoxin production and invasiveness of the organism. *Campylobacter* is probably the leading cause of bacterial diarrhea in the United States, exceeding both *Salmonella* and *Shigella.*[51]

Clinical Manifestations and Diagnosis. Gastrointestinal illness is characterized by abdominal cramping and pain, diarrhea, malaise, and fever.[52] Symptoms usually last 1 to 7 days or longer. Infants, pregnant women, and elderly individuals may be at increased risk; among older patients, predisposing debilitating illness is common. Clinical features of the disease are nonspecific and resemble both *Salmonella* and *Shigella*. Diagnosis is based on isolation of the organism from blood, stools, or body fluids. The vast majority of disease is gastrointestinal and caused by *C. jejuni.* Most bacteremias are caused by *C. fetus* and are seen most often in compromised hosts.

Treatment and Prognosis. The majority of gastrointestinal infections are self-limited and resolve within 7 days without treatment. For persisting bloody or severe diarrhea, erythromycin and ciprofloxacin have been used. In vitro susceptibility suggests that erythromycin, aminoglycosides, chloramphenicol, fluoroquinolones, and tetracyclines are active against the organism and that the organisms may be resistant to penicillins, cephalosporins, vancomycin, metronidazole, and trimethoprim-sulfamethoxazole. Patients who are bacteremic probably should receive an aminoglycoside such as gentamicin.

Acinetobacter calcoaceticus

Morphology and Identification. Two varieties of this organism cause disease in humans: *A. calcoaceticus* var. *anitratus* (formerly *Herellea vaginicola*) and *A. calcoaceticus* var. *lwoffi* (formerly *Mima polymorpha*). The organisms are short, plump, gram-negative rods or coccobacillary forms. They are strict aerobes, do not form spores, and grow readily on simple laboratory media without enrichment or supplementation.

Epidemiology and Pathogenesis. Acinetobacter calcoaceticus is a ubiquitous organism found in soil and water, in both wet and dry environments, and has been isolated from the normal skin, conjunctivae, genitourinary tract, and occasionally pharynx of people. Its pathogenic potential for debilitated and hospitalized patients has been realized only within the last 20 years.[53,54] Infections have been reported primarily from pulmonary sources, wounds, urinary tract, and occasionally cellulitis. Bacteremias have been reported from all these foci. Most patients have undergone instrumentation or manipulation of the respiratory or urinary tract or have had prior surgical procedures. The organism causing the infection is probably from the patient's own indigenous flora or is acquired from environmental sources or cross-contamination by hospital personnel or equipment.[54]

Clinical Manifestations and Diagnosis. Most patients with *A. calcoaceticus* infections have nosocomial respiratory, urinary, or wound infection and exhibit fever, chills, and occasionally hypotension that is indistinguishable from sepsis from other gram-negative organisms. Diagnosis is based on culture isolation of the organism from sputum, urine, blood, or body fluids.

Treatment and Prognosis. Acinetobacters are resistant to a large number of antimicrobials. Most are susceptible to the aminoglycosides, particularly tobramycin and amikacin, to imipenem, and may also be susceptible to trimethoprim-sulfamethoxazole, newer cephalosporins, minocycline, and tetracycline. Susceptibility testing should determine the therapy. Mortality in cases of pneumonia or septicemia ranges from 20 to 50 percent and is probably related to the underlying illnesses of the patients and the relative resistance of the organism to most antimicrobials.

Aeromonas Species

Morphology and Identification. The genus *Aeromonas* consists of motile, gram-negative, facultative, anaerobic organisms that are commonly isolated from water, soil, food, and a variety of environmental sources. Members of the genus *Aeromonas* use carbohydrates fermentatively but are oxidase positive, separating them from the Enterobacteriaceae.

Epidemiology and Pathogenesis. Aeromonas hydrophila is found in a variety of freshwater habitats. It has been known for some time as an opportunistic pathogen of immunocompromised hosts but more recently has been shown to cause pneumonia and traumatic wound infection in otherwise normal patients contaminated from freshwater sources.[55] Near-drownings in contaminated lakes, rivers, ditches, and ponds have been associated with *A. hydrophila* pneumonia.[55] *Aeromonas* species are also a likely cause of gastroenteritis, but the mechanism is not known.[56]

Clinical Manifestations and Diagnosis. Aeromonas hydrophila has been the cause of an increasing number of human infections, including infected traumatic wounds, pneumonia, septicemia, meningitis, osteomyelitis, diarrhea, and postoperative infections.[58] Because of the aquatic nature of these organisms, some infections have been related to trauma with a concomitant history of exposure to soil or water (eg, fish handlers). Surgeons should be particularly aware of the propensity of this organism to be present in traumatic wounds contaminated by fresh water.[57] Myonecrosis and gas formation in tissue may mimic clostridial infection.[57]

Treatment and Prognosis. Aeromonas hydrophila is susceptible to third-generation cephalosporins, imipenen, aztreonam, the aminoglycosides, trimethoprim-sulfamethoxazole, and ciprofloxacin.[57] Surgical drainage combined with antibiotic therapy is usually required for wound infections.[58] Diarrheal illness is usually acute and of short duration.

Moraxella (Branhamella) catarrhalis

Morphology and Identification. Moraxella (formerly *Branhamella*) *catarrhalis* is the type species of the subgenus *Branhamella* of the genus *Moraxella*. It is a gram-negative diplococcus formerly classified in the *Neisseria* genus. It is distinguished from the *Neisseria* species by its failure to produce acid from carbohydrates, its reduction of NO_2 and NO_3, and the presence of DNase.

Epidemiology and Pathogenesis. Moraxella catarrhalis is frequently an inhabitant of the nasopharynx of humans. It infrequently causes upper and lower respiratory infections including otitis, sinusitis, pharyngitis, bronchitis, and pneumonia (with bacteremia) in normal hosts.[59] Local spread from the sinuses, mastoids, and middle ear can produce meningitis. Patient-to-patient spread has not been described.

Clinical Manifestations and Diagnosis. Moraxella catarrhalis presents either as bacteremia in a compromised host, or as an upper or lower respiratory infection with purulent sputum, often in smokers or patients with chronic lung disease.[59] Diagnosis in lower respiratory infections is more certain if a transtracheal aspirate is performed, but sputum specimens that contain only *M. catarrhalis* or in which it is the predominant isolate have been used to make a diagnosis.[59]

Treatment and Prognosis. Many *M. catarrhalis* isolates produce beta-lactamase. Most are not susceptible to penicillin G and ampicillin or are variably susceptible to first-generation cephalosporins such as cephalothin, cephalexin, and cefazolin. In vitro, the following agents are usually active: aminoglycosides, tetracyclines, chloramphenicol, trimethoprim-sulfamethoxazole, ticarcillin, piperacillin, mezlocillin, ampicillin-sulbactum, amoxicillin-clavulonate, cefixime, cefuroxime, cefoxitin, the third-generation cephalosporins, the fluoroquinolones (eg, ofloxacin, ciprofloxacin), and the macrolides (erythromycin, clarithromycin, azithromycin).[60,61] Patients with respiratory infections usually do well with appropriate antimicrobial therapy.

Capnocytophaga Species

Morphology and Identification. Capnocytophaga is a proposed genus for a fastidious gram-negative gliding fusiform bacillus that grows anaerobically and aerobically in the presence of CO_2.

Epidemiology and Pathogenesis. Capnocytophaga species are frequent inhabitants of the oral cavity and have been isolated in high numbers from the periodontal lesions of patients with juvenile periodontitis. In the normal host they have been isolated from empyemas, lung abscesses, wound infections (including closed fist injuries) and bacteremias.[62] In the immunocompromised host most isolates have come from blood.[62,63] There is a high association between bacteremias in immunocompromised hosts and oral pathology including oral ulceration, gingivitis, and stomatitis.[62,63]

Clinical Manifestations and Diagnosis. Most patients present at a young age with periodontal symptoms of juvenile periodontitis and may be seen by oral surgeons. In immunocompromised (usually neutropenic) hosts the disease presents as a bacteremia in association with oral pathology. Traumatic injury to the fist from teeth leads to hand infections. The diagnosis is made by isolation of *Capnocytophaga* from appropriate clinical specimens including gingival swabs, wound cultures, and blood. Often the organism is present as part of a mixed bacterial population.[62]

Treatment and Prognosis. Optimal treatment for *Capnocytophaga* infection is not established, but penicillin, ampicillin, carbenicillin, clindamycin, erythromycin, cefoxitin, and tetracycline are active in vitro. Aminoglycosides, vancomycin, cephalothin, and cefazolin are not active in vitro. Most patients have recovered from *Capnocytophaga* infection, even when immunosuppressed and bacteremic, but mortality ranges from 10 to 35 percent in this group.[62,63]

Legionella pneumophila

Morphology and Identification. Legionella pneumophila was responsible for a large common-source outbreak of respiratory illness that occurred at the American Legion Convention in Philadelphia in July 1976, resulting in the first description of legionnaires' disease.[64] Similar outbreaks and sporadic cases of this illness have been found elsewhere. The organism is a gram-negative bacillus, 0.3 to 0.4 μm $\times$ 2 to 3 μm, with fastidious growth requirements, which were responsible for the initial failure to isolate it. The organisms grow optimally at 35C in air at 80 to 90 percent humidity. Growth of *Legionella* is slow and requires 2 to 3 days for detection.

Epidemiology. The epidemiology of legionnaires' disease has been actively researched. Evidence of both epidemic outbreaks and hyperendemic disease in certain geographic areas of the country has been established. Epidemic disease has occurred during the warm weather months from July through October, and sporadic cases in endemic areas have occurred throughout the year. Several outbreaks have implicated air-conditioning cooling towers as the possible source of the organism. Nosocomial infections, particularly in renal transplant recipients, have been traced to contamination of hospital potable water supplies. Potable water has also been the source of sporadic community-acquired cases.[66] Airborne inhalation of the organism is thought to be the usual mode of acquisition. Smokers seem to be more susceptible than nonsmokers to legionnaires' disease. The incubation period ranges from 2 to 10 days.

Pathogenesis. It is presumed that the organism is acquired by inhalation. The characteristic pathologic findings are limited to the lung, where either unilateral or bilateral lobar bronchopneumonia is most often found. The cellular exudate consists of polymorphonuclear neutrophils and macrophages with some areas of coagulative necrosis, but rarely formation of abscesses. Bacteria can be seen by using Dieterle or Gram stain of unfixed tissue imprints.

Clinical Manifestations. In the early phases of illness, legionnaires' disease cannot be distinguished from other respiratory infections. The patient complains of weakness, malaise, muscle aches, anorexia, mild headache, and occasional dry cough. This is usually followed within a day by the onset of rapidly rising fever, rigors, increasing nonproductive cough with pleuritic pain, and in some instances diarrhea. Altered mentation and obtundation may be a prominent feature in some patients. Rales are usually audible on chest examination, and chest roentgenograms reveal either patchy interstitial infiltrates or discrete areas of consolidation. About half the patients have unilateral involvement; small pleural effusions may be present; cavitation is usually not found. Leukocytosis is common, and hyponatremia, hypophosphatemia, and abnormal liver function tests have been described. Extrathoracic spread to heart, kidney, liver, and spleen has been reported in immunosuppressed or debilitated patients. Patients may present with no pulmonary manifestations of disease (Pontiac fever).

Diagnosis. In hyperendemic areas or during an epidemic the clinical presentation may be sufficiently distinctive to make the diagnosis; however, in sporadic cases diagnosis is difficult. Serologic conversion remains the mainstay of diagnosis, and the indirect fluorescent antibody test has been used most frequently. A fourfold rise in titer of paired serum specimens is required for unequivocal diagnosis. Diagnosis by means of direct culture of lung tissue or sputum is possible in over half of patients. Direct fluorescent antibody stain of sputum is a rapid but much less sensitive diagnostic test. In the nonepidemic situation, diseases such as psittacosis, Q fever, mycoplasma infection, and influenza can mimic the symptoms of legionnaires' disease.

Treatment and Prognosis. Mortality in the original Philadelphia outbreak was 16 percent. The number of deaths in subsequent epidemic outbreaks has been reduced because of more rapid recognition of the disease and institution of antimicrobial therapy. In vivo and in vitro susceptibility tests suggest that rifampin and erythromycin are the most effective antimicrobials.[67] Among clinical cases, erythromycin has been the mainstay of therapy, usually at a dosage of 2 to 4 g daily for at least 3 weeks.[67] Use of a combination of rifampin and erythromycin has been recommended for severely ill patients. A tetracycline such as doxycycline is recommended as alternative therapy.[68] Fluoroquinolones such as ciprofloxacin and newer macrolides such as clarithromycin are promising alternative agents with demonstrated clinical efficacy as well.

Other *Legionella* Species

Morphology and Identification. Additional species of *Legionella* that are thought to cause human disease include *L.* (*Tatlockia*) *micdadei* (Pittsburgh pneumonia agent), *L. bozemanii, L. dumoffii, L. gormanii, L. longbeachae,* and several other strains.[68] Direct examination of clinical specimens can be done with a number of stains including Gram, Gimenez, and Dieterle, and with direct fluorescent antibody tests, which contain antibody to most *Legionella* species. Modified acid-fast stains have been used for detection of *L. micdadei* in tissues.

Epidemiology and Pathogenesis. The means of acquisition and reservoirs of *Legionella* species are not as well known as for *L. pneumophila.* Most are thought to reside in water and moist environments, and some have been recovered from potable water.[69]

Clinical Manifestations and Diagnosis. Almost all reported patients have presented with pneumonia as their clinical manifestation of *Legionella* infection. *Legionella micdadei* has been reported to cause a nonpneumonic febrile illness. *Legionella micdadei* has occurred most often in immunosuppressed patients (particularly renal transplant recipients) and has been a nosocomial problem in some hospitals.[69] The symptoms and signs of *Legionella* species infection are indistinguishable from those due to *L. pneumophila.* Diagnosis is made by culture of the organism from sputum or lung tissue, by demonstration with direct fluorescent antibody, or by evidence of a fourfold rise in serum antibody titer.

Treatment and Prognosis. Therapeutic regimens have not been well evaluated for *Legionella* species. Erythromycin has been used to treat most cases, particularly *L. micdadei,* with good success.[69] In vitro, *L. micdadei* is more susceptible than *L. pneumophila* because of a lack of betalactamase, but there is little clinical experience with regimens other than erythromycin.[70] Rifampin plus erythromycin is also effective as are tetracyclines (doxycycline) and fluoroquinolones (ciprofloxacin), but experience is very limited.[69] Treatment with penicillins, cephalosporins, vancomycin, or clindamycin is not recommended.

ACID-FAST BACTERIA

Genus *Mycobacterium*

The diseases caused by *Mycobacterium* organisms are summarized in Table 9–1. Other saprophytic organisms exist but are rarely pathogenic except in highly immunosuppressed patients such as those with HIV infection.

Mycobacterium tuberculosis *and* Mycobacterium bovis

Morphology and Identification. Mycobacterium tuberculosis and *M. bovis* are slightly curved or straight rods that are 0.2 to 0.6 μm × 1 to 10 μm. With the other mycobacteria they exhibit the property of resistance to the decolorizing effect of acid-alcohol. The organisms do not stain readily by Gram method but are usually considered to be gram positive. Because of the slow growth characteristics of tubercle bacilli, special handling procedures are required to control contaminants. From 3 to 8 weeks may be required to detect growth of *M. tuberculosis* colonies, which are usually cream colored, dry, and wrinkled in appearance. Preliminary screening of cultures to separate *M. tuberculosis* from other mycobacteria is done by means of the niacin test. The identification of acid-fast bacilli in clinical specimens is an important diagnostic procedure but can be misleading if acid-fast contaminants are present. Newer direct fluorescent techniques on spectrum may be more sensitive than acid-fast stains and specific DNA probes have increased the rapidity of speciation of cultured organisms.

Epidemiology. Tuberculosis is contracted almost exclusively by airborne transmission of infected droplets from patients with active pulmonary disease. Although bovine tuberculosis may be acquired by the ingestion of contaminated milk, this risk has been all but eliminated by the practice of milk pasteurization. Although tuberculosis may be acquired from contact with infected animals, person-to-person infection is the most common mode of spread. Tuberculosis rates in the United States have been increasing since 1986 due to increased case rates in HIV-infected persons and an increase in immigrants from other areas endemic for tuberculosis such as Asia, Africa, the Caribbean, and Latin America. Tuberculosis occurs most frequently in

TABLE 9–1. MYCOBACTERIA MOST PATHOGENIC FOR HUMANS

Group[a]	Species	Disease Name	Primary Infection Site	Human Saphrophyte	Need for Surgical Treatment
Tuberculosis complex	*M. tuberculosis*	Tuberculosis	Pulmonary	No	Rare
	M. bovis	Bovine tuberculosis	Pulmonary	No	Rare
	M. ulcerans	Buruli ulcer	Skin	No	Rare
I Photochromogens	*M. kansasii*	None	Pulmonary	Yes	Occasional
	M. marinum	"Swimming pool granuloma"	Skin	No	Occasional
II Scotochromogens	*M. scrofulaceum*	Scrofula[b]	Cervical adenitis	Yes	Usual
III Nonphotochromogens	*M. avium complex* (*M. avium-intracellulare*)	None	Pulmonary (blood and GI in HIV)	Yes	Frequent (in non-HIV patients)
IV Rapid growers	*M. fortuitum*	None	Skin, wound	Yes	Usual
	M. chelonae	None	Skin, wound	Yes	Usual
Unclassified	*M. leprae*	Leprosy	Skin	No	Occasional

[a] Groups I to IV as classified by E. H. Runyon.
[b] Scrofula is also frequently caused by *M. kansasii, M. avium-intracellulare,* and *M. tuberculosis.*

major metropolitan areas, the southern United States, areas of high American Indian population, and among lower socioeconomic groups.[71]

Pathogenesis. Primary tuberculosis infection begins with the inhalation of tubercle bacilli into the alveoli of the lung, where local intracellular and extracellular multiplication takes place. This initial site of infection can be sufficiently prominent to be seen on chest x-ray but usually goes unrecognized. From the local pulmonary site of infection, organisms spread via the lymphatics to hilar lymph nodes and via the bloodstream to all parts of the body. The acute inflammatory cells are replaced by a lymphocytic and histiocytic response, which develops into the characteristic tubercle or granulomatous reaction, frequently with necrosis of central areas. The development of an active cellular immunity may be the rate-limiting factor in control of the initial infection.

Factors responsible for active dissemination and spread of tuberculosis at the time of initial infection are not clear. Some patients develop frank pulmonary infiltration or tuberculous pneumonia, while others develop widespread metastatic lesions that, because of their millet-seed appearance, have been called miliary tuberculosis. Patients who have initial hematogenous spread to distant organs usually have no symptoms with the initial infection but may activate disease in these areas at a much later date. Common sites of extrapulmonary involvement include bones, joints, kidneys, adrenal glands, and meninges. Production of cavities in the lung at the site of active infection is common and develops as a result of the emptying of a caseous pulmonary lesion. Pulmonary cavities are the source of large numbers of mycobacterial organisms. Although active disease in adults is most common in the apical and posterior segments of the upper lobes, disease in children may occur anywhere in the lung. The higher oxygen tension in the upper lobes of adults probably favors the growth of the organism in this area. In patients who have effectively controlled their primary infection, calcification of initial parenchymal lung lesions and lymph nodes occurs (Ghon's complex).

Clinical Manifestations and Diagnosis. Most patients with active tuberculosis initially have insidious nonspecific symptoms, which include general malaise and fatigue, anorexia, weight loss, low-grade fever, and night sweats. Patients seldom complain of cough during the early phase of the illness; however, as pulmonary lesions progress, cough becomes a more prominent symptom, and hemoptysis is common. Cavitary pulmonary tuberculosis can usually be established by the finding of acid-fast organisms in sputum, but in noncavitary disease the number of organisms expectorated may not be sufficient to be detected by smear.

Extrapulmonary tuberculosis may be even more insidious and difficult to diagnose than pulmonary disease. Patients with tuberculous meningitis usually have an indolent, semiacute course characterized by headache and stiff neck. Cerebrospinal fluid shows mononuclear cells, a low glucose, and an elevated protein, but acid-fast organisms are seen in only about 20 percent of cases. Diagnosis usually depends on evidence of tuberculous disease in other organ systems and the presence of a positive tuberculin skin test.

Patients with tuberculous genitourinary infection usually have asymptomatic pyuria for many years or may present with the acute onset of dysuria and hematuria. Parenchymal calcification of the kidney may be present but is overemphasized as a sign of renal tuberculosis. Cutures of urine are effective in confirming urinary tract infection, but slow growth of the organisms often makes initial empiric treatment necessary.

Female genital tract infections appear as low-grade chronic pelvic inflammatory disease.[72] The presentation of gastrointestinal tuberculosis is often confused with carcinoma of the colon or Crohn's disease. Patients have anorexia, weight loss, and signs of intermittent bowel obstruction. Radiographic gastrointestinal contrast studies may show either hypertrophy or ulceration, or both.[73] Tuberculous peritonitis is characterized by ascites and fever. Ascitic fluid shows mononuclear leukocytosis and elevated protein. Peritoneal biopsy is usually required for diagnosis, although a large volume of ascitic fluid may yield the organism on culture.[74] Skeletal tuberculosis usually involves chronic pain in the spinal area, although the disease can also involve the hips, pelvis, knees, or long bones. Diagnosis is best established by needle biopsy of bone or synovium.

The diagnosis of all forms of tuberculosis is heavily dependent on the establishment of a positive delayed hypersensitivity skin test. The test is normally applied with intermediate strength (5 tuberculin units) purified protein derivative (PPD), which is injected intradermally.

The presence of 5 mm or more of induration at 48 to 72 hours constitutes a positive result in persons with HIV infection, abnormal chest radiographs, and close contact of a tuberculosis patient. Induration of 10 mm or more is considered positive in intravenous drug users, nursing home residents, medically underserved and high-risk minorities, foreign-born persons from high-risk countries, and persons with other risk factors for active tuberculosis. For all other patients, induration of 15 mm or more is considered positive.[75] Negative skin test results have been found in up to 17 percent of patients with active tuberculosis.[76]

Treatment and Prognosis. The treatment of tuberculosis has been improved by effective chemotherapeutic drugs (Table 9–2 and Chap. 16). The organism has shown a propensity to develop resistance when single drugs are used for therapy. When a proper regimen of multiple chemotherapeutic drugs is prescribed and adhered to, however, an almost

TABLE 9–2. TREATMENT OF MYCOBACTERIAL DISEASE IN ADULTS

Drugs	Dosage[a] Daily	Dosage[a] Twice Weekly	Most Common Side Effects[b]	Tests for Side Effects[a]	Remarks[a]
First-line drugs					
Isoniazid	5–10 mg/kg up to 300 mg PO or IM	15 mg/kg PO or IM	Peripheral neuritis, hepatitis, hypersensitivity	SGOT/SGPT (not as a routine)	Bactericidal. Pyridoxine 10 mg as prophylaxis for neuritis; 50–100 mg as treatment
Pyrazinamide	15–30 mg/kg up to 2 g PO	50–70 mg/kg	Hyperuricemia, hepatotoxicity	Uric acid, SGOT/SGPT	Combination with an aminoglycoside is bactericidal
Ethambutol	15–25 mg/kg PO	50 mg/kg PO	Optic neuritis (reversible with discontinuation of drug; very rare at 15 mg/kg), skin rash	Red-green color discrimination and visual acuity[b]	Use with caution with renal disease or when eye testing is not feasible
Rifampin	10–20 mg/kg up to 600 mg PO	10 mg/kg maximum to 600 mg PO	Hepatitis, febrile reaction, purpura (rare)	SGOT/SGPT (not as a routine)	Bactericidal. Orange urine color. Negates effect of birth control pills
Streptomycin	15 mg/kg up to 1 g IM[c]	25–30 mg/kg	8th nerve damage, nephrotoxicity	Vestibular function, audiograms,[b] BUN and creatinine	Use with caution in older patients or those with renal disease
Second-line drugs					
Capreomycin	15–30 mg/kg up to 1 g IM		8th nerve damage, nephrotoxicity	Vestibular function, audiograms,[b] BUN and creatinine	Use with caution in older patients. Rarely used with renal disease
Kanamycin	15–30 mg/kg up to 1 g IM		Auditory toxicity, nephrotoxicity, vestibular toxicity (rare)	Vestibular function, audiograms,[b] BUN and creatinine	Use with caution in older patients. Rarely used with renal disease
Ethionamide	15–20 mg/kg up to 1 g PO		GI disturbance, hepatotoxicity, hypersensitivity	SGOT/SGPT	Divided dose may help GI side effects
Para-amino-salicylic acid	150 mg/kg up to 12 g PO		GI disturbance, hypersensitivity, hepatotoxicity, sodium load	SGOT/SGPT	GI side effects very frequent making cooperation difficult
Cycloserine	15–20 mg/kg up to 1 g PO		Psychosis, personality changes, convulsions, rash	Psychologic testing	Very difficult drug to use. Side effects may be blocked by pyridoxine, ataractic agents, or anticonvulsant drugs

[a] Check product labeling for detailed information on dose, contraindications, drug interaction, adverse reactions, and monitoring.
[b] Initial levels should be determined on start of treatment.
[c] Maximum dose 750 mg or 10 mg/kg in patients over age 60.
From Core Curriculum on Tuberculosis. U.S. Department of Health and Human Services, 1991.

uniformly successful result is achieved. Isoniazid (INH) coupled with rifampin has become the mainstay of antituberculous treatment, with pyrazinamide for the first 2 months.[75] Standard total treatment duration is now 9 months with the above regimen. Recommended treatment for extrapulmonary tuberculosis is the same as for pulmonary disease: 9 months of INH and rifampin with or without 2 months of ethambutol initially.[75] Resistance of *M. tuberculosis* to INH and rifampin has become frequent in certain urban centers such as New York and Miami, particularly in HIV-infected persons. In these areas it is recommended that four drugs (INH, rifampin, pyrazinamide, and ethambutol or streptomycin) be started initially and continued until susceptibilities are available. Duration of treatment is 9 months minimum.[75,77] The need for thoracic operations in the treatment of tuberculosis has decreased to almost negligible levels as the effectiveness of antimicrobial chemotherapy has increased. The present indications for surgical intervention in pulmonary and nonpulmonary tuberculosis have been summarized by Harrison.[78] Most operative intervention is performed for nonpulmonary tuberculosis, such as bowel obstruction or perforation in intestinal tuberculosis. In treatment of tuberculosis of the spine, operation may be required to decompress the spinal cord, for drainage of exceptionally large paravertebral abscesses, and occasionally to stabilize a badly destroyed weight-bearing joint. An operation to diagnose extrapulmonary tuberculosis is also frequently required, particularly for intestinal and skeletal disease. Pulmonary surgery for tuberculosis is usually indicated only for cavitary disease that has failed to respond to chemotherapy, uncontrolled hemoptysis, suspicion of neoplasm, or bronchopleural fistula.[77]

Mycobacteria Other than Tubercle Bacilli

Morphology and Identification. Nontuberculous mycobacteria, formerly called atypical mycobacteria, have been classified by Runyon into four distinct groups. The species most frequently pathogenic for humans are shown in Table 9–1 along with their disease name, the most frequent site of infection, their potential to be saprophytic in humans, and the need for surgical intervention. They can be differentiated in the laboratory by their pigmentation and growth characteristics. In addition to the species listed, a large number of mycobacterial species are probably strictly saprophytic, such as *M. gordonae* and *M. smegmatis*, which can be found in clinical specimens but are not known to be pathogenic for people except possibly in advanced HIV disease.[79] In addition, *M. simiae*, *M. szulgai*, and *M. xenopi* have also been found to be rare causes of pulmonary disease.

Epidemiology and Pathogenesis. In contrast to infection caused by members of the tuberculosis complex, people appear to become infected with these organisms either from their own saprophytic flora or from the widespread exposure to the organism in nature. Person-to-person spread has not been documented. *Mycobacterium marinum*, for example, has been found in a variety of water sources including seawater, aquariums, fish tanks, and swimming pools. Infection is probably acquired by abrasion of the skin and subsequent exposure to the organism, which causes disease in fish. *Mycobacterium avium-intracellulare* (MAI) has been found in soil as well as in cattle and swine; however, the exact mode of acquisition, particularly in the areas of high skin test reactivity in the southeastern coastal states, remains speculative. MAI has become a common opportunistic infection in the advanced stages of HIV infection. Similarly, *M. kansasii* has been isolated from water and raw milk, but specific vehicles of transmission in individual cases are usually obscure. *Mycobacterium scrofulaceum* and *M. gordonae* are commonly found in water, foods, and soil and are readily isolated from the respiratory secretions of normal people. *Mycobacterium fortuitum* has a widespread distribution similar to that of *M. scrofulaceum*. *Mycobacterium ulcerans*, the cause of Buruli ulcer, has been described only in Africa, Asia, Australia, and Mexico, where the organism is thought to be acquired from the soil. *Mycobacterium marinum* causes chronic granulomatous skin nodules and ulcers, which occur most frequently in the cooler extremities, and *M. scrofulaceum*, although occasionally a pulmonary pathogen, is usually the cause of cervical lymphadenitis in children. *Mycobacterium fortuitum* has been associated most often with cutaneous abscesses and wound infections, usually at the site of breaks in the skin, and *M. chelonae* has been associated with wound infections at the time of cardiovascular surgery, particularly sternal osteomyelitis, as well as contamination of porcine heart valves at the time of implantation. Abscesses at sites of injections have also been caused by *M. chelonae* in skin, and bone infections are also documented.[80,81]

Clinical Manifestations and Diagnosis. The clinical presentation of *M. kansasii* and MAI mimics that of pulmonary tuberculosis in non-HIV-infected patients. In HIV infection, MAI presents with diarrhea and fever with or without pulmonary lesions.[82]

Mycobacterium marinum causes chronic skin nodules and ulceration, which may be present for many years, and *M. ulcerans* produces extensive granulomatous ulceration of skin and underlying tissue. *Mycobacterium fortuitum* infections usually present as chronic nodules or draining ulcers at the site of previous trauma. *Mycobacterium scrofulaceum* shows remarkably little evidence of systemic infection and only a relatively asymptomatic cervical adenitis in children. Patients may develop disseminated MAI infection, which is particulary likely if advanced HIV infection is present. Infection involves lungs, gastrointestinal tract, blood and virtually any tissue in patients with AIDS and lung, lymph nodes, and bone marrow in patients without AIDS.[81]

Diagnosis of nontuberculous mycobacterial skin infection is best determined from biopsy samples from the margin of the lesion and from examination for acid-fast organisms and granulomas as well as culture for mycobacteria. The causative role of these organisms in pulmonary infection may be particularly difficult to demonstrate, because even the most pathogenic of the nontuberculous mycobacteria, *M. kansasii*, may be a saprophyte in the sputum. The presence of a nontuberculous mycobacteria in sputum must be correlated with the illness of the patient and with roentgenographic evidence for active pulmonary disease before a diagnosis can be made. Reactivity to the intermediate-strength 5 TU tuberculin skin test (PPD-S) is usually between 5 and 10 mm in diameter in patients with nontuberculous mycobacterial infection. Greater specificity of the skin test reaction may be achieved by using antigens specific for the mycobacterial species in question.

Treatment and Prognosis. The response to drug therapy of the nontuberculous mycobacteria is extremely variable. *Mycobacterium kansasii* is the most responsive; however, it is not as susceptible as *M. tuberculosis*. Multiple drug regimens that contain rifampin have been most successful in the treatment of *M. kansasii* pulmonary infections.[79] Triple drug therapy with rifampin and two other active agents is well tolerated and should be successful in more than 90 percent of cases. Duration of therapy is usually 18 months. Surgical intervention is only occasionally required as an adjunct to medical treatment. In contrast, MAI is often resistant to most antituberculous drugs. For life-threatening disseminated disease, newer agents such as ceprofloxacin, clofazimine, clarithromycin, or azithromycin should be included, but the prognosis is still poor.[82] Resection of residual diseased segments coupled with chemotherapy is usually recommended for progressive localized *M. avium-intracellulare* pulmonary infections in non-HIV-infected patients.[83] Infection caused by *M. scrofulaceum* and *M. fortuitum* usually requires resection because the organisms are highly resistant to antituberculous drugs. *Mycobacterium chelonei chelonei* is highly susceptible to clarithromycin, which is undergoing clinical trials.[81] The management of *M. marinum* is difficult to assess because the disease is frequently self-limited. A variety of chemotherapeutic, operative, and irradiation treatments have been applied; however, the results are difficult to evaluate. Successful regimens include traditional antituberculous drugs (rifampin and ethambutol) (see Table 9–2), trimethoprim-sulfamethoxazole, minocycline, and tetracycline (see Chap. 28).[79]

Mycobacterium leprae

Morphology and Identification. Mycobacterium leprae is the causative organism of leprosy (Hansen's disease). The organism is an obligate-intracellular, acid-fast bacillus, which is more readily decolored than tuberculosis organisms. Because of this the organism is not dependably stained by the Ziehl-Neelsen method. The Fite method or Fite-Faraco stain is recommended.[83] The organism has never been grown reliably on artificial media. Propagation of the organism in the footpads of mice has been achieved by the injection of infected human material and is a useful confirmatory diagnostic procedure.

Epidemiology and Pathogenesis. Leprosy is primarily a disease of tropical and subtropical areas. In the United States the majority of endemic cases are reported from Texas, California, Hawaii, and occasionally Louisiana. The average annual incidence in the United States is 0.67 cases per million population.[84] Most of the cases reported in the United States are acquired elsewhere, primarily in Mexico and the Philippines. Leprosy is probably spread directly from person to person, via either respiratory droplets or direct skin contact. Five classifications of the disease—tuberculoid, borderline-tuberculoid, borderline, borderline-lepromatous, and lepromatous—have been described. Histologically, patients with tuberculoid leprosy demonstrate typical granuloma formation. Those with borderline leprosy have both an epithelioid and histiocyte cellular response, while those with lepromatous leprosy have only a histiocytic response without demonstrable granulomas. Cellular invasion and destruction of nerves is commonly demonstrated in tuberculoid leprosy, while lepromatous leprosy demonstrates only the presence of organisms within the nerves. In the early stages of leprosy the disease may be indeterminate; that is, the type of reactivity is not yet apparent, and only a nonspecific perivascular mononuclear cell infiltrate may be present.[84]

Clinical Manifestations. The presence of skin lesions accompanied by sensory loss should arouse the suspicion of leprosy, particularly in patients from endemic areas. The organism has a propensity to involve the cooler areas of the body including the peripheral subcutaneous nerves, nasopharyngeal mucous membranes, testes, and the anterior third of the eye. The early sign of leprosy is a hypopigmented skin macule, which may or may not be associated with sensory loss. Patients with tuberculoid disease frequently have a large anesthetic single skin lesion that is raised and scaly and has a sharp, erythematous margin. In dimorphous or borderline leprosy, skin lesions are more widespread than in tuberculoid. In lepromatous leprosy, skin lesions are much smaller and more widely distributed, and diffuse nodular, macular, or plaque-like disease may be present.[84] Corneal nerves may be involved, as well as other structures of the anterior eye with potential loss of visual acuity, glaucoma, and blindness. In addition to the three basic types of leprosy, at least two types of reactive episodes have been described early in the course of treatment: the reversal reaction (fever, erythema, edema, neuritis) and erythema nodosum leprosum (red, hot, tender skin nodules).

Diagnosis. Material for diagnosis usually consists of skin scrapings or biopsies. Although nasal secretions are often positive for the organism, diagnosis of the disease depends on the demonstration of acid-fast organisms within the nerves on skin biopsies. The lepromin skin test is frequently used to differentiate the stage or type of leprosy; however, this test has not been useful in diagnosis. Patients with tuberculoid disease are normally reactive to lepromin, while those with lepromatous disease lack cutaneous reactivity.

Treatment and Prognosis. Because of the rapid emergence of resistance to dapsone, initial therapy with dapsone plus rifampin (tuberculoid) or with dapsone, rifampin, and clofazimine (lepromatous) is recommended. Plastic and reconstructive surgery is invaluable in the rehabilitation of patients with severe nerve involvement. Promising newer drugs include fluoroquinolones, minocycline, and macrolides.[85,86]

Nocardia asteroides

Morphology and Identification. Members of the genus *Nocardia* are of the family Nocardiaceae, which shares the order of Actinomycetales with both the Mycobacteriaceae and Actinomycetaceae. Nocardiae have previously been considered fungi; however, they are clearly bacteria. Although this discussion will focus on disease caused by *N. asteroides*, occasional infections caused by *N. caviae* and *N. brasiliensis* also occur in the United States. *Nocardia* organisms are aerobic, nonmotile, non-spore-forming, unencapsulated bacteria that are 0.5 to 1 μm in diameter and have a variable length. Classically, the organisms exhibit thin, filamentous morphology, frequently with branching. They are gram positive and are also acid fast.

Epidemiology and Pathogenesis. Nocardia organism are found in soil around the world. The primary route of organism acquisition is inhalation, and most patients develop pulmonary disease, but breaks in the skin may result in local inoculation of the organism. Widespread dissemination from the initial site of lung infection is common, particularly extension to the meninges and brain. Although healthy people can acquire nocardiosis, at least half the patients appear to have significant underlying predisposing disorders. The most frequent of these are corticosteroid therapy, chronic pulmonary disease or tuberculosis, leukemia, lymphoma, collagen-vascular disease, and renal and cardiac transplantation.[87–89] Localized pneumonitis frequently results in tissue necrosis with abscess formation. Direct extension from lung to chest wall is common, as is abscess formation at distant sites, particularly the brain.

Clinical Manifestations and Diagnosis. The classic presentation of pulmonary nocardiosis is a progressive necrotizing and cavity-forming infection. Patients usually have a subacute course characterized by fever and cough with purulent sputum. The appearance on chest roentgenogram is particularly variable, with manifestations that mimic tuberculosis, acute lobar consolidation, cavitary abscesses, pleural effusions, empyema, and hilar lymphadenopathy. In addition, solitary nodules may be present. Because of the nonspecificity of the presentation, diagnosis may be particularly difficult. If acid-fast smears and cultures of sputum are not productive, more invasive techniques should be pursued, particularly in immunosuppressed patients. Fiberoptic bronchoscopy with brushing and biopsy has been particularly useful, but percutaneous needle or open lung biopsy may be required.[88] Where subcutaneous nodules and abscesses are present, direct needle aspiration with microscopic examination and cultures should be performed. A brain abscess should be suspected in anyone with a *Nocardia* infection, and axial tomography or magnetic resonance imaging should be performed if symptoms suggest this possibility. A biopsy specimen from the brain will be needed if the diagnosis cannot be made from another site. Serologic tests have not been useful.

Treatment and Prognosis. The traditional treatment of nocardial infections has been sulfonamides, which should be administered in a dosage sufficient to result in peak serum concentrations of 12 to 15 mg/100 ml. Prolonged treatment is usually necessary, ranging from 6 to 12 months. More recently the combination trimethoprim-sulfamethoxazole has been successfully used.[89] Susceptibility testing suggests that minocycline, doxycycline, gentamicin, and amikacin may have activity, but only minocycline has been used sufficiently to evaluate clinical success.[90] Trimethoprim-sulfamethoxazole may be a particularly attractive choice for the treatment of brain abscess because both drugs penetrate well into cerebrospinal fluid. Although immunosuppressed patients can be successfully treated, even with adequate treatment, mortality was 25 to 45 percent.[91] However, a series of cardiac transplant recipients had no infectious mortality among 21 patients treated with sulfisoxazole for a mean of 13 months. Mortality has been higher in patients who have acute courses of infection, those treated with corticosteroids or other antineoplastic drugs, and those with widely disseminated disease.[91] Abscesses of the brain and other distant sites often must be drained surgically.

SPIROCHETES

Treponema pallidum

Morphology and Identification. Although this discussion will focus on *T. pallidum*, the causative organism of syphilis, two other *Treponema* organisms also cause disease in humans. They are *T. pertenue*, which is the cause of yaws, a communicable disease of skin and bones found in tropical regions, and *T. carateum*, which causes pinta, a communicable disease of the tropical Americas characterized by hypopigmented skin lesions. *Treponema pallidum* is a slender, tightly coiled helical organism 6 to 20 μm $\times$ 0.09 to 0.18 μm. The organism has not been successfully cultured in vitro, and identification depends on observation of typical motility on darkfield microscopy. The organism can be maintained in the laboratory by intratesticular injection in mature rabbits and can be stained by specific fluorescein-conjugated antisera as well as by silver impregnation methods on tissue specimens.

Epidemiology and Pathogenesis. Humans are believed to be the only natural host of *T. pallidum*, and infection is thought to occur only by direct contact with infected lesions, usually during sexual intercourse. Congenital syphilis is acquired by the fetus in utero. Most new syphilis cases occur in young persons in the sexually active age groups from 15 to 39. Reported cases of syphilis reached a low point in the United States in the late 1950s but since that time have been gradually increasing and have risen sharply since 1986 in concert with the rise in HIV infection in heterosexuals.[92] Organisms are thought to enter the body by direct inoculation through the skin or mucous membrane, from which lymphatic and hematogenous spread occurs. Infection is characterized by an endarteritis with vascular inflammatory cell-cuffing of a mononuclear cell type and, in some cases, development of frank granuloma formation, which may demonstrate necrosis.

Clinical Manifestations. Clinical disease is classically divided into three stages; primary, secondary, and tertiary syphilis. The chancre is the typical lesion of primary syphilis, which begins an average of 21 days after inoculation as a papule that eventually erodes and develops a smooth base with raised firm borders. Lesions are usually single, located on the skin or mucous membranes of the genital area, and painless. Primary lesions can occur at extragenital sites, usually the oral cavity, anus, breasts, and hands. Regional lymphadenopathy in the area of the chancre is common. The chancre usually heals within 3 to 6 weeks without treatment. A pelvic examination must be performed in females to locate the primary chancre, which is often asymptomatic.

Secondary syphilis occurs 6 weeks to 6 months following the primary chancre. Secondary syphilis is characterized by a variety of dermatologic manifestations, including macular, papular, and papulosquamous eruptions that are usually symmetric mucous membrane lesions, and by lymphadenopathy. The skin lesions on the plantar and volar aspects of the hands and feet are most characteristic. Condylomata lata are wartlike lesions of the anogenital area, which are highly infectious. Alopecia may occur, as well as localized infection of the eye, liver, or meninges.[92] The patient with secondary syphilis frequently exhibits nonspecific systemic symptoms such as malaise, headache, sore throat, arthralgias, and low-grade fever. Skin lesions heal without treatment in 4 to 12 weeks.

The patient then enters the latent phase of syphilis during which he or she remains infectious, probably for at least the first year. During the first 4 years of latency (early latency) the patient may have relapses with mucocutaneous lesions typical of secondary syphilis. In late latency the patient is considered noninfectious, except for the possibility of maternal-fetal transmission or blood transfusion.

Tertiary or late syphilis is the final stage of the disease and is considered noninfectious. Manifestations of tertiary syphilis are of three major types: (1) the gumma or granulomatous syphilitic lesion, which usually occurs in skin or bone; (2) cardiovascular syphilis, in which the basic lesion is aortitis; and (3) neurosyphilis, in which the manifestations may be either primarily meningovascular or general paresis. Patients with neurosyphilis can also have tabes dorsalis, in which degeneration of the posterior columns of the spinal cord occurs.

In addition, newborns with early congenital syphilis can have mucocutaneous lesions much like those of secondary syphilis, as well as nasal purulent discharge and bone lesions. Hepatosplenomegaly is common. Later manifestations of congenital syphilis include dental abnormalities (Hutchinson incisors) and skeletal abnormalities (saddle nose, saber shins, and perforated nasal septum).

Diagnosis. The diagnosis of syphilis can be established by positive dark-field microscopy of lesions of primary, secondary, or congenital syphilis. Although dark-field examination is the most certain way of diagnosis, it requires experience and skill in interpretation and is not generally available. Serologic tests therefore have become the most widespread method of syphilis diagnosis. The serologic tests are of two major types, the nontreponemal or reagin tests, such as the Venereal Disease Research Laboratory (VDRL) or rapid plasma reagin (RPR) tests, and the treponemal tests, of which the fluorescent treponemal antibody-absorption (FTA-ABS) test is the most frequently used. Although the nontreponemal tests are less specific than the treponemal tests, they continue to be used more frequently because of their low cost. They are also useful in following the course of the disease because the results become negative with treatment, whereas the FTA-ABS results do not. Because false-positive VDRL tests are common (leprosy, aging, collagen-vascular disease, and intravenous drug abuse), positive results should always be confirmed with the FTA-ABS. In general, false-positive reactions with the FTA-ABS are rare, but the test may be positive in nonsyphilitic treponemal diseases and in Lyme disease, leprosy, malaria, and infectious mononucleosis.[92]

Treatment and Prognosis. Recommended treatment regimens for the various stages of syphilis are available.[92] In general, early syphilis is treated with a long-acting penicillin, such as benzathine penicillin G, which is administered intramuscularly in a dosage of 2.4 million units. Alternate regimens include aqueous or procaine penicillin G, tetracycline (doxycycline) and erythromycin. For syphilis of more than one year's duration, benzathine penicillin G, 2.4 million units, is administered weekly for 3 weeks. The need for lumbar puncture to rule out central nervous system syphilis prior to treatment of asymptomatic late syphilis has been questioned.[93] Comparable cure rates are probably attainable by simply treating empirically with a total of 7.2 million units of benzathine penicillin G. Following treatment the patient should be followed every 3 months with quantitative VDRL to assure that treatment has been effective. Patients with early syphilis should be evaluated for 1 year, and those with late syphilis for 2 years. Follow-up of case contacts is the major mode of epidemiologic control of syphilis.

Borrelia burgdorferi

Morphology and Identification. Borrelia burgdorferi is a gram-negative, motile spirochete that causes Lyme disease in humans, an epidemic inflammatory disorder with a distinctive skin lesion, arthritis, and occasionally meningoencephalitis and myocarditis. The organism is 0.2×4 to 30 μm. Culture of the organism in vitro has been achieved on modified Kelly's medium, but culture yield of patient specimens of blood, skin, and spinal fluid has been very low. The organism can be cultivated in its arthropod vectors or in a variety of vertebrate host animals.

Epidemiology and Pathogenesis. In the United States, Lyme disease has been reported in 43 states, but the majority of cases are found in the Northeast coastal area, Minnesota and Wisconsin, and California and Oregon, following the same geographic distribution as the host vector ticks *Ixodes dammini* and *I. pacificus*. Disease has also been reported in western Europe where the tick *I. ricinus* is the vector. Erythema migrans (EM), the characteristic skin lesion of Lyme disease, was described in Sweden in 1909 but was not reported in the United States until 1970.

Clinical Manifestations and Diagnosis. The first sign of Lyme disease is usually the red macule or papule of EM, which expands centrifugally as an erythematous macule that may be slightly raised or flat.[95] Lesions may vary in size from 2 × 3 cm when seen early, to 20 × 40 cm for late lesions. About 75 percent of patients with Lyme disease have EM; 20 to 30 percent will have multiple lesions.[94] Only 34 percent of patients experienced symptoms (burning, itching) of their lesions. Fatigue, fever, malaise, headache, or arthralgias accompany the skin lesions in over 60 percent of patients. Later symptoms of Lyme disease include carditis, arthritis, and meningoencephalitis.[95] Diagnosis is most often based on the appearance of the skin lesion in a patient from an endemic area during the warmer months of the year. Serologic tests are the best way to confirm a clinical impression or resolve atypical cases or cases lacking a rash. Culture and direct tissue examination does not usually reveal the organism.

Treatment and Prognosis. Acute symptoms are best treated with oral doxycycline, in adults, 100 mg twice a day for 10 to 21 days. Oral amoxicillin, 500 mg three times a day, is also effective and is the preferred choice for children.[97] Erythromycin is also effective in cases of penicillin allergy, as is azithromycin and cefuroxime axetil. Late symptoms of arthritis, carditis, and meningitis also respond to treatment with high-dose intravenous penicillin or ceftriaxone for 14 to 21 days.[96] Acute symptoms respond well to antibiotic therapy, albeit with some residual flares of headache and joint symptoms. Resolution of neurologic symptoms requires 7 to 8 weeks, and some patients with arthritis do not respond to intravenous or oral regimens of treatment.

Other *Borrelia* Species

Morphology and Identification. Borrelia species cause relapsing fever. The causative organisms are gram negative and helical and measure 0.2 to 0.5 μm × 3 to 20 μm. They are considered microaerophilic or anaerobic and require complex special media for growth. *Borrelia recurrentis,* which is cosmopolitan in distribution, is spread by the human body louse. Three species in the United States are spread by ticks and are named after their respective tick vectors, *B. parkeri, B. turicatae,* and *B. hermsii.*

Epidemiology and Pathogenesis. Humans are infected by *Borrelia* through the bite of a tick or a louse. Lice acquire the organism by ingesting blood from an infected human and are carriers for life. Humans become infected when bitten by a louse that is subsequently crushed to release the organism into the abraded skin. A variety of mammalian animals, most often rodents, are probably the source of tick contamination with *Borrelia* organisms in the United States. Tick-borne relapsing fever is endemic to western and southwestern states.

Clinical Manifestations and Diagnosis. Tick-borne and louse-borne relapsing fevers have similar symptoms: the sudden onset of spiking fever up to 41C accompanied by headache, myalgias, and arthralgias. Gastrointestinal and upper respiratory symptoms may also be present. Splenomegaly and hepatomegaly are common. A macular truncal rash occurs in about one-fourth of the patients. Symptoms usually subside in 3 to 6 days but last as long as 17 days, followed by an afebrile interval that lasts an average of 6 to 10 days, at which time the patient once again experiences a febrile episode.[97] Antigenic variation of outer membrane proteins accounts for the organism's ability to repeatably relapse.[98] Wright- or Giemsa-stained blood smears are often positive on direct examination, but mouse inoculation may be necessary for diagnosis when numbers of organisms are low, as in relapses or afebrile intervals.

Treatment and Prognosis. Drugs currently recommended for the treatment of relapsing fever include tetracycline, erythromycin, and chloramphenicol. Single oral dose treatment regimens with tetracycline and erythromycin have been successful in the treatment of the *B. recurrentis* infection. Patients generally respond more slowly to penicillin G than to tetracycline or erythromycin. The Jarisch-Herxheimer reaction is frequent after the initial administration of an antibiotic, especially if the antibiotic is given during a febrile episode. This reaction is probably mediated by the release of leukocyte pyrogen. The reaction should be expected and can be fatal in louse-borne relapsing fever. Ninety-five percent or more of patients will recover with treatment.

Leptospira interrogans

Morphology and Identification. Only a single species of *Leptospira* pathogenic for humans, *L. interro-*

gans, is currently included in the genus *Leptospira* in *Bergey's Manual of Systematic Bacteriology*. The organisms are helical and tightly coiled, 6 to 20 μm × 0.1 μm, and have a characteristic hook at one or both ends. The organisms are faintly stained with most aniline dyes but can be seen by dark-field microscopy. Culture of the organisms requires special media containing 10 percent serum, such as Fletcher semisolid or Stuart liquid media.

Epidemiology and Pathogenesis. Leptospirosis is a disease of animals, and people acquire it by contact with animals or water contaminated by animal urine. Wild rodents, especially rats, and domestic animals (dog, cat, swine, cattle, horses) are usually responsible for infection in humans. Traditionally, the disease has occurred most often among those in occupations requiring high animal exposures (farmers, packing plant workers, and veterinarians). More recently, an increasing number of cases have been reported among campers, hikers, and swimmers, particularly those who swim in ponds and creeks potentially contaminated by animal urine. Approximately 100 cases per year are reported in the United States, mostly from the southern and southeastern states. In fatal cases, organisms are found in the kidney with destruction of tubular epithelium, and hepatocellular degeneration can also be found.

Clinical Manifestations and Diagnosis. Following an incubation period of 7 to 10 days, patients develop an acute febrile illness characterized by headache, severe myalgia, chills, and in some cases nausea, vomiting, and abdominal pain. Nuchal rigidity and meningismus occur frequently, and lumbar puncture reveals cerebrospinal fluid pleocytosis, as well as elevated protein. Severe cases with hepatic and renal dysfunction have been referred to as Weil's syndrome. The diagnosis of leptospirosis can be extremely difficult because of the nonspecificity of symptoms, particularly in mild cases. A history of exposure to animals should make the physician suspect the diagnosis. The presentation mimics influenza, viral meningitis, infectious hepatitis, mononucleosis, glomerulonephritis, and viral or mycoplasmal pneumonia.[99] Because of the difficulties in isolating the organism, all diagnostic tests are retrospective. The most frequently used serologic test is macroscopic agglutination, but indirect hemagglutination is also in use. Macroscopic agglutination titers should show either a fourfold rise or on single specimens a titer greater than 1:200. Of the serotypes currently reported in the United States, the most frequent are *icterohaemorrhagiae*, *canicola*, and *pomona*.

Treatment and Prognosis. In the past the benefits of antibiotic treatment for leptospirosis were debated. The disease is often not diagnosed until late in its course, when there appears to be little benefit from antimicrobial therapy. Two recent papers have documented the efficacy of doxycycline treatment both as a prophylactic agent at a dose of 200 mg once a week and as a therapeutic agent at a dose of 100 mg twice a day for 7 days when begun within the first three days of illness.[100] Intravenous treatment with penicillin G or ampicillin is also effective. In severe cases, with combined renal and hepatic failure, mortality may be as high as 10 to 40 percent.

RICKETTSIEAE

The genera of the tribe Rickettsieae that are pathogenic for humans are *Rickettsia* and *Coxiella*. A variety of worldwide illness is caused by these organisms, which are minute, 0.3 to 0.6 μm × 0.8 to 2 μm, gram-negative, coccobacillary, obligate intracellular parasites. Some characteristics of disease caused by these organisms are summarized in Table 9–3. All are transmitted by an arthropod vector, with the possible exception of Q fever, and all are associated with a nonhuman mammalian host for that vector. The organisms that are the most frequent causes of disease in the United States will be discussed. They are *R. rickettsii*, the cause of Rocky Mountain spotted fever; *R. typhi*, the cause of murine typhus; and *C. burnetti*, the cause of Q fever. *Ehrlichia canis*, the probable causative organism of human Ehrlichiosis, is increasingly reported in the southern United States and resembles Rocky Mountain spotted fever except for a lower frequency of rash.[101]

Rickettsia rickettsii

Morphology and Identification. Rickettsia rickettsii is the cause of Rocky Mountain spotted fever, probably the most important rickettsial illness in the United States. Because of the dangers and difficulties in identification of rickettsial organisms, isolation is not routinely performed in laboratories. Tissue diagnosis of rickettsial illness is usually made by demonstration of the organism in sections using immunofluorescent techniques or Giemsa or Gimenez stains.

Epidemiology and Pathogenesis. Rocky Mountain spotted fever is somewhat a misnomer in the United States, because the majority of cases occur in the Middle Atlantic states, Tennessee, Okla-

TABLE 9–3. CHARACTERISTICS OF HUMAN RICKETTSIAL DISEASES

Organism	Disease	Geographic Location	Arthropod Vector	Mammal Host	Weil-Felix Agglutination OX-19	OX-2	OX-K	Rash
Spotted fever group								
R. rickettsii	Rocky Mountain spotted fever	Western hemisphere	Tick	Rodents, dogs, foxes	+++[a]	+++[a]	0	+
R. sibirica	Tick typhus	Siberia, Mongolia	Tick	Rodents	+++[a]	+++[a]	0	+
R. australis	Tick typhus	Asia, Australia	Tick	Rodents, marsupials	+++[a]	+++[a]	0	+
R. akari	Rickettsialpox	North America, Russia, Africa, Korea	Mite	Mouse	0	0	0	+
Typhus fever group								
R. prowazekii	Epidemic typhus	Worldwide	Human body louse	Human	+++	+	0	+
R. prowazekii	Brill-Zinsser disease	North America, Europe	Reactivation of epidemic typhus years after first attack	Human	0 or +++	0	0	+
R. typhi	Murine typhus	Worldwide	Flea	Rodents	+++	0	0	+
Other Rickettsieae								
Coxiella burnetti	Q fever	Worldwide	Tick	Rodents, cattle, sheep, goats	0	0	0	0
Ehrlichia canis	Human Ehrlichiosis	Worldwide	Tick	Dogs	0	0	0	±

+++, Strong reaction (≥1:160 dilution).
[a] Either OX-19 or OX-2 agglutination can occur with Rocky Mountain spotted fever and tick typhus.

homa, Texas, and Arkansas. The usual mode of acquisition of the disease is by the bite of a tick. The common tick, *Dermacentor andersoni*, the dog tick, *D. variabilis*, and the Lone Star tick, *Amblyomma americanum*, are all capable of transmitting Rocky Mountain spotted fever and are distributed in virtually all parts of the United States.[101] The organism is passed transovarially within the ticks, and mammals serve only as supportive hosts for the tick population. The majority of disease occurs in children and young adults during the summer months when ticks are most active; however, in warm southern states the disease may also occur during the winter. Disease may also be acquired by skin abrasions, inhalation, and blood transfusion. The pathogenesis and pathology of all rickettsial diseases are similar because the organism proliferates in the endothelial cells that line the small blood vessels. This leads to perivascular infiltration and bleeding accompanied by thrombosis. Virtually any organ system can be affected, but the skin typically demonstrates a rash as a result of the vasculitic process.

Clinical Manifestations and Diagnosis. The initial presentation is nonspecific, consisting of fever, headache, myalgias, and often mental confusion, usually accompanied by a rash by the second or third day of the illness. The rash is typically maculopapular and petechial and begins on the extremities at the wrists and ankles and spreads proximally, typically involving both palms and soles. The symptoms are frequently confused with those of measles and meningococcal meningitis. Diagnosis may be delayed by the variability of symptoms, particularly a lack of rash. The disease should be suspected in anyone with a fever in endemic areas during spring and summer.[102,103] Diagnosis is usually made by serologic methods. Titers do not normally become positive for a week to 10 days, so diagnosis is frequently made on the basis of the clinical presentation. Biopsies of the skin lesions with staining by immunofluorescence technique may be positive as early as 4 to 5 days after the onset of the illness.[104]

Treatment and Prognosis. Although specific antimicrobial therapy is available for Rocky Mountain spotted fever, the difficulties and delays in making the diagnosis and initiating therapy are probably responsible for the relatively constant fatality rate, which remains at approximately 2 to 5 percent.

Both tetracycline and chloramphenicol have been effective and should be instituted promptly and at high dosages. Intravenous therapy is recommended in severe cases, but mild illness may be treated orally. The practice of taking prophylactic tetracycline before potential exposure does not seem to prevent Rocky Mountain spotted fever.

Rickettsia typhi

Morphology and Identification. Rickettsia typhi is the causative organism of murine or endemic typhus. The organism is similar to *R. prowazekii*, the causative organism of epidemic typhus (see Table 9–3).

Epidemiology and Pathogenesis. Murine typhus is an endemic disease of rodents and is transmitted to people by cat or rat flea bites.[104,105] Most cases in the United States are found in the South and Southwest, particularly South Texas. As with the other rickettsial diseases, the pathologic finding is a vasculitis; however, the extent and severity of the disease are generally milder than that of epidemic typhus.

Clinical Manifestations and Diagnosis. Patients typically develop a sudden onset of fever and headache. A pink macular rash appears in the truncal area between the fourth and eighth days of illness that, in contrast to Rocky Mountain spotted fever, spreads peripherally from the trunk. The rash usually remains maculopapular but in severe cases may become petechial. Muscular aches are common, and profound stupor and seizures can ensue.[105] Clinically the disease cannot be distinguished from epidemic typhus or Brill-Zinsser disease. The disease is usually diagnosed by Weil-Felix titer to *Proteus* OX 19 of 1:160 or greater or by indirect fluorescent antibody or complement-fixing antibody fourfold rises.[105]

Treatment and Prognosis. The best treatment is with either tetracycline or chloramphenicol, and in general the prognosis is excellent. Relapses, which can occur in patients treated early in the disease, respond to reinstitution of therapy. Mortality is 1 to 2 percent.

Coxiella burnetii

Morphology and Identification. Coxiella burnetii is the causative organism of Q fever. The organism differs somewhat from other rickettsiae in that it is resistant to physical and chemical agents and can survive in dust and excreta as well as water and milk. In addition, the Weil-Felix agglutinations fail to respond to infection with *C. burnetii.*

Epidemiology and Pathogenesis. Q fever is worldwide in distribution and is associated with cattle and sheep farms. Ticks are responsible for maintaining the disease in animals, but human infection is acquired primarily by inhalation of dust contaminated by infected animals, by drinking raw milk,[106,107] or by skin contact with infected animal products (eg, placenta). The disease probably spreads via the bloodstream, and pathologic findings are most frequent in the lung and liver. Peribronchial mononuclear infiltrates are seen in the lung with interstitial pneumonitis, and in the liver most of the infiltration is histiocytic with hepatic cell necrosis. In addition, frank granulomatous formation may be evident. Fibrin-ring granulomas are characteristic in bone marrow and liver.[107]

Clinical Manifestations. Q fever is an acute illness characterized by headache, chills, fever, myalgia, and malaise. Pneumonitis, hepatomegaly, and splenomegaly are present. In patients with atypical pneumonia or infectious hepatitis the diagnosis of Q fever should always be considered. In contrast to those with the other rickettsial illnesses, patients with Q fever do not have a rash. Severe cases may be complicated by endocarditis.

Diagnosis. Diagnosis is aided greatly by a history of contact with animals, particularly sheep, goats, or cattle; however, the disease may be difficult to differentiate from brucellosis or leptospirosis, which are also acquired from animals. Attempts to isolate the organism from blood or other tissues are usually not made because of the danger of laboratory infection. The most frequent mode of diagnosis is by complement-fixation or indirect fluorescence serologic titers to phase II antigen in acute disease. In patients with chronic infection such as endocarditis, complement-fixation titer to phase 1 antigen has been the most helpful diagnostic test.[107] Fourfold rises in serologic titers during convalescence are diagnostic.

Treatment and Prognosis. Most patients with acute Q fever have a self-limited illness, lasting 1 to 3 weeks, with a mortality under 1 percent. Both doxycycline and tetracycline are effective. Rifampin and fluroquinolones are alternative effective agents.[107,108]

Response to treatment is not as dramatic as with the other riskettsial diseases. Q fever endocarditis remains the most serious complication and requires long-term treatment for 1 to 3 years with tetracycline or doxycycline plus rifampin or a fluoroquinolone.[108] Even so, the prognosis is poor, and there is some question whether the disease can ever be cured. Prosthetic valve replacement is recommended for hemodynamic instability or uncontrollable or relapsing infection.

CHLAMYDIACEAE

Chlamydia psittaci

Morphology and Identification. Organisms of the genus *Chlamydia* are coccoid (0.2 to 1.5 μm diameter) gram-negative, obligate intracellular parasites. The chlamydial organisms have both DNA and RNA but are restricted to an intracellular existence because they are incapable of synthesizing ATP and must derive this energy source from their host cells. *Chlamydia psittaci* is the causative organism of human psittacosis and similar infections in nonpsittacine birds, in which it is called ornithosis. Isolation of the organism can be accomplished by use of embryonated eggs or cell culture lines; however, extreme caution should be exercised in performing these techniques because of danger of infection of laboratory personnel.

Epidemiology and Pathogenesis. Psittacosis is a disease acquired almost solely by contact with birds and bird products. The majority of cases in the United States occur in people with pet birds (parrots, parakeets, and cockatoos), pet shop workers, and poultry plant workers. Birds may transmit illness and still appear well. Human infection is acquired by inhalation of droplets or direct contact with infected bird tissues. The disease can also be spread from patient to patient during the acute illness. The organism spreads from the lung via the bloodstream to reticuloendothelial organs. Pathologic examination shows a lobar pneumonia, which is polymorphonuclear early in the disease but is later mononuclear. Cellular inclusions may be visible in large mononuclear cells and stain purple with Giemsa and red with Gimenez stain. Next to the lung, evidence of infection is seen most frequently in the liver and spleen.

Clinical Manifestations and Diagnosis. Patients develop chills, fever, malaise, and headaches usually 1 to 2 weeks after exposure. Cough is a prominent feature, but purulent sputum is not. Nausea, vomiting, mental confusion, and delirium may occur in severe cases. An interstitial pneumonitis is seen on x-rays of the chest.[109] Because of difficulties in isolating the psittacosis organism, diagnosis is normally made by complement-fixation serologic titers. Differential diagnosis is often difficult without evidence of exposure to birds and includes such diverse causes of pneumonia as Q fever, mycoplasmal pneumonia, influenza, blastomycosis, histoplasmosis, and *C. pneumoniae*.

Treatment and Prognosis. Tetracycline is the preferred drug for the treatment of psittacosis. Chloramphenicol and penicillin G have also been used, but they are not as effective as tetracycline. Treatment should be continued for 14 days. Mortality is 1 percent in treated patients.

Chlamydia trachomatis

Morphology and Identification. Isolation of *C. trachomatis* is usually accomplished in nonreplicating cell culture lines such as HeLa or McCoy cells, using antibiotics to inhibit other organisms. *Chlamydia trachomatis* cellular inclusions can be identified with the use of iodine stains, and this staining property distinguishes the organisms from *C. psittaci.*[110] Use of cell culture techniques has enhanced the ability of laboratories to isolate *C. trachomatis*, which is the causative organism of a number of clinical illnesses including trachoma, inclusion conjunctivitis, lymphogranuloma venereum, nongonococcal urethritis and other genital infections, and neonatal pneumonia. Development of a monoclonal antibody has greatly enhanced the laboratory diagnosis of *C. trachomatis* infections of mucosal surfaces through direct immunofluorescent examination.[111]

Epidemiology and Pathogenesis. The epidemiology of *C. trachomatis* infection varies with the type of infection. Specific serotypes have been implicated as the cause of lymphogranuloma venereum, while another group of serotypes is the cause of trachoma. Still a third group consisting of eight serotypes is associated with nongonococcal urethritis, cervicitis, salpingitis, proctitis, conjunctivitis, and neonatal pneumonia.[110]

TRACHOMA. Trachoma is thought to spread from person to person by direct contact with secretions from the eyes. It is a disease that is endemic in families in certain underdeveloped areas of Africa, Asia, and Latin America. In the United States the disease is most common in the Southwest. Trachoma begins as a hyperemic infiltrative lesion of the conjunctiva under the lids, usually in children under 10 years of age. Part of the pathologic development in trachoma may be related to secondary bacterial infections, which occur frequently. The classic cobblestone appearance of the palpebral conjunctiva is evident in well-established disease.

LYMPHOGRANULOMA VENEREUM. Lymphogranuloma venereum is transmitted by sexual contact and is most frequent in tropical areas of Africa and Asia. There are usually fewer than 1000 cases reported annually in the United States, most of which are acquired outside the country; however, the disease is endemic in the southeastern United States. Lymphogranuloma venereum usually begins with a nonspecific granulomatous genital vesicle or ulcer, from which the organisms spread to regional groin lymph nodes. Central radiating areas of necrosis are common in lymph nodes, which are usually filled with epithelioid cells and giant cells. Frank purulent drainage may occur in severe cases. Lymphatic obstruction may result in genital edema. Involvement of the rectum and perirectal tissues can lead to the formation of hemorrhagic mucosal lesions and eventually fibrotic stricture, mucosal ulceration, and fistula formation.

OTHER SEXUALLY TRANSMITTED INFECTIONS. Nongonococcal urethritis (the most common sexually transmitted disease in the United States) is also contracted by sexual contact, as are cervicitis, endometritis, salpingitis, proctitis, epididymitis and neonatal conjunctivitis, and pneumonia (acquired by direct contact at the time of birth).[112–115]

Clinical Manifestations and Diagnosis. Diagnosis of trachoma is usually established by typical clinical signs but should be confirmed with Giemsa, iodine, or immunofluorescent stains of conjunctival scrapings or by culture of the responsible agent.

Lymphogranuloma venereum is also diagnosed by the clinical appearance of inguinal adenopathy and isolation of *C. trachomatis* from lymph node aspirates. Direct Giemsa or iodine stain smears may be helpful where cultures are not available. The complement-fixation serologic test is the most widely used diagnostic test; however, it does cross-react with other *Chlamydia*. Single titers of 1:16 or greater are usually considered significant.

Complement-fixation titers are also elevated in *C. trachomatis* genital infections, conjunctivitis, and neonatal pneumonia. The only completely reliable diagnostic method is isolation of the organism in cell culture or embryonated eggs or direct visualization of elementary bodies by monoclonal antibody stains. Organisms that grow on cell culture are presumptively identified to be *C. trachomatis* by demonstrating iodine-stained cytoplasmic inclusions. In urethritis a serous discharge that contains few polymorphonuclear leukocytes favors a nongonococcal rather than a gonococcal cause.

Treatment and Prognosis. The treatment for trachoma has been difficult, largely because of the problem of regular administration of antibiotics to patients in underdeveloped countries. Tetracycline, erythromycin, rifampin, and sulfonamides are all effective against *C. trachomatis*, which differs from *C. psittaci* in its susceptibility to sulfonamides. Improvement in hygienic conditions is probably as important as the antimicrobial therapy in the control of trachoma. For lymphogranuloma venereum, treatment with either tetracycline or sulfonamides for 2 to 4 weeks has been recommended; however, the long-term complications of rectal stricture may not be prevented by these measures. Fluctuant lymph nodes should be drained by needle aspiration. For the treatment of chlamydial urethritis, tetracycline, doxycycline, or minocycline is recommended with a minimum course of 7 days. Some authors have recommended treatment with tetracycline or doxycycline for a minimum of 10 days for salpingitis and epididymitis. Erythromycin is also effective. The sexual partners of males with urethritis should also receive treatment.

Chlamydia pneumoniae

Morphology and Identification. Chlamydia pneumoniae is a third distinct strain of *Chlamydia* that is pathogenic for humans and can be distinguished clearly by serologic testing, DNA analysis, and appearance in cell culture (iodine stain negative).[116] Isolation of the organism, which was initially designated TWAR, is difficult and requires HeLa cell culture of embryonated chicken egg yolk sacs. Inclusion bodies in cell culture are identified by use of a fluorescenated monoclonal antibody.[116]

Epidemiology and Pathogenesis. Chlamydia pneumoniae is probably worldwide in distribution, producing respiratory illness in college students (pharyngitis, pneumonia, bronchitis), pneumonia in the community in Pittsburgh and Halifax,[116] outbreaks of epidemic pneumonia in military recruits in Finland,[117] and community- and hospital-acquired pneumonia in Seattle.[118] Serologic sampling of adult populations from Taiwan, Japan, Panama, Denmark, and the above-mentioned countries shows that 18 to 59 percent have IgG antibodies to TWAR.[117] Because of the association of pneumonia in groups with close contact (eg, college students and military recruits), spread is thought to occur from person to person via aerosol or droplets. The pneumonia may be diffuse or localized and is often mild in young patients. The mode of spread among hospital patients has not been determined.

Clinical Manifestations and Diagnosis. Patient manifestations range from asymptomatic to life-threatening pneumonia. Pharyngitis may present as an initial symptom followed in days to weeks by cough, bronchitis, and pneumonia, giving an appearance of biphasic illness. Onset of illness is subtle with rare fever, dry cough, and scanty or absent sputum. Sinusitis occurs in 5 to 10 percent of patients. Rales are heard on auscultation and chest x-ray most often shows single subsegmental infiltrates. Hospital-acquired infection is most frequent in intubated patients, often after injury, and is indistinguishable from other nosocomial pneumonias. Acute wheezing and asthma in adults have been associated with *C. pneumoniae* infection.[119] Diagnosis is based on isolation of *C. pneumoniae* in HeLa cell cultures or embryonated eggs, or a fourfold titer rise to greater than 1:16 by microimmunofluorescence serologic testing.[116]

Treatment and Prognosis. Chlamydia pneumoniae is susceptible to tetracycline (doxycycline) and erythromycin as well as the newer macrolides (azithromycin, clarithromycin).[120] No controlled clinical treatment data are available, but tetracycline or erythromycin at 2 g/d for 14 days has been recommended with tetracycline the preferred choice.[116] In young patients mortality is extremely low, but older patients and those with hospital-acquired infections have a mortality of up to 20 percent.[118]

MYCOPLASMATACEAE

Mycoplasma pneumoniae

Morphology and Identification. Although other *Mycoplasma* species have been implicated as potential causes of disease in the genitourinary tract, *M. pneumoniae* is primarily a respiratory tract pathogen. The mycoplasmas are the smallest organisms capable of independent existence and are about 0.3 to 0.8 μm in size. *M. pneumoniae* is filamentous. All *Mycoplasma* species lack a true cell wall and are enclosed only by a single triple-layered membrane. Special culture media are required for the isolation of *Mycoplasma* because cholesterol or other sterols are required. Serum and yeast extract is usually included in the medium. *Mycoplasma pneumoniae* grows aerobically but requires 2 to 3 weeks for isolation.

Epidemiology and Pathogenesis. Mycoplasma pneumoniae infections occur throughout the world's temperate zones. Most cases occur in people between the ages of 5 and 25 years and are unusual in preschool children and the elderly. High rates of mycoplasmal infection have typically been described in college students and military recruits, and case clustering occurs in families.[121] Inhalation of droplets from infected patients is the method of spread. An interstitial pneumonia with acute bronchiolitis accompanied by mononuclear cell infiltrates results.

Clinical Manifestations and Diagnosis. Patients usually have an insidious onset of upper respiratory symptoms (pharyngitis) accompanied by fever and cough. Occasionally there are chills. Fever persists for 8 to 10 days, and typically the cough remains dry and nonproductive. Headache and nausea and vomiting occur in 30 to 40 percent, but myalgias and arthralgias occur in only about 20 percent of patients. On physical examination, rales are heard in about three-fourths of the patients. About 20 percent have a rash. Bullous or hemorrhagic myringitis occurs in about 10 percent. Other manifestations of mycoplasmal infection include cold-agglutinin hemolytic anemia, gastroenteritis, hepatitis, pericarditis, myocarditis, and erythema multiforme.[122,123] Meningitis and meningoencephalitis are rarely described. The major differential diagnosis of *M. pneumoniae* is pneumonia caused by psittacosis, *C. pneumoniae*, Q fever, various viruses, and legionnaires' bacillus. Because of the difficulty and time required to culture the organism, presumptive diagnoses are frequently made on the basis of a positive cold-agglutinin titer of 1:32 or greater. More unusual manifestations of pulmonary mycoplasma infection include lung abscess and pleural effusion.

Treatment and Prognosis. Mycoplasma organisms are sensitive to erythromycin and the tetracyclines but are resistant to penicillin, cephalosporins, and chloramphenicol.[124] Clinical studies have shown that pneumonia resolves more rapidly in patients treated with either erythromycin or tetracyclines. Persistence of *Mycoplasma* organisms in the sputum of patients during antibiotic therapy has been described; in spite of this the patients appear to respond to treatment. The spectrum of mycoplasmal infection varies from asymptomatic infection to fatal pneumonia; however, most patients gradually recover after 7 to 10 days of illness whether antibiotic treatment is used or not.

REFERENCES

Gram-Positive Bacteria

Bacillus anthracis

1. Sirisanthana T, Navachareon N, Tharavichitkul P, et al: Outbreak of oral-oropharyngeal anthrax: an unusual manifestation of human infection with *Bacillus anthracis*. Am J Trop Med Hyg 33:144, 1984.

Bacillus *Species*

2. Farrar EW: Serious infections due to "non-pathogenic" organisms of the genus *Bacillus*. Am J Med 34:134, 1963.
3. Bekemeyer WB, Zimmerman GA: Life-threatening complications associated with *Bacillus cereus* pneumonia. Am Rev Respir Dis 131:466, 1985.
4. Tuazon CU, Murray HW, Levy C, et al: Serious infections from *Bacillus sp.* JAMA 241:1137, 1979.
5. Holmes JR, Plunkett T, Pate P, et al: Emetic food poisoning caused by *Bacillus cereus*. Arch Intern Med 141:766, 1981.
6. Wang MT, Dolan MJ: Significant infections due to *Bacillus* species following abrasions associated with motor-vehicle-related trauma. Clin Infect Dis 15: 855, 1992.

Genus *Corynebacterium*

7. Collier RJ: Diphtheria toxin: Mode of action and structure. Bacteriol Rev 39:54, 1975.
8. Groman NB: Conversion by corynephages and its role in the natural history of diphtheria. J Hyg Camb 93:405, 1984.
9. Bessman AS, Geiger PJ, Conawati H: Prevalence of corynebacteria in diabetic foot infections. Diabetes Care 15:1531, 1992.
10. Van Etta LL, Filice GA, Ferguson RM, Gerding DN: *Corynebacterium equi:* a review of 12 cases of human infection. Rev Infect Dis 5:1012, 1983.
11. Lipsky BA, Goldberger AC, Tompkins LS, Plorde JJ: Infections caused by nondiphtheria corynebacteria. Rev Infect Dis 4:1220, 1982.

Listeria

12. Greene KA, Clark RJ, Zabramski JM: Ventricular CSF shunt infections associated with *Corynebacterium jeikeium:* report of three cases and review. Clin Infect Dis 16:139, 1993.
13. Farber JM, Peterkin PI: *Listeria monocytogenes*, a food-borne pathogen. Microbiol Rev 55:476, 1991.
14. Ascher NL, Simmons RL, Marker S, Najarian JS: Listeria infection in transplant patients. Five cases and a review of the literature. Arch Surg 113:90, 1978.
15. Watson GW, Fuller TJ, Elms J, Kluge RM: *Listeria cerebritis:* relapse of infection in renal transplant patients. Arch Intern Med 138:83, 1978.

Erysipelothrix

16. Reboli AC, Farrar WE: *Erysipelothrix rhusiopathiae* an occupational pathogen. Clin Microbiol Rev 2:354, 1989.

Francisella tularensis

17. Guerrant RL, Humphries MK Jr, Butler JE, Jackson RS: Tickborne oculoglandular tularemia. Case report and review of seasonal and vectoral associations in 106 cases. Arch Intern Med 136:811, 1976.
18. Evans ME, Gregory DW, Schaffner W, McGee ZA: Tularemia: a 30-year experience with 88 cases. Medicine (Baltimore) 64:251, 1985.

Pasteurella multocida

19. Carter GR: Pasteurellosis. *Pasteurella multocida* and *Pasteurella haemolytica*. Adv Vet Sci 11:321, 1969.
20. Francis DP, Holmes MA, Brandon G: *Pasteurella multocida*. Infections after domestic animal bites and scratches. JAMA 233:42, 1975.
21. Webber DJ, Wolfson JS, Swartz MN, Hooper DC: *Pasteurella multocida* infections. Report of 34 cases and review of the literature. Medicine (Baltimore) 63:133, 1984.

Streptobacillus moniliformis *and* Spirillum minor

22. Shanson DC, Gazzard BG, Midgley J, et al: *Streptobacillus moniliformis* isolated from blood in four cases of Haverhill fever. Lancet 2:92, 1983.
23. Anderson LC, Leary SL, Manning PJ: Rat-bite fever in animal research laborator- personnel. Lab Anim Sci 33:292, 1983.

Eikenella corrodens

24. Dorff GJ, Jackson LJ, Rytel MW: Infections with *Eikenella corrodens*. A newly recognized human pathogen. Ann Intern Med 80:305, 1974.
25. Suwanagool S, Rothkopf MM, Smith SM, et al: Pathogenicity of *Eikenella corrodens* in humans. Arch Intern Med 143:2265, 1983.
26. Goldstein EJ, Citron DM: Susceptibility of *Eikenella*

corrodens to penicillin, apalcillin, and twelve new cephalosporins. Antimicrob Agents Chemother 26:947, 1984.

Bordetella pertussis

27. Nelson JD: The changing epidemiology of pertussis in young infants. The role of adults as reservoirs of infection. Am J Dis Child 132:371, 1978.
28. Olson LC: Pertussis. Medicine (Baltimore) 54:427, 1975.
29. Bass JW, Klenk EL, Kotheimer JB, et al: Antimicrobial treatment of pertussis. J Pediatr 75:768, 1969.

Haemophilus influenzae

30. Todd JK, Bruhn FW: Severe *Haemophilus influenzae* infections. Am J Dis Child 129:607, 1975.
31. Ward JI, Tsai TJ, Filice GA, Fraser DW: Prevalence of ampicillin- and chloramphenicol-resistant strains of *Haemophilus influenzae* causing meningitis and bacteremia: national survey of hospital laboratories (NY). J Infect Dis 138:421, 1978.
32. Overturf GD, Cable DC, Forthal DN, Shikuma C: Treatment of bacterial meningitis with ceftizoxime. Antimicrob Agents Chemother 25:258, 1984.
33. Congeni BL: Comparison of ceftriaxone and traditional therapy of bacterial meningitis. Antimicrob Agents Chemother 25:40, 1984.
34. Swedish Study Group: Cefuroxime versus ampicillin and chloramphenicol for the treatment of bacterial meningitis. Lancet 1:295, 1982.
35. Lecour H, Seara A, Miranda AM, et al: Treatment of 160 cases of acute bacterial meningitis with cefotaxime. J Antimicrob Chemother 14 (Suppl B):195, 1984.

Haemophilus ducreyi

36. Ronald AR, Plummer FA: Chancroid and *Haemophilus ducreyi*. Ann Intern Med 102:705, 1985.
37. Blackmore CA, Limpakarnjanarat K, Rigau-Perez JG, et al: An outbreak of chancroid in Orange County, California: descriptive epidemiology and disease-control measures. J Infect Dis 151:840, 1985.
38. Plummer FA, Nsanze H, D'Costa LJ, et al: Single-dose therapy of chancroid with trimethoprim-sulfamethoxazole. N Engl J Med 309:67, 1983.

Haemophilus *Species*

39. Bieger RC, Brewer NS, Washington JA II: *Haemophilus aphrophilus:* a new microbiologic and clinical review and report of 24 cases. Medicine (Baltimore) 57:345, 1978.
40. Albritton WL: Infections due to *Haemophilus* species other than *H. influenzae.* Annu Rev Microbiol 36:199, 1982.

Calymmatobacterium granulomatis

41. Lal S, Nicholas C: Epidemiological and clinical features in 165 cases of granuloma inguinale. Br J Vener Dis 46:461, 1970.
42. Stewart DB: The gynecological lesions of lymphogranuloma venereum and granuloma inguinale. Med Clin North Am 48:773, 1964.

Brucella *Species*

43. Polt SS, Dismukes WE, Flint A, Schaefer J: Human brucellosis caused by *Brucella canis:* clinical features and immune response. Ann Intern Med 97:717, 1982.
44. Elberg SS: Immunity to brucella infection. Medicine (Baltimore) 52:339, 1973.
45. Hall WH: Modern chemotherapy of brucellosis in humans. Rev Infect Dis 12:1060, 1990.

Vibrio Cholerae *and Non-O1* V. Cholerae

46. Morris JG Jr, Black RE: Cholera and other vibrioses in the United States. N Engl J Med 312:343, 1985.
47. Swerdlow DL, Ries AA: Cholera in the Americas. JAMA 267:1495, 1992.
48. Carpenter CCJ: The treatment of cholera: clinical science at the bedside. J Infect Dis 166:2, 1992.

Halophilic Vibrios

49. Koenig KL, Meuller J, Rose T: *Vibrio vulnificus:* hazard on the half shell. West J Med 155:400, 1991.
50. Johnston JM, Becker SF, McFarland LM: *Vibrio vulnificus,* man and the sea. JAMA 253:2850, 1985.

Campylobacter *Species*

51. Blaser MJ, Wells JG, Feldman RA, et al: *Campylobacter* enteritis in the United States. Ann Intern Med 98:360, 1983.
52. Blaser MJ, Reller LB: *Campylobacter* enteritis. N Engl J Med 305:1444, 1981.

Acinetobacter calcoaceticus

53. Glew RH, Moellering RC Jr, Kunz LJ: Infections with *Acinetobacter calcoaceticus* (*Herellea vaginicola*): clinical and laboratory studies. Medicine (Baltimore) 56:79, 1977.
54. Buxton AE, Anderson RL, Werdegar D, Atlas E: Nosocomial respiratory tract infection and colonization with *Acinetobacter calcoaceticus.* Epidemiologic characteristics. Am J Med 65:507, 1978.

Aeromonas *Species*

55. Reines HD, Cook FV: Pneumonia and bacteremia due to *Aeromonas hydrophila.* Chest 80:264, 1981.
56. Janda JM: Recent advances in the study of the taxonomy, pathogenicity, and infectious syndromes associated with the genus *Aeromonas.* Clin Microbiol Rev 4:397, 1991.
57. Gold WL, Salit IE: *Aeromonas hydrophila* infections of skin and soft tissue: report of 11 cases and review. Clin Infect Dis 16:69, 1993.
58. Davis WA II, Kane JG, Garagusi VF: Human *Aeromonas* infections. Medicine (Baltimore) 57:267, 1978.

Moraxella catarrhalis

59. Slevin NJ, Aitken J, Thornley PE: Clinical and microbiological features of *Branhamella catarrhalis* bronchopulmonary infections. Lancet 1:782, 1984.
60. Alvarez S, Jones M, Holtsclaw-Berk S, et al: *In vitro* susceptibilities and beta-lactamase production of 53 clinical isolates of *Branhamella catarrhalis*. Antimicrob Agents Chemother 27:646, 1985.
61. Verghese A, Berk SL: *Moraxella (Branhamella) catarrhalis.* Infect Dis Clin North Am 5:523, 1991.

Capnocytophaga *Species*

62. Parenti DM, Snydman DR: *Capnocytophaga* species: infections in nonimmunocompromised and immunocompromised hosts. J Infect Dis 151:140, 1985.
63. Forlenza SW, Newman MG, Lipsey AI, et al: *Capnocytophaga* sepsis: a newly recognised clinical entity in granulocytopenic patients. Lancet 1:567, 1980.

Legionella pneumophila

64. Fraser DW, Tsai TR, Orenstein W, et al: Legionnaires' disease: description of an epidemic of pneumonia. N Engl J Med 297:1189, 1977.
65. Shands KN, Ho JL, Meyer RD, et al: Potable water as a source of legionnaires' disease. JAMA 253:1412, 1985.
66. Stout JE, Yu VL, Maraca P, et al: Potable water as a cause of sporadic cases of community acquired legionnaires' disease. N Engl J Med 326:151, 1992.
67. Edelstein PH, Meyer RD: Susceptibility of *Legionella pneumophila* to twenty antimicrobial agents. Antimicrob Agents Chemother 18:403, 1980.
68. Meyer RD: *Legionella* infections: a review of five years of research. Rev Infect Dis 5:258, 1983.

Other Legionella *Species*

69. Farg GD, Yu VL, Vickers RM: Disease due to the Legionellaceae (other than *Legionella pneumophila*). Medicine (Baltimore) 68:116, 1989.
70. Pasculle AW, Dowling JN, Weyant RS, et al: Susceptibility of Pittsburgh pneumonia agent (*Legionella micdadei*) and other newly recognized members of the genus *Legionella* to nineteen antimicrobial agents. Antimicrob Agents Chemother 20:793, 1981.

Acid-Fast Bacteria

Mycobacterium tuberculosis *and* M. bovis

71. Glassroth J, Robins AG, Snider DE Jr: Tuberculosis in the 1980s. N Engl J Med 302:1441, 1980.
72. Ogawa SK, Smith MA, Brennessel DJ, Lowy FD: Tuberculous meningitis in an urban medical center. Medicine (Baltimore) 66:317, 1987.
73. Tabrisky J, Lindstrom RR, Peters R, Lachman RS: Tuberculous enteritis. Review of a protean disease. Am J Gastroenterol 63:49, 1975.
74. Dineen P, Homa WP, Grafe WR: Tuberculous peritonitis: 43 years experience in diagnosis and treatment. Ann Surg 184:717, 1976.
75. Centers for Disease Control, U.S. Public Health Service, Department of Health and Human Services: Core Curriculum on Tuberculosis, 2nd ed. Atlanta, GA, CDC, 1991.
76. Holden M, Dubin MR, Diamond PH: Frequency of negative intermediate-strength tuberculin sensitivity in patients with active tuberculosis. N Engl J Med 285:1506, 1971.
77. Barnes PF, Bloch A, Davidson PT, Snider DE Jr: Tuberculosis in patients with human immunodeficiency virus infection. N Engl J Med 324:1644, 1991.
78. Harrison LH Jr: Current aspects of the surgical management of tuberculosis. Surg Clin North Am 60:883, 1980.

Mycobacteria Other than Tubercle Bacilli

79. Wolinsky E: Nontuberculous mycobacteria and associated diseases. Am Rev Respir Dis 119:107, 1979.
80. Gremillion DH, Mursch SB, Lerner CJ: Injection site abscesses caused by *Mycobacterium chelonei.* Infect Control 4:25, 1983.
80. Greene JB, Sidhu GS, Lewin S, et al: *Mycobacterium avium-intracellulare:* a cause of disseminated life-threatening infection in homosexuals and drug abusers. Ann Intern Med 97:539, 1982.
81. Wallace RJ, Brown BA, Onyi GO: Skin, soft tissue and bone infections due to *Mycobacterium chelonei:* importance of prior corticosteroid therapy frequency of disseminated infections and resistance to oral antibiotics other than clarithromycin. J Infect Dis 166:485, 1992.
82. Benson CA, Ellner JJ: *Mycobacterium avium* complex infection and AIDS: advances in theory and practice. Clin Infect Dis 17:7, 1993.
83. Iseman MD, Corpe RF, O'Brien RJ, et al: National Consensus Conference on Tuberculosis: disease due to *Mycobacterium avium-intracellular.* Chest 87: S139, 1985.

Mycobacterium leprae

84. Meyers WM, Marty AM: Current concepts in the pathogenesis of leprosy. Drugs 41:832, 1991.
85. Ji B, Grosset JH: Recent advances in the chemotherapy of leprosy. Lepr Rev 61:313, 1990.
86. Gelber RH: Progress in the chemotherapy of leprosy: status, issues, and prospects. Progr Drug Res 34:421, 1990.

Nocardia asteroides

87. Frazier AR, Rosenow EC III, Roberts GD: Nocardiosis. A review of 25 cases occurring during 24 months. Mayo Clin Proc 50:657, 1975.
88. Simpson GL, Stinson EB, Egger MJ, Remington JS: Nocardial infections in the immunocompromised host: a detailed study in a defined population. Rev Infect Dis 3:492, 1981.
89. Wilson JP, Turner HR, Kirchner KA, Chapman SE:

Nocardial infections in renal transplant recipients. Medicine (Baltimore) 68:38, 1989.
90. Petersen EA, Nash ML, Mammana RB, Copeland JG: Minocycline treatment of pulmonary nocardiosis. JAMA 250:930, 1983.
91. Presant CA, Wiernick PH, Serpick AA: Factors affecting survival in nocardiosis. Am Rev Respir Dis 108:1444, 1973.

Spirochetes

Treponema pallidum

92. Hook EW III, Marra CM: Acquired syphilis in adults. N Engl J Med 326:1060, 1992.
93. Wiesel J, Rose DN, Silver AL, et al: Lumbar puncture in asymptomatic late syphilis. An analysis of the benefits and risks. Arch Intern Med 145:465, 1985.

Borrelia burgdorferi

94. Malone MS, Grant-Kels JM, Feder HM Jr, Luger SW: Diagnosis of Lyme disease based on dermatologic manifestations. Ann Intern Med 114:490, 1991.
95. Steere AC, Malawista SE, Bartenhagen NH, et al: The clinical spectrum and treatment of Lyme disease. Yale J Biol Med 57:453, 1984.
96. Rahn DW, Malawista SE: Lyme disease: recommendations for diagnosis and treatment. Ann Intern Med 114:472, 1991.

Other Borrelia *Species*

97. Southern PM Jr, Sanford JP: Relapsing fever. A clinical and microbiological review. Medicine (Baltimore) 48:129, 1969.
98. Barbour AG: Antigenic variation of a relapsing fever. *Borrelia* species. Annu Rev Microbiol 44:155, 1990.

Leptospira interrogans

99. Thorsteinsson SB, Sharp P, Musher DM, Martin RR: Leptospirosis: an underdiagnosed cause of febrile illness. South Med J 68:217, 1975.
100. Takafuji ET, Kirkpatrick JW, Miller RN, et al: An efficacy trial of doxycycline chemoprophylaxis against leptospirosis. N Engl J Med 310:497, 1984.

Rickettsieae

Rickettsia rickettsii

101. Walker DH, Fishbein DB: Epidemiology of rickettsial disease. Eur J Epidemiol 7:237, 1991.
102. Kirk JL, Fine DP, Sexton DJ, Muchmore HG: Rocky Mountain spotted fever. Medicine (Baltimore) 69:35, 1990.
103. Helmick CG, Bernard KW, D'Angelo LJ: Rocky Mountain spotted fever: clinical, laboratory, and epidemiological features of 262 cases. J Infect Dis 150:480, 1984.
104. Woodward TE, Pedersen CE Jr, Oster CN, et al: Prompt confirmation of Rocky Mountain spotted fever: identification of rickettsiae in skin tissues. J Infect Dis 134:297, 1976.

Rickettsia typhi

105. Dumler JS, Taylor JP, Walker DH: Clinical and laboratory features of murine typhus in South Texas, 1980 through 1987. JAMA 266:1365, 1991.
106. Dupont HT, Raoult D, Brouqui P, et al: Epidemiologic features and clinical presentation of acute Q fever in hospitalized patients: 323 French cases. Am J Med 93:427, 1992.

Coxiella burnetti

107. Sawyer LA, Fishbein BD, McDade JE: Q fever: current concepts. Rev Infect Dis 9:935, 1987.
108. Raoult D: Antibiotic treatment of rickettsiae, recent advances and current concepts. Eur J Epidemiol 7:276, 1991.

Chlamydiaceae

Chlamydia psittaci

109. Yung AP, Grayson ML: Psittacosis—a review of 135 cases. Med J Aust 148:228, 1988.

Chlamydia trachomatis

110. Schacter J: Chlamydial infections. N Engl J Med 298:428, 490, 540, 1978.
111. Tam MR, Stamm WE, Handsfield HH, et al: Culture-independent diagnosis of *Chlamydia trachomatis* using monoclonal antibodies. N Engl J Med 310:1146, 1984.
112. Mardh PA, Ripa T, Svensson L, Westrom L: *Chlamydia trachomatis* infection in patients with acute salpingitis. N Engl J Med 296:1377, 1977.
113. Berger RE, Alexander ER, Monda GD, et al: *Chlamydia trachomatis* as a cause of acute "idiopathic" epididymitis. N Engl J Med 298:301, 1978.
114. Quinn TC, Goodell SE, Mkrtichian E, et al: *Chlamydia trachomatis* proctitis. N Engl J Med 305:195, 1981.
115. Beem MO, Saxon EM: Respiratory-tract colonization and a distinctive pneumonia syndrome in infants infected with *Chlamydia trachomatis.* N Engl J Med 296:306, 1977.
116. Grayston JT, Wong SP, Kuo CC, Campbell LA: Current knowledge on *Chlamydia pneumoniae,* strain TWAR, an important cause of pneumonia and other acute respiratory diseases. Eur J Clin Microbiol Infect Dis 8:191, 1989.
117. Kleemola M, Saikku P, Visakorpi R, et al: Epidemics of pneumonia caused by TWAR, new *Chlamydia* organism in military trainees in Finland. J Infect Dis 157:230, 1988.
118. Grayston JT, Diwan VK, Cooney M, Wang S-P: Community and hospital-acquired pneumonia associated with *Chlamydia* TWAR infection demon-

strated serologically. Arch Intern Med 149:169, 1989.
119. Hahn DL, Dodge RW, Golubjatnikov R: Association of *Chlamydia pneumoniae* (strain TWAR) infection with wheezing, asthmatic bronchitis, and adult onset asthma. JAMA 266:225, 1991.
120. Cooper MA, Baldwin D, Matthews RS, et al: In-vito susceptibility of *Chlamydia pneumonia* (TWAR) to seven antibiotics. J Antimicrob Chemother 28:407, 1991.

Mycoplasmataceae

121. Taylor-Robinson D, McCormack WM: The genital mycoplasmas. N Engl J Med 302:1003, 1980.

Mycoplasma pneumoniae

122. Monsel JK, Rosenow EC III, Smith FT, Martin JW: *Mycoplasma pneumoniae* pneumonia. Chest 95:639, 1989.
123. Murray HW, Masur H, Senterfit LB, Roberts RB: The protean manifestations of *Mycoplasma pneumoniae* infection in adults. Am J Med 58:229, 1975.
124. Shames JM, George RB, Holliday WB, et al: Comparison of antibiotics in the treatment of mycoplasmal pneumonia. Arch Intern Med 125:680, 1970.

BIBLIOGRAPHY

Hoeprich PD (ed): Infectious Diseases, 3rd ed. Hagerstown, MD, Harper & Row, 1983.
Lennette EH, Balows A, Hausler WJ Jr, Shadomy HJ (eds): Manual of Clinical Microbiology, 4th ed. Washington, DC, American Society for Microbiology, 1985.
Mandell GL, Douglas RG Jr, Bennett JE (eds): Principles and Practice of Infectious Diseases, 3rd ed. New York, Wiley, 1990.
Sneath PHA, Mair NS, Sharpe ME, Holt JG (eds): Bergey's Manual of Systematic Bacteriology. Baltimore, Williams & Wilkins, 1986.

Fungi of Surgical Significance

CHAPTER 10

Scott F. Davies, George A. Sarosi

BIOLOGY OF THE FUNGI

Fungi are among the most primitive eukaryotic organisms.[1–3] They are classified as protists, as are algae and protozoa. These simple life forms do not show differentiation of cells into organs or specialized tissues; rather, a single cell is capable of regenerating the entire organism. Even large fungi are best thought of as collections of individual cells rather than as complex organisms.

Fungi require organic nutrients, so they must either live in organic debris or invade other living species. The majority live on decaying matter in soil or are pathogenic only to plants. Of the thousands of fungal species, only a few can cause disease in mammals. Even then, infection is an incidental part of the fungi's life cycle and the illness is usually mild.

The majority of fungi of medical importance grow as molds in nature. A mold is a fungus that is growing in long filaments called hyphae, often divided into cells by septae. The hyphae grow out from the surface of solid media as a tangled mass with many side branches and form an aerial growth called a mycelium; this is the visible fungus colony on a culture plate. Specialized branches of hyphae, called conidiophores, develop on the hyphae of most fungi; they are primarily reproductive structures and produce conidia, which are often referred to as spores. In general, spores are called microconidia if they are unicellular and macroconidia if they are multicellular, but there are a wide variety of names used for specific structures. The spores are small, easily aerosolized, and are usually the infectious particles.

Some fungi grow only yeasts, which are unicellular organisms that reproduce by budding. Buds may break off from the parent cell or remain attached, forming so-called pseudohyphae.

Many of the fungi of major medical importance are dimorphic. They can grow either as mycelia or as yeasts, depending on their environment. Thermal dimorphic fungi, including *Histoplasma capsulatum, Blastomyces dermatitidis, Paracoccidioides brasiliensis,* and *Sporothrix schenckii,* grow in soil at ambient temperatures as mycelia but within infected mammalian tissue at 37C as yeast. *Coccidioides immitis* is often referred to as a tissue dimorphic fungus. The mycelial phase is found in nature, but the tissue form consists of large spherules that rupture and release multiple endospores, each of which can mature into a new spherule.

GENERAL CLASSIFICATION OF FUNGAL DISEASE

The number of fungi that cause invasive disease in humans is small. These fungi are not easily classified but will be considered here in three major groups—according to the usual mechanism by which they cause infection.[4]

First are the *T cell opportunists.* These include the dimorphic endemic mycoses (histoplasmosis, coccidiodomycosis, and blastomycosis) plus cryptococcosis. They are acquired by inhalation of fungal spores. Specific cell-mediated immunity is required for recovery. All humans are susceptible to infection but most recover uneventfully once specific immunity is engaged. Occasional patients have unusually severe primary infections or have local complications from the brisk granulomatous inflammatory response. Patients with T cell defects—transplant patients, patients on chronic immunosuppressive drugs, and especially those with AIDS—have severe progressive infections requiring antifungal therapy.

Second are the *phagocyte opportunists.* Specific immunity is not necessary for defense. Intact barriers (mucosa and skin) and functioning phagocytes are sufficient to prevent infection. Defects in phagocyte number (especially neutropenia) or function (especially high-dose corticosteroids) are necessary before invasive disease can occur. Phagocyte opportunists include inhalational diseases due to ubiquitous environmental fungi with little or no ability to invade normal hosts. *Aspergillus* and *Mucor* species are most important but many essentially avirulent soil fungi can occasionally cause disease in defenseless hosts, including *Penicillium* species and *Fusarium* species. The latter are best thought of as aspergillus-like infections and will not be considered further. The phagocyte opportunists acquired by inhalation are not dimorphic: they are hyphae in nature and in infected tissue. *Candida* species are somewhat different from the other phagocyte opportunists. *Candida* are budding yeast in nature and in infected tissue. Serial budding can create pseudohyphae but there is no true mycelial phase. *Candida* are part of the normal flora found on mucosal surfaces and they also inhabit the gastrointestinal tract. They are not acquired by inhalation but invade across bowel mucosa or along intravascular catheters penetrating the skin. Rarely, they are acquired by aspiration of pharyngeal yeast, causing a primary pneumonia similar in pathogenesis to bacterial pneumonia. T cells are necessary to prevent local mucosal overgrowth (witness mucocutaneous candidiasis and especially *Candida* in AIDS). However, as long as phagocyte function and barrier function are intact, there is little opportunity for *Candida* to invade. Even in AIDS, systemic candidiasis is extremely unusual despite massive mucosal overgrowth (except in advanced disease with neutropenia from HIV infection, secondary infections, and/or effects of treatment including AZT and trimethoprim-sulfamethoxazole).

The third and last category include diseases ordinarily initiated by inoculation of fungal spores into subcutaneous tissues including sporotrichosis and mycetoma.

Introduction to the Diagnosis of Fungal Diseases

Only in rare instances can the diagnosis of an invasive fungal infection be made on clinical evidence alone. Rhinocerebral mucormycosis and lymphocutaneous sporotrichosis are two examples. In all other cases, a variety of diagnostic tests must be used to make a definitive diagnosis. A summary of the available diagnostic tests and their usefulness in specific fungal diseases is presented in Table 10–1.

Serology. Serologic tests measure the level of specific antibody to a fungal organism by complement-fixation assay, immunodiffusion, and other methods. Positive test results support a clinical impression but are rarely diagnostic. In general, the titer is proportional to the likelihood of infection by the particular organism. Negative results, however, seldom rule out the diagnosis. Cross-reactions between related fungi can also be confusing.

Immunodiagnostic testing for specific fungal antigens has greater diagnostic specificity. Testing of serum and cerebrospinal fluid (CSF) for cryptococcal antigen is the only example in wide clinical use. Detection of *Histoplasma* polysaccharide antigen is of use in diagnosis of AIDS patients with disseminated histoplasmosis and for monitoring treatment response and likelihood of relapse.[5]

Skin Tests. Intradermal skin tests were the first diagnostic tests used for fungal diseases. Skin tests are easy to perform, and the antigens for histoplasmosis and coccidioidomycosis are standardized. A positive skin test merely means that the patient has had an infection at some time. The frequency of positive results in an area endemic for a specific fungus is so high that these tests are more valuable in epidemiologic work than they are in making a specific diagnosis.

TABLE 10–1. VALUE OF DIAGNOSTIC TESTS IN CERTAIN MYCOTIC DISEASES

Disease	Culture	Smear (Sputum, Pus, etc)	Skin Test	Serology (CF Precipitin, etc)	Histopathology
Histoplasmosis	4+	0	2+	3+	3–4+
Blastomycosis	4+	4+	0	1+	4+
Coccidioidomycosis	4+	4+	4+	4+	4+
Paracoccidioidomycosis	4+	4+	2+	2+	4+
Cryptococcosis	4+	4+ (India ink)	0	4+ (Antigen)	3+
Aspergillus					
Invasive	2+	0	0	0	4+
Fungus ball	4+	2+	0	3+	4+
Mucormycosis	1+	0	0	0	3+
Candidiasis	1+	0	0	2+	3+
Sporotrichosis	4+	0	0	2+	1+

0, not useful; 1, rarely useful; 2, occasionally of some use; 3, useful; 4, very useful.

Pathologic Examination. Definitive diagnosis of a specific invasive fungal infection generally requires direct demonstration of the organism histopathologically or cultural isolation of the organisms from infected tissue. Examination of potassium hydroxide (KOH) digested sputum or pus from patients with possible fungal infections can be extremely helpful. The strong alkali dissolves the inflammatory cells and the mucus but leaves the fungal elements intact. This technique is especially useful in demonstrating the characteristic organisms of *B. dermatitidis* and *C. immitis* in freshly digested sputum or pus. Examination of KOH-treated CSF after addition of a drop of India ink is useful in the diagnosis of cryptococcosis.

Although such direct examination of specimens may sometimes be helpful, biopsy and histopathologic examination after fixation and staining adds greatly to the diagnostic yield. The routine hematoxylin and eosin stain fails to stain many of the fungi, but the demonstration of a granulomatous process may suggest a fungal infection and stimulate further diagnostic workup. Special stains greatly facilitate the histopathologic identification of specific organisms. The best available special stain for screening for fungi in tissue sections is the Gomori methenamine silver (GMS) stain, which colors all fungi and the filaments of *Actinomyces* and *Nocardia* a dark brown or black. It also stains old or dead (nonviable) fungal particles. In spite of the dark color of the stain, which can obscure the details of the various fungal elements, many of the fungi have specific morphologic features that allow recognition. Unfortunately, not everything that stains with GMS is a fungus. The parasite *Pneumocystic carinii* stains readily and, because of its size and avidity for the silver stain, has frequently been confused with *Histoplasma capsulatum* or with other yeast. Nuclear debris from degenerating cells can also take up silver stain.

Of other special stains available, Mayer's mucicarmine stain renders the mucopolysaccharide capsule of *Cryptococcus neoformans* a bright carmine. Because *C. neoformans* is the only encapsulated pathogenic fungus, the use of this stain is a specific diagnostic tool. Occasionally, the much larger yeasts of *B. dermatitidis* are also stained by this method, but the color is always a pale red and never the brilliant bright carmine seen with the cryptococcal capsule. The Gridley stain stains mucin and elastin as well as fungi; morphologic detail is good, but nonviable organisms are not stained. The periodic acid Schiff stain (PAS) is particularly useful for *B. dermatitidis;* it preserves fine detail and shows the multiple nuclei and the characteristic wide-necked single buds.

Culture. Although the direct identification of some fungi can be made by the preceding tests, identification by culture should be attempted whenever possible and may be the only means of making a specific diagnosis. Specimens are inoculated onto special fungal media and observed for at least 1 month because most fungi grow slowly. Most cultures are kept at room temperature for primary isolation of pathogenic fungi. Although it is usually more difficult, incubation and isolation may be attempted at 37C when the yeast form of a thermal dimorphic fungus is the suspected pathogen.

When growth begins, a tentative identification is made by examining teased and mounted specimens for the size, shape, and septation of the hyphae and the morphology of any spores or other specialized structures that are seen. Exoantigen testing can permit specific immunological identification of some clinical isolates faster than classical mycological methods.[6]

Because most pathogenic fungi are acquired by inhalation of spores, laboratory work with these organisms in the mycelial phase is hazardous and must be done only in biohazard hoods.

FUNGAL DISEASES CAUSED BY T CELL OPPORTUNISTS

Histoplasmosis

Histoplasma capsulatum induces a primary infection in the lung where the fungus replicates within the macrophages.[7] Fungemia is common and self-limited but results in seeding of reticuloendothelial organs throughout the body.[8] The ability of the organism to cause progressive disease in one or several sites results in a variety of clinical manifestations.

Etiology and Epidemiology. Histoplasma capsulatum is a thermal dimorphic fungus isolated from the soil. It is most common in temperate climates along river valleys and has been found in North, Central, and South America, India, and Southeast Asia. It is rare in Europe and in Australia. The center of endemic disease is in Ohio, Kentucky, Indiana, Illinois, Tennessee, Missouri, and Arkansas (ie, along the Ohio and Mississippi Rivers). Heavy concentrations are found in excrement of chickens and of pigeons, starlings, and other wild birds. Fungus-laden soil is most common in rural areas but may also be found in urban areas where starlings roost. Large outbreaks of histoplasmosis have been associated with excavation of infected soil for construction of roads or buildings. Progressive dissemination after a primary respiratory infection is rare. Infection is almost universal in highly endemic areas because any disturbance of the soil may scatter the infectious spores (microconidia) into the air. Over 90 percent of people living in some areas have had a primary pulmonary histoplasma infection before age 20.

Pathogenesis and Pathology. Inhalation of microconidia results in patchy areas of interstitial pneumonitis. The spores are engulfed by macrophages and multiply intracellularly in the yeast phase.[8] The draining lymph nodes are quickly involved, and hematogenous spread of the organism occurs with clearance by reticuloendothelial cells throughout the body.

The histology of individual lesions depends on the adequacy of the host cellular immune response. In disseminated infection, macrophages may be crowded with organisms and show no tendency to form aggregates. In contrast, the granulomas in the lung and in the reticuloendothelial organs after a normally limited primary spread are well developed with epitheloid histiocytes, giant cells, and central necrosis. Older lesions may show dense fibrosis and eventually may calcify.

Clinical Manifestations

PRIMARY PULMONARY HISTOPLASMOSIS. Primary pulmonary histoplasmosis usually has few symptoms.[9] Chest x-rays, even in asymptomatic cases, can show patchy nonsegmental areas of basal pneumonitis and prominent hilar adenopathy; pleural effusions are uncommon. Some patients, however, are symptomatic with onset 2 weeks after exposure. They have an influenza-like illness with fever, chills, myalgias, and a nonproductive cough. Regardless of the presence or absence of symptoms, a primary fungemia generally occurs; organisms can occasionally be recovered from blood and bone marrow at this time without implying progressive dissemination.

Following exposure to a large infecting inoculum, a more diffuse pulmonary involvement can occur, with an extensive nodular infiltrate on chest x-ray. Most of these patients are symptomatic, but they usually recover uneventfully. Rarely, the illness will continue for weeks to months, with a remitting and relapsing course.

The chest x-ray often reveals a return to normal after a primary pulmonary infection, but a variety of residual abnormalities can be seen. Initial soft infiltrates may "harden" and leave one or several nodules. Central necrosis may lead to a dense core of calcium (a target lesion), but this is not universal, especially in adults. Infrequently, alternate periods of activity followed by healing may result in characteristic concentric rings of calcium as the lesion slowly enlarges. Lymph node calcification, either in association with a parenchymal nodule or as a solitary finding, is common. Finally, small punctate "buckshot" calcifications may be scattered over both lung fields, a pattern characteristic of a heavy primary exposure with uneventful recovery (see Chap. 35).

Primary histoplasmosis has several uncommon local thoracic complications that lead to surgical consultations. Localized nodal masses (mediastinal granuloma) can compress soft structures including large veins and result in a superior venacaval syndrome. More extensive fibrotic reaction in the mediastinum (fibrosing mediastinitis) can obstruct bronchi, pulmonary arteries, and pulmonary veins. Clinical findings include hemoptysis, postobstructive pneumonia, and pulmonary hypertension.[10] Involvement of the pericardium may result in pericarditis and eventual constriction. Involvement of the esophagus can cause a traction diverticulum. A calcified node can erode through a bronchus, presenting as a broncholith. Clinical features include hemoptysis, lithoptysis, and postobstructive pneumonia.

CHRONIC CAVITARY HISTOPLASMOSIS. Upper lobe cavitary histoplasmosis closely resembles reinfection tuberculosis in its x-ray appearance. The mechanism of infection, however, is not endogenous reactivation; instead, it is the direct result of a primary infection in abnormal lungs, typically the lungs of middle aged, male smokers who have central lobular emphysema.[9] Acute pulmonary histoplasmosis in this setting usually resolves without sequelae, but infected air spaces persist in a few cases. A progressive fibrosing cavitary process then develops, which may gradually destroy adjacent areas of the lung. Specific antifungal chemotherapy is required. Although bilateral upper lobe involvement is characteristic, cavitary disease may occur in other parts of the lung. Chronic cough is a common clinical symptom, although some patients are asymptomatic. Constitutional symptoms, including weight loss, increase as the illness progresses, although fever need not be present. The coexistence of cavitary histoplasmosis with either tuberculosis or bronchogenic carcinoma is common.

DISSEMINATED HISTOPLASMOSIS. Disseminated histoplasmosis refers to any progressive extrapulmonary infection.[11] In children, it can occur as an overwhelming postprimary spread with no tendency to granuloma formation despite the presence of massive numbers of organisms in all reticuloendothelial tissues. High fever, lymphadenopathy, hepatosplenomegaly, disturbance of bone marrow function, and a fulminant course can cause death within weeks. Among adults, dissemination is most common in elderly men who have a smoldering, subacute, clinical illness many months long, with moderate fever, hepatosplenomegaly, skin and mucous membrane lesions, and weight loss. Disseminated histoplasmosis also occurs as an opportunistic infection in the immunosuppressed patient; high-dose glucocorticoid therapy is an important predisposing factor.[12] The degree of granulomatous response in the immunosuppressed patient can vary from almost nothing (the infantile form) to a considerable amount.

It is important to note that fewer than one-half of patients with disseminated histoplasmosis have a cough, dyspnea, or other pulmonary symptoms.[11,13] The chest x-ray may be normal or it may show a diffuse interstitial infiltrate that suggests a hematogenous process. Although at least one-third of nonimmunosuppressed patients will have a localized interstitial infiltrate on chest x-ray, such a finding is unusual in the immunosuppressed patient in whom there is usually no history of a preceding respiratory illness. The mechanism of infection may be endogenous reactivation. The clinical picture of disseminated histoplasmosis is extremely variable and nonspecific. Persistent fever is the only finding common to nearly all patients. Today progressive disseminated histoplasmosis is most common in patients with AIDS. Rapid progression of primary infection while immunosuppressed has been documented but late reactivation of remote latent disease is also a mechanism of infection. Diffuse infiltrates are common, but some patients have a nonspecific febrile illness, with a normal x-ray. Involvement of liver, spleen, bone marrow, and CNS is relatively common.

Diagnosis

MORPHOLOGY AND LABORATORY IDENTIFICATION. Histopathologic specimens that reveal macrophages crowded with small yeast are diagnostic of histoplasmosis. These organisms are easily seen in routine hematoxylin and eosin sections. With well-developed granulomas, the yeast forms may be rare, larger, and seen only in GMS-stained sections.

The organism can frequently be cultured from the sputum in primary or in chronic cavitary histoplasmosis, although it is almost never identified in KOH preparations. Bone marrow aspirate and fragments of liver biopsied by needle are frequently culture positive in disseminated histoplasmosis. If there are skin lesions, culture of a skin biopsy is easy and the results are reliable. Blood culture results may also be positive in disseminated histoplasmosis but should be requested specifically for fungal cultures, because they may have to be held for a longer time than routine bacterial cultures.

Although the organism is easy to grow from infected tissue specimens, identification may take several weeks. In suspected disseminated disease, this is too long and treatment must be instituted quickly. In AIDS, the organism can usually be grown from the blood and can sometimes be seen directly on the peripheral blood smear.[14]

SKIN TEST AND SEROLOGY. Skin testing is performed with mycelial (histoplasmin) or yeast antigens. The skin test is generally positive 2 to 3 weeks after a primary pulmonary infection and remains positive for many years. Most inhabitants of an endemic area will have a positive skin test, and therefore the test is not of diagnostic use in those areas.

Complement-fixing serologic reactions against yeast antigens become positive 3 to 4 weeks after primary infection. The titers usually decrease over 3 to 12 months but occasionally remain positive at a high dilution for years. Nonetheless, titers against the yeast antigen of 1:16 or greater in the appropriate clinical setting suggest a recent infection. A rising titer is diagnostic. Unfortunately, complement-fixation tests may be negative in 50 percent or more of the patients with disseminated histoplasmosis, although a high titer in an individual patient with an obscure febrile illness may suggest the diagnosis.

Immunodiffusion testing for precipitating antibodies to H or M antigens is specific for histoplasmosis, and positive reactions suggest recent infection. Immunodiffusion is less sensitive than complement fixation. In AIDS patients, histoplasma polysaccharide antigen can be measured in urine and in serum. Antigen testing is useful for diagnosis, assessing treatment response, and monitoring for relapse.[5]

Surgical Importance. Histoplasmosis is a common cause of a solitary pulmonary nodule. If it is noncalcified, thoracotomy is often required to exclude bronchogenic carcinoma. Amphotericin B is not required after the excision of such a nodule.

Specific antifungal chemotherapy is probably also unnecessary if a mediastinal mass has been biopsied to exclude lymphoma and histoplasmosis is documented. Large caseous masses should be removed.[15,16] Surgical therapy is generally not effective in cases when fibrosing mediastinitis has obstructed arteries, veins, and bronchi and has caused pulmonary hypertension. There is a significant risk of death and usually little of benefit can be done. Rarely, vascular bypass procedures have been performed in patients with severe symptoms, with limited success. If hemoptysis is caused by localized vascular obstruction without pulmonary hypertension, then appropriate resectional surgery can be beneficial. Treatment with amphotericin B is generally recommended only if operative specimens are culture positive. Operation should rarely be necessary if chronic cavitary histoplasmosis. An exception might be resectional surgery to control hemorrhage from a specific large cavity.

The diagnosis of disseminated histoplasmosis often depends on a biopsy of a skin lesion, a mucosal ulcer, or a vocal cord ulceration. The specimen should be cultured, as well as submitted for histopathology. Lapanoscopic or open liver biopsy may be indicated in some patients; however, bone marrow aspirate and bilateral trephine biopsy should precede laparotomy if a disseminated infection is suspected.

Disseminated histoplasmosis may also be of importance as an opportunistic infection among organ transplant recipients and other immunosuppressed patients.

Therapy. The usual primary pulmonary infection requires no therapy, but amphotericin B may be used for severe or prolonged infections.[17] A total course of 500 mg may be adequate in this situation.[18] Rarely, a massive primary exposure may result in an acute respiratory failure with marked hypoxia. Oxygenation and ventilatory support may be required, and use of amphotericin B is mandatory.

Progressive chronic cavitary histoplasmosis requires full therapy (a 2-g course) with amphotericin B, as does disseminated histoplasmosis. Itraconazole, 200 to 400 mg once daily for at least 6 months, can be used as an alternative to amphotericin B for patients with chronic cavitary histoplasmosis and for stable patients with chronic forms of disseminated histoplasmosis.[19]

AIDS patients require therapy to control the infection and then lifetime maintenance therapy to prevent relapse.[14] Amphotericin B is used for critically ill patients. Itraconazole is good maintenance therapy. (Ketoconazole doesn't work.) Itraconazole can be used from the onset in milder cases.

Blastomycosis

Blastomycosis, also known as North American blastomycosis to distinguish it from paracoccidioidomycosis or South American blastomycosis, refers to infection by *Blastomyces dermatitidis.* Primary infection is in the lung, where large central inflammatory masses can mimic carcinoma. Involvement of skin, bone, and prostate gland are prominent features of disseminated blastomycosis; unlike histoplasmosis, reticuloendothelial organs are seldom involved.

Etiology and Epidemiology. Blastomyces dermatitidis is a thermal dimorphic fungus. It is endemic in the southeastern and south central regions of the United States. Disease activity extends northward along the western shores of Lake Michigan and is also present in Minnesota, North Dakota, and bordering Canadian provinces. The organism is a soil saprophyte that infects only after direct, intimate exposure. The disease occurs most frequently in rural areas among those with outdoor jobs or interests, predominantly males aged 20 to 50.

Pathogenesis and Pathology. The infectious microconidia are inhaled into the lung, where a vigorous acute suppurative response occurs. Cell-mediated immunity develops later, and the tissue reaction at the time of diagnosis of pulmonary blastomycosis has a mixed pyogenic and granulomatous nature. Acute pulmonary blastomycosis is probably self-limited in many cases, although the tendency to heal is probably not as pronounced as it is with histoplasmosis.

Hematogenous spread does not always occur during pulmonary infection as it does in histoplasmosis; favored sites of spread are skin, bone, and prostate rather than liver and spleen.[20]

Clinical Manifestations

PRIMARY PULMONARY BLASTOMYCOSIS. Acute pulmonary blastomycosis is a variably symptomatic illness.[21] Patchy areas of alveolar consolidation usually affect one or both lower lobes. Hilar adenopathy may occur, but pleural involvement and cavitation are rare. If present, the symptoms are like acute pneumonia and include high fever, productive cough, pleuritic chest pain, and myalgias. Symptoms may vary in intensity and duration but usually last less than 2 weeks. Radiographic evidence often persists for up to 3 months (see Chap. 35).

CHRONIC PULMONARY BLASTOMYCOSIS WITH OR WITHOUT INVOLVEMENT OF DISTANT SITES. Most clinical cases of blastomycosis present as chronic pulmonary blastomycosis. Many of these patients give no history of an antecedent acute pneumonia but have chronic respiratory symptoms of weeks to months duration. Chronic cough, low-grade fever, night sweats, weight loss, and a variable amount of dyspnea are the common complaints. The chest x-ray may reveal a single large mass, often perihilar in location. This pattern is responsible for the fact that blastomycosis is misdiagnosed as probable carcinoma of the lung more often than any other fungal disease.[22] Other common findings on chest x-ray include focal or multifocal infiltrates and multiple nodules. Less commonly there are small cavities with stringy fibrosis extending toward the hilum. Several of these patterns resemble tuberculosis. A rare x-ray finding is a single large cavity, which may resemble a primary lung abscess (see Chap. 31).

Involvement of distant sites is common in chronic pulmonary blastomycosis; two-thirds of the patients have skin involvement, one-third have bone involvement, and one-fifth have genitourinary tract involvement. The occurrence of infection in these sites, in association with a chronic pulmonary infection, can be helpful in suggesting the presence of blastomycosis and in providing an easily accessible source of diagnostic material.

ISOLATED INVOLVEMENT OF DISTANT SITES. Isolated involvement of skin, bone, or genitourinary tract can occur without any history or evidence of respiratory tract infection. This probably represents reactivation of sites seeded during primary asymptomatic infection.

SKIN INFECTION. The characteristic lesions of skin infection are raised, warty, crusty lesions with irregular borders on the face and upper extremities. The lesions can mimic basal cell carcinoma, but the small microabscesses at the peripheral edges of the lesions are a distinguishing feature (see Fig. 27–29).

SKELETAL SYSTEM. Bone is the second most common distant site of infection in blastomycosis. The spine is most frequently involved, followed by the ribs, skull, and long bones.

GENITOURINARY SYSTEM. Unlike tuberculosis, blastomycosis rarely involves the kidney or ureter or any part of the female genitourinary tract. The prostate, epididymis, and, less frequently, testes, however, become involved and can result in a scrotal or prostatic mass, hematuria, pyuria, or bladder outlet obstruction.

Diagnosis

MORPHOLOGY AND LABORATORY IDENTIFICATION. The yeast can frequently be seen in the sputum, in aspirates of skin lesions, or in prostatic secretions. The organism can be positively identified in KOH preparations, although cytology specimens treated with Papanicolaou stain are superior.

Histopathologic examination of biopsy specimens of infected tissue also reveals the characteristic 8 to 20 μm yeast of blastomycosis with doubly refractile walls and wide-necked single budding. The organism is seldom seen in hematoxylin and eosin stained sections; silver and PAS stains are best for diagnosis.

In the laboratory, *B. dermatitidis* grows slowly, often requiring several weeks or even a month. Exoantigen testing of mycelial isolates can shorten the diagnostic interval.

SKIN TEST AND SEROLOGY. Skin testing is not useful. Serologic testing using new, more specific antigens (antigen A) is being evaluated. Complement-fixation tests, immunodiffusion, and enzyme immunoassay (EIA) tests are available. The EIA is very sensitive but is not specific (cross-reactions with histoplasmosis are common). Immunodiffusion is specific but only half as sensitive. A positive immunodiffusion test has predictive value, as does a negative EIA. A positive EIA should be confirmed by culture, histopathology, and serologic tests for the fungi. A negative immunodiffusion test has poor negative predictive value.

Surgical Importance. Blastomycosis can present as a mass (up to 10 cm) in the chest. Fever and night sweats suggest a chronic inflammation. If the diagnosis is confirmed from cytologic specimens, thoracotomy is not necessary. Itraconazole therapy will be required for a resected mass if proved to be chronic pulmonary blastomycosis (or even amphotericin B if the patient is very toxic and acutely ill).

Surgery is rarely necessary to drain a large abscess or an empyema.

Skin lesions can mimic basal cell carcinoma, but microabscesses at the periphery of the lesion should suggest the correct diagnosis. Aspiration of the lesion will ordinarily establish the diagnosis, and the lesions will respond to itraconazole.

Blastomycosis in the spine usually resembles tuberculosis, but an osteolytic lesion can suggest myeloma or other malignant disease. Aspiration of the bone lesions may be necessary.

If a needle biopsy of a prostate nodule reveals characteristic yeast forms, treatment with itraconazole is mandatory. Prostatic involvement can also cause bladder outlet obstruction. Testicular involvement can mimic a tumor, but more often the presence of tender swelling will indicate an infection.

Treatment. Acute pulmonary blastomycosis probably does not require treatment in all cases. Treatment with a total course of 2 g amphotericin B should be given if the patient is severely ill or if the illness progresses rapidly under observation. Itraconazole should be given if the patient is stable but unimproved after 2 or 3 weeks. Long-term evaluation of all untreated patients is always necessary because systemic disease can develop much later despite a self-limited primary infection. Patients with chronic pulmonary disease or disease at distant sites should all be treated. A 2-g course of amphotericin B is highly effective (see Chap. 24).[23] Itraconazole is an alternative treatment for chronic pulmonary and nonmeningeal disseminated infections if the patient is not severely ill. The initial dose is 200 to 400 mg once daily. Treatment should be continued at least 6 months. Itraconazole is effective treatment but takes weeks to work; it should never be used in place of amphotericin B for life-threatening pulmonary or disseminated infections.[19] However, itraconazole is sufficient for most cases of mild to moderate pulmonary and extrapulmonary blastomycosis—perhaps 90 percent of all clinically recognized cases. Amphotericin B is reserved for extreme toxicity, ARDS, edematous lobar pneumonia, and meningitis.

Coccidioidomycosis

Coccidioidomycosis is caused by the fungus *Coccidioides immitis.* Symptomatic pulmonary illnesses occur in almost half of all exposed people. Although the majority of primary infections resolve, a few patients develop disseminated disease with central nervous system, skeletal, and cutaneous involvement. Disseminated coccidioidomycosis is a chronic illness with many relapses.

Etiology. Coccidioides immitis is a tissue dimorphic fungus. In the soil and on laboratory culture media, the fungus grows as a septate mycelium with numerous side branches. Spore formation occurs along the hyphae; thick-walled arthrospores develop, which alternate with empty cells. When the infecting arthrospores are inhaled into the mammalian lung, they develop into spherules characteristic of the tissue phase of growth. Spherules are round, thick-walled structures, which grow to 30 to 80 μm in diameter and reproduce by progressive cleavage of the cytoplasm with formation of multiple endospores (as many as 10^5 per mature spherule). Each spherule eventually ruptures; the endospores are released into the tissue where each, again, has the potential to mature into another spherule and repeat the cycle.

Epidemiology. Coccidioides immitis is endemic in the southwestern United States, particularly in the San Joaquin Valley of California and in central and southern Arizona. The specific habitat favoring fungal growth is the desert soil in a semiarid climate with hot dry summers and mild winters with moderate rainfall.

The arthrospores are scattered long distances by the wind. Exposure to the fungus is an almost universal occurrence in highly endemic areas; 15 to 25 percent of nonimmune persons who move to such areas develop a primary pulmonary infection within 5 years.

Pathogenesis and Pathology. The infecting particle is the arthrospore, and infection occurs only by inhalation. The arthrospore is so infective that a casual exposure such as driving through an endemic area can cause a primary pulmonary infection. In exceptional cases, infection has occurred after exposure to arthrospore-contaminated articles shipped to nonendemic areas.

The arthrospore elicits an exudative response with polymorphonuclear cells predominating in the lung alveoli. Rupture of developing spherules liberates great numbers of endospores, most of which are phagocytosed and rapidly destroyed. Some of the endospores always survive and mature into new spherules.

Within 1 to 2 weeks, a specific cell-mediated immunity develops, which is directed against the maturing spherules. Such specific cell-mediated immunity is essential in arresting the infection. A mixed granulomatous and pyogenic tissue response is seen in histopathologic specimens obtained at this stage of the infection. If the cell-mediated response is inadequate, a fulminant miliary illness can result.

Clinical Manifestations

PRIMARY PULMONARY COCCIDIOIDOMYCOSES. Sixty percent of patients with a primary pulmonary infection have minimal or no symptoms.[24,25] The other 40 percent have a febrile pulmonary illness that resembles influenza and lasts 1 to 3 weeks. Chest pain, often pleuritic, is a common complaint but is often short-lived. Cough is usually quite mild. Weight loss and anorexia are common, as are myalgias, arthralgias, headache, and fatigue. Dyspnea is unusual in an uncomplicated pulmonary infection. The chest x-ray can show an alveolar infiltrate (usually at one of the lung bases) or a single nodular density.

Primary pulmonary infection resolves without any sequelae 95 percent of the time; the other 5 percent will have abnormal findings on chest x-rays, most commonly with solitary thin-walled cavities. Only one or two patients in 1000 will develop disseminated disease. Dissemination occurs most commonly in black and Filipino men, diabetics, and possibly in pregnant women.

DISSEMINATED COCCIDIOIDOMYCOSES. Persistent or recurrent fever can signal the onset of disseminated disease. Rapid progression with development of meningitis, multiple bony lesions, and verrucous cutaneous lesions like those of blastomycoses can occur (see Fig. 27–29).[26] Although it is rare, patients can have an even more fulminant postprimary miliary spread with diffuse nodular infiltrates and respiratory failure. Clinically recognizable defects in cell-mediated immunity are frequent in these patients; high-dose prednisone therapy is an important predisposing factor.[27]

Patients with AIDS are highly susceptible to coccidioidomycosis and rapidly disseminate. Diffuse nodular infiltrates occur in half the patients; meningeal spread occurs in one-quarter.[28]

For most other patients, however, the onset of disseminated infection with *C. immitis* is more insidious. Although it usually follows the primary pulmonary infection by either weeks or months, it may occur much later. Coccidioidal meningitis is the most frequent manifestation of extrapulmonary disease.[29] Skeletal disease occurs in 10 to 20 percent of patients with extrapulmonary disease.

Diagnosis

MORPHOLOGY AND LABORATORY IDENTIFICATION. Histopathologic specimens are diagnostic if large spherules or spherule fragments can be identified in hematoxylin and eosin or silver-stained sections. Spherules are also diagnostic if identified in KOH-treated specimens such as sputum or pus. The organisms can be cultured on Sabouraud agar or on blood agar without difficulty, but the arthrospores are highly infectious. Some saphrophytic fungi have similar arthrospores so that culture isolates showing arthrospores are not diagnostic of coccidiodomycosis. Confirmation of cultures was previously done by mouse inoculation with subsequent demonstration of the tissue phase of growth. Currently, cultures are confirmed by exoantigen testing, which is less hazardous. Because of all these difficulties and because cultures are seldom positive in coccidioidal meningitis (where they would be most helpful), culture identification is not of great clinical importance. Reliance on direct demonstration of organism and on skin tests and serology is adequate for management of most patients.

SKIN TEST AND SEROLOGY. Skin testing is performed with coccidioidin, prepared from the mycelial phase of growth, or with spherulin, derived from spherules. A positive test (5 mm induration) is present in most patients with primary disease from 10 to 20 days after infection. Failure to develop a positive test is predictive of progressive disseminated infection. Loss of established skin test reactivity often precedes late dissemination. Skin test positivity returns after successful chemotherapy, and relapse is likely if the skin test remains negative.

Complement-fixing antibodies are also of great clinical importance because patients with mild infections do not develop these antibodies. Patients with severe but self-limited primary infections in the lung may have a mild elevation in titer, which disappears in 6 months or persists at levels 1:8 or less. Persistent titers of 1:16 or greater, and especially gradually rising titers, are often seen in patients with dissemination or impending dissemination. Successful drug therapy results in a fall in complement-fixing antibody titers, which often happens as the skin test turns positive.

Complement-fixing serologic titers in the cerebrospinal fluid are of particular diagnostic importance in coccidioidal meningitis.

Precipitin tests identify antibodies that appear earlier and are quite specific. This type of antibody usually disappears within a month (see Table 10–1).

Surgical Importance. Coccidioidomycosis is a common cause of a solitary pulmonary nodule in endemic areas. Residual nodules rarely calcify, and thoracoscopy or thoracotomy may be required to exclude bronchogenic carcinoma.

Thin-walled cavities caused by coccidioidomycosis are common in endemic areas and ordinarily require no therapy. Resection of such cavities may be necessary, however, to control recurrent hemoptysis or symptomatic bacterial superinfection. Resection may be indicated for a growing cavity or one that is subpleural in location or crosses fissure lines. Such cavities can rupture into the pleural space, causing an empyema with bronchopleural fistula. This is a serious complication that requires pleural drainage and later operative closure of the bronchopleural fistula, under amphotericin B coverage. Growth of cavities and pleural rupture occur shortly after cavities form but almost never in stable, long-standing cavities.

A surgical procedure may be required for diagnosis. Biopsies of skin or bony lesions may be undertaken with a presumptive diagnosis of basal cell carcinoma or metastatic carcinoma, respectively.

Neurosurgical placement of an Ommaya reservoir may be needed to treat some patients with coccidioidal meningitis.[30]

Finally, immunosuppressed patients, including transplant recipients and other patients on high-dose prednisone, may develop disseminated coccidioidomycosis as a result of endogenous reactivation or progressive primary infection.

Therapy. Amphotericin B is less effective against *C. immitis* than against any other pathogenic fungi, but it is still the best available treatment.[23] Treatment is indicated in primary pulmonary coccidioidomycosis only in patients whose immune status or racial backgrounds place them at high risk of dissemination, that is, immunosuppressed patients, diabetics, pregnant women, and black and Filipino men. Treatment is especially advisable when pulmonary infection is severe, persistent, or progressive. The usual total dose of amphotericin B is 500 mg to 2 g.

Amphotericin B is not indicated after resection of a granuloma that proves to be coccidioidomycosis, unless caseous material is spilled during the procedure. A course of 1 g should be given postoperatively if this occurs. If a growing or subpleural cavity is resected, 500 mg of amphotericin B can be given before operation and an additional 500 mg afterward. This recommendation is anecdotal and is not supported by randomized prospective studies.

Disseminated disease always demands prompt and aggressive therapy. An initial course of 2.5 g is employed. If remission is not obtained, prolonged courses of 4 to 5 g are indicated.

Coccidioidal meningitis should be treated intrathecally with amphotericin B until complement-fixing antibody levels in the cerebrospinal fluid are negative. The skin test may revert to positive as well, although this is not always the case. Sclerosing complications may limit intrathecal administration of the drug at the lumbar site and an alternate route of administration (intracisternal or intraventricular via Ommaya reservoir) may have to be used.[30] Patients with isolated coccidioidal meningitis should also receive a total dose of 2 g of systemic amphotericin B.

The use of amphotericin B is not always successful.[23–32] Fluconazole is gaining a more important role in therapy. It is used for meningitis in place of combined systemic intrathecal amphotericin B, especially in milder cases and in patients with AIDS. It is used for persistent pulmonary infections in normal hosts and for mild to moderate disseminated disease in AIDS and non-AIDS patients. Mortality in patients with AIDS is very high (50% in 1 month). If there is an initial treatment response, suppressive therapy with fluconazole must be continued for life. There are a few 1- and 2-year survivors.

Further clinical studies are needed to fully define the role of fluconazole. For coccidioidal meningitis, recent practice has been to push the dose to 600 to 800 mg/d or even higher, as tolerated.

Paracoccidioidomycosis

Paracoccidioidomycosis (South American blastomycosis) is caused by *Paracoccidioides brasiliensis.* Symptomatic or asymptomatic pulmonary infection is produced when the organism is inhaled, and disseminated disease is characterized by involvement of the oral and pharyngeal mucosa and cervical adenopathy.

Etiology and Epidemiology. Paracoccidioides brasiliensis is a thermal dimorphic fungus. Endemic regions exist in Brazil, Colombia, and Venezuela with scattered cases from other areas of South and Central America. Most cases are asymptomatic.

Pathogenesis and Pathology. When inhaled, the infectious spores provoke an acute inflammatory response similar to that seen in blastomycosis. If progressive pulmonary disease occurs, the pathologic picture includes mixed granulomatous and suppurative processes. Mucocutaneous lesions demonstrate pseudoepitheliomatous hyperplasia with areas of granuloma formation, but also with microabscesses. Both the lung and skin pathologies resemble that seen in blastomycosis.

Clinical Manifestations. A primary asymptomatic self-limited illness is inferred by the frequency in endemic areas of positive skin tests and incidental findings at autopsy.[33,34] Progressive pulmonary disease presents with fever, weight loss, productive cough, and increasing shortness of breath over a period of weeks to months. The chest x-ray reveals nodular areas that may be confluent and most often involve the lower lobes. Another radiographic pattern is bilateral peri-hilar infiltrates. Fibrosis can occur as areas of the lung are destroyed. Cavitation occurs in one-third of the cases.

Disseminated paracoccidioidomycosis classically presents with multiple oral and pharyngeal ulcerations and cervical adenopathy. Widely disseminated disease also occurs with the lymph nodes, spleen, intestine, and skin as preferred sites. Bone and central nervous system involvement occurs only occasionally.

Diagnosis

MORPHOLOGY AND LABORATORY IDENTIFICATION. The mycelium grows slowly on yeast extract agar at 25C. It has no characteristic spores, and conversion to the typical yeast form by culture on blood agar at 37C is necessary before positive identification can be made. Culture isolation is the gold standard for diagnosis.

However, diagnosis often depends on the direct examination of sputum, purulent secretions, or tissue biopsies. The pathognomonic feature is a 15 to 25 μm yeast with multiple small peripheral buds, each with a narrow neck of attachment to the parent cell. The organism can be visualized on direct KOH-treated smears of sputum or other secretions or on silver-stained histopathologic sections.

SKIN TEST AND SEROLOGY. Skin testing has no important clinical role in paracoccidioidomycosis.

The complement-fixation test is positive in 80 percent of patients with active infection and generally negative after successful therapy. An immunodiffusion test developed by Restrepo is even more sensitive and specific.[34]

Surgical Importance. Biopsy of specimens from mucocutaneous lesions or of lymph nodes may be needed to make a specific diagnosis. Progressive pulmonary disease can generally be diagnosed from the sputum. Surgery has no major role in therapy.

Therapy. Previously, patients were treated with sulfonamides, with amphotericin B used for treatment failures. Oral imidazoles (itraconazole or ketoconazole) are now the treatment of choice.[35]

Cryptococcosis

Cryptococcosis is caused by the encapsulated yeast *Cryptococcus neoformans.* The primary pulmonary infection rarely produces a clinical illness, and most patients have subacute or chronic meningitis, which is associated with an underlying disease so often that it was formerly referred to in France as *signal malade.*

Etiology. Cryptococcus neoformans exists both in nature and in infected mammalian tissue as a 4 to 20 μm budding yeast. Its distinctive feature is its thick carbohydrate capsule; it is the only pathogenic yeast that is encapsulated.

Epidemiology. Cryptococcal organisms are distributed worldwide, in both urban and rural areas. They are most frequently associated with pigeon droppings.

Pathogenesis and Pathology. In the lung, the organism produces its carbohydrate capsule, which inhibits phagocytosis and the recruitment of inflammatory cells. Nonetheless, the innate infectivity of the organism is not great and the cellular immune response, although minimal, generally limits the local infection. In immunocompromised patients, hematogenous spread of organisms may occur so that cryptococcal infection later becomes active at a distant site, most commonly the meninges.

The lesions are either myxomatous or granulomatous. Myxomatous lesions have masses of encapsulated organisms lying free in the tissues, without inflammatory response.

Clinical Manifestations

PRIMARY PULMONARY CRYPTOCOCCOSIS. Patients usually have no symptoms, although if an active focus erodes into an airway there may be a transient heavy discharge of mucoid sputum laden with organisms. If present, fever is modest.

Chest x-rays usually show a localized discrete infiltrate in one of the lower lobes without hilar adenopathy. As a rule, the infiltrates completely resolve without cavitation or residual nodules.

CENTRAL NERVOUS SYSTEM CRYPTOCOCCOSIS. Eighty percent of diagnosed cases of cryptococcosis involve the central nervous system without a history of any respiratory illness.[36,37] Headaches that gradually increase in frequency and severity, together with mild fever and mild meningeal signs, are the usual presentation. Abnormal laboratory findings are usually confined to the cerebrospinal fluid with increased pressure, high protein, low glucose, and a variable lymphocytic pleocytosis, usually fewer than 200 cells. India ink preparation of spinal fluid is positive in half of the culture-proven cases.

Without specific treatment, progression and death will result. In the pre-AIDS era, about half the patients had an underlying immunosuppressive state, such as lymphoma, leukemia, diabetes, or any disorder treated with high-dose steroids.[38] These patients have a poor prognosis. Chronically immunosuppressed organ transplant patients develop an insidious chronic meningitis; if treated, recovery is the rule. Negative prognostic factors include fewer than 20 white blood cells per cubic millimeter in the cerebrospinal fluid, the presence of organisms on India ink preparation, positive cultures of blood or other extraneural specimens in association with meningitis, and high titers of cryptococcal antigen in cerebrospinal fluid or serum. The vast majority of serious cryptococcal infections now occur in patients with AIDS, who usually have meningitis and systemic infection.

Less commonly, patients have a single focus in the brain, a mass lesion, with signs of increased intracerebral pressure (nausea, vomiting, changes in level of consciousness) and focal neurologic signs.

BONE INVOLVEMENT. Although cryptococcosis can involve the skull, vertebrae, and long bones, it occurs much less frequently than in blastomycosis or coccidioidomycosis. X-rays show a destructive focus without much periosteal reaction, which is often indistinguishable from neoplasm.

CUTANEOUS INVOLVEMENT. A variety of skin lesions are produced by hematogenous spread rather than by inoculation and occur in conjunction with disseminated disease. Specific diagnosis is impossible without biopsy.

DISSEMINATED CRYPTOCOCCOSIS. Rapid hematogenous spread to many organs occurs primarily in immunosuppressed patients. High fever is common. Diffuse lung involvement can lead to respiratory insufficiency. Liver and bone marrow involvement can also be documented. The cerebrospinal fluid is usually involved. Diagnosis in these cases is usually made from a blood culture or on examination of the bone marrow.

Diagnosis

MORPHOLOGY AND LABORATORY IDENTIFICATION. Histopathologic material is diagnostic if a yeast form (4 to 20 μm) with a thick unstained halo can be demonstrated with hematoxylin and eosin stain or silver stain. The mucicarmine stain brightly colors the halo and shows that it is the carbohydrate capsule. India ink preparation permits rapid identification of an encapsulated yeast in the cerebrospinal fluid or other body fluids.

Cultures of cerebrospinal fluid, blood, urine, or aspirates of bony or skin lesions are diagnostic of cryptococcosis if an encapsulated yeast is recovered.

Interpretation of sputum cultures is more difficult because other cryptococcus species occasionally colonize the respiratory tract. Even *C. neoformans* can sometimes be recovered from the sputum of debilitated patients without an invasive infection.

Measurement of the fungal antigen in the spinal fluid in a patient with a compatible illness is diagnostic.

SKIN TEST AND SEROLOGY. No reliable skin test antigen is available for clinical use. The tube precipitin method, the best available serodiagnostic test for antibodies, is unreliable.

Cryptococcosis is the only fungal infection where measurement of a fungal antigen is important. Capsular material in serum and cerebrospinal fluid can be detected by a sensitive latex-fixation method, which is specific if controls for rheumatoid factor are included. Cryptococcal antigen is of diagnostic and also prognostic importance. Initial high levels of antigen, or failure of the antigen level to decrease during therapy, indicate the likelihood of treatment failure or early relapse. In AIDS (but not in non-AIDS patients) the *serum* cryptococcal antigen is invariably positive in cases of cryptococcal meningitis, usually in higher titer than simultaneous CSF titers.

Surgical Importance. A nodule resected to exclude the possibility of bronchogenic carcinoma can be a cryptococcal lesion. A spinal tap should be done in such patients to determine if the spinal fluid is involved, but treatment is not necessary if the CSF is negative.

Bone lesions can mimic neoplasm; diagnosis depends on aspiration or an open biopsy. Diagnosis of cutaneous cryptococcosis may also depend on biopsy.

Cryptococcal meningitis is an important opportunistic infection in renal transplant recipients and other immunosuppressed patients, so the onset of chronic headaches should prompt the performance of a spinal tap.[38,39] Disseminated cryptococcosis is also the differential diagnosis of generalized systemic infections in such patients and can mimic cytomegalovirus infection.

Therapy. All patients who have *C. neoformans* isolated from any site should have a spinal tap done to exclude meningeal involvement. Some patients will be asymptomatic when *Cryptococcus* has been identified in sputum or in a pulmonary nodule. These people do not require treatment if their CSF is free of the organism. All patients, however, who have extrapulmonary involvement require full treatment. The best treatment is combined therapy with amphotericin B, 0.3 to 0.5 mg/kg/d, and 5-fluorocytosine, 150 mg/kg/d in divided doses. Twelve of sixteen patients with culture-proven cryptococcal meningitis responded to this regimen, despite the presence of poor prognostic features in many cases.[40]

Intrathecal administration of amphotericin B is usually not required, but it can be tried in patients who are failing to respond to conventional therapy. AIDS patients cannot be cured. They require lifetime fluconazole to prevent relapse. Initial therapy is with fluconazole (if mental status is normal) or with amphotericin B plus 5-FC for more serious infections with decreased level of consciousness. Fluconazole from onset is also being evaluated for non-AIDS patients with milder infections.[41]

FUNGAL DISEASES CAUSED BY PHAGOCYTE OPPORTUNISTS

These opportunistic fungal diseases are caused by ubiquitous fungi, which are ordinarily nonpathogenic and invade tissue only under conditions of local or systemic host immunoincompetence. Defects in neutrophil number or function, together with barrier defects, are the major predisposition.

Aspergillosis

Aspergillosis refers to infection by any of the numerous members of the genus *Aspergillus.* These fungi have a low pathogenicity for healthy individuals. Although they can readily colonize mucosal surfaces, these organisms do not invade people unless the normal defense mechanisms are altered. Dissemination of the disease occurs only in severely immunosuppressed patients.

Etiology. There are more than 300 species of *Aspergillus.* The majority of human infections are caused by *A. fumigatus.* Occasionally, infections are caused by *A. niger, A. clavatus, A. flavus,* or *A. nidulans.*

The *Aspergillus* species are among the most common fungi. Spores are present in all environments, and any small source of organic debris serves as a nidus for growth.

Pathogenesis and Pathology. The organisms are inhaled and may be recovered from the sputum of uninfected patients after heavy exposure. In external otitis, the organism colonizes the superficial keratinized layer of the skin and evokes little or no inflammatory response. True invasive infections occur in the middle ear and the paranasal sinus, and the exudate is filled with acute and chronic inflammatory cells. As a rule, the density of the organism is low, and special stains must be used to find hyphae.

Perhaps the most characteristic lesion produced by *Aspergillus* species is the intracavitary fungus ball, or aspergilloma. Matted masses of aspergilli grow in preexisting cavities that communicate with airways. The cavity colonized by the fungus is usually an inactive residual lesion secondary to tuberculosis, fungal disease, sarcoidosis, carcinoma, or bronchiectasis. Although there may be some inflammatory infiltration (with many eosinophils) around the cavity, the fungus does not invade adjacent lung parenchyma.

In allergic bronchial aspergillosis, the bronchi are dilated and full of mucus plugs. Hyphae and eosinophils are seen within the inspissated mucus, but fungi never invade the dilated bronchial walls, which are heavily infiltrated with eosinophils and other inflammatory cells.

In chronic necrotizing aspergillosis, the organism grows in an abnormal lung and slowly invades adjacent areas. Fungus balls may form in new cavities caused by *Aspergillus* infection. The pathology shows chronic inflammation, fibrosis, and areas of cavitation. Overlying pleura is often involved.

In disseminated aspergillosis, widespread necrosis of tissue occurs, especially in the lung where there may be multiple wedge-shaped areas of bronchial pneumonia. Growth within blood vessels may cause thrombosis, with necrosis of further tissue and subsequent cavitation as the necrotic material is expectorated. Multiple metastatic abscesses may occur in the brain, liver, heart, skin, kidneys, and other organs.

Aspergillus endocarditis most commonly follows cardiac surgery. The vegetations are large, bulky, and friable and frequently embolize to major arteries.

Clinical Manifestations

EAR, PARANASAL SINUSES, AND ORBIT. Colonization of the oral pharynx causes no symptoms. Limited disease in the external ear causes pain and redness. When a paranasal sinus is invaded, local swelling and erythema result. Focal osteomyelitis should be considered when tenderness is severe. In the sinuses as well as in the nose and on the palate, the organism may grow as a large, bulky, soft tissue mass, which can bleed profusely. Once *Aspergillus* infection has become established in the paranasal sinuses, extension to the orbit and to the central nervous system is possible. Proptosis and ophthalmoplegia may be the dominant signs of orbital invasion. Sudden onset of a stroke indicates the involvement of an intracranial vessel, with distal hemorrhagic infarction. Patients who survive this complication usually develop brain abscesses with signs of increased intracranial pressure.

ASPERGILLOMA. The major clinical feature of intracavitary fungus balls is hemoptysis, which can be profuse and sometimes even life-threatening, especially if blood is aspirated.[42] In the absence of hemoptysis in the patient, symptoms are generally related to the underlying chronic cavitary pulmonary disease and are determined by the extent of pulmonary destruction present before the appearance of the fungus ball. The fungus ball will not invade deeply into the lung, nor will it lead to disseminated disease.

ALLERGIC BRONCHOPULMONARY ASPERGILLOSIS. Most patients with allergic bronchopulmonary aspergillosis have episodic dyspnea that is related to their underlying asthma. The clinical course of their asthma, however, is punctuated by intermittent bouts of increased anatomic obstruction of bronchi because the organisms proliferate in the thick mucus characteristic of asthma. When this happens, fever and cough are common and active infiltrates are usually seen on the chest x-ray. Mucous plugs are frequently expectorated, and pleuritic chest pain and peripheral blood eosinophilia are common. In the early stages of bronchopulmonary aspergillosis, the patients are relatively asymptomatic between acute exacerbations of bronchial plugging, except for the symptoms of their underlying asthma. Later on, however, the repeated attacks of bronchial plugging can result in gradual destruction of bronchial mucosa with eventual development of saccular bronchiectasis. When this occurs, the symptoms of infective bronchiectasis can dominate the clinical picture with continuous production of purulent sputum, even during the interval between episodes of bronchial plugging. Scanty hemoptysis comes from bronchiectatic lesions.

CHRONIC NECROTIZING ASPERGILLOSIS. This form of aspergillosis is intermediate between an aspergilloma and an invasive aspergillosis.[43] Infection occurs in middle-aged smokers with presumed centrilobular emphysema (similar to chronic cavitary histoplasmosis). The fungus grows in the abnormal air spaces and invades and destroys adjacent lung, producing a fibrocavitary upper lobe disease similar to tuberculosis. The adjacent pleura may be involved, but distant spread does not occur. Patients are chronically ill, and the disease progresses over several years. Many patients are mildly immunosuppressed. Symptoms include dyspnea, chronic cough, weight loss, night sweats, fever, and intermittent hemoptysis. Symptoms result from the severe underlying lung disease as well as the infection with aspergillosis.

INVASIVE ASPERGILLOSIS. The invasive form of aspergillosis has become common in patients on cancer chemotherapy or on glucocorticoid therapy. Clinical features may resemble bacterial pneumonia or pulmonary embolism with fever, cough, dyspnea, mild hemoptysis, and pleuritic pain. The chest x-ray may show focal peripheral infiltrates that sometimes rapidly cavitate. Because the fungus frequently grows intravascularly, chest radiograph and even perfusion lung scans may suggest pulmonary embolus, showing a wedge-shaped area of infarction. Dissemination to the central nervous system, heart, liver, and skin can occur.

Diagnosis

MORPHOLOGY AND LABORATORY IDENTIFICATION. The diagnosis of invasive infection often depends on the histopathologic demonstration of the organism in infected tissue. *Aspergillus* organisms grow in tissue as thick (5 to 8 μm) septate hyphae, which have an acute angle of branching. They may be evident in hematoxylin and eosin stained sections but are easier to see in silver-stained sections if the density of organisms is low.

The organisms are not fastidious, but a positive sputum culture does not necessarily indicate invasive infection and a negative culture does not preclude it. A positive culture of a bronchial plug from an asthmatic patient strongly suggests bronchopulmonary aspergillosis. A positive culture from a metastatic site is diagnostic of invasive aspergillosis. A positive sputum culture in an immunosuppressed patient with lesions consistent with pneumonia or brain abscess is highly suspicious and cannot be ignored. The results of blood cultures are almost uniformly negative, even in cases of endocarditis.

SKIN TEST AND SEROLOGY. Skin tests are of minimal use only in allergic bronchopulmonary aspergillosis: a wheal and flare reaction is elicited in asthmatics with or without the syndrome.

Serum precipitins are found in 70 to 90 percent of the patients with allergic bronchopulmonary aspergillosis and are also found in 15 to 20 percent of asthmatics without it. Precipitating antibodies, to one or more *Aspergillus* antigens, are almost always found in patients with aspergilloma but rarely in patients with invasive aspergillosis.

An increase in total IgE level (>1500 ng/ml) strongly suggests bronchopulmonary aspergillosis. High levels of specific IgE and IgG antibodies directed against aspergillosus antigens, as measured by radioimmunoassay, are diagnostic. Precipitins are usually positive in chronic necrotizing aspergillosis, similar to aspergilloma.

Surgical Importance. Invasive sino-orbital disease often requires aggressive debridement in combination with amphotericin B therapy. Similarly, a brain abscess such as those seen commonly after organ transplantation will rarely respond solely to drug therapy. Chronic necrotizing aspergillosis may or may not disappear on medical therapy and may require resection. Disseminated disease should be controlled prior to treatment by resection.

Significant hemoptysis is an indication for resection of a cavity with a fungus ball, if the underlying pulmonary disease is not too severe. Resection is curative, and amphotericin B is not required.[44,45] An operation is not indicated in an asymptomatic patient.

Although the diagnosis of invasive pulmonary aspergillosis can sometimes be made by transbronchial biopsy, an open biopsy of the lung may be needed for diagnosis. Aspiration or open biopsy of distant metastatic sites of infection may be required to establish the diagnosis in other instances.

Aspergillus endocarditis may present with occlusion of a major artery by a bulky embolus (eg, with a cold pulseless extremity) and thus may mimic other thromboembolic diseases. Endocarditis can occur on prosthetic valves as an early postoperative infection.

Ordinarily, operation is not used for either diagnosis or management of allergic bronchopulmonary aspergillosis.

Treatment. Invasive sino-orbital disease is treated with excision of the infected tissue. Concomitant amphotericin B may be of some value, but the drug probably does not have to be continued after the wound is healed.

Aspergillomas seldom require resection; most require no treatment.[44,45]

Amphotericin B is used for chronic necrotizing aspergillosis. It can reduce symptoms and control the infection but probably cannot cure. Resection of localized disease is curative but may be difficult because of the severity of the underlying lung abscess.

Amphotericin B is the only effective treatment of invasive pulmonary or widely disseminated aspergillosis.[46] When aggressive diagnostic methods have been used so that amphotericin B is started early, cure is possible. Glucocorticoid therapy, preferably on an alternate-day schedule, can be used successfully to treat allergic bronchopulmonary aspergillosis.[47] Liposomal amphotericin B is being evaluated.[48] It offers hope of higher doses with less toxicity. Itraconazole is the first oral agent with some activity against *Aspergillus*. It can be tried for milder nonoperable cases of chronic necrotizing aspergillosis. It has been used in small numbers of organ transplant recipients with invasive pulmonary disease.[49] Further experience is needed before it can be recommended for invasive aspergillosis.

Mucormycosis

Mucormycosis, a term used synonymously with phycomycosis and zygomycosis, refers to infection by any of several genera of fungi, including *Mucor, Rhizopus,* and *Absidia*. These organisms are ubiquitous in nature and lack any ability to invade a healthy person. Under special circumstances, these organisms invade the nose, sinuses, and other facial structures of ketoacidotic diabetics, the lungs of leukemics or transplant patients, or the necrotic body surface of burned patients.[50–52]

Etiology. Mucor, Rhizopus, and *Absidia* are the three genera of the family Mucoraceae that tend to cause human disease. Determination of the genus is done morphologically; speciation is extremely difficult. These fungi are found throughout the world and are commonly associated with decaying organic material.

Progressive facial infection in diabetics is caused by members of the genus *Rhizopus,* most commonly *R. arrhizus* or *R. oryzae*.

Pathogenesis and Pathology. Everyone is regularly exposed to airborne spores of these fungi, which settle on the skin or are inhaled. However, there is no tendency for invasion, except in the specialized settings of diabetic ketoacidosis, severe immunosuppression (especially hematologic malignancy), or severe burns. The histopathology of infected tissue reveals many polymorphonuclear cells and much necrosis. The organism tends to directly invade arteries, which causes infarction of tissue, adding to the area of necrosis. There is little granuloma formation.

Clinical Manifestations

RHINOCEREBRAL MUCORMYCOSIS. The most fulminant fungal infection of humans is rhinocerebral mucormycosis. Diabetic ketoacidosis provides a unique opportunity for *Rhizopus* species, which grow best at acid pH in a high-glucose environment.[50] Infection begins in the nose with a dark, blood-tinged discharge from both nostrils. Necrosis of the nasal septum and the turbinates occurs, with rapid spread to the paranasal sinuses. Ulceration and necrosis of the palate, periorbital cellulitis, and direct invasion of the orbit, eye, and brain can follow. Major arterial thrombosis adds to the extent of tissue destruction. Early focal neurologic findings include cranial nerve palsies. These are soon followed by generalized seizures and a deteriorating level of consciousness. The entire process may end in death within 1 week.

PULMONARY MUCORMYCOSIS. Pulmonary mucormycosis begins as acute pneumonia, with superimposed signs of pulmonary infarction. Fever, cough, and dyspnea are often accompanied by hemoptysis and pleuritic pain. The most characteristic x-ray finding is a wedge-shaped area of infiltration, which may cavitate. Most patients have had lymphoma or acute leukemia, but many cases also have been reported in transplant patients.[51,52] The disseminated disease most often presents as pulmonary disease with metastatic brain abscesses; liver, spleen, pancreas, kidney, and skin (ecthyma gangrenosum) may be involved.

CUTANEOUS MUCORMYCOSIS. Isolation of organisms from skin or wounds does not imply infection, although both local and invasive soft tissue infection has occurred. Contaminated Elastoplast has been implicated as a source of infection.[53] Patients with extensive burns can develop a rapidly fatal invasive infection.

GASTROINTESTINAL MUCORMYCOSIS. Gastrointestinal mucormycosis is a rare condition that is associated with severe protein malnutrition, especially in children. The organisms invade the bowel wall and eventually cause hemorrhage, bowel infarction, peritonitis, and death. Most cases have been discovered only at autopsy.

Diagnosis

MORPHOLOGY AND LABORATORY IDENTIFICATION. The diagnosis depends on the histologic demonstration of the broad nonseptate hyphae found in diseased tissue.

Positive cultures must be interpreted cautiously because the organisms are ubiquitous and can occasionally be recovered from the skin, sputum, and throat of healthy people.

SKIN TEST AND SEROLOGY. Skin or serologic tests are of no value in diagnosis.

Surgical Importance. Aggressive debridement of all necrotic tissue is an integral part of the management of rhinocerebral mucormycosis. It is often necessary to examine lung tissue to establish the diagnosis of pulmonary mucormycosis. The choice between transbronchial biopsy via a fiberoptic bronchoscope and open lung biopsy depends on the clinical situation.

Cutaneous mucormycosis is of particular importance in severely burned patients. Initial control of bacterial infection may be followed by invasive fungal disease. Cutaneous disease requires systemic treatment and total local debridement carried out daily until biopsies demonstrate the absence of the fungus. Reconstruction of the defect should be delayed to ensure control of the infection.

Treatment. Rhinocerebral mucormycosis has an 80 percent mortality. Successful therapy must include control of ketoacidosis, debridement of necrotic tissue, and use of amphotericin B.

Pulmonary mucormycosis is also usually fatal, although successful outcome after lung resection and amphotericin B therapy has been reported.

Candidiasis

Candidiasis refers to infection by any species of the genus *Candida*. *Candida* organisms are part of the normal bowel flora of humans and are also constant inhabitants of the mouth, pharynx, and upper airways. A wide variety of clinical illnesses can be caused by these organisms, including mucocutaneous infections, localized peritonitis, and invasive infections with septicemia and seeding of kidney, meninges, heart, joints, and other distant sites.[54,55] Invasive infections occur only in patients with altered local or systemic immunity. Defects of cell-mediated immunity predispose to mucocutaneous disease. Phagocytic defects (reduced neutrophil number or function often in concert with breaks in skin or mucosal barriers) are necessary for deep invasion.

Etiology. Clinical candidiasis is most frequently caused by *C. albicans*. Other *Candida* species, including *C. niger, C. glabrata, C. krusei, C. parapsilosis, C. tropicalis, C. stellatoidea,* and *C. guilliermondii,* can also be involved in human infections.

Pathogenesis and Pathology. Although *Candida* organisms ordinarily live in equilibrium with their host and do not cause disease, a variety of local or systemic factors can alter that harmony. The absence of competing bacterial flora permits local overgrowth of *Candida* in the oral cavity of infants, resulting in thrush. Alteration of vaginal flora by pregnancy, diabetes, or broad spectrum antibiotics may lead to vaginal candidiasis. Moist macerated skin in intertriginous areas is especially subject to *Candida* overgrowth, resulting in candidal dermatitis.

Invasive candidiasis is the most important clinical form of the disease. Recognized predisposing factors include malnutrition, broad spectrum antibiotics, systemic steroids, hyperalimentation, indwelling catheters, and immunosuppression. Invasion of the bloodstream can be transient and self-limited or can result in seeding of distant organs, establishment of multiple microabscesses, and death from progressive infection.

The organism normally grows on body surfaces as a yeast. When an overgrowth of yeast occurs in a given area, there is an associated acute inflammatory reaction. When tissue invasion occurs, sprout mycelia develop by serial budding and both yeast and pseudohyphae can be seen. In recently established microabscesses, yeast forms predominate and there is a polymorphonuclear response similar to the response to a bacterial abscess. In chronic ulcerations and more established metastatic foci of infection, pseudohyphae predominate and there may be some granulomatous response.

Clinical Manifestations

CUTANEOUS CANDIDIASIS. Cutaneous candidiasis involves the moist intertriginous areas of the groin, inframammary and gluteal folds, axillae, interdigital spaces, and adjacent areas of skin. Paronychial infection and chronic infection of the nails afflict those whose hands require frequent immersion. The lesions are generally moist, erythematous, and pruritic, with satellite vesicles surrounding the sharp margins.

MUCOCUTANEOUS CANDIDIASIS. Thrush consists of oral mucosal patches of a white exudate composed entirely of *Candida* yeast and hyphae. The mucosa underneath is red and oozing and may become ulcerated. Oral candidiasis occurs in people with diabetes, in asthmatics who are treated with inhalational steroids, and in patients being treated with systemic steroids, broad spectrum antibiotics, and antineoplastic drugs (who are at risk of developing invasive disease).

Candida esophagitis may occur as a direct extension of oral candidiasis; patients usually complain of dysphagia. The diagnosis can be confirmed by esophagoscopy or sometimes by barium swallow, which shows a ragged mucosa but no loss of esophageal distensibility.

Diabetes and antibiotic therapy also predispose to vaginal candidiasis, as do pregnancy and the postmenopausal state. The mucosa is red and covered with patches of whitish exudate. Pustular lesions and ulcerations occur in severe cases. Pruritis may be severe and there is a white to yellow vaginal discharge.

Candida organisms can be part of the bronchial flora in all chronic lung conditions including chronic bronchitis and bronchiectasis and may contribute to chronic productive cough in some instances. *Candida* yeast rarely cause severe pneumonia.[56]

Chronic mucocutaneous candidiasis is a distinct clinical syndrome with widespread superficial infection of nails, skin, and mucous membranes. It occurs primarily in children with immunodeficiency diseases or polyendocrine deficiencies.

INVASIVE CANDIDIASIS. Overgrowth of *Candida* organisms in the mouth, esophagus, bowel, bladder, or on the skin can result in deep penetration into the tissue and intermittent seeding of organisms into the bloodstream.[57] Indwelling plastic intravenous catheters, especially when used for hyperalimentation, may permit direct seeding. *Candida* esophagitis near the esophagogastric junction is common in diabetics who are also immunosuppressed.

Transient fungemia with *Candida* is probably of little significance in a normal host. However, the same patients who have overgrowth on mucosal surfaces or who require long-term intravenous therapy often have serious underlying diseases and are being treated with antibiotics, steroids, and immunosuppressive agents. In these patients, hematogenous spread of *Candida* organisms may result in the establishment of multiple microabscesses in multiple organs. About half of these patients have an underlying lymphoma or leukemia.[58] The clinical picture includes fever, chills, and renal failure. Macronodular skin lesions and endopthalmitis may be clues to the diagnosis. Seventy-five percent of these patients die despite therapy.

Patients with the septicemic form of candidiasis often have multiple cerebral microabscesses. Other patients may develop meningitis after an episode of candidemia. Any neurologic signs in patients at risk for systemic invasive candidiasis should be investigated to rule out infection of their central nervous system with *Candida.*

Candida endocarditis occurs among drug addicts, on the damaged valves of patients with previous bacterial endocarditis, and as an early postoperative infection on prosthetic valves. Vegetations are large and bulky, and embolic events often involve major arteries. Patients with *Candida* septicemia generally develop numerous cardiac microabscesses rather than endocarditis.

Intra-abdominal *Candida* infections may be a complication of peritoneal dialysis or of secondary bacterial peritonitis treated with broad spectrum antibiotics.[59,60] The prognosis is fair to good with relatively low doses of amphotericin B, but only if the perforation is recognized and surgically sealed and chemotherapy is promptly instituted. If the culture report of *Candida* is overlooked in the polymicrobial infection, lethal candidiasis can result.[61] Most complicated surgical patients who develop candidemia will have been treated with antibiotics and hyperalimentation and may have an underlying malignancy. Surveillance cultures will have revealed a drain tract, urinary catheter, or wound from which *Candida* could be cultured some time before candidemia occurred. Candidemia cannot be ignored under these circumstances. In fact, some investigators have encouraged beginning treatment when positive cultures have been obtained from multiple sites in susceptible patients.

Diagnosis

MORPHOLOGY AND LABORATORY IDENTIFICATION. The definitive diagnosis probably requires histopathologic confirmation of tissue invasion. The distinctive feature is the combination of yeast, pseudohyphae, and hyphae in the tissues.

This organism is relatively easy to culture. *Candida albicans* can be distinguished from other yeast by its ability to form sprout mycelium after incubation in serum for 2 hours.

Although cultural identification is easy, assessing the significance of a positive culture is extraordinarily difficult. *Candida* organisms are regularly found in stool, sputum, mouth, throat, bronchial washings, and also in the urine of patients with indwelling catheters—all without implying disease. Positive blood cultures most often indicate invasive disease, except when fungemia associated with an intravenous catheter disappears after removal of the device. *Candida* cultures from wounds and drain sites sometimes forecast deep tissue infections and should not be ignored.

SKIN TEST AND SEROLOGY. *Candida* organisms are part of our normal flora; therefore a positive skin test or serologic evidence of an antibody response to the organism has little meaning.

Surgical Importance. Invasive candidiasis is an important opportunistic infection and occurs in debilitated patients who are receiving hyperalimentation. It is especially common among patients who have had multiple abdominal operations and long courses of broad spectrum antibiotics.

Candida peritonitis is of obvious surgical importance. In the absence of peritoneal dialysis, it implies a breach in the integrity of the gastrointestinal tract.

Candida endocarditis occurs on prosthetic valves in the early postoperative period or on previously damaged valves.

Therapy. Oral candidiasis can be treated with oral nystatin or better with clotrimazole troches, which have a longer contact time with oral mucosa. *Candida* esophagitis can also be treated with topical therapy, but if there is no response after 48 hours, the infection should be treated with intravenous amphotericin B in doses of 0.25 to 0.5 mg/kg/day for 2 weeks. Vaginal or skin infections can be controlled with local topical therapy. *Candida* in the bladder can be treated by discontinuance of catheter drainage; when this cannot be done, irrigation with a solution of 50 mg of amphotericin B in a 1-liter solution of 5 percent glucose may be helpful.

Meningitis requires the use of amphotericin B. Endocarditis usually requires a combination of amphotericin B and operative removal of the valve. If there is clear-cut evidence of invasive candidiasis including hematogenous skin lesions, endophthalmitis, or multiple positive blood cultures, full treatment with amphotericin B is necessary. In systemic candidiasis, a combination of flucytosine and amphotericin B may be helpful, although this has not been well documented.[18]

Fluconazole is a nontoxic anti-*Candida* agent now available for oral and intravenous use. For three reasons its use in the Surgical Intensive Care Unit (SICU) is rapidly increasing: (1) many patients have risk factors for disseminated candidiasis and have persistent fevers; (2) cultures of sputum and urine are often positive, especially with Foley catheters and broad spectrum antibiotics—both nearly universal; and (3) there are no good diagnostic tests to prove or disprove invasive *Candida* infections. Whether the current enthusiastic widespread use of fluconazole in the SICU is warranted by the magnitude of the problem is controversial. Better diagnostic tests (not in sight) are greatly needed to better target therapy and to improve the quality of clinical studies. A 2-year study from the pre-fluconazole era found disseminated candidiasis in 14 of 1104 autopsies.[62] Eight of fourteen patients had positive blood and/or deep tissue cultures premortem. Only six patients without these premortem findings had disseminated candidiasis at autopsy. Fluconazole as routine therapy for all febrile SICU patients may not be indicated, especially since resistant *Candida* species, particularly *C. krusei,* can colonize patients treated with fluconazole. Better diagnostic tests for invasive candidiasis are badly needed to improve the quality of clinical studies.

Prevention. *Candida* seems to be an infection of endogenous origin that benefits from changes in ecologic balance between host defenses and competitive bacteria. Traditionally, one is advised to prevent candidiasis by avoidance of radiation, immunosuppression, antibiotics, indwelling catheters, and radical surgery. Sometimes these agents are necessary. Oral nystatin in high doses appears to be useful in reducing the numbers of *Candida* in the intestine and can reduce the incidence of fungemia in various populations of immunosuppressed patients. Oral imidazoles, especially fluconazole and itraconazole, may prove to be useful in preventing *Candida* colonization and subsequent deep *Candida* infections.[61] When fluconazole is used there is a potential for increased colonization with *C. krusei,* which has resistance.

FUNGAL DISEASES ACQUIRED BY SUBCUTANEOUS INOCULATION

Sporotrichosis

Sporotrichosis refers to any infection by the thermal dimorphic fungus *Sporothrix schenckii.* Suppuration, ulceration, and a slow proximal lymphatic spread follow subcutaneous inoculation of spores. A rare pulmonary form is caused by inhalation of the spores.

Etiology and Epidemiology. *Sporothrix schenckii* is a thermal dimorphic fungus. It is distributed worldwide in association with decaying vegetation, most notably rotting wood, sphagnum moss, and rich humus soil.

Pathogenesis and Pathology. The organism grows at the site of inoculation and spreads proximally along the lymphatic system. The skin overlying the nodules may reveal pseudoepithelioid proliferation. The nodules themselves have a mixed granulomatous and suppurative reaction similar to that seen in blastomycosis.

Clinical Manifestations

CUTANEOUS AND LYMPHATIC SPOROTRICHOSIS. Cutaneous and lymphatic sporotrichosis is an occupational disease of gardeners and others who are commonly traumatized by contaminated thorns, branches, and wood splinters. Epidemics among underground miners and forestry workers were caused by contaminated support timbers and sphagnum moss, respectively.[63]

A minor puncture wound, usually on the hand or foot, directly introduces the spores into the subcutaneous tissues. A small nodule develops, grows slowly, and attaches to the overlying skin as it becomes partially necrotic. Superficial ulceration (the sporotrichotic chancre) usually follows the initial inoculation by 2 to 3 weeks.

The course of the infection varies, often with periods of activity followed by regression. Eventually, spontaneous resolution may occur, especially in patients with fixed cutaneous sporotrichosis, with only a primary lesion.

PULMONARY SPOROTRICHOSIS. Inhalation of these spores occasionally results in a chronic pulmonary infection similar to other inhalational fungal infections.[64,65] Dissemination is rare.

Diagnosis

MORPHOLOGY AND LABORATORY IDENTIFICATION. Histopathologic specimens only rarely demonstrate the yeast, which are 3 to 5 μm in size and oval in shape. Although the clinical diagnosis of the lymphocutaneous form is easy, definitive diagnosis of all forms depends on culture of the organism.

SKIN TEST AND SEROLOGY. Sporotrichin is a skin test antigen that is not usually used in the diagnosis of individual cases, although it is useful in epidemiologic studies.

Available serologic tests include agglutination, immunodiffusion, and complement-fixation tests. High titers of agglutinating or complement-fixing antibody suggest an infection.

Surgical Importance. If the lymphocutaneous form of sporotrichosis is suspected, a biopsy of one of the nodules should not be taken. The yeast is seldom found histopathologically, and the increased tendency for spread after a biopsy is too great. The lesion should be aspirated for a culture.

Resection of chronically infected lung tissue has been part of the management of many successfully treated cases of pulmonary sporotrichosis.

Therapy. The lymphocutaneous form of the disease should be treated with a saturated solution of potassium iodide in doses of up to 10 drops three times a day for at least 4 weeks after the visible lesions have healed. Itraconazole may also be effective.

Pulmonary sporotrichosis may be treated with amphotericin B with variable efficacy. Itraconazole can also be tried. Resectional surgery may play a role in therapy of some localized infections. Cases are so few and available information is so anecdotal that it is difficult to make any strong recommendation about therapy.

Mycetoma

Mycetoma (maduromycosis) is the result of subcutaneous inoculation of some fungal spores. The resulting reaction produces swelling, multiple abscesses, and sinus tracts with purulent drainage that contains granules or grains.

Etiology. Mycetoma is caused by a wide variety of soil organisms including many true fungi (eumycotic mycetoma) and also several species of *Actinomyces* (actinomycotic mycetoma) (see Chap. 27).

Epidemiology. Mycetoma is primarily a tropical disease of India, Central Africa, and Mexico. *Allescheria boydii* is the most commonly reported agent in the southern United States. Mycetoma is initiated by the direct inoculation of spores into subcutaneous tissues. It is most common in rural areas among malnourished persons who go shoeless. Although mycetoma occurs most commonly on the foot (madura foot), it may also occur on the hand, the buttocks, and other areas.

Pathogenesis and Pathology. Purulent abscesses develop that burrow deeply into the involved tissues, invading soft tissue, fascia, and bone. Extensive fibrosis develops, and sinus tracts communicate between individual abscesses and also drain to the surface. Histopathologic examination shows multiple abscesses, which contain many neutrophils and occasional granules made up of the organisms themselves, the morphologic characteristics of which permit etiologic diagnosis. The tissue surrounding the abscesses contains granulomatous elements and much fibrosis.

Clinical Manifestations. The primary lesion is a small, painless, subcutaneous swelling, which slowly enlarges in a tumor-like fashion. Progression is slow, but eventually the swelling will suppurate and drain to the surface. When the lesion is on the foot, the entire foot eventually becomes swollen and studded with multiple sinus tracts. The pus expressed from the orifices of the sinus tracts reveals the small granules, which may be up to 5 mm in size. Eventually, the arch of the foot is lost and the sole becomes convex.

Mycetoma usually remains localized to an extremity. There are no constitutional symptoms nor even regional adenopathy. Extensive involvement, while it does not impair general health, can be disfiguring and disabling.

Diagnosis. Demonstration of granules permits a general diagnosis of mycetoma in a patient with a localized area of multiple abscesses and draining sinuses. Experienced laboratories can identify the exact agent. Of particular importance is the differentiation of actinomycotic from eumycotic mycetoma, because the former may respond to antibacterial therapy.

A deep biopsy sample is best for culture because superficial material is often contaminated by multiple bacteria and fungi. Granules obtained from such a biopsy are washed, crushed, and plated at 25C aerobically, and at 37C both aerobically and anaerobically.

Skin test and serology are not useful in the diagnosis of mycetoma.

Surgical Importance. Early cases of actinomycotic mycetoma can sometimes be cured with limited drainage and antibiotics. Because mycetoma can remain a localized process for a long time, a conservative approach is generally taken. Amputation is necessary for some advanced cases.

Therapy. Actinomycotic mycetoma may respond to penicillin or tetracycline. Eumycotic mycetoma is resistant to chemotherapy because the infection invades deep into the soft tissues and bone. Local excision is rarely helpful, even in early cases. Ketoconazole or the newer azoles may be helpful adjuncts.

REFERENCES

1. Conant NF, Smith DT, Baker RD, Callaway JD: Manual of Clinical Mycology. Philadelphia, Saunders, 1971.
2. Emmons CW, Binford CH, Utz JP: Medical Mycology, 3rd ed. Philadephia, Lea & Febiger, 1977.
3. Rippon JW: Medical Mycology: The Pathogenic Fungi and the Pathogenic Actinomycetes. Philadelphia, Saunders, 1974.
4. Schaffner A, Davis CE, Schaffner T, et al: In vitro susceptibility of fungi to killing by neutrophil granulocytes discriminates between primary pathogenicity and opportunism. J Clin Invest 78:511, 1986.
5. Wheat LJ, Connolly-Stringfield P, Kohler RB, et al: *Histoplasma capsulatum* polysaccharide antigen detection in diagnosis and management of disseminated histoplasmosis in patients with acquired immunodeficiency syndrome. Am J Med 87:396, 1989.
6. Kaufman L, Standard P, Padhye A: Exoantigen tests for the immunoidentification of fungal cultures. Mycopathologia 82:3, 1983.

Histoplasmosis

7. Howard DH: Intracellular growth of *Histoplasma capsulatum.* J Bacteriol 89:518, 1965.
8. Goodwin RA Jr, Des Prez RM: State of the art: histoplasmosis. Am Rev Respir Dis 117:929, 1978.
9. Goodwin RA Jr, Owens FT, Snell JD, et al: Chronic pulmonary histoplasmosis. Medicine (Baltimore) 55: 413, 1976.
10. Loyd JE, Tillman BF, Atkinson JB, et al: Mediastinal fibrosis complicating histoplasmosis. Medicine (Baltimore) 67:295, 1988.
11. Sarosi GA, Voth DW, Dahl BA, et al: Disseminated histoplasmosis: results of long-term follow-up. A Centers for Disease Control cooperative mycoses study. Ann Intern Med 75:511, 1971.
12. Davies SF, Khan M, Sarosi GA: Disseminated histoplasmosis in immunologically suppressed patients. Occurrence in a nonendemic area. Am J Med 64:94, 1978.
13. Smith JW, Utz JP: Progressive disseminated histoplasmosis: a prospective study of 26 patients. Ann Intern Med 76:557, 1972.
14. Sarosi GA, Johnson PC: Disseminated histoplasmosis in patients infected with human immunodeficiency virus. Clin Infect Dis 14:S60, 1992.
15. Dukes RJ, Grimlan CV, Dines DE, et al: Esophageal involvement with mediastinal granuloma. JAMA 236:2313, 1976.
16. Strimlan CV, Dines DE, Payne WS: Mediastinal granuloma. Mayo Clin Proc 50:702, 1975.
17. Parker JD, Sarosi GA, Doto IL, et al: Treatment of chronic pulmonary histoplasmosis. N Engl J Med 283:225, 1970.
18. Naylor BA: Low-dose amphotericin B therapy for acute pulmonary histoplasmosis. Chest 71:404, 1977.

19. Dismukes WE, Bradsher RW, Cloud GC, et al: Itraconazole therapy for blastomycosis and histoplasmosis. Am J Med 93:489, 1992.

Blastomycosis

20. Laskey W, Sarosi GA: Endogenous activation in blastomycosis. Ann Intern Med 88:50, 1978.
21. Sarosi GA, Hammerman KJ, Tosh FE, Kronenberg RC: Clinical features of acute pulmonary blastomycosis. N Engl J Med 290:540, 1974.
22. Poe RH, Vassallo CL, Plessinger VA, Witt RL: Pulmonary blastomycosis versus carcinoma—a challenging differential. Am J Med Sci 263:145, 1972.
23. Medoff G, Kobayashi GS: Strategies in the treatment of systemic fungal infections. N Engl J Med 302:145, 1980.

Coccidioidomycosis

24. Drutz DJ, Catanzaro A: Coccidioidomycosis. Part I. Am Rev Respir Dis 117:559, 1978.
25. Drutz DJ, Catanzaro A: Coccidioidomycosis. Part II. Am Rev Respir Dis 117:727, 1978.
26. Bayer AS, Yoshikawa TT, Galpin JE, Guze LB: Unusual syndromes of coccidioidomycosis: diagnostic and therapeutic considerations; a report of 10 cases and review of the English literature. Medicine (Baltimore) 55:131, 1976.
27. Rutala PJ, Smith JW: Coccidioidomycosis in potentially compromised hosts: the effect of immunosupressive therapy in dissemination. Am J Med Sci 275:283, 1978.
28. Fish DG, Mapel NM, Galgiani JN, et al: Coccidioidomycosis during human immunodeficiency virus infection. A review of 77 patients. Medicine (Baltimore) 69:384, 1990.
29. Ellner JJ, Bennett JE: Chronic meningitis. Medicine (Baltimore) 55:341, 1976.
30. Diamond RD, Bennett JE: A subcutaneous reservoir for intrathecal therapy of fungal meningitis. N Engl J Med 288:186, 1973.
31. Stevens D: Miconazole in the treatment of systemic fungal infections. Am Rev Respir Dis 116:801, 1977.
32. Catanzaro A, Einstein H, Levine B, et al: Ketoconazole for treatment of disseminated coccidioidomycosis. Ann Intern Med 96:436, 1982.

Paracoccidioidomycosis

33. Pan-American Health Organization 1972: First Pan-American Symposium on paracoccidioidomycosis. Medellin, Colombia 25–27 October 1971. Scientific Publication No 2540. Washington, DC, World Health Organization.
34. Restrepo A, Robledo M, Giraldo R, et al: The gamut of paracoccidioidomycosis. Am J Med 61:33, 1976.
35. Cuce LC, Wroclawski EL, Sampaio SAP: Treatment of paracoccidioidomycosis with ketoconazole. Rev Inst Med Trop Sao Paulo 23(2):82, 1981.

Cryptococcosis

36. Berger MP, Paz J: Diagnosis of cryptococcal meningitis. JAMA 236:2517, 1976.
37. Diamond RD, Bennett JE: Prognostic factors in cryptococcal meningitis. A study in 111 cases. Ann Intern Med 80:176, 1974.
38. Kaplan MH, Rosen PP, Armstrong D: Cryptococcosis in a cancer hospital: clinical and pathological correlates in 46 patients. Cancer 39:2265, 1977.
39. Schroter GPJ, Temple DR, Husberg BS, et al. Cryptococcosis after renal transplantation: report of ten cases. Surgery 79:268, 1976.
40. Bennett JE, Dismukes WE, Duma RJ: A comparison of amphotericin B alone and combined with flucytosine in the treatment of cryptococcal meningitis. N Engl J Med 310:126, 1979.
41. Larson RA, Leal MA, Chan LS: Fluconazole compared with amphotericin B plus flucytosine for cryptococcal meningitis in AIDS. A randomized trial. Ann Intern Med 113:183, 1990.

Aspergillosis

42. British Tuberculosis Association: Aspergillus in persistent lung cavities after tuberculosis. Tubercle (London) 49:1, 1968.
43. Binder RE, Faling LJ, Pugatch RD, et al: Chronic necrotizing pulmonary aspergillosis: a discrete clinical entity. Medicine (Baltimore) 60:109, 1982.
44. British Tuberculosis Association: Aspergilloma and residual tuberculosis cavities—the results of a resurvey. Tubercle (London) 51:227, 1970.
45. Varkey B, Rose HD: Pulmonary aspergilloma: a rational approach to treatment. Am J Med 61:626, 1976.
46. Aisner J, Wiernik PH, Schimpff SC: Treatment of invasive aspergillosis: relation of early diagnosis and treatment to response. Ann Intern Med 86:539, 1977.
47. Rosenberg M, Patterson R, Roberts M, Wang J: The assessment of immunologic and clinical changes occurring during corticosteroid therapy for allergic bronchopulmonary aspergillosis. Am J Med 64:599, 1978.
48. Ringden O, Meunier F, Tollemar J, et al: Efficacy of amphotericin B encapsulated in liposomes (AmBisome) in the treatment of invasive fungal infections in immunocompromised patients. J Antimicrob Chemother 28:73, 1991.
49. Denning D, Tucker RM, Hanson LH, et al: Treatment of invasive aspergillosis with itraconazole. Am J Med 86:791, 1989.

Mucormycosis

50. Abramson E, Wilson D, Arby RA: Rhinocerebral phycomycosis in association with diabetic ketoacidosis. Report of two cases and a review of clinical and experimental experience with amphotericin B therapy. Ann Intern Med 66:735, 1967.
51. Hammer GS, Bottone EJ, Hirschman SZ: Mucormycosis in a transplant recipient. Am J Clin Pathol 64:389, 1975.

52. Meyer RD, Rosen P, Armstrong D: Phycomycosis complicating leukemia and lymphoma. Ann Intern Med 77:871, 1972.
53. Gartenberg G, Bottone EJ, Keusch GT, Weitzman I: Hospital-acquired mucormycosis (*Rhizopus rhiaopodiformis*) of skin and subcutaneous tissue: epidemiology, mycology, and treatment. N Engl J Med 299:1115, 1978.

Candidial Infections

54. Edwards JE Jr, Lehrer RI, Stiehm ER, et al: Severe candidal infections: clinical perspective, immune defense mechanisms, and current concepts of therapy. Ann Intern Med 89:91, 1978.
55. Murray HW, Fialk MA, Roberts RB: *Candida* arthritis: a manifestation of disseminated candidiasis. Am J Med 60:587, 1976.
56. Masur H, Rosen PP, Armstrong D: Pulmonary disease caused by *Candida* species. Am J Med 63:914, 1977.
57. Gaines JD, Remington JS: Disseminated candidiasis in the surgical patient. Surgery 72:730, 1972.
58. Bodey GP: Fungal infections complicating acute leukemia. J Chronic Dis 19:667, 1966.
59. Bayer AS, Blumenkrantz MJ, Montgomerie JZ, et al: *Candida* peritonitis. Report of 22 cases and review of the English literature. Am J Med 61:832, 1976.
60. Solomkin JS, Flohr AB, Quie PG, Simmons RL: The role of *Candida* in intraperitoneal infections. Surgery 88:524, 1980.
61. Bernhardt HE, Orlando JC, Benfield JR, et al: Disseminated candidiasis in surgical patients. Surg Gynecol Obstet 134:819, 1972.
62. Goodman JL, Winston DJ, Greenfield RA, et al. A controlled trial of fluconazole to prevent fungal infections in patients undergoing bone marrow transplantation. N Engl J Med 326:845, 1992.

Sporotrichosis

63. Powell KE, Taylor A, Phillips BJ, et al: Cutaneous sporotrichosis in forestry workers. Epidemic due to contaminated *Sphagnum* moss. JAMA 240:232, 1978.
64. Jay SJ, Platt MR, Reynolds RC: Primary pulmonary sporotrichosis. Am Rev Respir Dis 115:1051, 1977.
65. Mohr JA, Patterson CD, Eaton BG, et al: Primary pulmonary sporotrichosis. Am Rev Respir Dis 106:260, 1972.

BIBLIOGRAPHY

Emmons CW, Binford CH, Utz JP: Medical Mycology, 3rd ed. Philadelphia, Lea & Febiger, 1977.

Mandell GL, Doublas RG Jr, Bennett JR (eds): Mycoses, Section F (Part III). In: Principles and Practice of Infectious Diseases, 2nd ed. New York, Wiley, 1985.

Medoff G, Kobayashi GS: Strategies in the treatment of systemic fungal infections. N Engl J Med 302:145, 1980.

Odds FC: Candida and Candidosis. Baltimore, University Park Press, 1979.

Rippon JW: Medical Mycology: The Pathogenic Fungi and the Pathogenic Actinomycetes. Philadelphia, Saunders, 1974.

Viral Infections

CHAPTER 11

Monto Ho

VIRUSES AND THEIR RELATIONSHIP TO SURGERY

Viruses are unique classes of infectious agents that infect both eukaryotes, prokaryotes, protozoa, plants, and animals. They were originally distinguished from bacteria by their small size and the fact that they were "filterable." The main characteristics of viruses are that they are obligate intracellular microbial agents that contain either DNA or RNA as genetic material, but not both. They lack the enzymatic and structural elements essential for their own replication and use the metabolic machinery of the host cell for the synthesis of the viral subunits. The genetic characteristics of the viruses are determined by their own nucleic acid and not that of the host cell. In that sense viruses are independent, continuously replicating, living agents.

Tremendous advances have been made in the basic molecular, structural, and functional understanding of animal viruses in the last 20 years.[1] In addition, viruses have also become more important in many clinical disciplines, including surgery. There are four reasons. (1) Antivirals, after a late start, have become useful in clinical practice and are producing an impact on it. (2) New viruses have been discovered to cause important diseases. The most dramatic example is the discovery of a completely new virus, the human immunodeficiency virus (HIV),[2] which causes HIV disease syndromes and AIDS. (3) New viral agents have been found to cause known diseases (eg, hepatitis C virus).[3] Previously well known viruses have gained importance as immunosuppressive agents and procedures have been introduced. Examples are diseases caused by members of the herpesviruses, such as cytomegalovirus and Epstein-Barr virus, parvoviruses (B17), rotovirus, and Norwalk virus. Steady progress has also been made in the discovery of other new virus agents of less importance to surgery in areas such as arthropod-borne viruses.

VIRUS-CELL INTERACTIONS AND PATHOGENESIS

Typically, viruses attach to susceptible host cells by a specific mechanism involving a virus attachment protein (VAP) (antireceptor) on virus surfaces and a receptor on the host cell surface. Receptor specificity is an important (but not the only) determinant of virus permissiveness for a particular cell, tissue, or organ. The specificity may at times be exquisite. Receptor proteins on host cells may be so specific that they can distinguish even different strains. The classification of staphylococcal strains may be based on their susceptibility patterns to specific phages or viruses.[4] A highly dynamic area of current research in human virology is the identification and characterization of viral receptors on host cells. The characteristics of such receptors are quite diverse. In a number of cases such proteins are truly important to the host.[5] For example, the complement 3D (C3D) receptor (CR2) on B lymphocytes is the receptor protein for Epstein-Barr virus. The receptor of HIV is an essential protein of a class of T lymphocytes, the CD4 protein. Rabies virus is thought to absorb via the acetylcholine receptor and intercellular adhesion molecule 1 (ICAM-1) is thought to be the receptor for the most important common cold virus group, the rhinoviruses. In other cases the VAP of cells may not have any defined cellular function such as receptors for the hemagglutinin of influenza virus or the VAPs of the picornaviruses. Attachment of a virus to the cell allows the virus or its nucleic acid to penetrate the cell membrane and initiate the replicative cycle. In some cases, attachment also initiates immediate reactions of biologic significance. In the case of HIV, attachment to a number of adjacent CD4 T cells by gp120 of HIV allows fusion of the membranes to be initiated, which is one mechanism by which such cells may be destroyed.[6] The destruction of T cells is the direct cause of immune system decompensation in HIV/AIDS.

Once the virus has attached and penetrated the cell, it may have to go through a series of conformational changes (uncoating) that prepare the virus for subsequent replication (for an example of the morphological aspect of viral replication in cells, see Fig. 11–1). Sometimes conformational changes require proteolytic enzymes, which may be important components of the virus, such as neuraminidase in the case of influenza virus.

After penetration and uncoating, the strategy of viral replication is dependent on the nucleic acid components of the virus. A *plus sense* RNA virus contains an RNA that can act directly as a messenger RNA in the cell. It can proceed to synthesize the necessary protein subunits for the virus using the available cellular structures and metabolites for protein synthesis. Examples of this are Picornaviridae, which includes the enteroviruses and rhinoviruses. A *negative sense* RNA virus, such as influenza and other myxoviruses, contains the complementary strand of functional messenger RNA (mRNA). An RNA-dependent RNA polymerase must be provided by the virus itself to transcribe the necessary plus strand. A third and very intriguing strategy of RNA replication is represented by HIV and other retroviruses. Its RNA cannot directly act as a mRNA or be directly transcribed to mRNA; instead it must first be transcribed to DNA through the operation of an RNA-dependent DNA polymerase, or *reverse transcriptase,* which is an important component of the virion. The virally encoded DNA is then translocated into the host cell nucleus where it becomes integrated into the chromosome DNA as a *provirus.* The infection may be arrested at this stage for an indefinite period, during which it becomes a true "latent" infection. Further processing of this provirus to mRNA, essential for initiating what is called a "productive" or "lytic" cycle of infection, is similar to the transcription of host DNA. The mRNA transcribed goes on to code for the synthesis of viral subunits, which results in the release of many progeny viruses. There is at present no

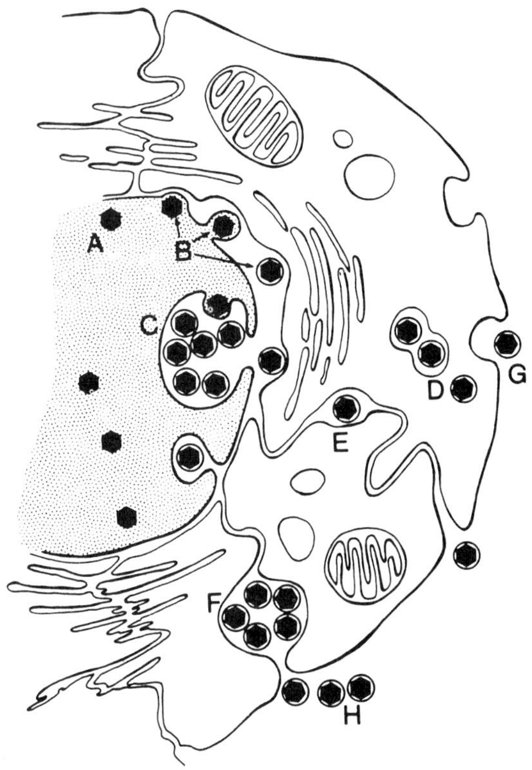

Figure 11–1. Envelopment and release of herpesvirus. Replication of viral DNA occurs in the nucleus. Viral proteins are synthesized in the cytoplasm and transported to the nucleus, where assembly takes place. Virus approaches the nuclear membrane (A), which thickens and progressively envelops the nucleocapsid (B). The viral envelope pinches off, leaving the nuclear membrane intact and the enveloped virus free in the perinuclear cisterna. The nucleocapsid can also acquire an envelope by budding into nuclear vacuoles (B). These vacuoles appear to be indentations of the nuclear membrane and are continuous with the perinuclear cisterna (C). The enveloped virus then is transported through the cytoplasm in vacuoles (D), which fuse with the surface membrane to release the virus to the extracellular space (G). Alternatively, the virus reaches the cell surface by traversing the cisternae of the endoplasmic reticulum (E, F) to the cell surface (H). *(From Jawetz E, Melnick JL, Adelberg EA: A Review of Medical Microbiology, 14th ed. Los Altos, CA, Lange Medical Publications, 1980.)*

way to attack or eliminate the DNA provirus, which remains latent and integrated in the chromosomes. In this situation, the host cell may show no outward signs of infection. But latent infection may be activated by poorly understood mechanisms to become a productive infection accompanied by virus production and destruction of host cells.

In the case of DNA viruses, host cell enzymes may be used to transcribe DNA to mRNA in the nucleus. Most such viruses (as herpesviruses) replicate in the nucleus. A unique exception is the vaccinia virus whose viral DNA can replicate in the cytoplasm.

Acute and Persistent Viral Infection

In the past, most viral diseases were considered acute infections which result in complete recovery and prolonged immunity (eg, measles, chickenpox, and rubella). A few viral diseases were known to result in permanent sequelae and others in death (eg, poliomyelitis and rabies). It is now apparent that most viruses produce acute or lytic infection resulting in the death (*lysis*) of the cell and production of virions. Other virus infections, however, may be nonproductive (Table 11–1). Complete virions are not produced but the virus genome may be partially expressed. That is, some virus directed cellular or virus structural proteins may be made. Such nonproductive infections are frequently persistent and chronic rather than acute. The nonproductive infection itself may be called latent, abortive, inapparent, or subclinical, depending on the parameter measured.

Latent viral infections are a specific form of persistent infection, which at the cellular level are characterized by the persistence of the viral genome in the infected cell and the replication of the genome along with the multiplying cell.

Translated into clinical manifestations in the host, acute lytic infections represent acute viral syndromes, with which we are most familiar. The virus replicates intensely in infected host cells, stimulates inflammatory responses, and produces a viral disease syndrome. Effective immunity, particularly neutralizing antibodies, stimulated by the large amounts of virus replicated, may then neutralize most or all of the viruses produced and the infection is terminated.

However, in some infections, not all viruses in the host are neutralized and some persist in specialized host cells. These persistent infections may later produce problems, particularly when the persistent infection is reactivated or triggered into the lytic cycle. Some clinically important syndromes caused by persistent viruses are listed in Table 11–2. A number of persistent infections by viruses of particular importance to surgery will be discussed further later: the herpesviruses, the hepatitis viruses, and HIV. Malignancies associated with EBV, HBV, and HCV are discussed in the sections on herpesviruses and on HBV and HCV. Human papillomavirus (HPV) types 16 and 18 genomes have been found to persist either as episomal forms or chromosomally integrated in carcinomas of the uterine cervix.

TABLE 11–1. TYPES OF VIRAL INFECTION: CELLULAR LEVEL

1. Productive infection: infection results in production of complete virions and lysis or death of cells (*lytic cycle*).
2. Nonproductive infections: complete virions not produced, but virus is absorbed and partial replication takes place, and infection *persists*.
   a. Latent infection: viral genome persists and replicates as cell multiplies. Varying degree of viral gene expression; characteristic *latency-associated genes* expressed.
   b. Other persistent viral infections: abortive infection, chronic infection, "slow" infection, etc

TABLE 11–2. CLINICALLY IMPORTANT SYNDROMES CAUSED BY PERSISTENT VIRUSES

I. Inflammatory diseases
   A. CMV—mononucleosis, pneumonitis, hepatitis, retinitis, etc
   B. HSV—oral herpes, genital herpes
   C. Hepatitis viruses—HBV, HCV, HDV
   D. "Slow" encephalopathic viruses:
      JC: progressive multifocal leukoencephalopathy
      Jakob–Creutzfeldt virus (kuru)
      measles virus: subacute sclerosing panencephalitis
   E. HIV/AIDS
II. Benign tumors
   A. Papillomaviruses; warts (genital warts and cervical cancer)
III. Malignant tumors
   A. EBV: Burkitt's lymphoma, nasopharyngeal carcinoma, lymphoproliferative syndromes including lymphomas in the immunosuppressed
   B. Hepatocellular carcinoma: HBV, HCV
   C. Carcinoma of the uterine cervix: HPV-16, -18

CMV, cytomegalovirus; HSV, herpes simplex virus; HBV, HCV, HDV, hepatitis virus B, C, D; EBV, Epstein-Barr virus; HPV, human papillomavirus.

How Viruses Cause Disease

The best understood and most graphic way by which a virus produces disease is through direct effects on cells that are infected. Infected cells may be killed by the virus. Such *cytolytic* viruses may show a great deal of variance in the speed of killing. For example, poliovirus and most picornaviruses will rapidly kill a cell within a day or two after infection. Polioviruses can uniquely kill the large motor neurons of the anterior horns of the spinal cord. After these irreplaceable neurons are eliminated, permanent paralysis of skeletal muscles innervated by the motor neurons can result because of lack of neuronal regeneration. HIV kills CD4 lymphocytes, which do regenerate but not well enough to maintain the numbers of such cells needed for the integrity of the immune system. In some cases viruses may cause slower cell death such as in the case of influenza and other myxoviruses. The rubella virus kills so slowly that its effects are not so much from direct killing, because viral cytopathology is minimal, as from the slower multiplication in affected embryonic cells and disruption of tissue and organ differentiation. This results in the well-known developmental defects and congenital deformities seen in the infected newborn child. Characteristically, such defects are more evident in newborns infected earlier during pregnancy, the first trimester.

Besides destroying cells, viruses may exert other profound effects. Some viruses are *transforming;* that is, they can change an arrested cell into a dividing one. In the case of B lymphocytes infected by EBV, such cells are picturesquely termed *immortalized cells.* Most immortalized B cells do not produce virus, but a small proportion of infected B lymphocytes will undergo a lytic or productive cycle and produce virus.[7] Immortalized B cells are thought to be "normal" cells. They do not grow in nude mice and produce metastasis like some cancer cells. However, in the severely immunosuppressed human or in severe combined immunodeficient (SCID) mice, they may produce lymphomas.[8] In the immunocompetent host, B cells or epithelial cells infected and immortalized by EBV are thought to play a role in the lymphoproliferative disorders of AIDS or after organ or bone marrow transplantation. Under some circumstances true B cell malignancies are seen in these patients, and EBV is the etiologic agent for Burkitt's lymphoma and nasopharyngeal carcinoma. Other viruses such as SV40 and many retroviruses will immortalize and transform cells into frankly cancerous cells even in some immunocompetent animals. Such direct tumor-producing viruses are less commonly observed in humans. Human T cell lymphotropic virus 1 (HTLV-1), which is associated with a T cell lymphoma, is an example.[9]

There are other more indirect effects of virus infection on cells and human organs that may be related to disease production. As in all infectious diseases, inflammation results from virus infection as from other microbial infections. Its precise determinants are manifold and not necessarily well worked out in individual cases. For example, it is thought that cytomegalovirus produces pneumonia in bone marrow recipients not only because the virus is cytolytic but because it stimulates immunopathologic processes as yet poorly understood.[10] Immunopathologic reactions in the form of cytotoxic T cells directed against hepatocytes are thought to be involved in the destruction of liver cells infected with HBV.[11]

Other direct or indirect viral effects are noninflammatory (see Table 11–2). Hepatitis B and C viruses have conclusively been implicated in the production of hepatocellular carcinoma[12–15] by as yet imperfectly understood mechanisms. These viruses as well as EBV and HPV are thought to be etiologically related to important human cancers.

MAJOR VIRUS GROUPS ACCORDING TO EPIDEMIOLOGIC CRITERIA

Viruses are now classified according to (1) the type and structure of viral nucleic acid and the method of its replication, (2) the type of symmetry of the virus capsid (helical versus icosahedral), and (3) the presence or absence of an envelope. This classification may be found in any current textbook on virology and microbiology and will not be presented here.[16] These technical criteria are also inadequate for the understanding of the biological, epidemiologic, and pathologic properties of viruses, particularly with respect to their relationship to surgery.

We present a biological scheme of classification based on the major epidemiologic characteristic of the virus and its method of transmission. In Table 11–3, five major categories of virus transmission are identified. Under each category, the virus families, as defined under the currently accepted terminology,[16] and some representative virus genera are listed. There is some overlap as members of a particular virus family may be transmitted by more than one method. Virus families, according to accepted classification convention, are major virus groups that consist of numerous genera and individual species. The names of all virus families end in *viridae.* Group 1 consists of five families of viruses that are transmitted by the oral-fecal route. Some of these viruses, as would be expected, cause important gastrointestinal infections but many viruses in this group affect other organ systems. For example, hepatitis A and E are major causes of epidemic and endemic hepatitis, and enteroviruses may affect the central nervous system. Polioviruses, coxsackieviruses, and echoviruses may cause

TABLE 11–3. MAJOR VIRUS GROUPS ACCORDING TO EPIDEMIOLOGIC CRITERIA

1. *Enteric viruses* (transmitted by oral-fecal route)
   - Picornaviridae (includes hepatitis A and E viruses, and enteroviruses, including poliovirus, echovirus, coxsackievirus)
   - Reoviridae (includes rotavirus)
   - Calciviridae (includes Norwalk virus)
   - Coronaviridae
   - Adenoviridae
2. *Respiratory viruses* (respiratory transmission)
   - Orthomyxoviridae (influenza viruses)
   - Paramyxoviridae (paramyxoviruses, measles, mumps, respiratory syncytial virus)
   - Picornaviridae (includes rhinoviruses)
   - Coronaviridae
   - Adenoviridae
   - Togaviridae (includes rubella virus)
   - Parvoviridae (parvovirus B-19)
   - Herpesviridae (varicella-zoster virus)
3. *Arthropod-borne viruses* (arboviruses)
   - Togaviridae (includes alphavirus, eg, eastern equine encephalitis virus)
   - Flaviridae (includes Japanese encephalitis, yellow fever, and dengue viruses)
   - Bunyaviridae (includes California encephalitis and sandfly fever viruses)
4. *Virus directly transmitted from animal bites*
   - Rhabdoviridae (rabies virus)
   - Bunyaviridae (Hataan virus)
5. *Viruses transmitted by body fluids, such as blood, saliva, and venereal secretions*
   - Herpesviridae (includes herpes simplex 1 and 2, cytomegalovirus, Epstein-Barr virus, herpesvirus 6)
   - Hepadnaviridae (hepatitis B)
   - Bunyaviridae (hepatitis C)
   - Unclassified (hepatitis D)
   - Arenaviridae (includes Lassa fever virus, Argentinian and Bolivian hemorrhagic fever viruses)
   - Papovaviridae (papillomaviruses)
   - Retroviridae (includes HIV 1, -2, HTLV-1, -2)

poliomyelitis, encephalomyelitis, and aseptic meningitis.

Group 2 represents respiratory transmission. Under this group, eight major virus families are represented. Included are influenza viruses, measles, mumps and the respiratory syncytial virus, and the common cold viruses, which encompass a number of virus families, such as rhinoviruses (Picornaviridae), Orthomyxoviridae, Paramyxoviridae, Coronaviridae, and Adenoviridae.

Group 3 consists of three major families of viruses, many of which are transmitted by arthropods, such as mosquitos, ticks, and mites. These used to be called the *arboviruses*[17] but are now divided among the Togaviridae, Flaviridae, and Bunyaviridae. These viruses are also characterized by specific geographic endemicity. For example, eastern equine encephalitis virus (a Togaviridae) is endemic in the eastern United States; Japanese encephalitis virus (a Flaviridae) is present only in the Far East, and yellow fever virus (a Flaviridae) is only present in the jungles of Africa and South America. The four types of dengue (a Flaviridae) are geographically more widespread (Mediterranean region, Caribbean region, Southeast Asia, and South America). Almost all the viruses in the original arbovirus groups cause zoonoses. *Zoonoses* are diseases that are transmitted from their normal animal reservoir to humans.

Zoonoses that are not transmitted by a *vector,* such as an arthropod, but that are directly transmitted from animals to humans and other hosts are listed in category 4. Rabies is endemic in certain animals and it may be transmitted to humans by animal bites from domestic dogs and cats or wild rodents such as bats, foxes, and skunks. A number of other zoonoses do not involve specific vectors. Hemorrhagic fever and renal syndrome caused by Hantaan virus is an example. The latter is a Bunyaviridae, which is widespread throughout the world and also known by the dramatic disease it produced during the Korean War, Korean hemorrhagic fever. In 1993, an outbreak of acute respiratory failure caused by this virus was first recognized in the United States.[17a] It is directly transmitted to humans via excreta of rodents.

Group 5 is a category of viruses transmitted by body fluids or transplants. Transmission may be facilitated by homosexual and heterosexual sex, transfusions, intravenous drug use, needle stick accidents, other occupational exposure, and perinatal infection of the newborn by the infected mother. Viruses in this group have become especially important since the discovery of AIDS[18] and HIV[2] and the increase in the number of immunosuppressed patients. They are also particularly important for clinical surgery because patients may be transfused with contaminated blood and other body fluids and they may contaminate surgeons and other health care workers in the course of their work. They are the group of viruses against which Universal Precautions have been instituted in American hospitals.[19]

Herpesviridae comprise the most numerous representatives of this group (see Table 11–3): herpes simplex virus (1 and 2), cytomegalovirus, Epstein-Barr virus, and herpesvirus 6 (Figs. 11–1 and 11–2). Varicella-zoster virus is also a herpesvirus but it is largely transmitted by the respiratory route. The herpesviruses infect large segments of the population without producing much clinical disease. Infections share certain biologic properties

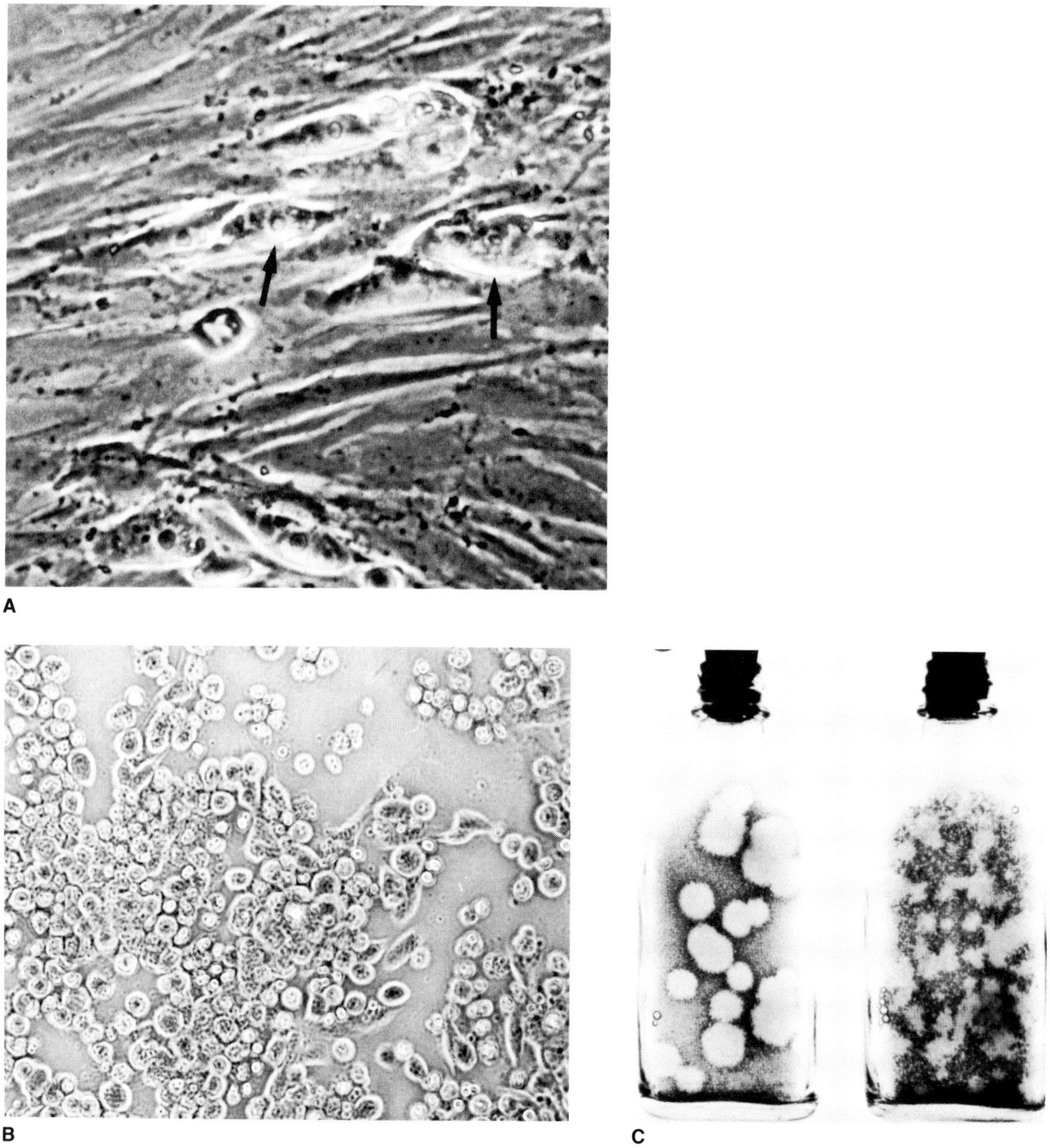

Figure 11–2. Cytopathic effects produced by herpesviruses. **A.** Cytomegalovirus-infected fibroblasts. Infected cells are enlarged and rounded (*arrows*) (×80). **B.** Rhesus monkey kidney cells infected with *Herpesvirus hominis.* The infected cells are rounded. Several cells have died and have lifted off the flask, leaving clear spaces where a confluent monolayer had been (×80). **C.** Plaques produced by poliovirus (*left*) and by an echovirus (*right*). *(From Jawetz E, Melnick JL, Adelberg EA: A Review of Medical Microbiology, 16th ed. Los Altos, CA, Lange Medical Publications, 1984.)*

(Table 11–4). Such infections are incurable; once a person is infected the virus persists even if symptoms are absent. They cannot be cured by host defenses and the virus remains latent indefinitely in the patient. Ordinarily, these latent infections are innocuous, but virus reactivation may result in symptomatic disease. Examples are recurrent oral and genital herpes. If the patient is immunosuppressed, such as a patient on immunosuppressants after transplantation, a patient on chemotherapy for cancer, or a patient with an immunosuppressive disease such as HIV/AIDS, both primary and reactivation infections caused by these viruses may greatly be increased in severity. By and large, the primary or original infection transmitted from outside the patient by body fluids is more severe than

TABLE 11–4. HUMAN HERPESVIRUSES

Name	Common Properties of All
Herpes simplex type 1	(1) Enveloped, ether sensitive, labile (120–180 mm)
Herpes simplex type 2	(2) Large double-strand DNA genome (100–150 × 10^8 daltons)
Cytomegalovirus	(3) Icosahedron (20 surfaces), 162 capsomes
Varicella-zoster virus	(4) "Once infected always infected" (incurable)
Epstein-Barr virus (EBV)	(5) Latency at specific sites; reactivation recurrences may occur
Human herpesvirus 6 (HHV-6)	(6) Primary and reactivation disease syndromes; primary syndromes more severe

secondary and reactivation infections, which take place in an immunized patient.

Group 5 viruses (see Table 11–3) include the hepatitis viruses. Except for hepatitis A and E viruses, which are enteroviruses that produce an acute disease from which one usually recovers completely, hepatitis viruses B, C, and D are transmitted by exchange of body fluids. All of them may produce persistent infections, cirrhosis, and cancer. Until recently, the best recognized one of this group was hepatitis B virus, which is endemic in large parts of the world where the chronic infection rate among the general population may be as high as 20 percent. Recently, infection by hepatitis C virus has been discovered, identified, and diagnosed in large numbers of people. Unfortunately, it is similar to hepatitis B in that it also causes chronic disease and may lead to hepatoma.[3,20] Hepatitis D virus is an incomplete virus that can only replicate in association with hepatitis B virus and aggravates severe hepatitis.

Human papillomaviruses (HPVs), of which there are more than 100 types, cause warts of the skin and of the genital and oral mucous membranes. Genital infection by papillomaviruses is the most common sexually transmitted virus. It ranges from condylomas and genital warts to subclinical infections and may be found in about 10 percent of men and women in the United States between 15 and 49 years of age.[21] HPV types 5 and 8 are latently present in a rare squamous cell carcinoma associated with epidermodysplasia verruciformis.[22] HPV types 16 and 18 DNA have been found to exist as episomes or chromosomally integrated DNA in cells of carcinomas of the uterine cervix. HPV is possibly an essential cofactor in the pathogenesis of cervical cancer but is not etiologic by itself.[23] Consistent with this hypothesis is the finding that the E6/E7 open reading frames of HPV 16 or 18 are always intact in cervical cancers, and the proteins of E6/E7 have been found to be the functionally transforming proteins that can immortalize keratinocytes.[24–26]

Recent discoveries prove that a number of retroviruses, which epidemiologically belong to group 5, cause serious disease in humans. HTLV-1 is an important cause of T cell lymphomas in certain populations such as the Japanese and Caribbean black population. In most cases, however, it produces an inapparent infection without proceeding to neoplasm. HTLV-2 may be associated with hairy cell leukemia.

The HIV pandemic that began in 1981 has now spread throughout the world.[18] Its epicenters are in Subsahara Africa and the United States but it is emerging in underdeveloped countries in Southeast Asia and Latin America. HIV is the most deadly of the viruses, which is transmitted by blood and body fluids. The most common means of transmission are venereal transmission and intravenous drug abuse. The many implications of retroviruses for surgeons and surgical diseases will be discussed later. HIV is further discussed in the section on HIV/AIDS.

DIAGNOSIS OF VIRAL INFECTIONS AND LABORATORY TESTS

In order to properly evaluate a patient for the presence of a viral infection it is essential to keep the principles of viral diagnosis in mind. A viral infection must first be suspected clinically on the basis of the history and physical examination before any steps toward laboratory diagnosis can be taken. A proper history includes ascertaining the epidemiologic background of the patient's disease. For example, if one suspects aseptic viral meningitis and that an enterovirus may be involved, one must keep in mind that such viruses are often epidemic during the summer and early fall in a particular community. This is all the more important because clinical diagnosis may have to suffice, as laboratory diagnosis of infections by this group of viruses may not be readily available under usual conditions of practice. In patients with enterovirus meningitis, a virus usually cannot be isolated from the spinal fluid and serologic methods are impractical because more than 100 agents may be involved. Serology directed by epidemiologic clues may be more useful, although results are rarely available in time to help the individual patient.

Epidemiologic clues may also be essential for the diagnosis of viral infections such as influenza, measles, arthropod-borne infections, and the more exotic infections such as those caused by Arenaviridae (see Table 11–3), for which the usual microbiology laboratory may be ill-equipped to be of assistance. Serum samples may be sent to the Centers for Disease Control (CDC) for confirmation.

Infections by the arthropod-borne viruses (see Table 11–3) must also be suspected primarily on clinical and epidemiologic grounds. They usually cannot be diagnosed by virus isolation, because of their rapid disappearance from blood or body fluids. One can collect serum samples for serologic confirmation in specialized laboratories.

Historical information is also critical in recognizing disease syndromes. Cytomegalovirus (CMV) mononucleosis is an important postsurgical complication associated with transfusion of large amounts of blood and organ transplants. It may present as fever of unknown origin. Once suspected, it is easy to confirm.

Laboratory tests used to diagnose a virus infection may be divided into three general types: demonstration of the virus or virus antigen in body fluid or tissue, serologic diagnosis, and specific histopathology.

Demonstration of the presence of virus is the simplest and most direct diagnostic test. This can be done by growing the virus in cell cultures or in an animal, such as the embryonated egg. Viruses are readily isolated from samples containing CMV, HSV, VZ, enteroviruses, influenza viruses, and the like (see Fig. 11–2). One must select judiciously the samples to be taken for culture because they vary with each virus and its disease. Usually the site of disease is the proper site from which to take a sample. For example, the responsible virus may readily be cultured from the skin or mucosal lesions of oral herpes, genital herpes, herpes zoster, or herpes esophagitis. To diagnose viral pneumonias, bronchoalveolar lavage fluid is best. Culture of involved tissue biopsies may prove necessary in some cases. But there are exceptions. One should try to isolate enteroviruses in cases of aseptic meningitis from the stool but *not* the apparent site of disease, the spinal fluid.

Serological diagnosis consists of demonstrating a specific serologic rise of antibodies to the virus in question during the course of infection or after convalescence, or conversion of the serologic state from one of being negative to one of having antibodies against the specific agent. Serologic diagnosis is excessively popular among some clinicians because the concept is simple. In practice, however, the usefulness of serological diagnosis is limited and it is often impractical. To demonstrate a change in the patient's antibody status requires the submission of a so-called acute and convalescent sera. Antibody changes are often only detected after recovery from the clinical disease and may be of little use for clinical management. The presence of antibodies in a single serum sample rarely diagnoses the presence of infection. It is rare indeed for the lab to receive properly paired specimens with a request for acute and convalescent antibody titers. Single specimens are sufficient to assay for specific IgM antibodies against a particular virus. Such antibodies, when present during an acute illness, are helpful. But they are rarely completely sensitive or specific. That is, IgM antibodies may be absent during many active infections, or they may be present when an infection has passed or when it is clinically insignificant.

From the point of view of the laboratory, many requests for serologic tests often cannot be fulfilled because too many agents are involved. The laboratory often receives requests for "viral studies." Even when specific clinical syndromes are indicated, the request for serological diagnosis cannot be fulfilled. This is the case in aseptic meningitis, upper respiratory infections, viral pneumonias, and viral encephalitis. One must indicate the suspected agent and its type, if relevant. One exception is viral hepatitis (see section on hepatitis). Some laboratories offer a panel of serologic tests that are useful in diagnosing or excluding hepatitis A, B, C, and D. Incidentally, these latter viruses can only be diagnosed by serologic means. Another example is EBV.

At this time molecular diagnostics are rapidly approaching widespread application. These diagnostic procedures make use of specific properties of a molecule of the virus itself or of an antibody stimulated by the virus. A few currently useful examples illustrate the value of these techniques.

Monoclonal antibodies against the immediate early (IE) antigens of the CMV virus are used to detect the presence of virus in cells. Such antigens appear within hours after inoculating a cell culture[27] and are excellent rapid markers for the presence of CMV.

Certain viruses cannot be cultivated in the laboratory at all, or only with difficulty. They may also be present in tissues in the latent, incomplete, or unculturable states. In these situations, detection of viral nucleic acid, either its DNA or RNA, may be a potent tool of diagnosis. There are now two major methods of detecting viral nucleic acid in tissues and body fluids: nucleic acid hybridization and polymerase chain reaction (PCR). In situ DNA hybridization can detect EBV genomes in tissues in EBV-related cancers and lymphoproliferative syndromes.[7] HPV genomes in tissues can also be found. PCR adds a new, major dimension to the detection of viral nucleic acid in clinical samples. This method amplifies viral nucleic acid so that the sensitivity of detection is increased to the point that it almost rivals viral culture (which technically is also an amplification method, ie, the whole virus is amplified). Not only is PCR specific and sensitive, but incomplete as well as latent viruses can be detected. Its present disadvantages are mainly technical ones. Because of its hypersensitivity, nonspecificity due to inadvertent contamination is a constant danger. One needs appropriate primers for each agent, of course. PCR has already proved its value in the detection of nonculturable virus, such as papillomaviruses, parvovirus B-19, and hepatitis C, the demonstration of HIV in infected patients before the appearance of specific antibody, or the detection of infection in the case of infants with suspected HIV, thus avoiding confounding antibody passively transferred from the mother.[28]

What viral infections are of interest to surgeons? Rabies and other zoonoses; virus infections that may lead to surgery; virus infections that affect patients who are candidates for surgery or who require or have recently had surgery; infections that may specifically affect health care workers (including surgeons) (ie, viruses transmitted by blood and body fluids); and, finally, viral infections that cause congenital malformations that may require surgical correction.

HERPESVIRUS INFECTIONS

Herpesviridae are 120 to 180 nm double-stranded DNA viruses with common characteristics listed in Table 11–4. They are enveloped viruses that are quite labile and do not persist in the physical environment (see Table 11–4). Each one of the six produces distinct diseases. All herpesviruses are capable of producing persistent as well as acute lytic infections (see Fig. 11–2). Translated to manifestations in the host, each virus produces its own specific acute viral syndrome after primary infection, for example, oral herpes (HSV-1), genital herpes (HSV-2), chickenpox (VZ virus), mononucleosis (CMV and EBV), and roseola (HHV-6). In addition, each virus is also able to persist in latent form at a particular site. Thus a person is never cured, even if asymptomatic. All herpesviruses are "forever."

Herpesviruses infect large segments of the population. Except for HSV-2, the viruses listed in Table 11–4 infect more than half of human adults, usually without apparent damage. Although primary infection by each one of the viruses is associated with a well-defined acute disease syndrome, most primary infections by these viruses are not noticed, and most adults have some degree of specific immunity. In the immunosuppressed patient, however, primary infection by HSV, CMV, and EBV may produce severe life-threatening diseases (see Chap. 51 on infections in the immunosuppressed).

The disease processes associated with persistent infection may be serious problems in both the immunologically competent as well as suppressed host.

Reactivated latent infection of cells may produce lytic cycles of infection. Typically acute inflammatory viral syndromes are produced. These are usually less severe than the primary disease, because the patient has some immunity. Like the primary infection, these episodes are self-limited in duration and extent. Herpes zoster is a good example. In zoster (shingles), the chickenpox localized to a dermatome corresponding to the sensory ganglion from which latent VZ virus was reactivated to enter the lytic cycle. Other examples include recurrent oral and recurrent genital herpes. None of these reactivation diseases is usually fatal, except that genital herpes in pregnant women may lead to herpes simplex infection of the newborn, in whom it may be severe or fatal.

The causes of reactivation of the above three conditions are not clear, particularly in the immune competent host. Reactivation disease is more frequent and more severe in immunosuppressed patients, such as patients on chemotherapy, after transplantation, or who have HIV/AIDS.

Reactivation of CMV is only seen in the immunosuppressed (see section on CMV and Chap. 51 on infections in the immunosuppressed). CMV retinitis in patients with HIV/AIDS is an example.

Persistent latent infection may also be associated with noninflammatory syndromes, such as malignancies. EBV is associated with two well-known tumors in the immunocompetent patient: Burkitt's lymphoma and nasopharyngeal carcinoma (NPC). In the immunocompromised host, EBV may produce a lymphoproliferative disease ranging from a severe mononucleosis syndrome to polyclonal and monoclonal B cell lymphomas. In the transplant recipient, these diseases are called post-transplant lymphoproliferative disorders (PTLDs).[29]

In Burkitt's lymphoma, NPC, and PTLDs, EBV genomes are latently present in the B cells (Burkitt's lymphoma and PTLDs) or in the epithelial tumor cells (nasopharyngeal carcinoma). Nine viral proteins, coded by so-called latency-associated genes, are synthesized and expressed to varying degrees by the tumor cells. These are EBNA (EBV nuclear antigen) 1, 2, 3a, 3b, 3c and LP, LMP, LMP-2, and EBERS. Some of these proteins (eg, LMP) have been shown to transform and immortalize B lymphocytes.[30]

The precise pathogenetic relationship between EBV infection and Burkitt's lymphoma and NPC is still unclear. However, in the case of PTLDs, several pertinent points lead to a workable hypothesis.[29] (1) Primary EBV infection after transplantation is a significant risk factor for the development of PTLD. It is more important than secondary or reactivation EBV infection.[31] (2) The B cells in the PTLD lesions are latently infected by EBV, but they resemble normal, immortalized B cells and do not usually have the typical chromosomal translocations seen in Burkitt's lymphoma cells, which account for the activation of the *myc* oncogene and their oncogenicity. (3) PTLD tumors in transplant patients may regress and even disappear if immunosuppressive drugs are reduced. (4) PTLD-type lymphomas may be produced in severe combined immunodeficient (SCID) mice by transfusion of normal human B lymphocytes infected with EBV.[8] These data are sufficient to suggest that most PTLD tumors are primarily conditioned by immune deficiency and that the lesions may consist of cells without any clear neoplastic characteristics.

HHV-6 is a newly discovered herpesvirus initially found in peripheral blood mononuclear cells.[32] Serologic studies suggest that infection occurs in most children by 3 years of age. Roseola (exanthema subitum) in infants has been associated with its infection,[33] as have nonspecific febrile illnesses in children less than 2 years of age.[34] The morbidity of primary or secondary infection by HHV-6 in immunosuppressed patients still awaits elucidation. HHV-7, similar to HHV-6 and cytomegalovirus, is a new herpesvirus that requires even further study.[34]

CYTOMEGALOVIRUS (CMV) INFECTION

CMV infection has become an important pathogen in immunosuppressed as well as in immunocompetent patients.[35] CMV disease in immunosuppressed patients and its treatment are discussed elsewhere (see Chap. 51) and will not be covered in detail here. We will concentrate on the basic medical biology of CMV, clinical manifestations in the immunocompetent, and its diagnosis.

CMV infection is common in the general population. About 50 to 90 percent of the adult population has been infected; that is, they have serum antibodies as evidence of some degree of immunity. At the same time they are persistently and inapparently infected with the virus. Primary infection with CMV occurs at two major time periods in life via transmission of infected body fluids. Babies can be infected by their seropositive mothers who may shed CMV in the cervix, urine, or breast milk. Toddlers sharing the virus with their playmates in day care centers are a likely source as well. The second major period of infection is during young adulthood, when transmission by heterosexual or homosexual contact with infected persons is probably the major route.

The discovery of CMV was associated with elucidation of a congenital disease in otherwise immunocompetent neonates—cytomegalic inclusion disease (CID).[36] CID and other forms of symptomatic neonatal CMV infection are relatively uncommon outcomes of an intrauterine fetal infection with CMV transmitted transplacentally from the mother undergoing a primary CMV infection. In a series of prospective studies analyzed by Ho,[37] primary CMV infection occurred in 0.4 percent of all pregnant women or in 13 percent of seronegative pregnant women. Congenital CMV infection occurred in 54 percent of mothers who were primarily infected, and 22 percent of infected neonates were symptomatic. The frequency of symptomatic CMV disease in neonates of all pregnant mothers was 0.06 percent (11 out of 19,522).

No CMV disease syndrome was recognized in adults until the CMV mononucleosis syndrome was described in 1965.[38] This syndrome may occur sporadically, after blood transfusions and frequently after transplantation. Sporadic cases account for about 10 percent of the mononucleosis syndromes in young adults, most of which is due to EBV.

Clinically, CMV mononucleosis is similar but not identical to EBV mononucleosis. It is characterized mainly by fever, chemical hepatitis, and atypical lymphocytosis. EBV mononucleosis has more pharyngitis, tonsillitis, splenomegaly, and lymphadenopathy. Leukopenia, pneumonitis, myocarditis, skin rashes, and Guillain-Barré syndrome have been reported as complications of CMV mononucleosis.[39] In many patients, prolonged fever alone may be the predominant manifestation. In a postsurgical patient whose CMV mononucleosis is caused by transfusion of CMV-infected whole blood, it may be the cause of fever of unknown origin lasting 3 to 4 weeks or longer.

In the sporadic case of CMV mononucleosis, as in the case of EBV mononucleosis, usually no specific source of infection is identified. It occurs in young adults as does EBV mononucleosis. EBV mononucleosis may occur in young adults of college age and CMV mononucleosis occurs in somewhat older young adults. The clinical manifestations are similar whether the syndrome occurs sporadically, in transfused subjects, or in immunosuppressed patients.

Asymptomatic and symptomatic CMV infections were discovered following cardiopulmonary bypass and open heart surgery around the same time.[40–42] The literature has recently been reviewed.[43] Blood, specifically the buffy coat, is the source of infection.[43] In a study of 119 children undergoing open heart bypass surgery at the University of Pittsburgh, we found 13 percent became infected as demonstrated by serologic changes or viremia.[44] Both seronegative as well as seropositive patients could be infected. None was symptomatic. The risk of infection was calculated to be 3.3 percent per unit of blood transfused. In most prospective studies, CMV infections were asymptomatic. When they occur, symptomatic infections are self-limited and without mortality. However, neonates, who are underdeveloped or premature, may suffer significant mortality from post-transfusion disease. In one well-known study,[45] neonates were infected primarily when a seronegative neonate received seropositive blood or secondarily when a seropositive recipient received seropositive blood. The frequency of infection was 15 to 18 percent, which was significantly higher than in older children or adults. CMV disease developed only after primary infection, and there was an outstanding 50 percent associated mortality. No infection resulted if a seronegative neonate received blood from a seronegative donor.

Studies such as those summarized above[43] have helped mold some of the current thinking regarding CMV infection and blood transfusions. In the immunocompetent well-developed child or adult, CMV infection may occur, but it is usually asymptomatic. With respect to immature neonates or immunosuppressed patients who undergo high infection risk transplantation procedures, such as bone marrow transplantation, the following may be concluded. (1) Primary CMV infection is the type that may be symptomatic after transfusion. Thus only CMV seronegative patients are at risk. Neonates reflect the serostatus of their mothers. Those who are born with passively transferred antibodies from their mothers appear to be protected from CMV disease. (2) One way to prevent primary CMV infection is to use only CMV seronegative blood for transfusions in babies born of seronegative mothers or in seronegative marrow recipients.

However, the situation regarding the danger of transfused blood transmitting CMV seems to have changed in recent years. In a summary of 15 studies, the risk of CMV infection was around 3 percent or greater per unit of blood from 1966 to 1982.[46] Studies since 1986 show the risk of infection per unit of blood to be significantly less than 1 percent per unit.[47,48] The high morbidity in neonates is also seen less often. The reason for these decreases in infection and morbidity is unknown. Possible reasons are changes in blood banking procedures and in the characteristics of donors. Infective CMV in banked blood may have decreased because, since the onset of the AIDS epidemic and routine HIV testing in 1984, highly infected donors, such as homosexual males and intravenous drug users, have largely been screened out.

Diagnosis of Cytomegalovirus Infection

As in evaluating most infections, infection must be carefully distinguished from disease. Infection or carriage of the virus is common. CMV disease has a characteristic, if somewhat variable, picture. In general, CMV disease is uncommon in adults unless the patient is immunocompromised or has been transfused.

Demonstration of the virus is the best method of CMV diagnosis. The virus is readily culturable in human fibroblast cell cultures. Within hours after inoculation, "shell vial" cultures produce diagnostic immediate early (IE) antigen specific for CMV.[27] This antigen can be detected by reaction with specific monoclonal antibodies against IE antigen using the immunofluorescent or immunoperoxidase test. This rapid assay obviates the need to observe the specific cytopathic effect of CMV in inoculated cells, which used to take 3 to 6 weeks of incubation and microscopic observation (see Fig. 11–2A).

To evaluate a positive CMV isolate, one should note that CMV may be isolated in normal immunocompetent asymptomatic subjects under the following conditions: (1) in the throat or urine of some neonates or toddlers who have recently acquired CMV infection; (2) in the uterine cervix of some sexually active women; and (3) in the semen and urine of sexually active males. However, in general, except for sexual secretions, CMV is not detectable in immunocompetent adults even if they are seropositive and latently infected.

In patients with CMV mononucleosis, the virus can usually be demonstrated either in the buffy coat of the blood, in the throat, or in urine. Demonstration of the virus at any one of these sites in a patient in whom one suspects CMV mononucleosis clinically is usually confirmation of such diagnosis.

In the immunosuppressed or HIV/AIDS patient, CMV disease may have other presentations, some of which may be serious. CMV may cause pneumonitis, gastrointestinal lesions anywhere in the gastrointestinal tract, and involvement of other organ systems such as the liver, gallbladder, skin, retina, and central nervous system. The required laboratory procedure for the diagnosis of these CMV diseases is ideally the demonstration of the virus or viral lesions (Fig. 11–3A) in the tissue that is clinically involved. The presence of virus in the buffy coat of the blood, throat washes, or urine from a patient who is immunosuppressed is not sufficient. Other infections are common in such patients, and a positive CMV culture may represent subclinical activation. The virus in bronchoalveolar lavage fluid in a patient with suspected CMV pneumonitis is diagnostic, as is the histopathologic demonstration in a biopsy of a gastrointestinal ulcer or liver.

Serology may be useful in management of acute CMV disease. The presence of antibodies against CMV is evidence for past infection. A negative serology, or absence of antibodies against CMV, unless it is very early in CMV infection, rules out CMV infection and disease. If by chance one had a serum specimen before the present illness and one can obtain a specimen during the illness and compare the two, the absence of antibody in the earlier serum and its presence in the later serum are useful to diagnose a case of primary CMV infection. This is quite helpful because primary infections are often clinically more severe. They produce disease not only in immunosuppressed patients but are also important in normal subjects. For example, CMV mononucleosis can be diagnosed by this method. In pregnant women, seroconversion or primary infection during pregnancy is a significant risk factor for the development of symptomatic congenital CMV infection in the neonate. Unfortunately, in most cases, a serum sample previous to pregnancy or early in pregnancy is not available to rule out a primary CMV infection. IgM antibodies indicate recent

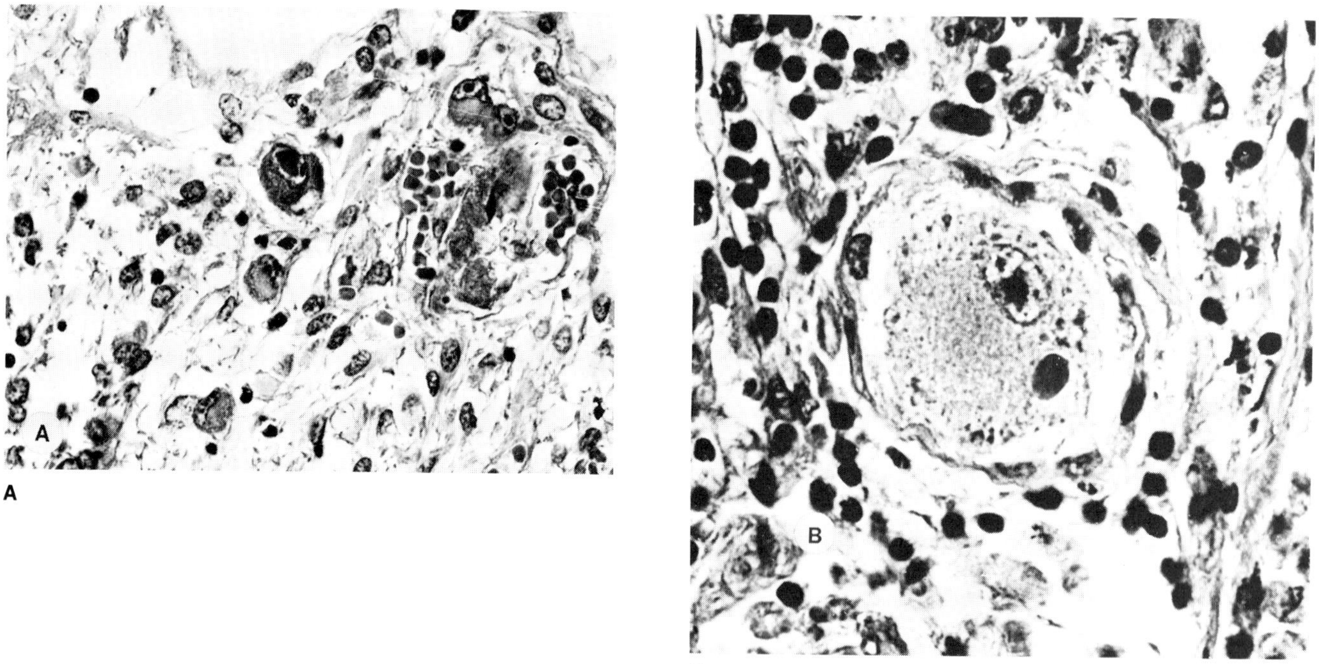

A

B

Figure 11–3. A. Intranuclear inclusions in glial cells infected with cytomegalovirus. The eosinophilic intranuclear inclusion is surrounded by a clear halo (×435). **B.** Cytoplasmic inclusion (Negri body) in ganglion cell infected with rabies virus (×696). *(Courtesy of Dr. JH Sung, Dept. of Neuropathology, University of Minnesota.)*

infection by CMV, and they help to some extent. However, one is often uncertain as to how long they have been present.

To diagnose primary CMV infection in an immunocompromised patient who just had an organ transplantation, one must demonstrate a negative serology before transplantation and the presence of antibody after transplantation. The distinction between primary and secondary infection cannot be made unless antibody studies can be done on pretransplant samples. We advise that routinely a sample of serum be saved from all transplant patients before transplantation, so that appropriate tests may be done later. Such samples are useful not only for the diagnosis of CMV but also for the diagnosis of primary infection by EBV, HSV, and other agents. The treatment of CMV infection is discussed in Chapters 28 and 51.

HIV/AIDS

HIV is a lentivirus belonging to the Retroviridae.[2] It causes a previously unknown infection of humans leading to the development of AIDS with a mean incubation period of 10 years and high mortality. It is transmitted by sexual activity, sharing of injection equipment among HIV-infected intravenous drug users, exposure to HIV-contaminated blood by transfusion or by contaminated needles, and perinatal infection of the newborn by an infected mother. The virus has the unusual property of persisting in blood and body fluids during the long incubation period, the prodromal symptomatic period preceding AIDS, and during all stages of AIDS.

There have been over 350,000 cases in this country alone from 1981 to 1994. This number is fairly reliable because AIDS is a notifiable disease. In addition, about 1.45 million HIV-infected individuals in this country have not yet developed AIDS.[49] Unfortunately, we do not have precise numbers for the number of infected.

HIV/AIDS has created a worldwide pandemic with separate component epidemics in different parts of the world. Bad as the situation is in this country, it is worse elsewhere. HIV/AIDS, like many other communicable diseases, has a propensity for the economically and socially underprivileged populations and nations of the world. There are now estimated to be about 17.5 million HIV-infected persons in the world. About 11.5 million or 66 percent are in Sub-Saharan Africa, 1.4 million (8 percent) are in Latin America, and 1.2 million (7 percent) are in Southeast Asia. AIDS was recognized early in Africa, where it remains the epicenter of the world pandemic. But other third world regions, particularly Southeast Asia and Latin America, are now witnessing an exponential increase in HIV-infected individuals, similar to what was seen a decade ago in the United States. However, unlike the earlier phases of the epidemic in the United States, which afflicted primarily homosexual males, the epidemic in third world nations extends to both females and males and is closely related to heterosexual prostitution and drug abuse. With involvement of the female population, a separate serious problem is created because neonates and children become affected.

In the United States, we now have a decline in, but not elimination of, HIV infection in gay men.[50] A parallel but somewhat later epidemic of HIV/AIDS due to intravenous drug use (IVDU), particularly evident on the East Coast, is in its accelerated phase. A related phenomenon is the change in the ethnic composition of the HIV/AIDS population in this country. The majority of infected gay males were middle class white men. With the shift toward more infection in the drug use group, more blacks and Hispanics are becoming affected.

Twelve years after the start of the AIDS pandemic, AIDS is spreading to groups of people who are least able to deal with it, that is, the poor and the uneducated. Estimates are that by the year 2000, instead of the present 17.5 million infected, 40 to 110 million people will be infected, the extremes representing estimates by WHO and the Harvard AIDS Institute.[49]

With the widespread distribution of cases, health care personnel, including surgeons, are at risk for occupational infection by needlestick and sharps accidents involving contaminated blood (see Chap. 27). The risk of infection is small but significant, about 5 in 1000.[51] Universal Precautions have been instituted in this country in most institutional health care settings.[19]

Biomedical Characteristics of HIV/AIDS

What are the biomedical characteristics of HIV/AIDS that allow this pandemic to last so long and to spread so widely? Table 11–5 lists the unique characteristics of HIV/AIDS, which set it apart from other major communicable diseases. The reason why other epidemics are aborted is the development of effective specific immunity. The preponderance of immune individuals aborts continued transmission of the responsible agent and terminates epidemics. However, effective immunity does not develop for HIV/AIDS. Specific immunity that

TABLE 11–5. CHARACTERISTICS OF HIV/AIDS INFECTED PATIENTS

1. All or almost all who become infected become diseased. (Contrary to other infectious diseases where most who get infected are *not* diseased but become *immune*.)
2. All or almost all who become diseased die. (Most infectious diseases have low mortality.)
3. All infected subjects are *infectious*. (This includes the 10-year incubation period before development of AIDS.)
4. Transmission from human to human by sex or IV drug abuse, routes that are difficult to control.

does develop after HIV infection is inadequate to terminate the virus infection in the individual or interdict its transmission. Paradoxically, the presence of specific immunity against HIV as determined by the ELISA and Western blot tests is used as evidence for the *presence* of infection.

The infected person remains potentially infectious as long as he/she lives, which may be as long as 10 to 20 years. Viremia (and probably HIV in other body fluids) is particularly high during the early months of infection and after development of AIDS,[52] times during which the infected individuals may be particularly infectious. It is possible for relatively few carriers to spread the virus extensively and over a long period of time.

The fact that all infected persons develop the disease and all diseased persons die makes AIDS (see Table 11–5) particularly devastating. Most highly communicable infections result only in a fraction who are actually diseased; the remainder become immune without becoming sick. In HIV/AIDS, there is no inapparent infection or herd immunity to interdict the chain of transmission.

Classically, the best way to control the spread of a communicable disease is to prevent it by interdicting the route or vehicle of transmission. Control is most economical and effective if preventive measures are feasible. Effective transmission of HIV (ie, by sex or IVDU) has so many stringent requirements that interdiction of transmission is theoretically simple. Added to this is the fact that the level of HIV infection in blood and fluids, while always present in the infected individual, is relatively low in concentration. HIV, for example, is much less sexually transmissible than hepatitis B virus, which has almost identical modes of transmission.[53] Practically, however, interdiction of transmission is very difficult because human behavior must be modified. It is remarkable that fear of a dreadful disease, even a lethal one, may not be adequate to significantly modify sexual behavior or drug dependency.

Theoretically, if there were an effective vaccine, prevention would be feasible. An excellent example of how effective vaccines can work is the control and global eradication of smallpox.[54] Herd immunity produced by the vaccine prevented infection and transmission, and eventually the virus died out because it had no place to replicate. As in the case of smallpox, HIV/AIDS is transmitted only from human to human, and there is no known reservoir for the virus outside the human being. Unfortunately, the development of an effective HIV vaccine is not yet in the offering.

Treatment may also be used as a method to control communicable diseases. Tuberculosis control is based on this method, as is the control of other sexually transmitted diseases such as syphilis and gonorrhea. To be effective as a control measure, treatment must result in a *cure*. So far there are no prospects that any antiviral therapy can cure HIV infection.

Treatment of HIV/AIDS

Zidovudine (azidothymidine, AZT) was the first and still is the most effective specific antiviral agent against HIV. AZT improved survival and reduced the number of major opportunistic infections in the initial trial in AIDS and AIDS-related complex (ARC).[55] HIV-infected subjects without evidence of AIDS whose CD4 counts were either less than 200 or less than 500 per mm^3 were also shown to benefit from AZT treatment.[56,57] It is effective against HIV-associated neurologic diseases[58,59] and HIV-related thrombocytopenia,[60,61] but it has no effect on AIDS-related tumors such as Kaposi's sarcoma.

Experience with AZT and related drugs also reveals significant problems. It must be taken for a long time. It is marrow-toxic, induces myopathy, and generates resistance.[62–65] This suggests that therapy for HIV infection might require combinations of two or more antivirals. Now two other nucleoside anti-reverse transcriptase drugs have been approved by the FDA—2′,3′-dideoxyinosine (ddI) and 2′,3′-dideoxycytidine (ddC)—and others are being tested.[66,67] ddI is not marrow-toxic but ddC is neurotoxic. Both are currently being tested in combination with AZT.

The major opportunistic infections that inevitably complicate HIV/AIDS require prophylaxis. These include pneumocystis pneumonia, tuberculosis, toxoplasmosis, cryptococcosis, CMV retinitis, and *Mycobacterium avium* complex infection. Prophylactic drug regimens have been developed for each of these infections once they have been diagnosed or after the CD4+ lymphocyte counts have reached a certain point.

Diagnosis of HIV/AIDS

HIV/AIDS may be suspected clinically from the presence of recurrent or severe opportunistic infections, a CD4+ lymphocyte count less than 800/mm^3, and the presence of what is called a risk factor for infection. Risk factors include male homosexuality, intravenous drug use, and heterosexual sex with a partner who abuses intravenous drugs. In the case of neonates, an HIV-infected pregnant mother is the only major risk factor. Health care workers who might have been exposed parenterally by infected body fluids have a small but significant increased "risk" (see Chap. 27).

The essential laboratory diagnosis for the presence of HIV is a positive ELISA test and a positive confirming Western blot test. This test for the antibody to HIV is highly sensitive and specific for infection with the virus. It may be demonstrated by more conventional means such as direct culture from blood leukocytes or from other tissue cells, but these approaches are technically difficult. One defect of the antibody test is that antibodies are not immediately demonstrable after infection. Molecular diagnostic methods are likely to become available.

Once the HIV serologic test has proved positive, a valuable parameter to follow is the CD4+ T lymphocyte count in order to diagnose AIDS and to evaluate the degree of immunodeficiency. A count of 200/mm^3 or less is diagnostic of AIDS.[68] Counts of 800/mm^3 or less provide a quantitative measure of the integrity of cellular immunity. With progressive decline of CD4+ counts, HIV/AIDS is associated with more and more manifestations of immunodeficiency such as minor and major opportunistic infections or opportunistic tumors such as Kaposi's sarcoma or lymphomas. It should be kept in mind that HIV is a very chronic infection and its protean clinical manifestations mandate that its existence be constantly suspected.

Health care workers stuck with a needle or sharp instrument contaminated with blood or body fluid from a patient known to have HIV/AIDS should provide blood samples immediately and at 1, 3, 6, and 12 months after the accident to demonstrate or rule out the presence of antibodies (infection).[51] The risk of getting the infection is relatively low (about 0.05 percent).[51] Whether or not one should treat such accidents with the administration of AZT is a controversial subject. This must be decided on an individual basis and the drug may be given if the physician and the patient both wish to do it.

VIRAL HEPATITIS

Hepatitis is caused by many different viruses. Herpesviruses, particularly CMV and HSV, may cause hepatitis, sometimes severe, in immunocompromised patients (see Chap. 5). However, in terms of infection of large numbers of people, the most important viruses are the hepatitis viruses A to E, that is, HAV, HBV, HCV, HDV, and HEV. It is likely that others will be discovered.

These five viruses are quite heterogeneous and belong to different virus families. HAV and HEV are Picornaviridae, HBV is a Hepadnaviridae, HCV is a Bunyaviridae, and HDV is an incomplete RNA virus. To understand their clinical and surgical importance, they may be approached by our epidemiologic classification (see Table 11–3).

Hepatitis A and the more recently characterized HEV are enteroviruses that cause acute hepatitis, which usually resolves in total recovery, with no associated latency, persistent infection, or late sequelae. They are transmitted by the oral-fecal route. Even though disease associated with HAV and HEV is associated with low mortality, both have been identified in major epidemic outbreaks of hepatitis usually caused by fecal contamination of the water supply or food stuffs.[69]

In contrast to HAV and HEV, HBV, HCV, and HDV are primarily transmitted by blood and body fluids (see Table 11–3) and are of special surgical significance. These will be discussed below.

The herpesviruses, such as CMV, HSV, and EBV, may also cause hepatitis. But this is usually of the milder kind. CMV and EBV usually cause only a chemical hepatitis as a part of disease syndromes caused by these agents in the immunologically normal subjects. In the neonate and in the immunosuppressed, CMV and herpes simplex may cause severe and life-threatening hepatitis.[70] Severe hepatitis by HSV and CMV is usually restricted to immunosuppressed patients, such as transplant recipients.

The delta agent, HDV, is a defective RNA virus that can only replicate together with hepatitis B virus. HDV infection occurs as either a coinfection with HBV or superinfection of a HBV carrier. The combination infection may result in fulminant life-threatening hepatitis.[1] Superinfection frequently

TABLE 11–6. HEPATITIS NOMENCLATURE

Abbreviation	Term	Comments
		Hepatitis A
HAV	Hepatitis A virus	Etiologic agent of infectious hepatitis; a picornavirus; single serotype
Anti-HAV	Antibody to HAV	Detectable at onset of symptoms; lifetime persistence
IgM anti-HAV	IgM class antibody to HAV	Indicates recent infection with hepatitis; positive up to 4–6 months after infection
		Hepatitis B
HBV	Hepatitis B virus	Etiologic agent of serum or long-incubation hepatitis; also known as Dane particle
HBsAg	Hepatitis B surface antigen	Surface antigen(s) of HBV detectable in large quantity in serum; several subtypes identified
HBeAg	Hepatitis B e antigen	Soluble antigen; correlates with HBV replication, high titer HBV in serum, and infectivity of serum
HBcAg	Hepatitis B core antigen	Not present in serum; detected only in liver with special stains
Anti-HBs	Antibody to HBsAg	Indicates past infection with and immunity to HBV, passive antibody from HBIG, or immune response from HBV vaccine
Anti-HBe	Antibody to HBeAg	Presence in serum of HBsAg carrier suggests lower titer of HBV
Anti-HBc	Antibody to HBcAg	Indicates past infection with HBV at some undefined time
IgM anti-HBc	IgM class antibody to HBcAg	Indicates recent infection with HBV; positive for 4–6 months after infection
HBV DNA	Hepatitis B virus DNA	Presence in serum is a marker of viral replication
		Hepatitis C
HCV	Hepatitis C virus	Accounts for 85–95% of bloodborne NANB
Anti-HCV	Antibody to HCV	First generation tests to C-100 antigen lacked specificity and sensitivity. Second generation tests detects several antigens and is more sensitive.
HCV-Ag	HCV antigen	No test currently available
		Hepatitis D (Delta Hepatitis)
HDV	Hepatitis D virus	Etiologic agent of hepatitis D; may only cause infection in presence of HBV
HD-Ag	Hepatitis D antigen	Detectable in early acute hepatitis D infection
Anti-HD	Antibody to hepatitis D antigen	Indicates past or present infection with hepatitis D virus
		Hepatitis E
HEV	Hepatitis E virus	Enterally transmitted non-A, non-B hepatitis (ET-NANB or ENANB) single-stranded RNA virus
Anti-HEV	Antibody to HEV	Detected by enzyme immunoassay
HEV-Ag	Hepatitis E antigen	One or more antigens may be present; correlates with viral replication; no test currently available
		Non-A, Non-B Hepatitis
NANB	Non-A, non-B hepatitis	Diagnosis of exclusion; hepatitis C and hepatitis E account for >90% of prior NANB

causes chronic HDV infection and chronic active hepatitis.

The nomenclature surrounding hepatitis can be confusing. Table 11–6 acts as a glossary of terms.

HEPATITIS B VIRUS

Hepatitis B virus belongs to the Hepadnaviridae group.[71] It contains a circular and incompletely double-stranded DNA molecule with single-strand gaps up to 50 percent of circle length. The virions are spherical particles of about 42 to 47 nm in diameter. The viral core contains a core antigen (HBcAg), the viral e antigen (HBeAg), the viral DNA, and enzymes including a DNA polymerase and a protein kinase that phosphorylates the major structural polypeptides of the viral core. The core is surrounded by lipid-containing envelope, which bears the viral surface (s) antigen (HBsAg). This important antigen is the antigen to which virus-neutralizing antibody is directed. Thus it is essential for infectivity of the virus, and, when isolated and purified, it makes an excellent vaccine.

Clinical Manifestations: Acute Hepatitis

The clinical course of hepatitis B is extremely variable. It can be completely asymptomatic or rapidly fatal. The incubation period of hepatitis B averages 75 days but can range from 40 to 180 days. Approximately 55 percent of adults infected with hepatitis B virus have no symptoms despite serologic documentation of infection.[72] This asymptomatic presentation is further reflected in the transmission of hepatitis B by blood donors who carry the virus but are in apparent good health. When symptoms are present, they may be so mild as to escape diagnosis. The patient may have only slight malaise, fatigability, and loss of appetite and may not even seek medical attention.

Approximately 45 percent of patients infected with hepatitis virus develop typical acute icteric hepatitis characterized by severe fatigue, anorexia, nausea, vomiting, jaundice, scleral icterus, and hepatomegaly. The onset is usually insidious. Arthritis, arthralgias, and skin rashes can also occur. A small proportion of these patients have a severe subacute course that may progress to coma and death over several weeks. Fulminant hepatitis, which may occur in coinfections with HDV, develops in approximately 1 percent of infected adults and is characterized by progressive hepatocellular destruction, encephalopathy, and deepening coma. Death occurs in 30 percent of children and 80 percent of adults with fulminant hepatitis. Liver transplantation is successful in individuals with acute fulminant hepatitis, but recurrence of the hepatitis is very frequent.

Persistent Carriers of HBV and Chronic Hepatitis

A certain proportion of patients who are infected with HBV, either symptomatically or asymptomatically, will go on to develop persistent infection.[72] Persistent infection with HBV has primary medical complications with significant long-term sequelae. Those who are persistently infected are chronic carriers of HBV, which is expressed by the presence of HBsAg in the bloodstream. In certain areas of the world most of the population become infected with HBV but as high as 10 to 20 percent will remain carriers of HBV. Such highly endemic areas exist in Southeast Asia and Sub-Saharan Africa. In this country the carrier rate is around 0.1 percent. About 10 percent of the carriers will go on to develop chronic hepatitis, of which a proportion will develop irreversible liver damage and cirrhosis. Furthermore, those with persistent infection and often with liver disease will go on to develop hepatocellular carcinoma. This cancer is frequently the number one cause of cancer in highly endemic areas. Epidemiologic as well as biological association of HBV and hepatocellular carcinoma is very strong.[13,72]

The epidemiology of HBV carriers varies depending on the method by which HBV is primarily transmitted. In highly endemic areas, HBV may primarily be transmitted perinatally from a chronically infected mother to the newborn.[73] The risk of such transmission ranges from 10 to 85 percent depending on the degree of viremia in the mother, which can be gauged by the presence of HBeAg. It is virtually 100 percent when the mother is HBeAg positive.[74,75] The risk of chronic infection is age dependent. It is inversely related to age. Young children 1 to 5 years of age have a 30 to 60 percent risk.[76] Perinatal transmission, in a population with a high frequency of chronic carriers, is a self-perpetuating situation unless prevented by immunization. It may account for as much as 50 percent of all persistent infections in highly endemic areas. In the United States, the carriers usually do not acquire their infection perinatally. Initially, infection is acquired during adulthood by transmission of blood or body fluids infected with HBV through venereal contacts, intravenous drug use, transfusions, or occupational accidents. Carrier frequency is higher in homosexual men and other highly sexually active groups. It is also an occupational hazard among health care workers who may contract HBV accidentally and become carriers by HBV-contaminated needle sticks.

Carriers may be totally asymptomatic or may have varying degrees of liver disease characterized by alterations in liver function tests or a pathologic picture of persistent or chronic active hepatitis. All HBV carriers characterized in the laboratory by the presence of HBsAg may have virus circulating in their bloodstreams and are potential transmitters of the virus. Patients with HBAg are usually transmitters.

Laboratory Diagnosis of HBV

Each of the three antigens mentioned—that is, the surface, core, and e antigens (HBsAg, HBcAg, and HBeAg)—stimulates antibodies after HBV infection, which are important in the diagnosis and evaluation of HBV infections. These antigens and their respective antibodies have patterns of appearance and disappearance from the bloodstream that vary during the phases of acute disease, recovery, and the chronic infective state (Table 11–7). The serologic diagnosis of HBV infection should be clearly understood, since this virus cannot be isolated in the laboratory in cell culture or in experimental an-

TABLE 11–7. SEROLOGIC PROFILES OF HBV HEPATITIS

HBsAg	Anti-HBcAg	Anti-HBsAg	Interpretation
Present	Absent	Absent	Acute hepatitis due to HBV
Absent	Present (IgM)	Absent	Recent or active infection
Absent	Present (IgG)	Absent	Past infection or chronic infection
Absent	Present (IgG)	Present	Past infection with immunity
Present	Present	Absent	Chronic infection, HBV carrier

HBV, hepatitis B virus; HBsAg, hepatitis B surface antigen; anti-HBsAg, antibody against HBsAg; anti-HBcAg, antibody against hepatitis B core antigen.

imals. The laboratory diagnosis therefore depends entirely on the characterization of the antigen and the respective antibodies found in blood. HBV virion particles (Dane particles) as well as HBV DNA polymerase may be present in the bloodstream in large concentrations in acute disease and in some chronic carriers. However, if present, these substances usually appear along with HBsAg, which is a sensitive surrogate marker for the virus. Neither Dane particles nor the enzymes are assayed in the usual diagnostic laboratory.

HBeAg (not shown in Table 11–7) may also be measured in the bloodstream during the acute infection and in some chronic infections. It is a marker for the presence of infective virus. It usually disappears before HBsAg in acute infection. The presence of HBeAg in a carrier who has HBsAg signifies that the patient's blood is heavily contaminated with virus particles and hence the blood and body fluids of this patient are more likely to be infectious. Antibodies against HBeAg may develop in the absence of HBeAg. The presence of anti-HBeAg and anti-HBcAg together may signify chronic infection with a small amount of viremia.

Like other virus infections, the acute disease by HBV may be aborted by the development of neutralizing antibodies (see Table 11–7). With recovery and convalescence from the acute disease, HBsAg disappears as anti-HBsAg develops. This occurs about 5 or 6 months after exposure. An earlier diagnostic antibody response, which can occur during acute disease, is the development of IgM antibodies against HBcAg. A single positive test for this particular antibody may be useful in diagnosing acute HBV hepatitis, particularly if HBsAg is not detected. HBsAg and anti-HBsAg are incompatible. Full recovery from HBV hepatitis is characterized by the absence of HBsAg and presence of anti-HBsAg, which signifies the presence of specific immunity and lack of chronic infection. This is also the desired response of successful immunization.

At times, both HBV and anti-HBsAg may be absent. In that case, the presence of anti-HBcAg is an indicator of past infection. But the presence of this antibody alone, which is not neutralizing, does not rule out the presence of chronic infection (see Table 11–7). The persistence of HBsAg 6 months to a year after infection and the lack of anti-HBsAg development mean that the patient may have persistent infection without development of immunity.

The clinical management of suspected carriers is (1) to determine whether there is a carrier state by defined laboratory tests and (2) to evaluate morbidity by assessing liver function including the liver function tests. Until recently there was no specific treatment for the carrier state or for chronic hepatitis due to HBV. At this time treatment with interferon (IFN-α) has been shown to be effective in certain cases. Stable, less advanced cases of chronic hepatitis due to HBV may benefit from courses of IFN-α. This drug can stabilize the hepatitis and occasionally reduce the viral burden and rarely may even eliminate HBsAg.

HBV Vaccines

The development of effective vaccines against HBV is one of the major biomedical achievements in the last 20 years.[72] The earlier vaccine consisted of HBsAg isolated from plasma of human carriers of HBV.[77] The production procedure employed a series of purification and inactivation steps designed to remove and partially purify HBsAg and to inactivate any residual infectious HBV. The critical virus inactivation steps involved pepsin digestion, denaturation with 8M urea, and inactivation with formalin. No known cases of accidental infection by HBV or any other virus have resulted from the extensive use of this vaccine.

The second and more recent vaccine, which is currently used in this country, consists of HBsAg produced by a yeast, *Saccharomyces cerevisiae*.[78] It carries a recombinant yeast expression vector (plasmid) consisting of specific promoter sequences and DNA containing the gene of HBsAg. The antigen is produced by the yeast and after release it is purified by ultrafiltration, chromatography, ultracentrifugation, and absorption to alum hydroxide. There is no possibility of any living human virus contaminating this vaccine.

Both types of vaccines are given in a three-dose series. The first two doses (1.0 ml IM) are given 1 month apart and the third dose 5 months after the second. Protection from these vaccines lasts at least 7 years among healthy adults. The possible need for booster doses to ensure further efficacy is still to be assessed.

Numerous studies have established the efficacy of HBV vaccine.[72,79,80] The CDC recommends that all neonates receive the HBV vaccine.[81] Immunization against HBV is recommended for adults in this country at increased risk of occupational, social, family, and environmental or illness-related exposure to HBV. These include homosexual men, intravenous drug users, persons with multiple sex partners, household or sexual contacts of HBV carriers, and workers in health-related fields that involve frequent exposure to blood and infected body fluids. At the moment this excellent vaccine is underutilized in most hospitals and clinical practices, and specifically by physicians and surgeons.

Targeting only high-risk population groups for immunization against HBV in this country has failed to reduce the number of HBV infections. The reported incidence of acute hepatitis B increased by 37 percent from 1979 to 1989 and an estimated 200,000 to 300,000 new cases occurred annually during the period from 1980 to 1991. The estimated 1 million to 1.5 million persons with chronic HBV infection in the United States are potentially infectious to others and are at risk for cirrhosis and primary hepatocellular carcinoma. Each year about 1000 to 5000 chronic carriers die from chronic liver disease.[82] The CDC has recommended a comprehensive strategy to eventually eliminate the HBV infection in the United States. This includes (1) prenatal testing of pregnant women for HBsAg; if the mother is positive, a newborn will require HBIG immunoprophylaxis along with immunization; and (2) routine vaccination without HBIG of children born to HBsAg negative mothers. This means that all newborns are to be immunized in this country in addition to risk groups (see above).

Immunoglobulin Prophylaxis

Human immunoglobulin is highly effective for prophylaxis against hepatitis A in relatively low doses. The proper dose for HBV is not clear. HBIG is similar to conventional immunoglobulin except that it is prepared from plasma preselected for high titer of anti-HBsAg and the absence of HBsAg.[72] In the United States, HBIG has an anti-HBsAg titer greater than 1:100,000 by radioimmunoassay. At this time postexposure prophylaxis with HBIG is recommended under the following circumstances: (1) exposure to HBV-containing material by percutaneous inoculation or direct mucosal contact; (2) intimate contact with an acutely infected individual; and (3) exposure of newborns to HBV infected mothers, specifically the use of HBIG in combination with active immunization with HBV vaccine. A normal series of immunizations with HBV vaccine, combined with a single dose of HBIG (0.06 ml/kg or 5 ml for adults) given at a different site from the vaccine is recommended for postexposure prophylaxis of previously unvaccinated health workers after accidental exposure, including needle sticks.

HEPATITIS C VIRAL INFECTION

After hepatitis B viral infection and transmission by blood transfusions could confidently be excluded by prior testing of blood donors, it became apparent that a significant group of patients who received blood developed hepatitis. This was called non-A non-B (NANB) hepatitis in the 1970s. It has now been determined that 79 to 91 percent of transfusion recipients with NANB hepatitis were infected with hepatitis C virus (HCV).[83–85] It is thus quite possible that still other hepatitis viruses besides HCV will be discovered that may cause post-transfusion hepatitis, but HCV probably represents the major culprit of this group.

The detection of HCV was not possible without an effective diagnostic test. The virus has not been isolated or grown, but a test was developed entirely by gene cloning and other molecular techniques. This test relied on the discovery of the C-100 antigen from material containing NANB virus. Nucleic acid was isolated from such materials, and a cDNA library was constructed in λgt 11 phage grown in bacteria. Fusion proteins expressed by the bacteria were screened by an antiserum known to react against the virus of NANB hepatitis. Rare clones of bacteria expressing reactive HCV antigen were isolated and a common open reading frame was identified. The isolated antigen was used to develop immunoassays. Later, the nucleotide sequence of the virus was elucidated and all its antigens were characterized. It is now believed that this virus belongs to the Bunyamwera virus group, which are double-stranded RNA viruses. Several other structural as well as nonstructural antigens besides C-100 have now been discovered and also can be used to detect antibodies. In addition it is now possible to search for the virus with polymerase chain reaction

(PCR), which is the most sensitive method to detect its presence.

Like HBV, HCV appears to be transmitted by parenteral routes, and it can lead to persistent and chronic hepatitis as well as hepatocellular carcinoma. The extent to which transmission can occur, its morbidity, pathogenicity, and epidemiology are still being worked out. It appears that hepatitis due to HCV may be milder than that due to HBV, but a significant proportion of patients with HCV hepatitis, which may be as high as 62 percent, can develop chronic infection.[86] What is not clear is how much morbidity this degree of chronic infection causes. In one study, transfusion recipients, who had by retrospective diagnosis NANB hepatitis in 1967, were found by comparison to matched controls not to have any increase in mortality. While this was a study of NANB hepatitis, one assumes that a significant number had HCV infection.[87]

OTHER HUMAN T-LYMPHOTROPIC VIRUSES (HTLV)

Besides HIV types 1 and 2, two other retroviruses, HTLV-1 and HTLV-2, have been found to infect humans and to produce disease as a result of infection. Because these viruses are transmitted by blood transfusion (they can also be found in other body fluids), blood donors in this country are routinely screened for these viruses.[88] HTLV-1 is the more prevalent and medically the more important one. It is endemic in southwestern Japan, the Caribbean basin, Melanesia, and parts of Africa. Prevalence rates as high as 15 percent have been reported. The prevalence in this country is estimated to be about 0.008 percent.[89]

HTLV-1 can be transmitted vertically from mother to child, or by sexual contact, blood transfusions, and sharing of contaminated needles. As in the case of HIV, the efficiency of sexual transmission is higher from infected men than women. Two diseases have been associated with HTLV-1: adult T cell leukemia and lymphoma, and HTLV-1 associated myelopathy/tropical spastic paraparesis (HAM/TSP). HTLV-1 associated lymphoma involves T cells, which extensively infiltrate lymph nodes, viscera, and skin. Hypercalcemia and bone lesions may be found. It occurs most frequently among persons 40 to 60 years of age in endemic areas, suggesting a long period of incubation. HAM/TSP is delineated by slowly progressive chronic spastic paraparesis, characterized by weakness, urinary incontinence, and sensory disturbances in the lower extremities. Adult T cell leukemia/lymphoma has been estimated to occur in about 2 to 4 percent of individuals infected with HTLV-1 in endemic areas. Thus in terms of morbidity, it is a significantly less virulent pathogen than HIV, even though the prevalence of infection in the U.S. population is similar to that of HIV.

HTLV-2 has not been clearly associated with any disease, although initially it was isolated from patients with hairy cell leukemia.[90]

Because of the differences in the epidemiologic and clinical implications of HTLV-1 and HTLV-2, an effort should be made to differentiate the two infections in subjects in whom the screening test is positive. This can be done by PCR and other research methods.

HTLV-1/2 is primarily a medical problem for blood banks. The test is not routinely done except for blood donors. Counseling on the nature of the infection and its method of transmission should be provided for patients or blood donors found to be positive. In monogamous relationships, the sexual partner should also be tested. If he/she is also positive, no further precautions need to be undertaken. However, if the partner is negative, barrier precautions to prevent sexual transmission should be considered.

RABIES

From none to five cases of human rabies occur each year in the United States, although animal rabies is fairly widespread and occurs in every state except Hawaii. In 1991, 6910 cases of animal rabies were reported by the CDC, the great majority occurring in wild animals.[91] Before 1950 more than 8000 cases of rabies in dogs occurred each year in the United States. This number is currently less than 150 per year. After a prodrome including fever, malaise, and headache, hyperactivity and diffuse cerebral dysfunction occur, followed by coma and death. Of individuals who contract rabies, 5 to 20 percent may show progressive paralysis. Occasionally, there is no history of animal bite. Diagnosis may be confirmed by virus culture from secretions, cerebrospinal fluid, or brain, demonstration of rabies antigen in cornea or skin, or rise in rabies antibody. It is incurable. At postmortem examination typical intracytoplasmic inclusions called Negri bodies can be seen in the brain (see Fig. 11–3B).

Surgeons may be called on to consider rabies prophylaxis in patients whom they treat for bite injuries. Local wound care is important. The wound should be thoroughly scrubbed with soap and water. The decision to give postexposure antirabies treatment should include the following considerations:

1. Type of exposure. Rabies is transmitted primarily by the bite of infected animals. It may also be transmitted by introducing the virus into open cuts or wounds in the skin or via mucous membranes by saliva. It can occasionally be transmitted by aeresol exposure—usually occurring in spelunkers who walk through caves in which rabid bats live. There is even one case that was transmitted by a cornea transplant that was removed from a patient dying of rabies.
2. Species of biting animals. Carnivorous wild animals (especially skunks, raccoons, and foxes) and bats are most commonly infected with rabies in the United States. The likelihood that domestic cats or dogs in the United States will be infected varies from region to region and depends largely on whether administration of one of the many rabies vaccines is required. A dog or cat that remains healthy for 10 days after a bite does not have rabies, and prophylaxis for a person bitten by that animal is not indicated. A negative fluorescent antibody examination of an animal brain in laboratory with staff experienced in the examination is reliable evidence that the animal did not have rabies. Rodents and lagomorphs (rabbits and hares) are rarely infected. Livestock occasionally can harbor rabies.
3. Circumstances of the biting incident. An unprovoked attack is more indicative of a rabid dog than a provoked attack. A properly immunized animal has only a minimal chance of transmitting the virus.[92]

If a person is bitten by a household pet such as a dog or cat and the animal is healthy, it should be observed for 10 days. If the animal remains healthy, no treatment need be given. If the animal shows signs of rabies, the patient should be treated with human rabies immune globulin (HRIG) and human diploid cell rabies vaccine (HDCV). The symptomatic animal should be killed and tested for rabies as soon as possible. HRIG and HDCV should be given as soon as possible if the household pet is rabid or suspect. If the animal escapes, public health officials should be consulted and HRIG and HDCV given if indicated. Wild animals such as skunks, bats, foxes, coyotes, raccoons, bobcats, and other carnivores should be regarded as rabid unless proved negative by laboratory testing. If available, the animal should be killed and tested. HRIG and HDCV should be given as soon as possible. Local and state health officials should be consulted on the need for prophylaxis for bites by livestock, rodents, and lagomorphs. Bites by squirrels, hamsters, guinea pigs, gerbils, chipmunks, rats, mice, other rodents, rabbits, and hares almost never call for antirabies prophylaxis.

Both HRIG and HDCV are used for postexposure prophylaxis. The recommended dose of HRIG is 20 IU/kg of body weight. If possible, up to one-half the dose of HRIG should be thoroughly infiltrated into the area around the wound, and the rest should be administered intramuscularly. Postexposure HDCV should be given in five 1-ml doses intramuscularly on days 0, 3, 7, 14, and 28. Persons who have had adequate preexposure rabies prophylaxis should receive two doses of HDCV, 1 ml intramuscularly on days 0 and 3.[92] The Centers for Disease Control recommends preexposure immunization be considered for high-risk groups: animal handlers, certain laboratory workers and field personnel, and persons planning to spend more than 1 month in areas of countries where rabies is a constant threat.[92]

Although there are few cases of clinical rabies per year in the United States, it remains a constant consideration, and approximately 18,000 people per year are given postexposure prophylaxis, and 10,000 persons receive preexposure prophylaxis.[92]

CONGENITAL MALFORMATIONS CAUSED BY VIRAL INFECTIONS REQUIRING SURGERY

Viruses may be transmitted transplacentally but may not cause malformations that require surgery. An important virus of this group is CMV, which is a primary cause of congenital viral infection, the most severe form of which is called cytomegalic inclusion disease (see section on CMV). Specific surgically correctable congenital malformations are usually not associated with this type of viral infection. In the severe cases the patient presents with intracranial calcifications, microcephaly, hepatosplenomegaly, and thrombocytopenia. There often may be late sequelae to congenital CMV infection, which include poor development and nerve deafness. Inguinal hernias, a surgically correctable condition, are more common in patients with congenital CMV disease. In one report, the frequency was 26 percent.[93]

Rubella is the most familiar virus that may cause congenital deformities.[94] This is a teratogenic virus that affects the fetus most critically in the first trimester when infection can retard and distort development. The newborn child may have cataracts, deafness, mental retardation, and congenital heart defects. Patent ductus arteriosus, pulmonary valve stenosis, supervalvular pulmonary stenosis, atrial septal defects, ventricular septal defects, and tetralogy of Fallot can occur. Some of these malformations are correctable by surgery. Infection by rubella virus as well as its sequelae are readily preventable by universal administration of the vaccine to infants.

VIRAL INFECTIONS AS CAUSE OF SURGICAL ILLNESS

Other viruses besides the ones mentioned in the previous sections are alleged to cause or participate in the pathogenesis of several illnesses that may require surgery, but the evidence is usually not convincing.[95,96] These diseases are listed in Table 11–8. Proving that a surgical illness is caused by a virus is not always easy. The most obvious method is to culture the virus from the tissues. Live virus may no longer be available, however, when operation or autopsy is performed. Some viruses may be present in latent form and may not be easily cultured or may be reactivated by the disease rather than cause it. Even finding culture or histologic evidence of tissue infection is not proof that the virus caused the illness. The virus may merely have found the diseased tissue suitable for propagation. Epidemiologic studies can establish a relationship between a viral infection and the occurrence of a disease, but they cannot prove causation.

TABLE 11–8. SURGICAL DISEASES IN WHICH A VIRAL PATHOGENESIS HAS BEEN PROPOSED

Disease	Virus
Appendicitis	Enterovirus Adenovirus Coxsackie B Hepatitis Other or unspecified
Mesenteric adenitis	Adenovirus Unspecified Measles
Ileocecal intussusception	Adenovirus Other
Pancreatitis	Mumps Hepatitis Cytomegalovirus Other
Gastrointestinal ulcers	Cytomegalovirus
Regional enteritis	Unidentified RNA virus
Ulcerative colitis	Cytomegalovirus
Constrictive pericarditis	Coxsackie B

VIRAL INFECTIONS IN TRANSPLANT RECIPIENTS

Viral infections are one of the most common infections that occur in organ transplant recipients.[97,98] These viral infections are almost always due to herpesviruses, of which cytomegalovirus (CMV) is the most common. Transplant patients may develop CMV infection with no sign of clinical illness, or it may cause severe illness and death. CMV can also be responsible for ulcers of the gastrointestinal tract, which can lead to bleeding or perforation requiring surgical therapy.[99,100] EBV-associated lymphoproliferative disorders including B cell lymphomas may present as a surgical problem in the abdomen, in the tonsils, or in lymph nodes anywhere[101,102] (see also section on herpesviruses). Infective disorders in the immunosuppressed are discussed in a separate chapter.

Acknowledgments. The author acknowledges Dr. Richard J. Howard, author of this chapter in the previous edition, for his contribution to the section on rabies and the sections thereafter, for Tables 11–6 and 11–8, and the figures.

REFERENCES

1. Fields BN (ed): Virology, 2nd ed. New York, Raven Press, 1990.
2. Barre-Sinoussi F, Chermann JC, Rey F, et al: Isolation of a T-lymphotropic retrovirus from a patient at risk for acquired immune deficiency syndrome (AIDS). Science 220:868, 1983.
3. Choo QL, Kus G, Weiner AJ, et al: Isolation of a cDNA clone derived from a blood-borne non-A non-B hepatitis genome. Science 244:359, 1989.
4. Wentworth BB: Bacteriophage typing of the staphylococci. Bacteriol Rev 27:253, 1963.
5. Tyler KL, Fields BN: Pathogenesis of viral infection, In Fields BN (ed): Virology, 2nd ed. New York, Raven Press, 1990, pp 191–239.
6. Stein BS, Gowda SD, Lifson SD, et al: pH independent HIV entry into CD4 positive T cells via virus envelope fusion to the plasma membrane. Cell 49:659, 1987.
7. Miller G: Epstein-Barr virus. In Fields BN (ed): Virology, 2nd ed. New York, Raven Press, 1990, pp 1921–1958.
8. Rowe M, Young LS, Crocker J, et al: Epstein-Barr virus (EBV)-associated lymphoproliferative disease in the SCID mouse model: implications for the

pathogenesis of EBV-positive lymphomas in man. J Exp Med 173:147, 1991.
9. Poiesz BJ, Ruscetti FW, Gazdar AF, et al: Detection and isolation of type C retrovirus particles from fresh and cultured lymphocytes of a patient with cutaneous T-cell lymphoma. Proc Natl Acad Sci USA 77:7415, 1980.
10. Grundy JE, Shanley JD, Griffiths PD: Is cytomegalovirus interstitial pneumonitis in transplant recipients an immunopathological condition? Lancet 2: 996, 1987.
11. Mondelli M, Eddleston ALWF: Mechanisms of liver cell injury in acute and chronic hepatitis B. Semin Liver Dis 4:47, 1984.
12. Sherlock S, Fox RA, Niazi SP, Schener PJ: Chronic liver disease and primary liver cell cancer with hepatitis associated (Australian) antigen in serum. Lancet 2:1243, 1970.
13. Beasly RP, Hwang L-Y, Lin GC-Y, Chien C-S: Hepatocellular carcinoma and hepatitis B virus: a prospective study of 22,707 men in Taiwan. Lancet 2:1129, 1981.
14. Bruix J, Calvet X, Costa J, et al: Prevalence of antibodies to hepatitis C virus in Spanish patients with hepatocellular carcinoma and hepatic cirrhosis. Lancet 2:1004, 1989.
15. Colombo M, Choo QL, Del Ninno E, et al: Prevalence of antibodies to hepatitis C virus in Italian patients with hepatocellular carcinoma. Lancet 2:1006, 1989.
16. Murphy FA, Kingsburg WA: Virus taxonomy. In Fields BN (ed): Virology, 2nd ed. New York, Raven Press, 1990, pp 9–36.
17. Horsfall FL, Tamm I: Viral and Rickettsial Infections of Man, 4th ed. Philadelphia, Lippincott, 1965, pp 580–650.
17a. Centers for Disease Control and Prevention (CDC): Outbreak of an acute illness—Southwestern United States. MMWR 42:422–424, 1993.
18. Centers for Disease Control: Pneumocystis pneumonia—Los Angeles. MMWR Morbid Mortal Wkly Rep 30:250, 1981.
19. Centers for Disease Control: Recommendation for preventing transmission of infection with human T-lymphotropic viruses type III/lymphadenopathy associated virus in the work place. MMWR Morbid Mortal Wkly Rep 34:681, 691, 1985.
20. Alter HJ: Descartes before the horse: I clone, therefore I am: the hepatitis C virus in current perspective. Ann Intern Med 115:644, 1991.
21. Koutsky LA, Galloway DA, Holmes KK: Epidemiology of genital human papillomavirus infection. Epidemiol Rev 10:122, 1988.
22. Orth G: Epidermodysplasia verruciformis. In Salzman NP, Howley PM (eds): The Papovaviridae, Vol 2. New York, Plenum Press, 1987, pp 199–243.
23. zur Hausen H: Intracellular surveillance of persisting viral infections. Human genital cancer results from deficient control of papillomavirus infection. Lancet 2:489, 1986.
24. Phelps WE, Yee CL, Munger K, Howley PM: The human papillomavirus type 16 E7 gene encodes transactivation and transformation functions similar to adenovirus E1A. Cell 53:539, 1988.
25. Wantanabe S, Kanda T, Yoshiike K: Human papillomavirus type 16 transformation of primary human embryonic fibroblasts requires expression of open reading frames E6 and E7. J Virol 63:965, 1989.
26. Durst M, Dzarlieva-Pertrusevzka P, Boukamp P, et al: Molecular and cytogenetic analysis of immortalized human primary keratinocytes obtained after transfection with human papilloma virus type 16 DNA. Oncogene 1:251, 1987.
27. Schuster EA, Beneke JS, Tegtmeier GF, et al: Monoclonal antibody for rapid laboratory detection of cytomegalovirus infections: characterization and diagnostic application. Mayo Clin Proc 60:577, 1985.
28. Cassol SA, Lapointe N, Salas T, et al: Diagnosis of vertical HIV-1 transmission using the polymerase chain reaction and dried blood spot specimens. J Acquir Immune Defic Syndr 5:113, 1992.
29. Ho M: EBV infection and post-transplant lymphoproliferative disorders. Transplant Sci 2:87, 1992.
30. Kieff E, Liebowitz D: Epstein-Barr virus and its replication. In Fields BN (ed): Virology, 2nd ed. New York, Raven Press, 1990, pp 1889–1920.
31. Ho M, Miller G, Atchison RW, et al: Epstein-Barr virus infections and DNA hybridization studies in post-transplantation lymphoma and lymphoproliferative lesions: Role of primary infection. J Infect Dis 152:876, 1985.
32. Salahuddin SZ, Ablashi DV, Markham PD, et al: Isolation of a new virus, HBLV, in patients with lymphoproliferative disorders. Science 234:596, 1986.
33. Yamanishi K, Okuno T, Shiraki K, et al: Identification of human herpesvirus-6 as a causal agent for exanthema subitum. Lancet 1:1065, 1988.
34. Pruksananonda P, Breese Hall C, Insel RA, et al: Primary human herpesvirus 6 infection in young children. N Engl J Med 326:1145, 1992.
34a. Frenkel N, Shirmer EC, Wyatt LS, et al: Isolation of a new herpesvirus from human CD4+ cells. Proc Natl Acad Sci 87:748, 1990.
35. Ho M: Cytomegalovirus: Biology and Infections, 2nd ed. New York, Plenum Medical, 1991.
36. Weller TH, McCauley JC, Craig JM, Wirth P: Isolation of intranuclear inclusion producing agents from infants with illnesses resembling cytomegalic inclusion disease. Proc Soc Exp Biol Med 94:4, 1957.
37. Ho M: Cytomegalovirus: Biology and Infections, 2nd ed. New York, Plenum Medical, 1991, pp 207–213.
38. Klemola E, Kaariainen L: Cytomegalovirus as a possible cause of a disease resembling infectious mononucleosis. Br Med J 2:1099, 1965.
39. Ho M: Cytomegalovirus: Biology and Infections, 2nd ed. New York, Plenum Medical, 1991, pp 229–247.
40. Kaariainen L, Klemola E, Paloheimo J: Rise of cytomegalovirus antibodies in an infectious-mononucle-

osis-like syndrome after transfusion. Br Med J 2:1270, 1966.
41. Lang DM, Scolnick EM, Willerson JT: Association of cytomegalovirus infection with the post-perfusion syndrome. N Engl J Med 278:1147, 1968.
42. Henle W, Henle G, Scriba M, et al: Antibody responses to the Epstein-Barr virus and cytomegalovirus after open-heart surgery. N Engl J Med 282:1068, 1970.
43. Ho M: Cytomegalovirus: Biology and Infections, 2nd ed. New York, Plenum Medical, 1991, pp 177–179.
44. Armstrong JA, Tarr GC, Ho M, et al: Cytomegalovirus infection in children undergoing open-heart surgery. Yale J Biol Med 49:83, 1976.
45. Yeager AS, Grumet FC, Hafleigh EB, et al: Prevention of transfusion-acquired cytomegalovirus infections in newborn infants. J Pediatr 98:281, 1981.
46. Ho M: Cytomegalovirus: Biology and Infections, 2nd ed. New York, Plenum Medical, 1991, pp 175–179.
47. Wilhelm JA, Matter L, Schopfer K: The risk of transmitting cytomegalovirus to patients receiving blood transfusions. J Infect Dis 154:169, 1986.
48. Preiksaitis JK, Brown L, McKenzie M: The risk of cytomegalovirus infection in seronegative transfusion recipients not receiving exogenous immunosuppression. J Infect Dis 157:523, 1988.
49. Mann J, Tarantola D, Netter TW: AIDS in the World, 1992. Cambridge, MA, Harvard University Press, 1992.
50. Centers for Disease Control: Acquired immunodeficiency syndrome, United States, 1981–1990. MMWR Morbid Mortal Wkly Rep 40:358, 1991.
51. Centers for Disease Control: Guidelines for prevention of transmission of HIV and HBV to health-care and public safety workers. MMWR Morbid Mortal Wkly Rep 38:1, 1989.
52. Pantaleo G, Graziosi C, Fauci AS: The immunopathogenesis of human immunodeficiency virus infection. N Engl J Med 328:327, 1993.
53. Kingsley LA, Rinaldo CR, Lyter DW, et al: Sexual transmission efficiency of hepatitis B virus and human immunodeficiency virus among homosexual men. JAMA 264:230, 1990.
54. World Health Organization: The Global Eradication of Smallpox, Final Report of the Global Commission for the Certification of Smallpox Eradication (History of International Public Health, No. 4). Geneva, World Health Organization, 1980.
55. Fischl MA, Richman DD, Grieco MH, et al: The efficacy of azidothymidine (AZT) in the treatment of patients with AIDS and AIDS-related complex: a double-blind, placebo-controlled trial. N Engl J Med 317:185, 1987.
56. Fischl MA, Richmann DD, Hansen N, et al: The safety and efficacy of zidovudine (AZT) in the treatment of subjects with mildly symptomatic human immunodeficiency virus type 1 (HIV) infection: a double-blind, placebo-controlled trial. Ann Intern Med 112:727, 1990.
57. Volberding PA, Lagakos SW, Koch MA, et al: Zidovudine in asymptomatic human immunodeficiency virus infection: a controlled trial in persons with fewer than 500 CD4 positive cells per cubic millimeter. N Engl J Med 322:941, 1990.
58. Yarchoan R, Thomas RV, Grafman J, et al: Long-term administration of 3′-azido-2′, 3′-dideoxythymidine to patients with AIDS-related neurological disease. Ann Neurol 23(Suppl):S82, 1988.
59. Schmitt FA, Bigley JW, McKinnis R, et al: Neuropsychological outcome of zidovudine (AZT) treatment of patients with AIDS and AIDS-related complex. N Engl J Med 319:1573, 1988.
60. Pottage JC Jr, Benson CA, Speak JB, et al: Treatment of human immunodeficiency virus-related thrombocytopenia with zidovudine. JAMA 260:3045, 1988.
61. Boyar A, Beall G: HIV-seropositive thrombocytopenia: the action of zidovudine. AIDS 5:1351, 1991.
62. McLeod GX, Hammer SM: Zidovudine: five years later. Ann Intern Med 117:487, 1992.
63. Bessen LJ, Greene JB, Louie E, et al: Severe polymyositis-like syndrome associated with zidovudine therapy of AIDS and AIDS-related complex. N Engl J Med 328:708, 1988.
64. Mhiri C, Baudrimont M, Bonne G, et al: Zidovudine myopathy: a distinctive disorder associated with mitochondrial dysfunction. Ann Neurol 29:606, 1991.
65. Larder BA, Darby G, Richman DD: HIV with reduced sensitivity to zidovudine (AZT) isolated during prolonged therapy. Science 243:1731, 1989.
66. Kahn JO, Lagakos SW, Richman DD, et al: A controlled trial comparing continued zidovudine with didanosine in human immunodeficiency virus infection. N Engl J Med 327:581, 1992.
67. Yarchoan R, Thomas RV, Allain JP, et al: Phase I studies of 2′,3′-dideoxycytidine in severe human immunodeficiency virus infection as a single agent and alternating with zidovudine (AZT). Lancet 1:175, 1988.
68. Centers for Disease Control: 1993 Revised classification system for HIV infection and expanded surveillance case definition for AIDS among adolescents and adults. MMWR Morbid Mortal Wkly Rep 41:1, 1992.
69. Bradley DW: Hepatitis non-A, non-B viruses become identified as hepatitus C and E Prog Med Virol 37:101, 1990.
70. Kusne S, Schwartz M, Breinig MK, et al: Herpes simplex virus hepatitis after solid organ transplantation in adults. J Infect Dis 163:1001, 1991.
71. Robinson WS: Hepadnaviridae and their replication. In Fields BN (ed): Virology, 2nd ed. New York, Raven Press, 1990, pp 2137–2170.
72. Hollinger FB: Hepatitis B virus. In Fields BN (ed): Virology, 2nd ed. New York, Raven Press, 1990, pp 2171–2236.
73. Stevens CE, Beasley RP, Tsui J, Lee W-C: Vertical transmission of hepatitis B antigen in Taiwan. N Engl J Med 292:771, 1975.
74. Beasley RP, Trepo C, Stevens CE, et al: The e anti-

gen and vertical transmission of hepatitis B surface antigen. Am J Epidemiol 105:94, 1977.
75. Lee AKY, Ip HMH, Wong VCW: Mechanisms of maternal-fetal transmission of hepatitis B virus. J Infect Dis 138:668, 1978.
76. Beasley RP, Hwang L-Y, Lin C-C, et al: Incidence of hepatitis B virus infections in preschool children in Taiwan. J Infect Dis 146:198, 1982.
77. Hilleman MR, Buynak EB, McAleer WJ, et al: Hepatitis A and hepatitis B vaccines. In Szumness W, Alter HJ, Maynard JE (eds): Viral Hepatitis—1981 International Symposium. Philadelphia, Franklin Institute Press, 1982, pp 385–398.
78. McAleer WJ, Buynak EB, Maigetter RZ, et al: Human hepatitis B vaccine from recombinant yeast. Nature 307:178, 1984.
79. Beasley RP, Hwang L-Y, Lee GC-Y, et al: Prevention of perinatally transmitted hepatitis B virus infections with hepatitis B immune globulin and hepatitis B vaccine. Lancet 2:1099, 1983.
80. Lo K-J, Tsai Y-T, Lee S-D, et al: Immunoprophylaxis of infection with hepatitis B virus in infants born to hepatitis B surface antigen positive carrier mothers. J Infect Dis 152:817, 1985.
81. Centers for Disease Control: HBV immunization policy. MMWR Morbid Mortal Wkly Rep 40:1, 1991.
82. Centers for Disease Control: Protection against viral hepatitis. MMWR Morbid Mortal Wkly Rep 39:1, 1990.
83. Miyamura T, Saito I, Katayama T, et al: Detection of antibody against antigen expressed by molecularly cloned hepatitis C virus cDNA: application to diagnosis and blood screening for posttransfusion hepatitis. Proc Natl Acad Sci USA 87:983, 1990.
84. Alter MJ, Margolis HS, Krawczynski K, et al: The natural history of community-acquired hepatitis C in the United States. N Engl J Med 327:1899, 1992.
85. Aach RD, Stevens CE, Hollinger B, et al: Hepatitis C virus infection in post-transfusion hepatitis: an analysis with first- and second-generation assays. N Engl J Med 325:1325, 1991.
86. Alter HJ: Chronic consequences of non-A, non-B hepatitis. In Seef LB, Lewis JH (eds): Current Perspectives in Hepatology. New York, Plenum Medical, 1989, pp 83–87.
87. Seeff LB, Buskell-Bales Z, Wright EC, et al: Long-term mortality after transfusion-associated non-A, non-B hepatitis. N Engl J Med 327:1906, 1992.
88. Centers for Disease Control: Guidelines for counseling persons infected with human T-lymphotropic virus type I (HTLV-I) and type II (HTLV-II). Ann Intern Med 118:448, 1993.
89. Centers for Disease Control: Human T-lymphotropic virus type-I screening in volunteer blood donors—U.S., 1989. MMWR Morbid Mortal Wkly Rep 39:915, 921, 1990.
90. Kalyanaraman VS, Sarngadharan MC, Robert-Guroff M, et al: A new subtype of human T-cell leukemia virus (HTLV-II) associated with a T-cell variant of hairy cell leukemia. Science 218:571, 1982.
91. Centers for Disease Control: Summary of notifiable diseases, United States. MMWR Morbid Mortal Wkly Rep 40:1, 1992.
92. Centers for Disease Control: Update on adult immunization. Recommendation of the immunization practices advisory committee (ACIP). MMWR Morbid Mortal Wkly Rep 40:37, 1991.
93. Pass RF, Stagno S, Myers GJ, et al: Outcome of symptomatic congenital cytomegalovirus infection: results of long-term longitudinal follow-up. Pediatrics 66:758, 1980.
94. Wolinsky JS: Rubella. In Fields BN (ed): Virology, 2nd ed. New York, Raven Press, 1990, pp 815–838.
95. Howard RJ, Balfour HH Jr, Simmon RL: The surgical significance of viruses. Curr Probl Surg 14:1, 1977.
96. Howard RJ: Virus infections in surgery. In Alexander JW (ed): Problems in General Surgery. Philadelphia, Lippincott, 1984, pp 522–542.
97. Ho M, Peterson PK, Simmons RL, Dummer JS: Risk factors and approaches to infections in transplant patients. In Mandell GL, Douglas R, Bennett JE (eds): Principles and Practice of Infectious Diseases, 3rd ed. New York, Wiley, 1989, pp 2294–2392.
98. Ho M: Laboratory evaluations of infections in immunosuppressed transplant patients. Clin Lab Med 211:715, 1991.
99. Peterson PK, Balfour HH Jr, Marker SC, et al: Cytomegalovirus disease in renal allograft recipients: a prospective study of the clinical features, risk factors and impact on renal transplantation. Medicine (Baltimore) 59:283, 1980.
100. Strayer DS, Phillips GB, Barker KH, et al: Gastric cytomegalovirus infection in bone marrow transplant patients: an indication of generalized disease. Cancer 48:1478, 1981.
101. Ho M, Jaffe R, Miller G, et al: The frequency of EBV infection and associated lymphoproliferative syndrome after transplantation and its manifestations in children. Transplantation 45:719, 1988.
102. Nalesnik MA, Makowka L, Starzl TE: The diagnosis and treatment of post-transplant lymphoproliferative disorders. Curr Probl Surg 25:370, 1988.

Barriers to Infection

CHAPTER 12

Jonathan L. Meakins

The natural history of each infection can be conceptualized on an anatomic basis, that is on the basis of the body's attempt to localize infection to the original site or, if that is not possible, to confine the process regionally. When regionalization fails, invasion of the bloodstream takes place, and bacteremia must be controlled using all homeostatic mechanisms.

At the site of injury, the body mounts the classic inflammatory response to contain invasion of bacteria. The usual result is control and resolution of the potential infection. When infection becomes established, the inflammatory response attempts to contain and localize the process. Suppuration and spontaneous drainage constitute an obviously successful resolution of this response, although suppuration is frequently not required for local control.

Failure to localize leads to cellulitis or some degree of lymphangitis. The infecting organism passes through the lymphatic channels, resulting in regional lymphadenopathy secondary to local inflammation and reactive edema, which effectively blocks lymph flow. Suppuration can occur in the attempt to regionalize the infection. Cutaneous and pulmonary infections are commonly controlled by these processes. Streptococcal lymphangitis and lymphadenitis, mesenteric lymphadenopathy with acute nonperforated appendicitis, and the Ghon complex in tuberculosis are common examples of the body's attempt to regionalize and contain an infection. Although in some situations this process cannot take place (eg, pleural cavity, brain), the concept is useful.

Some infections are not contained by these attempts to localize or regionalize, and systemic invasion results. When bacteremia does take place, there are a variety of responses, including fever, chills, and cardiovascular collapse. The reticuloendothelial system (RES) attempts to clear the bloodstream of opsonized bacteria by active phagocytosis and is the last line of defense against invasive infection. These echelons of defense are an integral part of homeostasis, just as the maintenance of cardiovascular stability is a homeostatic mechanism that prolongs life until the infection and its septic response can be controlled.

To be effective, host defense requires the integrated and efficient function of the component parts. The failure of any segment of the system can result in an infectious process, as is apparent in the congenital immunologic deficiencies that affect single-cell or cell enzyme systems and frequently result in persistent, recurrent, or lethal infection.

The inflammatory response is the basic delivery system. The classic signs of inflammation—rubor, dolor, tumor, and calor—can be explained by examining the vascular, cellular, and molecular components of the response. Inflammation is also the effector system, the final common pathway, of almost all aspects of immunologic injury. The trigger for the response can be quite variable: for example, injury, operation, bacteria, endotoxin, or fracture. The initiator triggers a cellular response that generates mediators, cytokines, which have autocrine, paracrine, and endocrine effects, leading to the coordinated generation of effectors that make up the local and systemic response and the nonspecific and specific responses to the infectious agent. Whether the initiator is live bacteria, endotoxin, or surgery, the sequence of cytokine production is tumor necrosis factor (TNF), interleukin 1 (IL-1), and interleukin 6 (IL-6).

The vascular changes are largely mediated through vasoactive amines, notably the kinin system, histamine, and serotonin through upregulation of the CD11/CD18 complex of endothelial leukocyte adherence molecules (ELAMs, selectins). The release of these substances is coordinated to produce the vascular and endothelial changes, which then allow delivery of the humoral and cellular components to the inflammatory response. The precise sequence of action is not completely understood, but a synthesis follows.

The vascular response, initially vasoconstriction, takes place within minutes of the insult and is then followed in 10 to 30 minutes by a persistent vasodilation. The overt cutaneous signs are the triple response of Lewis. The vasodilation is accompanied by changes in the vessel wall and, subsequently, blood flow. There is stasis of blood with increased margination and adherence to the endothelial lining by polymorphonuclear leukocytes. Endothelial changes allow diapedesis of the polymorphonuclear leukocytes into the inflammatory focus. The vessel wall changes, and increased capillary pressure produces increased vascular permeability allowing delivery of plasma proteins, notably immunoglobulins, complement, and fibrinogen. In addition, there is breakdown of some large protein molecules and increased fluidity of the tissue ground substance, all of which contribute to the "tumor" associated with inflammation.

The cellular exudate parallels the fluid exudate and initially is almost exclusively polymorphonuclear leukocytes. After the first 24 hours, monocytes tend to replace neutrophils as the predominant phagocytic cell. When activated, the monocyte becomes an activated macrophage and, as such, is a more effective phagocyte. However, the macrophage also processes bacterial and other antigens before delivery to the lymphocyte for production of specific antibody. As the inflammatory process develops, the lymphatics, in part secondary to local swelling, enlarge, and lymphatic flow increases, aiding delivery of antigen to the regional lymph nodes.

For purposes of this discussion, the inflammatory exudate is directed against microbial invasion. The humoral opsonic component is made up of complement and immunoglobulins. The role of complement is multifaceted; it aids immune adherence, bacterial cytolysis, polymorphonuclear leukocyte chemotaxis, and phagocytosis. Immunoglobulins, notably IgG and IgM, together with complement are involved in polymorphonuclear leukocyte bacterial phagocytosis. Bacterial cytolysis can be effected by complement and immunoglobulin, but these play a modest role in the control of invasive bacteria. The crucial role of complement is to attract polymorphonuclear leukocytes to the area of the bacteria and then together with IgG provide opsonization of the bacteria for effective polymorphonuclear leukocyte phagocytosis and subsequent bacterial killing (see Figs. 13–1 to 13–3). In the absence of complement or immunoglobulins, phagocytosis is substantially decreased. Fibrin polymerization facilitates localization of the infection in abscesses and also supplies a matrix against which neutrophils can phagocytize bacteria that are not opsonized; thus the humoral and cellular components work together to control bacterial growth.

Polymorphonuclear leukocytes are the initial cellular response to an insult. They are actively phagocytic when delivered to the inflammatory focus. With ingestion, the bacterium is encased in a membrane-lined sac, the phagosome, which becomes a phagolysosome when fused with the enzyme-rich contents of polymorphonuclear leukocyte lysosomes. These lysosomes contain the multiple enzymatic and metabolic processes that result in bactericidal action. The polymorphonuclear leukocyte is the initial killer cell and is essential to maintenance of intact host defense. The inability to contain the microbial invasion, whether because of decreased numbers (circulating or delivered) or efficacy, is a critical factor that allows active microbial invasion to take place.

The second line of phagocytic response is the monocyte, which is second at an area of inflammation to an aggressive phagocytic and bactericidal long-lived cell, the macrophage. As with polymorphonuclear leukocytes, macrophage chemotaxis and phagocytosis require antibody and complement. Following ingestion and digestion, the microbial antigen is processed by the macrophage and transported locally or regionally to lymphocytes for production of specific antibody. The involved cells can be derived from bone marrow (B) or thymus (T) lymphocytes. B cells are responsible for production of specific antibodies, and T cells for production of specifically sensitized lymphocytes. These lymphocytes play a major role in protection against intracellular parasites through the macrophage, which becomes the effective microbicidal cell when activated, and together they express antiparasite cell-mediated immunity.

The antimicrobial action of cell-mediated immunity takes place through a complex system of recognition and cell activation involving different cells and numerous humoral mediators. Simplified, the cell-mediated antimicrobial system is based on recognition of antigen by T lymphocytes and subsequent macrophage attraction and stimulation. If the body has not had previous experience with the specific organism, time is required before sensitized lymphocytes are produced. In this situation, the arc will work somewhat in reverse; that is, the bacterial antigen will be processed by macrophages and delivered to lymphocytes for production of specifically sensitized T cells, which will then deliver effector cells to the site of infection.

When the host has had experience with a specific microbe, specific T cells are attracted to the focus of infection where they are more specifically activated to produce lymphokines, a family of soluble humoral mediators and cytokines. The molecules, not all of which are described, coordinate the local and systemic responses to infection. The process and mechanism of intracellular killing are similar to polymorphonuclear leukocytes. Failure of T cell function or congenital absence of T cells results in failure to mount an effective antimicrobial response against intracellular parasites.

Cell-mediated immunity is a specific reaction to an antigen or to antigen on cell or microbe surfaces. Delayed hypersensitivity is a cell-mediated immune phenomenon. The failure to respond appropriately can be a reflection of an alteration of the specific cell-mediated immune reaction or of a nonspecific failure of the sequence required to produce the positive skin test reaction.

Humoral systems, phagocyte function, and cell-mediated immunity have specific organisms, or classes of organisms, against which they are most effective (Table 12–1). It should be made clear that usually two of the three listed compartments of host defense are involved against invading microbes and that the predominant system is listed. For example, in the absence of specific antibody, the pneumococcus is not phagocytized by polymorphonuclear leukocytes; however, once present, phagocytosis and intracellular killing proceed rapidly. The key to this defense is the specific antibody, although control of the actual infection is a two-compartment effort.

The above-described processes of systemic host responses are but one of the three important determinants of any infectious process (Fig. 12–1). The other two determinants are (1) the microbe or in-

TABLE 12–1. EFFICACY OF THREE COMPARTMENTS OF HOST DEFENSE IN COUNTERING INFECTIOUS ORGANISMS

Humoral	Cell-Mediated	Phagocytic
Bacteria	Bacteria	Bacteria
Pneumococcus	*Mycobacteria*	*Staphylococcus*[a]
Streptococcus	*Listeria*	*Klebsiella*
Haemophilus	*Brucella*	*Aerobacter*
Meningococcus	*Salmonella*	*Serratia*
Pseudomonas	*Staphylococcus*[a]	*Proteus*
		Probably most other enteric and anaerobic bacteria
Toxins	Fungi	Fungi
Diphtheria	*Candida*[a]	*Candida*[a]
Tetanus	*Aspergillus*	
	Histoplasma	
	Mucor	
Viruses	Viruses	
Polio	*Vaccinia*	
Hepatitis	Cytomegalic inclusion disease	
Rubella	Most others	
Others		
	Parasites	
	Pneumocystis carinii	

[a] Many infectious agents are attached by two compartments of host defense; selecting the predominant compartment may not be possible.

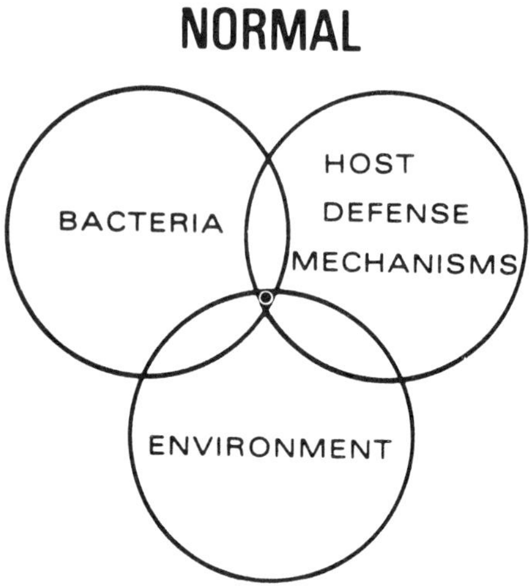

Figure 12–1. Schematic concept of interactions among host defense mechanisms, environment, and bacteria in determining whether infection occurs.

fecting organism, usually bacteria in surgical practice; and (2) the environment—local factors of resistance that are designed to prevent access of the microbe to the tissues in order to develop an infection. In all infectious processes these three determinants interact in the development of an infection. Separating the etiologic or determining factors of any process is important in the eventual approach in prevention.

The approach to wound infections has traditionally been based on a classification of the probability of bacterial contamination: clean, clean contaminated, contaminated, and infected. The recent study on the efficacy of nosocomial infection control (SENIC) analyzing the determinants of wound infection separates the contributing factors more clearly into bacterial factors and host-related factors. It is only by analyzing the host factors in this manner that further advances in control of this common problem can be achieved. Only one of the significant risk factors identified in the SENIC related solely to the bacterial determinant. The other three (abdominal operation, length of the procedure, and more than three diagnoses) all relate in part or completely to the host, either as local factors (ie, wound defenses) or as systemic ability to respond to the bacterial challenge. Christou and colleagues (see Chap. 17) have demonstrated that alterations in host physiology, host defense mechanisms, and bacterial inoculum bear directly and independently on infection-related deaths. Further evaluations will almost certainly demonstrate that altered physiology manifests its influence through secondary changes in resistance to bacteria.

Characteristics of the microbial determinant have already been discussed. This chapter shall address local and systemic responses to infection and how they may be abnormal in a surgical patient.

LOCAL HOST DEFENSES

The primary goal of the local host defense system is the *prevention of lodgement* of pathogenic microorganisms. The modified homunculus in Figure 12–2 indicates the routes of access of microbes to the body. All surfaces have highly specialized systems for regulation of their permanent and transient flora or for maintenance of their sterile environment. Although the components of this defense system vary for different organs, certain common factors are present: (1) a biologic wall (eg, skin and mucous membranes); (2) specialized surface cell functions (eg, macrophages, cilia); (3) local secretions, including those that provide specific local immunity; and (4) the normal microbial flora, which, by being more adapted to the environment, successfully compete with and thereby control colonization by pathogens.

The alteration of these protective interrelated systems in clinical practice is schematically represented by Figure 12–3. It is apparent that many routine therapeutic devices bypass or alter natural

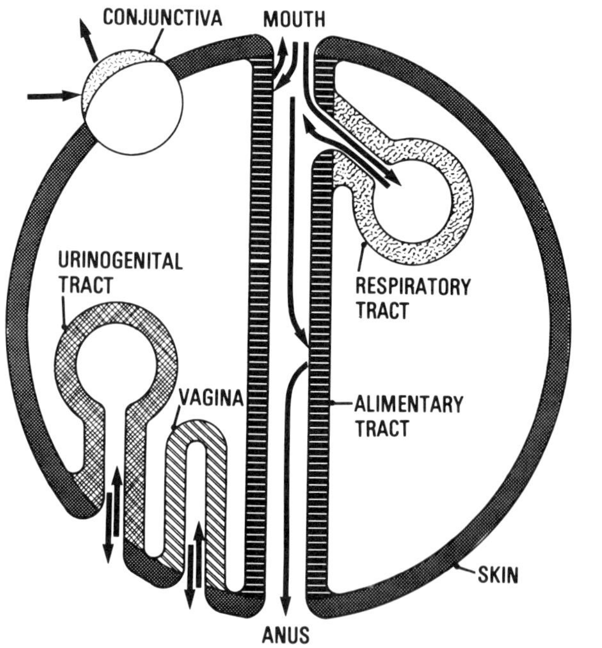

Figure 12–2. A modified homunculus, demonstrating the different epithelial surfaces and their relationship to the outside world.

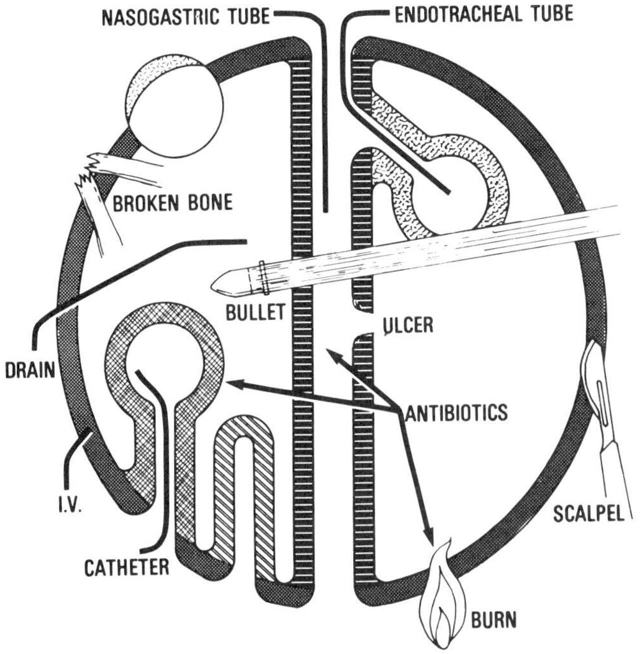

Figure 12–3. The epithelial disruptions induced by trauma, disease, and therapy, which permit microbial invasion.

environmental defenses, increasing the probability of infection.

SKIN

The skin presents a barrier to the external environment and has specific antibacterial mechanisms. Absorption of microorganisms through normal skin does not occur. At each juncture where the skin becomes internalized, a structural and functional alteration in the epithelium leads to a modification of the protective mechanisms.

The skin is in general a hostile environment for microbial growth (see Chaps. 3 and 31). Although there are sufficient nutrients for growth and survival, there is inadequate water. The pH of skin is normally between 5 and 6, and where bacteria flourish an alkaline environment is found. It is not clear if the alkalinity is a cause of bacterial growth or a result of it, but it is probably a combination of factors. The constant regeneration of skin and its desquamation contribute to elimination of transient or potentially pathogenic organisms.

The skin has specific antibacterial substances, although their precise nature is unclear.[1] Acetone extracts of normal skin lipids have some antimicrobial factors.[2] The free fatty acids on the skin, themselves products of bacterial degradation, also have antibacterial properties.[2] *Streptococcus pyogenes* is sensitive to some of these lipids and is rarely found on uninfected skin.

The resident flora lives in the stratum corneum and, in a limited way, in and around orifices of the glands of the skin. The sebum of sebaceous glands does not appear to have intrinsic major antibacterial properties.

The population density of the resident flora varies depending on environmental features. On skin of forearm and abdomen, there are 10^2 organisms/cm^2; on forehead, 10^4; and in most intertriginous areas such as the axilla, groin, and foot, 10^6. Wherever skin becomes moist, bacterial populations increase, so that skin adjacent to wet wounds, the perineum, and the backs of bedridden patients frequently develop an infective dermatitis. The addition of other factors that may damage skin, such as uncontrolled pancreatic, duodenal, gastric, or small bowel fistulas, produces environments conducive to infections. The skin is difficult to infect; both destruction of integrity and moisture are required and, of course, one leads to the other (see Chap. 31).

Interestingly, *Staphylococcus aureus* persists more effectively on fingertips and hands than in other areas.[3] Surgeons must maintain their own benign resident skin flora free from pathogenic transient flora, because hands are the most significant carriers of infection in hospitals. The sources of transient flora are the perineum and anterior nares of the personnel and the wounds of patients. Constant reminders regarding handwashing are required to develop this lost but valuable habit.

EYE

There is a modest indigenous bacterial flora in the conjunctival surface of the eye, largely *Staphylococcus epidermidis* and lactobacillus, with fewer *Haemophilus influenzae* and *S. aureus*.[4] Infections are unusual because of a combination of the mechanical, chemical, and immunologic properties of tears.[5,6]

Tears are isotonic, pH 7.35, and reflect blood urea and glucose levels. They are produced at about 12 μl/min, with about 6 μl in each eye. A flow rate greater than 100 μl/min will exceed the capacity of the eye. Blinking maintains an even wetness and promotes distribution of a tear film, which is structured into three layers: superficial lipid, middle aqueous, and deep mucous. The protein content is between 0.67 and 2 g per 100 ml divided relatively equally between albumin, globulin, and lysozyme. Lysozyme, which has both bacteriolytic and bacteriostatic properties, is found in highest concentration in tears.

The immunoglobulins IgA, IgG, and IgE are all found in tears, but IgA predominates. IgA is made by conjunctival and lacrimal plasma cells and acts to inhibit bacterial adherence to conjunctival epithelium. Tears can then wash away bacteria, reducing colonization.[6] IgG has an important but incompletely defined role in control of colonization and infection. Specific IgG picornavirus neutralizing antibody can be produced rapidly (1 to 3 days) by eye-associated lymphoid tissue in response to a specific local viral challenge. Its presence and concentration accurately parallel the course of the infection.[4]

RESPIRATORY TRACT

The respiratory tract, which extends from the anterior nares through the alveolus (Fig. 12–4), counteracts colonization by a variety of methods. Common to most parts are a moist surface, a mucous blanket, a mucociliary mechanism, and immunoglobulin A.

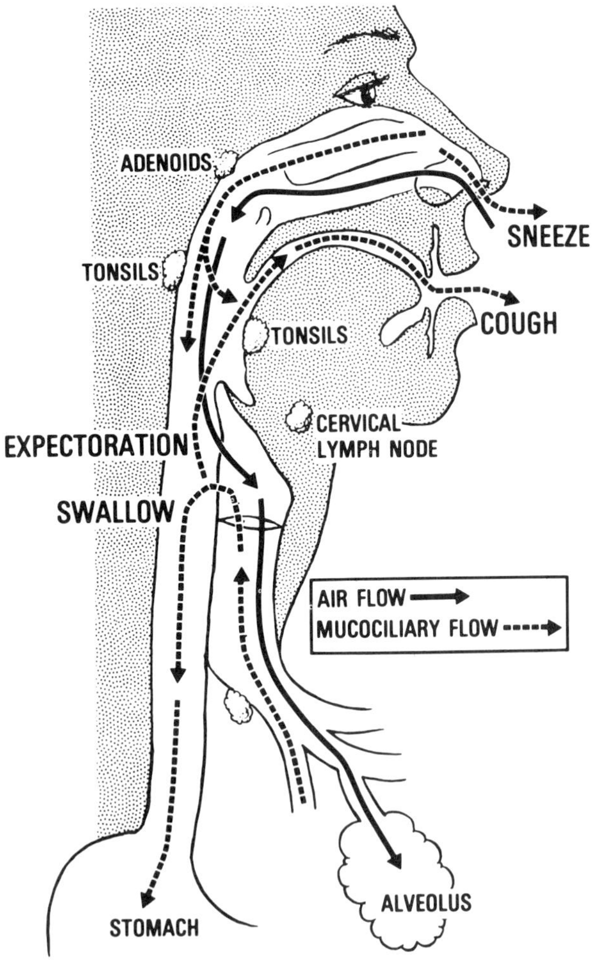

Figure 12–4. The natural environmental clearance mechanisms in the normal respiratory tract.

In addition to protecting itself from infection, the respiratory tract must cope with a considerable organic and nonorganic particulate matter. The respiratory tract provides innumerable convolutions and directional changes, providing opportunity for airborne particles to hit or settle onto the surface mucous layer overlying the respiratory epithelium. Once in contact with mucosa, they are moved toward the pharynx via mucociliary action (see Fig. 12–4) and coughing.

Nasopharynx

The nose is better designed to filter particulate matter including microbes from the air than is the mouth. The hairs, turbinates, and physical convolutions of the nose function to generate turbulence such that particulate matter of all sizes, but particularly those in the 10-μm range, strike the nasal and pharyngeal mucosa. They are then swept posteriorly by mucociliary action in the mucous blanket of the nasal mucosa to the pharynx. The mucociliary blanket clears the nose every 14 minutes.[7]

The anatomic arrangements to produce air turbulence around a richly vascularized mucosa provide for humidification and warming as well as filtration of inspired air. Dry air impairs ciliary action. In northern climates, artificial humidification of air in homes during the winter will reduce the incidence of colds. Bacterial infection of the nose is rare without a previous viral infection that damaged the mucosa. Viruses, the major infecting agents in the nose and pharynx, attach to receptors on the mucosal cells. As in the lower bronchopulmonary tree, bacterial invasion can follow viral infection after the mucociliary barrier is broken.

Larynx

The larynx, apart from its control over voice, acts essentially as an air conduit. All the defenses of the nasopharynx are present—the mucous blanket for entrapment, ciliary action, immune mechanisms, and normal flora to prevent colonization. In addition, irritants in the larynx are removed principally by an induced cough reflex.

A defective cough mechanism seriously impairs respiratory tract defenses, especially if an altered gag reflex is also present. Cough will be muted by the presence of an indwelling nasogastric tube and obliterated by an endotracheal tube or tracheostomy. Not only are the upper airway defenses bypassed, but aspiration and pooling of bronchial secretions will result (Fig. 12–5).

Tracheobronchial Tree

Particulates contaminating inhaled air are captured by the superficial mucous blanket, which glides over the ciliated respiratory epithelium. These cilia (200 per cell) beat regularly in coordinated sequence within a fluid medium.[8] The tips of the cilia push the gel-like mucous layer, guiding it toward the pharynx. In humans, the superficial mucous blanket moves at almost 15 μm per minute, with the proximal rates greater than more distal rates because of the greater volume of mucous within the larger bronchi.[9]

Matsuyama[10] used rabbit tracheal explants to show how ciliary action removes bacteria to the laryngeal end of the explant. Ultraviolet irradiation eliminates the ciliary action, allowing inoculated surface bacteria to invade. The logical extension of these studies suggests that any drug, process (viral infection), or mechanical device that interferes with mucociliary clearance places the patient severely at risk of infection.

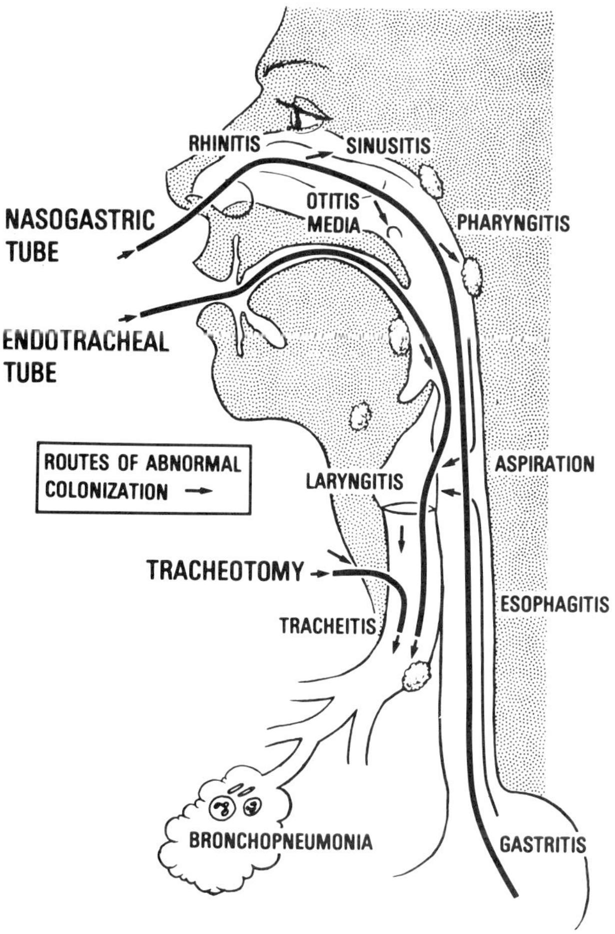

Figure 12–5. The alteration of anatomy and interference with natural bacterial clearance mechanisms in respiratory tract and their infectious complications.

The ciliated epithelium extends only into the terminal bronchiolar region. Material deposited in the terminal respiratory units is removed by alveolar macrophages, which function primarily to prevent lodgement of contaminants rather than to fight active infection. Alveolar macrophages behave as though they are in a perennially activated state.[11] Underlying cell-mediated immunity to a variety of airborne antigens may induce a high local concentration of macrophage-activating lymphokines.[12] After phagocytosis, macrophages migrate to the mucociliary area, after which they are swept upward.[13] The macrophage can also migrate through the interstitium to terminal respiratory bronchioles or to lymphatic channels, thence to lymph nodes. The lymphatic route is used least, generally when the other systems are overburdened. Some particulate matter (eg, silica particles) rests permanently in the alveoli because they injure macrophages. This is apparent when comparing the lungs of a city dweller to a country resident or a smoker to a nonsmoker.

Local Immunity

There are, in addition, immunologic antibacterial mechanisms that prevent microbial lodgement and clear the organisms that get through the mechanical and biologic barriers (see Chap. 15). In the upper respiratory tract, these include the immunoglobulins IgA and IgE and small molecular weight mediators; in the lower tract, IgG, IgM, and large molecular weight mediators are present.[14] IgA is the most important defense against new or transient bacteria in the nasopharynx and tracheobronchial tree, interfering with the ability of bacteria to adhere to mucosal cells. Protective local immunity can be present in excess of systemic immunity to previously encountered respiratory antigens.[12]

The defense mechanisms of the respiratory tract are not solely the physical, cellular, and immunologic characteristics of the mucociliary lining of the tracheobronchial tree. Some secretions have antibacterial or antiviral properties—lysozyme and interferon are probably the most important.

ALIMENTARY TRACT

Oropharynx

The squamous epithelium of the oropharynx generally provides a strong mechanical barrier against bacterial ingress. Two areas, however, have particularly thin epithelium, the gingival margin and the tonsillar crypts; invasive infection is most likely to originate in these areas. Considering the wealth of bacterial flora in the mouth, it is surprising that there are not more infections. It is also striking how well the mucous membranes within a mouth heal after ordinary trauma. This may be due to an epithelial growth factor in saliva.

Saliva constantly bathes the mouth to maintain a specific environment and contains mucin, lysozyme, and IgA. Lysozyme has antibacterial properties; bacteria become entrapped in the mucin and are thereby easily swallowed; and IgA has the ability to prevent adherence of bacteria to mucous membranes.[12] Postoperative parotitis was once a common problem. It has been eliminated by careful attention to systemic hydration, which facilitates salivary flow, and by adequate oral hygiene, which removes inspissated secretions behind which infection could develop.

The normal mixed flora of the mouth are an important defense mechanism. These flora do not, in general, cause disease except in lung abscesses, periodontal disease, and human bites. With adequate oral hygiene, the normal flora prevent colonization with more pathogenic bacteria. A clear example of the value of the normal oral flora was seen when penicillin lozenges became available for the treatment of (bacterial) pharyngitis. Rather than control the infection, the lozenges merely eliminated the normal flora and allowed *Candida* to flourish. One mechanism by which the normal flora inhibit fungal overgrowth is to reduce the salivary glucose to a level insufficient to support *Candida*.[15]

Esophagus

The esophagus is essentially a conduit that becomes infected only when obstructed or when systemic defenses are compromised. The swallowed bacteria are propelled more rapidly than they can reproduce.

Stomach

The pH of the stomach provides an inhospitable environment for the growth of bacteria. The stomach is generally sterile, and, as such, aspiration of gastric contents has generally been considered to be a chemical lesion rather than contamination with either endogenous or hospital-based bacteria. There is some electron microscopic evidence that bacteria may reside normally within the stomach. They appear attached to the mucosa, but their role and growth characteristics are as yet undefined. Because of the acid environment, even ulceration of the stomach in the face of systemic infection does not contribute to or permit bacterial invasion. *Helicobacter pylori* is not normal flora but the infectious agent associated with acid-peptic gastritis and gastroduodenal ulceration.

With the increased use of antacids and cimetidine not only in intensive care units but also throughout the hospital, we must change our concept of the stomach as a sterile environment. A study by Du Moulin et al[16] clearly demonstrates that, in the presence of antacids and cimetidine, bacteria are present in large numbers in the stomach and that the numbers of gram-negative organisms are directly related to the pH. The higher the pH the larger the number of colony-forming units per cubic millimeter. As the pH rises above 4, the number of colony-forming units increases from 10^3 to 10^6 at a pH of 7. The management of surgical patients, particularly use of the nasogastric tube, tends to break down the gastroesophageal barrier and permit relatively frequent aspiration of small amounts of gastric contents. The study by Du Moulin et al demonstrates very clearly that in 52 of their 60 patients the gram-negative flora in the stomach could be identified at the same time in the tracheobronchial tree and that at least half of their 60 patients developed a gram-negative pneumonia in association with this process of aspiration.

The second implication for this change in gastric flora will relate to the movement of these bacteria into what was previously a relatively privileged environment at the beginning of the gastrointestinal tract, with potential implications regarding translocation of bacteria and access of bacterial endotoxin or bacterial products to the portal or systemic circulation.[17,18]

Small and Large Bowel

An increasing gradient in the numbers of bacteria exists within the gastrointestinal tract from the ligament of Treitz to the anus. To a limited extent the mechanical barrier of the mucous membranes is effective in preventing bacterial invasion; however, some bacteria can penetrate the gastrointestinal epithelium (eg, tubercle bacilli, *Salmonella*). The propulsive motion of the gastrointestinal epithelium keeps the bacterial population of the small bowel in check, but in more stagnant areas of the distal ileum, proximal to the ileocecal valve or within the colon, bacterial numbers increase markedly. This is important in conditions in which small bowel functions deteriorates—ileus, obstruction, and the critically ill.[18,19] Bacteria make up a large part of the total weight of the intestinal contents (see Chap. 3).

The normal flora of the gastrointestinal tract are the most important factor inhibiting colonization by potential pathogens.[20] The anaerobic environment, the competition for nutrients, and a variety of antimicrobial substances produced by the normal flora all act to restrain the proliferation of pathogens. The ecologic balance is delicate, however; even hospitalization leads to colonization of the lower gastrointestinal tract with hospital organisms, particularly in the critically ill.[19] Antimicrobial agents, even a single dose for prophylaxis,[21] can facilitate the overgrowth of organisms that cause serious disease (eg, *Clostridium difficile* pseudomembranous colitis).[22]

In germ-free animals the anatomic structure of the gastrointestinal tract is markedly different from that seen in animals more normally colonized. The cecum attains only 50 percent of normal weight in these animals. It returns to its normal size and configuration after colonization. Without normal flora, there is no evidence of normal lymphoid maturation, and it is likely that the normal flora act as an immunologic stimulant for the submucosal lymphoid tissues. These lymphoid tissues secrete IgA (and to a lesser extent IgM). Although IgA cannot opsonize bacteria for lysis, bacteria coated with IgA cannot adhere to intestinal mucosa, a step necessary for invasion.

The mucosal barrier is critical to ensuring that the contents of the intestinal lumen do not have access to the host. The mucosa has specific nutritional requirements (eg, glutamine) and benefits from enteral rather than parenteral feeding.[23]

URINARY TRACT

The urinary tract is normally sterile except at the urethral orifice. The periodic mechanical flushing effect of urine flow usually keeps the proximal urethra clear. Urine itself has a mild bacteriostatic effect because of its high urea content, high osmolality, high ammonia concentration, urinary IgA, and acid pH.[24] Elevated urinary glucose levels support bacterial growth. Sodium, potassium, and organic acids have no inhibitory effect on bacterial growth.

Although urine contains IgG and IgA, the IgG probably has no antibacterial role. Secretory IgA acts primarily to prevent bacterial adherence to urothelium in the urethra, where colonization with fecal flora is common.[25] Both prostatic fluid and semen contain poorly characterized antimicrobial substances.

One of the most important defenses against urinary infection is anatomic. The male urethra is long, and the meatus is distant from the anus; urinary tract infections are unusual in normal men. In the female, the urethra is short and its orifice is close to the fecal stream, and normal women can have urinary tract infections. Trauma to the urethra from whatever cause, changes in urine and urinary dynamics during pregnancy, and heavy colonization easily overwhelm the other defenses.[27]

FEMALE GENITAL TRACT

Like other mucosal-lined spaces, the female genital tract offers a mechanical barrier to bacterial infection in the form of a thick squamous epithelium and a mucous plug within the cervix. IgA and lysozyme are among its secretions. In the adult (and newborn), an acid pH and a glycogen-rich desquamation foster the growth of lactobacilli (Döderlein's bacillus), which in turn compete successfully with pathogenic bacteria. The prepubertal vagina is alkaline, and its flora are made up of staphylococci, streptococci, coliforms, and diphtheroids.

REFERENCES

1. Aly R, Maibach HI, Shinefield HR, Strauss W: Survival of pathogenic microorganisms on human skin. J Invest Dermatol 58:205, 1972.
2. Aly R, Maibach HI, Rahman R, et al: Correlation of human in vivo and in vitro cutaneous antimicrobial factors. J Infect Dis 131:579, 1975.
3. William REO: Healthy carriage of *Staphylococcus aureus*: its prevalence and importance. Bacteriol Rev 27:56, 1963.
4. Langford MP, Stanton GJ, Barber JC, Baron S: Early-appearing antiviral activity in human tears during a case of picornavirus epidemic conjunctivitis. J Infect Dis 139:653, 1979.
5. Walter JB, Israel MS: General Pathology, 3rd ed. London, Churchill, 1970, p 414.
6. Newell FW: Physiology and biochemistry of the eye. In Newell FW (ed): Ophthalmology Principles and Concepts, 4th ed. St Louis, Mosby, 1978.
7. Proctor DF, Andersen I, Lundgvist G: Clearance of inhaled particles from the human nose. Arch Intern Med 131:132, 1973.
8. Rhodin JAG: Ultrastructure and function of the human tracheal mucosa. Am Rev Respir Dis 93 (Suppl):1, 1966.
9. Santa Crus R, Landa J, Hirsch J, Sackner M: Tra-

cheal mucosa velocity in normal man and patients with obstructive lung disease; effects of terbutaline. Am Rev Respir Dis 109:458, 1974.
10. Matsuyama T: Point inoculation of cultivated tracheal mucous membrane with bacteria. J Infect Dis 130:508, 1974.
11. LaForce FM: Effect of aerosol immunization with RE 595 *Salmonella minnesota* on lung bactericidal activity against *Serratin marcescens, Enterobacter cloacae* and *Pseudomonas aeruginosa.* Am Rev Respir Dis 116:241, 1977.
12. Ganguly C, Waldman RH: Local immunity and local immune defenses. Prog Allergy 27:1, 1980.
13. Hocking WG, Golde DW: The pulmonary-alveolar macrophage, I. N Engl J Med 301:580, 1979.
14. Cohan AB, Gold WM: Defense mechanisms of the lungs. Annu Rev Physiol 37:325, 1975.
15. Knight L, Fletcher J: Growth of *Candida albicans* in saliva: stimulation by glucose associated with antibiotics, corticosteroids and diabetes mellitus. J Infect Dis 123:371, 1971.
16. Du Moulin GC, Paterson DG, Hedley-White J, Lisbon A: Aspiration of gastric bacteria in antacid-treated patients: a frequent cause of post-operative colonization of the airway. Lancet 1:242, 1982.
17. Meakins JL, Marshall JC: The gut as the motor of multiple organ failure. In Marston A, Bulkley GB, Fiddian-Green RG, Haglund UH (eds): *Splanchnic Ischemia and Multiple Organ Failure.* London, Edward Arnold, 1989, pp 339–348.
18. Steinmetz OK, Meakins JL: Care of the gut in the surgical intensive care unit: fact or fashion? Can J Surg 34:207, 1991.
19. Marshall JC, Christou NV, McLean APH, Meakins JL: The gastrointestinal tract: the "undrained abscess" of multiple organ failure. Ann Surg 218: 111–119, 1993.
20. Donaldson RM Jr: Normal bacterial populations of the intestine and their relation to intestinal functions. N Engl J Med 270:938, 1964.
21. Yee J, Dixon CM, McLean APH, Meakins JL: *Clostridium difficile* disease in a department of surgery: the significance of prophylactic antibiotics. Arch Surg 126:241, 1991.
22. Bartlett JG, Gorbach SL: Pseudomembranous enterocolitis (antibiotic-related colitis). Adv Intern Med 22:455, 1977.
23. Wilmore DW, Smith RJ, O'Dwyer ST, et al: The gut: a central organ after surgical stress. Surgery 104:917, 1988.
24. Kaye D: Host defense mechanisms in the urinary tract. Urol Clin North Am 2:407, 1975.
25. Burden DE: Immunologic reaction to urinary infection: the nature and function of secretory immunoglobulins. In Williams DT, Chisholm GD (eds): Scientific Foundations or Urology, Chicago, Year Book Medical Publishers, 1976.
26. Stamey TA, Fair WR, Timothy MM, Chung HK: Antibacterial nature of prostatic fluid. Nature 218:444, 1968.
27. Stamey TA: Pathogenesis and Treatment of Urinary Tract Infections. Baltimore, Williams & Wilkins, 1980.

BIBLIOGRAPHY

Bellanti JH: Basic Immunology, 2nd ed. Philadelphia, Saunders, 1984.

Faist E, Meakins JL, Schildberg FW (eds): Host Defense Dysfunction in Trauma, Shock and Sepsis: Mechanisms and Therapeutic Approaches. Berlin, Springer-Verlag, 1993.

Ganguly R, Waldman RH: Local immunity and local immune responses. Prog Allergy 27:1, 1980.

Haley RW, Culver DH, Morgan WM, et al: Identifying patients at high risk of surgical wound infection. Am J Epidemiol 121:206, 1985

Howard RJ: Host defense against infection, I. Curr Probl Surg 17(5):267, 1980.

Howard RJ: Host defense against infection, II. Curr Probl Surg 17(6):319, 1980.

Myrvic QN (ed): Fundamentals of Immunology. Philadelphia, Lea & Febiger, 1984.

Root RK, Ryan JL: Humoral immunity and complement. In Mandell GL, Douglas RG Jr, Bennett JE (eds): Principles and Practice of Infectious Diseases, 2nd ed. New York, Wiley, 1985, pp 31–57.

Sites DP, Stobo JD, Fudenberg HH, Wells JV: Basic and Clinical Immunology, 5th ed. Los Altos, CA, Lange Medical Publications, 1984.

Phagocytes

CHAPTER 13

Sandra S. Kaplan

THE PHAGOCYTE

Phagocytes together with contributing humoral elements and cells of the immune system provide the main armamentarium for the suppression and elimination of invading microorganisms. Phagocytic cells include neutrophilic granulocytes and the blood monocytes. Monocytes can mature into the various tissue macrophages, which are present in all tissues and are especially numerous in the spleen, liver (Kupffer cells lining the sinusoids), and lung (alveolar macrophages lining the distal air sac). Monocytes/macrophages not only phagocytose and kill microbes, they also participate in all inflammatory reactions, regardless of the inciting cause, and are therefore central in the processes of wound healing and the disposal of immune complexes, injured cells, and foreign material. Under certain circumstances, phagocytes can themselves contribute to local tissue injury, for example, gouty arthritis, the adult respiratory distress syndrome (ARDS), and the systemic inflammatory response syndrome (SIRS), which accompanies multiple organ dysfunction.

Under ideal circumstances, disposal of bacteria, fungi, and parasites contaminating previously normal tissue is accomplished by phagocytosis followed by intracellular killing of the microbes. These two processes are therefore essential steps in the control of infection. Defects in these processes, either congenital and/or acquired, result in increased susceptibility to infection. Recognition that certain clinical syndromes are associated with defects in phagocytosis/killing has permitted targeted investigation of these processes (Table 13–1).[1–3]

THE GRANULOCYTE

The term granulocyte denotes a phagocytic leukocyte with cytoplasm filled with several types of granules. There are several classes of granulocytes, each classified according to the color the granules exhibit when the cells are stained with polychromic stains such as Wright or Giemsa. Neutrophilic granulocytes (neutrophils), the primary peripheral blood phagocytic cell, display small pink or pink-tan granules. Eosinophils display larger, more uniform orange-red granules; and basophils have large, somewhat irregular dark blue granules. All these granulocytes contain a nucleus that has undergone segmentation into lobes. Thus the cells may be referred to as polymorphonuclear cells (PMN, polys or segs), but these terms usually are reserved for neutrophilic granulocytes.

Granulopoiesis

Granulocytes originate and mature in the bone marrow in a maturation process that requires approximately 12 to 14 days with a turnover of

TABLE 13–1. NEUTROPHIL DEFECTS ASSOCIATED WITH IMPAIRED HOST DEFENSE

Congenital Cellular Defects	Impaired Function
Metabolic deficiency	Absence of oxidative radical formation associated with impaired killing
Chronic granulomatous disease	
Severe G6PD deficiency	
Granule absence/abnormalities	
Myeloperoxidase	Depressed bacterial killing
Cationic protein (defensins)	Depressed bacterial killing
Specific granule deficiency	Depressed bacterial killing
Chédiak-Higashi syndrome	Giant granules; decreased cell movement, decreased killing
Cell surface abnormalities	
Leukocyte adhesion deficiency (LAD)	Poor/absent cell movement and phagocytosis
Receptor abnormalities	Poor response to mediators
Cytoskeletal abnormalities	
Actin dysfunction	Depressed chemotaxis, phagocytosis
Microtubule dysfunction	Abnormal chemotaxis
Kartagener's syndrome (immotile cilia)	Depressed chemotaxis
Lazy leukocyte syndrome	Depressed chemotaxis
Congenital plasma defects	
Opsonin deficiency	
Antibody	Depressed phagocytosis
Complement	Depressed phagocytosis, generation of chemoattractant
Hyper-IgE syndrome	Depressed chemotaxis, resulting in cutaneous infections
Acquired host defense defects	
Malnutrition	Depressed phagocytosis, metabolic burst, killing
Cancer, solid organ	Depressed chemotaxis
Cancer, hematopoietic	Variably impaired movement, metabolism, killing
Inhibitors (complement fragments or activation)	Depressed chemotaxis
Immunoglobulin (polymer IgA)	Depressed chemotaxis
Immune complexes	Depressed chemotaxis, hypermetabolic PMNs
Hypophosphatemia	Depressed chemotaxis, phagocytosis
Diabetes	Depressed chemotaxis
Juvenile periodontitis	Depressed chemotaxis
Pharmacologic agents	Depressed chemotaxis
Alcohol	
Steroids	
Tetracyclines	
Amphotericin β	
Thermal injury	Depressed phagocytosis, killing
Developmental	
Newborn	Depressed chemotaxis

16×10^8 cells/kg/24 h. They develop from precursor cells (multipotent stem cells) under the influence of a variety of cell-derived growth factors (interleukins and cytokines) that regulate both the proliferative and maturational aspects of the hematopoietic growth cycle (Fig. 13–1).[4] The precursor cells are undifferentiated but are recognizable because of the emerging granularity of their cytoplasm and also because of proteins in the cell membrane, which permit immunophenotyping using monoclonal antibodies and flow cytometry. During the process of maturation, granules form in the Golgi apparatus, and these granules contain a variety of proteins synthesized by the endoplasmic reticulum. The earliest set of granules—primary granules—form during the promyelocyte stage and are metachromatically dark purple (azurophilic) with Wright's stain early in the maturation process. The secondary granules are formed and packaged in slightly more mature cells and are pink on Wright stain. A third class of granules, thought to contain gelatinase, is less well defined. The three granule types, their contents, and known functions are shown in Table 13–2. The granule membrane also serves as the repository for proteins that mediate essential functions of these cells. Adhesion molecules—such as the beta-2 integrins, receptors for peptide ligands and complement, and the components of the enzyme NADPH oxidase—are present on these granules.

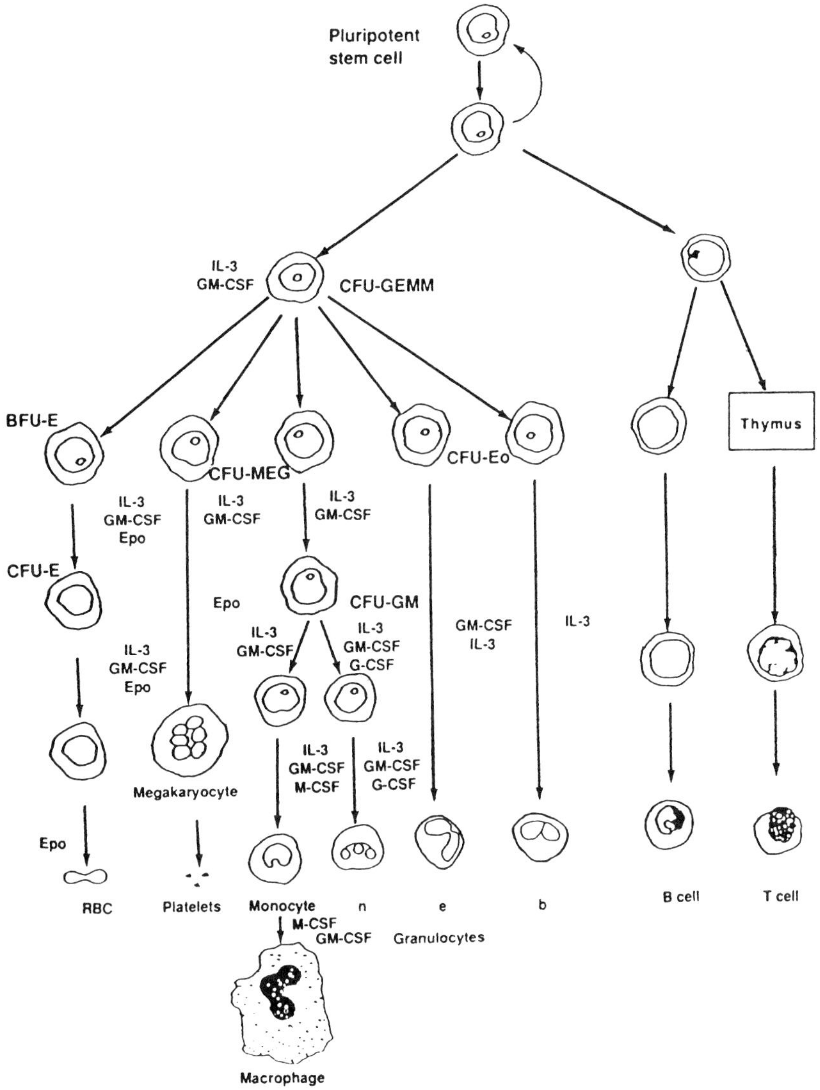

Figure 13–1. Model of hematopoietic differentiation and the effect of hematopoietic growth factors on progenitor cells. The growth factor list is incomplete but suggests complexity and redundancy of control. *(From Clark SC, Kamen R: Science 236:1229, 1987.)*

TABLE 13–2. CONTENTS AND CHARACTERISTICS OF NEUTROPHILIC GRANULES

Granule Type	Contents	Function
Primary or azurophilic	Myeloperoxidase	Host defense
	Defensins	Host defense
	Lysozyme	Host defense
	Acid hydrolases	Particle digestion
	Neutral proteases	Particle digestion
	Acid mucopolysaccharide	Particle digestion
	Elastase	Tissue degradation
Secondary or specific	Lysozyme	Host defense
	Lactoferrin	Host defense
	Membrane	Host defense
	Cytochrome b_{558}	Host defense
	Integrins	Host defense
	Other receptors	Host defense
	Collagenase	Inflammation
	Plasminogen activator	Inflammation
	Vitamin B_{12} binding protein	
	Monocyte chemotactic factor	Inflammation
	C3 and C5 cleaving proteases	Inflammation
Tertiary	Gelatinase	Inflammation

Granulocytes exhibit other maturational features. The precursor blasts have a round nucleus with finely dispersed chromatin and the capacity for cell division. During maturation, the nuclear chromatin condenses into irregular clumps and the nuclear shape flattens, becomes indented, elongates, and finally segments into two to five nuclear lobes. Mitosis becomes impossible.

There is also a reduction in mitochondrial content and an increase in glycogen stores. Energy metabolism changes, and the ATP necessary for cell movement and phagocytosis depends on anaerobic glycolysis. The maturing neutrophil also develops the metabolic machinery for the production of oxygen free radicals. These reactive oxygen intermediates (ROIs) together with the contents of the granules facilitate microbial killing and also mediate inflammatory responses. With maturation, the neutrophil membrane becomes more plastic and deformable, which permits egress of these cells from the marrow.[5]

After release of neutrophils from the marrow, the cells will have a circulation half-life of about 6 to 7 hours followed by a tissue survival after diapedesis of 1 to 2 additional days. About half the circulating neutrophils are normally adherent to vascular endothelium (marginated cells) and are exchangeable with cells in the circulating bloodstream. The bone marrow itself also retains a storage pool of unreleased, nearly mature neutrophils available to the circulation under conditions of infection, hypovolemic shock, or other stress. Neutrophil release from these two storage sites is under the influence of catecholamines, steroid hormones, and other cytokines. Catecholamines, for example, cause the release of marginated cells while steroids cause release of storage pool neutrophils, including less-than-fully-mature forms that may be less deformable, less motile, and less metabolically active.[5]

The other granulocytes (eosinophils and basophils) have specialized functions. Eosinophilic granules contain peroxidase, arylsulfatase, cationic proteins, and eosinophilic major basic protein. These cells respond to IL-5 and IL-3 and play a role in host defense against parasitic infections. Basophilic granulocytes contain large, irregular, dark blue granules that contain heparin, serotonin, histamine, lipids, and proteoglycans but do not contain hydrolytic enzymes. Basophils possess high-affinity cell surface receptors for IgE. When these receptors are engaged, not only are granule contents released, but metabolic activation of the cell leads to the production of active mediators such as leukotrienes, plasminogen activator, and proteases. This results in hypersensitivity reactions, contraction of smooth muscle, and increased vascular permeability.[6]

Components of the Host Defense System

Cell Number. Effective host defense requires first that neutrophil levels in the blood are maintained in sufficient quantity. The normal range for neutrophils is 1800 to 7000/μl, and morbidity due to infection does not become a problem until the number falls to below 1000/μl. Susceptibility to infection reaches critical levels when neutrophil counts fall to below 500/μl. Even then, host defenses can be maintained if the other professional phagocytes, the blood monocytes, are present in sufficient numbers to make up the difference.

The common causes of neutropenia are listed in Table 13–3.[7] Of special clinical importance are infectious and immune etiologies (both autoimmune and drug related), radiation, poisons, drugs (certain antibiotics, immunosuppressants, and chemotherapeutics), and primary dysplastic disorders of the bone marrow. A large variety of less common con-

TABLE 13–3. CAUSES OF NEUTROPENIA

Causes
Acquired neutropenias
Infection
Severe bacterial infection with hyperutilization
Chronic infection, especially typhoid
Viral—numerous, AIDS
Rickettsia
Protozoa
Physical, chemical agents
Inevitable
Benzyne
Alkylating agents
X-ray
Antimetabolites
Idiosyncratic/immune
Antibiotics
Phenothiozenes
Anticonvulsants
Antihistamines
Other agents
Neoplastic/dysplastic
Deficiency states
Pernicious anemia
Cachexia
Alcoholism
Mechanical
Hypersplenism
Congenital neutropenia
Kostmann's agranulocytosis
Cyclic neutropenia

Data from Athens JW: Neutropenia. In: Lee GR, Bilbell TC, Foerster J, et al (eds): Wintrobe's Clinical Hematology, Vol 2, 9th ed. Philadelphia, Lea & Febiger, 1993.

genital and familial disorders and hypersplenism also may be associated with neutropenia.

Activation of the Neutrophil

Adherence and Chemotaxis. Effective host defense also requires that neutrophils leave the circulation; phagocytosis and microbial killing take place in the tissues. This egress is a highly regulated process dependent on a coordinated series of events starting with the attachment of neutrophils to the endothelial cells of postcapillary venules and ending at the site of the initiating stimulus. The initiating stimulus may be an infection, tissue injury, an area of necrosis, an immune reaction, or any event that generates cytokines, which activate both neutrophils and endothelial cells. Such cytokines include interleukin 1 (IL-1), tumor necrosis factor (TNF), interferon gamma (IFN-γ), and the chemotaxins.

Adherence. Adherence is the first step, and it is mediated by a group of substances known as cellular adhesion molecules (CAM). These include both the molecules on the neutrophil and complementary molecules on endothelial cells and in the intercellular matrix. Three broad classes of adhesion molecules have been described—the integrins, the immunoglobulin superfamily, and the selectins. Each of these families is further divided into many subspecies (Table 13–4). Together, these molecules are responsible for the binding of the neutrophil to the intact or damaged endothelium and permit it to insinuate itself between the endothelial cells. However, this binding must be reversible if migration is to occur. One sequence of reactions appears especially important to this process. The beta-2 integrin heterodimer designated CD11b/CD18 on the neutrophil's surface binds to its ligand (a member of the immunoglobulin superfamily), an intercellular adhesion molecule 1 (ICAM-1), on the endothelial cell surface prior to migration. The ICAM-1 molecule is expressed in greater number and with enhanced activity on endothelial cells under the influence of the inflammatory cytokines such as IL-1, IFN-γ, and TNF. Thus stationary adherence occurs, followed by diapedesis and chemotaxis. In order for the CD11b/CD18 receptor to bind ICAM-1, however, the leukocyte must be rolling along the endothelium at the periphery of the flowing blood. The rolling process is mediated by a different group of adhesion molecules: selectins on neutrophils, most importantly L-selectin (leukocyte adhesion molecule 1, LAM-1) which binds to E selectin (endothelial leukocyte adhesion molecule 1, ELAM-1) by means of reversible interaction with their natural ligands, the carbohydrate moieties of glycoproteins.[8–13] (CD = cluster of differentiation).

It is important to note that bacterial lipopolysaccharide (LPS) has been known to play a particularly significant role in the adherence of neutrophils.[14] The mechanism of this effect is incompletely understood but could be related to LPS-induced complement activation or to LPS induction of cytokines like TNF or IL-1.[15] LPS, in addition, can exert its effect even in complement-depleted serum.[16] Recent work has demonstrated that LPS binding protein (LBP), normally present in serum and increased during inflammation, serves to augment the effectiveness of LPS by forming an LPS-LBP complex.[17] This complex then binds to CD14 molecules on both neutrophils and monocytes, and upregulates CD11b/CD18 expression.[18] Thus LPS acts to increase adherence directly on the phagocyte and concurrently stimulates TNF and IL-1. These mechanisms partially explain an old observation;

TABLE 13–4. IMPORTANT ADHESION MOLECULES FOR LEUKOCYTES

Class	Expressing Cell	Ligand
Integrins		
β1 (VLA-4)	Lymphocytes, eosinophils, monocytes	Endothelium, matrix (VCAM-1)
β2 (LFA-1, Mac-1) (gp150,95)	Phagocytes, lymphocytes	Endothelial cells, other cells (ICAM-1)
Selectins		
L (LAM-1)	Leukocytes	Vascular endothelium Carbohydrate moieties on leukocytes
P	Platelets, endothelial cells	
E (ELAM-1)	Endothelial cells	Sialylated Lewis X antigens on surface glycoproteins of leukocytes
Immunoglobulin superfamily		
ICAM-1, ICAM-2	Endothelial cells, matrix	Leukocyte β2 integrins
VCAM-1	Endothelial cells	Leukocyte β1 integrins

Data from Cronstein BN, Weissmann G: Arthritis Rheum 36:147, 1993.

namely, that endotoxemia is associated with multiple foci of neutrophil sequestration.

Chemotaxis. Neutrophils are motile cells that normally move in a random pattern. They can be induced to migrate in a given direction along a concentration gradient of certain chemicals called chemotaxins (Table 13–5). These chemotaxins include a wide range of substances derived from a variety of sources.[19] Some of these are small, bacterially derived formylated peptides, analogous to formyl methionyl-leucyl-phenylalanine (fMLP), a well-studied synthetic molecule. Others are substances derived from the activation of complement, especially C5a, and substances derived from cells such as neutrophils and monocytes. These include interleukin 8 (IL-8), monocyte chemotactic protein 1 (MCP-1), platelet-activating factor (PAF), and leukotriene B_4 (LTB_4), a product of the lipoxygenase pathway arachidonic acid metabolism. Chemotactic factors also can be generated by blood clotting, injury of tissues, interaction of injured tissues with bacteria, and antigen stimulation of lymphocytes.

The most important chemotaxin, however, is C5a, generated by both the classical and alternative pathways of complement activation. C5a is rapidly converted to C5a-des-arginine by carboxy peptidase; C5a-des-arg also is a potent chemotaxin, though approximately 100-fold less potent than native C5a. Antigen-stimulated lymphocytes indirectly enhance chemotaxis by the effect of lymphokines on monocytes and neutrophils, causing them to be more activatable (priming) and also inducing secretion of the phagocyte-derived chemotaxins LTB_4, MCP-1, and IL-8. The multiplicity of chemotaxins and the diverse origins of these chemotaxins provide for some cell migration even in hosts deficient in complement or in the ability to activate complement.

Chemotaxins serve to initiate neutrophil reactivity when chemotaxin-specific receptors on the neutrophil membrane are engaged by these ligands (Fig. 13–2). Receptor-ligand interaction sets into motion the process of transduction of the external signal or first messenger into other signals generated within the cell (the second messengers). The second messenger system ultimately induces a cellular action. These intracellular events have been best studied using the synthetic chemotaxin fMLP. The fMLP receptor and other receptors have extracellular, transmembrane, and intracellular domains, the last of which is linked to a heterotrimeric unit that binds guanine nucleotides (G-proteins). Receptor engagement results in activation of a G-protein, causing it to hydrolyze the polyphosphoinositide phosphatidyl-inositol 4,5-bisphosphate (PIP_2) into the second messengers diacylglycerol (DAG), which remains membrane associated, and inositol 1,4,5-trisphosphate (IP_3), which is released into the cytosol. DAG induces the translocation of protein kinase C (PKC) from the cytoplasm to the membrane. PKC-dependent phosphorylation and calcium-calmodulin dependent protein kinase-induced phosphorylations are necessary for activation of the critical neutrophil functions—chemotaxis, phagocytosis, and microbial killing.[20–22] IP_3 is re-

TABLE 13–5. CHEMOATTRACTANTS FOR PHAGOCYTES

Chemoattractant	Source
Exogenously derived	
N-formyl peptides	Bacterial metabolism
Endogenously derived	
C5a	Complement activation (classical/alternative)
Leukotriene B_4	Lipoxygenase metabolism of arachidonic acid
Platelet-activating factor	Lipid metabolite from activated leukocytes
Platelet factor 4	Release from platelet alpha granules
Neutrophil-activating proteins	
NAP-1 (IL-8)	Phagocytic cells and many other cells
NAP-2	Monocyte protease action on platelet and granule constituent
NAP-3	Stimulated monocytes
NAP-4	Platelets
Neuropeptides	
Substance P	Central and peripheral nervous system
Beta-endorphin	Central and peripheral nervous system
Laminin	Endothelial cells, neoplastic cells, basement membrane

Data from Harvath L: Neutrophil chemotactic factors. In Goldberg LD (ed): Cell Motility Factors. Basel, Switzerland, Birkhauser Verlag, 1991, pp 35–52.

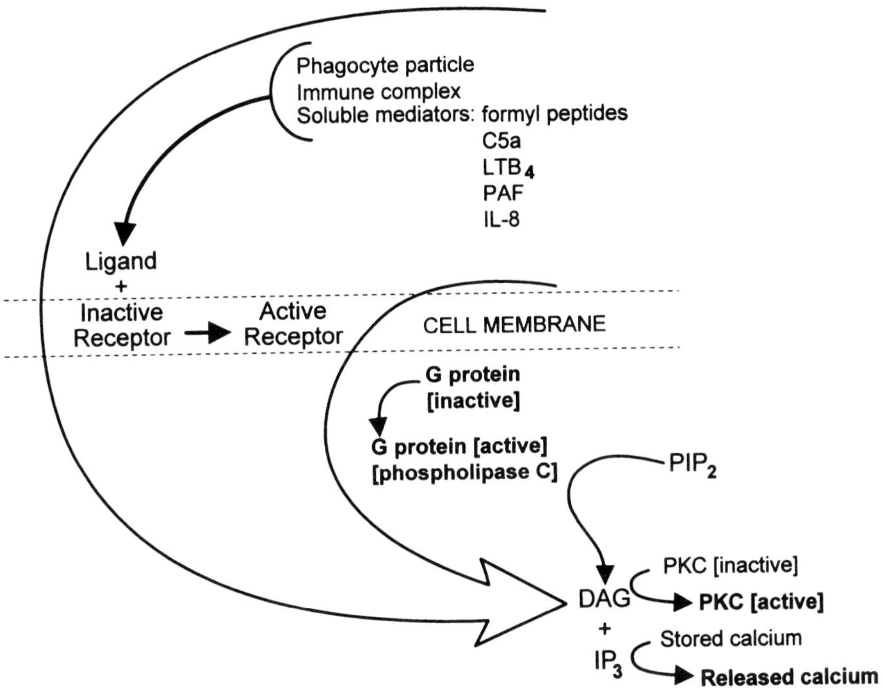

Figure 13–2. Receptor engagement by the first messenger (eg, the chemotaxin fMLP) induces an alteration in the receptor, which in turn activates a G-protein, causing it to have phospholipase C activity. This splits PIP_2, forming the second messengers IP_3 and DAG. IP_3 stimulates calcium release from intracellular storage sites. The increase in calcium stimulates calcium-calmodulin protein kinases, resulting in phosphorylation reactions (of unknown site and function), and also modulates actin filament length through its effect on gelsolin. Dynamic and focused changes in actin filament length are needed for cell shape changes and the cytoplasmic propulsion that results in cell movement. DAG activates protein kinase C, resulting in other essential phosphorylation reactions.

sponsible for further messenger elaboration by causing the release of calcium from intracellular storage sites, resulting in an early rise of intracellular free calcium.

These reactions are associated with institution of chemotaxis (directional motion in a concentration gradient). Neutrophils respond within seconds to low concentrations of these mediators and undergo a shape change from round to elongated with a broad ruffled leading edge (the lamellipodium) and a narrow pointed tail (the uropod). Inside the cell, the components of the cytoskeleton reorganize. Actin polymerizes into microfilaments, and tubulin polymerizes to form microtubules, which extend in a fan-shaped manner from the Golgi apparatus anterior to the nucleus toward the leading edge. These changes result in the crawling movement of the neutrophil, first in transendothelial egress from the circulation (extravasation) followed by movement in the tissues in the gradient of chemotaxin from lower to higher concentrations. Microtubules are believed to provide for structural rigidity and directionality and to provide a framework for transmigration of granules in the cytoplasm. The movement itself is a function of the force-generating mechanism of subcellular actin, which comprises 10 percent of the cellular protein and exists both as monomeric globular (G) actin and as the filamentous (F) form. In response to chemotactic stimuli, filament length increases both at the leading front (lamellipodium) and at the uropod. The filaments are cross-linked by actin-binding proteins, creating a lattice. This polymerization of actin is closely regulated by agonist-induced polyphosphoinositide changes, focal increases of calcium levels, and by a variety of filament-associated proteins that participate in this regulation.[23]

Neutrophils appear at sites of injury or infection within a few hours. Monocytes migrate by similar mechanisms, but more slowly. Experimental studies using the Rebuck skin window technique, in which a sterile coverslip is placed over a standard skin abrasion, show that large numbers of neutrophils are present at 4 hours and that monocytes are the predominant cell type at 12 to 24 hours. A similar pattern of leukocyte response is seen in surgical wounds.

Since neutrophils derive energy for chemotaxis by anaerobic glycolysis, migration can proceed under anoxic or hypoxic conditions. Motility can be maintained for several hours in glucose-free medium because neutrophils are rich in glycogen. Migration also appears to be unaffected by mild acidosis (pH 6.5). The intracellular pH of the neutrophil is more important. Intracellular acidification or inability of a stimulated cell to undergo alkalinization impairs chemotaxis and most other neutrophil functions. Anaerobic infection with production of short chain fatty acids impairs intracellular pH homeostasis and thereby acts to impair host defenses against the anaerobe itself as well as even more virulent copathogens.[24]

TABLE 13–6. LEUKOCYTE MOTILITY DISORDERS

Cellular defects
- Congenital
  - Leukocyte adhesion deficiency
  - Hyper-IgE syndrome
  - Lazy leukocyte syndrome
  - Chédiak-Higashi syndrome
  - Kartagener's syndrome
  - Increased microtubule assembly
  - Specific granule deficiency
  - Actin dysfunction
  - Localized juvenile periodontitis (LJP)
  - Newborn
- Acquired
  - Trauma and burns
  - Malnutrition
  - Tumors
  - Infections
  - Diabetes mellitus

Humoral defects
- Chemotactic factor deficiency
  - C3 deficiency
  - C5 deficiency or dysfunction
  - IgG deficiency
- Inhibitors of chemotactic factors
  - Cirrhosis
  - Hodgkin's disease
  - IgA
- Inhibitors of cell migration
  - Steroids
  - Serum inhibitors
  - Tumor factors
  - Viral and bacterial factors
  - Local anesthetics

Disorders of Leukocyte Migration

A variety of intrinsic and acquired disorders of leukocyte motility have been recognized (Table 13–6).[1,25] In these conditions, infections tend to be recurrent and prolonged, despite appropriate antibiotics. Such infections most commonly involve soft tissues, including the skin, while pulmonary, hepatic, and renal infections may also occur. Systemic septicemia and meningitis are uncommon in these patients. The pathogens seen in patients with chemotactic and granulocyte function defects are most often caused by *S. aureus,* but also by *S. epidermidis,* gram-negative enteric bacilli, and fungi. In contrast, patients with immunoglobulin abnormalities are subject to septicemia and meningitis with organisms such as *S. pneumoniae, H. influenzae,* and group A streptococci.[26] Chemotactic defects are frequently categorized as cellular disorders or humoral disorders. The cellular disorders are a consequence of an intrinsic cellular defect relating to adherence, granule content, deformability, or the cytoskeleton. The humoral disorders may be a result of a mediator deficiency or the result of a specific inhibitor. Both types may be congenital or acquired.

Cellular Defects. Patients with cellular defects may be referred to surgeons. Patients with leukocyte adhesion deficiency (LAD)[27,28] lack the invariant chain (CD18) of the beta-2 integrin heterodimer and therefore are unable to insert any of the alpha chains (CD11a, CD11b, CD11c) into the membrane. Affected patients exhibit a marked neutrophilia (up to 100,000/μl) because the cells are unable to adhere to vascular endothelium and therefore diapedesis into the tissues fails to occur. These cells exhibit chemotactic and phagocytic deficiencies, and affected patients are greatly susceptible to infection. Patients with the most severe forms of LAD survive only a few years. The only effective treatment is bone marrow transplantation.[29] Job's syndrome, or Hill-Quie syndrome, presents with severe pyoderma including "cold abscesses" and a cellular chemotactic defect plus elevated levels of IgE.[30] These patients display deficient production of interferon-gamma (IFN-γ) and therefore benefit from administration of IFN-γ.[31] Other cellular defects involve disorders of the cytoskeleton and several have been described that include actin dysfunction,[32–34] increased microtubule assembly,[35] and Kartagener's syndrome.[36] Granule abnormalities also can be associated with chemotactic abnormalities since there is decreased upregulation of necessary membrane factors. This defect occurs in the Chédiak-Higashi syndrome,[37] where granules are enlarged and move abnormally within the cell, and in specific granule deficiencies.[38] In juvenile peritonitis, the membrane lacks a 108 kD surface glycoprotein.[39]

Developmental Defects. The newborn displays a transient chemotactic defect, the pathogenesis of which remains controversial. Recently, IFN-γ was shown to enhance chemotaxis.[40,41]

Acquired Defects. Many conditions and numerous drugs have been shown to be associated with disordered host defense, frequently manifested as a chemotactic defect. Disordered leukocyte motility may partially explain the unusual susceptibility to infection seen in poorly controlled diabetics.[42,43] Transient impairment of chemotaxis has also been described in trauma, burns, malnutrition, and following administration of local anesthetics and is seen with malignant tumors as well (see Table 13–1).[44–49] Overwhelming infection may also cause impairment of the chemotactic response.

Deficiencies of chemotactic factor generation, or cellular inhibitors of chemotaxis are relatively

TABLE 13–7. EVALUATION OF CHEMOTACTIC DISORDERS

Morphology
Presence of giant granules of Chédiak-Higashi syndrome
Mediator evaluation
Complement activation
Immunoglobulin concentration
IgE determination
Cellular response
Determination of number of cells migrating or distance of migration
Stimulus-induced polarization
Actin content and function
Microtubule function
Ancillary determination
Clinical history, cancer, drugs, diabetes

uncommon. Inhibitors of chemotactic factor activity have been described in the sera of patients with cirrhosis or Hodgkin's disease and in anergic patients when levels of immunoglobulin A (IgA) are elevated. IgA may itself be an inhibitor.[50–52]

Patients with recurrent or persistent infections, particularly if there is a lifelong or family history, should be screened for genetically transmitted chemotactic disorders (Table 13–7). Vigorous nutritional therapy, aggressive management of serious infections, early skin grafting in burn patients, and avoidance wherever possible of the use of corticosteroids contribute to the preservation or restoration of leukocyte migration.

Phagocytosis

Although extracellular killing of microbes is possible, efficient killing requires that neutrophils must phagocytose (eat) them first (Fig. 13–3). The metabolic and physical changes are quite similar to those described for chemotaxis. Phagocytosis occurs in two phases—adherence of the microbe to the cell (recognition) and ingestion. The recognition phase is greatly facilitated if the organism is coated (opsonized) by substances for which the neutrophil has receptors (Fig. 13–4). Specific immune globulin will react with the organism via its Fab recognition sites, leaving the Fc portion of the immunoglobulin exposed and available for interaction with Fc receptors (CD16 and CD32) on neutrophils. If the immunoglobulin happens to be IgM or if the molecules of IgG are sufficiently close to each other on the surface of the microbe, complement is fixed and activated, resulting in disposition of C3b and iC3b (a breakdown product of C3b) on the bacterial surface. These molecules also are ligands for neutrophil receptors CD35 and CD11b, respectively, and facilitate adhesion of microbe to neutrophil.[26,53] In the absence of immunoglobulin, complement may be activated by the alternative pathway first discovered in the context of the lipopolysaccharide (LPS) of gram negative bacterial endotoxin, but also caused by polysaccharide peptidoglycan capsules of some microorganisms.[54] Gram-negative organisms can be opsonized via their LPS by a second mechanism, that is, binding the serum protein LPS binding protein (LBP). This opsonin permits binding of these organisms to neutrophils by the receptor,

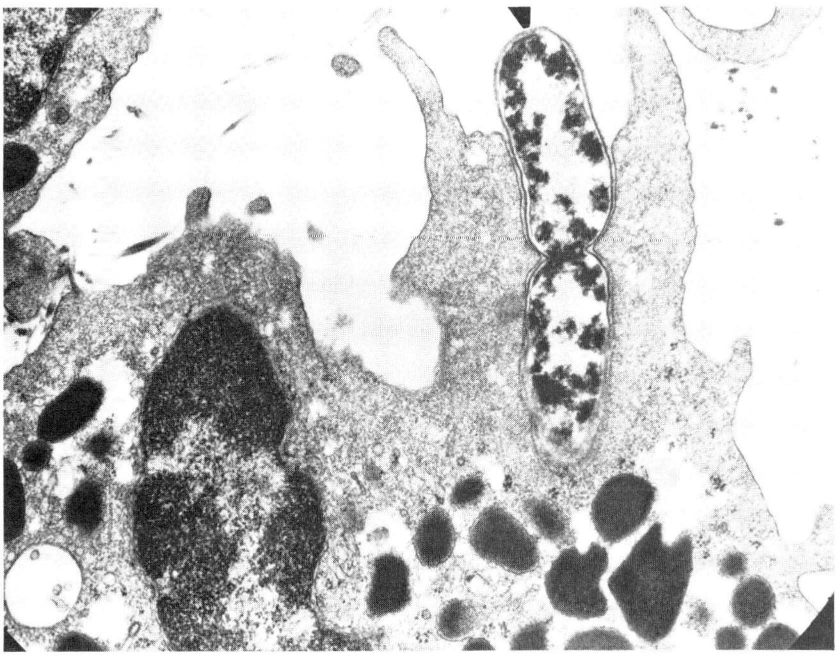

Figure 13–3. Bacteria (*arrow*) in the process of being ingested by a neutrophil. The electron-dense azurophil granules can be seen in the cytoplasm. *(From Hohn DC: The phagocytes. In Howard RJ, Simmons RL (eds): Surgical Infectious Diseases, 2nd ed. Norwalk, CT, Appleton & Lange, 1988, p 158.)*

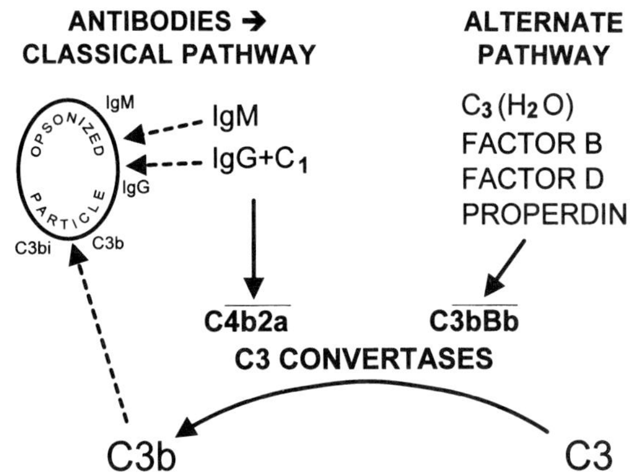

Figure 13–4. Opsonization of bacteria occurs when the organisms become coated with immunoglobulin and/or complement. Bacteria may activate complement when IgG or IgM antibodies bind to antigens on the cell surface, or complement may be activated via the alternate pathway when bacterial cell walls have repeating carbohydrate subunits. The complement fragments [especially C3b (CR1) or "inactive" C3b (C3bi or CR3)] on the surface of the organism engage receptors on neutrophils such as CD11b, which binds with C3bi and leads to attachment (recognition) of bacteria to neutrophils. When immunoglobulin specific for the microorganism binds to the microbe, the Fc portion of the immunoglobulin molecule attaches to neutrophils via Fc receptors on the surface of the neutrophil (CD16, CD32). Deposition of C3b and C3bi onto the microbial surface, together with immunoglobulin, intensifies the binding of microbe to neutrophil and facilitates ingestion.

CD14, and phagocytosis is potentiated by this mechanism.[15,55]

Other opsonic mechanisms have been described and include the fibronectin receptor,[56] believed to be a mechanism for clearance of wound and tissue debris, collagen fragments, and macroaggregates of fibrin by tissue macrophages. Fibronectin also binds to *S. aureus* and may participate in ingestion of this organism, but it does not bind to gram-negative organisms.[56] When bacteria adhere to neutrophils via neutrophil receptors, the extracellular signal is transduced in a manner similar to chemotaxin signaling, and organization of microtubules and actin filaments allows for pseudopod extension around the microbe with eventual fusion of the pseudopods distal to the organism.[26] This process, when complete, results in complete internalization of the microorganism, which is now contained in a space termed a phagosome, lined by what had been the external membrane of the cell.

Following phagocytosis and closure of the pseudopods, an integrated series of morphologic and metabolic changes occur that convert the phagosome into a microbicidal trap. These changes include movement of intracellular granules to the phagosome where they fuse with and discharge their contents into the phagosome (now termed a phagolysosome), augmenting the microbicidal effect of metabolic activation (Fig. 13–5). Phagocytosis, like chemotaxis, uses energy derived from anaerobic glycolysis.

Defects of Phagocytosis. Table 13–8 lists both congenital and acquired cellular or mediator defects

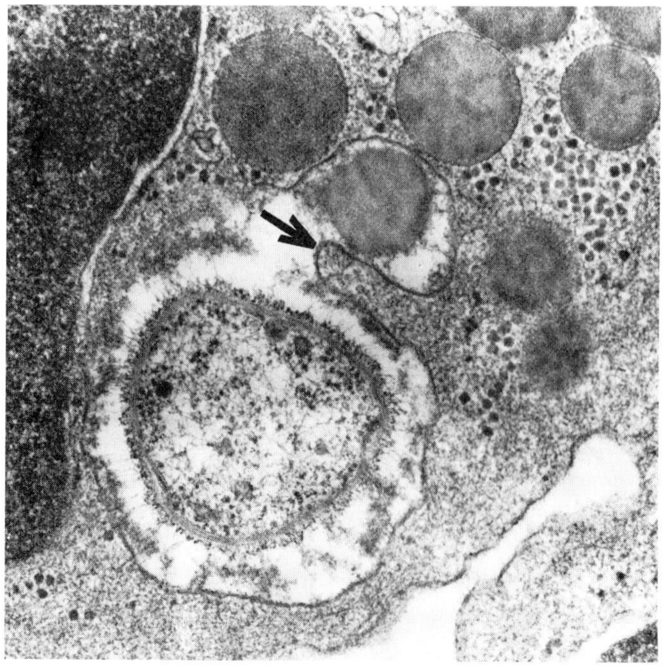

Figure 13–5. Neutrophil degranulation. *Arrow* indicates point of fusion between the granule membrane and that of the phagocytic vacuole. *(From Hohn DC: The phagocytes. In Howard RJ, Simmons RL (eds): Surgical Infectious Diseases, 2nd ed. Norwalk, CT, Appleton & Lange, 1988, p 162.)*

TABLE 13–8. DEFECTS OF PHAGOCYTOSIS

Cellular defects
Congenital
LAD
Actin dysfunction
Acquired
Thermal injury
Overwhelming infection
Malnutrition
Drugs
Opsonin defects
Congenital
Complement deficiencies
Immunoglobulin deficiencies
Acquired
Low birth weight infants
Immune complex disorders
Thermal injury
Overwhelming sepsis

of phagocytosis. Congenital cellular defects are uncommon and include adhesion receptor deficiencies and cytoskeletal defects of microtubules or microfilaments. Congenital mediator defects include opsonic deficiencies, which include low or absent immunoglobulin and low or absent complement components.[57] Patients with opsonin deficiencies develop severe infections with virulent encapsulated bacteria including pneumococci, *Pseudomonas aeruginosa,* streptococci, or *H. influenzae*. In contrast to patients with chemotactic disorders, these patients are typically susceptible to bacteremias, meningitis, and respiratory tract infections.[26]

A number of patients with genetic complement deficiency states have been identified and found to have defective opsonization and recurrent pyogenic infections (Table 13–8). The presence of adequate levels of C3 is particularly important in this regard, and patients with genetic C3 deficiency, hypercatabolism of C3, or defective C3 activation mechanisms may have opsonin deficiencies with associated infections. Patients with immune globulin deficiency or specific antibody deficiency may also opsonize bacteria ineffectively and be subject to infections.[52] Deficiencies of gamma globulin and certain of the complement constituents may be treated with immunoglobulin or infusions of fresh frozen plasma.

Alexander et al[58] have extensively studied the opsonic system following major burn injury, trauma, and infection. Depressed opsonic capacity has been found early in the burn injury period but there has been poor correlation between opsonic index and incidence of infection in burn patients. Patients with overwhelming infections have also been shown to be deficient in opsonic components, and it has been postulated that this is due to consumption of available opsonins. Others, however, have been unable to demonstrate convincingly that consumptive opsoninopathy is a clinical problem.

Although opsonins may not be totally depleted during infection, there is good evidence that complement is activated in the serum. C5a serum levels are increased in surgical infection, and C5a receptors on circulating leukocytes are lost in direct proportion to the loss of neutrophil function.[59] Similar events probably occur during cardiopulmonary bypass.[60] Acquired or transient defects are somewhat more common but are milder than congenital defects. These occur after severe thermal injury[58] with overwhelming infection[59] and secondary to drugs, alcohol, autoimmune disorders, and other systemic disorders. The reasons for poor phagocytosis in these acquired defects are likely to be multifactorial. Rarely, phagocytic defects are due to malnutrition as a function of abnormal ATP production by the neutrophil.

Activation of the Neutrophil

The various chemical stimuli that impinge on the neutrophil elicit a continuum of responses related to the intensity of the stimulus and the number of receptors occupied.[61] Low concentrations induce cell movement while higher concentrations during which the ligand is bound to about 10 percent of receptors induce secretion of granules and metabolic activation, resulting in the formation of reactive oxygen intermediates (ROIs).[62] The formation of ROIs and the combined lethal effect of ROIs and granule contents on the ingested microbe compose the centerpiece of phagocyte-mediated host defense against bacterial infection.

Formation of ROIs requires the transduction of first messengers into second messengers; this has been described in connection with induction of chemotaxis (Fig. 13–2).[20] In particular, DAG activation of protein kinase C, calcium-induced activation of calcium-calmodulin protein kinases, and calcium activation of phospholipase D and of phospholipase A2-associated arachidonic acid release serve to stimulate the activity cascade known as the *oxidative burst,* which generates ROIs. The ROIs include the superoxide anion, hydrogen peroxide, hydroxyl radicals, and singlet oxygen (Fig. 13–6). The release of arachidonic acid generates other important mediators of inflammation—the leukotrienes and the prostaglandins.

The oxidative burst first described by Baldridge and Gerard in 1933 as "the extra respiration of phagocytosis"[63] was shown by Sbarra and Karnovsky in 1959 to be independent of mitochondria,

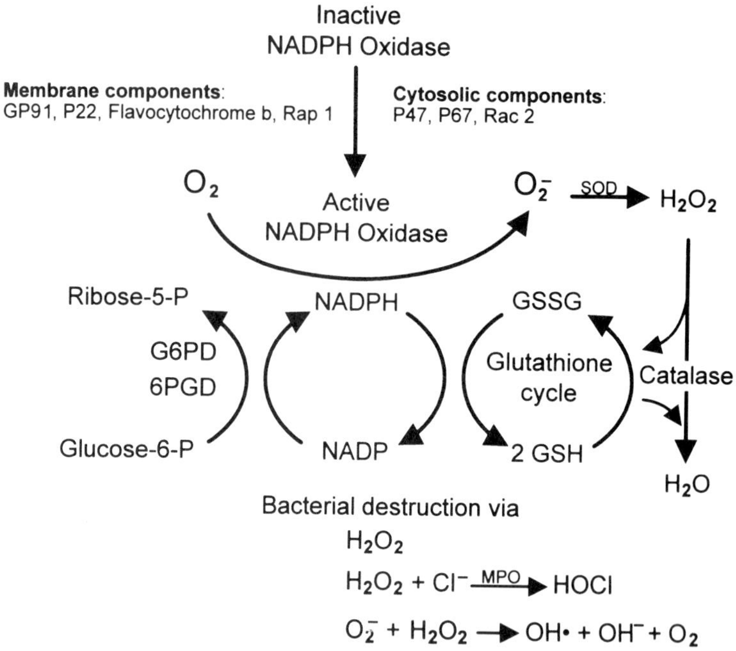

Figure 13–6. Generation of reactive oxygen intermediates (ROIs): ROIs are produced by the action of NADPH oxidase on the substrate NADPH, causing the one-electron reduction of oxygen to form superoxide (O_2^-). NADPH is generated during the pentose phosphate pathway where NADP is reduced to NADPH during the oxidation of glucose 6-phosphate to ribose 5-phosphate. The active NADPH oxidase is assembled from the interaction of membrane and cytosolic components. When superoxide is produced, it rapidly interacts with another superoxide molecule, forming hydrogen peroxide. Other ROIs are formed from the interaction of superoxide and H_2O_2.

cyanide resistant, and to occur via a subsidiary pathway, the pentose phosphate pathway.[64] Here, glucose 6-phosphate is oxidized to ribose 5-phosphate catalyzed by the enzymes glucose 6-phosphate dehydrogenase (G6PD) and 6-phosphogluconate dehydrogenase (6PGD) and is dependent on nicotinamide adenine dinucleotide phosphate (NADP) (see Fig. 13–6). In this reaction NADP is reduced to NADPH and, via a cascade of reactions, oxygen is consumed, accounting for the extra respiration.

Bacteria are not effectively killed by phagocytes unless oxygen is present.[65–67] This oxidative burst requires the activity of NADPH oxidase, which is latent in resting cells. NADPH oxidase is activated when surface membrane receptors are engaged. Receptor engagement results in formation of IP_3 and DAG, with activation of protein kinases, including protein kinase C (PKC) (see Fig. 13–2). The cytoskeletal microfilaments participate both structurally and functionally in this activation process, allowing for local activation by particulate stimuli.[68,69]

Activation of NADPH oxidase requires the assembly of the enzyme from its component parts, which include a membrane-associated heterodimer and several cytoplasmic constituents, including the p47 and p67 phagocyte oxidase proteins. This assembly is necessary for the formation of an electron transport chain from NADPH to molecular oxygen (see Fig. 13–6).[64,67] The putative terminal component of this electron transport chain is a unique low negative-redox-potential-b-type cytochrome, variably called cytochrome b_{245} or b_{558}.[70–74] The activated oxidase then catalyzes oxidation of NADPH, resulting in the one-electron reduction of oxygen forming the superoxide anion (O_2^-) (see Fig. 13–6):

$$2O_2 + NADPH \rightarrow 2O_2^- + NADP^+ + H^+$$

Superoxide is the precursor of other derivative ROIs. All these compounds are formed both at the surface and at the phagosome membranes so that these ROIs form the basis for the intraphagosomal killing of ingested microorganisms.

Microbicidal Mechanisms of Leukocytes

Microbial killing is the principal function of the phagocyte. Multiple mechanisms are present, but all can be classified into those that are oxygen dependent and those that are not. Oxygen-dependent

TABLE 13–9. LEUKOCYTE MICROBICIDAL MECHANISMS

Oxygen-dependent killing mechanisms
Hydrogen peroxide (H_2O_2)
H_2O_2 + halide + myeloperoxidase → HOCl
Superoxide anion (O_2^-)
Hydroxyl radicals (OH·)
Singlet oxygen ($'O_2$)
Nitric oxide ?
Oxygen-independent killing mechanisms
Acid (phagolysosome pH is 6)
Antimicrobial Polypeptides
See Table 13–10

Data from Klebanoff SJ: Phagocytic cells: products of oxygen metabolism. In Gallin JI, Goldstein IM, Snyderman R (eds): Inflammation: Basic Principles and Clinical Correlates. New York, Raven Press, 1988.

mechanisms are generally considered to be the most effective, but all the mechanisms are mutually supportive (Table 13–9).

Oxygen-Dependent Microbial Killing. Oxygen-dependent microbial killing is usually separated into two forms. In the simplest form, the reactive oxygen intermediates, derived from the superoxide anion: H_2O_2, and hydroxyl radical (OH·) are especially bactericidal.[75] H_2O_2 is formed from the dismutation (by superoxide dismutase) of superoxide; the hydroxyl radical (OH·) forms from the interaction of O_2^- and H_2O_2 in the presence of iron or copper. The hydroxyl radical is highly unstable and almost instantaneously reacts with most organic molecules.[66]

Another form of oxygen-dependent microbial killing requires the presence of an enzyme from the primary granules, myeloperoxidase (MPO). MPO has a broad spectrum of antimicrobial activity, and this enzyme, together with H_2O_2 and chloride, forms the highly reactive molecule hypochlorous acid[76,77]:

$$\text{MPO} + H_2O_2 + Cl^- \rightarrow \text{HOCl}$$

This reaction was shown to profoundly augment microbial killing by phagocytes, decreasing by 50-fold the level of H_2O_2 needed. MPO may not be essential, however, since asymptomatic MPO-deficient subjects are found with a frequency of as many as 1 per 4600 individuals.[78]

The mechanisms of bacterial death remain somewhat vague. In the MPO/H_2O_2/Cl^- system, halogenation of bacterial surface amino acids occurs. The ROIs themselves are likely to induce oxidation of sulfhydryl groups, which is incompatible with bacterial survival.[79]

Nitric oxide (NO) is a radical which is formed by the action of the enzyme nitric oxide synthase (NOS), acting on L-arginine.[80] NO formation seems to be important for neutrophil chemotaxis[81] but its role in microbial killing is relatively weak when compared to ROIs. It may play a role when other neutrophil microbicidal mechanisms are impaired or depleted.[82] Mechanisms requiring NO also require O_2 because NOS uses O_2 to oxidize the guanidino nitrogen on the arginine molecules. It is important to remember that O_2^- and NO interact to neutralize one another and might interfere with microbicidal activity. It is therefore likely that neutrophils do not utilize NO as a primary microbicidal mechanism. NO appears to play a relatively greater role in macrophage-mediated killing of difficult to kill organisms.[83]

Oxygen-Independent Microbial Killing. The oxygen-independent mechanisms of antimicrobial host defense involve approximately one dozen polypeptides that are contained in the neutrophil's granules.[84,85] These substances, the granules that contain them, and their host defense range are shown in Table 13–10.

Considerable attention has been focused recently on one of these granule classes—the defensins.[85,86] Defensins are small, cyclic, cysteine-rich peptides with a broad antimicrobial spectrum, which comprise 30 to 50 percent of the protein of the primary granules. They act on microorganisms to increase membrane permeability allowing ingress of other antibacterial substances such as lyso-

TABLE 13–10. OXYGEN-INDEPENDENT MICROBICIDAL SUBSTANCES OF NEUTROPHILIC GRANULES

Protein	Granule Type	Targets in Host Defense
BPI[a] proteins	Azurophilic	Rough gram-negative bacteria Homology with LPS binding protein
Cathepsin G	Azurophilic	Gram-positive and gram-negative bacteria and fungi
Elastase and proteinase 3	Azurophilic	Potentiates lytic action of lysozyme and cidal actin of cathepsin G
Azurocidin	Azurophilic	Coliforms, *S. faecalis, C. albicans*
CAP[b] 57 and 37	Azurophilic	*S. typhimurium* and other rough gram-negative organisms
Defensins HNP[c] 1,2,3,4	Azurophilic	Wide range of gram-negative and gram-positive bacteria, many fungi and some enveloped viruses
Lysozyme	Azurophilic	Some gram-positive organisms; synergistic with defensins, elastase, and proteinase 3
Lactoferrin	Specific	Some gram-positive and gram-negative organisms by chelating iron needed for bacterial growth

[a] Bacterial permeability increasing.
[b] Cationic antibacterial protein.
[c] Human neutrophilic protein.
Data from Lehrer RI, Ganz T: Blood *76:2169, 1990; and Lehrer RI, Lichtenstein AK, Ganz T: Annu Rev Immunol 11:105, 1993.*

zyme, and allowing egress of intracellular substances. These peptides, while not cytotoxic by themselves, synergize with other cytotoxic factors such as ROIs. Azurocidin, cathepsin G, proteinase 3, and elastase have been classified as serprocidins, which are homologous with serine proteases.[87] However, their antimicrobial activity is not dependent on their proteolytic activity. Cathepsin G, a glycosylated cationic protein, inhibits bacterial respiration and effectively kills gram-negative and gram-positive organisms as well as fungi. Elastase is another cationic protein that acts on the bacterial cell wall and permits entry of other active substances. Proteinase 3 also acts on elastin.

Disorders of Metabolic Activation and Microbicidal Activity

See Table 13–11 for a listing of some disorders.[1–3]

Congenital Defects. The discovery in the 1950s of chronic granulomatous disease (CGD) provoked investigations that opened the modern era of enlightenment pertaining to neutrophil behavior.[88] CGD is a group of conditions having as their common denominator the inability of the neutrophil to form ROIs with any stimulus. Affected patients usually present during infancy with recurrent severe infections including pneumonia, lymphadenitis, sometimes with spontaneous purulent drainage, hepatic abscesses, and osteomyelitis. Infections are usually caused by catalase-positive organisms (*S. aureus*) and often by organisms usually considered nonpathogenic, such as *Serratia marcescens*.[89]

Originally described as sex-linked, this form of CGD accounts for approximately 65 percent of cases and is due to the absence or abnormality of the larger of the heterodimeric NADPH oxidase membrane-associated components. Most other forms of CGD are of autosomal origin and can be due to deficiency or abnormality of any of the other components of the phagocytic oxidase.[90] An abnormality or absence of the smaller of two cytoplasmic components of the oxidase (the p47 phagocytic oxidase) accounts for about 30 percent of cases.[91]

Another mechanism of reduced or absent ROIs involves defects in the production of NADPH, the essential substrate of NADPH oxidase. Severe deficiency of G6PD has been shown to do this. These patients' neutrophils exhibit normal cell movement and phagocytosis but are unable to kill the same spectrum of microorganisms that affect patients with CGD.[92] Other enzymatic defects include abnormalities of the glutathione cycle, one of the mechanisms of free-radical detoxification that helps to prevent autologous damage. Myeloperoxidase deficiency is sometimes associated with a susceptibility to fungal infections, but, as indicated above, these patients do not seem to miss the presence of hypochlorite.[78] Abnormalities or deficiencies of other granule constituents also may impair phagocytic killing. Deficiencies of lysozyme, lactoferrin, and defensins have been described and are associated with a relatively mild host defense impairment.[38] Another type of granule abnormality occurs in the Chédiak-Higashi syndrome, a rare autosomal recessive disorder.[37,93] Here, the granules are present but are enlarged and abnormal, resulting in impaired fusion of granules with the phagosome and impaired microbial killing. These leukocytes also exhibit chemotactic defects. Other somatic cells exhibit abnormal lysosomes with associated functional impairment.

TABLE 13–11. SOME DISORDERS OF LEUKOCYTE INGESTION, DEGRANULATION, AND MICROBICIDAL FUNCTION

Congenital defects
Chronic granulomatous disease (CGD)
G6PD deficiency (severe)
Myeloperoxidase deficiency
Chédiak-Higashi syndrome (defective degranulation)
Other granule deficiencies
Acquired defects
Septicemia
Burn and traumatic injury
Malnutrition
Diabetes
Smoking
Myelodysplastic syndrome/leukemia
AIDS
Drugs
Cortisone
Alkylating agents/antimetabolites
Allergy medications
NSAIDs/retinoids
Local defects
Impaired killing due to tissue hypoxemia
Phagocytic engorgement
Biomaterial-induced phagocyte deactivation
Wounds

Acquired Defects. Many acquired defects have been described. Severe infection is associated with mild attenuation of neutrophil function, which may be a result of refractoriness following chronic stimulation.[1–3] For example, neutrophils stimulated with formyl peptides fail to respond to a second stimulus with a formyl peptide but are able to respond to an unrelated ligand. Thermal injuries also impair neutrophil function. Heated neutrophils are partially degranulated, and these may exhibit hyperadhesiveness as well as an impaired post-phagocytic granule release.[46–48] Malnutrition has been associated with impaired NADPH oxidase activity,[94] and total parenteral nutrition with low phosphate solutions may result in energy depletion with low ATP. Some acquired disease states are associated with impaired host defense. The best studied of these is diabetes mellitus in which impaired function appears to be related to poor control of the diabetes.[42,43] Cigarette smoking is associated with increased susceptibility to respiratory infections, and recently it has been shown that smoke-induced free-radical formation damages neutrophils and impairs their capacity for host defense functions.[95] Neutrophils in the myelodysplastic syndrome (MDS) and leukemia[96] and in acquired immune deficiency syndrome (AIDS) also exhibit variously impaired functions as well as deficient numbers of cells.[97] Some drugs have been shown to impair neutrophil function. Cortisone, for example, results in impaired NADPH oxidase activity and impairs other aspects of neutrophil activation.[98,99] Many other drugs adversely affect neutrophil reactivity including drugs used in cancer chemotherapy,[100] antiallergic drugs,[101] anti-inflammatory drugs, and retinoids.[102] Local impairment of host defense has been described following implantation of a variety of biomaterials. This is believed to occur due to gratuitous activation followed by depletion of the neutrophil's capacity to function effectively.[103–106] Wounding itself predisposes to infection, especially when contaminated. While contamination is an essential component, inflammatory constituents of phagocyte granules and production of mediators of inflammation, including cytokines and prostaglandins, together with the modulating effect of fluid and hemoglobin, create a witch's brew of compromised host defense.

Modulation of Phagocyte Responses

The idea that stimulating the phagocyte might enhance host defense was introduced by Metchnikoff[107] in his studies that formed the basis of modern leukocyte biology. This idea was reiterated by George Bernard Shaw in his play, "The Doctor's Dilemma," in which he declared that stimulating the phagocyte was the solution to all diseases and that drugs were a delusion.[108] Today, in fact, we know that certain substances (drugs, in fact) may stimulate the phagocyte, and the most important of these drugs are the cell-derived factors, cytokines, that both induce phagocyte proliferation through their effects on stem cells and also upregulate functional activities when these cells are in their fully mature state.[109,110] Table 13–12 lists some of these cytokines. They are produced by a broad range of cells,

TABLE 13–12. AGENTS THAT ENHANCE HOST DEFENSE

Colony-stimulating factors
Monocyte/macrophage-colony stimulating factor (M-CSF)
Granulocyte colony-stimulating factor (G-CSF)
Granulocyte-monocyte colony-stimulating factor (GM-CSF)
Interleukin 3 (IL-3)
Tumor necrosis factor (TNF)
Interferon gamma (IFN-γ)
Ascorbic acid
Vitamin D_3
Retinoids
Pentoxifylline (neonatal cells)

such as T lymphocytes (IL-3 and IFN-γ) and monocytes (GM-CSF, G-CSF, M-CSF, and TNF). Other cell types, including endothelial cells and fibroblasts, also produce some cytokines. In addition, other cytokines participate in a cellular network in which, for example, activated monocytes produce IL-1, which stimulates helper T cells to produce IL-2 and IFN-γ, which act on monocytes, lymphocytes, and other cells to produce other cytokines such as TNF, GM-CSF, and G-CSF.[111] Most of these cytokines are available in recombinant form and therefore are obtainable for clinical trials in conditions in which phagocyte numbers or function are suboptimal. GM-CSF and/or G-CSF have a salutary effect on phagocyte function in MDS[112] and AIDS[113] and attenuate the neutrophil nadir in congenital neutropenias,[114] including cyclic neutropenia[115] as well as chemotherapy-induced neutropenias.[116,117] Surgical infections are more likely to occur in neutropenic patients (marrow aplasia, cyclic neutropenia) and neutropenic colitis has been described. Although expression of the adhesion glycoprotein CR3 is enhanced on normal neutrophils after treatment with GM-CSF and IFN-γ,[118] this does not occur in patients with the leukocyte adhesion deficiency (LAD) syndrome even though their neutrophils do express more CR1.[1] LAD patients are helped mainly by supportive care or in some instances by bone marrow transplantation.[29]

IFN-γ has proved to be useful in the management of several neutrophil defects, that is, the chemotactic defect of neonatal neutrophils[40] and the hyperimmunoglobulin E syndrome.[31] Patients with chronic granulomatous disease also exhibit clinical improvement on IFN-γ treatment, despite the fact that no objective improvement in neutrophil function can be demonstrated.[119,120]

Several other agents have been shown to improve phagocyte activity, including ascorbic acid, which is associated with enhancement of chemotaxis and microbial killing in the Chédiak-Higashi syndrome.[93] Agents such as vitamin D_3 and retinoids induce maturation in instances of maturation arrest.[121] Pentoxifylline improves chemotaxis in neonatal neutrophils (see Table 13–12).[122]

Tissue-Toxic Harmful Effects of Neutrophils

While neutrophils are essential for host defense against microbial agents, they also mediate the acute inflammatory response; in that capacity, they can induce severe tissue injury. Examples include autoimmune disease,[123] the reperfusion injury associated with myocardial and cerebral infarcts,[124] the acute respiratory distress syndrome (ARDS),[125] and the systemic inflammatory response syndrome (SIRS) thought to terminate in multi-organ failure, currently the major cause of death in patients with and without septicemia who die in intensive care units[126] (Fig. 13–7). The current paradigm is that phagocytes, including both neutrophils and macrophages, become activated by cytokines produced as a response to injury or by infection. Tissue damage is then mediated by release of ROIs, prostaglandins, leukotrienes, and granule contents containing proteases such as collagenase and elastase. There are many routes to this final pathway; for example, LPS can activate complement, which primes phagocytes for enhanced response to other mediators.[127,128] LPS induces tumor necrosis factor (TNF), nitric oxide synthase, and secretion of IL-1 from monocytes. TNF amplifies the inflammatory response by further inducing cytokines such as IL-1 and by upregulating adhesion molecules both on neutrophils and endothelial cells. IL-1 has pleiotropic effects causing fever, hyperadhesiveness between neutrophils and endothelial cells, hypotension, and shock. Nitric oxide is probably responsible for vasodilation of

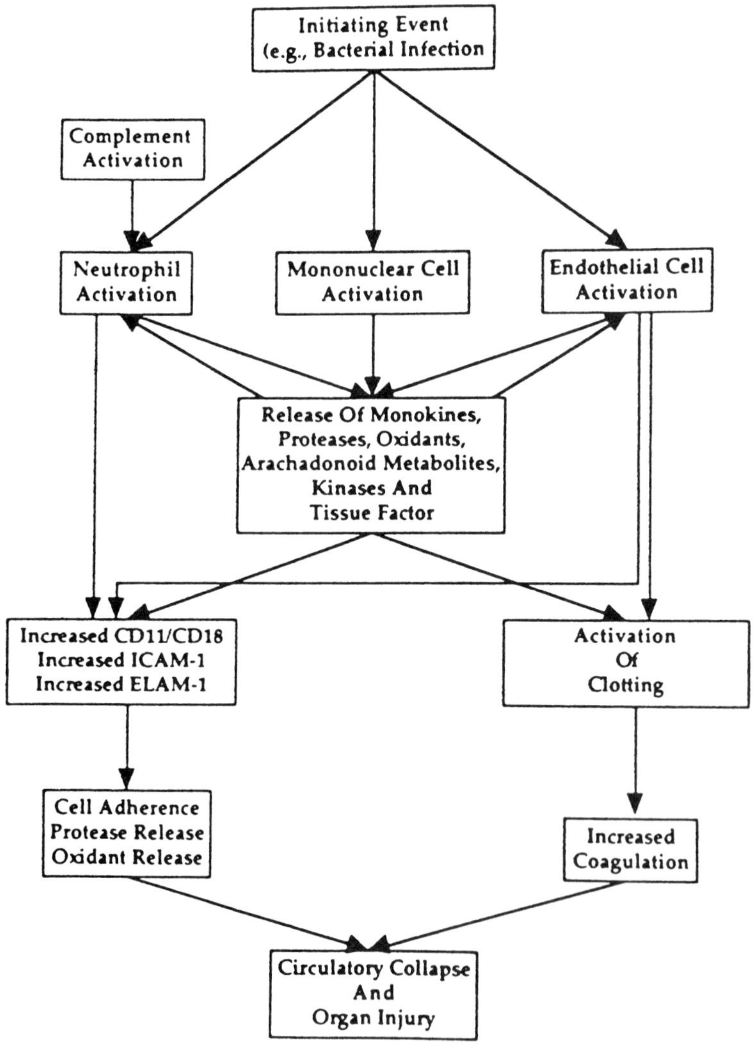

Figure 13–7. Proposed scheme for the pathogenesis of global microcirculatory failure. Following an initial insult (eg, bacterial infection), complement, inflammatory cells, and endothelial cells become activated. In response to these events, a host of inflammatory mediators (eg, monokines, proteases, oxidants, arachidonate metabolites, kinases, tissue factor) are released. The activation of the inflammatory cells and endothelial cells, coupled with the release of inflammatory mediators, leads to increased inflammatory cell-endothelial cell adherence, intravascular coagulation, and local tissue injury. The ultimate result of these interrelated events is circulatory collapse and multiple organ injury. *(From St John RC, Darinsky PM: Chest 103:932, 1993.)*

all the capillary beds in its vicinity and leads to hypotension and shock.[129] Recognition of the harmful effects of ROIs and other neutrophil products has generated intense study of means to attenuate these inflammatory effects without undermining the capacity for host defense.[126] These investigations have approached the problem in several ways, but all are based on the understanding of the mechanisms of neutrophil function, including those that are required for tissue localization, cytokines that affect phagocyte activity, and drugs that attenuate phagocyte activation.

The effects of LPS may be attenuated using monoclonal antibodies that block its activity.[130] Such antibodies can be directed against LPS itself and can act to prevent binding to its receptor, CD14. Alternatively, the CD14 receptor can be blocked by an antibody that would prevent LPS binding to cells so that the secretion of inflammatory mediators would be impaired. The effect of LPS on blood pressure also would be prevented. Studies using a polyclonal antibody to LPS[131,132] or using a monoclonal antibody[133,134] decreased mortality in patients with gram-negative bacteremia, but the cost effectiveness of this antibody has been questioned.

Since LPS acts in part to induce macrophage production and secretion of TNF, other work has explored the effect of monoclonal antibodies to TNF. These antibodies exert their action by binding to TNF and thus preventing the interaction of TNF with its receptor. Antibodies to the IL-1 receptor[135] also have been used and have been demonstrated to reduce the inflammatory response. The recombinant cytokine IL-1RA (receptor antagonist) is potentially useful in this regard.

The effects of blocking the adhesion receptors needed for phagocyte localization also are being investigated. These agents would serve to prevent inflammatory cells from adhering to vascular endothelium. Inflammatory cells therefore will not be able to extravasate or migrate to sites of injury or infection. Experimental reperfusion injury is greatly attenuated by such antibodies.[17] These observations are consistent with the hypothesis that reperfusion injury is mediated by neutrophils that swarm to the area of injury when circulation is restored. The injured site releases chemotaxins and cytokines, which upregulate neutrophil responses, including granule release of proteases (collagenase, elastase) and release of ROIs. However, it also has been shown that while the inflammatory response is reduced, so is host defense against bacterial infection; patients treated with monoclonal antibodies to the adhesion molecule CD18 exhibit increased mortality.[136] This secondary effect could have been predicted since patients without adhesion receptors exhibit profoundly compromised host defense and death at an early age.

There are still other approaches to this aspect of the inflammatory response. Agents that affect the endothelial cell cytoskeleton have been effective.[137–139] Studies have been presented showing that cytokine modulation of endothelial cells increases their adhesiveness for neutrophils and promotes diapedesis, and that this may be reduced by IL-8, which is an inhibitor of neutrophil adhesion to endothelium as well as being a chemoattractant.[140] This novel approach, directed at the endothelial cell rather than the inflammatory cell, exploits the requirement for first adherence to the endothelium and then extravasation. Inhibiting adherence with IL-8 would secondarily block extravasation and therefore would decrease the number of inflammatory cells coming to an injured area. Modulation of the endothelial cell cytoskeleton would impair extravasation because, in addition to adherence, egress between endothelial cells is facilitated by cytoskeletal-mediated retraction of cellular edges.

The anti-inflammatory property of certain drugs also has been exploited in this regard. Steroids, retinoids, nonsteroidal anti-inflammatory agents, and pentoxifylline all have been used to attenuate the inflammatory response.[126,141–143] Interestingly, while pentoxifylline decreases chemotaxis in adult neutrophils,[141] it enhances cell movement in neonatal cells.[122] These drugs act to decrease ROI production and to block secondary production of inflammatory mediators. Steroids, for example, decrease the action of phospholipase A2 and limit release of arachidonic acid. This results in decreased production of prostaglandins and of leukotrienes. Nonsteroidal anti-inflammatory drugs (NSAIDs) act by inhibiting metabolism of arachidonic acid. These issues are discussed further in Chapter 20.

MONOCYTE-MACROPHAGE SYSTEM

The mononuclear phagocyte system occupies a pivotal role in host defense against a wide range of microbial, viral, and facultative intracellular parasites. Not only do these phagocytes function in a manner similar to that of neutrophils, responding to chemotaxins, crawling to sites of infection, ingesting pathogenic substances, and killing these substances through ROI-associated phenomena, but because of their ability to produce and to be influenced by a vast network of cytokines, their capacity for function is exquisitely regulated.[144–148]

Maturation of Monocytes and Differentiation to Macrophages

These cells arise from the same stem cells that give rise to cells of the granulocytic series but comprise less than 3 percent of the nucleated marrow cells. During periods of microbial or cytokine stimulation, their numbers can increase and provide up to 70 percent of their marrow population to an inflammatory site. As monoblasts mature and form a complex Golgi apparatus with definite granule populations, they are identified as promonocytes. With maturation of promonocytes to monocytes, there is a reduced nuclear/cytoplasmic ratio, increased phagocytic capacity, and increased production of inflammatory mediators.[149] Later, maturing macrophages increase their size with the development of one or more large nuclei, numerous cytoplasmic lysosomes, and mitochondria. The intravascular half-life of blood monocytes is approximately 3 days followed by egress into tissues and organs, where they differentiate into mature tissue macrophages.[149] Tissue macrophages are also produced in situ through mitosis. The major types of tissue macrophages are listed in Table 13–13. Collectively, the monocyte-macrophage system is the functional equivalent of what originally was called the reticuloendothelial system (RES).

Functional and metabolic differentiation of maturing tissue macrophages is partially determined by the organ in which the cells reside. For example, variable quantities of myeloperoxidase are present in monocytes, depending on the degree of differentiation and the location of the cell. Circulating monocytes and most tissue macrophages, like neutrophils, depend largely on glycolytic energy metabolism and, like neutrophils, exhibit a cyanide-insensitive, NADPH oxidase-associated respiratory burst, generating ROIs after stimulation with soluble or particulate mediators. Alveolar macrophages, by contrast, are nearly devoid of peroxidase activity, lose phagocytic activity, develop numerous mitochondria, and depend predominantly on classical electron transport energy sources. Kupffer cells of the liver and splenic macrophages have particularly high phagocytic capacities.[150] All these macrophages respond to inflammatory and immunologic signals by producing and releasing numerous cytokines. These facilitate immunologic reactivity, repair tissue damage, and cause cytotoxicity against infectious and tumor cell targets. Tissue macrophages are capable of survival for several months.

TABLE 13–13. TYPES OF TISSUE MACROPHAGES

Macrophages of lymphoid tissue
Macrophages associated with serosa-lined spaces
Alveolar macrophages
Connective tissue macrophages (histiocytes)
Microglial cells of nervous system
Hepatic macrophages (Kupffer cells)
Macrophages of splenic sinusoids

Functions of Monocytes and Macrophages

The major functions of the monocyte-macrophage system are outlined in Table 13–14.[150–152]

Modulation of Immune Function. Monocyte-macrophage activities are modulated by substances in their environment. Conversely, they produce a vast array of molecules (more than 100) that act

TABLE 13–14. BIOLOGIC FUNCTIONS OF THE MONOCYTE-MACROPHAGE SYSTEM

- Cooperative immune function
  - Accessory function
    - Secretion
      - Cytokines
        - IL-1
        - IL-4
        - IL-6
        - IL-8
        - IL-10
        - TNFα
        - MCP-1
      - Growth factors
        - M-CSF
        - GM-CSF
        - G-CSF
        - TGF-β
        - FGF
      - Other mediators of inflammation
        - Complement components
        - Arachidonic acid metabolites
        - Plasminogen activator
        - Reactive oxygen intermediates (ROIs)
        - Reactive nitrogen intermediates (RNIs)
        - Coagulation factors
  - Regulation of proliferation
    - Wound repair
      - Collagen synthesis
      - Angiogenesis
- Scavenger function
  - Phagocytosis of particulate substances
    - Devitalized tissue
    - Microorganisms
    - Biomaterial wear debris
- Cytotoxicity
  - Host Defense
    - Bacteria
    - Fungi
    - Protozoa
    - Viruses
    - Tumor Cells

in an autocrine, paracrine, and even in a humoral fashion to regulate local and systemic inflammatory responses.[153,154] There are two main classes of substances that activate macrophages. The first are endogenous factors, that is, products of host cells—cytokines (of which IFN-γ, produced by T cells, is the most potent[155]), metabolic products such as ROIs, metabolites of arachidonic acid, and lysosomal substances such as proteases and hydrolases. The second are exogenous, that is, physical or chemical factors derived from nonhost sources; infectious agents and their products, such as LPS, are prime examples. As introduced above in the section on modulation of phagocyte responses, the substances produced by mononuclear phagocytes include modulators of inflammation such as the complement factors C2 and C3, plasminogen activator, prostaglandins, and cytokines. Many monokines have been identified: IL-1 and TNF (which are both pyrogens), IL-4, IL-6, IL-8, and IL-10 are some.[147,156] Mononuclear phagocyte growth factors such as GM-CSF, G-CSF, and M-CSF[157] not only induce and support hematopoiesis but also enhance the functional activity of the mature effector cells. These cells also secrete TGF-β and FGF, which induce fibroblast proliferation and collagen synthesis in healing wounds; such factors may be involved in stimulation of angiogenesis in wounds.[151,158]

Mononuclear phagocytes are essential for both humoral and cell-mediated immunity, and IFN-γ from T lymphocytes plays an essential role in their activation for this function.[139] It acts, at least in part, by means of its effect on induction of genes, which enhance nuclear transactivating factors that regulate the formation and secretion of histocompatibility antigens and cytokines like TNF and IL-1.[155,159,160] These histocompatibility proteins facilitate the interaction of mononuclear phagocytes with T cells via a surface molecule unique to T cells—the T cell receptor—which interacts with antigens inserted into the peptide binding cleft of the histocompatibility proteins. These T cells secrete cytokines (interleukins and interferons) capable of activating macrophage function[152,161,162] and of stimulating B lymphocytes for enhanced antibody production.[163] This process is initiated after macrophages are attracted to sites of inflammation by antigen-induced cytokines released from lymphocytes (lymphokines) and are maintained there by migration inhibitory factors (MIFs). Antigen binding to the macrophage's surface then occurs with little specificity, although opsonization may enhance binding. The antigens are then internalized by pinocytosis within minutes of cell association and become localized to acidic membrane-bound vesicles, the endosomes. Here, the proteins are broken down by proteases and then reinserted in the cell membrane as indicated. These phenomena are commonly referred to as antigen processing and presentation, and the macrophages performing this function are known as antigen processing cells, or APCs, and provide for delayed hypersensitivity responses as well as allograft rejection. Other cell types (eg, B cells) can also present antigens to T cells.

It is important to note that while macrophage activation involves a number of positive regulatory loops whereby LPS from bacteria and IFN-γ and IL-2 from T cells stimulate the production of mediators that further stimulate T cells, a system of negative regulators also is produced. IL-4 and IL-10, products of helper T-2 cells, for example, have both positive and negative effects. IL-4 induces C2 and plasminogen activator production, but IL-4 also is associated with depressed tumor cytotoxicity, decreased PGE_2, ROIs, IL-1, and TNF, as is IL-10.[164] Recently, it was shown that IL-4 induces increased production of the IL-1 receptor antagonist (RA) by macrophages and therefore suppresses IL-1-initiated inflammatory responses.[165] Another cytokine that has a suppressive effect on macrophages is transforming growth factor-beta (TGF-β). This cytokine is also produced by macrophages, and its effect is inhibitory on immature cells but stimulatory in mature cells.[166]

Thus, while a predominant biologic function of the monocyte-macrophage system involves defense against opportunistic infections, particularly in patients whose status is compromised by trauma, malnutrition, chronic infection, or immunosuppression, the system usually is highly regulated.[149,167] Some, but not all, of the modulators of mononuclear phagocyte response are summarized in Table 13–15.

TABLE 13–15. INDUCERS AND MODULATORS OF THE MONOCYTE-MACROPHAGE CYTOCIDAL RESPONSE

Inducers	Enhancers	Inhibitors
Soluble	Physiologic	IL-4
fMLP	IL-2	IL-6
C5a	IFNs	TGF-β
PMA	IL-3	IL-10
Arachidonic acid metabolites	Somatotropin	
Particulate	TNF	
Bacteria	M-CSF	
Fungi	GM-CSF	
Biomaterial wear debris	Environmental	
	LPS	
	fMLP	

Scavenger Function. Macrophages are involved in the removal of injured cells and tissue debris from wounds[168] and also the remodeling of tissue during embryogenesis.[151] Foreign substances are ingested by pinocytosis in the case of soluble materials such as macromolecules or of particles less than 0.1 μm. Phagocytic mechanisms are employed for larger particles. Lysosomal hydrolytic enzymes, including lipases and large quantities of lysozyme, are present in the cytoplasm, and these substances become markedly increased during the process of macrophage "activation." These enzymes are capable of digestion of most ingested substrates.[151] Phagocytosis or pinocytosis also normally precedes antigen processing and presentation.

Microbicidal Function. The clinical importance of the monocyte-macrophage system in resistance to infection is illustrated by the substantial antimicrobial resistance shown by patients with various neutropenic disorders. Although the rates of monocytic ingestion and killing of many common bacterial pathogens are substantially lower than for neutrophils, these phagocytes play the principal role for ingestion of pathogens such as *Pneumocystis carinii, Mycobacterium, Salmonella, Listeria, Cryptococcus, Toxoplasma, Plasmodium,* and *Brucella.*[153,169] Normal defenses result in microbial death, but the organisms have also developed mechanisms of survival there. Some (eg, tuberculosis), but not all, cause disease by escaping extracellular defenses by intracellular survival. Such organisms are obligate intracellular pathogens.

Like neutrophils, mononuclear phagocytes are motile cells and respond to chemoattractants such as formyl peptides C5a, foreign antigens, and other factors by transendothelial emigration into the tissues. Like neutrophils, these migrations are mediated by adhesive phenomena.[170-172] Monocytes migrate more slowly, but their movement can be sustained for rather prolonged periods.[173] Fixed macrophages in tissues retain migratory capacity. An autocrine chemoattractant, relatively specific for mononuclear phagocytes and also produced by mononuclear phagocytes, is monocyte chemoattractant protein 1 (MCP-1),[174] which, like other chemoattractants, induces ROI formation and calcium increases[175] and has been shown to enhance monocyte tumor cytotoxicity.[176]

Also like neutrophils, macrophages employ both oxygen-dependent and oxygen-independent microbicidal mechanisms (see Table 13–9, Fig. 13–6); the most important mechanisms are oxygen dependent. The first is the production of reactive oxygen intermediates (ROIs). The microbicidal cellular events for production of ROIs are remarkably similar to those that occur in the neutrophil (see Figs. 13–2 and 13–6), but ROI production in macrophages is dramatically elevated by activation stimuli. For example, while IL-2β receptors on macrophages are not upregulated by IFN-γ,[177] IL-2α receptors are[178]; thus IFN-γ "priming" leads to increased ROI production in association with IL-2.[179] Not only is ROI release increased, the primed macrophage also produces more IL-1, TNF, and IL-6.[180-182]

The second oxygen-dependent mechanism is the production of nitric oxide (NO) and other reactive nitrogen intermediates (RNIs) from molecular oxygen and the terminal guanidino group of arginine.[80] In macrophages, NO synthase (NOS) is not constitutive; it must be induced by cytokines which are known to activate macrophages. IFN-γ, IL-1, TNF, and LPS alone (and, to a much greater degree, in combination) induce NOS in macrophages. The enzyme has need for several cofactors: tetrahydrobiopterin, FAD, FMN, and thiol. Although RNI production depends on molecular oxygen, it is not part of the respiratory burst. RNIs play an important inhibitory role in the control of cryptococcus, schistosoma, leishmania, mycobacteria, and some viruses by mouse macrophages.[183] Its role in human macrophages has been difficult to show, but recently, NO-associated killing of intracellular *M. avium* has been demonstrated.[184] In hepatocytes, however, NO killing of malarial parasites has been demonstrated.[185]

RNI production parallels ROI production in several ways. Each system is made up of multiple enzyme components that utilize NADPH, molecular O_2, and flavin. Each produces a radical that reacts with oxygen to produce other potentially toxic substances. Nathan and Gabay have conceptualized the parallelisms in Figure 13–8.[186] Both O_2^- and NO are small lipophilic molecules that can penetrate microbial walls. The molecular targets for ROIs and RNIs are not completely clear but NO has a great avidity for heme enzymes and for Fe-S centers. For example, NO is effectively quenched by hemoglobin, perhaps accounting for the infection potentiation of heme compounds. NO inhibits ribonucleotide reductase, an enzyme essential in DNA synthesis, as well as the Krebs cycle enzyme aconitase and the mitochondrial electron transfer system.

The oxygen-independent microbicidal mechanisms of the neutrophil have been discussed (see Table 13–10). Almost all are mediated by proteins in the cytoplasmic granules. Macrophages have many fewer microbicidal proteins. Lysozyme is con-

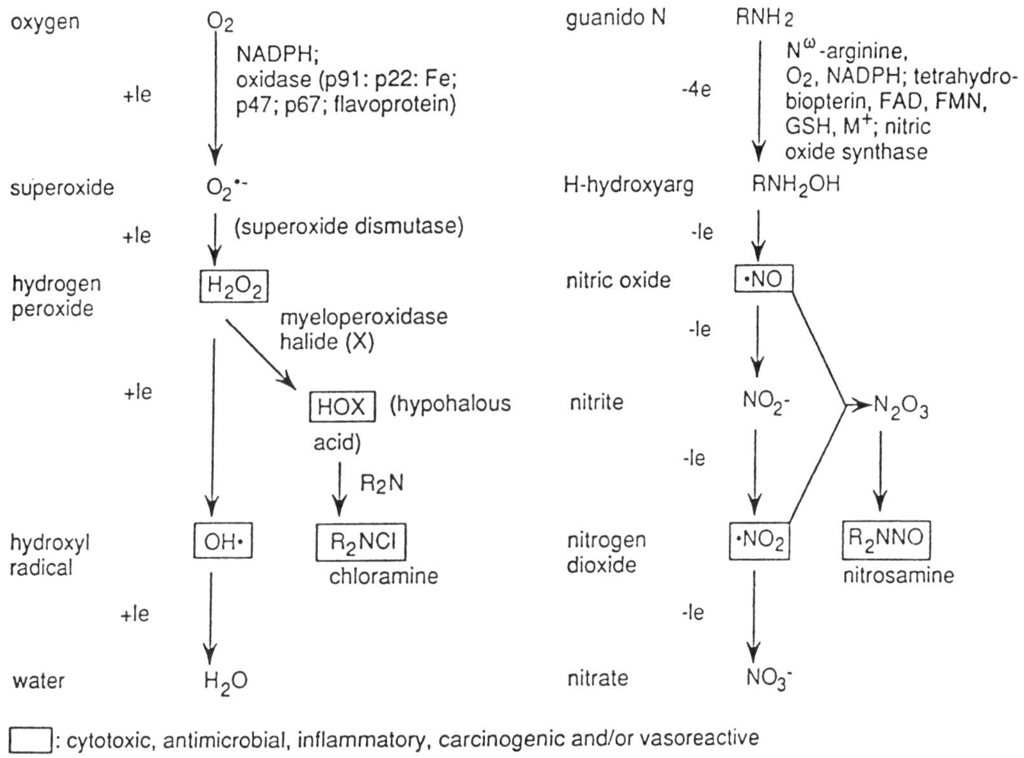

Figure 13–8. Reactive oxygen intermediates and reactive nitrogen intermediates—analogous but independent pathways for production of inorganic oxidants by activated macrophages. *(From Nathan C: Behring Inst Res Commun 88:200, 1991.)*

tained in mononuclear phagocytes as well as neutrophils, but the defensins have only been found in rabbit alveolar macrophages[86] and not in any human monocytes/macrophages. The serprocidins (cathepsin G, azurocidin, proteinase 3, elastase), which are potent as antibiotics but have broader spectrum, are found in few subsets of human monocytes although in low concentrations. Activation of macrophages does not upregulate their manufacture. Thus lysozyme appears to be the only nonoxidative microbicidal agent in most macrophages. However, other oxygen-independent mechanisms are present. For example, macrophages have the capacity to deplete the microenvironment of factors essential for certain microbes; specifically, *Toxoplasma gondii* requires tryptophan and depletion of tryptophan occurs by IFN-γ-induced indoleamine dioxygenase.[186–188] Legionella requires iron and IFN-γ also leads to a decrease in transferrin receptors in macrophages such that legionella within monocytes cannot grow. However, neither of these depleting effects is thought to be important. Macrophages also exhibit another, and apparently unique, second intracellular mechanism involving the conversion of tryptophan to picolinic acid[189,190]; its importance, however, is probably not great.

Nathan and Gabay have speculated on another, more closely targeted, system involving interaction between specifically sensitized T cells and macrophages.[186] It depends on the observation that cytolytic T cells bind to and kill macrophages infected by intracellular pathogens. The microbes die as well. This occurs because the specifically sensitized T cell releases perforans, which open pores in the macrophage membrane; T cell granzymes (serprocidins) then reach the microbe through the pores made into the macrophages.

Mononuclear phagocytic membranes also exhibit receptors for (1) the Fc fragments of two IgG subclasses (IgG1 and IgG3), (2) the derivatives of activated complement C3b (CR1) and C3bi (CR3), and (3) certain carbohydrates such as sugar conjugates terminating with mannose or fructose.[143] These receptors permit "recognition" of opsonizing substances on microbes or, in the case of mannose receptors, of the carohydrates on the outer coats of yeasts and pneumocystis themselves. By this means, attachment of the particulate material to the phagocyte acts as a prerequisite for phagocytosis, which occurs in a manner resembling that described for neutrophils. Ultimately, however, the magnitude of the response in terms of inflammation or host defense is a function of the numbers of mononuclear phagocytes recruited to the infected site together with their response to modulating cytokines, which may augment or inhibit inflammatory reactivity.

The enhanced tumoricidal activity of cytokine-stimulated mononuclear phagocytes (particularly IFN-γ, LPS, and TNF) is well known, and the differentiation of monocytes in culture with GM-CSF and 1,25-dehydroxy vitamin D_3 also enhances tumoricidal activity.[191] While this augmented cytotoxicity is not entirely understood, macrophages appear to kill tumor cells by means of secreted products, including ROIs, NO, lysosomal enzymes, and cytokines.[192] Recent work has shown that activation of macrophages for tumoricidal activity requires protein-tyrosine phosphorylation.[193]

Macrophages can also kill other selected mammalian cell targets,[194] including allogeneic targets and even host cells in autoimmune disorders. Some of these mechanisms require prior attachment of specific antibodies, while others depend on nonspecific macrophage activation. Intimate cell contact appears to be necessary,[195] but phagocytosis is not required for cytotoxicity.

TABLE 13–16. DISORDERS OF MONONUCLEAR PHAGOCYTES

Chemotaxis
Leukocyte adhesion deficiency
Newborn
Diabetes
Microcutaneous candidiasis
Burns
Cancer
AIDS
Chédiak-Hygashi syndrome
Immunosuppression (steroids)
Phagocytoses
Lupus
Leukocyte adhesion deficiency
End-stage renal disease
AIDS
Cytotoxicity
Chronic granulomatous disease
Steroids
Infections
Viral infection
Malaria
Yersinia
Tuberculosis
AIDS
Leishmanias
Newborn
Cancer/leukemia
Wiscott-Aldrich syndrome
Lipid storage diseases

Data from Johnston RB Jr: Monocytes and macrophages. In Lachmann PJ, Peters K, Rosen FS, Walport MJ (eds): Clinical Aspects of Immunology, 5th ed. Boston, Blackwell Scientific Publications, 1991, pp 467–479.

Abnormalities of Mononuclear Phagocytes

Many disease states have been associated with abnormalities of mononuclear phagocytes (as reviewed by Johnston and by Blaese),[145,146,148] and the more common or better known of these are listed in Table 13–16. Recently, it was shown that newborn T cells produce little IL-6[196] or IFN-γ,[197] and, in addition, newborn macrophages respond poorly to IFN-γ.[198] Newborn neutrophils, however, exhibit enhanced chemotaxis with IFN-γ.[40] These defects are transient, so that patients of this age must be managed with the understanding that scrupulous attention to prevention of infection and antibiotic therapy of sepsis are needed.

Numerous intracellular pathogens also have been shown to impair monocyte function. These include *Leishmania, Yersinia,* malaria, and the human immunodeficiency virus (HIV-1).[199–206] *Leishmania,* for example, require internalization in macrophages for replication. These organisms evade killing by macrophages at least in part because of *Leishmania* infection-induced reduction in IL-2.[201] Oliver et al[199,200] further show that this pathogen inhibits monocyte function by impairing intracellular signaling mechanisms involving protein kinase C and calcium shifts. This impaired killing of *Leishmania* may arise because of defective function of mononuclear phagocytes, of lymphoid cells, or of both. In the case of malaria, Schwarzer et al[205] demonstrated that malarial pigment is the cause of the toxic effect on macrophages, and they suggest that, specifically, the iron released from the pigment damages the macrophage, since stripping the iron from the pigment was associated with less inhibition of the oxidative burst. In patients with AIDS,[207] lepromatous leprosy,[208] and cutaneous leishmaniasis,[202,209] some improvement in cytotoxicity can be induced by treatment with IFN-γ.

In severe malnutrition, cell-mediated immunity is impaired, and these patients are often incapable of mounting delayed cutaneous hypersensitivity responses. This deficiency may arise because of defective function of mononuclear phagocytes, of lymphoid cells, or of both.[193] The causes of defective function in patients with neoplasms continue to be unclear. However, products of tumor cells are believed to be suppressive.[210,211]

Role of the Phagocyte in Multiple Organ Failure

While the professional phagocytes are essential for host defense and are known to mediate the inflammatory response, it has become increasingly clear that these same phagocytes were responsible for the syndrome of multiple organ failure (MOF) and the systemic inflammatory response syndrome (SIRS).[212] This syndrome is associated with considerable morbidity and a mortality rate of 40 to 70 percent.[213] It is characterized by a profound and often unresponsive hypotension, which appears to be a result of cytokine (especially IL-1 and IFN-γ) inducible NO formation.[129,214,215] Organ toxicity, however, including the adult respiratory distress syndrome,[126] may be a function of phagocyte activation including release of ROIs, RNIs, and granule enzymes together with the hypotension-associated ischemia. Both neutrophils and monocytes exhibit increased gene expression of TNF-α, IL-1α-β, IL-6, IFN-γ, IL-8 as a result of the LPS/LBP engagement of CD14. SIRS, however, also is associated with non-LPS-producing microorganisms as well as with severe trauma.[216] Cognizance of the role of cytokines that regulate the inflammatory response and knowledge of the function of matrix and adhesion molecules in this response have provoked innovative approaches designed to interrupt the inflammatory cascade, including agents that act on LPS, TNF, the IL-1 receptor, and the beta-2 integrins. These new approaches to MOF have been promising, but considerable additional study is needed to determine the most effective therapeutic regimen and to ensure that these therapies do not substitute infection for inflammation.

REFERENCES

1. Yang KD, Hill HR: Neutrophil function disorders: pathophysiology, prevention and therapy. J Pediatr 119:343, 1991.
2. Boogaerts MA: Acquired granulocyte dysfunction. Nouv Rev Fr Hematol 35:203, 1993.
3. Patriarca P, Menegazzi R, Dobrina A: Disorders of neutrophil function. In Peters TJ (ed): Subcellular Pathology of Systemic Disease. London, Chapman & Hall, 1987, pp 267–301.
4. Haig DM: Hematopoietic stem cells and the development of the blood cell repertoire. J Comp Pathol 106:121, 1992.
5. Trinchieri G: The hematopoietic system and hematopoiesis. In Knowles DM (ed): Neoplastic Hematopathology. Philadelphia, Williams & Wilkins, 1992, pp 1–25.
6. Serafin WE, Austin KF: Current concepts: mediation of immediate hypersensitivity reactions. N Engl J Med 317:30, 1987.
7. Athens JW; Neutropenia. In Lee GR, Bilbell TC, Foerster J, et al (eds): Wintrobe's Clinical Hematology, Vol 2, 9th ed. Philadelphia, Lea & Febiger, 1993, pp 1589–1612.
8. Cronstein BN, Weissmann G: The adhesion molecule of inflammation. Arthritis Rheum 36:147, 1993.
9. Long MW: Blood cell cytoadhesion molecules. Exp Hematol 20:288, 1992.
10. Bevilacqua MP, Nelson RM: Selectins. J Clin Invest 91:379, 1993.
11. Zimmerman GA, Prescott SM, McIntyre TM: Endothelial cell interactions with granulocytes: tethering and signaling molecules. Immunol Today 13:93, 1992.
12. Von Andrian UH, Hansell P, Chambers JD, et al: L-selection function is required for $\beta 2$ integrin mediated neutrophil adhesion at physiological shear rates in vivo. Am J Physiol 263:H1034, 1992.
13. Springer TA: Adhesion receptors of the immune system. Nature 346:425, 1990.
14. Cohn ZA, Morse SI: Functions and metabolic properties of polymorphonuclear leukocytes. II. The influence of a lipopolysaccharide endotoxin. J Exp Med 111:689, 1960.
15. Wright SD, Ramos RA, Tobias PS, et al: CD14 a receptor for complexes of lipopolysaccharide (LPS) and LPS binding protein. Science 249:1431, 1990.
16. Dahinden C, Galanos C, Fehr J: Granulocyte activation by endotoxin. I. Correlation between adherence and other granulocyte functions and the role of endotoxin structure on biologic activity. J Immunol 130:857, 1983.
17. Worthen GS, Avdi N, Vukajiovich S, Tobias PS: Neutrophil adherence induced by lipopolysaccharide in vitro: role of plasma component interaction with lipopolysaccharide. J Clin Invest 90:2526, 1992.
18. Wright SD, Ramos RA, Hermanowski-Vosatka A, et al: Activation of the adhesive capacity of CR3 on neutrophils by endotoxin: dependence on lipopolysaccharide binding protein and CD14. J Exp Med 173:1281, 1991.
19. Harvath L: Neutrophil chemotactic factors. In Goldberg LD (ed): Cell Motility Factors. Basel, Switzerland, Birkhauser Verlag, 1991, pp 35–52.
20. Freissmuth M, Casey PJ, Gilman AG: G-proteins control diverse pathway of transmembrane signaling. FASEB J 3:2125, 1989.
21. Baggiolini M, Wyman MP: Turning on the respiratory burst. TIBS 15:69, 1990.
22. Ding J, Badwey JA: Neutrophils stimulated with a chemotactic peptide or a phorbol ester exhibit different alterations in the activities of a battery of protein kinases. J Biol Chem 268:5234, 1993.
23. Stossel TP: On the crawling of animal cells. Science 260:1086, 1993.
24. Rotstein OD, Fiegel VD, Simmons RL, Knighton DR: The deleterious effect of reduced pH and hypoxia in neutrophil migration in vitro. J Surg Res 45:298, 1988.

25. Brown CC, Gallin JI: Chemotactic disorders. Hematol Oncol Clin North Am 2:61, 1988.
26. Stossel TP: Phagocytosis. N Engl J Med 290:717, 774, 833 (3 part series), 1974.
27. Arnaout MA: Leukocyte adhesion molecule deficiency: its structural basis, pathophysiology, and implications for modulation of the inflammatory response. Immunol Rev 114:145, 1990.
28. Anderson DC, Springer TA: Leukocyte adhesion deficiency: an inherited defect in the Mac-1, LFA-1, and p150,95 glycoproteins. Annu Rev Med 38:175, 1987.
29. Springer TA: Adhesion molecules of the immune system. Nature 346:425, 1990.
30. Hill HR, Estensen RD, Hogan NA, Quie PG: Severe staphylococcal disease associated with allergic manifestations, hyperimmunoglobulinemia E and defective neutrophil chemotaxis. J Lab Clin Med 88:796, 1976.
31. Jepson JD, Jaffe HW, Hill HR: Use of recombinant human interferon gamma enhances neutrophil chemotactic responses in Job syndrome of hyperimmunoglobulin E and recurrent infections. J Pediatr 118:383, 1991.
32. Southwick FS, Dabiri GA, Stossel TP: Neutrophil actin dysfunction is a genetic disorder associated with partial impairment of neutrophil actin assembly in three family members. J Clin Invest 82:1525, 1988.
33. Jung LKL: Association of aberrant F-actin formation with defective leukocyte chemotaxis and recurrent pyoderma. Clin Immunol Immunopathol 61:41, 1991.
34. Coates TD, Torkildson JC, Torres M, et al: An inherited defect of neutrophil motility and microfilamentous cytoskeleton associated with abnormalities in 47-Kd and 89-Kd proteins. Blood 78:1338, 1991.
35. Gallin JI, Malech HL, Wright DG, et al: Recurrent severe infection in a child with abnormal leukocyte function: possible relationship to increased microtubule assembly. Blood 51:919, 1978.
36. Malech HL, Englander L: Abnormal polymorphonuclear neutrophil function in Kartagener's syndrome. Clin Res 27:Abstr 590A, 1979.
37. Clark RA, Kimball HE: Defective granulocyte chemotaxis in the Chédiak-Higashi syndrome. J Clin Invest 50:2645, 1971.
38. Ganz T, Metcalf JA, Gallin JI, et al: Microbicidal/cytotoxic proteins of neutrophils are deficient in 2 disorders: Chédiak-Higashi syndrome and specific granule deficiency. J Clin Invest 82:552, 1988.
39. Van Dyke TE: Role of the neutrophil in oral disease: receptor deficiency in leukocytes from patients with juvenile periodontitis. Rev Infect Dis 7:419, 1985.
40. Hill HR, Augustine NH, Jaffe HS: Human recombinant interferon gamma enhances neonatal PMN activation and movement and increases free intracellular calcium. J Exp Med 173:767, 1991.
41. Hill HR: Modulation of host defenses with interferon-γ in pediatrics. J Infect Dis 167:S23, 1993.
42. Esman V: The polymorphonuclear leukocytes in diabetes mellitus. J Clin Chem Clin Biochem 21:561, 1983.
43. Markoffer W, Stein M, Maeser E, Federlin K: Impairment of polymorphonuclear leukocyte function and metabolic control of diabetes. Diabetes Care 15:256, 1992.
44. Clark RA: Disorders of granulocyte chemotaxis. In Gallin JI, Quie PG (eds): Leukocyte Chemotaxis: Methods, Physiology, and Clinical Implications. New York, Raven Press, 1978, p 329.
45. Meakins JL, McLean APH, Kelly R, et al: Delayed hypersensitivity and neutrophil chemotaxis: effect of trauma. J Trauma 18:240, 1978.
46. Damtew B, Marino JA, Fratianne RB, Spagnulo PJ: Neutrophil lipoxygenase metabolism and adhesive function following acute thermal injury. J Lab Clin Med 121:328, 1993.
47. Felix JC, Davis JM: Neutrophil function in thermally injured patients. In Gallin JD, Fauci AS (eds): Advances in Host Defense Mechanisms, Vol 6. New York, Raven Press, 1986, pp 63–75.
48. Hasslen Sharon R, Ahrenholz DH, Solem LD, Nelson RD: Actin polymerization contributes to neutrophil chemotaxis dysfunction following thermal injury. J Leukoc Biol 52:495, 1992.
49. Sasgawa S: Inhibitory effects of local anesthetics on migration, extracellular release of lysosomal enzyme and superoxide anion production in human polymorphonuclear leukocytes. Immunopharmacol Immunotoxicol 13:607, 1991.
50. Gallin JI: Abnormal phagocyte chemotaxis: pathophysiology, clinical manifestations, and management of patients. Rev Infect Dis 3:6, 1981.
51. NIH Conference Moderator: Gallin JI. Discussants: Wright DG, Malech HL, Davis JM, et al: Disorders of phagocyte chemotaxis. Ann Intern Med 92:520, 1980.
52. Van Epps DE, Palmer DL, Williams RC: Characterization of serum inhibitors of neutrophil chemotaxis associated with anergy. J Immunol 113:189, 1974.
53. Johnston RB Jr, Klemperer MR, Alper CA, Rosen FS: The enhancement of bacterial phagocytosis by serum: the role of complement components and two cofactors. J Exp Med 129:1275, 1969.
54. Verbrugh HA, Von Dijk WC, Peters R, et al: *Staphylococcus aureus* opsonization mediated via the classical and alternative complement pathways: a kinetic study using Mg EGTA chelated serum and human serum deficient in IgG and complement factors C1S and C2. Immunology 36:391, 1979.
55. Wright SD, Tobias PS, Ulevitch RJ, Ramos RA: Lipopolysaccharide (LPS) binding protein opsonizes LPS-bearing particles for recognition by a novel receptor on macrophages. J Exp Med 170:1231, 1991.
56. Doran JE: A critical assessment of fibronectins opsonic role of bacteria and microaggregates. Vox Sang 45:337, 1983.

57. Rosen FS, Alper CA, Janeway CA: The primary immunodeficiencies and the serum complement defects. In Nathan DG, Oski FA (eds): Hematology of Infancy and Childhood. Philadelphia, Saunders, 1974, p 529.
58. Alexander JW, Ogle CK, Stinnett JD, MacMillan BG: A sequential prospective analysis of immunoglobulin abnormalities and infection following severe thermal injury. Ann Surg 188:809, 1978.
59. Solomkin JS, Jenkins MD, Nelson RD, et al: Neutrophil dysfunction in sepsis. II. Evidence for the role of complement activation products in cellular deactivation. Surgery 90:319, 1981.
60. Gu YJ, van Oeveren W, Boonstra PW, et al: Leukocyte activation with increased expression of CR3 receptors during cardiopulmonary bypass. Ann Thorac Surg 53:839, 1992.
61. Sklar LA, Hyslop PA, Oades ZG, et al: Signal transduction and ligand-receptor dynamics in the human neutrophil. J Biol Chem 260:11461, 1985.
62. Snyderman R, Uhing RJ: Phagocytic cells: stimulus-response coupling mechanisms. In Gallin JI, Goldstein IM, Snyderman R (eds): Inflammation: Basic Principles and Clinical Correlates. New York, Raven Press, 1988, p 303.
63. Baldridge CW, Gerard RW: The extra respiration of phagocytosis. Am J Physiol 103:235, 1933.
64. Sbarra AJ, Karnovsky ML: The biochemical basis of phagocytosis. I. Metabolic changes during the ingestion of particles by polymorphonuclear leukocytes. J Biol Chem 234:1355, 1959.
65. Segal AW: The electron transfer chain of the microbicidal oxidase of phagocytic cells and its involvement in the molecular pathology of chronic granulomatous disease. J Clin Invest 83:1785, 1989.
66. Babior BM: Oxidants from phagocytes: agents of defense and destruction. Blood 64:959, 1984.
67. Clark RA: The human neutrophil respiratory burst oxidase. J Infect Dis 161:1140, 1990.
68. Ohno Y-I, Hirai K-I, Kanoh T, et al: Subcellular localization of H_2O_2 production in human neutrophils stimulated with particles and an effect of cytochalasin B on cells. Blood 60:253, 1982.
69. Woodman RC, Knedi JM, Jesaites AJ, et al: Respiratory burst oxidase and three of four oxidase related polypeptides are associated with the cytoskeleton of human neutrophils. J Clin Invest 87:1345, 1991.
70. Segal AW: Cytochrome b_{245} and its involvement in the molecular pathology of chronic granulomatous disease. In Phagocytic Defects II. Abnormalities of the respiratory burst. Hematol Oncol Clin North Am 2:213, 1988.
71. Segal AW, West I, Wientjes F, et al: Cytochrome b_{245} is a flavocytochrome containing FAD and the NADPH-binding site of the microbicidal oxidase of phagocytes. Biochem J 284:781, 1992.
72. Abo A, Boyhan A, West I, et al: Reconstitution of neutrophil NADPH oxidase activity in the cell free system by four components: p67-phox, P47-phox, P21 rac 1, and cytochrome b-245. J Biol Chem 267:16767, 1992.
73. Knaus UG, Heyworth PG, Evans T, et al: Regulation of phagocyte oxygen radical production by the GTP-binding protein Rac 2. Science 254:1512, 1992.
74. Quinn MT, Mullen ML, Jesaitis AL, Linner JG: Subcellular distribution of Rap-1A protein in human neutrophils: co-localization and co-translocation with cytochrome b559. Blood 79:1563, 1992.
75. McRipley RJ, Sbarra AJ: Role of the phagocyte in host parasite interactions. XII. Hydrogen peroxide-myeloperoxidase bactericidal system in the phagocyte. J Bacteriol 94:1425, 1968.
76. Klebanoff SJ: Phagocytic cells: products of oxygen metabolism. In: Gallin JI, Goldstein IM, Snyderman R (eds): Inflammation: Basic Principles and Clinical Correlates. New York, Raven Press, 1988.
77. Klebanoff SJ: Myeloperoxidase-halide-hydrogen peroxide peroxidase antibacterial system. J Bacteriol 95:2131, 1968.
78. Parry MF, Rost RK, Metcalf JA, et al: Myeloperoxidase deficiency: prevalence and clinical significance. Ann Intern Med 95:293, 1981.
79. Klebanoff SJ: Oxygen metabolism and the toxic properties of phagocytes. Ann Intern Med 93:480, 1980.
80. Moncada S, Higgs A, Hodson HF, et al: The L-arginine:nitric oxide pathway. J Cardiovasc Pharmacol 17:S1, 1991.
81. Kaplan SS, Billiar T, Curran RD, et al: Inhibition of chemotaxis with N^G-monomethyl-L-arginine: a role for cyclic GMP. Blood 74:1885, 1989.
82. Malawista SE, Montgomery RR, Van Blaricom G: Evidence of reactive nitrogen intermediates in killing of staphylococci by human neutrophil cytoplasts. J Clin Invest 90:631, 1992.
83. Murray HW, Teitelbaum RF: L-Arginine dependent reactive nitrogen intermediates and the antimicrobial effect of activated human mononuclear phagocytes. J Infect Dis 165:5134, 1992.
84. Lehrer RI, Ganz T: Antimicrobial polypeptides of human neutrophils. Blood 76:2169, 1990.
85. Lehrer RI, Lichtenstein AK, Ganz T: Defensins: antimicrobial and cytotoxic peptides of mammalian cells. Annu Rev Immunol 11:105, 1993.
86. Lehrer RI, Ganz T, Selsted ME: Defensins: endogenous antibiotic peptide of animal cells. Cell 64:229, 1991.
87. Gabay JE, Almeida RP: Antibiotic peptides and serine protease homologs in human polymorphonuclear leukocytes: defensins and azurocidin. Curr Opin Immunol 5:97, 1993.
88. Holmes B, Page AB, Good RA: Studies of metabolic activity of leukocytes from patients with a genetic abnormality of phagocyte function. J Clin Invest 46:1422, 1967.
89. Forrest CB, Forehand JR, Axtell RA, et al: Clinical features and current management of chronic granulomatous disease. In Phagocytic Defects II. Abnor-

malities of the respiratory burst. Hematol Oncol Clin North Am 2:253, 1988.
90. Segal AW: Variations on a theme of chronic granulomatous disease. Lancet 1:1378, 1985.
91. Babior BM, Woodman RC: Chronic granulomatous disease. Semin Hematol 27:247, 1990.
92. Bahner RL, Johnston RB, Nathan DG: Comparative study of the metabolic and bactericidal characteristics of severely glucose 6-phosphate dehydrogenase deficient polymorphonuclear leukocytes and leukocytes from children with chronic granulomatous disease. J Reticuloendo Soc 12:150, 1972.
93. Boxer LA, Watanabe AM, Rister M: Corrections of leukocyte function in Chédiak-Higashi syndrome by ascorbate. N Engl J Med 295:1041, 1976.
94. Suskind RM: The Phagocyte in Malnutrition and the Immune Response. New York, Raven Press, 1977, pp 209–293.
95. Tsuchiga M, Thompson DFT, Suzuki YJ, et al: Superoxide formed from cigarette smoke impairs polymorphonuclear leukocyte active oxygen generation activity. Arch Biochem Biophys 99:30, 1992.
96. Matzner Y: Granulocyte dysfunction in hematologic disorders. Cancer Invest 102:155, 1992.
97. Murphy PM, Love HC, Fauci AS, Gallin JI: Impairment of neutrophil bactericidal capacity in patients with AIDS. J Infect Dis 158:627, 1988.
98. Goldstein IM, Roos MD, Weissmann G, Kaplan HB: Influence of corticosteroids on human polymorphonuclear function in vitro: reduction of lysosomal enzyme release and superoxide production. Inflammation 1:305, 1976.
99. Umeki S, Soejima R: Hydrocortisone inhibits the respiratory burst oxidase from human neutrophils in whole blood and cell free systems. Biochem Biophys Acta 1052:211, 1990.
100. Hara N, Ichinose Y, Motohiro A, et al: Influence of chemotherapeutic agents on superoxide anion production by human polymorphonuclear leukocytes. Cancer 66:684, 1990.
101. Umeki S: Effects of anti-allergic drugs on human neutrophil superoxide-generating NADPH oxidase. Biochem Pharmacol 43:1109, 1992.
102. Fumarulo R, Conese M, Riccardi S, et al: Retinoids inhibit the respiratory burst and degranulation of stimulated human polymorphonuclear leukocytes. Agents Actions 34:339, 1991.
103. Zimmerli W, Lew PD, Waldvogel FA: Pathogenesis of foreign body infection: evidence for a local granulocyte defect. J Clin Invest 73:1191, 1984.
104. Gristina AG, Hobgood CD, Webb LX, Myrouk QN: Adhesive colonization of biomaterials and antibiotic resistance. Biomaterials 8:423, 1987.
105. Wang IW, Anderson JM, Marchant RE: *Staphylococcus epidermidis* adhesion to hydrophobic biomedical polymers is mediated by platelets. J Infect Dis 167:329, 1993.
106. Kaplan SS, Basford RE, Mora E, et al: Biomaterial-induced alterations of neutrophil superoxide production. J Biomed Mater Res 26:1039, 1992.
107. Metchnikoff E: Immunity in Infective Disease. Cambridge, Cambridge University Press, 1905.
108. Shaw GB: The Doctor's Dilemma. London, Constable & Co, 1911.
109. Rose RM: The role of colony-stimulating factors in infectious disease: current status, future challenges. Semin Oncol 19:415, 1992.
110. Khwaja A, Carver JE, Linch DG: Interaction of granulocyte-macrophage colony-stimulating factor (CSF), granulocyte CSF, and tumor necrosis factor in the priming of the neutrophil respiratory burst. Blood 79:745, 1992.
111. Konig W: Role of the immune system in recovery from infection. Respiration 60:16, 1993.
112. Vadhan-Raj S, Keating M, LeMaestre A, et al: Effects of recombinant human granulocyte-macrophage colony-stimulating factor in patients with myelodysplastic syndrome. N Engl J Med 317:1545, 1989.
113. Mitsuyasu RT: Hematopoietic growth factors in the treatment of patients with HIV infection. Biotherapy 2:173, 1990.
114. Ganser A, Ottmann OG, Erdmann H, et al: The effect of recombinant human granulocyte-macrophage colony-stimulating factor on neutropenia and related morbidity in chronic severe neutropenia. Ann Intern Med 111:887, 1989.
115. Boxer LA, Hutchinson R, Emerson S: Recombinant human granulocyte colony stimulating factor in the treatment of patients with neutropenia. Clin Immunol Immunopathol 62:S39, 1992.
116. Bronchud MH, Scarffe JH, Thatcher N, et al: Phase I/II study of recombinant human granulocyte colony-stimulating factor in patients receiving intensive chemotherapy for small cell lung cancer. Br J Cancer 56:809, 1987.
117. Brandt SJ, Peters WP, Atwater SK, et al: Effect of recombinant human granulocyte-macrophage colony-stimulating factor on hematopoietic reconstitution after high-dose chemotherapy and autologous bone marrow transplantation. N Engl J Med 318:869, 1988.
118. Arnaout MA, Wang EA, Clark SC, Sieff CA: Human recombinant granulocyte-macrophage colony-stimulating factor increases cell-to-cell adhesion and surface expression of adhesion-promoting surface glycoproteins on mature granulocytes. J Clin Invest 78:597, 1986.
119. Study Group: A phase III study establishing efficacy of recombinant human interferon gamma for infectious prophylaxis of chronic granulomatous disease. N Engl J Med 324:509, 1991.
120. Res JH, Bennett JE, Gallin JI, et al: In vivo interferon-γ therapy augments the in vitro ability of chronic granulomatous disease neutrophils to damage aspergillus hyphae. J Infect Dis 163:849, 1991.
121. Tobler A, Foeffler HP: Differentiation of human acute myelogenous leukemia cells: therapeutic possibilities. Acta Hematol 78:127, 1987.

122. Newton JA, Ashwood ER, Yang KD, et al: Effect of pentoxifylline on the developmental changes in neutrophil cell surface mobility and membrane fluidity. J Cell Physiol 140:427, 1989.
123. Weiss SJ: Tissue destruction by neutrophils. N Engl J Med 320:365, 1989.
124. McCord JM: Oxygen derived free-radicals in post ischemic tissue injury. J Vasc Surg 5:512, 1987.
125. Windsor AC, Mullen PG, Fowler AA, Sugerman HJ: Role of the neutrophil in adult respiratory distress syndrome. Br J Surg 80:10, 1993.
126. St John RC, Darinsky PM: Immunologic therapy for ARDS, septic shock and multiple organ failure. Chest 103:932, 1993.
127. Cybulsky M, Chan MKW, Movat HZ: Biology of disease, acute inflammation and microthrombosis induced by endotoxin, interleukin 1 and tumor necrosis factor and their implication in gram negative infection. Lab Invest 58:365, 1978.
128. Gough DB: Educate the phagocyte. Br J Surg 78:1, 1991.
129. Brady AJB, Poole-Wilson PA: Circulatory failure in septic shock. Nitric oxide: too much of a good thing? Br Heart J 70:103, 1993.
130. Ziegler EJ, Fisher CJ, Sprung CL, et al: Treatment of gram-negative bacteremia and septic shock with HA-IA human monoclonal antibody against endotoxin. N Engl J Med 324:429, 1991.
131. Ziegler EJ, McCutchan A, Fierer J, et al: Treatment of gram negative bacteremia and shock with human antiserums to a mutant *Escherichia coli*. N Engl J Med 307:1225, 1982.
132. Baumgartner JD, McCutcham JA, van Melle G, et al: Prevention of gram negative shock and death in surgical patients by antibody to endotoxin core glycolipid. Lancet 2:59, 1985.
133. Wolff SM. Monoclonal antibodies and the treatment of gram negative bacteremia and shock. N Engl J Med 324:486, 1991.
134. Warren HS, Donner RL, Mumford RS. Antiendotoxin monoclonal antibodies. N Engl J Med 326: 1153, 1992.
135. Exley AR, Cohen J, Buurman W, et al: Monoclonal antibody to TNF in severe septic shock. Lancet 335:1275, 1990.
136. Mileski WJ, Sikes P, Atiles L, et al: Inhibition of leukocyte adherence and susceptibility to infection. J Surg Res 54:349, 1993.
137. Goldman G, Welbourn R, Alexander S, et al: Modulation of pulmonary permeability in vivo with agents that affect the cytoskeleton. Surgery 109: 533, 1991.
138. Kortheus RJ, Carden DL, Kvietys PR, et al: Phalloidin attenuates post ischemic neutrophil infiltration and increases microvascular permeability. J Appl Physiol 71:1261, 1991.
139. Conti P, Panara MR, Barbacacone RC, et al: Human recombinant IL-1 receptor antagonist (Il-1Ra) inhibits leukotriene B4 generation from human monocyte suspensions stimulated by lipopolysaccharide (LPS). Clin Exp Immunol 91:526, 1993.
140. Westlin WF, Gembrone MA Jr: Neutrophil mediated damage to human vascular endothelium. Am J Pathol 142:117, 1993.
141. Roberts PJ, Yong KL, Khwaja A, et al: Pentoxifylline at clinically achievable levels inhibits fMLP-induced neutrophil response but not priming, up regulation of cell-adhesion molecules, or migration induced by GM-CSF. Eur J Hematol 50:1, 1993.
142. Fink M: Role of prostaglandins and related compounds in the pathophysiology of endotoxic and septic shock. Semin Respir Med 7:17, 1985.
143. Mileski WJ: Sepsis: what is it and how to recognize it. Surg Clin North Am 71:749, 1991.
144. Johnston RB Jr, Zucker-Franklin D: Monocytes and macrophages. In Zucker-Franklin D, Greaves MF, Grossi CE, Marmont AM (eds): Atlas of Blood Cells: Function and Pathology, 2nd ed. Philadelphia, Lea & Febiger, 1988, pp 321–357.
145. Johnston RB Jr: Monocytes and macrophages. N Engl J Med 318:747, 1988.
146. Johnston RB Jr: Monocytes and macrophages. In Lachmann PJ, Peters K, Rosen FS, Walport MJ (eds): Clinical Aspects of Immunology, 5th ed. Boston, Blackwell Scientific Publications, 1991, pp 467–479.
147. Takamatsu Y, Akashi K, Harada M, et al: Cytokine production by peripheral blood monocytes and T cells during haemopoietic recovery after intensive chemotherapy. Br J Haematol 83:21, 1993.
148. Blaese RM, Muchmore AV, Poplack DG: Disorders of the mononuclear phagocytic system. In Stichen ER (ed): Immunologic Disorders of Infants and Children, 3rd ed. Philadelphia, Saunders, 1989, pp 364–383.
149. Turpin JA, Lopez-Berestein G: Differentiation, maturation and activation of monocytes and macrophages: functional activity is controlled by a continuum of maturation. In Lopez-Berestein G, Klostergaard J (eds): *Mononuclear Phagocytes in Cell Biology*. Boca Raton, FL, CRC Press, 1993, pp 71–99.
150. Hamilton TA, Ohmari Y, Narumi S, Tannenbaum CS: Regulation of diversity of macrophage activation. In Lopez-Berestein G, Klostergaard J (eds): Mononuclear Phagocytes in Cell Biology. Boca Raton, FL, CRC Press, 1993, pp 47–70.
151. Rappolee DA, Mark D, Banda MJ, Werf Z: Wound macrophages express RGF-γ and other growth factors in vivo, analysis by mRNA phenotyping. Science 241:708, 1988.
152. Pierce CD: Macrophages: modulators of immunity. Am J Pathol 98:10, 1980.
153. Ziegler-Heitbrock HWL: The biology of the monocyte system. Eur J Cell Biol 49:1, 1989.
154. Nathan CF: Secretory products of macrophages. J Clin Invest 79:319, 1987.
155. Varesio L, Cox GW, Pulkki K, et al: Activation of macrophages and monocytes by interferon-γ and

IL-2. In Lopez-Berestein G, Klostergaard J (eds): Mononuclear Phagocytes in Cell Biology. Boca Raton, FL, CRC Press, 1993, pp 119–146.

156. Won SJ, Lin MT: Endogenous pyrogen formation by human blood monocytes stimulated by polyribocytidolyic acid. Experentia 49:157, 1993.
157. Metcalf D: Granulocyte macrophage colony stimulating factors. Science 229:16, 1985.
158. Leibovich SJ, Ross R: The role of the macrophage in wound repair. Am J Pathol 78:71, 1975.
159. Driggers PH, Ennist DL, Gleason SL, et al: An interferon gamma-regulated protein that binds the interferon-inducible enhancer element of major histocompatibility complex class I genes. Proc Natl Acad Sci USA 87:3743, 1990.
160. Collart MA, Baeuerle P, Vassalli P: Regulation of tumor necrosis factor alpha transcription in macrophages: involvement of four kB-like motifs and of constitutive and inducible forms of NF-kB. Mol Cell Biol 10:1498, 1990.
161. Germain RN, Margulies DH: The biochemistry and all biology of antigen processing and presentation. Annu Rev Immunol 11:403, 1993.
162. Allen PM, Unanue ER: Antigen processing and presentation at the molecular level. Adv Exp Med Biol 225:147, 1987.
163. Abbas AK: A reassessment of the mechanism of antigen-specific T cell-dependent B cell activation. Immunol Today 9:89, 1988.
164. Sieling PA, Abrams JS, Yamamura M, et al: Immunosuppressive roles for IL-10 and IL-4 in human infection. In vitro modulation of T cell responses in leprosy. J Immunol 150:5501, 1993.
165. Orino E, Sone S, Nil A, Ogura T: IL-4 up-regulates IL-1 receptor antagonist gene expression and its production in human blood monocytes. J Immunol 149:925, 1992.
166. Cilada A, Maki R: Transforming growth factor-B enhances the MCSF and GM-CSF proliferation of macrophages. J Immunol 148:1102, 1992.
167. Wilson CB: The cellular immune system and its role in host defense. In Mandell GL, Douglas RG Jr, Bennett JE (eds): Principles and Practice of Infectious Diseases. New York, Churchill Livingstone, 1990, p 101.
168. Savill JS, Wyllie AH, Hanson JE, et al: Macrophage phagocytosis of aging neutrophils in inflammation: programmed cell death in the neutrophil leads to its recognition by macrophages. J Clin Invest 83:865, 1989.
169. Sharma SD, Remington JS: Macrophage activation and resistance to intracellular infection. Lymphokines 3:181, 1981.
170. Arnaout MA, Lanier LL, Faller DV: Relative contribution of leukocyte molecules Mo1, LFA-1, and p150,95 (LeuM5) in adhesion of granulocytes and monocytes to vascular endothelium is tissue- and stimulus-specific. J Cell Physiol 137:305, 1988.
171. Springer TA: Adhesion receptors of the immune system. Nature 346:425, 1990.
172. Jiang Y, Beller DJ, Frendl G, Graves DT: Monocyte chemoattractant protein-1 regulates adhesion molecule expression and cytokine production in human monocytes. J Immunol 148:2423, 1992.
173. Chang ZL, Beezhold DH, Personius CD, Shen ZL: Fibronectin cell binding domain triggered transmembrane transduction in human monocytes. J Leukoc Biol 55:79, 1993.
174. Yoshimura T, Yuhki N, Moore SK, et al: Human monocyte chemoattractant protein-1 (MCP-1); full-length cDNA cloning, expression in mitogen-stimulated blood mononuclear leukocytes, and sequence similarity to mouse competence gene JE. FEBS Lett 244:487, 1989.
175. Rollins BJ, Warz A, Baggiolini M: Recombinant MCP-1/JE induces chemotaxis calcium flux and the respiratory burst in human monocytes. Blood 78:1112, 1991.
176. Rollins BJ, Sunday ME: Suppression of tumor formation in vivo by expression of JE gene in malignant cells. Mol Cell Biol 11:3125, 1991.
177. Espinoza-Delgado I, Longo DL, Gusella GL, Varesio L: Regulation of IL-2 receptor subunit genes in human monocytes: differential effects of IL-2 and IFN-gamma. J Immunol 149:2961, 1992.
178. Wahl SM, McCartney-Francis N, Hunt D, et al: Monocyte interleukin-2 receptor gene expression and interleukin-2 augmentation of microbicidal activity. J Immunol 139:1342, 1987.
179. Belosevic M, Finbloom DS, Meltzer MS, Nacy CA: IL-2, a cofactor for induction of activated macrophage resistance to infection. J Immunol 145:831, 1990.
180. Herrmann F, Cannistra SA, Lindemann A, et al: Functional consequences of monocyte IL-2 receptor expression: induction of IL-1 secretion by IFN and IL-2. J Immunol 142:139, 1989.
181. Strecter RM, Remick DG, Lynch JPL, et al: Interleukin-2-induced tumor necrosis factor alpha (TNFα) gene expression in human alveolar macrophages and blood monocytes. Annu Rev Respir Dis 139:335, 1989.
182. Musso T, Espinoza-Delgado I, Pulkki K, et al: IL-2 induces IL-6 production in human monocytes. J Immunol 148:795, 1992.
183. Nathan C, Hibbs JB Jr: Role of nitric oxide synthase in macrophage antimicrobial activity. Curr Opin Immunol 3:65, 1991.
184. Dennis M: Tumor necrosis factor and granulocyte macrophage colony stimulating factor stimulate human macrophages to restrict growth of virulent *Mycobacterium avium* and kill avirulent *M. avium:* killing effector mechanism depends on the generation of reactive nitrogen intermediates. J Leukoc Biol 49:380, 1991.
185. Nussler A, Drapier J-C, Renia L, et al: L-Arginine-dependent destruction of intrahepatic malaria para-

sites in response to tumor necrosis factor and/or interleukin-6 stimulation. Eur J Immunol 21:227, 1991.
186. Nathan CF, Gabay J: Antimicrobial mechanisms of macrophages. In van Furth R (ed): Mononuclear Phagocytes: Biology of Monocytes and Macrophages. Boston, Kluwer Academic Press, 1992, pp 259–267.
187. Pfefferkarn ER: Interferon-γ blocks the growth of *Toxoplasma gondii* in human fibroblasts by inducing the host cells to degrade tryptophane. Proc Natl Acad Sci USA 81:908, 1984.
188. Taylor MW, Feng F: Relationship between interferon-gamma, indoleamine 2,3-dioxygenase and tryptophane catabolism. FASEB J 5:2517, 1991.
189. Varesio L, Clayton M, Blasi E, et al: Picolinic acid, a catabolite of tryptophane, as the second signal in the activation of IFN-gamma primed macrophages. J Immunol 145:4265, 1990.
190. Taylor MW, Feng F: Relationship between interferon-gamma, indoleamine 2,3-dioxygenase and tryptophane catabolism. FASEB J 5:2517, 1991.
191. Chokari M, Lopez M, Aleron C, et al: Production of human macrophages with potent antitumor properties (MAK) by culture of monocytes in the presence of GM-CSF and 1,25 dehydroxy vitamin D_3. Anti Cancer Res 12:2257, 1992.
192. Wiltrout RH, Varesio L: Activation of macrophages for cytotoxic and suppressor effector function. In Oppenheim JJ, Shevach EM (eds): Immunopathology: The Role of Cells and Cytokines in Immunity and Inflammation. New York, Oxford University Press, 1991, pp 365–385.
193. Dong Z, O'Brien CA, Fidler IJ: Activation of tumoricidal properties in macrophages by lipopolysaccharide requires protein-tyrosine kinase activity. J Leukoc Biol 53:53, 1993.
194. Fidler IJ, Schroit AJ: Recognition and destruction of neoplastic cells by activated macrophages: discrimination of altered self. Biochem Biophys Acta 948:151, 1988.
195. Keller R: Cytostatic and cytocidal effects of activated macrophages. In: Nelson DS (ed): Immunobiology of the Macrophage. New York, Academic Press, 1976, p 487.
196. Schibler KL, Lichty KW, White WL, et al: Defective production of interleukin-6 by monocytes: a possible mechanism underlying several host defense deficiencies of neonates. Pediatr Res 31:18, 1992.
197. Wakasugi N, Vorelizier JL: Defective IFNγ production in the human neonate. I. Dysregulation rather than intrinsic abnormality. J Immunol 134:167, 1985.
198. Marodi L, Campbell DE, Polin RA, Johnston RB Jr: Protection against systemic candidal infection in the newborn: normal function of macrophage mannan receptor but deficient activation of newborn macrophages by IFNγ. Pediatr Res 31:269A, 1992.
199. Oliver M, Brownsley RW, Reiner NE: Defective stimulus-response coupling in human monocytes infected with *Leishmania donovani* is associated with altered activation and translocation of protein kinase C. Proc Natl Acad Sci USA 89:7481, 1992.
200. Oliver M, Baimbridge KG, Reiner NE: Stimulus-response coupling in monocytes infected with *Leishmania:* attenuation of calcium transients is related to defective agonist-induced accumulation of inositol phosphates. J Biol Chem 148:1188, 1992.
201. Nacy CA, Green SJ, Leiby DA, et al: Macrophages, cytokines, and leishmania. In Lopez-Berestein G, Klostergaard J (eds): Mononuclear Phagocytes in Cell Biology. Boca Raton, FL, CRC Press, 1993, pp 177–214.
202. Reiner NE, Ng W, Wilson CB, et al: Modulation of in vitro monocyte cytokine response to *Leishmania donovani:* interferon-γ prevents parasite-induced inhibition of interleukin-1 production and primes monocytes to respond to *Leishmania* by producing both tumor necrosis factor and interleukin-1. J Clin Invest 85:1914, 1990.
203. Pinching AJ, Nye KE: Defective signal transduction—a common pathway for cellular dysfunction in HIV infection? Immunol Today 1:256, 1990.
204. Baldwin GC, Fleishmann J, Chung Y, et al: Human immunodeficiency virus causes mononuclear phagocyte dysfunction. Proc Natl Acad Sci USA 87:3933, 1990.
205. Schwarzer E, Turrini F, Ulliero D, et al: Impairment of macrophage functions after ingestion of *Plasmodium falciparum*-infected erythrocytes or isolated malarial pigment. J Exp Med 176:1033, 1992.
206. Bliska JB, Guan KL, Dixon JE, Falkow S: Tyrosine phosphate hydrolysis of host proteins by an essential *Yersinia* virulence determinant. Proc Natl Acad Sci USA 88:1187, 1991.
207. Murray HW, Scavuzzo D, Jacobs JL, et al: In vitro and in vivo activation of human mononuclear phagocytes by interferon-gamma. Studies with normal and AIDS monocytes. J Immunol 138:2457, 1987.
208. Cohn ZA, Kaplan G: Hansen's disease, cell mediated immunity and recombinant lymphokines. J Infect Dis 163:1195, 1991.
209. Harms F, Zwengriberger K, Chebode AK: Effects of intradermal gamma-interferon in cutaneous leishmaniasis. Lancet 1:1287, 1989.
210. Cianciolo GJ: Anti-inflammatory effects of neoplasia. In Gallin JI, Goldstein IM, Snyderman R (eds): Inflammation: Basic Principles and Clinical Correlates. New York, Raven Press, 1988.
211. Szuro-Sudol A, Nathan CF: Suppression of macrophage oxidative metabolism by products of malignant and nonmalignant cells. J Exp Med 156:945, 1982.
212. Bone RC: The pathogenesis of sepsis. Ann Intern Med 115:457, 1991.

213. Martin MA, Wenzel RP, Gorelock KJ: Gram-negative bacterial sepsis in hospitals in the United States—natural history in the 1980s. Prog Clin Biol Res 367:111, 1991.
214. Kilbourn RG, Gross SS, Jubran A, et al: N^G-methyl-L-arginine inhibits tumor necrosis factor-induced hypotension: implications for the involvement of nitric oxide. Proc Natl Acad Sci USA 87:3629, 1990.
215. Wright CE, Rees DD, Moncada S: The protective and pathological roles of nitric oxide in endotoxin shock. Cardiovasc Res 26:48, 1992.
216. McCall CE, Grosso-Wilmoth LM, LaRue F, et al: Tolerance to endotoxin-induced expression of the interleukin-1 gene in blood neutrophils of humans with the sepsis syndrome. J Clin Invest 91:853, 1993.

Lymphocytes and Cell-Mediated Immunity

CHAPTER 14

Susan A. McCarthy

Many microbes, especially those that live within the host cell, cannot be efficiently eliminated by antibody-dependent opsonization and phagocytosis. The principal means of acquired resistance to these microbes resides in the action of specifically sensitized thymus-derived T lymphocytes (Table 14–1). Cell-mediated immunity refers to this system even though other immune cells (eg, antibody-producing B lymphocytes) and nonimmune cells (eg, phagocytes of all types) participate in all aspects of host defense. Indeed, specifically sensitized T lymphocytes cannot eliminate microbes by themselves but require many other specific and nonspecific cellular and humoral systems in performing their function.

THE IMMUNE APPARATUS

At birth, human beings are already immunologically competent to some degree and have undergone a complex developmental process. All lymphocytes are derived from a hematopoietic stem cell population, initially located in the embryonic yolk sac, that begins to proliferate early in embryonic life.[1,2] The resulting stem cells migrate to various centers of differentiation (Fig. 14–1), within which progenitor cells form erythrocytes, eosinophils, basophils, neutrophils, and lymphocytes depending on the local microenvironment (Fig. 14–2). Proliferation and differentiation of these progenitor cells are regulated by the action of cytokines (or growth factors),[3,4] which are the "hormones" of the immune system.

The lymphoid lineage develops as a dual system within two primary (or central) lymphoid tissues. The thymus governs the development of T lymphocytes, and of cellular immunity, in all vertebrates (Fig. 14–3). During ontogeny, committed T lymphocyte progenitors enter the thymus, where they undergo extensive proliferation and differentiation to produce mature T cells that emigrate to the peripheral lymphoid organs, that is, spleen, lymph nodes, and Peyer's patches.[5–7] The lymph node paracortical regions, between the cortical germinal centers and the medulla, are populated by T lymphocytes. Thymectomy early in the neonatal period in some mammals therefore results in failure of development of these regions of the lymph nodes. Humans populate their peripheral lymphoid depots long before birth, but the thymus maintains some immune functions.

The development of B lymphocytes and of humoral immunity is more difficult to assign to a particular tissue.[8–10] In birds, the bursa of Fabricius performs this function. In mammals, the fetal liver and the postnatal bone marrow appear to be the

TABLE 14–1. MICROBES CONTROLLED BY CELL-MEDIATED IMMUNITY

Bacteria	Fungi
Mycobacterium	*Candida* species
Listeria monocytogenes	*Histoplasma capsulatum*
Serratia marcescens	*Cryptococcus neoformans*
Nocardia species	Protozoa
Viruses	*Pneumocystis carinii*
Cytomegalovirus	*Toxoplasma gondii*
Epstein-Barr virus	*Cryptosporidium*
Herpes simplex	
Varicella-zoster	
Rotaviruses	

From Herrod HG: Cell-mediated immunity. In Patrick CC (ed): Infections in Immunocompromised Infants and Children. New York, Churchill Livingstone, 1992, p 70.

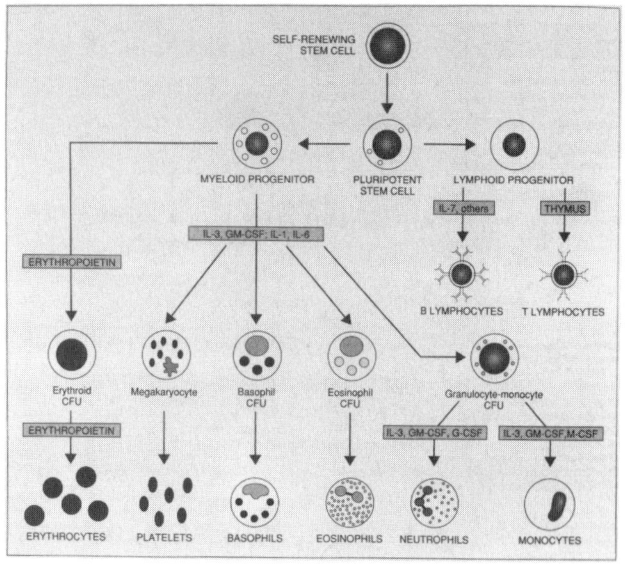

Figure 14–2. Maturation of blood cells: the hematopoietic "tree." The maturation of different lineages of blood cells is regulated by various cytokines. Note that the maturation of T and B lymphocytes is illustrated in summary form. CFU, colony-forming unit; IL, interleukin; GM-CSF, granulocyte-macrophage colony-stimulating factor. *(From Abbas AK, Lichtman AH, Pober JS: Cellular and Molecular Immunology. Philadelphia, Saunders, 1991, p 24.)*

major "bursal equivalents" in which pre-B lymphocytes undergo immunoglobulin gene rearrangement and become committed to immunoglobulin (antibody) synthesis before emigrating to the peripheral lymphoid organs. The lymph node germinal centers and the medullary cords contain B lymphocytes. In chickens, bursectomy therefore leads to the failure of development of these regions of the lymph nodes.

The combined function of the dual T and B lymphoid system is the basis of the body's specific immunologic response. Once the T and B cells have migrated to the peripheral lymphoid tissues, they are fully immunocompetent but are in a naive, unstimulated state prior to exposure to foreign antigen. As predicted by Burnet's clonal selection theory,[11] each cell (by virtue of its unique randomly produced antigen-specific receptor) can recognize and respond to a single conformationally related set of foreign antigens. Consequently, only a very small percentage of T and B lymphocytes in the body can recognize and respond to any particular foreign antigen. Upon antigen encounter, the lymphocytes specific for that antigen are activated and initiate a series of responses designed to eliminate the antigen (described in the following sections). The B cells appear to be relatively sessile, but their secreted antibodies can interact with foreign antigens at distant sites. In contrast, T cells are more peripatetic and must reside in, or migrate to, the site of antigen deposition to neutralize foreign antigens.

In addition to T and B cells, one other major population of lymphocytes has been identified. These are called natural killer (NK) cells because they are in an activated effector state prior to anti-

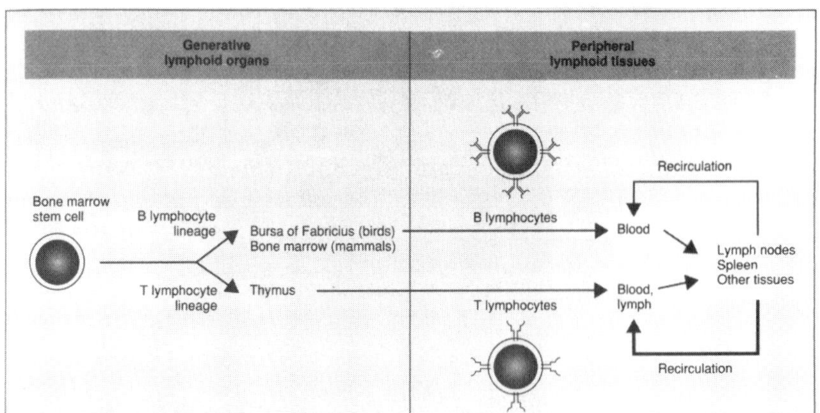

Figure 14–1. Maturation of lymphocytes. Development of mature lymphocytes prior to antigen exposure occurs in the generative lymphoid organs, and immune responses to foreign antigens occur in the peripheral lymphoid tissues. *(From Abbas AK, Lichtman AH, Pober JS: Cellular and Molecular Immunology. Philadelphia, Saunders, 1991, p 23.)*

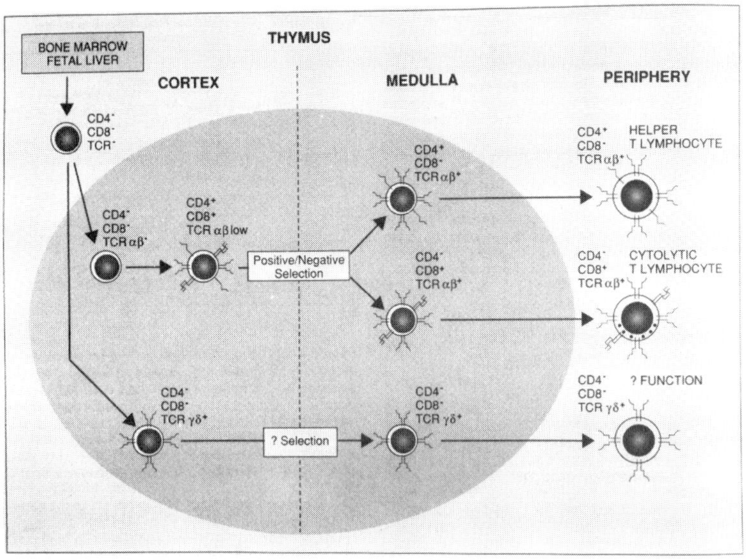

Figure 14–3. Ontogeny and lineage relationships of maturing T cells. TCR$\gamma\delta$- and TCR$\alpha\beta$-expressing cells are separate lineages that develop from a common precursor. In the $\alpha\beta$ lineage, the majority of thymocytes express both CD4 and CD8. TCR expression commences in this double-positive stage, beginning with low numbers of receptors on each cell and increasing as maturation proceeds. Single-positive, that is, CD4+ or CD8+, TCR$\alpha\beta$-expressing mature cells are selected from this population. Some $\gamma\beta$ cells express CD4 or CD8. *(From Abbas AK, Lichtman AH, Pober JS: Cellular and Molecular Immunology. Philadelphia, Saunders, 1991, p 178.)*

gen encounter and can kill antigen-bearing cells rapidly, without a requirement for further activation steps.[12,13] These cells may therefore play a critical role in the initial response to pathogens, before the antigen-specific T and B cell responses are fully activated.[14–16] NK cells also appear to have the capacity to kill certain tumor cells and may play an essential role in immune surveillance against cancer.[17,18] However, in contrast to T and B cells, NK cells exhibit little ability to discriminate among individual foreign antigens; each NK cell may only be able to recognize that a potential target cell is not a normal cell and is therefore a legitimate candidate for destruction. The nature of the antigen receptor on NK cells, which may or may not be identical on all NK cells, is still unclear.[19–21]

Table 14–2 lists some distinguishing characteristics of human T cells, NK cells, and macrophages, which are the major effector cells of cell-mediated immunity. Leukocytes (as well as all other cell types) express marker proteins on their surfaces, many of which identify functional subsets of cells. The common nomenclature for such marker proteins employs the designation CD for cluster of differentiation. These CD surface proteins, in many cases, actively contribute to the immune functions of the cells. For example, all T cells express the CD3 marker, which is physically associated with the T cell antigen receptor on the cell surface.[22,23] Each T cell may also express many different CD proteins that reflect the cell's lineage or state of activation.[24–27] The most useful markers for T cell analysis are the CD4 marker, which is expressed predominantly on helper T lymphocytes, and the CD8 marker, which is expressed predominantly on cytolytic T lymphocytes (CTLs). All differentiation markers can be used to experimentally delete (or enrich) cell subsets from mixed populations in order

TABLE 14–2. CHARACTERISTICS OF EFFECTOR CELLS FOR CELL-MEDIATED IMMUNITY

Cell Type	Surface Antigen	PBMC (%)
All T cells	CD3	75
T cell	$\alpha\beta$ TCR	75
T cell	$\gamma\delta$ TCR	1–2
Cytotoxic/suppressor T cell	CD3, DC8	25
All helper T cells	CD3, CD4	50
Memory helper T cell	CD3, CD4, CD45R−	25
Naive helper T cell	CD3, CD4, CD45R+	25
Natural killer cell	CD16, CD56	5–15
Monocyte/macrophage	CD14	5–10

From Markham RB: Cell-mediated immunity. In Gorbach SL, Bartlett JG, Blacklow NR (eds): Infectious Diseases. Philadelphia, Saunders, 1992, p 63.

to identify the cell types that perform well-defined immune functions (ie, proliferation or cell-mediated cytotoxicity in response to antigen).

INDUCTION OF IMMUNITY: T LYMPHOCYTE ACTIVATION

T lymphocytes are central to the cell-mediated immunity that is predominantly responsible for protection against intracellular pathogens. In order for T lymphocytes to be able to focus on antigens expressed in or on other cells, these lymphocytes must ignore soluble antigens in the serum or interstitial fluids; B lymphocytes and the antibodies they produce are responsible for clearing such soluble antigens. T cells focus on cell-bound antigens (and only on protein antigens) as a direct consequence of their special antigen-recognition requirements[28–30]; T cells can only recognize a foreign antigen when a peptide fragment of the antigen is physically associated with one of a family of normal cell surface proteins, the major histocompatibility complex (MHC) proteins, on another cell (Fig. 14–4). This requirement for recognition of an "MHC plus peptide" complex by T cells dictates that only those cell types able to create such a ligand can serve as stimulators or targets of T cell immunity. These cell types are different for different kinds of T cells, as outlined below.

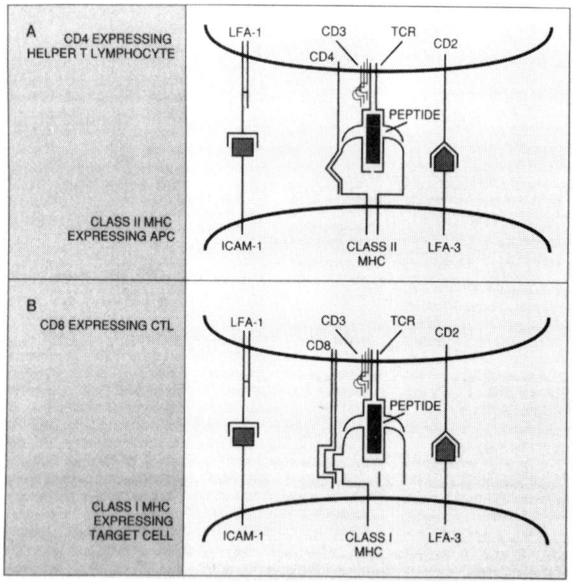

Figure 14–4. T lymphocyte surface molecules and their ligands involved in antigen recognition and T cell responses. Interactions between a CD4+ T cell and an antigen-presenting cell (APC) **(A)** or between a CD8+ cytolytic T lymphocyte (CTL) and a target cell **(B)** involve multiple T cell surface proteins that recognize different ligands on the APC or target cell. *(From Abbas AK, Lichtman AH, Pober JS: Cellular and Molecular Immunology. Philadelphia, Saunders, 1991, p 152.)*

Creation of the Immunogenic Ligand

Since foreign antigens must be associated with MHC proteins to stimulate T cell responses, the MHC proteins are central to cellular immunity. There are two subsets of MHC molecules, MHC class I and MHC class II (Figs. 14–4 and 14–5). These classes have genetic and physical homologies and are encoded by linked genetic loci. In humans, the main MHC class I proteins are called HLA-A, -B, and -C, while the main MHC class II proteins are called HLA-DR, -DP, and -DQ; the proteins are encoded by genes of the same names. MHC class I proteins are expressed by almost all nucleated cells, so that almost all nucleated cells can present antigenic peptides to the responsive CD8+ T cells. MHC class II proteins, by contrast, are normally expressed by cells of the immune system including macrophages, dendritic cells, and B lymphocytes, so that only such cells can present antigens to CD4 T cells. Other cell types can be induced to express MHC class II proteins, however, in response to inflammatory cytokines such as interferon gamma (IFN-γ) during an ongoing immune response and can therefore acquire stimulatory roles in immunity.

The MHC genes are codominantly expressed and are very polymorphic, with at least 50 alleles at each of the six loci. Each person is therefore heterozygous at all or most of the six loci and expresses six different MHC class I and six different MHC class II proteins. Each allelic MHC protein has different binding affinities for different antigen-derived peptides, determined by the amino acid sequences of the peptide-binding region of the MHC molecule (the *peptide cleft*) and the peptide itself (schematically represented in Figs. 14–4 and 14–5). The high variability of MHC proteins within an individual and among individuals in a population is very important because it virtually ensures that at least one peptide from a foreign pathogen will be able to associate with at least one MHC molecule in every normal immunocompetent individual to initiate a protective T cell immune response against the pathogen.

The T cells that coordinate and regulate cellular immunity are the CD4+ helper T cells. CD4+ T cells respond best to peptide antigens in association with MHC class II proteins. Macrophages and dendritic cells, which express MHC class II antigens, are the primary initial stimulators of these T cells.

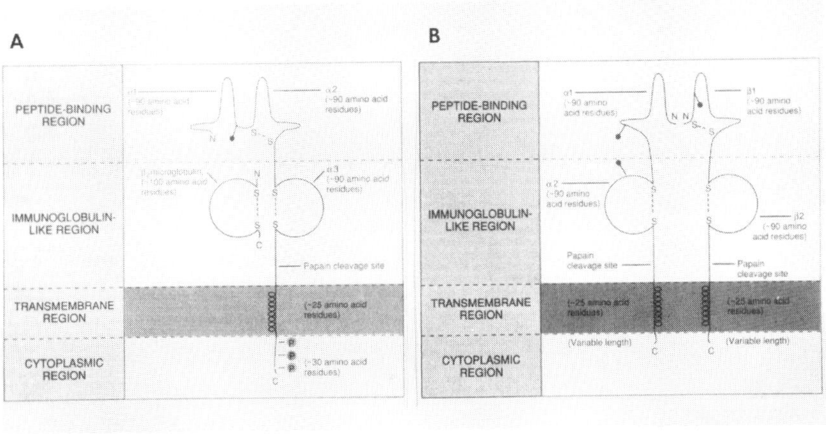

Figure 14–5. Schematic diagrams of a **(A)** class I MHC molecule and **(B)** class II MHC molecule. Different segments are not shown to scale. N and C refer to amino and carboxy termini of the polypeptide chains, respectively; S- - - -S, to intrachain disulfide bonds; —●, to carbohydrate; P to phosphorylation sites. *(From Abbas AK, Lichtman AH, Pober JS: Cellular and Molecular Immunology. Philadelphia, Saunders, 1991, pp 105, 108.)*

Macrophages and dendritic cells have therefore been called *professional* antigen-presenting cells (APCs), in recognition of this critical role. These APCs ingest soluble or particulate antigens (*exogenous antigen*) by pinocytosis, receptor-mediated endocytosis, or phagocytosis; it should be noted that even intracellular pathogens have portions of their life cycles that are extracellular and can provide exogenous antigens for the APCs. The APCs degrade the protein portions of the ingested antigen in acidic lysosomal-endosomal vesicles, then transport peptide fragments of the antigen (15 to 20 amino acids in length) to post-Golgi vesicles, where the antigenic peptides can be complexed with newly synthesized cellular MHC class II proteins and exported to the cell surface (Fig. 14–6). This cell surface [MHC class II plus foreign peptide] complex is then available to stimulate antigen-specific (CD4+) helper T cells.[31–34] Once stimulated, helper T cells can collaborate by means of cytokines with B cells, CD8+ CTLs, and phagocytic cells, to eliminate antigen, as described in the following section.

A parallel process allows any type of pathogen-infected cell to produce a [MHC plus foreign peptide] complex that can stimulate CD8+ CTLs, to render them competent to collaborate with helper T cells. In this case, the foreign antigen is actually produced from the pathogen within the infected cell (*endogenous antigen*), rather than being ingested from outside the cell, as described for professional APCs. Some of the newly synthesized foreign protein is partially degraded in the cytoplasm and actively transported into the endoplasmic reticulum, where antigenic peptides (8 to 10 amino acids in length) are complexed to newly synthesized cellular MHC class I proteins and then exported to the cell surface (see Fig. 14–6). This cell surface [MHC class I plus foreign peptide] complex identifies the cell as being infected and therefore an appropriate stimulus or target for a CTL.[35–38]

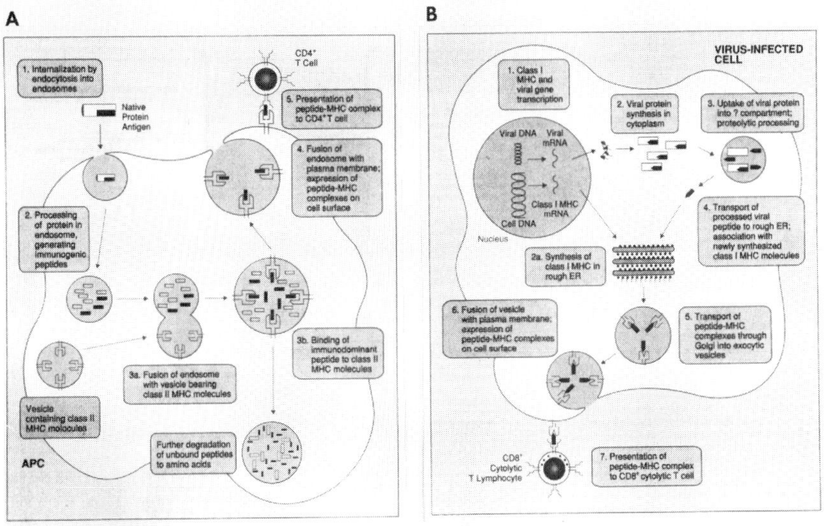

Figure 14–6. A. Pathway of class II MHC-restricted presentation of an extracellular protein antigen. **B.** Pathway of class I MHC-restricted presentation of an endogenously synthesized (eg, viral) antigen. *(From Abbas AK, Lichtman AH, Pober JS: Cellular and Molecular Immunology. Philadelphia, Saunders, 1991, pp 127, 133.)*

The close coordination of MHC class I and/or class II expression, antigen-presenting abilities, and T cell stimulating abilities among different types of cells in the body assures the proper functioning of cellular immunity. For the most part, only those professional APCs (usually phagocytes) that are designed to stimulate helper T cells can process and present exogenous foreign antigen and can express MHC class II molecules, to which CD4+ helper T cell recognition is directed. Conversely, all cells need to be able to stimulate CTLs, since all cells can potentially be infected by intracellular pathogens. Thus it is appropriate that all cells have the ability to process and present endogenous foreign antigens and express MHC class I molecules, to which CD8+ CTL recognition is directed. As in any biological system, these associations are not perfect; a minor subset of helper T cells is directed at [MHC class I plus peptide] complexes in some cases, and a subset of CTLs is directed at [MHC class II plus peptide] complexes.[39,40] The significance of these unusual T cell populations is not yet clear.

T Cell Recognition of Antigen

T cell recognition of [MHC plus peptide] complexes on other cells is mediated by antigen-specific T cell receptors (TCRs) on the T cells. The TCR contains two chains, usually the alpha and beta chains, and each contributes to binding of the receptor to the [MHC plus peptide] complex (see Fig. 14–4). Like the antigen-specific receptors on B lymphocytes (the surface immunoglobulins), TCRs on T cells are extremely variable among T cells, so that each T cell expresses a unique TCR and has a unique antigen fine specificity.[41,42] Even if two T cells are specific for the same protein of a particular pathogen, they are likely to recognize different peptides (epitopes) of that protein, in association with different MHC allelic proteins. This extremely high TCR variability is achieved by random genetic rearrangement of variable (V), diversity (D), and joining (J) region TCR gene segments, in analogy to the gene rearrangements that immunoglobulin genes undergo in B cells. This gene rearrangement and clonal TCR expression on T cells occur during their development in the thymus, prior to encounter with foreign antigen.[43–46] Thus each T cell is precommitted to its antigen specificity, and antigen only serves to activate those T cells with complementary TCR specific for the antigen.

The two variable, antigen-specific chains of the TCRs are noncovalently complexed on the T cell surface with a nonvariable signal-transducing protein complex, the CD3 complex. In addition, each mature T cell expresses either the CD4 or the CD8 protein on its surface (see Table 14–2). Almost all helper T cells express CD4, which has some binding affinity for nonpolymorphic portions of MHC class II proteins and so may contribute to T/APC avidity. Similarly, almost all CTLs express CD8, which has some binding affinity for MHC class I and so may contribute to T/stimulator avidity. When several/many copies of the TCR/CD3 complex, plus either CD4 or CD8, on a T cell are cross-linked by binding to several/many copies of the appropriate [MHC plus peptide] complex on an APC or infected cell, activation signals are initiated in the T cell.[47,48]

However, in most cases for most T cells, the intracellular signals initiated by TCR/CD3 (plus CD4 or CD8) cross-linking are not sufficient for full cellular activation. In fact, TCR/CD3 signals can instead ultimately lead to cellular inactivation, called *cellular anergy*, if they are not accompanied by additional signals induced in the T cell by other, antigen-nonspecific receptors.[49] This observation is consistent with the idea that each T cell needs two qualitatively different signals for activation[50,51]; signal 1 acts by way of the TCR and is antigen-specific, whereas signal 2 acts by way of one of the auxiliary receptors and is not antigen-specific but is produced when the T cell successfully interacts with an appropriate, competent partner cell such as an APC, a B cell, or another T cell (Fig. 14–7).

Different T cells appear to have different signal 2 requirements, reflecting their different normal activation scenarios.[52–55] Helper T cells typically receive signal 2 from professional APCs. Some helper T cells appear to require the soluble APC-derived cytokine IL-1, which binds to IL-1 receptors on the T cell.[56] Other helper T cells appear to require cross-linking of the CD28 protein on their cell surface by its ligand on the APC cell surface, a member of the B7 protein family.[57–59] In contrast to helper T cells, CTLs can interact with almost every cell type, many of which have no ability to activate signal 2 in the CTLs. Signal 2 for CTLs instead appears to be induced by cytokines such as IL-2 and IFN-γ produced and secreted by helper T cells.[60–63] Thus, whereas helper T cell activation requires T/APC collaboration, CTL activation requires T/T collaboration. Nevertheless, the principle that two signals are required for T cell activation is a unifying theme of modern immunology. As discussed below, this theme also applies to B cells, which require an antigen-specific signal 1 and an antigen-nonspecific signal 2 (induced by helper T cells) for activation.

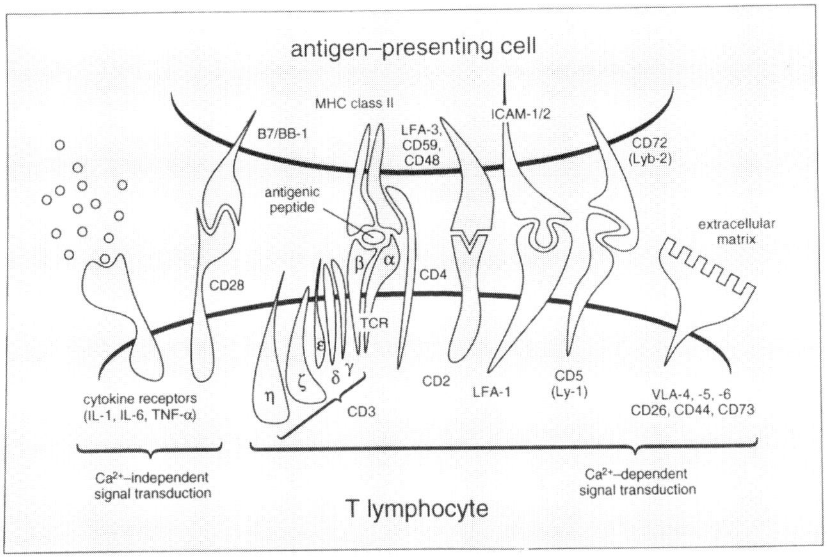

Figure 14–7. Both antigen-specific (signal 1) and antigen-nonspecific (signal 2) recognition events contribute to T cell activation. Signal 1 in the absence of signal 2 can result in T cell anergy. *(From Dendorfer U, Maslinski W, Remillard B, Strom TB: Transplant Sci 3:83, 1993.)*

Helper T Cell Activation and Function

Once a T cell has received a coordinated signal 1 plus signal 2 stimulus, intracellular second messengers such as calcium mobilization and protein kinase activation initiate a cascade that ultimately results in the transcription and translation of genes encoding the functional effector proteins of the cell.[64] The newly synthesized proteins are predominantly lytic molecules such as perforin and serine esterases in the case of CTLs (see below) and are predominantly cytokines in the case of helper T cells. The precise cytokines produced in each case define subcategories of helper T cells, the T_H1 and T_H2 cells. T_H1 cells produce IL-2 and IFN-γ, whereas T_H2 cells produce IL-4, IL-5, and IL-10; in addition, both helper T cell types produce cytokines such as IL-3 and GM-CSF. This difference in cytokine production leads to important differences in the functional activities of T_H1 and T_H2 cells; T_H1 cytokines activate primarily CTLs and macrophages and therefore promote cell-mediated immunity; whereas T_H2 cytokines activate primarily B cells and therefore promote humoral immunity.[65–69]

The cytokines produced and secreted by helper T cells (and by other cells) act by binding to cytokine receptors on the surface of CTLs, B cells, the helper T cells themselves, macrophages, and other cells.[70–72] Binding of cytokines to cytokine receptors induces activation signals in the cells that lead to new protein production, cellular proliferation, differentiation, and effector function. For example, IL-2 acts as a strong proliferative stimulus for all T cells as well as differentiative signal that may induce production of the "lytic machinery" in CTLs. IL-4 and IL-5 induce and regulate immunoglobulin production and synthesis in B cells. IFN-γ is a potent stimulus of phagocytic and microbicidal activity in macrophages. In addition, cytokines such as IL-1, TNF, and IL-6 promote inflammation by activating vascular endothelium and recruiting leukocytes to tissue sites of infection.

One particularly intriguing aspect of cytokine action is that some T_H1-derived cytokines have activities that downregulate T_H2 function, and some T_H2-derived cytokines have activities that downregulate T_H1 function.[73–75] The balance between T_H1-dependent cellular immunity and T_H2-dependent humoral immunity is therefore an active homeostatic process. This balance can be shifted in favor of cellular or humoral immunity by initial conditions of antigen exposure that preferentially induce T_H1 or T_H2, respectively.[76–80] The factors regulating the T_H1-T_H2 balance are not yet understood but are the subject of intense investigation.

Although each cytokine has a distinct receptor to which it binds, each cell type can express receptors for several distinct cytokines. As a result, one cytokine can act on several cell types (referred to as cytokine pleiotropy), and one cell type can respond to several cytokines. Furthermore, several distinct cytokines frequently have similar and/or overlapping activities (referred to as cytokine redundancy), which may reflect the fact that the receptors for these cytokines share intracellular signaling pathways.[81,82]

Cytokine receptors are usually expressed on lymphocytes only after they have been activated by antigen, which allows the cytokines secreted by antigen-specific helper T cells to preferentially act on neighboring antigen-specific T and B cells. In this way, cytokine-dependent triggering of immunity can be quite antigen-specific, even though the cytokines themselves are not antigen-specific, since neighboring unactivated lymphocytes will not respond to the cytokines. Nonlymphoid cells such as macrophages, dendritic cells, and many other cell types express some cytokine receptors constitutively, but they can also be induced to express other cytokine receptors after antigen encounter; the stimulus can be a bacterial cell wall product, infection by a virus, or phagocytosis of an antibody-coated microbe. These antigen-nonspecific cells play a critical role in the ultimate elimination of the antigen and thus serve as an essential complement to the antigen-specific lymphocytes (see below).

Excessive Stimulation in Cellular Immunity: Superantigens and Shock

Antigen-specific immune responses like those outlined above are of limited (but usually sufficient) intensity because each antigen stimulates only a tiny fraction of the T cells, due to the exquisite specificity of the cells' TCRs for antigen peptides complexed to MHC molecules on APCs. However, a second kind of immune response, involving many more T cells, is induced by *superantigens*.[83] Superantigens are molecules that stimulate entire sets of T cells expressing related TCRs (eg, all the cells expressing Vβ8 or Vβ11); they do so by cross-linking the variable regions of the TCR with MHC class II molecules on APCs or target cells (see Table 14–3). This TCR cross-linking mimics, in some respects, antigen-specific recognition to provide signal 1 to the T cells, but it may provide no signal 2 or an aberrant form of signal 2.

The most well-characterized superantigen is the *Staphylococcus* enterotoxin B (SEB), which is related to *S. aureus* and *S. pyogenes* enterotoxins.[84] However, there are many others including the *Mis* locus antigens in mice (encoded by endogenous retroviruses in the murine genomes)[85–89] and possibly HIV-encoded proteins.[90,91] The consequences of superantigen stimulation are manifold. Lymphocytes with susceptible TCR Vβ regions can be deleted by interaction with these microorganisms, thereby eliminating part of the lymphocyte pool (as in HIV infection perhaps). In mice, SEB and other superantigens lead to depletion of T cells after an initial expansion.[92–95] Cellular anergy can also be induced, with similar functional consequences.[96] Of greatest importance to clinicians, however, is the fact that superantigen stimulation may be responsible for shock in certain infections, because simultaneous stimulation of many lymphocytes by the microbe leads to the massive release of cytokines, especially TNF, that induce shock.[97–100] A similar mechanism may be responsible for the hypotension induced by agents like OKT3 (anti-CD3 monoclonal antibody), which massively stimulate CD3-bearing T cells.[101–103] Immunosuppressants that interrupt the cytokine amplification cascade can prevent shock.[104–106] The role of infection-induced shock syndromes in clinical staphylococcal infections has not yet been proved, but dissection of the cytokine pathways should reveal possible avenues for blockade or reversal of shock.

EXPRESSION OF IMMUNITY: MICROBIAL DESTRUCTION

Once helper T cells have completed their own activation program and have provided B cells, CTLs, NK cells, and macrophages with cytokines to activate or augment the effector mechanisms of those cells, the disposal of the foreign antigen by these effector cell types can proceed. Each of the four effector subsets can function individually, but they can also interact in some cases to provide additional

TABLE 14–3. SUPERANTIGEN RECOGNITION BY T CELLS

Enterotoxin	Mice	Humans
SEB	Vβ3, 7, 8.1–8.3, 17	Vβ3, 12, 14, 15, 17, 20
SEC 2	Vβ3, 8.2, 10, 17	Vβ12, 13.1, 13.2, 14, 15, 17, 20
SEE	Vβ11, 15, 17	Vβ5.1, 6.1–6.3, 8, 18
TSST	Vβ3, 15, 17	Vβ2

SE, staphylococcal enterotoxin; TSST, toxic shock syndrome toxin.
From Abbas AK, Lichtman AH, Pober JS: Cellular and Molecular Immunology. Philadelphia, Saunders, 1991, p 304.

means of antigen elimination. The primary role of B cells and the antibodies they produce will be discussed elsewhere in this book, although antibody-dependent facilitation of NK and macrophage activities will be briefly addressed below. Antibody-mediated immunity acts to augment complement in the opsonization of bacteria and fungi for phagocytic killing. Antibodies also play a primary role, without phagocytes, in the elimination of encapsulated bacteria, bacterial toxins, and some viruses. Cell-mediated (CTL, NK, and macrophage) immunity is most important in responses to the pathogens listed in Table 14–1.

Lymphocyte-Mediated Antigen Elimination

The major antigen-specific effector T cell is the CTL, which eliminates intracellular pathogens by killing the infected cells that harbor it.[107–109] This efferent phase of CTL activity has both an immunologically specific antigen recognition stage and an immunologically nonspecific lytic stage (Fig. 14–8). A CTL recognizes infected target cells that express the antigenic foreign peptide for which the CTL is specific, in association with an MHC molecule. The antigenic peptide is derived from the pathogen (usually but not necessarily a virus), physically complexes with the MHC molecule (usually but not necessarily an MHC class I molecule) inside the infected cell, and is then exported to the cell surface along with the MHC molecule. Recognition of this [MHC plus peptide] complex by the antigen-specific TCR of the CTL, in conjunction with auxiliary nonspecific CTL/target adhesion, initiates the lytic stage in the CTL.

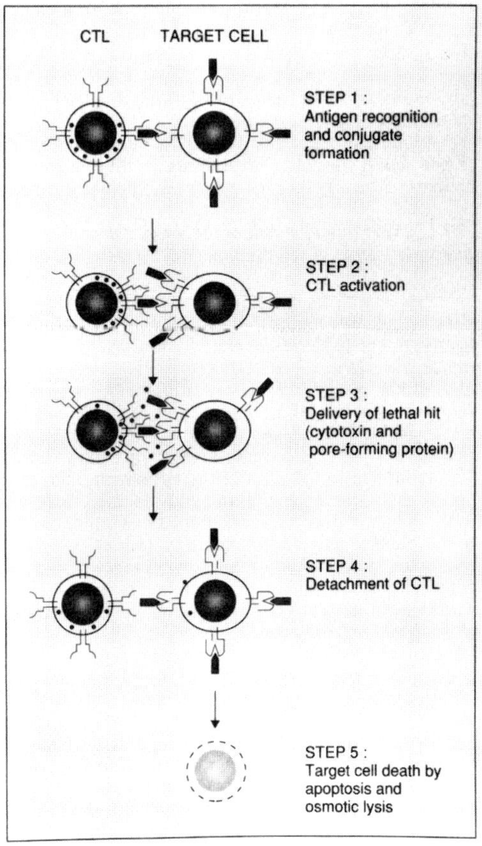

Figure 14–8. Steps in CTL-mediated lysis of target cells. Note that conjugate formation (step 1) also requires interactions between CTL accessory molecules (LFA-1, CD8) on the CTLs and their specific ligands on the target cell. *(From Abbas AK, Lichtman AH, Pober JS: Cellular and Molecular Immunology. Philadelphia, Saunders, 1991, p 255.)*

Activated CTLs are rich in intracellular cytoplasmic granules that contain proteins thought to be responsible for the ultimate lysis of the target cell.[110,111] Upon target cell recognition, the CTL granules are mobilized to the face of the CTL bound to the target cell. Some of the granules and their contents are then released into the narrow space between the CTLs and the target by a process called granule exocytosis, which resembles endocytosis in reverse. The granule proteins include a pore-forming protein related to the C9 component of the complement membrane attack complex. This protein, known as cytolysin or perforin, can insert into the target cell membrane, create a pore, and lead to osmotic lysis of the target cell.[112,113] The granules also contain a number of serine proteases whose function is unclear; these proteases may activate cytolysin, alter some target cell surface structure, and/or enter the target cell after it is perforated by the cytolysin.[114,115] This latter proposed action of the serine proteases may be central to another facet of target cell death. In some, but not all, instances of target lysis by CTLs, the target cell undergoes programmed cell death, or apoptosis.[116–119] Apoptotic cell death involves many intracellular reactions, most notably the extensive fragmentation of the cell's DNA by the cell's own nucleases. Serine proteases have been reported to activate apoptosis in membrane-permeabilized cells,[120] and these proteases may therefore function as mediators of target cell death via activation of nucleases. After delivery of its "lethal hit" to the target cell, the CTL disengages and can seek out and kill another infected target cell. A major continuing enigma is how the CTL itself is spared during the lytic event.

Although specifically sensitized CTLs can kill cells infected with intracellular pathogens, it is controversial whether this is a major method of control of infection. In order to halt virus replication and spread, lysis of target cells before the assembly of infectious virus within them would be necessary.

Thus assembly and export of [MHC plus viral peptide] complexes would have to occur early after infection. With some viruses this does happen. Ectromelia (mousepox) infected fibroblasts become susceptible to destruction by immune CTLs about 3 hours after infection. Similarly, vaccinia virus may not reproduce in the early hours after infection, and CTLs may therefore be able to kill virus-infected cells before more virus is produced. However, many viruses may not conform to this requirement. In those cases, the CTLs may kill the viral "factory," but they cannot kill pre-made viruses. Nevertheless, it would seem that repeated rounds of lysis of most or all of the viral factories would inevitably lead to a decline in viral loads in the body. The recent development of experimental mouse strains that are deficient in CD8+ CTLs[121,122] should allow a critical analysis of the relative importance of these CTLs in clearing viral infections in vivo.

NK cells can also contribute to elimination of infected cells. Although the precise nature of their target recognition specificity is not known, the nature of their effector mechanisms is well characterized.[123–126] NK cells can directly lyse target cells by a granule-dependent process that is very similar if not identical to that of CTLs. Like CTLs, the NK cells are protected from the lethal hit and can recycle to kill additional targets. Target cell killing by NK cells can be augmented in the presence of certain lymphokines produced by helper T cells and CTLs (particularly IFN-γ); the cytokines may render the targets more susceptible, or the NK cells more potent, or both. Because target cell recognition by NK cells has a limited specificity repertoire, and most or all NK cells might recognize any given infected target cell, the NK cell population could be a major quantitative component of direct target cell lysis in vivo, even though the NK subset is a quantitatively minor lymphocyte population. NK cells express Fc receptors for antibody and can therefore also bind to, and be triggered to lyse, antibody-coated cells in a process called antibody-dependent cellular cytotoxicity (ADCC). The relative importance of this mechanism of antigen elimination, which represents the interaction of humoral/specific and cellular/nonspecific immunity, is not yet known.

Macrophage-Mediated Antigen Elimination

Macrophages are critical participants in cell-mediated immunity to, and elimination of, certain microbes. Helper T cells produce and secrete cytokines that attract macrophages to the site of infection and then inhibit their escape, thereby increasing the number of effector cells available for antigen destruction.[127] Helper T cells also produce and secrete cytokines that activate the macrophages; IFN-γ is particularly effective in this regard.[128,129] Macrophages found at the site of delayed hypersensitivity reactions appear to be in an activated state. In the activated state, macrophage cytoplasm has the appearance of great activity both morphologically and enzymatically.[130] Many enzymes, including the digestive enzymes of the lysosomes, are elevated. Phagocytosis, pinocytosis, Fc receptor-mediated uptake of antibody-coated particles, bacteriostatic activity, and tumoricidal activity may all be increased. However, macrophages activated by different means may have different functional capacities. For example, certain populations of activated macrophages are capable of inhibiting tumor cells but lack the capacity to kill intracellular pathogens. For resistance to infection, the most important property of activated macrophages is their greatly increased capacity to inhibit or kill intracellular pathogens. The biochemical mechanisms used by macrophages to destroy pathogens include the halide-myeloperoxidase-H_2O_2 system and the nitric oxide ($\cdot N{=}O$) system.[131–135] Both of these systems produce reactive intermediates that interfere with the metabolism of the pathogen.

Excessive Effector Function in Cellular Immunity: Granulomatous Inflammations

In the same way that excessive initial stimulation of the immune system can lead to dysfunction (see discussion of superantigens, above), excessive or persistent immune effector function can lead to dysfunction. Granulomatous inflammations are chronic, predominantly mononuclear, host reactions to persisting, poorly degradable tissue irritants. The type, duration, and resolution of granulomatous inflammations depend on the physical characteristics, chemical reactivity, and biological activity of the irritant as well as the ensuing host response. Hypersensitivity granulomas, that is, those seen most commonly in granulomatous infections, are evoked by slowly released antigens, which induce cellular immunity.[136,137] Early in the process, microbial products or tissue- and plasma-derived chemical mediators may participate in cell recruitment and mobilization; however, in the subsequent phases, locally secreted cytokines mobilize, attract, and activate the various cellular components (neutrophils, macrophages, fibroblasts, T and B lymphocytes, plasma, cells, eosinophils, and basophils). The ultimate result of these cell-activation cascades is the containment, removal, and eventual elimination of antigens, antigen-antibody complexes, and replicating pathogens from the tissues. Such granulomatous inflammations thus represent a defense mechanism for aggregating cytokine-activated macrophages at the site of invasion by organisms not normally destroyed by opsonization and phagocytosis. Such organisms, if unchecked, tend to cause insidiously developing chronic disease, with parasitism of the mononuclear phagocytic system and miliary spread.

Although the granulomatous reaction is potentially a beneficial response against noxious irritants, the prolonged inflammation and inadvertent release of lysosomal enzymes can cause considerable tissue destruction, liquification, and severe organ derangement. Fibrotic tissue repair may often aggravate the disease to the point of becoming the major cause of pathological findings, as seen in schistosomiasis and the pneumonitides. Thus, whereas the granulomatous response is highly protective against replicating pathogens, it may be more detrimental than beneficial when it is formed in response to inanimate or noninvasive agents such as schistosome eggs. In any case, the key element in any granulomatous response seems to be the extent and duration of macrophage activation. Minimal or moderate activation will result in a quiescent lesion with minor or negligible tissue destruction and reparative fibrosis. Conversely, strong and/or prolonged macrophage activation, whether induced by inanimate silica or live tubercle bacilli, will result in lysosomal enzyme-mediated tissue damage and detrimental reparative fibrosis.

Mucosal Immunity

The mucosal surfaces frequently represent the first site of antigen encounter and elimination by the immune system.[138,139] Although cell-mediated immunity on secretory surfaces has been investigated for several years, the details of this aspect of the immune system are not well characterized. Immunity at secretory sites appears to operate at least partially independently of systemic cell-mediated immunity. The first convincing evidence that local cell-mediated immunity could be correlated with protection in vivo came from studies demonstrating that protection against tuberculosis in immunized mice correlated best with lung cell immunity rather than peritoneal cellular immunity.[140] Later, cell-mediated immunity to dinitrophenylated human IgG was identified in respiratory tract lymphocytes.[141] Such local cellular immunity appears to be mediated by T cells, and immunization to enhance the effects of local cellular immunity can be achieved with various aerosol immunizing agents. However, local cellular immunity may be relatively short-lived compared with antibody responses and may wane after several weeks.

All the known subsets of T lymphocytes are present in Peyer's patches and other gut-associated lymphoid tissue (GALT), and lymphocytes from the GALT have been shown to generate appropriate immune responses in vitro.[142,143] One candidate for the cells performing these functions is a subset of T cells expressing $\gamma\delta$ T cell receptors rather than $\alpha\beta$ T cell receptors.[144–148] These $\gamma\delta$ T cells constitute a rare T cell subset in most tissues but are relatively abundant in surface tissues such as the intraepithelial spaces of the gut,[149–152] the skin,[153] and the female reproductive tract.[154] Recent reports have implicated $\gamma\delta$ T cells as the dominant subset activated in cellular immune responses to specific mycobacterial antigens[155–157] and *heat shock proteins*, which are neoantigens induced in many types of infected or stressed cells.[158,159] Research on $\gamma\delta$ T cells has been facilitated by advances in their in vitro propagation and cloning,[160–165] and their role in antimicrobial immunity should become clearer in the not-too-distant future. The topic of mucosal immunity is covered more extensively in Chapter 15.

EVALUATION OF DEFICIENCIES IN CELL-MEDIATED IMMUNITY

Surgeons are only occasionally confronted with a primary problem of immunodeficiency, that is, patients with recurrent infections or with surgical complications of infections (eg, abscesses in chronic granulomatous disease). More frequently, surgeons encounter patients rendered immunodeficient by trauma, cancer, infection, age, or malnutrition. Prognosis is strongly associated with immunocompetence. Immune deficiency may or may not contribute directly to the poor prognosis, however, and the hope that simple immunostimulation would improve the prognosis is likely to be overly optimistic. Nevertheless, it is imperative that individuals susceptible to recurrent viral, protozoal, or intracellular bacterial infections be studied for defects in cell-mediated immunity.

Deficient cell-mediated immunity has been identified in a number of clinical conditions. Table 14–4 lists the major primary T cell deficiencies, and Table 14–5 lists some of the diseases that have been characterized as secondary T cell deficiency states, using one or more of the clinical tests described below.

INITIAL TESTS. Screening tests should include total peripheral blood lymphocyte counts as well as evaluation of T and B cell subset ratios and lymphocyte morphology and function. An x-ray study of the chest (PA and lateral) should show a thymic shadow; its absence suggests thymic hypoplasia. A

TABLE 14–4. PRIMARY T CELL IMMUNODEFICIENCIES

Disease	Functional Deficiencies	Presumed Mechanism of Defect
DiGeorge's syndrome	Decreased T cells; normal B cells; normal or decreased serum Ig	Anomalous development of third and fourth branchial pouches, leading to thymic hypoplasia
SCID		
X-linked	Markedly decreased T cells; normal or increased B cells; reduced serum Ig	Defective T cell maturation
Autosomal recessive	Decreased T and B cells; reduced serum Ig	Defective maturation of T and B cells
ADA deficiency	Progressive decrease in T and B cells (mostly T); reduced serum Ig	ADA deficiency leading to accumulation of toxic metabolites
PNP deficiency	Decreased T cells; normal B cells and serum Ig	PNP deficiency leading to accumulation of toxic metabolites in T cells
Class II MHC deficiency	Normal lymphocyte numbers; normal or decreased serum Ig; deficient cell-mediated immunity	Defective transcription of class II MHC genes
Reticular dysgenesis	Markedly decreased T and B cells and other blood cells; reduced serum Ig	Defective maturation of hematopoietic stem cells
Wiskott-Aldrich syndrome	Progressive decrease in T cells; normal B cells; decreased IgM; deficient antibody response to polysaccharide antigens	Defective glycosylation of membrane proteins; defective maturation of hematopoietic stem cells
Ataxia-telangiectasia	Decreased T cells; normal B cells; variable reduction in IgA, IgE, and IgG subclasses	?Defect in DNA repair

SCID, severe combined immunodeficiency disease; ADA, adenosine deaminase; PNP, purine nucleoside phosphorylase; Ig, immunoglobulin; MHC, major histocompatibility complex.
From Abbas AK, Lichtman AH, Pober JS: Cellular and Molecular Immunology. Philadelphia, Saunders, 1991, p 381.

right-sided aortic arch is also often seen in congenital thymic hypoplasia.

RECALL SKIN TESTS. Delayed skin tests can evaluate in vivo cellular immunity to microbial or vaccine agents. Antigens derived from mumps, trichophyton, purified protein derivative (PPD), *Candida albicans* (dermatophyton), tetanus toxoid, and streptokinase-streptodornase (SK:SD) are injected intradermally and the induration measured at 24 and 48 hours. Erythema without induration is not a good indication of reactivity. All adults and children over the age of 10 should exhibit a positive reaction to one or more antigens, but even normal infants

TABLE 14–5. ACQUIRED T CELL IMMUNODEFICIENCIES

Etiology	Comment
Malnutrition	Greatest effect on T cells; typically antibody response intact; susceptible of common pathogens (eg, measles, tuberculosis)
Immunosuppressive therapy	
Corticosteroids	Transient decrease in T cells
Radiation therapy	May produce a prolonged decrease in T cells, T cell function
Cyclosporine	Primarily inhibits synthesis of cytokines (eg, IL-2)
Cytotoxic drugs	Variable effect; usually affect both T and B cells
Infection	
HIV	Primarily infects CD4+ cells
Measles	Suppresses PHA response; DTH suppressed
Tuberculosis	Decreases T cell function
Others	
Malignancy	Abnormalities may be due to tumor-induced factors, malnutrition, or chemotherapy
Aging	Alterations in T cell function

From Herrod HG: Cell-mediated immunity. In Patrick CC (ed): Infections in Immunocompromised Infants and Children. New York, Churchill Livingstone, 1992, p 69.

will not respond in these tests. The DNCB skin sensitization test also has been found useful in screening programs.

LYMPH NODE BIOPSY. The morphologic appearance of a lymph node specimen obtained by biopsy also provides diagnostic information about the cellular immune system. However, a lymph node biopsy is unnecessary and contraindicated if there is unequivocal laboratory evidence of cellular immunodeficiency by the in vitro assays outlined below.

ENZYME ASSAYS FOR ADENOSINE DEAMINASE AND NUCLEOSIDE PHOSPHORYLASE. Patients with combined immunodeficiency defined by clinical parameters and the in vivo and in vitro assays outlined in this section should be analyzed for adenosine deaminase (ADA) and nucleoside phosphorylase in lysed erythrocytes, since absence of either of these enzymes identifies genetic variants of autosomal recessive combined immunodeficiency. Patients with deficiencies in ADA may be candidates for gene therapy protocols designed to restore functional ADA gene expression in circulating T cells.

T CELL ENUMERATION AND SUBSET ANALYSIS. The use of fluorescent-tagged monoclonal antibodies and fluorescence-activated flow cytometry have revolutionized leukocyte quantitation in the last 10 years. Monoclonal antibodies specific for all the major cell lineages—T cells (including antibodies that distinguish between helper T cells and CTLs), B cells, NK cells, macrophages, and neutrophils—are readily available for clinical laboratory screenings. Several different fluorescent labels (with different emission spectra) are available, which permits simultaneous quantitation of multiple markers on each cell in a population. For T cell analysis, mononuclear cell preparations from peripheral blood are incubated with one or more labeled antibodies at 4C, washed, and resuspended for analysis on the flow cytometer. In normal individuals, 55 to 75 percent of peripheral blood lymphocytes (PBLs) are T cells. Patients with T cell defects (eg, severe combined immunodeficiency) have few (less than 15 percent) T cells, a peripheral lymphopenia, and a very low absolute number of T cells. Patients with partial T cell defects (eg, Wiskott-Aldrich syndrome, Digeorge's syndrome) have moderately depressed T cell levels (15 to 40 percent). Patients with AIDS have selective defects of CD4+ helper T cells. Patients with secondary cellular immunodeficiency (eg, malnutrition, some viral diseases) have depression of T cell levels in proportion to the severity of their functional cellular immune defect.

LYMPHOCYTE PROLIFERATION ASSAYS. Cellular immunity can be evaluated by determining the ability of the patient's lymphocytes to proliferate in vitro in response to foreign recall antigens, foreign histocompatibility antigens on allogeneic cells (cells from another person), or mitogens such as phytohemagglutinin, pokeweed, or antibodies to the TCR/CD3 complex. Mitogens activate T cells nonspecifically by cross-linking their cell surface receptors to mimic antigen recognition. Lymphocyte responses can be assayed most easily and reproducibly by measuring incorporation of radioactive thymidine (utilized in DNA synthesis) into dividing cells. The radioactive counts incorporated in the stimulated cells and the ratio of those counts to the counts in unstimulated control cells—the stimulation index—are recorded.

Serum factors may influence the proliferative lymphocyte response to antigens or mitogens. Specific and nonspecific inhibitors have been reported. Specific inhibitors are usually antibodies to the antigen. Nonspecific inhibitors may be antibodies directed against lymphocytes or poorly characterized nonimmunoglobulin substances. These are seen in uremia, certain malignancies, leprosy, hepatitis, and ataxia-telangiectasia. Lymphocyte proliferation assays are routinely performed in the presence of a standardized pooled serum source, rather than in the patient's serum, to avoid possible inhibition by substances in the patient's serum.

CYTOKINE AND CYTOKINE-RECEPTOR ANALYSIS. The production of cytokines and the expression of cell surface receptors for cytokines can be assayed in vitro. Currently, these tests are of primarily research value but may acquire widespread clinical utility in the not-too-distant future.

REFERENCES

1. Abramson S, Miller RG, Phillips RA: The identification in the adult bone marrow of pluripotent and restricted stem cells of the myeloid and the lymphoid systems. J Exp Med 145:1587, 1979.
2. Spangrude GJ, Heimfeld S, Weissman IL: Purification and characterization of mouse hematopoietic stem cells. Science 241:58, 1988.
3. Heyworth C, Ponting ILO, Dexter TM: The response of haemopoietic cells to growth factors: developmental implications of synergistic interactions. J Cell Sci 91:239, 1988.
4. Testa NG, Dexter TM: Haemopoietic growth factors: their role in cell development and their clinical use. Cytotechnology 2:259, 1989.
5. Nikolic-Zugic J: Phenotypic and functional stages in

the intrathymic development of $\alpha\beta$-T cells. Immunol Today 12:65, 1991.
6. Boyd RL, Hugo P: Towards an integrated view of thymopoiesis. Immunol Today 12:71, 1991.
7. Finkel TR, Kubo RT, Cambier JC: T-cell development and transmembrane signaling: changing biological responses through an unchanging receptor. Immunol Today 12:79, 1991.
8. Hardy RR, Hayakawa K, Parks DR, et al: Murine B cell differentiation lineages. J Exp Med 159:1169, 1984.
9. Hardy RR, Carmack CE, Shinton SA, et al: Resolution and characterization of pro-B and pre-pro-B cell stages in normal mouse bone marrow. J Exp Med 173:1213, 1991.
10. Hardy RR, Hayakawa K: A developmental switch in B lymphopoiesis. Proc Natl Acad Sci USA 88:11550, 1992.
11. Burnet FM: The Clonal Selection Theory of Acquired Immunity. Cambridge, Cambridge University Press, 1959.
12. Roder JC, Karre K, Kiessling R: Natural killer cells. Prog Allergy 28:66, 1981.
13. Reynolds SC, Timonen T, Herberman RB: Natural killer (NK) cell activity in the rat. I. Isolation and characterization of the effector cells. J Immunol 127:282, 1981.
14. Stitz L, Althage A, Hengartner H, Zinkernagel R: Natural killer cells vs cytotoxic T cells in the peripheral blood of virus-infected mice. J Immunol 134:598, 1985.
15. Kohl S, Loo LS, Schmalstieg FS, Anderson DC: The genetic deficiency of leukocyte surface glycoprotein Mac-1, LFA-1, p150/95 in humans is associated with defective antibody-dependent cellular cytotoxicity in vitro and defective protection against herpes simplex virus infections in vivo. J Immunol 137:1688, 1986.
16. Welsh RM: Regulation of virus infections by natural killer cells. A review. Nat Immun Cell Growth Regul 5:169, 1986.
17. Hanna N, Fidler IJ: Role of natural killer cells in the destruction of circulating tumor emboli. J Natl Cancer Inst 65:801, 1980.
18. Masuyama K, Ochiani H, Ishizawa S, et al: Relations of H-2 expression on murine RCT (+) sarcoma cells to lung colonization and sensitivity to NK cells. J Cancer Res Clin Oncol 114:487, 1988.
19. Biron CA, van den Elsen P, Tutt MM, et al: Murine natural killer cells stimulated in vivo do not express the T cell receptor α, β, γ, T3δ, or T3ε genes. J Immunol 139:1704, 1987.
20. Ljunggren H-G, Karre K: In search of the "missing self": MHC molecules and NK cell recognition. Immunol Today 11:237, 1990.
21. Storkus WJ, Dawson JR: Target structures involved in natural killing: characteristics, distribution, and candidate molecules. CRC Crit Rev Immunol 10:393, 1991.
22. Davis MM, Bjorkman PJ: T-cell antigen receptor genes and T-cell recognition. Nature 334:395, 1988.
23. Moss PAH, Rosenberg WMC, Bell JI: The human T cell receptor in health and disease. Annu Rev Immunol 10:71, 1992.
24. Doyle C, Strominger JL: Interaction between CD4 and class II MHC molecules mediates cell adhesion. Nature 330:256, 1987.
25. Norment AN, Salter RD, Parham P, et al: Cell-cell adhesion mediated by CD8 and MHC class I molecules. Nature 336:79, 1988.
26. Rudd CE, Trevillyan JM, Dasgupta JD, et al: The CD4 receptor is complexed in detergent lysates to a protein-tyrosine kinase (pp58) from human T lymphocytes. Proc Natl Acad Sci USA 85:5190, 1988.
27. Veillette A, Bookman MA, Horak EM, Bolen JB: The CD4 and CD8 T cell surface antigens are associated with the internal membrane tyrosine-protein kinase $p56^{lck}$. Cell 55:301, 1988.
28. Zinkernagel RM, Doherty PC: Restriction of in vitro T cell-mediated cytotoxicity in lymphocytic choriomeningitis within a syngeneic or semi-allogeneic system. Nature 248:701, 1974.
29. Zinkernagel RM, Doherty PC: MHC-restricted cytotoxic T cells: studies on the biological role of polymorphic major transplantation antigens determining T-cell restriction-specificity, function, and responsiveness. Adv Immunol 27:52, 1979.
30. Swain SL: T cell subsets and the recognition of MHC class. Immunol Rev 71:129, 1983.
31. Kaufman JF, Auffray C, Korman AJ, et al: The class II molecules of the human and murine major histocompatibility complex. Cell 36:1, 1984.
32. Sette A, Buus S, Colon S, et al: The relation between major histocompatibility complex (MHC) restriction and the capacity of Ia to bind immunogenic peptides. Science 235:1353, 1987.
33. Neefjes JJ, Stollorz V, Peters PJ, et al: The biosynthetic pathway of MHC class II but not class I molecules intersects the endocytic route. Cell 61:171, 1990.
34. Germain RN, Hendrix LR: MHC class II structure, occupancy and surface expression determined by post-endoplasmic reticulum antigen binding. Nature 353:134, 1991.
35. Bjorkman PJ, Saper MA, Samraoui B, et al: Structure of the human class I histocompatibility antigen, HLA-A2. Nature 329:506, 1987.
36. Hosken NA, Bevan MJ: Defective presentation of endogenous antigen by a cell line expressing class I molecules. Science 248:367, 1990.
37. Otten GR, Bikoff E, Ribaudo R, Germain RN: Peptide and β2-MHC class I conformation and expression. J Immunol 148:3723, 1992.
38. Matsumura M, Fremont DH, Peterson PA, Wilson IA: Emerging principles for the recognition of peptide antigens by MHC class I molecules. Science 257:927, 1992.
39. Golding H, Mizuochi T, McCarthy SA, et al: Relationship among function, phenotype, and specificity in primary allospecific T cell populations: identifi-

cation of phenotypically identical but functionally distinct primary T cell subsets that differ in their recognition of MHC class I and class II allodeterminants. J Immunol 138:10, 1987.
40. Sprent J, Webb SL: Function and specificity of T cell subsets in the mouse. Adv Immunol 41:39, 1987.
41. Townsend ARM, Rothbard J, Gotch FM, et al: The epitopes of influenza nucleoprotein recognized by cytotoxic T lymphocytes can be defined by short synthetic peptides. Cell 44:959, 1986.
42. Bjorkman PJ, Saper MA, Samraoui B, et al: The foreign antigen binding site and the T cell recognition regions of class I histocompatibility antigens. Nature 329:512, 1987.
43. Havran WL, Poenie M, Kimura J, et al: Expression and function of the CD3-antigen receptor on murine $CD4^{+}8^{+}$ thymocytes. Nature 330:170, 1987.
44. Finkel TH, McDuffie M, Kappler JW, et al: Both immature and mature T cell mobilize Ca^{2+} in response to antigen receptor cross-linking. Nature 330:179, 1987.
45. Havran WL, Allison JP: Developmentally ordered appearance of thymocytes expressing different T-cell antigen receptors. Nature 335:443, 1988.
46. Strominger JL: Developmental biology of T cell receptors. Science 244:943, 1989.
47. Imboden JB, Stobo JD: Transmembrane signalling by the T cell antigen receptor. J Exp Med 161:446, 1985.
48. Desai DM, Newton ME, Kadlecek T, Weiss A: Stimulation of the phosphatidyl-inositol pathway can induce T-cell activation. Nature 348:66, 1990.
49. Bretscher P, Cohn M: A theory of self-nonself discrimination. Science 169:1042, 1970.
50. Jenkins MK, Pardoll M, Mizugushi J, et al: T cell unresponsiveness in vivo and in vitro: fine specificity of induction and molecular characterization of the unresponsive state. Immunol Rev 95:113, 1987.
51. Miller JFAP, Morahan G: Peripheral T cell tolerance. Annu Rev Immunol 10:51, 1992.
52. Magilavy DB, Fitch FW, Gajewski TF: Murine hepatic accessory cells support the proliferation of TH1 but not TH2 helper T lymphocyte clones. J Exp Med 170:985, 1989.
53. Chang T-L, Shea CM, Urioste S, et al: Heterogeneity of helper/inducer T lymphocytes. III. Responses of IL-2- and IL-4-producing (TH1 and TH2) clones to antigens presented by different accessory cells. J Immunol 145:2803, 1990.
54. Gajewski TF, Pinnas M, Wong T, Fitch FW: Murine TH1 and TH2 clones proliferate optimally in response to distinct antigen presenting cell populations. J Immunol 146:1750, 1991.
55. Croft M, Duncan DD, Swain SL: Response of naive antigen-specific $CD4^{+}$ T cells in vitro: characteristics and antigen-presenting cell requirements. J Exp Med 176:1431, 1992.
56. Stein PH, Singer A: Similar co-stimulation requirements of $CD4^{+}$ and $CD8^{+}$ primary T helper cells: role of IL-1 and IL-6 in inducing IL-2 secretion and subsequent proliferation. Int Immunol 4:327, 1992.
57. Hathcock KS, Laszlo G, Dickler HB, et al: Identification of an alternative CTLA-4 ligand costimulatory for T cell activation. Science 262:905, 1993.
58. Freeman GJ, Vorriello F, Hodes RJ, et al: Uncovering of functional alternative CTLA-4 counter-receptor in B7-deficient mice. Science 262:907, 1993.
59. Freeman GJ, Gribben JG, Boussiotis VA, et al: Cloning of B7-2: a CTLA-4 counter-receptor that costimulates human T cell proliferation. Science 262:909, 1993.
60. Keene J, Forman J: Helper activity is required for the in vivo generation of cytotoxic T lymphocytes. J Exp Med 155:768, 1982.
61. Wagner H, Hardt C, Rouse BT, et al: Dissection of the proliferative and differentiative signals controlling murine cytotoxic T lymphocyte responses. J Exp Med 155:1876, 1982.
62. Mizuochi T, Golding H, Rosenberg AS, et al: Both $L3T4^{+}$ and $Lyt2^{+}$ helper T cells initiate cytotoxic T lymphocyte responses against allogeneic major histocompatibility antigens but not against trinitrophenol modified self. J Exp Med 162:427, 1985.
63. Mizuochi T, Ono S, Malek TR, Singer A: Characterization of two distinct primary T cell populations that secrete interleukin-2 upon recognition of class I or class II major histocompatibility antigens. J Exp Med 163:603, 1986.
64. Crabtree GR: Contingent genetic regulatory events in T lymphocyte activation. Science 243:355, 1989.
65. Tamura SI, Chiba J, Kojima A, Uchida N: Properties of cloned T cells that mediate delayed-type hypersensitivity against ovalbumin in mice. Cell Immunol 76:156, 1983.
66. Kim J, Woods A, Becker-Dunn E, Bottomly K: Distinct functional phenotypes of cloned Ia-restricted helper T cells. J Exp Med 162:188, 1985.
67. Mosmann TR, Cherwinski H, Bond MW, et al: Two types of murine helper T cell clones. I. Definition according to profiles of lymphokine activities and secreted proteins. J Immunol 136:2348, 1986.
68. Kurt-Jones EA, Hamberg S, Ohara J, et al: Heterogeneity of helper/inducer T lymphocytes. I. Lymphokine production and lymphokine responsiveness. J Exp Med 166:1774, 1987.
69. Stout RD, Bottomly K: Antigen-specific activation of effector macrophages by IFNγ-producing (TH1) T cell clones. Failure of IL-4 producing (TH2) T cell clones to activate effector function in macrophages. J Immunol 142:760, 1989.
70. Bazan JF: Structural design and molecular evolution of a cytokine receptor superfamily. Proc Natl Acad Sci USA 87:6934, 1990.
71. Miyajima A, Kitamura T, Harada N, et al: Cytokine receptors and signal transduction. Annu Rev Immunol 10:295, 1992.
72. Minami Y, Kono T, Miyazaki T, Taniguchi T: The IL-2 receptor complex: its structure, function, and target genes. Annu Rev Immunol 11:245, 1993.

73. Fernandez-Botran R, Sanders VM, Mossman TR, Vitetta ES: Lymphokine-mediated regulation of the proliferative response of clones of T helper 1 and T helper 2 cells. J Exp Med 168:543, 1988.
74. Gajewski TF, Fitch FW: Anti-proliferative effect of IFNγ in immune regulation. I. IFNγ inhibits the proliferation of Th2 but not Th1 murine helper T lymphocyte clones. J Immunol 140:4245, 1988.
75. Fiorentino DF, Bond MW, Mosmann TR: Types of mouse T helper cell. IV. Th2 clones secrete a factor that inhibits cytokine production by Th1 clones. J Exp Med 170:2081, 1989.
76. Katsura Y: Cell-mediated and humoral immune responses in mice. III. Dynamic balance between delayed type hypersensitivity and antibody response. Immunology 32:227, 1977.
77. Yamamura M, Uymura K, Deans RJ, et al: Defining protective responses to pathogens: cytokine profiles in leprosy. Science 254:277, 1991.
78. Heinzel FP, Sadick MS, Mutha S, Locksley RM: Production of interferon-γ, interleukin-2, interleukin-4 and interleukin-10 by $CD4^+$ lymphocytes in vivo during healing and progressive murine leishmaniasis. Proc Natl Acad Sci USA 88:701, 1991.
79. Heath WR, Allison J, Hoffmann MW, et al: Autoimmune diabetes as a consequence of locally produced interleukin-2. Nature 359:547, 1992.
80. Salk J, Bretscher PA, Salk PL, et al: A strategy for prophylactic vaccination against HIV. Science 260:1270, 1993.
81. Karray S, Dautry-Varsat A, Tsudo M, et al: IL-4 inhibits the expression of high affinity IL-2 receptors on monoclonal human B cells. J Immunol 145:1152, 1990.
82. Gaya A, de la Calle O, Yague J, et al: IL-4 inhibits IL-2 synthesis and IL-2-induced up-regulation of IL-2R alpha but not IL-2R beta chain in CD4+ human T cells. J Immunol 146:4209, 1991.
83. Herman A, Kappler JW, Marrack P, Pullen AM: Superantigens: mechanism of T-cell stimulation and role in immune responses. Annu Rev Immunol 9:745, 1991.
84. Marrack P, Kappler J: The staphylococcal enterotoxins and their relatives. Science 248:705, 1990.
85. Marrack P, Kushnir E, Kappler J: A maternally inherited superantigen encoded by a mammary tumour virus. Nature 349:524, 1991.
86. Frankel WN, Rudy C, Coffin JM, Huber BT: Linkage of *Mis* genes to endogenous mammary tumour viruses of inbred mice. Nature 349:526, 1991.
87. Woodland DL, Happ MP, Gollob KJ, Palmer E: An endogenous retrovirus mediating deletion of $\alpha\beta$ T cells. Nature 349:529, 1991.
88. Dyson PJ, Knight AM, Fairchild S, et al: Genes encoding ligands for deletion of Vβ11 T cells cosegregate with mammary tumour virus genomes. Nature 349:531, 1991.
89. Acha-Orbea H, Shakhov AN, Scarpellino L, et al: Clonal deletion of Vβ14-bearing T cells in mice transgenic or mammary tumour virus. Nature 350:207, 1991.
90. Ameisen JC, Capron A: Cell dysfunction and depletion in AIDS: the programmed cell death hypothesis. Immunol Today 12:102, 1991.
91. Marx J: Clue found to T cell loss in AIDS. Science 254:798, 1991.
92. Takimoto H, Yoshikai Y, Kishihara K, et al: Stimulation of all T cell bearing Vβ1, Vβ3, Vβ11 and Vβ12 by staphylococcal enterotoxin A. Eur J Immunol 20:617, 1990.
93. Imberti L, Sottini A, Bettinardi A, et al: Selective depletion in HIV infection of T cells that bear specific T cell receptor V sequences. Science 254:860, 1991.
94. Groux H, Torpier G, Monte D, et al: Activation-induced death by apoptosis in $CD4^+$ T cells from human immunodeficiency virus-infected asymptomatic individuals. J Exp Med 175:331, 1992.
95. Meyaard L, Otto SA, Jonker RR, et al: Programmed death of T cells in HIV-1 infection. Science 257:217, 1992.
96. O'Hehir RE, Lamb JR: Induction of specific clonal anergy in human T lymphocytes by *Staphylococcus aureus* enterotoxins. Proc Natl Acad Sci USA 87:1, 1990.
97. Cone LA, Woodard DR, Schlievert PM, Tomory GS: Clinical and bacteriologic observations of a toxic shock-like syndrome due to *Streptococcus pyogenes.* N Engl J Med 317:146, 1987.
98. Stevens DL, Tanner MH, Winship J: Group A streptococcal infections associated with toxic shock-like syndrome and scarlet fever toxin A. N Engl J Med 321:1, 1989.
99. Fast DJ, Schlievert PM, Nelson RD: Toxic shock syndrome-associated staphylococcal and streptococcal pyrogenic toxins are potent inducers of tumor necrosis factor production. Infect Immun 57:291, 1989.
100. Marrack P, Blackman M, Kushnir E, Kappler J: The toxicity of staphylococcal enterotoxin B in mice is mediated by T cells. J Exp Med 171:455, 1990.
101. Chatenoud L, Ferran C, Legendre C, et al: Systemic reaction to the monoclonal antibody OKT3 in relation to serum levels of tumor necrosis factor and interferon γ. N Engl J Med 320:1420, 1989.
102. Ellenhorn JDI, Woodle ES, Ghobreal I, et al: Activation of human T cells in vivo following treatment of transplant recipients with OKT3. Transplantation 50:608, 1990.
103. Charpertier B, Hiesse C, Lantz O, et al: Evidence that antihuman tumor necrosis factor monoclonal antibody prevents OKT3-induced acute syndrome. Transplantation 54:992, 1992.
104. Chatenoud L, Ferran C, Legrendre C, et al: In vivo cell activation following OKT3 administration: systemic cytokine release and modulation by corticosteroids. Transplantation 49:697, 1990.
105. Ferran C, Dy M, Merite S, et al: Reduction of morbidity and cytokine release in anti-CD3 MoAb-treated mice by corticosteroids. Transplantation 50:642, 1990.
106. Chatenoud L, Legrendre C, Ferran C, et al: Cortico-

steroid inhibition of the OKT3-induced cytokine-related syndrome—dosage and kinetics prerequisites. Transplantation 51:334, 1991.
107. Lukacher AE, Braciale VL, Braciale TJ: In vivo effector function of influenza virus-specific cytotoxic T lymphocyte clones is highly specific. J Exp Med 160:814, 1984.
108. Henkart PA: Mechanism of lymphocyte-mediated cytotoxicity. Annu Rev Immunol 3:31, 1985.
109. Shu S, Chou T, Rosenberg SA: In vitro sensitization and expansion with viable tumor cells and interleukin 2 in the generation of specific therapeutic effector cells. J Immunol 136:3891, 1986.
110. Podack ER: The molecular mechanism of lymphocyte-mediated tumor cell lysis. Immunol Today 6:21, 1985.
111. Young JD-E, Cohn ZA: Cell-mediated killing: a common mechanism? Cell 46:641, 1986.
112. Masson D, Tschopp J: Isolation of a lytic, pore-forming protein (perforin) from cytolytic T-lymphocytes. J Biol Chem 260:9060, 1985.
113. Podack ER, Young JDE, Cohn ZA: Isolation and biochemical and functional characterization of perforin 1 from cytolytic T cell granules. Proc Natl Acad Sci USA 82:8629, 1985.
114. Masson D, Tschopp J: A family of serine esterases in lytic granules of cytolytic T lymphocytes. Cell 49:679, 1987.
115. Schmid J, Weissmann C: Induction of mRNA for a serine protease and a β-thrombo-globulin-like protein in mitogen-stimulated human leukocytes. J Immunol 139:250, 1987.
116. Don MM, Ablett G, Bishop CJ, et al: Death of cells by apoptosis following attachment of specifically allergized lymphocytes in vitro. Aust J Exp Biol Med Sci 55:407, 1977.
117. Russell JH, Dobos CB: Mechanisms of immune lysis 2. CTL-induced disintegration of the target begins within minutes of cell contact. J Immunol 125:1256, 1980.
118. Russell JH, Masakowski VR, Rucinsky T, Phillips G: Mechanisms of immune lysis 3. Characterization of the nature and kinetics of the cytotoxic T lymphocyte-induced nuclear lesion in the target. J Immunol 128:2087, 1982.
119. Duke RC, Chervenak R, Cohen JJ: Endogenous endonuclease-induced DNA fragmentation: an early event in cell-mediated cytolysis. Proc Natl Acad Sci USA 80:6361, 1983.
120. Hayes MP, Berrebi GA, Henkart PA: Induction of target cell DNA release by the cytotoxic T lymphocyte granule protease granzyme A. J Exp Med 170:933, 1989.
121. Zijlstra M, Bix M, Simister NE, et al: β2-microglobulin deficient mice lack $CD4^+8^+$ cytolytic T cells. Nature 344:742, 1990.
122. Koller BH, Marrack P, Kappler JW, Smithies O: Normal development of mice deficient in β2M, MHC class I proteins, and $CD8^+$ T cells. Science 248:1227, 1990.
123. Ullberg M, Jondal M: Recycling and target binding capacity of human natural killer cells. J Exp Med 153:615, 1981.
124. Quan P-C, Ishizaka T, Bloom BR: Studies on the mechanism of NK lysis. J Immunol 128:1786, 1982.
125. Hiserodt JC, Britvan LJ, Targan SR: Characterization of the cytolytic reaction mechanism of the human natural killer (NK) lymphocyte: resolution into binding, programming, and killer cell-independent steps. J Immunol 129:1782, 1982.
126. Carpen O, Virtanen I, Lehto V-P, Saksela E: Polarization of NK cell cytoskeleton upon conjugation with sensitive target cells. J Immunol 131:2695, 1983.
127. North RJ: The relative importance of blood monocytes and fixed macrophages to the expression of cell-mediated immunity to infection. J Exp Med 132:521, 1970.
128. Murray HW, Spitalny GL, Nathan CF: Activation of mouse peritoneal macrophages in vitro and in vivo by interferon-γ. J Immunol 134:1619, 1985.
129. Cher DJ, Mosmann TR: Two types of murine helper T cell clone II. Delayed-type hypersensitivity is mediated by TH1 clones. J Immunol 138:3688, 1987.
130. Wallis RS, Amir-Tahmasseb M, Ellner JJ: Induction of interleukin 1 and tumor necrosis factor by mycobacterial proteins: the monocyte Western blot. Proc Natl Acad Sci USA 87:3348, 1990.
131. Chan J, Xing Y, Magliozzo RS, Bloom BR: Killing of virulent *Mycobacterium tuberculosis* by reactive nitrogen intermediates produced by activated murine macrophages. J Exp Med 1111, 1975.
132. Stuehr DJ, Marletta MA: Induction of nitrite/nitrate synthesis in murine macrophages by BCG infection, lymphokines, or interferon-γ. J Immunol 139:518, 1987.
133. Denis M: Interferon-gamma-treated murine macrophages inhibit growth of tubercle bacilli via the generation of reactive nitrogen intermediates. Cell Immunol 132:150, 1991.
134. Flesch IEA, Kaufmann SHE: Mechanisms involved in mycobacterial growth inhibition by gamma-interferon activated bone marrow macrophages: role of reactive nitrogen intermediates. Infect Immun 59:3213, 1991.
135. Denis M: Tumor necrosis factor and granulocyte macrophage-colony stimulating factor stimulate human macrophages to restrict growth of virulent *Mycobacterium avium* and to kill avirulent *M. avium:* killing effector mechanism depends on the generation of reactive nitrogen intermediates. J Leukoc Biol 49:380, 1991.
136. Dannenberg AM Jr: Delayed-type hypersensitivity and cell-mediated immunity in the pathogenesis of tuberculosis. Immunol Today 12:228, 1991.
137. Mielke MEA, Rosen H, Brocke S, et al: Protective immunity and granuloma formation are mediated by two distinct tumor necrosis factor α- and γ-interferon-dependent T cell-phagocyte interactions in murine listeriosis: dissociation on the basis of phagocyte adhesion mechanisms. Infect Immun 60:1875, 1992.

138. Brandtzaeg P, Sollid LM, Thrane PS, et al: Lympho-epithelial interactions in the mucosal immune system. Gut 29:1116, 1988.
139. Reynolds HY: Immunologic system in the respiratory tract. Physiol Rev 71:1117, 1991.
140. Yamamoto K, Anacker RL, Ribi E: Macrophage migration inhibition studies with cells from mice vaccinated with cell walls of *Mycobacterium bovis* BCG: relationship between inhibitory activity of lung cells and resistance to airborne challenge with *Mycobacterium tuberculosis*, H37Rv. Infect Immun 1:595, 1970.
141. Henney CS, Waldman RH: Cell-mediated immunity shown by lymphocytes from the respiratory tract. Science 169:696, 1970.
142. Guy-Grand D, Cerf-Bensussan N, Malissen B, et al: Two gut intraepithelial $CD8^+$ lymphocyte populations with different T cell receptors: a role for the gut epithelium in T cell differentiation. J Exp Med 171:471, 1991.
143. Poussier P, Edouard P, Lee C, et al: Thymus-independent development and negative selection of T cells expression T cell receptor in the intestinal epithelium: evidence for distinct circulation patterns of gut- and thymus-derived T lymphocytes. J Exp Med 176:187, 1992.
144. Bank I, DePinho RA, Brenner MB, et al: A functional T3 molecule associated with a novel heterodimer on the surface of immature human thymocytes. Nature 344:179, 1986.
145. Lew AM, Pardoll DM, Maloy WL, et al: Characterization of T cell receptor gamma chain expression in a subset of murine thymocytes. Science 234:1401, 1986.
146. Lanier LL, Federspiel NA, Ruitenberg JJ, et al: The T cell antigen receptor complex expressed on normal peripheral blood $CD4^-$, $CD8^-$ T lymphocytes. J Exp Med 165:1076, 1987.
147. Nakanishi N, Maeda K, Ito K, et al: $T\gamma$ protein is expressed on murine fetal thymocytes as a disulfide-linked heterodimer. Nature 325:720, 1987.
148. Haas W, Pereira P, Tonegawa S: Gamma/delta cells. Annu Rev Immunol 11:637, 1993.
149. Mosley RL, Styre D, Klein JR: Differentiation and functional maturation of bone marrow-derived intestinal epithelial T-cells expression membrane T-cell receptor in athymic radiation chimeras. J Immunol 145:1369, 1990.
150. Lefrancous L, Lecorre R, Mayo J, et al: Extrathymic selection of TCR $\gamma\delta^+$ cells by class II major histocompatibility complex molecules. Cell 63:333, 1990.
151. Bandeira A, Itohara S, Bonneville M, et al: Extrathymic origin of intestinal cell antigen receptor $\gamma\delta$. Proc Natl Acad Sci USA 88:43, 1991.
152. Guy-Grand D, Cerf-Benussan N, Malissen B, et al: Two gut intraepithelial $CD8^+$ lymphocyte populations with different T cell receptors: a role for the gut epithelium in T cell differentiation. J Exp Med 173:471, 1991.
153. Asarnow DM, Kuziel WA, Bonyhadi M, et al: Limited diversity of γ/δ antigen receptor genes of Thy-1^+ dendritic epidermal cells. Cell 55:837, 1988.
154. Itohara S, Farr AG, Lafaille JJ, et al: Homing of a γ/δ thymocyte subset with homogenous T-cell receptors to mucosal epithelial. Nature 343:754, 1990.
155. Kabelitz D, Bender A, Schondelmaier S, et al: A large fraction of human peripheral blood $\gamma\delta$ T cells is activated by *Mycobacterium tuberculosis* but not by its 65-kD heat shock protein. J Exp Med 171:667, 1990.
156. Pfeffer K, Schoel B, Gulle H, et al: Primary responses of human T cells to mycobacteria: a frequent set of γ/δ T cells are stimulated by protease-resistant ligands. Eur J Immunol 20:1175, 1990.
157. Pfeffer K, Schoel B, Plesnila N, et al: A lectin-binding, protease-resistant mycobacterial ligand specifically activated $V\gamma9^+$ human $\gamma\delta$ T cells. J Immunol 148:575, 1992.
158. Haregewoin A, Soman G, Hom R: T cells respond to mycobacterial heat-shock protein. Nature 340:309, 1989.
159. O'Brien RL, Happ MP, Dallas A, et al: Stimulation of a major subset of lymphocytes expressing T cell receptor $\gamma\delta$ by an antigen derived from *Mycobacterium tuberculosis.* Cell 57:667, 1989.
160. Jitsukawa S, Trievel F, Faure F, et al: Cloned $CD3^+$ TcR α/β^- $TiaA^-$ peripheral blood lymphocytes compared to the $TiaA^+$ counterparts: structural differences of the γ/δ receptor and functional heterogeneity. Eur J Immunol 18:1671, 1988.
161. Ciccone E, Viale O, Pende D, et al: Specificity of human T lymphocytes expressing a $\gamma\delta$ T cell antigen receptor. Recognition of a polymorphic determinant of HLA class I molecules by a $\gamma\delta$ T cell clone. Eur J Immunol 19:1267, 1989.
162. Spits H, Paliard X, Engelhard VH, deVries JE: Cytotoxic activity and lymphokine production of T cell receptor (TCR)-$\alpha\beta^+$ and TCR-$\gamma\delta^+$ cytotoxic T lymphocyte (CTL) clones recognizing HLA-A2 and HLA-A2 mutants. J Immunol 144:4156, 1990.
163. Vandekerckhove BAE, Datema G, Koning F, et al: Analysis of the donor-specific cytotoxic T lymphocyte repertoire in a patient with a long-term surviving allograft. J Immunol 144:1288, 1990.
164. Bosnes V, Qvigstad E, Lundin KEA, Thorsky E: Recognition of a particular HLA-DQ heterodimer by a human $\gamma\delta$ T cell clone. Eur J Immunol 20:1429, 1990.
165. Holoshitz J, Vila LM, Keroack BJ, et al: Dual antigenic recognition of cloned human $\gamma\delta$ T-cells. J Clin Invest 89:308, 1992.

Humoral Immunity to Infection and the Complement System

CHAPTER 15

David L. Dunn, Jonathan L. Meakins

The preceding chapter discussed the cellular components of the immune response not only to infection but also to other foreign materials. This chapter will address the humoral components of the immune response, made up principally of immunoglobulins and complement. Historically, immunologists were divided into two camps. One, led by Metchnikov, championed the phagocytic cellular components as most important in the control of infection. The other, led by Ehrlich, proposed that humoral factors were more significant. Almroth Wright initiated resolution of the controversy in 1903 by demonstrating that neutrophil phagocytosis (cellular) was dependent on particle opsonization (humoral). The resolution of the early arguments as to which components of the immune response were most important was that they act in conjunction in support of one another. Although the immune response is presented as a series of separate components, they interact closely with one another.

IMMUNOGLOBULINS

All immunoglobulins (antibodies) are manufactured by lymphocytes of the B cell line, which terminates with the plasma cell. Interaction with a helper T (T_H) cell is required for active primary immunization of a B cell to most antigens (T-dependent), although some antigens are able to induce a B cell response without T cell interaction (T-independent). After sensitization, the clone of B cells that bear genetically programmed receptors for the antigens undergoes proliferative expansion with the concurrent manufacture and release of large quantities of immunoglobulin. The initial concept that a specific immunoglobulin was specifically produced for each antigenic molecule has been borne out, and this event occurs via somatic recombination of genes coding for the variable region of the molecule. Any given antigen, however, may generate the production of both highly specific antibody and antibody that reacts with other similar antigens (cross-reactive), corresponding to the various antigenic configurations or regions (epitopes) of a single complex molecule. So-called natural antibodies probably represent immunoglobulin generated against cross-reacting antigenic specificities elicited by previously encountered antigens.[1,2]

Immunoglobulin Structure

The basic immunoglobulin (Ig) molecule is a heterogeneous family of glycoproteins, which despite their diversity share many structural properties, biologic functions, and origins. There are five classes of immunoglobulins (see Table 15–1 on page 297), each defined by their heavy chain (α, μ, δ, ε). The basic structure of Ig molecules is made up of pairs of polypeptide chains of unequal size (Fig. 15–1). There are two light (L) and two heavy (H) chains, which are held together by strong noncovalent forces and interchain disulfide bonds. Each L chain is associated with an H chain, and the two H chains are bound together. Thus, the basic unit of the Ig molecule is L_2H_2, which may be considered as a monomer of two light and two heavy chains. This basic four-chain unit can form even larger units (sIgA, IgM) with utilization of further bonding of other molecular pieces (Fig. 15–2). The light and heavy chains are composed of domains, which are conformational regions formed of somewhat more than 100 amino acid residues.

The amino acid residues in the amino-terminal domain of each pair of light and heavy chains fold to form an antigen-binding site (see Fig. 15–1). The antigen-binding region within the amino-terminal domains is heterogeneous in primary structure and is termed the variable (V) region. The remaining domains, progressing to the carboxyl end of the molecule, are less variable and are called the constant (C) region. The carboxy-terminal domain of the molecule, termed the Fc (crystallizable fragment), is capable of binding to the Ig (Fc) receptors present on some leukocytes—a process that stimulates phagocytosis of the antibody and antigen to which it has bound. Complement activation sites also are present within the constant Fc region of the H chain; these are exposed after antigen-antibody binding occurs. The B cell clones that synthesize the immunoglobulins are genetically programmed to synthesize a single light-chain variable region and a single heavy-chain variable region. These domains determine the specificity of the antigen and are identical in each Ig molecule derived from a given clone.

There are five major classes of Ig molecules, and each has distinct physiochemical, physiologic, and antigenic properties (Tables 15–1 and 15–2). It is the constant region of the heavy chains that differs between classes and determines all class-specific properties. Different types of heavy chains are designated by Greek letters and correspond to the Ig class of immunoglobulin. The variable regions and light chains are not class specific, although an individual immunoglobulin molecule can only possess one type of light chain. In humans, there are two types of light chains, κ and λ.

The IgG molecule is susceptible to enzymatic attack (see Fig. 15–1), which produces specific mo-

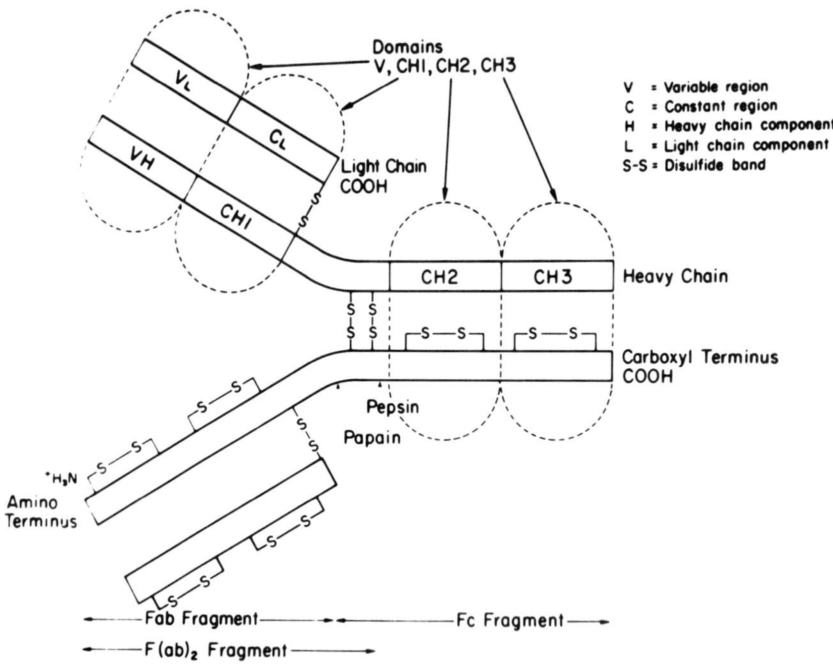

Figure 15–1. Four-chain structure of an IgG molecule. *(From Alexander JW, Good RA. Fundamentals of Clinical Immunology. Philadelphia, Saunders, 1977, p 69.)*

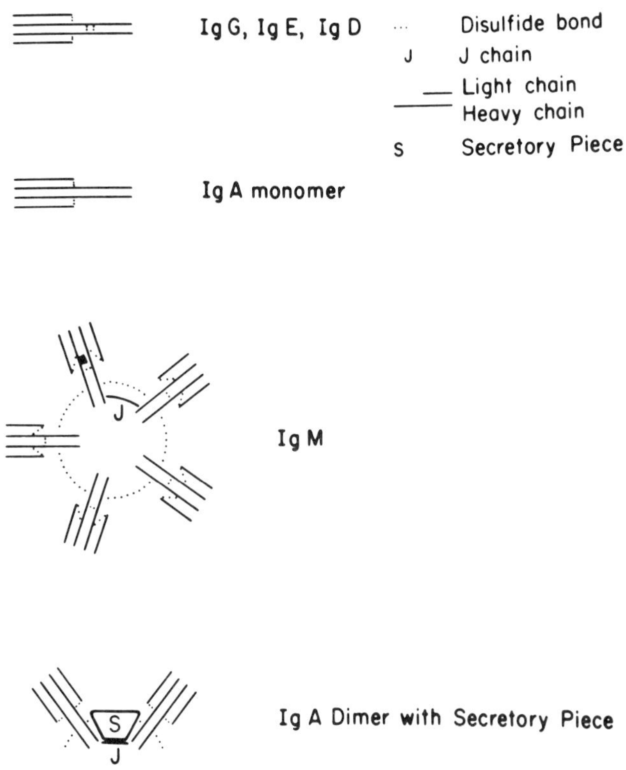

Figure 15–2. Schematic structures of the immunoglobulin classes. Disulfide bonds may differ from those shown for individual subclasses. *(From Alexander JW, Good RA: Fundamentals of Clinical Immunology. Philadelphia, Saunders, 1977, p 69.)*

lecular fragments made up of intact domains. The Fab, $F(ab)'_2$, and Fc fragments result from enzymatic reactions in the hinge region. Papain digestion produces the Fab and Fc fragments. The Fab has an intact light-chain and amino acid terminal as well as one constant heavy-chain domain. It contains a single intact antigen-combining site. The Fc fragment is the region that fixes to Fc cellular receptors and initiates complement activation. Pepsin digestion produces the $F(ab)'_2$ fragment, which is bivalent but lacks the Fc fragment that is degraded by this enzyme.

Immunoglobulin Classes (See Table 15–1)

Immunoglobulin G (IgG). IgG is the most abundant immunoglobulin (about 85 percent of serum Ig), comprising about 85 percent of the total Ig. IgG has a molecular weight of 150,000 and is widely distributed throughout the intravascular and extravascular spaces. Antibodies of the IgG class provide antiviral and antibacterial protection. They are used therapeutically against bacterial and viral infections, and for their antivenom and antitoxin activities.

In humans, IgG has four different subclasses (1 through 4 in order of abundance). Mice also have four subclasses (1, 2a, 2b, 3), but these are not strictly analogous to those in humans. The significance of each of these four subclasses is not clear. Antibodies of the IgG class bind to and are actively transported across the placenta to the fetus, accounting for the similarity of maternal and neonatal immunoglobulin levels. Maternal IgG levels subsequently decrease after the fourth month of life, at which time the normal child is producing IgG in adequate quantities. Serum IgG levels are in dynamic equilibrium throughout life, responding to various stimuli. Generally, levels progressively decrease with age. The biologic effectiveness of IgG resides in large part with its opsonic capacity. The Fab component binds to antigen, and the Fc component interacts with the Fc receptors on phagocytic cells—neutrophils, monocytes, or macrophages—with subsequent ingestion of the antigenic cell, particle, or antigen-antibody complex. Two or more molecules of IgG bound to a particulate antigen are able, in addition, to fix and activate the classic complement pathway (see Complement section).

Immunoglobulin M (IgM). IgM (see Fig. 15–2), originally referred to as macroglobulin, is the largest of the immunoglobulins, with a molecular weight in the region of 900,000 daltons. This antibody class accounts for 5 to 10 percent of serum Ig. The large size is a result of polymerization of five

TABLE 15–1. SELECTED PROPERTIES OF HUMAN IMMUNOGLOBULINS

Property	IgG	IgA	IgM	IgD	IgE
Molecular weight	150,000	160,000 and polymers	900,000	200,000	185,000
Normal serum concentration (μg/ml)	8–16	1.5–4	0.5–2	0.00004	0–0.4
Percent total immunoglobulin	80	13	6	0.002	1
Sedimentation coefficient	7S	7S, 9S, 11S	19S	8S	7S
Serum $T_{1/2}$ (days)	23	5.8	10	2.8	2.3
Valency for antigen binding	2	2	10	2	2

TABLE 15–2. BIOLOGIC PROPERTIES OF ANTIBODIES BY IMMUNOGLOBULIN CLASS

Property	IgG	IgA	IgM	IgD	IgE
Complement activation					
Classic pathway	++	−	++++	−	−
Alternate pathway	+	+	+	+	+
Opsonic activity	++++	−	+	−	−
Lytic activity[a]	++	−	++++	−	−
Inhibition of bacterial adherence	+	+++	+	?	?
Viral neutralization	+++	+++	++	?	?
Reaginic activity	−	−	−	−	++++
Placental transfer	++++	−	−	−	−

[a] Through activation of complement after combining with cellular antigens.
Adapted from Alexander JW, Meakins JL: Ann Surg 176:273, 1972.

Ig molecules into a pentamer $(L_2H_2)_5$ with a single J (joining) chain (see Fig. 15–2).[3] Because of its size, it is found only in the intravascular space. The 18-19S molecule is formed by polymerization of 5.7S subunits joined by disulfide bonds. It has a half-life of 5 to 6 days. IgM is the major component of the primary response to an antigen and comprises the first peak of immunoglobulin produced. IgM production declines on the basis of a feedback mechanism in response to increasing IgG production. Antibodies formed in response to T cell-independent antigens are usually of this class.

IgM is a potent activator of complement; a single molecule is able to initiate the classic complement sequence. Monomer subunits of IgM occur on the surface of many B lymphocytes and may have an important role as antigen receptors for these cells.

Immunoglobulin E (IgE). IgE, originally referred to as reagin (see Table 15–1), is present in minute amounts in the serum (about 0.003 mg/ml) and is an important mediator of acute allergic responses as exemplified by the Prausnitz-Kustner reaction in which passively transferred IgE antibody from an atopic individual elicits a wheal and erythema reaction in the test subject in response to antigen. It has the lowest synthetic rate of any known Ig class. Antibodies of this class are the chief antigen-specific mediators of immediate-type hypersensitivity reactions (reaginic) and therefore are extremely potent biologic effectors. The Fc portion of the molecule fixes specific Fc receptors on mast cells and basophils, which are thus sensitized to release histamine and other mediators when exposed to antigen. IgE is an important mediator of respiratory allergic disease. This type of immunoglobulin also may be important in protecting the respiratory tract against microbes.

Immunoglobulin D (IgD). IgD is present in relatively low concentrations in normal human plasma, less than 1 percent that of IgG. The structure of this immunoglobulin is similar to that of IgG. No distinct biologic function has been ascribed to circulating IgD, although it also serves as a surface marker on B cells.

Immunoglobulin A (IgA) and Local Mucosal Immunity. Antibodies can be produced by lymphoid tissues associated with mucosal surfaces, and IgA is secreted onto those surfaces. IgA in external secretions has a structure different from IgA in serum where it is a minor component. The contents of IgA in various mucosal fluids differ from site to site. Inflammation at the mucosal surface markedly changes those concentrations, especially during the transudation of serum proteins.

IgA AND SECRETORY IgA STRUCTURE. IgA exists as a monomer in serum. Secretory IgA (sIgA), however, exists in multiple polymeric forms with increasing sedimentation coefficients up to 18S. Most sIgA exists in the dimeric form with a molecular weight of 380,000 and possesses a unique secretory piece or component (SC), also called T component or transport piece (see Table 15–1 and Fig. 15–2). Secretory component is a nonimmunoglobulin glycoprotein (molecular weight 58,000) bound to the light immunoglobulin chains by disulfide bonds. Dimeric IgA also has a J chain (molecular weight 23,000 to 26,000) consisting of a single amino acid chain. These J chains also are found in dimeric serum IgA and IgM.

SC probably mediates transport of IgA (and probably IgM) across epithelial surfaces and may also be important in the absorption of antigens from mucosal surfaces. SC is also thought to be responsible for the greater resistance of sIgA to digestion by proteolytic enzymes. IgG does not possess SC and thus is not protected from proteolysis.

Most sIgA is synthesized locally in plasma cells within lymphoid tissue underlying the epithelium of secretory surfaces (eg, intestinal Peyer's patches). The dimeric IgA then reaches the mucosal surface by passing through intracellular channels or between the epithelial cells. SC is synthesized by the epithelial cells and combines with the dimeric IgA molecule. The sIgA molecule is thus produced.[3,4]

ANTIMICROBIAL ACTIVITY OF IgA. Secretory IgA can bind to viral and bacterial antigens to which the mammalian host has been exposed, but it can neither fix complement in the normal way nor serve as an opsonin for phagocytosis.[4] Burritt et al[5] have shown that the Fc fragment of IgA can bind complement and might, under proper conditions, have the capacity to activate complement and lyse bacteria. Adinolfi et al[6] demonstrated that secretory IgA antibody is capable of bacterial lysis in the presence of complement and lysozyme, while others have determined that a heat-stable component of complement is necessary for IgA-mediated bacterial lysis.[7] What is not known is whether complement is active within the complex milieu of intestinal and respiratory fluids. Equally as controversial as the role of IgA in the complement-mediated immunolysis of bacteria is the suggestion that IgA antibodies can function as opsonins.

However these controversies are resolved, most evidence currently supports the idea that IgA acts primarily to prevent the adherence of pathogenic bacteria to epithelium. The other immunoglobulin classes possess similar properties. This mechanism probably operates as a first line of defense against many, if not all, mucosal pathogens that normally invade by adhering to and colonizing the epithelium as a prelude to tissue invasion and dissemination.[8]

sIgA AND LOCAL IMMUNITY. Parenterally administered vaccines can elicit an sIgA response, but levels of local antibody are usually low and result in only partial protection against ingested pathogens. The direct application of vaccines to mucosal surfaces elicits a greater degree of local immunity as well as a moderate degree of systemic immunity.[9] The level of sIgA correlates with antimicrobial protection, but preexisting secretory antibody activity interferes with a secondary immunization response. In addition, the response of the mucosal immune system to bacterial antigens is so short lived that local immunity to *Neisseria gonorrhoeae,* for example, disappears within several weeks of its development, and there is often no booster effect following reinfection.

The local immunity achieved by the use of topical vaccines has been studied extensively and the results reviewed by Regamey et al[10]: (1) a higher dose of antigen is required compared with parenteral immunization; (2) repeated immunization is required; (3) dose of vaccine, size of particles and aerosol vaccines, living condition before exposure to antigen, and age of recipient influence the outcome of immunization; (4) attenuated nonparenteral vaccines are usually not transmissible to contacts, produce few side effects, and are suitable for mass application; and (5) serum antibodies do not always reflect the state of local mucosal immunity generated by nonparenteral vaccine.

SECRETORY HUMORAL IMMUNITY IN IgA DEFICIENCY STATES. IgA is not the only mucosal immunoglobulin. IgG-containing cells lie immediately below the surface epithelium of the nasal mucosa and the gingival tissues. Local synthesis of IgG also occurs in bladder, kidney, and urinary tract. In addition, IgM-producing cells predominate over IgG-producing cells within salivary glands and the gastrointestinal tract. In IgA deficiency, IgM usually predominates in mucosal secretion. IgE also is synthesized in secretory organs. The tonsils, adenoids, bronchial and mesenteric lymph nodes, and lamina propria of the gastrointestinal and respiratory tract mucosa contain a large number of IgE-producing cells.

IgA is the most commonly isolated immunoglobulin deficiency.[11] Most patients are healthy, without an increased incidence of mucosal infections and with humoral protection probably mediated by IgM. Patients with selective IgA deficiencies have IgA-bearing peripheral blood lymphocytes but lack IgA-producing plasma cells. IgA deficiency is associated with hereditary ataxia-telangectasia and partial deletion of chromosome 18, and recurrent viral and bacterial infections of the respiratory tract resulting in chronic bronchitis and bronchiectasis can occur. IgA deficiency is also frequently associated with allergic disorders, ear infections in children, autoimmune phenomena, malabsorption, and cancer. *Giardia lamblia* infections are particularly common in this group of patients. Patients deficient in secretory component can develop chronic intestinal candidiasis.[12]

Functions of the Circulating Immunoglobulins

Antibodies play almost no role in the eradication of intracellular pathogens once cells have become successfully invaded. The primary role, therefore, is directed against pathogens in an extracellular location. Specific antibodies promote the following events: (1) opsonization that promotes engulfment and intracellular destruction of microbes by phagocytic cells; (2) activation of the complement system with deposition of complement proteins on microbial cell membranes, leading to lysis and/or augmented opsonization and phagocytosis; (3) neutralization of microbial toxins and viruses; and (4) inhibition of attachment of microbes to susceptible host cells (see Table 15–2). IgG is the most abundant immunoglobulin in the extravascular fluids and is the most important immunoglobulin in tissue infection. IgM is a pentameric intravascular molecule and cannot leave normal vessels. It is an effective bacterial agglutinin and efficiently stimulates the classic complement-dependent cytolytic system. It functions as one of the first lines of specific systemic host immune defense.

Immunization

Active Immunization. Development of an immunoglobulin response by inoculation with a transmissible agent was the first form of immunotherapy against infection. Jenner's prevention of smallpox by vaccination with cowpox virus, which was probably attenuated and antigenically similar to the smallpox virus, was the first demonstration of the value of this approach in the control of infectious diseases. Pasteur's subsequent experiments to prevent anthrax with a killed vaccine ushered in a new era of immunotherapy. The near eradication of these diseases worldwide is testimony of the power of this form of prophylaxis. Active immunization can now be performed against tetanus, diphtheria, pertussis, poliomyelitis, measles, mumps, and rubella in the general population, as well as cholera, plague, rabies, Rocky Mountain spotted fever, typhoid, typhus, yellow fever, influenza, hepatitis B, and pneumococcus in selected persons. Thus the concept of manipulation of the natural defense systems of the infected host in order to promote host survival is by no means new. Yet because the pathophysiology of many types of infection is so complex and poorly comprehended, the results of augmentation of the humoral components of the host immune system either by direct vaccination or administration of exogenous antibody have been difficult to evaluate and therefore remain controversial for certain diseases. The goal of immunization is to raise available antibodies to the level that will allow eradication of an invading organism via enhanced opsonization, lysis, or neutralization in order to prevent, abort, or resolve the infectious process.

More recently, both pneumococcal and hepatitis vaccines have undergone extensive clinical testing. A number of studies have documented the occurrence of overwhelming sepsis due to encapsulated organisms such as *S. pneumoniae* after splenectomy or during splenic dysfunction (eg, sickle cell disease, lymphoma). The currently available vaccine contains 23 serotypes, which represent the most common strains encountered. Not all patients respond to each pneumococcal serotype in the polyvalent vaccine, and overwhelming sepsis has been reported even after vaccination. Thus while pneumococcal vaccination has been demonstrated to produce effective antibody titers in normal and asplenic persons, the response is often poor in patients with underlying malignancy or renal failure. Current evidence, however, indicates a distinct trend in reducing septic complications by vaccination.[13–16] Because of the low morbidity of vaccination it is therefore appropriate that all splenectomized patients should receive the polyvalent pneumococcal vaccine. Penicillin prophylaxis also may be administered daily as an adjunctive measure. Lifelong penicillin prophylaxis does require patient compliance, and some clinicians recommend that the asplenic individual self-administer penicillin only if chills, fever, or other symptoms of infection appear.

Hepatitis B vaccine has been tested in a number of trials and demonstrated to be efficacious in reducing the incidence of infection due to this agent by 80 to 95 percent when vaccinees receive all three recommended immunizations. Concern over the transmission of HIV by a form of the vaccine that was obtained by acetone treatment of a serum fraction obtained from infected individuals has not been borne out, and a human recombinant form of the vaccine currently is available. Lack of response in certain normal individuals as well as immunosuppressed and hemodialysis patients has been noted and may be eventually overcome by additional doses, higher dose vaccination, or vaccination with immunoenhancing agents concomitantly administered.[17–20] It is not entirely clear whether patients will require booster injections of either vaccine at various intervals to maintain protective antibody titers, although several recent studies indicate that this may be the case. Vaccination against cytomegalovirus and herpesvirus has demonstrated that antibody titers develop, but no consistent reduction in infection has been documented. The attenuated Towne strain of cytomegalovirus that was used for vaccination is no longer commercially available.

Prevention of the more prevalent problems of gram-negative bacterial sepsis and infection are also being attempted via immunotherapeutic means. Active immunization with rough mutant organisms (vide infra) has been demonstrated to be cross-protective in a variety of experimental animal models.[21-24] Active immunotherapy has not been extensively tested clinically for Enterobacteriaceae. Although several clinical trials demonstrated a reduction in sepsis and burn wound infection after vaccination with a polyvalent *Pseudomonas* lipopolysaccharide vaccine, other clinical trials could not demonstrate efficacy. Also, the incidence of adverse reactions to the vaccine in some studies was high.[25-29] For this form of therapy to have a salutary effect one must obviously be able to select those patients who are at high risk for gram-negative infections, immunize them before the septic insult, and simultaneously have their immune system able to respond sufficiently.

In the vast majority of cases, active immunization has been successful when (1) the organism exists as a single or limited series of antigenic forms, and (2) the disease occurs with reasonable frequency so that immunization before contact with the organism is feasible for a large number of individuals. Either cross-reactive antigenic or polyvalent vaccines must be used to combat those infectious agents that are antigenically diverse. The identification of specific virulence factors may allow specific immunogens to be produced without toxicity, either via detoxification or by the use of gene-cloning techniques. In the use of gene-cloning techniques, the gene sequence coding for the toxic factor is identified, sequenced, and either a portion or a modified sequence cloned so that the antigen produced lacks toxicity but still preserves antigenicity such that protective antibody levels are achieved with immunization. In addition, immunization with anti-idiotype antibodies, in which the binding site of the anti-idiotype Ig region mimics the initial antigen without incurring toxicity, may prove useful in certain situations.

Passive Immunization. Passive transfer of antibody (antibody immunotherapy, serotherapy) was once utilized in pneumococcal infection due to the lack of suitable antimicrobial agents and an inability to isolate specific bacterial antigens as immunogens. The administration of opsonizing antibody allowed the pneumococcus to be more readily ingested and killed by neutrophils. Before the availability of active poliomyelitis vaccines, IgG preparations were used as a protective measure with some success during poliomyelitis epidemics. Currently, passive immunoprophylaxis is useful for botulism, diphtheria, hepatitis A and B, measles, rabies, tetanus, and varicella-zoster. The ability of anticytomegalovirus immunoglobulin pooled from human sources to reduce cytomegalovirus-associated lethality when administered prophylactically to bone marrow allograft recipients also has been demonstrated.[30] In most cases, hyperimmune IgG of human origin is available. Monoclonal antibodies of both murine and human origin directed against a variety of bacterial and viral infectious agents are also becoming available and will find utility both as detection agents and in the treatment of many infectious diseases.

Obviously, antibody immunotherapy will be most efficacious in the immunocompromised host unable to mount a satisfactory antibody response, or in the immunologically naive host who develops a rapid, overwhelming infection in which the course of infection precludes even an initial antibody response. Gram-negative bacterial infections with the frequent sequelae of bacteremia with attendant shock, multiple system organ failure, and death typically occur in either setting. Many factors predispose patients to these infections: (1) underlying host disease processes (malignancy, renal insufficiency, diabetes mellitus); (2) old age and disability; (3) poor nutritional status; (4) prior or concurrent antimicrobial therapy; (5) major operations; (6) respiratory or urinary manipulation or intubation, and (7) immunosuppression, whether iatrogenic (eg, for allograft maintenance or cancer chemotherapy) or caused by defects in host defenses (eg, complement deficiency, leukocyte abnormalities). Even patients with no underlying disease state have a significant mortality rate (10 to 20 percent), and, considering the large patient population, this represents a large number of people dying from infectious complications. In the above-mentioned groups of immunosuppressed patients, the mortality rate is extremely high (greater than 30 percent).[31-34] The use of routine treatment modalities (antimicrobial agents, hemodynamic monitoring, aggressive fluid resuscitation, and metabolic support) has reduced but not eliminated the severe consequences of this disease process. Therefore, investigators have sought to determine how antibody immunotherapy might further ameliorate the lethal effects of gram-negative bacterial infections and gram-negative bacterial sepsis.

As described in Chapter 1, gram-negative bacteria possess a highly complex external antigenic structure that is extremely diverse even within a specific genus. Chemically, the outer membrane consists of (1) lipopolysaccharide (LPS, endotoxin), (2) lipoprotein, and (3) protein. Both the inner and outer membranes are lipid bilayers, and embedded within the external portion of the outer membrane are a variety of membrane proteins, as well as LPS. All of these outer membrane structures are presented to the external milieu and are thus available as bacterial antigens. This highly complex external antigenic structure, however, is extremely diverse even within a specific bacterial genus, accounting for the serotypic diversity of gram-negative microorganisms. This has been attributed in large part to the variability of polysaccharide residues in LPS and has been thought to be the reason that humoral immunity is ineffective during many gram-negative infections, since there is little chance that the host will have had prior experience with a particular serotype.[35] Although the presence of natural immunity before bacterial challenge in the form of existing antibody to microorganisms has been demonstrated by various investigators, it does not invariably occur at a level that will be immunoprotective. Attempts to develop a broadly reactive antiserum directed against a variety of gram-negative organisms have largely centered around the use of those portions of the gram-negative outer membrane shared by most gram-negative bacteria.

The toxic properties of LPS isolated from the outer membrane of gram-negative bacteria have produced great interest in its structure and biologic effects. It has been possible to demonstrate that LPS is composed of three integral components: (1) lipid A, a backbone of β-1,6 linked N-β-hydroxymyristoyl-D-glucosamine disaccharides with attached O-acylated β-hydroxymyristic acid and saturated C_{12-16} fatty acids; (2) core LPS, a series of saccharide residues that includes the sugar ketodeoxyoctonate (3-deoxy-D-mannooctulosonate) connecting the lipid A moiety with the O antigen; and (3) O antigen polysaccharide consisting of 30 to 180 identical units, each of which consists of four to six saccharides. Evidence has gradually accumulated that even smooth strains may express substantial amounts of unmodified core LPS on their cell surface, as well as O antigen residues of various chain length. In addition, in an intact host it has been postulated that serum enzymes exist that serve to cleave O antigens, exposing core determinants.[36]

Initial experimental studies demonstrated the ability of passive transfer of type-specific polyclonal antibody raised against a single O antigen serotype to provide potent, albeit limited, protection and served to confirm the importance of the role of humoral immunity in gram-negative bacillary infections. More recent studies using anti-O antigen polysaccharide monoclonal antibodies directed against LPS have confirmed the central role of LPS in the pathogenesis of sepsis and have substantiated the protective capacity of antibody during gram-negative bacteremia and endotoxemia.[37–39] More recent investigations have centered around the development of more broadly cross-reactive, cross-protective antibody preparations.

To produce cross-protective antibody, several components of the gram-negative outer membrane [eg, enterobacterial common antigen (ECA), lipid A, core LPS] have been identified as potential immunogens. ECA was first identified by Kunin and appears to be a complex of outer membrane amino sugars and lipids shared by many gram-negative microorganisms.[40] While in vitro cross-reactivity of this anti-ECA antiserum to various gram-negative bacteria has been demonstrated, passive transfer of this antiserum to mice did not protect against a lethal challenge of ECA containing gram-negative bacteria.[41] Although several studies have indicated that the lipid A antigen may reside in a cryptic position within the outer membrane of gram-negative bacteria, anti-lipid A antibody does form during experimental and clinical gram-negative bacterial infection. While several groups of investigators have demonstrated that the passive transfer of anti-lipid A rabbit antiserum does not protect against various bacterial infections nor an LPS challenge, others have indicated that anti-lipid A antiserum protects against some systemic effects of endotoxin.[21,42–44]

The core LPS region of endotoxin has been examined because structurally and antigenically it represents a region of the outer membrane common to many gram-negative microorganisms as well as being directly linked to the toxic lipid A component of LPS. Core LPS was initially defined by chemical analysis of the LPS extracted from a series of mutant organisms (*S. minnesota* Ra, Rb, Rc, Rd_1, Rd_2, and Re), each one of which was blocked at a more proximal step in the synthesis of core LPS. The colonial morphology of this series of mutants takes on a rougher, crinkled appearance from Ra to Re, hence the term *rough mutant*. Rough mutants of many genera have now been isolated and characterized, and at least six core LPS types have been defined, all of which are remarkably similar in their most proximal core structure.[45,46]

A large number of experimental studies have demonstrated the ability of anti-core LPS/lipid antibody to cross-react in vitro and cross-protect in vivo in a variety of models of gram-negative bacterial infection.[21,47–52] Not all investigators, however, have been able to demonstrate cross-protection against various gram-negative bacterial challenges. Several investigators have provided evidence that murine monoclonal antibodies directed against the core region of LPS demonstrate extensive serologic cross-reactivity with a variety of gram-negative bacteria.[53–58] It should be noted, however, that although the evidence that antibody directed against core LPS/lipid A can protect against gram-negative bacterial sepsis is supported by a number of studies, the following have yet to be established: (1) the antibody target site within the core LPS/lipid A region of the LPS molecule, (2) the antibody class or subclass, and (3) the monoclonal or polyclonal nature of the antibody preparation that can best maximize the protective effect.

The presence of an anti-core LPS antibody titer may be protective during clinical infection, as demonstrated in several retrospective clinical studies.[59–61] Law and Marks have demonstrated that antibody directed against the core region of LPS occurs naturally with an age-related prevalence, substantial IgM titers being present after the age of 2 in normal individuals.[62] Several investigators have demonstrated a reduction in mortality when anti-*E. coli* J5 human antiserum was administered to septic patients. Others, however, could not demonstrate protection when this antiserum was administered as a single-dose prophylaxis to neutropenic patients to prevent septic complications; yet another study demonstrated that this antiserum decreased the incidence of septic shock but did not alter the number of infectious complications in surgical patients.[63–66] Several large-scale, randomized blinded clinical trials have been performed using either E5, a murine monoclonal antibody, or HA-1A, a monoclonal antibody derived from a murine-human heteromyeloma cell line. Both antibodies are of the IgM class and appear to bind to the lipid A region of LPS. Unfortunately, controversy exists regarding the ability of these reagents to bind specifically and efficiently to LPS, and no reproducible survival benefit has been observed.[67–69]

Anti-gram-negative antibody may potentially be obtained from several sources: (1) immunization of large animals or humans with subsequent plasmaphoresis and antibody isolation, (2) murine or human monoclonal antibodies, (3) affinity purification of large amounts of normal antibody, and (4) pooling of prescreened lots of normal animal or human antibodies that react to a particular bacterial antigen. Additional clinical trials need to be undertaken to evaluate the efficacy of both monoclonal or polyclonal antibody preparations produced by these various methods.

B Cell Immunodeficiencies

Agammaglobulinemia was first diagnosed by Bruton in 1952, and this was the first description of any type of true immunodeficiency. This autosomal recessive condition responds well to the administration of immunoglobulins every 2 weeks. Similarly, patients with hypogammaglobulinemia of either an acquired or a congenital nature can be treated in this manner. Surgery in these patients can safely be conducted after preoperative administration of immunoglobulin and prophylactic administration of antibiotics. Some primary and secondary B cell immunodeficiency diseases are listed in Tables 15–3 and 15–4.

COMPLEMENT

Antibodies are highly efficient and highly specific methods for recognizing antigenic microorganisms. By themselves, they can sometimes inhibit clinical interactions between microbe and host necessary for bacterial virulence. By themselves, however, they are inefficient at eliminating invaders from the body. For this, antibodies require phagocytes to ingest and digest the opsonized organisms, and the

TABLE 15–3. PRIMARY B CELL IMMUNODEFICIENCIES

Isolated B Cell Immunodeficiency Diseases	Combined T Cell and B Cell Immunodeficiency Diseases
Sex-linked infantile hypogammaglobulinemia	Severe combined immunodeficiency
Transient hypogammaglobulinemia of infancy	Cellular immunodeficiency with abnormal immunoglobulin synthesis (Nezeloff's syndrome)
Sex-linked immunodeficiency with hyper-IgM	Immunodeficiency disease with enzyme deficiency
Selective IgA deficiency	Immunodeficiency with eczema and thrombocytopenia (Wiskott-Aldrich syndrome)
Selective IgM deficiency	Immunodeficiency with thymoma
Selective deficiencies of IgG subclasses	Immunodeficiency with ataxia-telangiectasia
	Immunodeficiency with short-limbed dwarfism
	Episodic lymphocytopenia with lymphotoxin (immunologic amnesia)

From Stiehm ER: Immunodeficiency disorders—general considerations. In Stiehm ER, Fulginiti VA (eds): Immunologic Disorders in Infants and Children, 2nd ed. Philadelphia, Saunders, 1980, p 183.

TABLE 15–4. SECONDARY B CELL DISORDERS

Disorder	B Cell
Infection	
Rubella (congenital)	May have hypogammaglobulinemia or selective immunoglobulin deficiencies; no response to rubella immunization; decreased response to multiple antigens
Leprosy	Decreased B cells in some, increased in others; increased antibody
Chronic infection	Increased immunoglobulins
Congenital cytomegalovirus	Elevated IgM, IgA
Malignancy	
Hodgkin's disease	Immunoglobulins normal to increased; decreased antibody response to certain antigens
Acute leukemia	Variable immunoglobulin levels
Chronic leukemia	Variable immunoglobulin levels
Nonlymphoid	Variable immunoglobulin levels
Myeloma	Impaired antibody response; decreased immunoglobulins
Autoimmune disease	
Systemic lupus erythematosus	Immunoglobulins usually elevated; increased antibody titers to multiple antigens
Rheumatoid arthritis	Immunoglobulin levels usually increased, normal antibody response to antigens
Chronic active hepatitis	Immunoglobulins increased
Protein-losing states	
Nephrotic syndrome	Decreased IgG; IgM and IgA may be decreased; antibody response decreased
Protein-losing enteropathy	Hypogammaglobulinemia frequent
Other disorders	
Burns	Decrease in all immunoglobulins; normal antibody response
Sarcoidosis	Increased immunoglobulins; normal antibody response
Splenectomy	Immunoglobulins normal; decreased antibody response to whole organisms; normal antibody response to purified antigens
Sickle cell disease	IgM may be decreased; decreased antibody response to whole organisms with normal response to purified antigens
Aging	Increased IgG (IgA in some); increased B cells; decreased IgG response to certain antigens

PHA, phytohemagglutinin stimulation of lymphocyte; MLC, allogeneic cell stimulation of lymphocytes.
Adapted from Ammann AJ: Immunodeficiency diseases. In Sites DP, Stubo JD, Fudenberg HH, Wells JW (eds): Basic and Clinical Immunology, 6th ed. Los Altos, CA, Appleton & Lange, 1987.

complement system to amplify opsonization or lysis. Antibodies have a second disadvantage: response to a new antigen requires a complicated cellular response, so that antibodies may not be detected for many days. A far more primitive and nonspecific humoral defense mechanism is the complement system. This comprises a number of components always present within the circulation, which can be activated by a variety of microbial and other stimuli. It can act independent of, as well as in concert with, the humoral and cellular immune systems.

Complement Components

Complement is not a single substance; it is a group of proteins in blood and interstitial fluid with smaller quantities on mucosal surfaces. The components themselves are listed in Table 15–5. All are inactive and without known biologic activity prior to activation.

Interaction of these normally inactive substances with microbial cell surfaces or antigen-antibody complexes leads to the formation of several proteolytic enzymes, which cleave other components, forming new enzymes until a cascade of reactive substances is produced. Two pathways of activation have been described—the classic pathway and the alternate (properdin) pathway. The early events in the two pathways are not the same but both converge at the third complement component (C3) to a final common pathway (Fig. 15–3). In the classic pathway, the initiators (see Table 15–5) interact with antigen-antibody complexes leading to C3 activation; in the alternate pathway, the initiators (see Table 15–5) interact with other plasma factors, which then activate C3. Figure 15–4 schematically outlines the classic pathways and the common pathway leading to cell lysis; however, most antimicrobial activity related to complement activation does not derive from direct bacteriolysis through either pathway. The ultimate effect of activation of the C3–9 terminal cascade is multifold: vasodilation, chemotaxis of phagocytic leukocytes into the contaminated region, and opsonization of

TABLE 15–5. MOLECULAR WEIGHTS AND SERUM CONCENTRATIONS OF COMPLEMENT COMPONENTS

Component	Molecular Weight (daltons)	Serum Concentration[a] (μg/ml)
Initiators		
Classic pathway		
C1q	400,000	180
C1r	180,000	?
C1s	86,000	110
C2	117,000	25
C4	206,000	640
Alternate pathway		
Initiating factor (IF)	150,000	?
Properdin	184,000	25
Properdin factor B	93,000	200
Properdin factor D	24,000	?
Effectors		
C3	180,000	1,600
C5	180,000	80
C6	95,000	75
C7	110,000	55
C8	163,000	80
C9	79,000	230
Inhibitors		
C1	90,000	180
C3b inactivator	100,000	25
C6	?	?
C3a, C5a inactivator	300,000	?

[a] Serum concentrations given are the means in adults.
From Root RK, Ryan JL: Humoral immunity and complement. In Mandell GL, Douglas RG Jr, Bennett JE (eds): Principles and Practice of Infectious Diseases, 2nd ed. New York, Wiley, 1985, p 31.

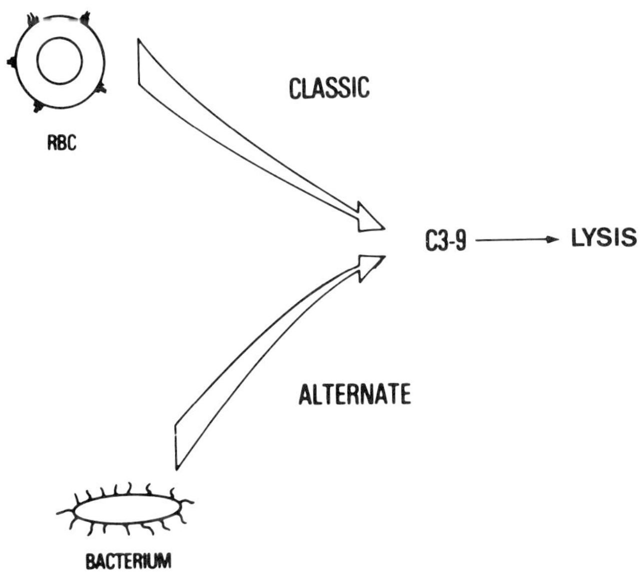

Figure 15–3. Two pathways of complement activation converge at the level of the complement component C3. These pathways then engage C5–C9 and lead to lysis of bacteria or sensitized erythrocytes (RBCs). *(Adapted from Frank MM. Rev Infect Dis 1:483, 1979.)*

the microbes so that augmented phagocytosis can take place (Fig. 15–5).

The Classic Pathway

The Initiating Events. Activation of complement components proceeds by a highly ordered sequence of events.[70,71] The usual initial event for activation of the classic pathway is the interaction of the components of Cl with the Fc fragment of one molecule of IgM combined with antigen on a cell surface, or two molecules of IgG side by side (a so-called antibody doublet) (Figs. 15–6 and 15–7). Binding of antibody to antigen effects a conformational change in the antibody molecule, exposing the complement-fixing domain of the Fc fragment for interaction with either Clq or Fc receptors on phagocytic cells. IgA, IgE, IgD, and some types of Ig do not bind Cl efficiently (human IgG_4 and IgA) and therefore do not activate the classic complement pathway. Although most microorganisms that activate complement do so directly through the alternative pathway (see Fig. 15–5) via their cell membranes, under some circumstances some microorganisms (lipid A or endotoxin, staphylococcal protein A) or plasmin may activate Cl and thus the classic pathway directly without participation of antibody.[72]

Cl is itself a complicated molecular complex, composed of three subunits termed Clq, Clr, and Cls. The complex interactions of Cl with C4 have been diagrammed by Frank (see Fig. 15–5). The activation of Cl leads to the activation of C2 in a manner similar to that by which C4 is activated (see Fig. 15–7). C2 is cleaved by enzymatic action of $C\bar{1}$ into two components, C2 and C2b. C2b is released into the environment, and C2a binds to C4b on the cell surface (see Fig. 15–6). The $\overline{C4b2a}$ complex (classic C3 convertase) in turn activates C3, leading to the release of C3a with its multiple biologic activities (chemotaxis, vasodilation) and to $C3\bar{b}$, which binds to the cell surface and is an opsonin for phagocytes (see Table 15–6).

One essential to the understanding of the complement cascade is the fact that the cascade itself acts as an amplification system, so that the binding of only a few molecules of antibody permits the activation of large amounts of the complement through enzymatic mechanisms. Amplification occurs at two important points along the cycle: (1) activated $C\bar{1}$ enzymatically cleaves many molecules of C4, so that many molecules of $C4\bar{b}$ are deposited on the cell membrane for each molecule of antibody; and (2) many C3b molecules are produced. C3b is the most critical molecule in the whole cascade [see Effectors of the Complement Cascade (C3–9)].

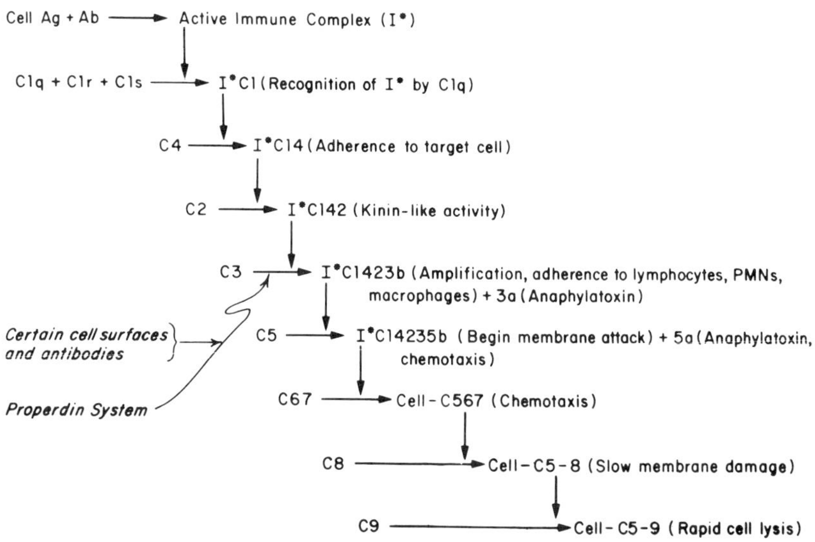

Figure 15–4. The complement pathways and the biologic activity released at each step. The classic pathway begins with a specific antigen-antibody reaction. The alternate pathway is triggered by a more nonspecific interaction between cell surfaces and the molecules that comprise the properdin system. Both pathways, however, converge at the C3 step, where most of the biologic activity associated with complement activation begins. Amplification also occurs at several steps, but it is greatest at C3. The subsequent steps lead to the molecular condensation of the target cell surface (I*), which ultimately results in membrane damage and lysis. There are several other important consequences of complement activation. The presence of these molecules on the target cell surface makes them adherent to other cells. Macrophages, platelets, polymorphonuclear leukocytes, and lymphocytes adhere and increase the damage to the target cells. The steps through C5 are largely enzymatic in nature; the C3 and C5 components, for example, are split during activation, releasing chemotactic and vasoactive molecules (anaphylatoxins). Attachment of the C5b molecule to the cell begins the condensation ending in membrane damage; this seems to occur away from the immune complex. Interaction of the C6, C7 components results additionally in the release of another chemotactic factor. The activation of the complement pathway therefore contributes to many of the features seen in infection: cellular infiltrates, adherent PMNs and platelets, thrombosed vessels, interstitial edema, and cellular damage. *(From Simmons RL, Foker JE, Lower RR, Najarian JS: Transportation. In Schwartz SI, Shires GT, Spencer FC, Storer EH (eds): Principles of Surgery, 3rd ed. New York, McGraw-Hill, 1979, pp 383–473.)*

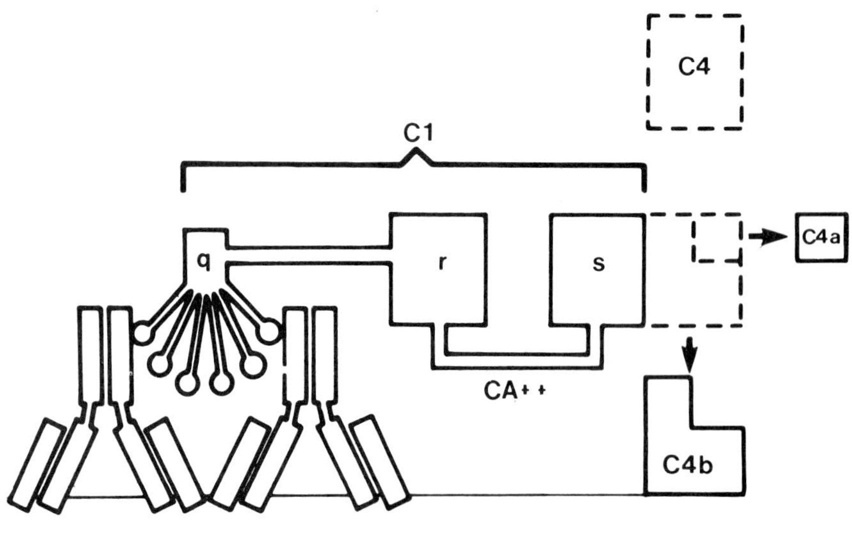

Figure 15–5. Detail of the earliest steps in the classic complement pathway. Shown is an IgG antibody doublet bound by its variable region combining sites to the membrane of a sensitized erythrocyte. The Fc fragments of the two IgG molecules are free to interact with a binding site on subunit q of C1. In the presence of calcium, subunits q, r, and s of C1 are held together in a macromolecular complex. Also shown is the fact that fluid-phase C4 can interact with C1s. This interaction leads to cleavage of C4 into a small fragment (C4a) and a larger fragment (C4b), which is bound by covalent bonds to the cell membrane. *(Adapted from Frank MM. Rev Infect Dis 1:483, 1979.)*

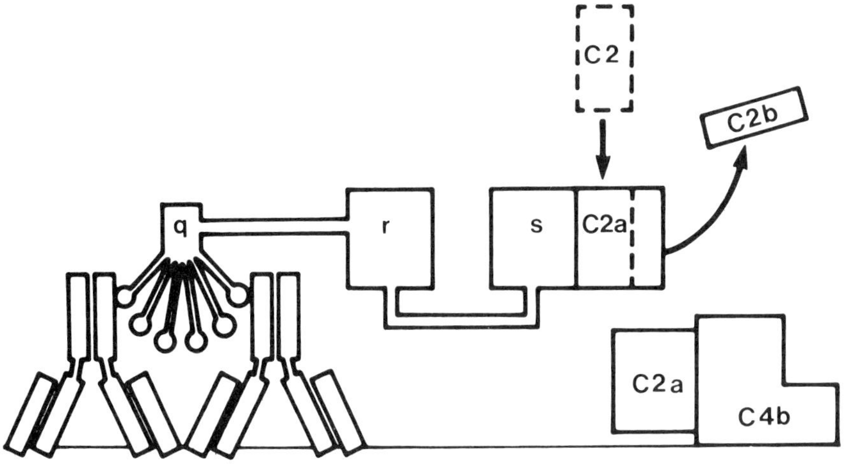

Figure 15–6. Further details of the activation of the classic complement pathway. In the presence of cell-bound C4b, the complex of immunoglobulin and activated C1 interacts with and cleaves C2 into two fragments. The smaller fragment, C2b, is released into the fluid phase. The larger fragment, C2a, associates with the cell-bound C4b to form a new enzyme complex composed of these two protein fragments and termed C3 convertase. *(From Frank MM. Rev Infect Dis 1:483, 1979.)*

The Alternate Pathway

Activators of the Alternate Complement Pathway. Microbial cell wall compounds (eg, gram-negative bacterial LPS, gram-positive bacterial polysaccharides, teichoic acid, and fungal zymosan and glucan), other types of complex polysaccharides, and aggregates of Ig have all been shown to be capable of activating this pathway. The alternate pathway is probably the major pathway of activation of the terminal complement components when antibody is absent.[73,74]

The Initiators. Table 15–5 includes a list of the four initiators of the alternate pathway. Each is somewhat analogous to one of the classic pathway initiators.

Properdin factor D is analogous to Cl; properdin factor B is analogous to C2. To activate D, one requires an initiating factor, properdin (P), in conjunction with one of the activators described in the previous section. In addition, $C3\bar{b}$ is required. It is obvious that some C3b must be formed before the alternate pathway can be initiated. This may be a function of other proteolytic enzymes, including plasmin and neutrophil lysozomal proteases. Thus small amounts of factor B are present owing to slow but continual cleavage by $\bar{D}$. This produces Bb, which binds to C3. The $\overline{C3Bb}$ complex also slowly produces ongoing low-level cleavage of C3 to produce small amounts of C3b. Figure 15–6 demonstrates the interaction of B, $\bar{D}$, and cell-bound $C3\bar{b}$. $\overline{C3bBb}$ (alternate C3 convertase) is capable of cleaving C3 into C3a and $C3\bar{b}$ as in the classic pathway. $\bar{D}$ and P act to stabilize the $\overline{C3bBb}$ complex.

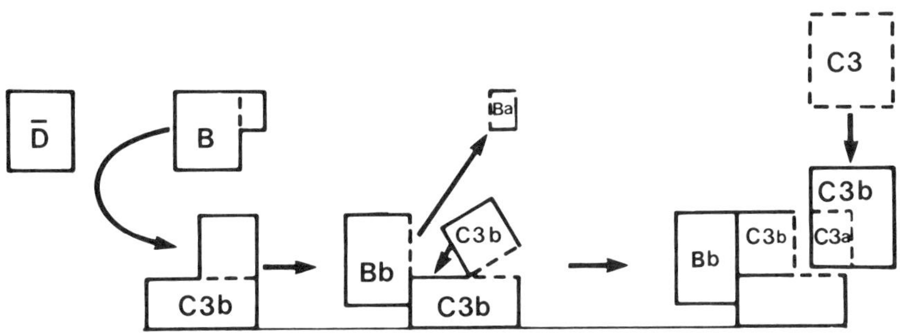

Figure 15–7. Schematic analysis of alternate pathway activation. Cell-bound C3b can interact with properdin factor B in the presence of activated properdin factor D. Activation is shown by a superscript bar. The factor B is cleaved into two fragments, Bb and Ba. The Ba is released into the fluid phase. Bb binds to C3b. Here, it is shown as causing an allosteric change in C3b such that the combination of Bb and C3b forms a protein configuration analogous to the complex of C4b and C2a. This complex, like the classic pathway convertase, is capable of coordinating with C3 and cleaving it into two fragments, C3a and C3b. *(From Frank MM. Rev Infect Dis 1:483, 1979.)*

TABLE 15–6. BIOLOGIC EFFECTS OF COMPLEMENT FRAGMENTS RELEASED DURING SEQUENTIAL ACTIVATION OF THE SYSTEM

Mediator	Effect
C4a	Release of serotonin
C2b	Kinin-like activity
C4b	Immune adherence
C3a	Anaphylatoxin, vascular effect; chemotaxis; leukocyte mobilization
C3b	Opsonization; immune adherence; release of platelet factor 3
C5a	Most potent chemotactic factor
C5b	May attach to platelets and cause platelet lysis
$\overline{C5b67}$	Chemotaxis
$\overline{C8}$	Initiates lytic process; inserted into membrane
$\overline{C9}$	Completes lytic process

Adapted from Alexander JW, Good RA: Fundamentals of Clinical Immunology. Philadelphia, Saunders, 1977, p 80.

Effectors of the Complement Cascade (C3–9) (See Table 15–6)

C3b. Although Clq and C4b may neutralize some viruses, the distal complement components are responsible for most of the biologic effects of the cascade. The C3b molecule is the critical one:

1. The C3b molecule acts to amplify the system by being produced in large quantity and serving as an enzyme cleaving further C3 molecules into C3a and C3b.
2. It serves as a key subcomponent with properdin factor $\overline{B}$, leading to even further formation of C3b through C3 cleavage via the alternate pathway (see Fig. 15–7).
3. It mounts a proteolytic attack on the C5 molecule, perpetuating the cascade.
4. Interaction of C3b with B lymphocytes may also mediate the release of lymphokines from the lymphocytes, thereby recruiting other cells into the inflammatory response.
5. Most importantly, $C3\overline{b}$ is the most potent biologic opsonin. Phagocytic neutrophils and both fixed tissue and wandering macrophages possess cell surface receptors for C3b, enabling bacteria to be phagocytosed and killed.

Despite the essential role of C3b in the opsonization of microbes for phagocytosis by phagocytes, the mere binding of C3b on the microbe to the C3b receptor does not guarantee that phagocytosis will occur. Even this process can be amplified by either activation of the macrophages or a few molecules of specific IgG or IgM bound to the cell surface. Otherwise, the presence of C3b inactivator can interfere with normal phagocytosis (see Inhibitors and Regulators of Complement Activation).

Lysis of Bacteria. When C3b is deposited on the surface of a microbe in proximity to $\overline{C4bC2a}$ (or the analogous $\overline{C3bBb}$) (see Fig. 15–7), C5 is cleaved into two fragments. C5a is released into the fluid phase, and C5b binds to the cell surface where it interacts with C6 and C7 to produce a $\overline{C5b67}$ complex on the cell membrane. This complex is not an enzyme but is actually inserted into the lipid bilayer of the cell membrane. This complex in turn binds C8 and then C9. The interaction leads to the formation of a damaged site or lesion in the surface of the cell, through which osmotically active materials are able to pass with ultimate osmotic lysis.

Inflammatory Mediators. C3a and C5a are soluble cleavage products of C3 and C5, respectively. They share similar properties: both are chemotactic for neutrophils and macrophages (C5a > C3a), and both are anaphylotoxins, acting as vasodilators and releasing histamine from basophils and most cells (C3a > C5a). In addition, C5a can trigger a respiratory burst from phagocytic cells. The $\overline{C5b67}$ complex seems to possess some chemotactic properties as well (see Table 15–6).

Inhibitors and Regulators of Complement Activation

At first glance, it would seem that complement activation would be a self-perpetuating system in which ultimate depletion of complement components would be an inevitable consequence. This does not normally occur. There are several mechanisms by which the complement cascade is regulated. For example, C4b is loosely bound to target cells, and, when released, it loses biologic activity. Its activity can be perpetuated only if it is continually produced by Cl esterase. In addition, there are inhibitors of the complement system within serum (see Table 15–5).

1. Cl esterase inhibitor can enzymatically disrupt $Cl\overline{qrs}$ by binding to Cls. If Cls esterase inhibitor is absent, hereditary angioneurotic edema results.[75]
2. C3b inactivator cleaves $C3\overline{b}$ into two inactive components, C3c and C3d. $C3\overline{b}$ can be attacked even when bound to cells. Since

C3̄b is the critical component in the perpetuation of the cascade, C3b inactivator is the most potent inhibitor of the system. When C3b inactivator is missing, C3 becomes depleted and is present only at very low levels, and such patients are severely susceptible to bacterial infections.

3. There are also inhibitors of C6, C3a, and C5a in serum (see Table 15–5).

Adverse Effects of Complement Activation

Similar to many other host defense mechanisms, activation of the complement cascade plays an important role in the pathogenesis of some of the secondary adverse effects of systemic infection. For example, the activation of complement within the blood can lead to a number of damaging effects: disseminated intravascular coagulation, vasodilation, and shock. Platelets and leukocytes become aggregated and adherent to blood vessel walls and are trapped within capillaries within critical areas of blood flow. Complement-stimulated leukocytes within the circulation or trapped within capillary beds release a variety of mediators (eg, lysosomal enzymes, superoxide and hydroxyl residues) that may exert deleterious effects on host tissues. This not only depletes essential complement components and leukocytes necessary for localization, opsonization, and lysis of the microbes but may be associated with the development of hypotension, altered pulmonary capillary permeability (shock lung), and intravascular disseminated coagulation. Furthermore, in diseases in which antigen-antibody complexes circulate, tissue damage occurs because of complement activation at sites of antigen-antibody deposition (eg, the renal glomerulae and joints). In short, many of the secondary effects of infections are mediated by the complement cascade being activated to an excessive degree.

Defects of the Complement System and the Consequences to Host Defense

Table 15–7 lists the known defects in the complement system as summarized by Root.[2] Patients with recurrent infections should be screened for complement deficiencies, the most serious of which is C3 deficiency.[76] Absence of this pivotal component results in recurrent infections with encapsulated and gram-negative bacteria—a picture similar to that seen in agammaglobulinemia. C3 deficiency is a rare congenital disorder, but acquired deficiencies caused by decreased production (eg, liver disease) or excessive utilization (eg, C3b inactivator deficiency, lupus erythematosus) have been described.

TABLE 15–7. DEFECTS OF THE COMPLEMENT SYSTEM AND CONSEQUENCES TO HOST DEFENSE

Component	Associated Diseases	Effects on Host Defenses[a]
C1		
C1q	Combined immunodeficiency	Major[b]
C1r	Systemic lupus erythematosus (SLE), glomerulonephritis	Minor[b]
C1s	SLE	Minor[b]
C1 inhibitor	Hereditary angioedema	None
C4	SLE	Minor[b]
C2	None, discoid lupus erythematosus, SLE, anaphylactoid purpura, Hodgkin's, dermatomyositis, congenital with bacterial infections	Minor[b] to none
C3	Hereditary deficiencies, cirrhosis, SLE, nephritis, immune complex disorders	Major[b,c]
C3b inactivator	Bacterial infections	Major[c]
C5	SLE, bacterial infections	Major[c]
C5 "dysfunction"	Bacterial infections, diarrhea, eczema (Leiner's syndrome)	Major[c]
C6	None, neisserial infections	Minor[b]
C7	None, Raynaud's, neisserial infections	Minor[c]
C8	None, SLE, neisserial infections	Minor[c]
Alternate pathway	Sickle cell disease, splenectomy (?)	Major[b,c]

[a] Major effects on host defenses are manifest by severe, recurrent bacterial infections, whereas minor effects are marked by infrequent infections.
[b] Effects on host defense appear to be mediated as much or more by the associated disease rather than by the complement deficiency per se.
[c] Effects on host defense are mediated primarily by the complement deficiency.
Adapted from Root RK, Ryan JL: Humoral immunity and complement. In Mandell GL, Douglas RG Jr, Bennett JE (eds): Principles and Practice of Infectious Diseases, 2nd ed. New York, Wiley, 1985, p 35.

C5 deficiency has been discovered in several patients who behave similar to patients with hypogammaglobulinemia with recurrent infections of the upper and lower respiratory tracts. Alexander et al[77] have described a state of consumptive opsonopathy, an acquired syndrome in which the opsonin is depleted by repeated or continuous gram-negative bacteremia.

REFERENCES

1. Fitch FW: Selective suppression of immune responses: regulation of antibody formation and cell-mediated immunity by antibody. Prog Allergy 19:195, 1975.
2. Root RK: Humoral immunity of complement. In Mandell GL, Douglas RG, Bennett JF (eds): Principles and Practice of Infectious Diseases, 2nd ed, New York, Wiley, 1985, p 21.
3. Alexander JW, Good RA (eds): The immunoglobulins. In Fundamentals of Clinical Immunology. Philadelphia, Saunders, 1977, p 69.
4. Ganguly R, Waldman RH: Local immunity and local immune responses. Prog Allergy 27:1, 1980.
5. Burritt MF, Calvanico NJ, Mehta S, Tomasi TB Jr: Activation of the classical complement pathway by Fc fragment of human IgA. J Immunol 118:723, 1977.
6. Adinolfi M, Glynn AA, Lindsay M, Milne CM: Serological properties of IgA antibodies to *Escherichia coli* present in human colostrum. Immunology 10:517, 1966.
7. Burdon DW: The bactericidal action of immunoglobulin. Am J Med Microbiol 6:131, 1973.
8. Freter R: Mechanism of action of intestinal antibody in experimental cholera, II. Antibody-mediated antibacterial reaction at the mucosal surface. Infect Immun 2:556, 1970.
9. Perkins JC, Tucker DN, Knopf HLS, et al: Comparison of protective effect of neutralizing antibody in serum and nasal secretions in experimental rhinovirus type 13 illness. Am J Epidemiol 90:519, 1969.
10. Regamey RH, Hennessen W, Hulse EC, Perkins FT: International symposium on vaccination of man and animals by the nonparenteral route. Proc 14th Int Congr Int Assoc of Biol Standardizations, Douglas, Isle of Man, 1975. Dev Biol Standard, Vol 33, Basel, Karger, 1976.
11. Ammann AJ, Hong R: Selective IgA deficiency and autoimmunity. Clin Exp Immunol 7:833, 1970.
12. Strober W, Krakauer R, Klaeveman HL, et al: Secretory component deficiency: a disorder of the IgA immune system. N Engl J Med 294:351, 1976.
13. Bolan G, Broome CV, Facklam RR, et al: Pneumococcal vaccine efficacy in selected populations in the United States. Ann Intern Med 104:1, 1986.
14. LaForce FM, Eickhoff TC: Pneumococcal vaccine: the evidence mounts. Ann Intern Med 104:110, 1986.
15. Schwartz JS: Pneumococcal vaccine: clinical efficacy and effectiveness. Ann Intern Med 96:208, 1982.
16. Shapiro ED, Clemens JD: A controlled evaluation of the protective efficacy of pneumococcal vaccine for patients at high risk of serious pneumococcal infections. Ann Intern Med 101:325, 1984.
17. Dienstag JL, Werner BG, Polk BF, et al: Hepatitis B vaccine in health care personnel: safety, immunogenicity, and indicators of efficacy. Ann Intern Med 101:34, 1984.
18. Stevens CE, Alter HJ, Taylor PE, et al: Hepatitis B vaccine in patients receiving hemodialysis: immunogenicity and efficacy. N Engl J Med 311:496, 1984.
19. Hepatitis B vaccine. Health and Public Policy Committee, American College of Physicians. Ann Intern Med 100:149, 1984.
20. Recommendations for protection against viral hepatitis: Recommendation of the Immunization Practices Advisory Committee, Centers for Disease Control, Department of Health and Human Services. Ann Intern Med 103:391, 1985.
21. McCabe WR, Bruins SC, Craven DE, Johns M: Cross-reactive antigens: their potential for immunization-induced immunity to gram-negative bacteria. J Infect Dis 136:S161, 1977.
22. Young LS, Stevens P: Cross-protective immunity to gram-negative bacilli: studies with core glycolipid of *Salmonella minnesota* and antigens of *Streptococcus pneumoniae.* J Infect Dis 136:S174, 1977.
23. Pennington JE, Menkes E: Type-specific vs. cross-protective vaccination for gram-negative bacterial pneumonia. J Infect Dis 144:599, 1981.
24. LaForce FM, Boose DS, Mills DM: Heightened lung bactericidal activity in mice after aerosol immunization with Re 595 *Salmonella minnesota:* importance of cellular rather than humoral factors. J Infect Dis 142:421, 1980.
25. Alexander JW, Fisher MW, MacMillan BG, Altemeier WA: Prevention of invasive pseudomonas infection in burns with a new vaccine. Arch Surg 99:249, 1969.
26. Jones RJ, Roe EA, Gupta JL: Low mortality in burned patients in a *Pseudomonas* vaccine trial. Lancet 2:401, 1972.
27. Pennington JE: Preliminary investigations of *Pseudomonas aeruginosa* vaccine in patients with leukemia and cystic fibrosis. J Infect Dis 130:S159, 1974.
28. Langford DT, Hiller J: Prospective, controlled study of a polyvalent pseudomonas vaccine in cystic fibrosis—three year results. Arch Dis Child 59:1131, 1984.
29. Polk HC Jr, Borden S, Aldrete JA: Prevention of pseudomonas respiratory infection in a surgical intensive care unit. Ann Surg 177:607, 1973.
30. Condie RM, O'Reilly RJ: Prevention of cytomegalovirus infection by prophylaxis with an intravenous, hyperimmune, native, unmodified cytomegalovirus globulin: randomized trial in bone marrow transplant recipients. Am J Med 76:134, 1984.
31. Kreger BE, Craven DE, Carling PC, McCabe WR: Gram-negative bacteremia, III. Reassessment of etiology, epidemiology and ecology in 612 patients. Am J Med 68:332, 1980.
32. Myerowitz RL, Medeiros AA, O'Brien TF: Recent experience with bacillemia due to gram-negative organisms. J Infect Dis 124:239, 1971.
33. Kreger BE, Craven DE, McCabe WR: Gram-negative bacteremia, IV. Re-evaluation of clinical features and treatment in 612 patients. Am J Med 68:344, 1980.
34. Bryan CS, Reynolds KL, Brenner ER: Analysis of

1,186 episodes of gram-negative bacteremia in non-university hospitals: the effects of antimicrobial therapy. Rev Infect Dis 5:629, 1983.
35. Wardlaw AC: Possible reasons for the inefficiency of gram-negative bacterial vaccines. Prog Immunobiol Standard 5:508, 1972.
36. Chedid L, Parant M, Boyer F: A proposed mechanism for natural immunity to enterobacterial pathogens. J Immunol 100:292, 1968.
37. Tate WJ, Douglas H, Braude AI: Protection against lethality of *E. coli* endotoxin with "O" antiserum. Ann NY Acad Sci 133:746, 1966.
38. Dunn DL, Bogard WC Jr, Cerra FB: Enhanced survival during murine gram-negative bacterial sepsis by use of a murine monoclonal antibody. Arch Surg 120:50, 1985.
39. Kirkland TN, Ziegler EJ: An immunoprotective monoclonal antibody to lipopolysaccharide. J Immunol 132:2590, 1984.
40. Kunin CM: Separation, characterization and biological significance of a common antigen in Enterobacteriaceae. J Exp Med 118:565, 1963.
41. McCabe WR, Greely A: Common enterobacterial antigen, II. Effect of immunization on challenge with heterologous bacilli. Infect Immun 7:386, 1973.
42. Mattsby-Baltzer I, Hanson LA, Olling S, Kaijser B: Experimental *Escherichia coli* ascending pyelonephritis in rats: active peroral immunization with live *Escherichia coli*. Infect Immun 35:647, 1982.
43. Mattsby-Baltzer I, Claesson I, Hanson LA, et al: Antibodies to lipid A during urinary tract infection. J Infect Dis 144:319, 1981.
44. Rietschel ET, Galanos C: Lipid A antiserum-mediated protection against lipopolysaccharide- and lipid A-induced fever and skin necrosis. Infect Immun 15:34, 1977.
45. Luderitz O, Staub AM, Westphal O: Immunochemistry of O and R antigens of *Salmonella* and related Enterobacteriaceae. Bacteriol Rev 30:192, 1966.
46. Schmidt G, Fromme I, Mayer H: Immunochemical studies on core lipopolysaccharides of Enterobacteriaceae of different genera. Eur J Biochem 14:357, 1970.
47. Braude AI, Ziegler EJ, Douglas H, McCutchan JA: Antibody to cell wall glycolipid of gram-negative bacteria: induction of immunity to bacteremia and endotoxemia. J Infect Dis 136:S167, 1977.
48. Dunn DL, Ferguson R: Immunotherapy of gram negative bacterial sepsis: enhanced survival in a guinea pig model by use of rabbit antiserum to *Escherichia coli* J-5. Surgery 92:212, 1982.
49. Dunn DL, Mach PA, Condie RM, Cerra FB: Anti-core endotoxin $(F(ab')_2$ equine immunoglobulin fragments protect against lethal effects of gram-negative bacterial sepsis. Surgery 96:440, 1984.
50. Johns M, Skehill A, McCabe WR: Immunization with rough mutants of *Salmonella minnesota*, IV. Protection by antisera to O and rough antigens against endotoxin. J Infect Dis 147:57, 1983.
51. Dunn DL, Mach PA, Cerra FB, Ferguson RM: The role of heparin in guinea pig gram negative bacterial sepsis. J Surg Res 34:479, 1983.
52. Dunn DL, Mach PA, Dalmasso AP, et al: Protection from the metabolic derangements of gram negative bacterial sepsis by use of *E. coli* J5 antiserum. J Surg Res 38:298, 1985.
53. Dunn DL, Mach PA, Cerra FB: Monoclonal antibodies protect against lethal effects of gram-negative bacterial sepsis. Surg Forum 32:142, 1983.
54. Dunn DL, Bogard WC, Cerra FB: Efficacy of type specific and cross-reactive murine monoclonal antibodies directed against endotoxin during experimental sepsis. Surgery 98:283, 1985.
55. Nelles JW, Niswander CA: Mouse monoclonal antibodies reactive with J5 lipopolysaccharide exhibit extensive serological cross-reactivity with a variety of gram-negative bacteria. Infect Immun 46:677, 1984.
56. Mutharia LM, Crockford G, Bogard WC Jr, Hancock REW: Monoclonal antibodies specific for *Escherichia coli* J5 lipopolysaccharide: cross-reaction with other gram-negative bacterial species. Infect Immun 45: 631, 1984.
57. Dunn D: Antibody immunotherapy of gram-negative bacterial sepsis in an immunosuppressed animal model. Transplantation 45:424, 1988.
58. Priest B, Brinson D, Schroeder D, Dunn D: Treatment of experimental gram-negative bacterial sepsis with murine monoclonal antibodies directed against lipopolysaccharide. Surgery 106:147, 1989.
59. Zinner SH, McCabe WR: Effects of IgM and IgG antibody in patients with bacteremia due to gram-negative bacilli. J Infect Dis 133:37, 1976.
60. Pollack M, Huang AI, Prescott RK, et al: Enhanced survival in *Pseudomonas aeruginosa* septicemia associated with high levels of circulating antibody to *Escherichia coli* endotoxin core. J Clin Invest 72:1874, 1983.
61. McCabe WR, Kreger BE, Johns M: Type-specific and cross-reactive antibodies in gram-negative bacteremia. N Engl J Med 287:261, 1972.
62. Law BJ, Marks MI: Age-related prevalence of human serum IgG and IgM antibody to the core glycolipid of *Escherichia coli* strain J5, as measured by ELISA. J Infect Dis 151:988, 1985.
63. Ziegler EJ, McCutchan JA, Fierer J, et al: Treatment of gram-negative bacteremia and shock with human antiserum to a mutant *Escherichia coli*. N Engl J Med 307:1225, 1982.
64. Lachman E, Pitsoe SB, Gaffin SL: Anti-lipopolysaccharide immunotherapy in management of septic shock of obstetric and gynaecological origin. Lancet 1:981, 1984.
65. McCutchan JA, Wolf JL, Ziegler EJ, Braude AI: Ineffectiveness of single-dose human antiserum to core glycolipid (*E. coli* J5) for prophylaxis of bacteremic, gram-negative infections in patients with prolonged neutropenia. Schweiz Med Wochenschr 113S:40, 1983.
66. Baumgartner JD, McCutchan JA, Van Melle G, et al:

Prevention of gram-negative shock and death in surgical patients by antibody to endotoxin core glycolipid. Lancet 1:59, 1985.
67. Ziegler E, Fisher C, Sprung C, et al: Treatment of gram-negative bacteremia and septic shock with HA-1A human monoclonal antibody against endotoxin. N Engl J Med 324:429, 1991.
68. Greenman R, Schein R, Martin M, et al: A controlled clinical trial of E5 murine monoclonal IgM antibody to endotoxin in the treatment of gram-negative sepsis. The XOMA Sepsis Study Group. JAMA 266:1097, 1991.
69. Wenzel R, Bone R, Fein A, et al: Results of a second double-blind, randomized, controlled trial of antiendotoxin antibody E5 in gram-negative sepsis, In: Program and Abstracts of the 31st Interscience Conference on Antimicrobial Agents and Chemotherapy. Chicago, American Society for Microbiology, 1991, p 294.
70. Dunn DL: Infection. In Greenfield LJ (ed): Surgery: Scientific Principles and Practice. Philadelphia, Lippincott, 1992, pp 148–170.
71. Dunn DL, Simmons RL: Surgical infections. In Fischer JE (ed): Surgical Basic Science. St. Louis, Mosby–Year Book, 1993, pp 171–203.
72. Cooper NR, Morrison DC: Binding and activation of the first component of human complement by the lipid A region of lipopolysaccharides. J Immunol 120:1862, 1978.
73. Frank MM: The complement system in host defense and inflammation. Rev Infect Dis 1:483, 1979.
74. Götze O, Müller-Eberhard HJ: The alternative pathway of complement activation. Adv Immunol 24:1, 1976.
75. Donaldson VH, Evans RR: A biochemical abnormality in hereditary angioneurotic edema: absence of serum inhibitor of Cl-esterase. Am J Med 35:37, 1963.
76. Alper CA, Abramson N, Johnston RB Jr, et al: Increased susceptibility to infection associated with abnormalities of complement-mediated functions and of the third component of complement (C3). N Engl J Med 282:349, 1970.
77. Alexander JW, McClellan MA, Ogle CK, Ogle JD: Consumptive opsoninopathy: possible pathogenesis in lethal and opportunistic infections. Ann Surg 184: 672, 1976.

BIBLIOGRAPHY

Burd RS, Cody CS, Dunn DL: Immunotherapy of Gram-Negative Bacterial Sepsis. Austin, TX, Medical Intelligence Unit. RG Landes Company, 1992.

Eisen HN: Immunology: An Introduction to Molecular and Cellular Principles of the Immune Response, 2nd ed. New York, Harper & Row, 1980.

Soluble Cytokine and Hormonal Mediators of Immunity and Inflammation

CHAPTER 16

Stephen F. Lowry, Steve E. Calvano

The protection afforded against infection includes physical barriers, circulating and tissue-fixed phagocytic cells, cytotoxic T lymphocytes, and soluble circulating molecules, which serve to orchestrate and maintain immune function (see Chaps. 12 to 15). Some defense mechanisms, generally termed innate or natural immunity, are present prior to infectious challenge and are not enhanced by single or repeated exposure to foreign molecules. Alternatively, other components of the immune response are induced or amplified by antigen exposure. This so-called specific or acquired immunity is specific to the challenging antigen and also exhibits the capacity to increase the magnitude of immune response with each succeeding exposure to antigen.

Phylogenetically, primitive host responses to foreign molecules were mediated predominantly by natural immune mechanisms consisting of phagocytic cells. The subsequent appearance of lymphocyte effector cells in the vertebrate species served to enhance natural immunity. In many respects, the specific immune response has retained many of the features of natural immunity while also incorporating additional properties necessary for defense of the delicate vertebrate species from a hostile internal and external milieu. Secretory products of the natural immune system serve to modify and direct phagocytic cells of the natural immune system and lymphocytes of the specific immune system to sites of antigen exposure. At such sites cognate and noncognate interactions occur among cells of the two systems. The hallmark of the specific immune system is the capacity to recall prior encounters with foreign antigens, which, when not otherwise compromised by disease, permits increasingly enhanced defensive activity.

The orchestration of interactions between natural and specific immune systems requires a mechanism for regulating both the magnitude and duration of their individual and complementary functions. This purpose is served by a variety of soluble mediators, with the effector phases of both natural and specific immunity being directed, to a large extent, by proteins now commonly known as cytokines. These proteins are produced largely by mononuclear phagocytes during natural immune responses, often in direct response to microbe phagocytosis. These proteins are also secreted by T cells stimulated by antigen presentation (see Chap. 14). Several cytokines secreted by stimulated T lymphocytes serve to regulate the activation and expansion of lymphocyte subpopulations, while other T cell derived cytokines direct the activity of other inflammatory cells. The use of these and other cytokines for therapy is discussed in Chapter 29.

CYTOKINE PROPERTIES

Cytokines are polypeptides or glycoproteins of relatively low molecular weight. Although their monomeric form is generally less than or equal to 25 to 30 kD (kilodaltons), some exert their biologic activity in higher molecular weight oligomeric forms. At present, it appears that the production and secretion of most cytokines are of limited duration and that basal (constitutive) production is usually absent or occurs at very low levels. Furthermore, most cytokines are not stored as preformed molecules; hence their production requires new gene transcription and translation. The transcription of many cytokine genes generally results in an unstable messenger RNA (mRNA), thereby providing a potential mechanism for tight regulation of their appearance.

All cytokines exert their action by binding to specific cell surface receptors (K_d usually of 10^{-9} to 10^{-12} M). As opposed to many other peptide hormones, cytokine activity is generally exerted over a short distance by binding to the cell of its origin (autocrine influence) or a neighboring target cell (paracrine influence). Cytokines can often exert an influence on distal target cells (endocrine influence), although in most cases the detection of such proteins in the circulation more likely reflects excessive production of these mediators at the tissue level.

Once bound to target cells, the postreceptor actions of cytokines are exerted through second messenger systems. Such events usually result in an altered pattern of gene expression. Most cellular responses to cytokines require new mRNA transcription and are relatively slow. Many of these activities include altered cell proliferation, differentiation, or differentiated function. Hence many cytokine species also serve as growth factors for the regulation of cell division and most exert some influence on hematopoietic cells. Additionally, cytokines may influence both the production and action of other cytokines, permitting an additional degree of regulation for attenuation or amplification of their influences. The information in Tables 16–1 and 16–2 emphasizes the diversity of individual cytokine activities and demonstrates the number of functional properties shared by these mediators. The discussion below catalogues those cytokines that have received sufficient study to depict documented in vitro and purported in vivo immune functions (Tables 16–1 and 16–2). It is important to note that most cytokines are pleiotropic (ie, act on many targets to achieve diverse effects) and are redundant (ie, many cytokines seem to have the same effects as other cytokines). For example, IL-2, IL-4, IL-7, and IL-12 are all promoters of T cell growth, but each has differing effects on the T cell as well.

Cytokines Predominantly Produced by Mononuclear Phagocytes

Tumor Necrosis Factor. Tumor necrosis factor (TNF)[1–9] is the first cytokine known to be activated in the natural immune response to bacterial lipopolysaccharide. Although several cells, including activated T, natural killer (NK), and mast cells, are capable of producing this potent mediator, those of mononuclear phagocyte lineage appear to be the principal sources of TNF production. This cytokine can exert activity as both a transmembrane, cell-associated species as well as a secreted one (polymorphism). TNF binds to either of two specific cell receptors (see Table 16–1) with relatively low avidity and may exhibit differing characteristics at varying concentrations. At lower levels (10^{-9} M) it activates inflammatory neutrophils and monocytes to affect microbial killing, stimulates T and B cell function, and increases expression of class I MHC molecules. TNF further stimulates the production of the proinflammatory cytokines (IL-1) and specialized cytokines (such as IL-6 and IL-8) and enhances endothelial cell adhesiveness for leukocytes, thereby contributing to the recruitment of these activated cells to sites of inflammation and infection. These characteristics of TNF underscore the significant role of this cytokine in the process of host containment and eradication of microbes. These functions may likewise serve to recognize and contain malignant cells by both direct tumor lysis and inducing thrombosis of tumor blood vessels.

The benefit of TNF's systemic effects are not as obvious. Circulating TNF does promote some beneficial responses such as increased core temperature and hepatic acute phase protein production. However, the adverse systemic responses to excess TNF activity include hemodynamic collapse due to reduced vascular smooth muscle tone, reduced myocardial contractility, and activation of the coagulation cascade with associated intravascular thrombosis. The importance of TNF in shock has

TABLE 16–1. IN VITRO NATURAL AND ACQUIRED IMMUNE CYTOKINE FUNCTIONS[a]

Cytokine	Cell Source	Cell Target	Primary Effects Target	Receptor MW (kD)
Tumor necrosis factor	Mononuclear phagocyte, T cell	Neutrophil Endothelial cell T, B cell	Activation (inflammation) Activation (inflammation, coagulation) Costimulator	55, 75
Lymphotoxin	T cell	Neutrophil Endothelial cell	Activation Activation	55, 75
Interleukin-1α Interleukin-1β	Mononuclear phagocyte	T cell, B cell Endothelial cell	Costimulator Activation (inflammation, coagulation)	60, 80 60, 80
Interleukin-2	T_H1 cell	T cell NK cell B cell	Growth; cytokine production Growth, activation Growth, antibody synthesis	50, 64, 75
Interleukin-4	T_H2 cell	T cell B cell	Growth Activation and growth; Ig isotype and class switching	120
Interleukin-5	T_H2 cell	Eosinophil B cell	Activation Growth and activation	60, 130
Interleukin-6	Mononuclear phagocyte, endothelial cell, T cell	T cell, B cell, Mature B cell	Costimulator Growth	80+ (gp/30)
Interleukin-8 (chemokines)	Mononuclear phagocyte, endothelial cell; fibroblast; T cell; platelet	Leukocytes	Leukocyte activation and chemotaxis	59, 67
Interleukin-10	T_H2 cell B cell	NK, T cell T cell Mononuclear phagocyte	Inhibits IFNγ production Inhibits IL-1 production Inhibits TNF production	
Interleukin-12	Mononuclear macrophage B cell	T cell NK cell	Activation	
Type I interferons α Type I interferons β	Mononuclear phagocyte, other (α); fibroblast, other (β)	Diverse NK cell	Antiviral, antiproliferative, increased class I MHC expression Activation	α 95–110 β 95–110
Interferon-γ	$T_H{}^1$ cell NK cell	Mononuclear phagocyte Endothelial cell NK cell All	Activation	90, 95
Transforming growth factor β	T cell, mononuclear phagocyte	T cell Mononuclear phagocyte	Inhibit activation and proliferation Inhibit activation	

[a] MHC, major histocompatibility complex; NK, natural killer; kD, kilodalton; IFN, interferon; IL, interleukin; Ig, immunoglobulin. Includes those cytokines for which sufficient data currently exist.

TABLE 16–2. IN VIVO RESPONSES POTENTIALLY ATTRIBUTABLE TO INDIVIDUAL CYTOKINES[a]

Response	TNF	LT	IL-1	IL-2	IL-4	IL-5	IL-6	IL-8	IL-10	IFN-γ
Induce fever	Y		Y	Y						Y
Induce acute phase proteins	Y		Y				Y			Y
Shock	Y		Y	Y			Y		N	Y
Cachexia	Y	Y		Y	?					Y

[a] Several cytokines with ill-defined in vivo functions are not included here. Y, established activity; N, no evidence of activity; ?, variably reported activities.

been well documented by the protective influence of anti-TNF antibodies (or free TNF receptor species).

Interleukin 1. Interleukin 1 (IL-1)[10–15] shares many functions with TNF that are directed toward natural immunity and inflammatory responses. While IL-1 may be produced from LPS-activated mononuclear phagocytes or by TNF stimulation, it also arises from epithelial and endothelial cells. Cognate interactions between mononuclear phagocyte antigen-presenting cells and antigen-specific CD4+ T cells are also efficient stimuli of IL-1 production. Two species of bioactive IL-1 are produced (α and β), although these distinct gene products share only limited amino acid sequence homology. Both IL-1 precursor molecules are proteolytically cleaved by an enzyme that may serve as a target for their regulation. IL-1α may be active in a larger molecular weight (33 kD) form as well as the mature 17 kD protein. IL-1α may also exert biologic activity through a membrane-associated species, whereas IL-1β is active only in the more mature soluble (17 kD) form. A mechanism for IL-1 secretion is not evident from the structure of the native proteins. Hence circulating forms of IL-1 in vivo may be more indicative of severe cell injury or lysis rather than endogenous secretion. Nevertheless, both IL-1 species bind to either of two cell surface receptors. The mechanisms for postreceptor IL-1 activation remain controversial and several potential biochemical pathways, including that resulting in prostaglandin synthesis, may be activated.

Proliferation of CD4+ T cells and B cells is observed at lower levels of IL-1 activity. IL-1s also stimulate the production of other cytokine mediators, including IL-2, IL-6, and IL-8, as well as being inherently pyrogenic and promoting components of the acute phase reaction. These cytokines do not increase expression of class I MHC complexes nor do they exert direct anti-tumor effects or elicit severe tissue injury and systemic hemodynamic collapse.

An additional member of the IL-1 family that shares some structural homology to IL-1α and IL-1β has also been identified. Although this IL-1 species binds to the same receptors as IL-1α and IL-1β, it does not exert an agonist influence. Preclinical data would suggest that this so-called IL-1 receptor antagonist (IL-1RA) may even prevent some sequalae of severe endotoxinemia or sepsis at sufficiently high doses.

Interleukin 6. Interleukin 6 (IL-6)[16–19] is also produced by mononuclear phagocytes and other cell types in response to IL-1 and TNF. Unlike most other cytokines, IL-6 is more readily detected systemically after local injury and thus serves a more classic endocrine function. For example, in minimal soft tissue injuries IL-6 regulates several distinct components of the hepatic acute phase response as well as promotes B cell differentiation and costimulation of T cells. Recent data regarding direct IL-6 influences on the adverse host response to severe infection are unclear. It would appear that activation of an additional cell surface receptor complex (gp130) is necessary for the complete induction of cellular responses to this cytokine. Prior activation by TNF and/or IL-1s hence is contributory to the full expression of IL-6 activity.

Interleukin 8. Interleukin 8 (IL-8)[20–22] is derived from activated mononuclear phagocytes and T cells as well as platelets. IL-8 is the best characterized of a family of so-called chemokinetic mediators and has been shown to be chemotactic and activating for neutrophils. Like IL-6, this cytokine exhibits no inherent toxicity when administered exogenously.

Interleukin 10. Interleukin 10 (IL-10)[23–25] is a 35 to 40 kD cytokine secreted by mononuclear phagocytes and a subset of helper T cells (T_H2). It was originally called cytokine synthesis inhibitory factor (CSIF) because of its ability to inhibit monocyte/macrophage production of most proinflammatory cytokines including TNF, IL-1, IL-6, and IL-8. IL-10 also markedly attenuates T cell IFN-γ and IL-2 synthesis/secretion by T_H1 cells. Associated with IL-10-induced decreases in IFN-γ is downregulation of monocyte/macrophage class II MHC and suboptimal antigen-presenting functions. In addition, IL-10 may cause upregulation of IL-1RA, further contributing to inhibition of proinflammatory cytokine responses.

Interleukin 12. Interleukin 12 (IL-12)[26–29] was originally identified as a 70 kD glycoprotein present in the culture supernatant of a human B lymphoblastoid cell line. Subsequent work has indicated that mononuclear phagocytes are a major source of IL-12. When added to cultures of normal human mononuclear cells, this protein increases T cell IFN-γ production, enhances NK cell cytotoxicity, and markedly increases T cell proliferation. Because of its enhancing effects on NK cells, IL-12 was originally called NK cell stimulating factor (NKSF).

It should be apparent from these brief descriptions of IL-10 and IL-12 that these cytokines have somewhat opposing regulatory effects. Indeed, as will be discussed in a subsequent section on cytokine modulation of the immune response, IL-10 and IL-12, along with IL-4, play major roles in determining the relative balance of two different types of helper T cell responses, so-called T_H1 and T_H2 responses.

Cytokines Predominantly Produced by Lymphocytes

Type I Interferons. Type I interferons (IFN-α, IFN-β)[30,31] include two distinct proteins, one of which, IFN-α, is a family of nearly 20 related peptides. Mononuclear cells represent the major source of these proteins (leukocyte IFNs), while fibroblasts and other cells produce IFN-β (fibroblast IFN). The synthesis of IFN-α and IFN-β is elicited by both viral infection and antigen responses. While structurally unrelated, these IFNs bind to the same receptor and result in inhibition of viral replication and normal cell replication. Like TNF, these cytokines may also increase class I MHC expression and enhance NK cell activity.

Immune Interferon. Immune interferon (IFN-γ)[32–34] exhibits many activities of IFN-α and IFN-β, including antiviral and antiproliferative influences. IFN-γ is produced by both CD4+ and CD8+ T cells in response to antigen activation and IL-2. It binds to a separate cell receptor than do IFN-α and IFN-β and varies functionally from them in several important respects, including its direct influence on mononuclear phagocyte activation. It serves to induce the synthesis of enzymes necessary for the respiratory burst and hence is also a macrophage-activating factor. IFN-γ increases class II MHC expression and promotes differentiation of T and B cells and activation of NK cells.

Interleukin 2. Interleukin 2 (IL-2)[35–38] is produced by CD4+ and CD8+ T cells. Known principally as a cytokine responsible for promoting T cell growth, it serves these functions by both autocrine and paracrine actions. The quantity of IL-2 production by CD4+ cells defines the magnitude of antigen-induced immune responses. This cytokine also stimulates NK cell growth and function, resulting in the generation of so-called lymphokine-activated killer (LAK) cells. This property has been widely adapted to ex vivo and in vivo adoptive immunotherapy of certain malignancies. IL-2 binds in a complex manner to three cell surface receptors (α, β, γ), although growth is maximal when IL-2 cross-links all three receptors. Chronic or excessive T cell stimulation leads to shedding of IL-2 receptors, a fact that has led to use of this as a marker (like that recently proposed for TNF receptors) for excessive antigen stimulation, as in transplant rejection and burn sepsis.

Interleukin 4. Interleukin 4 (IL-4)[39–41] is produced by CD4+ T lymphocytes yet human IL-4 does not share the variety of functions ascribed to the murine species. It induces switching of B cells to IgE and IgG4 production suggesting a role in hypersensitivity reactions. IL-4 may also induce endothelial cell binding of monocytes and lymphocytes. Recent data also suggest that IL-4 may regulate the production of proinflammatory cytokines such as TNF and serve to direct the clonal expansion of T_H2 cells (see below).

Transforming Growth Factor Beta. Transforming growth factor beta (TGF-β)[42,43] is secreted in active form predominantly by activated T cells and mononuclear phagocytes. TGF-β may variably inhibit or promote the growth of a variety of cell types and may also promote angiogenesis. This cytokine inhibits T cell proliferation to a number of stimuli as well as the maturation of cytotoxic T lymphocytes. TGF-β may serve as a mechanism to down-regulate the production and activity of the more potent proinflammatory species, thus serving as a "suppressor" of immune responses.

Lymphotoxin. Lymphotoxin (LT)[44] is secreted by activated T lymphocytes, often in conjunction with IFN-γ. Interestingly, LT shares a degree of structural homology with TNF (hence often termed TNF-β) and competes with TNF for binding to the same receptors. Although postreceptor functional responses to LT resemble those of TNF, this cytokine is produced in lesser quantities and probably serves only a local rather than systemic purpose. In this regard, it is an activator of neutrophils and vascular endothelial cells.

MEDIATOR INTERACTIONS FOR MODULATING THE SPECIFIC IMMUNE RESPONSE

Although sometimes called nonspecific immunity, natural immunity does involve specific recognitions between immune cell receptors and conserved molecules of pathogenic microorganisms. Because these receptors are encoded in the genome, however, this system has limited diversity and is only able to evolve via selection pressures of the pathogens themselves. Additionally, a case can be made that wide use of antibiotics has reduced these selection pressures because mortality from infection has, in part, been disassociated from individual variations in this genetically encoded immunity.

Specific immunity, by contrast, exhibits extremely high diversity owing to rearrangement of immunoglobulin and T cell receptor genes during development. In addition, clonal selection, whereby antigen induces proliferation and differentiation of only those B and T cells bearing immunoglobulin and T cell receptors, respectively, specific for that particular antigen, assures exponential amplification of the appropriate cells. In the face of continuing antigen stimulation, this process also results in the increasingly selective expansion of only those cells bearing the highest avidity immunoglobulins or T cell receptors. Thus specific immunity appears to have evolved with the potential to address the high and ever changing antigenic diversity of pathogenic microorganisms.

Mediators of Specific Immunity

It is increasingly clear that recognition of different types of pathogens by the specific immune system can result in qualitatively and quantitatively different immune responses. For example, CD4+ T_H1 cells appear to be more responsive to bacteria, protozoa, and viruses, but CD4+ T_H2 cells respond preferentially to metazoa and allergens.[29,45] When activated, CD4+ T_H1 cells produce IL-2 and IFN-γ, while CD4+ T_H2 cells produce IL-4, IL-5, and IL-10.[28,29,46–48] Thus the cytokine profile generated can vary with the type of infecting pathogen.

The mechanism underlying this differential responsiveness of T_H1 and T_H2 cells is not currently known, but it suggests an additional type of cognition by the immune system. However, it is known that generation of T_H1 and T_H2 responses is closely controlled by both monocyte/macrophage cytokines and cytokines produced by the T_H1 and T_H2 cells themselves (see Fig. 16–1). IL-12, TNF, and IL-1, derived from monocytes and macrophages, and IFN-γ, derived from NK and T_H1 cells, are upregulators of T_H1 cells and downregulators of T_H2 cells.[28,29] By contrast, IL-4, IL-5, IL-6, and IL-10 upregulate T_H2 cells and downregulate T_H1 cells.[28,29] Thus, since the cytokines produced by one subset upregulate that subset concomitant with downregulating the dichotomous subset, an inertia develops in which a T_H1 or T_H2 response begins to predominate and amplifies itself while inhibiting the opposing response (see Fig. 16–2).

T_H1 responses normally predominate in bacterial, viral, and protozoan infections.[29,45] The cytokine profile in response to injury suggests quite strongly that a predisposition for T_H2 responses occurs after injury although some important data are not currently available. Certainly, a T_H2 response to injury appears dysfunctional because it would leave the host relatively unprepared to deal with subsequent bacterial or viral challenges. One major reason T_H2 responses may be inefficient, particularly against bacterial infections, is that they induce B lymphocyte class switching such that the IgG1 (murine) and IgG4 (human) isotypes and IgE

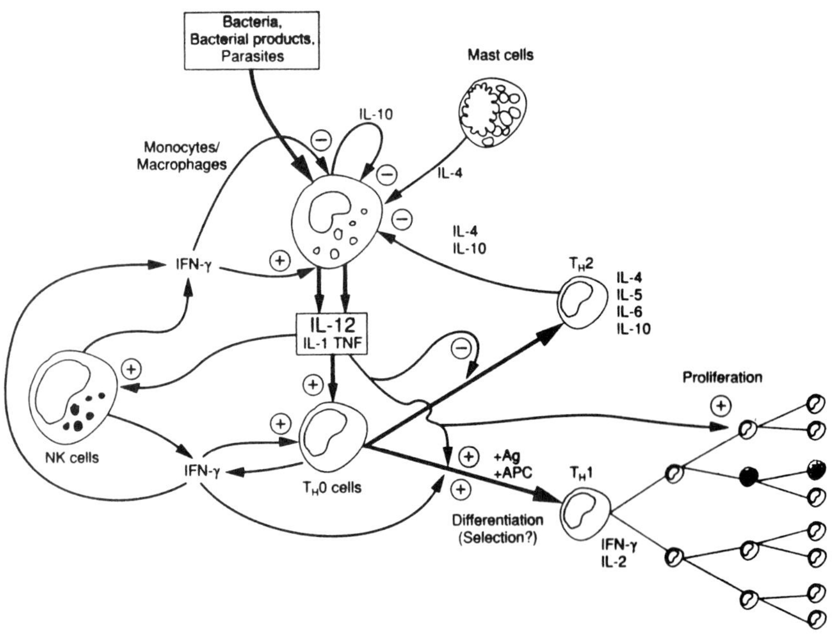

Figure 16–1. Role of cytokines in the generation of T_H1 and T_H2 cells. Negative (−) and positive (+) feedback mechanisms are indicated. *(From Trinchieri G: Immunol Today 14:335, 1993.)*

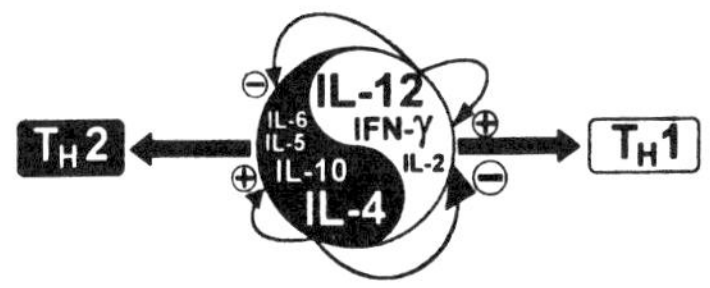

Figure 16–2. T_H1 and T_H2 cell generation is regulated by the equilibrium between different groups of cytokines, with dominant effects of IL-12 and IL-4. T_H1 and T_H2 responses are maintained by both positive (+) and negative (−) feedback mechanisms, with the effect of IL-4 probably being dominant over that of IL-12. *(From Trinchieri, G: Immunol Today 14:335, 1993.)*

immunoglobulins predominate.[39,41,49,50] IgG4 and IgE are not able to fix complement, and evidence suggests they are also among the least efficient opsonizing antibodies.[51] Because complement fixation (either for subsequent lysis or phagocyte adhesion) and antibody opsonization (for enhanced phagocytosis) are major host defenses against bacteria, a predominate T_H2 response to injury, with associated class switching to IgG4 isotype and IgE, would leave the host relatively susceptible to bacterial infections.

After injury, IL-2 and IFN-γ production are deficient.[52–56] These findings have been established by directly measuring these cytokines and by documenting decreased T cell proliferation in response to mitogens and antigens (which is dependent on IL-2) and decreased monocyte/macrophage expression of class II MHC (which is dependent, in part, on IFN-γ). It is likely that injury-associated decline in monocyte/macrophage class II MHC also contributes to defective T cell proliferation. The level of monocyte/macrophage expression of class II MHC is an important factor in the ability of these cells to present antigen in a class II-restricted fashion to CD4+ T cells. IL-2 and IFN-γ are important modulating cytokines for the development of T_H1 and the inhibition of T_H2 responses.[28] The decrease in IL-2 and IFN-γ after injury thus would appear to favor development along the T_H2 pathway (see Figs. 16–1 and 16–2).

Detection of some proinflammatory cytokines, such as TNF and IL-1, following injury is not consistent.[57,58] This must be contrasted with infection, with or without injury, where detectable levels of TNF and IL-1 occur with considerably greater frequency than after injury alone.[59,60] Failure to detect these cytokines systemically does not necessarily rule out increased production at the tissue level. Nonetheless, production of bioactive forms of these cytokines do not consistently increase after injury. Since increased TNF and IL-1 are associated with T_H1 responses, the failure to detect these cytokines after injury implies a lack of T_H1 activity. Unlike IL-2 and IFN-γ, TNF and IL-1 do not appear to actively downregulate T_H2 responses, but they do directly contribute to development of T_H1 responses.[28]

IL-4 is a major product of T_H2 cells and additionally plays an important role in upregulation of T_H2 responses and downregulation of T_H1 responses. Unfortunately, there are minimal data concerning the effect of injury of this cytokine, although inflammation caused by exposure to ultraviolet radiation leads to a reduction in T_H1 cytokines (IL-2, IFN-γ) and augmentation of T_H2 cytokines (IL-4).[61] Moreover, glucocorticoids (GCs) potently upregulate IL-4 production and downregulate IL-2 production.[62–64] Based on this cytokine profile, increases in GCs apparently favor T_H2-type responses. It has long been known that plasma levels of GCs are elevated after injury—sometimes for weeks. Additionally, the plasma GC binding proteins, corticosteroid-binding globulin and albumin, are significantly decreased after large injuries leading to chronic increases in free, biologically active GCs, which may be as much as ten-fold above normal values.[66–68] GCs also inhibit the elaboration of IFN-γ, TNF, and IL-1.[69–72] Thus elevations of GCs in humans after major injury may be important regulatory elements involved in directing the specific immune system preferentially to T_H2, rather than T_H1, responsiveness.

This does not preclude the necessity of GCs in the response to injury. Certainly, GCs are important, if not obligatory, for survival after major injury, since adrenal insufficiency is associated with an extremely labile clinical course.[73,74] Appropriate adrenocortical responses are especially important in the early postinjury ebb phase and, subsequently, if systemic inflammation or sepsis should occur. This is supported by numerous animal studies in which adrenalectomy or pretreatment with the GC receptor antagonist, RU 486, significantly decreases survival in acute models of endotoxemia or infection while GC pretreatment improves survival.[75–77] On the other hand, it can be argued that extreme and chronic elevations in GCs after major injury may lead to inhibition of critical phagocytic cellular functions and favor development of the less bactericidal T_H2 type of specific immunity.[28,29,45,62–64,78–87] But although these events may favor microbial colonization and growth, the GCs are essential acutely for gluconeogenesis, control of shock-inducing cytokine production, and inhibition of leukocyte adhesion and activation.

IL-12 and IL-10 also are key elements in the control of T_H1 and T_H2 responses (see Figs. 16–1 and 16–2). IL-12 appears to be a potent inducer of T_H1 development and an equally potent inhibitor of T_H2 development.[28,29] By contrast, IL-10 works in an opposite fashion, upregulating T_H2 and downregulating T_H1 responses.[23–25,28] Unfortunately, sufficient data are not available concerning the effects of injury on these recently characterized cytokines.

While IL-6 does not appear to be a major regulator of T_H1 or T_H2 responses, it nonetheless is a marker for T_H2 cell activation (see Figs. 16–1 and 16–2).[28,46–48] Furthermore, IL-6 is one of the few cytokines consistently elevated after injury.[18,19,76,88] IL-6 levels also correlate with the magnitude of injury and physiological status.[19,88]

Prostaglandins of the E series (PGE) are immunosuppressive for T cell function and are increased after injury.[89–92] Like GCs, they inhibit production of IL-2[93] and IFN-γ by T_H1 cells (Fig. 16–3),[94] but unlike GC, PGE apparently has no effect on IL-4 secreting T_H2 cells. This implies that PGE should be somewhat less robust than GCs in inducing T_H2 responses at the expense of T_H1 responses.

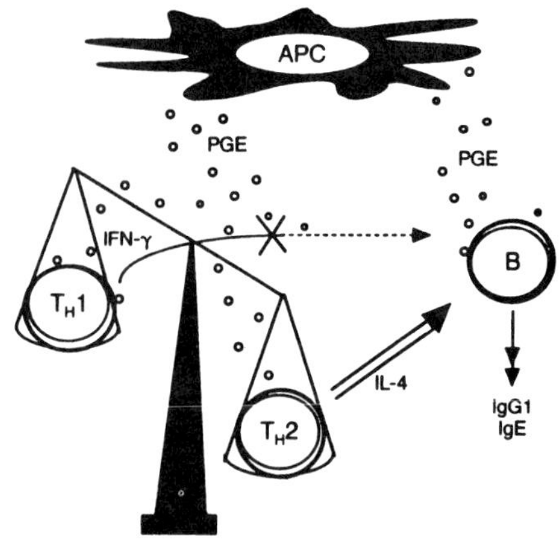

Figure 16–3. E series prostaglandins (PGE) regulate B and T cells. PGEs secreted by macrophages, fibroblasts, and dendritic cells can inhibit the synthesis of IFN-γ by T_H1 cells, but not the synthesis of IL-4 by T_H2 cells. Thus PGE secretion may tip the balance in favor of a T_H2-type response leading to B cell production of IgG1 and IgE. PGE also directly affects B cells by enhancing IL-4-induced class switching to IgG1 and IgE. *Note:* This figure is based on the murine system where IL-4 induces production of IgG1 (and IgE). In humans, IL-4 induces IgG4 (and IgE) as described in the text and in ref. 41. These Igs are not able to fix complement and are relatively poor opsonins.[51] *(From Phipps RP, Stein SH, Roper RL: Immunol Today 12:349, 1991.)*

CYTOKINE/GLUCOCORTICOID INTERACTIONS

Classic studies by Hume and Egdahl and others have shown that neural signaling, most likely nociceptive in nature, from a site of injury to the brain is a major stimulus for activation of the hypothalamic-pituitary-adrenal (HPA) axis.[95,96] However, more recent data indicate that there are additional mediator control mechanisms of activity of the HPA axis. The proinflammatory cytokine IL-1 and also probably TNF and IL-6 activate the hypothalamic and hypophyseal cells responsible for corticotropin releasing factor (CRF) and adrenocorticotropin hormone (ACTH) secretion, leading to increased plasma GC concentrations.[97–100] Because IL-1 does not readily cross the blood-brain barrier, it is unclear whether this is caused by the cytokines themselves or by an induced distal mediator. IL-1 receptors have been demonstrated in the rodent brain, but it is not known if these receptors exist to signal local or distant IL-1 production.[101] Certainly, elevated GCs are a consistent observation after administration of exogenous lipopolysaccharide (LPS), but there is controversy concerning whether this is mediated indirectly via the proinflammatory cytokines or directly by LPS.[102,103] Dunn administered LPS to mice with or without IL-1RA, antibody to TNF, or a combination of IL-1RA and antibody to TNF. Neither IL-1RA, antibody to TNF, nor the combination was able to block the elevation of plasma GCs measured 1 hour after LPS administration, suggesting a direct effect of LPS on the HPA axis.[104]

Another area of controversy concerns lymphocytes as a source of ACTH. Activated lymphocytes secrete ACTH and other peptides derived from proopiomelanocortin.[105,106] If lymphocytes do produce sufficient ACTH to activate adrenocortical GC secretion, are lymphocytes themselves able to modulate the immune response to different pathogens by modulation of GC concentrations? Blalock has argued that lymphocytes may be a "sensory organ" for pathogens, and GCs may be one way of signaling discrimination of one type of pathogen from another.[106,107] Certainly, this concept is consistent with the observation that GCs may play a key role in the balance between T_H1 and T_H2 responses.

GCs are omnibus inhibitors of mononuclear phagocyte-derived proinflammatory cytokines and arachidonic acid metabolites. The cellular basis for this inhibition has been extensively investigated for TNF and arachidonic acid metabolites. Han, Beutler, and their colleagues have shown that LPS, a potent secretagogue of TNF, causes both an increase in TNF gene transcription, leading to accumulation of TNF mRNA, and translational derepression of TNF mRNA, leading to far more efficient message utilization.[72] GCs inhibit this latter cellular event, preventing translational derepression while downregulating TNF gene transcription only slightly. Thus GCs allow accumulation of TNF mRNA in the cytosol of mononuclear phagocytes but prevent translation of this mRNA. Treatment of human volunteers with GCs either at the time or at 6 hours prior to LPS administration completely abrogated the plasma TNF response to LPS.[108] By contrast, if volunteers were given GCs 12 or even 144 hours prior to LPS, the TNF response to LPS was augmented three- to fourfold over that response observed with LPS alone (Fig. 16–4). This enhanced TNF response to LPS may be due to GC-induced accumulation of TNF mRNA in mononuclear phagocytes during the 12- or 144-hour interval before LPS. The ability of GCs to prevent translational derepression by LPS may have slowly eroded, leaving a larger than normal pool of untranslated TNF mRNA in the cytosol. This could then account for the enhanced TNF responses of these subjects upon exposure to LPS.

The basis for GC inhibition of arachidonic acid metabolite production by mononuclear phagocytes is well characterized. Elevation of GC causes an increase of lipocortin 1[109,110] for which mononuclear phagocytes and neutrophils possess specific receptors.[110] Furthermore, lipocortin 1 is a relatively potent inhibitor of phospholipase A_2 (PLA_2), a key enzyme responsible for release of arachidonic acid from membrane phospholipid pools.[109,110] Such inhibition of PLA_2 by lipocortin 1 may cause a decrease in the synthesis of both cyclooxygenase and lipoxygenase derived metabolites. Further complicating this system, the GC inhibitable proinflammatory cytokines TNF and IL-1 are capable of inducing synthesis of PLA_2. Thus GCs can inhibit production of arachidonic acid metabolites in two ways—via lipocortin 1[109–111] and by suppressing monokine production. In addition, PLA_2 can be released as an extracellular inflammatory mediator. Soluble PLA_2 may be increased up to 200-fold under conditions of severe injury/inflammation and exert a plethora of proinflammatory tissue responses including phagocyte activation, lung injury, increases in vascular permeability, hypotension, synovitis, and bowel inflammation.[111]

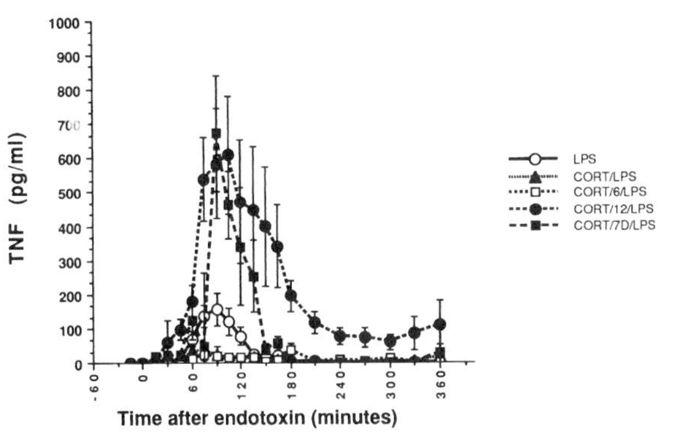

Figure 16–4. Circulating TNF levels following endotoxin without prior hypercortisolemia and after variable antecedent 6 hour periods of hypercortisolemia and normal (hour) intervals before LPS exposure (cort/xh/LPS). All studies were performed in healthy human subjects. The peaks achieved by subjects in the CORT/12/LPS and CORT/144/LPS are significantly higher than those following LPS alone. *(Adapted from Barber, AE, Coyle SM, Marano MA, et al: J Immunol 150:1999, 1993.)*

NATURALLY OCCURRING CYTOKINE ANTAGONISTS

Several endogenous factors capable of inhibiting cytokine function have been identified and later found in both the urine and serum of patients with febrile illnesses and malignancies. Some inhibitory proteins, such as uromodulin, bind nonspecifically to proinflammatory cytokines. Others are specific antagonists for TNF or IL-1.[112]

Two TNF inhibitors have been identified: both the 30-kD[113] and the 40-kD[114] species are actually the extracellular domains of p55 and p75 TNF receptors, respectively. Although the mechanisms for the regulation of these soluble TNF receptor (sTNFR) proteins are still poorly defined, they appear to be shed from the cell surface in response to many of the same inflammatory stimuli and induce TNF production.

The circulating half-life of sTNFR proteins is almost 20 minutes and both TNF bound and free sTNFR are rapidly eliminated through the kidney. Recent data would suggest that the presence of such sTNFR proteins may serve to diminish the toxicity of endogenously produced TNF.[115] It is likely that the shedding of cytokine receptors may be a common mechanism for local regulation of specific cytokine activity.

The specific IL-1 antagonist is not a soluble IL-1 receptor—it is another macrophage-derived cytokine called IL-1 receptor antagonist (IL-1RA).[13] The glycosylated form of the inhibitor competes with IL-1α and IL-1β for binding to the cell surface receptor. It has been shown to be effective in the prevention of the cardiovascular collapse attending bacteremia[116] when a molar excess of 100- to 1000-fold of IL-1RA over endogenous levels of IL-1 is achieved by exogenous infusion.[117]

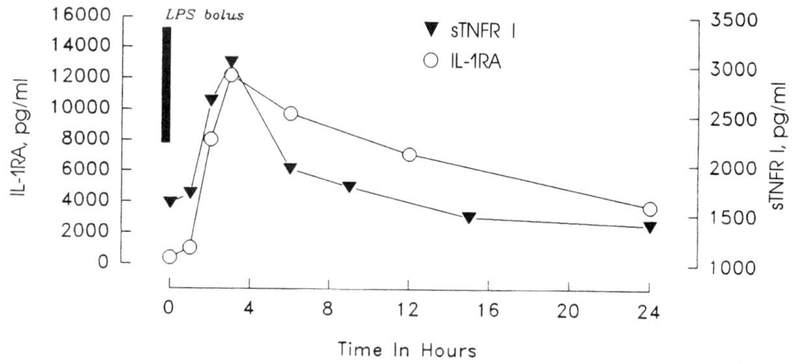

Figure 16–5. Concentrations of circulating soluble TNF receptor type I (sTNRFI) and of IL-1 receptor antagonist (IL-1RA) achieved in normal subjects receiving an intravenous bolus of lipopolysaccharide (LPS) at time 0. Note that both cytokine antagonists appear in the circulation within 1 to 2 hours after LPS infusion and remain detectable for ≤24 hours. The peak concentration achieved in these subjects are similar to those levels observed in critically ill patients with sepsis syndrome. *(From Lowry SF, New Horizons Sepsis Cell Physiol Alterations 1:120, 1993.)*

CLINICAL STUDIES DURING SEVERE INFECTION

There currently is little doubt that proinflammatory cytokines participate in the acute hemodynamic collapse attending severe endotoxemia or bacteremia. Such cytokines, however, may not be detectable. Much of the activity of these cytokines occurs at the tissue level; specific and nonspecific antagonists may neutralize them. Furthermore, they are inhibited by the glucocorticoid hormone response, so that their activity may well be episodic.

Recent evidence that endogenous antagonists may circulate over prolonged periods in such patients further complicates the assignment of cytokine-specific activity in critical illness beyond the earliest phases of infection. Both soluble TNF receptors and IL-1RA are found during endotoxin administration or in clinical infection (see Fig. 16–5). We have recently sought to determine the relationship between critical illness and the presence of the proinflammatory cytokines—TNF and IL-1—and of these natural antagonists. Patients admitted to a critical care unit because of major injury or infection most often had undetectable levels of circulating TNF and IL-1. Many had high levels of IL-6, sTNFR, and IL-1RA. While some cytokine levels, such as that of IL-6, correlate roughly with the magnitude of underlying injury and pathophysiological response,[18,19,88] no clear relationship existed between the clinical status and TNF and IL-1 nor for their respective antagonists.[118,119]

PRELIMINARY RESULTS FROM CLINICAL TRIALS OF ANTICYTOKINE THERAPIES

Clinical studies utilizing a variety of anticytokine therapies have been initiated within the past several years.[120] There are currently several prospective trials evaluating the response to TNF blockade utilizing various antibody constructs directed against this cytokine. These include a phase II trial of a murine IgG and a murine chimeric IgG. Two additional trials have also reached phase III testing, one with a humanized mouse IgG and another utilizing a murine IgG molecule. Preliminary results indicate that such agents have relatively little impact on long-term survival except in those patients presenting with septic shock. A report of one such agent suggests that improved biological re-

TABLE 16–3. RESULTS OF PHASE III TRIAL OF IL-1RA THERAPY IN HUMAN SEPSIS AND SEPTIC SHOCK

		Percent Mortality			
Illness	***n***	**Control**	**1 mg/kg/h**	**2 mg/kg/h**	***p***
Phase III (overall)	893	34	31	29	0.22
Shock	713	36	31	31	0.23
Shock or sepsis (baseline mortality risk[a] ≥24%)	595	45	37	35	0.03

[a] Based on retrospective analysis of patient variables using the APACHE III severity-of-illness scoring system.

sponses are more readily observed when circulating TNF is detectable at the outset of therapy.[121]

Additional strategies directed against TNF activity through the utilization of soluble p55 and p75 TNF receptor constructs (immunoadhesins) are also in early clinical trials. These unique molecules combine two extracellular receptor components with the Fc portion of IgG. In theory, such constructs promote both enhanced ligand binding as well as increased biologic half-lives of the antagonist. Phase II/III (p55) and phase III (p75) trials are currently being conducted.

A recently completed phase III trial of IL-1 receptor antagonist intervention in septic patients has also been presented. Preliminary results of this trial are outlined in Table 16–3. The prospective 28-day mortality from all causes did not demonstrate a statistically significant impact in this trial. Neither was a statistical improvement observed in survival of patients with shock at study entry. However, a retrospective analysis of these data based on a risk-prediction model demonstrated a benefit of the antagonist in those patients with higher risk of in-hospital mortality.

REFERENCES

1. Beutler B, Mahoney J, Le Trang N, et al: Purification of cachectin, a lipoprotein lipase secreted by endotoxin-induced RAW 264.7 cells. J Exp Med 161:984, 1985.
2. Aggarwal BB, Kohr WJ, Hass PE, et al: Human tumor necrosis factor, production, purification, and characterization. J Biol Chem 260:2345, 1985.
3. Loetscher H, Brockhaus M, Dembic Z, et al: Two distinct tumor necrosis factor receptors: members of a new cytokine receptor gene family. Oxf Surv Eukaryot Genes 7:119, 1991.
4. Wong GH, Tartaglia LA, Lee MS, Goeddel DV: Antiviral activity of tumor necrosis factor (TNF) is signalled through the 55kDa receptor, type I TNF. J Immunol 149:3350, 1992.
5. Vassalli P: The pathobiology of tumor necrosis factors. In Paul WE, Fathman CG, Metzger H (eds): Annual Review of Immunology, Vol 10. Palo Alto, CA, Annual Reviews, 1992, pp 411–452.
6. Hesse DG, Tracey KJ, Fong Y, et al: Cytokine appearance in human endotoxemia and primate bacteremia. Surg Gynecol Obstet 166:147, 1988.
7. Tracey KJ, Beutler B, Lowry SF, et al: Shock and tissue injury induced by recombinant human cachectin. Science 234:470, 1986.
8. Tracey KJ, Fong Y, Hesse DG, et al: Anti-cachectin/TNF monoclonal antibodies prevent septic shock during lethal bacteremia. Nature 330:662, 1987.
9. Van Zee KJ, Kohno T, Fischer E, et al: Tumor necrosis factor soluble receptors circulate during experimental and clinical inflammation and can protect against excessive tumor necrosis factor α in vitro and in vivo. Proc Natl Acad Sci USA 89:4845, 1992.
10. Dinarello CA: Interleukin-1 and its biologically related cytokines. Adv Immunol 44:153, 1989.
11. Dinarello CA: Biology of interleukin-1. FASEB J 2:108, 1988.
12. Dinarello CA: Role of interleukin-1 in infectious diseases. Immunol Rev 127:119, 1992.
13. Eisenberg SP, Evans RJ, Arend WP, et al: Primary structure and functional expression from complementary DNA of a human interleukin 1 receptor antagonist. Nature 343:341, 1990.
14. Hannum CH, Wilcox CJ, Arend WP, et al: Interleukin-1 receptor antagonist activity of a human interleukin-1 inhibitor. Nature 343:336, 1990.
15. Fischer E, Van Zee KJ, Marano MA, et al: Interleukin-1 receptor antagonist circulates in experimental inflammation and in human disease. Blood 79:2196, 1992.
16. Marinkovic S, Jahreis GP, Wong GG, Baumann H: IL-6 modulates the synthesis of a specific set of acute phase plasma proteins in vivo. J Immunol 142:808, 1989.
17. Gauldio J, Richards C, Baumann H: IL-6 and the acute phase response. Res Immunol 143:755, 1992.
18. Fong Y, Moldawer LL, Marano M, et al: Endotoxemia elicits increased circulating β_2-IFN/IL-6 in man. J Immunol 142:2321, 1989.
19. Guo Y, Dickerson C, Chrest FJ, et al: Increased levels of circulating interleukin-6 in burn patients. Clin Immunol Immunopathol 54:361, 1990.
20. Sticherling M, Schröder J-M, Christophers E: Production and characterization of monoclonal antibodies against the novel neutrophil activating peptide NAP/IL-8. J Immunol 143:1628, 1989.
21. Yoshimura T, Matsushima K, Tamaka S, et al: Purification of a human monocyte-derived neutrophil chemotactic factor that has peptide sequence similarity to other host defense cytokines. Proc Natl Acad Sci USA 84:9233, 1987.
22. Van Zee KJ, Fischer E, Hawes AS, et al: Effects of intravenous IL-8 administration in nonhuman primates. J Immunol 148:1746, 1992.
23. Fiorentino DF, Bond MW, Mosmann TR: Two types of mouse T helper cell. IV. Th2 clones secrete a factor that inhibits cytokine production by Th1 clones. J Exp Med 170:2081, 1989.
24. Howard M, O'Garra A: Biological properties of interleukin-10. Immunol Today 13:198, 1992.
25. Moore KW, O'Garra A, de Wall Malefyt R, et al: Interleukin-10. In Paul WE, Fathman CG, Metzger H (eds): Annual Review of Immunology, Vol 11. Palo Alto, CA, Annual Review, 1993, pp 165–190.
26. Kobayashi M, Fitz L, Ryan M, et al: Identification and purification of natural killer cell stimulatory factor (NKSF), a cytokine with multiple biologic effects on human lymphocytes. J Exp Med 170:827, 1989.

27. Stern AS, Podlaski FJ, Hulmes JD, et al: Purification to homogeneity and partial characterization of cytotoxic lymphocyte maturation factor from human B-lymphoblastoid cells. Proc Natl Acad Sci USA 87:6808, 1990.
28. Trinchieri G: Interleukin-12 and its role in the generation of T_H1 cells. Immunol Today 14:335, 1993.
29. Scott P: IL-12: initiation cytokine for cell-mediated immunity. Science 206:496, 1993.
30. Stewart WE: The Interferon System, 2nd ed. New York, Springer Verlag, 1979.
31. Kirchner H, Marcucci F: Interferon production in leukocytes. In Vilček J, DeMaeyer E (eds): Interferon 2: Interferons and the Immune System. Amsterdam, Elsevier, 1984, pp 7–34.
32. Adams DO, Hamilton TA: Molecular transductional mechanisms by which IFNγ and other signals regulate macrophage development. In Möller G (ed): Immunological Reviews, Vol 97, Gamma Interferon. Copenhagen, Munksgaard, 1987, pp 5–27.
33. Rubinstein M, Novick D, Fischer DG: The human interferon-γ receptor system. In Möller G (ed): Immunological Reviews, Vol 97, Gamma Interferon, Copenhagen, Munksgaard, 1987, pp 29–50.
34. Sandvig S, Laskay T, Andersson J, et al: Gamma-interferon is produced by CD3+ and CD3− lymphocytes. In Möller G (ed): Immunological Reviews, Vol 97, Gamma Interferon, Copenhagen, Munksgaard, 1987, pp 51–65.
35. Smith KA: T-cell growth factor. In Möller G (ed): Immunological Reviews, Vol 51, T Cell Stimulating Growth Factors. Copenhagen, Munksgaard, 1980, pp 337–357.
36. Robb RJ: Interleukin 2: the molecule and its function. Immunol Today 5:203, 1984.
37. Smith KA, Cantrell DA: Interleukin 2 regulates its own receptors. Proc Natl Acad Sci USA 82:864, 1985.
38. Minami Y, Kono T, Miyazako T, Taniguchi T: The IL-2 receptor complex: its structure, function and target genes. In Paul WE, Fathman CG, Metzger H (eds): Annual Review of Immunology, Vol 11. Palo Alto, CA, Annual Review, 1993, pp 245–268.
39. Snapper CM, Paul WE: B cell stimulatory factor-1 (interleukin 4) prepares resting murine B cells to secrete IgG1 upon subsequent stimulation with bacterial lipopolysaccharide. J Immunol 139:10, 1987.
40. Howard M, Farrar J, Hilfiker M, et al: Identification of a T cell-derived B cell growth factor distinct from interleukin 2. J Exp Med 155:914, 1982.
41. Snapper CM, Mond JJ: Towards a comprehensive view of immunoglobulin class switching. Immunol Today 14:15, 1993.
42. Wahl SM, McCartney-Francis N, Mergenhagen SE: Inflammatory and immunomodulatory roles of TGF-β. Immunol Today 10:258, 1989.
43. Kehrl JH, Wakefield LM, Roberts AB, et al: Production of transforming growth factor β by human T lymphocytes, and its potential role in the regulation of T cell growth. J Exp Med 163:1037, 1986.
44. Pennica D, Nedwin GE, Hayflick JS, et al: Human tumor necrosis factor: precursor, structure expression, and homology to lymphotoxin. Nature 312:724, 1984.
45. Scott P, Kaufmann SHE: The role of T cell subsets and cytokines in the regulation of infection. Immunol Today 12:346, 1991.
46. Mosmann TR, Cherwinski H, Bond MW, et al: Two types of murine helper T cell clone. I. Definition according to profiles of lymphokine activities and secreted proteins. J Immunol 136:2348, 1986.
47. Romagnami S: Human T_H1 and T_H2 subsets: doubt no more. Immunol Today 12:256, 1991.
48. Möller G (ed): Immunological Reviews, Vol 123, T-Helper Cell Subpopulations. Copenhagen, Munksgaard, 1991, pp. 5–229.
49. Coffmann RL, Seymour BWP, Lebman DA, et al: The role of helper T cell products in mouse B cell differentiation and isotype regulation. In Möller G (ed): Immunological Reviews, Vol 102, IL-4 and IL-5: Biology and Genetics. Copenhagen, Munksgaard, 1988, pp 5–28.
50. Snapper CM, Finkelmann FD, Paul WE: Regulation of IgG1 and IgE production by interleukin 4. In Möller G (ed): Immunological Reviews, Vol 102, IL-4 and IL-5: Biology and Genetics. Copenhagen, Munksgaard, 1988, pp. 51–76.
51. Morrison SL. In vitro antibodies: strategies for production and application. In Paul WE, Fathman CG, Metzger H (eds): Annual Review of Immunology, Vol 10. Palo Alto, CA, Annual Reviews, 1992, pp 248–249.
52. Antonacci AC, Calvano SE, Reaves LE, et al: Autologous and allogeneic mixed-lymphocyte responses following thermal injury in man: the immunomodulatory effects of interleukin-1, interleukin-2, and a prostaglandin inhibitor, WY-18251. Clin Immunol Immunopathol 30:304, 1984.
53. Wood JJ, Rodrick ML, O'Mahony JB, et al: Inadequate interleukin 2 production: a fundamental immunological deficiency in patients with major burns. Ann Surg 200:311, 1984.
54. Teodorczyk-Injeyan JH, Sparks BG, Mills GB, et al: Impairment of T cell activation in burn patients: a possible mechanism of thermal injury-induced immunosuppression. Clin Exp Immunol 65:570, 1986.
55. Hershman MJ, Appel SH, Wellhausen SR, et al: Interferon-gamma treatment increases HLA-DR expression on monocytes in severely injured patients. Clin Exp Immunol 77:67, 1989.
56. Hershman MJ, Cheadle WG, Wellhausen SR, et al: Monocyte HLA-DR antigen expression characterizes clinical outcome in the trauma patient. Br J Surg 77:204, 1990.
57. Stylianos S, Wakabayashi G, Gelfand JA, Harris BH: Experimental hemorrhage and blunt trauma do not increase circulating tumor necrosis factor. J Trauma 31:1063, 1991.
58. Ertel W, Morrison MH, Ayala A, Chaudry IH: Eico-

sanoids regulate tumor necrosis factor synthesis after hemorrhage in vitro and in vivo. J Trauma 31:609, 1991.
59. Fong Y, Moldawer LL, Shires GT, Lowry SF: The biological characteristics of cytokines and their implication in surgical injury. Surg Gynecol Obstet 170:363, 1990.
60. Marano MA, Fong Y, Moldawer LL, et al: Serum cachectin/tumor necrosis factor in critically ill patients with burns correlates with infection and mortality. Surg Gynecol Obstet 170:32, 1990.
61. Araneo BA, Dowell R, Moon HB, Daynes RA: Regulation of murine lymphokine production in vivo: UVR exposure depresses IL-2 and enhances IL-4 production by T cells through an IL-1-dependent mechanism. J Immunol 143:1737, 1989.
62. Daynes RA, Araneo BA: Contrasting effects of glucocorticoids on the capacity of T cells to produce the growth factors interleukin 2 and interleukin 4. Eur J Immunol 19:2319, 1989.
63. Daynes RA, Araneo BH, Dowell TA, et al: Regulation of murine lymphokine production in vivo. III. The lymphoid tissue microenvironment exerts regulatory influences over T helper cell function. J Exp Med 171:979, 1990.
64. Gillis S, Crabtree GR, Smith KA: Glucocorticoid-induced inhibition of T cell growth factor production. I. The effect on mitogen-induced lymphocyte proliferation. J Immunol 123:1624, 1979.
65. Vaughn GM, Becker RA, Allen JP, et al: Cortisol and corticotrophin in burned patients. J Trauma 22:263, 1982.
66. Calvano SE, Chiao J, Reaves LE, et al: Changes in free and total plasma cortisol and thyroxine following thermal injury in man. J Burn Care Rehabil 5:143, 1984.
67. Murray D: Cortisol binding to plasma proteins in man in health, stress, and at death. J Endocrinol 39:571, 1967.
68. Wise LW, Margraf HW, Ballinger WF: Adrenal cortical function in severe burns. Arch Surg 105:212, 1972.
69. Warren MK, Vogel SN: Opposing effects of glucocorticoids on interferon-γ-induced murine macrophage Fc receptor and Ia antigen expression. J Immunol 134:2462, 1985.
70. Knudsen PJ, Dinarello CA, Strom TB: Glucocorticoids inhibit transcriptional and post-transcriptional expression of interleukin-1 in U937 cells. J Immunol 139:4129, 1987.
71. Kern JA, Lamb RJ, Reed JC, et al: Dexamethasone inhibition of interleukin-1 beta production by human monocytes. Post-transcriptional mechanisms. J Clin Invest 81:237, 1988.
72. Han J, Thompson P, Beutler B: Dexamethasone and pentoxifylline inhibit endotoxin-induced cachectin/tumor necrosis factor synthesis at separate points in the signaling pathway. J Exp Med 172:391, 1990.
73. Kaplan EL, Lee RC: Acute postoperative hormonal insufficiency syndromes. In Condon RE, DeCosse JJ (eds): Surgical Care. A Physiologic Approach to Clinical Management. Philadelphia, Lea & Febiger, 1980, pp 370–384.
74. Murphy JF, Purdue GF, Hunt JL: Acute adrenal insufficiency in the patient with burns. J Burn Care Rehabil 14:155, 1993.
75. Bertini R, Bianchi M, Ghezzi P: Adrenalectomy sensitizes mice to the lethal effect of interleukin-1 and tumor necrosis factor. J Exp Med 167:1708, 1988.
76. Hawes AS, Rock CS, Keogh CV, et al: In vivo effects of the antiglucocorticoid RU 486 on glucocorticoid and cytokine responses to *Escherichia coli* endotoxin. Infect Immun 60:2641, 1992.
77. Hinshaw LB, Beller-Todd BK, Archer LT, et al: Effectiveness of steroid/antibiotic treatment in primates administered LD100 *Escherichia coli*. Ann Surg 194:51, 1981.
78. Dale DE, Fauci AS, Wolff SM: Alternate-day prednisone. Leukocyte kinetics and susceptibility to infections. N Engl J Med 291:1154, 1974.
79. Fauci AS: Mechanisms of corticosteroid action on lymphocyte subpopulations. II. Differential effects of in vivo hydrocortisone, prednisone, and dexamethasone on in vitro expression of lymphocyte function. Clin Exp Immunol 24:54, 1976.
80. Calvano SE, Albert JD, Legaspi A, et al: Comparison of numerical and phenotypic leukocyte changes during constant hydrocortisone infusion in normal humans with those in thermally injured patients. Surg Gynecol Obstet 164:509, 1987.
81. Fauci AS, Dale DC: The effect of hydrocortisone on the kinetics of normal human lymphocytes. Blood 46:235, 1975.
82. Webel ML, Ritts RE Jr, Taswell HF, et al: Cellular immunity after intravenous administration of methylprednisolone. J Lab Clin Med 83:383, 1974.
83. Cohen JJ. The effects of hydrocortisone on the immune response. Ann Allergy 29:358, 1971.
84. Butler WT, Rossen RD: Effects of corticosteroids on immunity in man. I. Decreased serum IgG concentration caused by 3 or 5 days of high doses of methylprednisolone. J Clin Invest 52:2629, 1973.
85. Rhinehart JJ, Balcerzak SP, Sagone AL, LoBuglio AF: Effects of corticosteroids on human monocyte function. J Clin Invest 54:1337, 1974.
86. Rhinehart JJ, Sagone AL, Balcerzak SP, et al: Effects of corticosteroid therapy on human monocyte functions. N Engl J Med 292:236, 1975.
87. Crabtree GR, Gillis S, Smith KA, Munck A: Glucocorticoids and immune responses. Arthritis Rheum 22:1246, 1979.
88. Meek M, Munster AM, Winchurch RH, Dickerson C: The Baltimore Sepsis Scale: measurement of sepsis in patients with burns using a new scoring system. J Burn Care Rehabil 12:564, 1991.
89. Faist E, Ertel W. Cohnert T, et al: Immunoprotective effects of cyclooxygenase inhibition in patients with major surgical trauma. J Trauma 30:8, 1990.
90. Wood JJ, Grbic JT, Rodrick ML, et al: Suppression of interleukin 2 production in an animal model of

thermal injury is related to prostaglandin synthesis. Arch Surg 122:179, 1987.
91. Ogle CK, Wu J, Wood S, et al: The increased release of prostaglandin E2 by Kupffer cells from burned guinea pigs. J Burn Care Rehabil 11:287, 1990.
92. Zapata-Sirvent RL, Hansbrough JF: Effect of indomethacin and impact liquid diet administration on inflammatory mediator production by murine splenocytes after burn injury. J Burn Care Rehabil 13:538, 1992.
93. Rappaport RS, Dodge GR: Prostaglandin E inhibits the production of human interleukin 2. J Exp Med 155:943, 1982.
94. Phipps RP, Stein SH, Roper RL: A new view of prostaglandin E regulation of the immune response. Immunol Today 12:349, 1991.
95. Hume DM, Egdahl RH: The importance of the brain in the neuroendocrine response to injury. Ann Surg 150:697, 1959.
96. Gann DS, Amaral JF: Endocrine and metabolic responses to injury. In Schwartz SI, Shires GT, Spencer FC (eds): Principles of Surgery, 5th ed. New York, McGraw-Hill, 1989, pp 1–68.
97. Besedovsky H, del Rey A, Sorkin E, Dinarello CA: Immunoregulatory feedback between interleukin-1 and glucocorticoid hormones. Science 233:652, 1986.
98. Bernton EW, Beach JE, Holaday JW, et al: Release of multiple hormones by a direct action of interleukin-1 on pituitary cells. Science 238:519, 1987.
99. Sapolsky, R, Rivier C, Yamamoto G, et al: Interleuken-1 stimulates the secretion of hypothalamic corticotropin-releasing factor. Science 238:522, 1987.
100. Warren RS, Starnes HF, Alcock N, et al: Hormonal and metabolic response to recombinant human tumor necrosis factor in rat: in vitro and in vivo. Am J Physiol 255:E206, 1988.
101. Cunningham ET Jr, DeSouza EB: Interleukin-1 receptors in the brain and endocrine tissues. Immunol Today 14:171, 1993.
102. Farmer TA Jr, Hill SR Jr, Pittman JA Jr, Herod JW Jr: The plasma 17-hydrocorticosteroid response to corticotropin, SU 4885 and lipopolysaccharide pyrogen. J Clin Endocrinol Metab 21:433, 1961.
103. Richardson RP, Rhyne CD, Fong Y, et al: Peripheral blood leukocyte kinetics following in vivo lipopolysaccharide (LPS) administration to normal human subjects: influence of elicited hormones and cytokines. Ann Surg 210:239, 1989.
104. Dunn AJ: Infection as a stressor: a cytokine mediated activation of the hypothalamo-pituitary-adrenal axis? In Chadwick DJ (ed): Corticotropin-Releasing Factor (Ciba Foundation Symposium 172). Chichester, Wiley, 1993, pp 226–242.
105. Smith EM, Blalock JE: Human lymphocyte production of ACTH and endorphin-like substances: association with leukocyte interferon. Proc Natl Acad Sci USA 78:7530, 1981.
106. Smith EM, Meyer WJ, Blalock JE: Virus induced increases in corticosterone in hypophysectomized mice: a possible lymphoid-adrenal axis. Science 218:1311, 1982.
107. Blalock JE: The immune system as a sensory organ. J Immunol 132:1067, 1984.
108. Barber AE, Coyle SM, Marano MA, et al: Glucocorticoid therapy alters hormonal and cytokine responses to endotoxin in man. J Immunol 150: 1999, 1993.
109. Flower RJ, Blackwell GJ: Anti-inflammatory steroids induce biosynthesis of a phospholipase A2 inhibitor which prevents prostaglandin generation. Nature 278:456, 1979.
110. Goulding NJ, Guyre PM: Regulation of inflammation by lipocortin-1. Immunol Today 13:295, 1992.
111. Pruzanski W, Vadas P: Phospholipase A2—a mediator between proximal and distal effectors of inflammation. Immunol Today 12:143, 1991.
112. Spinas GA, Bloesch D, Kaufmann M-T, et al: Induction of plasma inhibitors of interleukin 1 and TNF-α activity by endotoxin administration to normal humans. Am J Physiol 259:R993, 1990.
113. Engelmann H, Novick D, Wallach D: Two tumor necrosis factor-binding proteins purified from human urine. J Biol Chem 265:1531, 1990.
114. Kohno T, Brewer MT, Baker SL, et al: A second tumor necrosis factor receptor gene product can shed a naturally occurring tumor necrosis factor inhibitor. Proc Natl Acad Sci USA 87:8331, 1990.
115. Lesslauer W, Tabuchi H, Gentz R, et al: Recombinant soluble TNF receptor proteins protect mice from LPS-induced lethality. Eur J Immunol 21: 2883, 1991.
116. Ohlsson K, Björk P, Bergenfeldt M, et al: Interleukin 1 receptor antagonist reduces mortality from endotoxin shock. Nature 348:550, 1990.
117. Dinarello CA: The proinflammatory cytokines interleukin-1 and tumor necrosis factor and treatment of the septic shock syndrome. J Infect Dis 163:1177, 1991.
118. Lowry SF, Moldawer LL: Cytokines and cytokine antagonists in sepsis and critical illness. In Vincent J-L (ed): Yearbook of Intensive Care and Emergency Medicine, Update 1992. Berlin, Springer-Verlag, 1992, pp 36–43.
119. Rogy MA, Coyle SM, Rock CS, et al: Persistently elevated soluble TNF receptor and IL-1 receptor antagonist levels in critically ill patients. J Am Coll Surg 178:132, 1994.
120. Lowry SF: Anticytokine therapies in sepsis. New Horizons Sepsis Cell Physiol Alterations 1:120, 1993.
121. Fisher CJ, Opal SM, Dhainaut J-F, et al: Influence of an anti-tumor necrosis factor monoclonal antibody on cytokine levels in patients with sepsis. Crit Care Med 21:318, 1993.

Alterations of Host Defenses in the Surgical Patient

CHAPTER 17

Jonathan L. Meakins

The primary immunodeficiencies have been discussed in preceding chapters in their appropriate categories: (1) antibody or B cell deficiency, (2) cellular or T-cell deficiency, (3) phagocytic cell dysfunction, (4) disorders of complement, and (5) combined immunodeficiency disorders. A system of nomenclature has been proposed by a committee of the World Health Organization.[1]

ACQUIRED IMMUNE DEFICIENCY IN SURGICAL PATIENTS

Much more common and of greater general clinical significance but less well defined are acquired defects of host defense. As in patients with congenital defects, the characteristic feature of acquired defects is also recurrent infection, but it has been difficult to identify the cause of the susceptibility except that it is the result of injury or stress in its broadest sense. Unlike congenital defects, in which a single defect usually accounts for the clinical manifestations, acquired defects involve more than one component of host defense.

Burns

Recurrent infections, frequently life-threatening, are characteristic sequelae of thermal injury, and many of the components of the immune response are abnormal.[2] Thermal injury has, in fact, become the prototype of acquired derangement of host defenses because of the magnitude and breadth of the abnormalities. All defects return to normal following resolution and healing of the burn wound.

Humoral Responses. Immunoglobulins of all classes are reduced following thermal injury.[3,4] The early reductions are likely to be secondary to generalized catabolism, leakage into the burn wound and its underlying interstitial spaces, as well as some dilution by the enormous volumes of fluids required for resuscitation. Alexander and Moncrief[5] have shown that the primary humoral response to an antigen was reduced, although the anamnestic response to tetanus was earlier and greater than normal. Complement levels are only slightly reduced after burns but become increasingly depressed if infection supervenes.

Cellular Responses. Macrophage and reticuloendothelial system function is difficult to study in humans. Most animal studies indicate that reticuloendothelial function is somewhat depressed and that there is a reduced ability to deliver monocytes to an inflammatory focus after thermal injury.

Cell-mediated immunity is markedly altered following thermal injury. Both humans and experimental animals can accept skin allografts and even xenografts.[6,7] Pigskin xenografts have survived for prolonged periods in patients with burns over 30 percent of the body surface.[8] Burned patients are anergic to recall skin test antigens. Recovery of all these responses follows coverage of the burn wound.

Neutrophil function is similarly depressed following a major burn injury. Bactericidal function is abnormal, and such dysfunction sometimes coincides with the development of septic episodes.[2] Chemotaxis is defective in direct proportion to burn size and depth.[8] Neutrophil bactericidal function improves with nutritional support and the incidence of bacteremia falls.[9] Once the burn wound is covered, neutrophil function returns to normal.

The Transplant Patient

Transplantation became common clinical practice with the development of immunosuppressive regimens effective in preventing or treating rejection. The resultant pharmacologic immunosuppression induced a sizable risk of serious infection. Although more dexterous use of immunosuppression has reduced the risk of infection, it remains the major cause of death.[10,11]

The principal immunosuppressive agents utilized in transplantation are corticosteroids, cyclosporine, and azathioprine together with specific monoclonal antibodies for rejection. Steroid effects include reduced lymphoid proliferation, lympholysis of B and T cells in high concentrations, reductions in antibody formation, inhibition of neutrophil and monocyte chemotaxis, suppression of the inflammatory response, and prolongation of tissue allografts with concomitant effects on the efferent and afferent arcs of cell-mediated immunity. Cyclosporine inhibits T cell function. Azathioprine can reduce or abolish the delayed hypersensitivity response, the nonspecific inflammatory response, antigen processing, and the primary antibody and anamnestic response. Bone marrow suppression with significant leukopenia is the major potential complication leading to infection. The increased incidence of infection in this population is clearly a function of alteration of host defense mechanisms and includes all bacterial species as well as viral, fungal, and protozoal infestations (see Chap. 51).

Patients with Infections

Chapter 7 has reemphasized the interaction between various microbial agents and the effects produced by infection itself on the defenses against subsequent or superinfection (see Tables 7–1 to 7–3).[12]

All infected patients do not have reduced host defenses; in fact, many bear neutrophils with enhanced chemotactic and bactericidal activity.[13] Patients with more serious infections, however, show a depression in neutrophil function that is associated with increased susceptibility to subsequent infections.[14]

The abnormalities of skin test reactivity, neutrophil chemotaxis, and cell delivery all resolve with appropriate drainage of intraperitoneal abscesses or soft tissue infection.[15]

IDENTIFICATION OF THE SURGICAL PATIENT WITH ACQUIRED DEFECTS OF HOST DEFENSE

In clinical practice, there are a number of situations in which one could predict an increased probability of infection—advanced age, major operation, trauma, diabetes, uremia, cancer, poor nutrition, severe pancreatitis, hemorrhagic shock, and the septic or hyperdynamic response. Not every patient in these categories has detectable abnormalities of host defense, however, nor do they all develop infection. Identification of those likely to develop infection is an important task, in order to institute appropriate preventive measures and therapeutic adjustments. In addition, the development of a simple screening test to define a high-risk population would permit the selection of a population appropriate for further study of the critical defects. Selection of this population is difficult.

Investigations of primary immunodeficiencies involved a defined population of patients: those persons with recurrent infections. In surgical practice, investigations are usually instituted after the infection has already started. The discovered abnormalities may or may not have been present before the infectious episode and may be the result rather than the cause of the problem. Patients with potential for abnormalities of host defenses are a large and heterogeneous group. The approach of testing everyone is unrewarding and expensive.

Using the recall skin test antigens, defining the skin test results as in Tables 17–1 and 17–2, and infection as a positive blood culture or an abscess identified at surgery or autopsy, we have shown that patients who are anergic (A) and relatively anergic (RA) had a significantly increased incidence of sepsis and death compared with those whose skin tests were normal (N)[14–19] (Tables 17–1 and 17–2). The results have been confirmed.[20–23] These data show that skin testing preoperatively identified a group of patients at risk for increased infection and

TABLE 17–1. CLINICAL OUTCOME ACCORDING TO SKIN TEST RESPONSES IN TWO PROSPECTIVE STUDIES: INFECTION AND MORTALITY FOLLOWING INITIAL SKIN TEST

Patients Studied	Response	Number	Infection (%)	Mortality (%)
Preoperative (322)	Anergy	21	4 (19.0)	7 (33.3)
	Relative anergy	21	5 (23.8)	7 (33.3)
	Normal	280	13 (4.6)	12 (4.3)
Postoperative after trauma (115)	Anergy	71	44 (62.0)	24 (33.8)
	Relative anergy	25	15 (60.0)	6 (24.0)
	Normal	19	5 (26.3)	1 (5.3)
No operation (83)	Anergy	23	5 (21.7)	11 (47.8)
	Relative anergy	4	1 (25.0)	1 (25.0)
	Normal	56	0 (0.0)	1 (1.8)

mortality following surgery. Sequential skin testing indicates that patients who become anergic and recover normal responses have a higher ratio of infection *while* anergic but have a much improved mortality rate compared with those who *remain* anergic.[18]

Regardless of the patient population studied (preoperative, postoperative, intensive care,[16,17] trauma,[24,25] all general surgical, nonoperative surgical, cancer,[26,27] gastrointestinal bleeding[28]), the presence of altered responses to skin tests with recall antigens has predictive value for patient infection and mortality and identifies a patient population unusually sensitive to major infection.

Cutaneous responses to recall antigens—delayed hypersensitivity reactions (DHR)—are classically considered to be a reflection of cell-mediated immunity. The infections for which cell-mediated immunity is effective are rare in surgical patients, and the organisms that produce infection in anergic patients are common bacteria. Host response against these organisms is mediated via the humoral and phagocytic components of host defense. This suggests that even though the delayed hypersensitivity reaction is altered and correlates with increased rate and severity of infectious complications, the defect may be a general one and other anti-infective aspects of host defense are likely to be abnormal.

TABLE 17–2. CLINICAL OUTCOME ACCORDING TO SKIN TEST RESPONSES IN TWO PROSPECTIVE STUDIES: INFECTION AND MORTALITY IN 1776 PATIENTS BASED ON LEAST REACTIVE SKIN TEST

Skin Test	Patients	Infection (%)	Mortality (%)
Normal	1172	88 (7.5)	25 (2.1)
Relative anergy	178	57 (32)	27 (15)
Anergy	426	200 (47)	149 (35)

Despite the anomalous situation of a classically cell-mediated reaction and an association with bacterial infections, the evolving data are powerful and suggest a relationship. Christou[29] has developed an equation to identify risk of an infection-related death that is now used clinically in a prospective manner in our hospital. The original equation[30] of

$$P\ (\text{infection}) = 33.7 - 7.9 \ln\ (\text{DTH score})$$

has evolved to the equation presently used[29]:

$$P = 1 - \{1 + \exp\ (1.343 - 1.372\ (\text{albumin}) - 0.173\ (\ln\ [\text{DTH score}] + 0.0026\ (\text{age}) - 0.522\ (\text{sex})\}^{-1}$$

which becomes more powerful with incorporation of a contaminated status, thereby integrating the determinants of infection into the risk assessment process.

Immunologic Studies in Anergic Surgical Patients

In conjunction with skin testing, numerous measures of host defense have been assessed in normal and anergic patients. Mixed lymphocyte culture, lymphocyte response to the phytohemagglutinin[31] and pokeweed mitogens, cell-mediated lympholysis, and lymphocyte generation of blastogenic factor were all normal.[16] In four anergic patients, a serum inhibitor of their mixed lymphocyte culture was present.[16] Anergic patients had a reduction in the total lymphocyte count and number of rosetting T lymphocytes.[32]

Neutrophil chemotaxis is reduced in patients with altered skin test responses and returns toward normal with recovery of normal responses.[32–35] This evolution of chemotaxis to normal is more clearly seen in trauma patients. Following major injury, neutrophil chemotaxis is reduced to anergic levels within hours of the injury (Fig. 17–1). Recovery of

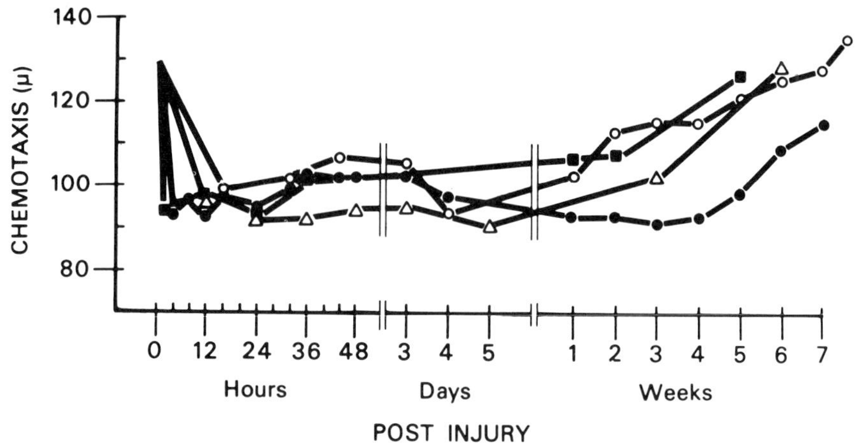

Figure 17–1. Neutrophil chemotaxis in four patients with blunt trauma from time of admission to recovery. Chemotaxis is abnormal at *first* examination 2 to 12 hours after injury. Recovery of normal chemotaxis takes weeks.

normal neutrophil chemotaxis can take weeks.[24,25] The prompt appearance of defective neutrophil chemotaxis suggests that it is mediated by a serum factor. Neutrophil adherence is significantly increased and is directly correlated with chemotaxis.[33]

Anergic serum was found consistently to inhibit the chemotactic responses of normal cells.[36] One inhibitor was found in all sera and has pI = 6.2, $S_{20,w}$ = 5.3, and molecular weight (MW)[36] = 110,000. The other was found only in anergic sera and has pI = 4.6, $S_{20,w}$ = 9.4, MW = 310,000. The data suggest that the decreased polymorphonuclear leukocyte (PML) chemotaxis observed in anergy is the result of the de novo appearance of the larger PML chemotaxis inhibitor and that decreased neutrophil chemotaxis and skin test anergy correlated highly with increased sepsis and mortality in the surgical patient.

Solomkin et al[37] have shown that defects in neutrophil chemotaxis in infected surgery patients are associated with both elevated C5a levels in plasma and loss of C5a receptors on neutrophils. Exposure of normal neutrophils to patient plasma reduces the number of C5a receptors on normal neutrophils and also impairs normal neutrophil function. Chenoweth et al[38] have shown similar results in patients undergoing open heart operations.

Lymphocyte chemotaxis[31] was studied to assess whether or not anergy might be caused by a failure of recruitment of lymphocytes to the area of antigen deposition. Lymphocytes from anergic patients migrated less well than did control lymphocytes. Simultaneous determinations of lymphocyte and neutrophil chemotaxis demonstrated that the two are highly correlated. Anergic sera, which decreased control neutrophil chemotaxis, also decreased normal lymphocyte chemotaxis. The failure of delayed hypersensitivity in surgical patients does not reflect classic defects in cell-mediated immunity.

Humoral immunity in response to tetanus toxoid has recently been demonstrated to be reduced in all surgical patients but particularly in those with anergy (Fig. 17–2). It is of note that these abnormalities are not present following vaccination with Pneumovax, a T cell independent antigen, suggesting that the active immunization programs discussed in Chapter 15 will have to ensure that their immunosuppressed surgical population can respond immunologically to the immunomodulators and vaccines we wish to utilize.

Immunologic defects are not uniformly distributed in anergic patients. It is clear that when the initiating disease or event is clinically controlled, immune abnormalities return to normal. It is likely that the defects are related to the host response to stress—hypovolemia, trauma, surgery—or to disease—cancer, cirrhosis, infection. As the cytokine and lymphokine regulatory influences on the immune system are defined, the acquired immunodeficiency in surgical patients will be better understood and more suitable to direct manipulation.

Etiologic Factors in Anergy

Studies of preoperative patients support the association of skin test anergy with the subsequent development of infection. In other patients, however, it becomes difficult to say that infection is a result rather than a cause of abnormal host defenses. In some patients, infection is obviously a major factor in the development of anergy and associated defects in host defense and its appropriate management is immediately followed by recovery of normal skin test reactions.[15]

The pathogenesis of anergy in surgical patients is difficult to sort out completely because multiple factors can contribute. Several clinical correlations

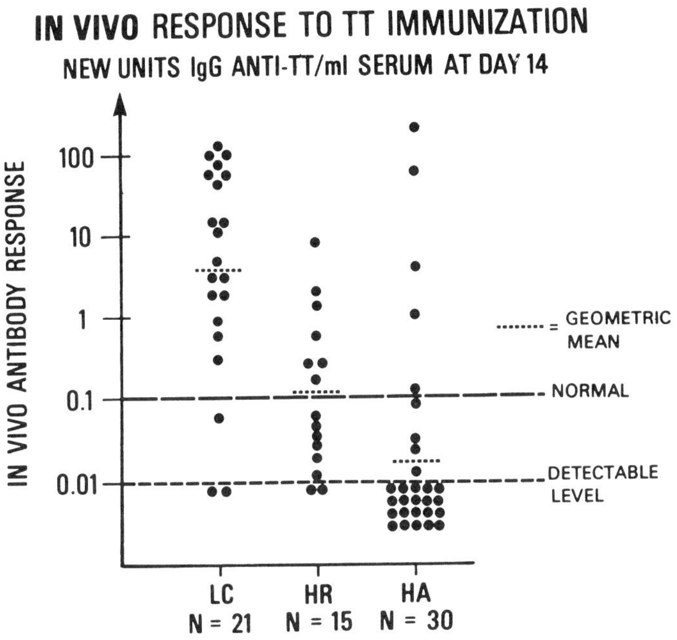

Figure 17–2. In vivo response to tetanus toxid (TT) immunization. Serum antibody response was determined as IU IgG anti-TT/ml at day 14 after TT immunization minus day 0. The detectable level is 0.01 IU/ml, a normal response ≥ 0.1 IU/ml. Healthy laboratory personnel were studied as controls (LC). Patients responding to two or more antigens were classified as hospital reactive (HR), and those responding to no antigens as hospital anergic (HA). *(From Nohr CW, Christon NV, Rode H, et al: Ann Surg 200:373, 1984.)*

can be made, however. Anergy following blunt trauma develops as a function of the age of the patient and the severity of injury. Neutrophil chemotaxis is reduced after major trauma, as a result of the action of a serum factor. The duration of abnormality is a function of the severity of the injury (Fig. 17–3). Following gastrointestinal hemorrhage, development of anergy is related to clinical measures of blood volume such as pulse and the total volume of blood and colloid solutions administered and is unrelated to nutrition or etiology of bleeding.[28] In cancer patients, on the other hand, nutritional measures seem more important in the anergic state than blood volume or site of origin.[26] In each of these patient populations, the anergic state precedes infection.

Malnutrition independently contributes to immune defects. In many of the patients with multifactorial problems, and frequently in those with sepsis, malnutrition is a component of the surgical illness. Abnormal body composition compatible with malnutrition is clearly associated with anergy. The restoration of body composition to normal with total parenteral nutrition is associated with restoration of skin test responses.[39] While not the only cause of anergy, malnutrition may be a significant contributing factor and, in some instances, the only etiologic factor. Other independent factors in generat-

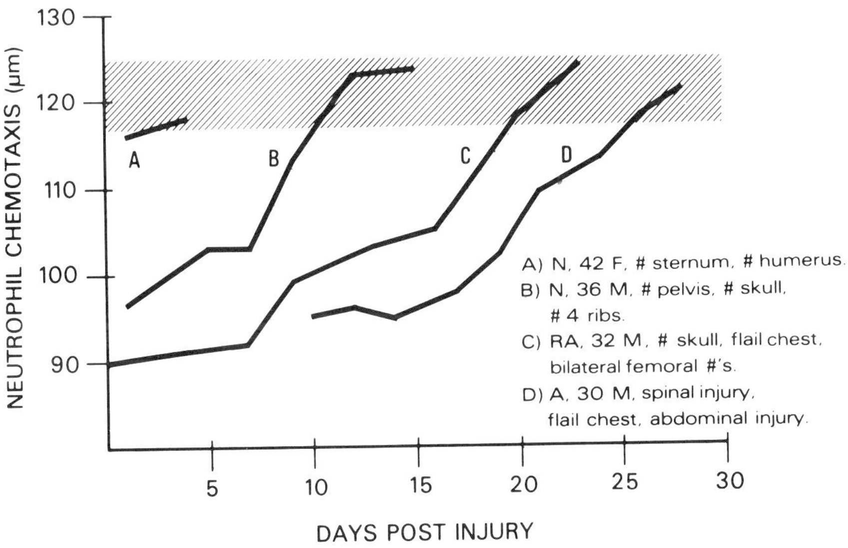

Figure 17–3. Recovery of neutrophil chemotaxis following injury of varying severity in patients of similar age. *(From Meakins JL, McLean API, Kelly R, et al. J Trauma 18:240, 1978.)*

ing acquired immunodeficiencies are related to hemorrhage[40] and the hyperdynamic response (whole-body inflammation) whatever the cause.[41]

OTHER FACTORS PRODUCING ACQUIRED IMMUNE DEFICIENCY

Operation and Anesthesia: Trauma

It becomes very difficult to separate the effects on the immune response of operation from that caused by anesthesia. Operation suppresses leukocyte counts and antibody production for 72 hours. Phagocytosis, allergic responses, and skin reactivity may be depressed. Neutrophil chemotaxis is not affected by anesthetics or superficial operation but is reduced by abdominal or cardiac operation.[41–44] At present, these cannot be related directly to the development of bacterial infection, although they may be important in the spread of tumor cells. Anesthetic gases do appear to affect adversely B cell, T cell, and phagocyte function. What this transient insult means for the patient is not clear.

The cytokine sequence following surgery is similar to that following trauma and endotoxin: TNF early followed by IL-1 and IL-6.[45] Interestingly, those patients who developed complications that manifested themselves days after surgery had an increased IL-6 response that was protracted, indicating that the biologic effect of the operative complication was present long before its clinical expression.

Immunosuppressive Effect of Pharmacologic Agents

Many drugs, by design or inadvertence, have immunosuppressive properties. The adrenocortical steroids, cancer chemotherapeutic agents, cyclosporin, imuran, monoclonal antibodies, and antilymphocytes have all been associated with infectious complications. Their influence is by cytolysis, dysregulation, inhibition, or bone marrow suppression.

Antibiotics may have immunosuppressive properties and may theoretically be working at odds with therapy.[46] The high incidence of superinfection in patients receiving antibiotic therapy, particularly the development of *Candida* infections, has been ascribed in part to antibiotic-mediated immunosuppression. The major practical difficulty relates to bone marrow suppression, which results occasionally from many antibiotics. The idiosyncratic irreversible bone marrow aplasia caused by chloramphenicol is the best known of these effects.

Other classes of drugs, of which the salicylates and NSAIDs are the best known and most important, may have some immunosuppressive activity as they interfere with arachidonic acid metabolism and the synthesis of various leukotrienes and prostaglandins.

Malnutrition and Acquired Immune Deficiency

A broad range of immunodeficiencies involving most components of the immune response are induced by malnutrition.[47–50] Their relationship to infection seems intuitively clear but has been difficult to prove. The question has been raised as to whether malnutrition decreases the immune response or infection precipitates malnutrition. The interaction of infection, malnutrition, and immunodeficiency is probably a vicious circle, each making the next stage worse.

Malnutrition can be shown to decrease phagocytic and bactericidal function, decrease complement levels and antibody responses, reduce lymphocyte response to mitogens, and obviate delayed hypersensitivity responses. The use of total parenteral nutrition[51–54] and enteral nutrition will maintain[55] or restore host defenses to normal and reduce the associated rates of infection. The malnourished patients are usually anergic, and restoration of body cell mass restores cutaneous responses to normal in about one-third of these patients.

Disease States Associated with Immunosuppression

Many disease states have a high incidence of infectious sequelae. Infections are even more common as treatment prolongs the life span of patients with metabolic derangements (diabetes, uremia), neoplastic disease (leukemias, lymphomas, advanced solid tumors), or altered physiologic states. An additional concern is that therapy may itself further reduce resistance, that is, cancer chemotherapy and immunosuppression. In advanced cancer or diabetes, there are secondary anatomic, physiologic, and nutritional alterations, all of which directly affect the local or systemic response to infection.

Today's surgeons are presented with a vastly different patient population from their predecessors. The natural histories of many illnesses are being altered, and new surgical situations constantly appear. The patient in end-stage renal failure is just one example. Transplantation, hemodialysis, and chronic ambulatory peritoneal dialysis have completely altered the inevitable outcome of kidney failure but have substituted a new set of potential problems. Alteration of host resistance is almost universal in these patient groups.

TREATMENT OF ACQUIRED IMMUNE DEFICIENCIES IN SURGICAL PATIENTS

General Physiologic Maintenance

Physiologic derangements are important in the development of infection, since such disturbances lead to acquired defects in host defense. Restoration of Bernard's "milieu interieure" has broader implications than simply the maintenance of vital signs. The restoration and maintenance of blood volume, good tissue perfusion, adequate Po_2, and a physiologic acid-base balance are essential for the delivery and adequate function of the humoral and cellular responses to infection. Similarly, clean, technically perfect operations have immunobiologic implications in the delivery and function of the mediators of host defense to the operative field.[56] Following recovery from the acute phase of injury and early respiratory insufficiency, infection is the major cause of death in the trauma patient. It is therefore of considerable significance that all aspects of a patient's physiology be supported with equal enthusiasm, starting from the moment he or she enters the emergency room.[57]

The Operation

Operative correction of the underlying disease frequently corrects the defects in host defense. Drainage of infection, control of hemorrhage, relief of bowel obstruction, and resection of cancer, with no other treatment, lead to conversions of skin test from anergy to relatively anergic or normal.[15,16] Al though the skin test responses are accompanied by improvement in a patient's general physiologic state, the effects are obviously due to changes at the cellular and molecular level. The persistence of anergy frequently indicates that there are complications that require attention.[15] In our experience,[15] anergy that continues after drainage of an abscess suggests inadequate drainage, another focus of infection, or both.

For this reason, major operations, when directed at the cause of the anergic state, must not be deferred "to build the patient up." Total parenteral nutrition is a valuable support for the catabolic septic patient. Cure of the primary disease is a better solution.[57]

Nutrition

For many reasons, one of them immunologic, total parenteral nutrition was probably the single most significant development in surgical care in the 1970s. However, it is as yet not possible to state the role of nutrition in maintenance and support of the immune system. Infection and malnutrition have been linked for centuries.

Each thrives on the other. Infection contributes or aggravates malnutrition, and malnutrition aids in providing the susceptible host for an infection. In our studies, infection and the septic response are both a cause and a result of malnutrition. The causative component relates primarily to the extraordinary metabolic demands of infected patients and their subsequent catabolism. In anergic patients, about one-third respond to total parenteral nutrition by converting skin tests to normal.[39] The balance of patients do not change skin tests and, significantly, their body composition remains the same. Total parenteral nutrition is therefore required to maintain body cell mass and presumably also helps to maintain, although not augment, host defense.

Studies in humans and animals have shown that malnutrition induces a variety of abnormalities of host defense, all of which can be corrected by nutritional replenishment. It is increasingly apparent that critical illness infection, shock, and trauma either deplete body reserves or consume extra building blocks, specific nutrients, and trace elements and maintenance of host defense and immune function will require supplementation[47,148] and by the appropriate route.[47] The route of nutritional support is important in burn[9] and trauma[55] patients where infection and mortality are reduced by enteral rather than total parenteral nutrition.

Immunomodulating Agents

We still do not have effective direct means of stimulating the immune system during an acute situation. Vaccines have not proved efficacious in most common bacterial diseases. The most active research in modulation of the immune response is in cancer therapy, where *C. parvum*, Bacille Calmette-Guerin (BCG), glucan, levamisole, and a host of other pharmacologic or microbial products are being tested (Table 17–3). The effort is directed toward stimulating immune responses, or restoration of abnormal immune response to normal, and as a means of controlling or curing cancer.

TABLE 17–3. ANERGIC PREOPERATIVE PATIENTS: COMPARISON OF OUTCOME WITH LEVAMISOLE OR PLACEBO

Outcome	Levamisole (19)	Placebo (20)
Infection	3 (16)	9 (45)
Mortality	2 (10)	5 (25)
Improved skin test	14 (74)	12 (60)
Improved chemotaxis	11/16 (69)	9/18 (50)

REFERENCES

1. Fudenberg HH, Good RA, Goodman HC, et al: Primary immunodeficiencies: report of a World Health Organization Committee. Pediatrics 47:927, 1971.
2. Alexander JW, Meakins JL: A physiologic basis for opportunistic infection. Ann Surg 176:273, 1972.
3. Arteison G, Hogman CF, Johnson SGO, Killander J: Changes in immunoglobulin levels in severely burned patients. Lancet 1:546, 1969.
4. Ritzmann SE, McLung C, Falls D: Immunoglobulin levels in burned patients. Lancet 1:1152, 1969.
5. Alexander JW, Moncrief JA: Alterations of the immune response following severe thermal injury. Arch Surg 93:75, 1966.
6. Kay GD: Prolonged survival of a skin homograft in a patient with very extensive burns. Ann NY Acad Sci 64:64, 1957.
7. Polk HC: Prolongation of xenograft survival in patients with pseudomonas sepsis: a clarification. Surg Forum 19:514, 1968.
8. Warden GD, Mason AD, Pruitt BA: Suppression of leukocyte chemotaxis in vitro by chemotherapeutic agents used in management of thermal injuries. Ann Surg 181:363, 1975.
9. Alexander JW: Emerging concepts in control of clinical infection. Surgery 75:934, 1974.
10. Matas A, Simmons RL, Najarian JS: Sepsis in renal transplant recipients. In Hardy JD (ed): Critical Surgical Illness. Philadelphia, Saunders, 1980, p 552.
11. Howard RJ: Infections associated with organ transplantation. In Sugarman B, Young EJ (eds): Infections Associated with Prosthetic Devices. Boca Raton, FL, CRC Press, 1984, p 251.
12. MacKowiak PA: Microbial synergism in human infections, II. N Engl J Med 298:83, 1978.
13. Barbour AG, Crain DA, Solberg CO, Hill HR: Chemiluminescence by polymorphonuclear leukocytes from patients with active bacterial infection. J Infect Dis 141:14, 1980.
14. Solomkin JS, Bauman MP, Nelson RD, Simmons RL: Neutrophil dysfunction during the course of intraabdominal infection. Ann Surg 194:9, 1981.
15. Meakins JL, Christou NV, Shizgal HM, MacLean LD: Therapeutic approaches to anergy in surgical patients: surgery and levamisole. Ann Surg 190:286, 1979.
16. MacLean LD, Meakins JL, Taguchi K, et al: Host resistance in sepsis and trauma. Ann Surg 182:207, 1975.
17. Pietsch JB, Meakins JL, MacLean LD: Delayed hypersensitivity response: application in clinical surgery. Surgery 82:349, 1977.
18. Christou NV: Alterations in host defense mechanisms of surgical and trauma patients with particular reference to polymorphonuclear function and predisposition to sepsis and mortality. PhD Thesis, McGill University, 1980.
19. Meakins JL: Clinical importance of host resistance to infection in surgical patients. Adv Surg 15:225, 1981.
20. Johnson WC, Ulrich F, Meguid MM, et al: Role of delayed hypersensitivity in predicting postoperative morbidity and mortality. Am J Surg 137:536, 1979.
21. George C, Robin M, Carlet J, et al: Tests cutanés explorant l'immunité cellulaire chez les malades en reanimation. Nouv Press Méd 7:2541, 1978.
22. McLoughlin GA, Wu AV, Saporoschetz I, et al: Correlation between anergy and a circulating immunosuppressive factor following major surgical trauma. Ann Surg 190:297, 1979.
23. Buzby GP, Mullen JL, Matthews DC, et al: Prognostic nutritional index in gastrointestinal surgery. Am J Surg 139:160, 1980.
24. Meakins JL, McLean APH, Kelly R, et al: Delayed hypersensitivity and neutrophil chemotaxis: effect of trauma. J Trauma 18:240, 1978.
25. Christou NV, McLean APH, Meakins JL: Host defense in blunt trauma: interrelationships between kinetics of anergy and depressed neutrophil function, nutritional status and sepsis. J Trauma 20:833, 1980.
26. Meakins JL, Christou NV, Hallé C, MacLean LD: Influence of cancer on host defense and susceptibility to infection. Surg Forum 30:115, 1979.
27. Christou NV, Rode H, Larsen H, et al: The walk-in anergic patient: how best to assess the risk of sepsis following elective surgery. Ann Surg 199:438, 1984.
28. Christou NV, Meakins JL, Gotto D, MacLean LD: Influence of gastrointestinal bleeding on host defense and susceptibility to infection. Surg Forum 30:46, 1979.
29. Christou NV: Predicting septic related mortality of the individual surgical patient based on admission host defense measurements. Can J Surg 29:424, 1986.
30. Christou NV, Boisvert G, Broadhead M, Meakins JL: Two techniques of measurement of a delayed hypersensitivity skin test response for the assessment of bacterial host resistance. World J Surg 9:798, 1985.
31. Christou NV, Meakins JL: Delayed hypersensitivity: a mechanism for anergy in surgical patients. Surgery 86:78, 1979.
32. Meakins JL, Pietsch JB, Bubenick O, et al: Delayed hypersensitivity: indicator of acquired failure of host defenses in sepsis and trauma. Ann Surg 186:241, 1977.
33. Christou NV, Meakins JL: Neutrophil function in surgical patients: neutrophil adherence and chemotaxis and cutaneous anergy. Ann Surg 190:557, 1979.
34. Zigmond SH, Hirsch JG: Leukocyte locomotion and chemotaxis. J Exp Med 137:387, 1973.
35. Christou NV: Host-defense mechanisms in surgical patients: a correlative study of the delayed hypersensitivity skin-test response, granulocyte function and sepsis. Can J Surg 28:39, 1985.
36. Christou NV, Meakins JL: Neutrophil function in surgical patients: two inhibitors of granulocyte chemotaxis associated with sepsis. J Surg Res 26:335, 1979.

37. Solomkin JS, Jenkins MD, Nelson RD, et al: Neutrophil dysfunction in sepsis, II. Evidence for the role of complement activation products in cellular deactivation. Surgery 90:319, 1981.
38. Chenoweth DE, Cooper SW, Hugli TE, et al: Complement activation during cardiopulmonary bypass: evidence of generation of C3a and C5a anaphylotoxins. N Engl J Med 304:497, 1981.
39. Spanier AH, Pietsch JB, Meakins JL, et al: The relationship between immune competence and nutrition. Surg Forum 27:332, 1976.
40. Chaudry IH, Ayala A, Meldrum D, Ertel W: Hemorrhage-induced alterations in cell-mediated immune function. In Faist E, Meakins JL, Schildberg FW (eds): Host Defense Dysfunction in Trauma, Shock and Sepsis: Mechanisms and Therapeutic Approaches. Berlin, Springer-Verlag, 1993, pp 149–159.
41. Goris RJA: Sepsis and multiple organ failure: the result of whole body inflammation. In Faist E, Meakins JL, Schildberg FW (eds): Host Defense Dysfunction in Trauma, Shock and Sepsis: Mechanisms and Therapeutic Approaches. Berlin, Springer-Verlag, 1993, pp 161–170.
42. Bubenik O, Meakins JL: Neutrophil chemotaxis in surgical patients: effect of cardiopulmonary bypass. Surg Forum 27:267, 1976.
43. Slade MS, Simmons RL, Yunis EJ, Greenberg LJ: Immunodepression after major surgery in normal patients. Surgery 78:363, 1975.
44. Howard RJ, Simmons RL: Acquired immunodeficiencies after trauma and surgical procedures. Surg Gynecol Obstet 139:771, 1974.
45. Baigre RJ, Lamont PM, Dallman MJ, Morris PJ: The response of interleukin-1 and interleukin-6 in patients undergoing surgery. In Faist E, Meakins JL, Schildberg FW (eds): Host Defense Dysfunction in Trauma, Shock and Sepsis: Mechanisms and Therapeutic Approaches. Berlin, Springer-Verlag, 1993, pp 665–672.
46. Faist E, Meakins JL, Schildberg FW (eds): Section 13 Antibiotic Interactions with Host Defense. In Faist E, Meakins JL, Schildberg FW (eds): Host Defense Dysfunction in Trauma, Shock and Sepsis: Mechanisms and Therapeutic Approaches. Berlin, Springer-Verlag, 1993, pp 943–991.
47. Zaloga GP: Nutrition and prevention of infection. In Taylor RW, Shoemaker WC (eds): Critical Care: State of the Art. Fullerton, Society of Critical Care Medicine, 1991, pp 31–79.
48. Alexander JW: Augmentation of host defense reactivity with special nutrients. In Faist E, Meakins JL, Schildberg FW (eds): Host Defense Dysfunction in Trauma, Shock, and Sepsis: Mechanisms and Therapeutic Approaches. Berlin, Springer-Verlag, 1993, pp 995–1001.
49. Susskind RM: Immune status of the malnourished host. In Dick G (ed): Immunological Aspects of Infectious Disease. Lancaster, England, MTP Press, 1979.
50. Christou NV, Superina R, Broadhead M, Meakins JL: Postoperative depression of host resistance: determinants and effect of peripheral protein-sparing therapy. Surgery 92:786, 1982.
51. Dionigi R, Zonta A, Dominioni L, et al: The effects of total parenteral nutrition on immunodepression due to malnutrition. Ann Surg 185:467, 1977.
52. Law DK, Dudrick SJ, Abdou NI: Immunocompetence of patients with protein-calorie malnutrition: the effects of nutritional repletion. Ann Intern Med 79:545, 1973.
53. Law DK, Dudrick SJ, Abdou NI: The effects of dietary protein depletion on immunocompetence: the importance of nutritional repletion prior to immunologic induction. Ann Surg 179:168, 1974.
54. Copeland EM, MacFadyen BV, Dudrick SJ: Effect of intravenous hyperalimentation on established delayed hypersensitivity in the cancer patient. Ann Surg 184:60, 1976.
55. Moore FA, Moore EE, Jones TN, et al: TEN versus TPN following major abdominal trauma—reduced septic morbidity. J. Trauma 29:916, 1989.
56. Edlich RF, Rodeheaver GT, Thacker JG, et al: Technical factors in wound management. In Hunt TK, Dunphy JE (eds): Fundamentals of Wound Management. New York, Appleton-Century-Crofts, 1979.
57. Meakins JL: Surgeons, surgery and immunomodulation. Arch Surg 126:494, 1991.

BIBLIOGRAPHY

Covino BG, Shires GT: Influence of anesthetic procedures on surgical sequelae: an update. Acta Chir Scand Suppl 550:1, 1989.

Faist E, Meakins JL, Schildberg FW (eds): Host Defense Dysfunction in Trauma, Shock, and Sepsis: Mechanisms and Therapeutic Approaches. Berlin, Springer-Verlag, 1993, pp 943–991.

Faist E, Ninnemann J, Green D (eds): Immune Consequences of Trauma, Shock, and Sepsis: Mechanism and Therapeutic Approaches. Berlin, Springer-Verlag, 1989.

Howard RJ: Effect of burn injury, mechanical trauma, and operation on immune defenses. Surg Clin North Am 59:199, 1979.

Simmons RL (ed): Surgical Aspects of Immunology (symposia). Surg Clin North Am 59(2):183, 1979.

NORMAL COMPENSATORY RESPONSES TO INFECTION

PART II

Hemodynamic Responses to Infection

CHAPTER 18

Mitchell P. Fink

Although the term *sepsis* has been defined as the systemic response to infection,[1,2] this definition is not entirely satisfactory for several reasons. First, the systemic manifestations of infection are very inconstant. For example, most infected patients are febrile, but some are hypothermic[3–6]; a few have neither fever nor hypothermia. Although most patients with sepsis have an elevated blood leukocyte count, profound leukopenia also can occur.[3,6,7] In view of the inconstancy of these and other key clinical findings, it is virtually impossible to define universally applicable criteria for establishing the diagnosis of sepsis.

Second, a variety of conditions are associated with the systemic release of proinflammatory mediators. These conditions can lead to the development of clinical findings, which are virtually identical to those characteristic of severe infection.[8,9] Indeed, many of systemic hemodynamic, hematologic, and hormonal responses to infection can be reproduced by infusing volunteers or patients with certain proinflammatory substances, such as TNF-α, IL-1 or IL-2.[10–14] Thus sepsis probably does not reflect the systemic response to infection per se, but rather the effects of proinflammatory mediators, which are released during infections as well as other conditions. Accordingly, a proposal has been made to adopt the cumbersome term *systemic inflammatory response syndrome* or *SIRS* to describe the clinical syndrome associated with the release of proinflammatory mediators, whatever the cause.[15]

Finally, considered one by one, most of the systemic signs of infection are very nonspecific. For example, tachycardia, which has been considered to be one of the cardinal features of both the *sepsis syndrome*[16] and the *systemic inflammatory response syndrome,*[15] can be caused by pain, anemia, hypovolemia, or many other conditions that are not necessarily related to the presence of infection (or even inflammation).

These considerations notwithstanding, the term *sepsis* in this chapter will be used to denote the continuum of acute and subacute responses by the host to the invasion of normally sterile tissues by microbes. The term *septic shock* will be used to denote circulatory collapse (ie, systemic arterial hypotension) due to overwhelming infection. The term *endotoxicosis* will be used to denote the syndrome induced in animals or human volunteers by the injection of lipopolysaccharide (LPS). The term *systemic inflammatory response* will be used to denote the complex (and variable) metabolic, hormonal, hemodynamic, and hematologic perturbations, which are associated with the exogenous administration or endogenous release of proinflammatory mediators (irrespective of cause).

SYSTEMIC HEMODYNAMICS IN SEPSIS

The hemodynamic response to sepsis is undoubtedly influenced greatly by commonly employed therapeutic interventions, such as intravascular volume expansion with crystalloid or colloid solutions, infusion of vasoactive drugs, or administration of inotropic agents. Therefore the data obtained in virtually all clinical studies of hemodynamics in septic patients are confounded to some extent by the therapeutic interventions employed. This fact alone may account for the discrepancies between the results obtained in certain animal models of sepsis and those recorded by clinical investigators studying patients.[17]

Role of the Infecting Organism

Although some studies have suggested that the hemodynamic profile of sepsis or septic shock depends on the nature of the infecting organism,[18–20] more recent analyses have reported that hemodynamic responses are similar for gram-positive and gram-negative infections.[21–23] Data obtained in a canine model of peritonitis further support the notion that the hemodynamic response to severe infection is host dependent and organism independent.[24] Even overwhelming viremia (due to cytomegalovirus infection) leads to hemodynamic perturbations similar to those observed in septic shock due to bacterial infections.[25,26]

Hemodynamic Response to Sepsis as a Determinant of Outcome

The "typical" patient with well-compensated sepsis is tachycardic (ie, heart rate greater than 90/min) and hyperthermic (ie, core temperature greater than 38.3C). Cardiac output indexed to body surface area (Q_T) is usually supranormal (ie, greater than 3.5 liters/min/M^2), whereas calculated systemic vascular resistance index (SVRI) is usually subnormal (ie, less than 2000 dyn $\times$ s $\times$ M^2/cm^5).[3,21,27,28] In well-compensated sepsis, mean arterial blood pressure (MAP) is normal; however, by definition, in septic shock, MAP is low (or there is a requirement for the infusion vasoactive drugs to preserve normal MAP). In the typical patient with septic shock, Q_T is normal[27,29] or elevated[4,25,26,30] and SVRI is very low.[4,25–27,30]

All septic patients, however, do not manifest these hemodynamic responses to the same degree. Accordingly, numerous investigators have attempted to correlate various hemodynamic profiles with outcome in patients with sepsis or septic shock. In a study of 42 patients with septic shock, Groeneveld et al[31] recorded hemodynamic data at three time points: within 12 hours of the diagnosis of septic shock (T1), at the time when Q_T was maximal (T2), and within 12 hours of death or discontinuation of pulmonary arterial catheterization (T3). These authors found that the hemodynamic profiles of survivors and nonsurvivors were similar at T1. At T2 and T3, however, MAP and SVRI were significantly lower in nonsurvivors than in survivors, whereas Q_T did not discriminate between these subgroups. These data suggest that dysregulation of peripheral vasomotor tone (ie, low SVRI) is a major factor contributing to mortality in septic shock.

Rackow et al[29] recorded hemodynamic data in 18 patients with septic shock before and after an intravascular volume challenge designed to raise pulmonary arterial wedge pressure (PAWP) to 12 mm Hg. In contrast to the results obtained by Groeneveld et al cited above, Rackow and colleagues found that commonly measured systemic hemodynamic parameters, including Q_T, SVRI, and calculated left ventricular stroke work index (LVSWI), did not differ between survivors and nonsurvivors.

Like Rackow et al,[29] D'Orio and colleagues[32] recorded hemodynamic parameters before and after intravascular volume loading in 26 patients with septic shock. D'Orio et al found that prior to intravascular volume expansion, nonsurvivors had lower Q_T and LVSWI and higher SVRI than did survivors. Furthermore, in response to a volume load, Q_T and LVSWI increased more in survivors than in nonsurvivors. Thus, in marked contradistinction to the data obtained by Groeneveld et al,[31] these results tend to minimize the importance of peripheral arteriolar dilation as a major predictor of mortality in septic shock but suggest that survival may depend on the adequacy of myocardial performance. Although several other studies also have obtained data suggesting that cardiac output and risk of mortality are inversely related in sepsis,[33,34] numerous investigators have failed to detect such a relationship.[31,35–37] The inconstancy among studies in the relationship between cardiac output and outcome may be explained by data obtained by Baumgartner et al,[3,35] which suggest that both relatively low Q_T (ie, less than 3.5 liters/min/M^2) or very high Q_T (ie, greater than 7.5 liters/min/M^2) predict a high likelihood of mortality in patients with sepsis. The association of very high Q_T with increased risk of mortality in sepsis may be because this particular hemodynamic pattern is very common in patients with underlying cirrhosis,[4,35] a clinical subgroup in which survival is uncommon.[4]

Parker et al[30] examined systemic hemodynamic parameters in 48 patients with septic shock. Data were recorded at two time points: within a few hours of diagnosis (T0) and 24 hours later (T24). In comparison to the patients who died, survivors manifested a greater decrease in heart rate and Q_T and greater increase in SVRI over the 24-hour period of observation. These data along with those obtained by others[31] tend to support the notion that impaired regulation of arteriolar tone is either an important causative factor leading to mortality in sepsis or is a marker for other physiologic phenomenona that bear importantly on outcome.

SYSTEMIC OXYGEN TRANSPORT AND UPTAKE IN SEPSIS

O_2 Regulators Versus O_2 Conformers

In mammals, different organs and tissues display differing metabolic responses to variations in oxygen delivery (Do_2).[38] In many tissues, which are termed *O_2 regulators*, oxygen uptake (Vo_2) is maintained or *regulated* by the cells at a nearly constant rate, unless oxygen availability falls to very low levels. Thus a plot of Vo_2 versus oxygen availability is biphasic, being characterized by a flat availability-independent region and a sloped availability-dependent region. The point of transition between these two regions has been termed the *critical Do_2* or Do_{2crit}. As Barcroft recognized in 1920,[39] diminished availability of oxygen at the cellular level can be the result of any of three processes: (1) inadequate arterial oxygen tension (*hypoxic hypoxia*), (2) inadequate circulating hemoglobin concentration (*anemic hypoxia*), or (3) inadequate blood flow (*stagnant hypoxia*). Obviously, these mechanisms are not mutually exclusive.

In some tissues, called *O_2 conformers,* Vo_2 is a function of oxygen availability over a wide range of values.[38] For example, some studies suggest that skeletal muscle can exhibit an O_2 conforming pattern.[40–42] Liver expresses an intermediate pattern, displaying evidence of O_2 regulation at high rates of oxygen delivery (Do_2), but shifting to a conforming pattern with even modest reductions in oxygen availability.[43]

In anesthetized animals and humans, the normal relationship between systemic Do_2 and systemic Vo_2 is one of O_2 regulation.[44–48] In anesthetized humans, the transition from the supply-independent to the supply-dependent region of the Do_2-Vo_2 diagram (ie, Do_{2crit}) seems to occur when systemic Do_2 decreases to less than about 300 to 330 ml/min/M^2.[47,48]

Pathologic Supply Dependence of Systemic VO_2 in Sepsis

In 1978, in a study of 11 patients with the adult respiratory distress syndrome (ARDS), Rhodes et al[49] examined the effects on systemic oxygen metabolism of acutely expanding circulating volume with an intravenous infusion of mannitol solution. Sepsis was the underlying cause of ARDS in six of the patients studied. Although Q_T and systemic Do_2 were supranormal prior to the volume challenge, infusing mannitol significantly increased both systemic Do_2 and systemic Vo_2. Thus the patients appeared to be O_2 conformers, or, stated another way, there was evidence of supply dependency of Vo_2 even at high rates of Do_2. Numerous subsequent studies, using a variety of means for manipulating systemic Do_2, have confirmed this observation in patients with sepsis and/or ARDS.[50–61] Cain[62] has termed this phenomenon *pathologic supply dependency* of oxygen uptake, implying that the normal relationship between systemic Do_2 and Vo_2 is one of O_2 regulation (rather than conformation) at normal or supranormal rates of Do_2.

If Vo_2 increases when Do_2 is increased, then utilization of oxygen is being determined by availability rather than metabolic demand. This has been interpreted as meaning that if one can demonstrate supply dependency of systemic Vo_2 in patients with sepsis, then an oxygen deficit must exist at the tissue level.[63] This notion is supported by studies showing that pathologic supply dependency in patients with sepsis occurs only in those with elevated circulating concentrations of lactate[64–68]; that is, pathologic supply dependency is associated with biochemical evidence of increased anaerobic metabolism. Other studies, however, have found evidence of supply dependency of Vo_2 in patients with sepsis and normal lactate levels[69] or have found that supply dependency is demonstrable irrespective of blood lactate concentration.[70]

Despite the large number of studies showing evidence of pathologic supply dependency in patients with sepsis or ARDS, it is becoming increasingly apparent that this phenomenon may be more artifactual than real. In most studies, systemic Vo_2 has not been measured directly but has been estimated using the following formula:

$$Vo_2 = Q_T \times (Cao_2 - Cvo_2)$$

where Cao_2 and Cvo_2 are the contents of oxygen in arterial and mixed venous (ie, pulmonary arterial) blood, respectively. Systemic Do_2 has been calculated as the product of Q_T multiplied by Cao_2. Thus relatively small errors in the measurement of either or both of the shared variables, Cao_2 and Q_T, will lead to artificial correlation of Do_2 and Vo_2, a methodological error, which has been termed mathematical coupling.[71,72] This methodological pitfall can be obviated by measuring systemic Vo_2 by a means, such as analysis of respiratory gases, that is completely independent from that used to calculate Do_2. Using this approach, several studies have found that systemic Vo_2 is independent of Do_2 in patients with sepsis and or ARDS.[73–77] Indeed, several carefully performed studies using indirect means to calculate systemic Vo_2 also have failed to find evidence of pathologic supply dependency.[65,78,79]

In addition to the issue of mathematical coupling, two other methodological problems have contributed to confusion regarding the issue of pathologic supply dependency of Vo_2 in sepsis. First, many investigators have performed regression analyses of Vo_2 as a function of Do_2 using pooled data obtained from multiple patients.[52,54,55,64] Since this sort of analysis ignores the contribution of interpatient variation in Do_2 and Vo_2, the strength of the dependence of the latter parameter of the former can be grossly overestimated.[80] Second, many investigators have failed to recognize that systemic Do_2 normally tracks Vo_2; that is, under normal circumstances, Do_2 (not Vo_2) is the dependent variable. Hence in order conclude that Vo_2 is dependent on Do_2, it is necessary to ensure that metabolic demand is constant over the period that the measurements are obtained. In many instances, spontaneous changes in systemic Vo_2, due, for example, to variations in the degree of stimulation or sedation of patients, can lead to the artifactual appearance of supply dependency of Vo_2.[81–83]

It is well known that the systemic oxygen extraction ratio (ie, the quotient of systemic Vo_2 divided by systemic Do_2) is often quite low in septic patients.[59,84,85] This observation, in conjunction with the apparent phenomenon of pathologic supply dependency, has suggested to numerous authors that sepsis leads to a defect in the extraction and utilization of oxygen by tissues.[53,55,86] Of course, if Q_T and systemic Do_2 are pathologically elevated out of proportion to metabolic demand by mechanism(s) unrelated to oxygen metabolism, then a low systemic oxygen extraction ratio may not be indicative of defective peripheral utilization of oxygen. In order to provide convincing evidence of impaired oxygen extraction by tissues, it is necessary to plot Vo_2 as a function of Do_2 at low rates of Do_2 and show that the slope of the resulting regression line is flatter than normal. Using this approach, some studies using experimental animal models have obtained evidence that sepsis or endotoxemia does indeed lead to both regional (eg, transmesenteric) and systemic defects in oxygen extraction.[87–91] Contrary results, however, have been obtained in other studies using different animal models of sepsis.[92–96] Consequently, the question of whether oxygen extraction is truly impaired in sepsis remains open.

Some studies have found that higher rates of systemic Do_2 and Vo_2 correlate with improved survival in patients with sepsis or ARDS.[97,98] This observation, along with the notion that Vo_2 is pathologically dependent on Do_2 in sepsis and ARDS, has prompted some clinicians to conclude that deliberate augmentation of systemic Do_2 (or Q_T) to supranormal levels will improve outcome in patients with these conditions. Two clinical studies have attempted to provide support for this hypothesis by comparing outcome in patients randomly allocated to receive standard therapy or therapy titrated to achieve supranormal values of Q_T, Do_2, and/or Vo_2. One of these trials, conducted by Shoemaker et al,[99] showed that survival was significantly better in the group of patients receiving therapy titrated to supranormal cardiorespiratory values. However, this study was not limited to patients with sepsis (or ARDS) and the treatment groups may not have been comparable with respect to severity or types of disease. The other trial, which was conducted by Tuchschmidt et al,[100] enrolled 51 patients with septic shock. Twenty-five were randomized to receive normal treatment (ie, colloid solution dopamine, and/or dobutamine titrated to maintain Q_T at 3 liters/min/M^2 or higher and systolic blood pressure at 90 mm Hg or higher). Twenty-six patients were randomized to receive treatment (colloid solution, dopamine, and/or dobutamine) titrated to maintain Q_T at 6 liters/min/M^2 or higher. When the results were analyzed on an intent-to-treat basis, mortality was 72 percent in the control arm as compared to 50 percent in the (*optimal treatment*) group receiving therapy titrated to a supranormal Q_T (P = 0.14). However, when results were analyzed by stratifying the patients into low (less than 4.5 liters/min/M^2) and high (4.5 liters/min/M^2 or higher) Q_T groups, both survival and systemic Do_2 were significantly ($P < 0.05$) higher in the high Q_T group than in the low Q_T group (60 percent versus 26 percent and 13.8 ml/min/kg versus 10.9 ml/min/kg, respectively). Thus it is unclear whether high Q_T and Do_2 are direct determinants of survival, or whether the ability to increase Q_T is a marker for better *physiologic reserve,* which portends a better outcome.

ALTERATIONS IN VASCULAR SMOOTH MUSCLE FUNCTION IN SEPSIS

Sepsis-Induced Vasodilation

As has been noted already, low calculated SVRI is a characteristic features of sepsis and septic shock in adequately resuscitated patients. Because dysregulation of arteriolar vasomotor tone might contribute to maldistribution of blood flow in sepsis (and hence regional tissue ischemia), this topic has been the focus of intensive investigation. Studies performed in animal models have provided clear evidence that vascular smooth muscle contractile function is impaired both in vivo and in vitro after a septic or endotoxic challenge.[101,102] Aortic rings obtained from septic rats and suspended in an organ bath generate significantly less contractile force in response to graded doses of norepinephrine than do rings obtained from nonseptic controls.[103] Similar results have been obtained when aortic rings were obtained from endotoxemic rats[104] or rats injected with a cytokine—tumor necrosis factor alpha—implicated in the pathogenesis of the septic response.[105] Data obtained using video microscopy indicate that sepsis[106,107] and endotoxicosis[108] are associated with vasodilation of small arterioles, the main site of vascular impedance, in vivo.

It seems likely that more than one mechanism accounts for the impairment of vascular smooth muscle contractile function in sepsis (Table 18–1). Moreover, many of the mechanisms appear to overlap. For example, certain cytokines have been shown to diminish vascular smooth muscle contractility via a cyclooxygenase-dependent pathway as well as via a pathway involving enhanced nitric oxide production and activation of guanylate cyclase. Some current notions regarding the mediators and mechanisms of altered vascular contractility in sepsis are discussed in the following paragraphs.

TABLE 18–1. POTENTIAL MEDIATORS AND MECHANISMS CAUSING EXCESSIVE VASODILATION OR VASOCONSTRICTION IN SEPSIS[a]

Excessive release of vasodilating mediators
Nitric oxide (or related endogenous nitrovasodilators)
Prostaglandins (PGI_2, PGE_2)
Calcitonin-gene related peptide
Excessive release of vasoconstricting mediators
Cysteinyl leukotrienes
Endothelin 1
Thromboxane A_2
Impaired adrenergic signal transduction
Increased sensitivity of vascular smooth muscle to cGMP
Opening of ATP-sensitive K^+ channels

[a] This list is not intended to be exhaustive. The mechanisms and mediators listed may overlap; for example, calcitonin-gene related peptide may induce vasodilation by activating ATP-sensitive K^+ channels.

Prostaglandins. Accumulating results suggest that vasodilating metabolites of arachidonic acid are among the mediators responsible for impaired vasomotor tone in sepsis. Extensive data from studies in both animals[109–112] and humans[113–115] indicate that production of vasodilating prostaglandins (ie, PGI_2 and PGE_2) is increased in sepsis and endotoxemia.

Several observations support the notion that the release of vasodilating prostaglandins, particularly prostacyclin, contributes to the loss of vasomotor tone in sepsis. In septic patients, very high levels of 6-keto-$PGF_{1\alpha}$ seem to correlate with hemodynamic decompensation.[113,115] Treatment of septic, hyperdynamic dogs with cyclooxygenase inhibitors (indomethacin or ibuprofen) normalizes Q_T and restores normal SVRI.[116] Treatment of septic rats with indomethacin normalizes the pressor response to bolus doses of norepinephrine.[101] Similar results also have been reported in models of acute endotoxemia by Auclair et al[117] and Gray et al,[118] although other authors have reported that inhibition of cyclooxygenase activity fails to reverse LPS-induced vascular hyporesponsiveness.[104,119] Recently, Cryer et al,[106] utilizing video microscopy to examine vasomotor responsiveness in rats with hyperdynamic bacteremia, have demonstrated that topical application of a cyclooxygenase inhibitor (meclofenamate) blunts or abrogates small arteriolar dilation in this model. Interestingly, the effect of inhibiting prostaglandin synthesis is much greater if meclofenamate is applied prior to rather than 60 minutes after initiating bacteremia, suggesting that release of prostaglandins triggers a secondary event, which is not completely blocked by this drug.[106]

Although some data suggest that vasodilating prostaglandins participate in the alterations in vasomotor function induced by sepsis or endotoxin, we found that inhibition of cyclooxygenase does not significantly affect SVRI in a rabbit model of normotensive, hyperdynamic sepsis[120] or a pig model of hypotensive, normodynamic septic shock.[112] Recently, Martich et al[121] confirmed these observations in human volunteers challenged with a low dose of LPS. Thus the importance of PGI_2 or PGE_2 as mediators of vasomotor dysfunction in sepsis remains an open question.

Nitric Oxide. In the past several years, it has become apparent that nitric oxide (NO), an inorganic free-radical gas, is an extraordinarily important secretory product of mammalian cells with diverse physiologic functions.[122] NO is derived from one of the guanidino nitrogens of the amino acid, L-arginine, via a five-electron oxidation reaction catalyzed by a group of enzymes called nitric oxide synthases (NOSs).[122] Two general classes of NOSs have been described. A constitutive form of the enzyme (cNOS) is expressed in a variety of tissues, including endothelium, brain, platelets, adrenal gland, retina, endocardium, and myocardium.[123] Inducible forms of NOS (iNOS) are present in macrophages, neutrophils, Kupffer cells, hepatocytes, vascular endothelium, vascular smooth muscle, endocardium, and myocardium.[123] Induction requires several hours exposure to inflammatory cytokines—especially IFN-γ, IL-1, TNF-α, and/or bacterial lipopolysaccharide. The iNOS produces much more NO than does cNOS.

Promotion of vasorelaxation is one of the many biologic actions of NO. This action occurs when NO forms an adduct with the heme moiety of soluble guanylate cyclase in vascular smooth cells, leading to activation of this enzyme and increased conversion of guanosine triphosphate (GTP) into guanosine-3′,5′-cyclic monophosphate (cGMP).[124] A cGMP-dependent protein kinase is then activated, ultimately resulting in dephosphorylation of myosin light chains and vasorelaxation.[124]

It has been known for a long time that a variety of agonists (eg, acetylcholine, bradykinin, histamine, serotonin, and thrombin) are capable of causing the relaxation of vascular rings, which have been preconstricted by exposure to a vasopressor (eg, potassium chloride, norepinephrine). Experiments in the early 1980s by Furchgott and Zawadzki[125] showed that this phenomenon requires the presence of intact endothelium and is mediated by a labile agent, called endothelial-derived relaxing factor (EDRF), that is not a prostaglandin. Subsequent experiments by Palmer et al[126] and Ignarro et al[127] identified NO as the EDRF, although it remains to be determined whether NO or some closely related reactive oxide of nitrogen or low molecular weight NO adduct is the true EDRF.[128–132]

It is increasingly apparent that excessive release of NO is a major factor contributing to the loss of vasomotor tone in patients with sepsis and septic shock and in experimental animal models of this syndrome. Several lines of evidence support this conclusion. First, inhibitors of NOS, including N^{ω}-amino-L-arginine,[133] N^{G}-monomethyl-L-arginine,[134,135] and N^{ω}-nitro-L-arginine,[136,137] reverse hypotension and lower SVRI in animals challenged with LPS or live bacteria. Indeed, anecdotal data suggest that blood pressure is increased when humans with septic shock are infused with an NOS inhibitor.[138] Second, hydroquinone, an agent that blocks NO-mediated phenomena by at least two mechanisms, prevents dilation of small arterioles in rats with hyperdynamic sepsis.[107] Third, in some[102,139–141] but not all[142] studies, treatment with either methylene blue, which blocks activation of guanylate cyclase, or an NOS inhibitor has been shown to restore normal contractility (measured in vitro) of vascular rings obtained from animals challenged with LPS. Fourth, agents, such as cycloheximide, actinomycin D, dexamethasone, or nifedipine, which block the induction of iNOS, ameliorate LPS-induced vascular hyporesponsiveness.[141,143–146] Fifth, urinary and plasma levels of nitrite and nitrate, end products of NO metabolism, are increased in endotoxic animals[147,148] and septic humans.[149,150] Moreover, in one clinical study, it was possible to show an inverse relationship between urinary nitrite/nitrate excretion and SVRI.[149]

NO, a very labile compound that is rapidly inactivated by hemoglobin, is thought to act exclusively as an autocrine or paracrine mediator. Initially, it was thought that the endothelium was the primary source of NO responsible for vasomotor hyporesponsiveness induced by sepsis or endotoxin.[151] However, several observations argue against this conclusion. Myers et al[152] have obtained data in a very carefully performed study, which indicate that, rather than stimulating NO release, LPS actually inhibits release of this mediator by cultured endothelial cells. This observation is consistent with results obtained by several investigators, which indicate that exposure to LPS or TNF-α blunts acetylcholine-induced vascular relaxation.[108,146,153–155] Since acetylcholine is a potent inducer for the release EDRF, these findings suggest that, at least under some conditions, LPS or TNF-α diminish (rather than increase) the release of NO or other EDRF-like mediators from the endothelium.

Vascular smooth muscle, rather than the endothelium, may be the key tissue responsible for impaired vasomotor regulation in sepsis. This notion is supported by the observation that LPS- or cytokine-induced vascular hyporesponsiveness to pressor agents can be demonstrated in both the presence and absence of endothelium,[102,105,144,146,156] although the presence of intact endothelium may accelerate the time course for the development of this phenomenon[145] or increase the magnitude of it.[157] Furthermore, an inducible NOS is present in vascular smooth muscle[158,159]; therefore NO might act in an autocrine fashion in sepsis to induce vasodilation. McKenna[160] has reported that the sensitivity of vascular smooth muscle to the vasorelaxant effects of cGMP is increased in aortic rings isolated from septic rats, suggesting that events distal to the release of NO also may be important in sepsis-induced vasomotor dysfunction.

Although NO (or a related compound) appears to contribute to the development of arterial vasodilation and hypotension in animals and patients with sepsis or endotoxemia, inhibition of NOS may have deleterious consequences under these conditions. NO not only acts as a vasodilator, it also neutralizes superoxide and deaggregates platelets. Inhibitors might well be expected to cause microvascular thrombosis and increase damage due to reactive oxygen intermediates. Broughton-Smith et al[161] reported that treatment of endotoxic rats with N^G-monomethyl-L-arginine exacerbates the development of jejunal mucosal lesions and increases LPS-induced jejunal microvascular hyperpermeability. Cobb et al[133] found that treatment of endotoxic canines with N^{ω}-amino-L-arginine results in diminished cardiac output, diminished systemic V_{O_2}, and increased mortality. Shultz and Raij[148] showed that treatment of endotoxic rats with a NOS inhibitor (N^{ω}-nitro-L-arginine methyl ester) improves arterial blood pressure and urine flow but also results in diminished renal creatinine clearance and the development of capillary thrombosis in glomeruli. Harbrecht et al[147] demonstrated that treatment of endotoxic mice with N^G-monomethyl-L-arginine worsens hepatic damage. In view of these results, the use of NOS inhibitors in the clinical setting should be approached with considerable caution until issues of dosage, timing, and perhaps tissue selectivity are more fully understood.

Cytokines. Recently, several studies have provided evidence that two cytokines, namely, tumor necrosis factor alpha (TNF-α) and interleukin 1 (IL-1), can induce vasodilation. Using an in vitro system, Hollenberg et al[157] have studied the effects of several cytokines on the contractility of rat aortic rings, which have been precontracted with phenylephrine. In this system, TNF-α diminishes the force of contraction in dose-dependent fashion, whereas IL-1 and interleukin 6 (IL-6) have minimal or no effect.[157] TNF-α also has been shown to cause arteriolar dilation in vivo.[162] Interestingly, this phenomenon is blocked by prior exposure to cyclooxygenase inhibitors, suggesting an intersection between cytokine- and prostanoid-dependent mechanisms.[162]

Whereas Hollenberg and colleagues found that IL-1 has minimal effects on vascular contractility in vitro, McKenna et al[163,164] and Beasley et al[146] have reported that IL-1 induces vascular hyporesponsiveness in arterial rings studied in organ bath. Moreover, incubation of vascular tissue with IL-1 increases content of cGMP,[165] suggesting that generation of NO is an important intermediate step in this phenomenon. This idea is supported by recent data showing that incubation of vascular tissue with IL-1 leads to increased nitrite release by smooth muscle cells,[158] a process that is inhibited by thrombin and potentiated by plasmin.[166,167]

Interleukin 2 (IL-2) is another cytokine that plays a central role in the network of mediators that includes TNF-α, IL-1, IL-6, and interferon gamma (IFN-γ). IL-2 has been used in the immunotherapy of cancer. Patients infused with IL-2 often develop fever, chills, hypotension, pulmonary edema, cholestatic jaundice, and other features of characteristic sepsis and the sepsis-induced multiple organ failure syndrome. Recently, patients receiving IL-2 were shown to have marked increases in circulating levels of nitrate and urinary excretion of nitrate.[168] These results provide clear evidence that increased synthesis of NO can be induced by a cytokine in humans.

Both IL-1 and TNF-α are thought to act predominantly as autocrine or paracrine hormones. It is noteworthy in this regard that McKenna[144] showed that in vitro incubation of rat aortic rings with LPS for 16 hours resulted in impaired contractility in response to graded doses of norepinephrine and the release of IL-1 and TNF-α into the tissue culture medium. Agents, such as dexamethasone, indomethacin, or actinomycin D, which blunted or blocked LPS-induced cytokine release by the vascular rings, also prevented LPS-induced vascular hyporesponsiveness.[144] In contrast, prior removal of the endothelium failed to block either the development of diminished contractility or the release of cytokines, suggesting that vascular smooth muscle may be the major source of IL-1 and TNF-α in this system.

ATP-Sensitive K^+ Channels. The ATP-sensitive K^+ channel recently has been identified as a key modulator of arteriolar vasomotor tone.[169] Opening of this channel permits potassium ions to exit the vascular smooth muscle cell. This hyperpolarizes the cell, thereby reducing the entry of calcium ions via voltage-gated Ca^{2+} channels. The resultant decrease in intracellular calcium ion concentration leads to relaxation of the contractile apparatus of the cell and vasodilation. Numerous factors tend to open the ATP-sensitive K^+ channel, including low intracellular ATP concentration,[170] cytosolic acidosis,[171,172] and increased concentration of lactate in the cytosol.[173] Since the conditions that tend to open the ATP-sensitive K^+ channel might be expected to occur in sepsis and septic shock, Landry and Oliver[174] hypothesized that this channel might play an important role in the pathogenesis of the low SVRI state characteristic of overwhelming infections. In order to test this hypothesis, these investigators took advantage of the availability of compounds (glyburide and glipizide), which have been shown to be selective ATP-sensitive K^+ channel antagonists.[175] In a canine model of acute endotoxicosis, treatment with these agents was shown to restore normal SVRI and arterial blood pressure.[174] These findings suggest that the ATP-sensitive K^+ channel is an important determinant of low vasomotor tone in septic shock, and that antagonists of this channel may find utility in the clinical management of patients with this condition.

Other observations support the notion that opening of ATP-sensitive K^+ channels may be important in the pathogenesis of sepsis-induced vasodilation. Several endogenous mediators that are known vasodilators, including prostacyclin,[176] calcitonin-gene related peptide,[177] and vasoactive intestinal peptide,[169] have been shown to act by opening the ATP-sensitive K^+ channel in vascular smooth muscle cells. Interestingly, elevated circulating levels of both prostacyclin[113,114] and calcitonin-gene related peptide[28] have been identified in patients with septic shock, and increases in levels of vasoactive intestinal peptide[178] have been demonstrated in animals with peritonitis.[178] Thus the ATP-sensitive K^+ channel may represent an important common pathway leading to the loss of vasomotor tone in sepsis and septic shock.

Adrenergic Signal Transduction. Another mechanism that might help account for vascular hyporesponsiveness in sepsis is impaired binding of adrenergic agonists to vascular smooth muscle cells or impaired signal transduction within the cell in response to receptor occupation by such agonists. Experimental data exist to support both of these possibilities. In rats, the induction of sepsis or endotoxemia is associated with a decreased number of hepatic and aortic alpha-1-adrenergic receptors.[179–181] Furthermore, alpha-1-adrenergically stimulated turnover of phosphoinositides is diminished in aortic tissue from septic rats[179]; that is, signal transduction is impaired.

Results from clinical studies also indicate that adrenoreceptor function is modified in septic patients, although no data have been presented as yet regarding vascular alpha-adrenergic receptor density or signal transduction. For example, Silverman et al[182] have shown that peripheral blood lymphocytes from septic patients manifest diminished stimulation of adenylate cyclase by isoproterenol, a beta-adrenergic agonist. Forse et al[183] have demonstrated that early in the course of the illness, alpha-2 and beta-1 receptors on adipocytes are modulated in different ways in survivors and nonsurvivors of intra-abdominal sepsis. In nonsurvivors, alpha-2 receptor density is unchanged but signal transduction is downregulated; in survivors, alpha-2 receptor sensitivity is upregulated. A similar pattern has been observed with respect to beta-1 receptors.

Sepsis-Induced Vasoconstriction

Although loss of vasomotor tone is the predominant hemodynamic manifestation of sepsis, a number of observations suggest that impaired vasodilation (or excessive vasoconstriction) also may occur, at least in some vascular beds. Numerous investigators have reported that acetylcholine-induced[108,155,184] or flow-induced[185] vascular smooth muscle relaxation is blunted after in vivo administration of LPS in experimental animals. Moreover, in a study of 23 patients with sepsis or septic shock, Astiz et al[186] showed that reactive hyperemia after 5 minutes of forearm ischemia is markedly attenuated, particular in patients with shock. Similar findings also have been reported by Hartl et al.[187]

In numerous animal models of sepsis and septic shock, vascular resistance in several vascular beds increases. However, in many of these models, Q_T decreases significantly and thus the relevance of these observations to clinical sepsis is debatable. Nevertheless, evidence of regional vasoconstriction has been demonstrated by several investigators using models of septic shock characterized by normal or even elevated Q_T. For example, mesenteric perfusion has been shown to diminish in both septic rats[188,189] and endotoxemic pigs,[112,190] even when Q_T is well maintained. In the pig, the early phase of LPS-induced mesenteric hypoperfusion appears to be mediated, at least in part, by a cyclooxygenase-derived metabolite of arachidonic acid (probably thromboxane A_2), since mesenteric blood flow can be preserved by using drugs to block prostanoid biosynthesis.[112] Leukotriene D_4 also appears to contribute to the early phase of LPS-induced mesenteric hypoperfusion.[190] Mediators other than thromboxane A_2 or leukotriene D_4, however, appear to be responsible for mesenteric hypoperfusion during the later phase of the porcine endotoxemia paradigm.[190,191]

Endothelin. Endothelin 1 (ET-1) is a 21 amino acid polypeptide, which is synthesized and released by endothelial cells.[192] ET-1 is a potent vasoconstrictor. Synthesis of ET-1 by endothelial cells is stimulated by LPS, TNF-α, and IL-1.[193–195] Increased circulating concentrations of ET-1 have been documented in several animal models of sepsis or endotoxemia.[195–197] Clinical studies have documented that plasma ET-1 levels are elevated in septic patients and are inversely correlated with Q_T and directly correlated with severity of illness as quantitated by APACHE II score.[7,198,199] Since ET-1-induced vasoconstriction tends to be more evident in the renal circulation than in the systemic circulation as a whole,[200,201] it is noteworthy that one clinical study showed a loose, but still significant, inverse relationship between ET-1 levels in plasma and creatinine clearance.[199] Thus it is possible that organ (eg, kidney, gut) dysfunction in sepsis is due in part to derangements in the release of two key counterbalancing regulators of vasomotor tone (ie, NO and ET-1).

Pulmonary Hypertension. Pulmonary hypertension is a characteristic feature of sepsis and the adult respiratory distress syndrome in humans. Pulmonary hypertension also is a prominent feature of experimental sepsis or endotoxemia in several animal species, including sheep and pigs. In these acute (ie, 2- to 6-hour) animal models, pulmonary artery pressure typically displays two phases: (1) an early spike peaking at about 30 minutes after the start of the septic or endotoxic challenge and (2) a delayed but persistent hypertension beginning about 2 hours after initiation of sepsis or endotoxemia. Several agents have been shown to abrogate or blunt the early phase of pulmonary hypertension in acute experimental sepsis or endotoxemia. Among these agents are cyclooxygenase inhibitors,[191,202] platelet-activating factor antagonists,[203–205] a leukotriene B_4 receptor antagonist,[206,207] leukotriene D_4 receptor antagonists,[190,208,209] thromboxane A_2 receptor antagonists,[210,211] thromboxane synthase inhibitors,[212,213] and 5-lipoxygenase inhibitors.[214,215] A serotonin receptor antagonist has been shown to ameliorate the delayed phase of increased pulmonary vascular resistance in porcine models of endotoxemia[216] and *Pseudomonas* bacteremia.[217]

In animal models of sepsis or endotoxemia, the early spike in pulmonary artery pressure occurs coincidently with the sudden appearance of large concentrations of thromboxane B_2 (thromboxane A_2 metabolite) in plasma and lung lymph.[210,218] In addition, agents that inhibit the synthesis of thromboxane A_2 or block its receptor are capable of blunting the rise in pulmonary artery pressure in animal models of bacteremia or endotoxemia. Therefore it seems likely that thromboxane A_2 is a particularly important mediator of the early phase of sepsis- or LPS-induced pulmonary hypertension. In limited clinical studies of septic patients, however, neither ibuprofen, a cyclooxygenase inhibitor, nor dazoxiben, a thromboxane synthase inhibitor, have had an effect on pulmonary hypertension.[219,220]

The failure to replicate in humans the findings obtained in acute models of sepsis may reflect the different time courses of the processes being studied. Persistent pulmonary hypertension in patients with the adult respiratory distress syndrome probably does not reflect the acute effects of vasoconstricting mediators, like thromboxane A_2, but rather anatomical narrowing and plugging of the pulmonary microvasculature due to subacute fibroproliferative changes.[120,221] Thus, in order to show beneficial effects on pulmonary hemodynamics, it is likely that cyclooxygenase inhibitors or thromboxane antagonists will need to be administered very early in the clinical course of sepsis. A multicenter prospective trial of ibuprofen for the adjuvant therapy of sepsis is in progress.

ALTERATIONS IN MYOCARDIAL PERFORMANCE IN SEPSIS

Although Q_T is typically normal or elevated in adequately resuscitated patients with septic shock, myocardial contractility is markedly diminished. The first truly convincing evidence for this concept was provided by Parker et al,[222] who performed serial radionuclide electrocardiographically gated blood pool scans to assess left ventricular (LV) ejection fraction (EF) in 20 patients with septic shock. In this study, these authors showed that LVEF was abnormally low (ie, less than 0.4) in 10/13 survivors. The nadir in LVEF typically occurred 1 or 2 days after the onset of septic shock. In most cases, LVEF normalized by 10 days after the beginning of the septic episode. Despite the observed (transient) decrease in LVEF, stroke volume and Q_T were well maintained because LV end-diastolic volume (EDV) was substantially increased; that is, septic shock was associated with the development of a reversible cardiomyopathy characterized by diastolic dilation and diminished LVEF. Interestingly, diminished LVEF and LV diastolic dilation were not observed in the seven patients in this study who died as a result of their illness, suggesting that diminished LVEF in sepsis might serve some compensatory function in sepsis.

Numerous subsequent studies have confirmed these major observations.[222] Parker et al[223] themselves subsequently extended their observations to 54 patients, including 33 survivors and 21 nonsurvivors. Results in these patients were contrasted with those obtained in 15 critically ill nonseptic patients (Table 18–2). LVEF was significantly depressed and LVEDV was significantly increased in septic patients who survived. Using similar methods, Raper et al[224] compared myocardial performance in 69 patients having sepsis with the performance in 18 nonseptic trauma victims.[224] Both the right and left ventricular EFs were significantly lower in septic patients than in trauma patients. Concurrently, mean EDVs for both the right and left ventricles were significantly larger for the septic group as compared to the trauma group. Thus these authors found evidence of right as well as left ventricular dysfunction in sepsis. This finding has also been noted in other clinical studies.[225,226]

Not all the findings obtained by Parker and her colleagues at the National Institutes of Health[222,223,226] have been confirmed in other studies. For example, Vincent et al[227] found that patients with fatal septic shock have lower right ventricular EFs and higher right ventricular EDVs than do survivors, suggesting that ventricular dilation is not a salutary compensatory phenomenon in sepsis. Whereas Parker and colleagues found that Q_T was well preserved even in patients with very profound myocardial depression, Jardin et al[228] reported that patients presenting with very low LVEFs (21 ± 8 percent) also present with low values for Q_T (2.2 ± 0.8 liters/min/M^2). The differences in the results obtained by these various investigators probably reflect differences in aspects of patient management, such as the use of vasopressors and/or inotropes and the end points for volume resuscitation.

Human patient data have been invaluable for establishing the existence of sepsis-induced myocardial depression. Nevertheless, some of the most rigorous methods for studying myocardial performance (eg, sonomicrometry) are too invasive for use in patients. Moreover, clinical data inevitably must be confounded, at least to some extent, by the necessity to provide patients with therapeutic agents, such as vasopressors, which can affect myocardial loading and performance. Therefore the results of studies in septic or endotoxemic animals are instructive, as are data obtained in human volunteers injected with small doses of LPS. Numerous studies, using a wide variety of methods, have demonstrated that sepsis[229–231] and endotoxicosis[232–235] lead to myocardial depression. In a canine model of intraperitoneal sepsis,[230] the depression in EF is maximal 24 to 48 hours after the onset of sepsis and resolves within 7 to 10 days, a time course that is very similar to that observed in the clinical setting. In another canine model of sepsis, systolic performance, assessed using a load-independent parameter (E_{max}), diminishes progressively over a 4-day period of observation.[231] In a classic study using human volunteers, Suffredini et al[236] showed that intravenous infusion of LPS (4 ng/kg) leads of cardiovascular derangements, including a decrease in left ventricular EF, that are reminiscent of those observed in compensated sepsis.

TABLE 18–2. DATA RESULTS FOR STUDY OF 54 PATIENTS WITH SEPTIC SHOCK AND 15 NONSEPTIC CRITICALLY ILL CONTROLS[a]

Parameter[b]	Critically Ill Nonseptic Controls	Septic Patients: Survivors	Septic Patients: Nonsurvivors
N	15	33	21
MAP	97 ± 3	76 ± 3[c]	72 ± 3[c,d]
PAWP	10.7 ± 1.1	11.7 ± 0.8	12.8 ± 1.0
Q_T	4.4 ± 0.3	4.4 ± 0.3	5.4 ± 0.5[c,d]
EF	0.53 ± 0.04	0.40 ± 0.03[c]	0.47 ± 0.04
LVEDV	90 ± 9	122 ± 8[c]	99 ± 9[d]

[a] Data obtained by Parker et al[223] at the time of patient enrollment in the study.
[b] N, number of patients studied; MAP, mean arterial pressure (mm Hg); PAWP, pulmonary artery wedge pressure (mm Hg); Q_T, cardiac output (liters/min/M^2); LVEF, left ventricular ejection fraction (dimensionless variable); LVEDV, left ventricular end-diastolic volume (ml/M^2). Results are expressed as means ± standard error.
[c] $P < 0.05$ versus critically ill nonseptic controls.
[d] $P < 0.05$ versus septic survivors.

The mechanisms responsible for myocardial depression in sepsis are incompletely understood. Numerous studies, however, suggest that myocardial ischemia is not an important factor. Using a coronary sinus thermodilution catheter, Cunnion et al[237] studied seven patients with septic shock and showed that coronary blood flow was at least as great as previously reported values for normal subjects. Furthermore, these investigators documented that lactate concentration was always greater in arterial than in coronary sinus blood, indicating that the heart was consuming lactate, rather than producing it (as is the case in myocardial ischemia).[237] Dhainaut et al[238] confirmed these findings in a study of 40 patients with septic shock and 13 control subjects. Numerous studies in animal models also have indicated that coronary perfusion tends to increase, rather than decrease, in septic states.[239–242]

The notion that sepsis is associated with the elaboration of circulating myocardial depressant factor(s) is an old one.[243–245] This idea, however, gained considerable currency in 1985, when Parrillo et al[246] reported that serum samples from patients with sepsis and low EF depressed the performance of spontaneously beating neonatal rat myocardial cells in vitro, whereas no such activity was demonstrable in serum samples from appropriate controls. Although only limited efforts were made in this study to characterize the sepsis-related myocardial depressant serum factor, the compound was shown to be water soluble and capable of passing through an Amicon filter with molecular weight cutoff of 5000 daltons but not a filter with a cutoff of 500 daltons.[246] In a subsequent report, Parrillo and colleagues[247] showed that there is an inverse relationship between EF and the extent of myocardial depression induced by septic serum in vitro.

More recent studies have suggested that TNF-α is capable of eliciting myocardial depression both in vivo and in vitro. Using a chronically instrumented, unanesthetized canine preparation, Pagani et al[248] showed that infusion of TNF-α resulted in reversible abnormalities in both left ventricular systolic and diastolic performance. The derangement in systolic performance was manifested as flattening of the preload recruitable stroke work relationship, a load-independent measure of myocardial contractility. The derangement in diastolic function was manifested by increased elastic stiffness of the left ventricle. These changes were not evident until 24 hours after the infusion of TNF-α and were completely reversible, being absent by 168 hours after injection of the cytokine. Heard et al[249] showed that in vivo administration of TNF-α in guinea pigs causes a decrement in maximal left atrial force and velocity of contraction in vitro and also diminishes left atrial responsiveness to the inotropic effects of norepinephrine. These changes were evident within 6 hours after the administration of TNF-α. Eichenholz et al[250] were able to observe TNF-α-induced depression of EF within 2 hours after infusing conscious dogs with the cytokine.

Several investigators have examined the effect of TNF-α and other cytokines on myocardial performance in vitro. Gulick et al[251] showed that supernatants from mixed lymphocyte cultures are capable of depressing contractility and beta-adrenergic agonist-induced cyclic adenosine monophosphate (cAMP) accumulation in cultured neonatal cardiac myocytes. Moreover, these authors showed that the depressant activities in the supernatants coeluted with IL-1 and TNF-α when the preparations were subjected to cation-exchange chromatography.[251] Gulick et al[251] also showed that recombinant IL-1 and TNF-α are capable of blunting the responsiveness of cardiac myocytes to the beta-adrenergic agonist isoproterenol. More recently, Finkel et al,[252] using a hamster papillary muscle preparation, showed that several cytokines (TNF-α, IL-6, IL-2) are capable of depressing myocardial contractility in vitro within minutes. Furthermore, these authors showed that cytokine-induced myocardial depression can be reversed by addition to the bath of the NOS inhibitor, N^G-monomethyl-L-arginine, implicating NO as a mediator of cytokine-induced myocardial depression.[252] Further support for this idea has been provided by Brady et al,[253] who have reported that myocardial depression (measured in vitro) induced by LPS (administered to guinea pigs) can be abrogated by blocking NO synthesis with N^G-nitro-L-arginine. Thus two of the most prominent cardiovascular manifestations of sepsis, vasodilation and myocardial depression, may be caused, at least in part, by the same mediator, NO.

In contrast to the results obtained by most other workers, DeMeules et al[254] have reported that in vivo administration of TNF-α leads to enhanced myocardial performance in vitro. Interestingly, in a related study utilizing appropriate controls, these authors reported that serum obtained from rats challenged 18 to 22 hours with TNF-α earlier depresses contractility in an isolated heart preparation in vitro.[254] This latter observation suggests that a factor distal to TNF-α in the inflammatory cascade may be responsible for the myocardial depression induced by this cytokine.

REGIONAL PERFUSION IN SEPSIS

Remarkably little is known about the effects of sepsis and septic shock on organ perfusion in humans. In most instances, reliable measurements of regional perfusion in humans require invasive methods, which often cannot be utilized in critically ill, unstable patients. Nevertheless, some data are available regarding coronary, renal, and hepatosplanchnic blood flow in patients with sepsis.

As already mentioned, there is good evidence that coronary blood flow is normal or supranormal in septic patients,[237,238] an observation that agrees with data obtained by numerous investigators using animal models of sepsis or endotoxemia.[239–242]

It has been known for many years that compensated sepsis or low-grade endotoxemia increases renal plasma flow in humans.[255,256] Recent data similarly suggest that perfusion to the kidneys is maintained even in patients with septic shock.[257] In animals, renal hemodynamic perturbations are very dependent on the model employed. In some models, renal blood flow increases[258,259]; in some models, renal blood flow is unchanged[241,242]; and in some models, renal blood flow decreases[239,240,260] following the induction of sepsis or endotoxicosis.

Total hepatosplanchnic (ie, hepatic portal plus hepatic arterial) blood flow increases in humans with normotensive sepsis.[84,261–263] Whether the same is true in patients with septic shock is not known. Also, it is not known whether total mesenteric perfusion or, even more important, blood flow to the intestinal mucosa is preserved in septic humans. Since sepsis has been associated with the development of gastrointestinal mucosal acidosis in both humans[264] and animals,[112,265] it seems likely that blood flow to the gut epithelium is inadequate to meet metabolic demands under these conditions. Numerous investigators using a variety of animal models have documented mesenteric hypoperfusion in acute models of sepsis or endotoxemia,[112,188,189,239] although in more chronic models, intestinal perfusion is typically normal or elevated.[241,242]

PRACTICAL CONSIDERATIONS REGARDING HEMODYNAMIC MONITORING AND THERAPY IN PATIENTS WITH SEPSIS AND SEPTIC SHOCK

It is undoubtedly true that improvements in our understanding of the pathophysiology of sepsis and septic shock will lead to major changes in our approach to the management of the hemodynamic derangements associated with these conditions. Nevertheless, at the present time, hemodynamic management is largely restricted to monitoring of conventional parameters (eg, arterial blood pressure and Q_T), expansion of intravascular volume, and treatment with drugs (usually catecholamines) that are vasopressors, inotropes, or both.

Although much of modern critical care medicine is devoted to the hemodynamic management of septic shock, there is a remarkable paucity of well-controlled, prospective data regarding the relative value of the various interventions that are commonly employed. For example, no clinical study has ever documented that infusion of pressors, such as dopamine or norepinephrine, improves outcome in human septic shock, although Natanson et al[266] have documented that treatment with appropriate antibiotics and administration of catecholamines (titrated to blood pressure) act synergistically to improve survival in a canine peritonitis model.

Despite intensive investigation, the appropriate end points (ie, therapeutic goals) for the resuscitation of patients with septic shock have not been established. As noted previously, some experts advocate titrating therapy to achieve "supranormal" values for Q_T, systemic Do_2, and systemic Vo_2, for example, 4.5 liters/min/M^2, 600 ml/min/M^2, and 160 ml/min/M^2, respectively.[99,100,267] However, the value of this approach has not been conclusively demonstrated by any study, and the aggressive volume loading that is necessitated by this approach may exacerbate pulmonary edema, prolong the necessity for mechanical ventilation, and worsen survival.[268,269] Moreover, infusing inotropic agents, such as dobutamine or dopamine, may increase tachycardia and myocardial oxygen demand, risking myocardial infarction in patients with fixed occlusive lesions in the coronary circulation. Accordingly, I currently advocate a moderate approach to therapy. After resuscitating intravascular volume to a moderate pulmonary artery wedge pressure (about 15 mm Hg), vasopressors are infused to support arterial blood pressure. Since sepsis leads to derangements in both myocardial performance and peripheral vasomotor regulation, I typically employ norepinephrine, a catecholamine with both inotropic and vasoconstrictor properties, to maintain mean systemic arterial pressure at about 80 mm Hg. Results from a recent prospective trial support the idea that norepinephrine is preferable to dopamine for increasing blood pressure, if lower blood lactate concentration and higher urine output are used as measures of therapeutic success.[270] In non-septic dogs infused with norepinephrine, adding a low dose of dopamine improves renal blood flow.[271]

Although I employ this practice in the clinical setting, the therapeutic value of adding "renal dose" dopamine (2 to 3 μg/kg/min) to norepinephrine has never been documented.

Recognizing that arterial blood pressure and/or global measures of oxygen metabolism may not be optimal parameters for guiding hemodynamic support of septic (or other critically ill patients), there has been increasing interest in other means for monitoring the adequacy of perfusion. One approach that has been attracting increasing attention is the use of gastrointestinal tonometry to estimate the tissue pH in the wall of a hollow visceral organ, usually the stomach.[272] In a porcine model of endotoxemia, we have shown that aggressive resuscitation with a colloid solution (hetastarch) and an inotropic agent (dobutamine) can ameliorate LPS-induced ileal mucosal acidosis and prevent the development of gut mucosal hyperpermeability.[273] Several studies have demonstrated that among critically ill patients, those with a low gastric mucosal pH have a higher mortality than those with normal gastric mucosal pH.[274,275] Recently, in a randomized, prospective, multicenter trial, Guitierrez et al[276] showed that titrating therapy to tonometrically estimated measurements of gastric mucosal pH can improve outcome in selected critically ill patients. Although this study is open to criticism on several fronts, it must be recognized for what it is: an important outcome-based evaluation of a novel form of hemodynamic monitoring that suggests that therapy guided by tissue-level indices of perfusion may be better than therapy guided by "conventional" measures of the adequacy of resuscitation.

SUMMARY

Sepsis and related systemic inflammatory states are associated with marked perturbations in circulatory function. Some of these hemodynamic changes are probably quite beneficial to the host, serving to increase the delivery of oxygen and endogenous antimicrobial factors to the site of infection and aiding in the development of salutary metabolic milieu. However, when excessive and inadequately regulated, the hemodynamic perturbations related to sepsis undoubtedly contribute to mortality. At present, our ability to intelligently and successfully modify the adverse effects of sepsis on perfusion are quite limited. However, in the very near future, it is almost certain that the hemodynamic management of sepsis and septic shock will be improved by the availability of (1) better means for monitoring the success of therapy and (2) agents that selectively correct the derangements in cardiac function and vasomotor regulation that are associated with the syndrome.

REFERENCES

1. Balk RA, Bone RC: The septic syndrome: definition and clinical implications. Crit Care Clin 5:1, 1989.
2. Pepe PE, Potkin RT, Reus DH, et al: Clinical predictors of the adult respiratory distress syndrome. Am J Surg 144:124, 1982.
3. Baumgartner J-D, Bula C, Vaney C, et al: A novel score for predicting the mortality of septic shock patients. Crit Care Med 20:953, 1992.
4. Moreau R, Hadengue A, Soupison T, et al: Septic shock in patients with cirrhosis: hemodynamic and metabolic characteristics and intensive care unit outcome. Crit Care Med 20:746, 1992.
5. Clemmer TP, Fisher CJ Jr, Bone RC, et al: Hypothermia in the sepsis syndrome and clinical outcome. Crit Care Med 20:1395, 1992.
6. Knaus WA, Sun X, Nystrom P-O, Wagner DP: Evaluation of definitions for sepsis. Chest 101:1656, 1992.
7. Pittet J-F, Morel DR, Hemsen A, et al: Elevated plasma endothelin-1 concentrations are associated with the severity of illness in patients with sepsis. Ann Surg 213:261, 1991.
8. Leatherman JW, Schmitz PG: Fever, hyperdynamic shock, and multiple-system organ failure: a pseudo-sepsis syndrome associated with chronic salicylate intoxication. Chest 100:1391, 1991.
9. Marshall J, Sweeney D: Microbial infection and the septic response in critical surgical illness. Arch Surg 125:17, 1990.
10. Siegel J, Puri R: Interleukin-2 toxicity. J Clin Oncol 9:694, 1991.
11. Smith J, Urba W, Steis R: Interleukin-1 alpha administered in a phase I trial to patients with advanced malignancies. J Clin Oncol 109:1141, 1992.
12. Wewers MD, Rinehart JJ, She Z-W, et al: Tumor necrosis factor infusions in humans prime neutrophils for hypochlorous acid production. Am J Physiol 259:L276, 1990.
13. Michie HR, Spriggs DR, Manogue KR, et al: Tumor necrosis factor and endotoxin induce similar metabolic responses in human beings. Surgery 104:280, 1988.
14. Starnes HF Jr, Warren RS, Jeevanandam M, et al: Tumor necrosis factor and the acute metabolic response to tissue injury in man. J Clin Invest 82:1321, 1988.
15. Members of the American College of Chest Physicians/Society of Critical Care Medicine Consensus Conference Committee: American College of Chest Physicians/Society of Critical Care Medicine Consensus Conference: definitions for sepsis and or-

gan failure and guidelines for the use of innovative therapies in sepsis. Crit Care Med 20:864, 1992.

16. Bone RC, Fisher CJ Jr, Clemmer TP, et al: Sepsis syndrome: a valid clinical entity. Crit Care Med 17:389, 1989.
17. Fink MP, Heard SO: Research review: laboratory models of sepsis and septic shock. J Surg Res 49:186, 1990.
18. Gunnar RM, Loeb HS, Winslow EJ, et al: Hemodynamic measurements in bacteremia and septic shock in man. J Infect Dis 128:S295, 1973.
19. Blain CM, Anderson TO, Pietras RJ, Gunnar RM: Immediate hemodynamic effects of gram-negative vs gram-positive bacteremia in man. Arch Intern Med 126:260, 1970.
20. Kwaan HM, Weil MH: Differences in the mechanism of shock caused by bacterial infection. Surg Gynecol Obstet 128:37, 1969.
21. Ahmed AJ, Kruse JA, Haupt MT, et al: Hemodynamic responses to gram-positive versus gram-negative sepsis in critically ill patients with and without circulatory shock. Crit Care Med 19:1520, 1991.
22. Peduzzi P, Shatney C, Sheagren J, et al: Predictors of bacteremia and gram-negative bacteremia in patients with sepsis. Arch Intern Med 152:529, 1992.
23. Wiles JB, Cerra FB, Siegel JH, Border JR: The systemic septic response: does the organism matter? Crit Care Med 8:55, 1980.
24. Natanson C, Danner RL, Elin RJ, et al: Role of endotoxemia in cardiovascular dysfunction and mortality: *Escherichia coli* and *Staphylococcus aureus* challenges in a canine model of human septic shock. J Clin Invest 83:243, 1989.
25. Okrent DG, Abraham E, Winston D: Cardiorespiratory patterns in viral septicemia. Am J Med 83:681, 1987.
26. Deutschmann CS, Konstantides FN, Tsai M, et al: Physiology and metabolism in isolated viral septicemia: further evidence of an organism-independent, host-dependent response. Arch Surg 122:21, 1987.
27. Abraham E, Shoemaker WC, Bland RD, Cobo JC: Sequential cardiorespiratory patterns in septic shock. Crit Care Med 11:799, 1983.
28. Joyce CD, Fiscus RR, Wang X, et al: Calcitonin gene-related peptide levels are elevated in patients with sepsis. Surgery 108:1097, 1990.
29. Rackow EC, Kaufman BS, Falk JL, et al: Hemodynamic response to fluid repletion in patients with septic shock: evidence for early depression of cardiac performance. Circ Shock 22:11, 1987.
30. Parker MM, Shelhamer JH, Natanson C, et al: Serial cardiovascular variables in survivors and nonsurvivors of human septic shock: heart rate as an early predictor of prognosis. Crit Care Med 15:923, 1987.
31. Groeneveld ABJ, Bronsveld W, Thijs LG: Hemodynamic determinants of mortality in human septic shock. Surgery 99:140, 1986.
32. D'Orio V, Mendes P, Saad G, Marcelle R: Accuracy in early prediction of prognosis of patients with septic shock by analysis of simple indices: prospective study. Crit Care Med 18:1339, 1990.
33. Nishijima H, Weil MH, Shubin H, Cavanilles J: Hemodynamic and metabolic studies on shock associated with gram-negative bacteremia. Medicine (Baltimore) 52:287, 1973.
34. Weil MH, Nishijima H: Cardiac output in bacterial shock. Am J Med 64:920, 1978.
35. Baumgartner JD, Varney C, Perret C: An extreme form of the hyperdynamic syndrome in septic shock. Intensive Care Med 10:245, 1984.
36. Weisel RD, Vito L, Dennis RC, et al: Myocardial depression during sepsis. Am J Surg 133:512, 1977.
37. Clowes GHA, Farrington GH, Zuschneid W, et al: Circulating factors in the etiology of pulmonary insufficiency and right heart failure accompanying severe sepsis (peritonitis). Ann Surg 171:663, 1970.
38. Hochachka PW: Metabolic suppression and oxygen availability. Can J Zool 66:152, 1987.
39. Barcroft J: On anoxaemia. Lancet 2:485, 1920.
40. Whalen DF, Buerk D, Thuning CA: Blood flow-limited oxygen consumption in resting cat skeletal muscle. Am J Physiol 224:763, 1973.
41. Gutierrez G, Pohil RJ, Strong R: Skeletal muscle oxygen consumption and energy metabolism during hypoxemia. J Appl Physiol 66:2117, 1989.
42. Duran WN, Renkin EM: Oxygen consumption and blood flow in resting mammalian skeletal muscle. Am J Physiol 226:173, 1974.
43. Edelstone DI, Paulone ME, Holzman IR: Hepatic oxygenation during arterial hypoxemia in neonatal lambs. Am J Obstet Gynecol 150:513, 1984.
44. Cain SM: Oxygen delivery and utilization in dogs with a sublethal dose of cobalt chloride. J Appl Physiol 38:20, 1975.
45. Cain SM: Oxygen delivery and uptake in dogs during anemic and hypoxic hypoxia. J Appl Physiol 42:228, 1977.
46. Adams RP, Dieleman LA, Cain SM: A critical value for O_2 transport in the rat. J Appl Physiol 53:660, 1982.
47. Komatsu T, Shibutani K, Okamoto K, et al: Critical level of oxygen delivery after cardiopulmonary bypass. Crit Care Med 15:194, 1987.
48. Shibutani K, Komatsu T, Kubal K, et al: Critical level of oxygen delivery in anesthetized man. Crit Care Med 11:640, 1983.
49. Rhodes GR, Newell JC, Shah D, et al: Increased oxygen consumption accompanying increased oxygen delivery with hypertonic mannitol in adult respiratory distress syndrome. Surgery 84:490, 1978.
50. Kaufman BS, Rackow EC, Falk JL: The relationship between oxygen delivery and consumption during fluid resuscitation of hypovolemic and septic shock. Chest 85:336, 1984.
51. Danek SJ, Lynch JP, Weg JG, Dantzker DR: The dependence of oxygen uptake on oxygen delivery in the adult respiratory distress syndrome. Am Rev Respir Dis 122:387, 1980.
52. Mohsenifar Z, Goldbach P, Tashkin DP, Campisi DJ: Relationship between O_2 delivery and O_2 con-

sumption in the adult respiratory distress syndrome. Chest 84:267, 1983.
53. Astiz ME, Rackow EC, Falk JL, et al: Oxygen delivery and consumption in patients with hyperdynamic septic shock. Crit Care Med 15:26, 1987.
54. Guitierrez G, Pohil RJ: Oxygen consumption is linearly related to O_2 supply in critically ill patients. J Crit Care 1:45, 1986.
55. Kariman K, Burns SR: Regulation of tissue oxygen extraction is disturbed in adult respiratory distress syndrome. Am Rev Respir Dis 132:109, 1985.
56. Palazzo MG, Suter PM: Delivery dependent oxygen consumption in patients with septic shock: daily variations, relationship with outcome and the sick-euthyroid syndrome. Intensive Care Med 17:325, 1991.
57. Clarke C, Edwards JD, Nightingale P, et al: Persistence of supply dependency of oxygen uptake at high levels of delivery in adult respiratory distress syndrome. Crit Care Med 19:497, 1991.
58. Lorente JA, Renes E, Gomez-Aguinaga MA, et al: Oxygen delivery-dependent oxygen consumption in acute respiratory failure. Crit Care Med 19:770, 1991.
59. Lucking SE, Williams TM, Chaten FC, et al: Dependence of oxygen consumption on oxygen delivery in children with hyperdynamic septic shock and low oxygen extraction. Crit Care Med 18:1316, 1990.
60. Ronco JJ, Montaner JSG, Fenwick JC, et al: Pathologic dependence of oxygen consumption on oxygen delivery in acute respiratory failure secondary to AIDS-related *Pneumocystis carinii* pneumonia. Chest 98:1463, 1990.
61. Wolf YG, Cotev S, Perel A, Manny J: Dependence of oxygen consumption on cardiac output in sepsis. Crit Care Med 15:198, 1987.
62. Cain SM: Supply dependency of oxygen uptake in ARDS: myth or reality? Am J Med Sci 288:119, 1984.
63. Bihari D, Smithies M, Gimson A, Tinker J: The effects of vasodilation with prostacyclin on oxygen delivery and uptake in critically ill patients. N Engl J Med 317:397, 1987.
64. Haupt MT, Gilbert EM, Carlson RW: Fluid loading increases oxygen consumption in septic patients with lactic acidosis. Am Rev Respir Dis 131:912, 1985.
65. Gilbert EM, Haupt MT, Mandanas RY, et al: The effect of fluid loading, blood transfusion, and catecholamine infusion on oxygen delivery and consumption in patients with sepsis. Am Rev Respir Dis 134:873, 1986.
66. Kruse JA, Haupt MT, Puri VK, Carlson RW: Lactate levels as predictors of the relationship between oxygen delivery and consumption in ARDS. Chest 98:959, 1990.
67. Fenwick JC, Dodek PM, Ronco JJ, et al: Increased concentrations of plasma lactate predict pathologic dependence of oxygen consumption on oxygen delivery in patients with adult respiratory distress syndrome. J Crit Care 5:81, 1990.
68. Vincent JL, Roman A, De Backer D, Kahn RJ: Oxygen uptake/supply dependency. Effects of short-term dobutamine infusion. Am Rev Respir Dis 142:2, 1990.
69. Steffes CP, Bender JS, Levison MA: Blood transfusion and oxygen consumption in surgical sepsis. Crit Care Med 19:512, 1991.
70. Bakker J, Coffernils M, Leon M, et al: Blood lactate levels are superior to oxygen-derived variables in predicting outcome in human septic shock. Chest 99:956, 1991.
71. Archie JP Jr: Mathematic coupling of data: a common source of error. Ann Surg 193:296, 1981.
72. Stratton HH, Feustel PJ, Newell JC: Regression of calculated variables in the presence of shared measurement error. J Appl Physiol 62:2083, 1987.
73. Ronco JJ, Fenwick JC, Wiggs BR, et al: Oxygen consumption is independent of increases in oxygen delivery by dobutamine in septic patients who have normal or increased plasma lactate. Am Rev Respir Dis 147:25, 1993.
74. Ronco JJ, Phang PT, Walley KR, et al: Oxygen consumption is independent of changes in oxygen delivery in severe adult respiratory distress syndrome. Am Rev Respir Dis 143:1267, 1991.
75. Vermeij CG, Feenstra BWA, Adrichem WJ, Bruining HA: Independent oxygen uptake and oxygen delivery in septic and postoperative patients. Chest 99:1438, 1991.
76. Carlile PV, Gray BA: Effect of opposite changes in cardiac output and arterial Po_2 on the relationship between mixed venous Po_2 and oxygen transport. Am Rev Respir Dis 140:891, 1989.
77. Vermeij CG, Feenstra BWA, Bruining HA: Oxygen delivery and oxygen uptake in postoperative and septic patients. Chest 98:415, 1990.
78. Dietrich KA, Conrad SA, Hebert CA, et al: Cardiovascular and metabolic response to red blood cell transfusion in critically ill volume-resuscitated nonsurgical patients. Crit Care Med 18:940, 1990.
79. Mink RB, Pollack MM: Effect of blood transfusion on oxygen consumption in pediatric septic shock. Crit Care Med 18:1087, 1990.
80. Feldman HA: Families of lines: random effects in linear regression analysis. J Appl Physiol 64:1721, 1988.
81. Weisman C, Kemper M: The oxygen uptake-oxygen delivery relationship during ICU interventions. Chest 99:430, 1991.
82. Villar J, Slutsky AS, Hew E, Aberman A: Oxygen transport and oxygen consumption in critically ill patients. Chest 98:687, 1990.
83. Boyd O, Grounds M, Bennett D: The dependency of oxygen consumption on oxygen delivery in critically ill postoperative patients is mimicked by variations in sedation. Chest 101:1619, 1992.
84. Dahn MS, Lange P, Lobdell K, et al: Splanchnic and total body oxygen consumption differences in septic and injured patients. Surgery 101:69, 1987.
85. Tuchschmidt J, Fried J, Swinney R, Sharma OP: Early hemodynamic correlates of survival in pa-

tients with septic shock. Crit Care Med 17:719, 1989.

86. Vincent J-L, Roman A, Kahn RJ: Dobutamine administration in septic shock: addition to a standard protocol. Crit Care Med 18:689, 1990.
87. Bredle DL, Cain SM: Systemic and muscle oxygen uptake/delivery after dopexamine infusion in endotoxic dogs. Crit Care Med 19:198, 1991.
88. Bredle DL, Samsel RW, Schumacker PT: Critical oxygen delivery to skeletal muscle at high and low Po_2 in endotoxemic dogs. J Appl Physiol 66:2553, 1989.
89. Nelson DP, Samsel RW, Wood LDH, Schumacker PT: Pathological supply dependence of systemic and intestinal O_2 uptake during endotoxemia. J Appl Physiol 64:2410, 1988.
90. Samsel RW, Nelson DP, Sanders WM, et al: Effect of endotoxin on systemic and skeletal muscle O_2 extraction. J Appl Physiol 65:1377, 1988.
91. Nelson DP, Beyer C, Samsel RW, et al: Pathological supply dependence of O_2 uptake during bacteremia in dogs. J Appl Physiol 63:1487, 1987.
92. Heard SO, Baum TD, Wang H, et al: Systemic and mesenteric O_2 metabolism in endotoxic pigs: effect of graded hemorrhage. Circ Shock 35:44, 1991.
93. Rackow EC, Astiz ME, Weil MH: Increases in oxygen extraction during rapidly fatal septic shock in rats. J Lab Clin Med 109:660, 1987.
94. Hurtado FJ, Gutierrez AM, Silva N, et al: Role of tissue hypoxia as the mechanism of lactic acidosis during *E. coli* endotoxemia. J Appl Physiol 72:1895, 1992.
95. Gutierrez G, Lund N, Palizas F: Rabbit skeletal muscle Po_2 during hypodynamic sepsis. Chest 99:224, 1991.
96. Hirschl RB, Heiss KF, Cilley RE, et al: Oxygen kinetics in experimental sepsis. Surgery 112:37, 1992.
97. Russell J, Ronco J, Lockhat D, et al: Oxygen delivery and consumption and ventricular preload are greater in survivors than in nonsurvivors of the adult respiratory distress syndrome. Am Rev Respir Dis 141:659, 1990.
98. Clowes CA, Vucinic M, Weidner M: Circulatory and metabolic alterations associated with survival or death in peritonitis. Ann Surg 163:866, 1966.
99. Shoemaker WC, Appel PL, Kram HB, et al: Prospective trial of supranormal values of survivors as therapeutic goals in high-risk surgical patients. Chest 94:1176, 1988.
100. Tuchschmidt J, Fried J, Astiz M, Rackow E: Elevation of cardiac output and oxygen improves outcome in septic shock. Chest 102:216, 1992.
101. Fink MP, Homer LD, Fletcher JR: Diminished pressor response to exogenous norepinephrine and angiotensin II in septic unanesthetized rats: evidence for a prostaglandin-mediated effect. J Surg Res 38:335, 1985.
102. Julou-Schaeffer G, Gray GA, Fleming I, et al: Loss of vascular responsiveness induced by endotoxin involves L-arginine pathway. Am J Physiol 259: H1038, 1990.
103. McKenna TM, Martin FM, Chernow B, Briglia FA: Vascular endothelium contributes to decreased aortic contractility in experimental sepsis. Circ Shock 19:267, 1986.
104. Pomerantz K, Casey L, Fletcher JR, Ramwell PW: Vascular reactivity in endotoxic shock: effect of lidocaine or indomethacin pretreatment. Adv Shock Res 7:191, 1982.
105. Takahashi K, Ando K, Ono A, et al: Tumor necrosis factor-α induces vascular hyporesponsiveness in Sprague-Dawley rats. Life Sci 50:1437, 1992.
106. Cryer HG, Garrison RN, Harris PD, et al: Prostaglandins mediate skeletal muscle arteriole dilation in hyperdynamic bacteremia. Am J Physiol 259: H728, 1990.
107. Lubbe AS, Garrison RN, Cryer HM, et al: EDRF as a possible mediator of sepsis-induced arteriolar dilation in skeletal muscle. Am J Physiol 262:H880, 1992.
108. Baker CH, Sutton ET: Arteriolar endothelium-dependent vasodilation occurs during endotoxic shock. Am J Physiol 264:H1118, 1993.
109. Fink MP, Gardiner WM, Roethel R, Fletcher JR: Plasma levels of 6-keto-PGF_{1a} but not TxB_2 increase in rats with peritonitis due to cecal ligation. Circ Shock 16:297, 1985.
110. Hanly PJ, Sienko A, Light RB: Role of prostacyclin and thromboxane in the circulatory changes of acute bacteremic *Pseudomonas* pneumonia in dogs. Am Rev Respir Dis 137:700, 1988.
111. Anderson FL, Jubiz W, Tsagaris TJ, Kuida H: Endotoxin-induced prostaglandin E and F release in dogs. Am J Physiol 22:410, 1975.
112. Fink MP, Rothschild HR, Deniz YF, et al: Systemic and mesenteric O_2 metabolism in endotoxic pigs: effect of ibuprofen and meclofenamate. J Appl Physiol 67:1950, 1989.
113. Halushka PV, Reines HD, Barrow SE, et al: Elevated plasma 6-keto-prostaglandin F_{1a} in patients in septic shock. Crit Care Med 13:451, 1985.
114. Bernard GR, Reines HD, Halushka PV, et al: Prostacyclin and thromboxane A_2 formation is increased in human sepsis syndrome: effects of cyclooxygenase inhibition. Am Rev Respir Dis 144:1095, 1991.
115. Oettinger W, Berger D, Beger HG: The clinical significance of prostaglandins and thromboxane as mediators of septic shock. Klin Wochenschr 65:61, 1987.
116. Fink MP, MacVittie TJ, Casey LC: Inhibition of prostaglandin synthesis restores normal hemodynamics in canine hyperdynamic sepsis. Ann Surg 200:619, 1984.
117. Auclair M-C, Carli A, Lechat P: Decrease of the hypertensive response to phenylephrine in the rat submitted to a sublethal dose of *E. coli* endotoxin. Restoration by indomethacin. J Pharmacol 13:341, 1982.
118. Gray GA, Furman BL, Parratt JR: Endotoxin-induced impairment of vascular reactivity in the pithed rat: role of arachidonic acid metabolites. Circ Shock 31:395, 1990.

119. Burnier M, Waeber B, Aubert JF, et al: Effect of nonhypotensive endotoxemia in conscious rats: role of prostaglandins. Am J Physiol 254:H509, 1988.
120. Fink MP, Morrissey PE, Stein KL, et al: Systemic and regional hemodynamic effects of cyclo-oxygenase and thromboxane synthetase inhibition in normal and hyperdynamic endotoxemic rabbits. Circ Shock 26:41, 1988.
121. Martich GD, Parker MM, Cunnion RE, Suffredini AF: Effects of ibuprofen and pentoxyfylline on the cardiovascular response of normal humans to endotoxin. J Appl Physiol 73:925, 1992.
122. Nathan C: Nitric oxide as a secretory product of mammalian cells. FASEB J 6:3051, 1992.
123. Palmer RMJ: The discovery of nitric oxide in the vessel wall: a unifying concept in the pathogenesis of sepsis. Arch Surg 128:396, 1993.
124. Brenner BM, Troy JL, Ballermann BJ: Endothelium-dependent vascular responses: mediators and mechanisms. J Clin Invest 84:1373, 1989.
125. Furchgott RF, Zawadzki JV: The obligatory role of endothelial cells in the relaxation of arterial smooth muscle by acetylcholine. Nature 288:373, 1980.
126. Palmer RMJ, Ferrige AG, Moncada S: Nitric oxide release accounts for the biological activity of endothelium-derived relaxing factor. Nature 327:524, 1987.
127. Ignarro LJ, Buga GM, Wood KS, et al: Endothelium-derived relaxing factor produced and released from artery and vein is nitric oxide. Proc Natl Acad Sci USA 84:9265, 1984.
128. Stamler JS, Simon DI, Osborne JA, et al: S-nitrosylation of protein with nitric oxide: synthesis and characterization of biologically active compounds. Proc Natl Acad Sci USA 89:444, 1992.
129. Myers PR, Minor RL Jr, Guerra R Jr, et al: Vasorelaxant properties of the endothelium-derived relaxing factor more closely resemble S-nitrocysteine than nitric oxide. Nature 345:161, 1990.
130. Fukoto JM, Chiang K, Hszieh R, et al: The pharmacological activity of nitroxyl: a potent vasodilator with activity similar to nitric oxide and/or endothelium-derived relaxing factor. J Pharmacol Exp Ther 263:546, 1992.
131. Uchizumi H, Hattori R, Sase K, et al: A stable L-arginine-dependent relaxing factor released from cytotoxic-activated macrophages. Am J Physiol 264:H1472, 1993.
132. Keaney JF Jr, Simon DI, Stamler JS, et al: NO forms an adduct with serum albumin that has endothelium-derived relaxing factor-like properties. J Clin Invest 91:1582, 1993.
133. Cobb JP, Natanson C, Hoffman WD, et al: N^{ω}amino-L-arginine, an inhibitor of nitric oxide synthase, raises vascular resistance but increases mortality rates in awake canines challenged with endotoxin. J Exp Med 176:1175, 1992.
134. Thiemermann C, Vane J: Inhibition of nitric oxide synthesis reduces the hypotension induced by bacterial lipopolysaccharides in the rat in vivo. Eur J Pharmacol 182:591, 1990.
135. Kilbourn RG, Jubran GA, Gross SS, et al: Reversal of endotoxin-mediated shock by N^G-methyl-L-arginine, an inhibitor of nitric oxide synthesis. Biochem Biophys Res Commun 172:1132, 1990.
136. Lorente JA, Landin L, Renes E, et al: Role of nitric oxide in the hemodynamic changes of sepsis. Crit Care Med 21:759, 1993.
137. Meyer J, Traber LD, Nelson S, et al: Reversal of hyperdynamic response to continuous endotoxin administration by inhibition of NO synthesis. J Appl Physiol 73:324, 1992.
138. Petros A, Bennett D, Vallance P: Effect of nitric oxide synthase inhibitors on hypotension in patients with septic shock. Lancet 338:1557, 1991.
139. Vallance P, Palmer RMJ, Moncada S: The role of induction of nitric oxide synthesis in the altered responses of jugular veins from endotoxaemic rabbits. Br J Pharmacol 106:459, 1992.
140. Auget M, Guillon J-M, Delaflotte S, et al: Endothelium independent protective effect of N^G-monomethyl-L-arginine on endotoxin-induced alterations of vascular reactivity. Life Sci 48:189, 1991.
141. Rees DD, Cellek S, Palmer RMJ, Moncada S: Dexamethasone prevents the induction by endotoxin of nitric oxide synthase and the associated effects on vascular tone. An insight into endotoxin shock. Biochem Biophys Res Commun 173:541, 1990.
142. Nelson S, Steward RH, Traber L, Traber D: Endotoxin-induced alterations in contractility of isolated blood vessels from sheep. Am J Physiol 260:H1790, 1991.
143. Szabo C, Mitchell JA, Gross SS, et al: Nifedipine inhibits the induction of nitric oxide synthase by bacterial lipopolysaccharide. J Pharmacol Exp Ther 265:674, 1993.
144. McKenna TM: Prolonged exposure of rat aorta to low levels of endotoxin in vitro results in impaired contractility. J Clin Invest 86:160, 1990.
145. Fleming I, Gray GA, Stoclet J-C: Influence of endothelium on induction of the L-arginine-nitric oxide pathway in rat aortas. Am J Physiol 264:H1200, 1993.
146. Beasley D, Cohen RA, Levinsky NG: Interleukin-1 inhibits contraction of vascular smooth muscle. J Clin Invest 83:331, 1989.
147. Harbrecht BG, Billiar TR, Stadler J, et al: Nitric oxide synthesis serves to reduce hepatic damage during acute murine endotoxemia. Crit Care Med 20:1568, 1992.
148. Shultz PJ, Raij L: Endogenously synthesized nitric oxide prevents endotoxin-induced glomerular thrombosis. J Clin Invest 90:1718, 1992.
149. Ochoa JB, Udekwu AO, Billiar TR, et al: Nitrogen oxide levels in patients after trauma and during sepsis. Ann Surg 214:621, 1991.
150. Green LC, Wagner DA, Ruiz de Luzuriaga K, et al: Nitrate biosynthesis in man. Proc Natl Acad Sci USA 78:7764, 1981.
151. Salvemini D, Korbut R, Anggard E, Vane J: Lipopolysaccharide increases release of a nitric oxide-

like factor from endothelial cells. Eur J Pharmacol 171:135, 1989.
152. Myers PR, Wright TF, Tanner MA, Adams HR: EDRF and nitric oxide production in cultured endothelial cells: direct inhibition by *E. coli* endotoxin. Am J Physiol 262:H710, 1992.
153. Parker J, Keller R, Defily D, et al: Coronary vascular smooth muscle function in *E. coli* endotoxemia in dogs. Am J Physiol 260:H832, 1991.
154. Aoki N, Siegfried M, Lefer A: Anti-EDRF effect of tumor necrosis factor in isolated, perfused cat carotid arteries. Am J Physiol 256:H1509, 1989.
155. Wylam ME, Samsel RW, Umans JG, et al: Endotoxin in vivo impairs endothelium-dependent relaxation of canine arteries in vitro. Am Rev Respir Dis 142:1263, 1990.
156. Beasley D, Cohen RA, Levinsky NG: Endotoxin inhibits contraction of vascular smooth muscle in vitro. Am J Physiol 258:H1187, 1990.
157. Hollenberg SM, Cunnion RE, Parrillo JE: The effect of tumor necrosis factor on vascular smooth muscle: in vitro studies using rat aortic rings. Chest 100:1133, 1991.
158. Beasley D, Schwartz JH, Brenner BM: Interleukin 1 induces prolonged L-arginine-dependent cyclic guanosine monophosphate and nitrite production in rat vascular smooth muscle cells. J Clin Invest 87:602, 1991.
159. Durante W, Schini VB, Scott-Burden T, et al: Platelet inhibition by an L-arginine-derived substance released by IL-1B-treated vascular smooth muscle cells. Am J Physiol 261:H2024, 1991.
160. McKenna TM: Enhanced vascular effects of cyclin GMP in septic rat aorta. Am J Physiol 254:R436, 1988.
161. Broughton-Smith NK, Hutcheson IR, Deakin AM, et al: Protective effect of S-nitroso-N-acetyl-penicillamine in endotoxin-induced acute intestinal damage in the rat. Eur J Pharmacol 191:485, 1990.
162. Vicaut E, Hou X, Payen D, et al: Acute effects of tumor necrosis factor on the microcirculation in rat cremaster muscle. J Clin Invest 87:1537, 1991.
163. McKenna TM, Reusch DW, Simpkins CO: Macrophage-conditioned medium and interleukin 1 suppress vascular contractility. Circ Shock 25:187, 1988.
164. McKenna TM, Lueders JE, Titius WAW: Monocyte-derived interleukin-1: effects on norepinephrine-stimulated aortic contraction and phosphoinositide turnover. Circ Shock 28:131, 1989.
165. Beasley D: Interleukin 1 and endotoxin activate soluble guanylate cyclase in vascular smooth muscle. Am J Physiol 259:R38, 1990.
166. Durante W, Schini VB, Catovsky S, et al: Plasmin potentiates induction of nitric oxide synthesis by interleukin-1B in vascular smooth muscle cells. Am J Physiol 264:H617, 1993.
167. Schini VB, Catovsky S, Durante W, et al: Thrombin inhibits induction of nitric oxide synthase in vascular smooth muscle cells. Am J Physiol 264:H611, 1993.
168. Hibbs JB Jr, Westenfelder C, Taintor R, et al: Evidence of cytokine-inducible nitric oxide synthesis from L-arginine in patients receiving interleukin-2 therapy. J Clin Invest 89:867, 1992.
169. Standen NB, Quayle JB, Davies NW, et al: Hyperpolarizing vasodilators activate ATP-sensitive K^+ channels in arterial smooth muscle. Science 245: 177, 1989.
170. Deutsch N, Klitzner TS, Lamp ST, Weiss JN: Activation of cardiac ATP-sensitive K^+ channels during hypoxia: correlation with tissue ATP levels. Am J Physiol 261:H671, 1991.
171. Davies NW: Modulation of ATP-sensitive K^+-sensitive potassium channels in skeletal muscle by intracellular protons. Nature 343:375, 1990.
172. Cuevas J, Bassett AL, Cameron JS, et al: Effect of H^+ on ATP-regulated K^+ channels in feline ventricular myocytes. Am J Physiol 261:H755, 1991.
173. Keung EC, Li Q: Lactate activates ATP-sensitive potassium channels in guinea pig ventricular myocytes. J Clin Invest 88:1772, 1991.
174. Landry DW, Oliver JA: The ATP-sensitive K^+ channel mediates hypotension in endotoxemia and hypoxic lactic acidosis in dog. J Clin Invest 89:2071, 1992.
175. Schmid-Antomarchi H, De Weille J, Fosset M, Lazdunski M: The receptor for antidiabetic sulfonylureas controls the activity of the ATP-modulated K^+ channel in insulin secreting cells. J Biol Chem 262:15840, 1987.
176. Jackson WF, Konig A, Dambacher T, Busse R: Prostacyclin-induced vasodilation in rabbit heart is mediated by ATP-sensitive potassium channels. Am J Physiol 264:H238, 1993.
177. Nelson MT, Huang Y, Brayden JE, et al: Arterial dilations in response to calcitonin gene-related peptide involve activation of K^+ channels. Nature 344:770, 1990.
178. Fuortes M, Blank MA, Scalea TM, et al: Release of vasoactive intestinal peptide during hyperdynamic sepsis in dogs. Surgery 104:894, 1988.
179. Carcillo JA, Litten RZ, Suba EA, Roth BL: Alterations in rat aortic $alpha_1$-adrenoreceptors and $alpha_1$-adrenergic stimulated phosphoinositide hydrolysis in intraperitoneal sepsis. Circ Shock 26:331, 1988.
180. Roth BL, Spitzer JA: Altered hepatic vasopressin and $alpha_1$-adrenergic receptors after chronic endotoxin infusion. Am J Physiol 252:E699, 1987.
181. McMillan M, Chernow B, Roth BL: Alterations in hepatic $alpha_1$-adrenergic receptors in a rat model of chronic sepsis. Circ Shock 19:185, 1986.
182. Silverman HJ, Penaranda R, Orens JB, Lee NH: Impaired beta-adrenergic receptor stimulation of cyclic adenosine monophosphate in human septic shock: association with myocardial hyporesponsiveness to catecholamines. Crit Care Med 21:31, 1992.

183. Forse RA, Saint-Vil D, Gagner M, Borlase BC: Intra-abdominal sepsis and adrenergic receptor response. J Trauma 32:564, 1992.
184. Young JS, Headrick JP, Berne RM: Endothelial-dependent and -independent responses in the thoracic aorta during endotoxic shock. Circ Shock 35:25, 1991.
185. Kuo L, Chilian WM, Davis MJ, Laughlin MH: Endotoxin impairs flow-induced vasodilation of porcine coronary arterioles. Am J Physiol 262:H1838, 1992.
186. Astiz ME, Tilly E, Rackow ED, Weil MH: Peripheral vascular tone in sepsis. Chest 99:1072, 1991.
187. Hartl GB, Inthorn D, Heberer G: Reactive hyperemia in patients with septic conditions. Surgery 103:440, 1988.
188. Whitworth PW, Cryer HM, Garrison RN, et al: Hypoperfusion of the intestinal microcirculation with decreased cardiac output during live *Escherichia coli* sepsis in rats. Circ Shock 27:111, 1989.
189. Steeb GD, Wilson MA, Garrison RN: Pentoxyfylline preserves small-intestine microvascular blood flow during bacteremia. Surgery 112:756, 1992.
190. Fink MP, Kruithoff KL, Antonsson JB, et al: Delayed treatment with an LTD_4/E_4 antagonist limits pulmonary edema in endotoxic pigs. Am J Physiol 260:R1007, 1991.
191. Fink MP, Kaups KL, Wang H, Rothschild HR: Ibuprofen improves survival but does not ameliorate increased gut mucosal permeability in endotoxic pigs. Arch Surg 127:49, 1992.
192. Yanagisawa M, Kuihara H, Kimura S, et al: A novel potent vasoconstrictor peptide produced by vascular endothelial cells. Nature 332:411, 1988.
193. Marsden PA, Brenner BM: Transcriptional regulation of endothelin-1 by tumor necrosis factor-alpha. Am J Physiol 262:C854, 1992.
194. Yoshizuma M, Kurihara H, Morita T, et al: Interleukin 1 increases the production of endothelin-1 by cultured endothelial cells. Biochem Biophys Res Commun 166:324, 1990.
195. Sugiura M, Inagami T, Kon V: Endotoxin stimulates endothelin release in vivo and in vitro as determined by radioimmunoassay. Biochem Biophys Res Commun 161:1220, 1989.
196. Takahashi K, Silva A, Cohen J: Endothelin immunoreactivity in mice with gram-negative bacteraemia: relation to tumour necrosis factor-alpha. Clin Sci 79:619, 1990.
197. Morel DR, Lacroix JS, Hemsen A: Increased plasma and pulmonary lymph levels of endothelin during endotoxin shock. Eur J Pharmacol 167:427, 1989.
198. Weitzberg E, Lundberg JM, Rudehill A: Elevated plasma endothelin levels of endothelin in patients with sepsis syndrome. Circ Shock 33:222, 1991.
199. Voerman HJ, Stehouwer CDA, van Kamp GJ, et al: Plasma endothelin levels are increased during septic shock. Crit Care Med 20:1097, 1992.
200. King AJ, Brenner BM, Anderson S: Endothelin: a potent renal and systemic vasoconstrictor peptide. Am J Physiol 256:F1051, 1989.
201. Pernow J, Hemsen A, Lundberg JM: Tissue specific distribution, clearance and vascular effects of endothelin in the pig. Biochem Biophys Res Commun 161:647, 1989.
202. Jenkins JK, Carey PD, Byrne K, et al: Sepsis-induced lung injury and the effects of ibuprofen pretreatment: analysis of early alveolar events via repetitive bronchoalveolar lavage. Am Rev Respir Dis 143:155, 1991.
203. Siebeck M, Weipert J, Keser C, et al: A triazolodiazepine platelet activating factor receptor antagonist (WEB 2086) reduces pulmonary dysfunction during endotoxin shock in swine. J Trauma 31:942, 1991.
204. Olson NC, Joyce PB, Fleisher LN: Role of platelet-activating factor and eicosanoids during endotoxin-induced lung injury in pigs. Am J Physiol 258: H1674, 1990.
205. Dobrowsky RT, Voyksner RD, Olson NC: Effect of SRI 63-675 on hemodynamics and blood PAF levels during porcine endotoxemia. Am J Physiol 260:H1455, 1991.
206. Wollert PS, Menconi MJ, O'Sullivan BP, et al: LY255283, a novel leukotriene B_4 receptor antagonist, limits activation of neutrophils and prevents acute lung injury induced by endotoxin in pigs. Surgery 114:191, 1993.
207. Fink MP, O'Sullivan BP, Menconi MJ, et al: LY255283, a novel leukotriene B_4 receptor antagonist, ameliorates hypoxemia and abrogates pulmonary edema in a porcine model of circulatory shock and acute lung injury caused by lipopolysaccharide. Crit Care Med 21:1825, 1993.
208. Olson NC, Kruse-Elliott KT, Johnson L: Effect of LY171883 on endotoxin-induced lung injury in pigs. J Appl Physiol 69:1315, 1990.
209. Gross D, Dahan JB, Landau EH, Krausz MM: Effect of leukotriene inhibitor LY-171883 on the pulmonary response to *Escherichia coli* endotoxemia. Crit Care Med 18:190, 1990.
210. Kuhl PG, Bolds JM, Loyd JE, et al: Thromboxane receptor-mediated bronchial and hemodynamic responses in ovine endotoxemia. Am J Physiol 254:R310, 1988.
211. Svartholm E, Bergqvist D, Hedner U, et al: Thromboxane A_2-receptor blockade and prostacyclin in porcine *Escherichia coli* shock. Arch Surg 124:669, 1989.
212. Henry CL, Ogletree ML, Brigham KL, Hammon JW Jr: Attenuation of pulmonary vascular response to endotoxin by a thromboxane synthesis inhibitor (UK-38485) in unanesthetized sheep. J Surg Res 50:77, 1991.
213. Redl G, Abdi S, Traber LD, et al: Inhibition of thromboxane synthesis reduces endotoxin-induced right ventricular failure in sheep. Crit Care Med 19:1294, 1991.
214. Coggeshall JW, Christman BW, Lefferts PL, et al: Effect of inhibition of 5-lipoxygenase metabolism of

arachidonic acid on response to endotoxemia in sheep. J Appl Physiol 65:1351, 1988.
215. Kuratomi Y, Lefferts PL, Christman BW, et al: Effect of a 5-lipoxygenase inhibitor on endotoxin-induced pulmonary dysfunction in awake sheep. J Appl Physiol 74:596, 1993.
216. Olson NC: Role of 5-hydroxytryptamine in endotoxin-induced respiratory failure in pigs. Am Rev Respir Dis 135:93, 1987.
217. Sielaff TD, Kellum JM, Sugerman HJ, et al: Serotonin receptor blockade improves cardiac output and hypoxia in porcine ARDS. J Surg Res 43:118, 1987.
218. Ogletree ML, Begley CJ, King GA, Brigham KL: Influence of steroidal and nonsteroidal anti-inflammatory agents on the accumulation of arachidonic acid metabolites in plasma and lung lymph after endotoxemia in awake sheep: measurements of prostacyclin and thromboxane metabolites and 12-HETE. Am Rev Respir Dis 133:55, 1986.
219. Reines HD, Halushaka PV, Olanoff LS, Hunt PS: Dazoxiben in human sepsis and adult respiratory distress syndrome. Clin Pharmacol Ther 37:391, 1985.
220. Leeman M, Boeynaema J, Degaute J, et al: Administration of dazoxiben, a selective thromboxane synthetase inhibitor, in the adult respiratory distress syndrome. Chest 87:726, 1985.
221. Snyder LS, Hertz MI, Harmon KR, Bitterman PB: Failure of lung repair following acute lung injury: regulation of the fibroproliferative response (part 1). Chest 98:733, 1990.
222. Parker MM, Shelhamer JH, Bacharach SL, et al: Profound but reversible myocardial depression in patients with septic shock. Ann Intern Med 100:483, 1984.
223. Parker MM, Suffredini AF, Natanson C, et al: Responses of left ventricular function in survivors and nonsurvivors of septic shock. J Crit Care 4:19, 1989.
224. Raper R, Sibbald WJ, Driedger AA, Gerow K: Relative myocardial depression in normotensive sepsis. J Crit Care 4:9, 1989.
225. Mitsuo T, Shimazaki S, Matsuda H: Right ventricular dysfunction in septic patients. Crit Care Med 20:630, 1992.
226. Parker MM, McCarthy KE, Ognibene FP, Parrillo JE: Right ventricular dysfunction and dilatation, similar to left ventricular changes, characterize the cardiac depression of septic shock in humans. Chest 97:126, 1990.
227. Vincent J-L, Gris P, Coffernils M, et al: Myocardial depression characterizes the fatal course of septic shock. Surgery 111:600, 1992.
228. Jardin F, Brun-Ney D, Auvert B, et al: Sepsis-related cardiogenic shock. Crit Care Med 18:1055, 1990.
229. Jha P, Jacobs H, Bose D, et al: Effects of *E. coli* sepsis and myocardial depressant factor on interval-force relations in dog ventricle. Am J Physiol 264:H1402, 1993.
230. Natanson C, Fink MP, Ballantyne HK, et al: Gram-negative bacteremia produces both severe systolic and diastolic cardiac dysfunction in a canine model that simulates human septic shock. J Clin Invest 78:259, 1986.
231. Stahl TJ, Alden PB, Ring WS, et al: Sepsis-induced diastolic dysfunction in chronic canine peritonitis. Am J Physiol 258:H625, 1990.
232. Shepherd RE, Lang CH, McDonough KH: Myocardial adrenergic responsiveness after lethal and nonlethal doses of endotoxin. Am J Physiol 252:H410, 1987.
233. Goldfarb RD, Nightingale LM, Kish P, et al: Left ventricular function during lethal and sublethal endotoxemia in swine. Am J Physiol 251:H364, 1986.
234. Baum TD, Heard SO, Feldman HS, et al: Endotoxin-induced myocardial depression in rats: effect of ibuprofen and SDZ 64-688, a platelet activating factor receptor antagonist. J Surg Res 48:629, 1990.
235. Guntheroth WG, Jacky JP, Kawabori I, et al: Left ventricular performance in endotoxin shock in dogs. Am J Physiol 242:H172, 1982.
236. Suffredini AF, Fromm RE, Parker MM, et al: The cardiovascular response of normal humans to administration of endotoxin. N Engl J Med 321:280, 1989.
237. Cunnion RE, Schaer GL, Parker MM, et al: The coronary circulation in human septic shock. Circulation 73:637, 1986.
238. Dhainaut J-F, Huyghebaert M-F, Monsallier JF, et al: Coronary hemodynamics and myocardial metabolism of lactate, free fatty acids, glucose, and ketones in patients with septic shock. Circulation 75:533, 1987.
239. Wyler F, Forsyth RP, Nies AS, et al: Endotoxin-induced regional circulatory changes in the unanesthetized monkey. Circ Res 24:777, 1969.
240. Breslow MJ, Miller CF, Parker SD, et al: Effect of vasopressors on organ blood flow during endotoxin shock in pigs. Am J Physiol 252:H291, 1987.
241. Lang CH, Bagby GJ, Ferguson JL, Spitzer JJ: Cardiac output and redistribution of organ blood flow in hypermetabolic sepsis. Am J Physiol 246:R331, 1984.
242. Fink MP, Fiallo V, Stein KL, Gardiner WM: Systemic and regional hemodynamic changes after intraperitoneal endotoxin in rabbits: development of a new model of the clinical syndrome of hyperdynamic sepsis. Circ Shock 22:73, 1987.
243. Maksad AK, Cha C-J, Stuart RC, et al: Myocardial depression in septic shock: physiologic and metabolic effects of a plasma factor on an isolated heart. Circ Shock Suppl 1:35, 1979.
244. Lefer AM: Mechanisms of cardiodepression in endotoxin shock. Circ Shock Suppl 1:1, 1979.
245. DeMeules JE: A physiologic explanation for cardiac deterioration in septic shock. J Surg Res 36:553, 1984.

246. Parrillo JE, Burch C, Shelhamer JH, et al: A circulating myocardial depressant substance in humans with septic shock: septic shock patients with a reduced ejection fraction have a circulating factor that depresses in vitro myocardial performance. J Clin Invest 76:1539, 1985.
247. Reilly JM, Cunnion RE, Burch-Whitman C, et al: A circulating myocardial depressant substance is associated with cardiac dysfunction and peripheral hypoperfusion (lactic acidemia) in patients with septic shock. Chest 95:1072, 1989.
248. Pagani FD, Baker LS, Hsi C, et al: Left ventricular systolic and diastolic dysfunction after infusion of tumor necrosis factor-α in conscious dogs. J Clin Invest 90:389, 1992.
249. Heard SO, Baum TD, Feldman HS, et al: Lipopolysaccharide-induced myocardial depression is not mediated by a cyclooxygenase product. Crit Care Med 19:723, 1991.
250. Eichenholz PW, Eichacker PQ, Hoffman WD, et al: Tumor necrosis factor challenges in canines: patterns of cardiovascular dysfunction. Am J Physiol 263:H668, 1992.
251. Gulick T, Chung MK, Pieper SJ, et al: Interleukin 1 and tumor necrosis factor inhibit cardiac myocyte β-adrenergic responsiveness. Proc Natl Acad Sci USA 86:6753, 1989.
252. Finkel MS, Oddis CV, Jacob TD, et al: Negative inotropic effects of cytokines on the heart mediated by nitric oxide. Science 257:387, 1992.
253. Brady AJB, Poole-Wilson PA, Harding SE, Warren JB: Nitric oxide production within cardiac myocytes reduces their contractility in endotoxemia. Am J Physiol 263:H1963, 1992.
254. DeMeules JE, Pigula FA, Mueller M, et al: Tumor necrosis factor and cardiac function. J Trauma 32:686, 1992.
255. Gombos EA, Lee TH, Solinas J, Mitrovic M: Renal response to pyrogen in normotensive and hypertensive man. Circulation 36:555, 1967.
256. Lucas CE, Rector FE, Werner M, Rosenberg IK: Altered renal homeostasis with acute sepsis: clinical significance. Arch Surg 106:444, 1973.
257. Brenner M, Schaer GL, Mallory DL, et al: Detection of renal blood flow abnormalities in septic and critically ill patients using a newly designed indwelling thermodilution renal vein catheter. Chest 98:170, 1990.
258. Ravikant T, Lucas CE: Renal blood flow distribution in septic hyperdynamic pigs. J Surg Res 22:294, 1977.
259. Gagnon JA, Ramwell PW, Flamenbaum W: Pyrogenic renal hyperemia: the role of prostaglandins. Nephron 22:29, 1978.
260. Haybron DM, Townsend MC, Hampton WW, et al: Alterations in renal perfusion and renal energy charge in murine peritonitis. Arch Surg 122:328, 1987.
261. Gump FE, Price JG, Kinney JM: Whole body and splanchnic blood flow in oxygen consumption measurements in patients with intraperitoneal infection. Ann Surg 171:321, 1970.
262. Wilmore DW, Goodwin CW, Aulick LH, et al: Effect of injury and infection on visceral metabolism and circulation. Ann Surg 192:491, 1980.
263. Dahn MS, Wilson RF, Lange P, et al: Hepatic parenchymal oxygen tension following injury and sepsis. Arch Surg 125:441, 1990.
264. Gys T, Hubens A, Neels H, et al: Prognostic value of gastric intramural pH in surgical intensive care patients. Crit Care Med 16:1222, 1988.
265. Rasmussen I, Haglund U: Early gut ischemia in experimental fecal peritonitis. Circ Shock 38:22, 1992.
266. Natanson C, Danner RL, Reilly JM: Antibiotics versus cardiovascular support in a canine model of human septic shock. Am J Physiol 259:H1440, 1990.
267. Edwards JD, Brown GCS, Nightingale P, et al: Use of survivors' cardiorespiratory values as therapeutic goals in septic shock. Crit Care Med 17:1098, 1989.
268. Mitchell JP, Schuller D, Calandrino FS, Schuster DP: Improved outcome based on fluid management in critically ill patients requiring pulmonary artery catheterization. Am Rev Respir Dis 145:990, 1992.
269. Humphrey H, Hall J, Sznajder I, et al: Improved survival in ARDS patients associated with a reduction in pulmonary capillary wedge pressure. Chest 97:1176, 1990.
270. Martin C, Papazian L, Perrin G, et al: Norepinephrine or dopamine for the treatment of hyperdynamic septic shock? Chest 103:1826, 1993.
271. Schaer GL, Fink MP, Parrillo JE: Norepinephrine alone versus norepinephrine plus low-dose dopamine: enhanced renal blood flow with combination pressor therapy. Crit Care Med 13:492, 1985.
272. Fiddian-Green RG: Splanchnic ischemia and multiple organ failure in the critically ill. Ann R Coll Surg Engl 70:128, 1988.
273. Fink MP, Kaups KL, Wang H, Rothschild HR: Maintenance of superior mesenteric arterial perfusion prevents increased intestinal mucosal permeability in endotoxic pigs. Surgery 110:154, 1991.
274. Gys T, Hubens A, Neels H, et al: Prognostic value of gastric intramural pH in surgical intensive care patients. Crit Care Med 16:122, 1988.
275. Doglio GR, Pusajo JF, Egurrola MA, et al: Gastric mucosal pH as a prognostic index of mortality in critically ill patients. Crit Care Med 19:1037, 1991.
276. Guitierrez G, Palizas F, Doglio G, et al: Gastric intramucosal pH as a therapeutic index of tissue oxygenation in critically ill patients. Lancet 339:195, 1992.

Thermoregulatory Responses to Infection

CHAPTER 19

Louis H. Aulick, Douglas W. Wilmore

The invasion of the body by microorganisms initiates a wide variety of host responses. First, local penetration of tissue stimulates mobilization of phagocytes, initiates an inflammatory response at the local site, and may activate additional local host immunologic mechanisms. If the infection progresses, fever, tachycardia, and other systemic responses occur; these more generalized reactions may reflect *direct* effects of the infective process on cellular function or *indirect* effects resulting from homeostatic adjustments to these alterations in function. These systemic events represent the interaction of all these processes and may be categorized into two general areas—thermoregulatory and metabolic adjustments. The predominant alteration in thermoregulation is fever, and the principal changes in metabolism relate to the regulation of glucose, nitrogen, and trace elements.

Several general characteristics describe the systemic events that occur after infection.

1. The systemic responses to infection appear rather stereotyped and can be produced after the administration of a wide variety of microorganisms or their toxins. The systemic responses to infection are similar in many respects to the events that follow injury.
2. The magnitude of the responses varies with the extent and duration of infection.
3. The complex sequence of systemic events that follow infection appears to be interrelated in time, and hence sequential studies must be performed to locate the response precisely within this time frame.
4. Although the systemic responses to infection are stereotyped, these processes are significantly modulated by the physiologic reserve of the individual. The magnitude of the responses to infection depends on age and sex of the individual, previous nutritional status, function of vital organs, immunologic memory, and associated disease processes. The classic responses to infection have been observed in young, previously healthy, well-nourished, active adults with no other associated medical problems. These patients, however, are rarely admitted to surgical services. Surgeons usually see patients at extremes of life who are hospitalized because of associated disease processes (degenerative disease, cancer, gastrointestinal disease, cardiovascular disease) and have additional stress (usually an operation or injury) that limits physiologic, biochemical, or immunologic responses to infection. Infection

complicating the recuperative course of surgical patients may not evoke the standard textbook systemic response. Limitations of a patient's capacity to respond to infection may greatly affect host recovery or survival.

5. As infection progresses, additional functional limitations may be imposed on one or more specific organs, which further impair the host systemic responses. This can be observed in patients in whom severe pneumonia and pulmonary dysfunction cause hypoxemia, and it can be associated with circulatory failure and hypotension related to severe gram-negative sepsis.

In spite of the complexities involved in unraveling and understanding the systemic responses to infection in critically ill surgical patients, a large body of investigative and clinical data is available to aid our understanding of these host defense mechanisms. This chapter will review the common systemic alterations associated with pyrogenic bacterial infections. These metabolic changes and the hemodynamic responses they invoke are discussed in Chapters 18 and 20.

FEVER

Body Temperature and Temperature Monitoring

The mechanisms for control of body temperature are extremely efficient, but alterations in the setpoint or derangements in sensitivity of the central thermostat are almost universally associated with infection or inflammation. Elevation of body temperature is such a sensitive and reliable indicator of the presence of disease that thermometry is one of the most common and frequent procedures used in hospitalized patients.

Core or central body temperature (the temperature of internal tissues) reflects the balance between metabolic heat production and surface heat loss. In general, physicians refer to a "normal body temperature" (37C, 98.6F), but this is not considered the true average or mean body temperature because of the wide variations in the temperature of various body tissues (eg, skin and subcutaneous tissue may be 2C to 6C cooler than visceral organs). Because there is no practical way to determine mean body temperature, clinicians rely for convenience on a single measurement of internal temperature and equate this value with body temperature.

Oral or rectal temperature taken in a group of healthy individuals demonstrates the usual bell-shaped distribution curve. The normal temperature for any one individual will vary as much as 1C throughout the day, and this temperature is affected by food intake and level of physical activity. The highest temperatures are usually observed in the afternoon; temperature falls with sleep and reaches its lowest value in the early morning. Oral (or axillary) temperatures average about 0.65C (1.2F) lower than rectal temperature, which is the accepted standard for clinical thermometry, but there are wide variations in this relationship. Although a normal active individual may demonstrate a central temperature ranging between 36C and 40C under ordinary conditions, a quiet person with a rectal temperature above 37.5C (99.5F) or an oral temperature above 37.0C (98.6F) should be suspected of harboring an inflammatory or infectious process until proved otherwise.[1]

What does rectal temperature really measure? The temperature of the rectum is determined by (1) local metabolism, (2) the temperature of the arterial blood delivered to this area and the rate of blood flow, and (3) conductive heat exchange between the rectum and surrounding tissue. Eichna et al[2] compared rectal temperatures of resting subjects with intracardiac and various intravascular temperatures. They found that rectal temperature was 0.2C to 0.3C higher than right heart temperature in afebrile individuals, but that it could exceed intracardiac temperature by as much as 0.8C in febrile patients. Femoral artery blood temperature was equivalent to intracardiac temperatures, and Eichna argued that these two intravascular temperatures offered the best index of average body temperature.

Cooper and Kenyon[3] placed thermocouples on the aorta during thoracic operations and compared para-aortic blood temperatures (an indirect measurement of central intravascular temperature) with rectal and esophageal temperatures. Esophageal temperature at the level of the heart was a more reliable index of aortic blood temperature than was rectal temperature. Moreover, rectal temperature was always higher than aortic temperature and responded slowly to rapid fluctuations in central blood temperatures. Molnar and Read[4] also confirmed that rectal temperature was slower than esophageal and stomach temperatures to respond to fluctuations in arterial temperature.

In spite of these limitations, rectal temperature (taken 5 to 10 cm above the anal sphincter) is the most practical method of monitoring core temperature in the critically ill patient. However, the rectal temperature response to alterations in body heat content is slow, and its relationship to that of the arterial blood that perfuses the temperature control center in the brain is altered in an unpredictable manner with the onset of a fever. Although the esophagus is a better location for more accurate central temperature monitoring, it is practical only in the operating room. Tympanic temperature has also been used as an index of central body temperature. Although it will follow body temperature changes more rapidly than will rectal measurements, it is more sensitive to variations in ambient temperatures, and the probe is difficult to position comfortably. With the use of thermal dilution cardiac output catheters, a central intravascular thermistor is available for continuous monitoring of mixed venous blood temperature. Rectal temperatures may range from 0.2C to 0.8C above these central intravascular values in both healthy individuals and febrile patients.[5] The temperature of venous blood from brain and liver will usually be higher than that observed in the right heart or aorta, reflecting the contribution of these particular organs to the heat input of the body.

Body Heat Balance

Body temperature reflects a balance between the heat produced and the heat lost, and under usual conditions this balance is a finely regulated physiologic process. Approximately two-thirds of the heat produced in the basal state occurs in the brain and visceral organs. Metabolic heat production will increase above basal levels for a variety of reasons. First, body metabolism increases slightly (10 to 15 percent) following food ingestion. This is known as the specific dynamic action of food. The effect lasts for several hours and uses approximately 10 percent of the ingested calories. Second, environmental cold stress or the rise in hypothalamic setpoint temperature with a fever will cause an increase in skeletal muscle activity (ranging from unconscious tensing to uncontrollable shivering and involuntary movements), which increases metabolic heat production. When stimulated by a cold environment, calorigenic hormones (primarily the catecholamines) are liberated to aid heat production and mobolize body fuels. Third, the greatest increase in metabolism occurs during physical exercise, when levels of heat production may reach four to five times basal rates.

To maintain thermal equilibrium, heat loss must equal metabolic and environmental heat gains. Body heat loss is regulated by physiologic adjustments in sweating and cutaneous blood flow as well as by behavioral means (eg, covering up with a blanket in a cool room or moving into the shade on a hot day). Because of the low thermal conductivity of deep body tissue, the body must rely heavily on the circulation to carry metabolic heat from the deeper tissues, where it is produced, to the skin and respiratory surfaces, where it can be dissipated. The wide range of vasomotor adjustments plus the high heat conductivity and specific heat of blood makes this system ideally adapted for thermoregulation. Cutaneous vasodilation will increase the rate of heat delivery to the body surface where, if skin temperatures exceed ambient temperatures, heat is dissipated primarily by radiation and convection. In warmer environments most, if not all, body heat is lost by the evaporation of sweat.

The primary means of heat conservation is vasoconstriction of the skin. The magnitude of cutaneous vasomotion is best appreciated in the fingers, where blood flow is primarily superficial. In response to a cold challenge, finger blood flow will drop to approximately one one-hundredth that occurring in a hot environment. Reduced surface circulation greatly increases the insulative layer of the body, causing a rise in body heat storage and central temperatures.

Many adaptations to alterations in internal temperature or to the external thermal environment are determined by behavioral changes. To retain heat, an individual will curl up to minimize exposed surface area and add clothing or bed covers to provide additional insulation. Conversely, if heat is to be lost, an individual will move into a cooler environment, remove clothing, drink cold liquids, and extend the extremities to maximize effective body surface area and promote heat exchange. Behavioral thermoregulation is available to most awake, alert hospitalized patients, but many individuals who are receiving critical care cannot make these important behavioral adjustments. Because these patients frequently have additional derangements of thermoregulation, they are extremely vulnerable to changes in the thermal environment.

Central Nervous System Control and Temperature Setpoint

Central control of body temperature resides predominantly within the hypothalamus. Cells within both the preoptic region of the anterior hypothalamus and the posterior hypothalamus receive a variety of extrinsic and intrinsic temperature information, integrate this sensory input, and initiate a coordinated effector response. Thermoreceptors in the skin and body core provide neurogenic afferents that ultimately reach and affect hypothalamic thermoregulatory activity. Thermosensitive cells have also been identified in the preoptic region of the hypothalamus; these alter their intrinsic firing rates with changes in local temperature. These cells are of two distinct populations: warm-sensitive cells will increase firing rates during a rise in local temperature, and cold-sensitive neurons will increase their firing frequency upon cooling. Like the rest of the body, hypothalamic temperature varies as a function of changes in local heat production and loss. Vascular heat transfer appears to be a primary means of reducing hypothalamic temperature. As a consequence, any variation in body heat content that changes arterial blood temperature can ultimately affect hypothalamic thermoregulatory activity. Circulatory as well as neurogenic factors, therefore, contribute to the afferent limb of hypothalamic temperature control.

Numerous mathematical and engineering models have been devised to explain the hypothalamic temperature controller. The most commonly used system involves a comparison between an intrinsic reference or setpoint signal and one from the sensor(s) of actual (eg, hypothalamic, core, mean) body temperature. The thermoregulatory output from such a controller would be qualitatively and quantitatively related to both the direction and the magnitude of the differences in these two signals.[6] Physiologic control of body temperature is, therefore, analogous to a thermostat, which compares room temperature to a set value and then activates either the heater or air conditioner until the thermal environment returns to the reference value of the thermostat. Likewise, the body's central reference temperature is not a fixed value can be adjusted up or down by seasonal or daily circadian rhythms, environmental stress, injury, and infection. Regardless of the cause for the shift in setpoint temperature, the body will continue to regulate temperature in a normal manner around this new central reference value.

Fever is explained by a rise in hypothalamic setpoint temperature, which initiates both physiologic and behavioral thermoregulatory mechanisms to elevate and hold central body temperature at a higher level. When the reference temperature is normal, the individual is considered *normothermic* when body temperature matches setpoint, *hypothermic* when it drops below setpoint, and *hyperthermic* when body temperature exceeds the normal central reference level.

Pyrogens: The Afferent Mediators of Fever

Fever is one of the earliest recognized signs of inflammation and infection. During the late eighteenth and early nineteenth centuries, it was realized that injection of a variety of solutions or putrified material into an animal caused fever. Clinical studies at this time also supported the relationship between fever and infection. Semmelweiss introduced endometrial secretions of patients with puerperal fever into female rabbits immediately after delivery and observed fever and lethal sepsis.[7] Billroth and his students demonstrated that the injection of filtrates of pus caused elevations in body temperature when administered to animals.

Following the discoveries of Lister and Pasteur concerning the germ theory of disease, scientists began to describe many features of the newly discovered microorganisms. A constant feature of the bacterial studies was that the organisms secreted a substance into the culture media that was regularly pyrogenic in animals and would often invoke a leukocyte response. By the early 20th century it was realized that bacteria produced pyrogenic factors in addition to the exotoxins that were excreted by the microorganisms into the culture media. A new toxin was described, which was tightly anchored to, if not a part of, the cell wall. This substance was called *endotoxin* and was later biochemically characterized as a lipopolysaccharide.

In addition to the pyrogenic substances associated with microorganisms, products secreted by the host's own cells serve as signals to stimulate fever. The first experimental evidence of an *endogenous pyrogen* (EP) was provided by Bennett and Beeson,[8] in 1953, when they isolated a product of rabbit granulocytes that differed in many respects from the pyrogen of microbial origin.[9] This particular EP was a 15 to 17 kD, heat-labile protein that subsequently proved to be the same compound that mediated many acute-phase responses to infection—hypoferremia, hypozincemia, hypercupremia, granulocytosis, hepatic acute-phase protein production, thymocyte proliferation, antibody production, fibroblast proliferation, and collagen production. When it became clear that this one molecule, or family of molecules, had multiple biologic properties, it was given the more generic title, interleukin 1 (IL-1).

IL-1's relative role in naturally occurring fever was called into question with the discovery of other EPs capable of causing fever when injected into experimental animals and humans. These other pyrogens are tumor necrosis factor/cachectin (TNF), interleukin 6 (IL-6), interferon alpha (IFN-α), and interferon gamma (IFN-γ), and macrophage inflammatory protein 1. In an effort to separate native from experimental EPs, Kluger[10] offered five criteria that must be satisfied before any putative

EP can be considered to be a native mediator of fever:

1. Application of the putative EP at the hypothetical site of action must result in a rise in body temperature.
2. When an exogenous pyrogen induces fever, the released EP has a quantitative relationship to the rise in body temperature, and the amount of EP released is similar to that which causes an equivalent rise in temperature when this same EP is given at the hypothetical site of action.
3. The rise in body temperature induced by the EP should be associated with appropriate thermoregulatory effector responses (eg, cutaneous vasoconstriction, shivering).
4. Substances that block production of the EP prevent the rise in body temperature.
5. Substances that block action of the EP prevent the rise in body temperature.

None of the putative EPs listed above fulfills all five criteria. Plasma IL-1 activity fails to correlate with LPS-induced changes in body temperature, and the intravenous dose of IL-1 required to produce fever raises plasma levels above those recorded in febrile animals. IL-1β antibodies block about half of LPS-induced fever, suggesting that IL-1 may act synergistically with other circulating pyrogens. Finally, cells in the brain make IL-1, so it is possible that central production of this EP is more critical to fever induction than its peripheral circulating level.

TNF satisfies more of the criteria as a putative EP than IL-1. When infused intravenously in cancer patients, TNF causes fevers at plasma concentrations similar to those observed in infected patients, and, in some cases, monoclonal antibodies reduce LPS-induced fevers in animals. One must be cautious about designating TNF a native EP, however, since the relationship between plasma TNF concentration and fever is not always clear. In addition, immunoassays for TNF are not well correlated with assays of its biologic activity. And, finally, there are studies that suggest that TNF is an endogenous cryogen.[11]

TNF and IL-1 induce cells to produce IL-6 and there is strong evidence to suggest that IL-6 is responsible for some of the pyrogenicity originally attributed to IL-1.[12] Plasma IL-6 concentration is correlated to body temperature of burn patients, but a relatively low r^2 defining this relationship indicates that most of the fever was the result of other factor(s).[13] Injections of IFN-α and IFN-γ raise body temperature of both animals and humans, but the persistent question is whether experimental doses were physiologic or pharmacologic. Macrophage inflammatory protein 1 (MIP-1) is a heparin-binding protein produced by LPS-activated macrophages and causing intense fevers when very small amounts are injected peripherally or centrally. Its role in naturally occurring fevers has not been extensively documented.

In summary, all data taken together suggest that exogenous pyrogens exert their thermoregulatory effects through the production of EPs, but exactly how this occurs is still unknown. The complexity of this problem is a function of many factors: (1) the pleiotropic nature of these cytokines, (2) the apparent redundancy of their biologic effects and the subsequent potential for synergistic/antagonistic interactions, and (3) the existence of numerous native inhibitors. Given all these variables and the evidence of species variations, it is not surprising that there is still no conclusive evidence that any of the putative EPs is a circulating mediator of fever.

How Pyrogens Affect the Central Thermostat

As previously noted, body temperature is maintained by a delicate balance between heat production and heat loss. The central thermostat located in the hypothalamus controls the physiologic, biochemical, and behavioral adjustments of the body to alterations in external and internal temperatures. Fever is the result of an upward adjustment of this central regulatory apparatus, and heat loss from the body is diminished or heat gain increased. When body temperature has risen to a new setpoint, thermoregulation occurs around this higher temperature (Fig. 19–1).

The central nervous system is essential for the febrile response, because fever is not observed in animals after selective ablation of the hypothalamic thermoregulatory center. Since the first evidence of EPs, the assumption has been that infectious agents did not act directly on the brain but caused phagocytic cells to produce pyrogens and that these "true mediators of fever" were delivered to the brain via the circulation. This is supported by the observation that the febrile response in humans does not occur after intravenous pyrogen administration if a proximal tourniquet prevents delivery of the substance to the brain. In rabbits the febrile response develops more rapidly and is more pronounced when the EP is infused in the carotid artery rather than given intravenously. Injections of EP directly into the anterior hypothalamus further

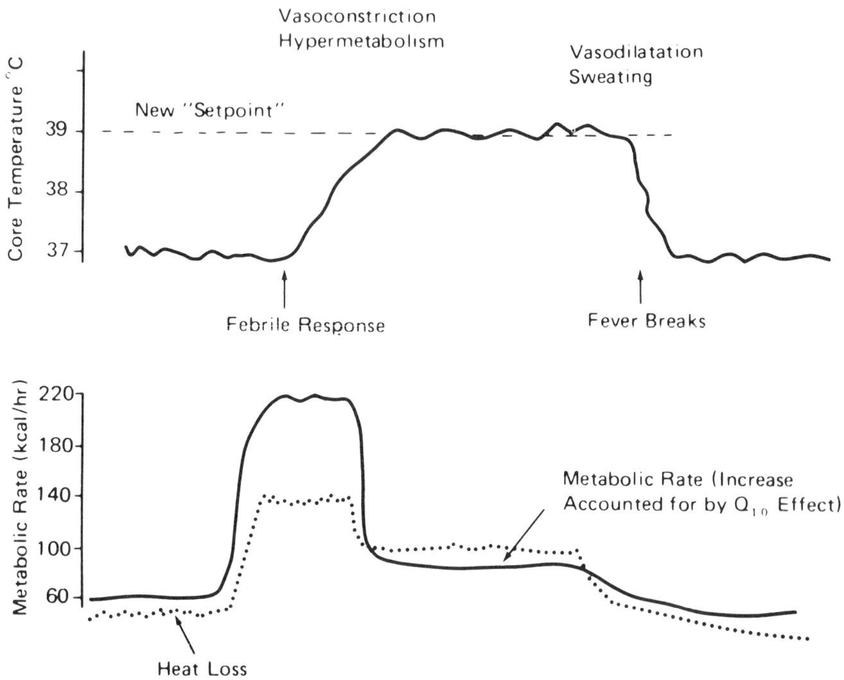

Figure 19–1. The response of body temperature, heat production (metabolic rate), and cutaneous heat loss to a pyrogenic fever.

accelerate and amplify the febrile response of rabbits. There is little evidence, however, that any of the EPs generated outside the brain actually enter the central nervous system. Most are too large to penetrate the blood-brain barrier without a specific carrier system and there is only one study providing any evidence of such carriers.[14] Thermosensitive neurons in the anterior hypothalamus have EP receptors and respond to microinjections of EP, but this does not obligate a blood-borne delivery scheme, because glial cells and astrocytes in the brain produce EPs.

There is increasing evidence to suggest that blood-borne EPs influence the hypothalamic thermoregulatory center through a circumventricular organ in the brain—the organum vasculosum laminae terminalis (OVLT). The OVLT is a highly vascularized structure with fenestrated capillaries lying on the anteroventral wall of the third ventricle adjacent to the thermosensitive preoptic area of the anterior hypothalamus. Electrolytic ablation of this wall or the capillary network in the OVLT decreases the fever evoked by intraperitoneal injections of exogenous pyrogens, indicating that the integrity of this region is required for a normal febrile response to circulating EP.[15,16] The EP may either pass through fenestrated capillaries into the perivascular spaces of the OVLT or bind to capillary endothelium to stimulate the release of other chemical messengers.[17] EPs passing through capillaries do not penetrate the tight junctions separating the OVLT from the brain but appear to stimulate phagocytic cells in the OVLT to synthesize and release prostaglandin E_2 (PGE_2) and possibly other transmitters. These substances either diffuse into the brain to affect thermosensitive cells directly or excite neurons in the OVLT that project into the thermoregulatory center. The relative significance of the OVLT as the site of signal transduction was emphasized by Stitt[18,19] when he found that cells in this area were more sensitive to injections of PGE_2 and IL-1β than cells in the anterior hypothalamus. Intravenous injections of EP increase PGE_2 concentration in the OVLT and the subsequent fever can be suppressed by intravenous injections of calcium channel blockers, verapamil and nifedipine, and cyclooxygenase inhibitors.[20] All these data suggest that the EP triggers PGE_2 production from cells in the OVLT (cells exposed to the blood) by opening calcium channels in the membrane and increasing intracellular free calcium levels. Cytosolic Ca^{2+} presumably activates phospholipases, which convert membrane phospholipids into arachidonic acid, which is then converted to PGE_2.

Neurochemical transmission initiated by the EP, in either the OVLT or the preoptic area of the anterior hypothalamus, appears to involve PGE_2 and/or non-PGE_2 mechanisms. The febrile response to intravenous infusion of LPS can be blocked by the PGE_2 synthetase inhibitor, indomethacin, when the latter is given systemically, but not when it is placed in the preoptic area of the hypothalamus.[21] Further evidence of separate PGE_2-dependent and PGE_2-independent transmission has been provided in rabbits responding to high-dose intravenous IL-1β.[22] One interpretation is that PGE_2 production may be involved in signal transduction outside the blood-brain barrier, and subsequent steps in the OVLT or inside the brain utilize other neurotransmitters. MIP-1, 5-hydroxytryptamine, and substance P have all been mentioned as other central neuromodulators.[21–23]

Although the exact biochemical mechanisms by which EPs and various neurotransmitters act on thermosensitive elements of the central temperature controller are unknown, the central thermostat is reset to an elevated level by reducing the activity of the warm-sensitive cells and increasing the firing rate of the cold-sensitive neurons. With the upward shift in hypothalamic setpoint, two mechanisms are used to achieve an increase in core temperature. Vasoconstriction by the cutaneous vessels limits heat loss. This may be the first and only adjustment made by individuals in a warm environment. Increased heat production, with or without distinct shivering, can also occur, especially if the thermal environment is inadequate. Frequently, both mechanisms operate together to increase body heat content and achieve the new setpoint temperature. Once this new reference temperature is achieved, temperature regulation will function in a normal manner around the elevated level. The metabolic rate at this new equilibrium (following the initial responses with the associated shivering) should be accounted for by the effect of the increased body temperature on metabolism (Q_{10} effect). When the infection clears, the setpoint returns to normal, and central nervous system mechanisms are activated to aid heat loss. Cutaneous vasodilation and sweating cause body temperature to fall, and the resting metabolic rate returns to normal. A new thermal equilibrium is achieved, and lower body temperatures are maintained around a normal hypothalamic setpoint.

The Bacteriostatic Effects of Fever

Although fever is a common sign of infection, it is not clear that an elevated body temperature itself provides any benefit to the host. Induced hyperthermia was once used in the treatment of poliomyelitis, neurosyphilis, and gonorrheal infection because of the in vitro sensitivity of the infecting organisms to elevated temperatures. More recently, the beneficial effects of fever have been demonstrated in fish and desert iguanas, ectotherms that adjust body temperatures by behavior. These species move into warm or cold environments to achieve higher or lower body temperatures. Iquanas were infected with live bacteria and then placed in incubators at 38C (their normal body temperature), 40C to 42C temperatures (fever response), and 34C and 36C (hypothermia).[24] A positive correlation existed between the lizard's temperature and survival rate following bacteremia. More than 80 percent of the warmest animals lived after infection, compared to survival rates of less than 40 percent in the group at normal (38C) temperature and less than 20 percent in the hypothermic animals. When the fever was reduced by sodium salicylate, seven of seven animals died following bacteremia.[25] In eight additional infected animals, salicylates were administered but the lizards were housed in a warm incubator, thereby preventing a fall in body temperature. Only one of eight warm animals died, demonstrating that the increased mortality after administration of salicylate was not the direct effect of the drug on the microorganisms but rather of the reduction of body temperature.

In similar studies in bacteremic rabbits, survival from infection increased as the magnitude of the fever increased up to 2.25C.[26] When the fever response was greater than 2.25C, the mortality rate increased. This evidence from mammals does not demonstrate a causal relationship between fever and survival, but the association between fever and survival is similar to that observed in humans: the lack of a febrile (and leukocyte) response after infection is, in general, associated with a poor prognosis.

The specific mechanisms augmented by fever to aid host defenses are unknown, but several nonspecific factors that may aid host immunity have been suggested. Van't Hoff described the physical law governing the relationship between the rate of biochemical reactions and heat. For ordinary temperatures, the velocity of chemical reactions increases approximately two- to threefold for every 10C rise in temperature (Q_{10} effect). The reaction rate of a variety of host defense mechanisms, therefore, may be accelerated by the febrile state. The half-life of endotoxin is reduced during fever. Fever in ectotherms increases the mobility of leukocytes into the site of infection, and fever appears to increase the iron requirements of pathogenic bacteria for growth.[24] Because serum iron levels fall during infection, this biochemical alteration caused by the febrile response decreases, in relative quantities, the iron available for metabolism by microorganisms.[27]

Other Effects of Fever and Requirements for Fever Treatment

In the past, marked increases in body catabolism and cardiac output have served as clinical indications for the need for antipyretics in infected febrile patients. Metabolism and body temperature are interdependent. As body temperature rises, there is an increase in the rate constant for chemical reactions. This Q_{10} effect accounts for a 10 to 13 percent increase in heat production for each degree centigrade rise in body temperature, although there is wide variation in this relationship in actual practice.[1] For example, the patient with a fever of 40C may demonstrate an increase in oxygen consumption of 30 to 35 percent because of the elevation in body temperature alone.

To distinguish between the direct effects of infectious disease and the effect of increased tissue temperature on body catabolism, Beisel and associates[28] studied healthy men placed in a hot chamber adjusted to increase the subject's rectal temperature over 18 hours to 39.4C and to maintain that temperature for 6 hours. The adrenal responses and alterations in nitrogen metabolism during artificial hyperthermia resembled changes during infectious disease. Negative balances of nitrogen, potassium, and magnesium were produced by a combination of reduced dietary intake, increased urinary excretion, and increased sweat losses. With induced hyperthermia, in contrast to the hyperthermia of infectious disease, surface electrolyte loss (through profuse sweating) was greater than cutaneous losses. In spite of the increase in body catabolism induced by fever, current methods of nutritional support are more than adequate to offset the wasting of body tissue during infectious illness.

There is a well-known effect of fever on heart rate. In general, with each 1C rise in body temperature, the pulse rate increases approximately 10 beats per minute. The accompanying increase in cardiac output reflects an increased burden on the circulation to support both rising metabolic demands and a thermoregulatory increase in surface blood flow.

The febrile course during an infectious disease is a valuable indicator of the effect of treatment, and it is argued that antipyretics interfere with this clinical indicator and thus hamper use of core temperatures as an accurate reflection of the course of the infection. If the febrile response does not impose great discomfort or strain the cardiovascular reserve of the patient, antipyretic treatment is rarely necessary. In trauma patients (with or without infection), we support the fever response by maintaining patients in a warm environment. We consider a normal (37C) or subnormal rectal temperature as one of the earliest indications of gram-negative bacteremia.

There are situations, however, when lowering the body temperature is of vital importance, specifically during heat stroke, postoperative or interoperative malignant hyperthermia, delirium or seizure activity associated with fever, and cardiocirculatory failure associated with hyperpyrexia. The body temperature can be lowered by sponging the body with alcohol, by increasing airflow over the body, or by using cooling blankets. *If these measures are taken without also pharmacologically altering the central setpoint (using aspirin, prostaglandin-synthesis inhibitors, chlorpromazine, or related medications, or morphine), additional vasoconstriction will be stimulated, and increased heat (through shivering) will be produced.* In cases of severe hyperthermia (>41C), rubbing the skin to promote vasodilation or immersion of the patient into an ice bath should be considered life-saving.

Clinical Manifestations of Fever

At one time many of the infectious diseases could be diagnosed by their characteristic fever patterns. In this era of sophisticated medical practice, diagnosis of specific infection is best made by microbiologic techniques. The fever pattern is unreliable. Several factors may affect the temperature of critically ill patients. First, the temperature of the room may affect the core temperature of the patient. Responsive, oriented individuals will inform the hospital staff if they are too hot or too cold. In critically ill patients, who are often unresponsive or sedated while receiving ventilatory support, behavioral adaptation to ambient temperature may not be possible. Air conditioning (<28C) is an additional stress for critically ill patients who have alterations in temperature regulation (such as sepsis, head injury, thermal trauma, or multiple injury).[29] Those patients who cannot communicate with the nursing staff should be cared for in thermally neutral (28C to 30C) environments. Shivering should never be allowed because of the added physiologic stress it places on the critically ill patient. If reduction of body temperature is a desired goal, drugs that lower central setpoint should be administered before ambient cooling is instituted.

Salicylates are the most common antipyretics administered to febrile patients. They are thought to act by altering prostaglandin synthesis. Alternatively, Myers and Tytell[30] have suggested that the salicylate effect in the central nervous system may be caused by alterations of the ionic balance across the cell membrane in the hypothalamic area. Other salicylate-like antipyretics are indomethacin, acetaminophen, phenacetin, antipyrine, and aminopyrine.

Some general anesthetics significantly diminish sympathetic outflow from the central nervous system. This is usually ascribed to the nonspecific depression of the central nervous system by the agent rather than to selective action on thermoregulatory centers. The hypothermia that frequently accompanies major operations is the combined result of decreased heat production that occurs secondary to general anesthesia and the increased heat loss that occurs in patients with depressed thermoregulatory capacities undergoing operations in the cool operating room.

Lomax[31] studied the effects of several drugs on body temperature. He found that morphine has a pronounced effect on decreasing heat production; narcotic administration may be associated with a prompt fall in body temperature. Although small doses of morphine exert minimal effects on heat production and heat loss, morphine can have a pronounced effect on sympathetic outflow from the brain and greatly diminish heat production when given in an anesthetic dose in the operating room or administered repeatedly to patients who are on artificial ventilation. Chlorpromazine and similar tranquilizers can also cause a fall in heat production. Amphetamines increase oxygen consumption, mainly by an increase in central nervous system activity rather than direct stimulation of the thermal regulatory areas. Other commonly used drugs can affect central setpoint: 1-methyl-dopa causes a slight reduction in core temperature of normal men studied in a cool room; atropine diminishes the rate of sweating and in large doses causes hyperthermia. It can also affect central thermal regulatory areas, resulting in a decrease in heat production.

Dehydration in infants is usually associated with fever (once referred to as inanition fever). The febrile response is greater if the dehydrated patient is hypertonic (ie, hypernatremic). Moyer[32] reproduced this finding in rats and found a decrease in oxygen consumption with hypo-osmolar dehydration, a rise in oxygen consumption during hyperosmolar dehydration, and no change in metabolic rate during isotonic dehydration. This effect may be mediated by the central nervous system, because injection of sodium into the thermoregulatory center causes a prompt rise in body temperature. A similar association between oxygen consumption and extracellular sodium concentration has been observed in vitro, presumably through the stimulation of the sodium-potassium membrane pumps that are accelerated by the increased sodium concentration in the medium.[33]

Alcohol ingestion is the most common cause of accidental hypothermia in the elderly patient. Alcohol causes cutaneous vasodilation and suppresses shivering, thereby increasing heat loss and decreasing heat production during cold exposure.[34] Alcohol also blocks hepatic gluconeogenesis, resulting in hypoglycemia and diminished glucose flow from the liver to peripheral tissues. The hypoglycemia is potentiated if the subject has been exercising or has partially or totally fasted. An unconscious hypothermic patient, therefore, may be somnolent not because of excess alcohol ingestion but because of hypoglycemia.

Hypothermia is frequently associated with gram-negative bacteremia. Cutaneous vasodilation may occur in patients with sepsis to promote increased heat loss. Gram-negative infection also blunts hepatic gluconeogenesis and other hepatic metabolic functions, which may account for a major reduction in the heat produced in support of the core temperature in traumatized patients. The hypoglycemia associated with severe infection[35] may also limit heat production, as the lack of available glucose substrate may create a significant fuel deficit.

REFERENCES

1. DuBoise EF: Fever and the Regulation of Body Temperature. Springfield, IL, CC Thomas, 1948.
2. Eichna LW, Berger AR, Rader B, Becker WH: Comparison of intracardiac and intravascular temperatures with rectal temperatures in man. J Clin Invest 30:353, 1951.
3. Cooper KE, Kenyon JR: A comparison of temperatures measured in the rectum, oesophagus and on the surface of the aorta during hypothermia in man. Br J Surg 44:616, 1957.
4. Molnar GW, Read RC: Studies during open-heart surgery on the special characteristics of rectal temperature. J Appl Physiol 36:333, 1974.
5. Wilmore DW, Aulick LH, Pruitt BA Jr: Metabolism during the hypermetabolic phase of thermal injury. In Rob C (ed): Advances in Surgery, Vol 12. Chicago, Year Book Medical Publisher, 1978, pp 193–225.
6. Hammell HT: Regulation of internal body temperature. Annu Rev Physiol 30:641, 1968.
7. Westphal O, Westphal U, Sommer T: The history of pyrogen research. In Schlessinger D (ed): Microbiology, Washington, DC, American Society for Microbiology, 1977, pp 221–238.
8. Bennett IL Jr, Beeson PB: Studies on the pathogenesis of fever, I. The effect of injection of extracts and suspensions of uninfected rabbit tissues upon the body temperature of normal rabbits. J Exp Med 98:477, 1953.
9. Atkins E, Bodel P: Fever. N Engl J Med 286:27, 1972.

10. Kluger MJ: Fever: role of pyrogens and cryogens. Physiol Rev 71:93, 1991.
11. Long NC, Kunkel SL, Vander AJ, et al: Antiserum against TNF enhances LPS fever in the rat. Am J Physiol 258(Regul Integrative Comp Physiol 27): R332, 1990.
12. LeMay LG, Otterness IG, Vander AJ, et al: In vivo evidence that the rise in plasma IL 6 following injection of a fever-inducing dose of LPS is mediated by IL 1β. Cytokine 2:199, 1990.
13. Nijsten MWN, De Groot ER, Ten Duis HJ, et al: Serum levels of interleukin-6 and the acute phase response. Lancet 2:921, 1987.
14. Banks WA, Kastin AJ, Durham DA: Bidirectional transport of interleukin-1α across the blood-brain barrier. Brain Res Bull 23:433, 1989.
15. Blatteis CM, Hales JRS, McKinley MJ, et al: Role of the anteroventral third ventricle in fever in sheep. Can J Physiol Pharmacol 65:1255, 1987.
16. Blatteis CM, Hunter WS, Wright JM, et al: Thermoregulatory response of guinea pigs with anteroventral third ventricle lesions. Can J Physiol Pharmacol 65:1261, 1987.
17. Hashimoto M, Ishikawa Y, Yokoto S, et al: Action site of circulating interleukin-1 on the rabbit brain. Brain Res 540:217, 1991.
18. Stitt JT: Prostaglandin E as the neural mediator of the febrile response. Yale J Biol Med 59:137, 1986.
19. Stitt JT: Febrile responses of rats to interleukin-1β, injected by three different routes. FASEB J 5:A1402, 1991.
20. Stitt JT, Shimada SG: Calcium channel blockers inhibit endogenous pyrogen fever in rats and rabbits. J Appl Physiol 71:951, 1991.
21. Blatteis CM, Xin L, Ungar AL, et al: Blockade of fever by intrapreoptically administered substance P but not indomethacin. Soc Neurosci Abstr 17:836, 1991.
22. Murakami N, Sakata Y, Watanabe T: Central action sites of interleukin-1β for inducing fever in rabbits. J Physiol 428:299, 1990.
23. Shibata M, Blatteis CM: Neurons in the organum vasculosum laminae terminalis respond to tumor necrosis factor and serotonin in slice preparations. In: Mercer JB (ed): Thermal Physiology, Amsterdam, Elsevier, 1989, p. 413.
24. Kluger MJ: The evolution and adaptive value of fever. Am Sci 66:38, 1978.
25. Bernheim HA, Kluger MJ: Fever: Effect of drug-induced antipyresis on survival. Science 192:237, 1976.
26. Kluger MJ, Vaughn LK: Fever and survival in rabbits infected with *Pasteurella multocida.* J Physiol 282:243, 1978.
27. Grieger TA, Kluger MJ: Fever and survival: the role of serum iron. J Physiol 279:187, 1978.
28. Beisel WR, Goldman RF, Joy RJT: Metabolic balance studies during induced hyperthermia in man. J Appl Physiol 24:1, 1968.
29. Liljedahl SO, Birke G: The nutrition of patients with extensive burns. Nutr Metab 14(Suppl):110, 1972.
30. Myers RD, Tytell M: Fever: Reciprocal shift in brain sodium to calcium ratio as the set-point temperature rises. Science 178:765, 1972.
31. Lomax P: Drugs and body temperature. Int Rev Neurobiol 12:1, 1970.
32. Moyer CA, Nissan S: Alterations in the basal oxygen consumptions of rats attendant upon three types of dehydration. Ann Surg 154:51, 1961.
33. Nissan S, Aviram A, Czaczkes JW, et al: Increased O_2 consumption of the rat diaphragm by elevated NaCl concentrations. Am J Physiol 210:1222, 1966.
34. Freinkel N, Arky RA, Singer DL, et al: Alcohol hypoglycemia. IV. Current concepts of its pathogenesis. Diabetes 14:350, 1965.
35. Wilmore DW, Mason AD Jr, Pruitt BA Jr: Impaired glucose flow in burned patients with gram negative sepsis. Surg Gynecol Obstet 143:720, 1976.

Metabolic Response to Infection

CHAPTER 20

Wiley W. Souba

Under normal circumstances bacteria and other microorganisms live within the body in a symbiotic manner, but following injury or during immunocompromised states these organisms can invade the body. A set of orchestrated responses are subsequently set into motion, which are designed to defend the host. The metabolic responses will be reviewed in this chapter. Sepsis involves a number of changes in protein, fat, and glucose metabolism, and these changes are regulated in large part by inflammatory cytokines.

GENERAL OVERVIEW OF THE METABOLIC RESPONSE TO INFECTION

The invasion of the body by microorganisms initiates a variety of host responses. Phagocytes are mobilized, inflammatory responses are set into motion at the site of invasion, and host immunologic mechanisms are activated. If the infection progresses, fever, tachycardia, malaise, anorexia, and other systemic responses are observed. These more generalized reactions can be categorized into those related to the host's immunologic defenses and into those related to the body's general metabolic and circulatory adjustments to the infection. The predominant alterations in host defense mechanisms include fever, leukocytosis, changes in acute-phase protein synthesis, and activation of a variety of immunologic reactions. The changes in metabolism relate to alterations in glucose, nitrogen, and fat metabolism, as well as those involving the redistribution of trace metals. Several general characteristics describe the systemic events that occur after infection: (1) the responses appear stereotyped and can be produced after administering many microorganisms or their toxins, indicating that common mediators are involved; (2) the magnitude of the responses is proportional to the extent and duration of the infection; (3) although the systemic responses to infection are stereotyped, these processes are modulated by the physiologic reserves of the individual, with the magnitude of the responses to infection depending in part on the patient's age and sex, nutritional status, and associated disease processes, and (4) as the infection progresses, additional functional limitations may be imposed on one or more specific organs, which may further impair the host systemic response.

The time course of metabolic and immunologic responses during the course of a typical febrile illness have been described.[1] Phagocytic activity is an early response that occurs shortly after the moment of exposure to the pathogen. The febrile period is the hallmark of systemic effects. With the onset of fever, negative nitrogen balance, accelerated losses of potassium, phosphate, and magnesium, and retention of salt and water are characteristic. Associated with the losses of certain elements from the body is an internal redistribution of specific macronutrients and trace metals. On resolution of the sepsis, a spontaneous diuresis is characteristic and a return to positive nitrogen and carbon balance is observed.

Systemic Metabolic Responses to Infection

Many of the metabolic responses to infection are similar to those observed following injury. Hence investigators have speculated that a final common pathway may apply to all catabolic states. It is likely that cytokines, complex polypeptide proteins elaborated in increased amounts in the patient with injury and/or infection, mediate the majority of the metabolic changes that develop during infection. Severe infection is characterized by persistent fever, hypermetabolism, diminished protein economy, altered glucose dynamics, and accelerated lipolysis. Anorexia is commonly associated with systemic infection and contributes to the loss of body mass.

Hypermetabolism. Oxygen consumption is usually elevated in the infected patient. The extent of this increase is related to the severity of infection, with peak elevations reaching approximately 50 percent above normal.[2] Such increases often occur in the postoperative and postinjury periods in response to severe pneumonia, intra-abdominal infection, or wound dehiscence. If the patient's metabolic rate is already elevated to a maximal extent because of severe injury, no further increase will be observed.[3] As a general rule, the hypermetabolism persists until the infection is adequately treated or controlled. In some infected patients, a diminished oxygen consumption is observed and this is usually associated with a poor outcome.

Altered Glucose Dynamics. Blood glucose levels are generally elevated in the infected patient, but the descriptive term *diabetes of infection* is inappropriate because plasma insulin concentrations are usually normal or elevated in previously healthy individuals who develop infection.[4] The elevated glucose production that develops in infected individuals appears to be additive with the augmented gluconeogenesis that occurs in noninfected injured patients.[5] For example, uninfected burn patients have an accelerated glucose production rate approximately 50 percent above normal; with the onset of bacteremia in similar individuals, hepatic glucose production increases to twice basal levels. Profound hypoglycemia and diminished hepatic glucose production have also been described in both animals and human patients.[6] This is often associated with more progressive stages of infection and may be related to alterations in splanchnic blood flow.[5]

Alterations in Protein Metabolism. Accelerated net proteolysis, increased nitrogen losses, and prolonged negative nitrogen balance occur following infection, and the response pattern is similar to that described for injury. Although net protein catabolism is accelerated in infected patients,[7] vigorous feeding can stimulate protein synthesis.[8] Amino acid flux from skeletal muscle is accelerated in patients with sepsis,[9] and this flux is matched by accelerated visceral amino acid uptake. In infected burn patients, splanchnic uptake of amino acids is increased 50 percent above rates in uninfected burn patients with injuries of comparable size.[5] These amino acids serve as glucose precursors and are used for synthesis of acute-phase proteins. In addition, acidosis frequently occurs in the patient with sepsis, and this stimulus serves as a signal for accelerated glutamine uptake by the kidney. Glutamine liberates an ammonia ion that combines with a hydrogen ion and is excreted in the urine, thus participating in acid-base homeostasis. Since the glutamine arises from skeletal muscle proteolysis, the acidosis associated with sepsis is yet another stimulus of heightened skeletal muscle breakdown.

During sepsis, amino acids are also released at an accelerated rate by the lungs, a response that is in part glucocorticoid mediated.[10] Like muscle, the majority of the amino acids liberated by the pulmonary bed are in the form of glutamine and alanine, the major vehicles for circulating nitrogen transfer between organs[11] (Figs. 20–1 and 20–2). Simultaneously, the liver exhibits increased amino acid uptake and appears to exceed the importance of the gut as a nitrogen processing station.[12] Accordingly, intestinal amino acid uptake, both from the lumen and from the bloodstream, is diminished. As glutamine is the principal fuel utilized by the small intestinal mucosa, the effects of sepsis on glutamine metabolism by the gastrointestinal tract have been studied in rodents and humans.[13] Despite a slight elevation of arterial glutamine in endotoxemic animals, gut glutamine uptake, extraction, and glutaminase activity were significantly depressed. In septic patients undergoing laparotomy for their primary disease there was a 70 percent reduction in gut glutamine extraction. Mucosal brush border transport of glutamine and several other amino

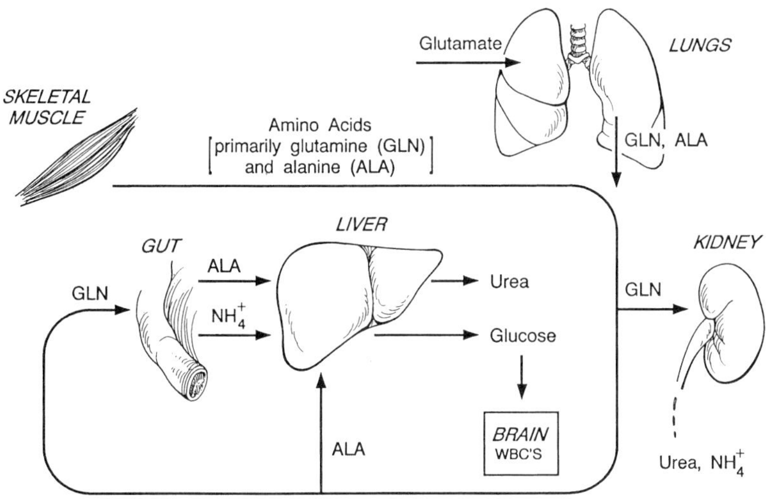

Figure 20–1. The interorgan flow and amino acids in the normal postabsorptive state. Skeletal muscle and the lungs are the principal releasers of amino acids, primarily in the form of glutamine and alanine. Glutamine is utilized by the kidney for ammoniagenesis and by the gut for energy. Alanine is the principal gluconeogenic amino acid utilized by the liver. In the basal state the central nervous system is the major organ of glucose consumption.

acids was also diminished during sepsis.[14] It has been suggested that sepsis and endotoxemia impair gut metabolism of glutamine, which may be related to the breakdown of the gut mucosal barrier and the development of bacterial translocation.

Alterations in Fat Metabolism. Fat is a major fuel oxidized in infected patients, and the increased metabolism of lipids from peripheral fat stores is especially prominent during a period of inadequate nutritional support. While accelerated lipolysis is probably mediated in part by the heightened sympathetic activity that is a potent stimulus for fat mobilization and accelerated oxidation, cytokines also appear to augment fat mobilization. Serum triglyceride levels reflect the balance between rates of triglyceride production by the liver and use and storage by peripheral tissues. Marked hypertriglyceridemia has been associated with gram-negative infection,[15] but plasma triglyceride concentrations may be normal or low. During simple starvation, hepatic uptake of free fatty acids is associated with ketosis, and concentrations of beta-hydroxybutyrate and acetoacetate rise. This change does not occur in infected patients, and it has been hypothesized that the accelerated proteolysis seen during infection is a consequence of this hypoketonemic state. However, when ketones were infused into infected animals the accelerated gluconeogenesis and proteolysis were not diminished, suggesting that the control of metabolism was more complex.[16] Other investigators have suggested that the hypoketonemic state of infection may be a consequence of the hyperinsulinemia associated with catabolic states.[17] Studies in rats and in human patients lend credence to this argument.[18]

Changes in Trace Mineral Metabolism. Changes in the whole-body balance and interorgan flow of magnesium, inorganic phosphate, zinc, and

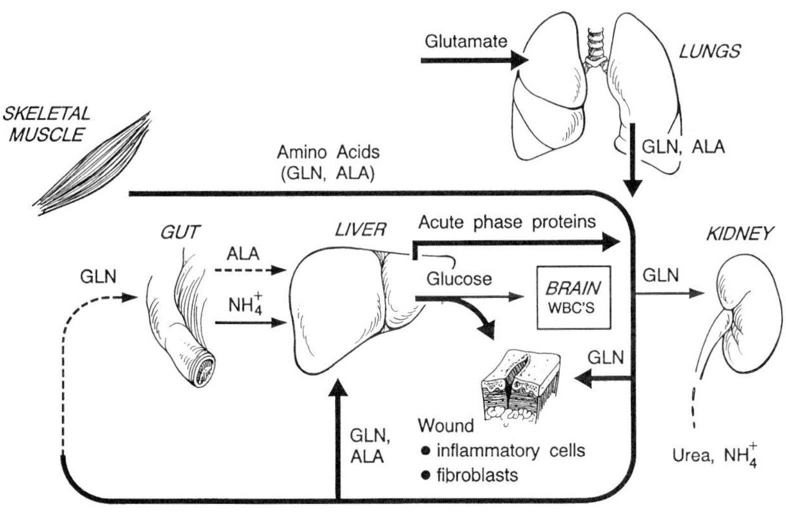

Figure 20–2. During sepsis glutamine and alanine release by muscle and lung are accelerated. The liver becomes the major organ of glutamine uptake at a time when intestinal glutamine utilization diminishes. Enhanced amino acid uptake by the liver supports gluconeogenesis and acute-phase protein synthesis. Inflammatory cells and/or associated wounds are also major consumers of glucose and glutamine. In the long run persistent catabolism leads to the loss of functional protein mass.

potassium are characteristic of sepsis.[19,20] Although the iron-binding capacity of transferrin is usually unchanged in early infection, iron disappears from the plasma, especially during severe pyrogenic infections. Similar alterations are observed with serum zinc levels. Both iron and zinc accumulate within the liver, and this accumulation appears to be another host defense mechanism since these trace metals are required by bacteria for function and their sequestration in the liver prevents their uptake by bacteria. The administration of iron to the infected host, especially early in the disease, is contraindicated because increased serum iron concentrations may impair resistance. Zinc may be required during a prolonged, infective illness because zinc is both sequestered in body tissues and excreted in the urine. Zinc deficiency, however, is not reflected in serum concentrations, which are usually diminished as an initial host response. Unlike iron and zinc, copper levels generally rise, and the increased plasma concentration is due principally to an increase in ceruloplasmin produced by the liver.

Role of Cytokines in Mediating the Metabolic Response to Infection

Cytokines are soluble protein molecules that are synthesized and released by the body's own cells in response to an inflammatory stimulus (see Chap. 14). It is clear that they, in combination with the counter-regulatory hormones, prostaglandins, and other mediators, orchestrate the body's response to infection. Historically, cytokines have been viewed as immune system modulators produced by monocytes and tissue macrophages in response to invading microorganisms. However, they also control the changes in substrate flow and metabolism that are characteristic of systemic infection (Fig. 20–3).

Under normal circumstances, these molecules appear to function as autocrine or paracrine modulators of cellular function, maintaining homeostasis in the microenvironment. Soon after an inflammatory insult, however, these mediators are produced both at the site of injury and by diverse cells throughout the body, generating a wide range of local and systemic effects of which metabolic alterations are an important component. Cytokines exert their biologic activities by binding to specific receptors on the cell membrane. They differ from classic endocrine hormones in that they are produced by a variety of cell types and have the capacity to exert the majority of their tissue effects locally via direct cell-to-cell communications in a paracrine fashion. In addition to specific target tissue effects, cytokines stimulate production of other cytokines, leading to important cascades that amplify, diversify, and regulate the effects of the proximal cytokine.

Cytokines can broadly be classified as tumor necrosis factors, interleukins, interferons, and colony-stimulating factors. Tumor necrosis factor (TNF) has been the most widely studied of the cytokines and is thought to be the most important proximal mediator of the inflammatory response. TNF induces the synthesis of cytokines, such as IL-1,[21,22] IL-6,[23] and interferons,[24] indicating that TNF is a proximal mediator of cytokine cascades. TNF is produced primarily by macrophages, but lymphocytes, natural killer (NK) cells, Kupffer cells, and a number of other cell types have been identified as

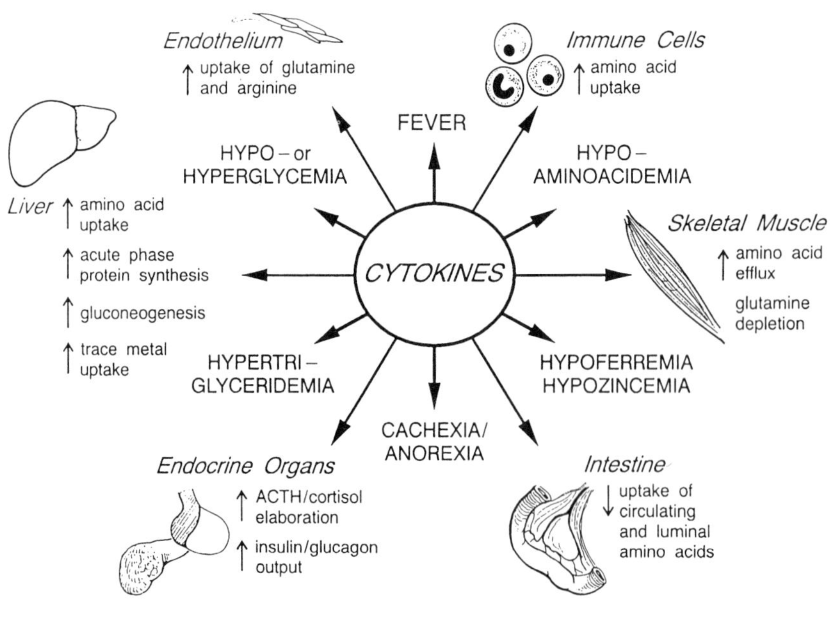

Figure 20–3. Influence of cytokines on interorgan metabolism and nutrition.

possible sources of TNF. The important role that TNF plays as the principal initial signal that mediates the septic response is apparent based on the following criteria.[25]

1. TNF can be detected in the bloodstream shortly after the onset of invasive systemic infection (Fig. 20–4). Although early attempts to detect circulating TNF during sepsis were often unsuccessful, this was due to the use of insensitive assays and the failure to appreciate the temporal nature of TNF secretion after bacterial invasion. It is now appreciated that the circulating TNF signal that appears during sepsis is a short-lived pulse that declines rapidly and is often undetectable when the patient develops symptoms such as tachycardia, fever, and malaise.
2. Administration of TNF to healthy individuals results in physiologic and metabolic abnormalities that are clinically indistinguishable from those that occur during invasive microbial infection.[26] The range of metabolic abnormalities is dose dependent, and the changes in muscle and hepatic amino acid metabolism are similar to those seen during endotoxemia.

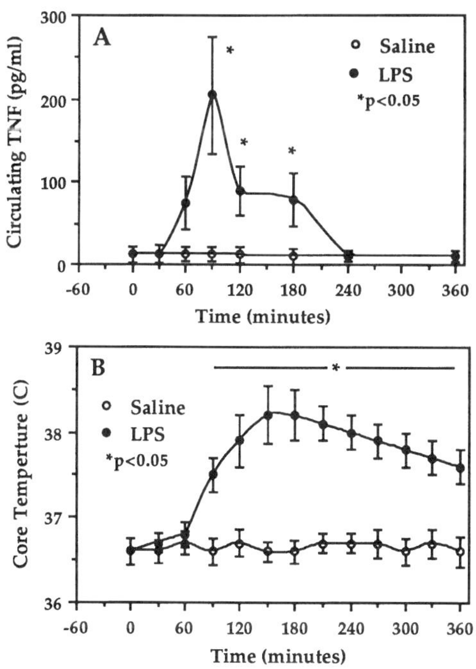

Figure 20–4. Changes in the circulating concentration of tumor necrosis factor (TNF) and in core temperature following endotoxin administration to healthy human volunteers. The increase in TNF levels preceded the development of fever. *$p < 0.05$ versus saline. *(Adapted from Michie et al: N Engl J Med 318:1481, 1988.)*

3. The production and appearance of TNF in the bloodstream of critically ill patients precede that of other known cytokines. Since TNF is known to stimulate the production of many other cytokines, it is possible that it is the most proximal cytokine elaborated in severe infection.
4. Neutralization of TNF with TNF antibodies prevents death following lethal gram-negative bacteremia and attenuates many of the metabolic responses that develop during sepsis.

Like TNF, interleukin 1 (IL-1) is produced by a wide variety of cells, with the monocyte/macrophage probably being the most important source. Endotoxin is the primary stimulus for IL-1 release, but TNF and IL-1 itself can stimulate IL-1 production. Treatment of animals with endotoxin produces an elevation of serum IL-1 levels within 1 hour with peak levels occurring at 2 hours. A single injection of IL-1 in animals results in fever, neutrophilia, increased hepatic acute-phase protein synthesis, anorexia, and release of ACTH, glucocorticoids, and insulin.[27]

Interleukin 6 (IL-6) was originally identified as a B cell differentiation factor that stimulated activated B cells to become mature immunoglobulin-producing plasma cells. IL-6 is now recognized as the primary mediator of altered hepatic protein synthesis known as the acute-phase protein synthetic response.[28,29,30] IL-6 is produced by a number of different cell types, and elevated levels of IL-6 are found in the circulation of patients with bacterial infections and sepsis[31–34] and trauma.[35] Serum IL-6 levels may also correlate with severity of illness in septic patients.

Although cytokines appear to be important determinants of outcome following severe infection, they have not been uniformly measurable in the bloodstream of septic patients. This inability to measure circulating cytokines may be due to several factors: (1) currently available assays may not be sensitive enough to detect low levels of cytokines, (2) cytokines may be elevated only during short periods early on in the course of the illness, and (3) tissue levels of cytokines may be increased without "spillover" into the systemic circulation. Occasionally, when produced in excess, cytokines may act as hormones and spill over into the systemic circulation and become detectable in the bloodstream. Under these circumstances, they may produce harmful systemic responses. It remains unclear why tighter control of these cytokine signals does not exist, and why on the one hand they are apparently life-saving, while on the other they are responsible for the death of the host following overwhelming microbial invasion.

Cytokine Regulation of Energy Metabolism and Nutrient Utilization

When energy intake exceeds energy expenditure a state of positive energy balance exists; weight is gained in the form of fat. When energy expenditure exceeds energy intake, the organism loses body fat and the host is said to be in negative energy balance. Under these latter circumstances, mobilization of host tissue stores (principally skeletal muscle) occurs so that lean body mass is lost as well. Administration of TNF to rodents and humans decreases food intake but the effect appears to be short-lived. In rats treated with chronic injections of TNF, voluntary food intake was markedly reduced for 2 days but had normalized by the sixth day of TNF administration.[36] In patients receiving TNF, food intake was also diminished but nitrogen losses were not accelerated, indicating that the resulting negative nitrogen balance was due to starvation alone. IL-1 also suppresses food intake and its effect, like that of TNF, appears to be a direct effect on the central nervous system. The long-term effects of cytokine administration on body weight have been thought to be due, for the most part, to reductions in food intake (partial starvation) since the degree of weight loss can be reproduced by feeding normal animals similar reduced quantities. In an elegant study by Oliff and colleagues,[37] mice implanted with tumors that secreted TNF showed marked reductions in weight loss compared to animals with non-TNF-secreting tumors. Therefore the effects of TNF on food intake and body composition are unlikely to be due to partial starvation alone, but rather may be due to the ability of TNF to stimulate basal metabolic rate (oxygen consumption).

Fat Metabolism. Altered fat metabolism is clinically apparent in septic patients from the observation that fat stores are diminished in association with weight loss. Similar observations have been made in cytokine-treated rodents. It is apparent that the loss of fat stores is due, in part, to the ability of TNF and IL-1 to mobilize fat stores. Bolus administration of TNF to rats causes an increase in serum triglyceride levels within 2 hours.[38] The increase in circulating triglyceride levels is due primarily to an increase in very low density lipoproteins, which are of normal size and composition. Starnes and colleagues[39] demonstrated a similar increase in plasma triglycerides in humans receiving TNF.

Lipoprotein lipase (LPL) plays an important role in adipocyte metabolism by hydrolyzing circulating triglycerides to fatty acids for subsequent storage as fat in the adipocyte. Accordingly, a reduction of LPL activity contributes to a decrease in total body fat stores. Both IL-6 and TNF reduced heparin-releasable LPL activity in 3T3-L1 adipocytes in a dose-dependent manner by 50 to 70 percent.[40] Incubation of cells with TNF decreased LPL activity by 90 percent. The experiments indicate that both TNF and IL-6 reduce adipocyte LPL activity and may contribute to the loss of body fat stores associated with critical illness. In a similar study, Patton and associates[41] investigated the effects of cytokines on lipid metabolism in 3T3-L1 mouse fibroblasts and adipocytes. Both TNF and interferon gamma. (IFN-γ) inhibited ^{3}H-acetate uptake and LPL activity in adipocytes.

Other investigators[42] have measured free fatty acid and ketone body kinetics in rats. TNF treatment increased the rate of free fatty acid appearance and concentration in the plasma. Despite this increased free fatty acid availability, ketogenesis was impaired after TNF injection, as shown by lower ketone body concentrations and appearance rates (Fig. 20–5). The percentage of free fatty acid flux used for ketogenesis was reduced by TNF. The increase in serum triglyceride levels observed after TNF administration is due not only to a reduction in adipocyte lipoprotein lipase activity, but also to stimulation of hepatic lipid secretion.[43]

Glucose Metabolism. Severe infection causes substantial changes in whole-body and regional glucose metabolism, and many of these alterations are cytokine mediated. It has been difficult to fully characterize the effects of a specific cytokine in vivo because of the multiplicity of other cytokines that are elaborated in response to parenteral administration. The variety of responses in glucose metabolism that are observed in critically ill patients attest to this complex interplay. Studies evaluating the effects of cytokine administration on the circulating glucose concentration indicate that the plasma glucose level will rise or fall depending on the cytokine, the dose administered, and the time of measurement. In rats, sublethal doses of TNF that did not produce hemodynamic changes resulted in the development of hyperglycemia within 1 hour of administration.[38] The increase in plasma glucose was only mild, however (20 percent increase) and was associated with an increase in the circulating concentration of glucagon, ACTH, corticosterone, and epinephrine, all of which can cause hyperglycemia. In contrast, relatively high doses of

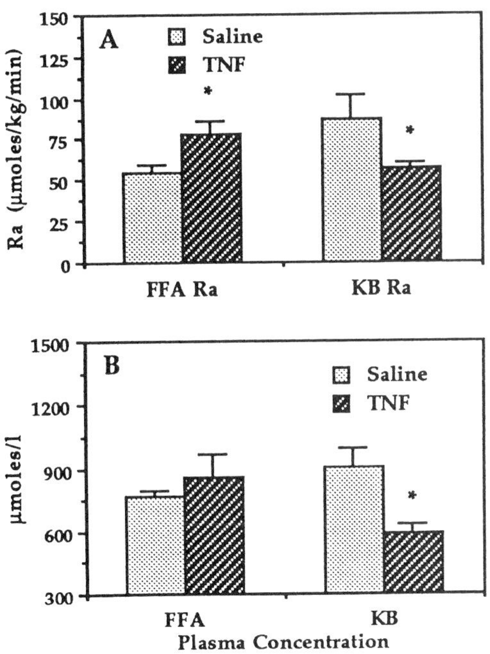

Figure 20–5. Influence of TNF on free fatty acid (FFA) and ketone body (KB) metabolism. Rats received TNF or saline. Six hours later the plasma concentrations **(A)** and plasma rate of appearance **(B)** of FFA and KB were measured. Hepatic FFA production was enhanced while ketogenesis was impaired. $*p < 0.05$ versus control. *(Adapted from Beylot et al: Am J Physiol 263:E897, 1992.)*

TNF infused into cancer patients did not alter the blood glucose concentration. Higher doses of circulating TNF are likely to cause hypoglycemia, although this may not be uniformly observed in septic patients who frequently receive glucose infusions. In dogs receiving a constant infusion of TNF-α, mild hypoglycemia developed.[44]

Similar complex changes in blood glucose levels are observed after IL-1 administration. At higher IL-1 doses, Fischer and colleagues[45] reported a rapid rise in blood glucose from 100 to 140 mg/dl within 1 hour, but this increase was transient with a return to baseline levels by the 2-hour mark. Simultaneously, there was a several-fold increase in hindquarter (most likely skeletal muscle) glucose consumption, which was also transient. In cultured muscle cells (L6 cell line), TNF-α stimulates glucose transport via a mechanism that involves de novo synthesis of glucose transporters, which are inserted into the plasma membrane.[46] Simultaneously, there is depletion of cellular glycogen stores and an increase in lactate efflux, all of which are consistent with stimulation of anaerobic glycolysis.

A characteristic response to systemic infection is accelerated gluconeogenesis, which is in part cytokine mediated. Hepatic gluconeogenesis from alanine is increased following IL-1 treatment.[47] In cultured hepatocytes incubated with cytokines, gluconeogenesis is not appreciably increased, indicating that TNF and IL-1 do not directly stimulate gluconeogenesis in vitro. It is likely that complex interactions between nonparenchymal cells (sinusoidal cells and Kupffer cells) and parenchymal cells (hepatocytes) occur in the liver during sepsis to augment gluconeogenesis. In addition, hormones such as dexamethasone and glucagon are likely to exert direct as well as permissive effects. Tumor necrosis factor stimulates hepatic acid transport in vivo and these precursors are used in part for the synthesis of new glucose. Tissue glucose utilization has been studied in vivo using the 2-deoxyglucose tracer technique in rats following infusion of a nonlethal dose of TNF.[48] Glucose uptake was increased in liver, kidney, spleen, skin, lung, and ileum. The largest increase was observed in diaphragm (150 percent). No significant increase was observed in skeletal muscle, testis, or brain. These data indicate a marked increase in whole-body glucose utilization following TNF administration (Fig. 20–6).

Protein/Amino Acid Metabolism. Marked changes in protein and amino acid metabolism are characteristic of sepsis. Cytokines are thought to mediate many, if not all, of the alterations that develop. Evidence of an important role for cytokines in the metabolic response to catabolic diseases is derived from studies that demonstrate that (1) cytokines are produced in increased amounts in patients with sepsis, (2) administration of cytokines to healthy humans or animals results in metabolic and nutritional derangements similar to those seen during critical illness, and (3) administration of antibodies to the various cytokines can attenuate or abrogate many of these responses.

A number of factors have impeded our ability to fully delineate how cytokines work. First, the production of cytokines generally occurs in a paracrine fashion such that elevated systemic concentrations are not always observed in ill patients. Second, numerous cytokines have now been identified and it is apparent that they network together in a complex manner. While alterations in whole-body metabolism may be apparent after in vivo cytokine administration, it is difficult, if not impossible, to sort out whether the effects are direct or mediated via some secondary or tertiary messenger molecule. Such information can only be obtained from in vitro cell culture studies in which the microenvironment is markedly different from that present in the body.

While it is clear that cytokine treatment causes hypoaminoacidemia (Fig. 20–7), studies evaluating the effects of cytokines on muscle protein metabo-

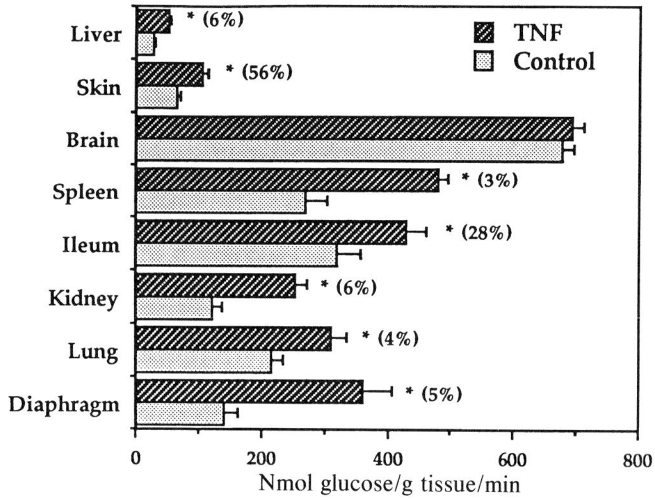

Figure 20–6. Effects of TNF on glucose utilization by different tissues in the rat. Consumption was measured using the 2-deoxyglucose tracer technique. Glucose utilization was increased 80 to 100 percent in spleen, liver, and kidney and by 150 percent in diaphragm. Numbers in parentheses indicate the percent contribution of the respective organ to the total increase in glucose utilization after TNF infusion. *$p < 0.05$ versus control. *(Adapted from Meszaros K, Lang CH, Bagby GJ: Biochem Biophys Res Commun 149:1, 1987.)*

lism are conflicting. When recombinant TNF was infused into cancer patients, forearm amino acid efflux was accelerated, consistent with net skeletal muscle proteolysis.[49] Similarly, when Flores and colleagues[50] infused radiolabeled leucine into rats receiving TNF and/or IL-1 and used tracer methodology techniques, they found an increase in muscle protein degradation in cytokine-treated animals. However, at low doses of TNF, protein breakdown is not stimulated, despite induction of fever.[51] Clowes and colleagues[52] identified a circulating protein factor in the plasma of septic patients, which was named proteolysis-inducing factor. It was suggested that this compound was a breakdown product of IL-1 and was responsible for the increased muscle proteolysis that was characteristic of sepsis.[53] However, when the IL-1 activity in activated monocyte supernatants was blocked with specific IL-1 antibodies, the accelerated protein breakdown was not attenuated, indicating a major role for other mediators. Thus, while it is generally agreed that cytokine administration in vivo (at sufficient doses) stimulates net muscle proteolysis, it is unclear which distal mediators in the cytokine cascade are the key signals.

In contrast to whole-animal studies, the majority of which indicate that in vivo administration of TNF or IL-1 results in net muscle proteolysis, in vitro studies have yielded negative results. Several investigators have incubated different types of skeletal muscles with a variety of cytokines and failed to demonstrate any effect on protein turnover. Goldberg and associates[54] incubated rat diaphragm with partially purified supernatant from stimulated macrophages and noted an increase in protein breakdown. The activity of the preparation was ascribed to IL-1 but it is likely that other cytokine mediators were also present. More recent studies have shown that when the IL-1 activity in activated monocyte preparations is blocked with specific IL-1

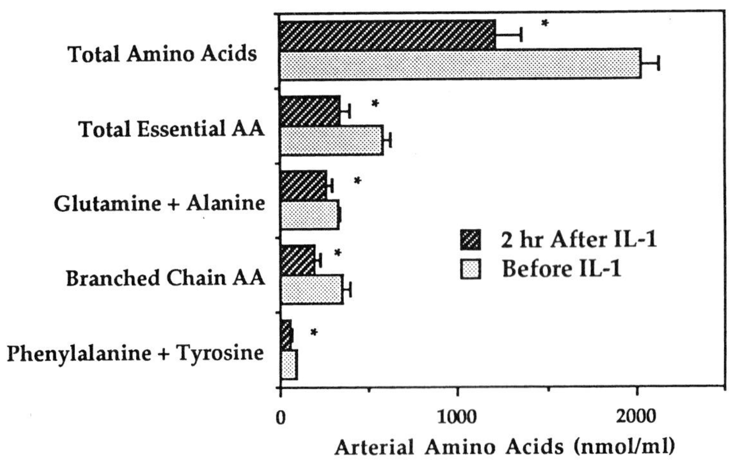

Figure 20–7. Influence of IL-1 administration on circulating amino acid concentrations. Generalized hypoaminoacidemia was observed. *$p < 0.05$ versus before IL-1. *(Adapted from Fischer et al: Am J Physiol 261:R442, 1991.)*

antibodies, the stimulation of protein breakdown was not attenuated, indicating that the proteolysis-inducing factor in crude monocyte preparations was not IL-1. The accelerated protein breakdown may be mediated by other cytokines or by combinations of cytokines that act synergistically or cooperatively. The majority of studies that have examined the effects of cytokines on muscle protein synthesis and degradation have used relatively short incubation times (less than 2 hours), and it may be that longer incubation times are necessary to demonstrate a response.

Other studies[55,56] indicate that secretory products in conditioned medium from cultured macrophages do not accelerate protein degradation. Addition of supernatant from cultured, endotoxin-stimulated rat peritoneal macrophages to incubated rat soleus muscles did not influence protein breakdown, despite the demonstration that IL-1 activity in the supernatants was high. On the other hand, when monocyte secretory products were added to cultured extensor digitorum longus muscles in the presence of fetal calf serum, an increase in protein degradation as measured by the release of tyrosine was observed (Fig. 20–8). Neither TNF nor IL-1

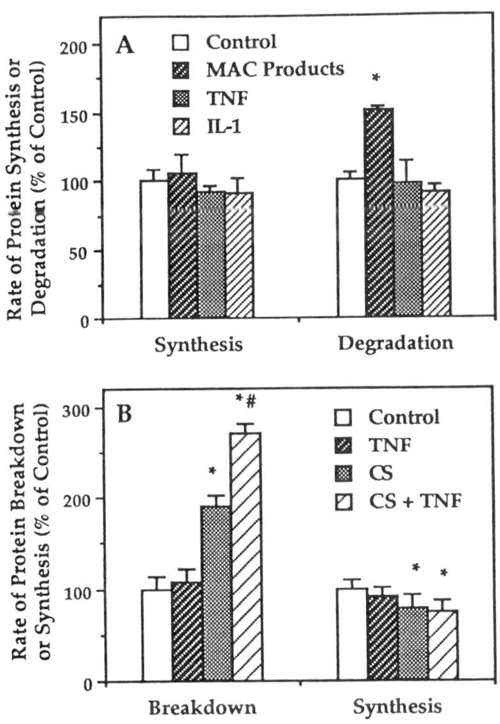

Figure 20–8. Rates of protein synthesis and breakdown in skeletal muscle in vitro incubated with macrophage-stimulated supernatant (MAC products), TNF, or IL-1. $*p < 0.05$ versus control. *(Adapted from Moldawer LL, Svanninger G, Gelin J, et al: Am J Physiol 253:C766, 1987.)*

had an effect on protein breakdown or on muscle amino acid uptake, while conditioned media from macrophages did increase proteolysis and inhibit amino acid transport.[57] In similar studies evaluating the effects of corticosterone on muscle protein breakdown, this glucocorticoid was noted to accelerate protein degradation and diminish protein synthesis. In combination with TNF, these steroid-mediated effects were augmented, but TNF alone did not alter protein turnover.[58]

In vitro and in vivo studies demonstrate that cytokines occupy an important role in mediating the hepatic metabolic response to sepsis. Following treatment with endotoxin, TNF, or IL-1, liver weight increases while muscle mass diminishes. Simultaneously, the expression of genes that control acute-phase protein synthesis is enhanced, a response that is TNF mediated. Administration of endotoxin to healthy animals stimulates a global increase in Na^+-dependent amino acid transport, a response that can be attenuated by pretreatment with a TNF antibody[59] (Souba et al, unpublished data) (Fig. 20–9). Similar observations were made in animals treated with a single dose of TNF. Stimulation of hepatic amino acid transport systems A, ASC, and N was noted within 4 hours of TNF administration.[60] Prior administration to TNF-treated animals with the glucocorticoid antagonist RU 386 diminished the increase in transport activity by approximately 50 percent, indicating that the glucocorticoid hormones play an important role in mediating this response.

Interleukin 6 and glucocorticoids have also been shown to work in a coordinated fashion to stimulate hepatic amino acid transport. Watkins and Souba[61] treated rats with dexamethasone followed 12 hours later by parenteral administration of varying doses of IL-6. Four hours after IL-6 treatment, hepatic plasma membrane vesicles were prepared and the activities of system N and system A were assayed. The investigators noted that IL-6 increased amino acid transport in a dose-dependent fashion. Dexamethasone alone had no effect on system N but enhanced the IL-6 effect. In contrast, dexamethasone increased system A activity but did not augment the IL-6 effect. These data indicate that IL-6 and glucocorticoids stimulate hepatic amino acid transport but their combined effects, be they independent, synergistic, or additive in nature, are different for each transport system.

Interpretation of in vivo studies is difficult because administration of a single cytokine can stimulate the release of glucocorticoids, insulin, glucagon, and other cytokines, all of which can regulate

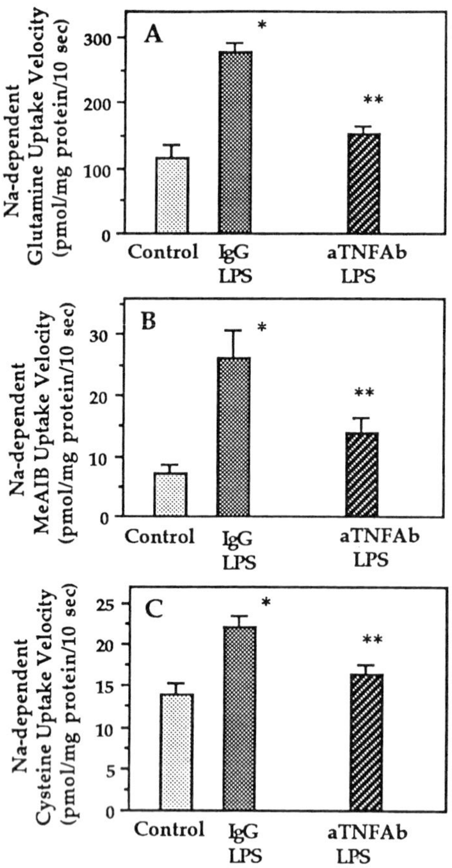

Figure 20–9. Attenuation of the endotoxin-induced increase in hepatic amino acid transport with an anti-TNF antibody (aTNFAb). Rats were pretreated with aTNFAb (4 mg/kg IP) 2 hours prior to receiving *E. coli* LPS (7.5 mg/kg BW). Hepatic plasma membrane vesicles were prepared. TNFAb blocked the transport of glutamine **(A)**, MeAIB **(B)**, and cysteine **(C)** by about 50 percent. Each amino acid is transported primarily by a different Na^+-dependent amino acid carrier, suggesting a global increase in hepatic amino acid transport activity during endotoxemia, which is part TNF mediated. *$p < 0.01$ versus control; **$p < 0.05$ versus both other groups. *(From Souba et al, unpublished data.)*

nitrogen metabolism in the liver. Studies in which cytokines were added to the culture medium of isolated hepatocytes in vitro have demonstrated that LPS (endotoxin), TNF, and IL-1 do not increase amino acid transport activity (Souba et al, unpublished data). IL-6, on the other hand, appears to stimulate hepatocyte glutamine transport after a 4-hour incubation, although the effect is only on the order of 30 percent. Although few cytokines directly stimulate amino acid transport in cultured hepatocytes, combinations of these cytokines do stimulate the acute-phase response, and IL-6 appears to be the most important cytokine in this capacity.

Glutamine

Glutamine occupies a special position in amino acid metabolism because it is the most abundant amino acid in the body and the one that becomes the most depleted in the course of critical illness. The majority of body glutamine stores are present in skeletal muscle, and profound muscle glutamine depletion is characteristic of catabolic diseases such as severe infection. Evidence suggests that the alterations in glutamine metabolism that occur during infection are, in large part, cytokine mediated. While increased circulating levels of these inflammatory mediators are not always detectable in critically ill patients, tissue expression of a variety of cytokine genes is enhanced in catabolic states, consistent with a primary paracrine role for these polypeptides.

When healthy rats were injected with TNF, there was a modest fall in the circulating glutamine concentration but there was no change in muscle glutamine efflux or tissue concentrations.[62] IL-1 treatment, on the other hand, induced a twofold increase in muscle glutamine release and a fall in the concentration of glutamine in muscle. Simultaneously, the activity of glutamine synthetase, the major enzyme of de novo glutamine biosynthesis, was increased by 30 percent. Teleologically, muscle responds to the fall in glutamine stores by increasing endogenous biosynthesis. Apparently the rate of biosynthesis is inadequate to match the rate of efflux, since some degree of glutamine depletion develops. These changes in muscle glutamine metabolism that occur after IL-1 administration are nearly identical to those that develop in endotoxin-treated animals.[63]

Cytokines also appear to play a key role in regulating glutamine utilization in the liver. Na^+-dependent glutamine transport in the liver of endotoxin-treated[64] rats is enhanced, and this response can be attenuated by pretreatment with a TNF antibody (Souba et al, unpublished data) (see Fig. 20–9). Predictably, administration of TNF to normal rats increases Na^+-dependent hepatic glutamine transport but does not alter Na^+-independent glutamine (efflux) transport.[60] The increase in glutamine transport was not due to an increase in carrier affinity but instead was due to an increase in maximal transport velocity. IL-1 also increases hepatic glutamine transport activity in vivo (Souba et al, unpublished data) as does IL-6.[61] As mentioned earlier, only IL-6 augments hepatocyte glutamine transport in vitro and the effect is modest. Glucocorticoids exert a permissive effect on this transport activity, possibly by increasing the expression of IL-6 receptors on the surface of the hepatocyte.

Cytokines also control the utilization of glutamine by the intestinal tract. Gut uptake of circulating glutamine is diminished in septic patients and in endotoxemic rats, and this is associated with a fall in mucosal glutaminase activity and the development of gram-negative bacteremia.[13] Interleukin 1 treatment also diminishes intestinal uptake of circulating glutamine,[64] while lymphocyte glutaminase activity in mesenteric lymph nodes is increased in septic rats.[65] In cultured Caco-2 cells, IFN-γ decreases glutamine transport across the brush border, while TNF and IL-1 do not alter transport.[66] In contrast, glutamine utilization is tenfold greater in proliferating lymphocytes as compared to resting cells.[67] Thus the reduced gut uptake of glutamine that occurs during sepsis may occur primarily in the mucosal cells, as opposed to lymphatic tissues that may actually consume more glutamine during stress states.

Glutaminase, the principal enzyme of glutamine hydrolysis, breaks down glutamine to supply energy and intermediates for cell growth. It is present in high concentrations in replicating tissues such as intestinal epithelium and malignant tumors. Sarantos and associates[69] investigated the influence of cytokines on mucosal glutaminase activity. Following a 12-hour incubation, glutaminase-specific activity and kinetic parameters (V_{max} and K_m) were determined. Glutaminase protein concentration was determined by Western blot analysis using a rabbit anti-rat polyclonal antibody. Total cellular RNA was extracted for Northern hybridization and radiolabeled with a glutaminase cDNA probe. Of the cytokines studied, only IFN-γ altered glutaminase activity. Kinetic studies indicated a decrease in activity secondary to a 25 percent decrease in V_{max} with no change in K_m, consistent with a reduction in the number of glutaminase molecules rather than a change in enzyme affinity. Glutaminase protein was decreased 50 percent in IFN-γ-treated cells when compared to controls. This decrease was dose independent and was associated with a concomitant 75 percent decrease in glutaminase mRNA levels. These reductions in message and protein translated into a 60 to 80 percent decrease in functional glutaminase-specific activity. This IFN-mediated decrease in glutaminase activity may be one mechanism by which gut glutamine metabolism is diminished as the tumor grows.

Like the hindquarter, lung glutamine release is also accelerated during sepsis, but the response is temporally different from that for muscle. Soon after an intravenous bolus of endotoxin, net lung glutamine efflux is increased but this augmented output is short-lived. These temporal observations have been made in rats[70] and in patients.[11] The accelerated release of glutamine from the lungs was limited to the time period directly after the onset of sepsis. The subsequent development of pulmonary edema in rats and the adult respiratory distress syndrome in patients resulted in elimination of this augmented response. The apparent reversion to net glutamine balance may be due to a simultaneous increase in glutamine uptake by pulmonary endothelial cells. Both endotoxin[71] and the cytokines TNF and IL-1[72] increase glutamine transport by the lung endothelium.

Despite these dramatic changes in interorgan exchange rates, the blood glutamine level remains fairly constant. Under these circumstances, the liver becomes the major glutamine consumer in the body,[12] exceeding gut glutamine uptake threefold. Hepatic glutamine uptake increases tenfold following endotoxin treatment secondary to increases in hepatic blood flow, in intracellular metabolism, and in transhepatocellular membrane transport. Inoue and colleagues[64] have examined the effects of endotoxin on glutamine transport activity (system N) in rat hepatic plasma membrane vesicles (HPMVs) from rats treated with *Escherichia coli* endotoxin in vivo. Endotoxemia resulted in a time-dependent two- to threefold increase in Na^+-dependent glutamine transport activity in HPMVs secondary to an increase in the transport V_{max}, consistent with the appearance of increased numbers of corresponding transporter proteins in the hepatocyte plasma membrane. Maximal increases in transport were observed 4 hours after exposure to endotoxin. This increase in transport activity represents an important mechanism underlying the accelerated hepatic amino acid uptake that occurs during critical illness.

Much like endotoxin, treatment of rats with TNF-α, IL-1, or IL-6 causes an increase in glutamine transport in the liver within 2 to 4 hours of administering the cytokine (Fig. 20–10). Pacitti and co-workers[60] investigated the activity of Na^+-dependent transport system N in HPMVs prepared from rats treated with TNF in vivo. TNF did not alter sodium uptake but resulted in time- and dose-dependent 50 percent maximal increases in system N activity, secondary to an increase in the transport V_{max}. Like endotoxin treatment, maximal increases in transport were observed 4 hours after exposure to TNF and had returned to basal levels within 24 hours. Incubation of HPMVs from normal rats in vitro with TNF did not alter transport activity, indicating that TNF-induced stimulation of glutamine uptake is not an event mediated by a direct action of TNF at the membrane surface (ie, cluster-

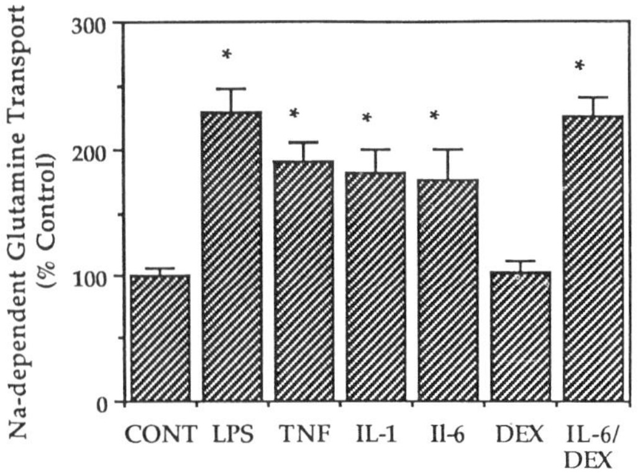

Figure 20–10. Effects of endotoxin and cytokines on hepatic glutamine transport. Glutamine transport was assayed in hepatic plasma membrane vesicles prepared from livers of animals treated with the indicated agents. $^*p < 0.01$ versus control. *(Data from refs. 59, 60, and 63.)*

ing of membrane proteins, changes in fluidity characteristics). The investigators showed that the marked increase in system N transport activity stimulated by TNF is mediated, in part, by the glucocorticoid hormones. Consistent with these results are studies by Gebhardt and Kleeman[73] that demonstrate that dexamethasone stimulates hepatocyte glutamine transport in vitro.

These investigations indicate that inflammatory-mediated increases in the activity of hepatic system N may play a major role in redirecting glutamine flow during sepsis and support glutamine-utilizing processes in the liver. However, it is not possible from these aforementioned in vivo studies to distinguish between direct and indirect effects of endotoxin or cytokines. In contrast to the in vivo results discussed earlier, incubation of hepatocytes from normal animals with endotoxin, TNF, or IL-1 does not alter Na^+-dependent amino acid transport (Dudrick and Souba, unpublished data), indicating that these mediators work through (or with) another mediator(s). IL-6, on the other hand, does increase system N activity by about 30 percent in cultured hepatocytes, a response that is accentuated when dexamethasone is added to the medium. It has been well established that endotoxin stimulates the release of multiple cytokines, which regulate metabolic responses via complex interrelationships with one another and with the classic endocrine hormones.

Previous studies in other cells have shown that endotoxin and cytokines modulate glutamine transport. For example, endotoxin,[71] TNF, and IL-1[72] stimulate glutamine uptake by endothelial cells, while high doses of TNF diminish glutamine transport in fibroblasts.[74] Here again we see that the effects of cytokines, whether direct or indirect, are diverse and tissue specific. This is in keeping with the concept that the body responds to prevailing metabolic pressures to redirect the flow of glutamine during critical illnesses and this is often accomplished at the plasma membrane level. It appears that hepatocytes, lymphocytes, and endothelial cells rank high on the body's list of cells that must have adequate amounts of glutamine after a septic insult. With time, requirements outstrip the body's ability to produce glutamine, and tissue and plasma levels fall.

The alterations in interorgan glutamine flow that occur following severe infection are profound and often of significant duration, depending on the magnitude and severity of the illness. Only when the disease process resolves or is effectively treated does glutamine homeostasis return to normal, assuming no permanent organ damage was sustained. The changes in organ flux that occur during critical illness may be affected by the prior nutritional status of the patient as well as the presence of other abnormalities such as metabolic acidosis. Nonetheless, many of the adaptive changes in glutamine metabolism that take place are mediated directly or indirectly by the glucocorticoid hormones, by endotoxin, by tumor necrosis factor, and by the interleukins.

Arginine

Considerable attention has also focused on the role of cytokines in the regulation of the metabolism of the amino acid arginine during critical illnesses. Arginine's significance in overall nitrogen metabolism is underscored by its key position as an intermediate in the urea cycle and its importance in amino acid biosynthesis. In addition, arginine is a precursor of creatine and polyamine biosynthesis. More recently, interest in arginine metabolism has increased due to its exclusive role as the precursor in nitric oxide (NO) biosynthesis. First identified in vascular endothelial cells,[75] NO production has been demonstrated in a variety of cell types including hepatocytes. NO is a potent, short-lived, bioregulatory molecule produced by a variety of cell types and thought to be a common final mediator of a host of physiologic and pathophysiologic responses. NO plays an important role in smooth muscle relaxation and platelet aggregation, and it may exert a protective effect on the hepatocellular damage associated with sepsis. NO production by several cell types is markedly stimulated by endotoxin and cytokines. The source of arginine precursor to support this sepsis-related NO synthesis is unclear.

The transport of arginine across the plasma membrane into the cytoplasm is mediated primarily by the Na^+-independent cationic amino acid transport system y^+.[76] System y^+ is likely to be a family of related proteins with different kinetic parameters, each isoform mediating arginine transport to a greater or lesser extent. Some of these carriers appear to be inducible by endotoxin and cytokines, and they appear to be structurally similar to NO synthase. In human liver, classic NO synthase inhibitors can also block arginine transport across the hepatocyte plasma membrane.[77] In the hepatocyte, the availability of the extracellular arginine pool to the hepatocyte is restricted to a large degree as a result of this low plasma membrane transport activity, which forms a kinetic barrier between extracellular arginine and the cytoplasmic space. In vivo studies have demonstrated that a single injection of TNF results in a stimulation of saturable, Na^+-independent, system y^+-mediated arginine transport activity in the liver in a time- and dose-dependent fashion.[78] Kinetic analysis of the TNF-induced stimulation of hepatic arginine transport revealed that the increase was due to a 78 percent increase in the V_{max}, or maximal transport velocity, with no alteration of transport affinity. Whether TNF stimulates system y^+-mediated transport directly or indirectly was unclear from this study. Future studies are necessary to further examine the actions and interactions of classic hormones and cytokines to delineate the precise mechanism whereby TNF stimulates system y^+. During sepsis, TNF-induced stimulation of hepatic arginine transport would serve to provide additional arginine precursor for polyamine production, in support of the sepsis-related acceleration of hepatic biosynthetic activity.

In some cultured cells, cytokines stimulate arginine transport directly. Sato and colleagues[79] demonstrated that system y^+ activity in mouse peritoneal macrophages was increased tenfold by endotoxin. Greene and colleagues[80] characterized arginine transport by pulmonary artery endothelial cells and demonstrated that it was mediated primarily by system y^+ and by the Na^+-dependent system $B^{o,+}$. Subsequent studies by this group demonstrated that system y^+ activity was enhanced in a dose-dependent fashion by *E. coli* endotoxin[81] (Fig. 20–11). When endotoxin was added to the endothelial cells in the presence of an anti-TNF antibody or in the presence of an IL-1 receptor antagonist, arginine transport was attenuated. TNF, IL-1, IL-6, and IFN-γ each stimulated arginine transport alone. These cytokines stimulated both system y^+ and system $B^{o,+}$ (Lind and Souba, unpublished data).

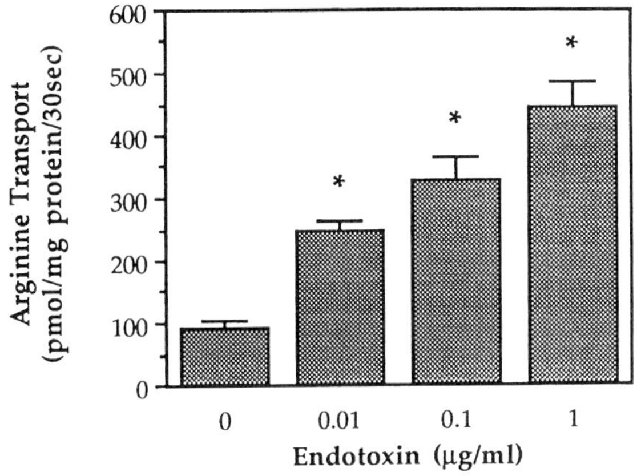

Figure 20–11. Effect of endotoxin on endothelial arginine transport. *(Data from ref. 80.)*

These studies and others suggest a relationship between arginine availability and NO production by several cell types. Nitrite formation is dependent on the extracellular arginine concentration and is stimulated by endotoxin and cytokines.[82] Further studies are necessary to delineate that precise role of plasma membrane arginine transport in regulating NO synthesis.

Summary of the Beneficial Metabolic Effects of Cytokines

Several studies indicate that cytokines, when produced in excess, are damaging to the host, leading to organ dysfunction and possibly death. If cytokines have detrimental effects, why do they exist? Why should the TNF gene be so strongly conserved if excessive production of the TNF protein results in hemodynamic manifestations of septic shock and death? The most likely and logical answer proposes that the genes that regulate cytokine biosynthesis are conserved because they exert effects that confer a survival advantage during infection and cancer. In general, cytokines exert a number of beneficial effects under the majority of circumstances, which appear to outweigh the detrimental effects that predominate in extreme pathophysiologic states. These helpful responses include the following.

Alterations in Substrate Flow and Regional Metabolism. Cytokines play a central role in coordinating the nutritional/metabolic response to critical illnesses. They act in conjunction with other mediators to promote mobilization of amino acids from skeletal muscle and fatty acids from adipose stores. These precursors support energy requirements in other tissues and support the acute-phase protein response in the liver. These responses also provide key nutrients to support cellular metabolism at a time when the animal generally cannot acquire food because of the associated immobility and anorexia. Both TNF and IL-1 have been demonstrated to promote proteolysis in skeletal muscle with release of amino acids. Concurrently, hepatic uptake of amino acids is increased by cytokines. The alterations in fat metabolism produced primarily by TNF result in the hyperlipidemia seen in sepsis.

Serum iron and zinc levels are also reduced in septic patients, an event that is cytokine mediated. The decrease in serum iron is probably important in protecting the host against various bacteria. The reduction of iron can inhibit the growth rate of both microorganisms and tumor cells that have a strict requirement for iron as a growth factor. Both TNF and IL-1 have been shown to mediate hypoferremia, hypozincemia, and other alterations in trace element metabolism. There is redistribution of zinc toward bone marrow and liver.

Acute-Phase Protein Synthesis. Cytokines, particularly TNF, IL-1, and IL-6, are the primary regulators of the hepatic acute-phase protein synthetic response, with augmentation by glucocorticoids.[83] Early observations on the effects of TNF and IL-1 on hepatic protein synthesis demonstrated a stimulation of protein synthesis and subsequent elevation in the elaboration of the acute-phase proteins. Recent data, however, have shown that TNF and IL-1 induce only a limited effect on liver gene expression in isolated hepatocyte cultures. IL-6 is now recognized as the cytokine primarily responsible for the alteration in hepatic protein synthesis recognized as the acute-phase response.

The primary metabolic component of the acute-phase response is a qualitative alteration in hepatic protein synthesis with a resulting alteration in plasma protein composition. Characteristically, proteins that serve as ubiquitous serum transport and binding molecules (albumin, transferrin) are reduced in quantity, and proteins that function to combat effects of injury and infection (fibrinogen, C-reactive protein, etc) are increased. Acute-phase proteins are elaborated, in part, for the purpose of reducing the systemic effects of tissue damage. While the true physiologic role of many of the acute-phase proteins remains unclear, many act as antiproteases, opsonins, or coagulation and wound-healing factors, and they likely inhibit the generalized tissue destruction that is associated with the local initiation of inflammation. For example, increases in fibrinogen and other clotting factors enhance thrombus formation, antiproteases reduce tissue damage caused by proteases released by dead or dying cells, hemopexin and haptoglobin bind heme and hemoglobin, respectively, released by erythrocyte lysis, and C-reactive protein has been hypothesized to have a scavenger function. This highly conserved hepatic response confers significant survival advantage in states of severe inflammation and sepsis.

Fever/Subjective Discomfort. Fever is the systemic response to invading microorganisms and their toxins and is elicited by changes in the microenvironment of the anterior hypothalamus. Specifically, induction of PGE_2 in the anterior hypothalamus raises the endogenous temperature setpoint and drives heat conservation mechanisms and heat-generating processes until blood and core temperatures match the setpoint.[84] This is classically described as a negative feedback loop. Fever has both beneficial and detrimental effects on the host, but it is generally believed that the generation of fever by endogenously produced substances has adaptive value and imparts a survival advantage on the host.[85] IL-1 initiates fever by increasing production of prostaglandins (primarily PGE_2) in the anterior hypothalamus. TNF also acts as an endogenous pyrogen, stimulating both the synthesis of PGE_2 in the anterior hypothalamus and the production of IL-1. Other cytokines, such as IL-2, IL-6, and the interferons, have been identified as endogenous pyrogens; however, either their effects are not as prominent as IL-1 and TNF or their pyrogenic mechanisms remain to be clearly defined.

Fever induced by the injection of cytokines in humans is associated with symptoms of malaise, myalgias, headaches, and joint pain. Thus cytokinemia can be implicated in the generation of the sick syndrome, which accompanies inflammatory states. These constitutional symptoms are likely to be beneficial since they encourage the "sick" animal to seek shelter, safety, and rest and to avoid additional stressful situations. Energy is conserved, and muscle switches from its role as an organ of locomotion to one that provides nitrogen in the form of amino acids to other tissues. A quiescent state is achieved with all efforts focused on combating the inflammatory process, healing the wound, and restoring homeostasis.

Localization of the Inflammatory Site. Events that are important in the localization or containment of tissue injury include vasodilation and increased capillary permeability, migration of neutrophils and monocytes to the wound and subsequent activation of these cells, initiation of the coagulation cascade (which involves proteins produced in the liver as part of the acute-phase response), activation of the immune system, and proliferation of fibroblasts in later stages of wound healing. These effects function to confine the insult as much as possible and activate defense mechanisms to minimize adverse systemic effects, such as cardiovascular collapse and subsequent organ failure. Cytokines are involved in all these functions. The wound becomes an organ of cytokine production in which local metabolism is controlled in part by cytokines. In addition, cytokines released into the circulation act as hormones on other organs such as the bone marrow, skeletal muscle, liver, and CNS. It has been suggested that vigorous resuscitation of septic patients may "wash" cytokines out of the wound and, on occasion, convert a local insult to a systemic one.

SUMMARY

Cytokines impact whole-body nutrition and metabolism. They are responsible for many of the clinically observed nutritional and metabolic effects of infection including fever, hypermetabolism, anorexia, protein catabolism, cachexia, and altered fat, glucose, and trace mineral metabolism. These nutritional/metabolic effects of cytokines are influenced by the nutritional status of the host, which is generally altered during the course of the critical illness. In the future, the use of specialized diets and the use of selective cytokine blockades are likely to be important components of the overall care of the catabolic patient.

REFERENCES

1. Beisel WR: Metabolic response to infection. Annu Rev Med 26:9, 1975.
2. Wilmore DW: The Metabolic Management of the Critically Ill. New York, Plenum Medical Book, 1977.
3. Wilmore DW, Goodwin CW, Audlick LH, et al: Effect of injury and infection on visceral metabolism and circulation. Ann Surg 192:491, 1980.
4. Gump FE, Long C, Killian P, et al: Studies on glucose intolerance in septic injured patients. J Trauma 14:378, 1974.
5. LaNoue KF, Mason AD, Daniels JP: The impairment of glucogenes by gram negative infections. Metabolism 17:606, 1968.
6. McFadzean AJS, Yeung RTT: Hypoglycaemia in suppurative pancholangitis due to *Clonorchis sinesis.* Trans R Soc Trop Med Hyg 59:179, 1965.
7. Long CL, Jeevanandam M, Kim BM, et al: Whole body protein synthesis and catabolism in septic man. Am J Clin Nutr 30:1340, 1977.
8. Herrmann VM, Clark D, Wilmore DW, et al: Protein metabolism: effect of disease and altered intake on the stable ^{15}N curve. Surg Forum 31:92, 1980.
9. Duff JH, Viidik T, Marchuk JB, et al: Femoral arteriovenous amino acid differences in septic patients. Surgery 85:344, 1979.
10. Sarantos PR, Howard D, Souba WW: Dexamethasone regulates glutamine synthetase expression in rat lung. Metabolism 42:795, 1993.
11. Plumley DA, Souba WW, Hautamaki RD, et al: Accelerated lung amino acid release in hyperdynamic septic surgical patients. Arch Surg 125:57, 1990.
12. Austgen TR, Salloum RM, Flynn TC, et al: The effects of endotoxin on splanchnic metabolism of glutamine and related substrates in vivo. J Trauma 31:742, 1991.
13. Souba WW, Herskowitz K, Klimberg VS, et al: The effects of sepsis and endotoxemia on gut glutamine metabolism. Ann Surg 211(5):543, 1990.
14. Salloum RM, Copeland EM III, Souba WW, et al: Brush border transport of glutamine and other substrates during sepsis and endotoxemia. Ann Surg 213:401, 1991.
15. Gallin JI, Kaye D, O'Leary WM: Serum lipids in infection. N Engl J Med 281:1081, 1969.
16. Radcliffe AG, Wolfe RR, Colpoys MF, et al: Ketone-glucose interaction in fed, fasted, and fasted-infected sheep. Am J Physiol 244:R667, 1983.
17. Neufeld HA, Kaminski MV, Wannemacher RW: Effect of inflammatory and noninflammatory stress on ketone bodies. Am J Clin Nutr 30:1357, 1977.
18. Watters JM, Wilmore DW: Role of catabolic hormones in the hypoketonaemia of injury. Br J Surg 73:108, 1986.
19. Huber KL, Cousins RJ: Maternal zinc deprivation and interleukin-1 influence on metallothionein gene expression and zinc metabolism of rats. J Nutr 118:1570, 1988.
20. Helyar L, Sherman AR: Iron deficiency and interleukin 1 production by rat leukocytes. Am J Clin Nutr 46:346, 1987.
21. Dinarello CA, Cannon JG, Wolff SM, et al: Tumor necrosis factor (cachectin) is an endogenous pyrogen and induces production of interleukin 1. J Exp Med 163:1433, 1986.
22. Libby P, Ordovas JM, Auger KR, et al: Endotoxin and tumor necrosis factor induce interleukin-1 gene expression in adult human vascular endothelial cells. Am J Pathol 124:179, 1986.
23. Akira S, Hirano T, Taga T, Kishimoto T: Biology of multifunctional cytokines: IL 6 and related molecules (IL 1 and TNF). FASEB J 4:2860, 1990.
24. Wherry JC, Schreiber RD, Unanue ER: Regulation of gamma interferon production by natural killer cells in SCID mice: roles of tumor necrosis factor and bacterial stimuli. Infect Immunol 59:1709, 1991.

25. Michie H, Wilmore DW: Sepsis and tumor necrosis factor; bedfellows that cannot be ignored (editorial). Arch Surg 125:653, 1990.
26. Michie HR, Manogue KR, Spriggs DR, et al: Detection of circulating tumor necrosis factor after endotoxin administration. N Engl J Med 318:1481, 1988.
27. Dinarello CA: Interleukin-1 and interleukin-1 antagonism. Blood 8:1627, 1991.
28. Gauldie J, Richards C, Harnish D, et al: Interferon $\beta 2$/B-cell stimulatory factor type 2 shares identity with monocyte-derived hepatocyte-stimulating factor and regulates the major acute phase protein response in liver cells. Proc Natl Acad Sci USA 84:7251, 1987.
29. Castell JV, Gomez-Lechon MJ, David M, et al: Interleukin-6 is the major regulator of acute phase protein synthesis in adult human hepatocytes. FEBS Lett 242:237, 1989.
30. Castell JV, Gomez-Lechon MJ, David M, et al: Acute-phase response of human hepatocytes: regulation of acute-phase protein synthesis by interleukin-6. Hepatology 12:1179, 1990.
31. Hack E, DeGroot E, Felt-Bersma R, et al: Increased plasma levels of interleukin 6 in sepsis. Blood 74:1704, 1989.
32. Damas P, Ledoux D, Nys M, et al: Cytokine serum level during severe sepsis in human IL-6 as a marker of severity. Ann Surg 215:356, 1992.
33. Ertel W, Morrison MH, Wang P, et al: The complex pattern of cytokines in sepsis: association between prostaglandins, cachectin, and interleukins. Ann Surg 214:141, 1991.
34. Starnes HF, Pearce MK, Tewari A, et al: Anti-IL-6 monoclonal antibodies protect against lethal *Escherichia coli* infection and lethal tumor necrosis factor challenge in mice. J Immunol 145:4185, 1990.
35. Ayala A, Wang P, Ba ZF, et al: Differential alterations in plasma IL-6 and TNF levels after trauma and hemorrhage. Am J Physiol 260:R167, 1991.
36. Michie HR, Sherman ML, Spriggs DR, et al: Chronic TNF infusion causes anorexia but not accelerated nitrogen loss. Ann Surg 209:19, 1989.
37. Oliff A, Defeo-Jones D, Boyer M, et al: Tumors secreting human TNF/cachectin induce cachexia in mice. Cell 50:555, 1987.
38. Darling G, Goldstein DS, Stull R, et al: Tumor necrosis factor: immune endocrine interaction. Surgery 106:1155, 1989.
39. Starnes HF, Warren RS, Jeevanandem M, et al: Tumor necrosis factor and the acute metabolic response to injury in man. J Clin Invest 82:1321, 1988.
40. Grunfeld C, Gulli R, Moser AH, et al: Effect of tumor necrosis factor administration in vivo on lipoprotein lipase activity in various tissues of the rat. J Lipid Res 30:579, 1989.
41. Patton JS, Shepard HM, Wilking H, et al: Interferons and tumor necrosis factors have similar catabolic effects on 3T3 L1 cells. Proc Natl Acad Sci USA 83:8313, 1986.
42. Beylot M, Vidal H, Mithieux G, et al: Inhibition of hepatic ketogenesis by tumor necrosis factor-α in rats. Am J Physiol 263:E897, 1992.
43. Memon RA, Feingold KR, Moser AH, et al: Differential effects of interleukin-1 and tumor necrosis factor on ketogenesis. Am J Physiol 263:E301, 1992.
44. Van Lanschot JJ, Mealy K, Wilmore DW: The effects of tumor necrosis factor on intestinal structure and metabolism. Ann Surg 212:663, 1990.
45. Fischer E, Marano M, Barber AE, et al: Comparison between effects of interleukin-1α administration and sublethal endotoxemia in primates. Am J Physiol 261:R442, 1991.
46. Lee MD, Zentella A, Pekala PH, et al: Effect of endotoxin-induced monokines on glucose metabolism in the muscle cell line L6. Proc Natl Acad Sci USA 84:2590, 1987.
47. Roh MS, Moldawer LL, Ekman LG, et al: Stimulatory effect of interleukin-1 upon hepatic metabolism. Metabolism 35:419, 1986.
48. Meszaros K, Lang CH, Bagby GJ: Tumor necrosis factor increases in vivo glucose utilization of macrophage-rich tissues. Biochem Biophys Res Commun 149:1, 1987.
49. Starnes HF, Warren RS, Jeevanandem M, et al: Tumor necrosis factor and the acute metabolic response to injury in man. J Clin Invest 82:1321, 1988.
50. Flores EA, Bistrian BR, Pomposelli JJ, et al: Infusion of tumor necrosis factor/cachectin promotes muscle catabolism in the rat. J Clin Invest 83:1614, 1989.
51. Kettelhut K, Goldberg AL: Tumor necrosis factor can induce fever in rats without activating protein breakdown in skeletal muscle or lypolysis in adipose tissue. J Clin Invest 81:1383, 1988.
52. Clowes GHA, George BC, Villee CA, et al: Muscle proteolysis induced by a circulating peptide in patients with trauma and sepsis. N Engl J Med 308:545, 1983.
53. Baracos V, Rodemann HP, Dinarello CA, et al: Stimulation of muscle protein degradation and prostaglandin E_2 release by leukocyte pyrogen (interleukin-1). N Engl J Med 308:553, 1983.
54. Goldberg AL, Kettelhut K, Furuno K, et al: Activation of protein breakdown and prostaglandin E_2 production in rat skeletal muscle in fever is signaled by a macrophage product distinct from interleukin-1 or other monokines. J Clin Invest 81:1378, 1988.
55. Hasselgren PO, James JH, Benson DW, et al: Is there a circulating proteolysis-inducing factor during sepsis? Arch Surg 125:510, 1990.
56. Zamir O, Hasselgren PO, vov Allmen D, et al: The effects of interleukin-1 and the glucocorticoid receptor blocker RU38486 on total and myofibrillar protein breakdown in skeletal muscle. J Surg Res 50:579, 1991.
57. Hummel RP, Warner B, Pedersen P, et al: In vitro effects of TNF, IL-1α, and other monokines on skeletal muscle amino acid uptake and protein degradation. Surg Forum 38:13, 1987.
58. Hall-Angeras M, Angeras U, Zamir O, et al. Interaction between corticosterone and tumor necrosis factor stimulated protein breakdown in rat skeletal muscle, similar to sepsis. Surgery 108:460, 1990.

59. Inoue Y, Bode BP, Souba WW: Antibody to TNFα blocks LPS-stimulated hepatic amino acid transport. Surg (in press).
60. Pacitti AJ, Inoue Y, Souba WW: Tumor necrosis factor stimulates Na^+-dependent amino acid uptake in plasma membrane vesicles. J Clin Invest 91:474, 1993.
61. Watkins KT, Dudrick PS, Copeland ES, et al: Interleukin–6 and dexamethasone work coordinately to augment hepatic amino acid transport. J. Trauma 36:523, 1994.
62. Austgen TR, Dudrick PS, Chen MK, et al: Early effects of cytokines on skeletal muscle glutamine metabolism. Surg Forum 42:90, 1991.
63. Austgen TR, Chakrabarti R, Chen MK, et al: Adaptive regulation in skeletal muscle glutamine metabolism in endotoxin-treated rats. J Trauma 32:600, 1992.
64. Inoue Y, Pacetti A, Souba WW: Endotoxin increases hepatic glutamine transport activity. J Surg Res 54:393, 1993.
65. Austgen TR, Chen MK, Dudrick PS, et al: Cytokine regulation of intestinal glutamine utilization. Am J Surg 163:174, 1991.
66. Sarantos P, Ockert K, Souba WW: Endotoxin stimulates lymphocyte glutaminase expression. Arch Surg 128:920, 1993.
67. Souba WW, Copeland EM: Cytokine modulation of brush border glutamine transport in monolayers of human Caco-2 cells. Ann Surg 215:536, 1992.
68. Brand K, Leibold W, Luppa P, et al: Metabolic alterations associated with proliferation of mitogen-activated lymphocytes and of lymphoblastoid cell lines: evaluation of glucose and glutamine metabolism. Immunobiology 173:23, 1986.
69. Sarantos P, Abouhamze, Copeland EM, et al: Interferon-γ decreases glutaminase expression in human intestinal epithelial cells. Ann Surg Oncol (in press).
70. Austgen TA, Chen MK, Salloum RM, et al: Glutamine metabolism by the endotoxin-injured lung. J Trauma 31:1068, 1991.
71. Herskowitz K, Bode BP, Block ER, Souba WW: The effects of endotoxin on glutamine transport by pulmonary artery endothelial cells. J Surg Res 50:356, 1991.
72. Souba WW, Salloum RM, Bode BP, Herskowitz K: Cytokine modulation of glutamine transport by pulmonary artery endothelial cells. Surgery 110:295, 1991.
73. Gebhardt R, Kleeman E: Hormonal regulation of amino acid transport system N in primary cultures of rat hepatocytes. Eur J Biochem 166:339, 1987.
74. Dudrick PS, Bland KI, Copeland EM, et al: Effects of tumor necrosis factor on system-ASC mediated transport by human fibroblasts. J Surg Res 52:347, 1992.
75. Palmer RMJ, Ferrige AG, Moncada S: Nitric oxide release accounts for the biologic activity of endothelium derived relaxing factor. Nature 257:524, 1987.
76. White MF: The transport of cationic amino acids across the plasma membrane of mammalian cells. Biochim Biophys Acta 822:355, 1985.
77. Inoue Y, Bode BP, Li AP, et al: Arginine transport in human liver: characterization and effects of nitric oxide synthase inhibitors. Ann Surg (in press).
78. Pacitti AJ, Copeland E, Souba WW: Stimulation of hepatocyte system y^+-mediated L-arginine transport by an inflammatory agent. Surgery 112:403, 1992.
79. Sato H, Ishii T, Sugita Y, et al: Induction of cationic amino acid transport activity in mouse peritoneal macrophages by lipopolysaccharide. Biochim Biophys Acta 1069:46, 1991.
80. Greene B, Pacitti AJ, Souba WW: Characterization of L-arginine transport by pulmonary artery endothelial cells. Am J Physiol XX:XX, 1993.
81. Lind DS, Copeland EM, Souba WW: Endotoxin stimulates arginine transport in pulmonary artery endothelial cells. Surgery 114:199, 1993.
82. Bogle RG, Baydoun AR, Pearson JD, et al: L-Arginine transport is increased in macrophages generating nitric oxide. Biochem J 284:15, 1992.
83. Baumann H, Prowse KR, Marinkovic S, et al: Stimulation of hepatic acute phase response by cytokines and glucocorticoids. Ann NY Acad Sci 557:280, 1989.
84. Dinarello CA, Wolff SM: Molecular basis of fever in humans. Am J Med 72:799, 1982.
85. Kluger M: The adaptive value of fever. In Mackowiak P (ed): Fever: Basic Mechanisms and Management. New York, Raven Press, 1991, pp 105–124.

Infection, the Inflammatory Response, and Multiple Organ Dysfunction

CHAPTER 21

Frank B. Cerra

Infection is currently viewed as an etiologic agent in the pathogenesis of the systemic inflammatory response and multiple organ dysfunction. Said another way, systemic inflammation and organ dysfunction are responses to infection that can persist after the infection is eradicated with antimicrobial agents and, occasionally, surgical intervention. In large part, the syndrome was recognized when modern critical care therapy retarded the process of dying. This clinical problem is now the major cause of morbidity, mortality, length of stay, and resource utilization in intensive care units treating surgical patients.[1]

This host response to infection appears to be a spectrum within which several basic patterns occur[2] (Fig. 21–1). With severe circulatory shock, death soon occurs, or circulatory resuscitation may be possible with death within a few days. At the other end of the spectrum, as in a single uncomplicated injury, the response peaks on day 3 to 5 postinjury and abates by day 7 to 10. In between these extremes, another pattern emerges. The patients continue on intensive care unit support with a persistent inflammatory response and varying degrees of organ dysfunction. In some cases, a complication is present; and recovery occurs when the complication is treated. In others, the response continues unabated even when a treatable problem is discovered, multiple organs fail, and the patient expires.

This response also appears to be somewhat nonspecific as a number of etiologies are capable of initiating it. Identified etiologies include infection, inadequate perfusion, direct soft tissue injury, and a persistent inflammatory focus such as pancreatitis and adult respiratory distress syndrome (ARDS).[2–6] Once initiated, the clinical alterations in vital signs, physiology, and metabolism are not discriminated by the etiology or, in the case of infection, by the kind of microorganisms involved. The responses generally are associated with fever, vasodilation (systemic rubor), pain, edema, and loss of function. Hence the concept of the systemic inflammatory response syndrome (SIRS) evolved, with the term sepsis reserved for SIRS where a diagnosable infection is present.[7]

Typically, the response is initiated with an episode of reduced tissue perfusion followed by a resuscitation intervention. Organ dysfunction, referred to as primary organ dysfunction, becomes manifest, as in acute lung injury or renal failure from acute tubular necrosis. The SIRS response then manifests itself. With time and persistence of

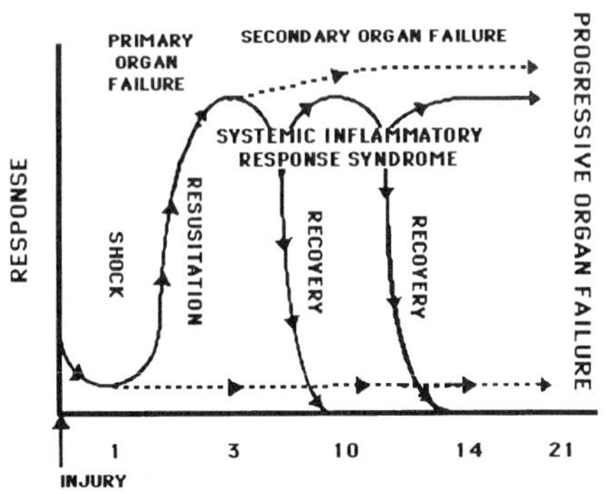

Figure 21–1. The systemic responses to infection are depicted. These responses appear to be relatively independent of the type of infecting organism. The responses of shock, resuscitation, systemic inflammation, and organ dysfunction represent a continuum in time.

SIRS, other organs begin to manifest dysfunction, referred to as secondary organ dysfunction.[1,8] In one pattern, frequently seen after a primary pulmonary initiating event such as aspiration, secondary organ dysfunction occurs very late (14 to 21 days). In another, commonly seen in septic shock with ARDS, multiple organ dysfunction is present from the time of injury. In both cases, the organ dysfunction can proceed to progressive multiple organ failure syndrome (MOFS) and death (Fig. 21–2).

Several risk factors are associated with the development of progressive organ failure.[3–6,9] These include a persistent perfusion deficit, a persistent focus of infection or inflammation, and the persistence of the inflammatory response itself. Patients who develop the progressive form of the disease manifest increasing jaundice, reduced hepatic amino acid extraction, a progressive failure of protein synthesis with increased ureagenesis in the presence of nutrition support, increased hepatic triglyceride production (predominantly very low density lipoproteins) with reduced peripheral triglyceride clearance, reduced mitochondrial redox potential, and, terminally, a failure of glucose release and hypoglycemia.[10–12]

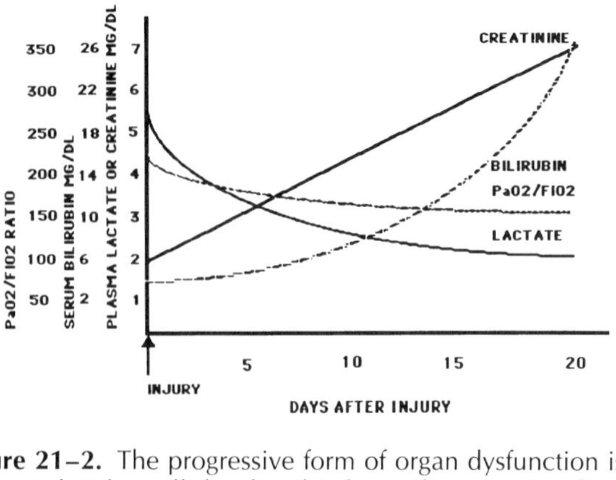

Figure 21–2. The progressive form of organ dysfunction is presented. Who will develop this form of progressive disease is poorly predicted by current risk assessment methods. Once developed, it usually results in mortality, even if the infection has been eradicated.

The transition to the progressive form of the disease heralds a change in mortality risk from 40 to 60 percent to 90 to 100 percent. Current risk assessment methodologies do not discriminate patients who will develop this problem.[13] In large part, this prediction failure appears to result from the emphasis on physiologic parameters that are treated or treatable, instead of on metabolic parameters that reflect the cell injury that appears to result in the organ dysfunction. Current technologic methods of organ support, such as hemodialysis or its hemoperfusion variants, have also not been demonstrated to improve outcome.[1,11]

PHYSIOLOGY AND METABOLISM

The initial physiology is one of reduced perfusion in the microcirculation (shock) that occurs in the area of injury and in regions of vasoconstriction (skin, kidney, and visceral compartment). With an invasive infection, reduced microcirculatory perfusion in the area of infection need not be initially present but may occur during the shock phase after the products of the local infection have "leaked" into the systemic circulation. As will be discussed in the section on pathogenesis, these products include factors derived from the microbial agent(s) such as endotoxin, exotoxins, tissue peptides, and multiple mediators induced by the infectious and shock processes. The onset of the postresuscitative systemic inflammatory response is usually heralded clinically by pulmonary insufficiency, frequently requiring mechanical ventilation, by a hyperdynamic physiologic response that may either be "warm" (vasodilated) or "cold" (vasoconstrictive), and by hypermetabolism.[1,2]

The pulmonary involvement occurs on at least three levels: primary lung injury or pathology, secondary lung involvement, and the mechanics of meeting the ventilatory demands of the systemic hypermetabolism. Primary lung injury is usually in the form of aspiration, lung contusion, or inhalation injury, all of which induce a local inflammatory response in the lung. Primary lung pathology usually occurs as a microbial pneumonitis, a frequent cause for an intensive care unit admission. The primary lung injury or pathology can be the event that triggers acute lung injury (ALI). Pneumonitis can also occur as a secondary infection during the course of SIRS-MODS (MOFS).

Secondary lung involvement occurs as acute lung injury induced by a variety of nonlung events including hemorrhagic shock, septic shock, severe sepsis, and noninfectious inflammatory events such as pancreatitis, acute intracranial hypertension, and soft tissue injury, particularly in muscle.[14,15] It typically occurs after resuscitation when systemic hypermetabolism is present and the oxygen and ventilatory demands are significantly increased. Typically 15 to 20 liters of minute ventilation is necessary and the oxygen consumption index exceeds 160 ml/m^2. A major component of the systemic response to infection appears to be an intrinsic reduction in skeletal muscle function that includes the muscle of respiration. The combination of the ventilatory demand and the intrinsic lung and muscle pathology usually necessitates mechanical ventilation.

The alterations in pulmonary physiology that result from acute lung injury are characterized by endothelial cell injury, increased permeability to crystalloid and colloid with an increase in lung water, destruction of alveolar type 1 pneumocytes, an acute inflammatory response that can be detected in bronchoalveolar lavage fluid, and a microcirculatory coagulopathy.[15] These phenomena result in physiologic alterations that include a decrease in lung compliance and an altered ventilation/perfusion relationship with increased lung shunt that results in decreased oxygenation. Ventilation (carbon dioxide removal) does not usually become a clinical problem until the disease is advanced. These alterations in physiology can be mild, referred to as acute lung injury; or they can be severe, referred to as ARDS. The presence of ARDS constitutes a major mortality risk. It is clear in most cases, however, that the systemic process is the primary determinant of outcome.[14,15]

The systemic physiology is dominated by a reduction in systemic vascular resistance, an increase in vascular capacitance, and an increase in oxygen consumption demand.[1,2] This increase in oxygen consumption demand must be met by an increase in supply if survival is to occur. The increase in supply results from increased cardiac output and an increase in minute ventilation to maintain oxygenation and facilitate carbon dioxide removal. The reduction in systemic vascular resistance and increase in vasoactive amines[16,17] and autonomic outflow induce a high cardiac output state.[18] The inability to achieve this balance of oxygen delivery and demand is associated with an increased mortality risk[19–22] and can occur for several reasons, including inadequate preload, preexisting cardiac disease, or acquired cardiac dysfunction, or as a manifestation of the underlying metabolic processes of organ dysfunction.

Preexisting cardiac disease that limits flow, such as stenotic valvular disease, or that precludes an adequate muscle response, such as previous scarring from myocardial infarction or a cardiomyopathy, necessitates interventional manipulation if there is to be adequate oxygen delivery. Acquired myocardial dysfunction is also common in the presence of systemic infection. The most common problem is usually reduced ventricular preload from inadequate fluid resuscitation. Acquired ventricular dysfunction is also frequently present and manifests as a disorder of diastolic compliance[23] and as reduced systolic contractile capacity.[24] The compliance dysfunction has two components: ventricular dilation with an increase in end-diastolic volume and a decrease in ventricular wall compliance, that is, the ventricle becomes stiff. This latter phenomenon is associated with inordinately high ventricular filling pressures and increased transmural wall tension. In these settings, adequate global cardiac function requires a high pulmonary capillary wedge pressure, an increase in ventricular preload, and sometimes inotropic support, occasionally with the addition of a systemic unloading agent. Frequently, both right and left ventricles are affected and manifest as *pseudotamponade,* with an equalization of filling pressures across the heart.

In patients with low cardiac output, flow-dependent oxygen consumption occurs during resuscitation.[19,20,25,26] In a subgroup of patients, usually with sepsis, flow-dependent oxygen consumption cannot be successfully treated,[13,14] and increases in oxygen delivery are met with increases in oxygen consumption. This group of patients is at very high risk to develop progressive organ failure and death. The origin of the phenomenon is unclear.

The decrease in systemic vascular resistance appears to be independent of the increased cardiac output and represents a primary alteration in vascular tone.[27] This reduction in vascular resistance, however, is not homogeneous in all vascular beds.[28] In the acute unresuscitated shock state, flow is markedly reduced in the skin, kidneys, and visceral compartment and can be increased in the muscle compartments. Flow to the cerebral and coronary arteries is generally maintained, except in the severest of shock states. In the adequately resuscitated state, major portions of the flow are going to skeletal muscle and visceral compartments. Current data indicate that visceral compartment resuscitation lags behind skeletal muscle and may take several days.[29] The clinical finding is one of delayed return of the plasma lactate to within a normal range. Even though total flow to an organ may be increased with resuscitation, distribution of flow within the organ may not satisfy increased tissue nutrient demand. Currently, there are limited clinical data on individual organ flow distribution during shock and resuscitation.

An extraction failure of oxygen in the peripheral microcirculation frequently occurs and is referred to as pathologic supply dependency.[27] The central venous hemoglobin becomes more saturated, and the arteriovenous oxygen content difference narrows so that there is less oxygen extracted per unit time per unit volume of blood as it passes through the microcirculation. This physiologic phenomenon is frequently monitored clinically in the oxygen extraction ratio (oxygen delivered/oxygen consumed), which is frequently reduced in these patients. Many consider that the elevated lactate frequently present in SIRS confirms the extraction defect. However, this increased lactate is not necessarily associated with the other metabolic characteristics of anaerobic metabolism and does not necessarily imply an energy deficit.

Physiology and metabolism are tightly correlated in time.[22] Metabolic responses depend on the degree of injury, type and severity of underlying disease, duration of shock, adequacy of resuscitation, and delay in definitive therapeutic interventions such as control of the source of infection. A number of mechanisms are known to regulate metabolism. They will be discussed in greater detail in the pathogenesis section and include neural responses, hormones, autocrines, paracrines, molecular mechanisms, and substrate induction. These mechanisms serve to regulate basic cell functions such as energy production, synthesis of structural and nonstructural compounds, biotransformation and detoxification reactions, and cell division.

This discussion of the metabolic responses assumes that adequate resuscitation has occurred. Inadequate resuscitation interferes with energy production and such energy-dependent functions as ion transport and protein synthesis, which potentiate cell injury and are associated with an increased mortality risk.[30,31]

One of the major clinical features in the postresuscitative phase of organ dysfunction is altered body composition.[16,17,32,33] Edema occurs and the skeletal muscle mass rapidly disappears, the latter process often being referred to as autocannibalism. The edema reflects an increase in total body water that is primarily located in the interstitial compartment. Variable increases in the intracellular compartment have also been observed. A number of variables appear to affect the magnitude of this response and include the degree and duration of shock (hypovolemic or septic), the timing and adequacy of resuscitation, and the prior nutritional status of the patient.

The lean body mass (LBM) disappears at a rate that exceeds that during bedrest or is associated with the use of paralyzing agents. This reduction in LBM closely correlates with the net nitrogen loss, frequently exceeding 20 to 30 g/day in such injuries as burns or closed head trauma. The use of nutrition support can ameliorate nitrogen loss but is unable to reclaim the LBM loss as long as the inflammatory process is active. Recent experience also indicates that the use of hormones such as insulin, anabolic steroids, and growth hormone during SIRS-MODS is also unable to abrogate or significantly ameliorate this response. Intravenous nutrition that incorporates glutamine, however, may lessen the accumulation of interstitial edema. The LBM is redistributed for use as substrate for energy production, glucose production in liver and kidney, and protein synthesis. Thus the LBM rapidly disappears (malnutrition), a process referred to as autocannibalism. It can occur after days to a few weeks, in contrast to the weeks to months observed in starvation in the absence of hypermetabolism.

Energy expenditure is increased proportionate to the degree of injury and is reflected in increased oxygen consumption and carbon dioxide production. In the absence of nutrition support, the respiratory quotient (R/Q) ranges from 0.78 to 0.85, reflecting mixed oxidation of carbohydrate, fat, and amino acids. Because of the increase in total energy expenditure to over 1.5 times the basal rate, an absolute increase in the amount of glucose and fat oxidized relative to a comparable period of starvation occurs. The fats oxidized are long, medium, and short chain fatty acids. The carbohydrate carbon sources include glucose, glycerol, and lactate. The amino acids that are oxidized for energy production include the branched chain amino acids in the Krebs cycle and such amino acids as glycine and serine in the glycolytic pathway. The production of ATP is maintained in the presence of adequate resuscitation except in the advanced stages of MODS.[2,27,34]

This increased energy expenditure appears to result from an oxidative process best described as aerobic glycolysis.[2,27,32] (Fig. 21–3). There are significant increases in plasma lactate and pyruvate with a normal lactate/pyruvate ratio and an increase in the release of lactate and pyruvate from muscle, wounds, and the mononuclear cell mass. In the presence of starvation, the liver can also release significant amounts of lactate. Thus the cytosol redox potential appears to be maintained. The mitochondrial redox potential as reflected in the ratio of beta-hydroxybutyrate to acetoacetate also remains within normal range. The oxidation of pyruvate appears to be reduced with an associated reduction in the activity of pyruvate dehydrogenase. There is increased oxidation of tricarboxylic acid cycle (TCA) fuels of two carbon fragments from amino acids and fatty acids. Alanine and glutamine synthesis is increased from the alpha amino group that is released when the amino acids enter the TCA cycle. The amino-nitrogen transaminates with lactate to form alanine and is processed with glutamate to form glutamine. In the case of alanine, this release is stoichiometric with the release of lactate and pyruvate. This constellation of metabolic events is not consistent with microcirculatory hypoxia or with vascular shunting of significant magnitude to affect energy availability. The Cori cycle is likewise very active (see Fig. 21–4). The lactate and alanine that are released are converted by the liver into glucose. There is no net energy production and no heat is generated. The lactate can also be used directly by cardiac muscle through the mitochondrial malate shuttle.

Within the limits of this regulated response, an excess of total calories or an excess of glucose calories can have a number of adverse effects: fat accumulation in the liver, hyperosmolar states, excess carbon dioxide production, increased oxygen consumption, stimulation of catecholamine release, increased lactate formation, and increased intestinal gas production and bowel distention when used enterally.[35–42] The recent experimental observation of reduced intestinal carbohydrate absorption capacity may explain this latter effect.

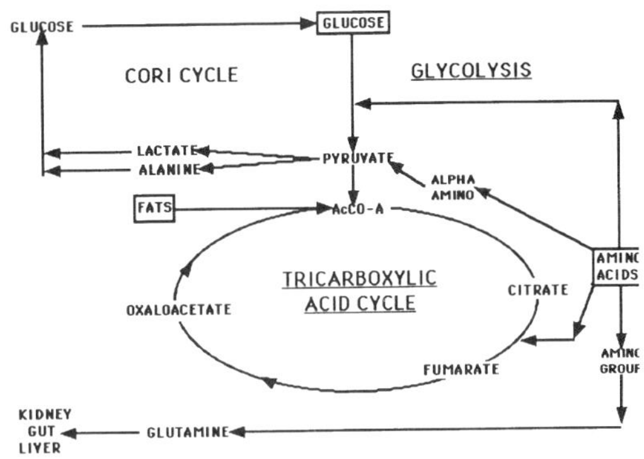

Figure 21–4. Infection causes tissue injury that activates the multiple response cascades. Mediator "leaks" into the systemic circulation and begins to initiate the inflammatory response.

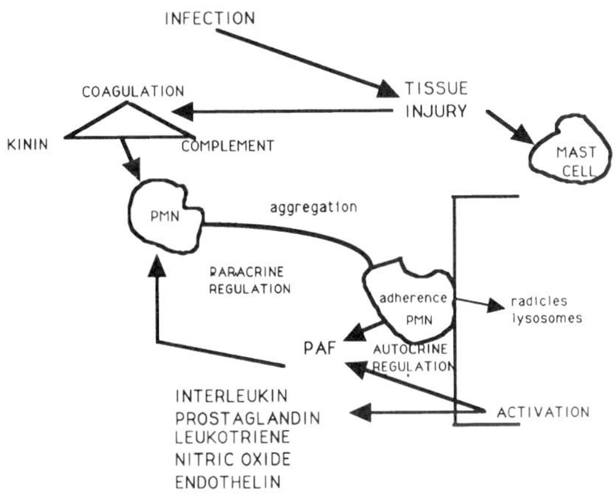

Figure 21–3. After adequate resuscitation, energy production appears to occur through aerobic glycolysis. This form of aerobic metabolism utilizes carbohydrate, fat, and amino acids as substrate. Adequate energy appears to be available during the inflammatory response.

Hepatic glucose release is increased, in part from increased gluconeogenesis and in part from increased glycogenolysis.[2] Gluconeogenic substrates include lactate, alanine, glutamine, glycine, serine, and glycerol. Gluconeogenesis is not efficiently suppressed by exogenous glucose and is driven by a number of mechanisms that include the amount of substrate presented, the existing hormone milieu, particularly a high glucagon/insulin ratio, and inflammatory mediators. Nitrogen released from the gluconeogenic amino acids entering into glucose production becomes substrate for urea production. Addition of insulin, where the levels of insulin are already high, serves to increase the peripheral uptake of glucose but does not appear to significantly change its oxidative use.

After resuscitation, lipolysis is increased, in part reflecting an increase in beta-adrenergic receptor stimulation.[2] Plasma ketones are very low and hepatic ketogenesis appears to be reduced, even though the peripheral mitochondria appear to have an increased capacity to oxidize two carbon fragments.[43–45] The intestine becomes a source of significant ketone body release. The turnover of medium and long chain fatty acids is also increased.[46,47] A picture of long chain fatty acid deficiency develops in the plasma immediately following injury.[48,49] The increase in oleic acid can be suppressed by administration of current fat emulsions, but the reductions in linoleic and arachidonic acid are not. Administering long chain fatty acid triglycerides can increase the metabolism of arachidonic acid with an increased production of its metabolites. Doses of long chain fatty acid triglyceride exceeding 1.5 g/kg/day have been associated with increased bacteremia rates, acute hypoxemia, and suppression of in vitro tests of lymphocyte function.[46,50]

As MODS progresses, the endogenous R/Q can exceed 1.0, reflecting a net total body lipogenesis that appears to occur primarily in the liver.[3] The peripheral clearance of triglyceride is also reduced, in part reflecting decreased lipoprotein lipase activity in skeletal muscle and adipose tissue. Tumor necrosis factor (TNF) has been implicated as one mechanism for this reduced lipase activity.[51] The plasma polyunsaturated fatty acid profile comes to resemble that reported for hepatic failure.

Total body protein and net protein catabolism are increased, reflecting an absolute catabolic rate that exceeds that of the absolute anabolic rate.[32,52,53] As mentioned, the clinical correlates of these phenomena are rapid loss of skeletal muscle mass, high urine nitrogen excretion, and rapid depletion of the LBM. The primary sites of amino acid efflux are from skeletal muscle, connective tissue, and unstimulated gut.[54] Uptake of amino acids by skeletal muscle is suppressed, further potentiating the net loss of LBM. Hepatic uptake of amino acids is increased and is reflected in increased hepatic protein synthesis. Certain proteins such as albumin and transferrin have relatively decreased synthesis, while others such as the acute-phase proteins are increased. Other locations of increased amino acid production are active sites of inflammation, wounds, and in mononuclear cells producing cytokines. Ureagenesis is increased and a prerenal azotemia can develop that becomes aggravated as the glomerular filtration falls.[2]

The catabolic rate is relatively unresponsive to exogenous amino acids.[2] Protein synthesis, however, does respond to increased amino acid supply. As the dose of amino acids is increased, the synthetic rate can increase until it equals the catabolic rate. At that point, nitrogen equilibrium is achieved and the rate of net catabolism is minimized by increasing the rate of synthesis and not so much by decreasing the rate of catabolism. Nitrogen retention is thereby increased, but the nitrogen does not accrue in the LBM. The dominant form of nitrogen in the urine is urea. As the catabolism increases, other forms of nitrogen appear in the urine, including uric acid, ammonia, and metabolic acids. In SIRS-MOFS, the total urine nitrogen excretion becomes poorly predicted from the urinary urea, an important nutritional assessment consideration.[55,56]

As MOFS progresses, total body and hepatic protein synthesis rates become less responsive to exogenous amino acids and fall, and the rates of absolute and relative catabolism increase. This is reflected in an increased rate of ureagenesis and an unrelenting prerenal azotemia. This response generally signifies a fatal outcome.[2,22,57]

PATHOGENESIS

Time is a key variable in the manifestation of the clinical response.[2] Within this time continuum one can identify clusters of clinically recognizable symptoms, signs, and laboratory tests (eg, shock, SIRS, MOFS). The pathogenic events in an earlier time most likely affect the pathogenic events in a later time. In addition, operator-dependent variables and the ability of the host to respond likely affect both pathogenesis and responses. The clinical time course implies that the pathogenic mechanisms change over time. Table 21–1 presents a scheme that coordinates the clinical events and manifestations with potential pathogenic mechanisms.

Tissue injury results from the products of infecting agents. This injury initiates multiple cascades of mediators that include the blood contact systems of coagulation, kininogen, and complement and the release of eicosinoids, nitric oxide, endothelin, and inflammatory mediators. Platelets and white blood cells become activated and adhere to endothelial cells, and endothelial cells release cytokines and eicosinoids.[58–61] With a "systemic leak" of these mediators and bacterial products such as endotoxin and exotoxins, the systemic response is initiated (Table 21–2). Alterations in systemic perfusion occur. These alterations are regional and depend on the degree and type of injury, the balance of local vasoactive mediators produced, and the adequacy of the cardiovascular response. Vasoconstriction occurs first in the sphlanchnic viscera and skin with preservation of the cardiocerebral axis until the low perfusion state becomes severe, at which time cardiocerebral perfusion can also be reduced. Within individual organs in the areas of reduced flow, total volume flow is reduced and the distribution of flow may also be altered. This altered flow distribution may take the form of corticomedullary shunting in the kidney or capillary dilatation in the viscera. In endotoxemia, this altered microcircula-

TABLE 21–1. SUMMARY OVERVIEW OF THE PATHOGENESIS OF SEPSIS

Clinical Presence	Reduced Microcirculatory Perfusion	Resuscitation	Systemic Inflammatory Response	Progressive Organ Failure
Pathogenesis/mechanisms of regulation and injury	1. Oxygen deprivation 2. Activation of complement, coagulation, PMNs, endothelial cells, eicosinoids 3. Macrohormone release 4. Mechanical effects of the injury	1. Local injury: oxygen radicals, cytokine, PG 2. Systemic injury: endothelial cells, macrophages, LPS release from gut, nitric oxide, eicosinoids	1. Macrohormone release 2. Cell-cell communication: endothelial cells, fixed macrophages, cytokines, eicosinoids 3. Molecular regulation	1. Dyshomeostatic cell regulation 2. Molecularly mediated death
Therapy	1. Source control	1. Restore oxygen transport 2. Antibody against LPS, cytokine effects	1. Nutrition support 2. ω-3 PUFA, Arg, RNA 3. Monoclonal/polyclonal antibody	1. Prevention

tory regulation manifests as a poor relationship between oxygen delivery and capillary recruitment. Thus there is microcirculatory stagnation, coagulation, initiation of inflammation, and injury to endothelial cells and associated parenchymal cells within both the area of primary injury and the systemic response areas.

There is also activation of the neurohumoral system by the microbial product and mediators released, even in the absence of bacteremia. Neurohumoral stimulation increases autonomic tone and releases ACTH, cortisol, catecholamine, aldosterone, antidiuretic hormone, glucagon, insulin, and other hormones.[62–65] This neurohumoral response mediates the systemic physiologic response and initiates the flow of metabolic substrate to support the metabolic response.

TABLE 21–2. CHARACTERISTICS OF THE INFLAMMATORY RESPONSE

Physiologic Response	Mediators
Vasodilation	Hageman factor, bradykinin, lactate, acidosis, nitric oxide, prostacyclin
Vasoconstriction	Thromboxane, leukotriene B4, C5a
Vascular permeability	PGE_2, C3a, C5a, leukotriene C and D, Hageman factor, bradykinin, prostacyclin
PMN chemotaxis, adherence, phagocytosis	IL-1, C3a, C5a, PAF, TNF, fibronectin, heparan, collagen fragments, leukotriene, laminin
Fever	TNF, interleukin, PGE_2
Pain	PGE_2

Resuscitation restores perfusion in the microcirculation. With reperfusion, new mechanisms of injury occur in both the local and systemic areas of injury. There are a number of mediators of reperfusion injury that include prostaglandins such as thromboxane/prostacycline, leukotrienes such as LTB_{4-6}, nitric oxide and endothelin, PMN adhesion and transmigration with oxygen radical release, platelet-activating factor, and endothelially released cytokines such as IL-1.[64–69] In the intestine, the mucosal barrier is altered. Mucosal permeability is increased and bacterial translocation rates increase.[70,71] There is little evidence to date in humans, however, that translocation is a pathogenic mechanism.[72,73]

Thus the local response products become systemic (Fig. 21–5). The effluent from the local injury site and visceral response areas appears to either cause or potentiate injury and dysfunction at distant organs such as heart and lung. The IL-1 released can induce systemic nitric oxide production from endothelial cells, either causing or potentiating a fall in systemic vascular resistance.[68,69,74–76] Platelet activating factor (PAF) and IL-1 together with PMNs primed for adherence may injure pulmonary endothelium and result in acute lung injury.[61] Leukotrienes released with liver reperfusion may also contribute to the altered cardiac contractile and compliance responses. TNF may also contribute to vasodilation and parenchymal cell injury.[35,77–79]

The macrophage populations become activated through a number of mechanisms that include lipopolysaccharide (LPS), bacteria, cytokines, hypoxia, PAF, and interferon.[80,81] This phenomenon initiates

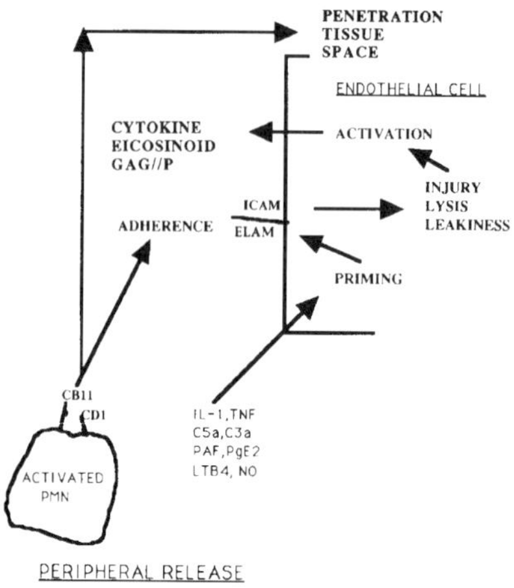

Figure 21–5. With resuscitation, the bacterial products, products of tissue injury, and mediators enter the systemic circulation. While one consequence is the systemic inflammatory response, another is the induction of tissue distant to the primary site of infection. Acute lung injury is felt to be an example of this phenomenon.

and may sustain the systemic inflammatory response. The activated macrophage populations modulate their associated parenchyme through autocrine/paracrine mechanisms (cell-cell interaction).[80–83] This phenomenon was modeled in Kupffer-liver cell cocultures evaluating the regulation of hepatocellular protein synthesis. The activated macrophage releases mediators that simulate total hepatocellular protein synthesis with a relative augmentation in acute-phase protein synthesis (eg, C-reactive protein). In the presence of LPS, total hepatocellular protein synthesis decreases, mainly due to a decrease in non-acute-phase protein synthesis (eg, albumin, transferrin). This decrease in total protein synthesis is associated with reduced mitochondrial proton transport and strongly correlates with nitric oxide formation by the liver cell.[84] Some of the products of macrophage activation also locally regulate release by the macrophage. One example is PAF, which appears to be an autocrine regulator of macrophage TNF release. The liver cell also releases a number of mediators that maintain Kupffer cell activation.[83,84] Thus a paracrine regulated system is present that amplifies itself once initiated.

This process is also influenced by a number of other mechanisms. Cortisol activates a soluble cell membrane receptor that stimulates gene transcription for a number of acute-phase reactants. LPS can directly stimulate certain acute-phase proteins.[80] It appears to act through the protein kinase C transduction system and appears to directly modulate transcription. Cytokines activate the G-protein signal transduction system, which modulates gene transcription through phosphorylation, protein kinase reactions, and nuclear protein release.

Another consequence of the inflammatory response is a compromised immune system and an increased susceptibility to infection. Hemorrhage, tissue injury, and bacterial products can produce alterations in T cell function.[85–87] The ability of CD4 and CD8 cells to respond to specific antigens is diminished. There is reduced release by CD4 T_H1 cells of TNF, IL-2, and IFN and an increased release by CD4 T_H2 cells of IL-4, IL-5, and IL-10. In addition, there are excessive amounts of prostaglandin E_2 in the cell-cell interaction milieu.[78] The net result of this altered signaling may be a reduced capacity of antigen processing and presentation functions and reduced proliferative responses by the T cell system.[85–88] One manifestation of these processes is the occurrence of nosocomial infections.

The major sites of nosocomial infections are the sinuses, lower respiratory tract, invasive lines or prosthetic devices, and urinary tract. The organisms involved tend to be those residing on the skin and in the gastrointestinal tract. The enteral flora rapidly colonize the skin, upper gut, and respiratory tract. Within 7 to 10 days of injury, up to 80 percent of those colonized will manifest a nosocomial infection with such organisms as *Pseudomonas* species, *Enterobacter* or *Klebsiella* species, *Candida* species, or *Staphylococcus epidermidis*.[89,90] Since the infecting agents seem to arise, in part, from the gut, selective gut decontamination (SDD) has been employed as a method to control them. The results of studies with SDD indicate a reduction of nosocomial infections by 50 to 80 percent, depending on the definitions used. However, the studies have not been associated with a reduction in organ failures, overall mortality, organ failure mortality, or infection-related mortality.[91,92] Thus a patient may expire with a nosocomial infection but not as a result of a nosocomial infection.

The transition to progressive MODS remains the most problematic area of investigation. Even though the persistent inflammatory response is felt to be a mechanism for organ dysfunction and failure, it has been difficult to prove that it is capable of inducing irreversible cell injury and dysfunction in a manner that reproduces the clinical syndrome of progressive MODS. Current thinking implicates molecular mechanisms as an explanation for the transition.[93–95] It has been hypothesized that the accumulated injuries eventually activate gene-mediated self-destruction (apoptosis). Another hypothesis takes into account the time-based pathogenesis of progressive MODS. During SIRS, the pathways of protein synthesis become upregulated and obligate the flow of energy and substrate away from the constitutive cell functions (eg, structural components). When a threshold of injury occurs, the heat shock genes become expressed and further divert the flow of energy and substrate. The result is a reduced constitutive capacity of the cell and a progressive loss of cell integrity. Experimentally, this process appears to be initiated, at least in part, by oxygen radicals released early in the injury process.[94,95] Eventually, sufficient cell metabolic dysfunction causes organ dysfunction. Interorgan balance then becomes upset, and the downward spiral resulting in death occurs.

THERAPEUTIC APPROACHES

Current therapy focuses on prevention of organ injury and supportive care. The approach emphasizes source control, restoration and maintenance of microcirculatory perfusion, and metabolic support. An untreated source of infection assures a high risk of progressive organ failure. Infections need to be treated as rapidly and effectively as possible with antimicrobial agents and appropriate surgical and radiological interventions. Eradicating the infection, however, does not necessarily assure survival. In iatrogenically immunosuppressed patients, minimizing the dose of immunosuppressive agents during critical illness can influence survival.

Mechanical ventilation is frequently required to support oxygenation and ventilation. There is increasing recognition that the method of mechanical ventilation can prolong the support interval, contribute to the lung pathology, and perhaps increase mortality. Modes of ventilation that utilize high peak inspiratory pressures, high inspiratory plateau pressures, and high mean pressures have been implicated in adverse outcomes. These observations have led to the development of alternate modes of ventilation that have minimized these pressure end points, such as pressure limited and inverse ratio ventilation.[96] Definitive demonstration that these new modes of ventilation improve outcome is still in clinical testing. In animal models, high inspired oxygen tensions are associated with pulmonary pathology similar to that seen in autopsy analysis of lungs from patients that have expired from ARDS. Evidence of inspired oxygen injury in humans has yet to be demonstrated. However, since ARDS is not a homogeneous disease and areas of normal lung are present, the feeling remains that the lowest possible inspired oxygen tension should be maintained.

Rapid and effective systemic resuscitation is a major therapeutic end point. The usual clinical criteria of resuscitation (ie, pulse, blood pressure, urine output, skin perfusion) do not appear sensitive enough to decide when oxygen delivery is equal to oxygen demand. Rather, invasive monitoring during the shock-resuscitation phase with measurements of oxygen delivery and consumption appear to be necessary.[97–99] The inability to achieve a balance of oxygen delivery and demand is associated with an increased mortality risk. In these settings, adequate cardiac function may require a higher than expected pulmonary capillary wedge pressure, increased volume administration, and inotropic support, frequently with the addition of a systemic unloading agent.

Flow-dependent oxygen consumption, when present, is treated with a comprehensive approach. Arterial blood oxygen content is increased by an oxygen tension that will maintain over 90 percent saturation of hemoglobin in the presence of a hemoglobin concentration in the 10 to 12 gram-percent range. Oxygen delivery is then increased until there is no clinically relevant increase in oxygen consumption and the plasma lactate returns to a normal range. Even though this approach can reduce morbidity and mortality, a significant percentage of patients will still develop SIRS-MOFS. The use of fluids for resuscitation usually raises concerns about the occurrence of interstitial edema, particularly in the lungs. Lower pulmonary capillary wedge pressures are associated with reduced lung water. When this reduced level of wedge pressure is associated with reduced volume perfusion, however, there is an increased incidence of organ failure. The controversy remains unresolved.

Starvation malnutrition can contribute to morbidity and mortality. It seems increasingly clear that current nutrition support does not alter the course of the disease process itself. Rather, standard nutritional support instituted after appropriate resuscitation can effectively manage single nutrient and generalized nutrient deficiencies and result in a small, but significant, reduction in morbidity and mortality (Table 21–3). More recent clinical research indicates that the enteral route of nutrition/metabolic support instituted after resuscitation and within 24 to 48 hours of injury is associated with improved disease-related and patient-related outcomes. These improvements include a reduction in acquired infectious complications, an attenuation of hormonal responses to injury, a reduction in the length of hospital stay for those patients who will survive the organ dysfunction process, and a more cost-effective use of resources.[100–104]

TABLE 21–3. GUIDELINES TO MAXIMIZE BENEFITS AND MINIMIZE COMPLICATIONS BY ADJUSTING NUTRIENT LOADS TO METABOLIC DEMANDS

1. Avoid calorie and glucose overload
   a. Total of 25–30 kcal/kg/d
   b. glucose not to exceed 5 g/kg/d
2. Avoid fat overload
   a. No more than 1.0 g/kg/d of current long chain fatty acid formulations as a continuous infusion
3. Adequate doses of amino acids or protein
   a. 1.5–2.0 g/kg/d
   b. Modified formulations are more efficient with less ureagenesis, more effective nitrogen retention, and protein synthesis
4. Multivitamins
   a. Balanced formula
   b. IV formulations require added vitamin K
5. Trace elements daily[a]
6. Minerals[a]
   a. Magnesium, 15–20 mEq/d
   b. Zinc, 15–20 mg/d

[a] Glomerular filtration greater than 20 ml/min assumed.

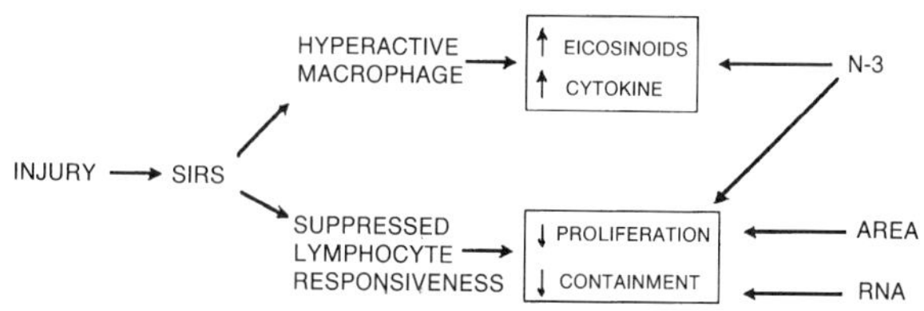

Figure 21–7. The nonspecific approach to modulating the inflammatory response attempts to alter the responses of the cells that are the targets of the mediators. Usually these targets are parenchymal cells such as hepatocytes, endothelial cells, glial cells, or pneumocytes.

Nutrients with antioxidant properties are now receiving attention. These include vitamins E and C, selenium, and glutamine.

In spite of these approaches to prevention and treatment, the morbidity and mortality rates in patients with persistent SIRS-MOFS remain high. With the concept that the response to injury may also contribute to the morbidity, mortality, and resource costs, new therapies are being directed at modulating the inflammatory response. Specific therapy is targeted against a defined mediator, such as endotoxin, IL-1 receptors, or TNF. Nonspecific therapy is directed at altering the responses to the mediators at the cellular level, such as second messenger generation (Figs. 21–6 and 21–7).

One of the specific therapies is the use of antibodies directed against endotoxin from gram-negative bacteria.[105,106] To date, the clinical trials have been disappointing and have generated a lot of new questions. At least two monoclonal antibodies targeted against LPS have not shown clinical efficacy and may have adverse effects in control populations. Experience with IL-1RA indicates that effectiveness may be related to the mortality risk of the patient.[107] Further clinical trials are pending. This may also be the case with antibodies directed against tumor necrosis factor. Currently, either in testing or planned for testing are a number of monoclonal antibodies targeted to interfere with PMN adherence and transmigration (anti-CD18 or CD11). Growth factors that stimulate white blood cell counts, such as G-CSF, are also of clinical interest. Questions concerning growth factors are related to dosing, the timing of use, and adverse reactions. Critically important are questions of whether there will be reasonable efficacy because they are too well targeted, thus leaving many alternate mediator pathways available; whether they will be associated with an increase in overall infection rate; and whether cost effectiveness will be demonstrated.

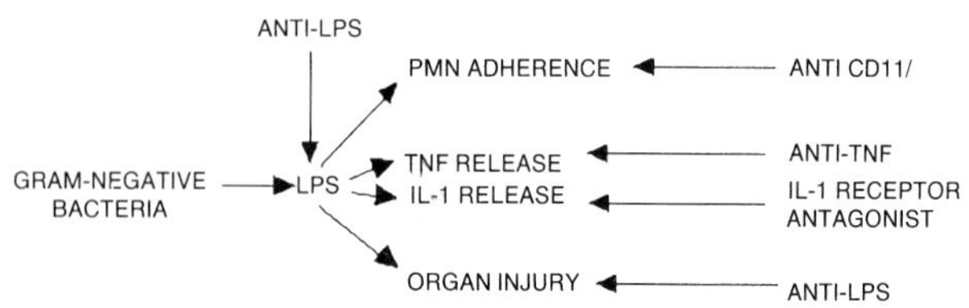

Figure 21–6. One approach to modulating the inflammatory response is with antibodies targeted against specific mediators of their receptors. To date, clinical trials with such therapy have been disappointing.

For those reasons, less-targeted therapies directed at the cells responding to the mediators are also being evaluated. Of great interest are nutrients whose use is designed to suppress the overactive macrophage and alter the output of interleukins, TNF, and eicosinoids such as PGE_2 and LTB, and stimulate lymphocyte proliferative responses. The former nutrients include omega-3 polyunsaturated fatty acids (ω-3 PUFA) such as eicosapentanoic acid (EPA) and docosahexanoic acid (DHA), and the latter include arginine, uracil, ribonucleic acid, and ω-3 PUFA. Such an approach has been termed nutrient pharmacology.

Arginine is a potent endocrine secretogogue and has been observed to restore antigen-induced lymphocyte blastogenesis.[108–110] Ribonucleotides are precursors of ribonucleic acids. Dietary nucleotides are effective in restoring macrophage activation of the T helper/inducer population and can restore delayed-type hypersensitivity responses, reduce abscess formation in mice, and reverse the immunosuppression associated with blood transfusion.[111–113] Lipid membrane composition is influenced by the type and quantity of exogenous lipid administration and can alter membrane fluidity, second messenger generation, and the pattern of eicosinoid synthesis and release.[114–117] The release of dienoic eicosinoids, TNF, and IL-1 by macrophages is directly related to the amount of ω-6 PUFA and the ω-3/n-6 PUFA ratio in the cell membrane. In T lymphocytes, n-3 PUFA incorporation is associated with enhanced proliferative responses to antigenic stimulation.[105] In animal models of sepsis, ω-3 PUFA incorporation into cell membranes was associated with a reduction in mortality.[46]

Clinical trials with these agents as part of an enteral nutrition regimen have demonstrated restoration and enhancement of the in vitro tests of immune function, improved nutritional outcomes, and significant reductions in length of hospital stay and complication rates.[101–104] These agents appeared to improve the survivability of those patients with sepsis who were going to survive, with little effect on those patients who were destined to expire.[104]

Combination therapies will be tested. These therapies will be designed to affect multiple points of the inflammatory response concurrently and sequentially, and specifically and nonspecifically. Whether they will improve outcome, alter the disease process itself, and be cost effective await the results of the clinical trials.

REFERENCES

1. Barton R, Cerra FB: The hypermetabolism multiple system organ failure. Chest 96:1153, 1989.
2. Cerra F: Hypermetabolism, organ failure, and metabolic support. Surgery 101(1):1, 1987.
3. Baue AE: Multiple, progressive or sequential systems failure: a syndrome of the 1970's. Arch Surg 110:779, 1975.
4. Pine RW, Wertz MJ, Lennard ES, et al: Determinants of organ malfunction or death in patients with intraabdominal sepsis. Arch Surg 118:242, 1983.
5. Tilney N, Bailey G, Morgan A: Sequential systems failure after rupture of abdominal aortic aneurysms. Ann Surg 118:117, 1973.
6. Goris RJA, Draisma J: Causes of death after blunt trauma. J Trauma 22:141, 1982.
7. ACCP-SCCM Consensus Conference: Definitions for sepsis and organ failure and guidelines for the use of innovative therapies in sepsis. Chest (in press).
8. Cerra FB, Negro F, Eyer S: Multiple organ failure syndrome: patterns and effect of current therapy. In Vincent JL (ed): Update in Intensive Care and Emergency Medicine. Berlin, Springer-Verlag, 1990, pp 22–31.
9. Moyer ED, Border JR, Cerra FB, et al: Multiple systems organ failure VI: death predictors in the trauma-septic state—the most critical determinants. J Trauma 21(10):862, 1981.
10. Cerra FB: Multiple organ failure syndrome. Disease-a-Month 38:843, 1992.
11. Siegel JH, Cerra FB, Border JR, et al: Physiological and metabolic correlation in human sepsis. Surgery 806:409, 1979.
12. Moyer ED, Border JR, Cerra FB, et al: Multiple systems organ failure VI: death predictors in the trauma-septic state—the most critical determinants. J Trauma 21(10):862, 1981.
13. Cerra FB, Abrams J, Negro F: APACHE II score does not predict MOFS or mortality in postoperative patients. Arch Surg 125:519, 1990.
14. Petty PE: ARDS: definition and historical perspective. Clin Chest Med 3:3, 1982.
15. Pepe PE, Porkin RT: Clinical predictors of ARDS. Am J Surg 144:124, 1982.
16. Cuthbertson D, Tilstone W: Metabolism during the post-injury period. Adv Clin Chem 12:1, 1977.
17. Wilmore DW, Orlick L: Systemic responses to injury and the healing wound. JPEN 4:147, 1980.
18. Parker MM, Parrillo JE: Septic shock: hemodynamics and pathogenesis. JAMA 250:3324, 1983.
19. Bihari D, Smithies M, Gimson A, et al: The effects of vasodilation with prostacyclin on oxygen delivery and uptake in critically ill patients. N Engl J Med 317:397, 1987.
20. Gutierrez G, Pohil R: Oxygen consumption is linearly related to the oxygen supply in critically ill patients. J Crit Care Med 1:45, 1986.
21. Danek S, Lynch J, Weg J, et al: The dependence of oxygen uptake on oxygen delivery in the adult respiratory distress syndrome. Am Rev Respir Dis 122:387, 1980.
22. Cerra FB, Siegel JH, Border JR, et al: Correlations between metabolic and cardiopulmonary measurements in patients after trauma, general surgery and sepsis. J Trauma 19:621, 1979.
23. Stahl TJ, Alden PB, Ring WS, et al: Sepsis induced diastolic dysfunction in chronic canine peritonitis. Am J Phys 27(3):H625, 1990.
24. Natanson H, Eichenholm PW, Danner RI, et al: Endotoxin and TNF challenges in dogs simulate the cardiovascular profile of human septic shock. J Exp Med 169:823, 1989.
25. Cain SM: Physiologic and pathologic oxygen supply dependency. In Gutierrez G, Vincent JL (eds): Up-

date in Intensive Care and Emergency Medicine: Tissue Oxygen Utilization. Berlin, Springer-Verlag, 1991, pp 114–124.
26. Thijs LG, Groenveld ABJ: Oxygen supply dependency in septic shock. In Gutierrez X, Vincent JL (eds): Update in Intensive Care and Emergency Medicine: Tissue Oxygen Utilization. Berlin, Springer-Verlag, 1991, pp 217–227.
27. Siegel JH, Cerra FB, Border JR, et al: Physiological and metabolic correlation in human sepsis. Surgery 806:409, 1979.
28. Schlichtig R, Snyder JV, Pinsky MR: Multiple organ oxygen supply-demand relationships in redistributional flow. In Gutierrez G, Vincent JL (eds): Update in Intensive Care and Emergency Medicine: Tissue Oxygen Utilization. Berlin, Springer-Verlag, 1991, pp 143–160.
29. Dahn MS, Lange P, Lobdell K, et al: Splanchnic and total body oxygen consumption in septic and injury patients. Surgery 101:69, 1987.
30. Shoemaker WC: Hemodynamic and oxygen transport patterns in septic shock: physiologic mechanisms and therapeutic implications. In Sibbald W, Sprung C (eds): New Horizons: Perspectives in Sepsis and Septic Shock. Fullerton, CA, Society of Critical Care Medicine, 1985, pp 203–234.
31. Shoemaker W, Appel PL, Kram HB: Tissue oxygen debt as a determinant of lethal and nonlethal postoperative organ failure. J Crit Care Med 16:1117, 1989.
32. Cerra FB, Siegel JH, Coleman B, et al: Septic atocannibalism, a failure of exogenous nutritional support. Ann Surg 192:570, 1980.
33. Giovannini I, Boldrini G, Castagnato B, et al: Respiratory quotient and patterns of substrate utilization in human sepsis and trauma. JPEN 7:226, 1983.
34. Chaudry IH, Herkema JM, Dean RE: Alterations in energy production: a manifestation of cell injuries. In Bihari DJ, Cerra FB (eds): New Horizons: Multiple Organ Failure. Fullerton, CA, Society of Critical Care Medicine, 1989, pp 277–297.
35. Elwyn D, Kinney JM, Juvanandum M: Influence of increasing carbohydrate intake on glucose kinetics in injured patients. Ann Surg 190:117, 1979.
36. Wolfe R, Allsop J, Burke J: Glucose metabolism in man: responses to intravenous glucose infusion. Metabolism 28:210, 1979.
37. Long C, Kinney J, Geiger J: Nonsuppressability of gluconeogenesis in septic patients. Metabolism 25:513, 1981.
38. Nordenstrom J, Jeevanandam M, Elwyn D, Kinney J: Increasing glucose intake during total parenteral nutrition increases norepinephrine excretion: in trauma and sepsis. Clin Physiol 1:525, 1981.
39. Askanazi J, Rosenbaum H, Hyman A, Elwyn D, Kinney J: Respiratory changes induced by high glucose loads of total parenteral nutrition. JAMA 243:1444, 1980.
40. Nordenstrom J, Askanazi J, Elwyn D, Kinney J: Nitrogen balance during total parenteral nutrition: glucose versus fat. Ann Surg 197:L27, 1983.
41. Shaw JHF, Wolfe RR: Glucose and urea kinetics in patients with early and advanced gastrointestinal cancer: the response to glucose infusion, parenteral feeding, and surgical resection. Surgery 101:181, 1987.
42. White RH, Frayn KN, Little RA, et al: Hormonal and metabolic responses to glucose infusion in sepsis studies by the hyperglycemic glucose clamp technique. JPEN 11:345, 1987.
43. Williamson CH: Regulation of ketone body metabolism and the effect of injury. Acta Chir Scand 507:22S, 1981.
44. Neufeld HA, Pace JG, Kaminski MV, et al: A probable endocrine basis for the depression of ketone bodies during infections or inflammatory states in rats. Endocrinology 107:596, 1980.
45. Neufeld HA, Pace JA, White FE: The effect of bacterial infections on ketone concentrations in rat liver and blood and on free fatty acid concentrations in rat blood. Metabolism 25:877, 1976.
46. Cerra FB, Alden PA, Negro F, et al: Sepsis and exogenous lipid modulation. JPEN 12(6):63S, 1988.
47. McGilvery RW, Goldstein G: The oxidation of fatty acids. In: Biochemistry: A Functional Approach, 2nd ed. Philadelphia, Saunders, 1979, p 434.
48. Alden PB, Svingen BA, Deutschman CS, et al: Essential fatty acid status in isolated closed head injury. J Trauma 27:1039, 1987.
49. Alden PB, Svingen BA, Johnson SB, et al: Partial correction by exogenous lipid of abnormal patterns of polyunsaturated fatty acids in plasma phospholipids of stressed and septic surgical patients. Surgery 100:671, 1986.
50. Frases I, Neoptolemos J, Darby H, et al: Effects of intralipid and heparin on human monocyte and lymphocyte function. JPEN 8:381, 1986.
51. Tracey KJ: Tumor necrosis factor (cachectin) in the biology of septic shock syndrome. Circ Shock 35:123, 1991.
52. Clowes GHA, O'Donnell TF, Blackburn G: Energy metabolism and proteolysis in traumatized and septic man. Surg Clin North Am 56:4469, 1976.
53. Waterlow JC, Golden M, Picou D: Measurement of rates of protein: turnover, synthesis and breakdown in man and effects of nutritional status and surgical injury. Am J Clin Nutr 30:1333, 1977.
54. Pearl RH, Clowes GHA, Hirsch EF, et al: Prognosis and survival as determined by visceral amino acid clearance in severe trauma. J Trauma 25:777, 1985.
55. Steinhorn D, Radmer W, Weisdorf SA: Altered urinary nitrogen excretion in sepsis and liver failure in critically-ill children. Pediatr Res 19:146A, 1985.
56. Williamson DH, Farrell R, Kerr A, et al: Muscle protein catabolism after injury in man, as measured by urinary excretion of 3-methylhistidine. Clin Sci Mol Med 52:527, 1979.
57. Cerra FB, Siegel JH, Border JR, et al: The hepatic

failure of sepsis: cellular vs. substrate. Surgery 86:409, 1979.

58. Burke JF, Gelfand JA: Events in early inflammation. In Howard RJ, Simmons RL (eds): Surgical Infectious Diseases. New York, Appleton-Century-Crofts, 1988, pp 201–208.
59. Taylor AE, Adkins WK, Moore T: Ischemia-reperfusion lung injury: repair of endothelial damage by adenosine and cAMP. In Vincent JL (ed): Yearbook of Intensive Care and Emergency Medicine. Berlin, Springer-Verlag, 1993, pp 12–20.
60. Ward PA, Warren JS, Remick, DG, et al: Cytokines and oxygen-radical-mediated tissue injury. In Bihari DJ, Cerra FB (eds): New Horizons: Multiple Organ Failure. Fullerton, CA, Society of Critical Care Medicine, 1989, pp 93–100.
61. Cook JA, Halushka, PV: Arachidonic acid metabolism in septic shock. In Bihari DJ, Cerra FB (eds): New Horizons: Multiple Organ Failure. Fullerton, CA, Society of Critical Care Medicine, 1989, pp 101–124.
62. Wilmore DW, Orlick L: Systemic responses to injury and the healing wound. JPEN 4:147, 1980.
63. Goetz KL, Wang BC: Secretion of vasopressin during hemorrhage: effects of receptors in the ventricles of the heart. In Crowley AW, Laird J-F, Ausiello DA: Vasopressin: Cellular and Integrative Functions. New York, Raven Press, 1988, p 399.
64. Clowes GHA: Stresses, mediators, and responses of survival. In Clowes GHA Jr (ed): Trauma, Sepsis and Shock: The Physiological Basis of Therapy. New York, Marcel Dekker, 1988, pp 1–53.
65. Davies CL, Newman RJ, Molyneux SG, Grahame-Smith DG: The relationship between plasma catecholamines and severity of injury in man. J Trauma 24:99, 1984.
66. Garrison RN, Cryer HM: Role of the microcirculation to skeletal muscle during shock. In Bond RF, Adams R, Chaudry IH (eds): Perspectives in Shock Research: Progress in Clinical and Biological Research, vol 264. New York, Alan R Liss, 1988, pp 43–52.
67. Dinarello C: Interleukin-1 and the pathogenesis of the acute-phase response. N Engl J Med 311:341, 1984.
68. Chang S, Feddersen CO, Henson PM, et al: Platelet-activating factor mediates hemodynamic changes and lung injury in endotoxin-treated rats. J Clin Invest 79:1498, 1987.
69. Vilcek LEJ: Biology of disease TNF and IL-1: cytokines with multiple overlapping biological activities. Lab Invest 56:234, 1987.
70. Deitch EA, Maejima K, Berg R: Effect of oral antibiotics and bacterial overgrowth on the translocation of the GI-tract microflora in burned rats. J Trauma 25:385, 1985.
71. Wells CL, Maddaus MA, Simmons RL: Proposed mechanism for the translocation of enteric bacteria. Rev Infect Dis 10:958, 1988.
72. Pittsman AB, Udekwu A, Ochva J, Smith S: Bacterial translocation in trauma patients. J Trauma 31:1083, 1991.
73. Moore FA, Moore EE, Poggetti R: Gut bacterial translocation via the portal vein: a clinical perspective in patients with major torso trauma. J Trauma 31:629, 1991.
74. Le J, Weinstein D, Gubler U, Vilcek J: Induction of membrane-associated interleukin-1 by tumor necrosis factor in human fibroblasts. J Immunol 138: 2137, 1987.
75. Mortensen RF, Shapiro J, Lin BF, et al: Interaction of recombinant IL-1 and recombinant tumor necrosis factor in the induction of mouse acute phase proteins. J Immunol 140:2260, 1988.
76. Okusawa S, Gelfand JA, Ikejima T, et al: Interleukin-1 induces a shock-like state in rabbits. J Clin Invest 81:1162, 1988.
77. Munro JM, Pober JS, Cotran RS: Tumor necrosis factor and interferon-gamma induce distinct patterns of endothelial activation and associated leukocyte accumulation in skin of *Papio anubis.* Am J Pathol 135(1):121, 1989.
78. Meyer JD, Yurt RW, Duhaney R, et al: Tumor necrosis factor-enhanced leukotriene B4 generation and chemotaxis in human neutrophils. Arch Surg 123(12):1454, 1988.
79. Beutler BA: Orchestration of septic shock by cytokines: the role of cachectin (tumor necrosis factor). In Roth BL, Nielsen TB, McKee AE (eds): Molecular and Cellular Mechanics of Septic Shock. New York, Alan R Liss, 1989, pp 219–235.
80. Mazuski JE, Platt JL, West MA, et al: Direct effects of endotoxin on hepatocytes. Arch Surg 123:340, 1988.
81. West MA, Keller G, Hyland B, et al: Hepatocyte function in sepsis: Kupffer cells mediate a biphasic protein synthesis response in hepatocytes after endotoxin and killed *E. coli.* Surgery 98:388, 1985.
82. Bankey P, Fiegel B, Singh R, et al: Hypoxia and endotoxin induce macrophage-mediated suppression of fibroblast proliferation. J Trauma 29(7):972, 1989.
83. Mazuski JE, Bankey PE, Carlson A, Cerra FB: Hepatocytes release factors that can modulate macrophage IL-1 secretion and proliferation. Surg Forum 39:13, 1988.
84. Curran RD, Finari FK, Kispert PH, et al: Effects of endogenous nitric oxide on mitochondrial respiration of rat hepatocytes. Arch Surg 126:186, 1991.
85. Munster AM, Winchurch RA, Birmingham WJ, et al: Longitudinal assay of lymphocyte responsiveness in patients with major burns. Ann Surg 192:772, 1980.
86. Abraham E, Chang Y-H: The effects of hemorrhage on mitogen-induced lymphocyte proliferation. Circ Shock 15:171, 1985.
87. Abraham E, Regan RF: The effects of hemorrhage and trauma on interleukin 2 production. Arch Surg 120:1341, 1985.
88. Kinsella JE, Lokesh B, Boughton S: Dietary PUFA

and eicosinoids potential effects on the modulation of inflammation and immune cells. Nutrition 6:24, 1990.
89. Atherton ST, White DJ: Stomach as a source of bacteria colonising respiratory tract during artificial ventilation. Lancet 2:968, 1983.
90. Driks M, Craven DE, Bartolome R, et al: Nosocomial pneumonia in intubated patients given sucralfate as compared with antacids or histamine type 2 blockers. N Engl J Med 317:1376, 1987.
91. Blair PHB, Rowlands K, Lowry H, et al: A stratified randomized prospective study in a mixed ICU. Surgery (in press).
92. Tetteroo GWM, Qagenvoort JHT, Castelein A, et al: SDD to reduce gram-negative colonization and infections after esophageal resection. Lancet 335: 704, 1990.
93. Barke RA, Brady PS, Brady LJ: The effect of peritoneal sepsis on hepatic gene expression and hepatic mitochondrial long chain fatty acid oxidation in rats. Surg Forum 42:62, 1991.
94. De Maio A, Buchman T: Molecular biology of circulatory shock. IV: Translation and secretion of HEP G2 cell proteins are independently attenuated during heat shock. Surgery 34:329, 1991.
95. Buchman TG, Cabin DE, Vickers S, et al: Molecular biology of circulatory shock. II: Expression of four groups of hepatic genes is enhanced following resuscitation from cardiogenic shock. Surgery 108:902, 1990.
96. Baum M, Mutz NJ, Hormann C: BIPAP, APRV, IMPRV: methodological concept and clinical impact. In Vincent JL (ed): Yearbook of Intensive Care and Emergency Medicine. Berlin, Springer-Verlag, 1993, pp 514–526.
97. Shoemaker WC: Hemodynamic and oxygen transport patterns in septic shock: physiologic mechanisms and therapeutic implications. In Sibbald W, Sprung C (eds): New Horizons: Perspectives in Sepsis and Septic Shock. Fullerton, CA, Society of Critical Care Medicine, 1985, pp 203–234.
98. Shoemaker W, Appel PL, Kram HB: Tissue oxygen debt as a determinant of lethal and nonlethal postoperative organ failure. J Crit Care Med 16:1117, 1989.
99. Tuchschmidt J, Fried F, Asitz M: Elevation of cardiac output and oxygen delivery improves outcome in septic shock. Chest 102:216, 1992.
100. Scheltinga MR, Young LS, Benfell K, et al: Glutamine-enriched intravenous feedings attenuate extracellular fluid expansion after a standard stress. Ann Surg 214:385, 1991.
101. Gottschlich MM, Jenkins M, Warden GD, et al: Differential effects of three enteral dietary regimens on selected outcome variables in burn patients. JPEN 14:255, 1990.
102. Cerra FB, Lehman S, Konstantinides N, et al: Effect of enteral nutrient on in vitro tests of immune function in ICU patients: a preliminary report. Nutrition 6:84, 1990.
103. Daly JM, Lieberman D, Goldfine MS, et al: Enteral nutrition with supplemental arginine, RNA, and omega 3 fatty acids in patients after operation: immunologic, metabolic, and clinical outcome. Surgery 112:56, 1992.
104. Bower RH, Lavin PT, Cerra FB, et al: A modified enteral formula reduces hospital lengths of stay (LOS) in patients in intensive care units (ICU). Crit Care Med 21:S275, 1993.
105. Dunn DL, Ferguson RM: Immunotherapy of gram-negative sepsis: enhanced survival in a guinea pig model by use of rabbit antiserum to *Escherichia coli* J5. Surgery 92:212, 1982.
106. Ziegler EJ, Fisher CJ, Sprung CL, HA-1A Study Group: Treatment of gram-negative bacteremia and septic shock with HA-1A human monoclonal antibody against endotoxin: a randomized, double-blind, placebo-controlled trial. N Engl J Med 324:429, 1991.
107. Fisher CJ: Administration of IL-1ra in patients with severe sepsis: results of a phase III trial. Presented at 13th International Symposium of Intensive Care and Emergency Medicine, Brussels, March 23–26, 1993.
108. Barbul A, Sisto DA, Wasserkrug HL, et al: Metabolic and immune effects of arginine in post-injury hyperalimentation. J Trauma 21:970, 1981.
109. Barbul A, Wasserkrug HL, Sisto DA, et al: Thymic and immune stimulatory actions of arginine. JPEN 4:446, 1980.
110. Reynolds JV, Thom AK, Zhang SM, et al: Arginine, protein calorie malnutrition and cancer. J Surg Res 45:513, 1988.
111. Zollner N, Grobner W: Dietary feedback regulation of purine and pyrimidine biosynthesis in man. In: Purine and Pyrimidine Metabolism. Amsterdam, Elsevier, 1977, pp 165–178.
112. Kulkarni AD, Fanslow WC, Rudolph FB, et al: Effect of dietary nucleotides on response to bacterial infections. JPEN 10:169, 1986.
113. Rudolph FB, Kulkarni AD, Fanslow WC, et al: Role of RNA as a dietary source of pyrimidines and purines in immune function. Nutrition 6:45, 1990.
114. Spector AA, Yorek MA: Membrane lipid composition and cellular functions. J Lipid Res 26:1015, 1985.
115. Holman RT: Nutritional and metabolic interrelationships between fatty acids. Fed Proc 23(5):1062, 1964.
116. Holman RT: Control of polyunsaturated acids in tissue lipids. J Am Coll Nutr 5:236, 1986.
117. Billiar TJ, Bankey PE, Svingen BA, et al: Fatty acid intake and Kupfer cell function alters eicosanoid and monokine production to endotoxin stimulation. Surgery 104:343, 1988.

WOUND INFECTION

PART III

Surgical Wound Infection: Epidemiology, Surveillance, and Clinical Management

CHAPTER 22

Richard J. Howard, James T. Lee, Jr.

HISTORICAL NOTE

A common impediment to normal wound healing is infection. Because relatively few operations were possible before the advent of anesthesia, most early data on wound infection rates pertain to amputation. Amputation was thought mandatory for gunshot or compound fractures and was performed more often than most other operations, especially in wartime. Mortality rates for amputation in military settings ranged from 50 to 90 percent, but for civilian amputation they were lower (10 to 50 percent).[1]

In 1867 Lister[2] published his first descriptions of antiseptic treatment of wounds. He successfully treated compound fracture, an injury previously thought to require amputation, with carbolic acid (phenol) dressings and was able to save most extremities. Although his treatment method was slowly accepted, even he did not practice asepsis until several years later.

Gradually Lister and others began to treat wounds aseptically. Over the latter years of the 19th century and the early 20th century, surgeons (frequently protesting) gradually adopted aseptic practices including use of gowns, masks, gloves, drapes, and sterile instruments.[3] The simultaneous development of the germ-theory of wound infection by Pasteur, Koch, and others gave scientific underpinning to the use of aseptic methods.[3,4] Wound infection rates have gradually fallen during the 20th century to the currently low levels. Nevertheless, wound infections continue to occur (and probably always will). All surgeons must regularly be reminded of methods for preventing and treating wound infections. Infections caused by less common organisms are discussed in Chapter 27.

DEFINITIONS

The Centers for Disease Control and Prevention (CDC) recently revised the definition of surgical wound infection.[5] In 1988 the CDC published a definition of surgical wound infection that divided wound infections into either incisional surgical wound infections or deep surgical wound infections.[6] This revision was made because "it was not clear in the 1988 definitions that specifying the anatomical location of the deep infection was necessary for deep surgical wound infection" and because *wound* connoted only the incision from skin to deep soft tissue. In the 1992 definition, the term *organ/*

space infection was introduced to define any part of the anatomy (organ or spaces) other than the incision opened or manipulated during the operative procedure. Thus a patient who developed a subphrenic abscess following elective cholecystectomy might not be classified under the previous definition as having a surgical wound infection but would meet new criteria for surgical site infection (SSI). The CDC changed terminology from *surgical wound infection* to *surgical site infection.* This new term, abbreviated SSI, covers the incision, regional extension, and organ or visceral infection but does not cover more distant infections (eg, postoperative pneumonia). These latter infections are considered complications but are not classified as surgical site infections because they are not directly associated with the surgical incision. An exception is a bloodstream infection arising from incisional or organ/space SSI.

For surveillance classification purposes, SSIs are divided into *incisional* SSIs and *organ/space* SSIs. Incisional SSIs are further classified as involving only the skin and subcutaneous tissue (*superficial incisional SSIs*) or involving deep soft tissues (eg, fascial and muscle layers) of the incision (*deep incisional SSIs*). Organ/space SSIs involve any part of the anatomy (organs or spaces) other than the incision opened or manipulated during the operative procedure (Fig. 22–1).

Superficial Incisional SSIs

Superficial incisional SSIs must meet the following criteria: infection occurs within 30 days after the operative procedure *and* involves only skin or subcutaneous tissue of the incision, *and* at least *one* of the following is present:

1. Purulent drainage from the superficial incision.
2. Organisms isolated from an aseptically obtained culture of fluid or tissue from the superficial incision.
3. At least one of the following signs or symptoms of infection: pain or tenderness, localized swelling, redness, or heat *and* superficial incision is deliberately opened by surgeon, *unless* culture of incision is negative.
4. Diagnosis of superficial incisional SSI by the surgeon or attending physician.

The following are *not* reported as superficial incisional SSIs: (1) stitch abscess (minimal inflammation and discharge confined to the points of suture penetration), (2) infection of an episiotomy or a neonate's circumcision site* [episiotomy and circumcision are not considered NNIS (National Nosocomial Infection Surveillance) operative procedures], (3) infected burn wound,† and (4) incisional SSI that extends into the fascial and muscle layers (see *deep incisional SSIs*).

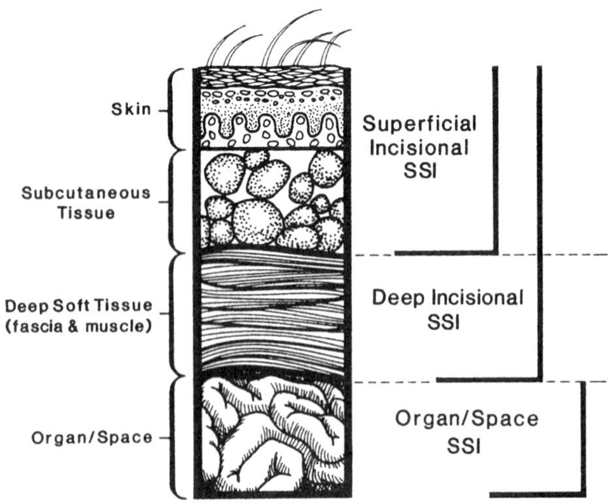

Figure 22–1. Schematic of surgical site infection and appropriate classification system. *(From Horan TC, Gaynes RP, Martone WJ, et al: Infect Control Hosp Epidemiol 13:606, 1992.)*

Deep Incisional SSIs

Deep incisional SSIs must meet the following criteria: infection occurs within 30 days after the operative procedure if no implant is left in place or within 1 year if implant is in place and the infection appears to be related to the operative procedure *and* infection involves deep soft tissues (eg, fascial and muscle layers) of the incision, *and* at least *one* of the following is present:

1. Purulent drainage from the deep incision but not from the organ/space component of the surgical site.
2. A deep incision spontaneously dehisces or is deliberately opened by a surgeon when the patient has at least one of the following signs or symptoms: fever (over 38C), localized pain, or tenderness, unless culture of the incision is negative.
3. An abscess or other evidence of infection involving the deep incision is found on direct

* Specific criteria are used for infected episiotomy and circumcision sites and for burn wounds.

† An implant is defined as a nonhuman-derived implantable foreign body (eg, prosthetic heart valve, nonhuman vascular graft, mechanical heart, hip prosthesis) that is permanently placed in a patient during operation.

examination, during reoperation, or by histopathologic or radiologic examination.

4. Diagnosis of a deep incisional SSI by a surgeon or attending physician.

Organ/Space SSIs

An organ/space SSI involves any part of the anatomy (eg, organs or spaces), other than the incision, opened or manipulated during the operative procedure. Specific sites are assigned to organ/space SSIs to identify the location of the infection. Table 22–1 lists the specific sites that must be used to differentiate organ/space SSIs. An example is appendectomy with subsequent subdiaphragmatic abscess, which would be reported as an organ/space SSI at the intra-abdominal site.

Organ/space SSIs must meet the following criteria: infection occurs within 30 days after the operative procedure if no implant is left in place or within 1 year if implant is in place and the infection appears to be related to the operative procedure *and* infection involves any part of the anatomy (eg, organs or spaces) other than the incision opened or manipulated during the operative procedure, *and* at least *one* of the following is present:

1. Purulent drainage from a drain placed through a stab wound* into an organ/space.
2. Organisms isolated from an aseptically obtained culture of fluid or tissue in the organ/space.
3. An abscess or other evidence of infection involving the organ/space on direct examination, during reoperation, or by histopathologic or radiologic examination.
4. Diagnosis of an organ/space SSI by a surgeon or attending physician.

For an SSI involving more than one specific site, the following criteria must be met:

1. Infection that involves *both* superficial and deep incision sites is classified as deep incisional SSI.
2. Occasionally an organ/space infection drains through the incision. Such infection generally does not involve reoperation and is considered a complication of the incision. It is therefore classified as a deep incisional SSI.[5]

As with all CDC definitions of nosocomial infections, a surgeon's or physician's diagnosis of infection is an accepted criterion of an SSI unless there is compelling evidence to the contrary.[5]

TABLE 22–1. CLASSIFICATION OF OPERATIVE WOUNDS IN RELATION TO CONTAMINATION AND INCREASING RISK OF INFECTION

Clean
Elective, primarily closed, and undrained
Nontraumatic, uninfected
No inflammation encountered
No break in aseptic technique
Respiratory, alimentary, genitourinary, or oropharyngeal tracts not entered
Clean-contaminated
Alimentary, respiratory, or genitourinary tracts entered under controlled conditions and with unusual contamination
Appendectomy
Oropharynx entered
Vagina entered
Genitourinary tract entered in absence of culture-positive urine
Biliary tract entered in absence of infected bile
Minor break in technique
Contaminated
Open, fresh traumatic wounds
Gross spillage from gastrointestinal tract
Entrance into genitourinary or biliary tracts in presence of infected urine or bile
Major break in technique
Incisions in which acute nonpurulent inflammation is present
Dirty and infected
Traumatic wound with retained devitalized tissue, foreign bodies, fecal contamination, or delayed treatment, or from a dirty source
Perforated viscus encountered
Acute bacterial inflammation with pus encountered during operation

From Altemeier WA, Burke JF, Pruitt BA Jr, Sandsky WR (eds): Manual on Control of Infection in Surgical Patients, 2nd ed. Philadelphia, Lippincott, 1984, p 28.

WOUND CLASSIFICATION

A wound classification system was developed in the National Academy of Sciences and National Research Council study of wound infection rates.[7] This system classes wounds according to intrinsic intraoperative bacterial contamination into clean, clean-contaminated, contaminated, and infected or dirty. The system continues to be used and has been the basis for comparing wound infection rates (see Table 22–1).

Table 22–2 shows wound infection rates from three large series using this wound classification system.

* If the area around a stab wound becomes infected, it is not an SSI but is considered a skin or soft tissue infection, depending on depth.

TABLE 22–2. WOUND INFECTION RATES

Wound Class	NAS-NRC[a] 1964 (n = 15,613)	Cruse and Foord[b] 1980 (n = 62,937)	SENIC[c] 1985 (n = 59,352)	Olson and Lee[d] 1990 (n = 36,439)	Culver et al[e] 1991 (n = 84,691)
Clean	5.1	1.5	2.9	1.3	2.1
Clean-contaminated	10.8	7.7	3.9	2.4	3.3
Contaminated	16.3	15.2	8.5	7.9	6.4
Dirty	28.0	40.0	12.6	—	7.1

[a] Reference 8.
[b] Reference 9.
[c] Reference 10.
[d] Reference 11.
[e] Reference 21. Includes contaminated and dirty wounds.

RISK FACTORS FOR POSTOPERATIVE WOUND INFECTION

Many factors influence the risk that a given patient will develop wound infection following an operation: (1) microbe-related factors (ie, the number and nature of the microorganisms contaminating the wound), (2) patient-related factors, and (3) operation-related factors.

Microbe-Related Risk Factors

The likelihood of infections is greater with an increasing number of bacteria placed into experimental wounds. This fact is the basis for the NAS-NRC wound classification system discussed above. Also important is the virulence of the bacteria contaminating the wound; some species are more infective than others. For instance, highly encapsulated strains of *Staphylococcus aureus* are more likely to cause experimental infections than unencapsulated strains. It is possible that, since gram-positive cocci such as *Staphylococcus* and *Streptococcus* are more likely to be encapsulated than gram-negative enteric bacteria, these gram-positive cocci are more likely to cause wound infection than are gram-negative bacteria. Aerobic bacteria are more likely to cause wound infections than anaerobic bacteria, because anaerobes cannot grow in the oxygen concentrations found in most wounds. Other bacteria-related factors pertain to elaboration of exotoxins, ability to resist host defenses (eg, capsules), and adherence to wound surfaces.

Host-Related Risk Factors

Certain host factors decrease the ability of a patient to resist infections. Various host-related factors have been implicated as increasing the risk of SSIs (Table 22–3).[10–17] Sherertz et al[12] and others[13] have suggested that certain factors are definitely associated with increased risk of surgical wound infection. These factors include morbid obesity, disease severity index, American Society of Anesthesiologist (ASA) class, old age, prolonged preoperative stay, and infection at other sites. Malnutrition and low serum albumin may be associated with increased risk of surgical wound infection; cancer and diabetes mellitus are possibly related to an increased risk of surgical wound infections.

Operation-Related Risk Factors

Many factors relating to the operation have been implicated in increasing the likelihood of surgical wound infection (Table 22–4).[10–18] Sherertz and others[12,13] have rated these risk factors as definite, likely, and possible. Definitely associated with an

TABLE 22–3. HOST-RELATED RISK FACTORS FOR SURGICAL WOUND INFECTION

Risk Factor	Relation to Wound Infection
Morbid obesity	Definite[a]
Old age	
Prolonged preoperative stay	
Infection at other sites	
ASA class	
Disease severity index	
Low albumin	Likely[a]
Malnutrition	
Cancer	Possible[a]
Diabetes mellitus	
Patient age (ref. 8)	Other possible
Having three or more discharge diagnoses (ref. 14)	
Immunosuppressive therapy	
Number of organs injured (blunt trauma) (ref. 17)	
Shock (gunshot wounds) (ref. 17)	

[a] From refs. 12 and 13.

TABLE 22–4. OPERATION-RELATED RISK FACTORS FOR SURGICAL WOUND INFECTION

Risk Factor	Relation to Wound Infection
Prolonged duration of surgery	Definite
Razor shaves	
Intraoperative microbial contamination	
Surgical wound class	
Low abdominal operative site	
Specific type of surgical procedure	
Tissue trauma	Likely
Prolonged hospital admission	
Multiple procedures	
Low procedure volume	Possible
Unskilled surgeon	
Foreign material	
Poor hemostasis	
Failure to obliterate dead space	
Number of people in operating room	
Emergency surgery	
No preoperative shower or scrub	
Drains	
Glove punctures	

increased risk of wound infection are surgical wound class, intraoperative microbial contamination, specific surgical procedure, failure to administer indicated prophylactic antibiotics, a low abdominal incision site, using a razor to shave the skin instead of clipping, and prolonged duration of the operation. Likely to be associated with an increased risk of surgical wound infection are prolonged hospital admission prior to operation, tissue trauma, and multiple procedures. These authors argue that poor hemostasis and foreign material in a wound are only "possibly associated" with increased risk of surgical wound infection; this position is surprising because, experimentally at least, foreign material and blood greatly increase the likelihood of infection by very small bacterial inocula.

Several operating room practices are traditionally thought to affect the surgical wound infection rate.[18] These practices include hand washing; wearing of masks, caps, gowns, and gloves; preoperative preparation of the patient's skin; type of draping material, use of plastic adhesive drapes; air exchange, talking in the operating room; and bringing drains through a surgical incision instead of a separate stab wound. Many of these practices have been rigidly honored for years, yet relatively few are supported by well-designed studies! Indeed, to examine a single parameter (eg, gown materials) would require such a large number of patients to control for all variables in a statistically valid comparison, that "proof" is unlikely to ever be forthcoming. Two studies (one controlled) have shown that wound infection rates are not affected by omitting face masks during operations.[19,20] Indeed, nasal and oral flora are rarely the etiology of wound infections.

RISK STRATIFICATION

Epidemiologists are concerned that the NAS-NRC wound classification alone may not be the best predictor of the risk of surgical wound infection. That classification does not take account of host-related risk factors or any operation-related risk factors.[14,16] Comparisons of wound infection rates among hospitals or surgeons on the basis of the NAS-NRC wound classification alone may be misleading because of hidden differences in host-related and operation-related risk factors. Haley and colleagues[14,16] have outlined the problems of developing a risk index and are wary about using "severity of illness measures" (eg, APACHE) developed for another purpose. Haley's CDC team derived a risk index in 1985,[14] developed by stepwise multiple logistic regression techniques to create a model for estimating the risk of surgical infection. Four factors were associated with increased risk of surgical wound infection, and these were of essentially equal weight. The factors included abdominal operation, operation time above 2 hours, contaminated or dirty-infected operation by NAS-NRC classification, and the presence of more than three diagnoses on the discharge face sheet. The simplified risk index, ranging from 0 to 4, was as good a predictor of surgical wound infection as the traditional scheme (Table 22–5). This risk stratification system is simple and can be managed by operating room personnel, with risk determined at the end of each operation.[10]

Obviously the number of discharge diagnoses, although easy to determine, can only be determined at discharge. Therefore the CDC,[21] using data from the National Nosocomial Infections Surveillance (NNIS) System, modified the Haley risk stratification index to include (1) the patient's wound class if contaminated or dirty; (2) the patient's assigned ASA score of 3, 4, or 5 as rated by an anesthesiologist before operation; and (3) procedure time over T hours, where T was the 75th percentile of the duration of surgery for particular procedures. In this risk index, the ASA score replaces the number of discharge diagnoses. These authors derived a risk

TABLE 22–5. SURGICAL WOUND INFECTION RATES AMONG 59,352 RANDOMLY SELECTED PATIENTS HOSPITALIZED IN 1975–1976, CATEGORIZED BY THE TRADITIONAL WOUND CLASSIFICATION SYSTEM AND BY THE SIMPLIFIED MULTIVARIATE RISK INDEX

Traditional Wound Classification System	Simplified Risk Index[a]					
	Low Risk	Medium Risk		High Risk		
	0	1	2	3	4	All
Clean	1.1	3.9	8.4	15.8	—	2.9
Clean-contaminated	0.6	2.8	8.4	17.7	—	3.9
Contaminated		4.5	8.3	11.0	23.9	8.5
Dirty		6.7	10.9	18.8	27.4	12.6
All	1.0	3.6	8.9	17.2	27.0	4.1

[a] Goodman-Kruskal nonparametric correlation statistic G (±SE), measuring the association between a patient's index value and whether he/she developed a surgical wound infection, is 0.666 (±0.010), and the partial G controlling for the traditional wound classification system is 0.638 (±0.012).
Adapted from Haley RW, Culver DH, Morgan WM, et al: Am J Epidemiol 121:206, 1985.

score method that yields values from 0 to 3, as determined by adding risk factors. Both Haley et al[14] and the CDC[21] found that risk stratified in this manner was as good a predictor of surgical wound infection as the standard NAS-NRC classification system. The ASA score is easily obtainable from operating room records and is known preoperatively (Table 22–6). The duration of a procedure that exceeds the 75th percentile value for selected operations can be determined from published NNIS data.[19,21,22] Using this risk index, wound infection rates for individual procedures have recently been published[21,22] (Table 22–7). Modified risk indexes will probably be in continuing development and may allow more realistic comparisons of wound infection data among hospitals and surgeons.

WOUND SURVEILLANCE

Surveillance involves ongoing systematic collection, analysis, and interpretation of data. Surveillance of surgical site (and other) infections is required by the Joint Commission on Health Care Organizations. It can be costly for hospitals to carry out surveillance because of the additional personnel required. However, some studies[23] have suggested that, by reducing the likelihood of wound infection, effective surveillance programs save money. The components of an effective surveillance program have been described.[12,13,24–26] These include (1) observations by a trained nurse/surveyor; (2) all specialties surveyed; (3) data reported directly to the chief of a surgical service; (4) all infected wounds and any suspected of harboring infection observed daily by a nurse/surveyor; (5) all wounds inspected periodically, such as on the third and seventh postoperative days, at hospital discharge, and at follow-up clinic; and (6) cultures being obtained from infected wounds.[24] With the tendency toward shorter hospital stays and outpatient surgery, many wound infections are only discovered in the outpatient setting.[27–33] Thus an increasing number of wounds may be unavailable for nurse/surveyor examinations. This has led to more difficulties for epidemiologists in determining the "true postoperative infection rate." Methods to detect wound infections presenting in outpatient settings include giving postcards to patients to allow them to report their own wound infections, telephone follow-up, or letters sent to patients' physicians. These techniques add to the cost of surveillance. Several studies have suggested that wound infection surveillance with data feedback to surgeons will lead to reduced infection rates.[9,10,26,34]

By whatever measure, the added cost of postoperative surgical wound infections is not trivial. Pa-

TABLE 22–6. SURGICAL WOUND INFECTION RATES[a] AMONG 84,691 OPERATIONS BY TRADITIONAL WOUND CLASSIFICATION AND NNIS RISK INDEX

Wound Class	Risk Category				(G[b])	All
	0	1	2	3		
Clean	1.0[a]	2.3	5.4	—	(0.47)	2.1
Clean-contaminated	2.1	4.0	9.5	—	(0.40)	3.3
Contaminated	—	3.4	6.8	13.2	(0.44)	6.4
Dirty	—	3.1	8.1	12.8	(0.43)	7.1
All operations	1.5	2.9	6.8	13.0		

[a] Number of surgical wound infections per 100 operations.
[b] Goodman-Kruskal correlation coefficient.
Adapted from Culver DH, Horan TC, Gaynes RD, et al: Am J Surg 91(Suppl 3B): 152S, 1991.

TABLE 22–7. SURGICAL WOUND INFECTION RATES BY OPERATIVE PROCEDURE CATEGORY AND RISK INDEX

	Number of Risk Factors								
	0		1		2		3		
Procedure Category	Number[a]	Rate[b]	Number	Rate	Number	Rate	Number	Rate	G[c]
Coronary artery bypass graft	381	1.05	5595	3.49	1574	6.67	3	33.33	0.37 (0.05)
Cardiac surgery	61	1.64	773	1.94	204	5.39	4	25.00	0.47 (0.16)
Other cardiovascular system	152	0.66	698	1.00	175	0.57	7	0.00	−0.06 (0.30)[d]
Thoracic surgery	351	0.57	641	2.18	195	4.62	4	0.00	0.52 (0.13)
Other respiratory system	9	0.00	108	3.70	50	10.00	3	0.00	0.49 (0.23)
Appendectomy	797	2.38	603	2.32	138	9.42	31	9.68	0.33 (0.12)
Bile duct, liver, or pancreatic surgery	67	0.00	109	11.93	31	29.03	3	0.00	0.74 (0.07)
Cholecystectomy	2506	1.36	1596	2.01	380	7.11	26	11.54	0.44 (0.08)
Colon surgery	754	3.18	1039	8.47	447	16.11	45	22.22	0.49 (0.05)
Gastric surgery	287	4.88	386	6.48	120	15.00	9	0.00	0.31 (0.11)
Small bowel surgery	150	4.00	219	6.85	141	11.35	23	13.04	0.33 (0.12)
Laparotomy	1202	1.50	1028	4.09	364	14.01	36	13.89	0.62 (0.05)
Other digestive system	243	0.82	311	5.79	82	8.54	2	50.00	0.61 (0.10)
Limb amputation	103	3.88	502	4.58	544	5.51	143	6.99	0.13 (0.10)[d]
Spinal fusion	3995	0.70	1380	1.88	278	3.96	4	50.00	0.53 (0.08)
Open reduction of fracture	1933	1.03	2062	1.84	397	3.53	27	3.70	0.34 (0.09)
Joint prosthesis	2895	1.21	2461	2.64	337	4.75	3	0.00	0.40 (0.07)
Other musculoskeletal system	2988	0.40	2153	0.65	384	2.34	27	0.00	0.41 (0.13)
Cesarean section	5400	4.22	1657	5.85	114	11.40	—	—	0.21 (0.06)
Abdominal hysterectomy	2634	1.37	1206	4.06	156	5.13	6	0.00	0.48 (0.07)
Vaginal hysterectomy	580	1.03	248	1.21	19	0.00	—	—	0.02 (0.34)[d]
Other obstetrical procedures	20	0.00	5	20.00	2	0.00	—	—	0.82 (0.12)
Nephrectomy	131	1.53	140	2.86	50	2.00	—	—	0.16 (0.29)[d]
Prostatectomy	201	1.00	161	3.73	40	5.00	—	—	0.51 (0.20)
Other genitourinary system	3360	0.65	1033	0.87	152	9.87	4	50.00	0.59 (0.09)
Head and neck surgery	475	1.26	348	3.45	111	9.01	1	100.00	0.58 (0.11)
Other ear, nose, mouth, pharynx	703	0.28	313	0.32	42	4.76	3	33.33	0.67 (0.23)
Craniotomy	358	0.56	651	2.46	234	2.56	4	0.00	0.36 (0.14)
Ventricular shunt	234	3.85	410	4.39	77	2.60	4	0.00	−0.04 (0.17)[d]
Other nervous system	334	0.90	150	1.33	34	2.94	3	0.00	0.29 (0.34)[d]
Herniorrhaphy	1789	0.95	1010	1.88	116	5.17	1	0.00	0.41 (0.12)
Mastectomy	905	0.77	791	2.40	82	1.22	1	0.00	0.43 (0.15)
Organ transplant	3	0.00	115	4.35	342	6.73	149	18.12	0.48 (0.11)
Skin graft	464	1.51	507	4.54	172	6.98	26	23.08	0.52 (0.09)
Splenectomy	52	1.92	87	1.15	31	16.13	2	50.00	0.72 (0.21)
Vascular surgery	967	1.55	2740	2.08	1248	6.09	27	14.81	0.46 (0.06)
Other endocrine system	163	0.00	143	0.70	29	3.45	—	—	0.89 (0.10)
Other eye	583	0.00	325	0.00	33	0.00	—	—	—
Other hemic and lymphatic systems	108	0.00	107	2.80	17	5.88	1	0.00	0.82 (0.08)
Other integumentary system	906	1.32	735	1.77	165	6.06	9	11.11	0.39 (0.13)

[a] Number of operations.
[b] Number of surgical wound infections per 100 operations.
[c] Goodman-Kruskal correlation coefficient (standard error).
[d] $Z = G/SE(G)$ not significant at $P = 0.05$.
From National Nosocomial Infections Surveillance System: Infect Control Hosp Epidemiol 12:609, 1991.

tient suffering and mortality aside, the estimated annual cost may be $1 to $2 billion in the United States.[28] With current payment through diagnostic related groups, hospitals will bear the brunt of increased costs when wound infections require longer inpatient stays. Estimated direct and indirect costs of postoperative wound infections are $6700 to $9500 per infection.[35]

CLINICAL CHARACTERISTICS OF WOUND INFECTION

Etiology

Virtually any bacterium can be cultured from infected wounds (Table 22–8). *Staphylococcus aureus* is the most common bacterium cultured from surgical wound infections. Gram-positive cocci, especially *Staphylococcus aureus,* are the most common organisms in upper-body clean operations and in thoracic operations. Gram-positive cocci are relatively more common in clean operations while gram-negative enteric aerobic and anaerobic bacteria are more common in contaminated and clean-contaminated surgical procedures. Gram-negative enteric bacteria are especially common in abdominal wound infections, and polymicrobial infections are common under these circumstances. Three to five percent of wound infections are due to yeasts, virtually all *Candida* species. The microbiologic evidence is that skin organisms, especially those of the patients themselves, and organisms colonizing the patients' own mucosal surfaces cause most SSIs.

Clinical Manifestations

The clinical presentation of wound (superficial surgical site) infections depends on the infecting organism and the tissue infected. All the manifestations and varieties of soft tissue infections (see Chap. 31) can be seen. The most common time for wound infection presentation is 4 to 6 days after operation but infections can be seen weeks or months later. Wound infections commonly present with edema, erythema, and increased pain at the incision site, followed by abscess formation. Gram-positive cocci frequently cause thick, creamy, odorless pus, which may occasionally have a yellow tinge. Fever and leukocytosis can be present. Toxic shock syndrome has occurred rarely following wound infection by *Staphylococcus aureus.* Infections due to gram-negative enteric bacteria may present later than those due to gram-positive cocci and may not be accompanied by the thick pus characteristic of gram-positive cocci. With anaerobic organisms and occasionally with enteric organisms, pus may not form. Finally, a wound infection can present only as cellulitis.

Some wound infections present very early and tend to run a fulminant course. *Streptococcus pyogenes* and clostridial infections can manifest within 1 day of operation. Streptococcal infections are characterized by diffuse cellulitis, lymphangitis, and lymphadenitis with blood-filled blebs around the wound. There is little tendency to abscess formation. Local tissue breakdown, gangrene, and necrotizing fasciitis can occur in untreated infections. A thin, watery, purulent exudate is characteristic; bacteremia is common.

Clostridial infections are rare and usually follow traumatic wounds or surgical procedures on the colon. Relatively little change may occur in the skin and yet the amount of necrosis of fascia and underlying subcutaneous adipose tissue can be extensive. Mixed anaerobic and aerobic bacteria can also cause necrotizing wound infections (see Chap. 31).

Prevention of Wound Infections

A landmark study by Polk and Lopez-Mayer[36] demonstrated that preoperative prophylactic antibiotics greatly reduce the likelihood of wound infection in patients having elective colectomy. Previous studies frequently failed to demonstrate this beneficial effect, because antibiotics had not been injected until operations were completed. Prophylactic antibiotics reduce the risk of postoperative wound infection for many clean and clean-contaminated operations (see Chap. 25). Prophylactic antibiotics are merely supplementary to aseptic methods and careful operative techniques that minimize bacterial contamination, tissue injury, collections of blood or serum, and foreign bodies. It is crucial to approximate tissues carefully and without tension. Guidelines for patient preparation, preparation of the surgical team, and wound care have been published.[18,37] Technical factors important in the prevention of wound infections are presented in Chapter 24.

TREATMENT OF SURGICAL WOUND INFECTIONS

Superficial Wound Infections

Most superficial SSIs can be treated in the office or at the bedside. If there is erythema at the wound margins and no fluid or pus can be expressed by gentle pressure (or aspirated by a needle), such a wound may be watched closely. Some surgeons "treat" such a patient with antibiotics if erythema is extensive.

TABLE 22–8. ORGANISMS CULTURED FROM 1032 INFECTED WOUNDS DURING 10-YEAR SURVEILLANCE PERIOD

Pathogen	Number of Isolates (Percent)	Wound Class Number		
		I	*II*	*III*
Staphylococcus aureus	240 (16.5)	140	51	49
Enterococcus	212 (14.6)	63	70	79
Pseudomonas species	183 (8.1)	38	52	93
Staphylococcus epidermidis	118 (8.1)	59	26	33
Proteus species	114 (7.9)	38	37	39
Escherichia coli	105 (7.2)	20	46	39
Enterobacter species	104 (7.2)	27	42	35
Serratia species	70 (4.8)	13	27	30
Klebsiella species	56 (3.9)	7	26	23
Yeast	49 (3.4)	13	16	20
Bacteroides species	34 (2.3)	3	17	14
Hemolytic *Streptococcus*	22 (1.5)	13	7	2
Citrobacter species	21 (1.5)	5	9	7
Anaerobic GPC[a]	20 (1.5)	4	15	1
Group A *β-Streptococcus*	15 (1.0)	8	5	2
Clostridium species	15 (1.0)	2	7	6
Amikancin-resistant organisms	15 (1.0)	4	7	4
Acinetobacter species	14 (1.0)	6	2	6
Other	44 (3.0)	8	29	7
All organisms	1451 (100.0)	471	491	489

[a] GPC indicates gram-positive cocci.
From Olson MM, Lee JT Jr: Arch Surg 125:794, 1990.

Wound cellulitis is usually caused by staphylococci and streptococci. An appropriate antibiotic is indicated. Wound cellulitis may occur without fluid collections or pus in the wound. Since cellulitis is frequently a sign of a fluid collection in the wound, such a wound should be aspirated. If a fluid collection is present, the wound is opened.

When pus or infected fluid leaks from a wound, or a wound fails to heal or opens spontaneously, the diagnosis of wound infection is obvious. While most recently closed wounds can be reopened easily, certain steps make the procedure more comfortable for patients. Infected wounds are usually tender and anesthesia is advisable. Local anesthesia is frequently difficult to obtain with agents such as lidocaine hydrochloride, but adequate analgesia can be provided by administering meperidine (Demerol) or morphine sulfate 20 to 30 minutes before the wound is manipulated. This is advisable so that the patient will permit the surgeon to examine the wound thoroughly.

"Failure to heal" frequently heralds wound infection, and removing sutures or staples may be all that is required to open the wound. If a wound can easily be inspected and dressed after it is opened, no analgesia or anesthesia is required. If the patient is extremely obese, in so much pain or so fearful that he or she cannot cooperate, or if the wound is complicated by necrosis of the soft tissue, fasciitis, deep wound infection, or intestinal fistula, the wound should be opened and explored in an operating room using general anesthesia.

The wound should be opened initially at sites at which pus is draining, fluctuance is greatest, tenderness is maximal, or induration is greatest. The wound site and surrounding skin should be prepared with an antiseptic solution and sterile towels and drapes should be used to isolate the area. It is helpful to remove one or two sutures or skin staples so that a cotton-tipped applicator can be inserted. The surgeon can thus determine if a wound needs to be opened further by sensing the extent of the underlying infection. This same swab can be used to obtain a specimen for bacterial culture.

A wound is opened to drain infected material. Whether a wound must be opened along its entire length is an individualized decision. Opening the wound fully permits better inspection of the fascia to determine if its closure is intact. Furthermore, fully opening a wound will afford better drainage and will ease debridement when that is necessary. Continuing drainage from inadequately opened wounds usually means greater difficulty in caring for wounds and longer times for healing.

After a wound is opened it should be inspected to determine if the fascial tissue is intact (when a fascial incision has been made) and to determine whether necrotic tissue must be debrided. Gentle examination with a cotton-tipped applicator or gloved finger can reveal sinus tracks and abscesses that are not initially obvious. Subcutaneous tissues will often be extremely tender; a digital examination must be gentle and brief. It is not necessary to remove all fibrin from a wound. Removal of fibrin and necrotic fat present only at the margins of a wound can be addressed on subsequent days. If there is extensive necrosis of skin and subcutaneous tissues, debridement is mandatory. It should take place in the operating room using general anesthesia.

The wound should be irrigated with sterile saline and dressed with sterile gauze. Dressing wounds is frequently referred to as "packing," an unfortunate term! Packing gauze tightly into the wound defeats the purpose of a dressing—to keep the margins of the wound separated so that drainage is facilitated. A dressing can promote debridement when adhering fibrin is removed at dressing changes. Another function of a dressing is to prevent further contamination of the wound. Finally, the dressing protects the clothes of the patient from being stained by the fluids emanating from the wound. With these goals in mind, the least amount of gauze should be placed into a wound to accomplish these purposes.

Some surgeons soak dressings in antiseptic solutions to reduce the number of bacteria. These solutions include povidone-iodine, acetic acid, and sodium hypochlorite (Dakins) solution. Antiseptic solutions, however, are more toxic to human cells than to most bacteria. Physiologic solutions (eg, saline) should be used. Some surgeons irrigate open wounds with hydrogen peroxide. While the bubbles of oxygen released when hydrogen peroxide touches human tissues are impressive, they do little to kill bacteria.

Some surgeons soak dressings in saline so that it will conform to the wound, then dry and contribute to debridement during the next dressing change. These "wet to dry" dressings help remove fibrin at wound margins but virtually never completely dry between dressing changes. Indeed, wound margins should not be allowed to desiccate. It is helpful to wet a dressing a few minutes before removal, especially if a wound is large, to lessen pain for the patient. After granulation tissue covers a wound, nerve endings are no longer exposed and dressing changes are painless. After a few days of open wound care, dry sterile dressings can be used.

Initially, dressings are usually changed two to four times a day. After drainage is diminished and the wound is cleaner, once or twice a day is sufficient. Showers are encouraged because they debride the wound further and improve comfort.

With earlier hospital discharge and rapid growth of outpatient surgery, patients are often asked to change their own dressings. Consequently, the process must be made simple. For complicated wounds, home health care nurses are available in most communities to perform dressing changes in the home. Wounds may be reclosed when their margins show no signs of infection and granulation is underway (generally after 4 to 5 days).

Deep Wound Infections

Infection of the fascia may present with wound dehiscence, fever, elevated white blood cell count, superficial wound infection, organ/space infection with pus draining between fascial sutures, or combinations of all signs. Deep wound infections that accompany superficial wound infections with fascial dehiscence or pus draining between fascial sutures frequently can be treated by removing fascial sutures and allowing pus to drain adequately. If the intestines herniate through the fascial margins, of course, it must be reclosed. The surgeon should make sure that no fascial necrosis has occurred and that fascia can be closed without tension. Otherwise, synthetic materials such as polypropylene mesh may have to be used. If there is minimal chance of intestinal herniation, the fascial defect may be allowed to persist so that drainage of any underlying infected collection can occur. The fascial defect that remains will almost always result in a hernia that can be repaired later.

Organ/Space Infections

Patients with fascia deep wound or fascia infections and even patients whose wounds seem to be healing well can develop abscess and organ/space infection. The reader is referred to Chapters 38 to 44 for detailed discussions of these deeper infections.

REFERENCES

1. Wangensteen OH, Smith J, Wangensteen SD: Some highlights in the history of amputation reflecting lessons in wound healing. Bull Hist Med 41:97, 1967.
2. Lister J: On a new method of treating compound fracture. Lancet 1:326, 1867.

3. Wangensteen OH, Wangensteen SD, Klinger CF: Some pre-Listerian and post-Listerian wound practices and the emergence of asepsis. Surg Gynecol Obstet 137:677, 1973.
4. Earle AS: The germ theory in America: antisepsis and asepsis (1867–1900). Surgery 65:508, 1969.
5. Horan TC, Gaynes RP, Martone WJ, et al: CDC definitions of nosocomial surgical site infections, 1992: a modification of CDC definitions of surgical wound infections. Infect Control Hosp Epidemiol 13:606, 1992.
6. Garner JS, Jarvis WR, Emori TG, et al: CDC definitions of nosocomial infections, 1988. Am J Infect Control 16:128, 1988.
7. Altemeier WA, Burke JF, Pruitt BA Jr, Sandsky WR (eds): Manual on Control of Infection in Surgical Patients, 2nd ed. Philadelphia, Lippincott, 1984, p 28.
8. Report of an ad hoc committee of Committee on Trauma, Division of Medical Sciences, National Academy of Sciences–National Research Council: Postoperative wound infections: the influence of ultraviolet irradiation of the operating room and of various other factors. Ann Surg 160(Suppl):1, 1964.
9. Cruse PJE, Foord R: The epidemiology of wound infection: a 10-year prospective study of 62,939 wounds. Surg Clin North Am 60:27, 1980.
10. Haley RW, Culver DG, White JW, et al: The efficacy of infection surveillance and control programs in preventing nosocomial infections in US hospitals. Am J Epidemiol 121:182, 1985.
11. Olson MM, Lee JT Jr: Continuous, 10-year wound infection surveillance. Results, advantages, and unanswered questions. Arch Surg 125:794, 1990.
12. Sherertz RJ, Garibaldi RA, Marosok RD, et al: Consensus paper on the surveillance of surgical wound infections. Am J Infect Control 20:263, 1992.
13. Society for Hospital Epidemiology of America, Association for Practitioners of Infections Control, Centers for Disease Control, Surgical Infections Society: Consensus paper on the surveillance of surgical wound infections. Infect Control Hosp Epidemiol 13:599, 1992.
14. Haley RW, Culver DH, Morgan WM, et al: Identifying patients at high risk of surgical wound infection. A simple multivariate index of patient susceptibility and wound contamination. Am J Epidemiol 121:206, 1985.
15. Garibaldi RA, Cushing D, Lerer T: Risk factors for postoperative infection. Am J Med 91(Suppl 3B): 1585, 1991.
16. Haley RW: Nosocomial infections in surgical patients: developing valid measures of intrinsic patient risk. Am J Med 91(Suppl 3B):1455, 1991.
17. Weigelt JA, Haley RW, Seibert B: Factors which influence the risk of wound infection in trauma patients. J Trauma 27:774, 1987.
18. Garner JS: CDC guideline for prevention of surgical wound infection, 1985. Infect Control 7:193, 1986.
19. Orr NWM: Is a mask necessary in the operating theater? Ann R Coll Surg Engl 63:390, 1981.
20. Tunnevall TG: Postoperative wound infections and face masks: a controlled study. World J Surg 15:383, 1991.
21. Culver DH, Horan TC, Gaynes RD, et al: Surgical wound infection rates by wound class, operative procedure, and patient risk index. Am J Surg 91(Suppl 3B):152S, 1991.
22. National Nosocomial Infections Surveillance System: Nosocomial infection rates for interhospital comparison: limitations and possible solutions. Infect Control Hosp Epidemiol 12:609, 1991.
23. Miller PJ, Farr BM, Gwaltney JM Jr: Economic benefits of an effective infection control program: case study and proposal. Rev Infect Dis 11:284, 1989.
24. Condon RE, Schulte WJ, Malangoni MA, et al: Effectiveness of a surgical wound surveillance program. Arch Surg 118:303, 1983.
25. Centers for Disease Control and Prevention: Guidelines for evaluating surveillance systems. MMWR Morb Mortal Wkly Rep 37(S-5):1, 1988.
26. Mead PB, Poues SE, Hall X, et al: Decreasing the incidence of surgical wound infections. Arch Surg 121:458, 1986.
27. Cardo DM, Falk PS, Mayhall CG: Validation of surgical wound surveillance. Infect Control Hosp Epidemiol 14:211, 1993.
28. Holty TH, Wenzel RP: Postdischarge surveillance for nosocomial wound infection: a review and commentary. Am J Infect Control 20:206, 1992.
29. Rosendorf LL, Octavio J, Estes JP: Effect of methods of postdischarge wound infection surveillance on reported infection rates. Am J Infect Control 11:226, 1983.
30. Flanders E, Hinant JR: Ambulatory surgery postoperative wound surveillance. Am J Infect Control 18:336, 1990.
31. Burns SJ, Diffe SE: Postoperative wound infections detected during hospitalization and after discharge in a community hospital. Am J Infect Control 10:60, 1982.
32. Surin VV: Effect of different surveillance methods on statistics of postoperative wound infection. J Hosp Infect 11:116, 1988.
33. Brown RB, Bradley S, Opitz E, et al: Surgical wound infections documented after hospital discharge. Am J Infect Control 15:54, 1987.
34. Condon RE, Haley RW, Lee JT Jr, Meakins JL: Does infection control control infection? Arch Surg 123: 250, 1988.
35. Cruse PJE: Wound infections, epidemiology and clinical characteristics. In Howard RJ, Simmons RL (eds): Surgical Infectious Diseases, 2nd ed. Norwalk, CT, Appleton & Lange, 1989, p 319.
36. Polk HC Jr, Lopez-Mayer JF: Postoperative wound infection: a prospective study of determinant factors and prevention. 66:97, 1969.
37. Polk HC Jr, Simpson CJ, Simmons BP, Alexander JW: Guidelines for prevention of surgical wound infections. Arch Surg 118:1213, 1983.

Defenses of the Wound

CHAPTER 23

Thomas K. Hunt, Daniel B. Allen, David R. Knighton

The preceding chapters have isolated and described the mechanisms of the phagocytic and immune host defenses. The clinical and epidemiologic factors that predict wound infections are discussed in Chapter 22. We attempt to describe how the individual host defense mechanisms combine to minimize the adverse consequences of minimal contamination of the wound. A greater understanding of these factors may permit the incidence of wound infections to be reduced.

NORMAL REPAIR

To understand fully the pathophysiology of wound infections, one must understand the repair processes and the microenvironmental changes associated with tissue injury.[1]

Immediate Consequences of Injury

Wounding disrupts microvasculature. Immediately, the normal flow of nutrients is interrupted. Transport of oxygen, glucose, and amino acids (and antibiotics) into the injured area and transport of carbon dioxide, lactate, and hydrogen ion out of it are inhibited. The transport problem becomes worse when ruptured microvessels then thrombose back to the nearest perfused capillary loops. In fascia and subcutaneous tissues, this creates a space of approximately 50 to 100 μm of unperfused tissue on each side of the injury even after a clean scalpel cut. This space in humans soon develops a unique microenvironment that is hypoxic (0 to 50 mm Hg), hypercarbic (40 to 100 mm Hg), acidotic (pH 6.9 to 7.3), hyperlactated (5 to 20 mmol), and hypoglycemic (2 to 4 mmol).[2,3] These conditions influence leukocyte, fibroblast, and endothelial cell functions.

Simultaneously, blood exposed to collagen generates Hageman factor, which together with injury translates the physical disruption of wounding into several biochemical amplification systems, including the complement, the coagulation, the kinin, and the plasminogen cascades. Each generates a number of potent biochemical signals that influence local and circulating cells.[4]

Inflammation and Coagulation

The complement cascade yields C5a and C3a, powerful chemoattractants for neutrophils and monocytes. The kinin cascade contributes bradykinin, which dilates local microvasculature. The coagulation cascade contributes thrombin and fibrinopeptides, which are chemotaxins for neutrophils and monocytes, and also mitogens. Platelets activated by thrombin release growth factors such as TGF-β, IGF-1, and PDGF from their alpha granules. Plasminogen activation leads to plasmin, which degrades fibrin into fibrin degradation products that are chemoattractants and activators of leukocytes.

Coagulation and inflammation interact. Macrophages activated by fibrin produce mitogens, chemoattractants, growth factors, and cytokines such as LDGF (leukocyte-derived growth factor), TGF-β, IGF-1, IL-1, IL-6, IL-8, and TNF, which act on fibroblasts and capillary endothelial cells, causing them to multiply and migrate toward the wound center.[5] Growth factors also enter from blood. EGF and IGF-1, for instance, normally circulate in appreciable amounts.

Many other undiscovered events probably also occur. The wound milieu is so complex that it seems best to regard it as a redundant growth environment, capable of many variations.

Granulocytes are the first leukocytes to enter wounds. Macrophages and lymphocytes follow. Granulocytes resist infection but only contribute lytic enzymes and lactate to the constructive aspects of repair. Macrophages and, to a lesser degree, lymphocytes, on the other hand, literally direct the repair process from the time of their entry. Macrophages not only release lactate aerobically (a critical factor in stimulating collagen deposition) but also release growth factors and proteolytic enzymes in aid of fibroplasia, angiogenesis, and debridement.

Corticosteroids prevent leukocyte entry and interfere with both healing and resistance to infection when given in the critical first 3 days after injury. Once inflammation is started, however, far greater amounts of steroid are required to slow or stop it. Steroids suppress the release of TGF-β in the wound. Vitamin A given locally or systemically restores TGF-β release, and matrix synthesis rises concomitantly. Details of the mechanism are unknown.

Granulocytes and macrophages are "primed" (see section on Nonspecific Host Defense System) in the process of entry into wounds and are "activated" by specific stimuli, often bacterial proteins or products of the complement cascade. They then consume large amounts of oxygen (up to 50-fold or more!) and glucose in the process of producing equally large amounts of superoxide (and other oxygen radicals) and lactate, in a complex set of reactions, which can be summarized as

$$O_2 + \text{glucose} \rightarrow O_2^- + \text{lactate} + H^+ \qquad (1)$$

All the terms in this equation are important. The oxygen radicals are important to bacterial killing. The lactate stimulates collagen synthesis and with the resultant hypoxia elicits release of growth factors and cytokines such as IL-1 and TGF-β from macrophages. IGF-1 and perhaps other growth factors released by platelets and macrophages cause fibroblasts to release more lactate. The resulting hypoxia, on the other hand (see below), also limits collagen synthesis and bacterial killing.

Connective Tissue Synthesis and Deposition

Collagen synthesis is suppressed under normal conditions and is released from suppression after injury. The shift from the "normal" to the wound phenotype is related to the oxyredox state, particularly the NAD^+ pool size.[6] Factors that reduce the NAD^+ pool will stimulate collagen synthesis.

Under normal, unwounded circumstances, several enzymes regulate the size of the NAD^+ pool. In addition to the well-known shuttling mechanism for hydrogens from the tricarboxylic acid cycle to the mitochondria, NAD^+ is reduced to NADH by lactate and lactate levels are increased in fresh wounds:

$$\text{lactate} + NAD^+ \rightarrow \text{pyruvate} + NADH \qquad (2)$$

NAD^+ itself plays little role in collagen synthesis, but NAD^+ can be metabolized:

$$NAD^+ \rightarrow ADPR + \text{nicotinamide} \qquad (3)$$

Several enzymes are responsible for this second step (3), each of which simply removes the nicotinamide from NAD^+, yielding one form of ADPR [adenosine diphosphoribose (NAD without the N)]. Two forms of ADPR, poly- and mono-ADPR, normally suppress collagen synthesis and deposition.[7] Therefore after injury the excess lactate (produced mainly by leukocytes) reduces the amount of NAD^+ in fibroblasts through the mass action effect mediated by lactate dehydrogenase. ADPR synthesis is therefore reduced, and the negative control over collagen synthesis is lifted.

When poly-ADPR (pADPR) concentration is reduced (as the lactate concentration rises), the intracellular level of mRNA for collagen abundance rises about fourfold. Synthesis of the rudimentary alpha chains of collagen then accelerates and proceeds by the usual rules of protein synthesis. However, in order for a collagen molecule to be released into the extracellular space, three alpha chains must be assembled into a triple helix, that is, into the final procollagen molecule. This is done in the endoplasmic reticulum and a crucial first step in this process is performed by prolyl hydroxylase, which hydroxylates selected collagen prolines and makes helix formation thermodynamically possible. This step, normally suppressed by mono-ADPR, has considerable clinical importance in that it cannot proceed without molecular oxygen as a substrate and ascorbate as a cofactor. Without them, collagen does not leave the cell and is reabsorbed instead. In a similar reaction, lysines are hydroxylated. This step is necessary for firm extracellular cross-linking and therefore strength. Thus ADPR exerts three controls on collagen: one on the synthesis of collagen peptides, one on the release of completed collagen molecules into the extracellular space, and one on the cross-linking potential to incorporate collagen molecules into fibers with tensile integrity.

In summary of this complex step, collagen synthesis is prompted by a low oxyredox potential in which lactate plays a prominent role. The critical "deinhibition" of collagen synthesis is mediated by two metabolites of NAD^+: mono- and poly-ADPR, which enhance collagen mRNA production and post-transcriptional modification. However, collagen can be released from fibroblasts *only* if oxygen is present at a relatively high Po_2.

This overall reaction, which invokes both lactate and oxygen, seems paradoxical; but the lactate in wounds is supplied by aerobic glycolysis in leukocytes [as noted in Eq. (1)], which release it in the process of generating superoxide. This lactate production is, in fact, generated by an oxygen-consuming process. Therefore collagen deposition can be speeded by supplying more oxygen without reducing the essential high lactate concentration.

Collagen synthesis is regulated by other signals as well. Both TGF-β[8] and IGF-1[9] "stimulate" it. TGF-β secretion in some macrophages is, in turn, enhanced by lactate, while exposure to IGF-1 or EGF increases lactate release by fibroblasts. It is not known whether these growth factors stimulate or merely aid in the derepression. Clearly, there are interconnecting mechanisms, but details are unknown.

Synthesis of collagen alpha chains can occur in virtual anoxia, but the vital last step, the prolyl hydroxylase reaction, which is crucial to extracellular deposition, absolutely requires oxygen (and ascorbate) and requires it at a rather high Po_2. The K_m (half maximal rate) with respect to oxygen concentration corresponds to a Po_2 of about 20 to 25 mm Hg.[6,10] The V_{max} corresponds to about 200 mm Hg. Therefore collagen deposition is dependent on Po_2 throughout the physiologic range. The effects of ascorbate deficiency (scurvy) are well known. The effect of hypoxia on wound healing is similar.

Nutritional needs for matrix synthesis also include arginine, lysine, methionine (or cysteine), vitamins A, C, and D, and trace metals including zinc, iron, copper (for prolyl hydroxylase), and cobalt. Large amounts of arginine accelerate collagen deposition in both normal healthy young men and aged volunteers.[11] Few of the mechanisms are known.

Angiogenesis

Current evidence indicates that the wound environment controls angiogenesis in much the same way that it controls collagen synthesis.[12] Lactated macrophages release angiogenic substance(s), one of which could be TGF-β in as much as we know that TGF-β is released by some macrophages when lactated. Similarly, IL-8 is released by hypoxic macrophages. IL-8 is a potent chemoattractant for inflammatory cells.[13] Almost certainly, a number of growth factors participate. For instance, new blood vessels migrate toward hypoxic and/or highly lactated tumors in which the mRNA for vascular endothelial cell growth factor, VEGF, is commonly seen. The gene for VEGF is activated to transcription by hypoxia.[14] However, new vessel growth and migration are much faster if the Po_2 of blood is so high that it exceeds full saturation of hemoglobin (greater than 100 mm Hg). Angiogenesis clearly proceeds best along a steep oxygen gradient.[15] This is likely to be important in management of human patients.

The end result of fibroplasia, angiogenesis, and connective tissue deposition is formation of a vascularized collagen-fibroblast mesh that eventually replaces the wound space with scar and provides a base for epithelialization.

Epithelialization

Epithelialization begins soon after injury, probably influenced by growth factors released by keratinocytes. If there is much of a gap between epithelial edges, epithelialization must await the production of the vascularized connective tissue bridge on which to grow. Epithelialization is also dependent on oxygen throughout the physiologic range, and it influences the underlying healing tissue probably via a keratinocyte-derived growth factor.[6] It is vulnerable to inhibition by anti-inflammatory steroids, and this inhibition is lifted by vitamin A[16] and by exogenous growth factors.[17]

WOUND HOST DEFENSES

There are no known immunologic defenses that are unique to wounds. Conversely, wounds probably employ almost all known immune defenses against infecting microorganisms depending on the circumstances. Wounds are unique, however, in their weaknesses. Injury impairs certain defenses, particularly ones that require oxygen.

The instant most wounds are made, the epithelial barrier to microorganisms is broken. Contamination of vulnerable tissues begins. Microcirculation and lymphatics, the pathways by which most major defenses operate, are damaged. Hemoglobin and excess iron, which impair host defenses, are introduced. The environment noted previously begins to dominate.

Both so-called specific and nonspecific host defenses participate in wound defenses. The lymphocyte and antibody-mediated specific defenses directed against viruses, many fungi, and some bacteria seem essentially unimpaired by local wounding unless the injury has been large enough to incur a major systemic response. Conversely, wound infection rates after minor or moderately major elective surgery are not materially changed by serious T cell deficiencies (ie, the presence of AIDS). Problems with specific defenses accumulate in seriously injured patients and these reflect on their wounds. Unfortunately, few therapies are known. On the other hand, the nonspecific immune system is seriously impaired even by small injuries, and the impairment increases as the degree of injury increases. Much of this impairment can be prevented with ordinary means in postoperative care. This requires some explanation.

Nonspecific (Phagocytic) Host Defense System

In contrast to the antibody-driven, specific host defense system, which requires prior exposure to a pathogen in order to kill it, the nonspecific host system clears pathogens without prior exposure. The predominant cells in the nonspecific defense system are polymorphonuclear neutrophils (granulocytes) and macrophages, and the common pathway of this system is phagocytosis with intracellular killing (see Chap. 13). The adequacy of this system rests on factors that control the delivery of granulocytes to the wound space, and how well they can find, engulf, and kill organisms in the abnormal environment they find there.[18]

Since each granulocyte or macrophage has a finite capacity to ingest and kill bacteria, the number of leukocytes available to wounds can be a limiting factor in host defenses[19] (see Chap. 13). Control of this system begins in the bone marrow, and any abnormality there, such as agranulocytosis, is likely to impair wound defenses. A few cases of infectability due to impaired leukocyte delivery because of congenital integrin deficiencies have been reported. More important but still rare are neutrophil abnormalities such as Chédiak-Higashi syndrome and lazy leukocyte syndrome and abnormalities caused by drugs that impair motility.[20,21] Local vascular obstruction impairs delivery but only when very severe. As a practical matter, vascular insufficiency of a severity capable of materially impeding leukocyte delivery is not compatible with survival of the tissue. The common clinical problems of leukocyte delivery include leukopenia due to chemotherapy (treatable with colony-stimulating factors) and suppression of inflammatory mechanism by corticosteroid therapy (treatable with vitamin A).[22]

Once in tissue, leukocytes seek out bacteria and foreign bodies and engulf them. This process is enhanced by complement factors and interleukins, especially IL-8. These processes function relatively normally even in anaerobic environments. Major deficiencies of chemoattraction and phagocytosis are often fatal through vulnerability to infection, but they are rare contributors to clinical wound infection.

If phagocytosed organisms survive inside leukocytes, infection will develop and persist. Phagocytic killing works through two major pathways, conveniently termed *oxidative* and *nonoxidative*. In the latter, killing is done by fusion of leukocyte granules, thus exposing bacteria to a variety of antibacterial substances including defensins, myeloperoxidase, cationic protein, and polysaccharidases (which digest bacterial capsules, making them more vulnerable to antibody attack).[23] This is such an effective system that bacteria which are materially sensitive to these substances rarely cause wound infections, and their names are unfamiliar to surgeons since they are "nonpathogens." Few defects of this system are known, and most are single deficiencies, such as myeloperoxidase deficiency, in which only a slight increase in infectability has been noted.[21,24]

The *oxidative* system is a study in contrast, and it seems to be the Achilles heel of wound immunity. It absolutely requires the presence of oxygen, which, as noted previously, is conspicuous by its relative absence from injured tissue. Organisms that are normally killed by well-oxygenated neutrophils, notably *Staphylococcus aureus, Escherichia coli,* and *Proteus,* are wound pathogens.[25] The mechanism is important to understand.

Phagocytosis triggers a series of metabolic events in which the components of an NADPH-linked, heme-containing enzyme are assembled and activated in the phagosomal membrane. The complex enzyme thus activated starts to convert O_2 to O_2^-, thus increasing the O_2 consumption by phagocytic cells 50- to 75-fold. The vast majority of the metabolic activity of the cell then becomes involved in producing this superoxide radical. Energy for this step is derived from metabolizing glucose, mainly to lactate. As noted before, these are not mitochondrial reactions, and lactate, not CO_2, is produced. The net result is

$$O_2 + \text{glucose} \rightarrow O_2^- + \text{lactate} + H^+ \quad (4)$$

The function of this metabolic or *oxidative burst* is to deposit superoxide anion into phagosomes where it can oxidize bacterial membranes and kill bacteria.[26] Any excess superoxide (which reaches the phagosomal membrane) is converted to hydrogen peroxide (another oxygen radical) by superoxide dismutase. The peroxide is then converted to hypochlorite by myeloperoxidase, which has been delivered to the site by granule fusion. Hypochlorite also is an oxidant and a component of bacterial killing.[27] Excess peroxide, particularly any that escapes from the phagosome, is quickly converted by catalase back to molecular oxygen, which is then available for reconversion to superoxide. This oxygen "cycle" and some of the radicals generated from it are shown in Figure 23–1. The relative importance of each radical is unknown. Nitric oxide (NO), one of the oxygen radical family, is clearly part of the defense system in some animals, but its role in human immunity is unestablished. NO and O_2 can react to form other nitroso radicals, which could also have antibacterial properties.

The rate at which these important oxygen radicals are generated depends on the tissue Po_2, which clearly depends on O_2 delivery. The K_m with respect to Po_2 of the NADPH-linked oxygenase, that is, the Po_2 at which this reaction proceeds at half maximal velocity, has variously been reported in the past to range from 8 mm Hg to approximately 30 mm Hg.[28,29] Our own estimate made by the latest instrumentation is approximately 50 mm Hg and is probably the most accurate. The V_{max}, the maximum rate of superoxide production when all other reactants are present at a surplus, probably occurs at a Po_2 of about 500 mm Hg. This finding has considerable clinical significance. It means that superoxide production is dependent on local tissue Po_2 from 0 to approximately 500 mm Hg. This, in turn, means that bacterial killing in most truncal and extremity wounds where Po_2 ranges from 0 to 50 mm Hg, with a mean of about 30 mm Hg, is occurring at only about one-quarter of maximal capacity. (Kinetics curves are hyperbolic.)

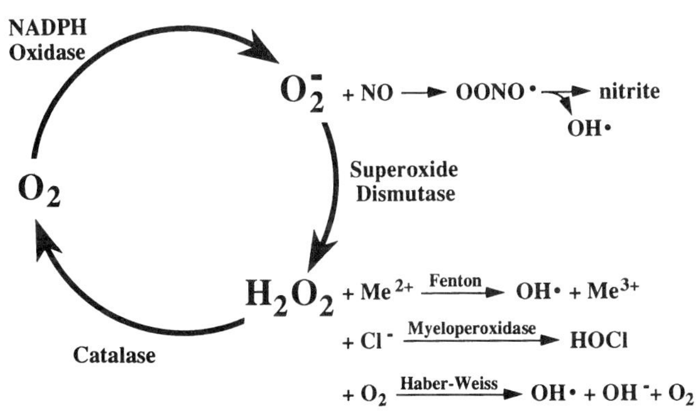

Figure 23–1. Schematic diagram of the oxygen cycle.

As noted, glucose concentration and pH are also low in wounds. Glucose is essential to radical generation. At first glance, one would expect the absence of insulin to limit the amount of glucose that reaches the phagosomal membrane. This might be expected to limit superoxide production since the metabolism of glucose in the hexose monophosphate shunt contributes the added electron, which is responsible for the conversion of oxygen to superoxide. Insulin is not necessary for glucose entry into leukocytes, but low pH and glucose slow radical formation as implied in Equation (4). The degree to which these contribute to wound vulnerability is unknown, but the importance of oxygen tension is highly significant and well demonstrated.

Vulnerability to infection is clearly a function of local Po_2. Experimental studies have shown a *critical inoculum* of about 100 bacteria per milliliter of fluid of the wound space in the skin of the trunk. If the bacterial inoculum is below this level, the normal nonspecific host defense system usually can clear it before significant bacterial proliferation has occurred. With greater bacterial challenges, clinically significant infections are progressively more probable.[30] On first thought, this would seem to be merely a problem of the number of leukocytes that are available. However, these same host defenses, when adequately supported by a more favorable wound environment, are obviously capable of dealing with even greater inocula as witnessed by the extraordinary resistance to infection found in wounds in the highly perfused face and anus and normal heart in which inocula several orders of magnitude larger fail to induce infections. As yet, surgical science has not determined how closely tissues of the trunk and extremities can approach this degree of resistance. Clearly, however, the difference in susceptibility lies in the tissue environment.

If oxidative killing is to continue at an effective level, oxygen tension and therefore blood perfusion must be maintained in order to supply oxygen and glucose and to carry away the lactate and hydrogen ions. In most wounds on the trunk and limbs, the disrupted circulation cannot meet those needs, and oxygen tension and pH fall while lactate concentration rises. Any additional impediment to perfusion or oxygenation will lower wound Po_2 and will increase vulnerability. For instance, that wound infections increase with respiratory insufficiencies has long been known.[31,32] In this sense, most wound infections might be called anaerobic, since hypoxia encourages growth of anaerobic bacteria and at the same time impairs defenses against aerobic pathogens. Furthermore, any event that unnecessarily increases the inflammatory cell population, such as unnecessary trauma at operation, will increase O_2 consumption, lower Po_2, glucose, and pH, and will contribute to infection.

Bactericidal oxygen radical formation can be hindered in numerous ways. Two ways that are intrinsic to wounds are illustrated by the presence of blood clot or infiltrated blood in wounded tissue. Any functional, extravascular hemoglobin competes for oxygen and assures a low Po_2 because of its affinity for oxygen. Hemoglobin impairs host defenses in several other ways: bacteria require iron for growth, and hemoglobin can provide this vital nutrient. Furthermore, iron released from hemoglobin acts as a powerful catalyst in the Fenton reaction, which converts molecular oxygen to radical oxygen intermediates (especially the hydroxyl radical) that are toxic to tissue. Indeed, hemoglobin itself may be a potent Fenton reagent. This probably occurs more frequently with increasing concentrations of extracellular superoxide, as this radical may reduce any ferric iron that may be present, thus favoring the Fenton reaction.

Vulnerability is also affected by the distribution pattern of oxygen in tissue. The hypoxic, hypercarbic, and acidotic wound conditions noted previously are spatially heterogenous. Explorations of "normal" wounds with microprobes have produced histograms that demonstrate frequent zones in which oxygen tension and glucose concentrations approach zero.[2] In poorly perfused wounds these zones are more frequent. As mean Po_2 falls, the number of zones in which $Po_2 = 0$ must rise and the chance of confluence must also increase. When enough of these hypoxic zones become confluent and coincide with contaminants, the chance of infection must increase.

The nonspecific system is clearly activated by injury, and in severe injury and shock, this becomes detrimental. Studies of neutrophils taken from the extracellular fluid of small, relatively atraumatic wounds reveal that they are activated during the transfer from blood to wound in the sense that their oxygen consumption has risen already above the baseline of cells taken from blood that have not migrated. They are also primed in the sense that their oxygen consumption will rise even more sharply when these cells encounter a second stimulus, such as bacteria, dead tissue, or foreign bodies.[33] In this condition they are intrinsically able to engulf and kill bacteria even more effectively than cells taken directly from the circulation, provided that their environment permits.[34] Mechanisms of activation and priming include several cytokines and IGF-1. Fibrin may play a role. This is usually a useful event. However, premature stimulation may exhaust killing capacity.

Defenses of Large Wounds and Burns

As the degree of trauma increases, the hemodynamic responses increasingly impinge on repair and resistance to infection. Severe shocking trauma, or even just prolonged shock due to simple blood loss or dehydration, activates the so-called reticuloendothelial system. Intravascular (premature) activation of leukocytes then occurs in another set of cascade mechanisms. After prolonged stimulation, neutrophils lose capacity to produce radicals, and, in this circumstance, neutrophils arrive in wounds with less capacity to respond to second challenges there.[35]

In its most extreme form, the reaction to major, shocking trauma leads to the systemic inflammatory response syndrome and multiple organ failure. There are many contributors: for example, the sympathetic nervous system, transfusion-induced immune suppression, cytokine release, activation of leukocyte and endothelial cell adhesion molecules or integrins, and abnormal manufacture and release of oxidant radicals. Most of these have deleterious effects on wound defenses as well. For instance wound defenses are regulated in part by cytokines. TGF-β, for example, is immunosuppressive in several senses in that it suppresses lymphocyte blastogenesis and prematurely (or perhaps excessively) stimulates the nonspecific immune system and thus contributes to exhausting it (see Chap. 16). The relevance to wound infections is simply that large wounds and wounds associated with severe or shocking trauma inherit these immune deficiencies. Consequently, infections due to more opportunistic infecting agents appear. Burn wounds are an excellent example. So far, only a small number of AIDS patients have been seriously burned. First experiences, however, have been dismal. It appears that HIV-positive patients become infected more frequently after major trauma.[36]

Large burn wounds also impose a number of additional burdens on patients. Nutritional depletion is common due to thermal and exudative losses. The glucose-lactate conversion, in which lactate synthesized by wounds is recirculated to the liver, reconverted to glucose, and sent back to the wound, imparts a metabolic inefficiency that is proportionate to wound size.[37]

Constant exposure to invading organisms constantly tests the capacities of the entire anti-infective immune system. Large burn wounds are constantly exposed for many weeks to ambient organisms such as fungi and saprophytes, which have only the duration of an operation to enter lesser surgical wounds. A vicious cycle ensues in which several scenarios may occur. Inflammatory mechanisms may be excessively activated, in which case excessive proteinase production accentuates the lysis that normally balances collagen synthesis. A net loss of wound substance (and hence of immunity) may occur in an astonishingly short time. Conversely, inflammatory mechanisms may become depleted or perhaps inadequately supported. In this case, healing may be prevented or delayed. The net result of delayed repair is, of course, a longer interval to wound closure, prolonged contamination, and a higher risk of infection.

One of the rules of healing is that wounds that heal quickly are generally the least productive of scar. Infection or its residua clearly delay repair and tend to increase residual scar. This is very clearly true of burn wounds.[38]

As healing progresses, the threat of infection diminishes. Healthy granulation tissue, except perhaps in large open wounds, is almost invulnerable. Nevertheless, the ultimate defense against a wound infection is a fully healed wound. Life-saving strategy for burn care is therefore to close wounds by excision and grafting as rapidly as possible. Even wounds that are healed to clinical examination, however, are not entirely free of the threat of infection. Wound infections may appear weeks after injury, and delayed infections have been reported even more than 30 years after ostensible healing.

CLINICAL APPLICATIONS

No new finding with respect to wound defenses changes in any way the fact that the extent of bacterial inoculation remains an important determinant of infection. Surgical discipline and aseptic surgical technique remain important! Similarly, the new findings do nothing but enhance the theoretical advantages of gentle surgical technique. Gentle surgery translates to well-perfused local tissues and absence of hematomas and dead spaces. The newer findings, however, do point out that the traditional, modest expectations of resistance to infection are lower than surgeons need to accept.

Wound Closure

The earliest possible closure of a wound is the best long-term defense against infection, but if the surgeon suspects that contamination is likely to overcome defenses, delayed primary closure is a useful preventive technique. In this technique, the wound is left open for 4 or 5 days and then closed. During the delay period, new vessels start to form, and local Po_2 rises, giving the tissue a stronger defense system. The open wound allows bacterial contamination to be diluted. If delayed closure is elected, certain rules should be followed. The open wound should carefully be protected from contamination and should not be dressed for 4 days. On either the fourth or fifth day it should be examined and closed preferably with skin tapes, but only if examination reveals a healthy wound. Any evidence of excess fibrin or ischemic tissue (vascularized tissue is slightly pink and moist) should prompt a decision not to close. Even delayed primary closure rarely works, however, when the wound is close to a colostomy, ileostomy, or draining abscess.

NUTRITION

Aspects of nutrition also affect immunity. This is based on a simple logic. Vulnerability decreases as healing advances. Healed wounds rarely become infected. Poorly nourished patients heal poorly. Therefore the nutritional needs of wound healing are also the nutritional needs of resistance to infection. Strangely, not as much is known about the specific details of wound nutrition as is often assumed.

Clearly, wounds are not always the highest priority in body economy. Current starvation affects wound closure profoundly. Slow chronic depletion is not as detrimental as has been thought until it becomes quite severe. New data demonstrate the relative importance of nutrition in the week or two preceding injury.[16] Unfortunately, the specifics are unknown. The converse also seems to be true. Nutritional needs for repair can be met rather quickly in response to any effective mode of repletion.[39]

In general, it is futile to seek specific nutritional deficiencies for wound problems. General nutrition is as effective as any specialized formula. It is useful, however, to know several facts. Vitamin A deficiency is common in Western cultures. Ascorbate deficiency is no longer common, but deficiencies are easily and inexpensively prevented in the most vulnerable patients—those with large open wounds. Amino acids (eg, cysteine, arginine, glutamine, lysine) seem to be exceptionally important. Early enteral feeding is highly desirable. Iron, zinc, copper, and manganese are important to repair.

PERFUSION

The major difference between vulnerable and invulnerable wounds clearly lies in their degree of blood perfusion. Hemorrhoids and oral mucosa, almost invulnerable to wound infections, are perfused so rapidly that their venous drainage is almost fully saturated with oxygen. On the other hand, the extreme hazards of infection in malperfused limbs and old scars have been noted for centuries.

There could be many reasons for the importance of perfusion, but tissue oxygenation and antibiotic distribution are the only two that are known in any detail. Antibiotics rapidly diffuse into normal tissue within a few minutes, but after an incision is made, the interval from intravenous injection to peak concentration rises by more than an hour. The highest levels in wounds are reached only after several bolus doses.

Three clinical factors control tissue P_{O_2}. They are the oxygen content and partial pressure of arterial blood, the rate of oxygen consumption by the wound, and the rate at which blood perfuses tissue. The basic rules by which they operate in injured tissues are often misunderstood. Clearly, the longer blood remains in an oxygen-consuming tissue, the more oxygen will be extracted from it, and the lower the oxygen tension in that tissue will fall. Conversely, it is axiomatic that tissue P_{O_2} must rise to approach P_{AO_2} as flow approaches infinity. The degree to which tissue P_{O_2} approaches that of P_{AO_2} in the clinically achievable range of perfusion depends on the rate at which the given tissue consumes oxygen. Wounds consume relatively little oxygen, and wound tissue P_{O_2} can approach P_{AO_2} rather closely as perfusion rises. In well-perfused surgical patients, P_{O_2} is often in the range of 100 to 150 mm Hg when P_{AO_2} is in the range of 200 to 250 mm Hg. Of the two variables—P_{AO_2} and oxygen content—P_{AO_2} is by far the most important to wounds, because wounds use relatively little O_2. Anemia becomes important when hematocrit falls below 15 percent, higher when cardiac output is restricted. Raising the oxygen-carrying capacity of blood does not raise tissue P_{O_2} or help healing or resistance to infection unless cardiac output or perfusion is limited. Mild to moderate anemia does not warrant transfusion.

Diffusion limits the flow of all gases in tissue and is particularly limiting in wounds where intercapillary distances are high. P_{AO_2} is the driving force behind oxygen distribution into tissue. In order to maintain a high P_{O_2} in the microvasculature, perfusion must be rapid, and P_{AO_2} must be high. When P_{AO_2} is held constant, wound tissue P_{O_2} is diminished by any decrement in perfusion. When perfusion is high and held constant, any change in P_{AO_2} is quickly reflected in tissue. When perfusion is low, the small changes that administering oxygen will add to normally saturated arterial blood will inevitably increase tissue P_{O_2}, but the change will be small and is, in fact, often undetectable. If, lastly, wound P_{O_2} is low due to arterial desaturation, and oxygen administration corrects the desaturation, a change in tissue P_{O_2} proportional to the change in P_{AO_2} and perfusion rate is detected. The clinical rule is simple. To maintain wound defenses, one must support both flow and P_{AO_2}.

Perfusion is determined by cardiac output, arterial and venous anatomy, the local vascularity, the tone of the autonomic nervous system, and an enormously complex set of locally and systemically active substances. Centrally, cardiac output controls the flow capacity. Patients with low cardiac output succumb to bacterial infections in wounds and elsewhere. More peripherally, arterial occlusion, for instance, inhibits regional flow resistance and flow. Ischemic limbs are notoriously vulnerable to infection.

The most common and least appreciated determinant of blood flow in tissue is the vascular muscle tone—and therefore microvascular flow. This is controlled by the sympathetic nervous system with catecholamines, vasopressin, angiotensin, and a variety of other factors including prostaglandins. The tone is balanced by the parasympathetic system, other prostaglandins, nitric oxide, and others. Some regions are controlled differently than others. For instance, precapillary tone in the intestine is controlled by angiotensin, whereas catecholamines and the sympathetic nervous system control it in most other tissues.[40] Since perfusion is so important to repair and resistance to infection, this area is vital and rather poorly understood from the point of view of clinical exploitation. Alpha-2 blockade is being investigated and at first look appears helpful in increasing local oxygen tension.

Sympathetic activity is controlled by four factors, all of which are almost universal features of surgical circumstances. They are pain, fear, cold, and loss of blood volume, each of which lowers tissue P_{O_2} and therefore impairs immunity. Control of sympathetic tone is not currently a part of most surgeons' postoperative management, though appreciation of its importance is growing. Pain, cold, fear, and contracted blood volume are each capable of producing vasoconstriction independently. Therefore, to prevent or correct vasoconstriction, all must be corrected, all at the same time. Several groups have now correlated surgical complications with postoperative or intraoperative tissue oxygen tension.[41,42] The authors have monitored wound tissue Po_2 in several hundred patients, and, in them, infection rates have been inversely proportional to wound Po_2. No infections have yet occurred, even in severely contaminated wounds, when subcutaneous wound Po_2 could be raised to 90 mm Hg or higher by breathing oxygen at sea level pressure.

Clearly, cardiopulmonary problems are significant to wound defenses. During clinical tissue oxygen monitoring, we have seen episodes of severe tissue hypoxia overlooked because they were not otherwise apparent. On the other hand, many peripheral flow problems, though subtle, are clinically detectable. One of the forefronts of infection control is clearly tissue Po_2 monitoring in the immediate postoperative period when hypothermia, volume deficits, and pain are most easily controlled. Pharmacologic control of perfusion is also part of the forefront. We have seen alpha-adrenergic blockers and removal of beta blockers clearly raise perfusion. One clear message from this work is that urine output cannot be equated to peripheral perfusion or blood volume state. Urine volume is, on the contrary, often misleading.[43] The best assessment of wound oxygenation is direct measurement, and methods are becoming available. Disorders of flow in the extremities are usually detectable by transcutaneous oximetry, a method available in most intensive care nurseries.

When perfusion cannot be increased, hyperbaric oxygen becomes a last resort to clear local infections without amputation, for instance. Tissues with intrinsically poor circulation, such as after irradiation and in scleroderma, present serious problems that can be treated with vasodilators or hyperbaric oxygen. A good response to hyperbaric oxygen can be predicted when tissue oxygen tension in the affected area is shown to be responsive to breathing oxygen.

SUMMARY

Prevention of contamination during operation is important, but contamination cannot always be controlled. Fortunately, wounds have defenses, and several of them can be preserved and protected by simply applied measures of clinical care.

REFERENCES

1. Barbul A, Caldwell M, Eaglstein W, et al: Wound Fluid: The Growth Environment. New York, Wiley, 1990.
2. Silver I: The measurement of oxygen tension in healing tissue. Prog Respir Res 3:124, 1969.
3. Niinikoski J, Grisilis G, Hunt T: Respiratory gas tensions and collagen in infected wounds. Ann Surg 175:588, 1972.
4. Barbul A, Regan M: Biology of Wound Healing. In Fischer J (ed): Surgical Basic Science. St Louis, Mosby, 1993, pp 67–73.
5. Simmons R, Steed D: Basic Science Review for Surgeons. Philadelphia, Saunders, 1992, pp 41–55.
6. Hunt T, Hussain M: Wound Microenvironment. In Cohen I, Diegelmann R, Lindblood W (eds): Wound Healing: Biochemical and Clinical Aspects. Philadelphia, Saunders, 1992, pp 274–281.
7. Hussain M, Ghani Q, Hunt T: Inhibition of prolyl hydroxylase by poly(ADP-ribose) and phosphoribosyl-AMP. Possible role of ADP-ribosylation in intracellular prolyl hydroxylase regulation. J Biol Chem 264(14):7850, 1989.
8. Beck L, Deguzman L, Lee W, et al: TGF-beta 1 accelerates wound healing: reversal of steroid-impaired healing in rats and rabbits. Growth Factors 5(4):295, 1991.
9. Spencer E, Skover G, Hunt T: Somatomedins: do they play a pivotal role in wound healing? Prog Clin Biol Res 266(103):103, 1988.
10. Hutton J, Tappel A, Udenfriend S: Cofactor and substrate requirements of collagen proline hydroxylase. Arch Biochem 118:231, 1967.
11. Barbul A, Lazarou S, Efron D: Arginine enhances wound healing in humans. Surgery 108:331, 1983.
12. Jensen J, Hunt T, Scheuenstuhl H, Banda M: Effect of lactate, pyruvate, and pH on secretion of angiogenesis and mitogenesis factors by macrophages. Lab Invest 54:574, 1986.
13. Metinko A, Kunkel S, Standiford T, Streiter R: Anoxia-hyperoxia induces monocyte-derived interleukin-8. J Clin Invest 90(3):791, 1992.
14. Ausprunk D, Folkman J: Migration and proliferation of endothelial cells in preformed and newly formed blood vessels during tumor angiogenesis. Microvasc Res 14:53, 1977.
15. Knighton D, Oredsson S, Banda M, Hunt T: Regulation of repair. Hypoxic control of macrophage-mediated angiogenesis. In Hunt T, Heppenstall R, Pines E, et al (eds): Soft and Hard Tissue Repair: Biological and Clinical Aspects. New York, Praeger Scientific Publications, 1984, pp 41–49.
16. Goodson WI, Hunt T: Wound healing and nutrition. In Kinney J, Jeejeebhoy K, Hill G, Owen O (eds): Nutrition and Metabolism in Patient Care. Philadelphia, Saunders, 1988, pp 635–642.
17. Brown G, Nanney L, Griffen J, et al: Enhancement of wound healing by topical treatment with epidermal growth factor. N Engl J Med 321(2):76, 1989.

18. Meakins J: Host defense mechanisms, wound healing, and infection. In Hunt T, Dunphy J (eds): Fundamentals of Wound Management. New York, Appleton-Century-Crofts, 1979, p 242.
19. Huizinga T, Roos D, von dem Borne A: Neutrophil Fc gamma receptors: a two-way bridge in the immune system. Blood 75:1211, 1990.
20. Meakins J: Alterations of host defenses in the surgical patient. In Simmons H (ed): Surgical Infectious Disease. Norwalk, CT, Appleton & Lange, 1988, pp 193–199.
21. Gallin J: Phagocytic cells: disorders of function. In Gallin J, Goldstein I, Snyderman R (eds): Inflammation: Basic Principles and Clinical Correlates. New York, Raven Press, 1988, pp 493–511.
22. Ehrlich H, Hunt T: Effects of cortisone and vitamin A on wound healing. Ann Surg 167:324, 1968.
23. Henson P, Henson J, Fittschen C, et al: Phagocytic granules: degranulation and secretion. In Gallin J, Goldstein I, Snyderman R (eds): Inflammation: Basic Principles and Clinical Correlates. New York, Raven Press, 1988, pp 363–390.
24. Klebanoff S: Myeloperoxidase-halide-hydrogen peroxide anti-bacterial system. J Bacteriol 95:2131, 1968.
25. Mandell G: Bactericidal activity of aerobic and anaerobic polymorphonuclear neutrophils. Infect Immun 9:337, 1974.
26. Babior B, Peters W: The superoxide-producing enzyme of human neutrophils. Further properties. J Biol Chem 256:2321, 1981.
27. Klebanoff S: Myeloperoxidase-mediated antimicrobial systems and their role in leukocyte functions. In Schultz J (ed): Biochemistry of the Phagocytic Process. Amsterdam, North Holland, 1970, pp 89–110.
28. Gabig T, Bearman S, Babior B: Effects of oxygen tension and pH on the respiratory burst of human neutrophils. Blood 53(6):1133, 1979.
29. Edwards S, Hallett M, Cambell A: Oxygen-radical production during inflammation may be limited by oxygen concentration. Biochem J 217(3):851, 1984.
30. Elek S: Experimental staphylococcal infections in the skin of man. Ann NY Acad Sci 65:85, 1956.
31. La Van F, Hunt T: Oxygen and wound healing. Clin Plast Surg 17(3):463, 1990.
32. Pollock A: Laparotomy. R Soc Med 74(7):480, 1981.
33. Paty P, Graeff R, Waldman F, et al: Biologic priming of neutrophils in subcutaneous wounds. Arch Surg 123(12):1509, 1988.
34. Hohn D, Ponce B, Burton R, Hunt T: Antimicrobial systems of the surgical wound, I. A comparison of oxidative metabolism and microbicidal capacity of phagocytes from wounds and from peripheral blood. Am J Surg 133:597, 1977.
35. Wakefield C, Carey P, Foulds S, et al: Polymorphonuclear leukocyte activation. An early marker of the postsurgical sepsis response. Arch Surg 128:390, 1993.
36. Paiement G, Hymes R, LaDouceur M, et al: Perioperative infections in asymptomatic HIV-seropositive orthopaedic patients. J Bone Joint Surg (in press).
37. Wilmore D, Goodwin C, Aulick L, et al: Effect of injury and infection on visceral metabolism and circulation. Ann Surg 192:491, 1980.
38. Deitch E, Wheelahan T, Rose M, et al: Hypertrophic burn scars: analysis of variables. J Trauma 23(10):895, 1983.
39. Windsor J, Knight G, Hill G: Wound healing response in surgical patients: recent food intake is more important than nutritional status. Br J Surg 75(2):135, 1988.
40. Reilly P, Bulkley G: Vasoactive mediators and splanchnic perfusion. Crit Care Med 21:S55, 1993.
41. Van Esbroeck G, Gys T, Hubens A: Evaluation of tissue oximetry in perioperative monitoring of colorectal surgery. Br J Surg 79(6):584, 1992.
42. Niinikoski J, Kutilla K: Adequacy of tissue oxygen in cardiac surgery: regional measurements. Crit Care Med 21(2 Suppl):S77, 1993.
43. Jensen J, Riggs K, Vasconez L, et al: Clinical assessment of postoperative peripheral perfusion. Surg Forum 38:66, 1987.

Technical Factors in the Prevention of Wound Infections*

CHAPTER 24

Richard F. Edlich, George T. Rodeheaver, John G. Thacker

The ultimate goal of the surgeon is to restore the physical integrity and function of injured or diseased tissue. Whether the tissue injury will be limited to the initial wound depends on the outcome of the interaction between the microbial contaminants and the traumatized tissue. A catastrophic outcome can be averted by well-devised surgical care in both the making of an operative wound and in the treatment of an accidental one. The major focus of this chapter is on traumatic soft tissue wounds, but the principles are applicable to all wounds.

MECHANISM OF INJURY

The outcome of both accidental and operative injury can be predicted by applying the physical concepts of power, work, and force. Surgery simply employs various principles of energy transfer in a planned procedure. Traumatic injuries are caused by the same energy source, even though the incidents are uncontrolled. If the surgeon does not control the sources of energy used, an operation becomes an assault similar to a traumatic injury. The surgeon must also be aware of the consequences of uncontrolled amounts of energy exerted on tissues, as occurs in accidental injury, and treat the resultant wound appropriately. Wounded tissue is more susceptible to infection than unwounded tissue.[1] The amount of susceptibility to infection will vary with the mechanism of wounding.

Mechanical Energy

Shear. Three mechanical forces can lead to soft tissue injury: shear, tension, and compression. To divide tissue with scissors, the surgeon applies a carefully controlled shearing force of equal magnitude, in opposite directions, in two adjacent parallel planes separated by a small distance. A scalpel cuts tissue by applying a shearing force in only one direction. Because the volume of tissue contacted by these instruments is extremely small, little total energy is required to produce tissue failure.

* This research has been supported by a generous grant from the Texaco Foundation, White Plains, NY.

A ritual practice in surgery has been to discard the sharp blade following its use on skin, in the fear that it introduces skin contaminants into the depths of the wound. Jacobs[2] reported that scalpels are almost always sterile subsequent to cutting skin and need not be discarded. The influence of the use of only one knife, instead of two knives, on the postoperative wound infection rate was not evaluated in this study. Hasselgren et al[3] initiated the first controlled clinical trial where the incidence of wound infections was recorded following the use of one or two knives for the skin incision. When the skin incision was made by only one knife, the incidence of infection in 277 patients was 3.6 percent. A comparable rate of infection (5.5 percent) was encountered in 309 patients whose skin incisions were made by two separate knives. This difference between the infection rates in these two groups of patients was not significant.

Despite the many technical advances in scalpel design, the ultimate performance of the scalpel rests with the surgeon. The experienced surgeon can cut to the desired depth with one sweep of the blade. One million or more bacteria are necessary to elicit infection in such a wound.[4] This level of host resistance is comparable to that encountered in nearly 80 percent of traumatic soft tissue injuries. Such injuries are caused by a piece of metal or glass and are recognized by their characteristic linear configuration. Wounds made with multiple strokes of the knife damage a greater volume of tissue, impair local defenses, and invite infection with much smaller microbial inocula.

Tension and Compression. When a wound is caused by a collision of two bodies, the mechanisms of injury are predominantly compression, tension, or both, rather than shear. In either case, two forces of equal magnitude are applied in opposite directions and act in the same plane. The injury is caused by tension force when a flat body hits soft tissue not supported by underlying bone. Compressive force operates when a flat body hits soft tissue overlying bone.

The energy required for tissue failure as a result of these forces is considerably greater than that for shear forces because the energy is distributed over a larger volume of tissue. The amount of energy absorbed by tissue during an impact can be calculated by the following equation:

$$T = \frac{MV^2}{2}$$

where T equals kinetic energy (joules, J), M equals mass of impacting object (kilograms, kg), V equals relative velocity between the impacting object and tissue (meters/second, m/s). Obviously, changes in the relative velocity of the object that impacts have a greater influence on the level of kinetic energy than do variations in the mass of the object.

Blunt Trauma

When the mechanism of injury is compression, tissue failure occurs at energy levels of 2.52 J/cm^2, which is comparable to the energy encountered with a car going 8 km/h strikes a tree[5]; the momentum of the collision causes the victim's head, weighing approximately 4 kg, to hit the dashboard with an area of impact approximately 8 cm^2. The absorbed level of energy disrupts the skin, resulting in a characteristic stellate laceration. In addition, the wound edges are damaged and rendered relatively ischemic. Wounds caused by impact injuries are 100 times more susceptible to infection than wounds caused by shear forces, and immediate antibiotic treatment is warranted to suppress the growth of the bacterial contaminants. Even then, antibiotic efficacy is substantially less than in contaminated wounds caused by shear forces.

Although impact injuries with energy levels lower than 2.54 J/cm^2 do not result in division of the skin, they can result in disruption of the vessels in the skin and underlying tissue. The vascular injury to the skin manifests clinically as ecchymosis. Disruption of vessels in the underlying tissue results in a hematoma. Some hematomas will resorb, but those that become encapsulated usually require surgical treatment. Left untreated, such hematomas may result in permanent subcutaneous deformity. When still in the currant jelly stage, a hematoma is best treated by incision and drainage. As further liquefaction occurs, aspiration with large-bore needle (18-gauge or larger) may be possible.

Missile Injury

A collision between a missile and the human body represents a considerably higher level of energy absorption per unit volume of tissue than that encountered in automobile accidents. The interaction of missile and human combines shear, tensile, and compressive forces. The two mechanisms of tissue disruption caused by a penetrating missile are the permanent and temporary cavities. The penetrating missile or fragment destroys tissue by crushing it during penetrating and punches a hole through the tissue. This hole or missile track is the permanent cavity. The cross-sectional area of the missile track is similar to the presenting area of the missile, and its dimensions are comparable for all soft tissues tested.

After passage of the missile, the walls of the permanent cavity are stretched outward radially. The maximum lateral tissue displacement delineates the temporary cavity. Tissue stretch is responsible for the damage of temporary cavitation. The tissue's resistance to stretch depends on tissue elasticity. The same stretch that causes moderate contusion and functional changes in relatively elastic muscle, skin, lung, and bowel wall can cause catastrophic disruption of the liver, heart, and brain. Muscle, skin, bowel wall, and lung are flexible and elastic, having the physical characteristics of good energy absorbers. These permanent and temporary activities are the sole wounding mechanisms of missiles. The sonic shock wave generated by supersonic missiles does not cause either tissue displacement or detectable damage. A method of capturing the entire projectile-tissue interaction in ordinance gelatin (25 cm × 25 cm × 50 cm blocks of a 10 percent by weight concentration shot at 4C), which has been calibrated to reproduce the crush and stretch encountered in living animal muscle, was developed at the Letterman Army Institute.[6] Comparison of the wound profiles in the gelatin tissue simulant showed the fallacy in attempting to judge wound severity with velocity alone because some low-velocity missiles produced substantial temporary cavities. Generalizations based on missile velocity do not recognize the basic fact that in the projectile-tissue interactions a minimum of five variables—projectile mass, projectile shape, projectile construction, projectile fragmentation, and target tissue type—are involved. Projectile fragmentation can greatly enhance the temporary cavity effects by providing points of weakness on which the stretching effects of cavitation are focused rather than being absorbed evenly by the tissue mass. A muscle, which tolerates a temporary cavity stretch from a nonfragmenting bullet with little gross disruption, is severely damaged when the stretch comes after it has been penetrated by a fragmenting bullet.[7]

Firearms include two basic types: rifled firearm and shotgun. A rifled firearm, pistol and rifle, has spiral grooves in its barrel and discharges hot gases, soot, powder grains, and a bullet. Rifled bullets are rotated around their long axes by the rifling of the barrel to give them sufficient gyroscopic stability to maintain the point-forward position traveling through air. Bullets fired from a properly designed rifled barrel yaw (the yaw angle is the angle between the bullet's long axis and the line of flight) no more than a few degrees in flight. This gyroscopic rotation, however, may be insufficient to stabilize bullet point-forward travel in tissue with the development of bullet yaw in tissue, which can be an important determinant of injury.

Most handgun projectiles strike tissue at a speed below 274 m/s. At this velocity, the predominant mechanism of tissue injury is the permanent cavity. There is some temporary cavitation, but tissue displacement is so small that there is no clinically detectable damage. Bullet shape, construction, and yaw make little difference at this velocity.

Rifle bullets are the nonexpanding and expanding types. The nonexpanding rifle bullets are designed primarily for military use and strike tissue at speeds between 610 and 914 m/s. No deformation of the bullet occurs unless bone is struck. Nonexpanding bullets make a 180-degree rotation around their short axes (yaw) and terminate by traveling in a base-forward position. The distance traveled in tissue by a particular bullet before it begins rotation around its short axis is a relatively constant characteristic. The increase in size of the permanent cavity by the yawing bullet is determined by how much tissue the bullet strikes traveling sideways. As the bullet yaws, there is also marked increase in the temporary cavitation.

Most bullets of the expanding variety (soft-point or hollow-point), used for hunting, are designed to deform on striking the tissue. They produce a marked increase in the size of the permanent cavity that occurs at a shallower depth. The expanding bullet also causes a large temporary cavity for the same reason as the yawing bullet. For expanding bullets striking at over 762 m/s, bullet fragmentation causes the major part of the permanent tissue destruction. As pieces of the bullet break off, they are flung radically outward by the centrifugal force of bullet rotation. Each fragment crushes its own path through tissue, ending up as far as 8 cm from its original path. This tissue, perforated multiple times, is stretched by temporary cavitation. This synergy between fragmentation and the temporary cavity causes massive tissue destruction.

Shotguns differ from rifles and pistols in that they have a smooth barrel that discharges hot gases, wad, and either multiple projectiles or a single projectile (rifle slug).[8] Shot charges containing multiple projectiles spread out from the muzzle in a cone-like pattern. The distance from the muzzle of the shotgun to the point of impact of the projectiles is a key determinant of the magnitude of injury. At a short range of less than 6 m, the shot charge containing multiple projectiles results predominantly in a single hole in shootwound (diameter of 6 cm or less) that communicates with a deep underlying wound with massive tissue destruction. At this short range, soft tissue impact deforms the individual pellets, increasing their original cross-section with concomitant increase in tissue crush or hole size. The multiple pellets result in severe disruption of anatomy by direct crush and in damage to the tissue blood supply between the multiple wound channels. A gradual decrease in the amount of pellet deformation and tissue destruction occurs as the distance of the impact range increases. When the impact range exceeds 7 m, the multiple projectiles result in numerous discrete wounds that are not associated with underlying massive tissue destruction.

Shotguns also can discharge rifled slugs that are designed for killing larger animals. The muzzle velocity of a rifled slug (487 m/s) is approximately half that of a nonexpanding, fully jacketed rifle projectile. The rifled slug will not hold the point orientation that it has as it propels from the muzzle of the gun but will drift toward a sideways orientation as it moves toward the target. The rifled slug experiences a 25 percent decrease in velocity as the impact range increases from 5 to 45 m. At short range (45 m or less), the slug deforms on striking the tissue, thereby enhancing the size of the permanent and temporary cavities.[9]

The surgeon is unlikely to know the properties of the wounding projectile (shape, mass, construction type, and striking velocity) and will have to base the treatment on an objective evaluation of the wound.[10] Even if the surgeon appreciates these properties, a point worth reiterating is that the surgeon is best advised to treat the wound and not the weapon. Gunshot wounds are managed in the same manner as in other trauma in that the amount and location of tissue disruption are determined by physical examination and appropriate radiographic studies. Determination of the missile's path through the body is a major concern. Because most penetrating projectiles follow a relatively straight course through the tissue, an estimate of the missile's path can be made from the location of the entrance and exit wounds or the position at which the expended projectile comes to rest within the body. In most cases, physical examination and biplanar x-ray films establish these points and allow clinical estimation of the structures that might have been damaged. In some cases, oblique x-ray films may be needed, and it may be impossible to establish with certainty whether penetration of a body cavity may have occurred. When it is uncertain whether the peritoneal cavity has been penetrated by abdominal wall wounds, it is prudent to perform a laparotomy rather than to wait and see. Bullet fragmentation and its correlative severe tissue destruction are especially useful x-ray signs. A rifle missile that causes extensive damage to the muscles of the shoulder girdle or that strikes the bone may be expected to cause a pulmonary contusion without penetration of the pleural cavity. The surgeon must be aware of this potentially life-threatening complication and must assure adequate follow-up observation and treatment.

Electrical Energy

Electricity is the flow of electrons from one atom to another, and electrons set in motion by electric force (voltage) collide with each other and generate heat. The amount of heat developed by a conductor varies directly with its resistance. The magnitude of resistance to electron flow varies widely in different tissues, for example, the high resistance of skin and low resistance of muscle to electron flow. The control and localization of the heating effect of electric current comprise the fundamental basis for electrosurgery.

The frequency of the current generated in electrosurgery is 250,000 to 2 million hertz (Hz), and its ability to damage tissue depends on its concentration or density. As the current density increases, its heating effect becomes more pronounced. For example, the size of the active monopolar electrode is deliberately kept small so that concentrated heating will occur at its point of contact with tissue. Following contact, the current is dispersed to the return (ground) electrode, which encounters low-current density and no tissue heating. The distribution of the current can be more carefully controlled by making the active electrode bipolar, usually in the form of forceps, so that the tissue through which the current will pass is precisely delineated. An equivalent current passed through a monopolar electrode causes approximately three times as much necrosis of the surrounding tissue as the use of bipolar coagulation.[11]

Wounds made by electrosurgery are approximately three times more susceptible to infection than wounds made with a stainless steel scalpel (Fig. 24–1).[12] In a prospective clinical study by Cruse and Foord,[13] the use of electrosurgery almost doubled the infection rates of operative wounds. Electrosurgery should not be used for cutting skin and subcutaneous tissue, because of the increased susceptibility of such wounds to infection.

In massive excisional operations (eg, large soft tissue tumors, debridement of third-degree burns), the threat of blood loss frequently outweighs the potential problems of subsequent infection. Levine et al[14] reported the blood loss and operating time were

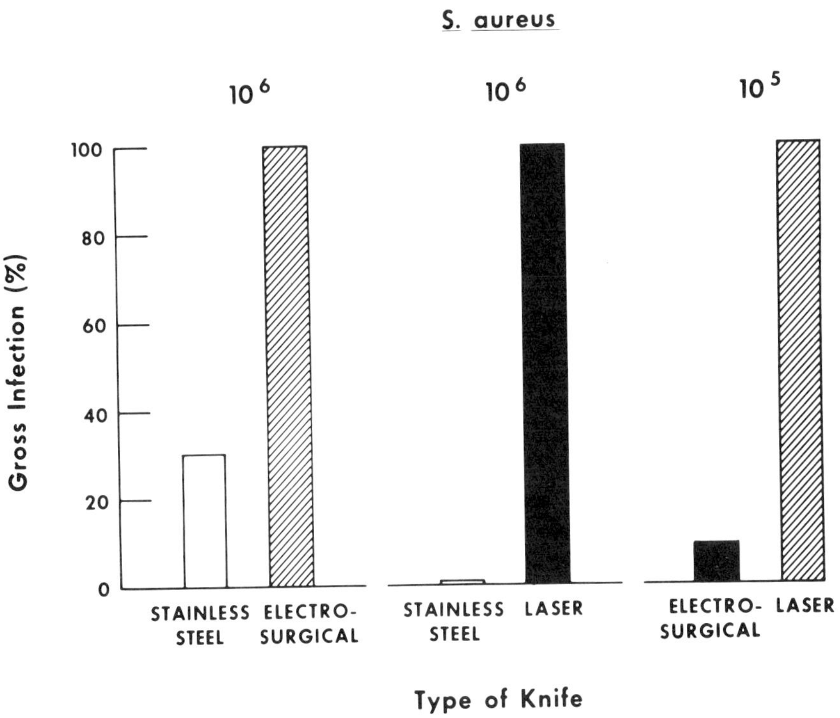

Figure 24–1. Standardized wounds made by either a stainless steel, electrosurgical, or laser knife were contaminated with a specified dose of *Staphylococcus aureus.* Four days later the incidence of gross infection was significantly greater in wounds made by the bloodless knives than those made by the stainless steel scalpel.

halved during electrosurgical excision of burn wounds when compared to scalpel excision.

When the oscillations are damped, hemostasis is achieved without cutting. This type of current causes a rapid dehydration of living cells, and the affected tissue is fused into a hyalinized mass. We prefer pinpoint electrosurgical coagulation of small bleeding vessels to suture ligation, but the power should be kept to the absolute minimum needed for vessel thrombosis.

Hemostasis must be accomplished with the least amount of electrocoagulation and suture material. The best method to control oozing and/or bleeding is to exert gentle continual pressure on the bleeding surface with sponges moistened with cool saline. Rubbing or abrading the tissue will dislodge thrombi and can cause further bleeding. Furthermore, hot (150F), wet sponges should never be used for hemostasis. In animals, this treatment causes hyperthermic injury to tissue and potentiates the development of infection.[15]

From surgery's beginning and well into the 19th century, cautery heated over a bed of hot coals was regularly prepared to control hemorrhage as well as to serve as an antiputrefactive agent. Modern surgeons can now cut tissue with a new heated scalpel whose temperature can be controlled within narrow limits. Levenson and colleagues[16] reported that the heated scalpel allowed excision of third-degree burns in pigs and human subjects with much smaller blood loss compared with the usually cold scalpel. Skin grafts applied immediately after excision had excellent rates of success similar to those of grafts applied immediately after excision with the unheated scalpel. These investigators[16] reported that the heated knife did not interfere with the wounds' ability to resist infection. In wounds in experimental animals made by either a heated or unheated scalpel and then contaminated with 100 million *Pseudomonas aeruginosa* or *Staphylococcus aureus*, no wound infection developed in either group. The absence of infection in wounds made either by the heated or unheated scalpel is difficult to explain because the inoculum used was 100 times greater than the infective dose for these pathogens in soft tissues. Consequently, inoculation of 100 million organisms should have resulted in gross evidence of infection in all wounds. Moreover, Levenson and colleagues[16] reported that the heated scalpel produced limited adverse effects on wound repair. Using a temperature of 180C, the breaking strengths of wounds made by the hot scalpel did not differ significantly from those in wounds made by the cold scalpel 7, 14, 25, 28, and 42 days after wounding. The only statistically significant difference ($P < 0.05$) between the breaking strengths of incision made by the unheated scalpel and the heated scalpel was noted at 21 days and was modestly in favor of the conventional scalpel. The innocuous effects of the heated scalpel could not be confirmed by our laboratory.[17] Using scalpels heated to a considerably lower temperature than that employed in the study of Levenson et al,[16] we found that the heated knife damaged the wound's resistance to infection and interfered with healing.

Radiant Energy

Radiant or electromagnetic energy can be used as a scalpel. This energy consists of photons that are both waves and particles. Once absorbed by tissue, radiant energy is converted into heat, which, applied to a small volume of tissue, divides it bloodlessly. The concept of light as a source of energy is realized in lasers.

The hemostatic effect of the laser scalpel makes it especially suitable for massive excisions. Blood loss encountered by scalpel excisions is nearly 3.3 times greater than the blood loss following the use of laser energy.[14] Electrosurgical excision has 1.67 times the blood loss of laser excision. The superior hemostatic effect of the laser over that of electrosurgery is associated with increased damage to the tissue defenses. Experimental wounds made by a laser are approximately tenfold more susceptible to infection than those made by electrosurgery (see Fig. 24–1).[12] Fortunately, the tissue damage resulting from either electrosurgery or the laser does not interfere with the take of either autografts or homografts on wound beds with low bacterial counts (less than 10^6 bacteria per gram of tissue).

BIOLOGY OF TISSUE INFECTION

The development of infection is a function of the interaction of several factors—the nature and degree of local contamination and both local and systemic resistance of the patient to infection.[18] The term *infected* refers to a wound that exhibits the classic signs of inflammation (calor, rubor, tumor, dolor) as a result of microbial contamination. In contrast, *contamination* refers only to the viable and nonviable foreign bodies within the wound that have as yet failed to elicit inflammation.

Influence of Bacterial Number

In experimental animals, the critical infective dose of a pure culture of obligate and facultative aerobic bacteria in wounds is 1 million bacteria, or greater, per gram of tissue; below this level, wounds heal without infection.[4] This remarkable resistance to infection has been identified in all soft tissues tested.[4] The type of aerobic bacteria contaminating a wound surface is less important in the development of infection than the number of bacteria. Apparent clinical differences in virulence may be based on ecologic advantages possessed by the pathogens and may not reflect specific differences in the host-parasite relationship.

In the presence of normal host defenses, pure cultures of obligate anaerobic bacteria rarely cause infection. The research of Kelly[19] and Ingham et al[20] clearly demonstrated that a bacterial synergy existed between obligate anaerobic bacteria and facultative organisms that resulted in serious infections. Kelly[19] found that guinea pig skin wounds were relatively susceptible to *Escherichia coli*, but not to *Bacteroides fragilis*. Inoculation of the skin wounds with 10^7 *E. coli* caused sepsis and death in 48 hours. Pure cultures (10^8) of *B. fragilis* never caused death. At 1 week, wounds contaminated by *B. fragilis* developed a moderate degree of wound induration.

Wound inoculation with fewer *E. coli* (10^4) caused minimal wound induration and no deaths. Wound challenged with 10^4 *B. fragilis* also caused minimal induration and no deaths. When these small inocula of *B. fragilis* and *E. coli* were added to the wound, they produced marked inflammation, purulent discharge, and clinical evidence of sepsis. The phenomenon of bacterial synergy was further evaluated by demonstrating that when pus had been formed, the wounds contained large and strikingly similar quantities of both organisms (10^7 to 10^9).

The mechanism of bacterial synergy has yet to be elucidated and may well depend on an interrelationship between the electrode potential (E_h) and induced inhibition of phagocytosis. Ingham et al[20] demonstrated that a variety of species of obligate anaerobes interfered with the phagocytosis measured in vitro by the uptake of *Proteus mirabilis* and other aerobic bacteria by human leukocytes. These studies help to explain why the prophylactic use of an essentially anti-anaerobic drug, such as metronidazole, has been successful despite its relative inactivity against the facultative component of mixed bacterial flora. Unless quantitative microbiologic techniques are performed under strict anaerobic conditions (rarely achieved in hospital laboratories), the presence and number of these organisms cannot be appreciated.

This relationship between bacterial counts and clinical wound infection has been a stimulus for the development of quantitative tissue bacteriologic techniques.[21,22] These measurements are initiated by excising a 2 cm × 1 cm × 0.5 cm sample of tissue, which weighs approximately 0.5 g. Because some anaerobic bacteria may not tolerate exposure to oxygen, the tissue specimen is placed immediately in an anaerobic transport vial. All fluids, including pus and exudates, are collected also in a sterile syringe that is introduced separately into the anaerobic transport vial. The specimens are taken promptly to the bacteriology laboratory for quantitative bacterial measurements and antibiotic sensitivity testing. The specimens are processed under anaerobic conditions, preferably in an anaerobic glove box. They are weighed in a measured amount of sterile prereduced salt solution that will also be used for the serial dilutions. The tissue specimens may be macerated with a knife, though homogenization with a sterile rotor knife blade is simpler.

Direct microscopic examination of an aliquot of the bacterial suspensions provides an estimate of the total number and morphology of the viable and dead bacteria in the suspension. The major advantage of this technique is the speed with which the results are available to the surgeon—within 20 minutes after obtaining the specimen. These findings will suggest appropriate antimicrobial therapy until the culture and antimicrobial susceptibility results are available and also provide an appropriate means of quality control. For example, if morphotypes observed in the smear do not appear in the culture, the collection, culturing, or subculturing procedures may have been defective. Results of the microscopic examination should be reported immediately to the surgeon.

This rapid technique gives accurate and reliable measurement when 400 or more bacteria are in the 0.01 ml suspension delivered to the slide (more than 2.5×10^5 organisms per gram of tissue). When less than this number of bacteria is added to the slide, bacteria are not detected on microscopic examination. The development of this technique does not replace quantitative serial dilution and plating techniques. These latter techniques are always performed concomitantly with the rapid slide technique because they allow specification of the pathogen and antibiotic sensitivity testing. Antibiotic susceptibility of cultured isolates then can be determined and species identification made. Quantitative bacteriology, consisting of the rapid slide technique as well as serial dilution and plating, is now used routinely by surgeons in our medical center to predict the safety of wound closure (both primary and delayed primary),[21] to determine graft bed receptivity, and to diagnose the onset of burn wound sepsis.[22]

Systemic Host Factors in the Resistance to Infection

The quantitative relationship between the host's resistance to infection and the number of bacteria can be upset by both systemic and local factors. Of the systemic factors, advancing age appears to be one of the most important, increasing infection rate. Infection rates are reported to be higher in patients with diabetes mellitus, obesity, or malnutrition and in those receiving steroid therapy.[18] Shock, remote trauma, or distant infection also enhance wound infection.[23–25] In addition, rare immunologic deficiencies, both primary and secondary, contribute to a diminished host resistance (see Chap. 51).[26]

Local Factors in Resistance to Infection

Local factors are especially important in determining the outcome of the interaction between the host and bacteria. Whether present by accident or intention, any foreign body in the wound damages the local tissue's defenses and invites infection. The magnitude of this damage appears to be related to the chemical reactivity of the foreign body. Soil and dirt are frequent contaminants in traumatic injuries. Although it has been recognized for centuries that severe bacterial infection often develops in wound containing dirt and soil, only recently has the role of these contaminants been clarified.[27] Specific infection-potentiating fractions have now been identified in soil, which include its organic components as well as inorganic clay fractions. For wounds contaminated by these fractions, only 100 bacteria per gram of tissue will elicit infection. The ability of these fractions to enhance the incidence of infection appears to be related to their damage to host defenses:

1. In the presence of these fractions, leukocytes are not able to ingest and kill bacteria[28]—a result of a direct interaction between the highly charged soil particles and white blood cells.
2. Soil infection-potentiating fractions also eliminate the nonspecific bactericidal activity in serum.
3. These highly charged anionic particles also react chemically with amphoteric and basic antibiotics, limiting their activity in contaminated wounds.

The concentration of these fractions in soil can be correlated with their location. Environmental conditions in swamps and marshes encourage the production of soil with as much as 98 percent organic infection-potentiating fractions. The major inorganic infection-potentiating particles are the clay fractions, which reside in heaviest concentration in the subsoil rather than in topsoil. Hence traumatic soft tissue injuries that occur in swamps or excavations run a high risk of being contaminated by these fractions, which predispose the wound to serious infection.

A corollary to these observations is that some soil contaminants, such as sand grains, are relatively innocuous. This fraction, which has a large particle size and a low level of chemical reactivity, causes considerably less damage to tissue defenses. Surprisingly, the black dirt on the surface of highways appears to have minimal chemical reactivity.

TECHNICAL FACTORS IN THE PREVENTION OF WOUND INFECTIONS

When caring for a traumatic wound, the surgeon must make judgments that frequently tip the balance in favor of either infection or healing per primum. The following specific recommendations for management of the surgical wound are based on the best currently available clinical and experimental studies.

Local Anesthesia

Cleansing of bacteria and other debris from traumatic injuries and debridement cannot be accomplished without the administration of anesthetics. The selection of the anesthetic agent for infiltration anesthesia is based on pharmacologic and toxicologic considerations.[29] The pharmacodynamic properties of these agents include severity of pain elicited by the injection of the agent, onset and duration of anesthetic activity, and frequency of satisfactory anesthesia. The toxicologic manifestations of local anesthetic agents are almost exclusively local complications (eg, damage to tissue defenses) because when these agents are absorbed systemically, they do not clinically affect organ systems other than the peripheral nerves. Because the amide type of local anesthetic agents appears to be relatively free of sensitivity and allergic reactions characteristic of the ester-type derivative, surgeons usually use amide-type agents (lidocaine and bupivacaine) for infiltration anesthesia. These anesthetic agents do not damage tissue defenses or invite infection. In addition, the pain of subdermal injection, the onset of anesthesia, and the frequency of satisfactory anesthesia are remarkably similar. Clinical studies by Christoph and colleagues[30] have demonstrated that the pain of administration of local anesthetics can be reduced dramatically by pH buffering of the local anesthetic agents before injection. Because the duration of local anesthesia induced by bupivacaine is nearly four times longer than that by lidocaine, bupivacaine is recommended for infiltration anesthesia.[29]

The duration of anesthetic activity of these agents can be enhanced by the addition of the vasoconstrictor epinephrine, which slows the clearance of the agent from the tissue, thereby prolonging the duration of anesthesia. This benefit must be weighed against its deleterious effects on tissue defenses; epinephrine will damage local tissue defenses. The infection-potentiating effect of this powerful local vasoconstrictor is proportional to its concentration and results from its vasoactivity.[31] As a result of its vasoconstrictive action, epinephrine may result in hypoxic conditions that limit white blood cell function. In vitro studies by Hohn and associates[32] and Mandell[33] demonstrated that hypoxia retards killing of *S. aureus* by wound leukocytes. Consequently, this increased infection rate of wounds treated with epinephrine may result from impaired killing of bacterial contaminants by wound leukocytes in the ischemic wounds. This damage to tissue defenses argues against the use of epinephrine in potentially heavily contaminated wounds.

Although infiltration and regional anesthesia remain the most common techniques, topical anesthesia of lacerations is gaining increasing popularity. Until the report of Pryor and his colleagues,[34] current clinical use of topical anesthetic agents had been limited to mucous membranes. In their clinical study, they indicated that skin lacerations should be anesthetized by a topical solution containing 0.5 percent tetracaine, 1:2000 epinephrine, and 11.8 percent cocaine (TEC). In their randomized prospective study involving a relatively small number of patients (138), TEC offered distinct advantages over infiltration anesthesia using 1 percent lidocaine. The most important advantage of this topical anesthetic agent was that it resulted in anesthesia without the discomfort associated with the injection of infiltration anesthesia. The injected anesthetic agent also caused considerable swelling and distortion of the wound, making meticulous approximation or the wound edges more difficult. An additional benefit of TEC was its intense vasoconstrictive effect that resulted in a bloodless wound. The vasoconstrictive effect was so profound that the investigators did not use this topical anesthetic agent in lacerations involving the ear, penis, and digits to avoid compromising their limited vascularity. This hemostatic effect of TEC may, however, limit access of the body's defenses to the wound and thereby decrease the wound's resistance to infection. This increased potential for infection of TEC-treated wounds was not evident in the small clinical study of Pryor et al.[34]

In a recent experimental study reported by Barker et al,[35] topical application of TEC damaged the local wound defenses and encouraged the development of infection. The increased incidence of infection in contaminated wounds treated with TEC was associated with necrosis of the wound edges. The infection-potentiating effect of TEC was probably related to its vasoconstrictive action, which was easily identified by the intravenous injection of fluorescein dye. This vasoconstrictive effect of TEC can be blocked by the addition of phentolamine to the solution. The potential dangers of the vasoconstrictive action of TEC is consistent with the toxicity of other vasoconstrictors studied in our laboratory.[1]

Hair Removal

The practice of hair removal may influence the likelihood of surgical infection. Since the days of Lister and Semmelweis, skin hair has been regarded as a source of contamination, and recent work supports this belief.[36] Removal of hair also facilitates operative surgery by preventing hair from becoming entangled in sutures and the wound during closure. However, the practice of razor preparation of the operative site has been challenged in recent studies.

In prospective clinical study, Seropian and Reynolds[37] reported that the infection rate of surgical patients after razor preparation was 5.6 percent as compared to 0.6 percent after a depilatory. These findings agree with those reported by Cruse and Foord.[13] In a 5-year prospective study of 23,649 surgical wounds the infection rate was 2.3 percent in the patients shaved. The incidence of infection fell to 0.9 percent in the patients who were not shaved or clipped.

In a recent study, Alexander and his colleagues[38] demonstrated that the technique and timing of hair removal have considerable influence on the incidence of postoperative infection. In their prospective study, Alexander et al[38] compared the wound infection rate in patients subjected to hair removal by either an electric clipper or razor. Patients were prospectively randomized to be either shaved or clipped the night before or the morning of the operation. Clipping the hair the morning of the operation was associated with significantly fewer infections than were encountered in patients whose hair was removed either by electric clippers the night before the operation or by shaving. These investigators concluded that preoperative shaving was deleterious and that the practice should be abandoned. Moreover, removal of hair with electric clippers immediately before surgery was recommended. The increased incidence of infection after razor shaves is probably related to the trauma inflicted by the razor. A safety razor consists of a blade held in a fixed position by the head. The exposure of the blade with respect to the razor head is the most important determinant of the blade's performance. The exposure of the surgical prep razor blade is so great that the infundibulum of the hair follicle is transected, so that the wounded hair follicles provide access and substrate for bacteria. In addition, the impermeable corneal layer is damaged and the exudate provides a moist field for bacterial proliferation. Inoculation of shaved skin results in dermatitis. In contrast, skin shaved with a recessed blade is refractory to bacterial contamination.

Hair removal by depilatories has been reported to be an effective method that does not enhance the risk of infection.[37] This potential benefit of depilatories, however, must be weighed against some shortcomings. A depilatory should not be used near a patient's eyes or genitalia because it can seriously irritate these tissues. Inadvertent spillage of the depilatory into the wound must be avoided because it can give rise to a prolonged inflammatory response and delayed healing.[39] In rare cases (1.3 percent), the depilatory causes severe dermatitis that necessitates postponement of surgery.[37]

Recent advances in the design of surgical clippers have made them especially suitable for preoperative hair removal. The clipper blade assembly can easily be removed from its mounting assembly on the electric motor so that it can be cleaned and sterilized. Sterilization of the clipper blade assemblies for electric clippers eliminates the high level of bacterial contamination encountered after repeated use that is a potential source of infection.[40] The fine teeth of its 0000 blade assembly cuts hair close to the skin surface without nicking the skin. Because this atraumatic removal of hair by electric clippers is associated with a lower incidence of infection, we now use electric clippers to remove hair before surgery and have abandoned the use of preoperative shaving.

Antisepsis

The term *antisepsis* refers to the use of antimicrobial chemicals on human tissue, while *disinfection* applies to the use of these agents on inanimate objects. In addition to an antiseptic agent, surgical scrub solutions contain a detergent or surface active agent, which facilitates removal of the surface contaminants. The clinical efficacy of an antiseptic agent can be evaluated by several parameters, including (1) the effect of storage, (2) its spectrum of activity, (3) its duration of antimicrobial activity, (4) the degree of local and systemic damage to the host, and (5) the influence of the carrier on the performance of the agent.

Not all antiseptic agents are used for the same purpose, nor should the requirements for their effectiveness be identical. Specific definitions for the antimicrobial product categories were established in a report by an advisory review panel on over-the-counter antimicrobial drug products for repeated daily use.[41] This report provides detailed information regarding hand washing, surgical skin wound cleansers, and patient preoperative skin preparation.

Hand Washing. Hands are the leading vector of pathogenic bacteria to the wound. Hands can transmit an infective dose of bacteria during any patient care activity (shaving, marking, lifting) conducted before and after the operation or through punctured gloves during the procedure. Glove punctures are found after 5 to 60 percent of all operations.[42]

Normally, the organisms are quite sparse on the palms and dorsa of the hands, numbering hundreds per square centimeter. Most organisms (10,000 to 100,000) on the hands reside beneath the distal end of the nail plate or adjacent to the proximal or lateral nail folds. These recesses frustrate efforts to disinfect the hands.

Before and after patient contact, hand washing is mandatory, even though the risk of acquiring an infective dose of bacteria from patients during routine physical examination seems to be negligible. Washing one's hands for 15 seconds with any of a variety of agents, including tap water, removes large numbers of bacteria and significantly reduces the bacterial count.[43] The hands should be rinsed and then dried. Because rings and chipped nail polish make removal of organisms more difficult, operating room personnel should wear neither.[44]

Repeated use of an antiseptic agent before and after patient contact appears to be unwarranted and may occasionally lead to the development of dermatitis.[45] Ordinary bar soap appears to be an excellent alternative to antiseptic agents for routine hand washings, as long as the bars are small and keep on drainage racks between uses.

We favor antiseptic agents for special circumstances in which invasive procedures will be performed.[45] Hand washing with antiseptic agents should last at least 15 seconds, while surgical procedures require the greatest degree of hand antisepsis.

A variety of agents can be employed. Semmelweis in 1861 decreased the incidence of puerperal fever by ordering the medical students to wash their hands in chlorinated lime.[46] Lister degermed his hands in a 1:20 solution of carbolic acid. Until the 1950s, tincture of green soap followed by an alcohol rinse was used. Currently, three antiseptic agents have been advocated for hand washing before operation as well as preoperative patient skin preparation—hexachlorophene, iodophor, and chlorhexidene. Surgical scrubs of hands and forearms of adults, five times a day, with a 3 percent hexachlorophene preparation leaves blood levels of 0.5 mg/ml or higher in selected individuals after 10 days.[47] Because these levels are potentially toxic, hexachlorophene should not be used routinely by operating room personnel and should be dispensed only by prescription. Fortunately, both other solutions appear to be safe.[48,49] After hand washing with iodophor or chlorhexidene solutions, the bacterial counts of the skin are suppressed, and the buildup of microbial counts under the occlusive surgical glove is limited. Neither agent is superior.

The surgical hand wash should begin by cleaning the fingernails with a plastic stick. The hands should then be scrubbed with a sponge or brush for 5 minutes with a chlorhexidene or iodophor solution. The sponge causes less irritation to the skin.[50,51]

Dermatitis from any cause, including washing, results in a high concentration of skin bacteria.[51] Afflicted personnel who are members of the operating team should be limited to patient care not directly related to the operative procedure. During patient contact, personnel with dermatitis should wear gloves. The best treatment of this condition is to refrain from using an antiseptic agent or wearing gloves for longer than 5 minutes. Emollients added to hand creams should decrease or prevent dermatitis and dry skin, but there have been reports of contaminated hand creams, associated with nosocomial infections.[45] Consistent use of emollients on the hands after hospital duty rather than during the workday might be efficacious in preventing dermatitis while reducing the risk of these infections.

Gloves. The choice of the surgical glove for use in surgery is another important consideration. Surgeons and manufacturers have long searched for the ideal glove lubricant to ease in the manufacture and donning of the surgical glove. Water was used for glove lubrication until a dry powder lubricant was found to be more effective.[52] Talc was the first powder used for glove lubrication until studies demonstrated postoperative complications associated with the presence of talcum powder in the surgical site. Most studies linked talc to the formation of granulomas, fistulas, chronic sinus tracts, and adhesions in the peritoneal cavity of patients operated on by surgeons wearing talcum-lubricated gloves.

In 1947, Lee and Lehman[53] introduced cornstarch as a replacement for talc. They maintained that cornstarch was completely absorbed by tissues and therefore should not lead to the complications associated with talc. Subsequent experimental studies and clinical reports demonstrated that cornstarch was far from benign. These investigations established that cornstarch resulted in granulomas, adhesions, fibrosis, "starch peritonitis," and the formation of fistulas in the peritoneal cavity.[52,54] Complications were not isolated to the peritoneal cavity alone, as many of these studies reported granulomatous reactions following surgery of the eye, middle ear, cranial cavity, thorax, and the head and neck. Cornstarch is currently the only powder used in the manufacture of surgical and examination gloves.

Our recent experimental study demonstrated that cornstarch used specifically for the manufacture and lubrication of surgical gloves damaged local tissue defenses, thereby increasing the rate of bacterial growth and inflammation in contaminated wounds.[55] Using a standard experimental wound, contaminated wounds containing cornstarch exhibited wider indurated margins and increased numbers of bacteria as compared to control wounds subjected to a comparable level of bacterial inoculum. Despite the vast literature showing the potential toxicity of this powder, cornstarch continues to be used as a glove lubricant. When powdered gloves are used during wound closure, inadvertent contamination of the wound with cornstarch is likely, inviting serious wound complications. Realizing the potential toxicity of cornstarch, manufacturers have prepared warning labels on each glove packet advising surgeons to wash off the powder before use in wounds. Unfortunately, this method of powder removal is ineffective. Jagelman and Ellis[56] reported that washing reduced the number of starch granules but left significant cornstarch on the glove that appeared to aggregate as clumps. They postulated that the development of clumps of cornstarch would delay absorption and enhance the foreign-body reaction. Tolbert and Brown[57] provided further evidence that glove washing left a large portion of the cornstarch on the glove surface.

With the advent of powder-free surgical gloves, the use of surgical gloves coated with cornstarch should be discontinued. Several powder-free gloves are commercially available. The London Rubber Company (now London International) manufactures a rubber surgical glove lubricated by a layer of Biogel hydrogel polymer used in the manufacture of "soft" contact lenses.[52] A new method of injection molding of gloves (World Medical Supply, Inc.) has been developed that also results in a smooth surface, free of powder and other foreign bodies.[58] The ease of donning and tactile sensitivity of the powder-free gloves are comparable to those of standard powdered surgical gloves.[58]

In addition to the problems associated with surgical glove powders, there is recent concern about the safety of latex. Latex is a naturally occurring substance found in the sap of the rubber tree, *Heavea brasiliarus*. It is composed primarily of long-chain molecules and small amounts of protein (2 to 3 percent), some of which are water soluble. During processing of the latex, much of this protein fraction is removed. The soluble fraction can be eluted from the glove surface during the leaching process, but inadequate leaching can result in high levels of soluble protein in the finished glove. It is believed that absorption of the remaining soluble proteins through intact mucosa or the surgical wound can elicit an IgE-mediated anaphylactic response in sensitive individuals.[59,60]

A number of recent reports of severe IgE-mediated anaphylactic reactions to latex include more than 50 fatalities. These cases have been reported in a variety of situations, including surgical procedures, vaginal examination, and rectal manometry.[61] Several anaphylactic reactions occurring during barium enema examination have resulted in the recall of all latex balloon-equipped enema tips.[62]

Certain populations appear to be at increased risk for reactions to latex. These groups include patients who have undergone multiple operations, those with atopic disease (frequency of atopy in the latex-allergic patient approaches 60 to 70 percent), children with spina bifida who are frequently exposed to latex products (prevalence of latex sensitivity approaches 40 percent in some studies), and people who frequently wear latex gloves, such as medical personnel.[63] Careful preoperative screening should identify patients who may be at increased risk for latex hypersensitivity.

Attempts to identify the responsible proteins have been successful. Carrillo[64] determined that the allergen responsible for the immediate hypersensitivity was a protein. Morales and his colleagues[65] later isolated four soluble polypeptides from latex that seemed responsible for the hypersensitivity reactions. They showed that these four proteins bind to IgE taken from patients who have experienced anaphylactic reactions to latex products. Furthermore, these four proteins resulted in a positive skin-prick test in individuals sensitive to latex.[65] Other soluble proteins isolated from latex gloves and chemical additives from latex processing did not elicit such a response in these patients.

Episodes of IgE-mediated anaphylaxis to latex proteins have prompted the Food and Drug Administration (FDA) and the Health Industry Manufacturers Association Latex Task Force to search for alternative glove materials, to develop screening tests to identify patients at risk for IgE-mediated anaphylactic response to latex, and to provide more efficient methods of protein elution. The FDA has established industry standards for the leaching of latex products. New methods of leaching for more efficient removal of the soluble latex proteins are being developed, and these appear to be quite successful at removing all but very small amounts of soluble protein. Techniques to measure accurately the amount of soluble protein in surgical gloves are being developed. The FDA and the Canadian Department of Health have urged hospital personnel to identify latex-sensitive individuals so that proper precautions can be instituted and severe reactions prevented. Diagnostic tests are being sought to screen for latex-sensitive patients. Skin-prick testing has shown accuracy in the identification of latex-sensitive patients, but the test can be dangerous in patients who are highly sensitive to latex.[66] When latex-sensitive patients are identified, the use of nonlatex gloves and prophylactic antihistamine medications has been advised.

It is important to point out that residual accelerators, such as thiurams and mercaptobenzothiazoles, used in the processing of latex have also been implicated in the allergic reactions to latex. In contrast to the soluble proteins, these chemicals cause contact dermatitis in sensitive individuals.[66]

Skin Wound Cleansers. Skin wound cleansers are designed to aid in the removal of bacterial and other contaminants from superficial wounds and may or may not contain an antimicrobial agent. While cleansing the wound, the agent must not damage the wound or the systemic defenses or deter healing.

Dilute solutions (1:750) of quaternary ammonium salts (quats) satisfy many of these requirements. These compounds are cationic surface active agents, which are basically organically substituted ammonium compounds. Although they affect cell membrane potential, the consequences are clinically apparent only at concentrations higher than those recommended for clinical use.

Gram-positive microorganisms are generally more susceptible to quats than gram-negative bacteria are. The gram-negative *Pseudomonas* species are usually resistant and even proliferate in the stored solution, accounting for occasional serious nosocomial outbreaks of gram-negative infection.[67]

In contrast, the commercially available surgical scrub solutions containing iodophors and hexachlorophene are not safe for use in surgical wounds. These solutions contain toxic anionic detergents that damage the tissue defenses and potentiate the development of infection.[68] Until this observation was made, detergents and surfactants in surgical scrub solutions were considered by many to be innocuous ingredients.

Pluronic polyol F-68, a nonionic surfactant, is an excellent substitute for toxic detergents. It belongs to a family of surfactants made of a series of block copolymers with a water-soluble polyoxyethylene group at both ends of a water-insoluble polyoxypropylene chain.[69] It has a molecular weight of 8350 and contains 80 percent ethylene oxide. Long-term toxicity studies in animals and people reveal it to be safe for intravenous use. Concentrated solutions containing as much as 40 percent Pluronic polyol F-68, when applied topically to the wound, do not damage resistance to infection. This surfactant also has negligible effect on bacterial viability.

Pluronic polyol F-68 has been approved by the FDA as a skin wound cleanser. Unlike all other commercial scrub solutions, this surfactant is so innocuous that it does not "bring tears to the baby's eye." Patients with painful, partial-thickness burns or abrasions washed with it find it soothing. In our emergency medical service, this agent has completely replaced all other surgical scrub solutions for use in traumatic wounds.

Topical iodophors, even without the addition of surfactant, would seem to be poor choices as skin wound cleansers. Application over a large surface area often results in a substantial elevation of free serum iodide.[70] Unexplained abnormalities have occurred in some patients, including renal failure, metabolic acidosis, and elevation of serum glutamic oxaloacetic transaminase. It is conceivable that large iodide loads were, at least in part, responsible for these abnormalities. Iodophors and many other antiseptics depend on an oxidative reaction between the antiseptic and the organism. But iodine reacts as easily with mammalian as with bacterial cells, and within seconds after instillation of a lethal dose of iodophor into the sterile peritoneal cavity the titratable iodine is undetectable, having reacted with the normal tissues.[71] In the heavily contaminated peritoneal cavity, bacterial counts are rapidly reduced by iodophors, but not all bacteria are killed.[72] The iodine can react with normal mesothelium and cause a chemical peritonitis, which is fatal in experimental animals even in the absence of bacteria. Repeated treatment of an open wound with this iodophor may delay healing.

Povidone-iodine (PVP-I) is cytocidal to human neutrophils at commercially available concentrations (1 percent titratable iodine). Even dilutions of 1:100 result in irreversible loss of a neutrophil's ability to respond to chemotactic stimuli. Topical antibiotics have a broad spectrum of activity without toxicity to mammalian tissue and continue to kill bacteria for prolonged periods. They appear to be safer agents for wound irrigation than antiseptics.

Unaware of these potential toxic manifestations of PVP-I complexes, many surgeons have continued to apply these agents to contaminated wounds with surprisingly good results. Gilmore and Martin[73] have made well-controlled studies of the efficacy of PVP-I powders in the treatment of contaminated wounds. In a series of 451 consecutive cases of appendectomy, topical PVP-I treatment reduced the wound infection rate and was found to be superior to an antiseptic spray. These beneficial effects of PVP-I in the treatment of contaminated wounds were later reported by Stokes and his associates[74] in a prospective randomized study of abdominal surgical patients. When topical prophylactic PVP-I was compared with topical cephaloridine in another series, however, antibiotic-treated wounds escaped infection far more often than those treated with the antiseptic.[75]

Patient Preoperative Skin Preparation. Immediately before the operative procedure, the site should be thoroughly cleansed with a sterile sponge soaked in solution containing 20 percent Pluronic F-68 to remove superficial flora and debris that could interfere with antisepsis. Then application of an antiseptic solution is necessary to kill or inhibit more adherent, deep, resident flora. Any of the agents used for antiseptic hand washing, except hexachlorophene, can be used to prepare the operative site, but tincture of chlorhexidine or iodophors offer advantages over the others.[76] Both have an excellent record of activity against bacteria. Tincture of chlorhexidine has a rapid onset of activity (due to alcohol) and persistent antibacterial activity. Iodophors also act rapidly and have persistent antibacterial activity if they are not wiped off. Tincture of iodine is also an excellent surgical prepping agent but can cause skin burns. Alcohols act rapidly but have no persistent effect after they evaporate.

The FDA has continued to receive reports of patients suffering thermal burns during electrosurgery after the skin has been prepared with an antimicrobial agent containing 0.5 percent chlorhexidine gluconate and 70 percent isopropyl alcohol.[77] Consequently, the skin must be completely dry without pooling of this antimicrobial agent before electrosurgery is started. Pooling of an iodophor solution should also be avoided because it can result in a chemical burn.

Hexachlorophene has been used as a preoperative skin preparation agent, but it has poor activity on gram-negative organisms and requires repeated use for maximum effectiveness. Hexachlorophene can be absorbed from the skin, and in large amounts it has toxic effects on the central nervous system, particularly in premature infants.

Surgical Debridement

Debridement is probably the most important single factor in the management of the contaminated wound.[78] First, it removes tissue heavily contaminated by soil infection-potentiating factors and bacteria, protecting the patient from invasive infection. Second, it removes permanently devitalized soft tissues that, if left in a wound, would damage its defenses and encourage the development of infection.[79] The capacity of devitalized fat, muscle, and skin to enhance bacterial infection is comparable. The infection-potentiating effect of skin is further enhanced by exposing it to a dry thermal injury. This change in the capacity of skin to damage the wound's defenses may be related to the development of a burn toxin. This observation is consistent with the experimental findings of Allgöwer et al,[80] who identified a toxin in skin that was subjected to dry heat. This toxin appears to be generated by a polymeric dehydration of substance(s) that occurs naturally in the skin.

There are at least three mechanisms by which devitalized soft tissue enhances infection: (1) it acts as a culture medium promoting bacterial growth, (2) it inhibits leukocyte phagocytosis and subsequent bacterial kill, and (3) the anaerobic environment within devitalized tissue must also limit leukocyte function. At low oxygen tension, the killing of certain bacteria by leukocytes is impaired.[32,33] Although the need for debridement of devitalized tissue is undisputed, identification of the exact limits of devitalized tissue in wounds remains a challenging problem, especially in muscle. Traditionally, the viability of muscle is determined by the "4C" guidelines (color, consistency, contraction, circulation). Generations of surgeons have accepted the assumption that nonviable muscle can be identified by its dark color, its "mushy" consistency, its failure to contract when pinched with forceps, and the absence of brisk bleeding from a cut surface. Although these classic signs do not always correlate with tissue viability, they have a useful clinical function. If there is doubt about the adequacy of debridement, the wound is reexplored 4 to 5 days after the initial operation.

The viability of skin is considerably easier to judge than that of muscle. At 24 hours after injury, a sharp line of demarcation is often apparent between the devitalized and viable skin. In fresh skin wounds in which this demarcation is not precise, the distribution of an intravenously injected fluorescein dye within the tissues may prove helpful.[81] Early staining of the injured skin by fluorescein is evidence of tissue viability. At times, active bleeding from the distal dermal margin may be present and indicates viability.

In some anatomic sites, such as the trunk, debridement is best accomplished by a more liberal excision of the skin and deep tissues. The soft tissue here is relatively free of tissues (eg, nerves, tendons) that perform important physical functions, and cosmetic considerations are less important.

The adequacy of debridement may be monitored by forcibly packing the wound with gauze or by coloring the wound surface with a vital dye. Flooding the field with a mixture of methylene blue and peroxide will encourage deep penetration of dye into distant cavities. Complete excision of the wound, back to a margin of normal tissue, is judged by dissecting in a plane that will not expose the gauze or the blue dye. Suturing the skin edges of the wound before excision may further minimize mechanical spread of the wound contaminants into uninjured tissue.

When a heavily contaminated wound contains specialized tissues, such as the tendon or nerve, complete excision is often not feasible. In such cases, high-pressure irrigation, followed by excision of all fragments of tissue that are not clearly viable, is indicated. In a compound wound of the abdominal cavity, selective debridement of nonviable fascia is tedious but essential, as the site constitutes a favorable environment for bacterial growth.

One must not debride certain specialized tissues that perform important physical functions, regardless of their viability.[82] Tissues such as dura, fascia, and tendon may survive as free grafts without living cells if immediately covered by healthy pedicle flaps. If these tissues can be rendered surgically clean, they should be left in the wound. Retraction of the wound edges during debridement is best accomplished by hooks. Kocher clamps or bulldog forceps should contact the wound only when the piece of tissue grasped is destined to be removed. Similarly, compressive retractors should be avoided; for prolonged exposure of the wound, its edges can be retracted by stay sutures placed in the dermis.

Prompt, adequate surgical debridement is also the cornerstone of therapy for war wounds. Because relief of tension is an important element of wound debridement, generous incisions of the wound should be made to relieve mechanical pressure, and open drainage must be established. The fascia should be incised parallel to the muscle fibers in both directions. The underlying muscle surrounding the missile tract should be opened in the direction of its fibers to the degree necessary to achieve exposure adequate to inspect the tract, remove foreign bodies, and excise nonviable tissue. Where one draws the line in excising muscle surrounding a missile path has been the subject of considerable debate in wound ballistics. Debridement of muscle should be rational rather than radical. The surgeon inclined to err in the direction of radical excision should bear in mind that in all studies in which animals were kept alive long enough to observe and measure healing objectivity or to evaluate the injury around the missile wound microscopically, there was less lasting tissue damage than estimated from observation of the wound in the first few hours after the wound was inflicted. In an experimental study of simple extremity wounds caused by the modern generation assault rifle, Fackler et al[83] found that wounds provided with adequate open drainage and systemic penicillin healed as rapidly as when an attempt was made to excise them surgically.

When the missile penetrates either the small or large intestine, the surgeon cuts across tissue where it appears normal. Missile perforations of the small bowel are managed by resecting the perforated bowel and reanastomosis. Gunshot wounds of the colon are excised in the same manner as those in the small bowel, but the ends are brought out as a double-barreled colostomy. The same management principle applies to penetrating gunshot wounds of blood vessels and other tissues; one cuts across tissue where it appears normal. There is no rational reason to excise an extra 1 to 2 cm in deference to the weapon's velocity or energy.

Mechanical Cleansing

The surgeon commonly uses mechanical forces to rid the wound of surface bacteria and other particulate matter retained by adhesive forces. Because these forces must exceed the adhesive forces of the contaminants, the two basic modes used are hydraulic forces and direct contact.

In irrigation, the hydraulic forces of the irrigating stream act on particulate matter in the wound. The total force component exerted on the particle by the moving stream is called drag. The total drag due to the fluid pressure and stress is expressed by the following equation:

$$\text{drag} = CA\rho\frac{V^2}{2}$$

where C is an experimentally derived drag coefficient dependent in part on the configuration of the particle; A is the projected area of the particle on a plane perpendicular to flow; ρ is the density of the fluid; and V is the relative velocity of the fluid with respect to the particle. It takes significantly lower hydraulic pressures to rid the wound of large foreign bodies than it does to remove bacteria.

Irrigation will be most efficient if the velocity of the irrigating stream is raised by increasing the pressure and enlarging the internal diameter of the needle. The pressure exerted by fluid delivered through a 19-gauge needle by the 35-ml syringe is 8 lb psi.[84] Such high-pressure irrigation (8 lb psi or more) successfully cleanses the wound of small particulate matter, bacteria, and soil infection-potentiating factors, thereby reducing the infection rate of experimentally contaminated wounds. In contrast, low-pressure syringe irrigation (as with a bulb syringe), even with large volumes of fluid, removes neither small nor large particulate matter.

Despite advantages of high-pressure irrigation, several objectives have been raised against its routine use. One commonly expressed concern is that foreign bodies on the surface of the wound may be disseminated more deeply into the wound as a result of high-pressure irrigation, although experimental studies indicate that this fear is unfounded.[85] After high-pressure irrigation, the bacteria remain at the surface of the wound even though the irrigant solution may disseminate deeply into the tissues. The tissue penetration of a high-pressure irrigating stream is predominantly lateral, similar to a jet parenteral injection.

The concern that high-pressure irrigation can damage tissue defenses, however, appears to be justified. Pulsatile or syringe irrigation results in trauma to the tissues, which makes the wound more susceptible to experimental infection. Therefore, high-pressure irrigation should not be performed indiscriminately, but should be reserved for use in heavily contaminated wounds.

In the clinical setting, high-pressure irrigation is accomplished with an inexpensive disposable irrigation assembly consisting of a 19-gauge plastic needle attached to a 35-ml syringe (Fig. 24–2). Sterile electrolyte solution (250 ml of 0.9 percent sodium chloride) is delivered through a one-way valve attached to the syringe barrel by standard intravenous plastic tubing. The tip of the needle, fastened to the syringe filled with saline, is placed perpendicular, and as close as possible, to the surface of the wound; then the surgeon exerts maximal force on the syringe plunger, delivering the irritant to the wound.

Another force used to cleanse a wound is direct mechanical contact. An example is scrubbing a dirty wound with a sponge. Although this technique removes bacteria from wounds, it does not decrease the incidence of infection. Also, trauma to the tissue, inflicted by the sponge, impairs the wound's ability to resist infection and allows the residual

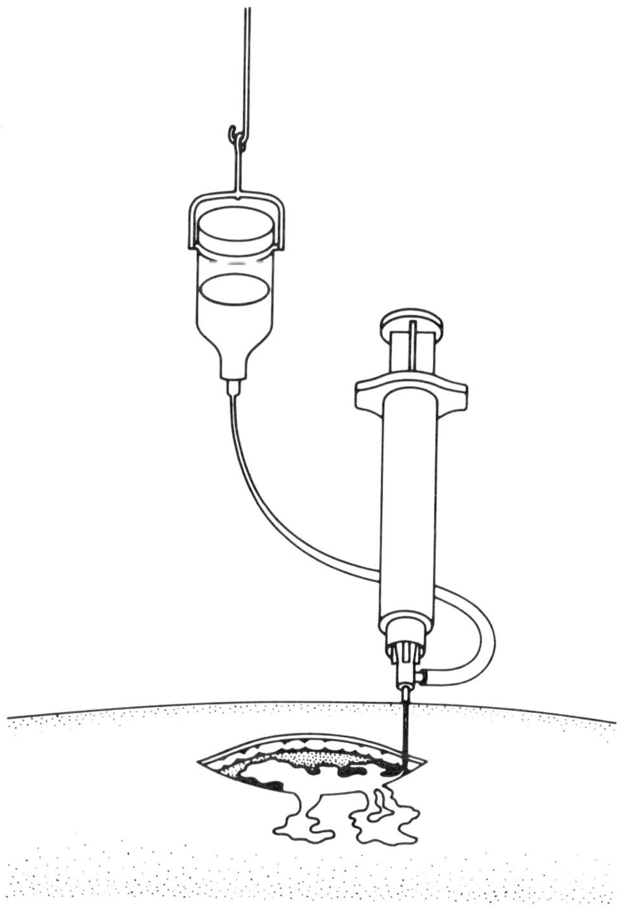

Figure 24–2. High-pressure wound irrigation assembly.

bacteria to elicit an inflammatory response.[86] The magnitude of the damage to the local tissue resistance is correlated with the porosity of the sponge: less porous sponges are more abrasive and cause more damage to the wound. The addition of a nontoxic surfactant, such as Pluronic polyol F-68, to a sponge minimizes the tissue damage it inflicts while maintaining the bacterial removal efficiency of mechanical cleansing. Consequently, the use of a surfactant-soaked sponge reduces the incidence of infection in contaminated wounds in experimental animals. Pluronic polyol F-68 has been used to cleanse traumatic lacerations in over 1 million patients without an adverse effect.

Fine pore-size sponges soaked in this surfactant, however, may not provide sufficient frictional forces to remove dirt and foreign bodies that are embedded in skin abrasions. The latter injury is due to shear forces applied almost parallel to the skin surface that disrupt the epidermis and papillary dermis. If the foreign body is not removed from the abrasion, wound repair will be accomplished by epithelial regeneration with the embedded foreign body becoming a pigmented tattoo.

Antibiotics

The relative success of antibiotic therapy in the prevention of infection in surgical wounds is influenced by the time of administration, the wound bacterial concentration, the presence of soil infection-potentiating factors, and the mechanism of injury. In laboratory and clinical studies, antibiotic therapy is significantly more effective when the drug is administered preoperatively rather than intraoperatively or postoperatively.[87] A delay in antibiotic treatment consistently diminishes its therapeutic merit. When there is an unavoidable delay in administering these drugs, the length of time during which the open wound is exposed plays an important role. As a result of this exposure, a sequence of events occurs that substantially limits the therapeutic value of antibiotics.[87]

When any wound is left open, its vessels exhibit a marked increase in vascular permeability. Fluids from the intravascular space extravasate and fill the wound crater. This exudate is rich in a wide variety of proteins, including fibrinogen. Once outside the vessels, much of the protein exudate is reabsorbed slowly by the lymphatic vessels, with the exception of fibrinogen, which partly polymerizes to form fibrin. It is our belief that the resulting fibrinous coagulum surrounds the bacteria and protects them from contact with the antibiotic.[87] The cause of this exaggerated inflammatory response in the open wound has not been defined. It may be related, however, to environmental conditions. The temperature of the operating room is usually considerably below the systemic body temperature, encouraging loss of heat from the wound. In addition, evaporation of fluid from the wound surface results in further heat loss and cooling of the tissues. A consequence of fluid loss from the wound is desiccation. Warming the operating room or covering the wound with wet sponges should reduce these environmental effects. Paradoxically, the fibrinous wound coagulum, which limits the effectiveness of antibiotics, may be a crucial positive factor in the host's defense against infection. The coagulum may serve as a plug in the open mouths of lymphatic vessels, preventing dissemination of bacteria. Occlusion of lymphatic vessels by the coagulum then becomes an obstacle to the invasion of bacteria and partly accounts for the resistance of an open wound to systemic sepsis.

This surface coagulum may be disrupted by a variety of mechanisms. Gentle scrubbing of the surface of the wound with a gauze sponge disturbs the fibrinous cover and allows an antibiotic to gain intimate contact with the bacteria.[88] Consequently, the therapeutic effectiveness of antibiotics is measurably enhanced by this treatment. Enzymatic digestion is a less traumatic and more selective means of disrupting the coagulum.[89,90] The in vitro fibrinolytic capacity of certain enzymes provides an accurate measure of their ability to potentiate antimicrobial activity. Travase (a proteolytic enzyme produced by *Bacillus subtilis*, the most potent fibrinolytic agent in vitro) is the most effective enzymatic adjunct to antibiotic treatment. Hydrolysis of the protein coagulum can be accomplished within 30 minutes by topical application of this proteolytic enzyme. Such a brief exposure to this fibrinolytic enzyme does not damage the wound's defenses or its healing capacity.

The presence of wound contaminants can influence the outcome of antibiotic therapy. When the wound is contaminated by exceedingly large numbers of organisms (more than 10^9), infection will develop despite antibiotic treatment. The circumstance is encountered when the wound surface is contacted by either pus or feces. The presence of soil infection-potentiating factors reacts chemically with amphoteric and basic antibiotics, limiting their activity in contaminated wounds.[91]

Antibiotic prophylaxis has therapeutic merit in several clinical settings. An antibiotic should be administered to all patients with wounds resulting from impact injuries.[5] In these wounds the weakened local tissue defense makes them susceptible to the development of infection by a relatively small inoculum (10^4 bacteria/g of tissue). It is indeed fortuitous that systemically administered antibiotics can gain contact with pathogens in the ischemic tissue of impact injuries.

Another indication for antibiotic treatment is a wound in which treatment has been delayed for 3 hours or more.[87] During this time interval, bacteria may proliferate to a level that will result in infection. This development is complicated by the gradual appearance of the fibrinous exudate, which becomes a protective barrier against topically or systemically administered antibiotics.

Antibiotic treatment is also mandatory in wounds containing an inflammatory exudate (pus), feces, saliva, and/or vaginal secretions. The bacterial inocula of such wounds markedly exceed the infective dose. Although antibiotic treatment significantly reduces this level of heavy contamination, the number of residual viable bacteria is often sufficient to elicit infection after primary closure. Consequently, open wound management of these heavily contaminated wounds must frequently supplement antibiotic treatment.

The presence of soil infection-potentiating factors in wounds also has considerable influence on the efficacy of specific antibiotics. The benefit of antibiotics in the presence of these fractions is predicted by the chemical composition of the antibiotic.[91] The basic antibiotic (eg, gentamicin) and amphoteric (eg, tetracycline) are inactivated by these highly charged anions. The acidic antibiotics, such as cephalosporins and penicillin, do not bind with these fractions and exert their antibacterial effect in wounds contaminated by these fractions.

Antibiotic treatment is recommended also in surgical patients who are prone to develop infective endocarditis. Because infective endocarditis causes significant morbidity and mortality, its prevention with antibiotic treatment has been a universally accepted and worthwhile goal. More than 100 case reports provide reasonably good evidence that bacteremias originating from the genitourinary tract may cause endocarditis, especially when urologic or gynecologic operations are preformed in the presence of urinary or pelvic infection.[92] Those underlying conditions that display a relatively high risk of developing endocarditis after a transient bacteremia include prosthetic valves, arteriovenous fistula, patent ductus arteriosus, Fallot's tetralogy, ventricular septal defect, coarctation of the aorta, aortic valve disease, mitral valve disease, Marfan's syndrome, and previous infective endocarditis. Antibiotic prophylaxis in such patients should include a combination of gentamicin and penicillin that is administered 30 to 60 minutes before the operative procedure (Table 24–1). Convincing cases of hematogenous infections of other prostheses are uncommon. Late hematogenous infections of arterial grafts (those appearing more than 60 days after surgery) are nearly unknown.[93] Instead, almost all reported infections have probably originated from contamination at surgery, from contiguous areas of purulence, or from the development of a fistula between the graft and gastrointestinal tract. Even in hip arthroplasties, the sources of infection have been distant sites of established suppuration, such as tonsillitis, cholecystitis, dental abscess, pyoderma, suppurative parotitis, or cystitis, rather than procedure-induced transient bacteremia.[94] These findings emphasize the importance of prompt and thorough treatment of distant infections in patients with indwelling prosthetic devices.

Lymphedematous patients are especially prone to develop infection. A streptococcus or less often a staphylococcus can be isolated from the infected tissue. Each infection produces more lymphatic destruction and edema. In patients with lymphedema and recurrent cellulitis, a generally accepted anti-

TABLE 24–1. ANTIBIOTIC PROPHYLAXIS OF INFECTIVE ENDOCARDITIS IN PATIENTS[a]

Adults	Aqueous crystalline penicillin G, 2 million units IM or IV or ampicillin, 1.0 g IV plus Gentamicin, 1.5 mg/kg IM or IV or streptomycin, 1.0 g IM. If gentamicin is used, give the same dosages of gentamicin and penicillin (ampicillin) every 8 h for two additional dosages. If streptomycin is used, give the same dosage of streptomycin and penicillin (or ampicillin) every 12 h for two additional dosages.
Children	Aqueous crystalline penicillin G, 30,000 units/kg IM or IV or ampicillin, 50 mg/kg IM or IV plus Gentamicin, 2.0 mg/kg IM or IV or streptomycin, 20 mg/kg IM
For patients allergic to penicillin	
Adults	Vancomycin, 0.5–1.0 g IV, infused slowly over 1 h plus Streptomycin, 1.0 g IM, given 30 min to 1 h before the procedure. Both drugs may be repeated once, 12 h later.
Children	Vancomycin, 20 mg/kg IV, infused slowly over 1 h plus Streptomycin, 20 mg/kg IM

[a] For brief procedures such as a change of urinary catheter or cystoscopy, one dose of these combination regimens will probably suffice. Conversely, in the case of unusually prolonged or repeated procedures or delayed healing, several additional doses may be given. IM, intramuscularly; IV, intravenously.

microbial prophylaxis includes 1.2 million units of penicillin G benzathine (Bicillin) administered intramuscularly per month. When a minor soft tissue laceration occurs in lymphedematous tissue, antimicrobial treatment should be initiated immediately before wound closure.

Antibiotics must be administered to patients with wounds in which the magnitude of tissue injury is extensive and difficult to ascertain accurately soon after injury. In such cases, open wound management is the method of choice with subsequent additional debridement as dictated by the appearance of the wound. It must be emphasized that antibiotic therapy is an adjunct to debridement rather than a replacement. In all missile injuries, adequate blood levels of penicillin or an antibiotic with a similar spectrum of activity (cephalosporin) should be established as soon as possible after wounding to prevent streptococcal bacteremia. Streptolysin, produced by the virulent streptococcal species, breaks down the fibrin that has been deposited in the body in an attempt to wall off collections of bacterial pathogens. Since the discovery of antibiotics, streptococcal bacteremia has all but disappeared from missile injuries.

The immediate selection of the specific antimicrobial agent is based on consideration of the results of direct microscopic examination of a wound biopsy, the normal bacterial flora harbored in different parts of the body, and the pathogens usually encountered in various diseases or conditions. Later, the results of immediate antibiotic sensitivity testing can also influence the surgeon's choice of antibiotic. In our laboratory, antibiotic sensitivity testing is performed directly on the bacterial suspension prepared from the wound biopsy specimen rather than on strains isolated from the tissue.[95]

Hemostatic Agents

Topical hemostatic agents have wide applications in a variety of bleeding sites. They can effectively control bleeding from large areas of cancellous bone.[96] These agents are often used to stop bleeding from vascular anastomoses before placing additional sutures.[97] Bleeding from renal, splenic, and hepatic injuries also can be arrested by application of these materials.[98–100]

Many topical hemostatic agents have been used clinically to reduce bleeding and include the following:

1. Beeswax (Ethicon, Inc.)
2. Stabilized fibrin and collagen paste (Ethnor, Ethicon, Ltd.)
3. Oxidized cellulose (OC) (Oxycel, Deseret Medical, Inc.)
4. Oxidized regenerated cellulose (ORC) (Surgicel, Johnson & Johnson Products, Inc.)
5. Absorbable gelatin foam (AGF) or powder (AGP) (Gelfoam, The Upjohn Co.)
6. Microfibrillary collagen (MC) (Avitene, American Critical Care)
7. Bovine thrombin (BT) (Thrombostat, Parke, Davis & Co.)
8. Fibrin glue

OC is an absorbable oxidized cellulose that is available in either cotton-type pledgets or gauze-like pads or strips. ORC is an absorbable knitted fabric prepared by the controlled oxidation of regenerated cellulose. AGF is a pliable, nonantigenic foam from specifically treated, purified gelatin solution and is capable of absorbing and holding within its mesh many times its weight of whole blood. This latter product is also available as a powder.

MC is an absorbable agent prepared as a dry, fibrous, water-insoluble, partial hydrochloric acid salt of purified bovine corium collagen. In its manufacture, swelling of the native collagen fibrils is controlled by ethyl alcohol to permit noncovalent attachment of hydrochloric acid to amine groups on the collagen molecule and preservation of its essential morphology. BT is produced through a conversion reaction in which prothrombin is activated by tissue thromboplastin in the presence of calcium chloride. After standardization of potency by dilution, thrombin solution is sterilized by filtration, poured into vials, dried from the frozen state, and sealed under aseptic conditions. BT can be combined with an equal volume of fibrinogen concentrate to produce fibrin glue by the following reaction:

$$\text{fibrinogen} \xrightarrow{\text{thrombin}} \text{fibrin monomer} \xrightarrow{\text{factor XIII},\ Ca^{2+}} \text{fibrin polymer}$$

This reaction can be enhanced by reconstitution of BT in 40 mM calcium chloride.

Beeswax has been used almost exclusively to arrest bleeding from the cut edges of cancellous bone. It was first described by Horsley in 1882. His antiseptic bone wax consisted of 7 parts beeswax, 1 part almond oil, and salicylic acid 1 percent. The most commonly used bone wax currently available has a formula of refined beeswax 88 percent (w/w) and isopropyl palmitate 12 percent (w/w). The hemostatic benefit occurs at the expense of a foreign-body giant cell response, persistence of wax at the bony site for years, and a physical barrier to bony union.[101] Thus the wax appears to be a nonabsorbable foreign body impermeable to components of healing tissue.[102] Acting as a foreign body, bone wax significantly impaired the ability of cancellous bone to kill bacteria.[103]

In 1977, Lawrie[104] reported a new absorbable bone hemostatic sealant containing stabilized fibrin, soluble collagen, glycerol, and dextran that had the consistency of "putty." Its hemostatic effect appears to be by tamponade, but both the fibrin and collagen may contribute to local hemostasis. It was a more efficient hemostatic agent than bone wax, and it did not interfere with bone healing.[105] Absorption was complete within 3 weeks. The effect of this stabilized fibrin and collagen paste on bacterial clearance has not been examined.

In experimental studies by Cobden and associates,[96] the efficacy of MC, BT-soaked AGF, and BT powder as topical hemostatic agents for bleeding cancellous bone was evaluated. All three agents significantly reduced bleeding compared with the controls, with MC being the most effective. At 3 months, there was no evidence that MC and BT-soaked AGF interfered with bone healing. Their influence on infection in this clinical setting was not investigated.

Most experimental studies have demonstrated that the absorbable hemostatic agents damaged tissue defenses and invited the development of infection. Jenkins and colleagues[106,107] pointed out that in the presence of contamination or infection AGF may act as a culture medium, which may influence the development and propagation of infection. The experiments of Cipolla and Narat[108] demonstrated that AGF and OC intensified infection caused by *S. aureus* in the subcutaneous tissue of dogs. Moistening these absorbable agents with penicillin was not able to prevent infection. Intramuscular administration of penicillin in oil, however, inhibited the potentiation of infection caused by absorbable hemostatic agents. Hinman and Babcock[109] reported that OC and AGF enhanced the incidence of infection of contaminated nephrotomy incisions as compared with control wounds without the hemostatic agent subjected to a comparable amount of the suspension of feces.

Hill[110] demonstrated that AGP and MC markedly increased the rate of experimental anaerobic infection when mixed with a normally subinfective dose of the bacterial inoculum that was injected into the peritoneal cavity. The degree to which these topical hemostatic agents enhanced infection did not differ significantly. With a standard subcutaneous wound infection model, Scher and Coil[111] demonstrated that both ORC and MC increased the frequency of infection as compared with the wound that did not contain any foreign body. The infection-potentiating property of these topical hemostats was more dramatic when MC was employed. It was possible to produce a dose-response curve for ORC by varying the quantity employed and by maintaining a constant bacterial inoculum. These data emphasize the importance of using the minimum amount of ORC consistent with satisfactory hemostasis. No such dose-response curve could be obtained for MC because significant infection occurred at even the smallest doses studies. Because ORC and MC were equally effective in controlling bleeding from raw surfaces,[112] the advantage of ORC over MC in terms of infection makes ORC the superior hemostatic agent.

Laufman and Method[113] showed deleterious effects of placing AGF and OC in contact with the anastomoses of the large intestine in dogs. They believed that the increased incidence of perforation and peritonitis with topical hemostatic agents was caused by their ability to act as a culture medium for bacteria. In another experimental study, Uhrich[114] demonstrated that OC did not prevent leakage from the large intestinal anastomotic line when a single through-and-through suture end-to-end anastomosis was performed in dogs. In addition, the presence of OC appeared to promote the growth of bacteria in the infected peritoneal cavity. Chamberlain and associates[115] demonstrated that AGF in apposition to intestinal anastomoses increased the risk of peritonitis and fetal perforation in dogs. Impregnation of this sponge with crystalline penicillin was effective in preventing perforation of the anastomosis and local abscess formation.

In contrast to the other investigations that document an infection-potentiating effect of topical hemostatic agents, Dineen[116] reported that ORC had an ability to reduce the bacterial population in vitro and in vivo. Its mode of antibacterial action was explained partly by its low pH. Most of its activity in vitro was blocked by the addition of sodium hydroxide. Dineen[116,117] and Kuchta and Dineen[118] demonstrated that ORC prevented infection with several different experimental models.

Dineen[119] reported that ORC also prevented sepsis after an intravenous bacterial challenge. In dogs with Teflon aortic patches, wrapping that area of the Teflon patch with ORC before the bacterial challenge reduced the bacterial contamination of the Teflon patches compared with animals without ORC. Similarly, ORC decreased the level of contamination in splenotomy sites as compared with AGF after an intravenous infection of a bacterial inoculum.[119] In another experimental model that simulated the clinical situation of infected subdiaphragmatic blood clots, animals treated with ORC showed longer survival times and no development of abscesses and/or peritonitis after an intravenous bacterial challenge compared with control animals or those treated with either AGF or MC who died within 5 days of frank peritonitis and/or abdominal abscess.[118]

European surgeons have a broad experience with a variety of surgical applications of fibrin glue, a biologic adhesive prepared from commercially pooled human plasma.[120,121] Hemostatic use of the glue can be facilitated by combination with AGF. The FDA has not approved the use of fibrin glue because of a high associated risk of hepatitis and acquired immunodeficiency syndrome from the pooled human plasma used in the production of fibrinogen, an essential component of the glue.

Wound Drainage

Use of surgical drainage requires a delicate weighing of potential benefits and harmful effects. The obvious beneficial effect of drainage is its ability to evacuate or at least provide tracts for the elimination of potentially harmful collections of certain fluids as pus, blood, bile, and gastric and pancreatic juices from wounds or body cavities. Pus is detrimental to the healing of wounds. Even sterile pus injected under the skin impairs healing of a distant wound.[122,123] Smith and Enquist[124] reported that subacute experimental staphylococcal wound infection in animals initiated profound gross, histologic, and biochemical changes in local and distant tissue. Pus within a wound or body cavity exerts many deleterious effects on the host and should be removed whenever a localized collection can be drained.

Sterile collections of blood per se are not major irritants to tissues, but hematomas enhance bacterial virulence.[125,126] Krizek and Davis[126] found that when red blood cells were injected into the same subcutaneous site as *E. coli*, a fatal infection often occurred, whereas the injection of bacteria alone was relatively innocuous. The precise mechanisms by which hemoglobins enhance infection have defied definition until the recent studies of Pruett and colleagues.[127] They demonstrated that leukotoxins resulted from *E. coli* growth in solutions of pure hemoglobin. These leukotoxins severely damaged neutrophils and accounted for the infection-potentiating effect of hemoglobin in experimental peritonitis. There was no experimental support for the hypothesis that hemoglobin provided a nutritional boost to the growth of *E. coli*.

The location and contents of the harmful collections of fluids will dictate which drainage technique is the treatment of choice. Surgical intervention in abdominal infections is indicated in the following conditions: an infected organized hematoma, a para-pancreatic phlegmon, thick fungal infections, and a necrotic infected tumor metastasis.[128] Successful management of these infections includes incision into the abscess cavity, debridement of devitalized tissue, postoperative drainage, and antimicrobial therapy appropriate for the pathogens in the abscess cavity. The efficacy of the postoperative drainage system is directly related to the efficacy of removing the collections of fluid in the abscess cavity. Nonvented suction drainage creates a vacuum that causes tissue encroachment on the holes of the drainage tube, resulting in impaired drainage and tissue damage. This problem was resolved by designing a drainage tube with an air vent that permitted access of air into the area of drainage.[129] A two-staged filter was attached to the vent lumen that removed particulate matter and bacteria from the air that passed through the filter. A clinical evaluation of this tube confirmed the superiority of the filtered sump tube as compared with closed suction drainage in the removal of fluids from wounds or cavities.

The performance of this drainage tube was improved further by coating the surfaces of the drain with a new hydrogel coating (Axiom Medical, Inc., Paramount, CA).[130] The hydrogel was formed by reacting polyvinylpyrrolidone with an isocyanate polymer. By absorbing water, the hydrogel created a drain surface with a low coefficient of friction. The results of our experimental studies demonstrated that the drain coating reduced the adherence of blood clots to the drain and facilitated the removal of the drain from the wound. On the basis of these studies, the FDA has allowed this hydrogel-coated drain to be used in clinical patients.

Recent advances in intraventional radiology have demonstrated the value of percutaneous aspiration and drainage in patients with abscesses. Catheter drainage is performed by a modified Seldinger technique, with the passage of the catheter being monitored by either ultrasound or computed tomography.[131] The indications for the technique can be diagnostic, palliative, and therapeutic. Cytologic and microbiologic examination of the aspirate can detect the presence of malignancy as well as the responsible pathogen. Palliation is defined as temporary control of the infection in which the clinical infection is relieved, but the infectious process is not cured until an elective operative procedure is performed. Percutaneous aspiration drainage is therapeutic in a well-localized, unilocular bacterial abscess with a success rate of 96 percent.[128] Although percutaneous aspiration drainage appears to be the preferred method of management of the latter abscess, it is uniformly unsuccessful in treating collections that contain semisolid particulate matter (eg, organized hematoma, parapancreatic phlegmon, fungal infections, necrotic infected tumor metastases).

In instances where no definite collection of fluid exists, drainage must be considered to be prophylactic. In these circumstances its potentially harmful effects become more important. Drains act as retrograde conduits through which skin contaminants gain entrance into the wound. Cerise and colleagues[132] performed a splenectomy in rabbits and inoculated the skin around the drain tract with type 6 *Streptococcus,* taking care not to incolate the drain. Twenty percent of the animals had positive intraperitoneal cultures at 24 hours and 56 percent at 72 hours, compared with positive culture results in only 5 percent of the undrained animals. Nora and colleagues[133] performed laparotomies in dogs and inserted Penrose drains separately into the splenic fossa and in Morison's pouch. Gross intra-abdominal infection was detected in nine of the ten dogs with drains in the splenic fossa. No infections occurred in the undrained dogs. In a clinical study the same investigators detected skin contaminants on the intra-abdominal portion of drainage tubes in 17 of 50 patients. *Staphylococcus epidermidis*, a skin contaminant, was found in 14 of the 17 cases. Of the 17 infected patients, 12 had minimum egress of fluid from the drain tract, and neither the gastrointestinal nor genitourinary tract had been opened at operation.

Raves and associates[134] initiated an experimental study that demonstrated that closed suction drainage was associated with less bacterial migration into the splenic bed than Penrose drains. After inoculating the drain skin exit site with a strain of *Streptococcus,* 90 percent of the cultures of the splenic bed were positive in animals with Penrose drains. Only 20 percent of the animals with closed suction drains had *Streptococcus* recovered from their splenic beds ($P < 0.001$).

The presence of drains impairs the resistance of tissues to infection. Drains placed within experimental wounds exposed to subinfective inoculations of bacteria enhanced the rate of infection.[135] Both Silastic and Penrose drains dramatically increased the infection rate of soft tissue wounds in guinea pigs. The rate of infection when the drain was brought out through the wound was similar to the rate when the drain lay entirely within the wound, suggesting a deleterious effect of the drain.

Studies of the impairment of wound healing in the presence of drains have been undertaken with intestinal anastomoses. Berliner and associates[136] performed proximal and distal intestinal anastomoses in dogs, draining one anastomosis in each dog. Three of the 20 undrained anastomoses leaked compared with 11 of 20 drained anastomoses; of these 11, anastomotic disruption proved fatal in four cases. Manz and associates[137] confirmed the damaging effects of drains on colonic anastomoses in dogs. Of 20 dogs with Penrose drainage at their anastomoses, nine died of anastomotic disruption and peritonitis, and the remainder had extensive adhesions, as well as varying degrees of stricture formation. All dogs with drainage had evidence of bacterial contamination at the site of the anastomosis; the control animals had only filmy adhesions and no stricture formation. In another experimental study, Crowson and Wilson[138] reported that low canine anastomosis healed best when bacterial contamination was minimal, the anastomosis was not drained, and the anastomosis was intraperitoneal. A drain made intraperitoneal sepsis worse and was harmful to the peritoneal cavity. Silastic drains were less harmful than either latex or vinyl drains.

It has been postulated that an adjacent drain may block the desquamated mesothelial cells from contacting the anastomosis, thereby interfering with its healing. The drain may also act as a retrograde conduit for bacteria, which then contaminate the anastomotic site, thereby predisposing to infection and leakage.

Dead Space

The importance of dead space in the potentiation of wound infection has long been recognized and can be demonstrated experimentally[139,140] (Fig. 24–3A). Although dead space is bad, suture closure of dead space is worse[139,140] (Fig. 24–3B). The mechanism by which dead space potentiates the infectivity of a subinfective bacterial inoculum is not clear. One possibility is that even a bloodless exudate potentiates wound infection. Wood and associates[141] noted that phagocytosis of bacteria suspended in a fluid medium was difficult unless the bacteria have been opsonized. In the same way, Ahrenholz and Simmons[71] demonstrated that sterile saline solution aggravated experimental peritonitis unless the bacteria were preopsonized. Alexander and associates[142] have reported that wound exudates were depleted of opsonins. Suspension of contaminating bacteria in opsonin-depleted exudate may well interfere with antibacterial phagocytosis.

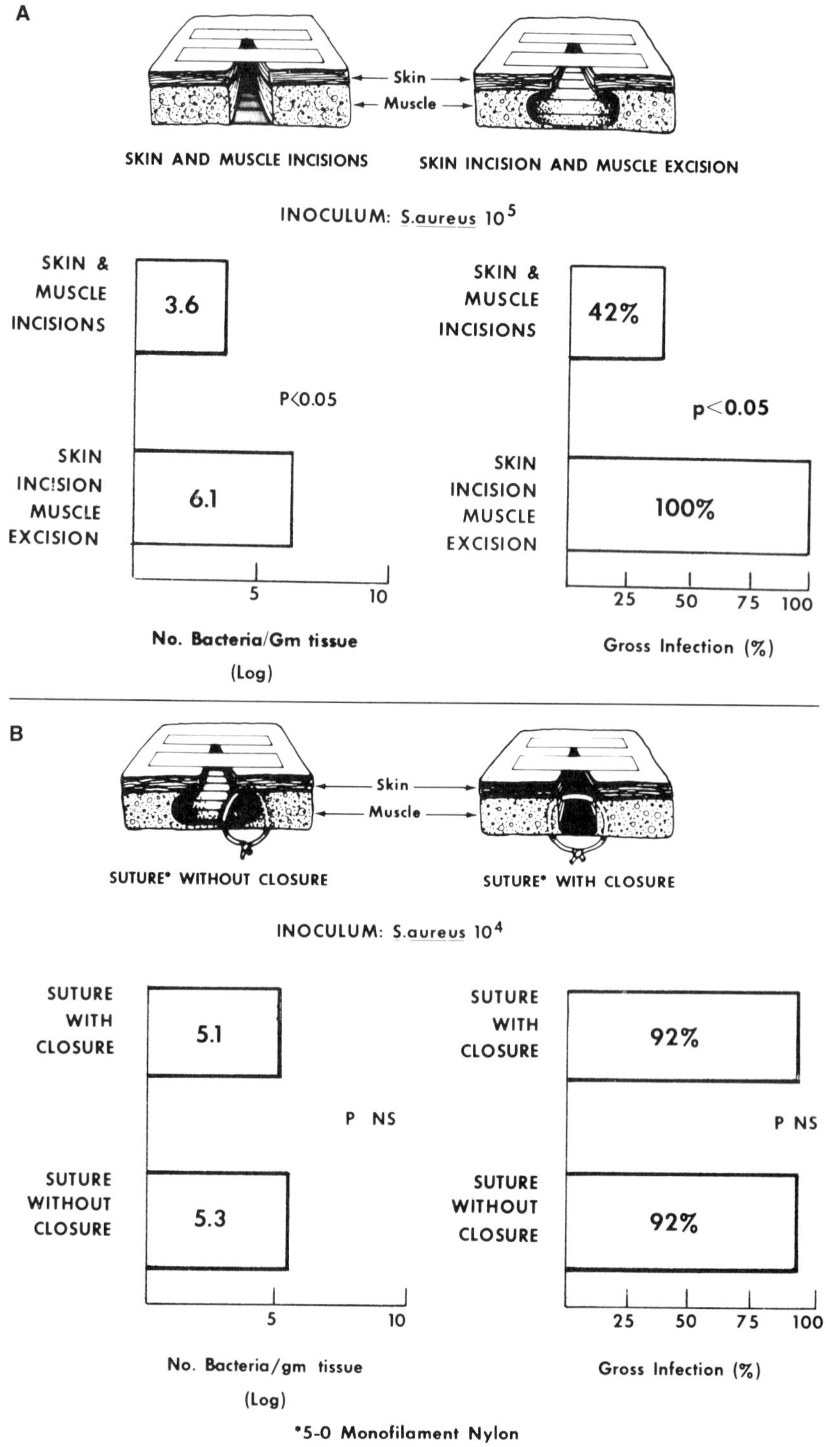

Figure 24–3. A. In experimental contaminated wounds, dead space was created by excising muscle adjacent to the wound edge. Four days later, the incidence of infection and the number of viable bacteria were significantly greater in wounds containing dead space than in wounds without muscle excision. **B.** Suture closure of the excised dead space did not eliminate the infection-potentiating effect of dead space. The infection rate of wounds and their viable bacteria following suture closure of dead space were comparable to that of wounds without dead space closure, but containing the same quantity of suture.

The presence of the suture material appears to potentiate the development of infection. The harmful effects of suture closure of dead space in experimental animals also occur in surgical incisions not involving muscle. Obliteration of the potential space between the cut edges of adipose tissue by sutures potentiated the incidence of infection (see Fig. 24–3C). The harmful effects of suture closure of dead space in experimental animals also occur in surgical incision not involving muscle (see Fig. 24–3D). Suturing that obliterated the potential space between the cut edges of adipose tissue potentiated infection.

These studies, combined with clinical observations, form the basis for the recommendation that suture closure of dead space should be avoided in

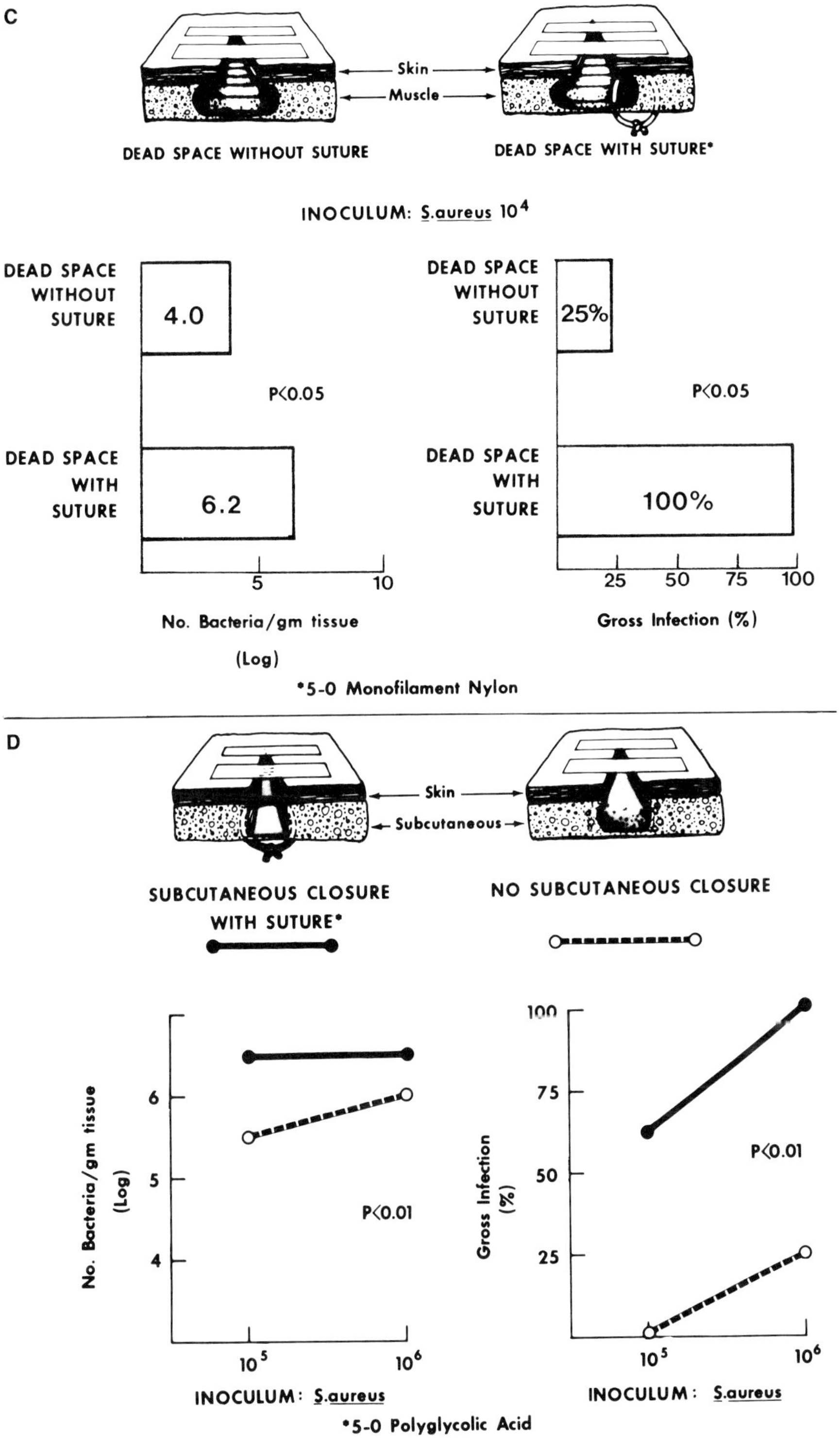

Figure 24–3. C. In the absence of dead space closure, the incidence of infection and level of bacterial contamination in wounds with sutures were higher than that in wounds without sutures. **D.** The gross infection rate and the number of bacteria in taped skin wounds subjected to suture closure of subcutaneous tissue were higher than that in wounds without suture closure.

contaminated wounds. Although dead spaces in wounds should definitely be avoided, the collapse of such space can be achieved by physiologic methods, such as relaxing incisions, rotation of distal flaps, and splinting dressings that may provide gentle surface pressure. The closure of dead space by sutures produces localized areas of wound ischemia and necrosis, and the presence of additional suture material adds further danger of wound complication. Whether suction drainage will achieve the known effect of drains to potentiate infection is unknown.[142]

Skin Closure

The technique of skin closure selected depends on the type of wounds. There are essentially two types of skin wounds. One type is characterized by a loss of tissue, whereas the other type has no evidence of tissue loss. In the latter, primary closure can be accomplished simply by reapproximating the divided skin edges by a variety of methods. For wounds with associated tissue loss, grafts or flaps are often required to close the defect.

A skin graft is a segment of epidermis that has been removed from its own blood supply and donor site attachment. It is transplanted to another area of the body that has less than 10^6 bacteria/g of tissue[143,144] and sufficient blood supply to vascularize the skin graft. Cortical bone denuded of its periosteum, cartilage without perichondrium, tendon without paratenon, and nerve without its perineurium do not have adequate blood supply to maintain the viability of skin grafts. The only exception to this rule is when skin grafts survive on a small (less than 0.5 cm) avascular area (bridging phenomenon).[145] In such cases, collateral circulation connects the vessels in the skin graft overlying the avascular area to the surrounding vascularized peripheral skin graft or granulation tissue.

Flaps are usually required for covering recipient site with poor vascularity; for padding bony prominences; for reconstructing full-thickness defects of eyelids, lips, ears, nose, and cheeks; and when it is necessary to reoperate through the wound at a later date to repair underlying structures. A flap is a composite of tissue attached by a vascular pedicle through which it receives its arterial blood supply and discharges venous effluent. The various types of flap include skin, omentum, muscle, and musculocutaneous tissue. A flap with arterialized tissue possessing a longitudinal vascular supply can have its blood supply detached and then reattached to a new anatomic area (free flap). The selection of a flap is based on the reliability of flap survival, its resultant function, the appearance at the site of coverage, and donor site availability.

When the area requiring coverage is heavily contaminated, it is of paramount importance that the flap chosen should have the capability to contain or eliminate local infection; otherwise the flap will succumb as a result of the underlying infection. In experimental studies, Chang and Mathes[146] demonstrated that musculocutaneous flaps showed a greater resistance to bacterial inoculation than random pattern skin flaps on both its cutaneous and muscular surfaces. Differences in the pattern of oxygen delivery to random pattern skin flaps and musculocutaneous flaps may partly explain the greater reliability of musculocutaneous flaps when transposed in the presence of infection. Gottrup and colleagues[147] reported that tissue oxygen tensions were significantly higher in the musculocutaneous flaps than in random pattern skin flaps up to 6 days after operation. They concluded that oxygen tension may govern the resistance of the tissue to infection. Efforts to enhance oxygen tension and resistance of tissue to infection by using musculocutaneous tissues are having direct clinical applications in the management of complicated infected wounds. May and associates[148] reported that radical debridement, intravenously administered antibiotics, and microvascular transfer of vascularized tissues for immediate closure resulted in resolution of the infection in 18 patients who had infected bone exposure wounds of the distal extremity. Another explanation for the success of muscle flaps in the treatment of long-standing infections has been provided by Russell and colleagues.[149] Their experimental study indicated that muscle flaps increased the concentration of antibiotics to the infected wound, which may kill the wound bacteria.

The gradual expansion of skin over 4 to 8 weeks with subcutaneously implanted silicone expander has become another accepted clinical means of providing local tissue for coverage of soft tissue defects.[150–152] The advantages of tissue expansion are several: (1) tissue is available from a local site without involving transfer over any distance, (2) an excellent color match is possible when the tissue is expanded in an area adjacent to the defect, (3) sensibility of the expanded tissue is preserved, and (4) the donor site does not require coverage because the expansion site can be closed primarily. Austad[153] indicated that the origin of the expanded tissue was the epidermis that had an increase in its total cell population. This thickening of the epidermis during expansion was associated with prominent thinning of the dermis. It is likely, however, that the dermis reconstitutes itself after the compressive forces caused by the expander have been removed. The relatively long time period involved in tissue expansion has limited the use of expanded skin flaps to elective reconstructive procedures. Because trauma patients frequently need coverage of soft tissue defects within days of injury, skin expansion has not been utilized often in this clinical setting.

Timing of Skin Closure. The timing of the closure is also critical. A decision must be made as to whether the closure should be immediate or delayed. Immediate closure should be reserved for (1) wounds resulting from elective procedures classified as being either refined-clean, clean, or clean-contaminated and (2) traumatic wounds that have not been contacted by feces, saliva, purulent exudate, or soil infection-potentiating factors. Immediate approximation of the skin edges of this group of wounds should be accompanied by an extremely low infection rate (less than 5 percent, regardless of the closure technique employed).

Open wound management with delayed primary closure is recommended for wounds that exhibit a high risk of infection after primary closure. The fundamental bases for delayed primary closure were the experiences of military surgeons who learned repeatedly over the centuries that immediate closure of battle wounds frequently resulted in infection.[154] These wounds were best left open until delayed primary closure could be undertaken. All wounds resulting from missile injuries, regardless of their appearance, are candidates for delayed primary closure. In these cases, the wound should be explored to remove foreign bodies, to rule out the presence of damage to specialized structures (eg, vessels, nerve), and to relieve increased compartmental pressure that may follow edema or slow bleeding into a fascia-enclosed muscle compartment. The removal of devitalized tissue is advisable, but in practice it is difficult as its identification is unclear. Wounds contacted by either feces, saliva, purulent exudates, or soil infection-potentiating factors are also candidates for open wound management. Because a delay in wound care that lasts longer than 6 hours is associated with an increased risk for infection, open wound management is also recommended.

The rationale for delayed primary closure is that the healing open wound will gain resistance to infection and permit an uncomplicated closure (Fig. 24–4). The reparative process of open wounds associated with this developing resistance to infection in the open wound undergoing delayed primary closure exhibits accelerated skin healing. In addition, Johnson and co-workers[155] showed that secondary closure of the subcutaneous tissue and skin resulted in stronger fascial strength than that encountered after primary closure.

In a group of patients with contaminated battle wounds in Vietnam, Surgeon General Heaton[154] reported an astoundingly low 2.5 percent incidence of infection. With experimental models, we have confirmed the superiority of delayed closure in the treatment of contaminated wounds.[156] The optimum time for closure of the contaminated wound is on or after the fourth postwounding day (see Fig. 24–4).

Although the type of open wound management must be individualized for each wound, aseptic

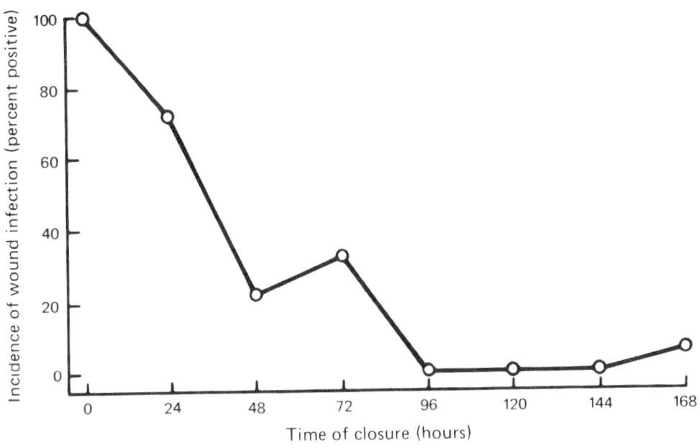

Figure 24–4. Optimal time for delayed primary closure. Experimental wounds were contaminated with an infective dose of bacteria and closed immediately or after a specified delay. Only delayed primary closure 96 hours (4 days) or more after wounding was associated with negligible infection.

technique is mandatory. For an infected wound filled with purulent discharge, the major objective is to remove the inflammatory exudate that will interfere with wound repair. Packing the wound with sterile coarse mesh gauze (type 8) is a reliable method of absorbing the purulent exudate from the crevices of the wound. Periodic dressing changes are usually necessary every 4 to 6 hours until a dry granulating wound bed becomes evident. The presence of residual necrotic tissue, foreign bodies, or soil infection-potentiating factors demands additional meticulous debridement in an operating room as dictated by the appearance of the wound. This reinspection of the wound with debridement must be continued until the wound is free of devitalized tissue and foreign bodies. Management of wounds heavily contaminated by bacteria is accomplished by packing the wound with sterile, dry, fine meshed gauze (type 1), which is then covered by a sterile dressing. This wound should not be disturbed for the first 4 days after operation, unless the patient develops an unexplained fever. Unnecessary inspection during this period increases the risk of contamination and subsequent infection. The selection of the technique for delayed primary closure will be based on the same considerations as used in primary closure. If percutaneous sutures are selected for wound closure, they should be passed through the wound edges at the end of the initial operation and left untied until the time of delayed primary closure. This step spares the patient the additional administration of a local or general anesthetic agent, which is required for sutural closure. The occasional wound that is destined to develop infection after delayed closure can be identified with quantitative microbiology. When the bacterial count of the tissue is lower than 10^5 organisms/g of tissue, delayed closure can be accomplished without infection.[157] With the proven merit of open wound management it is inconceivable that some surgeons resort to primary closure of contaminated, dirty wounds and risk life-threatening consequences.

Technique of Skin Wound Closure. There are several different methods to provide an accurate and secure approximation of the skin edges—tissue adhesives, staples, sutures, or tape. Ideally, the choice should be based on the biologic interaction of the materials employed, the tissue configuration, and the biomechanical properties of the wound. The tissue should be held in apposition until the tensile strength of the wound is sufficient to withstand stress. A common theme of the few reportable investigations is that all biomaterials placed within the tissue damage the host defenses and invite infection.

Adhesives. Cyanoacrylate tissue adhesives have been advocated for repair of injured tissue or as hemostatic agents.[158] Although the cyanoacrylates were first discovered in 1949, their use as tissue adhesives were described 10 years later. They are created through the reaction of cyanoacetate with formaldehyde, with variations in the alkyl group resulting in different compounds within the cyanoacrylate family. The cyanoacrylates are liquid monomers, similar to water in their appearance and viscosity. When exposed to water, they polymerize rapidly, releasing heat. The cyanoacrylates are thought to degrade through hydrolysis, the rate of which is determined by the length of the alkyl chain.[159] Studies using radioactively labeled cyanoacrylates have shown that small amounts are absorbed through skin and excreted in urine.[160]

Extensive experience with cyanoacrylates exists in many surgical fields.[161] They have been applied to skin, bone, and cartilage grafts, middle ear surgery, repair of cerebrospinal fluid leaks, as well as corneal ulcers. Methyl-2-cyanoacrylate was initially used the most widely, until its histotoxicity was recognized.[159] Longer alkyl chain derivatives were developed and found to produce a less acute inflammatory response with more rapid polymerization.[162] The optimal derivative is Histoacryl blue (N-butyl-2-cyanoacrylate).[163] Considerable clinical experience exists with this adhesive in the repair of skin lacerations.[164] It has been available for use in Canada since 1975. The FDA has not yet approved its use in humans.

Fibrin glue also has been used as an adhesive for burn wound repair. Ihara and colleagues[165] demonstrated the effects of fibrin sealant as a hemostatic and fixational agent in incisional skin wounds and transplants in burn patients. Jørgensen and co-workers[166] examined the mechanical strength of rat skin incisions treated with fibrin glue. Their results demonstrated that the fibrin sealant provided mechanical strength in the first days (0 to 4 days) of healing, whereas the control wounds possessed little independent strength. They also showed that the fibrin sealant delayed the development of mechanical strength at 20 days after wounding but did not interfere with wound repair after 42 days of healing.

Ellis and Shaikh[167] compared the tissue adhesive properties of Histoacryl blue to that of fibrin glue. The Histoacryl blue requires no preparation, while fibrin glue needed 20 minutes of preparation before each use. If the fibrin glue was not prepared properly, there was inadequate tissue bonding. They indicated that the tensile strength of wounds bonded by fibrin glue was much weaker than those approximated by Histoacryl blue. They favored Histoacryl blue over fibrin glue for closure of skin incisions.

Clips and Staples. The surgeon's burgeoning interest in clips and staples for wound closure has provided the impetus for an increasing number of scientific studies on the influence of staples and clips on the biology of wound repair and infection. Stephens and colleagues[168] compared the breaking strength of wounds closed by nickel-silver Michel clips with that of wounds approximated by continuous sutures of 4-0 monofilament stainless steel wire with rats as the experimental animal. Seven days after closure, the breaking strength of the wounds closed by Michel clips (602 ± 29.8 g) was significantly greater than that of wounds approximated by wire (488.8 ± 27.7 g) ($P < 0.01$). Early removal of wire sutures on the third postoperative day was associated with a greater breaking strength (674.0 ± 27.0 g) than that encountered in wounds in which the sutures were left for 7 days (506.7 ± 23.0 g) ($P < 0.001$). In similar studies, Myers and associates[169] reported that early removal of sutures was associated with an increase in breaking strength of the skin wounds.

The results of the investigation by Stephens and associates[168] contrasted dramatically with those reported by Harrison and colleagues,[170] demonstrating a deleterious effect on wound healing caused by skin clips in piglet wounds examined on postoperative days 5, 7, and 14. Wounds approximated by clips had a significantly lower tensile strength at all stages than those approximated by interrupted 2-0 monofilament nylon sutures. Comparison of the strength of 14-day wounds in which clips had been removed after only 7 days showed them to be significantly stronger than similar wounds in which the clips had been retained for the entire 14-day period. Retention of the nylon sutures during the second week of healing produced no significant change in strength as compared with similar wounds in which the sutures were removed early. Harrison and colleagues[170] noted progressive ulceration at the site of contact of clip teeth to the skin, which may account for its deleterious effects on wound healing.

More recent studies by Jewell and colleagues[171] compared the healing of sutured wounds with that of stapled wounds in the rat. The skin incisions in one experimental group were closed with regular-sized Proximate (Ethicon, Inc.) staples implanted at 5-mm intervals, whereas skin incisions in the remaining group were approximated by interrupted 4-0 monofilament nylon sutures placed at 5-mm intervals. Staples and sutures were removed from the wounds of postoperative day 7. They reported no significant difference between the mean breaking strength of wounds with either staples or sutures at 10, 42, and 80 days after closure. There was, however, a significant difference in the breaking strength at 21 days, with the sutured wounds being slightly stronger than the stapled wounds.

Chavpil[172] examined the influence of staple configuration on the magnitude of tissue injury and the biology of wound repair. The hypothesis that arcuate-shaped staples exerted different tissue reactions than rectangular staples was tested with finite-element and morphometric analyses of the staple tracks. The staples examined in this study were the arcuate-shaped wide Accustaple (Deknatel) and the rectangular-shaped wide Proximate and Premium (U.S. Surgical Co.) staples. Stress distribution of the rectangular and arcuate staples was made in a Swanson analysis system with infinite memory, using the linear static Ausys program. Finite-element analysis indicated a more uniform distribution of stresses in the nonlinear elastic environment around the arcuate staple and accumulation of stresses (crowding of the tissue elements) at the rectangular corner of the staple. The results of the finite-element analysis were in agreement with morphometric analysis of the tissue reactions to these samples. The magnitude and distribution of the inflammatory reaction along the staple tracks were characteristic for each staple. The Accustaple resulted in smooth, round staple tracks. A limited inflammatory reaction developed on the outside of this staple, mainly in its upper and lower portions. The rectangular staples inflicted an irregular-shaped track with evidence of tears. Inflammatory cells accumulated mostly along the outer side of the Proximate staple, being more abundant at the upper layer of skin and at the rectangular bend of the staple. The Premium staple caused a pronounced infiltration of inflammatory cells all along the staple, but mainly at the outer side of the staple. Chavpil[172] suggested that the limited tissue reaction to the Accustaple and Proximate staples may reflect the depth of penetration of the staple legs, which are shorter than that of the Premium staple.

It was surprising that Chavpil[172] reported that the magnitude of tissue injury inflicted by the staples did not correlate with the magnitude of the breaking strength of skin incisions in the neck, abdomen, and groin in pigs closed separately by the three different staples. Wounds closed by the Premium staple exhibited a significantly greater breaking strength than that of wounds approximated by either the Accustaple or Proximate staples, irrespective of the anatomic location of the incision.

The limited tissue damage inflicted by the arcuate staple as compared with that of the rectangular staple did not appear to minimize the pain of staple penetration or removal. In a clinical study by Silloway and colleagues,[173] rectangular and arcuate staples were implanted into the medial aspect of the forearms of eight healthy volunteers. After staple implantation and extraction, the patients were asked to grade the severity of the pain with a numerical scale. The pain associated with staple implantation was significantly greater than that caused by staple removal. The configuration of the staple, however, did not influence the magnitude of pain associated with either staple implantation or removal. Although the subjects tolerated implantation of four staples, they were reluctant to have implantation of additional staples without infiltration anesthesia.

There is uniform agreement that wounds closed by staples exhibit a superior resistance to infection than wounds contaminated by the least reactive suture. In an experimental study, Johnson and colleagues[174] compared the resistance to infection of contaminated wounds approximated by tapes, Premium staples, or sutures (Fig. 24–5). Wounds closed by tape exhibited the greatest degree of resistance to infection, followed by the stapled wounds and then the wounds approximated by sutures. The superiority of tape closure was evident at all levels of contamination except 5×10^7, at which all wounds were destined to develop infection regardless of the closure technique. In the presence of lower bacterial inocula, wounds approximated by staples exhibited a lower rate of infection than the least reactive nonabsorbable suture, monofilament nylon. The infection rate in these wounds correlated with the wound bacterial counts. Sutured wounds exhibited the highest bacterial counts, followed by stapled wounds and then taped wounds. When the infection rate of wounds reached 100 percent, the bacterial counts of the wounds did not differ significantly.

The superior resistance of stapled wounds to infection compared with sutured wounds was confirmed by the experimental study of Stillman and colleagues.[175] In contaminated wounds in mice, stapled wounds displayed a lower incidence of infection than wounds approximated by either percutaneous sutures (4-0 silk, 4-0 monofilament nylon, 4-0 polyglycolic acid suture) or subcuticular sutures (4-0 polyglycolic acid).

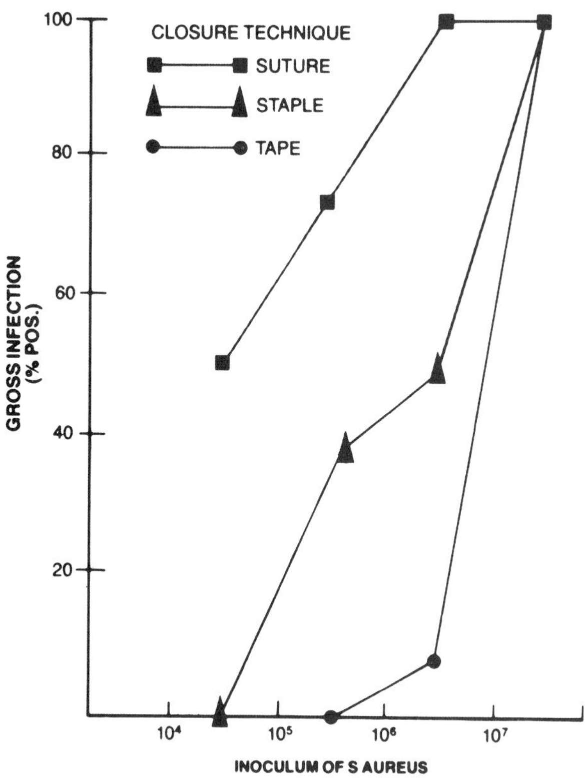

Figure 24–5. Effect of closure technique on wound infection. Standardized experimental wounds were subjected to graded doses of bacterial inocula before closure by either tape skin closures, staples, or nylon sutures. Four days later, the taped wounds displayed the least infection, followed by stapled wounds and then the sutured wounds.

In a recent study, we examined the influence of the staple configuration and its depth of implantation on the resistance of the wound to infection in experimental animals. The results of this investigation demonstrated that the configuration of the staple and its depth of implantation did not significantly alter the tissue's resistance to infection. Even though we were not able to demonstrate any deleterious effects of deeply implanted staples on the tissue's defenses, it is important to remember that staple cross-members that are flush with the skin can result in permanent transverse scars (*cross-hatching*).

A variety of disposable skin stapling devices are now commercially available for use in surgery. The selection of skin stapler by a surgeon will be determined primarily by its mechanical performance. Ideally, the device should be designed so that it does not obstruct the surgeon's view of the wound edge. Moreover, the stapler should have a prepositioning mechanism that permits the surgeon to hold the staple securely during its formation. The configuration of the stapler should also allow the position of its cartridge to be adjusted manually to facilitate placement of the staple. In addition, the stapler should have an ejector spring that automatically releases the staple. Finally, the handling characteristics of the stapler should be such that the surgeon can easily implant a large number of staples without becoming fatigued. The rotating head skin stapler manufactured by U.S. Surgical Co. (Norwalk, CT) meets these requirements.[176]

Sutures. Sutures remain the most common method of approximating the divided edges of tissue. Selection of a suture material is based on its biologic interaction with the wound as well as its mechanical performance in vivo and in vitro. Measurements of the in vivo degradation of sutures separate them into two general classes.[177] Sutures that undergo rapid degradation in tissues, losing their tensile strength within 60 days, are considered absorbable sutures. Those that maintain their tensile strength for longer than 60 days are nonabsorbable sutures. This terminology is somewhat misleading, because even some nonabsorbable sutures (eg, silk, cotton, nylon) lose some tensile strength during this 60-day interval. Postlethwait[178] measured the tensile strength of implanted nonabsorbable sutures during a period of 2 years. Silk lost approximately one-half of its tensile strength in 1 year and had no strength at the end of 2 years. Cotton lost 50 percent of its strength in 6 months, but still had 30 to 40 percent of its strength at the end of 2 years. Nylon lost approximately 25 percent of its original strength throughout the 2-year observation period.

Sutures may also be characterized by the physical configuration of the sutures. Sutures constructed from one filament are called monofilament sutures (nylon, polypropylene, polybutester, polytetrafluoroethylene, stainless steel). Sutures containing multiple fibers are called multifilament sutures (nylon, polyester, stainless steel, silk, cotton). Only nylon and stainless steel sutures are available as monofilament or multifilament sutures. Multifilament stainless steel and cotton sutures are formed by winding one filament around another, forming a twisted suture. Long continuous strands of stainless steel are twisted together to form different gauge sutures. Noncontinuous natural fibers of cotton are combined into plies. The plies are twisted together to form various cotton gauge sutures. The other multifilament sutures are formed by intertwining three or more filaments. Several fine silk fibers are twisted together to form plies, which are then braided. The number of silk fibers used regulates the suture gauge. With braids made from synthetic filaments, the large-gauge suture can be made either by increasing the number of filaments or by enhancing the size of the filaments.

The nonabsorbable sutures can be classified according to their origin. Nonabsorbable sutures made from natural fibers include silk, cotton, and linen. Metallic sutures are derived from stainless steel. Modern chemistry has developed a variety of synthetic fibers from polyamides (nylon), polyesters (Dacron), polyolefins (polyethylene, polypropylene), polytetrafluoroethylene, to polybutester. The latter suture is a block copolymer that contains poly (butylene) terephthalate (84 percent) and poly (tetramethylene ether) glycol terephthalate (16 percent). The polytetrafluoroethylene suture has been expanded to produce a porous microstructure that is approximately 50 percent air by volume.[179]

The absorbable sutures are made from either collagen or synthetic polymers. The collagen sutures are derived from the submucosa of sheep or bovine small intestine (gut). The collagenous tissue is treated in an aldehyde solution, which cross-links and strengthens the suture and makes it more resistant to enzymatic degradation. Suture materials treated in this way are called plain gut. If the suture is additionally treated in chromium trioxide, it becomes chromic gut, which is more highly cross-linked than plain gut and more resistant to absorption. The gut sutures are composed of several plies that have been twisted slightly, machine ground, and polished, yielding a relatively smooth surface and diameter that is monofilament-like in appearance. Salthouse and colleagues[180] demonstrated that the mechanism by which gut resorbs is the result of sequential attacks by lysosomal enzymes. In most locations, this degradation is started by acid phosphatase, with leucine aminopeptidase playing a more important role later in the absorption period. Collagenase is also thought to contribute to the enzymatic degradation of these collagen sutures.

A search for a synthetic substitute for collagen sutures began in the 1960s. Soon procedures were perfected for the synthesis of high molecular weight polyglycolic acid and the next homologue in this series of polyesters, polylactic acid, which led to the development of the polyglycolic acid and polyglactin 910 sutures.[181] The copolymers of polyglactin 910 were prepared by polymerizing nine parts of glycolide with one part of lactide, whereas the polyglycolic acid sutures were produced from the homopolymer. Because of the inherent rigidity of these copolymers, monofilament sutures produced from polyglactin 910 or polyglycolic acid sutures were too stiff for surgical use. These polymers can be used as a monofilament suture only in the finest size. Consequently, these high molecular weight polymers were extruded into thin filaments and braided. The polyglycolic acid and polyglactin 910 sutures degrade in an aqueous environment through hydrolysis of the ester linkage.

The surfaces of these synthetic sutures have been coated to decrease their coefficient characteristics.[182] The coating on the polyglycolic acid suture is an absorbable surface lubricant, poloxamer 188. The polyglactin 910 suture has been coated with an absorbable mixture of calcium stearate and copolymer of lactic acid (35 percent) and glycolic acid (35 percent).

A monofilament absorbable suture, polydioxanone, recently has been developed by polymerizing the monomer in the presence of a suitable catalyst.[182] This polymer is processed into small granules and melt extruded through appropriate dies into monofilaments of any desired size. Another new synthetic absorbable monofilament suture is glycolide trimethylene carbonate suture.[183] Glycolide trimethylene carbonate is a linear copolymer made by reacting trimethylene carbonate and glycolide with diethylene glycol as an initiator and stannous chloride dihydrate as the catalyst.

The strength of the synthetic monofilament absorbable sutures was maintained in vivo much longer than that of the braided synthetic absorbable sutures. These monofilament sutures retained approximately 70 percent of their breaking strength after implantation for 28 days and still retained 13 percent of their original strength at 56 days. In contrast, braided absorbable sutures retained only 1 to 5 percent of their strength at 28 days.[182]

The direct correlation of molecular weight breaking strength of the synthetic absorbable sutures with both in vivo and in vitro incubation implies a similar mechanism of degradation. Because in vitro incubation provides only a buffered aqueous environment, the chemical degradation of these sutures appears to be by nonenzymatic hydrolysis of the ester bonds. Hydrolysis would be expected to proceed until small, soluble products are formed when dissolved and removed from the implant site. In contrast, gut or collagen suture, being a proteinaceous substance, is degraded primarily by the action of proteolytic enzymes.

A distinction must be made between the rate of absorption and the rate of tensile strength loss of that material. The terms are not interchangeable. Although the rate of absorption is of some importance with regard to late suture complications, such as sinus tracts and granulomas, the rate of tensile strength loss is of much greater importance to the surgeon considering the primary function of the suture-maintaining tissue approximation during healing.

Herrmann[184] evaluated the tensile strength and knot security of knotted absorbable suture loops implanted in the subcutaneous tissue of rats and rabbits. Polyglycolic acid sutures possessed tensile strength and knot security almost equal to gut sutures after implantation. The polyglycolic acid sutures retained their strength superiority over comparable sizes of chromic gut during the first 20 days after implantation. Chromic gut and polyglycolic acid sutures had the same period of strength retention, lasting about 25 days. Plain gut had the lowest knot break strength of the absorbable sutures before implantation and had no detectable knot break strength at 14 days. Although knot security of the gut sutures was excellent in a dry state, the three throw square knots became insecure when exposed to body fluids.

The initial breaking strength of an absorbable suture is considerably influenced by the conditions of implant site that differ in various species. Postlethwait[185] reported that the rate of strength loss of two synthetic absorbable sutures in the canine stomach approximated their rate of loss in muscle, whereas the breaking strength of gut was markedly decreased in the stomach. Perey and Watier[186] reported that the breaking strength of chromic gut decreased rapidly within 1 day of exposure to human gastric or duodenal juices. Beyond 24 hours, gut had lost a large part of its initial strength, whereas the strength of polyglycolic acid remained relatively unchanged for at least 5 days. With baboons, Everett[187] measured the tensile strength of 00 chromic gut sutures in the sheath or rectus abdominis muscle, colon, and ileum. At 5 days after implantation, there was virtually no change in the strength of the gut sutures in the sheath of the rectus abdominis muscle, whereas the suture in the ileum had no strength at 3 days, and the colon suture exhibited only 15 to 20 percent of this original strength at 5 days.

Results of laboratory and clinical studies have shown that synthetic absorbable sutures maintain their strength and integrity when infection is present.[188] This is in contrast to the behavior of gut, which disintegrates and loses strength in infected tissues. Results of two investigations showed that bacterial growth is inhibited in the areas of absorbing polyglycolic acid suture.[177,189] Even though polyglycolic acid and its degradation products were not bactericidal, it was theorized that the pH at the polyglycolic acid suture sites was such that it retarded the growth of bacteria.

Higgins and associates,[190] Haxton,[191] Kirk,[192] Goligher and associates,[193] and Leaper and colleagues[194] found that fascial closure with chromic gut was associated with a significantly higher incidence of wound dehiscence than was encountered with closure with nonabsorbable sutures. Standeven[195] and Alexander and Prudden[196] noted that wound disruptions were usually caused by suture absorption or breakage. This dissolution of the chromic gut suture reduces its tensile strength, which accounts for the increased incidence of wound dehiscence. On the basis of this experience, the use of chromic catgut for fascial closure should be abandoned.

Since the advent of synthetic absorbable sutures, polyglycolic acid and polyglactin 910, several randomized prospective studies have demonstrated that they are equal to nonabsorbable sutures, including wire, in ensuring wound integrity. The recently introduced monofilament absorbable sutures may be suitable alternatives to nonabsorbable sutures because they retain approximately 50 percent of their tensile strength 5 weeks after implantation.

In a long-term experimental study, polydioxanone suture has provided a degree of protection against wound bursting that is comparable to that of polypropylene or Teflon-coated Dacron sutures.[197]

All sutures damage the local tissue defenses against infection, and several mechanisms are implicated:

1. The trauma of inserting a needle is sufficient to cause an inflammatory response.
2. The surgeon's suturing technique is crucial. Sutures tied too tightly impair blood supply and cause tissue necrosis.[198]
3. Sutures that penetrate the intact skin provide an avenue for wound contamination via the perisutural cuff.
4. The presence of the suture material itself increases the tissue's susceptibility to infection. The magnitude of this local injury to defenses is related to the quantity of suture within the wound (eg, diameter, length) and to its chemical composition.

The infection-potentiating effects of suture materials are listed in Table 24–2. Synthetic absorbable sutures elicit the least inflammatory response of the absorbable sutures, followed by plain gut and then chromic gut. Of the nonabsorbable sutures, nylon, polypropylene, and polytetrafluoroethylene sutures are the least reactive. The effect of polybutester sutures on tissue defenses has not been investigated.

The relatively high infection rates encountered with either monofilament or multifilament stainless steel sutures may be the result of their chemical or physical configuration. Stainless steel is not generally as inert as pure polymers and undergoes degradation in vivo. In addition, metallic sutures are so stiff that movement induces tissue damage and impairs the wound's ability to resist infection.

Sutures made of natural fibers potentiate infection more than any other nonabsorbable sutures, which correlates with the tissue's reaction to these sutures in clean wounds.[177] It would appear from these experimental studies that the use of silk and cotton should be avoided in wounds that had experienced gross bacterial contamination.

TABLE 24–2. INFECTION-POTENTIATING EFFECT ON SURGICAL SUTURES[a]

Absorbable	Nonabsorbable
Polyglycolic = polyglactin	Nylon = polypropylene
Plain gut	Dacron (coated = noncoated)
Chromic gut	Metal
	Silk = cotton

[a] The least reactive suture materials are listed first.

Surprisingly, our studies indicate that the physical configuration of the suture has a relatively insignificant role in the development of infection. Although the incidence of infection in contaminated tissues containing monofilament sutures was lower than in those containing multifilament sutures, these differences were not statistically significant.

With a model similar to that reported by our laboratory, Sharp and colleagues[199] reported that synthetic sutures potentiated less infection than the nonsynthetic sutures. The synthetic monofilament sutures were associated with less infection than encountered with the multifilament synthetic sutures exposed to the same bacterial inocula. The superiority of the synthetic absorbable sutures over that of naturally occurring gut sutures was also evident with this model.

In general, the techniques of sutural closure of skin can be divided into two types: percutaneous sutures and dermal (subcuticular) sutures. The selection of the technique for closure is influenced by the wound's configuration and biochemical properties as well as other special circumstances.

Percutaneous sutures of either monofilament nylon or polypropylene are excellent for closure of skin wounds because these suture materials exert the least damage to the wound's defenses.[177] The polybutester suture has unique performance characteristics that may be advantageous for wound closure.[200] This new monofilament suture exhibits distinct differences in elongation compared with other sutures. With the polybutester suture, low forces yield significantly greater elongation than that of other sutures. In addition, its elasticity is superior to that of other sutures, allowing the suture to return to its original length once the load is removed. In a clinical setting in which the tied suture loops are extended by the edema of the wound and yet are expected to return to their original length once the edema disappears, the performance of the polybutester suture would be expected to be superior to that of other sutures. Sutures with less extensibility under low forces, such as nylon, polypropylene, polyester, or silk, will frequently lacerate or necrose the encircled tissue, thereby increasing its susceptibility to infection.

In addition, percutaneous sutures are recommended for closure of stellate lacerations resulting from crush injuries. In these wounds, meticulous percutaneous suture closure of the skin edges approximates the wound more exactly than does tape. Closing these wounds often is like putting together a jigsaw puzzle, and tapes have little practical value. Undoubtedly, the more accurate approximation of skin edges by skillfully applied sutures leads to a more pleasing cosmetic result.

Because the magnitude of the suture's damage to the local tissue defenses is related to the quantity of the suture within the wound (eg, diameter, length), we employ the narrowest diameter suture (5-0 or 6-0) whose strength is sufficient to resist disruption of the skin wound. By approximating the middle portion and the bisected portions of the unclosed wound with percutaneous sutures, the least length of suture can be employed in the skin closure. An interrupted dermal suture placed in each quadrant of the wound subjected to strong static and dynamic skin tensions provides sufficient strength to permit early suture removal. Sutural closure of the adipose tissue beneath the skin should be avoided.[140] Obliteration of this potential dead space between the cut edge of adipose tissue by even the least reactive suture increases the incidence of infection.

When wounds of different thicknesses are to be reunited, the needle having passed through one edge of the wound should be drawn out before reentry through the other side of the wound. This maneuver will ensure that the needle will be inserted at comparable levels on each side of the wound. Unless appropriate adjustment of the bite is made on the thinner side, uneven coaptation of the skin will occur, resulting in a step-off scar. Grasping or crushing of the skin edges by forceps should be avoided during approximation of the wound.

Dermal (subcuticular) sutures can be used alone or as adjuncts to percutaneous sutures in wounds subjected to strong skin tensions; they serve as an added precaution against disruption of the wound. Dermal sutures are employed as either interrupted or continuous sutures. Some surgeons prefer a synthetic absorbable suture for dermal closure, whereas others favor a synthetic nonabsorbable suture. When continuous nonabsorbable sutures are employed, suture removal is recommended before the eighth day after wound closure to prevent the development of needle puncture scars.

In special circumstances, percutaneous sutures should be avoided in favor of dermal sutures: (1) infants frightened at the prospect of suture removal, (2) follow-up appointments are difficult to keep, (3) wounds covered by casts, and (4) patients prone to the development of keloids. When dermal closure alone is used, it is advisable to apply immediately tape skin closures to the wound edges to provide a more accurate approximation of the epidermis.

The influence of dermal suture closure on the wound infection rate is the subject of debate. Certainly dermal suture closure reduces or prevents totally the normal serosanguinous discharge noted on surgical dressings, which therefore may remain in the wound serving as a culture medium for bacteria. In a prospective clinical trial by Foster and colleagues[201] in 127 patients after appendectomy, wound infections were significantly more common after dermal polyglycolic acid sutures than wounds approximated by percutaneous interrupted nylon sutures. In another clinical study by Hopkinson and Bullen[202] involving 184 patients after appendectomy, the infection rate in wounds after interrupted polypropylene sutures did not differ from that of wounds approximated by continuous dermal polypropylene sutures. There is a general agreement, however, that wounds subjected to continuous dermal (subcuticular) closure are more resistant to exogenous bacterial contamination than wound closure by percutaneous sutures.[203] The percutaneous suture serves as an avenue for the migration of bacteria from the skin surface into the wound. After infection develops beneath the dermal skin closure, the collecting purulent exudate spreads preferentially between the divided edges of fat rather than penetrating the sutural closure. By the time infection becomes clinically apparent, it has involved the entire extent of the wound. This circumstance is distinct from the localized collections of purulent discharge encountered in infected, taped closed wounds. In the latter circumstance, the purulent discharge first exits between its wound edges before spreading between the divided layers of adipose tissue.

Another concern about continuous dermal nonabsorbable sutures is that suture pull-out may require considerable force that may break the suture and may be accompanied by patient discomfort. Several technical considerations may facilitate suture pull-out.[204] First, polypropylene sutures are advocated over other monofilament sutures because their surface displays the lowest coefficient of friction, facilitating suture removal. In addition, continuous dermal polypropylene sutures should be surfaced as a percutaneous suture every 5 to 6 cm to allow shorter segments of the suture to be removed. Suture pull-out by elastic traction applied over minutes to hours is considerably easier than manual traction. Despite the immediate aesthetically pleasing appearance of dermal skin closure, it does not improve the cosmetic appearance of the scar.[205]

The type of sutures used to approximate fascia (galea aponeurotica), however, has considerable influence on the width and depth of skin scars. In a study by Nordström and Nordström[206] of a group of patients undergoing scalp excision for correction of androgenic alopecia, polypropylene sutures reduced the postoperative stretching and depth of skin scars more than comparable size polyglycolic acid sutures. Another approach to reducing static skin tensions on the wound is to undermine its edges before closure. Despite common clinical usage of this technique, there has been only one experimental study that objectively evaluated its effects on wound closure. In this in vivo study, McGuire[207] identified the directional orientation of the static skin tensions by observing the oval distortion of 6-mm circular skin biopsy sites in pigs. At each location, the immediate change in the shape of the resulting defect indicated the magnitude and directional properties of the static skin tensions. The direction of the static skin tension lines corresponded to the long axis of the defects. Wounds parallel to these static skin tension lines required less force and work to close initially, retracted less with initial excision, and benefited more from undermining than similar wounds oriented perpendicularly to the static skin tension lines. Because undermining the wound margin decreased the forces required for wound closure, it should limit the width of the ultimate scar. This benefit, however, must be weighed against its potential damage to the skin blood supply, which may limit the host's defenses and invite infection. Consequently, we reserve undermining for wounds that are subjected to strong static and dynamic tensions with low levels of bacterial contamination during elective surgical procedures.

Regardless of the type of suture material, the surgeon's psychomotor skills have considerable influence on the security of the tied knot. When the recommended configuration of a knot, ascertained by mechanical performance tests, was compared to those used by board-certified general surgeons, only 25 percent of the surgeons correctly used the appropriate knot construction.[208] Of the 25 gynecologists, mostly department heads, who were polled about their knot-tying techniques, most were convinced that they made square knots, even though their tying resulted in slip knots that became untied.[209] When a knotted suture fails to perform its functions, the consequences may be disastrous. Massive bleeding may occur when the suture loop surrounding a vessel becomes untied. Wound dehiscence may also follow.

Surgical Needle and Needle Holders. The selection of a surgical needle and needle holder for use with a suture is an important consideration.[210] The biomechanical performance of surgical needles and needle holders has been characterized by quantitative measurements that record needle sharpness, needle resistance to bending and breakage, and needle holder clamping moment. These tests have documented important advances in the design, configuration, and performance of surgical needles and needle holders. High nickel maraging stainless steels have been used to produce surgical needles that exhibit an enhanced resistance to bending and breakage. The basic principle of high nickel maraging consists of strengthening Fe-Ni martensite matrices by the precipitation of fine intermetallic phases, such as Ni_3Ti. With the development of high nickel maraging stainless steels, the shape of the surgical needle can easily be changed without altering its resistance to breakage. Using this alloy, new compound curved needles have specifically been designed and developed for closure of thin, planar tissues (eg, skin, vessels).

Needle sharpening methods have been devised that produce needles with a narrow taper point geometry and sharper cutting edges. The needles are treated by electrohoning processes that polish the surfaces of the needles, while their edges are sharpened. The taper point geometry of needles made of high maraging stainless steels can be narrowed considerably, thereby enhancing their sharpness while maintaining substantial resistance to breakage. The sharpness of the needle's cutting edges can be increased further by reducing the angles of its cutting edges. Ideally, the sharpness of a surgical needle should be maintained after repeated passage through the tissue, which is a measure of the durability of the surgical needle. Coating a needle with silicone enhanced its sharpness and durability in tissue.

The site of attachment of the suture to the needle has received considerable attention by surgeons. Since 1914, the suture was attached to a drilled hole in larger diameter needles (more than 0.36 mm). Because a mechanical drill could not cut uniform holes in the swages of smaller diameter needles, a forming tool was used to create a channel in one-half of the diameter of the smaller needles. This channel became a receptacle for the attachment of the suture. This linear slit in the wall of the needle increased the drag forces encountered by the needle during the passage through tissue. With the advent of the laser, uniform holes can now be produced reliably in the swages of small needles that encountered lower drag forces than channel needles.

Ideally, the surgeon should select an atraumatic needle holder that holds the needle securely without damaging or deforming it. Selecting the appropriate needle holder for a designated needle can be accomplished by relating the clamping moment of the needle holder to the yield moment of the needle. The surgeon should use a needle holder whose clamping moment is less than the yield moment of the needle. Clamping a needle whose yield moment is greater than the clamping moment of the needle holder will result in reversible deformation of the needle. When the clamping moment of the needle holder exceeds the needle yield moment, clamping the needle between the jaws of the needle holder causes irreversible deformation of the needle.

Tape Skin Closure. Taped wounds demonstrate far superior resistance to infection when compared with sutured wounds.[211] The ease with which wounds can be closed by tape varies according to the anatomic and biomechanical properties of the wound site. Linear wounds in skin subjected to minimum static and dynamic tensions are easily approximated by tape. The relatively lax skin of the face and abdomen makes it amenable to wound closure by tape. Contrary to the usual expectation, approximation and eversion of the skin edges with tape are easily accomplished in obese patients. The taut skin of the extremities, subjected to frequent dynamic joint movements, requires that tape skin closures be supplemented with dermal sutures. The copious secretions from the skin of the axilla, palms, and soles also discourage tape adherence.

There are numerous advantages to tape closure of linear wounds subjected to weak skin tensions: (1) the cosmetic results are excellent, (2) the discomfort of suture removal is avoided, (3) suture puncture scars are eliminated, and (4) no local anesthetic agent is required for suturing. This closure technique is being used on approximately 10 percent of the patients with lacerations seen in our emergency medical service.

An ideal surgical wound closure tape should have the following performance characteristics. It should be strong enough, even when wet, to withstand the forces disrupting the wound. Its adhesive should be sufficiently aggressive to adhere securely to the skin and maintain approximation of the wound edges. Although a secure bond to skin is necessary for wound security, it also appears to be beneficial for the tape to stretch slightly under constant stress. This ability to elongate under moderate loads reduces the shear forces on the underlying edematous skin, thereby preventing blister formation. Finally, the tape construction should provide an environment on the skin surface that is antithetical to bacterial growth. Bacterial proliferation under a tape may be a source of infection during the time in which wound epidermization is incomplete.[212] On the basis of the results of in vivo and in vitro investigations, the nonwoven microporous tape (Curistrip, Kendall Co.) is recommended for skin closure.[213]

Even this tape will not adhere to excessively wet skin. An adhesive adjunct, such as compound benzoin tincture, if applied to the skin before tape application, reduces the chance for dislodgment. Inadvertent spillage of this adjunct will impair the wound's ability to resist infection.[214] To minimize the chance of contamination, the adhesive adjunct is applied with applicator sticks in a thin film at the wound edge.

Postoperative Wound Care

Postoperative wound care should optimize healing and should be tailored to the type of wound. In primarily closed wounds, the surgical dressing acts as a barrier against exogenous bacteria. Soaking dressing with serum permits passage of bacteria through the dressing. Saturation of a dressing with fluid that wets both inner and outer surfaces of the dressing is called fluid strike-through. As long as its outer surface remains dry, however, a dressing will remain an effective barrier to bacterial contamination.

The length of time that dry dressing should cover the closed wound is based on knowledge of the period during which the wound is susceptible to bacterial penetration. Sutured wounds, as they heal, become increasingly resistant to the development of infection after surface contamination.[212] Swabbing the surface of the wound with either *S. aureus* or *E. coli* during the first 48 hours after closure caused localized gross infections. Contamination after the third postoperative day did not produce gross infection in the sutured wound. Thus barrier dressings are useful to protect the fresh incision from surface contamination in the first few days. Thereafter, removal of the dressing permits daily inspection and palpation of the wound.

Wounds closed with tape had a greater capacity to resist infection than did sutured wounds.[212] Even immediate contamination seldom caused infection in any taped wounds. This resistance to infection of taped wounds after surface contamination reduces the need for protective dressings during the postoperative period in wounds free of sutures. In a real sense, the skin suture has the objectionable features of a small drain.

Another important purpose of some dressings is to exert pressure on the underlying tissues. A pressure dressing minimizes the accumulation of the intercellular fluid and limits the dead space. The application of pressure dressings is easiest on convex surfaces (ie, skull, extremity). Maximum pressure should be applied to the wound site as well as distal to it. Proximal to the wound, the pressure applied is decreased to minimize any chance of compromising the venous or lymphatic return.

A pressure dressing by the very nature of its bulk will immobilize what it covers. Immobilization of the site of injury is of great value; lymphatic flow is reduced, thereby minimizing the spread of the wound microflora. Furthermore, immobilized tissue demonstrates the best resistance to the growth of bacteria. Whenever possible, the site of injury should be elevated above the patient's heart to limit the accumulation of fluid in the wound's interstitial spaces. The injured wound with little edema proceeds more rapidly to complete rehabilitation than does the markedly edematous wound.

Most important, dressings must provide a physiologic environment that is conducive to epithelial migration from the wound edges across the surface of the fresh wound. When an area of epidermis is lost, water vapor begins at once to evaporate from the exposed dermal tissue. The exudate on the surface dries and becomes the outer layer of the scab, which does not prevent water from evaporating from the dermis underneath. The surface of the dermis progressively dries (within 18 hours). This dry scab and dermis resist migration of epidermal cells, which must seek the underlying fibrous tissue of the upper reticular layer of dermis where enough moisture remains to support cellular viability.[215]

When the wound is covered by a dressing that prevents or delays evaporation of water from the wound surface, the scab and underlying dermis remain moist. Epidermal cells can easily migrate through the moist scab over the surface of the dermis. Under such dressings, epithelialization is more rapid, and no dry dermis is sacrificed.

The water vapor permeable dressing would seem ideal for coverage of primarily closed wounds and has been employed in the treatment of donor sites, mesh grafts, and dermabraded skin.[216] Unfortunately, excessive exudate may make it difficult to keep the dressing in place, and the moist exudate, which provides an ideal medium for epidermal repair, is also a suitable culture medium for the multiplication of microorganisms.

In our clinical service, primarily closed wounds (with the exception of those located on the face) are covered by nonwoven microporous polypropylene dressings attached to surrounding skin by wide strips of microporous tape. In facial lacerations, the development of blood clots between the edges of the wounds are of more concern than the potential dangers of surface contamination. These clots will be replaced by a healing scar that can easily be avoided by swabbing the wound with half-strength hydrogen peroxide every 6 hours until the wound edge is free of blood. Because hydrogen peroxide causes the sutures to lose their color, the decolorized suture becomes a sign of patient compliance with the postoperative wound care regimen.

In abraded skin, this method of suture line care is ineffective. Despite washing the wound with hydrogen peroxide, a scab develops, which makes suture removal tedious and often painful to the patient. In such cases, we swab the wound and its adjacent edges with a water-soluble ointment, such as polyethylene glycol, which becomes dissolved by wound exudates, thereby encouraging their exodus from the wound. These percutaneous sutures must be removed before the eighth postoperative day because needle puncture scars can develop. The wound edges then should be supported by sterile tape skin closures until their adhesive tape bond weakens.

Ship and Weiss[217] indicated that abraded skin will develop permanent hyperpigmentation after exposure to the sun. Consequently, abraded skin should be protected with a sunblocking agent for at least 6 months after injury. Photoprotection against ultraviolet A in the past has been limited by the restricted range of ultraviolet A wavelengths absorbed by available sunscreen agents. With the introduction of Parsol 1789 in combination with padimate O (Photoplex, Herbert Laboratories, Santa Ana, CA), surgeons now have a full-spectrum absorbent sunscreen effective against the ultraviolet A and B wavebands.[218] This sunscreen should prove to be valuable in helping to prevent hyperpigmentation.

REFERENCES

Mechanism of Injury

1. Edlich RF, Rodeheaver GT, Thacker JG, Edgerton MT: Technical factors in wound management. In

Hunt TK, Dunphy JE (eds): Fundamentals of Wound Management. New York, Appleton-Century-Crofts, 1979.
2. Jacobs HB: Skin knife-deep knife: the ritual and practice of skin incisions. Ann Surg 179:102, 1974.
3. Hasselgren P-O, Hagberg E, Malmer H, et al: One instead of two knives for surgical incision. Does it increase the risk of postoperative wound infection? Arch Surg 119:917, 1984.
4. Roettinger W, Edgerton MT, Kurtz LD, et al: Role of inoculation site as a determinant of infection in soft tissue wounds. Am J Surg 126:354, 1973.
5. Cardany CR, Rodeheaver GT, Thacker JG, et al: The crush injury: a high risk wound. J Am Coll Emerg Physicians 5:965, 1976.
6. Fzckler ML: Ballistic injury. Ann Emerg Med 15:1451, 1986.
7. Fzckler ML, Surinchak JS, Malinowski JA, et al: Bullet fragmentation. A major cause of tissue disruption. J Trauma 24:35, 1984.
8. DeMuth WE Jr: The mechanism of shotgun wounds. J Trauma 11:219, 1971.
9. Sturdivan LM, Sacco WJ, Edgerton MT, Edlich RF: Firearm injuries: medicolegal considerations. In Wolcott BW, Rund DA (eds): Emergency Medicine Annual. Norwalk, CT, Appleton-Century-Crofts, 1984, p 125.
10. Dugas R, D'Ambrosia R: Civilian gunshot wounds. Orthopedics 8:1121, 1985.
11. Ferguson DJ: Advances in the management of surgical wounds. Surg Clin North Am 51:49, 1971.
12. Madden JE, Edlich RF, Custer JR, et al: Studies in the management of the contaminated wound. IV. Resistance to infection of surgical wounds made by knife, electrosurgery, and laser. Am J Surg 119:222, 1970.
13. Cruse PJE, Foord R: A five-year prospective study of 23,649 surgical wounds. Arch Surg 107:206, 1973.
14. Levine NS, Peterson HD, Hugh D, et al: Laser, scalpel, electrosurgical and tangential excisions of third degree burns. A preliminary report. Plast Reconstr Surg 56:286, 1975.
15. McDowell AJ: Wound infections resulting from the use of hot sponges. Plast Reconstr Surg 23:168, 1959.
16. Levenson SM, Gruber DK, Gruber C, et al: A hemostatic scalpel for burn debridement. Arch Surg 117:213, 1982.
17. Keenan KM, Rodeheaver GT, Kenney JG, Edlich RF: Surgical cautery revisited. Am J Surg 147:818, 1984.

Biology of Tissue Infection

18. Robson, MC, Krizek TJ, Heggers JP: Biology of surgical infection. Curr Probl Surg 10:1, 1973.
19. Kelly MJ: The quantitative and histological demonstration of pathogenic synergy between *Escherichia coli* and *Bacteroides fragilis* in guinea pig wounds. J Med Microbiol 11:513, 1978.
20. Ingham HR, Sisson PR, Tharagonnet D, et al: Inhibition of phagocytosis in vitro by obligate anaerobes. Lancet 2:1252, 1977.
21. Robson MC, Lea CE, Dalton JB, Heggers JP: Quantitative bacteriology and delayed wound closure. Surg Forum 19:501, 1968.
22. Edlich RF, Rodeheaver GT, Spengler M, et al: Practical bacteriologic monitoring of the burn victim. Clin Plast Surg 4:561, 1977.
23. Miles AA, Niven JSF: The enhancement of infection during shock produced by bacterial toxins and other agents. Br J Exp Pathol 31:73, 1950.
24. Conolly WB, Hunt TK, Soone M, Dunphy JE: Influence of distant trauma on local wound infection. Surg Gynecol Obstet 128:713, 1969.
25. Dineen P: A critical study of 100 consecutive wound infections. Surg Gynecol Obstet 113:91, 1961.
26. Alexander JW, Good RA: Immunobiology for Surgeons. Philadelphia, Saunders, 1970.
27. Rodeheaver GT, Pettry D, Turnbull V, et al: Identification of the wound infection-potentiating factors in soil. Am J Surg 128:8, 1974.
28. Haury BB, Rodeheaver GT, Pettry D, et al: Inhibition of nonspecific defenses by soil infection-potentiating factors. Surg Gynecol Obstet 144:19, 1977.

Technical Factors in the Prevention of Wound Infections

29. Fariss BL, Foresman PA, Rodeheaver GT, et al: Anesthetic properties and toxicity of bupivacaine and lidocaine in infiltration anesthesia. J Emerg Med 5:275, 1987.
30. Christoph RA, Buchanan L, Begalla K, et al: Pain reduction in local anesthesia administration through pH buffering. Ann Emerg Med 17:117, 1988.
31. Stevenson TR, Rodeheaver GT, Golden GT, et al: Damage to tissue defenses by vasoconstrictors. J Am Coll Emerg Physicians 4:532, 1975.
32. Hohn DC, MacKay RD, Halliday B, et al: Effect of O_2 tension on microbicidal function of leukocytes in wounds and in vitro. Surg Forum 27:18, 1976.
33. Mandell GL: Bacterial activity of aerobic and anaerobic polymorphonuclear neutrophils. Infect Immun 9:337, 1974.
34. Pryor GJ, Kilpatrick WR, Opp DR: Local anesthesia in minor lacerations: topical TAC versus lidocaine infiltration. Ann Emerg Med 9:568, 1980.
35. Barker W, Rodeheaver GT, Edgerton MT, Edlich RF: Damage to tissue defenses by a topical anesthetic agent. Ann Emerg Med 11:307, 1982.
36. Dineen P, Drusin L: Epidemics of postoperative wound infections associated with hair carriers. Lancet 2:1157, 1973.
37. Seropian R, Reynolds BM: Wound infections after preoperative depilatory versus razor preparation. Am J Surg 121:251, 1971.
38. Alexander JW, Fischer JE, Boyajian M, Palmquist J: The influence of hair-removal methods on wound infections. Arch Surg 133:355, 1967.

39. Almersjö O, Hulten L, Rydberg B, et al: Wound healing after depilation with a keratolytic cream. A tensiometric and histological study in the rat. Acta Chir Scand 133:355, 1967.
40. Masterson TS, Rodeheaver GT, Morgan RF, Edlich RF: Bacteriologic evaluation of electric clipper for surgical hair removal. Am J Surg 148:301, 1984.
41. Department of Health, Education, and Welfare, Food and Drug Administration: OTC topical antimicrobial products. Fed Reg 43:1210, 1978.
42. Walter CW, Kudsin RB: The bacteriologic study of surgical gloves from 250 operations. Surg Gynecol Obstet 129:949, 1969.
43. Sprunt K, Redman W, Leidy G: Antibacterial effectiveness of routine hand washing. Pediatrics 52:264, 1973.
44. A Report to the Medical Research Council by the Subcommittee on Aseptic Methods in Operating Theatres of their Committee on Hospital Infection: Aseptic methods in the operating suite. Lancet 1:705, 1968.
45. Steere AC, Mallison GF: Handwashing practices for the prevention of nosocomial infections. Ann Intern Med 83:683, 1975.
46. Slaughter FG: Immortal Magyar: Semmelweis Conqueror of Child-bed Fever. New York, Schuman, 1950, p 3.
47. US General Services Administration: O-T-C topical antimicrobial products and drug and cosmetic products. Fed Reg 39:33118, 1974.
48. Smylie HG, Logie JRC, Smith G: From PhisoHex to Hibiscrub. Br Med J 4:586, 1973.
49. Lowbury EJL, Lilly HA: Use of 4% chlorhexidine detergent solution (Hibiscrub) and other methods of skin disinfection. Br Med J 1:510, 1973.
50. Bornside GH, Crowder VH Jr, Cohn I Jr: A bactoriologic evaluation of surgical scrubbing with disposable iodophor-soap impregnated polyurethane scrub sponges. Surgery 64:742, 1968.
51. Michaud RN, McGrath MB, Goss WA: Improved experimental model for measuring skin degerming activity on the human hand. Antimicrob Agents Chemother 2:8, 1972.
52. Ellis H: The hazards of surgical glove dusting powders. Surg Gynecol Obstet 171:521,1990.
53. Lee CM, Lehman EP: Experiments with nonirritant glove powder. Surg Gynecol Obstet 84:689, 1947.
54. Norstrand K, Melhus O, Eide TJ: Intra-abdominal granuloma reaction in rats after introduction of maize-starch powder. Acta Pathol Microbiol Immunol Scand 95:93, 1987.
55. Ruhl CM, Urbancic JH, Foresman PA, et al: A new hazard of cornstarch, an absorbable dusting powder. J Emerg Med (in press).
56. Jagelman DG, Ellis H: Starch and intraperitoneal adhesion formation. Br J Surg 60:111, 1973.
57. Tolbert TW, Brown JL: Surface powders on surgical gloves. Arch Surg 115:729, 1980.
58. Villasenor RA, Harris DF II, Barron GJ, et al: Powder-free surgical gloves. Ophthalmic Surg 15:241, 1984.
59. Slater JE: Rubber anaphylaxis. N Engl J Med 320:1126, 1989.
60. Leynadier F, Pecquet C, Dry J: Anaphylaxis to latex during surgery. Anaesthesia 44:547, 1989.
61. Gerber AC, Jorg W, Zbinden S, et al: Severe intraoperative anaphylaxis to surgical gloves: latex allergy, an unfamiliar condition. Anesthesiology 71:800, 1989.
62. Owenby DR, Tomianovich M, Sammons N, McCullough J: Anaphylaxis associated with latex allergy during barium enema examinations. Am J Roentgenol 156:903, 1991.
63. Merguerian PA, Klein RB, Graven MA, Rozycki AA: Intraoperative anaphylactic reaction due to latex hypersensitivity. Urology 308:301, 1991.
64. Carrillo T: Contact urticaria and rhinitis from latex surgical gloves. Contact Dermatitis 15:69, 1986.
65. Morales C, Basomba A, Carriera J, Sastre A: Anaphylaxis produced by rubber glove contact: case reports and immunological identification of the antigens involved. Clin Exp Allergy 19:425, 1989.
66. Gonzalez E: Latex hypersensitivity: a new unexpected problem. Hosp Pract (Off Ed) 2:137, 1992.
67. Dixon RE, Kaslow RA, Mackel DC, et al: Aqueous quaternary ammonium antiseptics and disinfectants: use and misuse. JAMA 236:2415, 1976.
68. Custer J, Edlich RF, Prusak M, et al: Studies in the management of the contaminated wound. V. An assessment of the effectiveness of pHisoHex and Betadine surgical scrub solution. Am J Surg 121:572, 1971.
69. Edlich RF, Schmolka IR, Prusak MP, Edgerton MT: The molecular basis for the toxicity of surfactants in surgical wounds. I. EO:PO block polymers. J Surg Res 14:277, 1973.
70. Lavelle KJ, Doedens DJ, Kleit SA, Forney RB: Iodine absorption in burn patients treated topically with povidone-iodine. Clin Pharmacol Ther 17:355, 1975.
71. Ahrenholz D, Simmons RL: Povidone iodine in peritonitis. I. Adverse effects of local instillation in experimental *E. coli* peritonitis. J Surg Res 26:458, 1979.
72. Bolton JS, Bornside GH, Cohn I Jr: Intraperitoneal povidone-iodine in experimental canine and murine peritonitis. Am J Surg 137:780, 1979.
73. Gilmore OJA, Martin TDM: Aetiology and prevention of wound infection in appendectomy. Br J Surg 61:281, 1974.
74. Stokes EJ, Howard E, Peters JL, et al: Comparison of antibiotic and antiseptic prophylaxis of wound infection in acute abdominal surgery. World J Surg 1:777, 1977.
75. Pollock AV, Evans M: Povidone-iodine for the control of surgical wound infection: a controlled clinical trial against cephaloridone. Br J Surg 62:292, 1975.
76. Chlorhexidene and other antiseptics. Med Lett 18:21, 1976.

77. Food and Drug Administration: Burns with Hibitane tincture. FDA Drug Bull 15(1):9, 1985.
78. Jones RC, Shires GT: Principles in the management of wounds. In Schwartz SI (ed): Principles in Surgery. New York, McGraw-Hill, 1974, p 204.
79. Haury B, Rodeheaver G, Venski J, et al: Debridement: an essential component of traumatic wound care. Am J Surg 135:238, 1978.
80. Allgöwer M, Cueni LB, Stadtler K, et al: Burn toxin in mouse skin. J Trauma 13:95, 1973.
81. Myers MB: Prediction and prevention of skin sloughs in radical cancer surgery. Pacific Med Surg 73:315, 1967.
82. Peacock EE Jr, Van Winkle W Jr: Repair of skin wounds. In: Surgery and Biology of Wound Repair. Philadelphia, Saunders, 1970, p 71.
83. Fackler ML, Breteau JPL, Courbil LJ, et al: Open wound drainage versus wound excision in treating the modern assault rifle wound. Surgery 105:576, 1989.
84. Stevenson TR, Thacker JG, Rodeheaver GT, et al: Cleansing the traumatic wound by high pressure syringe irrigation. J Am Coll Emerg Physicians 5:17, 1976.
85. Wheeler CB, Rodeheaver GT, Thacker JG, et al: Side-effects of high pressure irrigation. Surg Gynecol Obstet 143:775, 1976.
86. Rodeheaver GT, Smith SL, Thacker JG, et al: Mechanical cleansing of contaminated wounds with a surfactant. Am J Surg 129:241, 1975.
87. Edlich RF, Smith QT, Edgerton MT: Resistance of the surgical wound to antimicrobial prophylaxis and its mechanisms of development. Am J Surg 126:583, 1973.
88. Edlich RF, Madden JE, Prusak M, et al: Studies in the management of contaminated wounds: VI. The therapeutic value of gentle scrubbing in prolonging the limited period of effectiveness of antibiotics in contaminated wounds. Am J Surg 121:668, 1971.
89. Rodeheaver GT, Edgerton MT, Elliott MB, et al: Proteolytic enzymes as adjuncts to antibiotic prophylaxis of surgical wounds. Am J Surg 127:564, 1974.
90. Rodeheaver GT, Marsh D, Edgerton MT, et al: Proteolytic enzymes as adjuncts to antimicrobial prophylaxis of contaminated wounds. Am J Surg 129:537, 1975.
91. Roberts AH, Rye GD, Edgerton MT, et al: Activity of antibiotics in contaminated wounds containing clay soil. Am J Surg 137:381, 1979.
92. Vosti KL: Special problems in prophylaxis of endocarditis following genitourinary tract and obstetrical and gynecological procedures. Am Heart Assoc Monograph 52:75, 1977.
93. Talkington CM, Thompson JE: Prevention and management of infected prostheses. Surg Clin North Am 62:515, 1982.
94. D'Ambrosia RD, Shoji H, Heater R: Secondarily infected total joint replacements by hematogenous spread. J Bone Joint Surg [Am] 58:450, 1976.
95. Verklin R, Rodeheaver GT, Hudson R, et al: Rapid antibiotic disk sensitivities of burn eschar and infected wounds. Surg Gynecol Obstet 144:507, 1977.
96. Cobden RH, Thrasher EL, Harris WH: Topical hemostatic agents to reduce bleeding from cancellous bone: a comparison of microcrystalline collagen, thrombin, and thrombin-soaked gelatin foam. J Bone Joint Surg [Am] 58:70, 1976.
97. Abbott WM, Austen WG: Microcrystalline collagen as a topical hemostatic agent for vascular surgery. Surgery 75:925, 1974.
98. Hanisch MG, Guerriero WG: The use of microfibrillar collagen hemostat for control of renal bleeding. J Urol 119:312, 1978.
99. Morgenstern L: Microcrystalline collagen used in experimental splenic injury: a new surface hemostatic agent. Arch Surg 109:44, 1974.
100. Morgenstern L, Michel SL, Austin E: Control of hepatic bleeding with microfibrillar collagen. Arch Surg 112:941, 1977.
101. Brightmore TGJ: Homeostasis and healing following median sternotomy. Br J Surg 62:152, 1975.
102. Howard TC, Kelley RR: The effect of bone wax on healing of experimental rat tibial lesions. Clin Orthop 63:226, 1969.
103. Johnson P, Fromm D: Effects of bone wax on bacterial clearance. Surgery 89:206, 1981.
104. Lawrie P: Unpublished work. Ethicon, Ltd, Research Unit, Edinburgh, 1977.
105. Harris P, Cappernauld I: Clinical experience in neurosurgery with Absele: a new absorbable homeostatic bone sealant. Surg Neurol 13:231, 1980.
106. Jenkins HP, Janda R, Clarke J: Clinical experimental observations on the use of gelatin sponge or foam. Surgery 20:124, 1946.
107. Jenkins HP, Senz EH, Owen HW, et al: Present status of gelatin sponge for the control of hemorrhage: with experimental data on its use of wounds of the great vessels and the heart. JAMA 132:614, 1946.
108. Cipolla AF, Narat JK: Effect of absorbable sponges on infection: experimental study. Surgery 24:828, 1948.
109. Hinman F Jr, Babcock KO: Local reaction to oxidized cellulose and gelatin hemostatic agents in experimentally contaminated renal wounds. Surgery 26:633, 1949.
110. Hill GB: Enhancement of experimental anaerobic infections by blood, hemoglobin, and hemostatic agents. Infect Immun 19:443, 1978.
111. Scher KS, Coil JA Jr: Effects of oxidized cellulose and microfibrillar collagen on infection. Surgery 91:301, 1982.
112. Hait MR, Robb CA, Baxter CR, et al: Comparative evaluation of Avitene microcrystalline collagen in experimental animal wounds. Am J Surg 125:284, 1973.
113. Laufman H, Method H: Effect of absorbable foreign substance on bowel anastomosis. Surg Gynecol Obstet 86:669, 1948.

114. Uhrich GI: Effect of oxidized cellulose in the protection of suture line in intestinal anastomoses in dogs. Arch Surg 59:326, 1949.
115. Chamberlain BE, Delmonico JE Jr, Gregg RO: Effect of Gelfoam on the integrity of intestinal anastomosis. Am J Surg 82:462, 1951.
116. Dineen P: Antibacterial activity of oxidized regenerated cellulose. Surg Gynecol Obstet 142:481, 1976.
117. Dineen P: The effect of oxidized regenerated cellulose on experimental infected splenotomies. J Surg Res 23:114, 1977.
118. Kuchta N, Dineen P: Effect of absorbable hemostats on intraabdominal sepsis. Infect Surg 2:441, 1983.
119. Dineen P: The effect of oxidized regenerated cellulose on experimental intravascular infection. Surgery 82:576, 1977.
120. Spotnitz WD, Dalton MS, Baker JW, et al: Reduction of perioperative hemorrhage by anterior mediastinal spray application of fibrin glue during cardiac operations. Ann Thorac Surg 44:529, 1987.
121. Spotnitz WD, Mintz PD, Avery N, et al: Fibrin glue from stored human plasma. An inexpensive and efficient method for local blood bank preparation. Am Surg 53:460, 1987.
122. Carrel A, Hartmann A: Cicatrization of wounds: I. The relation between the size of a wound and the rate of its cicatrization. J Exp Med 24:429, 1916.
123. Carrel A: Cicatrization of wounds: XII. Factors initiating regeneration. J Exp Med 34:425, 1921.
124. Smith M, Enquist IF: A quantitative study of impaired healing resulting from infection. Surg Gynecol Obstet 125:965, 1967.
125. Lee JT, Ahrenholz DH, Nelson RD, et al: Mechanism of the adjuvant effect of hemoglobin in experimental peritonitis: V. The significance of the coordinated iron components. Surgery 86:41, 1979.
126. Krizek TJ, Davis JH: The role of the red cell in subcutaneous infection. J Trauma 5:85, 1965.
127. Pruett TL, Rotstein OD, Fiegel VD, et al: Mechanism of the adjuvant effect of hemoglobin in experimental peritonitis. VIII. A leukotoxin is produced by *Escherichia coli* metabolism in hemoglobin. Surgery 96:375, 1984.
128. Pruett TL, Rotstein OD, Crass J, et al: Percutaneous aspiration and drainage for suspected abdominal infection. Surgery 96:731, 1984.
129. Edlich RF, Haines PC, Pearce RSC, et al: Evaluation of a new, improved surgical drainage system. Am J Surg 149:295, 1985.
130. Pearce RSC, West LR, Rodeheaver GT, et al: Evaluation of a new hydrogel coating for drainage tubes. Am J Surg 148:687, 1984.
131. Ferucci JT Jr, Meuller PR, Harbin WP: Percutaneous transhepatic biliary drainage. Techniques, results, and applications. Radiology 135:1, 1980.
132. Cerise EJ, Pierce WA, Diamond DL: Abdominal drains: their role as a source of infection following splenectomy. Ann Surg 171:764, 1970.
133. Nora PF, Vanecko RM, Bransfield JJ: Prophylactic abdominal drains. Arch Surg 105:173, 1972.
134. Raves JJ, Slifkin M, Diamond DL: A bacteriologic study comparing closed suction and simple conduit drainage. Am J Surg 148:618, 1984.
135. Magee C, Rodeheaver GT, Golden GT, et al: Potentiation of wound infection by surgical drains. Am J Surg 131:547, 1976.
136. Berliner SD, Burson LC, Lear PE: Use and abuse of intraperitoneal drains in colon surgery. Arch Surg 89:686, 1964.
137. Manz CW, LaTendresse C, Sako Y: The detrimental effects of drains on colonic anastomoses: an experimental study. Dis Colon Rectum 13:17, 1970.
138. Crowson WN, Wilson CS: An experimental study of the effects of drains on colon anastomoses. Am Surg 39:597, 1973.
139. Ferguson DJ: Clinical application of experimental relations between technique and wound infection. Surgery 63:377, 1968.
140. deHoll D, Rodeheaver G, Edgerton MT, et al: Potentiation of infection by suture closure of dead space. Am J Surg 127:716, 1974.
141. Wood WB Jr, Smith MR, Perry WD, et al: Studies on the cellular immunology of acute bacteremia: I. Intravascular leucocytic reaction and surface phagocytosis. J Exp Med 94:521, 1951.
142. Alexander JW, Kroelitz J, Alexander NS: Prevention of wound infections: a case of closed suction drainage to remove wound fluids deficient in opsonic proteins. Am J Surg 132:59, 1976.
143. Robson MC, Krizek TJ: Predicting skin graft survival. J Trauma 131:213, 1973.
144. Bacchetta CA, Magee W, Rodeheaver GT, et al: Biology of infection of split thickness skin grafts. Am J Surg 130:63, 1975.
145. Gingrass P, Grabb WC, Gingrass RP: Skin graft survival on avascular defects. Plast Reconstr Surg 55:65, 1975.
146. Chang N, Mathes SJ: Comparison of the effect of bacterial inoculation in the musculocutaneous and random flaps. Plast Reconstr Surg 70:1, 1982.
147. Gottrup F, Firmin R, Hunt TK, et al: The dynamic properties of tissue oxygen in healing flaps. Surgery 95:527, 1984.
148. May JW Jr, Gallico GG, Lukash FN: Microvascular transfer of free tissue for closure of bone wounds of distal lower extremity. N Engl J Med 306:253, 1982.
149. Russell RC, Graham DR, Feller AM, et al: Experimental evaluation of antibiotic carrying capacity of muscle flap into a fibrotic cavity. Plast Reconstr Surg 81:162, 1988.
150. Argenta LC: Controlled tissue expansion in reconstructive surgery. Br J Plast Surg 37:520, 1984.
151. Argenta LC, Marks MW, Pasyk KA: Advances in tissue expansion. Clin Plast Surg 12:159, 1985.
152. Manders EK, Schenden MJ, Furrey JA, et al: Soft-tissue expansion: concepts and complications. Plast Reconstr Surg 74:493, 1984.
153. Austad ED: The origin of expanded tissue. Clin Plast Surg 14:431, 1987.
154. Heaton LD, Hughes CW, Rosegay H, et al: Military

surgical practices of the United States Army in Viet Nam. Curr Probl Surg 3:19, 1966.
155. Johnson BW, Scott PG, Brunton JL, et al: Primary and secondary healing in infected wounds: an experimental study. Arch Surg 117:1189, 1982.
156. Edlich RF, Rogers W, Kasper G, et al: Studies in the management of the contaminated wound: I. Optimal time for closure of contaminated open wounds: II. Comparison of the resistance to infection of open and closed wounds during healing. Am J Surg 117:323, 1969.
157. Robson MC, Lea CE, Dalton JB, et al: Quantitative bacteriology and delayed wound closure. Surg Forum 19:501, 1968.
158. Coover HN, Joyner FB, Sheere NH, et al: Chemistry and performance of cyanoacrylate adhesive. J Soc Plast Surg Eng 15:5, 1959.
159. Pam KC, Gladieux G, Kulkarni RH, et al: The degradation of N-butyl-alpha cyanoacrylate tissue adhesive. Surgery 63:481, 1968.
160. Reynolds RC, Fassett DW, Astill BD, et al: Absorption of methyl-2-cyanoacrylate 2-14C from full thickness skin incisions in the guinea pig and its fate in vivo. J Surg Res 6:132, 1966.
161. Quinn JV, Drzewiecki A, Li MM, et al: A randomized, controlled trial comparing a tissue adhesive with suturing in the repair of pediatric facial lacerations. Ann Emerg Med 22:1130, 1993.
162. Leonard F: The N-alkylalphacyanoacrylate tissue adhesives. Ann NY Acad Sci 146:203, 1968.
163. Galil KA, Wright GZ, Schofield ID: The healing of hamster skin ulcers treated with N-butyl-2-cyanoacrylate. J Biomed Mater Res 18:601, 1984.
164. Kamer FM, Joseph JH: Histoacryl: its use in aesthetic facial plastic surgery. Arch Otolaryngol Head Neck Surg 115:193, 1989.
165. Ihara N, Suzuki K, Tanaka H, et al: Application of fibrin glue to burns. Its hemostatic and skin transplant fixation effect in the excised wound. Burns Incl Therm Injury 10:396, 1984.
166. Jørgensen PH, Jensen KH, Andreassen TT: Mechanical strength in rat skin incisional wounds treated with fibrin sealant. J Surg Res 42:237, 1987.
167. Ellis DA, Shaikh A: The ideal tissue adhesive in facial plastic and reconstructive surgery. J Otolaryngol 19:68, 1990.
168. Stephens FO, Hunt TK, Dunphy JE: Studies of traditional methods of care on the tensile strength of skin wounds in rats. Am J Surg 122:78, 1971.
169. Myers MB, Cherry G, Heinburger S: Augmentation of wound tensile strength by early removal of sutures. Am J Surg 117:338, 1969.
170. Harrison I, Williams DF, Cuschieri A: The effect of metal clips on the tensile properties of healing skin wounds. Br J Surg 62:945, 1975.
171. Jewell ML, Sato R, Rahija R: A comparison of wound healing in wounds closed with staples versus skin sutures. Contemp Surg 22:29, 1983.
172. Chavpil M: Personal communication, 1990.
173. Silloway KA, Morgan RF, Kenney JG, et al: Arcuate staple: its influence on pain of staple penetration and removal. Am J Surg 150:612, 1985.
174. Johnson A, Rodeheaver GT, Durand LS, et al: Automatic disposable stapling devices for wound closure. Ann Emerg Med 10:631, 1981.
175. Stillman RM, Marino CA, Seligman SJ: Skin staples in potentially contaminated wounds. Arch Surg 119:821, 1984.
176. Pfung D, Abidin MR, Thacker JG, et al: Evaluation of automatic disposable rotating cartridge skin staplers. J Burn Care Rehab 9:538, 1988.
177. Edlich RF, Panek PH, Rodeheaver GT, et al: Physical and chemical configuration of sutures in the development of surgical infection. Ann Surg 117: 679, 1973.
178. Postlethwait RW: Long term comparative study of nonabsorbable sutures. Ann Surg 171:892, 1970.
179. Dang M-C, Thacker JG, Hwang JC-S, et al: Some biomechanical considerations of polytetrafluoroethylene sutures for surgery. Arch Surg 125:647, 1990.
180. Salthouse TN, Williams JA, Willigan DA: Relationship of cellular enzyme activity to catgut and collagen suture absorption. Surg Gynecol Obstet 29:691, 1969.
181. Rodeheaver GT, Thacker JG, Owen J, et al: Knotting and handling characteristics of coated synthetic absorbable sutures. J Surg Res 35:525, 1983.
182. Ray JA, Doddi N, Regula D, et al: Polydioxanone (PDS), a novel monofilament synthetic absorbable suture. Surg Gynecol Obstet 153:497, 1981.
183. Katz AR, Mukherjee DP, Kaganov AL, et al: A new synthetic monofilament absorbable suture made from polytrimethylene carbonate. Surg Gynecol Obstet 161:213, 1985.
184. Herrmann JB: Changes in tensile strength and knot security of surgical sutures in vivo. Arch Surg 106:707, 1973.
185. Postlethwait RW: Rate of breaking strength of absorbable sutures in the stomach. Surgery 78:531, 1975.
186. Perey B, Watier A: Effect of human tissues on the breaking strength of catgut and polyglycolic acid sutures. Chir Gastroenterol 9:87, 1975.
187. Everett WG: Suture materials in general surgery. Prog Surg 8:14, 1970.
188. Laufman H, Rubel T: Synthetic absorbable sutures. Surg Gynecol Obstet 145:597, 1977.
189. Lilly GE, Obson DB, Hutchinson RA, et al: Clinical and bacteriologic aspects of polyglycolic acid sutures. J Oral Surg 31:103, 1973.
190. Higgins GA Jr, Antkowiak JG, Esterkyn SH: A clinical and laboratory study of abdominal wound closure and dehiscence. Arch Surg 98:421, 1969.
191. Haxton H: The influence of suture materials and methods on the healing of abdominal wounds. Br J Surg 52:372, 1965.
192. Kirk RM: Effect of method of opening and closing the abdomen on incidence of wound bursting. Lancet 2:352, 1972.
193. Goligher JC, Irvin TT, Johnston D, et al: A con-

trolled clinical trial of three methods of closure of laparotomy wounds. Br J Surg 62:823, 1975.
194. Leaper DJ, Rosenberg IL, Evans M, et al: The influence of suture material on abdominal wound healing assessed by controlled clinical trails. Eur Surg Res 8 (Suppl 1):75, 1976.
195. Standeven A: Rupture of laparotomy wounds. Lancet 1:533, 1955.
196. Alexander HC, Prudden JF: The causes of abdominal wound disruption. Surg Gynecol Obstet 122: 1223, 1966.
197. Kon ND, Meredith JW, Poole GV Jr, et al: Abdominal wound closure: a comparison of polydioxanone, polypropylene, and Teflon-coated braided Dacron sutures. Am Surg 50:549, 1984.
198. Edlich RF, Tsung MS, Rogers W, et al: Studies in the management of the contaminated wound. I. Technique of closure of such wounds together with a note on a reproducible model. J Surg Res 8:585, 1968.
199. Sharp WV, Belden TA, King PH, et al: Suture resistance to infection. Surgery 91:61, 1982.
200. Rodeheaver GT, Borzelleca DC, Thacker JG, et al: Unique performance characteristics of Novafil. Surg Gynecol Obstet 164:230, 1987.
201. Foster GE, Hardy EG, Hardcastle JD: Subcuticular suturing after appendicectomy. Lancet 1:1128, 1977.
202. Hopkinson GB, Bullen BR: Removable subcuticular skin suture in acute appendicitis: a prospective comparative study. Br Med J 284:859, 1982.
203. Polyglase A, Nayman J: A comparison of the incidence of wound infection following the use of percutaneous and subcuticular suture: an experimental study. Aust N Z J Surg 47:423, 1977.
204. Pham S, Rodeheaver GT, Dang MC, et al: Ease of continuous dermal suture removal. J Emerg Med 8:539, 1990.
205. Winn HR, Jane JA, Rodeheaver GT, et al: Influence of subcuticular sutures on scar formation. Am J Surg 133:257, 1977.
206. Nordström REA, Nordström RM: Absorbable versus nonabsorbable sutures to prevent postoperative stretching of wound area. Plast Reconstr Surg 78:186, 1986.
207. McGuire MF: Studies of the excisional wound: I. Biomechanical effects of undermining and wound orientation on closing tension and work. Plast Reconstr Surg 66:419, 1980.
208. Thacker JG, Rodeheaver GT, Kurtz L, et al: Mechanical performance of sutures in surgery. Am J Surg 133:713, 1977.
209. Trimbos JB: Security of surgical knots commonly used in surgical practice. Obstet Gynecol 64:274, 1984.
210. Edlich RF, Thacker JG, McGregor W, Rodeheaver GT: Past, present, & future for surgical needles and needle holders. Am J Surg 166:522, 1993.
211. Edlich RF, Rodeheaver GT, Kuphal J, et al: Technique of closure: contaminated wounds. J Am Coll Emerg Physicians 3:375, 1974.
212. Schauerhamer RA, Edlich RF, Panek P, et al: Studies in the management of the contaminated wound: VII. Susceptibility of surgical wounds to postoperative bacterial contamination. Am J Surg 122:74, 1971.
213. Rodeheaver GT, McLane M, West L, et al: Evaluation of surgical tapes for wound closure. J Surg Res 39:251, 1985.
214. Panek PH, Prusak MP, Bolt D, et al: Potentiation of wound infection by adhesive adjuncts. Am Surg 38:343, 1972.
215. Winter GD: Formation of the scab and the rate of epithelization of superficial wounds in the skin of the young domestic pig. Nature 193:293, 1962.
216. James JH, Watson ACH: The use Opsite, a vapour permeable dressing, on skin graft donor sites. Br J Plast Surg 28:107, 1975.
217. Ship AG, Weiss PR: Pigmentation after dermabrasion: an avoidable complication. Plast Reconstr Surg 75:528, 1985.
218. Lowe NJ, Dromgoole SH, Sefton J, et al: Indoor and outdoor efficacy testing of a broad-spectrum sunscreen against ultraviolet A radiation in psoralen sensitized subjects. J Am Acad Dermatol 17:224, 1987.

Chemoprophylaxis of Wound Infections

CHAPTER 25

Mark A. Malangoni

Few techniques of clinical surgery have excited as much controversy and produced as much conflicting data as the use of antimicrobial drugs to prevent incisional infection. Chemoprophylaxis can definitely decrease the incidence of wound infection after some operations. The risks of toxic and allergic side effects and the possible development of bacterial resistance and superinfections must be considered, however. Three methods of chemoprophylaxis—topical prophylaxis, systemic prophylaxis, and intestinal antisepsis with orally administered antibiotics—are discussed.

TOPICAL PROPHYLAXIS

Jensen et al[1] described their experience with the use of topical sulfanilamide for prophylaxis in the treatment of open fractures in 1939. They noted a reduction in the incidence of postoperative infection to less than 5 percent compared to a 27 percent incidence of infection in historical controls. Since that time, most antibiotic agents have been used at one time or another for direct application to wounds and body cavities. Although enthusiasm for such use has waxed and waned, there is a sound body of experimental and clinical data demonstrating effectiveness for some agents under specific circumstances. The rationale for topical antibiotic use in incisional and intraperitoneal infections is that concentrated antibacterial activity can be delivered directly to the site of actual or potential contamination in a greater concentration than could safely be achieved by systemic administration alone. The properties of an ideal topical antimicrobial agent are delineated in Table 25–1.[2,3]

One of the brightest chapters of near optimum application of these principles is the use of topical chemotherapy for the burn patient. Although the subject is not within the realm of this chapter, the regular use of effective surface antimicrobials has significantly increased survival of patients sustaining large burns (see Chap. 52).[4]

Local Use in the Surgical Wound

Experimental Studies. Consistently favorable reductions in wound infections have been reported when topical antibiotics are applied to experimentally contaminated wounds. Gray and Kidd[2] reported excellent results when Neosporin powder was used in wounds contaminated with *Staphylococcus, Pseudomonas pyocyanea, Clostridium perfringens,* or *Escherichia coli* and *Proteus vulgaris.* Hopson et al[5] and Singleton and Julian[6] reported significant reductions in the rate of experimental

TABLE 25–1. PROPERTIES OF AN IDEAL TOPICAL ANTIMICROBIAL AGENT FOR PROPHYLAXIS

Wide range of antimicrobial effect
Minimal local tissue irritation
Minimal systemic toxic effect
Minimal systemic absorption if toxicity is a hazard
Minimal allergenicity
Infrequent emergence of resistant microbial forms

Adapted from Gray FT, Kidd E: Surgery *54:891, 1963; and Poth EJ: JAMA 153:1516, 1953.*

wound infection treated with kanamycin (1 percent) or neomycin (1 percent) solutions. Cephalothin powder was effective when used by Waterman et al[7] for infections due to *S. aureus, S. pyogenes,* and *E. coli.* Hopson et al,[5] however, found that cephalothin solution (1 percent) was less effective than kanamycin solution (1 percent) in preventing staphylococcal infections in animals. DiGiglia et al[8] used kanamycin and bacitracin in combination in experimental wounds containing arterial prostheses, and found reductions in wound infections, graft infections, and graft failures.

Bergamini et al[9] have shown that there is a reduction in the wound infection rate when topical Neosporin spray is added to parenteral antibiotics given in the presence of a high degree of wound contamination with *S. aureus.* The combination of topical and systemic antibiotics was no better than systemic antibiotics alone in the presence of a lower inoculum, suggesting that the addition of topical treatment to systemic antibiotics is of greatest benefit when primary closure is used in the presence of substantial wound contamination.

If a streptomycin-mafenide combination is applied to crushed contaminated wounds more than 3 hours after injury, no protection occurs unless precise wound debridement is also employed,[10] an effect noted by others when hexachlorophene or neomycin solution is used.[6,11,12] Obviously the concept of the decisive period applies to all local wound manipulations, whether via systemic or topical routes.[13]

Iodine is a highly caustic, potent antimicrobial. Complexing iodine to a polymer (iodophor) renders it water soluble and stable. Recent experimental studies have focused on the usefulness of iodine-containing solutions as topical antiseptics in contaminated wounds.[14,15] Galland and colleagues[14] have reported a reduced infection rate in wounds with high levels of contamination when topical povidone-iodine is added to parenteral cephaloridine. Rodeheaver et al[16] performed experiments which suggest that the demonstrable antibacterial activity of povidone-iodine solutions in vitro may be partly related to the dilutional effects of large volumes of this compound. They were unable to show any clinical benefit when small volumes of this antiseptic were applied topically to contaminated wounds. Lineaweaver and co-workers[17] have shown that 1 percent povidone-iodine solution is cytotoxic to fibroblasts. These later studies suggest some theoretic drawbacks to iodine and iodophor compounds and question their usefulness as topical treatment. Although anecdotal clinical use supports its safety, the genuine efficacy of topical iodophors remains incompletely demonstrated.

Clinical Studies. Topical prophylaxis with single agents or antibiotic combinations in the forms of sprays, solutions, or powders has been used in a variety of clinical settings (see Table 25–2). Studies involving potentially contaminated or contaminated wounds have shown that topically applied Neosporin, neomycin, kanamycin, and cephaloridine are effective in reducing rates of wound infection. Stone and Hester[12,18] found that Neosporin spray and primary wound closure produced as good a result as delayed primary closure, a well-established procedure for dealing with contaminated emergency celiotomy incisions. Pollock and associates[19–21] found that topically applied cephaloridine reduced rates of wound sepsis in high-risk colorectal procedures and in obese patients more effectively than ampicillin or povidone-iodine did. The extensive studies of Cohn and DiVincenti[22,23] consistently documented the effectiveness of topically applied kanamycin. Clinical studies using cephalothin as a wound irrigant have produced conflicting results. Wound irrigation with the combination of cephalothin and kanamycin significantly reduced infections in clean vascular wounds[24] and after gas-

TABLE 25–2. CLASSIFICATION AND INDICATIONS FOR TOPICALLY APPLIED AGENTS AFTER POTENTIALLY CONTAMINATED OR CONTAMINATED OPERATIONS

Drug	Effective Dose
Neomycin[a]	1% solution as wound irrigant; avoid intraperitoneal use
Kanamycin[b]	0.5–1% solution for wound or intraperitoneal irrigation
Neosporin	Powder or spray in subcutaneous wounds
Kanamycin-bacitracin[a,b]	1 g or 50,000 units in 1 liter of saline for wound or intraperitoneal irrigation

[a] Aminoglycosides are absorbed from subcutaneous wounds; observe for potential ototoxic or nephrotoxic effects.
[b] Intraperitoneal aminoglycosides may produce respiratory depression.

tric, colonic, and biliary tract surgery.[25] However, the contribution of these agents is unclear, particularly if systemic antibiotics are also used.[26,27]

Raahave et al[28] studied the use of topical ampicillin powder in patients who had elective colorectal operations. All patients received a mechanical bowel cleansing and cefotaxime prior to operation as well as 6 and 12 hours later. There was no reduction in the incidence of wound infection when ampicillin powder (2 g) was added to that regimen.[28]

Povidone-iodine allows use of a nonantibiotic antiseptic with a wide antimicrobial spectrum.[19,21,29,30] Povidone-iodine spray yielding 0.5 percent available iodine was found to reduce wound infection rates significantly when compared with the propellant alone.[31] Povidone-iodine spray (0.5 percent) was compared to systemic tobramycin and lincomycin in 113 heterogeneous patients undergoing abdominal (including emergency) procedures. The spray was no more effective than no treatment at all, whereas parenteral lincomycin-tobramycin was associated with a significant reduction in wound infection.[29]

Significant amounts of neomycin (1 percent) can be absorbed via open hip wounds when it is used alone as a topical irrigant for wounds.[39] Although no adverse effects were seen, the potential exists for systemic nephrotoxicity or ototoxicity, as well as drug-induced respiratory depression resulting from potentiation of anesthetic ganglionic blockade. These adverse effects mitigate against the use of neomycin in these circumstances.

Neither Stone and Hester[12] nor Pollock et al[20] observed benefits when neomycin or Neosporin was applied to clean wounds. Existing data suggest that the use of topical antimicrobial agents in clean wounds is not justified,[19–21] although one report contradicts this thesis.[24] Topical antibiotics do not seem to provide additional reduction in the rate of infection of clean-contaminated or contaminated wounds when appropriate systemic antibiotics are also used unless contamination is severe.[26,27,32]

Polymethylmethacrylate (PMMA) bone cement impregnated with antibiotics was used in the past to prevent infection following total hip arthroplasty, but PMMA-impregnated beads have been used more recently to prevent wound infections in abdominal as well as head and neck operations.[33] This method has been shown to result in a high concentration of antibiotic at the wound site and there is some absorption of antibiotic that results in demonstrable concentrations in the bloodstream. Henry and colleagues[34] have used gentamicin-impregnated PMMA beads (Septopal) in addition to systemic antimicrobial treatment for prophylaxis in patients who sustained open extremity fractures. They found a statistically significant reduction of both acute wound infections and chronic osteomyelitis in patients who had Septopal beads placed in the wound at the time of the initial fracture treatment compared to a group of patients who received systemic antibiotics alone. This benefit was seen even in patients with grade III fractures, a group in which there was a fivefold reduction in overall infections compared to patients who received systemic antibiotics alone. Unfortunately, the parenteral antimicrobials used in these two groups of patients varied considerably and therefore it is difficult to conclude what benefit can be attributed to Septopal beads alone.

Incisional Infiltration

Taylor et al[35] have demonstrated a reduction in the incidence of wound infection with the use of preoperative intraincisional cefoxitin for clean and clean-contaminated cases. The authors injected 1 g of cefoxitin in 20 ml of water into the subcutaneous tissues along the proposed site of incision. This intraparietal injection reduced the wound infection rate to 4 percent compared to 17 percent in control patients. This same group has also noted that preincisional injection of 1 g of cefamandole results in serum levels comparable to those attained after intramuscular administration and has the added benefit that levels of antibiotic in the injected muscle, fat, and skin are higher than those reached with an identical dose given intravenously.[36] In a later randomized clinical trial comparing a single dose of 2 g of cefamandole administered either preincisionally or intravenously, Dixon and colleagues[37] have demonstrated a reduction in the rate of wound infection from 22 percent with no antibiotic to 12 percent with intravenous and to 1 percent with intraincisional cefamandole. Lazorthes et al[38] have reported that the infiltration of cefamandole along with the anesthetic solution reduced the infection rate from 4.6 percent to zero in a series of 308 patients undergoing primary inguinal hernia repair under a local anesthetic. Although this study has some faults in its design, it demonstrates a statistically significant reduction in wound infection and a cost savings compared to the control group. This method of antibiotic administration clearly merits further investigation.

Intraperitoneal Use

The use of antimicrobial agents in the peritoneal cavity to treat peritonitis and to prevent septic complications has produced conflicting results. Cohn[22] has succinctly detailed the history of intraperitoneal antibiotic use. Because some antibiotics (notably sulfonamides, tetracyclines, and streptomycin) have produced potentially severe toxic local and systemic side effects in animals, their use cannot be recommended. Emphasis in both experimental and clinical studies has been on agents effective against gram-negative bacteria. Aminoglycosides such as neomycin and kanamycin, as well as cephalothin, bacitracin (usually given in combination with an aminoglycoside), and povidone-iodine, may be useful in treating or preventing intraperitoneal infectious complications.

Experimental Studies. More than 40 years ago Poth[3] demonstrated that intraperitoneally administered neomycin protected the murine peritoneum from the lethal effects of fecal soiling. Intraperitoneal kanamycin reduced the 24-hour mortality rate in a canine model of experimental appendicitis. Cohn suggested that kanamycin is less toxic than neomycin and is associated with a lower risk of drug-induced respiratory depression.[22,23] Instillation of kanamycin (500 mg) intraperitoneally has produced significant intraperitoneal and serum concentrations. When kanamycin was given as a single intraperitoneal dose, peritoneal fluid and serum kanamycin concentrations were sustained for only about 4 hours, and the agent was eliminated within 12 hours. Therefore multiple intraperitoneal doses of kanamycin should be used.[23]

Dogs with gangrenous bowel segments that were treated with multiple peritoneal instillations of cephalothin (56 mg/kg) lived longer than those treated either with intravenous cephalothin or intraperitoneal saline.[40] Intraperitoneal kanamycin was compared to intraperitoneal cephalothin in experimental canine appendicitis.[40] Although no difference in infection rate was noted between the two antibiotic groups, both drugs were significantly more effective than saline. Hau and coauthors[41] have observed that the addition of peritoneal irrigation with saline significantly improved survival after experimental peritonitis in rats compared to another group of animals that received systemic antibiotics without irrigation. Supplementation of the irrigant with cephalothin did not further improve survival.

The effectiveness of intraperitoneal povidone-iodine was first studied in the rat.[42] Doses not exceeding 2.5 ml/kg of 10 percent povidone-iodine aqueous solution were uniformly nontoxic. A single intraperitoneal injection (2.5 ml/kg) protected rats inoculated with a lethal intraperitoneal challenge of *E. coli*. Povidone-iodine was effective only if given within 1 hour of microbial inoculation. Animals receiving the agent at 2 hours exhibited no improvement in survival when compared to controls.[42,43] Further, povidone-iodine was as effective as single intraperitoneal doses of cephalothin or kanamycin when given 1 hour after bacterial challenge.

Lagarde et al[43] administered povidone-iodine intraperitoneally to dogs with induced appendicitis. When animals were treated with 2 ml/kg of 10 percent povidone-iodine 24 hours after cecal ligation, mortality in the treated animals exceeded that of controls. Intraperitoneal administration of 10 percent povidone-iodine (2 ml/kg) 2 hours after intraperitoneal *E. coli* inoculation did not improve survival.

Flint et al[44] studied the effectiveness of povidone-iodine in a model of polymicrobial peritonitis. Ten percent povidone-iodine (2.5 ml/kg) as a single instillation failed to improve survival when given 2 hours after fecal soiling of the peritoneal cavity. Interestingly, lavage with 1.5 percent povidone-iodine in saline (600 ml/kg) resulted in a significant reduction in 24-hour mortality when compared with animals treated with sham operation alone. Peritoneal fluid cultures revealed that povidone-iodine 10 percent or 1.5 percent reduced bacterial counts, but the effect persisted only 3 hours; rapid intraperitoneal bacterial proliferation was noted by 6 hours. Povidone-iodine failed to control systemic infection; there was an improvement in survival if a single delayed intravenous dose of cephalothin (200 mg/kg) was given 1 hour after intraperitoneal administration of povidone-iodine. Thus povidone-iodine 10 percent used alone does not effectively treat established experimental peritonitis. In an elaborate set of experiments, McAvinchey et al[45] have demonstrated that 10 percent povidone-iodine irrigation of the rat abdominal cavity after induction of peritonitis is toxic and increases mortality compared to control animals.

Dilute povidone-iodine solutions (0.075 to 0.1 percent) were used in mouse and rat *E. coli* peritonitis.[46] In both models studied the dilute povidone-iodine given intraperitoneally exhibited a significant protective effect. These findings suggest that dilute intraperitoneal povidone-iodine may be a useful preventive adjunct in patients undergoing elective alimentary tract operation if it is given before peritonitis becomes established. The problem with povidone-iodine is that it may damage host tissues, so that if bacteria survive, their subsequent proliferation may be unopposed. As well, povidone-iodine may have associated toxic effects that are dose and species related.[16,17,44]

Lally et al[47] and Hau et al[41] have failed to show any benefit from intraperitoneal antibiotic irrigation when appropriate systemic antibiotics are given. The beneficial effects of antibiotic irrigation of the peritoneal cavity in these circumstances may be due to a mechanical effect.

Clinical Studies. Experimental studies[3,31] led to the clinical use of intraperitoneally administered neomycin. Initial enthusiasm for intraperitoneal neomycin waned in 1956 when Pridgen[48] reported four instances of respiratory arrest. Neomycin as well as other aminoglycosides possesses a nondepolarizing, postganglionic, neuromuscular blocking effect, which appeared to be enhanced by the concomitant presence of ether or neuromuscular blocking agents, such as curare. Consequently the intraperitoneal use of neomycin has been abandoned in favor of less toxic agents.

Kanamycin has been used extensively as an intraperitoneal topical agent[22,46,49,50] and has been alleged to cause less respiratory depression,[22,23] although sporadic reports of death or respiratory insufficiency have appeared.[51] Cohn and associates have studied both single- and multiple-dose regimens of kanamycin.[22,50] Multiple intraperitoneal instillations of kanamycin, (500 mg per dose), during a 72-hour intraoperative and postoperative period significantly reduced the incidence of infectious complications.[22]

Noon et al[49] compared intraperitoneal kanamycin-bacitracin in combination (1 g and 50,000 units, respectively) to saline irrigation in 404 individuals with spontaneous or traumatic perforative lesions of the gastrointestinal tract. Postoperative infectious complications occurred less frequently in patients treated with kanamycin-bacitracin than in those treated with saline irrigation (12 percent versus 24 percent). A report by Ericsson et al[52] cautions that bacitracin given by the intraperitoneal route undergoes systemic absorption and distribution. This is important since bacitracin possesses significant nephrotoxic potential.

Intraperitoneal cephalothin has also been popular, although objective assessment of its effect is difficult to make. McMullan and Barnett[53] treated a heterogeneous group of 32 patients undergoing abdominal operations. Most of these patients received multiple dose cephalothin via an intraperitoneal catheter postoperatively, and only three infectious complications resulted. When used as a single-dose intraperitoneal irrigation in 24 patients with contaminated peritoneal cavities, cephalothin provided no more protection than saline alone.[54]

The experimental data to support the use of intraperitoneal agents are conflicting and unclear, particularly when concomitant effective systemic antibiotics are given. Likewise, most clinical studies include the uncontrolled, concomitant use of systemic antibiotics. Thus the contention that topical antibiotics or povidone-iodine results in significant reductions in wound infection rates cannot be substantiated. Systemic and intestinal prophylactic regimens are associated with infection rates of 4 to 7 percent in well-designed, prospective, randomized studies. In no instance has topical prophylaxis been shown to be equivalent or superior to parenteral antibiotics when used alone. A report[55] by Stephen and Loewenthal provides clinical evidence in favor of a multiple drug attack upon organisms responsible for severe peritonitis using a combination of antibiotics given systemically and through continuous peritoneal lavage for 72 hours after operation. The low mortality using this regimen in selected patients with peritonitis is impressive; however, a controlled clinical trial is necessary to confirm the authors' initial observations.

Topical or intraperitoneal antibiotics may have value when delay in treatment is expected, such as in mass casualties or in combat wounds. The question that remains unanswered is whether local wound therapy is safer and more effective than systemic prophylaxis or, in the case of elective intestinal procedures, whether it is better than oral administration of poorly absorbed antibiotics. Furthermore, one cannot determine with certainty whether such methods may be additive; existing data suggest they are not. There is the additional fear that endorsement of topical prophylaxis may lead to a slackening of operative technique and the reliance upon topical therapy to "cover" otherwise preventable technical errors.

SYSTEMIC PROPHYLAXIS

The merit of specific antibacterial activity present within the tissues at the time of bacterial contamination is based on sound experimental data. The goal of systemic prophylaxis is to augment local incisional defense mechanisms by the suffusion of the wound with effective antibiotic concentrations (see Table 25–3).

Clinical evaluation of the efficacy of systemic prophylaxis has failed to consistently agree with experimental findings. Many early studies indicated that systemic antibiotic prophylaxis had no protective effect, and some even claimed that attempted prophylaxis increased wound infection rates. Many

TABLE 25–3. PRINCIPLES OF SYSTEMIC PROPHYLAXIS

Safe agent with low systemic toxicity
Antibacterial activity against expected pathogens
Administer immediately preoperatively
Short postoperative course
Use appropriate when infection is frequent or the consequences of infection are usually severe

reports have been inadequately designed or are not conclusive in their results.

The innate resistance of the operative wound to bacterial colonization and proliferation is a critical factor. Theoretically, this resistance may be enhanced by adequate antibiotic wound levels. The mere presence of bacteria within a wound does not necessarily lead to infection, as indicated by the 7 percent infection rate among patients initially surviving nonsterile thoracotomy for open cardiac massage.[56]

Experimental Studies. The natural host defense mechanisms are the most important factors in determining the outcome of wound contamination.[57] The temporal relationship between inhibition of host defenses and size of experimental bacterial lesions clearly shows that there is a decisive period during which enhancement of the size of lesions can be achieved.[57] The parenteral administration of an antibiotic reduces the maximal size of experimental lesions most effectively if given before contamination; if antibiotic is given later, progressively less effect is noted for up to 4 hours, after which none exists (Fig. 25–1). Indeed, if antibiotic is given before contamination, the effect is the same as that produced by the injection of autoclaved bacteria.

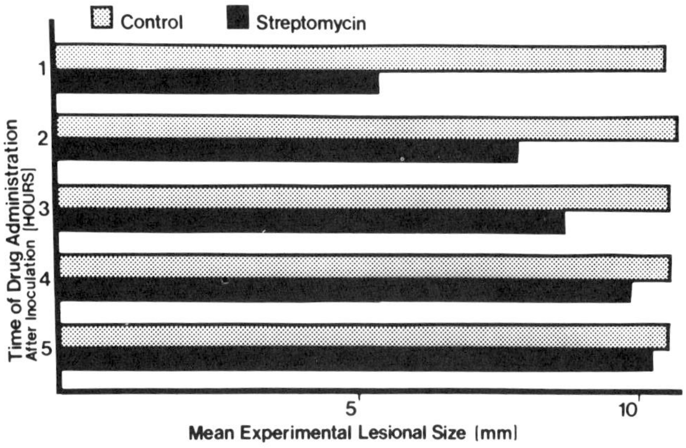

Figure 25–1. Decreasing susceptibility of experimental infectious lesions. Note that after 3 hours virtually no reduction in lesion size occurs despite administration of intravenous antibiotic.

The effectiveness of systemic antibiotics is so time dependent that antibiotics given 2 to 3 hours after staphylococcal wound contamination are ineffective.[58] These studies explain the routine failure of systemic prophylaxis given in the postoperative period. To be most effective, systemic prophylaxis must be administered before microbial wound contamination. Similarly, the drug selected must be appropriate for the most likely contaminating organisms. The benefits of prophylactic antimicrobial use can be negated by a large bacterial inoculum or by conditions such as hemorrhagic shock that can impair the systemic immunologic response.[59]

Clinical Studies. The first clinical study to confirm these experimental data was a report by Bernard and Cole.[60] A regimen of penicillin G, methicillin, and chloramphenicol was administered preoperatively, intraoperatively, and for 5 days postoperatively in a randomized trial of 145 patients undergoing potentially contaminated abdominal operations. Eight percent of the patients receiving antibiotic developed postoperative infections, whereas 27 percent of patients receiving the placebo became infected. A reduction in nonwound postoperative infectious complications (eg, pneumonia, urinary tract infection) was also observed. Unfortunately, additional antibiotics were also used in 27 patients, leaving the results of this trial subject to question.

Polk and Lopez-Mayor[61] reported 199 consecutive, potentially contaminated alimentary tract operations treated in a prospective, randomized, double-blind trial with either perioperative cephaloridine or placebo. Biliary and pancreatic operations were excluded. No patient received oral intestinal antibiotics or other preoperative or postoperative antibiotic therapy. A three-dose regimen of cephaloridine, 1 g intramuscularly, given on call to the operating room, and at 5 and 12 hours postoperatively was used. The group of patients receiving the systemic antibiotic had a 7 percent incidence of infection, while 29 percent of the patients receiving a placebo developed infections.

Since these initial studies there has been an explosive proliferation of both comparative and noncomparative studies of antibiotics. Reviews by Guglielmo and colleagues[62] and Conte et al[63] summarize the varied results of these studies, and a recent review[64] continues to support the use of systemic antibiotics in appropriate circumstances. In general, prophylactic systemic antibiotics have proved useful in those circumstances in which the numbers of contaminating organisms are greatest.

It has been relatively difficult to show in operations with lesser degrees of contamination and with lesser risk for clinical infection that benefits exist with the routine use of chemoprophylaxis. Systemic antibiotic prophylaxis will be reviewed in the context of those organs for which recommendations can be made.

Nichols and Smith[65] showed that the levels of endogenous intragastric flora were increased in patients in whom gastric pH was increased or gastric motility impaired because of treatment or disease. Patients with gastric ulcer or malignancy and bleeding or obstructing duodenal ulcer had high levels of colonization and postoperative infection rates greater than 20 percent.

Gatehouse et al[66] have reported a high correlation between the wound infection rate after gastric operations and preoperative bacterial counts in gastric aspirates. They noted that viable counts in the aspirates of patients with duodenal ulcer were low compared to patients with gastric ulcer or gastric carcinoma. In a follow-up study, Keighley et al[67] prescribed a perioperative antibiotic regimen based upon gastric aspirate bacterial contents. Patients who had fewer than 10^6 organisms per milliliter of aspirate received no antibiotics and had a wound infection rate of 9 percent. When there were more than 10^6 organisms per milliliter of aspirate, the use of a selective regimen of antibiotics (based on culture of the aspirate) reduced the rate of wound infection from 94 percent in control patients to 5 percent. Lewis et al[68] confirmed these observations in a prospective study in which perioperative cephaloridine given to patients at high risk for wound infection reduced the wound infection rate from 26 percent to zero. Nichols et al[69] reduced the rate of wound infection from 35 to 5 percent by using a perioperative regimen of cefamandole in a prospective, randomized trial of high-risk patients.

These studies suggest that the wound infection rate after elective surgery for duodenal ulcer disease is low and does not warrant prophylaxis unless treatment to increase gastric pH has been initiated. Most patients having gastroduodenal operations nowadays will have decreased gastric acid due to disease or treatment and should receive perioperative prophylaxis. This includes patients who undergo bariatric operations. In a prospective study of morbidly obese patients who underwent gastroplasty, Forse et al[70] showed that a greater dose of cefazolin (in this case, 2 g) was necessary to optimally reduce the rate of incisional infection.

The incidence of postoperative wound infection following biliary tract operation has been correlated with the presence of bacteria in the bile (bactibilia).[71,72] Patients who are 70 years of age or older, have choledocholithiasis, bile duct obstruction, acute cholecystitis, or previous biliary tract surgery have an increased likelihood of bactibilia.

Chetlin and Elliott[71] evaluated a perioperative antibiotic regimen of intramuscular cephaloridine in individuals at high risk for postoperative infection after biliary tract operations (older than 70 years, acute cholecystitis, obstructive jaundice, choledocholithiasis without jaundice). Such individuals have a significantly increased frequency of infected bile and are expected to have increased infectious complications. In a randomized, but not blinded, study of 84 patients the incidence of postoperative infectious complications was 4 percent in the group treated with cephaloridine and 27 percent in those not receiving antibiotics. Intraoperative bile cultures performed in all patients disclosed that the drug used had no effect in altering cultures in either treated or untreated groups. The significance of this study resides equally in demonstration of the effectiveness of prophylactic systemic antibiotics and in identification of a genuinely high-risk group of patients undergoing cholecystectomy. About 90 percent of these high-risk patients can be identified preoperatively, so that the groups most likely to benefit from prophylactic antibiotic therapy can be selected.

Strachan et al[73] showed a reduction in wound infection after cholecystectomy achieved with either a single preoperative dose of cefazolin (3 percent) or a 5-day course of the same antibiotic (6 percent). The clinical criteria of Chetlin and Elliott[71] have repeatedly been shown to predict patients who are at high risk for bactibilia and therefore would benefit from prophylactic administration of antibiotics. Since bactibilia can occur in 10 to 15 percent of patients without any risk factors, it seems wise to use antibiotic prophylaxis for all biliary tract procedures. The use of a single dose of cefazolin is as effective as any other antibiotic or combination of drugs for prophylaxis in this setting.[64] Recommendations for systemic chemoprophylaxis are similar for hepatic and pancreatic operations.

The incidence of postoperative wound infection following appendectomy is related to the pathologic state of the appendix and has been reported to be 7 percent, 31 percent, and greater than 50 percent for acute suppurative, gangrenous, and perforated appendicitis, respectively. In a prospective, randomized study comparing a single dose of cefoxitin (2 g) to placebo, the incidence of wound infection was reduced from 7 to 2 percent in patients with suppurative appendicitis and from 31 to 8 percent in patients with gangrenous appendicitis.[74] There was even a significant reduction in the rate of wound infection following removal of a normal appendix (from 5 to 1 percent).

Metronidazole, ticarcillin, and ampicillin are also effective in the control of wound infections after appendectomy.[75,76] Both cefotetan and cefmetazole have an antibacterial spectrum similar to cefoxitin and therefore would be expected to have similar efficacy for prophylaxis.[64]

Parenteral antimicrobial prophylaxis given along with mechanical bowel preparation has been demonstrated to reduce the incidence of wound infection following colorectal operations. In a review of clinical antibiotic trials published between 1965 and 1980, Baum et al[77] reported that colorectal procedures were associated with wound infection rates ranging from 30 to 60 percent when appropriate antibiotic prophylaxis was not used. The incidence of wound infection was reduced to 10 percent or less when an appropriate antimicrobial regimen was given. A variety of parenteral antibiotics have been shown to be effective prophylactic agents for operations on the colon and rectum.[78] Most experts agree that anaerobic antibacterial activity, particularly activity against *Bacteroides fragilis,* is essential in this setting.[79] Both parenteral and enteral agents have been demonstrated to be effective prophylaxis against wound infection following colorectal operations. Multiple dose parenteral antibiotic regimens have been demonstrated to be no better than a single dose of an appropriate drug.[80]

Perioperative antimicrobial chemoprophylaxis is recommended to decrease the incidence of wound infection in patients having clean-contaminated and contaminated operations done on the gastrointestinal tract. The choice of antibiotic should be made considering the specific organ to be operated on as well as the pathogens potentially encountered during operation. A first or second generation cephalosporin antibiotic is recommended for nearly every situation in which prophylaxis is needed. These agents have been shown to be as effective as other regimens that are more toxic, more expensive, or more likely to lead to the development of multiple-antibiotic-resistant bacteria.[81]

In an insightful study, Kaiser et al[82] compared parenteral cefoxitin to oral neomycin and erythromycin plus parenteral cefazolin, both regimens given perioperatively. Although both regimens gave wound infection rates of 4 to 5 percent in patients who had procedures lasting 4 hours or less, the latter regimen was superior to cefoxitin for protection against wound infection in patients who had longer operations (38 percent versus 0 percent). This obviously relates to the pharmacokinetic limitations of the duration of incisional effect of cefoxitin in the cases of greater duration; these studies further emphasize the importance of wound antibiotic activity in achieving optimal prophylaxis.[83]

Patients undergoing either vaginal or abdominal hysterectomy benefit from a decreased incidence of wound infection when antimicrobial prophylaxis is used.[84] Risk factors that increase the frequency of infection following hysterectomy include older age, diabetes mellitus, obesity, lower socioeconomic status, and previous instrumentation.[85] A recent review of 58 controlled clinical trials evaluating the use of prophylactic antibiotics in women having cesarean section demonstrated a 50 to 70 percent reduction in both wound infection and endometritis.[86]

The benefit of systemic prophylaxis in noncardiac thoracic operations cannot be determined from the available studies, which are conceptually or technically flawed.[87-89] Fallon and Wears[90] have analyzed the results of six clinical trials evaluating the use of antibiotics to prevent empyema following tube thoracostomy for trauma. Using the statistical technique of meta-analysis, they have concluded that prophylactic antibiotics are beneficial in this situation.

Prophylactic antibiotics are widely used in cardiac surgery without definitive clinical proof of their effectiveness. Because of the devastating consequences of prosthetic valve endocarditis, antibiotics are recommended for up to 48 hours after operation. The life-threatening nature of prosthesis-associated infections has led to the recommendation that perioperative antibiotic prophylaxis be given at the time of insertion of vascular grafts, orthopedic appliances, and other major foreign bodies.

There is no proven benefit for antibiotic use during elective craniotomy procedures. A recent review of this practice by Haines[91] suggests an advantage to the use of perioperative antibiotics for neurosurgical procedures. The postoperative wound infection rate is between 1 and 2 percent when antibiotics are used. Antibiotic prophylaxis reduces the incidence of postoperative urinary tract infection in patients with sterile urine, but it does not affect the incidence of bacteremia and other postoperative infectious complications.[63]

Systemic prophylaxis is generally not appropriate in clean operations. Because the risk of wound infection is sufficiently small, large numbers of patients need not receive unnecessary antibiotics. The risk of antibiotic side effects in such cases may be greater than the risk of infection. Nevertheless, in some clean and refined-clean operations a wound infection can lead to unusually severe complications, particularly in procedures where prosthetic devices are implanted.[84] The potentially disastrous consequences of prosthetic infection may outweigh the inherent risk of the antimicrobial agent. Ericson et al[92] demonstrated a significant benefit from prophylactic cloxicillin in patients undergoing prosthetic hip replacement. Nafcillin has been shown to be of prophylactic benefit in hip-nailing procedures.[93] The effectiveness of cefazolin (1 g intravenously) before operation and 4 doses after operation was studied in 462 patients undergoing peripheral vascular and abdominal aortic reconstructive procedures.[87] Among the 225 patients who received cefazolin, two infections occurred (0.8 percent). In the placebo (saline) group, 16 infections occurred (6.7 percent). The difference between these two groups is highly significant. No emergence of microbial resistance to the drug was noted. Graft infection occurred in four patients in the placebo group. In intrathoracic vascular procedures, no benefit from the use of cefazolin was shown, presumably because of the low infection rate in the placebo group. The effectiveness of either topical or systemic prophylactic cephalosporins in clean vascular surgery is now established.[26]

Beatty et al[94] have shown that the wound infection rate is increased when an interval occurs between breast biopsy and mastectomy. These authors note that the least rate of infection after mastectomy (3 percent) occurs when fine-needle aspiration biopsy is used. Waiting an interval of 1 to 27 days after biopsy to mastectomy increases the wound infection rate to 12 percent, compared to 5 percent when mastectomy immediately followed biopsy. When the interval between these procedures was from 4 to 7 days, the infection rate was 23 percent. This high risk of wound infection suggests that perioperative prophylactic antibiotics may be useful when this two-step approach cannot be avoided. Chemoprophylaxis has been shown to be of no benefit in women undergoing primary breast operations.[95,96]

Individuals who sustain penetrating wounds to the abdomen have a significantly increased incidence of infectious complications. A retrospective series of 295 patients were divided into those who received prophylactic penicillin-tetracycline or penicillin-chloramphenicol preoperatively, intraoperatively, and postoperatively.[97] A significant reduction in total infectious complications, deep infections, and wound infections occurred when antibiotic therapy was received preoperatively (in the emergency room). No protective effect could be detected if the antibiotic administration was delayed until the intraoperative or postoperative phase. When prophylaxis was delayed until the intraoperative or postoperative periods, the incidence of infection rose to 50 percent and 70 percent, respectively. While this study was retrospective, the results lend indirect support to the contention that individuals with penetrating trauma to the abdomen benefit significantly from the administration of preoperative prophylactic antibiotic therapy.

Oreskovich et al[98] prospectively randomized 82 patients with penetrating abdominal trauma to receive penicillin G and doxycycline for either a 12-hour or a 5-day course. Both regimens were similar in their capacity to prevent postoperative infectious complications. The infection rate nearly tripled in the presence of colon injury. Nichols et al[99] have identified patient age, the presence of colonic injury, the number of organs injured, and the extent of transfusion as risk factors for the development of wound infection following penetrating abdominal trauma. A recent study by Fabian and co-workers[100] found no difference in the rate of infection in patients sustaining penetrating intestinal injury who were treated with a second-generation cephalosporin for either 1 or 5 days. Dellinger[101] has reviewed selected reports totaling nearly 2400 patients with penetrating abdominal trauma who received prophylactic antibiotics for varying periods of time. He concluded that there was no advantage to administration of antibiotics for more than 24 hours after injury. Cefoxitin, cefotetam, or cefmetazole are generally considered the antibiotics of choice for chemoprophylaxis of abdominal injury.[102]

In a prospective, but nonrandomized and not blinded study of 499 patients with simple lacerations closed in the emergency room setting, Thirlby and Thal[103] compared the use of oral cephalexin, 250 mg four times daily for 3 days, to placebo. They could not demonstrate any benefit of antibiotic administration in this series even when contaminated lacerations were selectively reviewed. Thus oral administration of antibiotics for prophylaxis of simple lacerations is not justified.

ENTERAL PROPHYLAXIS

Operative procedures that require opening the colon have long been associated with a high risk of wound infection. Mechanical cleansing, while an important part of preparing the colon for operation, does not eliminate bacteria. Therefore residual colonic bacterial concentration is only slightly altered.[104] Large numbers of both aerobic and anaerobic bacteria exist in the normal and mechanically cleansed colon.

Optimum oral antimicrobial therapy produces a 100- to 1000-fold reduction in colonic bacterial concentration but regularly leaves bacterial densities of 10^5 to 10^6 organisms per gram of feces. The goal of intestinal antisepsis is to reduce the flora in the lumen, expecting ultimately to reduce proportionately the number of organisms that reach the incision. Numerous agents have been used singly or in combination in an attempt to protect the operative wound.

Poth[3] originally characterized the ideal intestinal antiseptic. Studies in the early 1940s suggested a possible role for sulfa derivatives. Enteral administration of succinylsulfathiazole was found by Sarnoff and Poth[105] to exert a protective effect in a canine model of peritonitis. They found significant protection from intraluminal sulfonamides only when blood supply was impaired. From these limited observations, far-reaching applications were suggested and widely practiced. Sulfonamides were subsequently shown to have variable effects on colonic aerobes and no effect on anaerobes.[104]

Poth[3] found that orally administered neomycin, given every 4 hours in 1-g doses for 3 days preoperatively, suppressed all the easily cultured aerobic fecal organisms. He therefore advocated this drug for the preoperative preparation of the colon. The subsequent observation of overgrowth of *Enterobacter aerogenes* in 10 percent of patients so treated led to a recommendation of the addition of sulfathalidine. Dearing and Needham[106] demonstrated that neomycin effectively reduced aerobic bacterial concentration but failed to reduce the numbers of anaerobic organisms recovered, particularly *Bacteroides* species.

The advantages of neomycin are rapid onset of action, broad-spectrum effectiveness against fecal aerobic organisms, and the need for administration only during the 24-hour period before operation. However, the lack of significant effectiveness against the predominantly anaerobic flora of the colon, in theory, precluded its use as the sole agent for intestinal antibiotic preparation. Other single agent regimens have been tried but have not proved useful, generally because of a limited antibacterial spectrum or the emergence of resistant bacteria.

In the period from 1945 to 1974, antibiotic preparation of the colon was used extensively. The popularity of these agents was based, however, on poorly designed and largely uncontrolled studies, in which concomitant systemic antibiotic therapy frequently was given. Such studies contributed little to genuine insight into the role of preoperative antibiotic preparation of the colon. Excessively prolonged preoperative oral therapy or concomitant systemic therapy may help explain the sporadic appearance of pseudomembranous enterocolitis. No controlled or randomized trials had demonstrated the clear effectiveness and safety of these regimens in preventing operative wound infection, nor had there been careful determination of which agents have the lowest incidence of systemic toxicity or emergence of resistant organisms.

In 1974 the first well-designed, prospective, randomized, double-blind study was published in which oral antibiotic preparation of the colon was compared to mechanical cleansing alone.[107] Neomycin alone, neomycin and tetracycline in combination, and placebo were compared in patients undergoing elective colon procedures. The combined use of neomycin-tetracycline was associated with a significantly reduced incidence of infectious complications. Neomycin alone, however, did not significantly reduce the incidence of operative wound infection or other infectious complications. Altemeier[108] and others have suggested that the benefits observed are largely the result of absorption of the tetracycline and consequent systemic activity.

The use of neomycin and erythromycin base was proposed because each agent is allegedly poorly absorbed, and benefit was demonstrated in a small pilot trial.[109] This combination, which effectively suppresses both aerobic and anaerobic organisms, has been shown to be better than placebo in reducing the rate of overall systemic and abdominal wound infectious complications after elective colonic surgery.[110] Importantly, all patients underwent a 3-day mechanical bowel preparation. The placebo group had a 43 percent incidence of septic complications and a 35 percent incidence of wound infections. The antibiotic-treated group exhibited 9 percent wound infections, which constituted all their infectious complications. Anaerobic infection was observed in five placebo-treated patients and only one antibiotic-treated patient. Quantitative cultures of colonic content showed a 10,000- to 100,000-fold decrease in the concentration of both aerobic and anaerobic organisms in the antibiotic group when compared to the group treated with placebo.

Metronidazole is quite effective against anaerobic organisms and against *Bacteroides* species in particular.[111] The use of metronidazole has been advocated for the preoperative preparation of the colon for elective operation.[108,109] Goldring et al[112] evaluated the effect of a 3-day preoperative regimen of kanamycin (1 g) and metronidazole (200 mg) administered every 6 hours in conjunction with mechanical cleansing. No other preoperative, intraoperative, or postoperative antibiotics were given. Fifty patients undergoing elective colon procedures were divided into two groups, those treated with kanamycin-metronidazole and those receiving purgative alone. There was a highly significant difference in postoperative infectious complications. In the group receiving the antibiotics, two patients developed staphylococcal infections. Eleven of the patients treated with mechanical cleansing alone developed postoperative infections, which were generally caused by coliforms. Two deaths occurred in this group; one patient had *Bacteroides* septicemia.

The double-blind, prospective, randomized series of 70 patients reported by Brass et al[113] had either neomycin-erythromycin base or neomycin-metronidazole as oral preparation for elective colon surgery. All patients received mechanical cleansing. Metronidazole was given in 750-mg doses three times a day for 2 days before operation. Erythromycin base and neomycin were given three times a day in 1-g doses, each during a 24-hour period preoperatively. In addition, all patients received a three-dose perioperative regimen of 1-g doses of cephalothin intravenously. Ordinarily the use of systemic drugs would fatally flaw such a study; however, systemic cephalothin is rapidly excreted and achieves low wound antibiotic levels and appears to exert minimal, if any, effect on the overall results of this study. All ten infections in the neomycin-erythromycin group of 40 patients were associated with coliform organisms. The two infections in the group treated with metronidazole were due to staphylococcal organisms; no coliform organisms were observed.

Beggs et al[114] were unable to show a difference between oral and intravenous administration of identical doses of metronidazole (500 mg every 8 hours) given along with oral neomycin as prophylaxis in colorectal operations. Intravenous administration produced effective serum levels of antibiotics at the end of the operation while oral antibiotics gave suboptimal serum levels. Wound and tissue concentrations of antibiotics were not measured. Gram-positive wound infections were common in the 6 of 46 patients who failed prophylaxis in the oral antibiotic group.

Although these studies clearly demonstrate the effectiveness of metronidazole in suppressing anaerobic flora, a comparison with the report by Clarke and associates[110] is difficult to make because of the certain absorption and therefore concomitant systemic activity of both metronidazole and erythromycin. The perioperative use of cephalothin, an agent with low prophylactic effectiveness in this situation, contributes another major difference from the study by Clarke. Lewis et al[115] have demonstrated that neomycin may not be a necessary component of enteral prophylaxis. These authors showed no difference in the incidence of wound infection between patients who received neomycin and erythromycin and those who were given erythromycin with metronidazole.

Various studies have attempted to evaluate the effect of adding parenteral antibiotics to the oral neomycin-erythromycin base regimen.[115–118] The addition of either the combination of gentamicin and clindamycin[115] or cephalothin[117] did not significantly affect the incidence of wound infection after colorectal operations. Coppa et al[118] have reported a reduction in wound infections by adding a perioperative regimen of cefoxitin to neomycin-erythromycin oral prophylaxis. The results of this study have been controversial since the wound infection rate in the patient group that received neomycin-erythromycin was 18 percent, a higher incidence than in earlier studies by other investigators who used this regimen. Schoetz and colleagues[119] observed similar results. No difference in the risk of wound infection was observed when intravenous cefoxitin was added to the standard neomycin erythromycin base regimen described above in patients who underwent elective colorectal operations or colectomy with ileal pouch-anal anastomosis.[120,121]

Hojer and Wetterfors[122] used oral doxycycline for prophylaxis in patients undergoing colonic operations. Doxycycline possesses antibacterial activity against both aerobes and anaerobes and has a high affinity for intestinal tissue. In a double-blind, prospective, randomized study, doxycycline was administered as a 200-mg oral loading dose during the 24-hour preoperative period and was continued parenterally for 5 days postoperatively at 100 mg/day. Abdominal wound sepsis occurred in 8 percent of patients receiving the doxycycline and 41 percent of those receiving placebo. Mean serum doxycycline levels were often exceeded by doxycycline levels in intestinal mucosa. Eighty-three percent of anaerobes and 71 percent of aerobes were classified as being sensitive to this agent. However, overall aerobic resistance to doxycycline increased from 22 percent in the controls to 50 percent in the experimental group.

Both systemic prophylaxis and enteral prophylaxis appear to reduce the rate of infectious complications following operation upon the colon. A randomized study by Lewis et al[123] compared these two regimens in patients undergoing elective colon operation. Systemic therapy was accomplished by using perioperative cephaloridine, and enteral prophylaxis was completed using neomycin-erythromycin base. The patient populations in both groups were well matched. In the total group of 79 patients, no significant difference was observed in the rate of infectious complications after elective colon operation. The distribution of anaerobic organisms in stool culture specimens was essentially the same, and each group had one episode of anaerobic wound infection.

Edmondson and Rissing[124] have compared systemic and enteral prophylaxis along with mechanical bowel preparation in colon procedures. They found perioperative intramuscular cephaloridine to be inferior to preoperative oral neomycin and erythromycin base. Five of the eight patients who developed wound infection after cephaloridine administration had *B. fragilis* isolated on culture. This study confirms the principles advocated by Cohn, that the primary role of the intestinal antibiotics is to decrease the concentration of intraluminal bacteria within the colon. Patient accession to this study was sporadic and raises questions as to its reproducibility.

It is apparent that in the presence of adequate mechanical bowel preparation, either systemic or enteral antibiotic prophylaxis for colorectal operations is adequate. Enteral antibiotic use is not effective when mechanical bowel preparation cannot be done, when the oral agents are given incorrectly or are not tolerated (particularly erythromycin base), or when the duration of the operation exceeds 3 hours. Also, the substitution of polyethylene-glycol solution lavage for the traditional 3-day mechanical bowel preparation has affected the usefulness of the standard neomycin-erythromycin base enteral regimen. When whole gut lavage is used, an alternative enteral regimen of neomycin (2 g) and metronidazole (2 g) given at 7 p.m. and 11 p.m. on the day prior to operation has been demonstrated to be effective.[125] The use of enteral prophylaxis regimens may have begun to decrease due to a trend toward outpatient mechanical bowel cleansing and admission of patients on the same day as operation. It remains doubtful whether this benefit is augmented by combined systemic-oral prophylaxis.

CHEMOPROPHYLAXIS: PRINCIPLES AND PRACTICE

The principles of chemoprophylaxis are distinctly different from the principles used to guide therapeutic antibiotic use and selection. In order to be successful, chemoprophylaxis must be given before or at the time of contamination.[13,57,126–129] Prophylactic antibiotic therapy is not indicated, nor will it be beneficial, in all surgical wounds. In most clean operative wounds (eg, herniorrhaphy, thyroidectomy) the risk of infection approaches 1 percent. It is, at best, questionable whether the routine use of systemic or topical chemoprophylaxis can successfully reduce this rate further. The risks of drug reactions (2 to 3 percent) and the tendency toward selection of resistant organisms outweigh the potential benefit of topical or systemic antibiotics in low-risk patients. Many studies have disclosed no benefit associated with the use of topical or systemic agents in clean operative wounds.[12,18–21,29] The major exception is in clean procedures in which prosthetic devices are implanted where infection introduces the risk of unusually severe complication.[24,26,93,97] The primary indication for prophylactic agents is in cases associated with a high frequency of, or unusually severe, sequelae of infection[60,61,71] (Table 25–4).

The selection of an antimicrobial agent must also be based on the sensitivity of the expected flora. Current recommendations for parenteral prophylaxis are listed in Table 25–4.

Topical therapy allows the use of poorly absorbed, but potentially more toxic agents in higher local concentrations than can be safely achieved by systemic administration alone. In addition, local therapy has been advocated because there may be fewer antibiotic-induced alterations in granulocyte function, a concern of as yet undetermined clinical significance. No studies show that topical therapy fully obviates the problem of systemic absorption; topical neomycin is absorbed in significant quantities.[122] Curiously, no studies appear to have compared topical therapy in a controlled fashion to either systemic or intestinal prophylactic methods. Aminoglycosides are absorbed from the peritoneal cavity, and the use of intraperitoneal antibiotics, while possibly effective, requires that precautions be taken to prevent respiratory complications or nephrotoxic or ototoxic effects. Effective topical agents are delineated in Table 25–2. A major determining factor in successful systemic prophylaxis is the ability of parenterally administered agents to penetrate the tissues in sufficiently high concentrations to exceed the minimal inhibitory concentration of expected contaminating flora.

TABLE 25–4. RECOMMENDATIONS FOR PROPHYLACTIC ANTIBIOTICS TO PREVENT WOUND INFECTION

Operation	Common Pathogens	Recommended Drugs	Dosage Before Operation
Clean			
Cardiac—prosthetic valve, coronary artery bypass, etc	*S. aureus, S. epidermidis, Corynebacterium*; enteric gram-negative bacilli	Cefazolin or vancomycin	1 g IV 1 g IV
Neurosurgery—craniotomy	*S. aureus, S. epidermidis*	Cefazolin or vancomycin	1 g IV 1 g IV
Orthopedic—internal fracture fixation, prosthetic joint replacement	*S. aureus, S. epidermidis*	Cefazolin	1 g IV
Vascular—aortic surgery, prosthetic graft insertion, groin incision, amputation for ischemia	*S. aureus, S. epidermidis*	Cefazolin	1 g IV
Clean-contaminated			
Appendectomy	Enteric gram-negative bacilli; anaerobes	Cefoxitin or cefotetan or cefmetazole	2 g IV 1–2 g IV 1–2 g IV
Biliary tract, hepatic, or pancreatic surgery	Enteric gram-negative bacilli; enterococci, *C. perfringens*	Cefazolin	1 g IV
Colorectal/distal ileum	Enteric gram-negative bacilli; anaerobes	Neomycin, erythromycin base or cefoxitin or cefotetan or cefmetazole	1 g each PO at 1, 2, 11 p.m. on day prior to operation 2 g IV 1–2 g IV 1–2 g IV
Gastroduodenal; proximal small intestine—includes gastric bypass, gastrostomy	Enteric gram-negative bacilli; gram-positive cocci	Cefazolin	1 g IV
Head and neck—operations involving aerodigestive tract	*S. aureus*, streptococci anaerobes	Cefazolin or clindamycin	1 g IV 600 mg IV
Hysterectomy	Enteric gram-negative bacilli; anaerobes, group B streptococci, enterococci	Cefazolin	1 g IV
Cesarean section	Enteric gram-negative bacilli; anaerobes, group B streptococci, enterococci	Cefazolin	1 g IV after clamping of umbilical cord
Thoracic—pulmonary; esophageal surgery	*S. aureus*, anaerobes, streptococci; gram-negative enteric bacilli	Cefazolin	1 g IV
Urologic	Gram-negative enteric bacilli; enterococci	Cefazolin	1 g IV
Contaminated			
Penetrating trauma	Gram-negative enteric bacilli; anaerobes	Cefoxitin or cefotetan or cefmetazole	2 g IV 1–2 g IV 1–2 g IV
Blunt trauma	Gram-negative enteric bacilli	Cefazolin	1 g IV

Several clear points emerge from these data: (1) wound antibiotic activity is probably the primary mechanism of action of systemic prophylaxis; (2) accordingly, maintaining such levels is crucial (via redosing or continuous infusion, depending on the pharmacology of a given drug[130]); and (3) the degree and duration of wound antibiotic activity are those characteristics that best define drugs likely to be effective prophylactic agents.[131]

Although some orally administered intestinal antibiotics are effective in reducing infectious complications after colon operation, there is no clear benefit of oral or systemic agents, one over the other, for prophylaxis in colon operations.

The experimental work of Miles et al[57] and Burke[126] have demonstrated the importance of timing of antibiotic administration in order to achieve an optimal effect. Stone and co-workers[132] have shown that no benefit was recognized when antimicrobials were given for 24 hours prior to operation compared to a single preoperative dose given properly. In fact, when an antibiotic is given more than 1 hour before the incision is made, the incidence of wound infection may actually be increased.[133] A recent report by the Antimicrobial Agents Committee of the Surgical Infection Society has recommended that "on call" antimicrobial administration prior to operation is not acceptable practice.[134] Classen and co-workers[135] reported that prophylactic administration of antibiotics in the 2-hour interval before operation reduced the risk of wound infection. Antimicrobials given more than 2 hours preceding operation or postoperatively were much less effective. The prolonged use of antibiotics for more than 24 hours following operation has not reduced the incidence of wound infection following clean-contaminated and contaminated abdominal procedures.[132]

In view of the effectiveness of these methods in reducing infectious complications, the question of the appropriateness of using a combination of drugs for prophylaxis warrants discussion. Pitt et al[26] found no benefit when topical drug use was added to systemic administration, or vice versa; they did, however, confirm the advantages of one or the other over untreated control vascular operations. Similarly, Dion et al[136] found no difference between oral and parenteral use of metronidazole in colon operations, but this use did have an antimicrobial effect on bacteria in the colon following systemic therapy. Newer parenteral cephalosporins appear to add little benefit to prophylaxis in spite of a broader antimicrobial spectrum.[81] Likewise the structure of many clinical comparative trials of antibiotics is such that results should be interpreted with caution.[137]

REFERENCES

1. Jensen NK, Johnsrud LW, Nelson MC: Local implantation of sulfanilomide in compound fractures. Surgery 6:1, 1939.
2. Gray FJ, Kidd E: Topical chemotherapy in prevention of wound infection. Surgery 54:891, 1963.
3. Poth EJ: Intestinal antisepsis in surgery. JAMA 153:1516, 1953.
4. Polk HC Jr, Stone HH (eds): Contemporary Burn Management. Boston, Little, Brown, 1971, pp 171–244.
5. Hopson WB Jr, Britt LG, Sherman RT, Ledes CP: The use of topical antibiotic in the prevention of experimental wound infection. J Surg Res 8:261, 1968.
6. Singleton AO, Julian J: An experimental evaluation of methods used to prevent infection in wounds which have been contaminated with feces. Ann Surg 151:912, 1960.
7. Waterman NG, Howell RS, Babich M: The effect of a prophylactic topical antibiotic (cephalothin) on the incidence of wound infection. Arch Surg 97:365, 1968.
8. DiGiglia JW, Leonard GL, Ochsner JL: Local irrigation with an antibiotic solution in the prevention of infection in vascular prostheses. Surgery 67:836, 1970.
9. Bergamini TM, Lamont PM, Cheadle WG, Polk HC Jr: Combined topical and systemic antibiotic prophylaxis in experimental wound infection. Am J Surg 147:753, 1984.
10. Howes EL: Topical use of streptomycin in wounds. Am J Med 2:449, 1947.
11. Gingrass RP, Close AS, Ellison EH: The effect of various topical and parenteral agents on the prevention of infection in experimental contaminated wounds. J Trauma 4:763, 1964.
12. Stone HH, Hester TR Jr: Incisional and peritoneal infection after emergency celiotomy. Ann Surg 177:699, 1973.
13. Polk HC Jr, Miles AA: The decisive period in the primary infection of muscle by *Escherichia coli*. Br J Exp Pathol 54:99, 1973.
14. Galland RB, Heine KJ, Trachtenberg LS, Polk HC Jr: Reduction of surgical wound infection rates in contaminated wounds treated with antiseptics combined with systemic antibiotics: an experimental study. Surgery 91:329, 1982.
15. Scher KS: Prevention of wound infection—the comparative effectiveness of topical and systemic cefazolin and povidone-iodine. Am Surg 48:268, 1982.
16. Rodeheaver G, Bellamy W, Kody M, et al: Bacterial activity and toxicity of iodine-containing solutions in wounds. Arch Surg 117:181, 1982.
17. Lineaweaver W, Howard R, Soucy D, et al: Topical antimicrobial toxicity. Arch Surg 120:267, 1985.
18. Stone HH, Hester TR Jr: Topical antibiotic and delayed primary closure in the management of contaminated surgical incisions. J Surg Res 12:70, 1972.
19. Pollock AV, Evans M: Povidone-iodine for the control of surgical wound infection: a controlled clinical trial against cephaloridine. Br J Surg 62:292, 1975.
20. Pollock AV, Leaper DJ, Evans M: Single dose intra-incisional antibiotic prophylaxis of surgical wound sepsis: a controlled trial of cephaloridine and ampicillin. Br J Surg 64:322, 1977.
21. Pollock AV, Froome K, Evans M: The bacteriology of primary wound sepsis in potentially contaminated abdominal operations: the effect of irrigation, povidone-iodine and cephaloridine on the sepsis rate assessed in a clinical trial. Br J Surg 65:76, 1978.
22. Cohn I Jr: Intraperitoneal antibiotic administration. Surg Gynecol Obstet 114:309, 1962.
23. DiVincenti FC, Cohn I Jr: Intraperitoneal kanamy-

cin in advanced peritonitis. Am J Surg 111:147, 1966.
24. Lord JW Jr, Rossi G, Daliana M: Intraoperative antibiotic wound lavage: an attempt to eliminate postoperative infection in arterial and clean general surgical procedures. Ann Surg 185:634, 1977.
25. Lord JW, LaRaja RD, Daliana M, Gordon MT: Prophylactic antibiotic wound irrigation in gastric, biliary, and colonic surgery. Am J Surg 145:209, 1983.
26. Pitt HA, Postier RG, MacGowan WAL, et al: Prophylactic antibiotics in vascular surgery—topical, systemic, or both? Ann Surg 192:356, 1980.
27. Freischlag J, McGrattan M, Busuttil RW: Topical versus systemic cephalosporin administration in elective biliary operations. Surgery 96:686, 1984.
28. Raahave D, Hesselfeldt P, Pedersen T, et al: No effect of topical ampicillin prophylaxis in elective operations of the colon or rectum. Surg Gynecol Obstet 168:112, 1989.
29. Galland RB, Saunders JH, Mosley JG, Darrell JH: Prevention of wound infection in abdominal operations by perioperative antibiotics or povidone-iodine: a controlled trial. Lancet 2:1043, 1977.
30. Gilmore OJ, Martin TD: Aetiology and prevention of wound infection in appendicectomy. Br J Surg 61:281, 1974.
31. Gilmore OJ, Sanderson PJ: Prophylactic intraparietal povidone-iodine in abdominal surgery. Br J Surg 62:792, 1975.
32. Pitt HA, Postier RG, Gadacz TR, Cameron JL: The role of topical antibiotics and "high-risk" biliary surgery. Surgery 91:518, 1982.
33. Calhoun JH, Mader JT: Antibiotic beads in the management of surgical infections. Am J Surg 157.443, 1989.
34. Henry SL, Ostermann PAW, Seligson D: The prophylactic use of antibiotic impregnated beads in open fractures. J Trauma 30:1231, 1990.
35. Taylor TV, Walker WS, Mason RC, et al: Preoperative intraparietal (intraincisional) cefoxitin in abdominal surgery. Br J Surg 69:461, 1982.
36. Armstrong CP, Taylor TV, Reeves DS: Preincisional intraparietal injection of cephamandole: a new approach to wound infection prophylaxis. Br J Surg 69:459, 1982.
37. Dixon JM, Armstrong JP, Duffy SW, et al: A randomized prospective trial comparing the value of intravenous and preincisional cefamandole in reducing postoperative sepsis after operations upon the gastrointestinal tract. Surg Gynecol Obstet 158:303, 1984.
38. Lazorthes F, Chiotasso P, Massip P, et al: Local antibiotic prophylaxis in hernia repair. Surg Gynecol Obstet 175:569, 1992.
39. Weinstein AJ, McHenry MC, Gavan TL: Systemic absorption of neomycin irrigating solution. JAMA 238:152, 1977.
40. Crook JN, Cotlar AM, Bornside GH, Cohn I Jr: Intraperitoneal cephalothin in the treatment of experimental appendiceal peritonitis. Am Surg 34:736, 1968.
41. Hau T, Nishikawa R, Phuangsab A: Irrigation of the peritoneal cavity and local antibiotics in the treatment of peritonitis. Surg Gynecol Obstet 156:25, 1983.
42. Lavigne JE, Brown CS, Machiedo GW, et al: The treatment of experimental peritonitis with intraperitoneal Betadine solution. J Surg Res 16:307, 1974.
43. Lagarde MC, Bolton JS, Cohn I Jr: Intraperitoneal povidone-iodine in experimental peritonitis. Ann Surg 187:613, 1978.
44. Flint LM Jr, Beasley DJ, Richardson JD, Polk HC Jr: Topical povidone-iodine reduces mortality from bacterial peritonitis. J Surg Res 26:280, 1979.
45. McAvinchey DJ, McCollum PT, McElearney NG, et al: Antiseptics in the treatment of bacterial peritonitis in rats. Br J Surg 70:158, 1983.
46. Gilmore OJA, Reid C, Houang ET, Shaw EJ: Prophylactic intraperitoneal povidone-iodine in alimentary tract surgery. Am J Surg 135:156, 1978.
47. Lally KP, Trettin JC, Torma JM: Adjunctive antibiotic lavage in experimental peritonitis. Surg Gynecol Obstet 156:605, 1983.
48. Pridgen A: Respiratory arrest thought to be due to intraperitoneal neomycin. Surgery 40:571, 1956.
49. Noon GP, Beall AC Jr, Jordan GL Jr, et al: Clinical evaluation of peritoneal irrigation with antibiotic solution. Surgery 62:73, 1967.
50. DiVincenti FC, Cohn I Jr: Prolonged administration of intraperitoneal kanamycin in the treatment of peritonitis. Am Surg 37:177, 1971.
51. Mullett RD, Keats AS: Apnea and respiratory insufficiency after intraperitoneal administration of kanamycin. Surgery 49:530, 1961.
52. Ericsson CD, Duke JH Jr, Pickering LK, Qadri SMH: Systemic absorption of bacitracin after peritoneal lavage. Am J Surg 137:65, 1979.
53. McMullan MH, Barnett WO: The clinical use of intraperitoneal cephalothin. Surgery 67:432, 1970.
54. Rambo W: Irrigation of the peritoneal cavity with cephalothin. Am J Surg 123:192, 1972.
55. Stephen M, Loewenthal J: Continuing peritoneal lavage in high-risk peritonitis. Surgery 85:603, 1979.
56. Altemeier WA, Todd J: Studies on the incidence of infection following open chest cardiac massage for cardiac arrest. Ann Surg 158:596, 1963.
57. Miles AA, Miles EM, Burke J: The value and duration of defense reactions of the skin to the primary lodgement of bacteria. Br J Exp Pathol 38:79, 1957.
58. Burke JF: The effective period of preventive antibiotic action in experimental incisions and dermal lesions. Surgery 50:161, 1961.
59. Livingston DH, Malangoni MA: An experimental study of susceptibility to infection after hemorrhagic shock. Surg Gynecol Obstet 168:138, 1988.
60. Bernard HR, Cole WR: The prophylaxis of surgical infection: the effect of prophylactic antimicrobial

drugs on the incidence of infection following potentially contaminated operations. Surgery 56:151, 1964.
61. Polk HC Jr, Lopez-Mayor JF: Postoperative wound infection: a prospective study of determinant factors and prevention. Surgery 66:97, 1969.
62. Guglielmo BJ, Hohn DC, Koo PJ, et al: Antibiotic prophylaxis in surgical procedures—a critical analysis of the literature. Arch Surg 118:943, 1983.
63. Conte JE, Jacob LS, Polk HC Jr: Antibiotic Prophylaxis in Surgery—A Comprehensive Review. Philadelphia, Lippincott, 1984.
64. Antimicrobial prophylaxis in surgery: Med Lett, 35:91, 1993.
65. Nichols RL, Smith JW: Intragastric microbial colonization in common disease states of the stomach and duodenum. Ann Surg 182:557, 1975.
66. Gatehouse D, Dimock F, Burdon DW, et al: Prediction of wound sepsis following gastric operations. Br J Surg 65:551, 1978.
67. Keighley MRB, Burdon DW, Gatehouse D: Rate of wound sepsis with "selective" short-term antibiotic prophylaxis in gastric surgery. World J Surg 6:445, 1982.
68. Lewis RT, Allan CM, Goodall RG, et al: Discriminate use of antibiotic prophylaxis in gastroduodenal surgery. Am J Surg 138:640, 1979.
69. Nichols RL, Webb WR, Jones JW, et al: Efficacy of antibiotic prophylaxis in high risk gastroduodenal operations. Am J Surg 143:94, 1982.
70. Forse RA, Karam B, MacLean LD, Christou NV: Antibiotic prophylaxis for surgery in morbidly obese patients. Surgery 106:750, 1989.
71. Chetlin SH, Elliott DW: Preoperative antibiotics in biliary surgery. Arch Surg 107:319, 1973.
72. Keighley MRB, Flinn R, Alexander-Williams J: Multivariate analysis of clinical and operative findings associated with biliary sepsis. Br J Surg 63:528, 1976.
73. Strachan CJ, Black J, Powis SJ, et al: Prophylactic use of cephazolin against wound sepsis after cholecystectomy. Br Med J 1:1254, 1977.
74. Bauer T, Vennits B, Holm B, et al: Antibiotic prophylaxis in acute nonperforated appendicitis: the Danish multicenter study group 111. Ann Surg 209:307, 1989.
75. Ambrose NS, Donovan IA, Wise R, et al: Metronidazole and ticarcillin in the prevention of sepsis after appendicectomy. Am J Surg 146:346, 1983.
76. Lau WY, Fan ST, Yiu TF, et al: Prophylaxis of post-appendicectomy sepsis by metronidazole and ampicillin: a randomized, prospective and double-blinded trial. Br J Surg 70:155, 1983.
77. Baum ML, Anish DS, Chalmers TC, et al: A survey of clinical trials of antibiotic prophylaxis in colon surgery: evidence against further use of no-treatment controls. N Engl J Med 305:795, 1986.
78. Gorbach SL: Antimicrobial prophylaxis for appendectomy and colorectal surgery. Rev Infect Dis 13(Suppl 10):S815, 1991.
79. The Norwegian Study Group for Colorectal Surgery: Should antimicrobial prophylaxis in colorectal surgery include agents effective against both anaerobic and aerobic microorganisms? A double-blind, multicenter study. Surgery 97:402, 1985.
80. Polk HC Jr, Trachtenberg L, George CD: A randomized, double-blind trial of single dose piperacillin versus multidose cefoxitin in alimentary tract operations. Am J Surg 152:517, 1986.
81. DiPiro JT, Bowden TA, Hooks VH: Prophylactic parenteral cephalosporins in surgery—are the newer agents better? JAMA 252:3277, 1984.
82. Kaiser AB, Herrington JL, Jacobs JK, et al: Cefoxitin versus erythromycin, neomycin, and cefazolin in colorectal operations. Ann Surg 198:525, 1983.
83. Nix DE, DiPiro JR, Bowden TA Jr, Vallner JJ: Cephalosporins for surgical prophylaxis: computer projections of intraoperative availability. South Med J 78:962, 1985.
84. Polk BF, Tager IB, Shapiro M: Randomized clinical trial of perioperative cefazolin in preventing infection after hysterectomy. Lancet 1:437, 1980.
85. Hempsell DL, Heard MC, Nobles BJ: Single dose prophylaxis for vaginal and abdominal hysterectomy. Am J Obstet Gynecol 157:498, 1987.
86. Mugford M, Kingston J, Chalmers I: Reducing the incidence of infection after caesarean section: implications of prophylaxis with antibiotics for hospital resources. BMJ 299:1003, 1989.
87. Kaiser AB, Clayson KR, Mulherin JL, et al: Antibiotic prophylaxis in vascular surgery. Ann Surg 188:283, 1978.
88. Kvale PA, Ranga V, Kopacz M, et al: Pulmonary resection. South Med J 70(Suppl 1):64, 1977.
89. Truesdale R, D'Alessandri R, Manuel V, et al: Antimicrobial vs. placebo prophylaxis in noncardiac thoracic surgery. JAMA 241:1254, 1979.
90. Fallon WF Jr, Wears RL: Prophylactic antibiotics for the prevention of infectious complications including empyema following tube thoracostomy for trauma: results of meta-analysis. J Trauma 33:110, 1992.
91. Haines SJ: Efficacy of antibiotic prophylaxis in clean neurosurgical operations. Neurosurgery 24:401, 1989.
92. Ericson C, Lidgren L, Lindberg L: Cloxacillin in prophylaxis of postoperative infections of the hip. J Bone Joint Surg (Am) 55(1):808, 1973.
93. Boyd RJ, Burke JF, Colton T: A double blind clinical trial of prophylactic antibiotics in hip fractures. J Bone Joint Surg (Am) 55:1251, 1973.
94. Beatty JD, Robinson GV, Zaia JA, et al: A prospective analysis of nosocomial wound infection after mastectomy. Arch Surg 118:1421, 1983.
95. Platt R, Zalenznik DF, Hopkins CC, et al: Perioperative antibiotic prophylaxis for herniorrhaphy and breast surgery. N Engl J Med 322:153, 1990.
96. Wagman LD, Tegtmeier B, Beatty JD: A prospective, randomized double-blind study of the use of an-

tibiotics at the time of mastectomy. Surg Gynecol Obstet 170:12, 1990.
97. Fullen WD, Hunt J, Altemeier WA: Prophylactic antibiotics in penetrating wounds of the abdomen. J Trauma 12:282, 1972.
98. Oreskovich MR, Dellinger EP, Lennard ES, et al: Duration of preventive antibiotic administration for penetrating abdominal trauma. Arch Surg 117:200, 1982.
99. Nichols RL, Smith JW, Klein DB, et al: Risk of infection after penetrating abdominal trauma. N Engl J Med 311:1065, 1984.
100. Fabian TC, Croce MA, Payne LW, et al: Duration of antibiotic therapy for penetrating abdominal trauma: a prospective trial. Surgery 112:788, 1992.
101. Dellinger EP: Antibiotic prophylaxis in trauma: penetrating abdominal injuries and open fractures. Rev Infect Dis 13(Suppl 10): S847, 1991.
102. Malangoni MA, Jacobs DG: Antibiotic prophylaxis for injured patients. Infect Dis Clin North Am 6:627, 1992.
103. Thirlby RC, Thal ER: The value of prophylactic antibiotics for simple lacerations. Surg Gynecol Obstet 156:212, 1983.
104. Nichols RL, Condon RE: Preoperative preparation of the colon. Surg Gynecol Obstet 132:323, 1971.
105. Sarnoff SJ, Poth EJ: Intestinal obstruction. I. The protective action of succinylsulfathiazole following simple venous occlusion. Surgery 16:927, 1944.
106. Dearing WH, Needham GM: The effect of oral administration of neomycin on intestinal bacterial flora of man. Mayo Clin Proc 28:502, 1953.
107. Washington JA II, Dearing WH, Judd ES, Elvebach LR: Effect of preoperative antibiotic regimen on development of infection after intestinal surgery: prospective, randomized, double-blind study. Ann Surg 180:567, 1974.
108. Altemeier WA: Discussion of Whelan JP, Hale JH: Bactericidal activity of metronidazole against *Bacteroides fragilis*. J Clin Pathol 26:393, 1973.
109. Nichols RL, Broido P, Condon RE, et al: Effect of preoperative neomycin-erythromycin intestinal preparation on the incidence of infectious complications following colon surgery. Ann Surg 178:453, 1973.
110. Clarke JS, Condon RE, Bartlett JG, et al: Preoperative oral antibiotics reduce septic complications of colon operations: results of prospective, randomized, double-blind clinical study. Ann Surg 186:251, 1977.
111. Whelan JP, Hale JH: Bactericidal activity of metronidazole against *Bacteroides fragilis*. J Clin Pathol 26:393, 1973.
112. Goldring J, McNaught W, Scott A, Gillespie G: Prophylactic oral antimicrobial agents in elective colonic surgery: a controlled trial. Lancet 2:997, 1975.
113. Brass C, Richards GK, Ruedy J, et al: The effect of metronidazole on the incidence of postoperative wound infection in elective colon surgery. Am J Surg 135:91, 1978.
114. Beggs FD, Jobanputra RS, Holmes JT: A comparison of intravenous and oral metronidazole as prophylactic in colorectal surgery. Br J Surg 69:226, 1982.
115. Lewis RT, Goodall RG, Marien B, et al: Is neomycin necessary for bowel preparation in surgery of the colon? Oral neomycin plus erythromycin versus erythromycin-metronidazole. Can J Surg 32:265, 1989.
116. Barber MS, Hirschbert BC, Rice CL, et al: Parenteral antibiotics in elective colon surgery? A prospective, controlled and clinical study. Surgery 86:23, 1979.
117. Condon RE, Bartlett JG, Greenlee H, et al: Efficacy of oral and systemic antibiotic prophylaxis in colorectal operations. Arch Surg 118:496, 1983.
118. Coppa GF, Eng K, Gouge TH, et al: Parenteral and oral antibiotics in elective colon and rectal surgery. Am J Surg 145:62, 1983.
119. Schoetz DJ, Roberts PL, Murray JJ, et al: Addition of parenteral cefoxitin to regimen of oral antibiotics for elective colorectal operations. Ann Surg 212:209, 1990.
120. Becker JM, Alexander DP: Colectomy, mucosal proctectomy, and ileal pouch-anal anastomosis: a prospective trial of optimal antibiotic management. Ann Surg 213:242, 1991.
121. Stellato TA, Danziger LH, Gordon N, et al: Antibiotics in elective colon surgery: a randomized trial of oral, systemic, and oral/systemic antibiotics for prophylaxis. Am Surg 56:251, 1990.
122. Hojer H, Wetterfors J: Systemic prophylaxis with doxycycline in surgery of the colon and rectum. Ann Surg 187:362, 1978.
123. Lewis RT, Allan CM, Goodall RG, et al: Antibiotics in surgery of the colon. Can J Surg 21:339, 1978.
124. Edmondson HT, Rissing JP: Prophylactic antibiotics in colon surgery. Arch Surg 118:227, 1983.
125. Wolff BG, Beart RW Jr, Dozois RR, et al: A new bowel preparation for elective color and rectal surgery: a prospective, randomized clinical trial. Arch Surg 123:895, 1988.
126. Burke J: The effective period of preventive antibiotic action in experimental incisions and dermal lesions. Surgery 50:161, 1961.
127. Waterman NG, Raff MJ, Scharfenberger L, Barnwell P: Antibiotic concentrations in hepatic interstitial and wound fluid. Surg Gynecol Obstet 142:235, 1976.
128. Waterman NG, Raff MJ, Scharfenberger I, Barnwell P: Protein binding and concentrations of cephaloridine and cefazolin in serum and interstitial fluid of dogs. J Infect Dis 133:642, 1976.
129. Bagley DH, MacLowry J, Beazley RM, et al: Antibiotic concentration in human wound fluid after intravenous administration. Ann Surg 188:202, 1978.
130. Goldman DA, Hopkins CC, Karchmer AW, et al: Cephalothin prophylaxis in cardiac valve surgery: a prospective, double-blind comparison of two-day and six-day regimens. J Thorac Cardiovasc Surg 73:470, 1977.

131. Polk HC Jr, Trachtenberg L, Finn MP: Antibiotic activity in surgical incisions. The basis for prophylaxis in selected operations. JAMA 244:1353, 1980.
132. Stone HH, Harper CA, Kolb LD, et al: Antibiotic prophylaxis in gastric, biliary, and colonic surgery. Ann Surg 184:443, 1976.
133. Galandiuk S, Polk HC Jr, Jagelman DG, Fazio VW: Reemphasis of priorities in surgical antibiotic prophylaxis. Surg Gynecol Obstet 169:219, 1989.
134. Page CP, Bohnen JMA, Fletcher JR, et al: Antimicrobial prophylaxis for surgical wounds: guidelines for clinical care. Arch Surg 128:79, 1993.
135. Classen DC, Evans RS, Pestotnik SL, et al: The timing of prophylactic administration of antibiotics and the risk of surgical-wound infection. N Engl J Med 326:281, 1992.
136. Dion YM, Richards GK, Prentis FML, Hinchey EJ: The influence of oral versus parenteral preoperative metronidazole on sepsis following colon surgery. Ann Surg 192:221, 1980.
137. Evans M, Pollock AV: Trials on trial—a review of trials of antibiotic prophylaxis. Arch Surg 119:109, 1984.

INFECTIONS ARISING IN THE HOSPITAL

PART IV

Hospital-Acquired Infections in Surgical Patients

CHAPTER 26

Richard J. Howard

Hospital-acquired or nosocomial infections are infections that develop within a hospital or are caused by microorganisms acquired within a hospital. Although patients are usually the center of interest, physicians, hospital staff, visitors, workers, salespeople, and delivery personnel can also acquire infections within a hospital. These infections occur in every hospital in the country, and hospitals that report extraordinarily low rates of nosocomial infections probably have no or poor surveillance techniques. Nosocomial infections are expensive both in terms of the suffering and even death they can cause patients and their families and in terms of the economic costs of the increased hospital stay and time lost from work. Each year in the United States, there are over 2 million hospital-acquired infections, which result in 150,000 deaths.[1]

INCIDENCE OF HOSPITAL-ACQUIRED INFECTIONS

The National Nosocomial Infections Study (NNIS), carried out by the Centers for Disease Control and Prevention (CDC) surveys many hospitals throughout the country for hospital-acquired infections. The nosocomial infection rate in this study for 1984, the most recent year reported, was 33.5 infections per 1000 discharges, which is similar to the infection rate for 1980 to 1983.[2] These data probably underestimate the true incidence of nosocomial infections in these hospitals. The Study on the Efficacy of Nosocomial Infection Control programs (SENIC Project) found that between 5 and 6 percent of hospitalized patients develop nosocomial infections,[3] the same figure that was generally accepted a decade ago. In a recent NNIS report on surgical patients for 1986 to 1992, there were 52,388 nosocomial infections among 42,509 surgical patients from 95 hospitals using a comprehensive protocol.[4] In this report surgical site infection was the most common (37 percent). Specific nosocomial infections (ie, urinary tract, wound, pneumonia) varied widely by type of operation.

The most recently published NNIS report studies 51 of the 6375 acute care hospitals in the United States. The hospitals are categorized as nonteaching hospitals, small (less than 500 beds) teaching hospitals, and large (greater than 500 beds) teaching hospitals. Patients on the surgical services had a higher rate of hospital-acquired infections than did other services (Table 26–1), but this higher infection rate largely reflects surgical wound infections, which do not occur on medical service. Urinary tract infections were the most common,

TABLE 26–1. INFECTION RATES (CASES/1000 DISCHARGES) BY HOSPITAL CATEGORY AND SERVICE, 1984

	Service[a]					
Hospital Category	SURG	MED	GYN	OB	NEW	PED
Nonteaching	30.8	23.3	8.6	5.6	8.6	1.2
Small teaching	47.3	38.1	35.2	14.9	14.7	14.6
Large teaching	59.3	46.9	31.7	20.3	17.3	16.6
Total	46.7	36.5	28.1	15.3	14.4	13.3

[a] SURG, surgery; MED, medicine; GYN, gynecology; OB, obstetrics; NEW, newborn; PED, pediatrics.
From Horan TC, White JW, Jarvis WR, et al. Morb Mortal Wkly Rep 35(1SS):17SS, 1986.

followed by wound infections and lower respiratory tract infections (Table 26–2).

Escherichia coli was the pathogen most commonly cultured from urinary tract infections in surgical patients (Table 26–3). *Staphylococcus aureus* was most frequently cultured from surgical wounds, and *Pseudomonas aeruginosa* was most commonly isolated from patients with lower urinary tract infections.

COST OF HOSPITAL-ACQUIRED INFECTIONS

Hospital-acquired infections cause additional hospitalization and costs. The costs of nosocomial infections may vary depending on how they are estimated: whether costs or charges are included, whether only marginal costs are considered, whether extra days in the hospital are the basis for calculating costs or whether extra costs only are included, and whether nondirect costs are included such as time lost from work.[5] Whatever factors are used in calculating costs attributable to nosocomial infections, the costs are great. One estimate places the extra charges for each nosocomial infection at $680 for urinary tract infection and $5683 for pneumonia (Table 26–4).[6] And these costs do not take into account pain and suffering or morbidity and mortality of hospital-acquired infections. The increased length of hospitalization due to nosocomial infections varies from 1.0 day for patients who de-

TABLE 26–2. SITE-SPECIFIC INFECTION RATES (CASES/1000 DISCHARGES) BY SERVICE, 1984

	Site						
Service	UTI	SWI	LRI	BACT	CUT	Other	All Sites
1. Nonteaching Hospitals							
SURG	12.1	8.5	5.4	1.3	1.4	2.0	30.8
MED	12.6	0.4	5.2	1.9	0.8	2.3	23.3
GYN	5.8	1.6	0.1	0.1	0.1	0.8	8.6
OB	1.1	2.4	0.1	0.1	0.5	1.4	5.6
PED	0.0	0.1	0.1	0.0	0.1	0.9	1.2
NEW	0.5	0.2	1.8	0.6	2.6	2.9	8.6
Total	9.9	3.6	4.2	1.3	1.1	2.0	22.2
2. Small Teaching Hospitals							
SURG	17.7	13.6	7.8	1.8	1.6	4.7	47.3
MED	20.1	0.6	7.5	2.8	1.7	5.3	38.1
GYN	19.9	11.1	1.3	0.4	0.2	2.2	35.2
OB	3.8	6.8	0.3	0.2	0.5	3.4	14.9
PED	2.0	0.6	2.0	2.4	2.3	5.2	14.6
NEW	0.6	0.2	1.4	2.0	4.8	5.6	14.7
Total	13.9	6.0	5.4	1.9	1.8	4.7	33.8
3. Large Teaching Hospitals							
SURG	19.5	15.0	11.2	4.2	3.3	6.1	59.3
MED	19.5	1.2	10.2	5.7	3.0	7.3	46.9
GYN	14.4	10.2	2.6	0.9	0.6	3.1	31.7
OB	4.2	6.6	0.5	0.9	0.5	7.5	20.3
PED	2.8	1.6	3.9	2.1	1.2	4.9	16.6
NEW	1.0	0.3	2.9	3.6	3.7	5.6	17.4
Total	14.2	6.6	7.7	3.9	2.6	6.4	41.4

From Horan TC, White JW, Jarvis WR, et al: Morb Mortal Wkly Rep 35(1SS):17SS, 1986.

TABLE 26–3. FIVE MOST COMMON PATHOGENS ISOLATED AND PERCENTAGE OF TOTAL WITHIN EACH SITE AND SERVICE, 1984

	Site									
	UTI		SWI		LRI		BACT		CUT	
Service	Pathogen	%	Pathogen	%	Pathogen	%	Pathogen	%	Pathogen	%
Medicine	*E. coli*	30.6	*S. aureus*	19.7	*P. aeruginosa*	16.6	*S. aureus*	14.4	*S. aureus*	26.3
	Enterococci	14.2	Enterococci	12.1	*S. aureus*	14.8	Coag-neg *Staphylococcus*	13.8	Coag-neg *Staphylococcus*	11.8
	P. aeruginosa	11.3	*P. aeruginosa*	9.3	*Klebsiella* species	12.2	*E. coli*	12.2	*P. aeruginosa*	11.0
	Klebsiella species	9.4	Coag-neg *Staphylococcus*	9.0	*Enterobacter* species	7.7	*P. aeruginosa*	9.2	Enterococci	9.1
	Proteus species	8.1	*E. coli*	6.9	*E. coli*	7.3	*Klebsiella* species	8.5	*Candida* species	6.6
Surgery	*E. coli*	29.2	*S. aureus*	19.0	*P. aeruginosa*	16.5	Coag-neg *Staphylococcus*	14.0	*S. aureus*	19.0
	P. aeruginosa	16.1	Enterococci	12.1	*S. aureus*	11.5	*S. aureus*	10.2	*P. aeruginosa*	12.9
	Enterococci	13.4	*E. coli*	11.5	*Enterobacter* species	11.4	*Enterobacter* species	9.2	Enterococci	10.7
	Proteus species	7.4	*P. aeruginosa*	9.7	*Klebsiella* species	11.2	Enterococci	9.1	Coag-neg *Staphylococcus*	10.1
	Klebsiella species	6.7	Coag-neg *Staphylococcus*	7.9	*Serratia* species	6.9	*Klebsiella* species	7.5	*E. coli*	7.9
Gynecology	*E. coli*	40.7	*E. coli*	15.1	*P. aeruginosa*	15.6	*E. coli*	16.0	*S. aureus*	18.8
	Enterococci	23.5	*S. aureus*	12.9	*Enterobacter* species	9.4	*Bacteroides* species	16.0	Coag-neg *Staphylococcus*	12.5
	Klebsiella species	6.7	Enterococci	12.9	*S. aureus*	6.3	Coag-neg *Staphylococcus*	8.0	*Morganella* species	12.5
	Proteus species	5.0	Coag-neg *Staphylococcus*	11.5	*Candida* species	6.3	*S. aureus*	8.0	Viruses	12.5
	P. aeruginosa	4.5	*Bacteroides* species	6.8	*Klebsiella* species	3.1	*Klebsiella* species	4.0	Other anaerobes	12.5
Obstetrics	*E. coli*	36.3	*S. aureus*	13.7	*P. aeruginosa*	7.7	*S. aureus*	14.3	*E. coli*	25.6
	Enterococci	28.8	*E. coli*	13.7	*S. aureus*	7.7	Other anaerobes	12.2	*S. aureus*	23.1
	Group B *Streptococcus*	6.0	Enterococci	12.5	*Klebsiella* species	7.7	*E. coli*	8.2	Enterococci	10.3
	Coag-neg *Staphylococcus*	3.6	Coag-neg *Staphylococcus*	9.6	*E. coli*	7.7	Coag-neg *Staphylococcus*	6.1	Coag-neg *Staphylococcus*	7.7
	Proteus species	3.3	*Bacteroides* species	8.3	*Candida* species	7.7	Enterococci	6.1	Group B *Streptococcus*	5.1
Pediatrics	*E. coli*	30.4	*S. aureus*	34.8	*P. aeruginosa*	19.8	Coag-neg *Staphylococcus*	29.0	*S. aureus*	40.3
	P. aeruginosa	13.4	*E. coli*	10.6	*S. aureus*	11.6	*S. aureus*	14.0	Coag-neg *Staphylococcus*	19.4
	Enterococci	10.7	*P. aeruginosa*	10.6	*Klebsiella* species	9.3	*E. coli*	10.8	*E. coli*	10.4
	Klebsiella species	10.7	Coag-neg *Staphylococcus*	10.6	*Enterobacter* species	7.0	*Klebsiella* species	6.5	*Candida* species	7.5
	Candida species	10.7	Enterococci	7.6	*Candida* species	3.5	*Candida* species	6.5	Enterococci	4.5
Newborn	*E. coli*	35.2	*S. aureus*	23.1	*P. aeruginosa*	29.5	Coag-neg *Staphylococcus*	20.8	*S. aureus*	54.5
	Klebsiella species	15.5	Coag-neg *Staphylococcus*	23.1	*Klebsiella* species	15.2	Group B *Streptococcus*	15.3	Coag-neg *Staphylococcus*	12.6
	Coag-neg *Staphylococcus*	9.9	*P. aeruginosa*	15.4	Coag-neg *Staphylococcus*	9.8	Enterococci	9.9	*E. coli*	6.1
	Enterococci	8.5	Enterococci	7.7	*E. coli*	8.0	*E. coli*	9.4	Enterococci	4.8
	Candida species	8.5	*Klebsiella* species	7.7	*S. aureus*	7.1	*Klebsiella* species	8.4	*Enterobacter* species	4.2

From Horan TC, White JW, Jarvis WR, et al: Morb Mortal Wkly Rep 35(1SS):17SS, 1936.

TABLE 26–4. ESTIMATED EXTRA DAYS, EXTRA CHARGES, AND DEATHS ATTRIBUTABLE TO NOSOCOMIAL INFECTIONS ANNUALLY IN U.S. HOSPITALS

	Extra Days		Extra Charges			Deaths Directly Caused by Infections		Deaths to Which Infections Contributed	
	Average per Infection[a]	Estimated U.S. Total[b]	Average Extra Charges per Infection in 1975 Dollars[a]	Average Extra Charges per Infection in 1992 Dollars[c]	Estimated U.S. Total in 1992 Dollars[b]	Percentage[d]	Estimated U.S. Total[b]	Percentage[d]	Estimated U.S. Total[b]
Surgical wound infection	7.3	3,726,000	838	3,152	1,609,000,000	0.64	3,251	1.91	9,726
Pneumonia	5.9	1,339,000	1,511	5,683	1,290,000,000	3.12	7,087	10.13	22,983
Bacteremia	7.4	762,000	935	3,517	362,000,000	4.37	4,496	8.59	8,844
Urinary tract infection	1.0	903,000	181	680	615,000,000	0.10	947	0.72	6,503
Other site	4.8	1,946,000	430	1,617	656,000,000	0.80	3,246	2.48	10,036
All sites	4.0[e]	8,676,000	560[e]	2,100	4,532,000,000	0.90[e]	19,027	2.70[e]	58,092

[a] *Adapted from Haley RW, et al: Am J Med 70:51, 1981,* by pooling data from the three SENIC pilot study hospitals.
[b] Estimated by multiplying the total number of nosocomial infections estimated in the SENIC Project (*Haley RW, et al: Am J Epidemiol 121:159, 1985*) by the average extra days, average extra charges, or percentage of infections causing or contributing to death, respectively.
[c] 1992 Dollars *estimated from Haley RW, et al: Am J Med 70:51, 1981,* by pooling data from the three hospitals and adjusting for the annual rate of inflation of hospital expenses from 1976 to 1992 (range 5.0 to 12.3 percent) obtained from the American Hospital Association's National Panel Survey. Estimates for inflation rates in 1991 and 1992 were projected 1987-to-1990 trend.
[d] Unpublished analyses of data reported to the National Nosocomial Infections Surveillance (NNIS) System in 1980–1982 (*Hughes JM, et al: Abstracts of the Twenty-Second Interscience Conference on Antimicrobial Agents and Chemotherapy, Miami Beach, FL, October 4–6, 1982*).
[e] Nationwide estimate obtained by summing the products of the site-specific estimate of the average extra days, average extra charges, or the percentage of infections causing or contributing to death, respectively from the SENIC pilot studies (*Haley RW, et al: Am J Med 70:51, 1981*), and the nationwide estimate of the proportion of nosocomia infections affecting the site from the main SENIC analysis (*Haley RW, et al: Am J Epidemiol 121:159, 1985*).
From Martone WJ, Jarvis WR, Culver DH, Haley RW: Incidence and nature of endemic and epidemic nosocomial infections. In Bennett JV, Brachman PS (eds): Hospital Infections, *3rd ed. Boston, Little, Brown, 1992, p 593.*

velop urinary tract infections to 7.3 days for patients with surgical wound infections and 7.4 days for patients with bacteremia.[4]

TYPES OF HOSPITAL-ACQUIRED INFECTIONS IN SURGICAL PATIENTS

Surgical patients are generally not more susceptible to hospital-acquired infections than the rest of the hospital population, but some important differences do exist. The most obvious difference is that most surgical patients have operations that subject them to wound infections. Patients on the other services who do not have operations cannot develop these infections. Operations usually necessitate inserting an intravenous catheter and an endotracheal tube and often a urinary and arterial catheter, all of which predispose to nosocomial infections. In addition, patients with extensive trauma or burns, who have severely compromised host defenses, are almost always housed on the surgical service.

Wound infections are the nosocomial infections that have been of greatest interest to surgeons. It is such an important subject that four chapters (22 through 25) are devoted to a discussion of wound infections and their prevention. This section will discuss other types of hospital-acquired infections that occur in surgical patients.

Urinary Tract Infections

Infections of the urinary tract are the most common nosocomial infections. They account for approximately 40 percent of all hospital-acquired infections (see Table 26–2) and involve an estimated 400,000 patients each year. For all hospitals the infection rate for urinary tract infections is 12.9 cases per 1000 discharges. This rate is higher on the surgical service, up to 19.5 cases per 1000 discharges (see Table 26–2). Others have shown that up to 10 percent of hospital patients develop a urinary tract infection sometime during their hospital course.

Urinary tract infections in surgical patients occur most commonly because of instrumentation. Approximately 80 percent of nosocomial urinary tract infections today are attributable to the use of indwelling urinary catheters and 20 percent occur after other types of transient urological instrumentation.[7]

Virtually every urinary tract infection is associated with a colony count of 100,000 organisms per milliliter or more. There are few exceptions to this rule. If the urine is obtained directly from the bladder by suprapubic bladder puncture, a colony count of 100 bacteria per milliliter is considered sufficient for diagnosing a urinary tract infection. In addition, large numbers of bacteria and neutrophils found in the microscopic examination of the urinary sediment are considered presumptive evidence of a urinary tract infection. Culture of the tip of the urinary catheter has been advocated, but studies show that most patients with positive catheter tip cultures do not have significant bacteriuria.

Organisms Causing Urinary Tract Infections. Most urinary tract infections are due to gram-negative aerobic bacteria found in the gastrointestinal tract. The most common organisms found to cause urinary tract infections in the National Nosocomial Infections Study were *E. coli, Enterococcus, Klebsiella, Proteus,* and *Pseudomonas* organisms (see Table 26–3). No doubt the high frequency of infection with fecal flora is due to the close approximation of the urethra and anus and the likely contamination of the nearby skin by fecal organisms.

Risks of Catheterization. Most nosocomial urinary tract infections in surgical patients are due to the use of indwelling urinary catheters. Ten to 25 percent of catheterized patients develop bacteriuria.[7] Bacteriuria is seen in 1 to 5 percent of patients after a single short-term catheterization.[8] The risk is higher in pregnant females, elderly or debilitated patients, and patients with urologic abnormalities.[9] Single catheterizations are done to relieve overdistension of the bladder or temporary obstruction that might occur after an operative procedure, to obtain roentgenographic studies of the bladder and urethra, to determine residual urine, or to obtain a clean specimen for culture.

Urinary tract infections are much more common following the use of indwelling catheters, which are commonly used on surgical wards to prevent overdistention of the bladder and to monitor urinary output. They are required for patients having urologic procedures, especially operations on the urethra to facilitate repair, and for operations on the rectum. They are also used for severely injured patients who cannot void, burn patients, patients with fractures who may have difficulty voiding, and neurologically injured patients who cannot void because of the injury.

Patients with a normal lower urinary tract are usually able to rid themselves of the infection spontaneously following removal of the urinary catheter. Many, however, remain infected. In these patients and in patients who have continued need for urinary catheterization there is always the risk of sepsis, shock, and death. Urinary catheterization is the predisposing factor most frequently associated with gram-negative bacteremia. The rate of gram-negative bacteremia secondary to urinary tract infection is twice the rate of gram-negative bacteremia due to infection at any other site.

The costs and possible side effects of antimicrobial therapy and the costs of hospitalization required all add to the cost of unnecessary urinary catheterization. One study showed that only 8 to 10 percent of patients on catheter drainage for 2 to 7 days had significant bacteriuria once the catheter was removed, and only 0.7 percent had subsequent clinical infections after the catheter was removed.[10] Nevertheless, because of the large number of patients who have urinary catheters sometime during their hospital course and because of the large number of patients on surgical wards and in hospitals, the number of patients with significant bacteriuria attributed to catheter use and the consequent costs in terms of increased hospital stay, further diagnostic tests, and antimicrobial therapy, as well as such effects as bacteremia, shock, and death are substantial. The risk of developing a urinary tract infection increases with the duration of catheterization, and the risk of developing bacteriuria is 5 to 10 percent for each day of catheterization.[9]

Modes of Contamination of Bladder in Patients with Urinary Catheters. Before the use of closed drainage systems, patients with indwelling catheters had open drainage systems in which the catheter was merely drained into a bottle or other receptacle. With such open drainage systems, 95 to 100 percent of patients with indwelling catheters had bacteriuria within 3 to 4 days. The advent of closed drainage systems has greatly reduced the incidence of bacteriuria in catheterized patients. Nevertheless, there are many routes by which bacteria can still find their way into the urine. First, the periurethral area in the male and introitus and periurethral area in the female may not be adequately prepared before the insertion of the catheter. These areas, especially that of the female, are frequently contaminated by the fecal flora. Poor aseptic technique in introducing catheters or other instruments introduced into the urethra or inadequate cleaning of these instruments may also lead to bacteriuria. Bacteria can also enter the bladder from the urethral meatus, going up the urethra around the outside of the urinary catheter. This problem is usually not seen until late and is more common in females. The urinary tract can also become contaminated at any site where there is a break in the closed drainage system. Thus, contamination of the end of the urinary catheter where it connects to the drainage tube can also lead to urinary tract infections. Contamination of the collection vessel lower down may also lead to retrograde infection via the urinary stream. Irrigation of the bladder with contaminated irrigating solutions is another source of potential urinary tract infections. The use of a urinary collection bag that is presealed to the urinary catheter can lower the rate of urinary tract infection and death from these infections.[11]

Prevention of Urinary Tract Infection. Condom catheter drainages and suprapubic catheters can be used to try to reduce the incidence of urinary tract infections. These are especially appropriate where prolonged urinary catheterization would be required, such as in comatose patients, incontinent males, or spine-injured patients. The condom and its attached collection tube should be changed daily, and the penis should be carefully cleaned and dried to avoid maceration. Suprapubic drainage is becoming more popular because it does not lead to obstruction of the urethral glands by the urethral catheter. This type of drainage has most often been used for patients having gynecologic surgery, but it could also be used for other surgical and general medical patients as well. Preliminary results have shown a delayed onset of infection and a reduced incidence of infection in patients with suprapubic urinary catheters. Antibiotic or silver-coated urinary catheters do not decrease the incidence of urinary tract infections.[7,12] But systemic antimicrobials can reduce the incidence of urinary tract infections in the first 4 to 5 days of catheterization.[12]

Infections Associated with Intravascular Catheters

Up to 12 percent of hospital patients have some type of intravascular infusion catheter. This rate is much higher in surgical patients, since every patient having a general or spinal anesthetic requires an intravenous cannula. Intravenous catheters are used for the administration of intravenous fluids, drugs, blood and blood products, and total parenteral nutrition. Most intravenous catheters are left in place for only a few days, but some may be left in place indefinitely for prolonged administration of total parenteral nutrition or chemotherapeutic agents. In addition, arterial catheters are used for blood pressure monitoring, and Swan-Ganz catheters are used for hemodynamic measurements in seriously ill patients.

Incidence of Intravenous Cannula-Associated Infections. Reports vary widely on the incidence of positive cultures from intravenous cannulas, all the way from 4 to 64 percent.[13] The incidence varies according to the type of cannula (see Table 26–5). Steel needle or scalp intravenous catheters have the lowest incidence of cannula-tipped contamination (14.6 percent), whereas subclavian catheters have the highest incidence (26.3 percent).[14] Data in Table 26–5 are not strictly comparable, however, because plastic catheters are the ones most often inserted in emergency situations and are usually inserted by physicians rather than by trained intravenous teams. They also tend to remain in place longer than steel needles and are more likely to be used in sicker patients. Finding a positive cannula culture does not necessarily mean the patient had a cannula-associated infection.

The definition of intravenous catheter-associated infection may vary from one study to another. It is clear that when purulent thrombophlebitis occurs in a vein that has an intravenous catheter, there is a catheter-associated infection, but when inflammation occurs only around the site of the intravenous catheter or when a thick cord develops or thrombophlebitis develops, it is more difficult to say that there is an intravenous catheter-associated infection. Some studies of cannula-related infections have not found a correlation between phlebitis and intravenous cannula infection, but others have suggested such a relationship does indeed exist.[15] It can be difficult to determine whether bacteremia is due to a vascular catheter. Removing the catheter and culturing the tip in broth does not mean the catheter itself was infected. The catheter may have become contaminated with bacteria in the blood or the catheter may have become contaminated from the skin or tract during its removal, since theoretically a contamination with a single organism can produce a positive broth culture. Maki and co-workers[16,17] have developed a semiquantitative technique for culturing vascular catheters. With this technique a 5- to 6-cm length of catheter that has been removed after aseptic preparation of the skin exit site is rolled at least four times across the surface of an agar culture plate. If at least 15 colonies grow on the plate, the catheter is considered to be positive. More than 1000 colonies can be cultured from most catheters associated with bacteremia.

TABLE 26–5. INFECTIONS ASSOCIATED WITH INTRAVENOUS CANNULAS

Types	Percentage of Contaminated Cannula Tips	Percentage of Cannula-Associated Septicemia
Plastic cannulas		
Percutaneous	17.9	0.5
Peripheral	17.9	0.5
Subclavian	26.3	3.8
Umbilical	23.3	6.5
Cutdowns	24.2	6.5
Steel needles	14.6	0.2

From Rhame FS, Maki DG, Bennett JV: Intravenous cannula-associated infections. In Bennett JV, Brachman PS (eds): Hospital Infections. Boston, Little, Brown, 1979.

Central venous catheters are being used more frequently—especially for patients requiring long-term vascular access for total parenteral nutrition and for patients receiving chemotherapy. These catheters are associated with the highest rate of infection and are frequently used in patients (the neutropenic patient with leukemia receiving chemotherapy) who are most susceptible to infection.

Percutaneous placement of polyethylene catheters for total parenteral nutrition is associated with a catheter-associated sepsis incidence as high as 27 percent.[14] The use of Silastic catheters and subcutaneous tunnels has reduced the rate of catheter-associated sepsis to 11.5 to 14 percent.[18,19] Catheter sepsis is associated with a 3 percent mortality rate.[18] Rigorous aseptic nursing care of the exit site is the most important factor in reducing central venous catheter sepsis.[19] Most investigators now believe that the source of catheter sepsis is microorganisms at the skin exit site that follow the catheter into the vein rather than originating from intravenous fluids, connections, or a distant site that colonizes the catheter via the bloodstream. The organisms most commonly isolated from patients with central intravenous catheter-related sepsis are *S. epidermidis* (20 percent), *Candida* (7 percent), and *P. aeruginosa* (6 percent).[18]

Arterial catheters used for hemodynamic monitoring can also be the source of bacteremia (0.85 to 7.8 percent) and are frequently associated with contamination of the transducer dome or sampling stopcock.[20,21] Swan-Ganz pulmonary artery catheters have a 5.8 percent incidence of positive catheter tip cultures.[22] The infection usually results from a distant focus of infection.

Preventing Intravenous Catheter-Associated Infections. Cutdown should be avoided insofar as possible because of the higher risk of sepsis. Steel needles rather than indwelling plastic cannulas should be used when short-term intravenous therapy is to be used. Intravenous catheters should be placed above the waist; the saphenous vein or femoral vessels should be used only in emergency situations; and the catheter should be removed as soon as the emergency is over. The skin should be thoroughly cleansed with chlorhexidine, an iodine-containing disinfectant or 70 percent ethanol. All cutdowns should be done in the operating room unless there is an emergency. Where cannulas have been inserted with suboptimal asepsis, they should be removed and replaced as soon as possible.

Central venous catheters used for total parenteral nutrition or chemotherapy should be placed in the operating room. Silastic central venous cannulas that require tunneling and all central lines that will remain in place more than 48 hours are best placed in the operating room. Sterile conditions are optimal there, and fluoroscopy can be used there to assure proper position. All Silastic catheters currently used for long-term central venous access have a Dacron cuff that is placed in the subcutaneous tunnel near the skin exit site. Fibrous tissue grows into the cuff and prevents bacteria from tracking around the outside of the catheter from the skin to the vein. Some catheters also have a second silver-impregnated cuff between the Dacron cuff and the skin exit site to further reduce the risk of infection, since the silver in the cuff exerts antibacterial activity. Aseptic cleaning and application of an antimicrobial ointment at the skin-cannula junction by a specially trained nurse every 24 to 48 hours can significantly reduce the incidence of catheter-related sepsis.[14,19]

Any evidence of phlebitis, cellulitis, or suspicion of septic complications due to intravenous cannulas should lead to prompt removal of the cannula. The CDC recommends that all peripheral intravenous cannulas be replaced every 48 to 72 hours. This policy is difficult to adhere to for children and for adult patients with no or few remaining peripheral sites for vascular access. Others have shown leaving peripheral intravenous catheters in place for up to 96 hours in low-risk patients is safe.[15]

Central venous cannulas, especially Silastic cannulas, are used long term for the administration of chemotherapy and total parenteral nutrition in patients who are compromised hosts, with lymphoreticular malignancies and low white counts. These patients frequently have fevers and septic episodes. More often than not, the fever is not due to the cannula. Because only a limited number of sites are available for insertion of such cannulas and because they are so valuable for the therapy of the patient, a judicious search should be made for all other sites of infection. If, finally, no infection stemming from any other site can be identified, these cannulas probably should be removed. As long as there is no indication of infection, these catheters can be left in for prolonged periods, probably indefinitely. Thrombosis of the subclavian vein and superior vena cava is being recognized increasingly in patients who have these catheters in for prolonged periods (up to 11.5 percent).

If central venous catheter sepsis is strongly suspected or cannot be ruled out, the catheter should be removed and another placed after 24 to 48 hours. This policy has led to the unnecessary removal of 80 to 85 percent of central venous catheters.[23] Exchanging central venous catheters suspected of causing sepsis over a guidewire does not lead to contamination of the new catheter and greatly lowers the hazards of a new cannulation.[24]

Because contamination can occur at virtually every point in an intravenous infusion system, addition of medications to the intravenous fluid container, injections into the tubing, piggyback administration catheters, and introduction of stopcock manometers and other devices into the lines should be kept to an absolute minimum. Changes in bottles and administration sets and irrigation of clotted catheters increase the risk of contamination.

Nosocomial infections stemming from infection or contamination of the intravenous fluid is most frequently seen with total parenteral nutrition therapy. These nosocomial infections can be reduced by changing all bottles and intravenous infusion lines daily and by having a micropore filter in line with the intravenous fluids so that the total parenteral nutrition fluid is filtered before it is administered to the patient.

Lower Respiratory Tract Infections

Lower respiratory tract infections are the second most common hospital-acquired infection according to the National Nosocomial Infections Study, occurring in 5.4 to 11.2 cases per 1000 discharges on surgical services, depending on the type of hospital.[2]

Susceptibility to Lower Respiratory Tract Infections in Surgical Patients. Variables independently associated with nosocomial pneumonia include age greater than 70 years, chronic lung disease, mechanical ventilation, depressed consciousness, large-volume aspiration, chest surgery, the presence of an intracranial pressure monitor, the use of histamine type 2 (H_2) blockers with and without antacids, frequent chances of ventilator circuits (every 24 versus 48 hours), and the fall or winter seasons.[25] Risk factors for pneumonia may also include presence in an intensive care unit, treatment for pneumonia, and immunosuppression.

Although the lower respiratory tract has a variety of defense mechanisms that protect the lungs from infections, many of these defense mechanisms are compromised in surgical patients by their basic disease, metabolic status, or operations. Preexisting pulmonary disease and bronchitis further predispose to postoperative respiratory infections. Anesthesia, alcohol, and operations on the head and neck can interfere with the normal protective cough reflex and may permit aspiration of infected material. The pain associated with trauma or operations to the chest and upper abdomen may also interfere with coughing and breathing and thus allow accumulation of secretions within the tracheobronchial tree. Patients with thoracic and upper abdominal operations have a higher incidence of postoperative pneumonia than do patients having operations at other sites. This pain can interfere with deep breathing and normal alveolar expansion, leading to atelectasis of the lungs, a condition that predisposes to pulmonary infections. Trauma or operations involving any site on the body may interfere with movement and with deep breathing and normal alveolar expansion. The basic disease processes and the aftereffects of any operation frequently lead to a depressed central nervous system that also interferes with deep breathing and predisposes to aspiration of infected material.

Pulmonary edema resulting from injudicious use of intravenous fluids, cardiac failure, chest injuries, bacterial sepsis, renal failure, or inhalation of hot or irritant gases by burn patients also leads to pulmonary infection. The fluid that accumulates in the alveoli prevents normal phagocytic activity of alveolar macrophages. On the other hand, if patients are dehydrated or are on a respirator and receive the normal anhydrous oxygen as it comes out of most lines without adequate humidification, the cilia and the tracheobronchial tree do not function normally to clear bronchial secretions.

Spread of Microbes to Lower Respiratory Tract. Microbes may invade the lower respiratory tract by one of four routes: (1) aspiration from the oropharynx, (2) direct entrance through tracheostomies, (3) from respiratory care devices, and (4) from the blood.

Aspiration from Oropharynx. Only 2 to 6 percent of physiologically normal subjects have gram-negative bacteria in their oropharynxes. Johanson et al[26] found that gram-negative bacteria can be cultured from the oropharynxes of 35 percent of moderately ill patients and 73 percent of moribund patients. The prevalence of gram-negative bacteria was not related to the duration of hospitalization. In a subsequent study these authors prospectively examined 213 patients.[27] Twenty-two percent became colonized on their first hospital day, and 45 percent became colonized sometime during their hospital stay. Seventy-six percent of the patients who became persistently colonized were colonized on the first hospital day, and 12.2 percent of these patients developed nosocomial respiratory infections. Patients were predisposed to develop gram-negative colonization if they had coma, hypotension, sputum production, tracheal intubation, acidosis, azotemia, abnormal white blood cell counts, or received antimicrobial drugs. Glover and Jolly[28] reported a 40 to 63.2 percent gram-negative bacterial colonization rate of the respiratory tract of hospitalized patients, depending on the number of cultures taken.

Surgical patients periodically aspirate small but unrecognized quantities of material from the oropharynx and gastrointestinal tract that are contaminated with microorganisms. Probably this unrecognized aspiration occurs much more frequently than does the gross aspiration of gastrointestinal contents that occurs occasionally with vomiting episodes. Culver et al[29] placed Evans blue dye into the stomach of 300 surgical patients before induction of anesthesia. After completion of anesthesia the mouth, pharynx, larynx, trachea, and main bronchi were examined by laryngoscopy and bronchoscopy. Regurgitation (dye detected in the pharynx) occurred in 26.3 percent of the patients, and 16.3 percent aspirated (dye detected below the vocal cords). Unsuspected aspiration (no vomiting) occurred in 8.3 percent of patients. Aspiration was more common when nasogastric tubes were not used (23.9 percent of cases) than when they were used (5.6 percent). Aspiration occurred with all anesthetics used. Aspiration even occurs in normal individuals during sleep.[30]

Thus the oropharynxes of surgical patients are frequently contaminated by gram-negative bacteria, and aspiration occurs during anesthesia and surgery—both conditions favoring the development of nosocomial respiratory infections.

Entrance of Microorganisms Through Tracheostomies. Respiratory infections occur in 5 to 26 percent of patients following tracheostomy, and pneumonia is frequently the cause of death.[31] Tracheostomy leads to drying of the tracheal mucosa because the inhaled air bypasses the humidification provided by the nasal mucosa. Drying leads to decreased ciliary movement, with increased likelihood of colonization. Tracheostomy also prevents the buildup of airway pressure required for effective coughing. Inability to cough increases the likelihood of aspirating oropharyngeal secretions. Finally, the microorganisms colonizing the skin and tracheostomy would have direct access to the bronchial tree. All these factors favor respiratory tract infections.

Respiratory Care Devices. Patients exposed to respiratory care devices have an increased risk of acquiring nosocomial pneumonia although it is frequently difficult to separate this exposure from intrinsic host susceptibility. Patients receiving respirator or ventilator support have 7 to 25 times the incidence of nosocomial pneumonia compared to patients not exposed to such therapy.[31–33] The highest incidence of pneumonia occurs in patients having tracheostomy plus respirator care (66.7 percent). Lower rates are seen in patients with tracheostomy alone (25 percent), intubation plus respirator therapy (3.7 percent), and intubation alone (1.3 percent). The risk of acquiring pneumonia is directly related to the duration of respiratory assistance.

When respiratory care devices came into prominent use in the 1950s and 1960s, the incidence of gram-negative necrotizing pneumonias increased markedly. The components of the respirators—especially the nebulizers—that were implicated were often heavily contaminated with gram-negative bacteria, generally with strains that caused epidemics of gram-negative pneumonias. Contamination was found in aerosolized medications, ultrasonic nebulizers, room humidifiers, and in the condensate in tubes between the patient and ventilator.[34] As a result of such findings, techniques for decontaminating and maintaining respiratory care equipment were developed and widely adopted. Contaminated respiratory care devices now seem to be relatively unimportant sources for infection in the United States.

To keep bacterial contamination to a minimum, components of such systems should be changed daily. Nebulization equipment should be cleaned daily and filled with sterile water. Exposure to aerosolized tap water contaminated with *Legionella pneumophila* was associated with acquisition of nosocomial legionnaires' disease.[35,36] All lines through which gases flow from ventilator to patient should also be changed daily. The ventilator circuit becomes contaminated as early as 2 hours after use, and 80 percent are contaminated at 24 hours.[37] The source of this bacterial contamination is the host's own oropharyngeal flora. No more contamination is found at 48 hours than at 24 hours, which has led some to advocate changing the tubing only every 48 hours.[38]

Hematogenous Spread. Invasion of the lungs via the bloodstream is a theoretical cause of pneumonia. It can occur when there is bacteremia, and this may lead to pneumonia, but it is probably an uncommon source. Septic thrombophlebitis can also lead to a septic pulmonary embolism that might lead to septic infarct and pulmonary abscess. Septic thrombophlebitis especially may occur with the use of indwelling venous catheters. *Pseudomonas aeruginosa* pneumonia may occur via hematogenous spread from burn wounds.

Prevention of Nosocomial Pneumonia. The CDC has published guidelines for the prevention of nosocomial pneumonias.[39,40] These recommendations discuss preoperative measures, hand washing, maintenance of respiratory therapy equipment, fluid use for nebulizers and humidifiers, processing reusable equipment, microbiologic monitoring, patients with tracheostomy, suctioning of the respiratory tract, and protection of patients from other infected patients and staff. Others have also recently reviewed data and made recommendations.[41–43] Because of the relationship between gastric bacterial colonization and oropharyngeal and tracheal colonization, strategies have been developed to prevent or reduce gastric colonization.[41–43] Patients in intensive care units are frequently given agents to lower gastric acidity as a method of reducing stress gastric bleeding. This reduced acidity, however, increases gastric colonization and with it the likelihood of pneumonia. Sucralfate can reduce the risk of stress ulcer bleeding without altering gastric pH. Sucralfate therapy led to a 12 percent (7 of 61 patients) incidence of nosocomial pneumonia compared to a 23 percent (16 of 69 patients) incidence in patients treated with antacids or cimetidine.[44] Similar results were noted in ventilator patients who had a 10 percent (3 of 29 patients) incidence of nosocomial pneumonia compared to a 32 percent (11 of 34 patients) incidence when treated with antacids.[45]

Another strategy to reduce gastric colonization is administration of oral, nonabsorbed antibiotics to reduce bacterial colonization and known as selection decontamination of the digestive tract (SSD) (see Chap. 38). Several regimens have been used. A typical antibiotic regimen would include polymyxin B, tobramycin, and amphotericin B. Some regimens also add an intravenous antibiotic or local oropharyngeal application of antibiotics. Such regimens can result in a marked reduction of oropharyngeal colonization and lower the incidence of pneumonia in intensive care unit patients from 45 to 85 percent for control patients to 5 to 15 percent[46–50] for patients receiving SDD. SDD can also lower the incidence of other infections as well but does not alter the mortality rate.

Infections Associated with Blood Transfusions

The adoption of safe blood transfusion practices in the early part of this century did more to reduce the mortality of surgery than did aseptic practices or the introduction of antibiotics. More than 11 million units of blood and components are administered yearly in the United States with a remarkable record of safety.

Nevertheless, blood transfusions can be a source of infection in surgical patients.[51] Hepatitis is the most common transfusion-associated infection. Other viral illness including cytomegalovirus, Epstein-Barr virus, and human immunodeficiency virus (HIV), the etiologic agent of the acquired immune deficiency syndrome (AIDS) can also be transmitted by blood transfusion. Bacterial contamination from improperly sterilized equipment or errors in technique in drawing blood can cause sporadic infections. Parasites can also be transmitted by transfusion. Malaria transmission is rare in the United States, but five to nine cases per year occurred from 1968 to 1971 as soldiers returned from Vietnam. It does occur in Europe because of travel from malarial areas.[52] Transmission of malaria can occur after infusion of blood components such as platelets, leukocytes, and cryoprecipitates, as well as after whole blood transfusion. *Toxoplasma gondii* infection has occurred after granulocyte transfusion. *Trypanosoma cruzi* infection following transfusion is common in Latin America.

Hepatitis. Before the introduction of serologic testing for hepatitis B, as many as 60 percent of posttransfusion hepatitis cases were due to hepatitis B.[53] Although the precise prevalence of hepatitis B-infected blood donors whose blood has a negative test for HB_sAg is not known, it is estimated to be 0.6 percent of the population, based on a 3 percent rate of hepatitis B in recipients of 1 to 5 units of blood.[54] Following development of serologic testing for hepatitis B in the 1970s, the incidence of post-transfusion hepatitis B dropped dramatically from approximately 60 percent to 5 to 10 percent. Serologic testing all blood for hepatitis B and eliminating paid donors have led to a marked decrease in the risk of transfusion-transmitted hepatitis B from approximately 5 to 7 percent to between 1 in 200 and 1 in 300.[55] Ninety to 95 percent of hepatitis was due to an unidentified virus, which was neither hepatitis A nor hepatitis B and was called non-A, non-B hepatitis. In the 1980s hepatitis C virus was identified and a test for antibody to hepatitis C became available. Hepatitis C accounts for an estimated 60 to 80 percent of post-transfusion non-A, non-B hepatitis. The remaining non-A, non-B, non-C hepatitis cases may be due to an as yet unidentified virus(es) or may be due to hepatitis C not detected by the first-generation test for antibody to the C-100 epitope. As a recently available second-generation test and testing for viral DNA by the polymerase chain reaction becomes more widely applied, probably an even greater percentage of post-transfusion hepatitis will be attributed to hepatitis C. Current regulations require that all blood and blood products be screened for evidence of hepatitis B, hepatitis C, and non-A, non-B, non-C hepatitis (using elevated amino-leucine transferase levels as a surrogate test), as well as HIV and HTLV-I. All units with evidence of viral infection must be discarded. The ability to screen donors for hepatitis C can reduce the estimated risk per transfusion from 1 in 100 to between 1 in 300 and 1 in 900. One study from Japan found that the incidence of post-transfusion hepatitis C in recipients of 1 to 10 unit transfusions was 4.9 percent before screening compared to 1.9 percent after screening for hepatitis C.[56] Cytomegalovirus and Epstein-Barr virus can also cause post-transfusion hepatitis.

Reducing the number of paid blood donors has lowered the incidence of post-transfusion hepatitis, because blood from paid donors is more likely to transmit hepatitis than is blood from volunteer donors. Since 1978, all blood for transfusion in the United States has been required by federal regulation to be labeled "paid" or "volunteer" according to its source. Many states prohibit paid blood donors altogether.

The incidence of hepatitis in the United States is approximately 0.06 to 0.12 percent of the population.[57,58] Most cases of post-transfusion hepatitis, however, are asymptomatic. Where recipients of blood transfusions are tested prospectively for abnormal liver function tests, the incidence of post-transfusion hepatitis rises to 0.24 cases per 1000 transfusions. Blood products such as washed red blood cells, factor VIII concentrates, factor IX concentrates, and fibrinogen can also transmit hepatitis.

Hepatitis and Health Personnel. Physicians and other hospital personnel can become infected by patients with hepatitis, and they can also transmit hepatitis to their patients (see Chap. 27). Nineteen percent of physicians have antibody to hepatitis B, indicating earlier exposure to the virus compared to a 3.5 percent prevalence among volunteer blood donors.[59] Among physicians, surgeons had the highest prevalence (28 percent) of anti-HB_s. The prevalence of anti-HB_s increases with age and with the number of years in practice. These are old data. With the widespread use of hepatitis B vaccine, current hepatitis B prevalence rates in health care workers are difficult to ascertain.

Sporadic outbreaks of hepatitis transmission from hospital personnel to patients occur. Oral surgeons are most frequently implicated, but surgeons and gynecologists can also transmit hepatitis.

Human Immunodeficiency Virus. Testing of blood and blood products for HIV become mandatory in 1985. The CDC estimates that 12,000 Americans have or will ultimately develop the acquired immunodeficiency syndrome from blood transfused before 1985. Hemophiliacs who require factor VIII concentrates, cryoprecipitate plasma, or other blood products have a very high prevalence rate of HIV (approximately 75 percent) because pooled plasma (from up to 10,000 donors) was used to make factor VIII concentrates. Currently, factor VIII is made using recombinant DNA technology, which eliminates transmission of HIV and other viruses. Cryoprecipitate is pasteurized, which eliminates transmission of HIV and other viruses. Even though all transfused blood is screened for antibody to HIV and individuals with risk factors for HIV infection are not allowed to donate blood even if their blood tests negative, transmission of HIV by blood transfusion can still occur. There is a period of approximately 12 weeks between HIV infection and the development of anti-HIV antibodies when the test becomes positive. During this window a donor is potentially infectious because he/she has HIV in his/her blood and yet serologic testing for HIV is negative. Thus blood can still potentially transmit HIV even though tests are negative. Several published studies have estimated the risk of acquiring HIV infection from blood donors to be between 1 in 36,282 and 1 in 153,000 per component unit transfused.[60–66]

Patient's blood-borne diseases can also be transmitted to hospital personnel, and over 100 health care workers have become infected with HIV since 1981 (see Chap. 27). The CDC estimates that in 1991 alone over 5000 health care workers were infected with hepatitis B from exposure to patient's blood or other body fluids.

Cytomegalovirus. Cytomegalovirus infection can also be transfusion associated. It is a herpes virus that exists in a latent form in the white blood cells. Posttransfusion cytomegaloviral infection is most frequently seen after open heart procedures with extracorporeal perfusion. A syndrome resembling infectious mononucleosis and characterized by fever, erythematous rash, hepatomegaly, splenomegaly, eosinophilia, and atypical lymphocytosis appears 3 to 5 weeks after operation. It is variously called the postperfusion syndrome, the postpump syndrome, and the posttransfusion syndrome. The disease is almost always self-limited. It is unusual in adults but can affect 10 percent of children and young adults.

The postperfusion syndrome has been attributed to both cytomegalovirus and to Epstein-Barr virus. Most cases have been attributed to cytomegalovirus, and the transfused blood is almost certainly the source of the virus.

THE ENVIRONMENT AND THE HOST

Surveillance

Surveillance, when applied to disease, may be defined as "the systematic, active, ongoing observation of the occurrence and distribution of disease within a population and of the events or conditions that increase or decrease the risk of such disease occurrence."[67] Surveillance of disease includes the selection, recording, analyzing, and dissemination of data about that disease. It facilitates the early detection of outbreaks of infection, especially when an uncommon source is at fault, something that would be difficult in the absence of baseline surveillance data. The effectiveness of old and newly instituted infection control measures can only be assessed if adequate surveillance data are available. Surveillance data are also useful for detecting problems within the hospital that contribute to nosocomial infections, and which departments or what part of a patient's hospital stay is most likely to result in a nosocomial infection. Surveillance is required for determining baseline information about nosocomial infections so that deviations can be recognized. It can also be used as a continuing reminder to medical and nursing personnel of the importance of adhering to good infection control practices.[67,68] For these reasons, the Joint Commission on Accreditation of Healthcare Organizations requires that each hospital have a practical surveillance system carried out under the direction of an infection control committee.

The Infection Control Committee. The Joint Commission on the Accreditation of Healthcare Organizations has published guidelines and standards for infection prevention, control, surveillance, and reporting.[69] The American Hospital Association[70] and the Committee on Control of Surgical Infections of the Pre- and Postoperative Care Committee of the American College of Surgeons[71] agree with the guidelines and standards. Each hospital should provide (1) the appointment of an infection control committee; (2) procedures and techniques for meeting established sanitation and asepsis standards that are evaluated and revised on a continuing basis; (3) a practical surveillance system for reporting, evaluating, and keeping records of infections among patients and personnel; (4) policies and procedures for isolation of infected patients; (5) the development of written standards for hospital sanitation and medical asepsis and proper instruction of hospital personnel in medical and surgical asepsis; (6) an adequate microbiology service; (7) adequate measures against contamination of food; and (8) periodic review of antibiotic usage.[71]

The Infection Control Practitioner. The infection control practitioner or infection control nurse (nurse epidemiologist) is usually the only hospital employee whose full-time activity is devoted to infection control, although there is a tendency for large hospitals to employ a full-time physician epidemiologist also. While most hospitals have one infection control nurse, a large, active surgical service may justify a full-time surgical infection control nurse. The major responsibility of the infection control nurse is to carry out hospital surveillance of nosocomial infections. The nurse should detect and record data about nosocomial infections in a systematic and current manner, analyze such data, and prepare monthly reports for the infection control committee.

Determinants of Nosocomial Infections. The development of nosocomial infections is determined by several factors, among which are the source of infection, the microbial agent, the route of transmission, the susceptibility of the host, and the environment.

Sources of Infection. The sources of microorganisms in the hospital are persons, inanimate objects, food, animals, and arthropods. All persons in the hospital, whether they are patients, hospital personnel, or visitors, are potential sources of infection. Many patients who develop wound infections or intra-abdominal abscesses after intestinal surgery are themselves the sources of infection. Their own endogenous organisms frequently cause wound infections or other postoperative infections.

Inanimate objects (fomites) other than food, such as anesthesia equipment, nebulizers, intravenous catheters and solutions, furniture, and linen supplies, can also be sources of nosocomial infections. Occasionally, food and water may be contaminated with bacteria—especially *Clostridium* and *Salmonella*—and may also be sources of nosocomial infections. Infrequently, animals, such as rats and other vermin, and insects are important sources of infections in hospitals.

The Microbial Agent. Patients may be exposed to many types of pathogens during hospitalization. The likelihood of infection depends on several microbe-determined factors: the type of pathogen, its virulence or disease-producing ability, and the numbers introduced into the patient. Many microbes normally of low virulence can cause infections if the patient is a compromised host (see Chap. 51), if sufficient numbers are introduced into the patient, and if they are introduced by the correct route.

Route of Transmission. Microorganisms can be transmitted within the hospital by four routes: contact, a common vehicle, air, or a vector. More than one route may be operative for a given pathogen.

CONTACT TRANSMISSION. Contact transmission occurs when the patient acquires the infection by contact with the source. Contact-spread infection is either direct, indirect, or by droplets. Direct contact occurs when there is actual physical contact between the person or object harboring the infectious agent and the patient. Infections (wound infections, abscesses) in which the patient is the source of the bacteria are direct autogenous infections. Hepatitis A, gonorrhea, and syphilis also occur by direct contact spread.

Indirect contact spread occurs when the patient comes in contact with an intermediate object, usually inanimate, from which there is transfer of an infectious agent. Hepatitis B can be spread in this manner by contaminated needles and syringes. Contact contamination can occur from virtually any inanimate object, for example, endoscopes, cystoscopes, dialyzers, nebulizers, anesthesia equipment, thermometers, venous arterial catheters, pressure transducers, antiseptics, suction equipment, bedpans, urinals, and barium enema equipment. Medicine, blood, food, and water are additional sources, and there are numerous other sources as well.

Droplet spread refers to brief spread of the infectious agent through the air in contaminated droplets when the source and victim are relatively near each other. Talking, sneezing, and coughing can result in droplet spread of streptococcal pharyngitis and measles.

COMMON-VEHICLE TRANSMISSION. In common-vehicle spread infection, multiple cases of the same infection are transmitted from a common source. Medicine, blood and blood products, food, and water are the most common sources of common-vehicle spread. Other sources, such as intravenous fluids, contaminated eye drops, diagnostic dyes, cosmetics, and bronchodilators have been responsible for common-vehicle spread of nosocomial infections.

AIRBORNE TRANSMISSION. Airborne spread refers to transmission of microorganisms through the air for more than the several feet between source and victim. The organisms are contained in droplet nuclei or dust particles whose small size (less than 5 μm) permits them to remain suspended in the air for a prolonged time. Examples of nosocomial infections that can be transmitted by airborne spread include chickenpox, tuberculosis, and influenza. Dust from a variety of sources can also cause nosocomial infections. *Aspergillus* infections have been attributed to fireproofing materials in a new hospital,[72] and an outbreak of salmonellosis occurred because of contaminated dust in a vaccum cleaner bag. Each time the vacuum cleaner was used, the dust was resuspended.[73]

VECTORBORNE TRANSMISSION. Vectorborne spread of nosocomial infections no longer occurs in the United States, but spread by flies or cockroaches, which are frequently found in hospitals, theoretically could occur.

Host Susceptibility. More and more surgeons are dealing with compromised hosts (Chap. 51). Patients at the extremes of age and patients with certain diseases, especially leukemia, lymphoma, and other types of cancers, uremia, and diabetes mellitus, and those receiving immunosuppressive therapy, radiation therapy, and chemotherapy have decreased resistance to infection. Anesthesia and surgery themselves inhibit a host's immune response.[74]

The Environment. The environment is yet another factor that can affect infection. Overcrowding of patients, especially in intensive care units, favors patient-to-patient spread of infections. The humidity and temperature can affect the persistence of a microbe at its source, its transmission through the air, and the effectiveness of the host's mucous membranes. Routinely taking cultures from environmental sources (walls, floors, furniture) is not helpful in reducing hospital-acquired infections.

Nosocomial Infections Related to Different Hospital Departments

Each department within the hospital is a potential source of nosocomial infection, frequently of a specific type. Although many departments, such as the food preparation service, laundry service, and pharmacy, are a potential source of hospital-acquired infection to all patients within the hospital, some departments, such as the operating room, intensive care ward, and dialysis unit, are of particular concern to surgical patients.

The Operating Room. Because bacterial contamination of host tissues most often occurs in the operating room, infection control practices in this area are of great importance. Many wound infections are due to contamination of the wound with the patient's own bacteria, frequently from the intestine during gastrointestinal or gynecologic procedures. Few operating room infection control practices can alter this type of wound contamination, but certain techniques of patient preparation, operative care, and antibiotic use can help. Infection control measures in the operating room can reduce nosocomial infections due to environmental contamination.

Many sites in the operating room are potential sources of nosocomial infections. Operating room personnel are one potential source. Small holes in surgeons' gloves commonly develop during operative procedures, and the wound infection rate is higher where such punctures occur. The contamination comes from the hands of the surgeon. Even the soap that the surgeon uses to wash his or her hands can be contaminated with bacteria.

Personnel who are nasal carriers of *S. aureus* can disseminate these organisms into the operating room air so that they cause wound infections, even if they are not standing directly at the operating table.[75] Airflow systems are designed to reduce the possibility of airborne contamination.[76] Orthopedic surgeons who implant joint prostheses have been instrumental in promoting clean air systems, including laminar flow operating rooms with microbially filtered air and even total body exhaust gowns.

The inanimate objects in the operating room, blood and blood products, intravenous catheters and solutions, urinary catheters, and anesthesia equipment, are also potential sources of nosocomial infections. Inanimate objects, such as oxygenators used for open heart surgery, surgical instruments, cystoscopes, drapes and linens, sutures, gloves, and sponges, may not be sterile. Blood, blood products, and intravenous fluids may be contaminated with bacteria or hepatitis virus. Anesthesia equipment and anesthesia can give rise to bacteremia and aspiration. There is a 16 percent incidence of bacteremia following nasotracheal intubation compared to no bacteremia with orotracheal intubation.[77] The organisms isolated were oral and nasal bacteria, such as alpha-hemolytic streptococci.

The Intensive Care Unit. Intensive care units are designed to give special care to critically ill patients and to certain patients with special needs. The most seriously ill patients who may have compromised host defenses and who usually have invasive monitoring devices, multiple catheters, and surgical wounds are placed in a setting where the hospital's most resistant bacteria frequently are found. No wonder nosocomial infections are extremely common in this setting. Infection control measures should be adequately stressed. In most community hospitals, surgical intensive care units admit all postsurgical and injured patients requiring special care. In many larger hospitals, intensive care units are specialized into general surgery units, cardiac surgery units, burn units, respiratory units, neuro surgery units, coronary-care units, oncology units, transplantation units, and neonatal units.

The intensive care unit brings in close proximity many patients who are highly susceptible to infection. Their illnesses, operations, burns, and trauma suppress their host defenses.[74] They are frequently treated with antibiotics, thus favoring the emergence of resistant bacteria, and they undergo a variety of invasive procedures in addition to operations, such as central nervous system catheters, arterial catheters, Swan-Ganz catheters, chest tubes, tracheostomies, endotracheal tubes, and urinary catheters. Often, these invasive procedures must be done in the intensive care ward during a medical emergency, and proper sterile precautions are compromised.

Several recommendations have been made to reduce the incidence of nosocomial infections in intensive care unit settings, but only vigorous vascular access care and transducer care, ventilator care, and selective decontaminating consistently reduce infection rates.[78]

Partial separation of patients can be important in suppressing cross-infection. Single rooms can provide barriers between patients, but observing patients closely can be difficult even with remote monitoring devices, especially if there is a nursing shortage. Physical barriers can also be placed between patients so that they are separated on three sides. Such a system retards cross-infection but still allows close observation. United States government standards require at least 7 feet between beds and a clear area of 120 square feet around each bed.

Placement of patients in a unit can also be important. In some intensive care units, it is common practice to place patients with similar problems (ie, endotracheal tubes, tracheostomies, urinary catheters) near each other, but the risk of transmission of microbes on the hands of personnel is increased if patients with similar tubes or catheters are placed near one another. Rather than grouping patients, they should be spread out as much as possible.

Contact transmission is the most likely method of spread of most nosocomial infections within intensive care facilities. Organisms are spread from patient to patient on the hands of hospital personnel. The most effective method of preventing such spread is diligent handwashing between patient contacts. To encourage handwashing, sinks must be readily available. Only 14 percent of physicians in private hospitals and 28 percent of physicians in university hospitals, however, wash their hands after patient contact in intensive care units.[79] Of total personnel in the intensive care units, only 28 percent in private hospitals and 41 percent in university hospitals wash their hands after patient contact, still better than the rate for physicians. Multiple bed units should have one sink for every six beds, and every isolation room should have its own sink.[1] Wearing gloves is more effective than hand washing. Personnel should be encouraged to wear gloves when handling intravenous or arterial catheters, wounds, dressings, and urinary catheters. Wearing gloves should be required when handling or suctioning tracheostomies or endotracheal tubes.

Other Departments. Nosocomial infections in surgical patients can originate in other hospital departments as well.

Admitting and Outpatient Departments. The admitting office and outpatient departments are often overlooked in the infection control policies of a hospital because they are frequently not regarded as integral parts of the hospital itself. Insofar as infection control is concerned, the admitting office and outpatient facilities should be considered as inpatient facilities. An attempt should be made in both of these departments to judiciously separate infected patients from uninfected patients, especially those whose infections might be spread through the air to other persons. Infected patients should perhaps bypass the admissions office and should not be allowed to come into close contact with uninfected patients or with those who are going to have surgical procedures during their hospital admission.

Laundry. Linens from both hospital wards and the operating room frequently are contaminated by infectious materials, and diseases can be transmitted by soiled linens. *Salmonella typhimurium* and Q fever have been transmitted to hospital employees handling soiled linens.[80]

All soiled linen should be bagged and put in covered carts where they should remain until taken to the laundry. In the laundry, linen should be washed in hot water to kill contaminating microorganisms. Water temperature above 71C for 25 minutes kills almost all microorganisms except spores. Even with the potential for transmission of pathogens, nosocomial infections related to linen supplies are extremely rare.

Central Supply Service. The central supply service is responsible for processing, storing, and dispensing supplies and equipment required for all aspects of patient care, diagnosis, and treatment. The central supply service is thus responsible for cleaning and disinfecting contaminated reusable items, such as endoscopic equipment, thermometers, bedpans, urinals, respiratory therapy equipment, anesthesia supplies, and procedure trays used for cutdowns on the wards. They are also responsible for cleaning diagnostic equipment, such as sigmoidoscopes, anoscopes, vaginal speculums, and laryngoscopy instruments.

Hospitals have found it economically advantageous to have all reusable supplies and equipment requiring specialized cleaning, disinfection, and sterilization handled by the central supply service whenever possible. Therefore much equipment that could be a potential source of transmitting infections passes through the central supply service. Therefore it is essential that the central supply service have adequate facilities for decontaminating items that have been used by hospital patients, for washing and cleaning this equipment, and finally for disinfecting it or sterilizing it and packaging it for reuse. In addition, the central supply service should have adequate storage areas for equipment. These areas should be ventilated with at least two air changes per hour, and the temperature should be maintained between 18C and 25C.

Pharmacy. The pharmacy is frequently not thought of as a potential source of disseminating infection within the hospital. However, pharmacies are currently responsible for mixing solutions for total parenteral nutrition therapy. These solutions are easily contaminated with bacteria and provide growth media for many kinds of organisms. Because hyperalimentation solutions do not come prepared from the manufacturer but have to be mixed in the pharmacy, contamination can occur. In addition, some medications purchased from commercial sources have been found to be contaminated with such potential pathogens as *E. coli, Pseudomonas, Proteus,* and *Salmonella.* These drugs have included digitalis alkaloids, barbiturates, and oral tranquilizers. The hospital pharmacy is also a good place for surveillance for antimicrobial usage within the hospital.

Food Service. The food service has the task of providing attractively prepared, wholesome, appetizing food that is safe to eat. Because such a high percentage of patients and staff eat hospital food, the food service is a potential source of widespread nosocomial infections.

Foodborne illnesses have been caused by staphylococcal enterotoxins, *Clostridium perfringens, Salmonella, Shigella,* and hepatitis A.[81] The most common responsible agents are *C. perfringens* and *Salmonella,*[82] and these types of illnesses can be responsible for patient death, especially in old and frail patients. The major factors leading to outbreaks of foodborne illnesses are inadequate refrigeration (46 percent of outbreaks), preparing food far in advance of planned service (22 percent), handling of food by infected persons who practice poor personal hygiene (21 percent), inadequate cooking or heat processing (19 percent), holding food in warming devices at bacteria-incubation temperatures (16 percent), uncooked foods contaminated by raw ingredients (12 percent), and inadequate reheating (9 percent).[81]

Hospital food can become contaminated before, during, and after preparation. Meat and poultry are frequently contaminated with *C. perfringens* and *Salmonella* at the time of purchase; up to 50 percent of poultry is contaminated by *Salmonella.* The external surface of unprocessed eggs can be contaminated with fecal matter containing *Salmonella.* Raw seafood can be contaminated with *C. perfringens* and *Vibrio* species.

Prevention of foodborne transmission involves proper handling of food and personal hygiene by foodhandlers. Food must be adequately cleaned, refrigerated or stored, and adequately cooked. Prepared foods and foods that are to be reused must also be adequately stored, stored at cold enough temperatures, and adequately reheated prior to use.

Foodhandlers and kitchen personnel should be instructed in infection control measures. Handwashing facilities should be convenient, because the hands are probably the chief mode of transmission of nosocomial infections by foodhandlers.

Universal Precautions and Isolation Procedures

Following the development of a test for HIV in 1985 the CDC and others considered whether testing all patients would reduce HIV transmission. Because of other considerations such as patient confidentiality, possible HIV transmission before the development of anti-HIV antibody, and inability to predict the patients' risk for transmission of hepatitis B, hepatitis C, and other blood-borne pathogens in 1987 the CDC published guidelines known as universal precautions that assume that blood and other body fluids from *all* patients are potentially infections and therefore pecautions should be used for all patients.[83] Since all patients are treated the same, there is no need for testing. A discussion of universal precautions can be found in Chapter 27.

CDC Systems for Isolation Precautions. The CDC currently recommends that hospitals use either category-specific or disease-specific isolation precaution methods.[84] Category-specific isolation precautions have been recommended by the CDC since 1970. This system groups diseases for which similar isolation precautions are indicated. In 1983 the CDC adopted disease-specific isolation precautions. These precautions considered each infectious individual so that only those precautions such as private rooms, masks, gowns, and gloves that are indicated to interrupt transmission of that particular disease need be used. There are no data concerning the efficacy of the traditional category-specific isolation precautions and the more recently recommended disease-specific isolation precautions.

The category-specific system is simpler and is easier for personnel to learn since they need learn only a few established routines. Because many different diseases are grouped into six categories, unnecessary precaution will be applied to some diseases. The disease-specific system is designed so that the only isolation precautions applied are those required to interrupt transmission of a specific infection. Because this set of precautions is individualized to each disease, it requires more special training and a higher level of attention from health care personnel. Both systems use a card displayed near the patient to alert personnel what specific precautions are required. Six isolation categories are currently used in the category-specific system: strict isolation, contact isolation, respiratory isolation, tuberculosis isolation, enteric precautions, and drainage secretion precautions. A previous category—blood and body fluid precautions—was superseded by CDC recommendations for universal precautions in 1987. In general, the term isolation is used when a private room is indicated and the term precaution is used when a private room is optional but not indicated.

Isolation procedures are designed to prevent the spread of microorganisms among patients, hospital personnel, and visitors. Because microorganisms and host factors are difficult to control, isolation procedures are directed at the chain of transmission to interrupt the chain of infection. Isolation procedures are difficult, time consuming, and costly, and they should be suited to both the patient and to the infection to be controlled. Furthermore, isolation makes frequent visits by physicians, nurses, and other hospital personnel inconvenient and may discourage the hospital from giving the best possible care. In addition, the requirement for a private room might necessitate using space designed to accommodate additional patients, thus causing an economic loss for the hospital. Thus isolation procedures should not be used when not required.

The infection control committee is responsible for developing isolation policies and procedures. The policies and procedures should be reviewed from time to time and modified as necessary. The infection control nurse should be knowledgeable about isolation procedures and should serve as a consultant on isolation policies and procedures.

REFERENCES

1. Bennett JV: Human infections: economic implications and prevention. Ann Intern Med 89:761, 1978.
2. Horan TC, White JW, Jarvis WR, et al: Nosocomial infection surveillance, 1984. MMWR 35(1SS):17SS, 1986.
3. Haley RW, Hooton TM, Culver DH: Nosocomial infections in U.S. hospitals, 1975–1976. Estimated frequency by selected characteristics of patients. Am J Med 70:947, 1981.

4. Horan TC, Culver DH, Gaynes RP, et al: Nosocomial infections in surgical patients in the United States, January 1986–June 1992. Infect Control Hosp Epidemiol 14:73, 1993.
5. Haley RW: Measuring the costs of nosocomial infections: methods for estimating economic burden on the hospital. Am J Med 91(Suppl 3B):32S, 1991.
6. Haley RW, Culver DH, White JW, et al: The nationwide nosocomial infection rate: a new need for vital statistics. Am J Epidemiol 121:159, 1985.
7. Johnson JR, Roberts PL, Olsen RJ, et al: Prevention of catheter-associated urinary tract infections with a silver oxide-coated urinary catheter: clinical and microbiological correlates. J Infect Dis 162:1145, 1990.
8. Stamm WE: Guidelines for prevention of catheter-associated urinary tract infections. Ann Intern Med 82:386, 1975.
9. Kunin CM: Detection, Prevention and Management of Urinary Tract Infections. Philadelphia, Lea & Febiger, 1972.
10. Guinan PD, Bayley BC, Metzger WI, et al: The case against "The case against the catheter": initial report. J Urol 101:909, 1969.
11. Platt R, Murdock B, Polk BF, Rosner B: Reduction of mortality associated with nosocomial urinary tract infection. Lancet 1:893, 1983.
12. Stamm WE. Catheter-associated urinary tract infections: epidemiology, pathogenesis, and prevention. Am J Med 91(Suppl 3B):65S, 1991.
13. Maki DG, Goldmann DA, Rhame FS: Infection control in intravenous therapy. Ann Intern Med 79:867, 1973.
14. Rhame FS, Maki DG, Bennett JV: Intravenous cannula-associated infections. In Bennett JV, Brachman PS (eds): Hospital Infections. Boston, Little, Brown, 1979, p 433.
15. Tager IB, Ginsberg MB, Ellis SE, et al: An epidemiological study of the risks associated with peripheral intravenous catheters. Am J Epidemiology 118:839, 1983.
16. Maki DG, Weise CE, Sarafin HW: A semiquantitative culture method for identifying intravenous-catheter-related infection. N Engl J Med 296:1305, 1977.
17. Band JD, Alvarado CJ, Maki DG: A semiquantitative culture technique for identifying infection due to steel needles used for intravenous therapy. Am J Clin Pathol 72:980, 1979.
18. Press OW, Ramsey PG, Larson EB, et al: Hickman catheter infections in patients with malignancies. Medicine 63:189, 1984.
19. Keohane PP, Attrill H, Northover J, et al: Effect of catheter tunnelling and a nutrition nurse on catheter sepsis during parenteral nutrition. A controlled trial. Lancet 2:1388, 1983.
20. Maki DG, Hassemer CA: Endemic rate of fluid contamination and related septicemia in arterial pressure monitoring. Am J Med 70:733, 1981.
21. Shinozaki T, Deane RS, Mazuzan JE Jr., et al: Bacterial contamination of arterial lines. A prospective study. JAMA 249:223, 1983.
22. Myers ML, Austin TW, Sibbald WJ: Pulmonary artery catheter infections. A prospective study. Ann Surg 201:237, 1985.
23. Padberg FT Jr., Ruggiero J, Blackburn, Bristrian BR: Central venous catheterization for parenteral nutrition. Ann Surg 193:264, 1981.
24. Bozzetti F, Terno G, Bonfanti G, et al: Prevention and treatment of central venous catheter sepsis by exchange via a guidewire. A prospective controlled trial. Ann Surg 198:48, 1983.
25. Craven DE, Steger KA, Barber TW: Preventing nosocomial pneumonia: state of the art and perspectives for the 1990s. Am J Med 91(Suppl 3B):44S, 1991.
26. Johanson WE Jr, Pierce AK, Sanford JP: Changing pharyngeal bacterial flora of hospitalized patients. Emergence of gram-negative bacilli. N Engl J Med 281:1137, 1969.
27. Johanson WE Jr, Pierce AK, Sanford JP, Thomas GD: Nosocomial respiratory infections with gram-negative bacilli: the significance of colonization of the respiratory tract. Ann Intern Med 77:701, 1972.
28. Glover JL, Jolly L: Colonization of the respiratory tract by gram-negative bacilli in hospitalized patients. Exp Med Surg 29:114, 1971.
29. Culver GA, Makel HP, Beecher HK: Frequency of aspiration of gastric contents by the lungs during anesthesia and surgery. Ann Surg 133:289, 1951.
30. Huxley EJ, Voroslau J, Gray WR: Pharyngeal aspiration in normal adults and patients with depressed consciousness. Am J Med 64:564, 1978.
31. Bryant LR, Trinkle JK, Mobin-Uddin K, et al: Bacterial colonization profile with tracheal intubation and mechanical ventilation. Arch Surg 104:647,1972.
32. Haley RW, Hooten TM, Culver DH, et al: Nosocomial infections in U.S. Hospitals, 1975–1976. Estimated frequency by selected characteristics in patients. Am J Med 70:947, 1981.
33. Craven DE, Kunches LM, Kilinsky V, et al: Risk factors for pneumonia and fatality in patients receiving continuous mechanical ventilation. Am Rev Respir Dis 133:792, 1986.
34. Cross AS, Roup B: Role of respiratory assistance devices in endemic nosocomial pneumonia. Am J Med 70:681, 1981.
35. Tubin TO, Beare J, Dunhill MS, et al: Legionnaires' disease in a transplant unit: isolation of the causative agent from shower baths. Lancet 2:118, 1980.
36. Arrow PM, Chou T, Weil D: Nosocomial legionnaires' disease caused by aerosolized tap water from respiratory devices. J Infect Dis 146:460, 1982.
37. Craven DE, Goularte TA, Make BJ: Contaminated condensole in mechanical ventilator circuits. A risk factor. Ann Rev Respir Dis 129:625, 1984.
38. Craveb DF, Connoly MG Jr, Lechtenberg DA, et al: Contamination of mechanical ventilators with tubing changes every 24 to 48 hours. N Engl J Med 306:1505, 1982.
39. Simmons BP, Wong EP: Guidelines for prevention of nosocomial pneumonia. Infect Control 3:327, 1982.
40. Simmons BP, Wong EP: CDC guidelines for the pre-

vention of nosocomial pneumonia. Am J Infect Control Hosp Epidemiol 17:230, 1983.
41. Hamer DH, Barza M: Prevention of hospital-acquired pneumonia. Antimicrob Agents Chemother 37:931, 1993.
42. Acourt C, Garrard CS: Nosocomial pneumonia in the intensive care unit: mechanisms and significance. Thorax 47:465, 1992.
43. Mahol P, Auboyer C, Jospe R, et al: Prevention of nosocomial pneumonia in intubated patients: respective role of mechanical subglottic secretion drainage and ulcer prophylaxis. Intensive Care Med 18:20, 1992.
44. Driks MR, Craven DE, Cell BR, et al: Nosocomial pneumonia in intubated patients given sucralfate as compared with antacids or histamine type 2 blockers. N Engl J Med 317:1376, 1987.
45. Tryba M: Risk of acute stress bleeding and nosocomial pneumonia in ventilated patients and nosocomial pneumonia in ventilated intensive care unit patients: sucralfate versus antacids. Am J Med 83:117, 1987.
46. Unertl K, Ruckdeschel G, Selbmann HE, et al: Prevention of colonization and respiratory infections in long-term ventilated patients by local antimicrobial prophylaxis. Intensive Care Med 13:106, 1987.
47. Ledingham MA I, Alcock SR, Eastaway AT, et al: Triple regimen of selective decontamination of the digestive tract, systemic cefotaxime, and microbiologic surveillance for prevention of acquired infection in intensive care. Lancet 1:785, 1988.
48. Kerver AJH, Rommes JH, Mevissen Verhage EAE, et al: Prevention of colonization and infection in critically ill patients: a prospective randomized study. Crit Care Med 16:1087, 1988.
49. Ulrich C, de Weerd W, Bakker NC, et al: Selective decontamination of the digestive tract with norfloxacin in the prevention of ICU-acquired infections: a prospective randomized study. Intensive Care Med 15:424, 1989.
50. Flaherty J, Nathan C, Kabins A, et al: Nonabsorbable antibiotics versus sucralfate in preventing colonization and infection in a cardiac surgery intensive care unit. J Infect Dis 162:1393, 1990.
51. Holland PV: Transfusion transmitted infectious diseases. J Fla Med Assoc 80:33, 1993.
52. Wells L, Ala FA: Malaria and blood transfusion. Lancet 1:1317, 1985.
53. Alter HJ, Holland PV, Purcell RH: The emerging pattern of post-transfusion hepatitis. Am J Med Sci 270:329, 1975.
54. Aach RJ, Lander JJ, Sherman LA, et al: Transfusion-transmitted viruses: interim analysis of hepatitis among transfused and nontransfused patients. In Vyas GN, Cohen SN, Schmid R (eds): Viral Hepatitis. Philadelphia, Franklin Institute Press, 1978, pp 383–396.
55. Welch HG, Meehan KR, Goodnough LT: Prudent strategies for elective red blood cell transfusion. Ann Intern Med 166:393, 1992.
56. Japanese Red Cross non-A, non-B Hepatitis Research Group: Effect of screening for hepatitis C virus antibody and hepatitis B core antibody on incidence of post-transfusion hepatitis. Lancet 338:1040, 1991.
57. Schmidt P: Post-transfusion hepatitis in Florida. J Fla Med Assoc 67:999, 1980.
58. Huestis DW, Bove JR, Busch S: Hazards of transfusion. In Huestis DW, Bove JR, Busch S (eds): Practical Blood Transfusion. Boston, Little, Brown, 1981, pp 249–285.
59. Denes AE, Smith JL, Maynard JG: Hepatitis B infections in physicians. JAMA 239:210, 1978.
60. Kleinman S, Secord K: Risk of human immunodeficiency virus (HIV) transmission by anti-HIV negative blood. Estimates using the look back methodology. Transfusion 28:499, 1988.
61. Cohen ND, Muñoz A, Reitz BA, et al: Transmission of retroviruses by transfusion of screened blood in patients undergoing cardiac surgery. N Engl J Med 320:1172, 1989.
62. Busch MP, Eble BE, Khayam-Bashi H, et al: Evaluation of screened blood donations for human immunodeficiency virus type 1 infection by culture and DNA amplification of pooled cells. N Engl J Med 325:1, 1991.
63. Cumming PD, Wallace EL, Schorr JB, et al: Exposure of patients to human immunodeficiency virus through the transfusion of blood components that test antibody-negative. N Engl J Med 321:941, 1989.
64. Busch M, Eble B, Heilbron D, et al: Risk associated with transfusion of HIV-antibody-negative blood (letter). N Engl J Med 322:850, 1990.
65. Donahoe JG, Nelson KE, Muñoz A, et al: Transmission of HIV by transfusion of screened blood (letter). N Engl Med 323:1709, 1990.
66. Nelson KE, Donahue JG, Muñoz A, et al: Transmission of retrovirus from seronegative donors by transfusion during cardiac surgery. A multicenter study of HIV-1 and HTLV I/II infections. Ann Intern Med 117:554, 1992.
67. Aber RC, Bennett JV: Surveillance of nosocomial infections. In Bennett JV, Brachman PS: Hospital Infections. Boston, Little, Brown, 1979, p 53.
68. Mulholland SG, Creed J, Cierauf LA, et al: Analysis and significance of nosocomial infection rates. Ann Surg 180:827, 1974.
69. Joint Commission on Accreditation of Healthcare Organizations: 1994 Accreditation Manual for Hospitals. 1993, Joint Commission on Accreditation of Healthcare Organizations, Oakbrook, IL.
70. American Hospital Association, Committee on Infections Within Hospitals: Infection Control in the Hospital, 5th ed. Chicago, American Hospital Association, 1983.
71. Altemeier WA, Burke JF, Pruitt BA Jr, Sandusky WR (eds): Manual on Control of Infection in Surgical Patients. Philadelphia, Lippincott, 1984.
72. Aisner J, Schimpff SC, Bennett JE, et al: *Aspergillus* infections in cancer patients. Association with fire-

proofing materials in a new hospital. JAMA 235:411, 1976.
73. Bate JG, James U: *Salmonella typhimurium* infection dustborne in a children's ward. Lancet 2:713, 1958.
74. Howard RJ: Host defense against infection. I. Curr Probl Surg 17:267, 1980.
75. Dineen P, Drusin L: Epidemics of postoperative wound infections associated with hair carriers. Lancet 2:1157, 1973.
76. Howorth FH: Prevention of airborne infection during surgery. Lancet 1:386, 1985.
77. Berry FA Jr, Blankenbaker WL, Ball CG: A comparison of bacteremia occurring with nasotracheal and orotracheal intubation. Anesth Analg 52:873, 1973.
78. Weinstein RA: Epidemiology and control of nosocomial infections in adult intensive care units. Am J Med 91(Suppl 3B):179S, 1991.
79. Albert RK, Condre F: Hand washing patterns in medical intensive care units. N Engl J Med 304:1465, 1981.
80. Steere AC, Craven PJ, Hall WJ III, et al: Person-to-person spread of *Salmonella typhimurium* after a hospital common-source outbreak. Lancet 1:319, 1975.
81. Bryan FL: Status of food borne disease in the United States. J Environ Health 38:74, 1975.
82. Editorial: Food poisoning in hospitals. Lancet 1:576; 1980.
83. Centers for Disease Control: Recommendations for prevention of HIV transmission in healthcare settings. MMWR 36(Suppl 2S):1S, 1987.
84. Garner JS: Universal precautions and isolation systems. In Bennet JV, Brachman PS (eds): Hospital Infections, 3rd ed. Boston, Little, Brown, 1992, p 231.

BIBLIOGRAPHY

Altemeier WA, Burke JF, Pruitt BA Jr, Sandusky WR: Manual on Control of Infection in Surgical Patients, 2nd ed. Philadelphia, Lippincott, 1984.

American Hospital Association, Committee on Infections Within Hospitals: Infection Control in the Hospital, 5th ed. Chicago, American Hospital Association, 1983.

Bennett JV, Brachman PS: Hospital Infections, 3rd ed. Boston, Little, Brown, 1992.

Transmissible Infections Between Patients and Health Care Workers

CHAPTER 27

Richard J. Howard

HISTORICAL NOTE

Physicians have realized for centuries that disease could be transmitted from one person to another. The vehicle of transmission was termed a contagion, but physicians had no clear idea what it was. Bacteria were discovered only in the last half of the 19th century and viruses were unknown until the 20th.

Physicians also knew that diseases that passed from patient to patient could also be passed to them. During the plague years in the 14th century and during subsequent recurrences, many physicians selflessly cared for patients and put themselves at risk. Some died. Others simply left town and sought refuge in the countryside. To reduce the risk of transmission physicians wore gloves, long gowns, hats, and head covers with a long beak-like container in the front into which they could place a perfumed cloth to overcome the stench of death.

Physicians were subject to serious infection and death if they sustained a minor wound while draining an abscess or during an autopsy, a tragedy that led Rudyard Kipling to write: "They took their lives in their lancet hand."[1]

Oliver Wendell Holmes (1809 to 1894) and Ignaz Semmelweis (1818 to 1865) showed that physicians could be a source of infection for their patients and introduced hand washing to prevent puerperal sepsis. The German gynecologist, Alfred Hegar (1830 to 1914), first introduced routine hand washing in his practice of abdominal surgery. When asked what was new in surgery in 1882, Ernst von Bergman (1836 to 1907) replied, "today we wash our hands before operation."[1]

Barriers were only gradually introduced to reduce the risk of the physician transmitting infection to a patient, because many surgeons resisted. Face masks that covered the mouth and nose were an innovation of Johann von Mikulicz-Radecki (1850 to 1905) of Breslau in 1897 after his microbiologist colleague demonstrated that droplet contamination of wounds could occur during speech.

Other barrier techniques were accepted in the first quarter of the 20th century. In 1889 William S. Halsted (1852 to 1922) obtained rubber gloves for his operating room nurse (and future wife), Caroline Hampton, because of reactions on her hands to the corrosive sublimate hand rinse.[2] But it was his student, Joseph Bloodgood (1867 to 1935), who first wore gloves as a routine practice in nearly all clean operations. Gowns, caps, and sterile drapes were introduced to further prevent contamination of surgical wounds by exogenous sources. Although originally developed to prevent transmission of disease from physician to patient, interest in microbiologic barriers has been renewed because of concern of transmission of infectious agents especially human immunodeficiency virus type 1 (HIV-1) from patient to physician.

Tuberculosis is another infection that is readily transferred from patients to physicians. Before antimycobacterial agents were available, tuberculosis was responsible for a large number of patients in many hospitals. Those with pulmonary infection could pass the infection by coughing and creating airborne particles that could pass the infecting agent to health care workers. Some physicians developed tuberculosis and became patients themselves. If surgeons or pathologists sustained cuts while working on tuberculous patients or tissues, they often developed cutaneous tuberculous nodules.

Disease transmission from patient to physician and from physician to patient remains a problem. Although, the current focus is on viral illnesses, especially HIV-1, hepatitis B virus (HBV), non-A, non-B hepatitis, and hepatitis C virus (HCV), infections with bacteria and fungi continue to pose a threat.

ROUTES OF INFECTION

There are two potential sources of infection between patient and physician and between physician and patient: (1) airborne particles and (2) direct inoculation from instruments or other sharp objects that are contaminated with blood and other body fluids that contain infectious agents.

Airborne Particles

Tuberculosis. Coughing patients with pulmonary infections can generate numerous tiny droplets containing infectious agents. Patients with pulmonary or laryngeal tuberculosis have long been known to pass infection to health care workers. Before antimycobacterial agents were available and patients with active pulmonary tuberculosis were congregated in sanatoriums, many health care workers who cared for them developed tuberculosis or converted their skin test responses. Since surgery was used to treat tuberculosis, surgeons were also at risk, especially if they were cut by contaminated instruments. Pathologists were similarly subject to inoculation. Passage of tuberculosis to health care workers became much less prevalent following the introduction of antimycobacterial agents.

There has recently been a resurgence in tuberculosis among persons infected with HIV-1. These patients have frequently been infected with multidrug-resistant strains of *Mycobacterium tuberculosis* or with *M. avium-intercellulare,* which is not very susceptible to current antimycobacterial agents. Transmission to health care workers is a serious risk[3–9] (Table 27–1). The risk may be higher in areas where patients are provided care before diagnosis (eg, clinic waiting areas and emergency rooms). Nosocomial transmission of tuberculosis has occurred in association with close contact with infectious patients and with procedures such as bronchoscopy, endotracheal intubation and suctioning, open abscess irrigation,[7] and autopsy.[3,8] Sputum induction and aerosol treatments (eg, pentamidine) that induce cough may also increase the potential for transmission of tuberculosis.[3,9]

As recently as 10 years ago tuberculosis seemed to be disappearing from the United States. Cases of tuberculosis seem to be decreasing at a rate of approximately 6 percent per year from over 84,000 cases in 1953 to more than 22,000 cases in 1984.[10] Between 1985 and 1991, however, the number of new cases of tuberculosis has increased to more than 26,000. Many of these newly diagnosed cases occur in individuals who are infected with HIV. Furthermore, the isolates have often proved to be resistant to one or more chemotherapeutic agents. Mortality among patients with multidrug-resistant tuberculosis ranges from 72 to 89 percent and is associated with rapid progression from diagnosis to death (median interval, 4 to 6 weeks). Over 80 percent of cases of multidrug-resistant tuberculosis occur in HIV-infected individuals. Because tuberculosis is spread by aerosols, one infected patient could theoretically infect many health care workers as well as other patients. In contrast, HIV, HBV, and HCV are spread sporadically through accidental exposure to blood and other body fluids.

Most instances of transmission of tuberculosis from patients to health care workers have been documented by tuberculin skin test conversions, but some cases of active pulmonary tuberculosis and even death have occurred. Because the interval from infection to development of active tuberculosis can range from a few weeks to decades, the occurrence of active tuberculosis in health care workers may not be attributed to contact with a patient in the remote past, a period during which exposure and infection may have occurred.

TABLE 27–1. TRANSMISSION OF TUBERCULOSIS FROM PATIENTS TO HEALTH CARE WORKERS

Location	Number of HCWs with Tuberculosis/Number Tested (%)	Reference
Hospital (Miami, FL)		
HIV ward	13/39 (33)[a]	11
Control ward	0/15 (0)[a]	
Hospital—Infection Disease Unit (Italy)		
Exposed to HIV-positive patients	7/85 (8.2)[b]	12
Not exposed to HIV-positive patients	1/1079 (0.2)[b]	
Hospital—Pediatric ward (Louisville, KY)	3/78 (3.8)[a]	13
Hospital (Amarillo, TX)	19/93 (20)[a]	14
Hospice (Amarillo, TX)	11/65 (17)[a]	
Hospital (San Juan, PR)		
Nurses—HIV unit	9/19 (56)[c]	15
Nurses—Internal Medicine ward	45/90 (50)[c]	
Clerical personnel—other floors	35/188 (17)[c]	
Hospital (New York, NY)		
Wards housing patients with TB	11/32 (34)[a]	16
Other wards	1/47 (2.1)[a]	

[a] PPD conversion.
[b] Active tuberculosis.
[c] Positive PPD skin test.

The resurgence of tuberculosis necessitates careful infection control programs on wards where patients with tuberculosis are treated. Four basic approaches are used in health care settings to prevent tuberculosis transmission: (1) prevention of the generation of infectious airborne particles (droplet nuclei) by early identification and treatment of persons with tuberculosis infection and active tuberculosis, (2) prevention of the spread of infectious droplet nuclei into the general air circulation, (3) reduction of the number of infectious droplet nuclei, and (4) surveillance of health care personnel for tuberculosis and tuberculous infection.

The Centers for Disease Control and Prevention (CDC) has published guidelines for prevention of tuberculosis in health care settings. All health care workers should have a baseline PPD test placed at the time of employment so that later conversion can be documented. Patients with suspected or confirmed infectious tuberculosis should be placed in tuberculosis isolation in a private room with negative air pressure relative to adjacent areas. Isolation precautions should be maintained until the patient improves clinically, until the cough has substantially decreased, and until the number of acid-fast bacilli on sequential sputum smears decreases, which usually does not occur until 2 to 3 weeks after beginning effective antituberculosis therapy. Isolation precautions should be used in everyone suspected of having multidrug-resistant tuberculosis until the patient improves clinically and until the sputum is negative for acid-fast bacilli.

Protection of staff requires prevention of mycobacterial contamination of the air through early identification of patients with tuberculosis and initiation of chemotherapy. Patients removed from their rooms should be required to wear masks and to cover the nose and mouth while coughing to prevent the spread of aerosolized *M. tuberculosis.*

Staphylococcus aureus. Some individuals harbor *S. aureus* in their nasopharynx as part of the residential bacterial flora. Generated airborne particles can contain these bacteria, as can contaminated surgical wounds leading to wound infections.

Sporadic outbreaks of wound infections due to *S. aureus* have occurred, which have been attributed to operating room personnel, but clinical infection of health care workers is hard to document.[17,18] Up to 80 percent of adults harbor *S. aureus* in the anterior nares one time or another, but the carrier state is usually transient. Twenty to 40 percent of individuals may harbor *S. aureus* for months. Surveillance cultures and treatment for staphylococcal carriage are not worthwhile unless it is demonstrated that a person actually is responsible for nosocomial infection. The carrier state can be treated effectively in several ways. Rifampin, 600 mg PO daily for 5 days, combined with a second oral antistaphylococcal drug (eg, dicloxacillin or trimethoprim-sulfamethoxazole) or a topical agent to the nares is the standard. Mupricin in a 2 percent ointment applied to the nares for 5 days is a simple, equally effective regimen. Recurrence and the need for retreatment are common. Surveillance cultures of the anterior nares should be repeated at monthly intervals in carriers.

Streptococcus. Several outbreaks of group A beta-hemolytic streptococcal wound infection have been attributed to airborne transmission from surgical personnel who were carriers.[19]

Other Microorganisms. Other microbes may cause pulmonary, wound, or other infections if aerosols are generated. These types of infections rarely are transferred from patients to health care workers or from health care workers to patients but theoretically can occur. Thus a physician with herpes zoster caused by varicella-zoster virus could cause chickenpox in a child without antibodies or in an immunosuppressed patient even if the patient has had chickenpox previously. *Salmonella* and cryptosporidiosis have been transmitted from patient to health care workers presumably via the fecal-oral route. One cannot overemphasize the need for hand disinfection after every patient contact.

Direct Inoculation

Injuries with needles, bone, or sharp instruments are common among surgeons, dental workers, and other hospital personnel.[20–27] Contaminated "sharps" are always dangerous, even if these injuries are sporadic and rare. They rarely cause severe morbidity in the recipients because of modern antibiotic therapy. Before antibiotics were available, bacterial infection caused substantial morbidity and even death among health care workers. Surgeons draining abscesses and pathologists performing autopsies were most at risk. Currently, technicians in microbiology laboratories are probably at greatest risk for infection due to airborne particles and direct inoculation.[28]

Blood and other body fluids may harbor infection, which can be exchanged between patient and health care workers. Health care workers can be exposed to blood and other body fluids of patients percutaneously by punctures and cuts, from splashes to eyes and mucous membranes, and by direct exposure of skin. Patients can be exposed to blood of health care workers, usually those who perform invasive procedures, if a needle or other sharp instrument that has become contaminated with blood by a percutaneous injury to the operator is allowed to recontact the patient percutaneously. The most common place for this event to occur is when a surgeon accidentally punctures himself/herself with a suture needle that then recontacts the wound.

Any infectious agent in the blood can possibly be transmitted from patient to health care worker and from health care worker to patient. Several infections can be transmitted by blood transfusion[29,30] (Table 27–2). Only viral infections, however, have actually been transmitted from patient to health care worker and from health care worker to patient through blood. All donors of blood and blood products, and of tissue and organ grafts as well, in the United States are currently screened for evidence of HIV-1, hepatitis B virus, and hepatitis C virus and are excluded from donation if such evidence is found. Such screening greatly reduces but does not eliminate the risk of these viral infections being transmitted.[31,32] Patients and health care workers, however, are usually not screened for these infections.

HUMAN IMMUNODEFICIENCY VIRUS

Epidemiology

The CDC estimate that between 415,000 and 535,000 cases of acquired immunodeficiency syndrome (AIDS) will have been diagnosed in the United States through 1994[33] (see Chap. 11). Between 330,000 and 385,000 of these patients will have died. The CDC does not collect data on the number of individuals infected with HIV-1 but estimate that for every person with AIDS there are approximately eight individuals with HIV-1 infection who have not yet developed clinical AIDS. The CDC estimate there are approximately 1,000,000 infected with HIV-1 in the United States.[33,34] Approximately 14,000,000 people are believed to be infected with HIV-1 worldwide. The average time between HIV-1 infection and development of AIDS (from transfusion- acquired HIV-1 infection) is 7 years and the time between onset of AIDS and death is approximately 2 years.[35]

HIV-1 has been isolated from blood, semen, saliva, tears, vaginal secretions, alveolar fluid, cerebrospinal fluid, breast milk, synovial fluid, and amniotic fluid. Only blood and blood products, semen, vaginal secretions, and breast milk have been linked to transmission.[36]

Groups at highest risk for HIV-1 infection are (1) homosexual and bisexual men, (2) intravenous drug abusers, (3) persons with hemophilia or other coagulation disorders, (4) heterosexual contacts of the individuals in the three previous categories,

TABLE 27–2. TRANSFUSION-TRANSMITTED INFECTIONS

Infection	Comments
Viruses	
NANB (non-A, non-B hepatitis)	90% of transfusion-associated hepatitis, probably more than one agent, no specific test; mean incubation 7–8 weeks
HBC (hepatitis C virus)	Accounts for approximately 50% of NANB hepatitis; with approval of commercial test, more information will become available
HBV	Decreasing as cause of transfusion-associated hepatitis since HB_sAg testing (1972); mean incubation 11–12 weeks
HDV (delta agent)	Transfusion-associated HDV has occurred in multiply transfused individuals
HB_sAg-positive patients	HDV can only occur in HB_sAg-positive individuals
HAV (hepatitis A virus)	Only four cases reported
HIV-1 (human immunodeficiency virus)	Approximately 2500 cases reported, virtually all occurring before HIV-1 antibody testing of blood (1985)
CMV (cytomegalovirus)	Heterophile negative (postperfusion syndrome)
EBV (Epstein-Barr virus)	Mononucleosis, postperfusion syndrome
HTLV-1	Human T cell leukemia virus
Parasites	
Plasmodium (malaria)	Rare in the United States
Toxoplasma gondii	Toxoplasmosis has occurred after granulocyte transfusion
Babesia microti	Nantucket fever (hemolytic anemia, renal failure), usually asymptomatic; transmitted by blood donors in northeastern United States who have become infected by deer ticks
Trypanosoma cruzi	Chagas' disease (American trypanosomiasis) is spread by transfusion in Central and South America; can remain infective in refrigerated blood for 3 weeks
Filaria	Microfilariae can survive in refrigerated citrated blood for at least 14 days; *Wuchereria bancrofti* and *Acanthocheilonema perstans* (tropical Africa and Latin America), *Mansonella ozzardi* (Latin America), *Loa* (Africa), and *Brugia malayi* (Southeast Asia) can be transmitted by blood transfusion from donors from these regions
Spirochetes	
Treponema pallidum	Killed by storage of blood at 4C; syphilis tests routine on donor blood
Bacteria	
General	Contamination from improperly sterilized equipment, technique errors in drawing or infusing blood; cool growing organisms can be a problem
Pseudomonas cepacia	Contamination in thawing or pooling blood components

From Polesky HF: Transfusion-transmitted infections. In Howard RJ (ed): Infectious Risks in Surgery. Norwalk, CT, Appleton & Lange, 1991, p 1.

and (5) children born to HIV-1-positive mothers. Recipients of transfusions of blood and blood products from HIV-1-positive donors have approximately a 95 percent chance of developing HIV-1 infection and over 5000 cases of transfusion-acquired AIDS have been reported to the CDC.[37] This number could eventually reach 12,000 due to HIV-1-positive transfusion recipients who are thought to exist but who have not yet developed AIDS.[38] Since testing of blood donors for evidence of HIV-1 became mandatory in 1985, new cases of transfusion-acquired HIV-1 infection have virtually been eliminated.

HIV-1 seroprevalence among different populations varies greatly depending on the specific population studied, the location of the population, sex, race and ethnic origin, and year of study.[34] The lowest HIV-1 seropositive rates are found among blood donors (0.0041 percent for repeat female donors, 0.0189 percent for repeat male donors) and are highest among hemophiliacs (50 to 100 percent positive), intravenous drug users (20 to 60 percent positive), and homosexual and bisexual men (30 to 60 percent positive).[34]

Relatively few seroprevalence studies have been done among hospital or emergency room patients[39–55] (Table 27–3). One can expect that type of hospital, location, and specific hospital population will greatly affect HIV-1-seropositivity rates. According to a sentinel hospital study of 195,829 blood specimens from hospitalized patients conducted by the CDC, the overall seropositivity was 4.7 percent, but the HIV-1-seropositive rate of individual hospitals ranged from 0.2 to 14.2 percent.[43] Hospitals in the Northeast had a higher seropositive rate than hospitals in other parts of the United States.

TABLE 27–3. HIV-1 SEROPREVALENCE IN PATIENT POPULATIONS

Population	Location	Year	Number Tested	Number of HIV-1 Positive	Percentage	Reference
Hospital patients	Harborview Medical Center, Seattle, WA	1987	506	15	3.0	39
Hospital patients	St. Paul-Ramsey Medical Center, St. Paul, MN	1985–1986	275	25	9.1	40
Hospital patients	Sentinel Hospitals	1986–1988	26,275	—	0.24	41
Hospital patients	Sentinel Hospitals United States	1988–1989	89,547	—	1.3	42
Hospital patients	Sentinel Hospitals	1989–1991	195,829	9286	4.7	43
Hospital patients	Veterans Administration Hospital, Washington, DC	1987	616	23	3.7	44
Hospital patients	Lubbock, TX	1988–1989	2458	12	0.5	45
Emergency room patients	Johns Hopkins Hospital Emergency Department, Baltimore, MD	1987	126	9	7.1	46
Emergency room patients	Johns Hopkins Hospital Emergency Department, Baltimore, MD	1986	203	6	3.0	47
Emergency room patients	Johns Hopkins Hospital Emergency Department, Baltimore, MD	1988	2544	152	6.0	48
Emergency room patients	Johns Hopkins Hospital Emergency Department, Baltimore, MD	1986	2302	119	5.2	49
Acutely injured patients	Peoria, IL	1987	262	1	0.4	50
Burn patients	Miami, FL	1987	90	2	2.2	51
Acutely injured patients	San Antonio, TX	1988–1989	146	0	0	52
Surgery patients	Baltimore, MD	1988–1989	4087	18	0.4	53
Surgery patients	Strasbourg, France	1989–1991	4119	3	0.07	54
Surgery patients	Sydney, Australia	1990	1171	30	2.6	55

HIV-1 and AIDS in Health Care Workers

More than 7000 health care workers with AIDS have been reported to the CDC. There may be more than 50,000 health care workers infected with HIV-1 based on an estimate of eight persons infected with HIV-1 for every patient with AIDS.

Health care workers with AIDS comprise approximately 5 percent of the total number of patients with AIDS in the United States.[56] Approximately 5.7 percent of the labor force in the United States is comprised of health care workers. Most health care workers with AIDS are homosexual or bisexual men[57] (Table 27–4). Significantly fewer, however, are intravenous drug abusers. A large "undetermined" category accounts for 5.9 percent of health care workers with AIDS. On further examination, one-half of these patients can be classified under one of the risk factors, one-fourth are dead or refused to be interviewed, and the remaining one-fourth are still being investigated.

More than 100 health care workers have developed HIV-1 infection as a result of exposure to blood from HIV-1-infected patients. One-third of the health care workers had the patient-acquired infection confirmed by being seronegative at the time of exposure and becoming seropositive after exposure. Two-thirds did not have a blood specimen obtained at the time of exposure, but other risk factors were excluded. Two of these health care workers are surgeons. Not all health care workers with occupationally acquired HIV-1 infection may be included in the CDC data set, however.[58,59]

HIV-1 Seroprevalence Studies of Health Care Workers. Several studies have reported HIV-1 seroprevalence among health care workers[60–78] (Table 27–5). The low seroprevalence rates, especially among those who did not have community risk factors, attest to the low risk for HIV-1 transmission in the health care setting.

TABLE 27–4. COMPARISON OF HEALTH CARE WORKERS AND NON-HEALTH CARE WORKERS WITH AIDS BY TRANSMISSION CATEGORY

Transmission Category	Health Care Workers (%)	Non-Health Care Workers (%)
Male homosexual/bisexual contact	71.8	61.1[a]
Heterosexual intravenous drug user	6.6	21.1[a]
Male homosexual/bisexual contact and intravenous drug user	7.4	7.0
Heterosexual contact	5.3	4.5
Recipient of blood/blood product	3.0	3.3
Other	<1.0	0.0
Undetermined	5.9	2.9[a]

[a] $P < 0.001$.

Adapted from Panlilio AL, Bell DM: HIV infection in health care workers: assessment of risk. In Howard RJ (ed): Infectious Risks in Surgery. Norwalk, CT, Appleton & Lange, 1991, pp 65–81.

Risk of HIV-1 Seroconversion in Health Care Workers. Surgeons and other health care workers are naturally concerned about their risk of acquiring HIV-1 and other blood-borne infections from their exposure to patients' blood and other body fluids. Both theoretical estimates and prospective surveillance studies are available to enable health care workers to assess this risk.

Wormser et al[79] estimated the probability of HIV seroconversion based on the total number of hospital days for HIV-infected patients and on the expected number of needle-stick injuries. They estimated that there was a 50 percent chance at least one health care worker would seroconvert for every 105,000 HIV-infected patient days during which time there would be 200 needle-stick injuries. The probability would increase to 95 percent for 440,000 HIV-infected patient days when 836 needle-stick injuries could be expected to occur. Hagen et al[80] arrived at a risk to the surgeon of acquiring HIV infection from operating on an HIV-infected patient to be between 1/130,000 and 1/4500. Since the percentage of HIV-infected patients in most hospitals is likely to be less than 1 percent, the risk of operating on a patient whose HIV status is unknown is 1/100 of the previous numbers. Howard[81] calculated the risk of seroconversion based on the number of needle-stick injuries, HIV seropositivity of patient population, and the risk of seroconversion if a surgeon sustains a percutaneous injury with a needle or instrument contaminated with HIV-infected blood. If a surgeon operates on patients with a 1 percent HIV-seroprevalence rate and sustains

TABLE 27–5. HIV-SEROPREVALENCE STUDIES AMONG HEALTH CARE WORKERS

Country	Year of Report	Occupation	Number Tested	Number Positive	Positive (%)	Reference
United States	1985	Hospital workers	85	0	0	71
United States	1985	Hospital workers	359	8	2.2	7
United States	1985	Hospital workers	188	0	0	72
United Kingdom	1985		151	1	0.66	73
Denmark	1986	Dental personnel	961	0	0	74
Denmark	1986	Dental professionals, household contact of HIV-1	10	0	0	75
Denmark	1986	Infected persons	325	0	0	76
Denmark	1986	Nurses	45	0	0	77
Canada	1986	Hospital workers	1590	2	0.13	78
Zaire	1986	Hospital workers	2492	152	6.4	79
United States	1987	Hospital workers	270	0	0	80
United States	1987	Dentists, hygienists, assistants	266	0	0	81
United States	1987	Dentists, paradental employees	255	0	0	82
United States	1988	Dental professionals	1309	1	0.08	83
Zaire	1988	Hospital workers	2193	191	8.7	84
United States	1988	Hospital workers	860	4	0.47	85
United States	1988	Lab workers	265	1	0.38	86
United States	1990	Hospital workers	1344	7	0.52	68
United States	1991	Orthopedic surgery	3420	2	0.6	87

TABLE 27–6. PROSPECTIVE SURVEILLANCE STUDIES OF THE RISK OF HIV-1 INFECTION IN HEALTH CARE WORKERS FOLLOWING PERCUTANEOUS EXPOSURE TO BLOOD AND BLOOD-CONTAINING BODY FLUIDS

Country	Year of Report	Number of Exposures	Number of Health Care Workers	Seroconversion	Seroconversion Rate (% per exposure)	Reference
United States	1987	129	168	0	0	71
United States	1987	10	48	0	0	82
United Kingdom	1987	76	76	0	0	83
Canada	1987	165	165	0	0	84
United States	1988	31	53	1	3.2	85
Spain	1988	58	58	0	0	86
Italy	1988	77	77	0	0	87
United States	1988	860	860	3	0.35	60
Italy	1989	97	97	0	0	89
Italy	1989	63	63	0	0	90
Norway	1989	183	183	0	0	91
Sweden	1989	40	40	0	0	92
United States	1990	179	159	1	0.56	61
Total		1968	1879	5	0.25	

250 needle-stick injuries during a surgical career, he/she has a 1.24 percent lifetime chance of becoming infected with HIV.

Fourteen prospective studies have examined the actual risk of health care workers becoming infected with HIV-1 after sustaining a percutaneous exposure to blood or blood-containing body fluids from patients with HIV-1 infection[60,61,71,82–92] (Table 27–6). Six (0.29 percent) of 1948 health care workers who sustained 2042 percutaneous exposures seroconverted to HIV-1.

On the other hand, none of 668 health care workers in 12 reports, who sustained a total of 1051 mucous membrane exposures to blood or blood-containing body fluids from HIV-1-infected patients, seroconverted[60,61,71,82–85,88–92] (Table 27–7).

Exposure of Surgeons to Blood. Surgeons are frequently exposed to patient's blood and other body fluids, but until recently there were no studies documenting the actual risk of blood exposure to operating room personnel[23,24,26,27,92–95] (Table 27–8). Most exposures are to the skin and can be decreased by wearing two pairs of gloves and face shields.[23,25] The percutaneous injury rate from sur-

TABLE 27–7. PROSPECTIVE SURVEILLANCE STUDIES OF THE RISK OF HIV-1 INFECTION IN HEALTH CARE WORKERS FOLLOWING MUCOUS MEMBRANE EXPOSURE TO BLOOD AND BLOOD-CONTAINING BODY FLUIDS

Country	Year of Report	Number of Exposures	Number of Health Care Workers	Seroconversions	Seroconversion Rate (% per exposure)	Reference
United States	1987	213	55	0	0	71
United States	1987	15	15	0	0	82
United Kingdom	1987	24	24	0	0	83
Canada	1987	28	28	0	0	84
United States	1988	27	27	0	0	60
Italy	1989	7	7	0	0	89
Italy	1989	20	20	0	0	90
Norway	1989	72	72	0	0	91
Sweden	1989	15	15	0	0	92
United States	1990	346	243	0	0	61
Total		767	506	0	0	

Adapted from Henderson DK, Fahey BJ, Willy M, et al: Ann Intern Med 113:740, 1990.

TABLE 27–8. EXPOSURE TO PATIENTS' BLOOD DURING SURGICAL PROCEDURES

Location	Year of Report	Number of Operations	Operations with Blood Contact to OR Personnel	Number of OR Personnel with Blood Contact	Total Exposures	Parenteral	Skin	Eye Splash or Mucous Membrane	Reference
Albuquerque, NM[a]	1991	684	190	293	NS	21	NS	NS	26
Atlanta, GA[b]	1991	206	62	96	147	10	133	4	23
San Francisco, CA[c]	1990	1307	84	NS	117	18	95	4	25
London, UK[d]	1989	427 (123 open, 304 endoscopic procedures)	136	NS	139	15	93	31	92
Milwaukee, WI	1991	234	118	194	NS	NS	118	NS	95
United States	1992	1382	NS	95	95	95	NS	NS	27

[a] Risk factors: cardiothoracic, trauma, cesarean section procedures, increased operating time.
[b] Risk factors: trauma, burn, orthopedic emergency surgery, blood loss >250 ml, operation >1 hour.
[c] Risk factors: operating > 3 hours, blood loss > 300 ml.
[d] Risk factors: all urologic operations, all parenteral exposures occurred during open procedures.
NS, not stated.

vey studies is also high with injuries occurring in 5.6 percent of operations and 86 percent of surgeons reporting one percutaneous injury per year.[22,93]

None of these studies attempted to assess the risk of transmission of HIV-1 or hepatitis or the amount of blood transferred to operating room personnel during percutaneous injury. Most percutaneous injuries to operating room personnel are due to solid suture needles. Number 22 and 19 phlebotomy needles result in an inoculation of 1.4 and 2.1 μl of blood, respectively, when a puncture is simulated.[96,97] A solid suture needle inoculates 1.4 μl of blood when inserted to a depth of 0.5 cm and only 0.4 μl when it is first passed through a latex glove.[98]

HEPATITIS B VIRUS

Hepatitis B virus is a hepadnavirus (hepatitis DNA virus). The complete virion has a diameter of 42 nm. The double-stranded DNA-containing core particle is surrounded by the lipoprotein surface antigen (HB_sAg, formerly called Australia antigen). The e antigen is a breakdown product of the core particle; in blood it indicates infectivity. HB_sAg is not a marker for the complete virus. Antibody to the core particle (anti-HB_c or HB_cAb) is present in all patients with current or past infections. Antibody to HB_sAg (anti-HB_s or HB_sAb) indicates immunity to HBV as a result of vaccination or past infection.

In contrast to HIV-1 infection, in which 10^2 to 10^4 virus particles/ml are found in the blood of patients with AIDS and even fewer in patients with HIV-1 infection without AIDS,[99] up to 10^{12} to 10^{14} HB_sAg particles/ml of blood are found in patients with HBV infection.[100] Sera from non-A, non-B hepatitis infected animals contain up to 10^6 infection units per milliliter.[101] This greater virus load with HBV makes it more likely that one will become infected following needle-stick injury. Whereas the risk of infection following needle-stick exposure to HIV-1 is approximately 0.3 percent (see Table 27–6), 10 to 20 percent of individuals develop HBV infection following needle-stick injury contaminated with HB_sAg-positive blood if the source is also HB_eAg-positive.[102,103] If the source is HB_eAg-negative, the risk of HBV infection after needle-stick injury is approximately 5 percent.

Epidemiology

The global impact of HBV infection is enormous. It is estimated that 200 million people worldwide, 5 percent of the earth's population, are chronically infected with HBV.[104] Twenty percent of the adult population in Sub-Sahara Africa and the Far East are chronically infected with HBV.[105] It is estimated that as many as 25 percent of these chronically infected individuals may die of cirrhosis or hepatocellular carcinoma.[105]

Approximately 0.1 percent of the adult population in North America and western Europe has chronic HBV infection.[103] The prevalence of chronic HBV infection in the United States is approximately 0.5 percent, suggesting more than 1 million Americans are chronic carriers.[106] Approximately 3 to 5 percent of the general population in the United States and blood donors have antibody to HB_sAg, however, indicating previous infection.[107,108] These chronic carriers form a reservoir that results in persistence of HBV infection and from which an estimated 300,000 new cases of HBV occur yearly in the United States.[100]

HBV was formerly thought to be transferred solely by percutaneous inoculation, hence the former name "serum hepatitis." Currently, only 5 percent of cases of hepatitis B occur following penetration of the skin by contaminated instruments or from other blood exposure. The majority of cases are transmitted sexually or by neonatal exposure.

HBV is transmitted mainly by (1) percutaneous inoculation of blood, blood products, or other body fluids; (2) sexual intimacy; and (3) perinatal transmission from an HB_sAg-positive mother to her offspring. This last mode of transmission accounts for spread in Sub-Sahara Africa and the Far East and is the most important on a global level. These individuals who acquire chronic HBV infection as neonates or infants have the greatest relative risk for hepatocellular carcinoma, greater than 200 : 1.[109]

Surgeons and other health care workers are most concerned about percutaneous transmission because that is the method by which both they and their patients are most likely to acquire hepatitis B. HB_sAg can be found in all current blood and blood products except albumin and immune globulins (the virus is destroyed by the alcohol used in Cohn fractionation) and plasmanate (the virus is inactivated by radiation). It can also be found in saliva, tears, sweat, semen, vaginal secretions, breast milk, cerebrospinal fluid, ascites, pleural fluid, synovial fluid, gastric juice, urine, and, rarely, feces of HB_sAg-positive persons.[105] But saliva and semen are the only body fluids other than blood and blood products that have been shown to contain infectious HBV by experimental transmission studies.[110,111] Nevertheless, *all* body fluids from HB_sAg-positive persons should be regarded as being infectious.

A survey of 6216 adult hospital patients revealed an HB_sAg carriage rate of 0.9 percent.[112] It was 1.2 percent among 1656 surgical patients. Only 17 percent of the HB_sAg-positive patients, however, were admitted with a diagnosis of hepatitis or had an order for determination of HB_sAg status.

Hepatitis from Blood Transfusions

Several viruses can cause transfusion-associated hepatitis, and hepatitis B is not the most common. Hepatitis B transmission from blood transfusions has greatly decreased since 1972, when testing of blood for evidence of HB_sAg became mandatory. It is currently estimated that 85 to 95 percent of post-transfusion hepatitis in the United States is due to non-A, non-B hepatitis.[113] Testing blood for antibody to hepatitis C, available since 1990, and alanine aminotransferase concentrations as a surrogate test for non-A, non-B hepatitis may further reduce the risk of this type of post-transfusion hepatitis.

Studies done before these tests were required suggested 10 percent of blood recipients developed hepatitis.[114] More recent studies, however, suggest it occurs in less than 1 to 2 percent of recipients.[115] It is difficult to determine the precise incidence of transfusion-associated hepatitis in the United States, however, because of incomplete reporting and because only one-third to one-half of persons with non-A, non-B hepatitis have clinical disease. Nevertheless, with approximately 3,000,000 patients being transfused with 12,000,000 blood component units yearly and with 5 to 10 percent of blood recipients developing non-A, non-B hepatitis, one could expect 150,000 to 300,000 cases of non-A, non-B hepatitis as a result of blood transfusion.[116,117] The reported transfusion-associated non-A, non-B hepatitis, however, occurs in only 7500 to 15,000 patients per year. Approximately half of all infected individuals acquired chronic liver disease.

Transfusion-associated hepatitis can vary by location. In the prospective transfusion-transmitted virus study, the incidence of transfusion associated hepatitis was 4.7 percent (91 percent non-A, non-B hepatitis) in St. Louis and 19.5 percent (89 percent non-A, non-B hepatitis) in Houston.[116,118] In Minneapolis the incidence of transfusion-associated hepatitis was 0.2 to 0.47 cases per 1000 patients and 66 percent were caused by hepatitis C.[116] Hepatitis C causes almost all cases of transfusion-associated non-A, non-B hepatitis.[101,104,105] As better tests for hepatitis C are developed, the risk of transfusion-associated transmission will be reduced further.[116,119,120] Hepatitis D (the delta agent) can also be transmitted by transfusion and rare cases of hepatitis A have been transmitted by this route when the donor was incubating the disease.

Epidemiology of Hepatitis B in Health Care Workers and Patients

Every year 12,000 health care workers whose jobs entail exposure to blood become infected with HBV.[116] As a result of that infection 500 to 600 are

TABLE 27–9. PREVALENCE OF HEPATITIS B SEROLOGIC MARKERS IN VARIOUS POPULATION GROUPS

Population Group	Prevalence of Serologic Markers of HBV Infection	
	HB_sAg (%)	All Markers (%)
High risk		
Immigrants/refugees from areas of high HBV endemicity	13	70–85
Clients of institutions for the mentally retarded	10–20	35–80
Users of illicit parenteral drugs	7	60–80
Homosexually active men	6	35–80
Household contacts of HBV carriers	3–6	30–60
Patients of hemodialysis units	3–10	20–80
Intermediate risk		
Health care workers with frequent blood contacts	1–2	15–30
Prisoners (male)	1–8	10–80
Staff of institutions for the mentally retarded	1	10–25
Low risk		
Health care workers with no or infrequent blood contacts	0.3	3–10
Healthy adults (first-time volunteer blood donors)	0.3	3–5

From Centers for Disease Control: Morb Mortal Wkly Rep 34:313, 1985.

hospitalized, and 700 to 1200 of those infected become chronic carriers. Approximately 250 of infected health care workers die each year, 12 to 15 from fulminant hepatitis, 170 to 200 from cirrhosis, and 40 to 50 from liver cancer. Hepatitis in health care workers has decreased during the past 20 years[121,122]; these data are based on CDC estimates for 1987 and should be updated for the 1990s. The incidence of hepatitis B among health care workers is likely decreasing because of wider use of hepatitis B vaccine, increased use of universal precautions, and increased reporting of exposure incidents with subsequent greater use of hepatitis B vaccine and immune globulin. Whereas 85 to 95 percent of transfusion-associated hepatitis is due to non-A, non-B hepatitis, 80 percent of hepatitis acquired by health care workers is due to hepatitis B and 20 percent is caused by non-A, non-B hepatitis.

Most studies have measured the prevalence of past HBV infection by determining the prevalence of serologic markers in populations[108] (Table 27–9). The prevalence of HBV serologic markers in surgeons and other health care workers depends on variables other than the number of HB_sAg-positive patients encountered. Other factors that affect the prevalence of HBV serologic markers include specific job category, frequency of exposure to blood and other body fluids, and years in practice.[107] The prevalence of hepatitis B serologic markers is higher in hospital personnel in the emergency department (27.9 percent) and operating room (25.2 percent) than in the hemodialysis unit (17.2 percent) or intensive care units (12.7 percent).[123] HBV-seroprevalence markers in community hospital personnel are unrelated to section of the United States, size of hospital or community, or whether the hospital was rural or suburban.[124]

Prevalence and incidence studies of HBV serologic markers (HB_sAg or anti-HB_s) in hospital personnel and physicians were reported in the late 1970s and early 1980s[92,125–143] (Tables 27–10 and 27–11). Incidence studies among health care personnel have shown a range of 3.2 to 32.0 events per 1000 person-years for clinical laboratory personnel and 11.3 to 105.8 events per 1000 person-years for dialysis personnel.[131–138] For physicians (surgeons were not studied separately) the incidence of hepatitis B has ranged from 2.5 to 23 events per 1000 person-years.[133,134,136,139]

TABLE 27–10. PREVALENCE OF HB_sAg AND ANTI-HB_s IN VARIOUS GROUPS OF HEALTH PERSONNEL

Profession	Year of Report	Number Tested	Percentage with HBV Markers	Reference
Administration Hospital	1982	32	16.0	107
Dietician	1982	19	5.0	107
Housekeeper	1975	56	13.0	125
Nurse–LPN	1975	41	22.0	125
Nurse–RN	1975	77	12.0	125
Nurse				
Emergency ward	1982	30	30.0	104
Intravenous	1982	68	22.0	104
Intensive care	1982	94	10.0	104
General duty	1982	68	5.0	104
Hospital health care workers	1977–1982	837	14	126

TABLE 27–11. PREVALENCE OF HB_sAg AND ANTI-HB_s AMONG PHYSICIANS

Profession	Year of Report	No. Tested	% With HBV Markers	Reference
Physician (hospital)	1975	52	12.0	125
Physician (hospital)	1978	80	10.0	127
Physician (Dialysis Unit)	1979	37	35.1	128
Physician	1978	176	28.4	129
Surgery				
Pathology	1978	37	27.0	129
Pediatrics	1978	63	20.6	129
Internal Medicine	1978	259	17.8	129
Anesthesiology	1978	59	16.9	129
Ob-Gyn	1978	63	15.9	129
Family Practice	1978	341	15.8	129
Non-patient care	1978	25	4.0	129
Others	1978	169	15.4	129
All		1192	18.5	138–141
Dentists	1975–1981	2723	13.6–26.5	122–125
Hospital physicians	1992	231	6.1	142

These data are old. Newer data on the prevalence of HBV serologic markers that reflect past HBV infection are not available. These data would be difficult to evaluate anyway, since HBV vaccination renders the recipient positive for anti-HB_s. Extrapolating from the data, available in 1984, Lemmer[144] estimated the risk of infection from hepatitis (acute symptomatic or subclinical) during a surgical career to be 30 to 40 percent. The probability of a surgeon becoming a chronic carrier during 40 years of practice is 4 percent. The decreasing prevalence of hepatitis B among hospital personnel (including surgeons) and the availability of an effective hepatitis B vaccine probably have lowered this risk.

HEPATITIS C (NON-A, NON-B HEPATITIS)

Hepatitis virus(es) that was neither hepatitis A nor hepatitis B (non-A, non-B) was hypothesized in the early 1970s when many cases of hepatitis, especially post-transfusion hepatitis, could not be accounted for by hepatitis A or hepatitis B viruses. It was not until 1988 that the hepatitis C virus, which accounts for 90 to 95 percent of cases of post-transfusion non-A, non-B hepatitis, was identified.[116,119,120,145] Hepatitis C virus (HCV) is an RNA virus and has structural and genomic similarities to the flaviviruses or pestiviruses.[145] It can be transmitted by transfusion of blood or blood products (eg, factor VIII, factor IX, platelets, fibrinogen, washed red blood cells, fresh frozen plasma) but, like hepatitis B, not by albumin, gamma globulin, or plasmanate.

The CDC estimates that approximately 150,000 non-A, non-B hepatitis infections occur annually and only 7500 to 15,000 are due to transfusions.[146] Of those infected, half may develop biochemical evidence of chronic liver disease or cirrhosis.

A serologic test for antibody to HCV has been available since the spring of 1990, and since that time all transfused blood has been screened for this virus. The test has a high number of false-positives (up to 50 percent) and false-negatives (up to 30 percent).[147] Antibody to HCV is not detected until an average of 21.9 weeks (range, 10 to 39 weeks) after transfusion or 15 weeks (range, 4 to 32 weeks) after the onset of clinical hepatitis.[148] It is not clear whether antibody is protective. At least some blood donors with anti-HCV antibody can transmit hepatitis.[149]

Recently, a second-generation test has been approved by the Food and Drug Administration that is more sensitive and more specific than first-generation tests that measured antibody to the HCV protein antigen, C-100. The second-generation tests measure antibodies to additional HCV antigens as well as the C-100 antigen. The new assays identify HCV as the etiologic agent in approximately 20 to 30 percent more cases of non-A, non-B hepatitis than are identified by first-generation assays. Second-generation tests also identify HCV in the circulation 1 to 3 months earlier than first-generation tests. Circulating HCV RNA can be detected by the polymerase chain reaction, but this technology remains primarily a research tool. Seroprevalence studies using second-generation tests usually find a higher prevalence of HCV in most groups than do first-generation tests. Several seroprevalence studies of anti-HCV antibodies in different populations have now been published[150–153] (Table 27–12).

Health care workers, in general, do not have much higher prevalence rates than blood donors. Furthermore, health care workers who are at high risk for blood exposure have anti-HCV antibody seroprevalence rates similar to health care workers who are not commonly exposed to blood.

Transmission of HCV Between Patients and Health Care Workers

There are many individual case reports of parenteral transmission of HCV from patients to health care workers.[156–160] The only large study of needlestick transmission of HCV from HCV-positive source patients to exposed health care workers showed that the rate of HCV transmission was low.[156] Of 110 health care workers exposed to blood from patients infected with HCV, only four (3.6 percent) developed hepatitis and only three (2.7 percent) seroconverted to HCV. One other study followed 98 HCV-seronegative health care workers who had experienced parenteral exposure to blood of HIV-infected patients. Sixty-four of the 98 health care workers were exposed to blood of HIV-infected intravenous drug users, a group with an HCV-seroprevalence rate in excess of 50 percent. No seroconversions to HCV were observed during an average follow-up of 17.6 months.

Even though the risk of transmission of HCV is low, somewhere between that of HIV and hepatitis B, it is a dangerous virus and should be taken seriously. Approximately 50 percent of individuals who are infected by blood transfusions or who acquire infection in the community setting become HCV carriers. A significant proportion of HCV carriers develop chronic liver disease with the attendant long-term risk of cirrhosis and primary hepatocellular carcinoma.

PREVENTION OF BLOOD-BORNE INFECTIONS IN HEALTH CARE WORKERS

The AIDS epidemic brought into focus a problem that has always existed, that health care workers could become infected with disease harbored by

TABLE 27–12. ANTI-HCV ANTIBODY SEROPREVALENCE IN VARIOUS POPULATIONS

Population	Anti-HCV Antibody Seroprevalence (%)	Reference
Chronic non-A, non-B hepatitis after transfusion	85–95	150
Sporadic non-A, non-B hepatitis without obvious transmission	54–72	
Intravenous drug abusers	50–90	150
Hemophiliacs	60–83	153
Homosexual males	8–18	150, 151
Military recruits	0.3	
Blood donors	0.5–1.5	150, 154
Elderly, long-term care facility residents	1.4	
Dialysis patients	3–51	
Emergency room patients (Baltimore, MD)	18	
Cardiac surgery patients (Baltimore, MD)		
Preoperatively	2.4	151
8–12 months postoperatively	3.9	
Hospital patients (Toronto, Canada)	0.5	
Health care workers	1.1–2.2	
Health care workers with high risk of blood exposure	1.6	152
Health care workers, high-risk ER and OR staff	1.0	
Dentists (New York City)	1.75	153
Oral surgeons	9.3	
Other dentists	0.97	
Health care workers (Vienna, Austria)	2	
Physicians	4.3	155

their patients. The CDC and several other authorities have published recommendations for infection control precautions in caring for AIDS patients.[26,88,116,161–172] While there were naturally some differences in approach, the recommendations were designed to minimize the exposure of health care workers to blood and other body fluids of patients. The motivation for some of these proposals came from the desire of some health care workers to test patients for HIV, a very controversial subject (see below).

Universal Precautions

In August 1987, the CDC issued new guidelines, which have come to be called "Universal Precautions," designed to minimize the risk of transmission of HIV in the health care setting.[36] These guidelines have been updated and extended but not substantially altered[116,172] (Table 27–13). They are applicable to clinical and laboratory staffs, workers in health care settings, emergency service personnel, and health care workers performing invasive procedures as well as those who are not included in direct patient care (eg, housekeeping personnel, kitchen staff, laundry workers).[36,116,172] Although universal precautions were issued to reduce the transmission of HIV in health care settings, they are also appropriate for reducing the transmission of other blood-borne viruses including HBV, non-A, non-B hepatitis, and HCV. The Office of Safety and Health Administration (OSHA) has made the CDC (which have no regulatory authority) guidelines mandatory.

The intent of the CDC guidelines is that *all* patients should be regarded as potentially harboring blood-borne pathogens, because the medical his-

TABLE 27–13. GUIDELINES TO PREVENT TRANSMISSION OF HIV

Universal Precautions

1. All health care workers should use appropriate barrier precautions routinely to prevent skin and mucous membrane exposure when contact with blood or other body fluids of any patient is anticipated. Gloves should be worn for touching blood and body fluids, mucous membranes, or nonintact skin of all patients; for handling items or surfaces soiled with blood or body fluids; and for performing venipuncture and other vascular-access procedures. Gloves should be changed after contact with each patient. During procedures that are likely to generate aerosolized droplets of blood or other body fluids, masks and protective eyewear or face shields should be worn to prevent exposure of mucous membranes of the mouth, nose, and eyes. Gowns or aprons should be worn during procedures that are likely to generate splashes of blood or other body fluids.
2. Hands and other skin surfaces should be washed immediately and thoroughly if contaminated with blood or other body fluids. Hands should be washed immediately and thoroughly if contaminated with blood or other body fluids. Hands should be washed immediately after gloves are removed.
3. All health care workers should take precautions to prevent injuries caused by needles, scalpels, and other sharp instruments or devices during procedures; when cleaning used instruments; during disposal of used needles; and when handling sharp instruments after procedures. To prevent needle-stick injuries, needles should not be recapped, purposely bent or broken by hand, removed from disposable syringes, or otherwise manipulated by hand. After they are used, disposable syringes and needles, scalpel blades, and other sharp items should be placed in puncture-resistant containers for disposal; the puncture-resistant containers should be located as close as practical to the area of use. Large-bore reusable needles should be placed in a puncture-resistant container for transport to the reprocessing area.
4. Although saliva has not been implicated in HIV transmission, to minimize the need for emergency mouth-to-mouth resuscitation, mouth-pieces, resuscitation bags, or other ventilation devices should be available for use in areas in which the need for resuscitation is predictable.
5. Health care workers who have exudative lesions or weeping dermatitis should refrain from all direct patient care and from handling patient care equipment until condition resolves.
6. Pregnant health care workers are not known to be at greater risk for contracting HIV infection than health care workers who are not pregnant; however, if a health care worker acquires HIV infection during pregnancy, the infant is at risk for infection resulting from perinatal transmission. Because of this risk, pregnant health care workers should be especially familiar with and strictly adhere to precautions to minimize the risk of HIV transmission.

Additional Precautions for Invasive Procedures

1. All health care workers who participate in invasive procedures must use appropriate barrier precautions routinely to prevent skin and mucous membrane contact with blood and other body fluids of all patients. Gloves and surgical mask must be worn for all invasive procedures. Protective eyeware or face shields should be worn for procedures that commonly result in the generation of aerosolized droplets, splashing of blood or other body fluids, or the generation of bone chips. Gowns or aprons made of materials that provide an effective barrier should be worn during invasive procedures that are likely to result in the splashing of blood or other body fluids. All health care workers who perform or assist in vaginal or cesarean deliveries should wear gloves and gowns when handling the placenta or the infant until blood and amniotic fluid have been removed from the infant's skin and should wear gloves during postdelivery care of the umbilical cord.
2. If a glove is torn or a needle stick or other injury occurs, the glove should be removed and a new glove used as promptly as patient safety permits; the needle or instrument involved in the incident should also be removed from the sterile field.

From Centers for Disease Control: Morb Mortal Wkly Rep 36(2S):1S, 1987; 37:377, 1988; 38(S-6):1037, 1989.

tory, physical examination, and laboratory testing cannot identify all patients infected with HIV or other blood-borne pathogens and because in emergencies there may be no time for testing patients for various pathogens. Since all patients should be treated alike (as if they potentially have a transmissible blood-borne infection), there is no need for testing patients since it will not alter health care worker behavior.

Compliance with universal precautions has been examined in the emergency room and hospital environment.[173–176] Hammond et al[173] found that compliance with universal precautions was only 18 percent in a large inner city hospital emergency room and compliance fell to 5 percent if the patient was bleeding from an external injury. Courington et al[174] found the rates of noncompliance with universal precautions to be 74 percent on the surgical care unit. The noncompliance rate fell to 43 percent in the intensive care unit after an educational program about universal precautions but did not change on the surgical wards. On the other hand, Wong et al[176] found that frequency of barrier use increased from 54 percent to 73 percent on a medical service after universal precautions were put into effect. But 84 percent of teaching staff on medical services were observed not using universal precautions.[177]

There are several reasons why there has been resistance among some health care workers in putting universal precautions into effect. The risk is perceived by many as being low, the "it would never happen to me" attitude. Surgeons are frequently exposed to blood; so not following CDC guidelines is "doing what we have always done." A low priority is given to infection control practices in many hospitals and by many chiefs-of-staff, and physicians frequently do not want to take the extra time required to put on gloves, gowns, masks, and other barriers where appropriate. In the 1990s, we must adopt a new attitude: it is unacceptable not to use universal precautions. Universal precautions and the reasons for using them should be taught in medical school, and every responsible physician should insist they be strictly followed. We must not think of not using universal precautions any less than we would think of operating on a patient without cap, mask, gown, and gloves.

Testing Patients for Blood-Borne Pathogens

Ever since serologic testing for antibodies to HIV became available in 1985, there has been considerable heated discussion among physicians, medical ethicists, and lay groups about the effectiveness, ethics, and social consequences of testing patients.[166,178–186] Surgeons have generally favored patient testing, believing they could take special precautions with HIV-positive patients.[187–194] Some surgeons have developed special protocols for the operating room, believing universal precautions to be insufficient for that high-risk environment[187,188] (Table 27–14). Others[195] have argued against testing.[162] The reasons for and against testing patients for HIV or hepatitis are given in Table 27–15.

The CDC does not recommend routine HIV testing of all patients.[36,116,172] HIV testing of patients is recommended for management of health care workers who sustain parenteral or mucous membrane exposure to blood or other body fluids from a patient, for patient diagnosis and management, and for counseling associated with efforts to prevent and control HIV transmission in the community.[36,116]

If hospitals, physicians, or other health care agencies choose to perform HIV testing, the CDC advocates certain principles: (1) obtain patient consent for testing, (2) inform patients of results and provide counseling for seropositive patients, (3) ensure confidentiality, (4) ensure that seropositive patients will not receive compromised care, and (5) prospectively evaluate the efficacy of the program in reducing the incidence of exposure of health care workers to blood or other body fluids of patients who are infected with HIV. Most states have laws regulating testing of patients for HIV. Many of these laws require written informed consent of the patient with pretest and post-test counseling for both HIV-positive and HIV-negative patients.

Management of Health Care Workers Exposed to Patients' Blood and Other Body Fluids

The CDC[36,116,171,172] and others[88,161,196] have issued recommendations for the management of health care workers exposed to patients' blood and other body fluids. Hospitals, physicians' offices, and other employers of health care workers should establish a systematic approach for managing adverse exposures that is consistent with CDC and Department of Labor guidelines and state laws. The Department of Labor and CDC have published detailed employer responsibilities in protecting workers from acquisition of blood-borne diseases in the workplace.[36,116,163,172,197] Employers should develop standard operating procedures for all activities having the potential for exposure and should provide an initial and a periodic worker education program.

The CDC guidelines recommend that, if an exposure occurs, a blood sample should be drawn

TABLE 27–14. PROPOSED PROTOCOL FOR PATIENTS WITH BLOOD-BORNE INFECTIONS IN THE OPERATING ROOM

1. Only the minimum number of surgeons and nurses needed for an operation are allowed in the operating room; no observers are permitted.
2. Inexperienced persons—medical, nursing, and technical students—are barred from the operating room.
3. Pregnant persons also are barred because of the possibility of transmission to them of opportunistic infections.
4. Personnel with skin lesions or dermatitis are barred from the operating room.
5. No residents act as the operating surgeon unless thoroughly qualified to perform the indicated procedure; no resident teaching is done.
6. Preoperative discussion and notification of operating room personnel and pathologists of the diagnosis and operative plans are ensured.
7. Disposable scrub suits, gowns, drapes, and other barriers are used.
8. Rubber-soled canvas shoes that can be decontaminated with bleach are worn by all persons entering the operating room.
9. An impervious apron under the gown or a completely impervious gown is worn in trauma or ascites cases.
10. An intermediary "sharps" table is used. Only the surgeon and scrub nurse touch sharps. There is no direct passing of sharps, and assistants keep their hands clear when sharps are in the field.
11. Disposable knives are used in order to reduce risk to the scrub nurse from mounting blades.
12. Cautery and scissors rather than a sharp knife are used for incision and dissection.
13. Contaminated masks, gowns, and gloves are changed immediately, and any member of the team whose skin becomes contaminated rescrubs after thoroughly cleansing the area with antiseptic soap.
14. Hands and arms are washed after the operation, a shower is taken if other areas have been contaminated, and antiseptic soap is always used.
15. Instruments are cleaned and decontaminated and then autoclaved before being returned to central supply for reprocessing.
16. All disposables are bagged, labeled, and then autoclaved.
17. After completion of the operation, the operating room and permanent equipment are cleaned and decontaminated with dilute (1:10) chlorine bleach solution.

From Centers for Disease Control: Morb Mortal Wkly Rep 35:376, 1986.

TABLE 27–15. ARGUMENTS FOR AND AGAINST TESTING OF PATIENTS FOR BLOOD-BORNE PATHOGENS, ESPECIALLY HIV-1

For Testing	Against Testing
1. Physicians have a right to know of infections their patients may have.	1. Confidentiality of test results cannot be maintained.
2. Knowing will allow physicians to take proper precautions.	2. Informed consent is unlikely to be obtained.
3. Valuable epidemiologic data can be collected.	3. Psychological and social consequences of being found to be seropositive can be devastating.
4. Treatment of infected patients can be instituted.	4. Insurance may be impossible to obtain for seropositive patients.
5. Others at risk (eg, sexual partners, needle sharers) can be warned or appropriate precautions can be taken.	5. A seronegative result does not assure the physician the patient cannot transmit disease because it takes from 2 weeks to 6 months, and even longer in some cases, to develop HIV-1 antibodies.
6. Universal precautions and additional appropriate precautions—especially in the operating room—are too cumbersome and are impractical to be taken for every patient. Knowing who harbors disease would allow intense, focused precautions to be taken for individuals most at risk of spreading infections.	6. There are some false-positive and false-negative tests for HIV-1.
7. While universal precautions are to be taken for all patients, additional precautions are taken for patients known to be HIV-1, HB_sAg, or HCV positive.	7. Seropositive patients will likely be denied medical and dental care.
8. No matter how much a surgeon says only universal precautions alone are sufficient, his/her behavior is likely to be different when operating on seropositive patients (ie, the surgeon is likely to take additional care, move more slowly and deliberately).	8. For low prevalence populations the cost of screening and confirmatory tests is great for every positive test result.
9. HIV-1 testing is currently so reliable that false-positive tests are extremely unlikely.	9. If the health care worker adheres to universal precautions, there is no need for testing because it will not change behavior.
	10. At least one has shown that knowing a person is seropositive does not affect the rate of percutaneous blood exposure.
	11. A false sense of security may be instilled in caring for seronegative patients who may still transmit HIV-1 and other blood-borne pathogens.

after consent is obtained from the individual from whom the exposure occurred and tested for Hb_sAg and antibody to HIV.[116] Local laws regarding consent for testing source individuals should be followed. Policies should be available for testing source individuals when consent cannot be obtained (eg, an unconscious patient). Pretest counseling, post-test counseling, and referral for treatment, if appropriate, of the source individual should be provided.

HIV Postexposure Management. If a health care worker is exposed percutaneously or by a splash to the eye or mucous membrane from a patient who has HIV infection or AIDS, or who refuses to be tested, the worker should be counseled regarding the risk of infection and be evaluated clinically and serologically for evidence of HIV infection as soon as possible after the exposure. The worker should be advised to report and seek medical evaluation for any acute febrile illness that occurs within 12 weeks after exposure. Following the initial test at the time of exposure, seronegative workers should be retested 6 weeks, 12 weeks, and 6 months after exposure to determine whether transmission has occurred. During this period the worker should refrain from blood or semen donation and should use appropriate protection (condoms and spermicides) during sexual intercourse.

If the source individual is found to be seronegative, baseline testing of the exposed worker with follow-up 12 weeks later may be performed if desired or recommended by the health care provider.

Zidovudine (AZT) is used to treat patients with HIV infection and has been proposed as chemoprophylaxis to prevent occupational infection in health care workers. There are no data that indicate prophylactic AZT therapy can prevent HIV infection in humans, although AZT given immediately after exposure can alter the course of animal retroviral (not HIV) infection.[198,199] The use of AZT for chemoprophylaxis in health care workers has been reviewed.[198,199] There are no clear indications for AZT prophylaxis but some institutions recommend it for employees sustaining massive exposures (eg, injections or transfusions of HIV-containing blood), endorse it for serious parenteral exposures (eg, deep needle sticks), and have it available but do not recommend it for less severe exposure.[175] The final decision is left to the employee after he/she is counseled about the toxicity and applicable data. AZT should be given within 24 hours, preferably as soon as possible, after exposure. If the HIV status of the source patient is unknown, AZT therapy can be begun until test results are available. A dilemma arises when the source individual refuses to be tested.

AZT prophylaxis protocols generally advise administering 200 mg AZT every 4 hours for 28 to 42 days.[198,199] Some protocols skip the 4 a.m. dose. Since an adverse exposure can occur anytime, AZT should be available 24 hours a day.

Hepatitis B. The CDC has issued recommendations for hepatitis B prophylaxis after percutaneous, mucous membrane, or ocular exposure to blood[108,200] (Table 27–16). These recommendations are based on consideration of (1) whether the source of the exposure is available, (2) the HB_sAg status of the source, and (3) the hepatitis B vaccination and vaccination-response status of the exposed person. After exposure, a blood sample should be obtained from the person who was the source of the exposure. It should be tested for HIV, HB_sAg, HCV, and AST and ALT (as an indication of non-A, non-B hepatitis). The hepatitis B vaccination status and the anti-HB_s response status (if known) should be reviewed or determined. The serologic status of the source and exposed health care worker should be used in considering whether to give active or passive immunoprophylaxis. Hepatitis B immune globulin (HBIG), if indicated, should be given within 7 days of exposure. HBIG does not inhibit the response to hepatitis B vaccine.

The U.S. Public Health Service recommends that persons at risk for exposure to hepatitis B receive hepatitis B vaccine.[108,200] Health care workers who are at increased risk for acquiring hepatitis B include physicians (especially surgeons), dentists, and laboratory and support personnel such as nurses and technicians who work in the operating room or who have contact with infected patients, blood or blood products, or excreta. Because of their frequent contact with blood and their high risk of acquiring hepatitis B, all surgeons should receive the hepatitis B vaccine. Two safe, effective recombinant vaccines are currently available, Recombivax-HB® and Engerix®. Yet only 30 to 50 percent of surgeons have been vaccinated. The standard vaccination regimen provides almost 100 percent effective immunity in children but less in adults older than 40. Immunosuppressed persons respond poorly. For unvaccinated health care workers, combined passive-active immunization is recommended with immediate HBIG (0.06 mg/kg IM) and conventional vaccination.

Hepatitis C (Non-A, Non-B Hepatitis). There is no hepatitis C vaccine as yet. Studies assessing the

TABLE 27–16. RECOMMENDATIONS FOR HEPATITIS B PROPHYLAXIS AFTER PERCUTANEOUS OR PERMUCOSAL EXPOSURE

Hepatitis B Vaccination Status of Exposed Person	HB_sAg Status of Source of Exposure		
	HB_sAg-Positive	HB_sAg-Negative	Untested or Unknown
Unvaccinated	Give single doses of HBIG; initiate HB vaccine series	Initiate HB vaccine series	Initiate HB vaccine series
Previously vaccinated Known responder	Test exposed person for anti-HB_s; if anti-HB_s levels are adequate[a] no treatment is needed; if they are inadequate, give an HB vaccine booster dose	No treatment is needed	No treatment is needed
Known nonresponder	Give two doses of HBIG or one dose of HBIG plus one dose of HB vaccine	No treatment is needed	If source is at high risk for hepatitis B infection, consider proceeding as if it had been demonstrated to be HB_sAg-positive
Response unknown	Test exposed person for anti-HB_s; if anti-HB_s levels are adequate,[a] no treatment is needed; if they are inadequate, give one dose of HBIG plus an HB vaccine booster dose	No treatment is needed	Test exposed person for anti-HB_s; if anti-HB_s levels are adequate,[a] no treatment is needed; if they are inadequate, give an HB vaccine booster dose

[a] An adequate anti-HB_s level is ≥10 mIU/ml, which is approximately equivalent to 10 sample ratio units (SRU) on radioimmunoassay or positive result on enzyme immunoassay.

From Centers for Disease Control: Morb Mortal Wkly Rep 39(RR-2):1, 1990.

value of immunoglobulin prophylaxis for non-A, non-B hepatitis or hepatitis C have produced equivocal results. The U.S. Public Health Service has stated that it may be reasonable to administer immune globulin (0.06 ml/kg) as soon as possible to persons exposed to blood from a patient with parenterally transmitted non-A, non-B hepatitis,[200] but there is no evidence that any immune globulin preparation is effective. If it is not clear whether the patient who is the source of the exposure definitely has non-A, non-B hepatitis, no specific recommendations can be made.

TRANSMISSION OF BLOOD-BORNE PATHOGENS FROM HEALTH CARE WORKERS TO PATIENTS

Blood-borne pathogens can also be transmitted from health care workers to patients. HIV, HBV, and non-A, non-B hepatitis (HCV) can potentially be transmitted from surgeon to patient during invasive procedures when the surgeon sustains a percutaneous injury with a needle or sharp instrument, which then recontacts the patient. Only HBV has been demonstrated to be transmitted from physicians to patients, but HIV has been transmitted from a dentist to several patients.

Hepatitis B Virus

Experience with HBV suggests that transmission from physicians to patient is uncommon. There are reports of 15 physicians who transmitted HBV to a total of 135 patients, five family members, and one laboratory technician[201–213] (Table 27–17). Twelve of the 15 physicians were surgeons. The other physician was a family practitioner from rural Switzerland who never performed invasive procedures, even venipuncture.[206] He accounted for 41 of the 125 cases transmitted to patients. All physicians who were tested were HB_eAg-positive. Some gynecologists transmitted hepatitis when performing vaginal hysterectomy but not when hysterectomy was done transabdominally. Using the fingers to palpate the invisible suturing needles is frequently required during vaginal hysterectomy.

Seven of the health care workers who passed HBV to their patients were allowed to continue performing invasive procedures following modification of techniques (eg, double gloving and restriction of certain high-risk procedures).[214] No further transmission occurred for five health care workers. In two instances involving an obstetrician-gynecologist and an oral surgeon, however, HBV was transmitted to patients even after techniques were modified. No doubt many other physicians have also infected their patients with hepatitis B, but the cases have not been reported.

Four studies have prospectively followed 784 patients cared for by 16 HB_sAg-positive health care workers (two surgeons) and compared them with 556 control patients[215–219] (Table 27–18). No patient developed overt hepatitis or became HB_sAg-positive. Eight (1.0 percent) patients from the HB_sAg-positive health care worker group developed anti-HB_s, but so did six (1.1 percent) of the control patients.

There are also several reports of HBV transmission from dentists, especially oral surgeons, to patients[220–225] and one report each of transmission by an inhalation therapist and a cardiopulmonary-bypass technician. There are no reported cases of transmission of HCV from an infected surgeon to a patient.

Human Immunodeficiency Virus

One dentist has transmitted HIV to six patients.[226,227] There are no other reports of transmission of HIV from a health care worker to a patient. Thirty-seven unpublished and six published studies have followed approximately 3500 patients cared for by 21 dentists, 19 physicians, and three nurses with HIV infection.[189] Except for the six patients described above, no other patient has developed HIV infection.

There are six reports following patients of surgeons with AIDS[228–233] (Table 27–19). None of a total of 1167 patients developed HIV infection as a result of being cared for by HIV-infected surgeons. Other investigations are currently in progress. Serologic testing was done in only 767 of the 1167 patients. The other patients were simply matched with the state AIDS registry to determine whether they were reported.[228] Because of the considerable lag time between HIV infection and development of AIDS, it is possible that potential cases of transmission could have been missed.

The CDC reported[227] that "as of March 31, 1993, HIV tests were completed for 19,036 persons treated by 57 HIV-infected HCWs. No seropositive persons were reported among 11,529 patients tested from the practices of 46 HCWs, including 23 dentists and dental students, 12 physicians and medical students, seven surgeons and obstetricians, and four others. For the remaining 11 HCWs (six dentists and five surgeons and obstetricians), 7507 patients were tested, and 92 seropositive patients were identified. Follow-up investigations have been completed for 86 (94 percent) of these 92 patients: eight patients were documented to be infected before receiving care from the HIV-infected HCW; 54 had established risk factors for HIV; 19 may have had other opportunities for exposure to HIV (ie, exchange of sex for drugs or money and/or multiple sex partners); and five had no risks identified. Investigations are in progress for six patients of two HCWs."

"Genetic sequencing was performed on HIV strains from 29 of the 92 seropositive patients from the practices of three HCWs. . . . The degree of genetic similarity of viruses from the patients and the infected HCWs was in the range previously reported for persons with epidemiologically unrelated infections. . . . Thus, follow-up to date has not demonstrated transmission from an HCW as a source of HIV infection for any of the patients tested."

Undoubtedly, future reports will appear. Some may even report the transmission of HIV to a patient from a surgeon. But the likelihood of such an occurrence is extremely small.

Management of the HIV or HB_sAG-Positive Health Care Worker

The report of a dentist passing HIV to his patients sparked considerable discussion in the scientific and popular press about the HIV-positive health care worker, especially surgeons and dentists since they were most likely to participate in invasive procedures. The CDC first issued guidelines for the management of HIV-infected personnel in 1985.[171] The CDC subsequently issued guidelines for management of HIV-infected health care workers who participate in invasive procedures.[161] In the early guidelines the CDC recommended that health care personnel who are otherwise fit for duty and who do not participate in invasive procedures be allowed to perform their regular duties.[171] In the subsequent guidelines the CDC recommended that HIV-infected personnel who do participate in invasive procedures be evaluated on a case-by-case basis.[161] These recommendations were consolidated in 1987 with the suggestion that whether health care workers could perform their regular duties be decided on an individual basis.[36]

Following the report of transmission of HIV by a dentist, the CDC issued recommendations for

TABLE 27–17. TRANSMISSION OF HEPATITIS B FROM PHYSICIANS TO PATIENTS

Place	Year	HB_eAg Status of Physicians	Number of Patients Tested or Operated on	Handling of Needle Tip	Outbreak Cases	Procedure	Outcome	Reference
London	1985–1987	+	247	Unknown	5 Clinical 17 Clinical	10 Cesarian sections 10 Hysterectomies 2 Not stated	Surgeon stopped operating	201
Georgia	1983–1984	+	207	Denied	6 Clinical 11 Serologic	4 Major gynecologic 2 Cesarian sections	Surgeon stopped operating; resumed after initiating barrier techniques; informed consent of patient required	202
England	1977–1978	+	158 Major gynecologic 300 Minor gynecologic 136 Obstetric	Yes	8 Clinical 0 0	All major gynecologic	Surgeon stopped operating	203
Minnesota	1978–1979	+	Not stated	Yes	3 Clinical 2 Serologic	All major gynecologic	Unknown	202
Mississippi	1979–1980	+	Not stated; 58 after technique modified	Yes	4 Clinical 0	All major gynecologic	Suspended practice; resumed modified technique	204
Louisiana	1980–1982	+	Not stated	Yes	5 Clinical	4 Major gynecologic 1 Orthopedic	Unknown	202

Amsterdam	1979	Unknown	Not done	Unknown	3 Clinical	All cardiac operations	Surgeon resumed operating	205
Switzerland	1973–1977	+	Not done	Unknown	41 Clinical	Family practitioner, no operating; possible transmission during venipuncture	Doctor died 1977	206
Seattle	1976	Unknown	30	Unknown	1 Clinical	Major orthopedic	Surgeon recovered; developed anti-HB_s; continued operating	207
Oslo	1981	Unknown	72	Unknown	5 Patients 3 Relatives of patients 1 Laboratory technician 2 Surgeon's family members	Cardiac surgery	Surgeon recovered	208
United Kingdom	1976–1979	+	1020	Unknown	8 Clinical 1 Serologic 3 Cesarian sections 1 Minor gynecologic	5 Major gynecologic	Unknown	209
United Kingdom	1980–1983	Unknown	Not stated	Unknown	5 Clinical	5 Cardiac surgeries	Surgeon recovered	210
Orange County, CA	1987	+	Not stated	Unknown	5 Clinical	Unknown	Stopped operating	211
Canada	1991	+	Not stated	Unknown	2 Clinical	Orthopedic procedure	Stopped operating	212
United Kingdom	1991	+	Not stated	Unknown	3 Clinical	General surgery	Stopped operating	213

From Heseltine PNR: The HIV- or HBV-infected professional. In Howard R; (ed): Infectious Risks in Surgery. Norwalk, CT, Appleton & Lange, 1991, pp 139–156.

TABLE 27–18. HEPATITIS AND HEPATITIS B SEROLOGIC EVENTS IN PERSONS PROSPECTIVELY FOLLOWED AFTER EXPOSURE TO HB_sAg-POSITIVE HEALTH CARE WORKERS

Number of HB_sAg-Positive HCWs	Number of Surgeons	Number of Persons Followed	Number Developed: Overt Hepatitis	Elevated SGPT	HB_sAg	Anti-HB_s	Reference
5	0	228	0	5	0	1	212
2	0	237	0	NT	0	3	213
1	0	24	0	NT	0	0	214
2	0	49	0	9	0	4	215
6	2	246	0	NT	0	0	215
Total 16	2	784	0		0	8	
Control							
		167	0	2	0	2	212
		245	0	NT	0	4	213
		144	0	NT	0	0	216
Total		556	0		0	6	

NT, not tested; SGPT, serum glutamic pyruvic transaminase.
From Heseltine PNR: The HIV- or HBV-infected professional. In Howard RJ (ed): Infectious Risks in Surgery. Norwalk, CT, Appleton & Lange, 1991, pp 139–156.

TABLE 27–19. HIV-1 TRANSMISSION FROM HIV-1–INFECTED SURGEONS TO THEIR PATIENTS

Location	Number of Patients Exposed	Number Tested for HIV-1	Number Positive	Reference
Miami, FL	400	0[a]	0	225
Nashville, TN	2160	616	1[b]	226
Brooks Air Force Base, TX	1804	75	0	227
London, UK	339	76	0	228
Baltimore, MD	1131	413	0	229
New Hampshire	2317	1174	0	230

[a] Patients were not tested for HIV-1, but names were compared with those on the state AIDS registry.
[b] This patient had risk factors for HIV-1 infection.

health care workers infected with HIV or HBV[214] (Table 27–20). Defining "exposure-prone" procedures has met with resistance from the medical community.[234] These recommendations do not require testing of health care workers for HIV or HBV but suggest that they should voluntarily be tested. Health care workers who are infected with HIV or HBV should not perform exposure-prone procedures unless they have sought counsel from an expert panel, and their patients should be informed of their seropositivity. The recommendations specify the composition of the panel but provide no guidelines for the panel on which to base their decisions.

It is conceivable that an infected surgeon or other health care worker could be allowed to perform "exposure-prone" invasive procedure by one review panel and not by another. How can such a panel fully evaluate levels of risks? Available data—that no surgeon has yet been shown to pass HIV to a patient—indicate the risk is extremely low. Forcing a surgeon to disclose his/her seropositivity to patients would destroy his/her practice. There is obviously a tension over a surgeon's right to privacy when he/she has an infection that poses minimal, if any, risk to patients. These issues are currently being vigorously debated. Because of opposition to defining "exposure-prone" procedures, the CDC seems to have abandoned efforts and left it up to the individual states to define these procedures. So far no state has done so.

TABLE 27–20. RECOMMENDATIONS FOR HEALTH CARE WORKERS INFECTED WITH HIV OR HBV

Investigations of HIV and HBV transmission from HCWs to patients indicate that, when HCWs adhere to recommended infection-control procedures, the risk of transmitting HBV from an infected HCW to a patient is small, and the risk of transmitting HIV is likely to be even smaller. However, the likelihood of exposure of the patient to the HCW's blood is greater for certain procedures designated as exposure-prone. To minimize the risk of HIV or HBV transmission, the following measures are recommended:

- All HCWs should adhere to universal precautions, including the appropriate use of hand washing, protective barriers, and care in the use and disposal of needles and other sharp instruments. HCWs who have exudative lesions or weeping dermatitis should refrain from all direct patient care and from handling patient-care equipment and devices used in performing invasive procedures until the condition resolves. HCWs should also comply with current guidelines for disinfection and sterilization of reusable devices used in invasive procedures.
- Currently available data provide no basis for recommendations to restrict the practice of HCWs infected with HIV or HBV who perform invasive procedures not identified as exposure-prone, provided the infected HCWs practice recommended surgical or dental techniques and comply with universal precautions and current recommendations for sterilization/disinfection.
- Exposure-prone procedures should be identified by medical/surgical/dental organizations and institutions at which the procedures are performed.
- HCWs who perform exposure-prone procedures should know their HIV antibody status. HCWs who perform exposure-prone procedures and who do not have serologic evidence of immunity to HBV from vaccination or from previous infection should know their HB_sAg status and, if that is positive, should also know their HB_eAg status.
- HCWs who are infected with HIV or HBV (and are HB_eAg positive) should not perform exposure-prone procedures unless they have sought counsel from an expert review panel and been advised under what circumstances, if any, they may continue to perform these procedures.[a] Such circumstances would include notifying prospective patients of the HCW's seropositivity before they undergo exposure-prone invasive procedures.
- Mandatory testing of HCWs for HIV antibody, HB_sAg, or HB_eAg is not recommended. The current assessment of the risk that infected HCWs will transmit HIV or HBV to patients during exposure-prone procedures does not support the diversion of resources that would be required to implement mandatory testing programs. Compliance by HCWs with recommendations can be increased through education, training, and appropriate confidentiality safeguards.

[a] The review panel should include experts who represent a balanced perspective. Such experts might include all of the following: (1) the HCW's personal physician(s), (2) an infectious disease specialist with expertise in the epidemiology of HIV and HBV transmission, (3) a health professional with expertise in the procedures performed by the HCW, and (4) state or local public health official(s). If the HCW's practice is institutionally based, the expert review panel might also include a member of the infection-control committee, preferably a hospital epidemiologist. HCWs who perform exposure-prone procedures outside the hospital/institutional setting should seek advice from appropriate state and local public health officials regarding the review process. Panels must recognize the importance of confidentiality and the privacy rights of infected HCWs.

From Centers for Disease Control: Morb Mortal Wkly Rep 40(RR-8):1, 1991.

REFERENCES

1. Wangensteen OH, Wangensteen SD, Klinger CF: Some pre-Listerian and post-Listerian wound practices and the emergence of asepsis. Surg Gynecol Obstet 137:677, 1973.
2. Wangensteen OH, Wangensteen SD: The Rise of Surgery from Empiric Craft to Scientific Discipline. Minneapolis, University of Minnesota Press, 1978, p 7.
3. Dooley SW Jr, Castro KG, Hutton MD, et al: Guidelines for preventing the transmission of tuberculosis in health care settings, with special focus on HIV-related issues. Morb Mortal Wkly Rep 39(RR-17):1, 1990.
4. Barrett-Connor E: The epidemiology of tuberculosis in physicians. JAMA 241:33, 1979.
5. Goldman KP: Tuberculosis in hospital doctors. Tubercle 69:237, 1988.
6. Haley CE, McDonald RC, Rossi L, et al: Tuberculosis epidemic among hospital personnel. Infect Control Hosp Epidemiol 10:204, 1989.
7. Hutton MD, Stead WW, Cauthen GM, et al: Nosocomial transmission of tuberculosis associated with a draining tuberculosis abscess. J Infect Dis 161:286, 1990.
8. Kantor HS, Poblete R, Pusateria SL: Nosocomial transmission of tuberculosis from unsuspected disease. Am J Med 84:833, 1988.
9. Centers for Disease Control: Mycobacterium tuberculosis transmission in a health clinic—Florida, 1988. Morb Mortal Wkly Rep 38:256, 1989.
10. Centers for Disease Control: National action plan to combat multidrug-resistant tuberculosis. Morb Mortal Wkly Rep 41(RR-11):1, 1992.
11. Beck-Sagué C, Dooley SW, Hutton MD, et al: Hospital outbreak of multidrug-resistant *Mycobacterium tuberculosis* infections. Factors in transmission to staff and HIV-infected patients. JAMA 268:1280, 1992.
12. Di Perri G, Cadeo GP, Castell F, et al: Transmission of HIV-associated tuberculosis to health care workers. Lancet 340:682, 1992.
13. Rabalais G, Adams G, Stover B: PPD skin test conversion in health care workers after exposure to *Mycobacterium tuberculosis* infection in infants. Lancet 338:826, 1991.
14. Pierce JR Jr, Sims SL, Holman GH: Transmission of tuberculosis to hospital workers by a patient with AIDS. Chest 101:581, 1992.

15. Dooley SW, Villarino ME, Lawrence M, et al: Nosocomial transmission of tuberculosis in a hospital unit for HIV-infected patients. JAMA 267:2632, 1992.
16. Pearson ML, Jereb JA, Frieden TR, et al: Nosocomial transmission of multidrug-resistant *Mycobacterium tuberculosis.* Ann Intern Med 117:191, 1992.
17. Gaynes R, Marosok R, Mowry-Hanley J, et al: Mediastinitis following coronary artery bypass surgery: a 3-year review. J Infect Dis 163:117, 1991.
18. Bassett HFM, Ferguson WG, Hoffman E, et al: Sources of staphylococcal infection in surgical sound sepsis. J Hyg 61:83, 1963.
19. Richman DD, Breton SJ, Goldmann DA: Scarlet fever and group A streptococcal surgical wound infection traced to an anal carrier. J Pediatr 90:387, 1977.
20. Porter D, Scully C, Theyer Y, Porter S: Occupational injuries to dental personnel. J Dent 18:258, 1990.
21. Jagger J, Pearson RD: Sharp object injuries in the hospital: causes and strategies for prevention. Am J Infect Control 18:227, 1990.
22. Lowenfels AB, Wormser GP, Jain R: Frequency of puncture injuries in surgeons and estimated risk of HIV infection. Arch Surg 124:1284, 1989.
23. Panlilio AL, Foy DR, Edwards JR, et al: Blood contact during surgical procedures. JAMA 265:1533, 1991.
24. McCormick RD, Mak DG: Epidemiology of needlestick injuries in hospital personnel. Am J Med 70:928, 1981.
25. Gerberding JL, Littell C, Tarkington A, et al: Risk of exposure of surgical personnel to patients' blood during surgery at San Francisco General Hospital. N Engl J Med 322:1788, 1990.
26. Popejoy SL, Fry DE: Blood contact and exposure in the operating room. Surg Gynecol Obstet 172:480, 1991.
27. Tokars JI, Bell DM, Culver DH, et al: Percutaneous injuries during surgical procedures. JAMA 267: 2899, 1992.
28. Pike RM: Past and present hazards of working with infectious agents. Arch Pathol Lab Med 102:333, 1978.
29. Polesky HF: Transfusion-transmitted infections. In Howard RJ (ed): Infectious Risks in Surgery. Norwalk, CT, Appleton & Lange, 1991, p 1.
30. Seidl S, Kühnl P: Transmission of disease by blood transfusion. World J Surg 11:30, 1978.
31. Cumming PD, Wallace EL, Schorr JB, Dood RY: Exposure of patients to human immunodeficiency virus through the transfusion of blood components that test antibody-negative. N Engl J Med 321:941, 1989.
32. Bove JR: Transfusion-associated hepatitis and AIDS. What is the risk? N Engl J Med 317:242, 1987.
33. Centers for Disease Control: Projections of the number of persons diagnosed with AIDS and the number of immunosuppressed HIV-infected persons—United States, 1992–1994. Morb Mortal Wkly Rep 41(RR-18):1, 1992.
34. Centers for Disease Control: Human immunodeficiency virus infection in the United States. A review of current knowledge. Morb Mortal Wkly Rep 36(5–6):1, 1987.
35. Ward JW, Bush TJ, Perkins HA, et al: The natural history of transfusion-associated infection with human immunodeficiency virus. Factors influencing the rate of progression to disease. N Engl J Med 321:947, 1989.
36. Centers for Disease Control: Recommendations for prevention of HIV transmission in health care settings. Morb Mortal Wkly Rep 36(2S):1S, 1987.
37. Centers for Disease Control: The HIV/AIDS epidemic: the first 10 years. Morb Mortal Wkly Rep 40:357, 1991.
38. Centers for Disease Control: Human immunodeficiency virus infection in transfusion recipients and their family members. Morb Mortal Wkly Rep 36:137, 1987.
39. Handsfield HH, Cummings J, Swenson PD: Prevalence of antibody to human immunodeficiency virus and hepatitis B surface antigen in blood samples submitted to a hospital laboratory. Implications for handling specimens. JAMA 258:3395, 1987.
40. Henry K, Maki M, Crossley K: Analysis of the use of HIV antibody testing in a Minnesota hospital. JAMA 259:229, 1988.
41. Centers for Disease Control: AIDS and human immunodeficiency infection in the United States: 1988 update. Morb Mortal Wkly Rep 38(S-4):1, 1989.
42. St Louis ME, Rauch KJ, Peterson LR, et al: Seroprevalence rates of human immunodeficiency virus infection at sentinel hospital in the United States. The Sentinel Hospital Surveillance Group. N Engl J Med 323:213, 1990.
43. Janssen RS, St Louis ME, Satten GA, et al: HIV infection among patients in US acute care hospital. Strategies for the counseling and testing of the hospital patients. N Engl J Med 327:486, 1992.
44. Gordin FM, Gilbert C, Hawley HP, et al: Prevalence of human immunodeficiency virus and hepatitis B virus in unselected hospital admissions: implications for mandatory testing and universal precautions. J Infect Dis 161:14, 1990.
45. Butler T, Sawyer J: Prevalence of human immunodeficiency virus infection in hospitalized adults at a teaching hospital in West Texas. Tex Med 88:66, 1992.
46. Kelen GD, Fritz S, Qaquish B, et al: Substantial increase in human immunodeficiency virus (HIV-1) infection in critically ill emergency patients; 1986 and 1987 compared. Ann Emerg Med 18:378, 1989.
47. Baker JL, Kelen GD, Silvertson KT, et al: Unsuspected human immunodeficiency virus in critically ill emergency patients. JAMA 257:2609, 1987.
48. Kelen GD, D'Giovanna T, Bisson L, et al: Human immunodeficiency virus infection in emergency department patients. Epidemiology, clinical presenta-

tions, and risk to health care workers: the Johns Hopkins experience. JAMA 262:516, 1989.
49. Kelen GD, Fritz S, Qaquish B, et al: Unrecognized human immunodeficiency virus infection in emergency department patients. JAMA 318:1645, 1988.
50. Zeman MG, Mahue FE: Human immunodeficiency virus (HIV) seropositivity in a midwestern community trauma population. Ann Emerg Med 17:409, 1988.
51. Hammond J, Ward CG: The occurrence of acquired immunodeficiency syndrome and unsuspected human immunodeficiency virus in burn patients. J Burn Care Rehabil 10:156, 1989.
52. Orr MD, Hoos A, Riester DE, et al: HIV-1 infection in patients with penetrating trauma in San Antonio, TX, letter. N Engl J Med 262:1629, 1989.
53. Charache P, Cameron JL, Maters AW, et al: Prevalence of infection with human immunodeficiency virus in elective surgery patients. Ann Surg 214: 562, 1991.
54. Reid CB, Kaldor JM, Lord RS, et al: HIV risk factors and seroprevalence in surgical patients. Med J Aust 158:21, 1993.
55. Evraro S, Meyer P, van Haaften K, et al: Occupational risk to surgeons of unrecognized HIV infections in a low-prevalence area. World J Surg 17:232, 1993.
56. Panlilio AL, Bell DM: HIV infection in health care workers: assessment of risk. In Howard RJ (ed): Infectious Risks in Surgery. Norwalk, CT, Appleton & Lange, 1991, pp 65–81.
57. Bureau of Labor Statistics: Employment and Earning, Vol 35. Washington, DC, US Department of Labor, Bureau of Labor Statistics, 1988, pp 13, 93, 194.
58. Aoun H: When a house officer gets AIDS. N Engl J Med 321:693, 1989.
59. Ciesielski CA, Bell DM, Chamberland ME, et al: When a house officer gets AIDS (letter). N Engl J Med 322:1156, 1990.
60. Marcus R, The Cooperative Needlestick Surveillance Group: Surveillance of health care workers exposed to blood from patients infected with the human immunodeficiency virus. N Engl J Med 319:1118, 1988.
61. Henderson DK, Fahey BJ, Willy M, et al: Risk of occupational transmission of human immunodeficiency virus type 1 (HIV-1) associated with clinical exposure: a prospective evaluation. Ann Intern Med 113:740, 1990.
62. Hirsch MS, Wormser GP, Schooley RT, et al: Risk of nosocomial infection with human T-cell lymphotropic virus III (HTLV-III). N Engl J Med 312:1, 1985.
63. Weiss SH, Goedert JJ, Sarngadharan MG, et al: Screening test for HTLV-III (AIDS) agent antibodies. Specificity, sensitivity, and applications. JAMA 253:221, 1985.
64. Shanson DC, Evans R, Lai L: Incidence and risk of transmission of HTLV-III infection to a staff at a London hospital, 1982–85. J Hosp Infect Suppl C:15, 22, 1985.
65. Ebbesen P, Milbye M, Scheutz F, et al: Lack of antibodies to HTLV-III/LAV in Danish dentists (letter). JAMA 256:2199, 1986.
66. Lubick HA, Schaeffer LD: Occupational risk of dental personnel survey (letter). J Am Dent Assoc 113:10, 1986.
67. Harper S, Flynn N, VanHorne J, et al: Absence of HIV antibody among dental professions, surgeons, and household contacts exposed to persons with HIV infection (abstract). Abstract THP.215. Presented at the 3rd International Conference on AIDS, Washington, DC, June 1986.
68. Boland M, Keresztes J, Evans P, et al: HIV seroprevalence among nurses caring for children with AIDS/ARC (abstract). Abstract THP.212. Presented at the 3rd International Conference on AIDS, Washington, DC, June 1986.
69. Gilmore N, Ballachey M-L, O'Shaughnessy M, et al: HTLV-II/LAV serologic survey of health care workers in a Canadian teaching hospital (abstract 200). Presented at the 2nd International Conference on AIDS, Paris, France, June 1986.
70. Mann JM, Francis H, Quinn TC, et al: HIV seroprevalence among hospital workers in Kinshasa, Zaire: lack of association with occupational exposure. JAMA 256:3099, 1986.
71. Gerberding JL, Bryant-LeBlanc CE, Nelson K, et al: Risk of transmitting the human immunodeficiency virus, cytomegalovirus, and hepatitis B virus to health care workers exposed to patients with AIDS and AIDS-related conditions. J Infect Dis 156:1, 1987.
72. Gerberding JL, Nelson K, Greenspan D, et al: Risk to dentists from exposure to patients infected with AIDS virus (AV) (abstract 698). Program and Abstracts of the Twenty-seventh Interscience Conference on Antimicrobial Agents and Chemotherapy, New York, October 4–7, 1987.
73. Flynn NM, Pollet SM, Van Horne JR, et al: Absence of HIV antibody among dental professional exposed to infected patients. West J Med 146:439, 1987.
74. Klein RS, Phelan JA, Freeman E, et al: Low occupational risk of human immunodeficiency virus infection among dental professionals. N Engl J Med 318:86, 1988.
75. N'Galy B, Ryder RW, Bila K, et al: Human immunodeficiency virus infection among employees in an African hospital. N Engl J Med 319:1123, 1988.
76. Weiss SH, Goedert JJ, Gartner S, et al: Risk of human immunodeficiency virus (HIV-1) infection among laboratory workers. Science 239:68, 1988.
77. Weiss SH, Saxinger WC, Rechtman D, et al: HLTV-III infection among health care workers. Association with needle-stick injuries. JAMA 254:2089, 1985.
78. Centers for Disease Control: Preliminary analysis: HIV serosurvey of orthopedic surgeons, 1991. Morb Mortal Wkly Rep 40:309, 1991.
79. Wormser GP, Rubkin CS, Joline C: Frequency of

nosocomial transmission of HIV infection among health care workers (letter). N Engl J Med 319:307, 1988.

80. Hagen MD, Meyer KB, Parker SG: Routine preoperative screening for HIV. Does the risk to the surgeon outweigh the risk to the patient? JAMA 259:1357, 1988.
81. Howard RJ: Human immunodeficiency virus testing and the risk to the surgeon of acquiring HIV. Surg Gynecol Obstet 171:22, 1990.
82. Kuhls TL, Viker S, Parris NB, et al: Occupational risk of HIV, HBV, and HSV-2 infections in health care personnel caring for AIDS patients. Am J Public Health 77:1306, 1987.
83. McEvoy M, Porter K, Mortimer P, et al: Prospective study of clinical, laboratory, and ancillary staff with accidental exposures to blood or body fluids from patients infected with HIV. Br Med J 294:1595, 1987.
84. Elmslie K, O'Shaughnessy JV: National surveillance program on occupational exposure to HIV among health care workers in Canada. Can Dis Wkly Rep 13:163, 1987.
85. Ramsey KM, Smith EN, Reinarz JA: Prospective evaluation of 44 health care workers exposed to human immunodeficiency virus-1 with one seroconversion (abstract). Clin Res 36:22A, 1988.
86. Hernandez E, Gatell JM, Puyvelo T, et al: Risk of transmitting the HIV to health care workers (HCW) exposed to HIV infected body fluids (abstract 9003). IV International Conference on AIDS, Stockholm, Sweden, June 1988, p 476.
87. Pizzocolo G, Stellini R, Cadeo GP, et al: Risk of HIV and HBV infection after accidental needlestick (abstract 9012). IV International Conference on AIDS, Stockholm, Sweden, June 1988, p 478.
88. Wormser GP, Joline C, Sivak S, Arlin ZA: Human immunodeficiency virus infections: considerations for health care workers. Bull NY Acad Med 64:203, 1988.
89. Rastrelli M, Ferrazzi D, Vigo B, et al: Risk of HIV transmission to health care workers and comparison with viral hepatitides (abstract A.503). Abstracts from V International Conference on AIDS, Montreal, June 4–9, 1989.
90. Francavilla E, Cadrobbi P, Scaggiante R, et al: Surveillance on occupational exposure to HIV among health care workers in Italy (abstract D623). V International Conference on AIDS, Montreal, 1989, p 795.
91. Ippolito G, Cadrobbi P, Carosi G, et al: Risk of occupational exposure to HIV-infected body fluids and transmission of HIV among health care workers: a multicenter study (abstract MDP72). V International Conference on AIDS, Montreal, 1989, p 722.
92. Jorbeck H, Marland M, Steinkeller E: Accidental exposures to HIV-positive blood among health care workers in 2 Swedish hospitals (abstract A517). V International Conference on AIDS, Montreal, 1989, p 163.
93. McNicholas A, Jones DJ, Sibley GNA: AIDS: the contamination risk in urologic surgery. Br J Urol 63:565, 1989.
94. Hussain SA, Latif ABA, Choudhary AAAA: Risk to surgeons: a survey of accidental injuries during operations. Br J Surg 75:314, 1988.
95. Quebbeman EJ, Telford GL, Hubbard S, et al: Risk of blood contamination and injury to operating room personnel. Ann Surg 214:614, 1991.
96. Napoli VM, McGowan VM Jr: How much blood in a needlestick? J Infect Dis 155:828, 1987.
97. Mast ST, Gerberding JL: Factors predicting infectivity following needlestick exposure to HIV: an in vitro model (abstract). Clin Res 39:58A, 1991.
98. Bennett NT, Howard RJ: How much blood is inoculated in a needlestick injury from a suture needle? Surg Gynecol Obstet 178:107, 1994.
99. Ho DD, Mordgil T, Alan M: Quantitation of human immunodeficiency virus type 1 in the blood of infected persons. N Engl J Med 321:1621, 1989.
100. Kim CY, Tilles JG: Purification and biophysical characterization of the hepatitis B antigen. J Clin Invest 52:1176, 1970.
101. Feinstone SM, Alter HJ, Dienes HP, et al: Non-A, non-B hepatitis in chimpanzees and marmosets. J Infect Dis 144:588, 1981.
102. Werner BG, Grady GF: Accidental hepatitis-B surface antigen positive inoculations: use of e antigen to estimate infectivity. Ann Intern Med 97:367, 1982.
103. Friedman LS, Dienstag JL: Recent developments in viral hepatitis. DM 32:320, 1986.
104. Prince AM, Brotman B, Inchaupé G, et al: Patterns and prevalence of hepatitis C infection in posttransfusion non-A, non-B hepatitis. J Infect Dis 167:1296, 1993.
105. Beasley RP, Hwang L-Y, Lan CC, et al: Prevention of perinatally transmitted hepatitis B virus infections with hepatitis B immune globulin and hepatitis B vaccine. Lancet 2:1099, 1983.
106. Rogers ML, Davis GL: Infectious risks to the surgeon: viral hepatitis. In Howard RJ (ed): Infectious Risks in Surgery. Norwalk, CT, Appleton & Lange, 1991, p 53.
107. Dienstage JL, Ryan DM: Occupational exposure to hepatitis B virus in hospital personnel: infection or immunization. Am J Epidemiol 115:26, 1982.
108. Centers for Disease Control: Recommendations for protection against viral hepatitis. Morb Mortal Wkly Rep 34:313, 1985.
109. Beasley RP, Hwang L-Y, Lin C-C, Chien CS: Hepatocellular carcinoma and hepatitis B virus: a prospective study of 22,707 men in Taiwan. Lancet 2:1129, 1981.
110. Scott RM, Snitbhn R, Bancroft WH, et al: Experimental transmission of hepatitis B virus by semen and saliva. J Infect Dis 142:67, 1980.
111. Alter HJ, Purcell RH, Gerin JL, et al: Transmission of hepatitis B to chimpanzees by hepatitis B surface antigen-positive saliva and semen. Infect Immunol 16:928, 1977.

112. Maynard JG: Nosocomial viral hepatitis. Am J Med 70:439, 1981.
113. Bove JR: Transfusion-associated hepatitis. What is the risk? N Engl J Med 317:242, 1987.
114. Wick MR, Moore S, Taswell HF: Non-A, non-B hepatitis associated with blood transfusion. Transfusion 25:93, 1985.
115. Polesky HF, Hanson MR: Transfusion-associated hepatitis C virus (non-A, non-B) infection. Arch Pathol Lab Med 113:232, 1989.
116. Centers for Disease Control: Guidelines for prevention of transmission of human immunodeficiency virus and hepatitis B virus to health care and public-safety workers. MMWR Morb Mortal Wkly Rep 38(S-6):1037, 1989.
117. Surgenor DM, Wallace EL, Hao SHA, et al: Collection and transfusion of blood in the United States, 1982–1988. N Engl J Med 322:1646, 1990.
118. Alter HJ, Holland PV, Purcell RH: The emerging pattern of post-transfusion hepatitis. Am J Med Sci 270:329, 1975.
119. Alter HJ, Purcell RH, Shih JW, et al: Detection of antibody to hepatitis C virus in prospectively followed transfusion recipients with acute and chronic non-A, non-B hepatitis. N Engl J Med 321:1494, 1989.
120. Cuthbert JA: Southwestern internal medicine conference: hepatitis C. Am J Med Sci 299:346, 1990.
121. Alter MJ, Hadler SC, Margolis HS, et al: The changing epidemiology of hepatitis B in the United States. Need for alternative vaccination strategies. JAMA 263:1218, 1990.
122. Osterterholm MT, Garayalde SM: Clinical viral hepatitis B among Minnesota hospital personnel. Results of a ten-year statewide survey. JAMA 242: 3207, 1985.
123. Jovanovich JF, Saravolatz LD, Arking LM: The risk of hepatitis B among select employee groups in an urban hospital. JAMA 250:1893, 1983.
124. McLean AA, Monahan GR, Finkelstein DM: Prevalence of hepatitis B serologic markers in community hospital personnel. Am J Public Health 77:998, 1987.
125. Pattison CP, Maynard JE, Berquist KR, et al: Epidemiology of hepatitis B in hospital personnel. Am J Epidemiol 101:59, 1975.
126. Gibas A, Blewett DR, Schoenfeld DA, et al: Prevalence and incidence of viral hepatitis in health workers in the prehepatitis B vaccination era. Am J Epidemiol 136:603, 1992.
127. Krugman S, Friedman H, Lattimer C: Hepatitis A and B. Serologic survey of various population groups. Am J Med Sci 275:249, 1978.
128. Szmuness W: Large-scale efficacy trials of hepatitis B vaccines in the USA: baseline data and protocols. J Med Virol 4:327, 1979.
129. Denes AE, Smith JL, Maynard JE, et al: Hepatitis B infection in physicians. Results of a nationwide seroepidemiologic survey. JAMA 239:210, 1978.
130. Hirschowitz BI, Dasher CA, Whitt FJ, et al: Hepatitis B antigen and antibody and tests of liver function. A prospective study of 310 hospital laboratory workers. Am J Clin Pathol 73:63, 1980.
131. Levy BS, Harris JC, Smith JL, et al: Hepatitis B in ward and clinical laboratory employees of a general hospital. Am J Epidemiol 106:330, 1977.
132. Pantelick EL, Steere AC, Lewis HD, et al: Hepatitis B infection in hospital personnel during an eight-year period. Policies for screening and pregnancy in high risk area. Am J Med 70:924, 1981.
133. Snydman DR, Bryan JA, Hanson B: Hemodialysis-associated hepatitis in the United States—1972. J Infect Dis 132:109, 1975.
134. Osterholm M, Andrews JS Jr: Viral hepatitis in hospital personnel in Minnesota. Report of a statewide survey. Minn Med 62:683, 1979.
135. Najem GR, Louria DB, Thind IS, et al: Control of hepatitis B infection. The role of surveillance and an isolation hemodialysis center. JAMA 245:153, 1981.
136. Favero MS, Deane N, Leger RT, et al: Effect of multiple use of dialyzers on hepatitis B incidence in patients and staff. JAMA 245:166, 1981.
137. Polesky HF, Hanson M: AABB-CAP survey data on hepatitis—incidence, surveillance, and prevention. Am J Clin Pathol 74:565, 1980.
138. Smith JL, Maynard JE, Berquist KR, et al: Comparative risk of hepatitis B among physicians and dentists. J Infect Dis 133:705, 1976.
139. Weil RB, Lyman DO, Jackson RJ, et al: A hepatitis serosurvey of New York dentists. NY State Dent J 43:587, 1977.
140. Mosley JW, Edwards VM, Casey G, et al: Hepatitis B virus infection in dentists. N Engl J Med 293:729, 1975.
141. Mosley JW, Edwards VM: The risk of hepatitis B virus infection among dentists. Paper presented at a meeting of the American Dental Association in Kansas City, October 1981.
142. Norrgren H, Flodman-Norrlund I, Lindholm T, et al: Prevalence of antibodies against hepatitis B and C viruses among different groups of medical staff. Scand J Infect Dis 24:553, 1992.
143. West DJ: The risk of hepatitis B infection among health professionals in the United States: a review. Am J Med Sci 287:26, 1984.
144. Lemmer JH: Hepatitis B as an occupational disease of surgeons. Surg Gynecol Obstet 159:91, 1984.
145. Choo QL, Kuo G, Weiner AL: Isolation of a cDNA clone derived from a blood-borne non-A, non-B viral hepatitis genome. Science 244:362, 1989.
146. Alter MA, Sampliner RE: Hepatitis C: and miles to go before we sleep. N Engl J Med 321:1538, 1989.
147. Goldsmith ME: Blood bank officials hope donor altruism will pass new (anti-HCV) test. JAMA 263:1749, 1990.
148. Alter HJ, Purcell RH, Shih JW, et al: Detection of antibody to hepatitis C virus in prospectively followed transfusion recipients with acute and chronic non-A, non-B hepatitis. N Engl J Med 321:1494, 1989.

149. Garson JA, Tedder RS, Briggs M, et al: Detection of hepatitis C viral sequences in blood donations by "nested" polymerase chain reaction and prediction of infectivity. Lancet 335:1419, 1990.
150. Weiland O, Schuarcz: Hepatitis C: virology, epidemiology, clinical course, and treatment. Scand J Gastroenterol 27:337, 1992.
151. Donahue JG, Nelson KE, Muñoz A, et al: Antibody to hepatitis C virus among cardiac surgery patients, homosexual men, and intravenous drug abusers in Baltimore, Maryland. Am J Epidemiol 134:1206, 1991.
152. Cooper BW, Krusell A, Tilton RC, et al: Seroprevalence of antibodies to hepatitis C virus in high-risk hospital personnel. Infect Control Hosp Epidemiol 13:82, 1992.
153. Klein RS, Freeman K, Taylor PE, et al: Occupational risk for hepatitis C virus infection among New York City dentists. Lancet 338:1539, 1991.
154. Williams NP, Takatsuki K, Kawano F, et al: Antibodies to hepatitis C virus in Japanese blood donors and in hospital personnel (letter). Transfusion 30: 667, 1990.
155. Hofmann H, Kunz C: Low risk of health care workers for infection with hepatitis C. Infection 18:286, 1990.
156. Kiyosawa K, Sodeyama T, Tanaka E, et al: Hepatitis C in hospital employees with needlestick injuries. Ann Intern Med 115:367, 1991.
157. Tsude K, Fujiyamn S, Sota S, et al: Two cases of accidental transmission of hepatitis C to medical staff. Hepatogastroenterology 39:73, 1992.
158. Jochen ABB: Occupationally acquired hepatitis C virus infection. Lancet 339:304, 1992.
159. Vagilia A, Nicolin R, Puro V, et al: Needlestick hepatitis C virus seroconversion in a surgeon. Lancet 336:1315, 1990.
160. Vaglia A, Nicolin R, Puro V, et al: Needlestick hepatitis C virus seroconversion in a surgeon. Lancet 336:1315, 1990.
161. Centers for Disease Control: Recommendations for preventing transmission of infection with human T-lymphotropic virus type III/lymphadenopathy-associated virus during invasive procedures. Morb Mortal Wkly Rep 35:221, 1986.
162. Centers for Disease Control: Prevention of acquired immune deficiency syndrome. Morb Mortal Wkly Rep 32:101, 1983.
163. Centers for Disease Control: Acquired immunodeficiency syndrome (AIDS): precautions for health care workers and allied professionals. Morb Mortal Wkly Rep 32:450, 1983.
164. Centers for Disease Control: Recommendations for providing dialysis treatment to patients infected with human T-lymphotropic virus type III/lymphadenopathy-associated virus. Morb Mortal Wkly Rep 35:376, 1986.
165. Centers for Disease Control: Recommendations infection-control practices for dentistry. Morb Mortal Wkly Rep 35:237, 1985.
166. Gerberding JL, Henderson DK: Design of rational infection control policies for human immunodeficiency virus infection. J Infect Dis 156:861, 1987.
167. Adams A, Lowry FD: Infection control and the hospitalized AIDS patient. Infect Control 6:200, 1985.
168. Conte JE Jr: Infection with human immunodeficiency virus in the hospital. Ann Intern Med 105: 730, 1986.
169. Gerberding JL: The UCSF Task Force on AIDS. Recommendations for infection control policies for patients with human immunodeficiency virus infection. N Engl J Med 315:1562, 1986.
170. Lynch P, Jackson MM, Cummings MJ, et al: Rethinking the role of isolation practices in the prevention of nosocomial infection. Ann Intern Med. 107:243, 1986.
171. Centers for Disease Control: Recommendations for preventing transmission of infection with human T-lymphocyte type III/lymphadenopathy-associated virus in the work place. Morb Mortal Wkly Rep 34:681, 1985.
172. Centers for Disease Control: Update: universal precautions for prevention of transmission of human immunodeficiency virus, hepatitis B virus, and other blood-borne pathogens in health-care settings. Morb Mortal Wkly Rep 37:377, 1988.
173. Hammond JS, Eckes JM, Gomez GA, et al: HIV trauma, and infection control: universal precautions are universally ignored. J Trauma 30:555, 1990.
174. Courington K, Patterson SL, Howard RJ: Universal precautions are not universally followed. Arch Surg 126:93, 1991.
175. Williams DS, Stuart CG, Markowitz SM: Are universal precautions effective in reducing the number of occupational exposures among health care workers? A prospective study of physicians on a medical service. JAMA 265:1123, 1991.
176. Wong ES, Stoka JL, Chinchilli VE, et al: Are universal precautions effective in reducing the number of occupational exposures among health care workers? A prospective study of physicians on a medical service. JAMA 265:1123, 1991.
177. Huff JS, Basala M: Universal precautions in emergency medicine residencies. Ann Emerg Med 18:798, 1989.
178. Rhame F, Maki D: The case for wider use of testing for HIV infection. N Engl J Med 320:1248, 1989.
179. Nolan K, Bayer R: AIDS: the responsibilities of health professionals. Hastings Cent Rep 18:1, 1988.
180. Dudley HAF, Sim A: AIDS: a bill of rights for the surgical team? BMJ 295:1447, 1988.
181. Emanuel EJ: Do physicians have an obligation to treat patients with AIDS? N Engl J Med 318:1686, 1985.
182. Meyer KB, Pauker SG: Screening for HIV: can we afford the false positive rate? N Engl J Med 317:238, 1987.
183. Gillon R: Refusal to treat AIDS and HIV positive patients. BMJ 294:1332, 1987.
184. Dickey NW: Physicians and the acquired immuno-

deficiency syndrome: a reply to patients. JAMA 262:2002, 1989.

185. Gerbert B, Maguire BT, Hulley SB, Coates TJ: Physicians and acquired immunodeficiency syndrome: what patients think about human immunodeficiency virus in medical practice. JAMA 262:1969, 1989.
186. Blendor RJ, Donelon K: Discrimination against people with AIDS: the public's perspective. N Engl J Med 319:1022, 1988.
187. Quebbeman EJ, Telford GL, Condon RE: Should patients or health care workers be screened for human immunodeficiency viruses? In Howard RJ (ed): Infectious Risks in Surgery. Norwalk, CT, Appleton & Lange, 1991, pp 117–124.
188. Bessinger CD Jr: Preventing transmission of human immunodeficiency virus during operations. Surg Gynecol Obstet 167:287, 1988.
189. Shelley GA, Howard RJ: Surgeons' attitudes about patients with HIV-1 infection and AIDS: a national survey. Arch Surg 127:206, 1992.
190. Searle ES: Knowledge, attitudes, and behavior of health professionals in relation to AIDS. Lancet 1:26, 1987.
191. Richardson JL, Lochner T, McGuigan K, Levine AM: Physician attitudes and experience regarding the care of patients with acquired immunodeficiency syndrome (AIDS) and related disorders (ARC). Med Care 25:675, 1987.
192. Condit D, Frater RWM: Human immunodeficiency virus and the cardiac surgeon: a survey of attitudes. Ann Thorac Surg 47:182, 1989.
193. Mandelbrot DA, Smythe WR, Norman SA, et al: A survey of exposures, practices and recommendations of surgeons in the care of patients with human immunodeficiency virus. Surg Gynecol Obstet 171: 99, 1990.
194. Arnow PM, Pottenger LA, Stocking CB, et al: Orthopedic surgeons' attitudes and practices concerning treatment of patients with HIV infection. Public Health Rep 104:121, 1989.
195. Fry DE: Patients and physicians should not be screened for HIV or hepatitis. In Howard RJ (ed): Infectious Risks in Surgery. Norwalk, CT, Appleton & Lange, 1991, pp 111–116.
196. Kuhls TL, Cherry JD: The management of health care workers' accidental parenteral exposures to biological specimens of HIV seropositive individuals. Infect Control 8:211, 1987.
197. Department of Labor: Joint Advisory Notice: Department of Labor/Department of Health and Human Services. Fed Reg 52:41818, 1987.
198. Hendersen DK, Gerberding JL: Prophylactic zidovudine after occupational exposure to the human immunodeficiency virus: an interim analysis. J Infect Dis 160:321, 1989.
199. Centers for Disease Control: Public Health Service statement on management of occupational exposure to human immunodeficiency virus, including considerations regarding zidovudine postexposure use. Morb Mortal Wkly Rep 39(RR-1):1, 1990.
200. Centers for Disease Control: Protection against viral hepatitis. Recommendations of the Immunization Practices Advisory Committee (ACIP). Morb Mortal Wkly Rep 39(RR-2):1, 1990.
201. Welch J, Tilzey A, Webster M, et al: Hepatitis B after gynecological surgery. Lancet 1:205, 1989.
202. Lettau LA, Smith JD, Williams D, et al: Transmission of hepatitis B with resultant restriction of surgical practice. JAMA 255:934, 1986.
203. Communicable Disease Surveillance Centre: Acute hepatitis B associated with gynecological surgery. Lancet 1:1, 1980.
204. Carl M, Francis DP, Blakey DL, et al: Interruption of hepatitis B transmission by modification of a gynaecologist's surgical technique. Lancet 1:731, 1982.
205. Coutinho RA, Albrecht-Van Lent P, Stoutjesdi JKL, et al: Hepatitis B from doctors (letter). Lancet 1:345, 1982.
206. Grob PJ, Bischoff B, Naeff F: Cluster of hepatitis B transmitted by physician. Lancet 2:1218, 1981.
207. Meyers JD, Stamm WE, Kerr MM, et al: Lack of transmission of hepatitis B after surgical exposure. JAMA 240:1725, 1978.
208. Haerem JW, Siebke JC, Ulstrup J, et al: HB_sAg transmission from a cardiac surgeon incubating hepatitis B resulting in chronic antigenemia in four patients. Acta Med Scand 210:389, 1981.
209. A District Control Infection Officer: Acute hepatitis B following gynecological surgery. J Hosp Infect 9:23, 1987.
210. Polakoff S: Acute hepatitis B in patients in Britain related to previous operations and dental treatment. Br J Med 293:33, 1986.
211. Prendergast TJ Jr, Teitelbaum S, Pock B: Transmission of hepatitis B by a surgeon. West J Med 154:353, 1991.
212. Anonymous: Surgeons who are hepatitis B carriers. BMJ 303:184, 1991.
213. Jones D: Hepatitis leaves Halifax surgeon an operating room outcast. Can Med Assoc J 145:1345, 1991.
214. Centers for Disease Control: Recommendations for preventing transmission of human immunodeficiency virus and hepatitis B virus to patients during exposure-prone invasive procedures. Morb Mortal Wkly Rep 40(RR-8):1, 1991.
215. Alter HJ, Chalmers TC, Freeman BM, et al: Health care workers positive for hepatitis B surface antigen. Are their contacts at risk? N Engl J Med 292:454, 1975.
216. Williams SV, Pattison CP, Berquist KR: Dental infection with hepatitis B. JAMA 232:1231, 1975.
217. Gerber MA, Lewm EB, Gerety RJ, et al: The lack of nurse-infant transmission of type B hepatitis in a special care nursery. J Pediatr 91:120, 1977.
218. LaBrecque DR, Dhand AK: The risk of hepatitis B transmission from staff to patients in hemodialysis

units—an overrated problem? Hepatology 1:398, 1981.
219. LaBrecque DR, Muhs JM, Lutwick LI, et al: The risk of hepatitis B transmission from health care workers to patients in a hospital setting—a prospective study. Hepatology 6:205, 1986.
220. Polakoff S: Acute hepatitis B in patients in Britain related to previous operations and dental treatment. BMJ 293:33, 1986.
221. Levin ML, Maddrey WC, Wands JR, Mendeloff AI: Hepatitis B transmission by dentist. JAMA 228:1139, 1974.
222. Reingold AL, Kane MA, Murphy BL, et al: Transmission of hepatitis B by an oral surgeon. J Infect Dis 145:262, 1982.
223. Kane MA, Lettau LA: Transmission of HBV from dental personnel to patients. JAMA 110:634, 1985.
224. Shaw FE Jr, Barrett CL, Hamm R, et al: Lethal outbreak of hepatitis B in a dental practice. JAMA 255:3260, 1986.
225. Heseltine PNR: The HIV- or HBV-infected professional. In Howard RJ (ed): Infectious Risks in Surgery. Norwalk, CT, Appleton & Lange, 1991, pp 139–156.
226. Centers for Disease Control: Update: transmission of HIV infection during an invasive dental procedure—Florida. Morb Mortal Wkly Rep 40:21, 1991.
227. Centers for Disease Control and Prevention: Update: investigations of persons treated by HIV-infected health care workers—United States. Morb Mortal Wkly Rep 42:329, 1993.
228. Sacks JJ: Correspondence: AIDS in a surgeon. N Engl Med 313(16):1017, 1985.
229. Mishu B, Schaffner W, Horan JN, et al: A surgeon with AIDS: lack of evidence of transmission to patients. JAMA 264:467, 1990.
230. Armstrong FP, Miner JC, Wolfe WH, et al. Investigation of health care workers with symptomatic human immunodeficiency virus infection: an epidemiologic approach. Mil Med 152:414, 1987.
231. Porter JD, Cruickshank JG, Gental PH, et al: Management of patients treated by surgeon with HIV infection (letter). Lancet 335:113, 1990.
232. Rogers AS, Froggatt JW III, Townsend T, et al: Investigation of potential HIV transmission to the patients of an HIV-infected surgeon. JAMA 269: 1795, 1993.
233. Von Reyn CF, Gilbert TT, Shaw FE Jr, et al: Absence of HIV transmission from an infected orthopedic surgeon. A 13-year look-back study. JAMA 269:1807, 1993.
234. Altman LK: Rules for AIDS-infected workers are resisted by medical groups. New York Times 140:A1,AB, 1991.

ANTIMICROBIAL THERAPY PART V

Antimicrobial Agents CHAPTER 28

Joseph S. Solomkin, Richard J. Howard

PRINCIPLES OF THERAPY

Antimicrobial therapy is an essential component of surgical practice. Prophylactic usage of antibiotics has not only reduced infection rates following elective and emergency operation but has also allowed the development and application of extended surgical procedures. Appropriate antibiotic therapy for established infection, in conjunction with early diagnosis, a well-conceived and executed operative procedure, and hemodynamic, respiratory, and nutritional support, reduces the incidence of failure and death from intra-abdominal, soft tissue, and other forms of infection requiring physical intervention. The principles of antimicrobial therapy for infections treated by operative or percutaneous intervention are similar to those for other forms of infection.

The past decade has seen an extraordinary number of new antibiotics released. The four major classes of these antibacterial agents include extended spectrum penicillin derivatives and beta-lactamase inhibitors, cephalosporins, carbapenems, and quinolones. Imidazole therapy for fungal infections has also been developed to the point of replacing amphotericin B in some clinical situations. These newer agents have challenged traditional concepts of anti-infective therapy and in many clinical settings have become agents of choice. Table 28–1 lists appropriate antimicrobial drugs for common pathogens.

The downside of progress has been an increasing incidence of multidrug-resistant organisms causing nosocomial infections, particularly *Enterobacter* species, *Pseudomonas aeruginosa,* and methicillin-resistant *Staphylococcus aureus* and *S. epidermidis.* Nosocomial infections caused by *Enterococcus* and *Candida* species are also increasingly common, due in part to potent broad spectrum antibiotic therapy. The emergence of these organisms has complicated management of nosocomial infection.

Viral infections in transplant, chemotherapy, and acquired immunodeficiency syndrome (AIDS) patients have also moved into the arena of surgical infections, as have a range of previously uncommon fungal infections.

Value of Precise Identification of Infecting Organism(s)

In vitro data, especially antimicrobial susceptibility tests, are predictive of the in vivo response of infecting bacteria to particular antibacterial agents. Such data also allow selection of a specific agent or combination regimen and obviate the need for broad spectrum therapy. These are the primary reasons to obtain cultures of sites of infection. In many infections, equally important information can

TABLE 28–1. ANTIBACTERIAL DRUGS OF CHOICE

Infecting Organism	Drug of First Choice	Alternative Drugs
Gram-positive Cocci		
Enterococcus[a]		
Endocarditis or other severe infection	Penicillin G or ampicillin with gentamicin or amikacin	Vancomycin with gentamicin or amikacin
Uncomplicated urinary tract infection	Ampicillin or amoxicillin	Nitrofurantoin; a fluoroquinolone[b]
Staphylococcus aureus or *epidermidis*[c]		
Non-penicillinase producing	Penicillin G or V[d]	A cephalosporin[e,f]; vancomycin; imipenem; clindamycin; a fluoroquinolone[b]
Penicillinase-producing	A penicillinase-resistant penicillin[g]	A cephalosporin[e,f]; vancomycin; amoxicillin-clavulanic acid; ticarcillin-clavulanic acid; ampicillin-sulbactam; piperacillin-tazobactam; imipenem; clindamycin; a fluoroquinolone[2]
Methicillin-resistant[h]	Vancomycin, with or without gentamicin, and/or rifampin	Trimethoprim-sulfamethoxazole; minocycline[i]
Streptococcus pyogenes (Group A) and Groups C and G	Penicillin G or V[d]	An erythromycin[j]; a cephalosporin[e,f]; vancomycin; clarithromycin; azithromycin; clindamycin[j]
Streptococcus, Group B[c]	Penicillin G or ampicillin	A cephalosporin[e,f]; vancomycin; an erythromycin
Streptococcus, viridans group[a]	Penicillin G with or without gentamicin	A cephalosporin[e,f]; vancomycin
Streptococcus bovis[a]	Penicillin G	A cephalosporin[e,f]; vancomycin
Streptococcus, anaerobic or *Peptostreptococcus*	Penicillin G	Clindamycin; a cephalosporin[e,f]; vancomycin
Streptococcus pneumoniae[c,k] (pneumococcus)	Penicillin G or V[d]	An erythromycin; a cephalosporin[e,f]; chloramphenicol[l]; vancomycin with or without rifampin
Gram-negative Cocci		
Moraxella (*Branhamella*) *catarrhalis*	Trimethoprim-sulfamethoxazole	Amoxicillin-clavulanic acid; an erythromycin; clarithromycin; azithromycin; a tetracycline[i]; cefuroxime[e]; cefotaxime[e]; ceftizoxime[e]; ceftriaxone[e]; cefuroxime axetil[e]; cefixime[e]
Neisseria gonorrhoeae[c,m] (gonococcus)	Ceftriaxone[e]	Spectinomycin; a fluoroquinolone[b]; penicillin G; amoxicillin with probenecid; cefotaxime[e]; cefoxitin[e]; cefixime[e]; trimethoprim-sulfamethoxazole; chloramphenicol[l]
Neisseria meningitidis[n] (meningococcus)	Penicillin G	Cefotaxime[e]; ceftizoxime[e]; ceftriaxone[e]; chloramphenicol[l]; a sulfonamide[o]
Gram-positive Bacilli		
Bacillus anthracis (anthrax)	Penicillin G	An erythromycin; a tetracycline[i]
Clostridium perfringens[p]	Penicillin G	Chloramphenicol[l]; metronidazole; clindamycin; a tetracycline[i]
Clostridium tetani[q]	Penicillin G	A tetracycline[i]
Clostridium difficile[r]	Vancomycin or metronidazole	Bacitracin
Corynebacterium diphtheriae[s]	An erythromycin	Penicillin G
Corynebacterium, JK group	Vancomycin	Penicillin G plus gentamicin
Listeria monocytogenes	Ampicillin with or without gentamicin	Trimethoprim-sulfamethoxazole
Enteric Gram-negative Bacilli		
Bacteroides[c]		
Oropharyngeal strains	Penicillin G[t]	Clindamycin; cefoxitin[e]; metronidazole; chloramphenicol[l]; cefotetan[e]

TABLE 28–1. *(continued)*

Infecting Organism	Drug of First Choice	Alternative Drugs
Gastrointestinal strains[u]	Metronidazole	Clindamycin; imipenem; ticarcillin-clavulanic acid; cefoxitin[e]; cefotetan[e]; ampicillin-sulbactam; piperacillin-tazobactam; chloramphenicol[l]; ceftizoxime[e]; cefmetazole[e]
Campylobacter jejuni[c]	A fluoroquinolone[b] or an erythromycin	A tetracycline[i]; gentamicin
Enterobacter[c]	Imipenem[v]	Cefotaxime,[e,v] ceftizoxime,[e,v] ceftriaxone,[e,v] or ceftazidime[e,v]; gentamicin, tobramycin, or amikacin; trimethoprim-sulfamethoxazole; carbenicillin,[w] ticarcillin,[w] mezlocillin,[w] or piperacillin[w]; aztreonam[v]; a fluoroquinolone[b]
Escherichia coli[c,x]	Cefotaxime, ceftizoxime, ceftriaxone, or ceftazidime[e,v]	Ampicillin with or without gentamicin, tobramycin, or amikacin; ticarcillin,[w] mezlocillin,[w] or piperacillin[w]; gentamicin, tobramycin, or amikacin; amoxicillin-clavulanic acid[v]; ticarcillin-clavulanic acid[w]; ampicillin-sulbactam[v]; piperacillin-tazobactam; trimethoprim-sulfamethoxazole; imipenem[v]; aztreonam[v]; a fluoroquinolone[b]; another cephalosporin[e,f]
Helicobacter pylori[c]	A tetracycline[i] plus metronidazole plus bismuth subsalicylate[y]	
Klebsiella pneumoniae[c,x]	Cefotaxime, ceftizoxime, ceftriaxone, or ceftazidime[e,v]	Gentamicin, tobramycin, or amikacin; amoxicillin-clavulanic acid[v]; ticarcillin-clavulanic acid[w]; ampicillin-sulbactam[v]; piperacillin-tazobactam; trimethoprim-sulfamethoxazole; imipenem[v]; aztreonam[v]; a fluoroquinolone[b]; mezlocillin[w] or piperacillin[w]; another cephalosporin[e,f]
Proteus mirabilis[c,x]	Ampicillin[z]	A cephalosporin[e,f,v]; ticarcillin,[w] mezlocillin,[w] or piperacillin[w]; gentamicin, tobramycin, or amikacin; trimethoprim-sulfamethoxazole; aztreonam[v]; a fluoroquinolone[b]; chloramphenicol[l]
Proteus,[c] indole-positive (including *Providencia rettgeri, Morganella morganii,* and *Proteus vulgaris*)	Cefotaxime, ceftizoxime, ceftriaxone, or ceftazidime[e,v]	Imipenem[v]; gentamicin, tobramycin, or amikacin; carbenicillin,[w] ticarcillin,[w] mezlocillin,[w] or piperacillin[w]; amoxicillin-clavulanic acid[v]; ticarcillin-clavulanic acid[w]; ampicillin-sulbactam[v]; piperacillin-tazobactam; aztreonam[v]; trimethoprim-sulfamethoxazole; a fluoroquinolone[b]
Providencia stuartii[c]	Cefotaxime, ceftizoxime, ceftriaxone, or ceftazidime[e,v]	Imipenem[v]; ticarcillin-clavulanic acid[w]; gentamicin, tobramycin, or amikacin; ticarcillin,[w] mezlocillin,[w] or piperacillin[w]; aztreonam[v]; trimethoprim-sulfamethoxazole; a fluoroquinolone[b]
Salmonella typhi[c,aa]	Ceftriaxone[e]	Chloramphenicol[l]; ampicillin; amoxicillin; trimethoprim-sulfamethoxazole; a fluoroquinolone[b]
Other *Salmonella*[c,bb]	Cefotaxime[e] or ceftriaxone[e]	Ampicillin or amoxicillin; trimethoprim-sulfamethoxazole; a fluoroquinolone[b]; chloramphenicol[l]
Serratia[c]	Cefotaxime, ceftizoxime, ceftriaxone, or ceftazidime[e,cc]	Gentamicin or amikacin; imipenem[cc]; aztreonam[cc]; trimethoprim-sulfamethoxazole; carbenicillin,[dd] ticarcillin,[dd] mezlocillin,[dd] or piperacillin[dd]; a fluoroquinolone[b]

TABLE 28–1. *(continued)*

Infecting Organism	Drug of First Choice	Alternative Drugs
Shigella[c]	A fluoroquinolone[b]	Trimethoprim-sulfamethoxazole; ampicillin; ceftriaxone[e]
Yersinia enterocolitica[c]	Trimethoprim-sulfamethoxazole	A fluoroquinolone[b]; gentamicin, tobramycin, or amikacin; cefotaxmine[e] or ceftizoxime[e]
Other Gram-negative Bacilli		
Acinetobacter[c]	Imipenem[v]	Tobramycin, gentamicin, or amikacin; ticarcillin,[w] mezlocillin,[w] or piperacillin[w]; trimethoprim-sulfamethoxazole; minocycline[i]; doxycycline[i]
Aeromonas[c]	Trimethoprim-sulfamethoxazole	Gentamicin or tobramycin; imipenem; a fluoroquinolone[b]
Bordetella pertussis (whooping cough)	An erythromycin	Trimethoprim-sulfamethoxazole; ampicillin
Brucella[c]	A tetracycline[i] with gentamicin	Chloramphenicol[l] with or without streptomycin; trimethoprim-sulfamethoxazole; rifampin with a tetracycline[i]
Calymmatobacterium granulomatis (granuloma inguinale)	A tetracycline[i]	Streptomycin; trimethoprim-sulfamethoxazole; an erythromycin
Eikenella corrodens[c]	Ampicillin	An erythromycin; a tetracycline[i]; amoxicillin-clavulanic acid; ampicillin-sulbactam; ceftriaxone
Francisella tularensis (tularemia)[c]	Streptomycin or gentamicin	A tetracycline[i]; chloramphenicol[l]
Fusobacterium[c]	Penicillin G	Metronidazole; clindamycin; chloramphenicol[l]
Gardnerella (Haemophilus) vaginalis[ee]	Metronidazole	Ampicillin
Haemophilus ducreyi (chancroid)[c]	Ceftriaxone[e] or an erythromycin	Ciprofloxacin[ff]
Haemophilus influenzae[c]		
Meningitis, epiglottitis, arthritis, and other serious infections	Cefotaxime or ceftriaxone[e]	Cefuroxime[e] (for pneumonia); chloramphenicol[l]
Upper respiratory infections and bronchitis	Trimethoprim-sulfamethoxazole	Ampicillin or amoxicillin; cefuroxime[e]; a sulfonamide with or without an erythromycin; amoxicillin-clavulanic acid; cefuroxime axetil[e]; cefaclor[e]; cefotaxime[e]; ceftizoxime[e]; ceftriaxone[e]; cefixime[e]; a tetracycline[i]; clarithromycin; azithromycin
Legionella species	An erythromycin plus rifampin	Trimethoprim-sulfamethoxazole; clarithromycin; azithromycin; ciprofloxacin[ff]
Leptotrichia buccalis	Penicillin G	A tetracycline[i]; clindamycin; an erythromycin
Pasteurella multocida	Penicillin G	A tetracycline[i]; a cephalosporin[e,f]; amoxicillin-clavulanic acid; ampicillin-sulbactam
Pseudomonas aeruginosa[c]		
Urinary tract infection	Ciprofloxacin[ff]	Carbenicillin, ticarcillin, piperacillin, or mezlocillin; ceftazidime[e]; imipenem; aztreonam; gentamicin; tobramycin; amikacin
Other infections	Ticarcillin, mezlocillin, or piperacillin plus tobramycin, gentamicin, or amikacin[gg]	Ceftazidime,[e] imipenem, or aztreonam plus tobramycin, gentamicin, or amikacin; ciprofloxacin[ff]
Pseudomonas mallei (glanders)	Streptomycin with a tetracycline[i]	Streptomycin with chloramphenicol[l]
Pseudomonas pseudomallei[c] (melioidosis)	Ceftazidime[e]	Chloramphenicol[l] with doxycycline[i] and trimethoprim-sulfamethoxazole; amoxicillin-clavulanic acid
Pseudomonas cepacia[c]	Trimethoprim-sulfamethoxazole	Chloramphenicol[l]; ceftazidime[e]

TABLE 28–1. *(continued)*

Infecting Organism	Drug of First Choice	Alternative Drugs
Spirillum minus (rat bite fever)	Penicillin G	A tetracycline[i]; streptomycin
Streptobacillus moniliformis (rat bite fever; Haverhill fever)	Penicillin G	A tetracycline[i]; streptomycin
Vibrio cholerae (cholera)	A tetracycline[i]	Trimethoprim-sulfamethoxazole; a fluoroquinolone[b]
Vibrio vulnificus	A tetracycline[i]	Cefotaxime[e]
Xanthomonas maltophilia[c] (Pseudomonas maltophilia)	Trimethoprim-sulfamethoxazole	Minocycline[i]; ceftazidime[e]; a fluoroquinolone[b]
Yersinia pestis (plague)	Streptomycin	A tetracycline[i]; chloramphenicol[l]; gentamicin
Acid-fast Bacilli		
Mycobacterium tuberculosis[c,ii]	Isoniazid with rifampin and pyrazinamide with or without ethambutol	Ethambutol; streptomycin[l]; cycloserine[l]; ethionamide[l]; kanamycin[l]; capreomycin[l]; ciprofloxacin[ff]; ofloxacin[ff]
Mycobacterium kansasii[c]	Isoniazid with rifampin with or without ethambutol or streptomycin[l]	Ethionamide[l]; cycloserine[l]
Mycobacterium avium complex[c]	Clarithromycin[jj] ± rifampin ± ethambutol ± clofazimine	Rifampin with ethambutol, ciprofloxacin,[ff] and clofazimine, with or without amikacin[l]; azithromycin[jj]; ethionamide[l]; cycloserine[l]; rifabutin (ansamycin)[kk]; imipenem
Mycobacterium fortuitum[c] complex	Amikacin[l] and doxycycline[i]	Cefoxitin[e]; rifampin; an erythromycin; a sulfonamide
Mycobacterium marinum (balnei)[ll]	Minocycline[i]	Trimethoprim-sulfamethoxazole; rifampin; clarithromycin
Mycobacterium leprae (leprosy)	Dapsone with rifampin with or without clofazimine	Minocycline[i]; protionamide[l,kk]; ofloxacin[ff,mm]
Actinomycetes		
Actinomyces israelii (actinomycosis)	Penicillin G	A tetracycline[i]
Nocardia	Trimethoprim-sulfamethoxazole	Sulfisoxazole; amikacin[l]; minocycline[i]; imipenem; cycloserine[l]
Chlamydiae		
Chlamydia psittaci (psittacosis; ornithosis)	A tetracycline[i]	Chloramphenicol[l]
Chlamydia trachomatis (trachoma)	A tetracycline[i] (topical plus oral)	A sulfonamide (topical plus oral)
Inclusion conjunctivitis	An erythromycin (oral or IV)	A sulfonamide
Pneumonia	An erythromycin	A sulfonamide
Urethritis, cervicitis	A tetracycline[i] or an erythromycin	Azithromycin; ofloxacin[ff]; sulfisoxazole
Lymphogranuloma venereum	A tetracycline[i] or an erythromycin	
Chlamydia pneumoniae (TWAR strain)	A tetracycline[i]	An erythromycin; clarithromycin
Mycoplasma		
Mycoplasma pneumoniae	An erythromycin or a tetracycline[i]	Clarithromycin
Ureaplasma urealyticum	An erythromycin	A tetracycline[i]; clarithromycin
Rickettsia		
Rocky Mountain spotted fever, endemic typhus (murine), epidemic typhus (louse-borne), scrub typhus, trench fever, Q fever, human ehrlichiosis[nn]	A tetracycline[i]	Chloramphenicol[l,oo]; a fluoroquinolone[b]
Spirochetes		
Borrelia burgdorferi[pp] (Lyme disease)	A tetracycline[i]	Ceftriaxone[e]; cefotaxime[e]; penicillin G or V; amoxicillin; an erythromycin; azithromycin; clarithromycin
Borrelia recurrentis (relapsing fever)	A tetracycline[i]	Penicillin G
Leptospira	Penicillin G	A tetracycline[i]

TABLE 28–1. *(continued)*

Infecting Organism	Drug of First Choice	Alternative Drugs
Treponema pallidum[m]	Penicillin G	A tetracycline[i]; ceftriaxone[e]
Treponema pertenue (yaws)	Penicillin G	A tetracycline[i]
Miscellaneous		
Agent of bacillary angiomatosis (*Rochalimaea henselae*)	An erythromycin	A tetracycline[i]
Cat scratch bacillus (*Afipia felis*)	Ciprofloxacin[qq]	Trimethoprim-sulfamethoxazole; gentamicin

[a] Disk sensitivity testing may not provide adequate information; beta-lactamase assays and dilution tests for susceptibility should be used in serious infections, and in endocarditis should assess bactericidal as well as inhibitory end points.
[b] Ciprofloxacin or ofloxacin. Norfloxacin or lomefloxacin should only be used for treatment of urinary tract infections. Only ciprofloxacin is available for intravenous use. None of these agents is recommended for children.
[c] Resistance may be a problem; susceptibility tests should be performed.
[d] Penicillin V is preferred for oral treatment of infections caused by non-penicillinase-producing staphylococci and other gram-positive cocci. For initial therapy of severe infections, penicillin G, administered parenterally, is first choice. For somewhat longer action in less severe infections due to group A streptococci, pneumococci, or *Treponema pallidum,* procaine penicillin G, an intramuscular formulation, is given once or twice daily. Benzathine penicillin G, a slowly absorbed preparation, is usually given in a single monthly injection for prophylaxis of rheumatic fever, once for treatment of group A streptococcal pharyngitis, and once or more for treatment of syphilis.
[e] The cephalosporins have been used as alternatives to penicillins in patients allergic to penicillins, but such patients may also have allergic reactions to cephalosporins.
[f] For parenteral treatment of staphylococcal or non-enterococcal streptococcal infections, a first-generation cephalosporin such as cephalothin or cefazolin can be used; for staphylococcal endocarditis, some *Medical Letter* consultants prefer cephalothin. For oral therapy, cephalexin or cephradine can be used. The second-generation cephalosporins, cefamandole, cefuroxime, cefuroxime axetil, cefonicid, cefotetan, cefmetazole, and cefoxitin, are more active than the first-generation drugs against gram-negative bacteria. Cefuroxime and cefamandole are active against ampicillin-resistant strains of *H. influenzae,* but cefamandole has been associated with prothrombin deficiency and occasional bleeding. Cefoxitin, cefotetan, and cefmetazole have moderate activity against *B. fragilis.* The third-generation cephalosporins, cefotaxime, cefoperazone, ceftizoxime, ceftriaxone, and ceftazidime, have greater activity than the second-generation drugs against enteric gram-negative bacilli. Moxalactam, another third-generation cephalosporin, has been associated with serious, sometimes fatal, bleeding disorders, and *Medical Letter* consultants now advise against its use; in any case, it should not be used to treat infections caused by gram-positive organisms. Cefixime is an oral cephalosporin with more activity than second-generation cephalosporins against facultative gram-negative bacilli, but no useful activity against staphylococci, anaerobes, or *Pseudomonas aeruginosa* (*Med Lett 31:73, 1989*). With the exception of cefoperazone (which can also cause bleeding) and ceftazidime, the activity of all currently available cephalosporins against *Pseudomonas aeruginosa* is poor or inconsistent.
[g] For oral use against penicillinase-producing staphylococci, cloxacillin or dicloxacillin is preferred; for severe infections, a parenteral formulation of methicillin, nafcillin, or oxacillin should be used. Neither ampicillin, amoxicillin, bacampicillin, cyclacillin, hetacillin, carbenicillin, ticarcillin, mezlocillin, nor piperacillin is effective against penicillinase-producing staphylococci. The combinations of clavulanic acid with amoxicillin or ticarcillin of sulbactam with ampicillin and piperacillin with tazobactam are, however, active against these organisms.
[h] Occasional strains of coagulase-positive staphylococci and many strains of coagulase-negative staphylococci are resistant to penicillinase-resistant penicillins; these strains are also resistant to cephalosporins and imipenem. Some of these strains are susceptible to ciprofloxacin, which may be useful when the organism is resistant to other oral antimicrobials.
[i] Tetracyclines are generally not recommended for pregnant women or children less than eight years old.
[j] Occasional strains of group A streptococci may be resistant to erythromycins and clindamycin (*Seppälä H, et al: N Engl J Med 326:292, 1992*).
[k] In patients allergic to penicillin, an erythromycin is preferred for respiratory infections and chloramphenicol is generally recommended for meningitis. Rare strains of *Streptococcus pneumoniae* may be resistant to chloramphenicol, and rare strains may be relatively resistant or resistant to penicillin. These strains are susceptible to vancomycin, but in some patients vancomycin may not reach effective levels in spinal fluid (*Viladrick PF, et al: Antimicrob Agents Chemother 35:2467, 1991*). The addition of rifampin or substitution of ceftriaxone may be useful for such patients.
[l] Because of the possibility of serious adverse effects, this drug should be used only for severe infections when less hazardous drugs are ineffective.
[m] For more details, see *Med Lett 33:119, 1991.*
[n] Rare strains of *N. meningitidis* are resistant or relatively resistant to penicillin (*Riley G, et al: N Engl J Med 324:997, 1991*). Rifampin is recommended for prophylaxis in close contacts of patients infected by sulfonamide-resistant organisms.
[o] Sulfonamide-resistant strains are frequent in the United States and sulfonamides should be used only when susceptibility is established by susceptibility tests.
[p] Debridement is primary. Large doses of penicillin G are required. Hyperbaric oxygen therapy may be a useful adjunct to surgical debridement in management of the spreading, necrotic type.
[q] For prophylaxis, a tetanus toxoid booster and, for some patients, tetanus immune globulin (human) are required.
[r] For more details, see *Med Lett 31:94, 1989.*
[s] Antitoxin is primary; antimicrobials are used only to halt further toxin production and to prevent the carrier state.
[t] *Bacteroides* species from the oropharynx may be resistant to penicillin; for patients seriously ill with infections that may be due to these organisms, or when response to penicillin is delayed, clindamycin is preferred.
[u] When infection is in the central nervous system, either intravenous metronidazole or chloramphenicol is recommended.
[v] In severely ill patients, some *Medical Letter* consultants would add gentamicin, tobramycin, or amikacin.
[w] In severely ill patients, some *Medical Letter* consultants would add gentamicin, tobramycin, or amikacin (but see footnote gg).
[x] For an acute, uncomplicated urinary tract infection, before the infecting organism is known, the drug of first choice is trimethoprim-sulfamethoxazole.
[y] *Graham DY, et al: Ann Intern Med 116:705, 1992.*
[z] Large doses (6 g or more daily) are usually necessary for systemic infections. In severely ill patients, some *Medical Letter* consultants would add gentamicin, tobramycin, or amikacin.
[aa] Ampicillin or amoxicillin may be effective in milder cases. Ciprofloxacin or ampicillin is the drug of choice for *S. typhi* carriers.
[bb] Most cases of *Salmonella* gastroenteritis subside spontaneously without antimicrobial therapy.

TABLE 28–1. *(continued)*

[cc] In severely ill patients, some *Medical Letter* consultants would add gentamicin or amikacin.
[dd] In severely ill patients, some *Medical Letter* consultants would add gentamicin or amikacin (but see footnote gg).
[ee] Metronidazole is effective for bacterial vaginosis even though it is not active against *Gardnerella* in vitro. Ampicillin should be used for sepsis.
[ff] Not recommended for use in children.
[gg] Neither gentamicin, tobramycin, netilmicin, nor amikacin should be mixed in the same bottle with carbenicillin, ticarcillin, mezlocillin, or piperacillin for intravenous administration. When used in high concentrations or in patients with renal failure, carbenicillin or ticarcillin may inactivate the aminoglycosides.
[hh] Antibiotic therapy is an adjunct to and not a substitute for prompt fluid and electrolyte replacement.
[ii] For more details, see *Med Lett 34:10, 1992.*
[jj] Because of the rapid emergence of resistance in *M. avium* infections, neither clarithromycin nor azithromycin should be used alone.
[kk] An investigational drug in the United States.
[ll] Most infections are self-limited without drug treatment.
[mm] *Ji B, Grosset J: Acta Leprol 7:321, 1991.*
[nn] *Raoult D, Drancourt M: Antimicrob Agents Chemother 35:2457, 1991.*
[oo] Not recommended for human ehrlichiosis.
[pp] For treatment of early infection in nonpregnant adults, tetracycline is preferred; for fully developed infection with arthritis or meningitis, ceftriaxone is preferred.
[qq] *Holley HP Jr: JAMA, 265:1563, 1991.* Ciprofloxacin is not recommended for use in children.
From Med Lett 34:49, 1992.

be gained from Gram stains of infected fluid collections or, in certain circumstances, in other forms of direct examinations such as KOH or India ink preparations of cerebrospinal fluid for *Cryptococcus* or bronchoalveolar lavage fluid for other fungi.

While a variety of susceptibility testing techniques are available, automated testing is appropriate for bacteria isolated from most infections except in extraordinary circumstances (see Chap. 2). Tables 28–2 and 28–3 summarize the in vitro susceptibilities of acquired pathogens to commonly used anti-infective agents. Certain organisms do not require routine susceptibility testing. Nonenterococcal streptococci are routinely susceptible to penicillin. Because of the technical problems of performing anaerobic susceptibility tests, we believe it best for such isolates to be identified and then batch-tested on a yearly basis for changes in otherwise predictable susceptibilities. This particularly applies to *Bacteroides fragilis* group isolates. Local

TABLE 28–2. ANTIBIOTIC SUSCEPTIBILITIES OF GRAM-NEGATIVE BACTERIA AT THE UNIVERSITY OF FLORIDA, SHANDS HOSPITAL

Gram Negative	Number of Isolates	Amikacin	Ampicillin	Aztreonam	Cefazolin	Cefotetan	Cefuroxime	Ciprofloxacin	Ceftazidime	Ceftriaxone	Gentamicin	Imipenem	Mezlocillin	Timentin	Tobramycin	Trimethoprim/ Sulfamethoxazole
Acinetobacter species	151	78[a]		52	3	19	20	73	82	85	64	94	73	79	74	52
Citrobacter freundii	77	100	39	83	3	77	51	92	61	81	97	100	70	55	97	78
Citrobacter diversus	40	100	5	94	85	82	90	98	100	100	100	100	41	94	100	95
Enterobacter cloaceae	257	99	21	67	1	45	39	93	57	63	95	97	57	56	96	87
Enterobacter aerogenes	79	100	32	95	6	61	54	97	73	88	97	100	69	73	97	94
Escherichia coli	638	99	56	99	87	99	98	99	100	100	97	100	72	96	98	82
Klebsiella pneumoniae	275	100	?	98	92	99	95	97	98	97	96	100	20	94	96	87
Klebsiella oxytoca	29	100	3	100	31	94	86	100	100	100	90	100	18	88	90	90
Morganella morganii	27	96	4	100	0	93	37	100	89	100	96	93	87	100	100	96
Proteus mirabilis	144	99	90	97	92	99	97	99	100	98	94	78	89	95	94	92
Providencia stuartii	17	94	12	92	0	92	59	88	94	100	59	100	100	92	53	88
Providencia rettgeri	10	100	60	100	30		90	100	90	100	100				100	60
Pseudomonas aeruginosa	777	91		82	1	6	2	86	86	62	79	90	74	81	95	22
Salmonella enteriditis	22	100	86	95	95	100	95	100	100	100	95	95	86	91	100	100
Serratia marcescens	91	97	39	83	0	96	14	99	79	93	97	70	88	97	87	99
Xanthomonas maltophilia	64	48		25	6	79	6	63	72	21	40	14	65	91	30	95

[a] Percentage of isolates susceptible.

TABLE 28–3. ANTIBIOTIC SUSCEPTIBILITIES OF GRAM-POSITIVE COCCI AT THE UNIVERSITY OF FLORIDA, SHANDS HOSPITAL

Gram Positive	Number of Isolates	Ampicillin	Augmentin	Cefazolin	Ciprofloxacin	Clindamycin	Erythromycin	Gentamicin	Imipenem	Oxacillin (NF)	Penicillin G	Rifampin	Tetracycline	Trimethoprim/Sulfamethoxazole	Vancomycin
Staphylococcus aureus	426	11[a]	87	87	86	86	51	89	87	87	12	99	92	93	100
Staphylococcus epidermidis	323	7	32	32	76	60	35	54	32	32	8	98	78	93	100
Enterococcus faecalis		51	100	100							100				100

[a] Percentage of isolates susceptible.

or regional hospital antimicrobial susceptibility patterns should be heeded in selecting initial empiric therapy.[1,2]

Fluid collections, particularly if purulent, should be obtained for Gram smear and culture. Specimens of infected fluid are sent to the laboratory either in a capped airless syringe with no needle or in appropriate separate aerobic and anaerobic transport media. If the Gram stain reveals a predominance of gram-positive cocci, which may indicate that the *Enterococcus* or other fecal streptococci are significant copathogens, the clinician should consider alterations in the antibiotic regime to include agents specifically active against *Enterococcus*.

If the smear reveals gram-negative bacilli, failure to isolate either facultative or obligate anaerobes on culture does not obviate the need to continue to provide antimicrobial agents against both. Conversely, failure to identify organisms on Gram stain in the presence of purulence will occur if organisms are present at a density less than 10^5/ml. A negative Gram stain should not prompt discontinuance of antibiotics until culture results are available and a clinical response has been achieved.

Antibiotic Susceptibility Testing

The disk-diffusion method provides qualitative data about the susceptibility of an organism to a given agent. Quantitative data require serial solutions of the antimicrobial agent media. The lowest concentration of the agent that prevents visible growth after an 18- to 24-hour incubation period is known as the minimum inhibitory concentration (MIC). The minimal bactericidal concentration (MBC) can be determined by subculturing on antibiotic-free medium those tubes that show no growth in the determination of the MIC.

There are a number of common errors in the interpretation of sensitivity results from hospital laboratories. Certain agents are tested at concentrations achievable only in urine. Such agents include nalidixic acid, nitrofurantoin, and norfloxacin. Susceptibility results for such agents are not meaningful for the management of systemic infections and treatment failure may result if used. Conversely, some nontoxic antibiotics for urinary tract infections, such as ampicillin, are not tested at the high concentrations achieved in urine and may be effective even though "resistance" is reported. Intravascular infections such as endocarditis or catheter-related bacteremia may be treated inadequately by bacteriostatic agents despite in vitro susceptibility testing suggesting efficacy.

Perhaps the most important caveat is the fact that concentrations of bacteria employed in susceptibility testing are considerably below those found in clinical situations. Antibiotics effective at the lower bacterial concentrations may not necessarily be effective at the higher inoculum. This bacterial concentration dependence of antibiotic efficacy is termed the inoculum effect and is prominent for beta-lactam antibiotics.

Treatment Failure and Its Prevention

Treatment response is defined as a diminution in the physical signs of infection including decrease in fever, tachycardia, and local findings of tenderness and organ dysfunction (such as ileus). The more localized the initial infection, the more rapidly response will occur; conversely, extensive infections such as peritonitis or multilobar pneumonia may respond only slowly. As a general rule, infections should show definite evidence of response within 72 hours of initiation of treatment. The absence of such a response is not an automatic indication that the wrong antibiotic was selected. In fact, most cases of apparent treatment failure call for continuation of the same antibiotic. Potential bases for inadequate response are detailed in Table 28–4. A

TABLE 28–4. POSSIBLE CAUSES OF ANTIBIOTIC TREATMENT FAILURE

Inappropriate Antibiotic
1. Organism not susceptible to antibiotic at concentrations achievable in focus of infection.
2. Superinfection (or erroneous initial diagnosis).
3. New, unrelated infection elsewhere in body.
4. Failure of drug to reach site of infection (eg, because of shock or poor penetration of drug into appropriate body compartment such as not passing into central nervous system and cerebrospinal fluid).
5. Bacteria in a dormant state or present as wall-deficient form when growth of cell wall must be present for antibiotic action.
6. Inactivation of antibiotic (penicillins, cephalosporins) by bacterial enzymes (beta-lactamases).
Appropriate Antibiotic but Insufficient Treatment
7. Too small a dose of drug given or dose given too infrequently.
8. Course of therapy too short.
9. Drug administered by inappropriate route (eg, orally rather than intravenously).
10. Wrong preparation of appropriate drug (eg, procaine benzylpenicillin, which yields very low blood levels, rather than aqueous crystalline penicillin, which yields very high serum levels, when high levels are required).
Appropriate Antibiotic but Other Therapy Required
11. Failure to institute appropriate measures in addition to prescribing antibiotics (eg, surgical drainage, debridement, replace blood volume, correct metabolic disorders).
12. Failure to prescribe necessary adjuvant medication (eg, acidifying or alkalinizing medication in certain instances of urinary tract infections).
13. Presence of substances (indigenous or prescribed) that antagonize the antibacterial activity of the drug being used.
14. Impaired host defenses (cellular, humoral, or nutritional, naturally occurring or secondary to physical or chemical injury).
15. Treatment started too late, that is, after changes had been initiated that cannot be stopped or reversed by effective chemotherapy.

diligent search should be made for a septic focus requiring drainage, debridement, or excision.

Enhancing the Activity of Antibiotics. In some special situations, the conventional activity of an antibiotic may be increased or decreased. For example, in urinary tract infections, the pH of the urine can easily be changed. The aminoglycosides and erythromycins are much more active in an alkaline medium, whereas others are more active in an acidic medium (tetracyclines, mandelamine, nitrofurantoin). NH_4Cl or ascorbic acid (usually 4 to 8 g/day) can be given to acidify the urine, or $NaHCO_3$ (8 to 18 g/day) or acetazolamide (0.5 to 2.0 g/day) to alkalinize the urine. The activity of the antibiotic may frequently be increased 100-fold, and in some instances 500-fold.[3] Obviously, evaluation of the patient's overall condition must be made to determine whether administration of these acidifying or alkalinizing agents would be contraindicated. With these techniques, erythromycin plus alkali can be as effective as conventional therapy in urinary tract infections caused by gram-negative bacilli,[4] or the dose of potentially toxic agents (eg, gentamicin) can be drastically reduced if the urine is made alkaline.[3]

A second technique for enhancing antibacterial activity is to combine antibiotics for a synergistic effect, such as treating enterococcal or staphylococcal endocarditis with a penicillin plus an aminoglycoside. A similar synergistic effect is achieved by carbenicillin plus gentamicin against *Pseudomonas aeruginosa.*[5]

A third technique for increasing the activity of a given dose of antibiotic is to delay its excretion. By administering probenecid, 0.5 g, every 6 hours to an average-weight adult, the peak serum concentrations of most penicillins and cephalosporins can be doubled, and the duration of effective serum antibiotic concentrations can be prolonged. Probenecid competes with the penicillins for the active transport mechanism in the renal tubules, which are responsible for 80 percent of the excretion. We usually prescribe probenecid along with benzylpenicillin for adults with normal renal function in whom 10 million or more units of benzylpenicillin per day (or comparable amounts of other penicillins or cephalosporins) are recommended.

A fourth method for increasing the activity of a given antibiotic is to increase its dose. Increasing the dose of the cephalosporins, for example, which after standard doses achieve levels of 50 to 100 μ/ml in the blood, have greatly augmented their spectrum, especially with respect to *Bacteroides fragilis.* Doses of many nontoxic drugs can be safely increased—especially the penicillins and cephalosporins. A fifth method for increasing activity is to give an agent (eg, clavulanic acid, sulbactam, tazobactam) that inhibits enzymes (eg, beta-lactamases) responsible for inactivating the penicillins. Clavulanic acid combined with amoxicillin (Augmentin), ticarcillin (Timentin), or sulbactam combined with ampicillin (Urasyn), or tazobactam combined with piperacillin (Tazosyn) are currently available.

An additional method of increasing the total dose is to prolong the therapy. Effective therapy should not be arbitrarily discontinued unless the infection is under control. By similar reasoning, systemic intravenous therapy should not be prematurely changed to oral therapy with its resultant lower serum levels. Determining the point of discontinuation of therapy is difficult—the lack of febrile response does not necessarily indicate a cure.

Continuing therapy for arbitrarily prolonged periods may sometimes be necessary to prevent relapse of fungal or more chronic infections. Unfortunately, rigid data on the proper duration of therapy are lacking.

Responses to appropriate antibiotics may be improved by changing the route of administration. Oral administration is seldom sufficient in patients with serious deep tissue infections. Intramuscular therapy may fail to achieve adequate serum levels in patients with unstable hemodynamic responses. Intravenous therapy should, therefore, be used in patients with severe life-threatening infections, and maintained until the patient is clearly improved.

Presumptive or Empiric Therapy: Community-Acquired Versus Nosocomial Infections

Because of the effectiveness of antibiotic treatment for infection, antimicrobials are often begun if infection is even a remote possibility in the differential diagnosis for a particular patient. The wisdom of this approach depends on the evidence suggesting an infection, taken against the background risk of harm to the patient. Antimicrobial treatment is not without potential adverse effects, but these generally are perceived as temporally remote, such as changes in hospital- or unit-specific susceptibility patterns.

For patients with suspected community-acquired infection, recent onset of malaise, symptoms referable to a specific anatomic area, and physical findings of fever and localizing tenderness, mass, or evidence of organ dysfunction, are often sufficient to begin antimicrobial therapy after appropriate cultures are obtained. Except for certain forms of meningitis, the timing of initiation of antibiotic therapy is not critical. In patients with localized abscesses, antibiotics will reduce fever and other manifestations of systemic response, but over a 24- to 36-hour interval. Antibiotics should be administered after fluid resuscitation has begun to provide better distribution of the drug(s).

In the case of suspected community-acquired infection, knowledge of the endogenous flora giving rise to infection is a valuable guide to selection of antibiotic therapy while awaiting the results of cultures (see Chap. 3). The gastrointestinal tract is the primary reservoir for organisms causing infection, ranging from aspiration of oral flora (pneumonia) to gastrointestinal perforation (intra-abdominal abscess or peritonitis). The identity and density of microorganisms depend on the level of the gastrointestinal tract. In general, gastric, duodenal, and proximal jejunal contents include small numbers of gram-positive aerobic and gram-negative anaerobic organisms. These organisms are generally susceptible to beta-lactam antibiotics and are rapidly eradicated by host defense mechanisms in intact hosts. About 20 percent of patients with acute perforations of the gastrointestinal tract will release *Candida albicans* or other fungi.[6] Unless the patient has recently received immunosuppressive therapy for neoplasm, transplantation, or inflammatory disease or has recurrent intra-abdominal infection, no specific therapy needs to be given. The distal small bowel harbors gram-negative facultative organisms with variable density. Colonic anaerobes such as *Bacteroides fragilis* are variably present. Patients with colon-derived intra-abdominal infections contaminate the peritoneal cavity with large numbers of facultative and anaerobic gram-negative organisms.

Infections in hospitalized patients, particularly in the intensive care unit, require a different set of criteria for beginning antimicrobial therapy. Such patients have often undergone extensive operative procedures and have numerous potential causes for fever not due to infection. Conversely, infection may be masked by immunosuppression associated with the condition (or treatment) resulting in hospitalization. Perhaps more importantly, such patients become colonized and cultures of sputum, wounds, and drain tracts are often positive in the absence of infection. Interpretation of culture results is therefore quite difficult unless positive cultures are obtained from a routinely sterile site such as blood, pleural fluid, or peritoneal fluid.

Rationale for Selection of Antibacterial Agents

The primary issue is whether currently available single agents are adequate for the empiric treatment of various infections or whether combination treatment still remains appropriate.

Perhaps the most common circumstance for surgeons is empiric treatment for suspected mixed flora infections, including intra-abdominal and soft tissue infections. The combination of evidence from in vitro data, animal studies, and clinical trials has led to widespread acceptance of the need to provide empiric antimicrobial therapy directed against *Escherichia coli* and other common members of the family Enterobacteriaceae and *B. fragilis*.[7,8] *Bacteroides fragilis* and *E. coli* are the most common isolates from intra-abdominal infections and are the organisms most likely to cause bacteremia in abdominal sepsis, further attesting to their pathogenicity.

The evidence in support of broadening therapy to cover organisms other than common facultative and obligate anaerobes such as *E. coli* and *B. fragilis* is more controversial. Initial empiric coverage of *Pseudomonas aeruginosa* is associated with a decreased likelihood of persistent or recurrent abdominal infection if these organisms are isolated from the site of infection.[9] Other clinical trials using anti-infectives not effective against *P. aeruginosa* have not found a high incidence of treatment failure with this organism.[10]

There are a large number of agents that are broadly active against the bacteria found in intra-abdominal infection. These are best discussed as classes of drugs and include aminoglycosides, carbapenems, cephalosporins, penicillins plus beta-lactamase inhibitors, and quinolones. Aztreonam will be considered as a cephalosporin-class agent.

Combination Therapy Employed for Serious Infections

One result of the availability of multiple classes of effective antibiotics is the possibility of combination therapy with two effective agents. Combination therapy has several theoretical advantages. A broader spectrum of pathogens may be covered, of particular importance when treatment is initiated for suspected sepsis without an identified source. Use of agents with differing mechanisms of action may also delay or prevent emergence of resistance and superinfection. Combinations of such agents may act synergistically to enhance killing organisms.

The time-honored tradition of providing an aminoglycoside along with a beta-lactam has recently gained support from two recent studies of gram-negative bacteremia. These studies indicate that improved survival occurs in patients with severe acute illness treated with combination therapy as opposed to those treated with a single agent.[11] In a similarly constructed study of *Klebsiella* bacteremia, a similar improvement in severely ill patients treated with combination therapy was noted.[12] In both studies, survival approximated 70 percent in the combination therapy group versus 50 percent in the monotherapy group.

Regimens employing two beta-lactams have been tried, primarily in the setting of febrile neutropenia. No benefit has been found, and there is concern that coverage with such regimens is not as broad as that obtained with an aminoglycoside-based regimen since beta-lactams have similar mechanisms of action.[13,14]

Tissue Penetration by Antibiotics

Treatment of localized infections with systemic antimicrobial agents demands that an adequate concentration of drug be delivered to the site. Ideally, the tissue concentration of antibiotics should exceed the minimum inhibitory concentration even though there is evidence that subinhibitory concentrations of antimicrobials may occasionally result in clinical cure (eg, subinhibitory concentrations of some penicillins enhance the phagocytosis of *S. aureus*).

Tissue penetration appears to depend in part on antibiotic protein binding. Only the unbound form of antibiotic will pass the capillary wall in vivo[15] or act to inhibit bacterial growth in vitro. The penetration of antibiotics into fibrin clots—an important factor in the capacity of antimicrobial agents to penetrate areas of tissue injury—depends on the concentration of free antibiotics. Therapeutic outcome, on the other hand, seems not to correlate with protein affinity, presumably because protein binding is easily reversible.

The lipid solubility of an antibiotic is an important factor in its tissue penetration. It determines its capacity to pass through membranes by nonionic diffusion or into wounds, bone, cerebrospinal fluid, aqueous and vitreous humor of the eye, endolymph of the ear, or into the vegetations of bacterial endocarditis, abscesses, and other areas of devitalized tissue. Prolonged high-dose systemic therapy or even local therapy is required for antibiotics with poor penetration into the infected areas. Table 28–5[15] lists the factors thought to be important in the tissue penetration of a hypothetical antibiotic agent.

Even when therapeutic concentrations are achieved at the sites of tissue infections, local factors may influence the antimicrobial activity. For example, aminoglycosides and polymyxins are inactivated by purulent material, whereas carbenicillin does not lose activity in pus. For this as well as other reasons, drainage of purulent secretions is sometimes necessary. It is also important to recognize that infections caused by mixed species, one

TABLE 28–5. IMPORTANT FACTORS IN TISSUE PENETRATION BY ANTIBIOTICS

1. Maximum level of concentration in the blood
2. Duration of that maximum blood level
3. Serum protein binding
4. Serum factors that influence protein binding
5. Active transport mechanisms and secretory organs (especially kidney and liver)
6. Electrical charge on the antibiotic
7. Lipid solubility
8. Urine pH
9. Barriers to diffusion
10. Biotransformation of antibiotic
11. Circulating or local antibiotic inactivators
12. Tissue binding of antibiotic

of which produces beta-lactamase, will render the hydrolyzable penicillins ineffective against even sensitive organisms within the infection. Penicillins and tetracyclines are also bound by hemoglobin and may be less effective in the presence of hematomas.[16] Similarly, *P. aeruginosa* is protected from the action of aminoglycosides by high concentrations of calcium and magnesium in the culture medium.[17] Local decreases in oxygen tension, such as occur within abscesses, will render certain antimicrobial agents less effective. For example, aminoglycosides are much less effective in anaerobic environments because oxygen is required for transport of these agents into the bacterial cell. Similarly, phagocytic and killing cellular mechanisms are inhibited in an anaerobic environment, so that bacteriostatic agents are also less effective.[18]

Tissue Distribution of Antibiotics[15]

Blood. The concentration of an antibiotic in the blood or any other compartment is the difference between what has entered and what has left or been inactivated. The rapidity of excretion is therefore an important clinical consideration. Nitrofurantoin is excreted so rapidly that no antimicrobial effect can be achieved in the blood. In contrast, cefazolin is excreted slowly, and higher blood levels are obtained than with an equivalent dose of cephalosporins, which are excreted more rapidly.

Urine. Most antibiotics in common use (sulfonamides, penicillins, cephalosporins, aminoglycosides, vancomycin, the tetracyclines, polymyxins, nitrofurans, flucytosine) are excreted appreciably, if not principally, in urine. Prominent exceptions are erythromycin and chloramphenicol. Many antimicrobial substances used for treating urinary tract infections usually appear in the urine at 50 to 200 times the concentration at which they are found in blood. Indeed, their efficacy is often dependent on that special body distribution; consequently, in severe renal disease, treatment of infection within the urinary tract becomes more difficult.

Central Nervous System. Distribution of antimicrobial compounds in cerebrospinal fluid is related not only to the nature of the antimicrobial agent but also to the extent of inflammation. The most important practical matter is that the partially lipid-soluble agents chloramphenicol, isoniazid, rifampin, sulfonamides, and flucytosine enter the cerebrospinal fluid especially well, the aminoglycosides and polymyxins enter with great difficulty, and amphotericin B does not enter at all. Therefore, when amphotericin B must be used for infection of the central nervous system, it must usually be administered directly into the cerebrospinal fluid (*Cryptococcus* meningitis does not require direct amphotericin B instillation). Of the tetracyclines, doxycycline and minocycline enter most readily because of their lipid solubility.

Interstitial Fluid. In general, high prolonged blood levels and freedom from protein binding favor diffusion of antibiotic into extravascular tissues. Absolute levels in a particular tissue may not accurately represent the therapeutic potential of the drug, however, because the drug may be so tightly bound to the tissue that it is not available for binding to bacteria.

Bile. Only urine and bile regularly contain higher concentrations of antibiotic than does serum. Table 28–6 lists the concentration factors (bile concentration, blood concentration) for a variety of antibiotics. Nafcillin and rifampin may reach concentrations in bile 500 times their serum concentrations. The penicillins, cephalosporins, tetracyclines, and clindamycin are also concentrated in bile to varying degrees. Chloramphenicol, although not concentrated in bile, readily enters bile and has been frequently used successfully in biliary tree infections. Aminoglycoside antibiotics enter the bile less well, especially when liver disease is present (see Table 28–6).

Prostate, Seminal Vesicles, and Epididymis. Using a split ejaculate technique, and measuring zinc content (which indicates prostate origin), pH, and antibiotic, investigators have found that the ampicillin, erythromycin, and doxycycline present in ejaculate

TABLE 28–6. BILIARY EXCRETION OF ANTIBIOTICS

Antibiotic	Bile Concentration/Serum Concentration (>1.0 Means Bile Concentration Exceeds Serum)
Penicillins	
Penicillin G	1.0–1.5
Ampicillin	1.0–10
Methicillin	0.1–0.5
Nafcillin	19–60
Carbenicillin	0.7
Mezlocillin	8.0
Azlocillin	5.6–15
Piperacillin	6.0
Cephalosporins	
Cephalothin	0.5–1.0
Cefazolin	1.0–7.0
Cefamandole	6–30
Ceforanide	2.0–2.6
Cefoxitin	4.0
Moxalactam	1.1–1.5
Cefuroxime	0.2–0.3
Cefoperazone	4.0–8.0
Cefotaxime	0.5
Ceftazidime	0.3
Cephalexin	0.2
Ceftizoxime	0.3
Cephradine	4
Cefadroxil	0.8
Cefmetazole	10
Cefotetan	10
Cefonicid	<0.1
Other beta-lactams	
Imipenem	<0.1
Aztreonam	0.6–1.0
Quinolones	
Ciprofloxacin	5–10
Ofloxacin	2.5
Enoxacin	9
Perfloxacin	2–16
Aminoglycosides	
Gentamicin	0.3–0.8
Amikacin	0.2–0.3
Tobramycin	0.1–0.2
Tetracyclines	
Tetracycline	7.3
Doxycycline	4.4
Chlortetracycline	3.3
Other	
Chloramphenicol	2.2
Clindamycin	2.9
Metronidazole	1.0
Rifampin	100
Vancomycin	0.5
Erythromycin	3.9

primarily originate from the prostate and seminal vesicle in about equal concentrations. Some variation in results has been noted with both sulfonamides and metronidazole, although the latter appears to enter mainly via the prostate.[15]

Abscesses. There are only few data of clinical relevance concerning the distribution of antibiotics into abscesses. Clearly, however, the generalization that antibiotics do not penetrate abscesses is untrue. The penicillins and cephalosporins seem to penetrate mature abscess cavities poorly[19,20] whereas metronidazole, chloramphenicol, and clindamycin can achieve inhibitory concentrations.[21,22]

A separate problem is whether, after penetration and concentration, an antibiotic can retain antimicrobial efficacy under the conditions of pH and low redox potential and high concentration of both microbial and mammalian tissue products. Metronidazole and clindamycin both penetrate and retain antimicrobial potency in such environments.[22] The apparent failure of the penicillins and cephalosporins to penetrate may be related to the concurrent presence within the abscess of beta-lactamase, which inactivates the antibiotic. Chloramphenicol can penetrate an abscess[23] but can be inactivated in vivo by organisms (eg, *B. fragilis*) that are usually sensitive to it, so that treatment failure is common.

It is possible that the ability of antibiotics to penetrate and be concentrated in abscesses is related to their ability to be concentrated in leukocytes. Rifampin has the ability to be concentrated in neutrophils, and clindamycin becomes concentrated in alveolar macrophages.[24]

Use of Antibiotics for Prophylaxis

The concept of using essentially harmless drugs for one or a few days to prevent enormous morbidity or even mortality seems attractive enough, and the belief that it is easier to treat an incipient disease than a well-established one seems sound. Unfortunately, the potential harm—sometimes substantial—that may result from the use of any drug must be recognized. The prophylactic use of antibiotics against the danger of wound infections is discussed in Chapter 25.

Use of Antibiotics in Patients with Hepatic and Renal Failure

Hepatic Failure. Although numerous antibiotics are partially excreted via the hepatobiliary system (Table 28–6), and some are primarily metabolized by the liver (tetracycline, chloramphenicol, sulfonamides, p-aminosulfonic acid, isoniazid), there are few data about how these antibiotics should be used—or avoided—in patients with abnormalities of the hepatobiliary system. A summary of reasonable practices appears in Table 28–7. Because penicillins, cephalosporins, and aminoglycosides are ex-

TABLE 28–7. USE OF ANTIBIOTICS IN PATIENTS WITH SEVERE HEPATIC DYSFUNCTION OR CHOLECYSTASIS

Avoid, if possible:	
Sulfonamides	
Pyrazinamide	
Tetracycline	
Reduce dosage if prolonged use (>3 days) necessary:	
Cefoperozone	Clindamycin
Rifampin	Erythromycin
Metronidazole	Chloramphenicol
Nafcillin	
No change in normal dosage:	
Penicillins	Ethambutal
Vancomycin	Isoniazid
Nitrofurantoin	Amphotericin B

creted mainly by the kidneys and have low direct toxicity, there is no reason to decrease their dosage in patients with liver disease. Although one would expect that chloramphenicol, lincomycin, clindamycin, and erythromycin would accumulate in patients with obstructive or hepatocellular disease, the evidence is lacking. Initially, therefore, it would seem advisable to use normal doses of these antibiotics in such patients (if reasonable alternative antibiotics are not likely to be effective) but to measure serum or plasma concentrations every 3 to 7 days and to reduce doses if excessive concentrations are present.

Renal Failure. Antibiotics normally excreted primarily by the kidneys accumulate in the sera of patients with impaired renal function. The dosage should, therefore, be reduced or the interval between doses should be lengthened. There are many schedules that detail how to estimate dosage of antibiotics normally excreted by the kidneys,[25–27] but all such compendia, including that shown in Table 28–8, are unreliable. One must not use the data in Table 28–8 without frequently obtaining direct measurements of serum or plasma antibiotic concentrations to verify that the appropriate doses are

TABLE 28–8. DOSAGE OF ANTIMICROBIAL DRUGS IN ADULT PATIENTS WITH RENAL IMPAIRMENT

Drug	Dose for GFR >90 mL/min	Adjustment for Renal Failure by GFR, mL/min			Supplement for Dialysis	
		>50–90	10–50	<10	Hemo	CAPD
Aminoglycosides						
Amikacin	7.5 mg/kg q12h	q12h	q12–18h	q24–48h	4–5 mg/kg	15–20 mg/liter(d)[a]
Gentamicin	1.7 mg/kg q8h	q8–12h	q12h	q24–48h	1–2 mg/kg	3–4 mg/liter(d)[a]
Netilmicin	2–2.2 mg/kg q8h	q8–12h	q12h	q24–48h	1.5–2 mg/kg	4–5 mg/liter(d)[a]
Tobramycin	1.7 mg/kg q8h	q8–12h	q12h	q24–48h	1–2 mg/kg	3–4 mg/liter(d)[a]
Cephalosporins						
Cefaclor	250 mg PO tid	tid	tid	q12h	250 mg	250 q8–12h
Cefadroxil	0.5–1 g PO q12h	q12h	q24h	q48h	0.5–1 g	0.5 g/d
Cefamandole	0.5–1 g q4–8h	q6h	q6–8h	q12h	0.5–1 g	0.5–1 g q12h
Cefazolin	0.5–1.5 g q6h	q8h	q12h	q24–48h	0.5–1 g	0.5 g q12h
Cefixime	200 mg PO q12h	q12h	300 q24h	200 q24h	300 mg	200 mg/d
Cefmenoxime	1 g q6h	q8h	q12h	q24h	750 mg	750 mg q12h
Cefonicid	1 g q24h	q24h	q24h	q48h	None	None
Cefoperazone	1–2 g q12h	q12h	q12h	q12h	1 g	None
Cefotaxime	1 g q6h	q6h	q8–12h	q24h	1 g	1 g/d
Cefotetan	1–2 g q12h	q6h	q24h	q48h	1 g	1 g/d
Cefoxitin	1–2 g q6–8h	q8h	q8–12h	q24–48h	1 g	1 g/d
Ceftazidime	1–2 g q8–12h	q8–12h	q24–48h	q48–72h	1 g	0.5 g/d
Ceftizoxime	1–2 g q8–12h	q8–12h	q48h	q72h	1 g	0.5–1 g/d
Ceftriaxone	1–2 g q12–24h	q24h	q24h	q24h	1 g	750 mg q12h
Cefuroxime	0.75–1.5 g q8h	q8h	q8–12h	q24h	1 g	1 g
Cephalexin	250–500 mg PO q6h	q6h	q8h	q12h	250 mg	250 mg tid
Cephalothin	2 g q4h	q6h	q6–8h	q12h	2 g	1 g q12h
Cephapirin	2 g q4h	q6h	q8h	q12h	2 g	1 g q12h
Cephradine	0.5 g q6h	q8h	q12h	q24h	500 mg	250 mg
Moxalactam	2 g q8h	q12h	q24h	q48h	2 g	2 g
Penicillins						
Amoxicillin	500 mg q8h	q8h	q12h	q24h	500 mg	500 mg
Ampicillin	500 mg q6h	q6h	q6–12h	q12–24h	500 mg	500 mg
Dicloxacillin	500 mg PO q6h	q6h	q6h	q6h	None	None
Methicillin	2 g q4h	q4–6h	q6–8h	q8–12h	None	None
Mezlocillin	3 g q4h	q4h	q6–8h	q8h	None	None

TABLE 28–8. *(continued)*

Drug	Dose for GFR >90 mL/min	Adjustment for Renal Failure by GFR, mL/min			Supplement for Dialysis	
		>50–90	10–50	<10	Hemo	CAPD
Nafcillin	2 g q4h	q4h	q4h	q4h	None	None
Penicillin G	0.5–5 mU q6h	q6h	q8h	q12h	≤5 mU	≤5 mU
Piperacillin	3 g q4h	q4–6h	q6–8h	q8h	3 g	3 g
Ticarcillin	3 g q4h	q4h	q8h	q12h	3 g	3 g
Other beta-lactams and beta-lactamase inhibitors						
Aztreonam	1–2 g q8–12h	q8–12 h	q12–24h	q24h	0.5 g	0.5–1 g
Imipenem	500 mg q6h	q6h	q12h	q24h	10.5 g	10.5 g
Trimentin	3.1 g q4h	q4h	q8h	q12h	3.1 g	3.1 g
Unasyn	3.0 g q6h	q6h	q6–12h	q12–24h	3.1 g	3.1 g
Miscellaneous antimicrobials						
Chloramphenicol	max 750 mg q6h	q6h	q6h	q6h	None	None
Clindamycin	150–450 mg q6h	q6h	q6h	q6h	None	None
Metronidazole	7.5 mg/kg q6h	q6h	q6h	q12h	7.5 mg/kg	7.5 mg/kg
Sulfamethoxazole	1 g q8h	q12h	q18h	q24h	1 g	1 g q24h
Trimethoprim	100 mg q12h	q12h	q12–24h	q24h	100 mg	100 mg
Vancomycin	500 mg q6h	q24–72h	q72–240h	q240h	None	None
Teicoplanin	6–15 mg/kg/d	q24h	q48h	q72h	None	None
TMP/SMX	160/800 mg q12h	q12h	80/400	80/400	80/400 mg	80/400 mg q12h q24h
Tetracyclines						
Doxycycline	100 mg q12h	q12h	q12h	q12h	None	None
Fluoroquinolones						
Ciprofloxacin	500–750 mg q12h	q12h	q12–24h	q24h	250 mg q12h	250 mg q12h
Ofloxacin	400 mg q12h	q12h	q12–24h	q48h	100 mg bid	400 mg q48h
Temafloxacin	400 mg q12h	q12h	q24h	q24–48h	None	None
Macrolide antibiotics						
Azithromycin	500 mg PO day 1, 250 mg qd	q24h	q24h	q24h	None	None
Clarithromycin	250–500 mg q12h	q12h	q12h	q24h	Insufficient data	
Erythromycin	250–500 mg q6h	q6h	q6h	q8h	None	None
Antifungal antibiotics						
Amphotericin B	0.4–1 mg/kg q24h	q24h	q24h	q24h	None	None
Fluconazole	100–200 mg q24h	q24h	q24–48h	q48–72h	200 mg	q48–72h
Flucytosine	0.5–1 g q6h	q6–8h	q12–24h	q24–48h	0.5–1 g	0.5–1 g
Griseofulvin	125–500 mg q6h	q6h	q6h	q6h	None	None
Itraconazole	100–200 mg q12h	q12h	q12h	q12h	None	None
Ketoconazole	200 mg q24h	q24h	q24h	q24h	None	None
Miconazole	200–1200 mg q8h	q8h	q8h	q8h	None	None
Antiparasitic drugs						
Chloroquine	1.5 g over 3 d	None	None	½	None	None
Pentamidine	4 mg/kg q24h	q24h	q24–36h	q48h	None	None
Pyrimethamine	50–75 mg q24h	q24h	q24h	q24h	None	None
Quinidine	600 mg load then 0.02 mg/kg/min	None	None	0.015 mg/kg/min	100–200 mg	None
Quinine	650 mg q8h	q8h	q8–12h	q24h	650 mg	650 mg q24h
Antituberculous drugs						
Ethambutol	15 mg/kg q24h	q24h	q24–36h	q48h	15 mg/kg	15 mg/kg q48h
Isoniazid	5 mg/kg q24h	q24h	q24h	q48h	5 mg/kg	q48h
Rifampin	600 mg q24h	q24h	q24h	q24h	None	None
Antiviral drugs						
Acyclovir	5–12.4 mg/kg q8h	q8h	q12–24h	q24h	5–12.4 mg/kg	q24h
Amantidine	100 mg q12h	q24–48h	q48–72h	q1 week	None	None
Ganciclovir	5 mg/kg q12h	q12–24h	q24–48h	q48–72h	2.5 mg/kg	No data
Ribavirin	200 mg q8h	q8h	q8h	100 mg q8h	200 mg	100 mg q8h
Zidovudine (AZT)	200 mg q8h	q8h	q8h	q12–24h	100 mg	q12–24h

[a] mg/liter(d), milligrams per liter of dialysate.
Agents that should not be used (patients with GFR < 50 ml/min): bacitracin, methenamine mandelate, nalidixic acid, nitrofurantoin, pyrazinamide, tetracycline.
Agents for which data are insufficient/inadequate: dapsone, primaquine, didanosine (ddI), zalcitabine (ddC), foscarnet.
From Sanford JP: Guide to Antimicrobiol Therapy. Dallas, TX, Antimocrobial Therapy, Inc., 1992, p 108.

being administered. The obvious dangers to the patient of too little antibiotic (leaving the infection virtually untreated) or too much (possibly resulting in toxicity to the kidneys, and often to the 8th nerve) are much greater than the cost of obtaining frequent antibiotic determinations.

The general approach to antibiotic usage in patients with renal failure is to give a first dose of 80 to 100 percent the usual amount and then to estimate the timing and amount of the second dose according to the schedule in Table 28–8. Peak levels (1½ to 2 hours after the second intramuscular dose or immediately at the end of the second intravenous dose) should be taken, and the third dose can be adjusted (regarding timing and amount) on the basis of the results. In patients with severe infections and rapidly changing renal function, it may be advisable to assay peak serum concentrations once daily after injection of an antibiotic. In less severely ill patients, or in those with stable renal function, only one or two assays may be required. Trough concentrations may help detect incipient toxicity.

Anuric patients or those in whom the creatinine clearance is less than 10 ml per minute will invariably have toxic serum or plasma levels of aminoglycosides if they continue to receive average doses for 24 hours; the second dose must be tailored to individual requirements. Although such patients can usually be prevented from receiving toxic concentrations of antibiotic by being given half the usual dose every half-life of the antibiotic, patients with long antibiotic half-lives (greater than 24 hours) should receive somewhat smaller doses more frequently to keep serum or plasma concentrations above required inhibitory levels. This is especially desirable if there is a life-threatening infection, when it would seem inadvisable to have the patient go many hours with antibiotic concentrations well below the concentration required to inhibit the infecting organism.

Allergy to Antibacterial Agents

All antibiotics have been accused of initiating allergic reactions. Persistence or recurrence of fever in a patient whose infection has been controlled as indicated by all other clinical criteria should always be considered a possible manifestation of allergy to the antibiotics. The problem is obviously complicated in patients who are receiving multiple drugs if several are common causes of allergic reactions. In such circumstances, all drugs should be stopped if the condition permits. After the putative allergic signs or symptoms have subsided, the drugs are instituted (over a period of days) one at a time until the offending agent is identified (unless the possible consequences are unacceptable).

It is far better to avoid an allergic reaction than to encounter it. Avoidance is best done by eliciting a medical history of previous adverse reactions. Obviously, the primary allergic response cannot be anticipated by history taking. The only accurate predictor of an allergic reaction is a prior anaphylactoid response.

A safe test, which would help detect the allergy-prone patient before the antibiotic is used, is obviously desirable. Despite encouraging early reports that in vivo or in vitro tests would identify patients allergic to penicillin, no reliable clinically applicable test is currently available. Many experts in infectious diseases use only the patient's statement as a means of detecting penicillin allergy.

Penicillin Allergy. Penicillin allergy occurs in about 3 percent of the population, and is most commonly of the delayed type (fever, erythema, urticaria, rash, arthritis), which rarely causes significant morbidity or mortality. A majority of patients with documented histories of previous delayed reactions to penicillin G can receive it again without any adverse response, and it is rare for such patients to develop immediate anaphylactic-type reactions. Nonetheless, patients with previous delayed reactions should receive therapy with unrelated compounds whenever possible. Although antihistamines plus steroids are sometimes required to suppress the allergy, there is usually no adverse effect.

After there has been an immediate (anaphylactic) reaction to a penicillin, all penicillins and cephalosporins must be avoided. Although the matter of "cross-allergenicity" between penicillins and cephalosporins is unsettled, most investigators agree that there is cross-allergenicity among the beta lactams.

Chloramphenicol Reactions. Although penicillin allergy is the most frequent antibiotic allergy, it is rarely a catastrophe. In contrast, allergic or idiosyncratic reactions to chloramphenicol may lead to irreversibly fatal aplastic anemia. Fortunately, the incidence is only 1 per 30,000 or more courses of therapy.

Other Allergies. Two other characteristic allergic reactions to antimicrobial agents are (1) bullous eruptions (fortunately rare) following the use of sulfonamides, which can develop to a fatal Stevens-Johnson syndrome; and (2) cholestatic jaundice associated with use of the esters of erythromycin, which is reversible after stopping use of the drug.

Sometimes, there is also right upper quadrant tenderness and fever, which simulate acute cholecystitis.

Any of the antibiotics is capable of producing fever or rashes, neither of which is diagnostic.

Special Problems in Antibiotic Administration

Age

Penicillin Absorption. The gastrointestinal absorption of antimicrobial agents partly depends on their acid stability in the stomach. The oral absorption of penicillin G is reduced by gastric acid, but adequate levels can be achieved in children and in elderly patients who have reduced gastric acid secretion. Penicillin V is not necessary in these patients.

Renal Function. The serum half-lives of drugs primarily excreted by the kidneys are increased in neonates and the elderly. The doses of many antimicrobial agents must therefore be altered (see Table 28–8). Failure to take these facts into consideration will increase antimicrobial toxicity.

Both nephrotoxic reactions and true hypersensitivity reactions to these drugs are more common in the elderly. In part, these reactions are due to declining renal function in the elderly, which is aggravated by secondary drug-induced nephrotoxicity. Prior exposure may sensitize older patients to previously received antibiotics.

Hepatic Function in the Neonate. The neonatal liver is underdeveloped. Chloramphenicol is normally conjugated to the inactive glucuronide form in the liver, but neonatal hepatic levels of glucuronyl transferase are insufficient. High levels of unconjugated chloramphenicol can produce shock, cardiovascular collapse, and death (the gray syndrome).[28] For this reason, chloramphenicol can be safely administered only in reduced dosage.[28]

Sulfonamides should not be given to neonates because the sulfonamides compete with bilirubin for binding sites on serum albumin. Kernicterus can be induced by increased serum levels of unbound bilirubin. A similar problem may follow the use of novobiocin, which inhibits hepatic glucuronyl transferase, which normally conjugates bilirubin.

Hepatic toxicity caused by isoniazid increases with age, apparently the result of poorly defined abnormalities in the livers of older patients. For this reason, prophylactic isoniazid should not be given to patients older than 35 who have had positive tuberculin test results, unless they have recently converted.[29]

Tetracyclines should be avoided in young children because the tetracyclines bind to developing teeth (resulting in stained teeth) and bone.

Critically Ill Patients. The large interpatient variability in pharmacokinetics is not surprising given the markedly different physiologic characteristics between noncritically ill patients and critically ill patients.[30] Septic and postsurgical patients in intensive care units often require large volumes of fluid for resuscitation and have large intravascular fluid shifts.[30,31] Alterations in the concentrations of hormones and vasoactive substances may affect blood flow and organ perfusion and function.[30,31] Cardiac, respiratory, renal, and hepatic failure occur frequently, alone and in combination, and can significantly alter the absorption, distribution, metabolism, and elimination of many drugs.[32–36] The critically ill patient presents a major challenge to clinicians in regard to appropriate management of drug therapy.

Traditional aminoglycoside dosing methods (manufacturer's recommendations, nomograms) are based on the assumption that pharmacokinetic parameters such as volume of distribution (Vd) and clearance (Cl) are similar from patient to patient, regardless of their severity of illness.[37] Since there is a wide interpatient variability of these parameters among noncritically ill and critically ill patients,[37,38] utilization of traditional dosing methods can result in inappropriate aminoglycoside regimens.

Pregnancy. Tetracycline should also be avoided in pregnancy, not only because of its adverse effects on fetal dentition, but also because pregnant women appear to be vulnerable to the hepatotoxic effects.[39]

Pregnancy poses certain problems for the administration of any drug. For example, all suspected teratogenic drugs should be avoided. Metronidazole and ticarcillin are teratogenic in rodents, and the teratogenic potential of many other antibiotics has not been ruled out.

It is possible that antimicrobial clearance is greater during pregnancy, so that the doses may need to be revised upward. Although this is clear for ampicillin, data on other antimicrobial agents is not available.

Most antimicrobial agents appear in breast milk in low concentration. Sulfonamides in breast milk may be dangerous to premature babies, because they predispose the child to kernicterus. Nalidixic acid and the sulfonamides in breast milk can cause hemolysis in infants with glucose 6-phosphate dehydrogenase deficiency.[40]

Drug Incompatibilities

Antibiotics should not be mixed with other drugs in syringes or intravenous bottles. Some incompatible drug combinations form insoluble precipitates, which inactivate the antibiotic—other combinations inactivate one another without forming a distinctive precipitate. In other instances, one drug may antagonize the action of a second, or prolong or shorten the duration of the activity, leading to serious problems of apparent over- or underdosage.

Another important problem is drug instability in solution. This most commonly occurs with penicillins, which are shipped as dry powders for parenteral use. If the drug is dissolved many hours in advance, there may be significant deterioration of activity before or during administration—if given over many hours. Instability is a well-documented problem for methicillin (which is unstable in acidic fluids) dissolved in saline or other unbuffered fluids with low pII, and most penicillins in fluids that contain carbohydrate. Most of these problems can be avoided by dissolving the penicillin immediately before use and making up no more than will be given over the next 1 to 2 hours. The pH of fluids that contain methicillin should be checked and adjusted to approximately 7.0 with sterile $NaHCO_3$. Of particular note is the increased toxicity of drugs normally metabolized in the liver (warfarin, barbiturates, tolbutamide, phenytoin) when combined with antibiotics that are also metabolized in the liver (chloramphenicol, sulfonamides, INH, rifampin). Alternatively, these drugs may induce microsomal enzymes (tolbutamide, oral contraceptives), which then reduce the effectiveness of the drug by accelerating its metabolism.

Bacterial Resistance

Bacteria can become resistant to antibiotics through genetically mediated mechanisms that result in inactivation of the antibiotic, ineffective binding of antibiotic, or a change in the permeability of the bacterial cell wall to the antibiotic. Antibiotic resistance factors can be mediated by genes on the bacterial chromosomes or plasmids. The most important resistance factor is beta-lactamase, which can inactivate beta-lactam antibiotics.

Overview of Beta-lactamases in Bacterial Resistance. Beta-lactamases are ubiquitous, and therapeutic use of beta-lactam antibiotics has selected strains with increased amounts of enzymes and/or selected enzymes with an extended spectrum of activity. The most important chromosomal enzymes are the class I enzymes, occurring in Enterobacteriaceae and *Pseudomonas* species.[41–45] These enzymes have high affinity for beta-lactams but hydrolyze the drugs only slowly. Some bacteria are able to synthesize large amounts of beta-lactamases if challenged with a beta-lactam. This induced expression is important for *Pseudomonas aeruginosa, Enterobacter, Citrobacter, Serratia, Morganella,* and *Providenica* species, for *Proteus vulgaris,* and in bacteria in which enzyme activity is stably depressed.[46–49] Once selected, derepressed mutants remain sensitive to carbapenems, cafepime, cefpirome, quinolones, and aminoglycosides.

TEM-1 is now the commonest plasmid-mediated beta-lactamase. This is followed in frequency by SHV-1, PSE-1, and PSE-4, which confer resistance to ampicillin, amoxicillin, ticarcillin, piperacillin, mezlocillin, cefamandole, and cefoperazone. Mutants have been identified in clinical isolates which have even broader substrate profiles, including most penicillins, cephalosporins, and aztreonam.[50]

Most beta-lactamases function as shown in Figure 28–1. A serine in the active site forms a noncovalent complex with the beta-lactam, followed by acylation. During this reaction the lactam ring is opened, destroying the drug's activity. This reaction also occurs with the drug's true target, the penicillin binding proteins (PBPs). In this case, drug binding to the PBPs inactivates it and prevents cell replication. For beta-lactamases, hydrolysis is much more rapid than for PBPs and liberates the enzyme and results in drug inactivation. It was initially thought that many beta-lactams were resistant to inactivation. It has since been recognized that in vivo susceptibility to hydrolysis depends on the pericytoplasmic concentration of the antibiotic, which often is quite low.[51–53]

ANTIBACTERIAL AGENTS

Penicillins

Chemistry. Benzylpenicillin (penicillin G) is produced by strains of *Aspergillus* and *Penicillium* (particularly *P. notatum* and *P. chrysogenum*). Fleming first isolated penicillin in 1929, but not until 1941 did it come into clinical use. Chemical modification of the basic penicillin structure has dramatically altered the pharmacokinetic and antibacterial properties (Fig. 28–2).

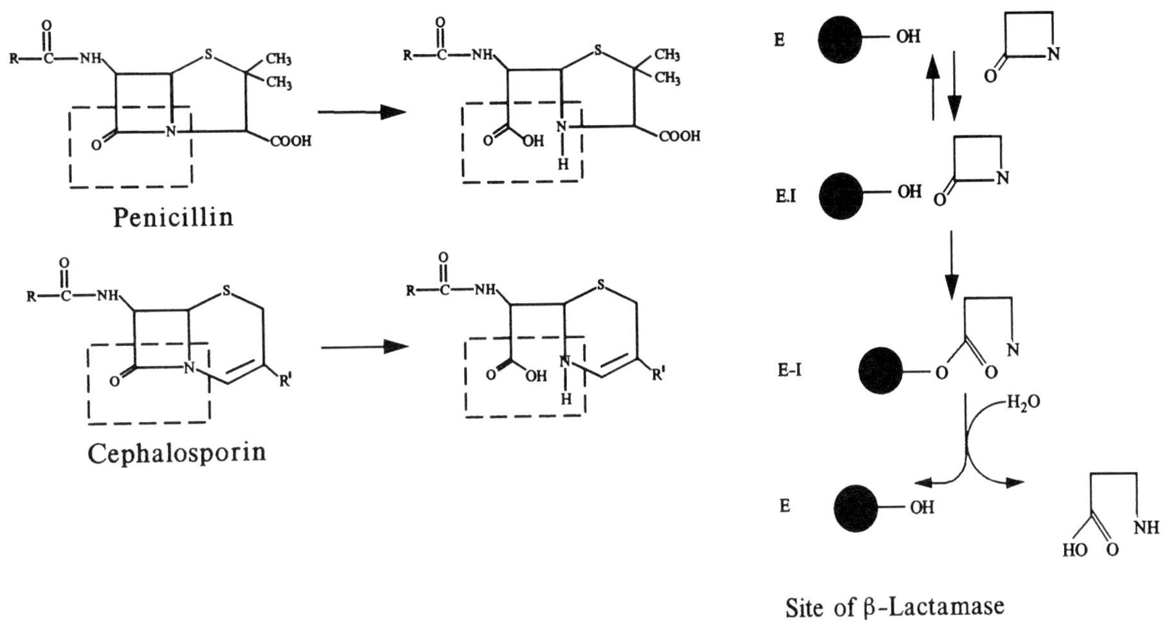

Figure 28–1. **A.** Mechanism of action of serine beta-lactamases and their effects on penicillin and cephalosporin molecules. *(From Livermore J:* Antimicrob Chemother *31(Suppl A):9, 1993.)* **B.** Suicide inhibitors (E-I) are not hydrolyzed and irreversibly inhibit enzyme activity. *(From Dever LA, Dermody TS: Mechanism of bacterial resistance to antibiotics, Arch Intern Med 151:886, 1991.)*

Pharmacology. Penicillin V, ampicillin, amoxicillin, and cyclacillin are well absorbed from the gastrointestinal tract, whereas the other penicillins are degraded by the acidic environment of the stomach.[54] Penicillins given intravenously immediately reach high blood levels and are distributed quickly to most body compartments, including interstitial fluid, bone, and placenta. Ampicillin penetrates best into the cerebrospinal fluid, achieving about 50 percent of the blood level when the meninges are inflamed. Because the most penicillins are excreted unchanged by rapid glomerular filtration and tubular secretion (average half-life of 0.5 to 1.5 hours), they must be administered every 4 to 6 hours to

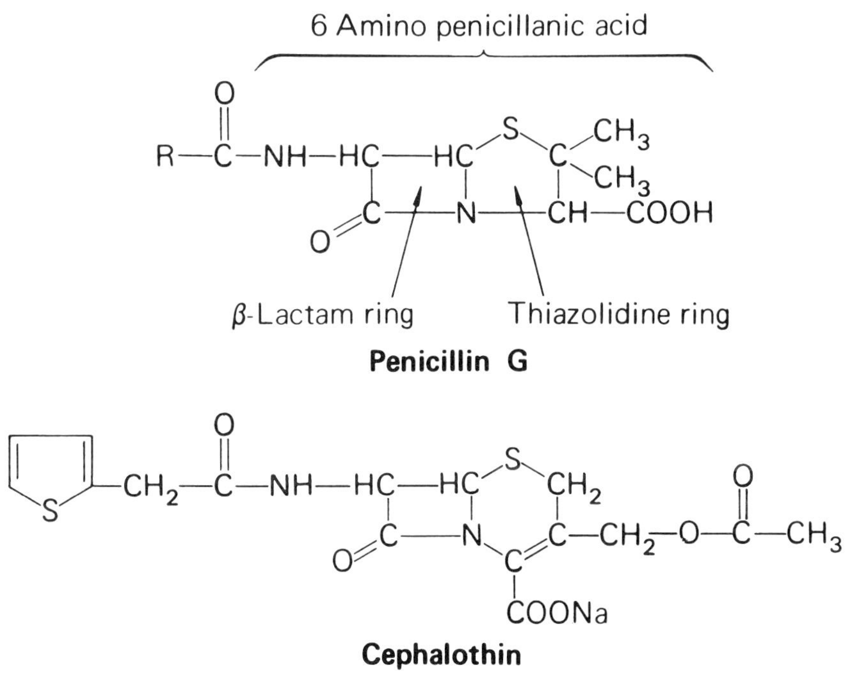

Figure 28–2. Structure of beta-lactam antibiotics. *(From Pratt WB: The inhibitors of cell wall synthesis. In Pratt WB (ed): Chemotherapy of Infection. New York, Oxford University Press, 1977, p 22.)*

maintain effective blood levels. Dosage of all penicillins, except nafcillin, should be somewhat decreased in patients with impaired renal function—nafcillin is cleared by the liver. Most penicillins are secreted into bile in amounts exceeding serum concentrations. When penicillin G is given intramuscularly as a procaine or benzathine suspension, low peak levels are achieved but with sustained antibacterial activity (48 hours and 2 to 4 weeks, respectively).

Antimicrobial Spectrum and Clinical Uses. The penicillins have antibacterial activity against most gram-positive, gram-negative, and anaerobic organisms. Table 28–9 lists the usual spectrum for each of the penicillins. Sensitivity is so variable, however, that it is important to know the antibiotic sensitivity pattern for each organism in one's own institution and area of practice.

Structural changes in the cephalosporins have made these agents as active as many penicillins, but with broader spectrums of antibacterial coverage. This must be considered when selecting antibiotic therapy, especially for surgical patients, who often have mixed infections that require a broader spectrum.

Penicillins G and V have limited bacterial coverage compared to the semisynthetic agents. The penicillinase-resistant penicillins are useful only in proved *S. aureus* infections, although they are moderately active against streptococci, pneumococci, and anaerobic cocci. All the penicillinase-resistant penicillins are similar; methicillin should be avoided, because it is likely to cause interstitial nephritis.

Ampicillin is active against most gram-positive cocci including *Enterococcus*, except those *S. aureus* strains that produce penicillinase. Ampicillin kills three common gram-negative rods—*Haemophilus influenzae, Escherichia coli,* and *Proteus mirabilis*—but the rest are usually resistant.

Carbenicillin and ticarcillin have the broadest gram-positive antibacterial activity of the penicillins, killing most organisms except for penicillinase-producing *Staphylococcus* and *Enterococcus*. Carbenicillin and ticarcillin are also active against many gram-negative rods, including *Pseudomonas,* although *Klebsiella* and *Serratia* tend to be resistant. Anaerobic bacteria including *B. fragilis* and *Clostridium* are generally sensitive to either of these agents when large doses are given.

The acylureido-penicillins, piperacillin, pirbenicillin, mezlocillin, aplocillin, and azlocillin are similar to carbenicillin and ticarcillin in antibacterial spectrum. They have greater antibacterial activity at similar dosage, especially against *P. aeruginosa,* but are still beta-lactamase sensitive.[55]

Clavulanic acid, sulbactam, and tazobactam are potent inhibitors of beta-lactamases. These inhibitors increase the activity of penicillins against resistant bacteria that produce beta-lactamases but do not alter activity against bacteria that do not produce beta-lactamase or against bacteria that have another mechanism of resistance to penicillins. These beta-lactamase inhibitors also bind to PBPs and have weak antibacterial properties of their own. Combinations of penicillins and beta-lactamase inhibitors have increased antibacterial spectra so that many gram-negative bacteria are sensitive to these agents and formerly resistant gram-positive bacteria are frequently sensitive. The combinations currently available include amoxicillin-clavulanic acid (Augmentin), ticarcillin-clavulanic acid (Timentin), ampicillin-sulbactam (Unasyn), and piperacillin-tazobactam (Zosyn).

Mechanisms of Antibacterial Action. Penicillins and cephalosporins appear to have similar mechanisms of antibacterial action—they alter bacterial cell wall synthesis and activate the endogenous autolytic system. Specifically, they block multiple bacterial enzymes (PBPs) that the organism uses to build peptidoglycan polymers. The penicillins inhibit enzymes responsible for cross-linking peptide chains, thereby preventing development of the normal peptidoglycan structure. These enzymes (transpeptidase, carboxypeptidase, endopeptidase) are located beneath the cell wall and are termed penicillin-binding proteins (PBPs).[54]

Mechanisms of Bacterial Resistance. The synthesis of beta-lactamase by bacteria, which opens the beta-lactam ring, is the major mechanism of bacterial resistance. Bacteria also alter the cell wall enzymes to disrupt the effective interaction of the penicillins (see subsequent section on cephalosporin).

Bacteria may also develop resistance to the penicillins by decreasing the permeability of their cell walls to penicillins or by developing PBPs that have decreased affinity for penicillins.[54] Gonococci can develop resistance by the former mechanism while *S. aureus* and *Streptococcus pneumoniae* can develop resistance by the latter mechanism.

Preparations and Doses. Table 28–10 lists the usual doses of the penicillins. The low toxicity of these drugs permits higher doses to be given in appropriate circumstances.

TABLE 28–9. ANTIMICROBIAL SPECTRUM OF THE PENICILLINS

			Broad Spectrum Penicillins			
	Natural Penicillins	Penicillinase Resistant	Aminopenicillins	Carboxypenicillins	Ureidopenicillins	Penicillin + Beta-lactamase Inhibitor
Organism	Penicillin G Penicillin V Phenithicillin	Methicil in Nafcillin Oxacillin Cloxacil in Dicloxacillin	Ampicillin Amoxicillin	Carbenicillin Ticarcillin	Azlocillin Mezlocillin Piperacillin	Ampicillin-Sulbactam Ticarcillin-Clavulanic Acid Amoxicillin-Clavulanic Acid Piperacillin-Tazobactam
Gram-positive cocci						
S. aureus (penicillin-sensitive)	+++	+++	+++	+++	+++	+++
S. aureus (penicillin-resistant)	−	+++	−	−	−	++
S. epidermidis	−	++	−	−	+	++
S. pyogenes	+++	++	+++	+++	++	++
Streptococcus pneumoniae	+++	++	+++	+++	+++	+++
Enterococcus	+	±	++	±	++	++
Gram-negative cocci						
Meningococcus	+++	+	+++	+++	+++	+++
Gonococcus	+++ (not pen V⁺)	+	+++	++	+++	+++
Gram-positive rods						
C. diphtheriae	+++	++	+++	+++	++	+++
Gram-negative rods						
E. coli	±	−	++	++	++	+++
Klebsiella	−	−	−	−	++	+++
Enterobacter	−	−	−	±	++	+++
P. mirabilis	−	−	+++	+++	+++	+++
Other *Proteus*	−	−	−	±	±	±
Pseudomonas	−	−	−	++	++	±
Serratia	−	−	−	−	−	−
H. influenzae	+	−	++	++	++	++
Anaerobes						
B. fragilis	±	−	−	++	++	++
Clostridium	+++	++	+++	+++	+++	+++
Anaerobic cocci	+++	++	+++	+++	+++	+++
Listeria	++	?	++	++	+++	+++

+++, highly susceptible; ++, moderately susceptible; +, weakly susceptible; ±, weakly resistant; −, resistant.

TABLE 28–10. PENICILLIN PREPARATIONS AND DOSES

Generic Name	Usual Dose: Pediatric	Usual Dose: Adult
Natural penicillins		
Penicillin G	25,000–3,000,000 units/kg/d in 4–6 doses IV	2–24 million units in 6 doses
Penicillin V	125–250 mg/d in 4 doses; 50 mg/kg/d in 3 doses	250 mg to 2 g in 4 doses
Penicillinase-resistant penicillins		
Methicillin	50–200 mg/kg/d in 4–6 doses IV, IM	4–12 g in 4–6 doses IV or IM
Nafcillin	50–200 mg/kg/d in 4 doses	1–6 g/d in 4 doses
	25–100 mg/kg/d in 4 doses IV	500 mg to 6 g in 4 doses IV maximum dose 12 g/d
Oxacillin	50–150 mg/kg/d in 4 doses	1–6 g/d in 4 doses
	50–300 mg/kg/d in 6 doses IM, IV	4–12 g in 6 doses IV
Dicloxacillin	25–100 mg/kg/d in 4 doses	500 mg to 4 g/d in 4 doses
Cloxacillin	25–100 mg/kg/d in 4 doses	1–4 g/d in 4 doses PO in 4 doses
Broad spectrum penicillins		
Ampicillin	75–300 mg/kg/d in 4 doses PO	2–12 g/d in 4 doses
	75–300 mg/kg/d in 4 doses IV, IM	2–12 g/d in 4 doses, IV, IM
Amoxicillin	20–100 mg/kg/d in 4 doses	1–4 g/d in 4 doses
Carbenicillin	400–600 mg/kg/d in 4 or 6 doses IV	4–30 g/d in 4 or 6 doses IV
Indanyl carbenicillin	10–30 mg/kg/d in 4 doses	1–2 tablets q6h
Ticarcillin	100–300 mg/kg/d in 4 or 6 doses	4–24 g/d in 4 or 6 doses
Piperacillin	50–300 mg/kg/d in 4 or 6 doses	4–24 g/d in 4 or 6 doses
Mezlocillin	300 mg/kg/d in 6 doses	4–24 g/d in 4 doses IV
Azlocillin	450 mg/kg/d in 6 doses	8–24 g/d in 6 doses IV
Penicillin + beta-lactamase inhibitor		
Ampicillin-sulbactam		1.5–3 g q6h IV
Ticarcillin-clavulanic acid		3.1 g q4–6h IV
Amoxicillin-clavulanic acid	20–40 mg/kg/d in 3 doses PO	250–500 mg tid PO
Piperacillin-tazobactam		4.5 g q4–6h IV

Cephalosporins

Chemistry. Most cephalosporins are derivatives of the fungus *Cephalosporium acremonium,* and the cephalomycins are derived from *Streptomyces* species. Cephalosporin C, the basic compound, resembles penicillin with a beta-lactam structure in which the five-member thiazolidine ring (characteristic of penicillin) is replaced by a six-member dihydrothiazine ring (see Fig. 28–2). The antibacterial activity of this compound can be modified by substitutions at position 7 of the beta-lactam ring. Changes in pharmacokinetics and metabolic parameters are achieved by substitution at position 3 of the dehydrothiazine ring.

Pharmacology. Table 28–11 lists the cephalosporins.[56] All the oral agents are similar in pharmacology to cephalexin. Only one agent, cephradine, is effective by both parenteral and oral routes; most cephalosporins require parenteral administration. Most cephalosporins are metabolized in the liver to the inactive lactone, then excreted by the kidney. Dosages should be altered in patients with renal insufficiency (Table 28–8). High concentrations are achieved in the fetus and in synovial, pericardial, pleural, and peritoneal cavities. Bile levels are usually high.

Classification and Antimicrobial Spectrum. Cephalosporins are classified by generations based on general features of antimicrobial activity (see Table 28–11). First-generation cephalosporins have good activity against gram-positive bacteria. Penicillins are generally more specific and less expensive and should be used as first-line agents. They also have modest activity for gram-negative bacteria.[57]

The second-generation cephalosporins have increased activity against gram-negative bacteria but are less active than third-generation agents.

Third-generation cephalosporins are more active against the Enterobacteriaceae, and some have activity against *B. fragilis*. Ceftazidime and cefsulodin are also active against *P. aeruginosa*. These antibiotics are less effective than first-generation agents against gram-positive cocci.

Second- and third-generation cephalosporins have less activity against gram-positive cocci than first-generation agents do and should not be used for these infections. Cephalosporins also have good activity against most streptococci, but enterococci are resistant to all members of this group.

Clinical Uses. Cephalosporins are broad-spectrum antibiotics with a high therapeutic/toxic ratio. They are frequently used empirically to treat infections due to gram-positive and gram-negative bacteria. The third-generation cephalosporins—ceftriaxone, cefotaxime, and moxalactam—are currently regarded by many physicians as the drugs of choice for meningitis due to gram-negative enteric bacilli.

Perhaps the greatest use of the cephalosporins in surgery is to prevent rather than to treat infections. Their use as perioperative prophylaxis is discussed in Chapter 25.

TABLE 28–11. CEPHALOSPORINS

Generic Name (Trade Name)	Routes of Administration	Usual Dose: Pediatric	Usual Dose: Adult
First generation			
Cephalothin (Keflin)	IV	180–160 mg/kg/d in 4 doses	0.5 2.0 g q4 6h
Cefazolin (Kefzol, Ancef)	IM, IV	25–50 mg/kg/d in 3–4 doses	0.25–1.0 g q6–12h
Cephapirin (Cefadyl)	IM, IV		0.5–2.0 g q4–6h
Cephradine (Anspor, Velosef)	PO, IV	50–100 mg/kg/d in 4 doses	0.5–1.0 g q6h
Cephalexin (Keflex)	PO	25–50 mg/kg/d in 2–4 doses	0.25–1.0 g q6h
Cefadroxil (Duricef)	PO	30 mg/kg/d in 2 doses	1.0–2.0 g qd or q12h
Second generation			
Cefamandole (Mandol)	IM, IV	50–100 mg/kg/d in 3–6 doses	0.5–1.0 g q4–8h
Cefoxitin (Mefoxin)	IM, IV	80–160 mg/kg/d in 4–6 doses	1.0–2.0 g q6–8h
Ceforanide (Precef)	IM, IV	20–40 mg/kg/d in 2 doses	0.5–1.0 g q12h
Cefuroxime (Zinacef, Kefurox)	IM, IV	50–100 mg/kg/d in 3–4 doses	0.75–1.5 g q8h
Cefonicid (Monocid)	IM, IV	—	1.0 g q24h
Cefaclor (Celor)	PO	20 mg/kg/d in 3 doses	0.25 g q8h
Cefmetazole (Zefazone)	IV	—	2.0 g q6–12h
Cefotetan (Cefotan)	IM, IV	—	0.5–3 g q12–24 h
Third generation			
Cefmenoxime (Cefmax)	IM, IV		
Moxalactam (Moxam)	IV	200 mg/kg/d in 3–4 doses	1.0–2.0 g q8–12h
Cefoperazone (Cefobid)	IV	150–200 mg/kg/d in 3–4 doses	1.0–2.0 g q8–12h
Cefotaxime (Claforan)	IM, IV	50–180 mg/kg/d in 4–6 doses	1.0–2.0 g q4–12h
Cefotetan (Cefotan)	IM, IV	—	1.0–2.0 g q12h
Cefsulodin (Cefomonil)	IM, IV	—	0.5–3.0 g q6h
Ceftazidime (Fortaz, Tazididime, Tazicef)	IV	90–150 mg/kg/d in 3 doses	0.5–2 g q8–12h
Ceftriaxone (Rocephin)	IM, IV	50–75 mg/kg/d in 2 doses	1.0–2.0 g q12–24h
Ceftizoxime (Cefizox)	IM, IV	150–200 mg/kg/d in 3–4 doses	1.0–2.0 g q8–12h
Cefixime (Suprax)	PO	8 mg/kg/d in 1–2 doses	0.4 g qd

The cephalosporins can also be used to treat infections due to susceptible Enterobacteriaceae. Hospital-acquired strains of these bacteria are frequently resistant to older antibiotics, and most are sensitive to third-generation agents. The response rate for treating gram-positive and gram-negative bacteria is 90 percent.[57,58] They can also be used to treat pneumonia due to these gram-negative bacteria.

Cefoxitin and the third-generation cephalosporins can also be used to treat intra-abdominal infections and polymicrobial soft tissue infections. They are as effective as an aminoglycoside plus clindamycin for treating intra-abdominal infections, but strict criteria for entrance into most studies have eliminated the sickest patients.[57,58] There is no evidence one of these agents is better than another when used for these infections. Third-generation cephalosporins may be most appropriate when there is concern about renal toxicity of aminoglycosides. *Bacteroides fragilis* plays a part in virtually all mixed aerobic-anaerobic infections. Cephalosporins are not as active as metronidazole, clindamycin, or chloramphenicol against *B. fragilis*. Therefore, where *B. fragilis* is thought to play a major role, one of these other agents should perhaps be used.

Cefazolin, cefoxitin, and the third-generation cephalosporins are useful in hepatobiliary infections. Several are excreted in the bile in concentrations equal to or higher than serum levels. Because surgical therapy is often required, and the bile is drained or gallbladder removed, high tissue penetration is a more important consideration than high bile concentration.

Most soft tissue infections are due to gram-positive cocci and are best treated with penicillins. In polymicrobial soft tissue infections—especially when tissue necrosis is present—cefoxitin or third-generation cephalosporins can be used.

Third-generation cephalosporins are also used as empiric therapy for the febrile neutropenic patient or immunocompromised host, usually in combination with an aminoglycoside or vancomycin.

Urinary tract infections are widely treated by oral cephalosporins. Ampicillin, amoxicillin, sulfisoxazole, or cotrimoxazole are preferable, however, for single-dose therapy of lower urinary tract infections. The third-generation cephalosporins are alternatives to aminoglycosides for hospital-acquired, multiply resistant Enterobacteriaceae. The cure rates for pseudomonal urinary tract infections with agents that have antipseudomonal activity is around 70 percent.

Mechanisms of Antimicrobial Action. Until recently, all beta-lactam antibiotics were thought to have the same mechanism of action—interference with cell wall structure by disruption of the cross-linking of the peptidoglycan polymer. Now it is known that beta-lactam antibiotics block enzymes that govern important steps in the biosynthesis of peptidoglycan. In addition, beta-lactam antibiotics may also inhibit the inhibitor of a bacterial autolysin, which is then free to damage the bacterial cell itself.

Mechanisms of Bacterial Resistance. The most important mode of bacterial resistance to the cephalosporins is the hydrolysis of the beta-lactam ring by bacterial beta-lactamases. Whereas most gram-positive organisms secrete their beta-lactamase into the environment, gram-negative organisms retain most beta-lactamase within the cell and are therefore far more effective in resisting cephalosporins.[59] In general, however, cephalosporins are all relatively more resistant to beta-lactamases than the penicillins.

Additional modes of resistance include (1) poor penetration of beta-lactam antibiotics through gram-negative cell walls; gram-positive bacteria, by contrast, have accessible sites of antibiotic binding and (2) tolerance, defined as dissociation of inhibitory and killing actions. The mechanism may be related to the deficiency of autolytic enzymes in the cells, so that the antibiotic becomes bacteriostatic rather than bactericidal.

Adverse Reactions. The cephalosporins are among the safest of drugs, although thrombophlebitis frequently occurs after intravenous administration. The most common side effects are delayed allergic reactions (anaphylaxis and bronchospasm are relatively rare), such as a maculopapular rash that appears after several days of therapy. Although immunologic cross-reactivity with penicillin is found in 20 percent of penicillin-allergic patients, clinical cross-reactivity occurs in only 5 to 10 percent of patients. Patients with a history of a recent severe and immediate reaction to penicillin should not be given cephalosporins. Rare adverse reactions include hemolysis, granulocytopenia, thrombocytopenia, and defects in platelet aggregation.

More controversial are the reports that cephalosporins are potentially nephrotoxic, which is true of cephaloridine. There is some evidence that the combination of cephalothin plus gentamicin or tobramycin is synergistically nephrotoxic, especially in older patients or patients with other causes for renal insufficiency. A moderate dose reduction is

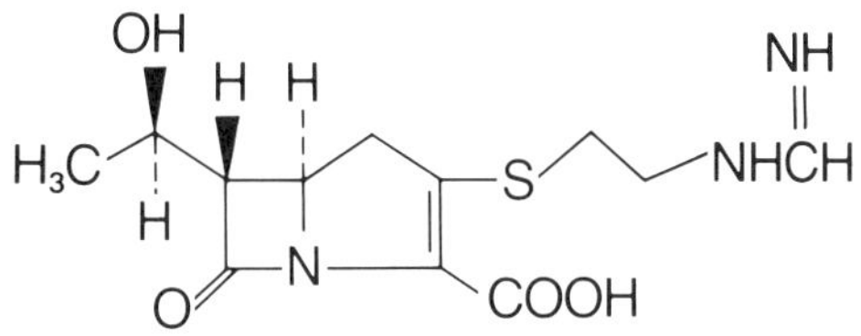

Figure 28–3. N-formidimidoyl thienamycin.

necessary in patients with renal insufficiency, and an increase in dose is required during dialysis (see Table 28–8).

Other Beta-Lactam Antibiotics: Carbepenems and Monobactams

Imipenem

Chemistry. The structure of imipenem, the *N*-formidimidoyl derivative of thienamycin, is shown in Figure 28–3. Biochemically, the thienamycins are carbapenems, which differ from the penicillins by the substitution of a carbon atom for a sulfur atom and by the presence of a double bond in the five-membered ring of the penicillin nucleus.

Antibacterial Spectrum. Imipenem has excellent activity against a wide range of gram-positive and gram-negative anaerobic and aerobic bacteria. The minimal inhibitory concentration (MIC) for most bacteria is less than 1 μg/ml.[60] Beta-lactamase-producing strains of *S. aureus* are inhibited by imipenem. *Staphylococcus epidermidis* and *Streptococcus faecalis* are also sensitive. The majority of the Enterobacteriaceae are also sensitive. Some *Proteus* species have minimal inhibitory concentrations of 3 to 4 μm/ml. *Serratia marcescens* has an MIC of 1.9 to 6.3 μm/ml. The MIC for *P. aeruginosa* is 5 to 12.5 μg/ml. *Pseudomonas maltophilia* and *Pseudomonas cepacia* are resistant.

Imipenem inhibits most anaerobes, including *B. fragilis,* and other *Bacteroides* species at concentrations less than 0.5 μg/ml. Gram-positive cocci, *Clostridium* species, *Fusobacterium* species, and *Veillonella* species are also sensitive.

Mechanism of Action. Like the penicillins and cephalosporins, imipenem is bactericidal by inhibiting cell wall synthesis. It binds to an enzyme (penicillin-binding protein 2) involved in cell wall synthesis. It causes rapid death and there is little difference between the minimal inhibitory concentration and the minimal bactericidal concentration. It is not inhibited by beta-lactamases.

Pharmacology. High serum concentrations are achieved following intravenous administration with plasma levels of 20 μg/ml after an intravenous bolus of 12.5 mg/kg. The serum half-life is 45 minutes and rises to 4 hours in patients with a creatinine clearance of less than 10 ml/min. The dosage must be reduced for individuals with compromised renal function. Imipenem is not destroyed and is distributed widely in body compartments. There is virtually no biliary secretion.

Extensive renal metabolism due to dehydropeptidase-1, which is found on the brush border of the renal tubules, results in low urinary levels. To achieve adequate urine levels, cilastatin dehydropeptidase is added to imipenem for clinical use. Cilastatin has no antibacterial effect nor does it alter the antibacterial effect of imipenem.

Clinical Uses. Imipenem is effective against a wide variety of infections including bacteremia, respiratory tract infections, skin and soft tissue infections, intra-abdominal infections, gynecologic infections, joint and bone infections, endocarditis, and urinary tract infections.[61,62] It may be most useful in febrile neutropenic patients and in patients with hospital-acquired infections—especially those due to *P. aeruginosa*—that are resistant to other antibiotics. Most other infections can be effectively treated with less-expensive antibiotics.

Adverse Reactions. Nausea, vomiting, diarrhea, and rash or drug fever occur in approximately 3 percent of patients treated with imipenem. Seizures, the side effect of greatest concern, occur in 1 to 3 percent of patients. To prevent seizures, the dosage of imipenem should be no greater than 2.0 g or 25 mg/kg/day in patients with normal renal function. The dosage should be reduced in patients with renal insufficiency. In addition to renal insufficiency, other risk factors for the development of seizures are lesions of the central nervous system, history of seizures, and too high doses of imipenem.

Aztreonam. Aztreonam is a beta-lactam antibiotic that is the first monobactam. It is highly resistant to the hydrolytic action of beta-lactamases.

Chemistry. Aztreonam is a monocyclic beta-lactam antibiotic. It is termed a monobactam because it is a monocyclic bacterially produced beta-lactam agent. In contrast to the penicillins, cephalosporins, and carbepenems, which are bicyclic beta-lactams, aztreonam has only a beta-lactam ring. In addition, unlike other beta-lactames, aztreonam has a sulfonic acid group on the nitrogen at the N-1 position. It also has an acyl side chain at position 3 and a methyl group at position 4. It has a sulfate group of nitrogen at position 1, an acyl side chain at position 3, and a methyl group at position 4.

Antibacterial Spectrum. Aztreonam is highly effective against most Enterobacteriaceae especially *E. coli, Klebsiella* species, *Serratia marcescens,* and the *Proteus-Providencia* group. It has significant activity against *Pseudomonas aeruginosa.* It is highly active against many other gram-negative bacteria including *H. influenzae, Neisseria* species, *Salmonella* species, *Shigella* species, *Aeromonas hydrophila,* and *Yersenia enterocolitica.* It has almost no activity against gram-positive bacteria or anaerobic bacteria.

Mechanism of Action. Aztreonam has a high affinity for the penicillin-binding protein 3 of gram-negative bacteria. It causes growth of long filamentous structures that are not viable. Aztreonam does not bind to the penicillin-binding proteins of gram-positive or anaerobic bacteria, hence its lack of activity.

Pharmacology. Aztreonam must be given parenterally. It has a half-life of approximately 1.7 hours. After a 30-minute infusion of a 2-g dose, the peak serum level is 204 μg/ml. Most sensitive bacteria have an in vitro MIC of less than 2 μg/ml. For *P. aeruginusa* the MIC is 16 μg/ml.

Aztreonam is primarily excreted by the kidney. The dose must be decreased in patients with renal insufficiency. This antibiotic is removed by both hemodialysis and peritoneal dialysis.

Clinical Uses. Aztreonam can be used to treat a variety of serious infections caused by susceptible bacteria, including intra-abdominal infection, soft tissue infections, bone and joint infections, pulmonary infections, urinary tract infections, and septicemia. For mixed infections it must be combined with an agent effective against anaerobic organisms (clindamycin or metronidazole) or with an agent active against gram-positive infections (clindamycin or vancomycin).

Because aztreonam is associated with so few side effects it may be useful in place of aminoglycosides in seriously ill patients with renal dysfunction. The usual adult dose can range from 1.5 to 8 g/day.

Adverse Reactions. Aztreonam is extremely safe. It can cause nausea, vomiting, and a rash.

The Quinolones

The quinolones are the newest class of antibiotics and are having a major impact on the chemotherapy of infections. They may become important as the beta-lactam antibiotics. Several fluoroquinolones have recently been released and others will be released in the future.

Chemistry. The quinolones are all fluorinated derivatives of nalidixic acid. The fluoroquinolones have greatly increased antibacterial and pharmacology properties compared to the weak antibacterial activity and the rapid development of antibacterial resistance of nalidixic acid.

All fluoroquinolones have a fluorine atom at the number 6 position of the quinolone ring[63,64] (Fig. 28–4). Substitutions of a carboxyl group at position 3 and of a keto group at position 4 are thought to be important to its antibacterial activity.[64] These 3-carboxyl and 4-keto groups may also be important in passage through bacterial outer membranes.[64] Substitutions at positions 7 and 8 affect the microbiologic activity and pharmacologic properties of the fluoroquinolones.

Mechanism of Action. The fluoroquinolones exert their bacterial activity by inhibiting DNA gyrase, a type-2 topoisomerase composed of two A subunits and two B subunits. These enzymes are involved in DNA replication, recombination, and repair. Binding of quinolones to the DNA gyrase inhibits rejoining after DNA breaks have occurred. Quinolone resistance is attributed to mutations of the A or B subunits, but it occurs infrequently (less than 1 per 10^9 to 10^{11} bacteria) for most bacteria and 1000-fold more frequently for *P. aeruginosa* and mycobacteria.[63,65]

Pharmacology. All fluoroquinolones are absorbed from the gastrointestinal tract. Peak serum concentrations usually are achieved 1 to 2 hours after ingestion in a fasting state and after 2 hours when taken after a meal. Peak serum concentrations may be delayed in the elderly and in some patients with very depressed renal function.[63]

The quinolones differ from one another in their predominant clearance pathways. Almost all are

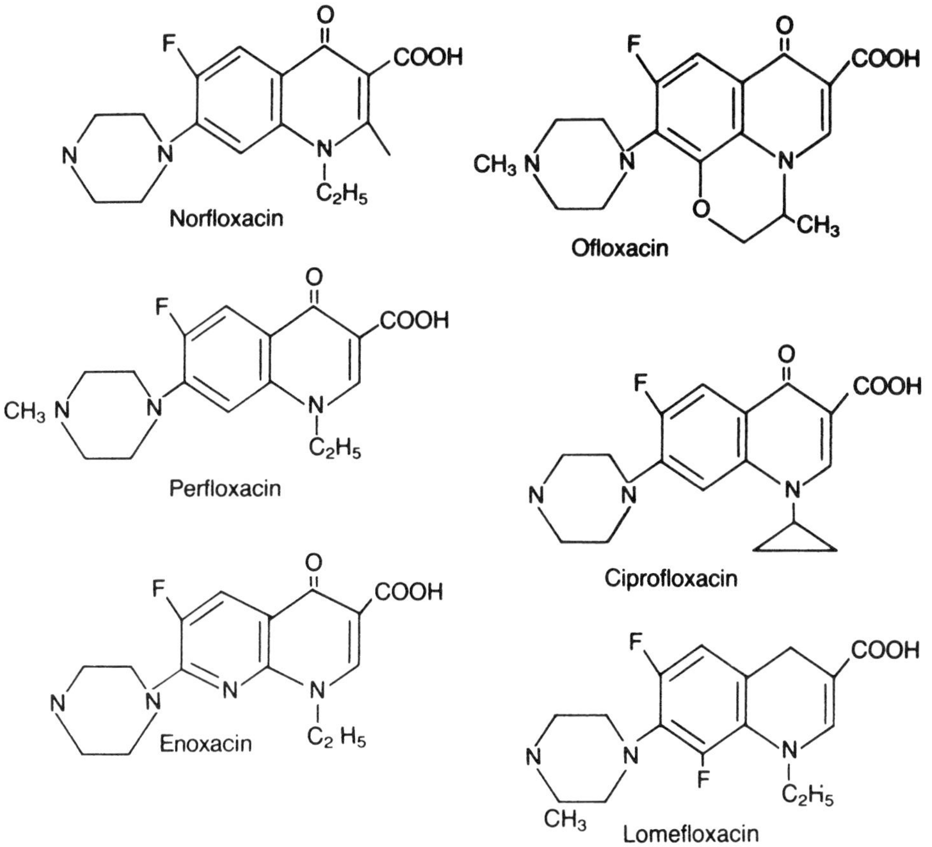

Figure 28–4. Chemical structures of various quinolones. *(From Neu HC: Infect Dis Clin North Am 3:625, 1989.)*

excreted through the kidneys and achieve high urinary concentrations. For others (eg, perfloxacin), hepatic clearance pathways predominant. Norfloxacin and ciprofloxacin are excreted via an enterohepatic pathway and therefore achieve very high (greater than 1000 μg/ml) fecal concentrations. Both renal and hepatic routes of clearance occur for norfloxacin, ciprofloxacin, enoxacin, and lomefloxacin.[64] The dose must be reduced for ofloxacin in patients with renal failure where clearance is almost entirely via the result route. Norfloxacin, ciprofloxacin, and enoxacin, which are also cleared by the hepatic route, have only modest increases in half-lives in patients with renal failure—from 4 to 5 hours to 8 to 9 hours.[64]

The quinolones are widely distributed in the body including central nervous system, bone, and prostate.[63,64] They concentrate up to ten fold in human leukocytes, which may promote killing of intracellular pathogens.

Antimicrobial Activity. The fluoroquinolones have a broad spectrum of activity against gram-negative and gram-positive bacteria, although each agent has certain gaps (Table 28–12). All agents in use clinically have excellent activity against the Enterobacteriaceae with 90 percent of isolates inhibited by less than 2 μg/ml.[63,65] Ciprofloxacin is the most active against the Enterobacteriaceae with 90 percent of isolates inhibited by 0.25 μg/ml or less.[63]

The fluoroquinolones also have excellent activity against other gram-negative bacteria as well, in cluding *S. typhi, Shigella* species, *Yersinia enterocolitica, Campylobacter jejuni, Haemophilis, Brucella, Legionella, Neisseria, Branhamella, Vibrio,* and *Aeromonas* species.[63,64] *Pseudomonas aeruginosa* is susceptible to ciprofloxacin, where 90 percent of isolates are sensitive to concentrations of less than 1.0 μg/ml. Ofloxacin and perfloxacin have higher MIC values than ciprofloxacin but also achieve higher serum concentrations.

The quinolones also inhibit *Mycoplasma hominis* and *Ureaplasma urealyticum* at concentrations of 2 to 8 μg/ml and *Chlamydia trachomatis* at concentrations less than 2 μg/ml.[63] New quinolones such as ciprofloxacin inhibit rickettsia at concentrations as low as 25 μg/ml.

The fluoroquinolones are also active against gram-positive bacteria. Staphylococci, including most methicillin-resistant *S. aure* and *S. epidermidis,* streptococci, especially *S. pneumoniae,* and *Enterococcus faecalis* are less susceptible to most

TABLE 28–12. COMPARATIVE IN VITRO ACTIVITY OF QUINOLONE ANTIBIOTICS[a]

	Minimum Inhibitory Concentrations (MIC_{90}) (μg/ml)							
Organism	**Ciprofloxacin**	**Norfloxacin**	**Ofloxacin**	**Enoxacin**	**Lomefloxacin**	**Fleroxacin**	**Temafloxacin**	**Tosufloxacin**
Escherichia coli	0.12	0.25	0.25	0.25	0.25	0.25	0.25	0.12
Klebsiella pneumoniae	0.12	0.5	0.25	0.25	0.5	0.5	0.5	0.06
Enterobacter species	0.12	1	0.25	0.5	0.5	0.5	0.25	0.25
Citrobacter species	0.12	1	0.25	0.25	1	0.5	2	0.12
Serratia marcescens	0.25	2	2	2	2	2	4	0.25
Shigella species	0.12	0.25	0.25	0.25	0.25	0.25	0.5	0.12
Proteus mirabilis	0.12	0.25	0.25	0.25	0.25	0.25	0.5	0.12
Proteus, other	0.25	0.5	0.5	0.5	1	0.5	1	0.12
Morganella morganii	0.12	0.5	0.12	2	0.5	0.5	1	0.25
Providencia species	0.25	2	0.5	2	0.25	0.25	1	0.12
Yersinia enterocolitica	0.12	0.25	0.12	0.25	4	4	4	0.25
Pseudomonas aeruginosa	0.5	8	4	2	0.5	0.5	0.25	0.12
Acinetobacter species	1	8	1	8	4	4	4	0.5
Staphylococcus aureus methicillin-susceptible	0.5	1	0.5	2	4	2	1	0.12
Staphylococcus aureus methicillin-resistant	0.5	4	0.5	4	2	2	0.5	0.12
Staphylococcus epidermidis	0.5	2	2	8	2	2	0.5	0.25
Enterococcus	2	8	4	6	1	2	0.5	0.5
Streptococcus (group A)	1	4	2	8	16	8	2	0.12
Streptococcus (group B)	1	8	2	16	8	8	0.5	0.25
Streptococcus pneumoniae	2	8	2	16	16	16	1	0.25
Haemophilus influenzae	<0.06	<0.12	<0.12	<0.12	8	8	0.25	<0.12
Neisseria gonorrhoeae	<0.06	<0.12	<0.12	<0.12	0.12	0.12	0.12	<0.12
Neisseria meningitidis	<0.06	<0.12	<0.12	<0.12	0.12	0.12	0.12	<0.12
Campylobacter species	0.05	0.05	1	1	0.12	0.12	0.12	<0.12
Bacteroides fragilis	16	>32	8	>32	—	—	4	1
Bacteroides melaninogenicus	8	>32	8	>32	64		4	2
Peptostreptococcus	4	>32	2	>32	16		4	2
Mycobacterium tuberculosis	1	—	1	—	16		—	—
Branhamella catarrhalis	<0.12	<0.12	<0.12	<0.12	—		<0.12	<0.12
Brucella species	1	8	2	8	0.12		—	—
Listeria monocytogenes	2	4	2	8	—		0.25	0.25
Corynebacterium JK	1	4	1	8	8		0.25	0.25
Legionella species	<0.12	0.5	<0.25	0.5	—		0.25	0.25
Chlamydia trachomatis	2	8	1	8	0.25		0.12	0.25
Mycoplasma hominis	0.5	32	1	64	1		—	0.5
Ureaplasma	2	32	2	64	—		—	—
Mycoplasma pneumoniae	1	8	1	8	—		—	—

[a] Median MIC_{90} of the new quinolone antibiotics was 1 μg/ml. Based on published results from multiple studies.
From Neu HC: Infect Dis Clin North Am 3:625, 1989.

fluoroquinolones, but some of the newer agents have increased activity against these bacteria.

Ciprofloxacin and ofloxacin have activity against *Mycobacterium* species including *M. tuberculosis, M. fortuitum,* and *M. kansasii* at concentrations of 2 μg/ml or lower. Other mycobacterial species such as *M. avium-intracellulare* and *M. chelonei* are less sensitive.[63]

Bacterial Resistance. Despite their relatively recent introduction, resistance to fluoroquinolones is already becoming a problem due to mutations in DNA gyrase, which occurs with a frequency of from 10^{12} to 10^5 when bacteria are exposed to concentrations close to the MICs.[63,65] Spontaneous mutants revert to susceptible in the absence of drug.

Clinical resistance has been noted most frequently in infections caused by *S. aureus, P. aeruginosa,* and *S. marcescens* and less commonly in infections caused by *Citrobacter freundii* and rarely by *K. pneumoniae*. This emerging resistance points to the need to not use the fluoroquinolones indiscriminately.

Clinical Uses. Appropriate clinical uses of the fluoroquinolones—especially in the treatment of surgical infections—are still being defined. They have been used longer, and hence more clinical trials have been performed, in Europe and Japan than in the United States. Currently, they are seldom the antibiotic of choice in treating most infections, something that may change as more clinical data are reported. Many experts believe they are currently overused, which may lead to antibacterial resistance and loss of clinical effectiveness. They are effective in treating urinary tract infections, sexually transmitted diseases including *N. gonorrheae* and *C. trachomatis* genital infections, lower respiratory tract infections, and gastrointestinal tract infections due to enterotoxigenic *E. coli, Shigella, Salmonella, Aeromonas, Pleisomonas,* and *Campylobacter* species.[63,64] The fluoroquinolones are also effective in treating osteomyelitis and soft tissue infections and may prove useful in treating intra-abdominal infections as well. Trials are currently underway.

Adverse Reactions. The fluoroquinolones are safe and toxic effects are rare. But like all antimicrobial agents, adverse reactions do occur. Gastrointestinal side effects such as nausea, vomiting, anorexia, and abdominal pain occur in 1 to 5 percent of patients.[63,64] Central nervous system symptoms include headache, dizziness, confusion, sleep disturbances, mood alterations such as anxiety and depression, tremors, and hallucinations. Seizures have been reported in a few patients with underlying brain disorders. Fluoroquinolones also cause hypersensitivity reactions such as rash, fever, pruritus, urticaria, and anaphylaxis.

Aminoglycosides

The aminoglycoside antibiotics share many pharmacologic and antimicrobial properties. All are primarily useful in the treatment of aerobic gram-negative enteric bacteria and can be used in combination with other antimicrobial agents in the treatment of staphylococcal and enterococcal infections. In addition, all except tobramycin and sisomicin are active against mycobacterial species, including tuberculosis. The gram-positive organisms, except for staphylococci, are generally resistant, and anaerobic organisms are almost all resistant. The differences in spelling between "mycin" or "micin" depends on whether these compounds were isolated from *Streptomyces* or *Micromonospora* species, respectively.[66]

Chemistry. Aminoglycoside antibiotics contain at least two aminosugars joined by glycosidic linkage to a central hexose (streptidine or deoxystreptidine). Aminocyclitols are related compounds.

Pharmacology. None of the aminoglycosides can be absorbed from the gastrointestinal tract and all must be administered parenterally. All are excreted, unchanged, in the urine, so that doses must be modified in patients with renal functional impairment (see Table 28–8). Although they are not absorbed from the gastrointestinal tract in large quantities, their absorption in patients with renal failure can produce toxic levels. Absorption from the peritoneal cavity and other tissue sites is complete, so that toxic levels can be achieved easily after topical use.

Penetration into the cerebrospinal fluid, eye, biliary tree, and tracheal-bronchial secretions is poor after systemic administration. An intrathecal or subconjunctival injection yields high levels in cerebrospinal fluid and aqueous fluid respectively. Penetration into serous cavities yields levels equal to about one-half the peak plasma level.

Antimicrobial Spectrum and Clinical Uses. Aminoglycosides have been the mainstay of therapy for serious gram-negative infections for the last 30 years. Due to their potential for nephrotoxicity and ototoxicity, there has been considerable movement away from aminoglycosides as first-choice agents for community-acquired infections. The use of beta-lactam antibiotics with clindamycin or metronidazole, beta-lactams combined with beta-lactamase inhibitors, or single agent imipenem/cilastatin in mixed flora infections has resulted in clinical results equivalent to or better than those seen with aminoglycoside-based combinations.[67] Aminoglycosides no longer represent a "gold standard" of comparison and need not be used for community-acquired intra-abdominal infections.

The caveat to this statement is the growing body of evidence that hypotensive patients with gram-negative bacteremia have higher survival rates if treated at least initially with aminoglycoside-based combination therapy.[68] Approximately one-third of patients with nonappendiceal intra-abdominal infection are bacteremic. While gram-negative organisms do not represent the same risk of endocarditis on normal valves or of metastatic abscess formation seen with *Staphylococcus aureus,* combination bactericidal therapy may result in more rapid clearance of organisms and abbreviate host deterioration. We believe aminoglycosides should specifically be used in the initial treatment of patients with major intra-abdominal infection and hypotension in combination with a beta-lactam agent effective against the anticipated gram-negative organisms.

Aminoglycoside antibiotics are active against aerobic gram-negative bacilli and *S. aureus*. They are virtually inactive against anaerobes. Sensitivity is defined as inhibition by easily achievable serum concentrations, ie. less than 4 μg/ml for gentamicin, tobramycin, and netilmicin, and less than 16 μg/ml for amikacin and kanamycin. Certain differences in antimicrobial spectrum between the aminoglycosides should be emphasized. Tobramycin and gentamicin, the most commonly useful antimicrobial agents, have similar spectra, except that tobramycin is more active against strains of *Proteus* and especially *P. aeruginosa*. Streptomycin is no longer a clinically useful parenteral antibiotic for the treatment of gram-negative aerobic infections except in isolated circumstances (ie, tularemia, plague, brucellosis, myobacterial infections). Netilmicin is similar to gentamicin except that it shows almost no activity against *Serratia,* and netilmicin is poorly active against *Proteus* species.

All the aminoglycosides can be useful for staphylococcal infections, but not for other gram-positive organisms. Enterococci are relatively resistant, but gentamicin is synergistic for enterococcal endocarditis in combination with penicillin.

Mycobacterium tuberculosis is highly sensitive to streptomycin, but this agent is not useful for atypical mycobacteria. Amikacin is active against both *M. tuberculosis* and the atypical mycobacteria.

ANTIMICROBIAL COMBINATIONS. The beta-lactam antibiotics act synergistically or additively with aminoglycosides against staphylococci, enterococci, the enteric bacteria, and pseudomonads. Carbenicillin (or ticarcillin) plus tobramycin is a particularly useful combination against *P. aeruginosa,* but one must not mix them in the same infusion since carbenicillin can inactivate the aminoglycoside.

Neomycin is too toxic for parenteral use, and the toxic serum levels that can occur after peritoneal instillation, wound irrigation, or cutaneous application seriously restrict this indication. Neomycin should be restricted to oral use for the suppression of intestinal flora in preoperative preparation of the colon and in the treatment of hepatic failure.

Kanamycin is no longer indicated for the initial treatment of suspected gram-negative infections because resistance is common. It is still useful in the reduction of bacterial flora in the bowel before intestinal operations and in patients with hepatic coma, but neomycin is cheaper.

Amikacin has a broad spectrum of activity against gram-negative bacilli including *Serratia,* indole-positive *Proteus, Pseudomonas,* and *Providencia*. It is not susceptible to bacterial enzymes that inactivate other aminoglycosides and consequently is useful against gentamicin and tobramycin-resistant strains of enteric bacteria.[69] Resistance to amikacin seldom occurs because of infrequent use. Most authorities advocate the restriction of amikacin use to specific indications, in order to minimize the emergence of resistant mutants.

Spectinomycin is an aminocyclitol with pharmacologic activities similar to aminoglycosides. Its only use is the treatment of uncomplicated gonococcal urethritis, cervicitis, or proctitis in patients unresponsive or allergic to penicillin (a single 2-g dose IM). It is not useful for pharyngeal gonococcal infections because it is not secreted into saliva. In doses of 2 to 4 g/day for 5 days it may be useful for the treatment of pelvic inflammatory disease.

Spectinomycin is inactive against *Chlamydia*. It is also inactive against *Treponema pallidum,* so that serologic tests for syphilis should be performed at the initial examination and 3 months later in all patients treated with spectinomycin for gonococcal infections.

Pharmacokinetics: Maximizing Aminoglycoside Efficacy. In contrast to the beta-lactams, the efficacy of aminoglycosides depends on the maximal concentration achieved. As the ratio of the concentration of aminoglycoside to the minimum inhibitory concentration (peak concentration to MIC ratio) is increased, the rate and extent of killing are also increased.[70,71] Moore et al[72,73] examined the relationship between plasma aminoglycoside concentration, MICs for the infecting organisms, and therapeutic outcome. Higher peak and mean peak aminoglycoside concentration to MIC ratios (6:1) were strongly associated with a positive clinical response.

In addition to concentration-dependent bactericidal activity, aminoglycosides, like other antimicrobials that affect protein, DNA, or RNA synthesis, exhibit persistent suppression of bacterial growth after antimicrobial exposure, or a postantibiotic effect (PAE).[74] This phenomenon allows killing to continue despite drug concentrations well below the MIC of the infecting organism. Clinical application of this PAE translates into prolonged dosing intervals. Cell-wall-active agents such as penicillins and cephalosporins exert only a PAE against gram-positive bacteria and none against gram-negative organisms.[74,75] Imipenem exerts a modest PAE against gram-negative bacteria. In general, the less frequently aminoglycosides are administered, the lower the risk of aminoglycoside toxicity.[76]

The preceding two pharmacodynamic characteristics have provided the rationale for once-daily dosing of aminoglycosides. The usual total daily dose (2 mg/kg three times a day) is administered as a single dose (6 mg/kg). The PAE should maintain a sufficient killing effect to allow this dose to be given once a day (every 24 hours) instead of the traditional every 8 or 12 hours.[76] Once-daily aminoglycoside dosing may provide more rapid killing, a decrease in the emergence of aminoglycoside-resistant subpopulations, and reduced nephrotoxicity and ototoxicity.[77,78]

There has been considerable movement toward high-dose intermittent therapy with aminoglycosides. Patients with major infections have expanded volumes of distribution for aminoglycosides. If cultures reveal organisms sensitive to the non-aminoglycoside used, single agent anti-gram-negative therapy may be continued after 48 hours. Once-daily dosing of aminoglycosides provides effective therapy for a variety of infections.[82–93]

The immunocompetence of the individual may affect utility of this regimen. In one experimental study, once-daily tobramycin reduced the mean bacterial titer in the lungs significantly more than the every 4 hours regimen in non-neutropenic animals.[71] In neutropenic animals, however, the once-daily regimen proved to be less effective than the every 4 hours regimen as evidenced by a rapid regrowth of bacteria during the latter 12 to 16 hours of the 24-hour dosing interval.

USE OF AMINOGLYCOSIDES IN RENAL FAILURE. Aminoglycoside nephrotoxicity is believed to be caused by accumulation of the antimicrobial within the proximal renal tubular cell by the process of adsorptive pinocytosis.[92] Once in the cell, the antimicrobial is taken up by cellular lysosomes. This process is diminished when aminoglycoside tubular fluid concentrations fall below a critical value and become saturated at higher concentrations. Neither of these limiting values is known precisely, but 2 and 12 mg/dl appear to be of the right order of magnitude.

Historically, clinicians have advocated allowing serum aminoglycoside concentrations to decline below 2 mg/dl ("trough level") before administering the next scheduled dose. In individuals with normal renal function, once-daily dosing of gentamicin and netilmicin routinely results in serum trough concentrations less than 0.5 mg/dl. Animal studies in dogs, rats, and rabbits suggest that multiple daily doses of aminoglycosides result in more frequent or more severe nephrotoxicity (based on creatinine clearance, serum creatinine, urinary enzymes, insulin clearance, renal histology) than do less frequent or once-daily doses of these agents.[91,94–97]

A number of clinical trials have evaluated the effect of once-daily dosing on renal function as assessed by changes in serum creatinine concentration and/or measured 24-hour urines for creatinine clearance.[82,83,85,86,93,98,99] Comparative human trials examining alterations in enzymuria or proteinuria have not been performed. The majority of trials have been small, randomized, and nonblinded in design. Many administered aminoglycosides for at least 7 days (range, 5.3 to 10 days). Eight of nine trials reported no significant differences in serial serum creatinine concentrations between the two groups. Labowitz et al[99] were the only investigators to find a significant difference in favor of multiple daily doses.

When renal function is impaired, the doses of all aminoglycosides must be modified (see Table 28–8). No theoretical method is totally satisfactory, despite the widespread availability of dosage nomograms that have been devised, including those shown in Table 28–8. An estimate of the dose reduction in patients with renal dysfunction can be made from an estimate of the percentage of normal creatinine clearance (ml/min) = (140 − age) × weight (kg) ÷ serum creatine × 72. The result is multiplied by 0.85 for female patients. Assuming a normal creatinine clearance of 100 ml/min, the estimated creatinine clearance is the percentage of normal: a calculated clearance of 25 ml//min represents 25 percent of normal renal function and only 25 percent of the normal dose of aminoglycoside is given. Alternatively, the dosage interval can be increased. The most accurate guide to therapy is the determination of serum aminoglycoside levels. Both peak levels and trough levels should be obtained to assure adequate blood levels and to minimize the possibility of toxicity. For patients in renal failure a "loading dose" of 1.5 mg/kg for gentamicin, tobramycin, and netilmicin and 7.5 to 15 mg/kg for amikacin is advisable in critically ill patients. A blood sample is obtained for the peak level 30 minutes after completion of a 30-minute intravenous infusion. Trough levels should be determined before the next dose. Recommended peak and trough levels are 4 to 6 μg/ml and 1 to 2 μg/ml for gentamicin and netilmicin, respectively. For amikacin and streptomycin, recommended peak concentrations are 20 to 30 μg/ml. The recommended trough concentration for amikacin is 5 to 10 μg/ml, and for streptomycin it is less than 5 μg/ml. Serum antibiotic concentrations should be monitored frequently and at least once 24 hours after any change of dose scheduling.

Aminoglycosides are easily removed both by peritoneal dialysis and hemodialysis. Approximately one-half of initial loading dose should reestablish adequate serum concentration after an efficient hemodialysis run. During peritoneal dialysis, it is best to add the desired serum level of aminoglycoside to the peritoneal dialysis fluid to maintain the serum levels.

Mechanism of Antimicrobial Action. Aminoglycosides are bactericidal antibiotics because they interfere with the synthesis of essential proteins. They bind irreversibly to the 30S subunit of bacterial ribosomes, which leads to misreading of mRNA codons. A nonsense sequence of amino acids results in an abnormal protein.

Mechanisms of Bacterial Resistance to Aminoglycosides. Three mechanisms are responsible for the resistance of bacteria to aminoglycoside antibiotics. The most common type is due to extranuclear plasmids, which code for enzymes that can acetylate, adenylate, or phosphorylate hydroxyl or amino groups on the aminoglycoside molecule. The modified aminoglycoside does not penetrate the microbe or bind to the ribosome in sufficient quantity. Resistance to kanamycin and streptomycin have made these antibiotics obsolete for parenteral administration. Gentamicin and tobramycin cross-resistance is common, except that some gentamicin-resistant strains of *Pseudomonas* are still susceptible to tobramycin. Amikacin has so few sites for enzyme modification that resistant strains are relatively infrequent.

The second mechanism of bacterial resistance to aminoglycosides is the emergence of bacterial mutants, which prevent aminoglycoside transport into bacteria. Most instances of amikacin resistance are the result of such mutants.

A rare cause of bacterial resistance is the emergence of bacterial chromosomal mutants, which are deficient in binding sites.[66]

Adverse Effects. There are three major adverse effects of the aminoglycoside antibiotics.

OTOTOXICITY. Permanent and irreversible deafness can appear without warning, and nystagmus, vertigo, nausea, vomiting, and acute Menière's syndrome can also occur. Audiograms and electronystagmograms suggest a high rate of subclinical nerve damage—especially high-frequency tone loss. The risk is increased with increasing age, duration of therapy, total dose, preexisting renal impairment with high serum antibiotic concentration, preexposure to other aminoglycosides, and concurrent administration of other ototoxic agents, particularly furosemide.

RENAL TOXICITY. Neomycin is the most nephrotoxic agent, and streptomycin the least. The true incidence is difficult to determine because infection, hypotension, and other effects on renal function are difficult to assess. All levels of nephrotoxicity can be observed—oliguric of nonoliguric renal failure, proteinuria, cylindruria, and hematuria.

NEUROMUSCULAR BLOCKADE. Flaccid paralysis of skeletal muscle sometimes follows local irrigation with large doses of aminoglycosides during the use of anesthesia. Respiratory arrest has been reported. The paralytic effects can be reversed by anticholinesterases (neostigmine) and calcium.

Other toxic reactions include local pain, erythema, and occasionally hypersensitivity rashes. Prolonged oral administration of poorly absorbed antimicrobial agents can precipitate or aggravate the development of pseudomembranous enterocolitis, as can almost any antibiotic.

Tetracyclines

Tetracyclines are broad spectrum bacteriostatic antibiotics.

Chemistry. The basic structure consists of the hydronaphthacene nucleus, which contains four fused rings.

Pharmacology. Because the longer-acting tetracyclines are more readily absorbed from the gastrointestinal tract, lower doses are required. Food impairs the absorption of the tetracyclines, especially by complexing with divalent and trivalent cations—calcium, magnesium, and aluminum. Milk, iron, or antacids should not be administered with tetracyclines. Intravenous preparations are available, but thrombophlebitis is a common complication.

Penetration of most tissues is excellent, but cerebrospinal fluid levels are low. The tetracyclines cross the placenta and are incorporated into fetal bone and teeth. Because they are excreted in the milk, they should not be given during pregnancy or lactation. The drug concentrates in the bile and urinary levels are sufficient for the treatment of susceptible organisms within the urinary tract.

Only one tetracycline, doxycycline, can be used in patients with renal failure, because it can be excreted via the gastrointestinal tract under these circumstances.

Antimicrobial Spectrum and Clinical Uses. All tetracyclines share a similar antimicrobial spectrum, and a tetracycline disk is used for susceptibility testing. Minocycline and doxycycline are the most active analogues. Most gram-positive and gram-negative aerobic and anaerobic organisms are susceptible to the tetracyclines, including *S. aureus, Streptococcus pyogenes, Streptococcus pneumoniae, H. influenzae,* and the gram-negative enteric bacteria, but newer agents have replaced them for the treatment of infections due to these bacteria because many bacterial strains are resistant to the tetracyclines. The tetracyclines find few indications in the treatment of serious life-threatening surgical diseases because of the gaps in the spectrum (see Tables 28–2 and 28–3). For this reason, tetracyclines can rarely be presumed to be effective therapy for common bacterial infections until sensitivity testing is done. Tetracyclines are effective in the treatment of sexually transmitted diseases due to *Chlamydia*. Doxycycline and a cephalosporin are usually administered in combination.[100] Tetracyclines provide effective therapy for treating other infections caused by *Chlamydia* species including lymphogranuloma venereum, psittacosis, trachoma, inclusion conjunctivitis, and pneumonitis caused by the TWAR strain.[100]

Tetracyclines are effective therapy for Lyme disease. They are the drug of choice in combination with erythromycin for treating *Mycoplasma pneumoniae.* The tetracyclines can also be used for gonococcal infection in patients who cannot tolerate penicillin. Finally, doxycycline provides effective prophylaxis for traveler's diarrhea caused by toxigenic strains of *E. coli.*[100,101]

Because tetracycline is active against *B. fragilis* at concentrations that can be achieved in the gastrointestinal tract following oral administration, the combination of neomycin and tetracycline or doxycycline alone can be used as an oral, preoperative bowel preparation.

Mechanism of Antimicrobial Action. The tetracyclines inhibit protein synthesis by binding to the 30S ribosomal subunit, which interferes with the addition of amino acids to the growing peptide chain.[100]

Mechanism of Resistance. The principal mechanism of resistance is the development of impermeability of a bacteria to the antibiotic. Enteric organisms become resistant by means of R factors.

Adverse Reactions. The principal adverse reactions are the irritative effects on the upper gastrointestinal tract—esophageal ulcerations, nausea, vomiting, epigastric distress. Diarrhea is caused by alteration of enteric flora, and pseudomembranous colitis has been reported.

Incorporation of tetracycline into teeth and bones during the deposition of tooth enamel (ie, in children up to age 8) will result in permanent discoloration of the teeth. Hypersensitivity reactions are unusual. Tetracycline can aggravate the azotemia of renal failure by inhibiting protein synthesis, but doxycycline is safe in renal failure.

Vertigo, a unique side effect of minocycline, is so common in women (70 percent) that it has seriously limited the use of this drug. Vestibular toxicity usually subsides within 48 hours of discontinuing minocycline therapy.

Effectiveness of the tetracyclines is reduced by concurrent administration of diphenylhydantoin and barbiturates, which induce enzymes capable of metabolizing the drug.

Chloramphenicol

Chloramphenicol is virtually never used in the United States because of its history of irreversible bone marrow suppression, it is still used in many parts of the world because of its broad spectrum of activity and low cost.

Pharmacology. Oral administration results in higher levels than intravenous administration because (1) the drug is almost totally absorbed in active form and (2) intravenous chloramphenicol succinate must be hydrolyzed to biologically active chloramphenicol. The intramuscular route results in even lower levels and is not recommended. Adequate therapeutic levels are found in all tissues and body fluids, including the brain and cerebrospinal fluid.

Chloramphenicol is metabolized in the liver, where it is conjugated with glucuronic acid and excreted in the kidneys. Newborn infants require half the recommended adult dose because they metabolize it slowly. Renal excretion of the unchanged drug is low, and no alteration is necessary in renal insufficiency, although metabolites continue to accumulate in the blood. The dose must be reduced for patients with hepatic failure to avoid suppression of the bone marrow.

Antimicrobial Activity and Clinical Uses. Chloramphenicol is active against bacteria, spirochetes, rickettsiae, chlamydiae, and mycoplasmas. Almost all gram-positive and gram-negative bacteria, whether aerobes or anaerobes, are susceptible. The notable exceptions are most of the methicillin-resistant *S. aureus, P. aeruginosa, S. marcescens,* and indole-positive *Proteus organisms*; many *Enterobacter* species are also resistant. Many more active and less toxic therapeutic agents are available for the pathogens that are susceptible to chloramphenicol. Despite its broad spectrum, chloramphenicol is the best drug in a relatively narrow set of indications. It is, however, effective alternative therapy in many mixed infections of gram-positive and gram-negative organisms, and in selected patients with bacteria proved to be susceptible by susceptibility testing studies.

Because of its high penetration into cerebrospinal fluid and cerebral tissue, it is the drug of choice for many central nervous system infections, including the three most common causes of meningitis in childhood (*H. influenzae, S. pneumoniae,* and *Neisseria meningitidis*).[100] Because of its activity against *B. fragilis*, chloramphenicol is a good second choice in the treatment of mixed aerobic and anaerobic enteric infections, such as peritonitis, or the soft tissue infections caused by fecal contamination (necrotizing fascitis).

Mechanism of Antimicrobial Action. Chloramphenicol inhibits protein synthesis and is bacteriostatic. The drug binds to the 50S ribosomal subunit that interferes with peptide formation.

Mechanisms of Microbial Resistance. Bacteria become resistant to chloramphenicol by becoming impermeable to the drug or by R factors capable of inducing an enzyme that degrades the antibiotic to the inactive derivative.

Adverse Reactions. The principal adverse reaction is suppression of the bone marrow, which can take one of two forms: (1) a reversible, dose-related bone marrow depression caused by an inhibition of protein synthesis, and (2) an idiosyncratic, irreversible, generally fatal aplastic anemia unrelated to dose.[102] Irreversible, fatal aplastic anemia can occur either during or after therapy. A few cases have been reported after parenteral administration.[103] Leukocyte counts should be carried out in all patients who receive chloramphenicol, and the drug should be stopped if levels below 2500 mm^3 are found.

Hemolytic anemias occasionally occur in patients with a severe form of glucose 6-phosphate dehydrogenase (G6PD) deficiency.

Other toxic manifestations include the gray syndrome in neonates—abdominal distension, vomiting, flaccidity, cyanosis, circulatory collapse, and death—the result of the incapacity of neonates to detoxify chloramphenicol.

Coumadin toxicity can be induced by the concurrent dose of chloramphenicol, which can inhibit hepatic metabolism of this and other drugs. Chloramphenicol is a bacteriostatic agent and, theoretically, should antagonize bactericidal activity of the penicillins, cephalosporins, or the aminoglycoside antibiotics. This has doubtful clinical significance. Bacteriostatic agents should not be used, however, in granulocytopenic and other immunodepressed subjects.

Erythromycin

Erythromycin is an extremely safe antibiotic that, in addition to its usefulness as an alternative to penicillin G, has important primary indications.

Chemistry. Erythromycin is a macrolide compound that contains macrocyclin lactone ring to which are attached one or more deoxy sugars. For the erythromycin base, an agent commonly used for oral prophylaxis for colon surgery, two sugars—desosamine and cladinose—are attached to an erythronolide lactone ring.

Pharmacology. Erythromycin is rapidly inactivated by gastric acid and must be protected during oral administration. Gastrointestinal absorption of all oral preparations is good, but much higher levels can be obtained by intravenous administration. Tissue distribution is excellent everywhere except in the cerebrospinal fluid, middle ear, and synovial fluid. Urine concentrations are variable. Erythromycin is concentrated in the liver and excreted in the bile; fecal excretion can be high. Erythromycin base and neomycin are a popular and effective antimicrobial bowel preparation because the erythromycin base is only partially absorbed. In such high concentrations, it exerts a potent antianaerobic effect on the gut flora.

Antimicrobial Spectrum and Clinical Uses. Erythromycin has a broad spectrum against gram-positive bacteria and is active in vitro against *Actinomyces, Mycobacterium, Treponema, Mycoplasma, Chlamydia,* and *Rickettsia*. Erythromycin is the drug of choice for treating infections caused by *Mycoplasma pneumonia* and *Legionella* species. Its main use in surgery is oral prophylaxis in combination with a neomycin base for colon surgery. It is bactericidal in high concentration and under circumstances of rapid bacterial growth. Its activity in urine is accelerated by increasing the pH into the alkaline range of 8.5. At that level, it is active even against Enterobacteriaceae, which are otherwise quite resistant. Unfortunately, *Enterococcus, S. aureus, S. epidermidis, Clostridium perfringens, H. influenzae,* and *B. fragilis* have unpredictable susceptibility at achievable serum concentrations, so that erythromycin cannot be used as empiric therapy of infections that are frequently caused by these organisms until sensitivity testing is done. Infections for which erythromycin can occasionally be used are *Actinomyces israelii, Mycobacterium scrofulaceum,* and *Mycobacterium kansasii,*[100] and combined with ampicillin against *N. asteroides*.

MECHANISMS OF ANTIMICROBIAL ACTION. Erythromycin is a bacteriostatic drug that inhibits RNA-dependent protein synthesis of binding to the 50S ribosomal subunit.

MECHANISMS OF BACTERIAL RESISTANCE. Resistance to erythromycin is sometimes due to (1) decreased permeability of the cell wall (gram-negative enterics), (2) alteration of the 50S ribosomal protein receptor site (chromosomal mutation), or (3) alteration in the 23S ribosomal RNA of the 50S ribosomal subunit by methylation of adenine. This resistance is mediated by a plasmid. Cross-resistance with lincomycin and clindamycin is common.

ADVERSE REACTIONS. Erythromycin is one of the safest antibiotics, although gastrointestinal irritation, occasional allergic reactions, and superinfection have been reported. Cholestatic hepatitis is rare and reversible. Transient hearing losses have been reported with large intravenous doses of drug, especially if other ototoxic drugs are in concurrent use (eg, aminoglycosides).

Clindamycin

The lincosamide antibiotics are chemically unrelated to erythromycin but share pharmacologic and antimicrobial properties.

Pharmacology. Adequate serum and tissue levels are reached with the usual doses of 600 to 2400 mg/day in three or four equal doses for parenteral administration or 150 to 600 mg every 6 hours for oral administration. The cerebrospinal fluid has inadequate concentrations, and most of the absorbed drug is metabolized in the liver. The dose need not be reduced in renal failure; the drug is not dialyzed (see Table 28–8).

Antimicrobial Spectrum. Clindamycin has a broad spectrum of activity against the gram-positive cocci, especially streptococci and pneumococci. Most strains of staphylococci are sensitive, but enterococci, gonococci, and meningococci are resistant. Almost all anaerobic organisms, including most clostridial species and *B. fragilis,* are susceptible. Gram-negative enteric organisms are resistant. Of the anaerobes, a few peptococcus and clostridial species[104] are resistant to clindamycin. Consequently, resistant strains of *Clostridium difficile* can induce pseudomembranous enterocolitis after clindamycin therapy.[105]

Most authorities agree that clindamycin should be limited in its indications to only those infections that are likely to involve *B. fragilis* and that are outside the central nervous system. It is an extremely useful drug in combination with an aminoglycoside for the treatment of mixed intra-abdominal, gynecologic, or necrotizing soft tissue infections caused by facultative and anaerobic gram-negative and gram-positive bacteria.

Clindamycin is occasionally useful as an alternative to penicillin G for anaerobic necrotizing pulmonary infections. Some authorities have suggested that clindamycin may be superior to penicillin for the treatment of anaerobic pulmonary abscess.[100,106] Clindamycin is also useful as an alternative to, or in combination with, penicillin in the treatment of *C. perfringens* infections. Although high concentrations of clindamycin are achieved in bone, no clinical advantage of clindamycin for the treatment of osteomyelitis has been established.

Mechanisms of Action. The lincosamide antibiotics bind to 50S ribosomal binding sites as do the macrolides and chloramphenicol. Protein synthesis is thereby inhibited.

Mechanisms of Resistance. Failure of clindamycin, like erythromycin, to penetrate the gram-negative organisms results in resistance. Some resistant bacteria are mutants with changes in the binding site on the 50S ribosomal protein.

Adverse Reactions. Minor adverse reactions of the allergic type and mild hepatotoxicity have been noted; however, the principal toxic effect of lincosamide antibiotics is diarrhea. Most evidence supports the idea that clindamycin-associated diarrhea is usually caused by an enterotoxin elaborated by colonic *C. difficile*. In the more severe cases, a true pseudomembranous enterocolitis is produced. True pseudomembranous enterocolitis has been reported in up to 10 percent of clindamycin recipients followed prospectively,[107] but a much lower incidence of this complication has been reported after parenteral administration. Pseudomembranous enterocolitis, its pathogenesis and treatment, is discussed extensively in Chapter 42. Whenever possible, the appearance of antibiotic-associated diarrhea should prompt discontinuation of the responsible antibiotic—most cases are mild and will resolve spontaneously. The most severe cases of pseudomembranous enterocolitis will respond to oral vancomycin or metronidazole, even though relapses after treatment occasionally occur. Cholestyramine, which can bind the *C. difficile* toxin, has been suggested as well.

Bacitracin

Bacitracin was originally isolated from *Bacillus licheniformis (subtilis)* and was formally used for the treatment of severe staphylococcal infections. Because of its nephrotoxicity, it is rarely administered systemically but it can be used, without serious side effects, as a topical antibiotic. Toxicity due to systemic absorption has not been reported even when used in large doses to irrigate the peritoneal cavity.[108] Bacitracin is a peptide antibiotic composed of peptide-linked aminoacids. It is highly active against most gram-positive bacteria including *S. pyogenes,* group A beta-hemolytic streptococci, and C and G beta-hemolytic streptococci. Group B streptococci are usually resistant, however, as are gram-negative bacilli. Other pyogenic cocci such as the *Neisseria* are sensitive. Acquired bacterial resistance is unusual although some resistant *S. pyogenes* strains have been found.

Bacitracin interferes with bacterial cell wall synthesis by inhibiting the dephosphorylation of a lipid pyrophosphate. In addition, it damages the bacterial cytoplasmic membrane and is active against protoplasts.

Bacitracin is most often used topically as creams, ointments, antibiotic sprays and powders, and in solutions for wound irrigation or bladder instillation. Most commonly, it is combined with both neomycin and polymyxin B to provide an effective cover for gram-negative bacilli and *Pseudomonas* in addition to its own activity against gram-positive cocci.

Polymyxins

Polymyxins are cyclic basic polypeptides that are much too toxic for routine clinical use. Only polymyxin B and E (colistin) are available.

Pharmacology. Polymyxin is not absorbed from the gastrointestinal tract, and intramuscular injections are painful. Topical preparations (0.1 percent polymyxin) in combination with other antibiotics (bacitracin, neomycin) have been found useful in the prophylaxis of wound infections and in the treatment of superficial infections of skin and mucous membranes. Continuous irrigation of serous or wound cavities is contraindicated because absorption can produce nephrotoxicity and apnea.

Antimicrobial Spectrum and Clinical Uses. Polymyxins are only active against gram-negative bacilli, especially *Pseudomonas,* and they are used intravenously, almost exclusively, for serious life-threatening *Pseudomonas* infection when other drugs cannot be used (1.5 to 2.5 mg/kg/day by continuous IV infusion).

Even so, the polymyxins are poor drugs for the treatment of deep-seated infections and immunocompromised patients. The best results have been obtained in urinary tract infections or in cases of septicemia that arise from the urinary tract. Intrathecal administration is necessary for the treatment of meningitis.

Polymyxins are of principal clinical use in the topical treatment of superficial infections (eg, external otitis, corneal ulcers). Bladder infections can be treated by continuous irrigation with a solution of neomycin (40 mg/liter) and polymyxin B (20 mg/liter).[109]

Combinations of the polymyxins with sulfamethoxazole and trimethoprim are said to be synergistic in the treatment of serious infections with multiple drug-resistant *Serratia, Pseudomonas cepacia, P. maltophilia,* or *P. aeuruginosa.* A combination of polymyxin B and rifampin has been used to treat patients with *Serratia* infections.[110] Experience with both combinations is limited.

Adverse Reactions. The two important side effects of the polymyxins, nephrotoxicity and neurotoxicity, are reversible and can be reduced by reducing the dosage. Neurotoxicity manifests itself as paresthesias with flushing, dizziness, vertigo, ataxia, slurred speech, drowsiness, or confusion. In addition, the polymyxins have a curare-like action on striated muscles and block neuromuscular transmission. If apnea occurs it can be treated with intravenous calcium chloride.

Vancomycin

Chemistry. Vancomycin is a complex glycopolypeptide unrelated to any other antibiotic.[111] Vancomycin exerts its major antibacterial effect by inhibiting synthesis of peptidoglycan, the major structural component of bacterial cell walls but at a different site than the penicillins. Thus there is no cross-resistance. In addition, it also affects the permeability of plasma membranes and may impair RNA synthesis.[111]

Pharmacology. It is usually given intravenously, because it is not absorbed by mouth and is painful on intramuscular injection. It is excreted almost exclusively by the kidney. Organisms susceptible to less than 10 μg/ml (the peak serum concentration after intravenous administration of a 500-mg dose) are considered susceptible. Vancomycin yields peak serum concentrations of 20 to 50 μg/ml and trough levels of 5 to 10 μg/ml after a 1-g dose in patients with normal renal function. There is some penetration into the cerebrospinal fluid of patients with meningitis, but penetration through uninflamed meninges is poor. It is irritating in serous cavities. Because it is excreted in the kidney, the dose must be reduced in patients with renal malfunction—hemodialysis does not adequately remove it. It is best to monitor the serum levels in uremic patients to prevent excessive accumulation in the serum, even though formulas for reduction of dose are available.

Antimicrobial Spectrum and Clinical Uses. Gram-negative organisms (*S. aureus, S. epidermidis, Streptococcus pyogenes, Streptococcus pneumoniae,* anaerobic streptococci, *N. gonorrhoeae*), *Clostridium, B. anthracis, Actinomyces,* and *Corynebacterium diphtheriae* are usually susceptible. Streptococci of the viridans group, *S. bovis,* and *E. faecalis,* although inhibited, resist killing. Vancomycin plus an aminoglycoside may be synergistic against *E. faecalis.* Gram-negative bacilli, *Mycobacterium, Bacteroides,* and fungi are not susceptible. The development of resistance is rare during treatment.[111]

The clinical uses of vancomycin are listed in Table 28–13. Because of its toxicity, vancomycin is prescribed only for the treatment of serious gram-positive infections in patients who are allergic to penicillin or for organisms not susceptible to penicillin or cephalosporins. Appropriate doses are listed in Table 28–14.

Adverse Reactions. The most common side effects of its parenteral administration are fever, chills, and thrombophlebitis. Shock, leukopenia, and rashes are rare complications. The most important adverse reaction is neurotoxicity as manifested by auditory nerve damage and hearing loss. Nephrotoxicity is now unusual since the impurities in the prepara-

TABLE 28–13. THERAPEUTIC INDICATIONS FOR VANCOMYCIN

1. Serious infections caused by methicillin-resistant strains of *Staphylococcus aureus* and coagulase-negative staphylococci
2. Serious infections caused by *S. aureus* or streptococci in patients intolerant of β-lactam antibiotics
3. Endocarditis treatment—as alternative therapy in beta-lactam-intolerant patients
   - *S. aureus*
   - Coagulase-negative staphylococci
   - Streptococci
   - Beta-hemolytic streptococci
   - Viridans streptococci
   - Nonenterococcal group D streptococci
   - Enterococci (in combination with gentamicin)
4. Infections caused by multiply resistant gram-positive organisms (eg, *Corynebacterium jeikeium* and resistant strains of *Streptococcus pneumoniae*)
5. *Clostridium difficile* colitis (oral administration)
6. Endocarditis prophylaxis (in combination with gentamicin) for selected genitourinary and gastrointestinal procedures in penicillin-intolerant patients

From Wilhelm MP: Mayo Clin Proc 66:1165, 1991.

TABLE 28–14. PRIMARY INDICATIONS FOR ANTIFUNGAL AGENTS IN DEEP FUNGAL INFECTIONS[a]

Indication	Drug of Choice	Alternate	Possibly Effective, Awaiting Comparative Trials
Candidiasis (deep-seated)	Amphotericin B (± flucytosine)	—	Fluconazole
Histoplasmosis			
Mild or moderate	Ketoconazole	Amphotericin B	Itraconazole
Severe, meningeal, or ICH	Amphotericin B	—	—
AIDS: Initial	Amphotericin B	—	Itraconazole
Maintenance	Amphotericin B	—	Itraconazole
Cryptococcosis			
Meningeal	Amphotericin B + flucytosine	—	—
Other deep-seated	Amphotericin B (+ flucytosine ?)	—	—
AIDS: Meningeal or acute	Amphotericin B (+ flucytosine ?)	—	Fluconazole, itraconazole
Maintenance	Fluconazole	Amphotericin B	Itraconazole
Coccidioidomycosis			
Meningeal	Amphotericin B (IV + intrathecal)	—	Fluconazole, itraconazole
Other deep-seated	Amphotericin B	—	Fluconazole, itraconazole
AIDS: Initial	Amphotericin B (IV + intrathecal)	—	Fluconazole, itraconazole
Maintenance	Amphotericin B	—	Fluconazole, itraconazole
Blastomycosis			
Mild or moderate	Ketoconazole	Amphotericin B	Itraconazole
Severe, meningeal, GU, or ICH	Amphotericin B	—	—
Aspergillosis (invasive)	Amphotericin B (+ flucytosine ?)	—	Itraconazole
Sporotrichosis			
Lymphocutaneous	Potassium iodide	—	Itraconazole, fluconazole
Deep-seated	Amphotericin B	Ketoconazole	Itraconazole
Pseudallescheria boydii infection	Miconazole	Amphotericin B	—
Mucormycosis	Amphotericin B	—	—

[a] See text for details of antifungal therapy for specific sites of infection. AIDS, acquired immunodeficiency syndrome; GU, genitourinary; ICH, immunocompromised host; IV, intravenous.
From Terrell CL, Hughes CE: Mayo Clin Proc 67:69, 1992.

tion have been removed. The major "toxicity" of oral administration is its disagreeable taste.

Sulfonamides

Chemistry and Classification. The sulfonamides have a structure similar to that of para-aminobenzoic acid (PABA), a factor necessary for bacterial folic acid synthesis. Substitutions of the 4-amino group result in decreased gastrointestinal absorption. Substitutions at the SO_2NH_2 group alter the pharmacologic properties of the drug, but the antimicrobial spectrum remains the same. Zinner and Mayer[112] have classified the sulfonamides into (1) short- or medium-acting sulfonamides useful for urinary tract infections, (2) long-acting sulfonamides (sulfamethoxypyridazine and sulfameter), (3) sulfonamides limited to the gastrointestinal tract (sulfaguanidine, sulfathalidine, salicylazosulfapyridine), and (4) topical sulfonamides (mafenide acetate, silver sulfadiazine). Topical preparations applied to extensive burns are absorbed.

Pharmacology. Intravenous administration of sulfadiazine, sulfisoxazole, and cotrimoxazole is possible, but most sulfonamides are administered orally or topically. After absorption from the gastrointestinal tract, they are distributed throughout the body, including the cerebrospinal fluid and serous cavities. The drugs undergo acetylation and glucuronidation in the liver, and both free and metabolized drugs are excreted in the urine. The doses should be reduced during renal failure (see Table 28–8).

Antimicrobial Spectrum and Clinical Uses. Sulfonamides are active in vitro against a broad spectrum of gram-positive and gram-negative aerobic bacteria plus *Actinomyces, Chlamydia, Plasmodium*, and *Toxoplasma* (see Tables 28–2 and 28–3). But the activity is irregular, and certain organisms,

S. marcescens, P. aeruginosa, Enterococci, and anaerobes, are frequently resistant at serum levels that can easily be obtained after oral administration.

Antimicrobial Resistance. Susceptible organisms may develop resistance by mutations, which result in overproduction of para-aminobenzoic acid, or a structural change in folic acid synthesizing enzyme so that it has lower affinity for sulfonamide.[113] The resistance can be mediated by R factors.

Adverse Reactions. Sulfonamides are known to cause nausea, vomiting, diarrhea, rash, fever, headache, depression, jaundice, hepatic necrosis, and a serum sickness-like syndrome. Soluble sulfonamides rarely produce crystalluria anymore. Acute hemolytic anemia (associated with G6PD deficiency), aplastic anemia, agranulocytosis, thrombocytopenia, and leukopenia have all been reported. Serious hypersensitivity reactions (ie, erythema nodosum, erythema multiforme) are more common in children. Because the sulfonamides compete with bilirubin-binding sites on plasma albumin, they may increase the chances of kernicterus and therefore should not be administered during the last month of pregnancy.

Sulfonamides interact with many other drugs. They increase the effect of activity of warfarin by displacing it from albumin-binding sites; anticoagulant dosage should be reduced during sulfonamide therapy. Numerous other drug interactions have been described by Zimmer and Mayer.[112]

Trimethoprim and Sulfamethoxazole (Co-Trimoxazole)

The sulfonamides act in synergy with trimethoprim, and a fixed drug combination is available (cotrimoxazole). Trimethoprim itself is useful in the treatment of urinary tract infections.

Mechanism of Action. Trimethoprim inhibits bacterial dihydrofolate reductase, the enzymatic step that follows the step in bacterial folic acid metabolism-inhibited sulfonamides. Because both drugs block the same biosynthetic pathway at different sites, their combination acts synergistically against a wide spectrum of microorganisms. Since mammals do not synthesize folic acid, purine synthesis is not affected significantly.

Pharmacology. Trimethoprim plus sulfamethoxazole (co-trimoxazole) in a ratio of 1:5 is available for oral use, and an intravenous preparation will probably soon be available. Trimethoprim (like sulfamethoxazole) is readily absorbed from the gastrointestinal tract, and after the usual dose (160 mg trimethoprim, 800 mg sulfamethoxazole), the serum levels are 1.6 to 3.2 μg/ml. It is widely distributed in tissues, and the levels reached in the cerebrospinal fluid are therapeutic. Trimethoprim is concentrated in prostatic fluid. It is excreted by the kidney, and its half-life is prolonged by renal insufficiency. The concentrations in the urine are usually far in excess of the maximum inhibitory concentration for most urinary pathogens. In severe uremia, a loading dose followed by half the dose once or twice daily has been recommended.

Antimicrobial Spectrum and Clinical Uses. Most gram-positive cocci and most gram-negative rods, except *P. aeruginosa* and *Bacteorides* species, are susceptible. Synergy with sulfamethoxazole (see Tables 28–2 and 28–3) and with the polymyxins and the aminoglycosides has been reported.[113,114] The optimal ratio for in vitro synergy of trimethoprim and sulfamethoxazole in combinations is 1:20. This ratio is achieved by having an oral or intravenous combination of 1:5 (trimethoprim: sulfamethoxazole). Even strains resistant to sulfamethoxazole will become sensitive to the combination in many cases, although this cannot be universally predicted.[115]

The principal clinical use of trimethoprim is in combination with sulfamethoxazole (co-trimoxazole) for the treatment of acute and chronic urinary tract infections. This combination is also useful for long-term suppressive therapy of recurrent or chronic urinary tract infections—it can control bacteria in vaginal secretions and in stool flora.

Co-trimoxazole is useful in the treatment of pneumonia or bronchitis caused by sensitive organisms, but parenteral therapy with other agents is currently preferred. It may also be useful in the prophylaxis of acute exacerbations in patients with chronic bronchitis. It is the drug of choice for treating infections due to *Pneumocystis carinii.* Prophylaxis against *P. carinii* pneumonia in patients infected with the human immunodeficiency virus and in other immunosuppressed patients can be achieved by long-term, daily therapy with 150 mg/m^2 of trimethoprim and 750 mg/m^2 of sulfamethoxazole.[116] Co-trimoxazole is useful in reducing the incidence of gram-negative rod bacteremia in neutropenic patients (two tablets twice a day, or more, until stools are free of enteric organisms). Gastrointestinal anaerobes are not affected by this prophylaxis, so that the aerobes are seldom replaced by resistant organisms.

Adverse Reactions. The adverse reactions of the sulfonamides are seen with the use of co-trimoxazole—a megaloblastic marrow with hypersegmented polymorphonuclear leukocytes, leukopenia, thrombocytopenia, and granulocytopenia can result. The administration of folic acid usually prevents or treats the side effects, and the antibacterial efficacies (except possibly against enterococci) are not impaired by such prophylaxis.

Metronidazole

Chemistry and Pharmacology. Metronidazole is a nitroimidazole derivative that is rapidly absorbed orally, with peak levels occurring 1 to 3 hours after ingestion. Blood levels after intravenous injection approximate those following oral, rectal, or vaginal administration. Two-thirds of the drug is excreted unchanged in the urine, with only trace quantities identifiable in the feces. Tissue penetration is excellent and therapeutic levels are found in the cerebrospinal fluid, abscesses, bile, bone, breast milk, and placenta. The serum half-life is 8 hours.[100]

Antimicrobial Spectrum and Clinical Uses. Metronidazole is active against the protozoa *Trichomonas vaginalis, Giardia lamblia,* and *Entamoeba histolytica.* It is the drug of choice for trichomoniases and of use in intestinal amebiasis and amebic liver abscess. Metronidazole shows marked activity against almost all anaerobic bacteria, especially *B. fragilis.*

Metronidazole is effective in the treatment of antibiotic-associated colitis caused by *C. difficile.* The potent antianaerobic bacterial activity makes this agent effective in reducing wound infections when given in combination with neomycin for preparation of the bowel before colorectal surgery (see Chap. 43).[100]

Metronidazole in combination with an aminoglycoside is as effective as clindamycin-aminoglycoside in treating mixed aerobic-anaerobic intra-abdominal and pelvic infections. It is also useful in combination with an aminoglycoside for treating severe polymicrobial soft tissue infections.[100] It does seem superior to other agents in treating anaerobic cerebral abscess where penetration into the abscess cavity is excellent.

Adverse Effects. Gastrointestinal distress with symptoms of anorexia, nausea, diarrhea, and abdominal cramps are common complaints. Less common side effects are skin rashes, leukopenia, and central nervous system symptoms (dizziness, vertigo, ataxia tremor). Darkening of the urine to a reddish-brown color is of no significance. Patients should not drink alcohol while taking metronidazole because this agent has disulfiram-like properties and will cause flushing, vomiting, and abdominal cramping.

Studies in animals suggest that metronidazole has an oncogenic potential. The human significance of this finding has yet to be determined.

Rifampin

Chemistry. The rifamycins are a group of antibacterial agents isolated from cultures of *Streptomyces mediterranei.* Rifamycin B is the active parent compound that yields rifamide and rifampin after chemical modification.

Pharmacology. Rifampin is lipid soluble and is rapidly absorbed orally with peak serum levels of 5 to 10 μg/ml after a 600-mg oral dose 1 to 3 hours before. Rifampin penetrates liver, lung, placenta, bone, ascitic fluid, pleural exudates, and other intracellular and extracellular spaces in concentrations equal to or greater than that in the serum. The cerebrospinal fluid concentrations are greatest when the meninges are inflamed. Eighty percent of the drug is protein bound in plasma, and deacetylation takes place in the liver with 60 percent excretion in the feces. Bile concentrations of rifampin are about 100 times that of simultaneous serum levels. Urine concentrations are about ten times those in the serum.

Spectrum. Gram-positive bacteria are usually sensitive to rifampin, including *Staphylococcus* strains (penicillin- and methicillin-resistant strains), pneumococcus, most *Streptococcus* (enterococcus is moderately sensitive), and *Clostridium.* Many gram-negative organisms are also sensitive including gonococci, meningococci, *H. influenzae, E. coli, Enterobacter, Klebsiella, Proteus, P. aeruginosa, Salmonella, Shigella,* and *Bacteroides* species. *Mycobacterium tuberculosis, M. kansasii, M. ulcerans, M. marinum, M. phlei,* and *M. leprae* are usually sensitive, but *M. avium-intracellularis, M. smegmatis,* and *M. fortuitum* are resistant. Rifampin shows in vitro activity against *Chlamydia* and some viruses, including cytomegalovirus, vaccinia, and adenoviruses.

Clinical Uses. Rifampin is a first-line agent, in combination with others, for the treatment of tuberculosis and asymptomatic pharyngeal carriers of *N. meningitidis.* In general, rifampin should not be used alone, because resistance develops rapidly.[117] Because of its broad spectrum, however, it is becoming increasingly useful in combination with other antibiotics (trimethoprim, nafcillin) for the treatment of resistant staphylococci.

Mechanism of Action. RNA synthesis is blocked by rifampin by inhibiting DNA-dependent RNA polymerase. The human RNA polymerase is much less sensitive than the bacteria and thus is unaffected.

Adverse Effects. Flushing, itching, and rash of the face can occur after taking large doses of rifampin. Liver damage is the most serious effect. Thrombocytopenia has also been reported. Rifampin colors the urine red, as it does other body fluids.

Urinary Tract Antiseptics

Urinary tract antiseptics are drugs that are concentrated in the urine but are not useful for the treatment of systemic infections. Nalidixic acid, oxolinic acid, and nitrofurantoin are useful for acute or recurrent infections and methenamine for chronic urinary tract suppression.

Nalidixic Acid and Oxolinic Acid. These compounds are chemically related and have similar pharmacologic characteristics and clinical uses. Both inhibit DNA synthesis in bacterial cells and have a broad spectrum against gram-negative bacteria, but *Pseudomonas* species and gram-positive bacteria are resistant. Cross-resistance has been demonstrated between the two agents.

Both drugs are absorbed after oral administration and are excreted primarily by the kidneys. Both can be used in moderate or advanced renal failure,[118] although metabolites may accumulate in the blood.

Most adverse reactions are minor and disappear with discontinuation of the drug. These include gastrointestinal side effects, dermatologic reactions, and occasional visual abnormalities. Central nervous system reactions with excitation, headache, restlessness, insomnia, and dizziness have been observed with both drugs.

Nitrofurantoin. Nitrofurantoin is a useful drug in the treatment of acute urinary tract infections because it inhibits multiple enzymes within bacterial cells. It is effective against most strains of *E. coli* and other enteric gram-negative rods, but many *Klebsiella, Enterobacter,* and *Proteus* strains are resistant—*Pseudomonas* is almost always resistant. Gram-positive cocci including enterococci are generally sensitive.

Nitrofurantoin is administered orally and is rapidly absorbed from the gastrointestinal tract and excreted in the urine after some metabolic changes. Secretion into the urine of patients with renal malfunction is decreased so that it is not useful in patients with renal failure.

The common adverse reactions are minor, and most are reversed by cessation of drug therapy. Gastrointestinal irritation is the most common side effect; hypersensitivity reactions, and dermatologic allergic manifestations are generally mild and infrequent. Acute or chronic hypersensitivity and interstitial pneumonitis occur in elderly patients and may require steroid therapy. The most serious side effects of nitrofurantoin therapy are neurologic reactions, especially polyneuritis, which occurs primarily in patients with renal failure and patients who receive prolonged therapeutic courses. Demyelination and degeneration of both sensory and motor nerves occur. Use of the drug should be stopped at the earliest signs of paresthesias.

Methenamine. Methenamine has no antibacterial action by itself but is metabolized in acid pH to formaldehyde. The normal urine pH is sufficient for this transformation although various attempts to increase the acidity of urine have been tried using mandelic acid, hippuric acid, ascorbic acid, or cranberry juice. Methenamine is virtually useless, therefore, for the treatment of urea-splitting organisms such as *Proteus* species. All gram-positive and gram-negative bacteria and fungi are equally susceptible to formaldehyde at concentrations of 20 mg/liter.[119]

Although the drug is rapidly absorbed from the gastrointestinal tract, it is inactive until excreted into acid urine. Only bladder urine contains adequate levels of formaldehyde. For this reason, the only toxic effects are upper gastrointestinal distress and bladder irritation. Methenamine is useful primarily as a chronic suppressive agent and is not useful for acute upper or lower urinary tract infections.

Of the four agents, nitrofurantoin is the most versatile, since it is effective in treating both upper and lower urinary tract infections and recurrent bacteriuria. It can also be used as a long-term suppressive agent in children and pregnant women.

ANTIMYCOBACTERIAL AGENTS[120]

Mycobacterium tuberculosis, other mycobacteria, and treatment regimens are discussed in Chapter 9. Following a steady decline in the incidence of tuberculosis in the United States, it began to increase in 1986, most likely due to the number of individuals infected with human immunodeficiency virus who have an increased susceptibility to infections with *M. tuberculosis* and other atypical mycobacteria. These individuals are frequently infected with mycobacterial strains resistant to antimycobacterial agents, and those individuals who are also intravenous drug abusers frequently are noncompliant with therapeutic regimens.

Antituberculous drugs and treatment regimens have been reviewed[120] (see Chap. 9). Six- and 9-month treatment regimens are recommended. A 6-month regimen uses a combination of isoniazid, rifampin, and pyrazinamide daily for 2 months and then isoniazid and rifampin either daily or twice weekly for an additional 4 months.[120] The 9-month regimen consists of isoniazid and rifampin daily for 2 months followed by daily or twice weekly for isoniazid and rifampin for an additional 7 months.

According to Van Scoy and Wilkowske[120] the 6- and 9-month regimens can be used when (1) the organism is known to be sensitive to the drugs used, (2) patients are monitored for compliance and adverse reactions, (3) ethambutol or streptomycin is added if resistant organisms are suspected or if life-threatening or extensive disease is suspected, (4) HIV-infected patients are treated with three or four drugs during the first 2 months of therapy, and (5) the duration of treatment in HIV-infected patients is at least 9 months and is continued for at least 6 months beyond substantiated conversion of cultures (negative cultures). Prophylactic therapy is recommended in susceptible individuals with positive PPD reactions[120] (see Chap. 9).

Isoniazid. Isoniazid is a bactericidal drug that is active against growing *M. tuberculosis* but static against resting organisms. Resistance to the drug develops rapidly when it is administered alone. It is absorbed after oral or intramuscular administration and distributed through the body, and achieves adequate cerebrospinal fluid levels. It is acetylated in the body with acetylation affected by the genetic status of the recipient (ie, a fast acetylator or a slow acetylator). Dosage modification is not necessary in hepatic or renal failure unless the patient is a slow acetylator.

Isoniazid is a safe drug, except that the acetylhydrazine metabolite sometimes causes hepatitis, especially in the elderly. No longer is routine isoniazid prophylaxis advised for adult PPD skin test converters.

The second toxic reaction is a peripheral neuropathy, which can be ameliorated and prevented by concurrent pyridoxine administration. Other hypersensitivity phenomena are unusual. Liver toxicity is increased when rifampin is concurrently used, and isoniazid serum levels are increased by concurrent para-amino-salicyclic acid administration.

Ethambutol. Ethambutol is tuberculostatic through an action on RNA synthesis. It is absorbed through the gastrointestinal tract and distributed into the cerebrospinal fluid, as well as other tissues, in patients with meningitis. Since it is excreted in the urine, dosage must be reduced in patients with renal malfunction. Resistance is unusual.

The principal toxicity of ethambutol is a retrobulbar neuritis with impairment of visual acuity or color vision and constriction of visual fields. Those changes are reversible on drug cessation. Other toxicities are unusual. Ethambutol has replaced para-amino-salicylic acid as a companion drug for isoniazid.

Rifampin. The pharmacology and spectrum of rifampin are discussed in a preceding section. Rifampin is a potent tuberculocidal drug, which is excreted primarily in bile and consequently does not require dosage reduction in renal failure. Resistance to *M. tuberculosis* develops fairly frequently.[121] The only serious adverse reaction is its additive hepatic toxicity to isoniazid and its intrinsic mild hepatotoxicity with other hepatotoxic drugs. In addition, it is mildly immunosuppressive and colors all body secretions orange, including urine, serum, semen, saliva, feces, and cerebrospinal fluid—patients should be warned.

Streptomycin. Streptomycin and amikacin are tuberculocidal aminoglycosides.[122] Streptomycin is used as part of multiple drug therapy for *M. tuberculosis* infections. Combination regimens delay development of resistance to streptomycin, which would otherwise develop rapidly. The other properties of the aminoglycosides are discussed in a preceding section.

Quinolones. The quinolones are promising new agents with in vitro activity against mycobacteria.[63,64] Their role in treating these clinical infections is not yet established.

Pyrazinamide. Pyrazinamide is a tuberculostatic drug that is absorbed from the gastrointestinal tract and achieves therapeutic levels in the cerebrospinal fluid when the meninges are inflamed. Its high incidence of severe hepatotoxicity has severely limited its use in the United States to the treatment of resistant disease. However, because it is a cheap, effective agent and can be administered in once-weekly doses (90 mg/kg), it has been useful in developing countries (usual adult doses; 20 to 35 mg/kg per day by mouth or two or three divided doses.)

ANTIFUNGAL AGENTS

Amphotericin B

Chemistry. Amphotericin is a polyene macrolide antibiotic obtained from *Streptomyces nodosus.* Amphotericin B exerts its action by its ability to combine with cytoplasmic membrane sterols, principally ergosterol in fungi. Resistant mutants with abnormal membrane sterols are rare in clinical practice.[123]

Pharmacology. Amphotericin B is poorly soluble in water at neutral pH, so that a colloidal suspension in 5 percent glucose is used intravenously. The infusion bottle does not have to be shielded from the light. Saline solutions cause the colloid to aggregate, resulting in suboptimal therapeutic effects. Even without aggregation, the colloidal solution is partially retained by a 0.22-μm membrane filter.

Following intravenous infusion, more than 95 percent of the drug is bound to beta-lipoproteins, presumably as a result of the cholesterol carried on this protein. The majority of the drug then promptly leaves the circulation. The reservoir of the drug is unknown, but it slowly reenters the circulation. It is apparently degraded in situ, and only a small amount is excreted in the bile or urine. Blood levels are not influenced by renal function or hemodialysis. The amphotericin B concentrations and fluids obtained from an inflamed area, such as the pleuroperitoneum or joint and aqueous humor, are approximately two-thirds of the serum levels. Amphotericin B cannot, however, penetrate into the cerebrospinal fluid, vitreous humor, or amniotic fluid. Therefore, to treat fungal meningitis, intrathecal or intercisternal administration is recommended. The peak serum concentrations with the usual intravenous administration are 1.2 to 2.0 μg/ml, but these concentrations rapidly fall to a plateau of approximately 0.5 μg/ml.[124]

Antimicrobial Spectrum. Amphotericin B is useful for infection with almost all fungal pathogens, including *Cryptococcus neoformans, Candida albicans, Blastomyces dermatitidis, Sporothrix schenckii, Paracoccidioides brasiliensis, Histoplasma capsulatum, Coccidioides immitis, Aspergillus* species, *Torulopsis glabrata,* and *Phycomycetes,* which cause mucormycosis (see Table 28–14 and Chap. 10). Because of their lower toxicity and availability as oral agents, the azole antifungal agents have replaced amphotericin B as first-line agents to treat some fungal infections.

Adverse Effects. The toxicity of amphotericin B represents the most serious limitation to its use. These toxic effects are so notorious that inexperienced physicians, who fear the toxicity more than the infection, frequently withhold it from needy patients. Despite the fact that some toxic effects are almost inevitable, almost all patients can complete a conventional course of therapy.

Fever (sometimes with shaking chills), headache, nausea and vomiting, anorexia, malaise, and muscle and joint pains are frequent problems at the onset of therapy. Therapy should not be curtailed, however, because these effects usually abate as therapy progresses. Ibuprophen, hydrocortisone, diphenhydramine, and salicylates are frequently used to control the side effects. Tolerance to the febrile reactions develops with time, allowing diminution in the hydrocortisone and diphenhydramine. Frequently, they can be discontinued altogether. Patients who are already receiving steroid therapy, such as renal transplant recipients, get little benefit from additional steroids.[123–125]

Renal toxicity is the most serious problem associated with amphotericin B therapy. A dose-related decrease in renal blood flow and glomerular filtration occurs, and changes in the glomerular basement membranes and tubules are produced. Hypokalemia may require potassium supplementation, and a mild renal tubular acidosis can be produced. Renal function improves when amphotericin B is stopped, but permanent deterioration of clearance occurs in patients who receive extremely high doses. The hope that mannitol or alkali infusion could reduce nephrotoxicity has not been borne out. Administration of amphotericin B on alternate days, rather than daily, will reduce nephrotoxicity, but only if the cumulative rate of administration is halved.

The other toxic reactions associated with amphotericin B include thrombophlebitis and local pain at the injection site, normocytic anemia usually accompanied by a normal bone marrow, and hypokalemia. Less frequent side effects are cardiovascular toxicity including arrhythmias, hypertension, thrombocytopenia, leukopenia, and burning sensations on the soles of the feet. These side effects, which disappear slowly during the first 3 months after therapy, reflect slow catabolism of the drug.

The dosage schedule of amphotericin administration has been manipulated in an attempt to reduce its toxicity. To obviate the nausea, vomiting, fever, and chills, the infusion can be given over a longer period than the usual 6 hours. Some patients have fewer reactions if the dose is given during 2 hours, and others have shown that the drug can be given safely with no increase in side effects over 45 minutes or even 10 minutes. Short-term infusion has been reported to decrease the incidence of nausea and chills, to reduce the premedication needed, and to shorten the length of clinic visits for outpatients who are receiving amphotericin B.[125]

Doses. The usual daily maintenance dose ranges from 0.4 to 0.6 mg/kg. These doses are decreased somewhat from the previously recommended daily dose of 1 to 1.5 mg/kg. The duration of therapy is two weeks for Candida, longer for other mycoses, with a total adult dose equaling 1 to 3 g depending on the mycosis treated, but no reliable guidelines for duration of therapy exist. After initially treating patients in the hospital and establishing their tolerance to the drug, one can treat them as outpatients if their clinical status permits. These rather arbitrary dose schedules appear to be necessary for the eradication of chronic histoplasmosis, aspergillosis, and cryptococcal meningitis. Such prolonged high-dose therapy is probably not necessary in cases of infected wounds, empyema, or fungal peritonitis, in which cases short courses of therapy (total dose approximately 6 to 8 mg/kg) are probably adequate.[126]

Cerebrospinal fluid levels are inadequate, and intrathecal or intracisternal injections via Omaya reservoirs are occasionally used in patients with fungal meningitis. When given intrathecally, the lumbar injections may cause temporary radicular pain and loss of motor function in the legs, rectum, and bladder. Use of 10 percent glucose as a diluent, and positioning the patient during injection to permit hyperbaric flow toward the brain, may decrease this local myopathy. Bladder irrigations with amphotericin 50 μg/ml in distilled water have been used in *Candida* cystitis. The cornea may be bathed with a solution containing 1 mg per ml of amphotericin. The solution is irritating but is beneficial in keratomycosis. Local infusion into joints and other body cavities has been useful.

Other Amphotericin B Preparations. In order to decrease its toxicity and increase its bioavailability, alternative approaches to administering amphotericin B have been tried. These approaches have been to complex amphotericin B with liposomes. Liposomes are lipid bilayers that contain amphotericin B in their interiors. Higher serum levels of liposomal amphotericin B can be obtained together with an improved toxicity profile compared to the standard amphotericin B deoxycholate.[123] Liposomal preparations are unstable and the need for daily preparation of liposomal amphotericin B has made it commercially unavailable in the past. Newer formulations, however, result in more stable liposomes and clinical trials with these preparations are currently underway.

Amphotericin B in Combination with Other Drugs. Amphotericin B has been used in combination with other antifungal agents in an effort to reduce its toxicity and increase its therapeutic effect. Because amphotericin B combines with the cell membranes of fungi and increases permeability, these other agents may be able to gain entrance into the fungal cell in larger quantities. For this reason, antibiotics such as tetracycline and rifampin appear to have an amphotericin-sparing effect,[127] but clinical experience is limited.

Flucytosine has increased antifungal activity against *Candida* and *Cryptococcus* when combined with amphotericin. Flucytosine should not be administered alone because of the rapid emergence of resistant organisms.

Some new antifungal agents have also been tried in combination with amphotericin B. Clotrimazole enhances the effectiveness of amphotericin B against *Candida* species in vitro, but it is antagonistic against *Torulopsis* in vitro. Similarly, miconazole is antagonistic with amphotericin B against *Candida*.

Nystatin. Nystatin is a polyene macrolide antibiotic, which is both fungistatic and fungicidal like amphotericin B. Because of its toxicity after parenteral administration, it is used only topically and orally. It is not absorbed from the gastrointestinal tract and is currently used most often for the prophylaxis and therapy of esophageal, gastrointestinal, vaginal, or cutaneous candidiasis. Its efficacy is proportional to its concentration and dose. Higher doses (up to 1 million units) have been recommended for prophylaxis of oral candidiasis in severely immunodepressed patients. Even higher doses (4 million units every 4 hours) have prevented *Candida* sepsis in neutropenic children during leukemia chemotherapy. Theoretically, candidemia in such patients originates in gastrointestinal overgrowth and persorption of the yeasts through the intestinal wall. Reduction of the yeast count in the intestine by high-dose nystatin may prevent this complication. There is as yet, however, no evidence to support this concept in general surgical patients, on broad-spectrum antibiotics, who have high *Candida* counts in their gastrointestinal tract, even though the practice is common.

Flucytosine. Flucytosine (5-fluorocytosine) was first synthesized as a cytosine antimetabolite for the treatment of leukemia. The drug proved ineffective for this purpose but was found to be effective as an antifungal agent.[128]

Pharmacology. Flucytosine is absorbed from the gastrointestinal tract, and peak serum levels are reached in 2 to 6 hours. Because it is excreted unchanged by glomerular filtration, the dose must be reduced in patients with renal failure. The appropriate dose is best monitored by measuring the drug in serum 2 hours after the last dose and immediately before the next dose. These values should range between 50 and 100 μg/ml. The drug is removed by hemodialysis. In patients on hemodialysis, therapeutic nontoxic serum levels of flucytosine can usually be maintained by administering a single dose (25 to 50 mg/kg) after each dialysis.

5-Fluorocytosine is well distributed in body tissues and fluids, including the cerebrospinal fluid.

Antifungal Properties and Clinical Uses. Flucytosine is currently recommended for cryptococcosis, candidiasis, torulopsis, and chromoblastomycosis. Because of the tendency of resistant strains to emerge, and the greater efficacy when combined with amphotericin, it is never used as a sole agent (see Table 28–14).

Mechanisms of Action. Flucytosine enters a cell by way of permease enzymes located on the cell membrane and is believed to exert its effect by deamination in the fungal cells to the antimetabolite 5-fluorouracil, which inhibits synthesis of DNA and RNA. Resistance of fungi to 5-fluorocytosine may be due to a change in their plasma membrane that prevents penetration of the drug into the cell. The synergistic effect of 5-fluorocytosine and amphotericin B against some fungi probably results from the action of amphotericin B, which permits more flucytosine to enter the cell.

Adverse Effects. Flucytosine has relatively few toxic side effects. Nausea and diarrhea can occur but are uncommon. Skin rashes have also occasionally been seen. Because so many of the patients who receive flucytosine have underlying hematopoietic disorders and have also been receiving amphotericin B, its toxicity on the bone marrow alone is difficult to assess, but individual reports of bone marrow depression and aplastic anemia have been reported. Anemia, neutropenia, thrombocytopenia, and eosinophilia have also been described. Transient liver enlargement associated with elevated transaminase levels has been noted in a few patients. Nephrotoxicity has not been ascribed to 5-fluorocytosine.

Imidazole and Azole Antifungal Agents

The imidazole and triazole antifungal agents promise effective therapy for the treatment of fungal infections that is as effective as amphotericin B but without the toxic side effects.[123] Furthermore, they are available in oral preparations. Four imidazole antifungal agents, miconazole, ketoconazole, fluconazole, and intraconazole, are currently available for routine clinical use. Others are currently in clinical trial.

Chemistry. This class of antifungal agents has one imidazole or two triazole rings attached to other groups that alter their pharmacologic properties (Fig. 28–5).

Mechanism of Action. The azole antifungal agents bind to the iron in and inhibit the cytochrome P450 enzyme, 14-alpha-demethylase, responsible for conversion of lanosterol to ergosterol. The resulting deficiency in ergosterol results in damage to the fungal cell membrane, which inhibits growth.

Ketoconazole, but not fluconazole or itraconazole, also inhibits mammalian cytochrome P450 enzymes, leading to hormone suppression, with decreased testosterone and cortical concentrations occurring in humans. All azoles interfere with hepatic cytochrome P450 enzymes and can result in an elevation of concomitantly administered drugs, a decrease in azole drug levels, or both. This inhibition of hepatic P450 enzymes is actually put to use by administering ketoconazole to organ transplant recipients in order to inhibit the metabolism of cyclosporine so that less of the costly immunosuppressive agent is required.

Pharmacologic Properties. The azoles differ in their pharmacologic properties because of marked differences in their nonazole structures. Ketoconazole is water soluble only at a pH of less than 3 and therefore is not available in parenteral form. Normal gastric acidity is required for its absorption from the gastrointestinal tract. Similarly, itraconazole is highly lipid soluble and well absorbed orally, which is enhanced by the presence of food in the stomach.

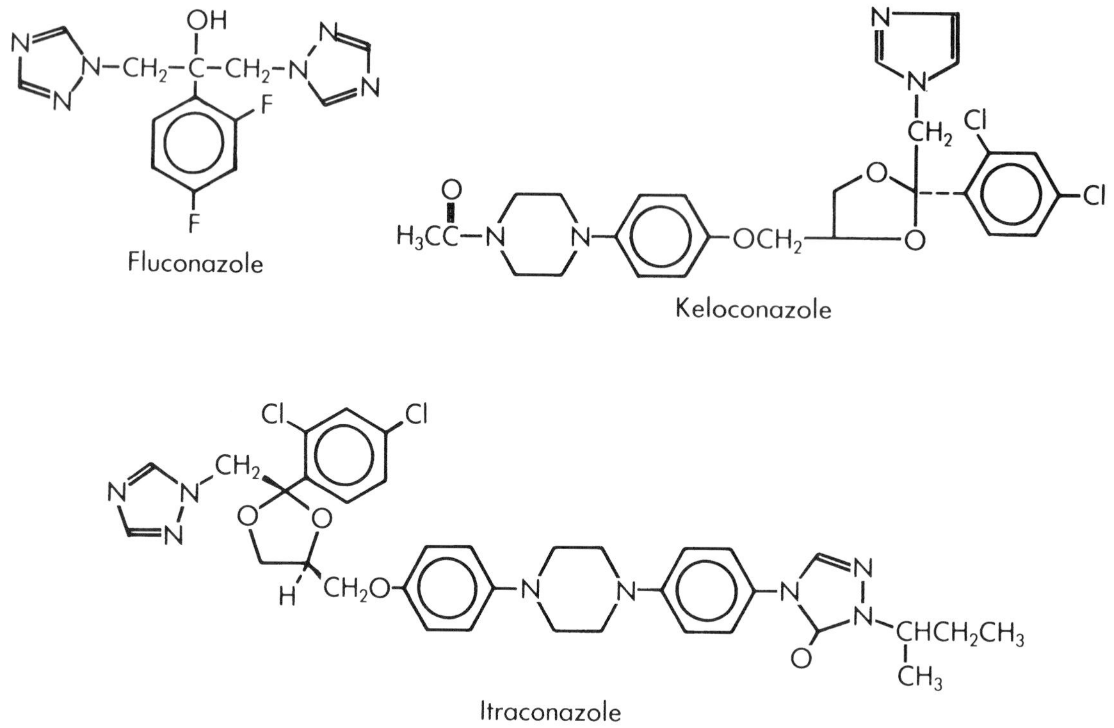

Figure 28–5. Structures of ketoconazole, fluconazole, and itraconazole. *(From Mandell GL, Douglas RG Jr, Bennett JE (eds): Principles and Practice of Infectious Diseases, 3rd ed, update 11. New York, Churchill Livingstone, 1991, p 3.)*

Absorption is erratic in some patients, which has led to treatment failures.[123,129,130] Fluconazole and miconazole, on the other hand, are water soluble, which makes them available for intravenous administration. Intravenous miconazole administration results in peak serum concentrations of 2 to 6 μg/ml that are maintained for only 2 to 5 hours and oral absorption is poor.[123] Thus miconazole is primarily used as a topical antifungal agent.

The azoles also differ with respect to other properties such as protein binding, tissue distribution, and metabolism. Because they are almost entirely metabolized by the liver and excreted in bile, with no excretion by the kidneys, ketoconazole and itraconazole do not require dose adjustments in patients with renal dysfunctions. Fluconazole, on the other hand, is excreted primarily by the kidneys and thus dose adjustments are needed for patients with compromised renal function.

Spectrum of Activity. The azoles have in vitro activity and are effective in vivo in animal models against most pathogenic fungi but they are seldom the drug of choice (see Table 28–14). Ketoconazole is the drug of choice for treatment of nonmeningeal, non-life-threatening histoplasmosis and blastomycosis in immunocompromised patients.[123] Ketoconazole is also the drug of choice for chronic mucocutaneous candidiasis and is as effective a prophylaxis as other agents in preventing superficial candidiasis in neutropenic patients. Itraconazole promises to replace ketoconazole as the agent of choice in the treatment of these immunocompromised patients because of its decreased risk of adverse reactions. Miconazole is the drug of choice in the treatment of invasive infections due to *Pseudallescheria boydii.*

The main indications for fluconazole are oropharyngeal, esophageal, vaginal, and other more serious deep infections due to *Candida* (eg, peritonitis, genitourinary tract infections), cryptococcal meningitis (but the relapse rate is high), and sporotrichosis. Fluconazole provides effective prophylaxis against oral candidiasis in patients with cancer who are having chemotherapy.[123,131]

Itraconazole is more effective against *Aspergillus* than ketoconazole or fluconazole. It holds promise for treating cryptococcal meningitis and coccidioidomycosis (including meningitis).[123] Itraconazole is also effective against cutaneous and lymphangitic sporotrichosis, chromomycosis, and paracoccidioidomycosis.[123] It provided more effective prophylaxis than ketoconazole against *Aspergillus* in patients with leukemia.

The appropriate place for the treatment of fungal infections with the azoles is still being established. Few controlled trials have been carried out comparing their efficacy to amphotericin B or to each other. They have the advantage over amphotericin B of having less toxicity and being available in oral preparations, but in many instances it is not clear that they provide as effective a therapy as amphotericin B. The decision to use one azole over another has as much to do with side effects as with efficacy of therapy.

Adverse Effects. The most common side effects of the azoles involve the gastrointestinal tract. Anorexia, nausea, and vomiting occur in approximately 20 to 40 percent of patients taking ketoconazole.[123] Abdominal pain and diarrhea can occasionally occur. Gastrointestinal side effects occur much less commonly in patients taking fluconazole or itraconazole. Because it inhibits testosterone synthesis, ketoconazole can cause decreased libido, impotence, and gynecomastia in men. In women it can cause menstrual irregularities and alopecia. Rash and puritis occur in 5 to 10 percent of patients receiving ketoconazole.[123] Fluconazole—in addition to gastrointestinal symptoms—can cause rash, headache, and transiently increased hepatic enzymes. Pruritis, headache, dizziness, and transiently increased hepatic enzymes can occasionally occur in patients taking itraconazole.

Antiviral Agents

The few available chemotherapeutic antiviral agents stand in sharp contrast to the numerous antibacterial drugs that have been developed during the past 50 years. The unique structural and metabolic machinery of bacteria has allowed numerous antibiotics to be developed that are both toxic to the bacteria and yet safe for human cells. In contrast, viruses use the host cell's metabolic machinery for their replication. Thus antiviral agents frequently are toxic to the host cells and have narrow therapeutic indices.

Targets for antiviral chemotherapy include interference of attachment to the host cell membrane and entry into the host cell commune, inhibition of transcription or translation, and interference with virus assembly. All these steps important in viral replication involve active metabolism that is subject to attack. There is currently no effective therapy for latent viruses.

For many years, amantadine, useful against influenza virus, was the only approved antiviral agent. In the last decade, several other agents have been approved including acyclovir, ganciclovir, ribavirin, zidovudine, and interferon alpha-2b.

Antiviral Activity. In cell cultures, amantadine prevents infection with RNA viruses of several groups (myxovirus, paramyxoviruses, togaviruses) (see Table 28–15). Its only clinical application is against influenza A viruses. Many influenza A virus strains are sensitive to less than 0.4 μg/ml. Resistance can be induced in vitro, however, by serial passage of influenza A virus strains in low concentrations of amantadine. Much higher and more toxic concentrations of amantadine (25 to 50 μg/ml) are inhibitory for some other viruses.

The mechanism of the antiviral activity is not fully appreciated. Amantidine interferes with successful penetration of the cell by influenza virus, and it blocks uncoating of the virus and release of the viral nucleic acid into the cell.[132] It does not directly inactivate the virus, nor does it inhibit the viral neuramidinase. When added 1.5 hours after virus inoculation, amantadine no longer inhibits virus multiplication.

Pharmacology and Toxicity. Amantadine is rapidly absorbed from the gastrointestinal tract, and peak serum levels of approximately 0.3 μg/ml are achieved 2 to 4 hours after a dose of 2.5 mg/kg body weight. The half-life in serum is approximately 20 hours. With the usual adult dose of 100 mg every 12 hours, 48 hours are required to reach maximum tissue concentration. Almost all the drug is excreted unchanged in the urine, so that if renal function is compromised, the dose must be reduced. Most side effects occur in patients with compromised renal function.

Side effects occur in 3 to 7 percent of healthy adults and usually include insomnia and difficulty in concentration. Confusion, hallucinations, convulsions, anxiety, and coma have also been reported. Symptoms of toxicity usually occur shortly after amantadine is begun as peak blood levels are reached, and the effects are reversible when the drug is discontinued. Insomnia may be minimized by giving the full daily dose of 200 mg in the morning rather than 100 mg every 12 hours.

Clinical Indications. The prophylactic efficacy of amantadine has been clearly demonstrated. The drug reduced morbidity by 50 percent during an ep-

TABLE 28–15. RECOMMENDED TREATMENT OF SPECIFIC VIRAL INFECTIONS

Infection and Site	Agent	Route of Administration	Dosage	Duration
Herpes simplex				
Primary genital	Acyclovir	Oral	200 mg 5 times/d	10 d
Recurrent genital	Acyclovir	Oral	200 mg 5 times/d	5 d
Chronic recurrent genital	Acyclovir	Oral	400 mg 2 times/d	Up to 1 yr
Encephalitis	Acyclovir	Intravenous	10 mg/kg every 8 h	10 d
Keratoconjunctivitis	Trifluridine	Topical	1 drop of 1% solution every 2 h	[b]
Mucocutaneous in ICH[a]	Acyclovir	Oral[c]	400 mg 5 times/d	7 d
		Intravenous	5 mg/kg every 8 h	7 d
Cytomegalovirus				
Retinitis	Ganciclovir	Intravenous	5 mg/kg every 12 h	14–21 d[d]
Varicella-zoster				
Varicella in ICH[c]	Acyclovir	Intravenous	500 mg/m^2 every 8 h	7 d
Herpes zoster in ICH	Acyclovir	Intravenous	10 mg/kg every 8 h	7 d
Herpes zoster in normal host[e]	Acyclovir	Oral	800 mg 5 times/day	7–10 d
Herpes zoster ophthalmicus in normal host[c]	Acyclovir	Oral	600–800 mg 5 times/d	10 d
Influenza A	Amantadine	Oral	200 mg/d	5–7 d
Respiratory syncytial virus	Ribavirin	Aerosol	12–18 h/d	3–7 d
Papillomavirus	Interferon alpha-2b	Intralesional	1 million U/0.1 ml in up to 5 warts 3 times/wk	3 wk
Human immunodeficiency virus	Zidovudine	Oral	100 mg 5 times/day	Indefinitely
Chronic hepatitis C	Interferon alpha-2b	Subcutaneous or intramuscular	3 million U 3 times/wk	24 wk

[a] ICH, immunocompromised host.
[b] Therapy should be monitored by an ophthalmologist.
[c] Not approved by the Food and Drug Administration for this indication.
[d] In patients with acquired immunodeficiency syndrome (AIDS), maintenance therapy at 5 mg/kg daily or 6 mg/kg daily for 5 days/week is recommended.
[e] No antiviral treatment is an alternative approach in the normal host with herpes zoster.
From Keating MR: Mayo Clin Proc 67:160, 1992.

idemic of influenza As/Hong Kong, and 100 percent in an epidemic of a H_3N_2 strain (80 percent reduction in seroconversion). Amantadine is effective against H_2N_2, H_3N_2, and H_1N_1 subtypes of influenza A in doses of 200 mg per day (see Table 28–15). Dose-response curves have not been established in clinical studies. When deciding on its use, however, one must remember that influenza A virus attack rates are only 10 to 20 percent, so therefore amantadine given to 100 persons will prevent influenza in only 7 to 16 of them; at the same time, it will cause minor central nervous system side effects in five or six people who would not be expected to contract the disease. Other problems with the use of prophylactic administration of amantadine has been the lack of virologic facilities to find the cause of many outbreaks of respiratory illnesses in scattered communities and the inability to rapidly distribute amantadine among the population.[133]

When given therapeutically in controlled studies, amantadine causes a decrease in fever and a shortening of the illness.[134]

Amantadine is approved for use in the United States for both prevention and treatment of influenza A virus infections. Prophylactic use is appropriate in certain circumstances: if there is virologic epidemiologic confirmation of an outbreak of influenza A and if vaccination cannot be carried out. Prophylaxis is then indicated for unvaccinated persons at high risk of serious complications because of underlying immunodeficiency, pulmonary, metabolic, or cardiovascular disease. In addition, older persons who have not received influenza vaccine and unimmunized adults whose activity is essential to the community should be vaccinated. Prophylaxis should be begun as soon as influenza is identified in the region, and it should be continued throughout the risk period because any beneficial effect ceases within 48 hours after the drug is discontinued. Since amantadine does not interfere with immunogenicity of an inactivated vaccine, the drug can be started in conjunction with immunization and continued for 2 weeks until protective antibody develops.

For amantadine to be effective therapeutically, it must be administered within the first 24 to 48 hours of the onset of symptoms. Patients for whom such therapy should be considered are those at high risk for developing serious problems from influenza, such as the elderly, those with immunodeficiency disorders, and those with pulmonary disease.

Acyclovir. Acyclovir (acycloquanosine) is an acyclic analog of the natural nucleoside 2′-deoxyguanosine with activity against the herpesviruses.[135] A variety of nucleosides have been developed and approved for treatment of herpesviruses such as adenine arabinoside and idoxuridine (5-iodo-2-deoxyuridine, IUdR). Because of the low effectiveness and high toxicity, these latter nucleoside derivatives are rarely used with currently available agents. Acyclovir and ganciclovir have largely replaced them for treating herpesviruses.

Pharmacology and Toxicity. Renal toxicity is usually caused by precipitation and crystallization of the drug in the renal tubules and may be prevented with adequate hydration.[136] It does not seem to occur after oral use of acyclovir. Neurologic symptoms include confusion, delirium, lethargy, tremors, and seizures. The dose of acyclovir must be adjusted for patients with decreased renal function.[135,136]

The half-life after an intravenous dose is 3 hours in patients with normal renal function. Clearance of acyclovir is predominantly through the kidneys, resulting in a half-life of 20 hours in end-stage renal failure. Approximately 60 percent of the drug is removed by hemodialysis. Peritoneal dialysis is much less effective.

Clinical Uses. Acyclovir shortens the period of viral shedding, duration of acute pain, time of new vesicle formation, and time to healing of lesions of mucocutaneous herpes simplex virus infection in both normal and immunocompromised hosts[135,136] (see Table 28–15). The recommended dose is 200 mg five times a day for 10 days for primary genital herpes and for 5 days for recurrent genital herpes. It may be given for a prolonged period, up to a year, for chronic recurrent genital herpes. For treating encephalitis it can be given as an intravenous infusion of 10 mg/kg every 8 hours for 10 days. Intravenous therapy for mucocutaneous herpes is generally reserved for individuals with more serious infections.

Topical administration of acyclovir is effective in patients for the initial episodes of genital herpes simplex virus infection but not in patients with recurrent infection. Oral therapy is nevertheless recommended because of its more pronounced response and it remains the treatment of choice.

Acyclovir both intravenously and orally leads to significantly reduced viral shedding, local symptoms including pain, and time of healing in immunocompromised patients with varicella-zoster infection. In immunocompromised patients, intravenous doses of 500 mg/m^2 every 8 hours and oral doses of 800 mg five times a day for 7 to 10 days are recommended.[135,136]

The place of acyclovir in the treatment of varicella-zoster infection in the normal host remains controversial. Zoster in healthy patients responds to oral therapy with 800 mg acyclovir five times daily for 7 to 10 days.[136,137] This regimen can significantly shorten the duration of viral shedding, accelerate the time of scabbing and healing, decrease the formation of new lesions, and reduce the duration of pain. Lower doses, however, are not effective. While there is a trend toward overall reduction of postherpetic neuralgia in acyclovir-treated patients, there is no significant difference compared to placebo-treated patients. No consensus currently exists about the use of acyclovir in the treatment of herpes zoster in normal hosts. The benefits must be weighed against the potential toxicity. Because older immunocompromised patients are more likely to experience acute pain of longer duration, oral treatment should be considered. Otherwise, most healthy patients probably should not be treated.

Similarly, acyclovir given within 24 hours of the onset of rash in otherwise healthy children can promote healing, decrease new lesion formation, and reduce systemic symptoms, particularly fever.[135,136] Nevertheless, because of its potential toxicity, most experts currently do not recommend a routine use of oral acyclovir in children with chickenpox. Because the disease is more severe in adolescents and adults, error on the side of treatment may be prudent.

Acyclovir should generally be used to treat chickenpox and zoster in immunocompromised patients because of the concern of dissemination, especially encephalitis. Generally, intravenous acyclovir 500 mg/m^2 every 8 hours for 7 to 10 days will reduce the cutaneous and visceral dissemination in patients with herpes zoster or in children with chickenpox.

While not effective against the established cytomegalovirus (CMV) infections, high-dose, early intravenous prophylaxis with acyclovir may decrease the incidence of CMV disease in bone marrow transplant recipients. High-dose oral acyclovir, 200 mg four times a day, similarly decreases the incidence and severity of CMV disease in renal transplant recipients, although preexisting reductions in renal function yield elevated plasma levels following oral dosing in this population.[135,136] Prophylactic ganciclovir may be more effective.

Ganciclovir. Ganciclovir, like acyclovir, is an acyclic nucleoside analog of guanine, but it differs from acyclovir in that it has a carbon and hydroxyl group at the 3′ position of the acyclic side chain. Ganciclovir is at least ten times more potent than acyclovir in vitro in inhibiting CMV and Epstein-Barr virus and is equal to acyclovir in the inhibition of herpes simplex virus and varicella-zoster virus.[136] It is also active against human herpesvirus 6.[138]

Like other nucleoside analogs, the active form is a triphosphate. This conversion is achieved by a CMV-specific protein kinase that has not yet been characterized. It is both an inhibitor of and faulty substrate for CMV DNA polymerase, resulting in chain termination.[135]

Pharmacology and Toxicity. The half-life of intravenous ganciclovir is approximately 4.2 hours. It is excreted almost exclusively by the kidney; so dosage adjustment is mandatory in renal failure.[135,136] The drug is removed by hemodialysis. Intravenous doses achieve intraocular drug levels that exceed the LD_{50} for most strains of CMV. The oral bioavailability is less than 5 percent so it must be given intravenously.

Clinically resistant virus strains resulting in refractory CMV disease do occur. This viral resistance is thought to be due to reduced phosphorylation ability of the resistant strain.[139]

Neutropenia is the most common dose-limiting side effect. Neutropenia (fewer than 1000 cells/mm^3) occurs in approximately 30 percent of patients. Severe neutropenia (fewer than 500 cell/mm^3) occurs in approximately 15 percent.[136] Thrombocytopenia occurs in less than 10 percent of patients. Neutropenia usually occurs during the second week of therapy and is usually reversible after the dosage is decreased or treatment is discontinued. Other adverse effects are reported in less than 2 percent of patients and include nausea, vomiting, diarrhea, fever, rash, infusion site reactions, anemia, and eosinophilia.

Clinical Uses. The only approved indication for ganciclovir is the treatment of CMV retinitis in immunocompromised hosts, including patients with acquired immune deficiency syndrome (AIDS) (see Table 28–15). The usual dosage is 5 mg/kg twice daily for 14 to 21 days. Maintenance therapy of 5 or 6 mg/kg daily for 5 days each week is recommended, because recurrences are common in AIDS patients.[136,140]

Although not approved for use, ganciclovir is also used extensively for CMV infections in AIDS patients and other immunocompromised hosts, especially bone marrow and organ transplant recipients. It has been used to treat CMV infection of the gastrointestinal tract, liver, and lungs.[135,136] In these patients, doses of 7.5 to 10 mg/kg/day for 10 to 14 days are generally recommended.

Ganciclovir is also used as a prophylactic agent in preventing CMV disease after bone marrow and organ transplantation, and many centers have replaced acyclovir for this purpose. It has the disadvantage of requiring intravenous administration; so it is inconvenient to administer ganciclovir outside the hospital.

Foscarnet. Foscarnet is an inorganic phosphate analog that has been approved for use in several European countries and is currently being reviewed for approval in the United States by the Food and Drug Administration. It does not have to be phosphorylated into an active form by viral or host cell enzymes.[136] It acts by selectively inhibiting viral DNA polymerases and reverse transcriptases without appreciable inhibition of host cell enzymes. It is active in vitro against herpesviruses, HIV, and hepatitis B virus. Like all other antiviral agents, it is virustatic. Because foscarnet does not require phosphorylation, viral resistance may be decreased because phosphorylation is the most common site of mutation-induced resistance to nucleoside analogs.

Pharmacology and Toxicity. Foscarnet is cleared unchanged by the kidneys, with more than 80 percent of the dose excreted as the parent compound. Accumulation of the drug occurs in renal failure and dose adjustment is mandatory. Most of the rest of the drug is probably deposited into bone.

The most common significant side effect is renal toxicity. This is usually reversible but may progress to full-blown renal failure, especially in dehydrated patients or in those receiving other nephrotoxic drugs. Anemia and, less frequently, thrombocytopenia and neutropenia may also occur.[141] Changes in serum calcium and phosphorus levels have also been documented.[136] Painful erosive mucocutaneous lesions of the penis have been well described and attributed to high concentrations in the urine. Oral ulcerations have also been described in a few patients. Other side effects include nausea, vomiting, diarrhea, headache, fatigue, malaise, and seizures in patients with high blood levels associated with renal failure.

Clinical Uses. Foscarnet must be administrated intravenously at a dosage of 60 mg/kg three times a day for induction therapy and 90 to 120 mg/kg daily for maintenance therapy. The dose must be adjusted for patients with renal failure. It is effective in the treatment of CMV retinitis in patients with AIDS.[136] No comparative studies have demonstrated that foscarnet offers advantages over ganciclovir. Foscarnet in uncontrolled trials of 40 to 60 mg/kg every 8 hours has also been effective in treating resistant herpes simplex virus infections in AIDS patients.

Zidovudine. Zidovudine (azidothymidine, AZT) is a thymidine analog that inhibits reverse transcriptase and is active against HIV-1.[142] Some activity has also been reported against human T cell lymphotropic virus type 1 (HTLV-1), HIV-2, and Epstein-Barr virus.[136] Zidovudine must be phosphorylated to the triphosphate form inside host cells by host kinases. Zidovudine triphosphate is then incorporated into the nascent DNA chain by viral reverse transcriptase.

Zidovudine is currently used to treat patients with advanced, symptomatic HIV infection with CD4 lymphocyte counts less than 200/mm^3 and in patients with AIDS (see Table 28–15).[143] The mortality rate and frequency of opportunist infections were significantly decreased among patients given 250 mg zidovudine every 4 hours compared to control subjects who received a placebo. Subsequent studies showed that a reduced daily dosage of 500 mg (100 mg every 4 hours), while the patients were awake, was associated with equal efficacy and less toxicity. Even lower doses may be effective. Zidovudine has also been advocated for mildly symptomatic HIV infection and for chemoprophylaxis after occupation nosocomial exposure. Double-blind, placebo controlled studies have demonstrated that zidovudine is effective in delaying the progression to advanced AIDS related complex (ARC) or AIDS in patients with CD4 counts less than 500/mm^3. But there is no evidence of benefit for patients with CD4 counts between 500 and 800/mm^3.[136] Zidovudine is thus indicated for the treatment of patients with AIDS and those with symptomatic or asymptomatic HIV infections and CD4 counts less than 500/mm^3.

While zidovudine has been advocated as chemoprophylaxis following occupational exposure to HIV, there are no human data that suggest it is effective. The U.S. Public Health Service offers no definitive recommendation for or against the use of zidovudine as prophylaxis after exposure to HIV. There are several individual reports of failure of zidovudine prophylaxis after HIV exposure.

The adverse side effects attributed to zidovudine have limited its use. The major side effects include macrocytic anemia and granulocytopenia.[136] Anemia occasionally occurs in the first month of treatment but is most common after 8 weeks of therapy. Many patients require maintenance transfusions. The likelihood of developing anemia is related to the dose and duration of zidovudine therapy.

Other side effects include headache, insomnia, myalgia, and nausea, which seem to be dose related. Central nervous system effects include agitation, confusion, and seizures.

Dideoxyinosine (ddI). Dideoxyinosine was recently approved for the treatment of AIDS. It inhibits HIV and retains in vitro potency against strains that have decreased sensitivity to AZT. It has fewer adverse side effects than does AZT and a longer intracellular half-life, allowing less frequent oral administration.[136,144] Its most serious side effect is a painful peripheral neuropathy.[145] It can also cause rash, increased hepatic transaminases, pancreatitis, and hyperuricemia.[136,145]

Interferon. The interferons are a family of cytokines, which are glycoproteins that have antiviral activity.[136] They also have many other actions. They are not viral specific and are neither virucidal or virustatic. Rather, they induce changes in infected or exposed cells that promote resistance to subsequent virus infection. Recently, recombinant DNA technology has enabled large quantities of purified interferons to be produced for investigational purposes. They have been used to treat virus infections, malignant lesions, and other conditions. There are three major classes of interferons—interferon alpha (IFN-α), interferon beta (IFN-β), and interferon gamma IFN-γ); they differ in the type of cell that produces it. Only IFN-α-2b has been approved for clinical use.

Pharmacology and Toxicity. Recombinant DNA technology has permitted the insertion of the gene coding for interferon into bacteria, resulting in production of large quantities of interferon for clinical trials. The subcutaneous or intramuscular routes are usually used because of the ease of administration and because the presence of interferon in the serum is prolonged (half-life, 4 to 6 hours). Adverse reactions include fever, myalgia, headache, diarrhea, and alopecia.[136]

Clinical Indications. Subcutaneous IFN-α-2b is approved for treatment of chronic hepatitis C.[146] Among patients treated with 3 million units subcutaneously three times a week for 24 weeks, 46 percent had normalization or near normalization of the serum alanine amino transferase level in comparison with 28 percent treated with 1 million units three times a week and 8 percent in untreated patients. Histologic improvements were demonstrated on liver biopsy in patients receiving the higher dosage.

Interferon alpha-2b has also been approved for treating condyloma acuminatum due to human papillomavirus. A double-blind study demonstrated that intralesion injection three times weekly for 3 weeks resulted in a significantly decreased mean wart area after 13 weeks of therapy.[147] Interferon has also been used to treat chronic hepatitis B. While 37 percent of patients treated with IFN-α-2b responded compared to 7 percent of untreated control subjects, almost two-thirds of the patients did not respond.[148]

Ribavirin. Ribavirin is a purine nucleoside analog that has antiviral activity in vitro against many viruses including respiratory syncytial virus, influenza virus, herpes simplex virus, mumps virus, measles virus, coxsackievirus, and several other viruses.[136] Clinical efficacy has been reported against influenza A and B viruses, respiratory syncytial virus infection, and Lassa fever virus, but it has only been approved by the Food and Drug Administration for aerosolized use in treating respiratory syncytial virus in infants and young children.

Pharmacology and Toxicity. When administrated by aerosol, ribavirin is absorbed systemically. The plasma half-life is 9.5 hours.

Ribavirin is teratogenic, mutagenic, embryotoxic, and gonadotoxic in small animals, and therefore its use is contraindicated in pregnancy.[136] These toxicities were not seen in primates, however, prolonged use can cause anemia. Increased serum bilirubin and uric acid, nausea, headache, and fatigue have been reported after oral administration of ribavirin.

Clinical Use. Ribavirin is approved for use in infants and young children with severe respiratory syncytial virus pulmonary infections. These children are treated with aerosolized ribavirin for delivery directly into the pulmonary tissue. Ribavirin is given at 20 mg/ml of sterile water and is administered 12 to 18 hours per day for 3 to 7 days. Infants so treated showed faster rates of improvement and more rapid clearance of respiratory syncytial virus from respiratory secretions and higher arterial oxygen saturation compared to placebo-treated control subjects.[136] It is also recommended for treatment of infants with severe underlying chronic disease such as chronic cardiac, pulmonary, or immunosuppressive illnesses.

Vidarabine. Vidarabine (adenine arabinoside) is one of several nucleoside derivatives that are effective against the herpesvirus family. This agent is currently approved in the United States for treatment of herpes simplex encephalitis and herpes simplex catarrhal conjunctivitis.

Antiviral Activity. Vidarabine has activity against the herpes group viruses, pox viruses, and even possibly hepatitis B viruses. Vidarabine and its less active metabolic product arabinosyl hypoxanthine are converted within the cell to monophosphates, diphosphates, and triphosphates, which may in turn selectively and competitively inhibit the activity of the herpesvirus DNA polymerase. The phosphorylated drug is then incorporated into both cellular and viral DNA. Incorporated viral vidarabine has been reported to act as a chain terminator for newly synthesized herpes simplex DNA strains. Antiviral activity is greatest against herpes simplex virus types I and II, cytomegalovirus, varicella-zoster virus, vaccinia, and variola virus.[149] Other DNA viruses, such as adenoviruses and papovaviruses, are not inhibited, apparently because they lack a DNA polymerase.

Pharmacology and Toxicity. The plasma half-life of vidarabine is approximately 4 hours in adults, and nearly 60 percent of the dose is recovered in the urine, principally as hypoxanthine arabinoside. It must be given in reduced doses to patients with decreased renal function. Administration to patients with compromised renal function is further complicated by its poor solubility, which requires that it be diluted in large fluid volumes.

Little toxicity is seen at doses of 5 to 15 mg/kg/day given by 12-hour intravenous infusion. Nausea, vomiting, and diarrhea have been observed in a small percentage of patients. Large doses, 20 mg/kg, cause tremors, weight loss, and bone marrow megaloblastosis. Other adverse reactions include anorexia, nausea, vomiting, diarrhea, skin rash, thrombophlebitis at the intravenous site, and weakness. Central nervous system side effects include tremor, dizziness, hallucinations, psychosis, ataxias, and electroencephalogram changes. Rapid mental deterioration with agitation, tremulousness, facial grimacing, and eventual coma and death occurred in four renal transplant patients who each received 10 mg/kg/day vidarabine for cytomegalovirus infections.[150]

Clinical Indications. In a randomized crossover study vidarabine was effective treatment for 87 immunocompromised patients with zoster. Vidarabine is also as effective as idoxuridine against herpes simplex catarrhal conjunctivitis, even in patients who cannot take idoxuridine because of allergy, toxicity, or drug resistance.

In a double-blind treatment study of 28 biopsy-proven cases of herpes simplex encephalitis, the mortality was reduced from 70 to 28 percent. Survival in patients with herpes simplex encephalitis who were treated with vidarabine was enhanced if the patient (1) had a minimally altered level of consciousness at the start of therapy, (2) was under 40 years of age, or (3) had low virus titers in the brain. Although neurologic sequelae often occur in survivors, about 40 percent of these patients resumed normal activity after vidarabine therapy. However, patients who are already in a coma at the onset of drug therapy did not benefit from the drug.[151]

Other controlled studies show that vidarabine was not effective for smallpox or for cytomegalovirus infections in renal transplant recipients. Uncontrolled studies with patients with congenital cytomegalovirus and the cytomegalovirus mononucleosis syndrome, however, showed that vidarabine transiently suppressed virus excretion in the urine. Similarly, serum DNA polymerase activity was suppressed in two patients with chronic active hepatitis.[152]

Vidarabine is presently recommended only for the treatment of biopsy-proven herpes simplex encephalitis (15 mg/kg per day for 10 days by slow infusion) and for herpes simplex catarrhal conjunctivitis (a 3 percent ophthalmic ointment applied every 3 hours). Culture-proven disseminated or central nervous system herpes simplex infection will also respond to a 10-day course of intravenous vidarabine, although this indication has not yet been formally approved by the Food and Drug Administration.

GERMICIDES, ANTISEPTICS, AND DISINFECTANTS

A germicide is a general term for any agent that destroys microorganisms. Germicides may be further divided according to their antimicrobial spectrum—bactericides, fungicides, virucides—or use.

An antiseptic is a germicide that is usually applied to living tissue, and disinfectant is usually applied to inanimate objects. Such agents tend to denature protein and are not licensed for use in body cavities or wounds.

Desirable Properties of Antiseptics and Disinfectants

Antiseptics. One of the most important properties of antiseptics, of course, is germicidal potency. An agent that is lethal to microorganisms is superior to one that merely inhibits growth. A broad antimicrobial spectrum is essential, especially for microorganisms that inhabit the skin or wounds. Bactericidal and fungicidal properties are much more important than virucidal or protozoacidal actions. Antiseptics should spread over the skin or wound surfaces and therefore should have a low surface tension. These agents should also retain their potency in the presence of inflammatory exudates in infected regions. The action of antiseptics should be both rapid and sustained so that bacteria and fungi are killed rapidly during hand washing or skin preparation to minimize the time required for these activities and yet continue to exert their antimicrobial effect throughout an operation. They should not be inactivated by soaps used for cleansing the skin. Antiseptic agents should not cause irritation of skin or tissues and should not interfere with mechanisms of healing and tissue repair. They also should not cause hypersensitivity reactions and should not be systemically absorbed.

Disinfectants. Disinfectants should also have high germicidal efficacy, a wide antimicrobial spectrum, rapid action, and the ability to penetrate into crevices and cavities and beneath films of organic matter. It is essential that lethal concentrations of the agent can be obtained in the presence of organic matter such as blood, sputum, pus, and fecal matter. Disinfectants should be compatible with soaps and other chemical substances that are likely to be present on the material to be disinfected. The disinfecting agent should be stable for prolonged periods and should not corrode surgical instruments or injure other materials. Other important considerations in choosing a disinfectant include odor, staining qualities, and cost.

Levels of Disinfection

Different materials require different levels of disinfection, depending on their intended use. For instance, some surgical instruments and prosthetic devices must be sterile but cannot be autoclaved.

Four high-level germicides that will ensure destruction of all bacteria and spores are 20 percent formalin, 2 percent alkalinized aqueous glutaraldehyde, gaseous ethylene chloride, and a 10 to 20 percent stabilized aqueous solution of hydrogen peroxide.

Intermediate-level disinfectants include, those that are not sporicidal but do kill tubercle bacilli, fungi, and non-lipid-containing viruses. Low-level disinfectants do not kill tubercle bacilli or resistant non-lipid-containing viruses. They do, however, kill vegetable forms of bacteria, many fungi, and the more susceptible viruses.

The level of disinfection required also varies according to the use intended for the item. Internal prosthetic devices must be sterile. For endoscopes contaminated by mucosal surfaces, on the other hand, the level of disinfection should only be high enough to destroy viruses, fungi, and bacteria; spores need not be killed. Other items can be contaminated with nonpathogenic bacteria and fungi, and hence only a low level of disinfection is required.

Commonly Used Antiseptics and Disinfectants

Phenols and Phenol Derivatives. Phenol (carbolic acid) was first used by Lister in 1867. Phenol is also of historical interest because in 1903 Rideal and Walker[153] developed the phenol coefficient test, which allowed the comparison of various germicides to the standard phenol in their ability to kill selected bacteria. Because of its toxicity, however, it is rarely used today. Instead, less toxic and more bactericidal derivatives of phenol are in use. Phenol causes leakage of essential intracellular metabolites through the cell wall and also inactivates many intracellular enzymes.

Hexachlorophene. The chlorine-substituted bis-phenol, hexachlorophene, is the most commonly used phenol derivative. It is more effective against gram-positive than against gram-negative organisms. Hexachlorophene is highly bacteriostatic, but prolonged contact is required to kill microorganisms. The growth of pathogenic fungi is also inhibited by this agent.

Organic matter such as pus and serum reduces it efficiency, but it does not lose potency in the presence of soap. Three percent hexachlorophene is a synthetic detergent vehicle. Hexachlorophene liquid soap, USP, and other hexachlorophene preparations are frequently used as operative scrubs and as germicidal soaps for hand washing. Maximal reduction of skin flora is attained only after several days of hand washing because the chemical only gradually builds up on the skin and reaches optimal concentrations. To gain this thin film of hexachlorophene on the skin with its continuous degerming action, it is necessary to wash the hands with hexachlorophene exclusively and frequently.[154] Because repeated use of hexachlorophene is required for maximal efficiency, it is less effective as an antiseptic for the operative site.

Hexachlorophene can be absorbed through the skin where it can produce neurologic symptoms, especially after repeated use. For this reason the Food and Drug Administration banned over-the-counter sales of products containing more than 0.1 percent hexachlorophene. Its use on burned or denuded skin, mucous membranes, newborn infants, or for total body bathing is contraindicated. Use is now limited to surgical scrubbing and hand washing.

Alcohols. Alcohols are bactericidal, cheap, have a cleansing action, and evaporate readily. They are colorless, but dyes can easily be added when required. Their bactericidal activity increases with molecular weight, but only ethyl and isopropyl alcohol are extensively used clinically.

Alcohols are believed to exert their antibacterial action by denaturing proteins. Proteins are not as easily denatured in the absence of water as when water is present, which explains why absolute ethyl alcohol is less bactericidal than mixtures of alcohol and water. Alcohol in a 0.41 M concentration also interferes with bacterial metabolism and may account for some of the bacteriostatic action of alcohols. Ethyl alcohol also exerts substantial fungicidal and virucidal activity.

Ethyl Alcohol. Ethyl alcohol is widely used as an antiseptic before venipuncture, hypodermic injections, and finger pricks. It is also used before surgery for degerming the operative site and hands after washing, although it is currently being used much less frequently for these purposes. For skin degerming, alcohol concentrations between 70 and 92 percent by weight are equally effective.[155]

Alcohol is also an effective disinfectant when killing spores is not required, but it is not completely reliable.[156] *Clostridium tetani* and *C. perfringens* are not killed after an exposure of 18 hours.[156] Alcohol is useful, however, for disinfecting instruments such as clinical thermometers, where sterilization is not required.

Isopropyl Alcohol. The alcohol most commonly used clinically is isopropyl alcohol. It is the highest molecular weight alcohol miscible with water in all proportions, and it is not subject to the legal restrictions and taxation of ethyl alcohol. Isopropyl alcohol is nonpotable and does not have to be denatured. It is more bactericidal than ethanol, but like ethyl alcohol, it has no effect on spores. It has no harmful effects on human skin, although its vapors can be absorbed through the lungs and produce toxic side effects—usually narcosis in children. For skin degerming, solutions of 70 percent or more are recommended. The bactericidal action of isopropyl alcohol increases with its concentration.

Iodine. Iodine is one of the oldest antiseptics. Tincture of iodine was used as an antiseptic by a French surgeon as early as 1839 and for treating battle wounds in the Civil War.

Elemental iodine is bactericidal and sporicidal over a wide pH range against bacteria, fungi, viruses, and protozoa. Acid solutions markedly increase germicidal efficiency. It kills extremely rapidly. A 1:20,000 solution of iodine kills almost all bacteria within 1 minute; 15 minutes is required to kill spores with this concentration.

Because toxicity of iodine is extremely low in relation to its germicidal capacity, it is a safe antiseptic agent. Strong iodine solutions (above 5 percent iodine), however, can cause burns if placed on large areas of the skin.

Iodine Preparations Containing Free Iodine. The 2 percent iodine tincture, USP, contains 2 percent iodine and 2 percent sodium iodide in 44 to 55 percent ethyl alcohol. Using 70 percent alcohol instead may provide a superior solution; it spreads evenly, dries slowly, does not burn the skin, and rarely causes any patient discomfort. Iodine is also an effective antiseptic and disinfectant in aqueous solution. An iodide salt must be added to solubilize the iodine. Iodine solution, NF, contains 2 g iodine and 2.4 g sodium iodide dissolved in distilled water to make a 100 ml solution. The use of this solution avoids alcohol in cases where it may harm the object to be disinfected.

Stronger iodine solutions, such as Lugol solution, which contains 5 percent iodine, and strong tincture of iodine, NF, which contains 16.5 percent iodine, are used occasionally to prepare solutions with lower concentrations of free iodine for antiseptic purposes.

Iodophors. An iodophor is the combination of iodine and a solubilizing agent or carrier that liberates free iodine in solution. Povidone-iodine is a complex of iodine and polyvinylpyrrolidone. The compound slowly releases free iodine when dissolved in water. It is claimed that povidone-iodine is more effective and less toxic than aqueous or alcoholic solutions of free iodine, but definite proof is lacking. Blatt and Maloney[157] found that the germicidal properties of three different iodophors were similar to those of iodine solutions of equivalent iodine content. King and Price,[158] however, showed that 1 percent iodine in 70 percent alcohol was superior as a skin antiseptic to any of five iodophors tested, including povidone-iodine. Iodophors produce less pain when applied around wounds and abrasions. There is also no allergic response to iodine even in sensitive individuals when applied in the form of an iodophor.

Iodophors have broad-spectrum antimicrobial activity. They are nonirritating to the eyes, skin, nose, mouth, and vaginal mucosa. They are marketed in a variety of forms—solutions, ointments, aerosol sprays, skin cleansers, swabsticks, gauze pads, surgical scrubs, douches, and other disposable forms. In dilutions, they do not permanently stain skin or natural fabrics. Their stability permits easy storage. A variety of solubilizing agents other than povidone are also used.

Chlorine. Chlorine is widely used in treating municipal water supplies, swimming pool water, utensils and equipment in dairy and food processing industries, and in sewage and waste water treatment. It is used considerably less in the hospital setting. Dakin's solution, a buffered solution of sodium hypochlorite, was introduced in World War I as an antiseptic irrigant for wounds. It is injurious to tissues. Modified Dakin's solution contains 0.5 percent instead of 5 percent sodium hypochlorite and is much less injurious to tissues. As a disinfectant in hospitals, chlorine has limited use. Yet sodium hypochlorite solution is still one of the best germicides for spot disinfection. It is a particularly effective germicide for spills contaminated with hepatitis B virus.

Chlorine appears to exert its antibacterial action in the form of undissociated hypochlorous acid. Chlorine combines with water to form HOCl and dissociated HCl. HOCl is undissociated in neutral or acid solutions and exerts a strong bactericidal effect. In alkaline solutions, it dissociates, and the hypochlorite ion is much less effective.

Chlorhexidine. Chlorhexidine is a biquanidine used extensively for skin degerming before operative procedures. Gram-positive bacteria are inhibited by concentrations below 10 μg/ml, and most gram-negative bacteria are inhibited at concentrations below 50 μg/ml. The lowest recommended concentration in practice is 200 μg/ml. Its effectiveness is not adversely affected by organic matter including pus or blood.

There is no absorption through intact skin, and it has a low potential for causing skin reactions. It can be used many times for hand degerming without causing dryness, irritation, or discomfort. It is reported not to cause additional tissue injury or delayed healing when used for cleaning superficial wounds.

Chlorhexidine is for topical use only. It is irritating to the eyes and may cause deafness if instilled into the middle ear of a patient with a perforated tympanic membrane.

Its rapidity of action is a major advantage when used for hand washing. Only 15 to 30 seconds are required to achieve a 99 to 99.99 percent reduction in skin bacterial counts. Because of its strong affinity for skin, it remains on the skin for several hours where it retains its activity.[159]

Quaternary Ammonium Compounds. Quaternary ammonium compounds were for many years the most popular disinfectants because of their blandness and low cost. Unfortunately, however, they are relatively inactive against gram-negative bacteria. They are rapidly inactivated by traces of soap or inanimate objects that may be left on the skin by regular washing, and they form a thin film on the skin under which bacteria can remain viable. They can become contaminated by *Pseudomonas* if allowed to stand, and have been the source of some hospital-acquired infections.[160]

Commonly used commercial preparations include benzalkonium chloride (Zephiran) and cetylpyridinium chloride (Ceepryn). Tincture of benzalkonium chloride is more effective than an aqueous solution; indeed, a considerable portion of the benefit is attributed to the alcohol-acetone solvent. A 1:1000 tincture is recommended for degerming the unbroken skin. A 1:10,000 to 1:2000 aqueous concentration is used for denuded skin and mucous membranes. A 1:20,000 aqueous concentration is used for bladder irrigation and a 1:40,000 concentration for retention lavage.

Heavy Metals and Their Salts

Mercurials. Inorganic mercury compounds were among the earliest antiseptics used. Mercurials—both organic and inorganic—are bacteriostatic compounds, which combine with sulfhydryl groups on enzymes either on the cell wall or in the cytoplasm. Growth of mercury-inhibited bacteria can be reactivated by exposing the bacteria to sulfhydryl groups. Because numerous sulfhydryl groups are readily available in the body, organisms inhibited by mercury can become reactivated when introduced into the body. Because mercury also inactivates enzymes in tissues, mercurials are toxic and have a low therapeutic index.

Organic mercurial compounds are more bacteriostatic, less irritating, and less toxic than the inorganic mercurial salts. Merbromin (Mercurochrome) is a fluorescein derivative. It is only feebly active—its bacteriostatic activity is greatly reduced by organic matter, and it is relatively inactive at the pH of body fluids. Thimerosal (Merthiolate) is commonly applied to cuts and abrasions. Tinctures of organic mercurials are more effective than aqueous solutions but not as effective as 70 percent ethyl alcohol.

Mercurials should not be used to prepare the skin or as disinfectants for instruments because more effective agents are available.

Silver. Silver, like mercury, appears to exert its antimicrobial activity by inhibiting cellular enzymes. It also binds to DNA and blocks replication. Silver compounds are bactericidal in high (10 percent) concentrations but only bacteriostatic in lower concentrations. Silver nitrate solutions are applied as antiseptics to mucous membranes for ulcers of the mouth. Weak (0.5 percent) solutions were formerly applied to second- and third-degree burns to protect against contamination of the burn wound by gram-negative bacteria. One percent silver nitrate is used as eyedrops at birth to prevent ophthalmia neonatorum.

Currently, silver sulfadiazine, administered as 1 percent cream, is applied to burns to prevent bacterial infections (see Chap. 52). This compound is bactericidal and is easier to work with than silver nitrate. Rooms do not become stained black because of spilled silver nitrate and subsequent precipitation of silver salts during use. Silver sulfadiazine is painful (burns) when it is applied to third-degree burns. Furthermore, it is a carbonic anhydrase inhibitor and can cause a metabolic acidosis.

Other silver salts of acetate, citrate, and lactate are used for eye lotion, treating burn wounds, and dusting on wounds. Silver proteinates are colloidal preparations of silver. They are used for eyedrops, urethral irrigations, throat and nose sprays, and vaginal and rectal suppositories.

Other Antiseptics and Detergents

Soaps. Soap is a poor antiseptic. While a bar of soap will quickly sterilize itself after it has been used, it is relatively ineffective in degerming skin. Its value lies in its ability to remove gross dirt, grease, and oils, and other surface debris that might contain microorganisms. Soap can be used as an initial skin cleanser but cannot be relied on to remove the bacteria on the skin.

Organic Agents. Organic agents such as ether, acetone, chloroform, and xylene have also been used to degerm the skin but are somewhat injurious, and especially drying, to skin. In addition, because ether and acetone are extremely flammable, they are banned from many operating rooms.

Formalin. Formalin is a solution of formaldehyde gas dissolved in water. Eight percent formaldehyde dissolved in water makes a solution of 20 percent formalin. It is a high-level germicide. A combination of 20 percent formalin and 65 to 70 percent isopropyl alcohol is rapidly bactericidal and even kills tubercule bacilli. It is also sporicidal, but the time required may be 24 hours or more. Formalin is extremely toxic to tissues, so disinfected materials must be thoroughly rinsed before use.

Glutaraldehyde. Glutaraldehyde is a high-level bactericidal disinfectant. When combined with alcohol, it is also tuberculocidal. At the present time, aqueous buffered glutaraldehyde is the only highly effective chemical sterilant recommended by the Centers for Disease Control for disinfecting respiratory therapy equipment.

Hydrogen Peroxide. Hydrogen peroxide has long been used as an antiseptic and disinfectant. It is frequently used in granulating and other open wounds to reduce bacterial contamination. Low concentrations of unstable preparations, however, are usually applied to tissues, and these are rapidly inactivated by catalase in the tissues. Consequently, numerous bubbles of oxygen gas are formed when the hydrogen peroxide is placed into open tissues, which makes the physician and the patient think the agent is extremely active. The bubbles, however, only signify rapid inactivation of the hydrogen peroxide. It is almost totally ineffective as an antiseptic, and has been generally abandoned.

Recently, hydrogen peroxide has been available in pure stabilized preparations with a long shelf-life. Experimental tests have shown it to be an extremely effective germicide, but it has not achieved widespread use. It has been used to some degree to sterilize drinking water but has not received wide attention in hospital settings. Still, hydrogen peroxide in relatively high (10 to 25 percent) concentrations is a promising sporicidal agent. It has been recommended for the disinfection of acrylic resin sections used as surgical implants. It is also used for disinfection of hydrophil soft contact lenses.

REFERENCES

1. Thornsberry C: Review of in vitro activity of third-generation cephalosporins and other newer beta-lactam antibiotics against clinically important bacteria. Am J Med 79(2A):14, 1985.
2. Cornick NA, Cuchural GJ, Snydman DR, et al: The antimicrobial susceptibility patterns of the *Bacteroides fragilis* group in the United States, 1987. J Antimicrob Chemother 25:1011, 1990.
3. Sabath LD, Gerstein DA, Leaf CD, Finland M: Increasing the usefulness of antibiotics: treatment of infections caused by gram-negative bacilli. Clin Pharmacol Ther 11:161, 1970.
4. Klastersky J, Debusscher L, Daneau D: Effectiveness of erythromycin plus alkalinization and nitrofurantoin in the treatment of urinary tract infections. Curr Ther Res 13:427, 1971.
5. Brumfitt W, Percival A, Leigh DA: Clinical and laboratory studies with carbenicillin. A new penicillin active against *Pseudomonas pyocyanea.* Lancet 1:1289, 1967.
6. Solomkin JS: Pathogenesis and management of *Candida* infection syndromes in non-neutropenic patients. In Solomkin JS (ed): New Horizons. Baltimore, Williams & Wilkins, 1993, pp 202–213.
7. National Committee for Clinical Laboratory Standards: Approved Standard M7-A. Methods for Dilution Antimicrobial Susceptibility Tests for Bacteria that Grow Aerobically. Villanova, PA, National Committee for Clinical Laboratory Standards, 1985.
8. Lau WY, Fan ST, Yiu TF, et al: Prophylaxis of post-appendicectomy sepsis by metronidazole and cefotaxime; a randomized, prospective and double blind trial. Br J Surg 70:670, 1983.
9. Yellin AE, Heseltine PN, Berne TV, et al: The role of *Pseudomonas* species in patients treated with ampicillin and sulbactam for gangrenous and perforated appendicitis. Surg Gynecol Obstet 161:303, 1985.
10. Malangoni MA, Condon RE, Spiegel CA: Treatment of intra-abdominal infections is appropriate with single-agent or combination antibiotic therapy. Surgery 98:648, 1985.
11. Chow JW, Fine MJ, Shlaes DM, et al: *Enterobacter* bacteremia: clinical features and emergence of antibiotic resistance during therapy. Ann Intern Med 115:585, 1991.
12. Hilf M, Yu VL, Sharp J, et al: Antibiotic therapy for *Pseudomonas aeruginosa* bactermia: outcome correlations in a prospective study of 200 patients. Am J Med 87:540, 1989.

13. Sanders CC: New β-lactams: new problems for the internist. Ann Intern Med 115:650, 1991.
14. Gutmann L, Williamson R, Kitzis MD, et al: Synergism and antagonism in double beta-lactam antibiotic combinations. Am J Med 80(Suppl 5C):21, 1986.
15. Sabath LD: Body distribution of antibiotics. J Surg Prac 8:56, 1979.
16. Craig WA, Kunin CM: Significance of serum protein and tissue binding of antimicrobial agents. Annu Rev Med 27:287, 1976.
17. Zimelis VM, Jackson GG: Activity of aminoglycoside antibiotics against *Pseudomonas aeruginosa:* specificity and site of calcium and magnesium antagonism. J Infect Dis 127:663, 1973.
18. Bryan LE, Van DenElzen HM: Streptomycin accumulation in susceptible and resistant strains of *Escherichia coli* and *Pseudomonas aeruginosa.* Antimicrob Agent Chemother 9:928, 1976.
19. Louie T, Onderdonk AB, Bartlett JG, Gorbach SL: Failure of penicillin in experimental intra-abdominal sepsis (abstract 62). Interscience Conference on Antimicrobial Agents and Chemotherapy, 1975.
20. Louie T, Onderdonk AB, Bartlett JG, Gorbach SL: Failure of penicillin in experimental *Bacteroides fragilis* infections. Clin Res 23(3):307A, 1975.
21. Lewis C, Stern K, Zurenko GE: A comparison in mice of blood and *Bacteroides fragilis*-induced abscess levels of antibiotics (abstract A-18). 80th Annual Meeting, American Society for Microbiology, 1980.
22. Joiner K, Lowe B, Dzink J, et al: Antibiotic levels and efficacy in mouse abscess model (abstract A-19). 80th Annual Meeting, American Society for Microbiology, 1980.
23. Thadepalli H, Gorbach SL, Bartlett JG: Apparent failure of chloramphenicol in the treatment of anaerobic infections. Curr Ther Res 22:421, 1977.
24. Francis JB, Corwin RW, Johnson JD, Hand WL: Antibiotic uptake by alveolar macrophages. Clin Res 26:394A, 1978.
25. Van Scoy RE, Wilson WR: Antimicrobial agents in patients with renal insufficiency. Mayo Clin Proc 58:246, 1983.
26. Gilbert DN, Bennett WM: Use of antimicrobial agents in renal failure. Infect Dis Clin North Am 3:517, 1989.
27. St Peter WL, Redic-Kill KA, Halstenson CE: Clinical pharmacokinetics of antibiotics in patients with impaired renal function. Clin Pharmacokinet 22: 169, 1992.
28. McCracken GH Jr: Pharmacological basis for antimicrobial therapy in newborn infants. Am J Dis Child 128:407, 1974.
29. Moellering RC Jr: Factors influencing the clinical use of antimicrobial agents in elderly patients. Geriatrics 33:83, 1978.
30. Wilson RF: Science and shock: a clinical perspective. Ann Emerg Med 14:714, 1985.
31. Bodenham A, Shelly MP, Park GR: The altered pharmacokinetics and pharmacodynamics of drugs commonly used in critically ill patients. Clin Pharmacokinet 14:347, 1988.
32. Slaughter RL, Hassett JM: Hepatic drug clearance following traumatic injury. Drug Intell Clin Pharmacol 19:799, 1985.
33. Davey PG: Pharmacokinetics in liver disease. J Antimicrob Chemother 21:1, 1988.
34. Hawker F: Liver dysfunction in critical illness. Anaesth Intensive Care 19:165, 1991.
35. Corwin HL, Bonventre JV: Acute renal failure in the intensive care unit. Part 1. Intensive Care Med 14:10, 1988.
36. Corwin HL, Bonventre JV: Acute renal failure in the intensive care unit. Part 2. Intensive Care Med 14:86, 1988.
37. Zaske DE, Cipolle RJ, Strate RJ: Gentamicin dosage requirements: wide interpatient variations in 242 surgery patients with normal renal function. Surgery 87:64, 1980.
38. Sawchuk RJ, Zaske DE, Cipolle RJ, et al: Kinetic model for gentamicin dosing with the use of individual patient parameters. Clin Pharmacol Ther 21: 362, 1976.
39. Weinstein L, Dalton AC: Host determinants of response to antimicrobial agents. N Engl J Med 279:467, 1968.
40. Vorherr H: Drug excretion in breast milk. Postgrad Med 56:97, 1974.
41. Richmond MH, Sykes RB: The beta-lactamases of gram-negative bacteria and their possible physiological role. Adv Microb Physiol 9:31, 1973.
42. Sanders CC: Beta-lactamases of gram-negative bacteria: new challenges for new drugs. Clin Infect Dis 14:1089, 1992.
43. Bush K: Characterization of beta-lactamases. Antimicrob Agents Chemother 33:259, 1989.
44. Bush K: Classification of beta-lactamases: groups 1, 2a, 2b, and 2b′. Antimicrob Agents Chemother 33:264, 1989.
45. Bush K: Classification of beta-lactamases: groups 2c, 2d, 2e, 3 and 4. Antimicrob Agents Chemother 33:271, 1989.
46. Lipman B, Neu HC: Imipenem: a new carbapenem antibiotic. Med Clin North Am 72:567, 1988.
47. Phillips I, Shannon K: Importance of beta-lactamase induction. Eur J Clin Microbiol Infect Dis 12(Suppl 1):S19, 1993.
48. Livermore DM: Interplay of impermeability and chromosomal beta-lactamase activity in imipenem-resistant *Pseudomonas aeruginosa.* Antimicrob Agents Chemother 36:2046, 1992.
49. Sanders WE Jr, Sanders CC: Inducible beta-lactamases: clinical and epidemiologic implications for use of newer cephalosporins. Rev Infect Dis 10:830, 1988.
50. Philippon A, Labia R, Jacoby G: Extended-spectrum

beta-lactamases. Antimicrob Agents Chemother 33:1131, 1989.
51. Hiraoka M, Inoue M, Mitsuhashi S: Hydrolytic rate at low drug concentration as a limiting factor in resistance to newer cephalosporins. Rev Infect Dis 10:746, 1988.
52. Charnas RL, Then RL: Mechanism of inhibition of chromosomal β-lactamases by third-generation cephalosporins. Rev Infect Dis 10:752, 1988.
53. Hewinson RG, Cartwright SJ, Slack MPE, et al: Permeability to cefsulodin of the outer membrane of *Pseudomonas aeruginosa* and discrimination between β-lactamase-mediated trapping and hydrolysis as mechanisms of resistance. Eur J Biochem 179:667, 1989.
54. Wright AJ, Wilkowske CJ: The penicillins. Mayo Clin Proc 66:1047, 1991.
55. Spicehandler JR, Bernhardt L, Simberkoff MS, Rahal JJ Jr: Mezlocillin and piperacillin: a comparative clinical evaluation. In Nelson JD, Grassi C (eds): Current Chemotherapy and Infectious Disease, Vol I. Washington, DC, American Society for Microbiology, 1980, pp 293–294.
56. Wise R: Penicillins and cephalosporins: antimicrobial and pharmacological properties. Lancet 2:140, 1982.
57. Gustaferro CA, Steckelberg JM: Cephalosporin antimicrobial agents and related compounds. Mayo Clin Proc 66:1064, 1991.
58. Nev HC: Clinical uses of cephalosporins. Lancet 2:252, 1982.
59. Richmond MH, Sykes RB: The beta-lactamases of gram-negative bacteria and their possible physiological role. Adv Microb Physiol 9:31, 1973.
60. Birnbaum J, Kahan FM, Kropp H, MacDonald JS. Carbapenems: a new class of beta lactam antibiotics. Am J Med 78(6A):3, 1985.
61. Remington JS (ed): Carbapenems: a new class of antibiotics. Am J Med 78(6A):1, 1985.
62. Hellinger WC, Brewer NS: Imipenem. Mayo Clin Proc 66:1074, 1991.
63. Neu HC: The quinolones. Infect Dis Clin North Am 3:625, 1989.
64. Walker RC, Wright AJ: The fluoroquinolones. Mayo Clin Proc 66:1249, 1991.
65. Bergon T: Pharmacokinetics of the fluorinated quinolones. In Andriole VT (ed): The Quinolones. London, Academic Press, 1988, pp 119–154.
66. Edson RS, Keys TF: The aminoglycosides. Mayo Clin Proc 66:1158, 1991.
67. Solomkin JS, Dellinger EP, Christou NV, Busuttil RW: Results of a multicenter trial comparing imipenem/cilastatin to tobramycin/clindamycin for intra-abdominal infections. Ann Surg 212:581, 1990.
68. Salacata A, Chow JW: Cephalosporin therapeutics for intensive care infection. In Solomkin JS (ed): New Horizons. Baltimore, Williams & Wilkins, 1993, pp 181–186.
69. Yu VL, Rhame FS, Pesanti EL, Axline SG: Amikacin therapy: use against infections caused by gentamicin- and tobramycin-resistant organisms. JAMA 238:943, 1977.
70. Pechere M, Letarte R, Pechere JC: Efficacy of different dosing schedules of tobramycin for treating a murine *Klebsiella* broncho-pneumonia. J Antimicrob Chemother 19:487, 1987.
71. Kapusnik JR, Hackbarth CJ, Chambers HF, et al: Single large daily dosing versus intermittent dosing of tobramycin for treating experimental *Pseudomonas* pneumonia. J Infect Dis 158:7, 1988.
72. Moore RD, Smith CR, Lietman PS: Risk factors for the development of auditory toxicity in patients receiving aminoglycosides. J Infect Dis 149:23, 1984.
73. Moore RD, Smith CR, Lietman PS: Association of aminoglycoside plasma levels with therapeutic outcome in gram-negative pneumonia. Am J Med 77:657, 1984.
74. Vogelman B, Gudmundsson S, Leggett J, et al: Correlation of antimicrobial pharmacokinetic parameters with therapeutic efficacy in an animal model. J Infect Dis 158:831, 1988.
75. Vogelman B, Gudmundsson S, Turnidge J, et al: In vivo postantibiotic effect in a thigh infection in neutropenic mice. J Infect Dis 157:287, 1988.
76. Gilbert DN: Once-daily aminoglycoside therapy. Antimicrob Agents Chemother 35:399, 1991.
77. Blazer J, Stone BB, Zinner SH: Efficacy of intermittent versus continuous administration of netilmicin in a two-compartment in-vitro model. Antimicrob Agents Chemother 27:343, 1985.
78. Blaser J, Stone BB, Groner MC, et al: Comparative study with enoxacin and netilmicin in a pharmacodynamic model to determine importance of ratio of antibiotic peak concentration to MIC for bactericidal activity and emergence of resistance. Antimicrob Agents Chemother 31:1054, 1987.
79. Niederman MS, Fein AM: The interaction of infection and the adult respiratory distress syndrome. Crit Care Clin 2:471,1986.
80. Spitzer JJ, Bagby GJ, Meszaros K, Lang CH: Altered control of carbohydrate metabolism in endotoxemia. Prog Clin Biol Res 286:145, 1989.
81. Dickersin K: Reference bias in reports of drug trials (letter). Br Med J [Clin Res] 295:1066, 1987.
82. Fan ST, Lau WY, Teoh-Chan CH, et al: Once daily administration of netilmicin compared with thrice daily, both in combination with metronidazole, in gangrenous and perforated appendicitis. J Antimicrob Chemother 22:69, 1988.
83. Hollender LF, Bahnini LFJ, DeManzini N, et al: A multicentric study of netilmicin once daily versus thrice daily in patients with appendicitis and other intra-abdominal infections. J Antimicrob Chemother 23:773, 1989.
84. Nordstrom LH, Ringberg S, Cromberg O, et al: Does administration of an aminoglycoside in a single

daily dose affect its efficacy and toxicity? J Antimicrob Chemother 25:159, 1990.
85. Sturm AW: Netilmicin in the treatment of gram-negative bacteremia: single daily versus multiple daily dosage. J Infect Dis 159:931, 1989.
86. Tulkens PM: Pharmacokinetic and toxicological evaluation of a once-daily regimen versus conventional schedules of netilmicin and amikacin. J Antimicrob Chemother 27(Suppl C):49, 1991.
87. VanderAuwera P, Meunier F, Ibrahim S, et al: Pharmacodynamic parameters and toxicity of netilmicin (6 milligrams/kilogram/day) given once daily or in three divided doses to cancer patients with urinary tract infection. Antimicrob Agents Chemother 35:640, 1991.
88. Giamarellou H, Yiallouros K, Petrikkos G: Comparative kinetics and efficacy of amikacin administered once or twice daily in the treatment of systemic gram-negative infections. J Antimicrob Chemother 27(Suppl C):73, 1991.
89. Marik PE, Havlik I, Moneaagudo FSE, et al: The pharmacokinetics of amikacin in critically ill adult and paediatric patients. Comparison of once- versus twice-daily dosing regimens. J Antimicrob Chemother 27(Suppl C):81, 1991.
90. VanderAuwera P: Pharmacokinetics evaluation of single daily dose amikacin. J Antimicrob Chemother 27(Suppl C):63, 1991.
91. Powell SH, Thompson WL, Luthe MA, et al: Once-daily vs. continuous aminoglycoside dosing: efficacy and toxicity in animal and clinical studies of gentamicin, netilmicin, and tobramycin. J Infect Dis 147:918, 1983.
92. Tulkens PM: Experimental studies on nephrotoxicity of aminoglycosides at low doses. Am J Med 80(Suppl 6B):105, 1986.
93. TerBraak EW, DeVries PJ, Bouter KP, et al: Once-daily dosing regimen for aminoglycoside plus beta-lactam combination therapy of serious infections: comparative trial with netilmicin plus ceftriaxone. Am J Med 89:58, 1990.
94. Wood CA, Norton DR, Kohlhepp SJ, et al: The influence of tobramycin dosage regimens on nephrotoxicity, ototoxicity, and antibacterial efficacy in a rat model of subcutaneous abscess. J Infect Dis 158:13, 1988.
95. Reiner NE, Bloxham DD, Thompson WL: Nephrotoxicity of gentamicin and tobramycin given once daily or continuously in dogs. J Antimicrob Chemother 4(Suppl A):85, 1978.
96. Bennett WM, Plamp CE, Gilbert DN, et al: The influence of dosage regimen on experimental gentamicin nephrotoxicity: dissociation of peak serum levels from renal failure. J Infect Dis 140:576, 1979.
97. Herscovici L, Grise G, Thauvin C: Efficacy and safety of once daily versus intermittent dosing of tobramycin in rabbits with acute pyelonephritis. Scand J Infect Dis 20:205, 1988.
98. Shankar A, Sharma SD: Gentamicin as once daily dose therapy in recurrent urinary tract infections in children. Curr Ther Res 41:599, 1987.
99. Labowitz E, Levison ME, Kay D: Single dose daily gentamicin therapy in urinary tract infection. Antimicrob Agents Chemother 6:465, 1974.
100. Smilack JD, Wilson WR, McKerill FR III: Tetracyclines, chloramphenicol, erythromycin, clindamycin, and metronidazole. Mayo Clin Proc 66:1270, 1991.
101. Sack DA, Kaminsky DC, Sack RB, et al: Prophylactic doxycycline for travelers' diarrhea: results of a prospective double-blind study of Peace Corps volunteers in Kenya. N Engl J Med 298:758, 1978.
102. Best WR: Chloramphenicol-associated blood dyscrasias. A review of cases submitted to the American Medical Association Registry. JAMA 201:181, 1967.
103. Polin HB, Plaut ME: Chloramphenicol. NY State J Med 77:378, 1977.
104. Sutter VL: In vitro susceptibility of anaerobes: comparison of clindamycin and other antimicrobial agents. J Infect Dis 135(S):S7, 1977.
105. Nastro LJ, Finegold SM: Bactericidal activity of five antimicrobial agents against *Bacteroides fragilis.* J Infect Dis 126:104, 1972.
106. Guidiol F, Manresa F, Pallares P, et al: Clindamycin vs penicillin for anaerobic lung infections: high rate of penicillin failures associated with penicillin-resistant *Bacteroides melaninogenicis.* Arch Intern Med 150:2525, 1990.
107. Tedesco FJ: Clindamycin and colitis: a review. J Infect Dis 135(S):S95, 1977.
108. Noon GB, Beall AC, Jordan GL, et al: Clinical evaluation of peritoneal irrigation with antibiotic solution. Surgery 62:73, 1967.
109. Martin CM, Brookrajian EN: Bacteriuria prevention after indwelling urinary catheterization. Arch Intern Med 110:703, 1962.
110. Ostenson RC, Fields BT, Nolan CM: Polymyxin B and rifampin: new regimen for multiresistant *Serratia marcescens* infections. Antimicrob Agents Chemother 12:655, 1977.
111. Wilhelm MP: Vancomycin. Mayo Clin Proc 66:1165, 1991.
112. Zinner SH, Mayer KH: Sulfonamides and trimethoprim. In Mandell GL, Douglas RC Jr, Bennett JE (eds): Principles and Practice of Infectious Diseases, 3rd ed. New York, Churchill Livingstone, 1990, p 325.
113. Reeves D: Sulphonamides and trimethoprim. Lancet 2:370, 1982.
114. Parsley TL, Provonchee RB, Glicksman C, Zinner SH: Synergistic activity of trimethoprim and amikacin against gram-negative bacilli. Antimicrob Agents Chemother 12:349, 1977.
115. Bach MC, Finland M, Gold O, Wilcox C: Susceptibility of recently isolated pathogenic bacteria to trimethoprim and sulfamethoxazole separately and combined. J Infect Dis 128:S508, 1973.
116. Hughes WT, Kuhn S, Chaudhary S, et al: Successful

chemoprophylaxis for *Pneumocystis carinii* pneumonitis. N Engl J Med 297:1419, 1977.

117. Kunin C, Brandt D, Wood H: Bacteriologic studies of rifampin, a new semisynthetic antibiotic. J Infect Dis 119:132, 1969.
118. Stamey TA, Nemoy NJ, Higgins M: The clinical use of nalidixic acid. A review of some observations. Invest Urol 6:582, 1969.
119. Stamey TA (ed): Urinary Infections. Baltimore, Williams & Wilkins, 1980.
120. Van Scoy RE, Wilkowske CJ: Antituberculous agents. Mayo Clin Proc 67:179, 1992.
121. Stottmeir KD: Emergence of rifampin-resistant *Mycobacterium tuberculosis* in Massachusetts. J Infect Dis 133:88, 1976.
122. Sanders WE Jr, Cacciatore R, Valdez H, et al: Activity of amikacin against mycobacteria in vitro and in experimental infections with *M. tuberculosis*. Am Rev Respir Dis 113:59, 1976.
123. Terrell CL, Hughes CE: Antifungal agents used for deep-seated mycotic infections. Mayo Clin Proc 67:69, 1992.
124. Atkinson AJ Jr, Bennet JE: Amphotericin B pharmacokinetics in humans. Antimicrob Agents Chemother 13:271, 1978.
125. Medoff G, Kobayashi GS: Strategies in the treatment of systemic fungal infections. N Engl J Med 302:145, 1980.
126. Solomkin JS, Simmons RL: *Candida* infections in surgical patients. World J Surg 4:381, 1980.
127. Arroyo J, Medoff G, Kobayashi GS: Therapy of murine aspergillosis with amphotericin B in combination with rifampin or 5-fluorocytosine. Antimicrob Agents Chemother 11:21, 1977.
128. Bennett JE: Flucytosine. Ann Intern Med 86:319, 1977.
129. Denning DU, Tucker RM, Hansan LH, et al: Treatment of invasive aspergillosis with itraconazole. Am J Med 86:791, 1989.
130. Hardin TC, Graybill JR, Fetchick R, et al: Pharmacokinetics of itraconazole following oral administration to normal volunteers. Antimicrob Agents Chemother 32:1310, 1988.
131. Walsh TJ, Lee J, Aoki S, et al: Experimental basis for use of fluconazole for preventive or early treatment of disseminated candidiasis in granulocytopenic hosts. Rev Infect Dis 12(Suppl 3):S307, 1990.
132. Hirsch MS, Swartz MN: Antiviral agents (2 parts). N Engl J Med 302:903, 949, 1980.
133. Monto AS, Gunn RA, Bandyk MG, King CL: Prevention of Russian influenza by amantadine. JAMA 241:1003, 1979.
134. Little JW, Hall WJ. Douglas RG Jr, et al: Airway hyperreactivity and peripheral dysfunction in influenza A infection. Am Rev Respir Dis 118:295, 1978.
135. Sasadeusz JJ, Sacks SL: Systemic antivirals in herpesvirus infections. Dermatol Clin 11:171, 1993.
136. Keating MR: Antiviral agents. Mayo Clin Proc 67:160, 1992.
137. McKendrick MW, McGill JI, White JE, et al: Oral acyclovir in acute herpes zoster. Am J Med 85(Suppl 2A):90, 1988.
138. Burns WH, Sanford GR: Susceptibility of human herpesvirus 6 to antivirals in vitro. J Infect Dis 162:634, 1990.
139. Chatis PA, Crumpacker CS: Resistance of herpesviruses to antiviral drugs. Antimicrob Agents Chemother 36:1589, 1992.
140. Jabs DA, Enger C, Bartlett JG: Cytomegalovirus retinitis and acquired immunodeficiency syndrome. Arch Ophthalmol 67:75, 1989.
141. Safrin S, Assaykeen T, Fallansbee S, et al: Foscarnet therapy for acyclovir-resistant mucocutaneous herpes simplex virus infection in 26 AIDS patients: preliminary data. J Infect Dis 161:1078, 1990.
142. Broder S, Mitsuya H, Yarchoan R, et al: Antiretroviral therapy in AIDS. Ann Intern Med 113:604, 1990.
143. Fischl MA, Richman DD, Grieco MH, AZT Collaborative Working Group: The efficacy of azidothymidine (AZT) in the treatment of patients with AIDS and AIDS-related complex: a double-blind, placebo-controlled trial. N Engl J Med 317:185, 1987.
144. Yar Choan R, Mitsuyo H, Myers CE, et al: Clinical pharmacology of 3′-azido-2′,3′-dideoxythymidine (zidovudine) and related dideoxynucleosides. N Engl J Med 321:726, 1989.
145. Rosensweig M, McClaren C, Beltaugady M, et al: Overview of phase I trials of 2′,3′-dideoxyinosine (ddI) conducted on adult patients. Rev Infect Dis 12(Suppl 5):S570, 1990.
146. Davis GL, Balact LA, Schiff ER, et al: Treatment of chronic hepatitis C with recombinant interferon alpha: a multicenter randomized controlled trial. N Engl J Med 321:1501, 1989.
147. Eran LJ, Judson F, Tucker S, et al: Interferon therapy for condylomata acuminate. N Engl J Med 315:1059, 1986.
148. Perrillo RP, Schiff ER, Davis GL, et al: A randomized, controlled trial of interferon alpha-2b alone and after prednisone withdrawal for the treatment of chronic hepatitis B. N Engl J Med 323:295, 1990.
149. Champney K, Lauter CB, Bailey EJ, Lerner AM: Antiherpesvirus activity in human sera and urines after administration of adenine arabinoside. In vitro and in vivo synergy of adenine arabinoside and arabinosylhpoxanthine in combination. J Clin Invest 62:1142, 1978.
150. Marker SC, Howard RJ, Groth KE, et al: A trial of vidarabine for cytomegalovirus infection in renal transplant patient. Arch Intern Med 140:1441, 1980.
151. Whitley RJ, Soong SJ, Dolin R, et al: Adenine arabinoside therapy of biopsy-proved herpes simplex encephalitis. National Institute of Allergy and Infectious Diseases Collaborative Antiviral Study. N Engl J Med 297:289, 1977.
152. Hayden FG, Douglas RG Jr: Antiviral agents. In Mandell GL, Douglas RG Jr, Bennett JE (eds): Prin-

ciples and Practice of Infectious Diseases, 2nd ed. New York, Wiley, 1985, p 270.
153. Rideal S, Walker JTA: Standardization of disinfectants. JR Sanit Inst 24:424, 1903.
154. Price PB: Fallacy of a current surgical fad—the three-minute preoperative scrub with hexachlorophene soap. Ann Surg 134:476, 1951.
155. Price PB: Ethyl alcohol as a germicide. Arch Surg 38:528, 1939.
156. Block SS: Disinfection, Sterilization and Preservation, 2nd ed. Philadelphia, Lea & Febiger, 1977.
157. Blatt R, Maloney JV Jr: Evaluation of the iodophor compounds as surgical germicides. Surg Gynecol Obstet 113:699, 1961.
158. King TC, Price PB: An evaluation of iodophors as skin antiseptics. Surg Gynecol Obstet 116:361, 1963.
159. Ojaväri J: An evaluation of antiseptics used for hand disinfection in wards. J Hyg 76:75, 1976.
160. Sanford JP: Disinfectants that don't. Ann Intern Med 72:282, 1970.

Biologic Response Modifiers and Infectious Diseases

CHAPTER 29

Michael T. Lotze

Most immunologists believe that the major function of the adaptive immune system is to respond to microbial pathogens. Concurrently, the immune response[1] also serves to police the internal cellular milieu in multicellular organisms. Actually, both of these roles require regulatory cytokines, which alter the growth and modulate the function of cells both within the immune system proper (B cells, T cells, etc) and those not traditionally found within it (hepatocytes, endothelial cells). Not only do cytokines serve homeostatic and regulatory functions, but they also mediate destruction of tissues at appropriate times and alter the growth and differentiative functions at others.

Recently, it has been demonstrated that many pathogens[2] have developed quite ingenious mechanisms, which decrease the effectiveness of individual cytokines (see below). Mammalian hosts, in turn, have evolved multiple "backup systems" to control the spread of pathogens. Thus cytokines are characterized by *pleiotropy* (the ability of a single cytokine to mediate multiple biologic effects), *redundancy* (the ability of many different cytokines to mediate the same or similar effects such as T cell growth), and *synergy* (the ability of many different cytokines to work together in a coordinate fashion).

DEFINITION OF BIOLOGIC RESPONSE MODIFIERS

The term *biologic response modifier* was originally designed to encompass those agents that were capable of enhancing host defense as distinguished from cytotoxic drugs that directly caused tumor destruction. Part of the premise of the Biologic Response Modifiers Program of the National Cancer Institute was that there was a difference between the maximum tolerated dose and the so called optimal biological dose required to mediate important antitumor effects. The same notions may be thought to exist in treating infectious diseases. Certain general principles evolved prior to the testing of interferon alpha (IFN-α) in cancer trials; similar principles can be applied to the therapy of microbial diseases. (1) A clear statement of the underlying immunologic paradigm is necessary in order to apply an agent; empiricism must then guide the evaluation of any single cytokine. (2) Effectiveness may be limited because of immune responses to nonglycosylated or minor modified recombinant proteins. This is particularly true[3] for IFN-α. (3) Successful therapy may require prolonged treatment at lower doses. (4) Natural products with multiple different biologic activities are difficult to characterize and may give different results from those obtained with purified recombinant products. (5) The availability of large amounts of recombinant cytokines requires both empirical evaluation as well as targeted therapy for some desired biologic effect in individual diseases.

Cytokines are generally defined as soluble products of monocytes and lymphocytes (thus monokines and lymphokines), which regulate immune reactivity between individual cells within the immune system as well as cells outside it. *Interleukins* are broadly defined as cytokines made by one white cell and acting on another. This is not strictly true since some cytokines such as interleukin 6 (IL-6) can be produced by a variety of cell types and can also act on many others. The *colony-stimulating factors* (CSFs) are produced by a number of cell types and act on bone marrow-derived progenitors and act singly or frequently in combinations to enhance the growth and maturation of the hematopoietic cells (IL-1, IL-3, IL-6, M-CSF, G-CSF, GM-CSF). Other growth factors exist for other tissues and cells. The *interferons*, which currently include IFN-α, IFN-β, IFN-ω, and IFN-γ subtypes, have the common ability to interfere with viral replication. *Tumor necrosis factor* alpha and beta (TNF-α, TNF-β) as well as transforming growth factors alpha and beta (TGF-α, TGF-β) have diverse biologic properties that subsume their initial description. More recently, a variety of stromal derived factors have been defined (IL-7, IL-6, TGF-β), suggesting another broader category of so-called stromalkines or otherkines. The availability of recombinant molecules produced in *Escherichia coli*, yeast, or mammalian expression systems has lead to the widespread availability of many cytokines for testing in cancer and infectious diseases.[4–6] Although there has to be an upper limit to the number of molecules whose major purpose is to subserve intracellular communication (which is a broad definition of cytokines), each year still brings two to five new cytokines. IL-14 has recently been described as a B cell growth factor and the term IL-15 has been assigned to a recently described epithelial derived T cell growth factor.[6] As a general principle, each of these individual cytokines are pleiotropic, having multiple biologic effects, with occasional exceptions (erythropoietin). The currently identified major cytokines and their alternative names are listed in Table 29–1 as well as their molecular weight and major biologic effects.

Serum Levels During Infectious Diseases

During most viral infections serum levels of IL-6 are detectable. Only occasionally are elevations of TNF-α or IFN-γ identified, although it is clear that such cytokines can be identified within responding tissues.[2] Furthermore, some cytokines such as TNF and IL-6 actually upregulate viral expression at the transcriptional and post-transcriptional level (HIV). This is thought to be mediated in part by the pleiotropic transcription factor NFκB.

Microbial Subversion of Cytokine Function

It has recently been found that many cytokines have their function subverted by individual viruses.[7–13] This is best exemplified by identification of a truncated human IL-10 gene within the open reading frame, BCRF-1, in the Epstein-Barr virus (EBV)[7,8] This protein, like its human homolog, inhibits production of IFN-γ and IL-2 but does not promote T cell growth. Many other examples currently exist (Table 29–2). The Shope fibroma virus, for example, produces a TNF receptor[9] that is soluble and capable of binding TNF in solution. The human herpesvirus 6 replicates only in activated T cells. Transcription of the human immunodeficiency virus (HIV) is enhanced following binding of TNF or IL-6 to an infected cell. Cowpox is capable of producing a serine protease inhibitor, SPI-2, which in-

TABLE 29–1. IDENTIFIED RECOMBINANT CYTOKINES

Cytokine	Molecular Weight (kD)	Alternative Names/Biologic Activities
IL-1α or IL-β1	14–17	B cell activating factor (BAF); B cell differentiation factor (BDF); catabolin; endogenous pyrogen (EP); hematopoietin 1 (HP1); lymphocyte activating factor (LAF); leukocyte endogenous mediator (LEM); mitogenic protein (MP); mononuclear cell factor (MCF); proteolysis inducing factor (PIF); serum amyloid A (SAA) inducer; T cell replacing factor III (TRF-III)—costimulates T cells, induces IL-2 production, induces acute phase responses
IL-2	15	Killer helper factor (KHF); T cell-derived growth factor (TCGF); T cell maturation/stimulating factor (TMF/TSF); T cell replacing factor (TRF)—activates cytolitic response in T cells and NK cells [LAK (lymphokine activated killer) activity], cofactor for B cell growth and differentiation

TABLE 29–1. *(continued)*

Cytokine	Molecular Weight (kD)	Alternative Names/Biologic Activities
IL-3	28	Burst promoting activity (BPA); eosinophil colony-stimulating factor (Eo-CSF); erythroid colony-stimulating factor (E-CSF); hematopoietic cell growth factor (HPGF); hematopoietin 2 (HP2); mast cell growth factor (MCGF); megakaryocyte colony-stimulating factor (MEG-CSF); multipotential colony-stimulating factor (Multi-CSF); persisting cell stimulating factor (PSF)
IL-4	15–20 (>60 hyper-glycosylated)	B cell growth factor (BCGF); B cell stimulating factor 1 (BSF-1); macrophage fusion factor (MFF); mast cell growth factor II (MCGF-II); T cell growth factor II (TCGF-II): immunoglobulin switch factor (increase Ig61 and IgE)—activates endothelium to express VCAM, a docking molecule for T cells, eosinophils and macrophages; decreases unstimulated or enhances IL-2 stimulated NK activity
IL-5	12–18	B cell growth factor II (BCGF-II); eosinophil colony-stimulating factor (Eo-CSF); eosinophil differentiation factor (EDF); IgA-enhancing factor (IgA-EF); killer helper factor (KHF); T cell replacing factor (TRF)
IL-6	21–29	B cell differentiation factor (BCDF); B cell stimulatory factor 2 (BSF-2); B cell stimulatory factor p2 (BSFp2); HP-1; cytotic T cell differentiation factor (CDF); hepatocyte stimulating factor (HSF); hybridoma/plasmacytoma growth factor (HPGF); interferon beta-2 (IFN-β2); 26-kD protein—induces acute phase response proteins by liver
IL-7	25	Pre-B cell growth factor (pBCGF)—costimulates purified T cells, induces LAK activity, induces cytokine secretion by human monocytes, a lymphopoietin
IL-8 (PF4 super-family)	8–16	Monocyte-derived neutrophil chemotactic factor (MDNCF); neutrophil activating factor/protein (NAF/NAP); neutrophil chemotactic factor (NCF); T cell chemotactic factor (TCF)
RANTES/SIS (PF4 super-family)	8–16	Family members include the cytokines: RANTES (regulated on activation, normal T expressed and secreted); I-309; macrophage inflammatory protein 1α or 1β (MIP-1α or 1β); monocyte chemotactic protein (MCP-1; HC14)
IL-9	32–39	40-kD protein (P40) stimulates antigen-specific T cell, mast cells, and erythroid colony formation
IL-10	17–21	Cytokine synthesis inhibitory factor (CSIF); B cell-derived T cell growth factor (B-TOGF); mast cell growth factor III (MCGF-III)
IL-11	24	No alternative names associated with this cytokine; stimulates plasma cells and, with IL-3, megakaryocyte colony formation; stimulates gut crypt cell proliferation
IL-12	75	Cytoxic lymphocyte maturation factor (CLMF); natural killer cell stimulatory factor (NKSF)—promotes T_H1 type cytokine release from NK cells and T cells, T cell growth factor for activated cells; inhibits leishmania and viral infections
IL-13	10	P600—induces monocyte and B cell differentiation, CD23 expression, and IgG4 and IgE switching
IL-14	53	High molecular weight B cell growth factor—induces B cell proliferation, inhibits immunoglobulin production
IL-15	14–15	T-cell growth factor produced by a wide variety of cells and tissues interacting with β and α chains of the IL-2 receptor; a separate α chain has been identified in gut crypt cells
IFN-α or IFN-β	16–27	No alternative names associated—antiviral activity, increases NK activity, increases class I and β2 microglobulin expression; and antiproliferative
IFN-γ	15.5	Macrophage activating factor (MAF); T cell replacing factor (TRF)—antiviral activity, increase NK activities, expression of class I and class II molecules
TNF-α	17	Cachectin—stimulates T cell proliferation, induces acute phase response, activates acute phase response, activates endothelium, activates PMNs, activates clotting cascade (procoagulant)
TNF-β	25	Lymphotoxin (LT)—30% homologous with TNF-α, antiproliferative, other properties shared with TNF-α
G-CSF	20–25	Colony-stimulating factor beta (CSF-β)—stimulates growth of and activates granulocytes; increases ADCC
GM-CSF	18–30	Colony-stimulating factor alpha (CSF-α); neutrophil inhibition factor (NIF); pluripoietin—stimulates growth of granulocytes, monocytes, early erythoid and some megakaryocyte progenitors; stimulates dendritic cells
M-CSF	45–70	Colony-stimulating factor 1 (CSF-1)—stimulates monocyte growth, ADCC, pinocytoses, and chemotaxis

Adapted from Mule JJ, Rosenberg SA, Catalogue of cytokines. I DeVita VT, Hellman S, Rosenberg SA (eds): Biologic Therapy Updates. Philadelphia, Lippincott, 1993.

TABLE 29–2. MICROBIAL SUBVERSION OF CYTOKINE FUNCTION

Cytokine	Virus	Activity
vIL-10	Epstein-Barr virus; equine herpesvirus	Suppress IL-2, IFN-γ production
Soluble TNF-α/βR	Shope fibroma virus, variola virus, vaccinia virus	Produced by virus and binds TNF
TNF	Human immunodeficiency virus	Upregulates transcription HIV
TNF-α	Adenovirus	14.7-kD protein in E3 region protects infected human cells from TNF-mediated cytolysis
IL-8R	Malaria (*Plasmodium vivax*)	Malaria binds to this receptor on RBC
IL-6	Human immunodeficiency virus	Upregulates transcription HIV
IL-2	Human herpesvirus 6	Replicates in *activated* T-cells, NK cells
IL-1	Cowpox, vaccinia, variola viruses, *Streptococcus pyrogenes*	SPI-2 and SPEβ protein inhibit processing of pro-IL-1β to mature IL-1β by IL-1β converting enzyme, produce secreted IL-1 binding protein
Soluble IFN-γR	Vaccinia, variola, myxoma viruses	B14R and B15R secreted viral proteins bind IFN-γ

hibits the processing of pro-IL-1β to mature IL-1β by the IL-1 converting enzyme (ICE). Both vaccinia and variola encode genes that confer IFN-α resistance. Adenovirus encodes a gene for resistance to TNF-α by infected cells. Resistance to bacterial pathogens such as *Salmonella typhimurium, Leishmania donovani*, and mycobacterium in the mouse are related to bacterial inhibition of IFN-γ production.

There are a variety of other mechanism that are involved with escape from immune recognition. This includes the well-known ability of certain adenovirus proteins to inhibit export of class I molecules from the endoplasmic reticulum; certain cytomegalovirus proteins serve to mimic major histocompatibility complex (MHC) class I molecules and bind endogenous peptides. The herpes simplex virus protein expresses an immediate early protein. ICP47 blocks transport of class I proteins presumably by inhibiting the production of peptides or translocation into the endoplasmic reticulum or cis golgi.[13] Furthermore, there are a variety of viruses that are capable of blocking the production and activity of the interferons.[14] Viruses can block the action of interferon (Table 29–3) induced antiviral enzymes. The double-stranded RNA-dependent protein kinase (DAI) is inhibited by a number of different viruses, suggesting its major role in inhibiting viral infection. These findings, which are dictated by genetic sequences in the viral genome, are perhaps the best indirect evidence that cytokines play a major role in vivo in modulating viral replication.

Adoptive Transfer of Antiviral Cells

One potential mechanism for employing immunologic reagents against microbial diseases is the adoptive transfer of T cells specifically sensitized to certain viruses. Adoptive transfer of activated natural killer (NK) cells appears to play little role in enhancing the immune response to viruses. Re-

TABLE 29–3. VIRAL SUBVERSION OF IFN-α FUNCTION

Vaccinia (K3L), variola (C3L), reovirus (σ3), influenza, poliovirus, EBV, adenovirus (VAI)	Inhibits dsRNA-dependent protein kinase (DAI) phosphorylation of eukaryotic initiation factor 2 (eIF-2) that inhibits protein synthesis in infected cells
Vaccina virus, encephalomyocarditis virus	Inhibit interferon induced 2', 5' A synthetase (or binding), which produces oligodenylates, degrading viral RNA and inhibiting replication
HIV	Tat protein inhibits 2', 5' A synthetase
HIV, HBV (core protein), adenovirus (EIA)	Inhibit IFN-α production

cently, Riddell et al[15] have shown that the adoptive transfer of cytomegalovirus (CMV) specific T cell clones is associated with immunity and decreased complications in the setting of bone marrow transplantation. Similar findings have recently been reported with transfer of EBV specific T cells in patients with transplantation associated lymphoproliferative disorder.[16]

Other Host Factors in Infectious Diseases

Cytokines clearly do not act directly on most pathogens; other nonprotein mediators and effector molecules have been discussed (see Chap. 16). These include arachidonic acid metabolites as well as nitric oxide (NO). For example, it is clear that cytokines (especially IFN-γ) induce NO synthase in macrophages; NO is critical to the intracellular killing of a variety of organisms including *Legionella, Pneumophila, Toxoplasma gondii, Leishmania* species, *Francisella tularensis, Mycobacterium tuberculosis* and *Mycobacterium leprae, Cryptococcus neoformans, Schistosoma mansoni, Mycobacterium avium* and *Candida albicans.*[17–19] IFN-γ knockout mice or animals made resistant to the effects of IFN-γ by targeted disruption of the IFN-γ receptor are susceptible to multiple intracellular pathogens. Colonies of these animals are troubled with persistent parasitic infections as well.[20–22] This suggests that a major role of IFN-γ is the regulation of both NO production and protection from these pathogens. How NO acts to kill these pathogens is unknown, but it probably acts by combining with radical oxygen intermediates to produce peroxynitrite anion and hydroxyl radicals. These species are among the most powerful oxidants in nature and disrupt many processes essential for cellular viability. Some additional biological effects are thought to be mediated by eliminating the availability of intracellular iron. IL-4 and IL-10 both inhibit the induction of NO synthase and IFN-γ so that T_H2 cytokines seem to be detrimental to antimicrobial defense (see Chap. 16).

Recombinant Proteins Administered to Humans

Many recombinant cytokines as well as other recombinant proteins have been administered to humans as therapeutic agents (Table 29–4). Clinical trials are usually begun with the intent to determine the maximum tolerated dose as well as the optimal biological dose. A variety of steps are important to develop new biologic response modifiers.[23] These include (1) early preclinical studies with identification, cloning, and expression of the gene and production of the protein to define its physiologic role in animal models; (2) preclinical studies designed to develop an agent for clinical use; these include scale-up production under good manufacturing practice (GMP) conditions, studies of formulation, purification, and stability, and preclinical toxicology, pharmacology, and therapeutic studies; and (3) Individual New Drug (IND) submission to the Food and Drug Administration (FDA) requirements; these include pre-IND meetings as well as preparation of an initial clinical protocol. Monitoring during treatment is particularly important to determine whether the appropriate surrogate markers (increase in nonspecific killing,

TABLE 29–4. RECOMBINANT PROTEINS ADMINISTERED TO HUMANS

Year	Protein
1980	Growth hormone[a]
1981	Leukocyte interferon (IFN-α)[a]
1983	Insulin[a]
1984	Tissue plaminogen activator[a]
1985	Interleukin 2[a]
1986	Immune interferon (IFN-γ)[a]
1987	Hepatitis B surface antigen[a]
1987	Fibroblast interferon (IFN-β)
1987	Erythropoietin[a]
1987	Granulocyte-macrophage colony-stimulating factor[a]
1987	Insulin-like growth factor I
1988	Granulocyte colony-stimulating factor[a]
1988	Interleukin 1α
1988	Interleukin 3
1988	Luteinizing hormone (primates)
1988	Interleukin 4
1989	Soluble CD4 (and variants)
1989	Macrophage colony-stimulating factor
1990	Interleukin 1 receptor antagonist
1990	Basic fibroblast growth factor
1990	Factor VIII
1991	Hepatitis B S and pre-S2 antigens
1991	Platelet-derived growth factor BB
1991	Hirudin
1992	Interleukin 6
1992	Atrial natriuretic factor peptide
1992	Interleukin 1 receptor antagonist
1992	Epidermal growth factor
1993	PIXY 321 (IL-3/GM-CSF fusion)
1993	Factor IX
1994	Interleukin 12

[a] Licensed by FDA for clinical use.

increased expression of MHC molecules etc) or specific assays of microbial killing in vitro or in vivo are enhanced.

TYPE 1 INTERFERONS (IFN-α, IFN-β, IFN-ω)

General Information

There are at least 22 genes encoding human IFN-α but only a single identified IFN-β and IFN-ω gene. IFN-γ shares about 30 percent of the amino acids with IFN-α and binds to a common receptor (Table 29–5). Disulfide bonds between residues are important for biologic activity. There are a variety of factors that induce interferon production: double-stranded RNA, viral infection itself, and other cytokines [platelet-derived growth factor (PDGF), TNF, M-CSF, IL-1].

When interferon binds to a specific receptor, a number of intracellular proteins are induced within hours. These include induction of the human analog of the MX-protein, which has direct antiviral function and two major enzymes—2',5'-oligoadenylate synthetase and a double-stranded RNA-dependent protein kinase (DAI). DAI phosphorylates eukaryotic initiation factor 2 (eIF-2), which in turn inhibits protein synthesis in infected cells. 2', 5', A-synthetase produces oligoadenylates that induce enzymes to degrade viral RNA. IFN-α also activates NK cells and T cells and induces enhanced expression of MHC class I antigens. It has direct antiproliferative activity, inhibits angiogenesis, and regulates differentiation.

IFN-α also induces a phosphodiesterase that catalyzes transfer-RNA degradation, an enzyme that degrades intracellular tryptophan, and an enzyme that impairs methylation of newly synthesized mRNA from retroviruses. IFN-α1 and IFN-α2 as well as IFN-β1 production is observed in human peripheral blood leukocytes following viral infection. Three interferons are currently commercially available for clinical treatment (from Schering-Plough, Hoffmann-LaRoche, and Interferon Sciences). IFN-α2C is available under an experimental IND from Boeringer-Ingelheim.

Clinical Efficacy

IFN-α has been shown to be efficacious in a variety of different infectious diseases including those caused by rhinovirus,[24] papillomavirus, cytomegalovirus, varicella zoster, herpes simplex, and vaccinia viruses (Table 29–6). It has been approved by the FDA for the treatment of Kaposi's sarcoma in acquired immunodeficiency syndrome (AIDS) patients and is currently being tested for antiviral activity in patients with HIV infection. A variety of chronic papillomavirus infections, including those associated with respiratory (laryngeal) papillomatosis, condyloma acuminatum, and common warts, have been shown to be responsive to IFN-α. IFN-α has recently been demonstrated to have efficacy in 25 to 40 percent of hepatitis B and hepatitis C infections. IFN-α is cleared rapidly from the serum with a half-life of 2 to 3 hours after IV administration, 3 to 8 hours after IM administration, and 20 minutes after intranasal administration. Side effects are frequent and include fatigue, fever, chills, anorexia, malaise, hepatitis, cardiomyopathy with congestive heart failure, and psychologic problems including disorientation and frank psychosis. Interferon is given for most viral diseases at doses of 1 to 15 million units SC, three to seven times weekly. Antibodies against IFN-α, which may be neutralizing, have been observed in 1 to 40 percent of patients and may limit response. Sometimes switching to another interferon formulation including IFN-β allows renewed responsiveness. Volunteers pretreated with IFN-α and given rhinovirus do not shed virus after challenge. Unless interferon is given within a few hours of challenge, however, no effect is observed. INF-α also inhibits the growth of a number of retroviruses including HIV in vitro but has little effect against HIV in patients.

TABLE 29–5. INTERFERONS

Type	Number of Genes	MW (kD)	Amino Acids	Cell Source	Chromosomal Location of IFN Gene	Chromosomal Location of IFN-R Gene
IFN-α	22 (13 structural)	16–27	166	Macrophages, NK and B cells	9p21pter	21q 22.1
IFN-β	1	20	166	Fibroblasts, epithelial cells	9p21pter	21q 22.1
IFN-ω	1	16–27	172	Macrophages	9p21pter	21q 22.1
IFN-γ	1	15.5–25	146	T and NK cells	12q24	6q

TABLE 29–6. CHRONIC VIRAL INFECTIONS TREATABLE WITH TYPE 1 INTERFERON

Cytomegalovirus
Hepatitis B
Hepatitis C
HIV infection (Kaposi's sarcoma)
Papillomavirus infections (laryngeal papillomatosis, condyloma acuminatum, common warts)
Rhinovirus
Varicella-zoster

TYPE 2 INTERFERON (IFN-γ)

General Information

IFN-γ is the acid labile interferon that is, hydrolysis at acid pH causes loss of antiviral activity. Interferon may act as either a dimer or a tetramer. Most of the properties of IFN-α and IFN-β are shared with IFN-γ due to common interferon responsive elements (IREs) being activated upstream of several interferon-inducible genes. Different properties mediated by IFN-γ include activation of monocyte cytolytic activity, enhanced nitric oxide production, and the ability to upregulate class II MHC molecules on many cell types. Induction of enhanced immunoglobulin production by B cells and induction of IL-2 receptors on macrophages is stimulated by IFN-γ. The antimicrobial activity induced by IFN-γ is believed in part to be due to induction of nitric oxide production and a variety of infectious disorders have been associated with defective IFN-γ production.[25] (Table 29–7).

Use in Chronic Granulomatous Disease (CGD)

The inherited disorder chronic granulomatous disease is associated with a defect in the membrane-associated NADPH oxidase responsible for production of oxygen intermediates required for microbicidal activities in neutrophils and macrophages. This enzyme is rapidly upregulated by IFN-γ and inhibited by IFN-α. These individuals have frequent catalase-positive microbial infections such as *S. aureus* and *Aspergillus* species. Other infecting organisms include *Escherichia coli* and *Nocardia* as well as *Chromobacterium violaceum, Pseudomonas cepacia, Klebsiella,* and *Serratia marcescens*. Chronic IFN-γ administration substantially improves the expression of this enzyme in vitro in patients with the disease and decreases the number and severity of bacterial infections.[26,27] Side effects include fever, headache, chills, and erythema, which can be relieved by administration of acetaminophen or giving the drug at bedtime. Neutralizing antibodies to IFN-γ are not usually detected. The recommended dosage is 50 μg/m^2 (1.5 × 10^6 U/m^2) given SC three times weekly. IFN-γ is produced in *E. coli* by Genentech, Inc. IFN-γ has recently also been tried with success in treating osteoporosis and rheumatoid arthritis,[28,29] but without major success in cancer patients.

Antiviral Mechanisms

IFN-γ mediated antiviral effects also appear to be related, like IFN-α, to decreased viral replication as well as through its ability to activate NK cells and macrophages. IFN-γ upregulates the receptor for TNF-α and induces its production from macrophages. TNF, in turn, has strong antiviral activities and synergizes with the interferons.[30] Interestingly, the antiviral effects of IFN-γ require local persistence of the cytokine, which is abrogated by rapid diffusion away from its source of production.[31] INF-γ is strongly induced by both IL-2 and IL-12 (see below) with the latter being perhaps most potent in inducing it from stimulated T cells or NK cells especially following intracellular parasitic infection.[32] IFN-γ has been given to animals infected with a variety of different intracellular organisms including protozoa (*Toxoplasma gondii, Leishmania,* and *Toxoplasma cruzi*), bacteria (*Listeria monocytogenes, Brucella* and *Salmonella* species, and *Legionella pneumophila*), mycobacteria (*Mycobacterium tuberculosis, Mycobacterium avium-intracellulare, Mycobacterium kansasi, Mycobacterium leprae*), fungi (*Histoplasma capsulatum, Cryptococcus neoformans, Coccidioides immitis, Paracoccidioides brasiliensis, Blastomyces dermatitidis*), and viruses (herpes simplex, cytomegalovirus, varicella-zoster, human immunodeficiency virus, Epstein-Barr virus, and rubeola). IFN-γ given to animals infected with these microbes prior to the time of infection leads to resolution. Furthermore, pretreatment of animals with antibodies to IFN-γ or TNF makes these animals more susceptible to infection.

TABLE 29–7. INFECTIOUS CONDITIONS WITH DEFECTIVE IFN-γ PRODUCTION

Malaria	Filariasis
Cytomegalovirus	Condyloma acuminatum
Leprosy	Chronic hepatitis B infection
Leishmaniasis	Human immunodeficiency virus
Tuberculosis	Chronic herpes simplex virus infection

INTERLEUKIN 1 (IL-1)

IL-1, primarily a macrophage product, mediates a variety of important biologic effects (Table 29–8). Enhanced resistance of mice to bacterial infections has been noted with administration of recombinant hIL-1α.[33] IL-1α and IL-1β, although only modestly related, each appear to interact with two separate receptors on the cell surface (type I and II) and are members of a family of molecules that includes the IL-1 receptor antagonist (IL-1RA). Administration of IL-1α to patients with cancer is associated with an increase in the total white blood cell count, increase in bone marrow cellularity, increases in serum triglycerides, serum cortisol, C reactive protein, and thyroid-stimulating hormone, and decreases in cholesterol, testosterone, and protein C.[34] Major toxicities, including hypotension due to decreases in systemic vascular resistance, are noted at doses of 0.3 to 1.0 μg/kg given daily over 7 days. Myocardial infarction, confusion, severe abdominal pain, and renal insufficiency were also noted in some patients. IL-1RA administration may reduce the mortality from endotoxin shock.[35,36]

IL-1 also induces a series of proinflammatory cytokines, members of the so-called intercrine family, which includes IL-8, IP-10, and GRO.[37] These molecules are important for regulating neutrophil and other inflammatory cell chemotaxis across endothelial barriers. IL-1 also appears to cause alteration in vascular tumor blood flow primarily by inducing hemorrhagic necrosis.[38,39] *Streptococcus pyrogenes* exotoxin (SPE-β) is a cysteine protease that mimics IL-1 converting enzyme (ICE) and converts the inactive precursor of IL-1 to biologically active IL-1, perhaps contributing to the tissue necrosis observed with infection by this organism.[40] IL-1 function has also been subverted by other microbial pathogens: IL-1 binds to an IL-1-like receptor on the surface and enhances the growth of only virulent strains of *E. coli*.[39]

TABLE 29–8. INTERLEUKIN 1 MEDIATED EFFECTS

Activate T cells and B cells
Activate NK cells
Potentiate hematopoiesis
Activate vascular endothelium
Stimulate fibroblast proliferation
Antiproliferative activity against human tumors
Induce other cytokines (TNF-α)
Protect from radiation, chemotherapy, or IL-2 toxicity
Anti-infection properties

INTERLEUKIN 2 (IL-2)

IL-2 is a 15,000-dalton protein produced primarily by T cells and in particular by T_H1 cells. It is the prototypic T cell growth factor that is released following antigen or mitogen stimulation and the major cytokine inhibited by the immunosuppressive agents cyclosporin and FK506. IL-2 has recently been approved by the FDA for the treatment of metastatic renal cell carcinoma,[41] and it has activity in melanoma or lymphoma. Although activity[42–54] has been observed in a variety of murine infectious diseases (Table 29–9), systemic administration for human infections is not yet adequately studied. By contrast, adoptively transferred immune cells expanded in IL-2 and stimulated with viral antigen have been shown to be efficacious for herpes simplex virus infection[42] and cytomegalovirus infection in mice. Similarly IL-2 activated NK cells (lymphokine activated killer cells or LAK) appear to home to sites of viral infection.[55,56] Recently, restoration of viral immunity in humans made immunodeficient following cytotoxic chemotherapy and bone marrow transplantation was accomplished by adoptive transfer of IL-2 expanded T cell clones specific for cytomegalovirus.[15] Adoptive transfer of T cells in murine models has also been effective in protection against malaria.[57]

IL-2 activation of LAK cells induces profound cytolytic activity against cells infected with *Toxoplasma gondii*.[58] Lack of NK cells in vivo is associated with repetitive herpes infections[59] and papillomavirus infections.[60] Administration of IL-2 enhances survival against a lethal challenge with *T. gondii* in mice.[42] IL-2 also protects mice from lethal challenge with gram-negative bacteria[47] but does not enhance the response to visceral leishmaniasis.[48] Prophylactic administration of IL-2 in the setting of challenge with gram-negative bacteria *Klebsiella pneumonia* is effective in limiting morbidity and mortality.[49] It appears to have some potential therapeutic role in *E. coli* sepsis[52] and limits the induction of parasitemia in experimental Chagas' disease.[53] A neutralizing antibody to a T_H2 cytokine, IL-4, can induce systemic protection and enhance T_H1 immunity in a murine model of candidiasis.[61] The susceptibility to *C. albicans* correlates with a T_H2 type response.[62] A single patient with Epstein-Barr virus infection has been reported who responded to recombinant IL-2 treatment.[63]

Production of both IL-1 and IL-2 by peripheral blood mononuclear cells of patients with obstructive jaundice is markedly decreased[64] and increases with effective measures that restore normal biliru-

TABLE 29–9. IL-2 THERAPY OF INFECTIOUS DISEASES IN ANIMAL MODELS

Observation	Reference	Dose
Enhances activity of adoptively transferred immune cells to herpes simplex virus	142	200 U × 1 d (IV)
Enhances survival against a lethal challenge with *T. gondii*	142, 143	100 U/d × 3–5 d
Results in lower rates of infection and increased healing of herpes simplex genital lesions	144, 145	8×10^4–8×10^5 U/kg × 4 d
Enhances effectiveness of the adoptive transfer of immune cells to cytomegalovirus	146	10^4 U IP bid × 4 d
Prophylactic administration protects mice from lethal challenge with gram-negative bacteria	147	1.8–7 × 10^6 U/kg IV/IP × 1 d
Does not enhance response to visceral leishmaniasis (IFN-γ did)	148	10^2–10^5 U IP 1–3 times/d × 5–10 d
Prophylactic and therapeutic effect on respiratory tract infection with *K. pneumoniae*	149	2–20 μg/d SQ × 7–14 d
Overcomes genetic nonresponsiveness to malaria sporozoite peptides	150	5 × 10^4 U IL-2 emulsified with antigen
Protects neonatal mice from lethal herpes simplex virus infection (macrophage mediated, IFN-γ induced)	151	50–200 U IP × 1 d
Therapeutic effect/protection against fatal *E. coli* sepsis	152	5 × 10^5 U/kg IP × 1 d
Reduces paresitemia and myocarditis by *Trypanosoma cruzi* (Chagas' disease)	153	1.5–10 × 10^3 U IP/d × 3 d
Systemic adjuvant with IL-2 or PEG-IL-2 increases the potency of inactivated rabies virus vaccine	154	3×10^4–3×10^6 U/kg SQ bid × 5 d × 2 or 1.5 × 10^5 U/kg of PEG-IL-2 SQ QD × 5 d × 2

Adapted from Lotze MT: Interleukin 2: basic principles. In Devita VT, Hellman S, Rosenberg SA (eds): Biologic Therapy of Cancer. Philadelphia, Lippincott, 1991, pp 123–141. All results shown in murine models except Weinberg studies with herpes simplex performed in guinea pigs.[44,45]

bin levels. This may explain the depressed immune reactivity observed in patients with jaundice. IL-2 administration to patients with *Mycobacterium leprae* enhances the responsiveness of skin tests to tuberculosis (TB). The major toxicity observed with IL-2 administration in humans is the induction of a "vascular leak" syndrome, presumably secondary to the elaboration of other cytokines including TNF-α and IL-1. This toxicity can be mimicked in experimental models and reduced by systemic administration of steroids.[65,66] Interestingly, IL-2 therapy is also associated with a chemotactic defect[67,68] in neutrophils and an associated marked increase in infection (as high as 30 percent) with gram-positive organisms, primarily due to central line related sepsis. Prophylactic antibiotics are capable of largely preventing this complication.[69,70]

TUMOR NECROSIS FACTOR

General Information

In the early 1900s, William B. Coley demonstrated that certain tumors were potentially susceptible to treatment by systemic administration of bacterial toxins. Coley's toxins used several strains of *Streptococcus* and *Bacillus prodigious.*[71] Subsequently, Carswell et al[72] demonstrated a serum factor in mice stimulated by lipopolysaccharide (LPS) in BCG infected mice, which, when administered to other mice, induced hemorrhagic necrosis in transplanted tumors. It is now known that TNF-α is released by macrophages following LPS interaction with LPS binding protein and subsequent binding to CD14 on the macrophage membrane. LPS also binds to the plasma LPS binding protein and soluble CD14 in plasma. This trimolecular complex binds a receptor on the cell surface leading to production of a variety of other factors by reactive endothelial and epithelial cells.[73] TNF-β (lymphotoxin) is a molecule 30 percent homologous to TNF-α, which is produced by T, B, and NK lymphocytes, and binds to TNF receptors. In combination with IL-1 and IL-6, TNF-β regulates the acute phase response so critical to many antimicrobial responses. TNF-α has a variety of important biological functions (Table 29–10). Animals given a combination of IFN-γ and TNF are able to reduce abscess size when inoculated with live bacteria.[74] Sepsis appears to alter the function of a variety of leukocytes including polymorphonuclear neutrophils and may do this through the production of factors such as

TABLE 29–10. BIOLOGIC ACTIVITIES OF TNF

Endothelium
Hemorrhagic necrosis
T cells and NK cells
Increase proliferation
Enhance cytolytic activity
Tumors
Direct cytolysis
Induction of apoptosis
Neutrophils
Increase adherence to endothelium
Decrease mobility
Activate PMN respiratory burst
Macrophages
Produced concurrently with NO
Stimulate other monokines (TNF itself, IL-1, IL-6), M-CSF, G-CSF, PGE_2, TxB_2, and PAF
Fibroblasts
Enhance proliferation

TNF.[75] These properties are discussed in Chapter 14 and summarized in Table 29–10.

Clearly, TNF is an important mediator in infection, and many attempts have been made to exploit the therapeutic potential of TNF biology. Treatment of animals with either steroids[76] or an antibody to TNF prevents tumor hemorrhagic necrosis induced by TNF. Glucocorticoid administration markedly decreases TNF production by LPS activated macrophages in vivo and prevents LPS induced lethality, but corticosteroids administered concurrently with TNF administration do not protect.[76] Small doses of TNF induce tolerance to subsequent lethal doses of LPS.[77] It appears that small doses of TNF induce enzymes responsible for cellular resistance to its cytolytic activity; one such enzyme is manganous superoxide dismutase.[78] Tolerance to TNF reduces both the toxicity as well as the therapeutic efficacy of TNF in tumor models.[79]

The hypotensive effects of endotoxin are to a large extent dependent on TNF release, as well as other cytokines. Anti-TNF antibodies protect mice and rabbits from endotoxemia and prevent the septic shock syndrome in baboons. Antibodies to TNF also reduce the IL-1β and IL-6 appearance following infusion of bacteria[80–84] Antibodies to TNF have been tested in the setting of sepsis in a recently completed phase II study at doses of 0.1 to 10 mg/kg given once or twice.[85] Antibodies to the murine anti-TNF were observed in 98 percent of patients. No survival benefit was found for the total study population. Patients with increased circulating TNF at study entry appear to possibly have benefited, with decreased mortality and length of hospitalization. Increased IL-6 levels predicted a fatal outcome ($P = 0.003$).[85]

Although TNF was originally identified as a cachectin and transfection of murine tumors with human TNF could indeed induce cachexia, only variable ability of reduction of cachexia by antibodies to TNF was observed.[86–88] In fact, antibodies to IFN-γ appeared to have the greatest effect in reducing cancer cachexia.[88] Other pharmacologic means of reducing TNF include systemic administration of agents such as pentoxifylline, thalidomide, and hydroxyzine.

TNF-α, like other cytokines, has pleiotropic effects and although a variety of manifestations of systemic sepsis are indeed manifested by the activities of TNF, it also appears to have a critical role in the induction of immune reactivity. The dendritic cells found in virtually every tissue are thought to be the most potent antigen presenting cells. Both GM-CSF and TNF-α appear to stimulate and enhance the generation of these critically important cells.[89] Reducing TNF production may adversely affect immunity.

TNF Receptors

Two types of TNF receptors are expressed on a variety of cell types. Both soluble TNF-α (17 kD) and a 26-kD membrane bound form of TNF bind these receptors but interaction of TNF with a variety of different cell types induces quite different end effects. Both proliferation and cytolysis (see Table 29–10) are observed. A soluble TNF binding protein can also be found in the serum,[90] which represents the proteolytic product of the cell membrane receptor. These are a number of members of the TNF receptor family—a gene within the Shope fibroma virus, the nerve growth factor receptor, human CD40 and a murine clone with an as yet unidentified function, and 4-1BB.[91] Other members include the lymphoid activation antigen CD30, the rat T cell antigen OX40 and the surface antigen Fas/APO-1 associated with apoptotic cell death, a poxvirus gene product (T2), and, most recently, CD27, a surface antigen found on T cells and B cells.[92] This antigen when cross-linked by antibody or by interaction with its ligand (recently cloned from an Epstein-Barr virus cell line) causes the proliferation and cytolytic induction of human T cells. Thus members of the TNF/TNF receptor family subserve a variety of important functions including those designed to enhance both proliferation and differentiation as well as apoptotic cell death.[93–95]

Sensitivity of Cells to TNF

It is well known that the sensitivity of cells to lysis by TNF is enhanced by blocking new protein synthesis. This may indeed be due to the lack of protective effects when molecules such as manganous superoxide dismutase are inhibited. This may represent one of the means by which virally infected targets can be identified by the host since viruses often infect cells with concomitant decrease of host protein synthesis.[96–98]

TNF Administration

TNF administration in human clinical trials for the treatment of cancer is associated with a relatively short half-life of 13 to 25 minutes and disappointing antitumor effects.[99] Inhibition of granulopoietic differentiation and proliferation, which has been observed in vitro[100], has also been observed following TNF administration in vivo.[101] The leukopenia observed in vivo may also be due in part to enhanced expression of the granulocyte adhesion protein CD11B on neutrophils, which causes enhanced binding and emigration from the circulation. TNF has not been proposed as a biologic response modifier useful for the treatment of infections. But the possible adverse effects of TNF administration in cancer immunotherapy need to be borne in mind. TNF delivery for cancer gene therapy is under development.[102–104]

COLONY-STIMULATING FACTORS

General Information

One of the major advances in current cancer therapeutics has been the availability of recombinant colony-stimulating factors to enhance the number and activity of monocytes and granulocytes.[105–107] G-CSF and GM-CSF have been approved for human clinical use in the context of intensive chemotherapy administration, of cyclic neutropenia, and with bone marrow transplantation. In most studies, decreased number of days of hospitalization, decreased number of infections, and occasionally increased survival is observed. IL-3 and the IL-3 GM-CSF fusion protein, PIXY 321, have entered clinical trials and have shown similar effects with decreased infection. M-CSF may be important in the treatment of fungal infections, in particular in combination with more traditional antifungal agents. Other hematopoietic growth factors include IL-1, erythropoietin (which stimulates red cell production), IL-6, and stem cell factor (also known as C-kit ligand). These factors are believed to act within the context of the bone marrow stromal environment although some have other activities. For example, GM-CSF serves as a factor capable of supporting the viability of mature polymorphonuclear leukocytes in the tissues and as an activating agent for dendritic cells. The two colony-stimulating factors that are now approved for clinical use include GM-CSF and G-CSF, the latter enjoying somewhat greater use because of the decreased spectrum of side effects.

Granulocyte CSF

G-CSF is a 174 amino acid (molecular weight = 20,000) factor produced by endothelial cells, fibroblasts, macrophages, and some neutrophils, G-CSF appears to promote maturation more distally in hematopoietic differentiation, increasing polymorphonuclear leucocyte number and function. Recombinant G-CSF (filgrastim) has been effective in the treatment of patients undergoing chemotherapy.[108] Patients have been shown to have decreased periods of neutropenia, fewer hospital days, and a decreased use of antibiotics due to decreased incidence of neutropenic fever.

Only minimal toxicities are observed with administration of G-CSF. These include transient mild bone pain and occasional cellulitis at the site of infusion. Therapy is usually given later than 24 hours following chemotherapy. A daily dose of 5 mg/kg/day (SC or IV) can be doubled or tripled for inadequate responses. G-CSF, however, is not useful for established *Pseudomonas aeruginosa* bacteremia during cytotoxic treatment of hematologic malignancy.[114] G-CSF has also been useful in preventing infection in cyclic neutropenia[109] and severe chronic neutropenia.[110,111] Acceleration of neutrophil recovery occurs after bone marrow transplantation.[172] G-CSF can be used favorably to treat patients with chronic benign granulocytopenia and congenital agranulocytosis (Kostmann's syndrome)[113] but increased doses of up to 100 to 200 mg/m^2/day may be required.

Granulocyte-Macrophage Colony-Stimulating Factor (GM-CSF)

GM-CSF has a molecular weight of between 18 and 30 kD due to a wide variation in the degree of glycosylation of this molecule. GM-CSF appears to function perfectly well when nonglycosylated in biologic assays. Its range of activities are far greater than G-CSF in that it stimulates CFU-GM, CFU-M, and CFU-EO, as well as BFU-E. It appears to stimulate cells of the megakaryocytic pathway as well as having a direct effect on stem cells. Like G-CSF it stimulates antibody-dependent cellular cytotoxicity[115] superoxide generation and serves as a chemoattractant inducing many of these activities (unlike G-CSF) in macrophages.[116] It also induces the production of IL-1 and TNF and is a potent stimulator of dendritic cells, an important cell in antigen processing and presentation. GM-CSF can be produced in murine models of *E. coli*, yeast, or in Cos cells where the specific activity ranges from approximately 1×10^7 to 1×10^8 units/mg of protein. GM-CSF is naturally produced by T lymphocytes, fibroblasts, and endothelial, epithelial, and macrophage cell lines.

The currently available recombinant human GM-CSF differs only slightly from the natural protein. Side effects observed infrequently include dyspnea, a vascular leak syndrome, and phlebitis at the site of injection. It generally is administered no sooner than 24 hours after chemotherapy. Bone pain, like that observed with G-CSF, may occur. Daily infusions over a period of 2 hours of 250 $\mu g/m^2$ for periods of 14 to 21 days are currently used. Its only FDA approved indication is to enhance myeloid reconstitution after bone marrow transplantation but it is frequently used in patients with aplastic syndromes, for leukopenia secondary to HIV patient treatment with azidothymidine or other chemotherapeutic agents, and after cancer chemotherapy.[117–130] In general, such studies have shown an increased ability to deliver chemotherapy with decreased infectious complications and periods of neutropenia.

Monocyte-Colony-Stimulating Factor (M-CSF)

M-CSF or CSF-1 (70,000 to 90,000-dalton dimer) is produced naturally by macrophages, fibroblasts, and endothelial cells. M-CSF enhances macrophage colony stimulation, appears to enhance tumoricidal activity as well ADCC activity,[131] and may play a role in vitro in controlling fungal infections.[132] Doses up to 100,000 $\mu g/m^2$/day have been well tolerated with toxicities primarily of iritis and malaise in patients with cancer.[133–135] Although M-CSF has been evaluated in combination with other antifungal agents for patients with invasive fungal infections,[136] its efficacy in this role has yet to be demonstrated. Although both GM-CSF and IL-3 enhance infectivity of human stem cells by HIV, far less deleterious effects are noted in vitro for M-CSF, G-CSF, and IL-3.[137] In vivo administration of M-CSF does appear to enhance monocyte function, increasing the response to F-met-leu-phe (FMLP) and increasing the number of *Candida* organisms ingested.[138] Its precise role in treatment of patients with cancer and infectious diseases remains to be demonstrated.

Interleukin 3 (IL-3)

IL-3 or multi-CSF is variably glycosylated with a molecular weight of 15 to 30 kD. The primary cell source is the T lymphocyte. It stimulates broadly across many cell lineages as well as acting on the pluripotent stem cell. It also has more distal effects activating certain cellular subsets such as monocytes to enhance antimicrobial activity. In a variety of human clinical trials, stimulatory effects on neutrophils, eosinophils, monocytes, and platelets have been observed.[139,140] Doses of up to 15 μg/kg/day lude headache, fever, flu-like symptoms, nausea, skin rash, flushing facial erythema, and urticaria. Combinations with GM-CSF have also been carried out[141,142] with some apparent improvement in terms of neutrophil recovery. A fusion protein termed PIXY 321, encompassing both the GM-CSF and IL-3 molecules, is currently undergoing testing.

INTERLEUKIN 12 (IL-12)

IL-12 entered human cancer and HIV clinical trials in 1994. It is a macrophage product first described as a natural killer stimulating factor (NKSF) and as a cytotoxic lymphocyte maturation factor (CLMF).[143] Human IL-12 does not act on murine cells, but murine IL-12 stimulates human cells. Recombinant IL-12, like the natural product, stimulates IFN-γ production[144] and enhances the antigen-dependent proliferation of activated T cells.[145] It enhances primarily a T_H1 response, being released by macrophages shortly after stimulation with bacteria, protozoa, viruses, or helminths and is thus an initiation cytokine for cell-mediated immunity against infections.[146–149] It improves survival in animals with leishmaniasis and in mice injected with murine lymphocytic choriomeningitis virus. This appears to be due in part to stimulation of cytolytic activity as well as the profound induction of IFN-γ. It will be tested in a wide variety of malignancies and infectious states including AIDS in the next few years.

CYTOKINE TREATMENT OF SPECIFIC INFECTIOUS DISEASES

Epstein-Barr Virus

The control of Epstein-Barr virus infection is readily accomplished in most individuals[150] but not those with certain inborn errors of immunity.[151] Viral escape from immune recognition may be due to the production of a unique viral sequence homologous to the human IL-10 gene (vIL-10). EBV enters cells through binding to the receptor for complement fragment C3d. Following binding to this receptor,[152] EBV induces capping and then endocytosis, thus gaining entry to the cell. IFN-α appears to inhibit the capping of this molecule and may be one of the mechanisms by which it exerts its antiviral effects. Interestingly, EBV also induces the endogenous production of IL-10[153] as well as other nominal T cell cytokines (IL-4, IFN-γ, IL-2) by transformed B cells.[154] T cells may also compete with EBV for a variety of different growth factors.[155] Since EBV is usually a self-limited illness, treatment protocols have largely been limited to those individuals with chronic EBV infection or those with EBV-associated malignancies. IL-2 has been used successfully in a single patient with chronic EBV syndrome.[63] Administration of IFN-α and IFN-γ has also met with minimal success in patients with EBV-associated nasopharyngeal carcinoma.[156–158]

Hepatitis B

Chronic hepatitis B is responsive to IFN-α treatment and seroconversion occurs in 25 to 40 percent of those treated[159–164] (Table 29–11). The loss of hepatitis B DNA in the sera correlates well with the disappearance of hepatitis B core antigen from liver cells. IFN-α therapy has not been as successful in preventing recurrence after liver transplantation (T. Starzl, personal communication). In fact, rapid reinfection of the donor liver in most individuals precludes successful transplantation in such patients.

The addition of IFN-γ or zidovudine appears not to improve the effects of IFN-α[160,161] in chronic hepatitis B or HIV. The glomerulonephritis observed with chronic hepatitis B virus infection, however, appears to be improved with a 4-month course of IFN-α,[162] even in the presence of HIV infection.[163]

Hepatitis C

Hepatitis C is caused by a flavivirus and is associated with a chronic carriage state. Treatment with IFN-α for approximately 24 weeks at doses of 1 to 3 million units is associated with a response rate of about 50 percent, but half of the responders will relapse.[165–171]

Retreatment of relapsed patients, who had previously been successfully treated, also fails.[172–174] Variations in the treatment regimens[170] suggest that a decrescendo regimen starting with very high doses of IFN and a prolonged maintenance period using lower doses may be the most efficacious cause of treatment. An early clearance of virus by PCR

TABLE 29–11. RECENT TREATMENT RESULTS IN HEPATITIS B AND HEPATITIS C INFECTION WITH IFN-α

Investigator	Location	Reference	Number of Patients	Comments
Wong/Hep B	Toronto, Meta-analysis studies 1966–1992	164	837	Fifteen randomized studies with at least 3 months of treatment; seroconversion more frequent (7.8% vs 1.8%, P = 0.0001) and loss of viral replication more frequent (33% vs 12%, P = 0.0001) in interferon-treated patients.
Shindo/Hep C	NIH, United States	166	10	Six patients seroconverted with maintenance for 3–6 yr
Viladomiv/Hep C	Barcelona, Spain	167	28	Randomized study showed benefit of treatment only at end of 3-month treatment
Douglas/Hep C	Mayo Clinic, United States	168	32	Randomized study showed benefit of treatment at end of 6-month treatment; 86% of responders relapsed
Shibata/Hep C	Nagoya, Japan	169	13	Serum HCV by PCR disappeared in 9 patients after 3 months of treatment; 60% of patients relapsed
Iino/Hep C	Multicenter, Japan	170	126	Randomized study showed that intensive therapy administered at 10^7/U/d × 6 d for 2 weeks followed by 3 ×/wk for 12 wk produced sustained responses in 48.3% of patients
Kleter/Hep C	Rotterdam, Amsterdam	171	24	Study demonstrated that benefit of IFN-α apparent at 4 wk, no response by PCR occurred later

appears to define those individuals who are most likely to benefit from treatment.[171]

Human Immunodeficiency Virus (HIV)

Most cytokine therapy in patients with AIDS and AIDS related complex (ARC) is experimental. IFN-α, however, has been approved for the treatment of Kaposi's sarcoma associated with HIV infection. A 20 to 40 percent tumor response has been observed with IFN-α.[175] Similar responses have been observed with IFN-β administration.[176]

Of great potential interest is the effect that a variety of cytokines have on HIV replication. In asymptomatic HIV-infected individuals, a switch to a T_H2 phenotype appears to be observed; IL-4[177,178] and IL-10 production is seen and IL-2 and IFN-γ production falls. The role of cytokines in modulating HIV expression has been well reviewed by Poli and Fauci.[179,180] IL-1, IL-2, IL-4, TGF-β, and TNF all appear to enhance HIV replication, whereas IFN-α, IFN-β, and IFN-γ appear to decrease HIV replication. The mechanism by which this occurs is increasingly well understood. Some of these effects appear to be mediated through enhancing tat and rev binding to viral RNA target sequences known as TAR RRE. Transcriptional regulatory factors such as NFκB, NFAT-1, and Sp-1 are induced subsequent to stimulation with many of the cytokines noted above. They appear also to activate HIV transcription. It has recently been suggested that IL-12 may be effective in the treatment of patients with HIV since it promotes primarily a T_H1 response and since decreases in IL-12 are one of the earliest observed findings in asymptomatic individuals following HIV infection (S. Wolf, personal communication). IL-13 (a T_H2 cytokine) has recently been demonstrated to inhibit HIV production in macrophages but not lymphocytes obtained from peripheral blood.[181] This suggests that IL-13 might be useful for this function in in vivo treatment.

Herpesviruses

Currently, IFN is not used routinely in the treatment of patients with herpes infections.[182] It has been shown to be effective in enhancing the rate of clearance of viral lesions due to reactivation of herpes zoster as well as in patients with oral and genital herpes. More effective antiviral agents (acyclovir), however, are available. Combinations of IFN-α and IFN-γ are thought to be effective in herpes keratitis[183] and potentially in varicella-zoster reactivation.[184] IFN-α has also been shown, when used perioperatively, to prevent the reactivation of oral herpes occurring after sectioning of the trigeminal ganglia.[182]

Leishmaniasis

The combinations of pentavalent antimony and recombinant IFN-γ (0.1 mg/m^2 IM for 14 days) is associated with improvement in most patients.[185] Interestingly, IL-2 appears to be required for progression of the disease in murine hosts,[186] suggesting that this cytokine will probably not be useful for treatment of this disorder. Production of T_H1 cytokines, in murine models and humans, presumably promoted by IL-12, appears to be associated with disease resistance (Table 29–12), with susceptibility dictated by production of T_H2 cytokines.[187]

Leprosy

Leprosy is caused by chronic infection with the intracellular parasite *Mycobacterium leprae*. Treatment with injection intradermally of IFN-γ is associated with accumulation of mononuclear phagocytes and T lymphocytes as well as a reduction in the bacillary burden.[188–190] This has also been observed with IL-2 treatment.[64] IL-4 and IL-10 production is enhanced in the lesions of patients with lepromatous as opposed to tuberculoid lesions.[191] Inhibitors of IL-4 and IL-10 may reverse the clinical pattern of expression of leprosy infection.

TABLE 29–12. CYTOKINES IN MURINE LEISHMANIASIS

Effect	IL-12	IL-2	IFN-γ	GM-CSF	TNF-α	IL-3	IL-4	IL-10	TGF-β
Curative effects in vivo	+++		++		+				
Intracellular *Leishmania* killing			++		+				
Associated with healing	+++	+	++		+				
T_H1 promoting	+++		++	+					
T_H2 promoting		+							++
Associated with disease		+			+	+	+	+	+

Adapted from Reed SG, Scott P: Curr Opin Immunol 5: 524, 1993.

Papillomavirus Infection

Condyloma acuminata is caused by one of more than 50 different subtypes of human papillomavirus and may be one of the most common sexually transmitted diseases. Direct injection of IFN-α (1 $\times$ 10^6 IU/day into a maximum of five lesions three times a week or systemic administration of 1 $\times$ 10^6 to 5 $\times$ 10^6 IU daily, two to three times per week) has led to clearance in upward of 82 percent of patients.[192] Adverse side effects include fever, chills, and malaise and required dose reduction or discontinuation in approximately 5 to 15 percent of patients. The FDA approved intralesional therapy requires multiple visits to the physician. These therapies, however, appear to be comparable to other therapies[193,194] available to patients, which are less costly. Cryotherapy may be the treatment of choice for these disorders.[194] Treatment with other cytokines has not been described.

Acknowledgment. This work was supported in part by a grant from the National Cancer Institute Program Project #1PO1 CA 59371-01. Careful preparation of the manuscript for this chapter by Kathy Rakow is much appreciated.

REFERENCES

1. Cohen N, Haynes L: The phylogenetic conservation of cytokines. In Warr GW, Cohen N (eds): Phylogenetics of Immune Functions. Boca Raton, CRC Press. 1991, pp 241–260.
2. Campbell IL: Cytokines in viral diseases. Curr Opin Immunol 3:486, 1991.
3. Finter NB, Chapman S, Dowd P, et al: The use of interferon-α in virus infections. Drugs 42:749, 1991.
4. Wittek AE, Quinnan GV: Immunology of viral infections. In Belshe RB (ed): Textbook of Human Virology. St Louis, Mosby/Year Book, 1991, pp 116–132.
5. Mule JJ, Rosenberg SA: Catalogue of cytokines. In DeVita VT, Hellman S, Rosenberg SA (eds): Biologic Therapy Updates, Philadelphia, Lippincott, 1993.
6. Grabstein KH, Eisenman J, Shanebeck K, et al: Cloning of a T cell growth factor that interacts with the β chain of the interleukin–2 receptor. Science 264:965, 1994.
7. Moore KW, Viera P, Fiorentino DF, et al: Homology of cytokine synthesis inhibitory factor (IL-10) to the Epstein-Barr virus gene BCRF1. Science 248:1230, 1990.
8. Viera P, De Waal-Malefyt R, Johnson MN, et al: Isolation and expression of human cytokine synthesis inhibitory factor cDNA clones homologous to Epstein-Barr virus open reading frame BCRF1. Proc Natl Acad Sci USA 88:1172, 1991.
9. Smith CA, Davis T, Anderson D, et al: A receptor for tumor necrosis factor defines an unusual family of cellular and viral proteins. Science 248:1019, 1991.
10. Schelkunov SN, Blinov VM, Sandakchiev LS: Genes of variola and vaccinia viruses necessary to overcome the host protective mechanisms. Fed Eur Biochem Soc 319:80, 1993.
11. Ranheim TS, Shisler J, Horton TM, et al: Characterization of mutants within the gene for the adenovirus E3 14.7 kilodalton protein which prevents cytolysis by tumor necrosis factor. J Virol 67:2159, 1993.
12. Ramarathinam L, Niesel DW, Klimpel GR: Ity influences the production of IFN-γ by murine spenocytes stimulated in vitro with *Salmonella typhimurium*. J Immunol 150:3965, 1993.
13. McNair ANB, Kerr IM: Viral inhibition of the interferon system. Pharmacol Ther 56:79, 1992.
14. York IA, Troop C, Andrews DW, et al: A cystosolic herpes simplex virus protein inhibits antigen presentation to CD8+ T lymphocytes. Cell 77:525, 1994.
15. Riddell SR, Watanabe KS, Goodrich JM, et al: Restoration of viral immunity in immunodeficient humans by the adoptive transfer of T cell clones. Science 257:238, 1992.
16. Papadopoulos EB, Ladanyi M, Emanuel D, et al: Infusions of donor leukocytes to treat Epstein–Barr virus-associated lymphoproliferative disorders after allogenic bone marrow transplantation. N Engl J Med 330:1185–1191, 1994.
17. Summersgill JT, Powell LA, Buster BL, et al: Killing of *Legionella pneumophila* by nitric oxide in γ-interferon-activated macrophages. J Leukoc Biol 52:625, 1992.
18. Doi T, Ando M, Akaike T, et al: Resistance to nitric oxide in *Mycobacterium avium* complex and its implication in pathogenesis. Infect Immun 62:1980, 1993.
19. Cenci E, Romani L, Mencacci A, et al: Interleukin-4 and interleukin-10 inhibit nitric oxide-dependent macrophage killing of *Candida albicans*. Eur J Immunol 23:1034, 1993.
20. Del Prete G, De Carli M, Almerigogna F, et al: Human IL-10 is produced by both type 1 helper (Th1) and type 2 helper (Th2) T cell clones and inhibits their antigen-specific proliferation and cytokine production. J Immunol 150:353, 1993.
21. Dalton DK, Pitts-Meek S, Keshav S, et al: Multiple defects of immune cell function in mice with disrupted interferon-γ genes. Science 259:1739, 1993.
22. Kamijo R, Shapiro D, Le J, et al: Generation of nitric oxide and induction of major histocompatibility complex class II antigen in macrophages from mice lacking the interferon-γ receptor. Proc Natl Acad Sci USA 90:6626, 1993.
23. Creekmore SP, Urba WJ, Longo DL: Principles of the clinical evaluation of biologic agents. In DeVita

VT, Hellman S, Rosenberg SA (eds): Biologic Therapy of Cancer. Philadelphia, Lippincott, 1991, pp 67–86.
24. Scott GM, Philpotts RJ, Wallace J, et al: Purified interferon as protection against rhinovirus infection. Br Med J 284:1822, 1982.
25. Murray HW: Interferon-γ, the activated macrophage and host defense against microbial challenge. Ann Intern Med 1908:595, 1988.
26. Todd PA, Goa KL: Interferon gamma-1b. Drugs 43:111, 1992.
27. Mulebach TJ, Gabay J, Nathan CF, et al: Treatment of patients with chronic granulomatous disease with recombinant human interferon-gamma does not improve neutrophil oxidative metabolism, cytochrome *b*558 content or levels of four anti-microbial proteins. Clin Immunol 88:203, 1992.
28. Key LL, Ries W, Rodriguiz RM, Hatcher HC: Recombinant human interferon gamma therapy for osteopetrosis. J Pediatr 121:119, 1992.
29. Machold KP, Neumann K, Smolen JS: Recombinant human interferon in the treatment of rheumatoid arthritis: double blind placebo controlled study. Rheum Dis 54:1038, 1992.
30. Wong GHW, Goeddel DV: Tumour necrosis factors α and β inhibit virus replication and synergize with interferons. Nature 323:819, 1986.
31. Kundig TM, Hengartner H, Zinkernagel RM: T cell-dependent IFN-γ exerts an antiviral effect in the central nervous system but not in peripheral solid organs. J Immunol 150:2316, 1993.
32. Gazzinelli RT, Hieny S, Wynn TA, et al: Interleukin 12 is required for the T-lymphocyte dependent induction of interferon γ by an intracellular parasite and induces resistance in T-cell-deficient hosts. Proc Natl Acad Sci USA 90:6115, 1993.
33. Osaki Y, Ohashi T, Minami A, et al: Enhanced resistance of mice to bacterial infection induced by recombinant human interleukin-1α. Infect Immunol 55:1436, 1987.
34. Smith JW, Urba WJ, Curti BD, et al: The toxic and hematologic effects of interleukin-1 alpha administered in phase I trial to patients with advanced malignancies. J Clin Oncol 10:1141, 1992.
35. Uhlsson K, Bjork P, Bergenfeldt M, et al: Interleukin-1 receptor antagonist reduces mortality from endotoxin shock. Nature 348:550, 1990.
36. Alexander HR, Doherty GM, Buresh CM, et al: A recombinant human receptor antagonist to interleukin 1 improves survival after lethal endotoxemia in mice. J Exp Med 173:1029, 1991.
37. Oppenheim JJ, Zachariae COC, Mukaida N, Matsushima K: Properties of the novel proinflammatory supergene "intercrine" cytokine family. Annu Rev Immunol 9:617, 1991.
38. Braunschweiger PG, Kumar N, Constantinidis I, et al: Potentiation of interleukin-1α mediated antitumor effects by ketoconazole. Cancer Res 50:4709, 1990.
39. Porat R, Clark BD, Wolff SM, Dinarello CA: Enhancement of growth of virulent strains of *Escherichia coli* by interleukin-1. Science 254:430, 1991.
40. Kapur V, Majesky MW, Li LL, et al: Cleavage of interleukin 1β (IL-1β) precursor to produce active IL-1β by a conserved extracellular cysteine protease from *Streptococcus pyogenes*. Proc Natl Acad Sci USA 90:7676, 1993.
41. Lotze MT: Interleukin 2: basic principles. In DeVita VT, Hellman S, Rosenberg SA (eds): Biologic Therapy of Cancer. Philadelphia, Lippincott, 1991, pp 123–141.
42. Rouse BT, Miller LS, Turtunen L, et al: Augmentation of immunity to herpes simplex virus by in vivo administration of interleukin-2. J Immunol 134:924, 1985.
43. Sharma SD, Hofflin JM, Remington JS: In vivo recombinant interleukin-2 administration enhances survival against a lethal challenge with *Toxoplasma gondii*. J Immunol 134:926, 1985.
44. Weinberg A, Rausmussen L, Merigan TC: Acute genital infection in guinea pigs: effect of recombinant interleukin-2 on herpes simplex virus type 2. J Infect Dis 154:134, 1986.
45. Weinberg A, Basham TY, Merigan TC: Regulation of guinea-pig immune functions by interleukin-2: critical role of natural killer activity in acute HSV-2 genital infection. J Immunol 137:3310, 1986.
46. Reddehase MJ, Mutter W, Koszinowski UH: In vivo application of recombinant interleukin-2 in the immunotherapy of established cytomegalovirus infection. J Exp Med 165:650, 1989.
47. Chong K-T: Prophylactic administration of interleukin-2 protects mice from lethal challenge with gram-negative bacteria. Infect Immun 55:668, 1987.
48. Murray HW, Stern JJ, Welte K, et al: Experimental visceral leishmaniasis production of interleukin-2 and interferon-gamma, tissue immune reaction, and response to treatment with interleukin-2 and interferon-gamma. J Immunol 138:2290, 1987.
49. Lizawa Y, Nishi T, Kondo M, et al: Effect of recombinant human interleukin-2 on the course of experimental chronic respiratory tract infection caused by *Klebsiella pneumoniae* in mice. Infect Immun 56:45, 1988.
50. Good MF, Pombo S, Lunde MN, et al: Recombinant human IL-2 overcomes genetic nonresponsiveness to malaria sporozoite peptides. J Immunol 141:972, 1988.
51. Kohl S, Loo LS, Drath DB, et al: Interleukin-2 protects neonatal mice from lethal herpes simplex virus infection: a macrophage-mediated, gamma interferon-induced mechanism. J Infect Dis 159:239, 1989.
52. Goronzy J, Weyand C, Quan J, et al: Enhanced cell-mediated protection against fatal *Escherichia coli* septicemia induced by treatment with recombinant IL-2. J Immunol 142:1134, 1989.
53. Hulsebos LH, Choromanski L, Kuhn RE: The effect

of interleukin-2 on parasitemia and myocarditis in experimental Chagas' disease. J Protozool 36:293, 1989.
54. Nunberg JH, Doyle MV, York SM: Interleukin-2 acts as an adjuvant to increase the potency of inactivated rabies virus vaccine. Proc Natl Acad Sci USA 86:4240, 1989.
55. Natuk RJ, Bukowski JF, Brubaker JO, Welsh RM: Antiviral effect of lymphokine-activated killer cells: chemotaxis and homing to sites of virus infection. Am Soc Microbiol 65:4969, 1989.
56. Kaplan G, Sampaio EP, Walsh GP, et al: Influence of *Mycobacterium leprae* and its soluble products on the cutaneous responsiveness of leprosy patients to antigen and recombinant interleukin 2. Proc Natl Acad Sci USA 86:6269, 1989.
57. Romero P, Maryanski JL, Corradin G, et al: Cloned cytotoxic T cells recognize an epitope in the circumsporozoite protein and protect against malaria. Nature 341:323, 1989.
58. Sabauste CS, Dawson L, Remington JS: Human lymphokine-activated killer cells are cytotoxic against cells infected with *Toxoplasma* gondii. J Exp Med 176:1511, 1992.
59. Biron CA, Byron S, Sullivan K: Severe herpes virus infection in an adolescent without natural killer cells. N Engl J Med 320:1731, 1989.
60. Ballas ZK, Turner JM, Turner DA, et al: A patient with simultaneous absence of "classical" natural killer cells (CD3−, CD16+, and NKH1+) and expansion of CD3+, CD4−, CD8−, NKH1+ subset. J Allery Clin Immunol 85:453, 1990.
61. Romani L, Mencacci A, Grohmann U, et al: Neutralizing antibody to interleukin 4 induces systemic protection and T helper type 1-associated immunity in murine candidiasis. II: Susceptibility to *Candida albicans* infection correlates with the induction of a biased Th_2 like antifungal response. J Exp Med 176:19, 1992.
62. Mencacci A, Romani L, Mosci P, et al: Low-dose streptozotocin-induced diabetes in mice. Cell Immunol 150:36, 1993.
63. Kawa-ha K, Franco E, Doi S, et al: Successful treatment of chronic active Epstein-Barr virus infection with recombinant interleukin-2. Lancet 62:154, 1987.
64. Haga Y, Sakamoto K, Egami H, et al: Changes in production of interleukin-1 and interleukin-2 associated with obstructive jaundice and biliary drainage in patients with gastrointestinal cancer. Surgery 106:842, 1989.
65. Morse ED, Gunther RA, Jesmok GJ, Hughes KS: Steroid pretreatment reduces interleukin-2 toxicity in sheep. Surgery 107:639, 1990.
66. Goldblum SE, Yoneda K, Cibull M, et al: Human recombinant interleukin-2 provokes acute pulmonary vascular endothelial injury in rabbits. J Biol Res Mod 9:127, 1990.
67. Klempner MS, Noring R, Mier JW, Atkins MB: An acquired chemotactic defect in neutrophils from patients receiving interleukin-2 immunotherapy. N Engl J Med 322:959, 1990.
68. Jablons D, Bolton E, Mertins S, et al: IL-2 based immunotherapy alters circulating neutrophil Fc receptor expression and chemotaxis. J Immunol 144: 3630, 1990.
69. Hartman LC, Urba WJ: Use of prophylactic antibiotics for prevention of intravascular catheter-related infections in interleukin-2-treated patients. J Natl Cancer Inst 81:1190, 1989.
70. Bock SN, Lee RE, Fisher B, et al: A prospective randomized trial evaluating the prophylactic antibiotics to prevent catheter-related sepsis in patients treated with immunotherapy. J Clin Oncol 8:161, 1990.
71. Coley WB: The treatment of inoperable sarcoma by bacterial toxins (the mixed toxins of the *Streptococcus erysipelas* and the *Bacillus prodigiosus*). In: Reprinted Proceedings of the Royal Society of Medicine. London, John Bale, Sons and Danielsson, Ltd, 1909.
72. Carswell EA, Old LJ, Kassel RL, et al: An endotoxin induced serum factor which causes necrosis of tumors. Proc Natl Acad Sci USA 72:3666, 1975.
73. Pugin J, Schurer-Maly CC, Leturcz D, et al: Lipopolysaccharide activation of human endothelial and epithelial cells is mediated by lipopolysaccharide-binding protein and soluble CD14. Proc Natl Acad Sci USA 90:2744, 1993.
74. Malangoni MA, Livingston DH, Sonnenfeld G, Polk HC: Interferon gamma and tumor necrosis factor alpha: use in gram-negative infection after shock. Arch Surg 125:444, 1990.
75. Christou NV, Tellado JM: In vitro polymorphonuclear neutrophil function in surgical patients does not correlate with anergy but with "activating" processes such as sepsis or trauma. Surgery 106:718, 1989.
76. North RJ, Havell EA: Glucocorticoid-mediated inhibition of endotoxin-induced intratumor tumor necrosis factor production and tumor hemorrhagic necrosis and regression. J Exp Med 170:703, 1989.
77. Sheppard BC, Fraker DL, Norton JA: Prevention and treatment of endotoxin and sepsis lethality with recombinant human tumor necrosis factor. Surgery 106:156, 1989.
78. Wong GHW, Elwell JH, Oberley LW, Goeddel DV: Manganous superoxide dismutase is essential for cellular resistance to cytotoxicity of tumor necrosis factor. Cell 58:923, 1989.
79. Fraker DL, Sheppard BC, Norton JA: Impact of tolerance on antitumor efficacy of tumor necrosis factor in mice. Cancer Res 50:2261, 1990.
80. Jansen NJG, van Oeveren W, Gu J, et al: Endotoxin release and tumor necrosis factor formation during cardiopulmonary bypass. Ann Thorac Surg 54:744, 1992.
81. Kinkhabwala M, Sephajpal P, Skolnik E, et al: A

novel addition to the T cell repertory. Cell surface expression of tumor necrosis factor/cachectin by activated normal human T-cells. J Exp Med 171:941, 1990.
82. Salomon GD, Kasid A, Director E, et al: Effects of local tumor necrosis factor on wound healing. Surg Forum 60:637, 1989.
83. Gerlach H, Lieberman H, Bach R, et al: Enhanced responsiveness of endothelium in the growing/motile state to tumor necrosis factor/cachectin. J Exp Med 170:913, 1989.
84. Fong Y, Tracey KJ, Moldawer LL, et al: Antibodies to cachectin/tumor necrosis factor reduce interleukin 1β and interleukin 6 appearance during lethal bacteremia. J Exp Med 170:1627, 1989.
85. Fisher CJ, Opal SM, Dhainaut JF, et al: Influence of an anti-tumor necrosis factor monoclonal antibody on cytokine levels in patients with sepsis. Crit Care Med 21:318, 1993.
86. Oliff A, Defeo-Jones D, Boyer M, et al: Tumors secreting human TNF-cachectin induce cachexia in mice. Cell 50:555, 1987.
87. Sherry BA, Gelin J, Fong Y, et al: Anticachectin/tumor necrosis factor-α antibodies attenuate development of cachexia in tumor models. FASEB 3:1956, 1989.
88. Langstein HN, Fraker DL, Norton JA: Reversal of cancer cachexia by antibodies to interferon-gamma but not cachectin/tumor necrosis factor. Surg Forum 60:408, 1989.
89. Loetscher H, Pan YCE, Lahm HW, et al: Molecular cloning and expression of the human 55 kd tumor necrosis factor receptor. Cell 61:351, 1990.
90. Schall TJ, Lewis M, Koller KJ, et al: Molecular cloning and expression of a receptor for human tumor necrosis factor. Cell 61:361, 1990.
91. Smith CA, Davis T, Anderson D, et al: A receptor for tumor necrosis factor defines an unusual family of cellular and viral proteins. Science 248:1019, 1990.
92. Goodwin RG, Alderson MR, Smith CA, et al: Molecular and biological characterization of a ligand for CD27 defines a new family of cytokines with homology to tumor necrosis factor. Cell 73:447, 1993.
93. Banner DW, D'Arcy A, Janes W, et al: Crystal structure of the soluble human 55 kd TNF receptor-human TNFβ complex: implications for TNF receptor activation. Cell 73:431, 1993.
94. Van Ostade X, Vandenabeele P, Everaerdt B, et al: Human TNF mutants with selective activity on the p55 receptor. Nature 361:266, 1993.
95. Scheurich P, Kobrich G, Pfizenmaier K: Antagonistic control of tumor necrosis factor receptors by protein kinases A and C. J Exp Med 170:947, 1989.
96. Woods KM, Chapes SK: Three distinct cell phenotypes of induced-TNF cytotoxicity and their relationship to apoptosis. J Leukoc Biol 53:37, 1993.
97. Pogrebniak HW, Matthews W, Pass HL: Chemotherapy amplifies production of tumor necrosis factor. Surgery 110:231, 1991.
98. Kyprianou N, Alexander RB, Issacs JT: Activation of programmed cell death by recombinant human tumor necrosis factor plus topisomerase II-targeted drugs in L929 tumor cells. J Natl Cancer Inst 83:346, 1991.
99. Gamm H, Lindemann A, Mertelsmann R, Herrmann F: Phase I trial of recombinant human tumour necrosis factor α in patients with advanced malignancy. Eur J Cancer 27:856, 1991.
100. Caux C, Favre C, Saeland S, et al: Potentiation of early hematopoiesis by tumor necrosis factor-α is followed by inhibition of granulopoietic differentiation and proliferation. Blood 78:635, 1991.
101. Logan TF, Kaplan SS, Bryant JL, et al: Granulocytopenia in cancer patients treated in a phase I trial with recombinant human tumor necrosis factor. J Immunol 10:84, 1991.
102. Asher AL, Mule JJ, Kasid A, et al: Murine tumor cells transduced with the gene for tumor necrosis factor-α. J Immunol 146:3227, 1991.
103. Hwu P, Yannelli J, Kriegler M, et al: Functional and molecular characterization of tumor-infiltrating lymphocytes transduced with tumor necrosis factor-α cDNA for the gene therapy of cancer in humans. J Immunol 150:4104, 1991.
104. Orosz P, Echtenacher B, Falk W, et al: Enhancement of experimental metastasis by tumor necrosis factor. J Exp Med 177:1391, 1993.
105. Gabrilove JL: Introduction and overview of hematopoietic growth factors. Semin Hematol 26:1, 1989.
106. Morstyn G, Campbell L, Lieschke G, et al: Treatment of chemotherapy-induced neutropenia by subcutaneously administered granulocyte colony-stimulating factor with optimization of dose and duration of therapy. J Clin Oncol 7:1554, 1989.
107. Neidhart J, Mangalik A, Kohler W, et al: Granulocyte colony-stimulating factor stimulates recovery of granulocytes in patients receiving dose-intensive chemotherapy without bone marrow transplantation. J Clin Oncol 7:1685, 1989.
108. Sarosy G, Kohn E, Stone DA, et al: Phase I study of taxol and granulocyte colony-stimulating factor in patients with refractory ovarian cancer. J Clin Oncol 10:1165, 1992.
109. Ferrero D, Pregno P, Omede P, et al: Cyclic neutropenia and severe hypogammaglobulinemia in a patient with excess of CD8+ T lymphocytes: response to G-CSF therapy. Haematologica 78:59, 1993.
110. Dale DC, Bonilla MA, Davis MW, et al: A randomized controlled phase III trial of recombinant human granulocyte colony-stimulating factor (filgrastim) for treatment of severe chronic neutropenia. Blood 81:2496, 1993.
111. Linch DC, Scarffe H, Proctor S, et al: Randomized vehicle-controlled dose-finding study of glycosylated recombinant human granulocyte colony-stimulating factor after bone marrow transplantation. Bone Marrow Transplant 11:307, 1993.

112. Chao NJ, Schriber JR, Grimes K, et al: Granulocyte colony stimulating factor "mobilized" peripheral blood progenitor cells accelerate granulocyte and platelet recovery after high-dose chemotherapy. Blood 81:2031, 1993.
113. Imashuku S, Tsuchida M, Sasaki M, et al: Recombinant human granulocyte-colony stimulating factor in the treatment of patients with chronic benign granulocytopenia and congenital agranulocytosis (Kostmann's syndrome). Acta Paediatr Jpn 81:133, 1992.
114. Funada H, Machi T, Ohtake S, et al: Effect of recombinant human granulocyte colony-stimulating factor (G-CSF) in the treatment of *Pseudomonas aeruginosa* bacteremia complicating hematologic malignancy—a preliminary study. J Jpn Assoc Infect Dis 66:76, 1992.
115. Masucci G, Wersall P, Ragnhammar P, Mellstedt H: Granulocyte-monocyte-colony-stimulating factor augments the cytotoxic capacity of lymphocytes and monocytes in antibody-dependent cellular cytotoxicity. Cancer Immunol Immunother 29:288, 1989.
116. Gamble JR, Elliott MJ, Jaipargas E, et al: Regulation of human monocyte adherence by granulocyte-macrophage colony-stimulating factor. Proc Natl Acad Sci USA 86:7169, 1989.
117. Dorr TR: Clinical properties of yeast-derived versus *Escherichia coli*-derived granulocyte-macrophage colony-stimulating factor. Clin Ther 15:19, 1993.
118. Lieschke GJ, Maher D, O'Connor M, et al: Phase I study of intravenously administered bacterially synthesized granulocyte-macrophage colony-stimulating factor and comparison with subcutaneous administration. Cancer Res 50:606, 1990.
119. LaPorte JPH, Fouillard L, Douay L, et al: GM-CSF instead of autologous bone-marrow transplantation after the BEAM regimen. Lancet 338:601, 1991.
120. Ardizzoni A, Venturini M, Crino L, et al: High dose-intensity chemotherapy, with accelerated cyclophosphamide-dosorubicin-etoposide and granulocyte-macrophage-etoposide and granulocyte-macrophage colony stimulating factor, in the treatment of small cell lung cancer. Eur J Cancer 29A:687, 1993.
121. Pene R, Appelbaum FR, Fisher L, et al: Use of granulocyte-macrophage colony-stimulating factor and erythropoietin in combination after autologous marrow transplantation. Bone Marrow Transplant 11:219, 1993.
122. Rabinowe SN, Neuberg D, Bierman PJ, et al: Long-term follow-up of a phase III study of recombinant human granulocyte-macrophage colony-stimulating factor after autologous bone marrow transplantation for lymphoid malignancies. Blood 81:1903, 1993.
123. Peters WP, Rosner G, Ross M, et al: Comparative effects of granulocyte-macrophage colony-stimulating factor (GM-CSF) and granulocyte colony-stimulating factor (G-CSF) on priming peripheral blood progenitor cells for use with autologous bone marrow after high-dose chemotherapy. Blood 81:1709, 1993.
124. Wolf M, Havemann K: Experience with GM-CSF in the treatment of solid tumors. Infection 2:S111, 1992.
125. Ajani JA, Roth JA, Ryan MB, et al: Intensive preoperative chemotherapy with colony-stimulating factor for resectable adenocarcinoma of the esophagus or gastroesophageal junction. J Clin Oncol 11:22, 1993.
126. Gorin NC, Coiffier B, Hayat M, et al: Recombinant human granulocyte-macrophage colony-stimulating factor after high-dose chemotherapy and autologous bone marrow transplantation with unpurged and purged marrow in non-Hodgkin's lymphoma: a double-blind placebo-controlled trial. Blood 80:1149, 1992.
127. O'Dwyer PJ, LaCreta FP, Schilder R, et al: Phase I trial of thiotepa in combination with recombinant human granulocyte-macrophage colony-stimulating factor. J Clin Oncol 10:1352, 1992.
128. Neidhart JA, Mangalik A, Stidley CA, et al: Dosing regimen of granulocyte-macrophage colony-stimulating factor to support dose-intensive chemotherapy. J Clin Oncol 10:1460, 1992.
129. Kaiser U, Klausmann M, Kolb G, et al: Felty's syndrome: favorable response to granulocyte-macrophage colony-stimulating factor in the acute phase. Acta Haematol 87:190, 1992.
130. Scodden DT: The use of GM-CSF in AIDS. Infection 2:S103, 1992.
131. Munn DH, Cheung NKV: Antibody-dependent antitumor cytotoxicity by human monocytes cultured with recombinant macrophage colony-stimulating factor. J Exp Med 170:511, 1989.
132. Gregory SH, Wing EJ, Twcardy DJ, et al: Primary listerial infections are exacerbated in mice administered neutralizing antibody to macrophage colony-stimulating factor. J Immunol 149:188, 1992.
133. Sanda MG, Yang JC, Topalian SL, et al: Intravenous administration of recombinant human macrophage colony-stimulating factor to patients with metastatic cancer: a phase I study. J Clin Oncol 10:1643, 1992.
134. Redman BG, Flaherty L, Chou TH, et al: Phase I trial of recombinant macrophage colony-stimulating factor by rapid intravenous infusion in patients with cancer. J Immunother 12:50, 1992.
135. Zamkoff KW, Hudson J, Groves ES, et al: A phase I trial of recombinant human macrophage colony-stimulating factor by rapid intravenous infusion in patients with refractory malignancy. J Immunother 11:103, 1992.
136. Nemunaitis J, Meyers JD, Buckner CD, et al: Phase I trial of recombinant human macrophage colony-stimulating factor in patients with invasive fungal infections. Blood 78:907, 1991.
137. Kitano K, Abbound CN, Ryan DH, et al: Macrophage-active colony-stimulating factors enhance hu-

man immunodeficiency virus type 1 infection in bone marrow stem cells. Blood 77:1699, 1991.

138. Khawaja A, Johnson B, Addison IE, et al: In vivo effects of macrophage colony-stimulating factor on human monocyte function. Br J Haematol 77:25, 1991.
139. Biesma B, Willemse PH, Mulder NH, et al: Effects of interleukin-3 after chemotherapy for advanced ovarian cancer. Blood 80:1141, 1992.
140. deVries EG, van Gameren MM, Willemse PH: Recombinant human interleukin 3 in clinical oncology. Int Rev Exp Pathol 11:72, 1993.
141. Brugger W, Frisch J, Schulz G, et al: Sequential administration of interleukin-3 and granulocyte-macrophage colony-stimulating factor following standard-dose combination chemotherapy with etoposide, ifofamide and cisplatin. J Clin Oncol 10:1452, 1992.
142. Crump M, Couture F, Kovacs M, et al: Interleukin-3 followed by GM-CSF for delayed engraftment after autologous bone marrow transplantation. Exp Hematol 21:405, 1993.
143. Wolf SF, Temple PA, Kobayashi M, et al: Cloning of cDNA for natural killer cell stimulatory factor, a heterodimeric cytokine with multiple biologic effects on T and natural killer cells. J Immunol 146:3074, 1991.
144. Chan SH, Perussia B, Gupta JW, et al: Induction of interferon γ production by natural killer cell stimulatory factor: characterization of the responder cell and synergy with other inducers. J Exp Med 173:869, 1991.
145. Bertagnolli MM, Lin BY, Young D, Herrmann SH: IL-12 augments antigen-dependent proliferation of activated T lymphocytes. J Immunol 148:3778, 1992.
146. Manetti R, Parronchi P, Giudizi MG, et al: Natural killer cell stimulatory factor [interleukin-12 (IL-12)] induces T helper type 1 (Th_1)-specific immune responses and inhibits the development of IL-4 producing Th cells. J Exp Med 177:1199, 1993.
147. Hsieh CS, Macatonia SE, Tripp CS, et al: Development of Th1 CD4+ T cells through IL-12 produced by *Listeria*-induced macrophages. Science 260:547, 1993.
148. Scott P. IL-12: initiation cytokine for cell-mediated immunity. Science 260:496, 1993.
149. Locksley RM: Interleukin 12 in host defense against microbial pathogens. Proc Natl Acad Sci USA 90:5879, 1993.
150. Straus SD, Cohen JI, Tosato G, Meier J: Epstein-Barr virus infections: biology, pathogenesis and management. Ann Intern Med 118:45, 1993.
151. Purtilo DT: X-linked lymphoproliferative disease manifests immune deficiency to Epstein-Barr virus which results in diverse diseases. Med Virol 2:153, 1992.
152. Delcayre AX, Lotz M, Lernhardt W: Inhibition of Epstein-Barr virus-mediated capping of CD21/CR2 by alpha interferon (IFN-α): immediate antiviral activity of IFN-α during the early phase of infection. J Virol 67:2918–2921, 1993.
153. Burdin N, Peronne C, Banchereau J, Rousset F. Epstein-Barr virus transformation induces B lymphocytes to produce human interleukin 10. J Exp Med 177:295, 1993.
154. Tang H, Matthes T, Carballido-Perrig N, et al: Differential induction of T cell cytokine mRNA in Epstein-Barr virus-transformed B cell clones: constitutive and inducible expression of interleukin-4 mRNA. Eur J Immunol 23:899, 1993.
155. Frugoni P, Pike SF, Tosato G: A mechanism of T cell regulation of Epstein-Barr virus latency. Cell Immunol 147:256, 1993.
156. Mahjoubi R, Bachouchi M, Munck JN, et al: Phase II trial of recombinant interferon gamma in refractory undifferentiated carcinoma of the nasopharynx. Head Neck 15:115, 1993.
157. Treuner Y, Niethammer D, Dannecker G, et al: Successful treatment of nasopharyngeal carcinoma with interferon. Lancet 1:817, 1980.
158. Connors JM, Andurian WA, Howarth CB, et al: Treatment of nasopharyngeal carcinoma with human leucocyte interferon. J Clin Oncol 3:813, 1985.
159. Perillo RB, Schiff ER, Davis GI, et al: A randomized controlled trial of interferon alpha-2B alone and after prednisolone withdrawal for the treatment of chronic hepatitis B. N Engl J Med 109:95, 1990.
160. Janssen HLA, Berk L, Heijtink RA, et al: Interferon-α and zidovudine combination therapy for chronic hepatitis B: results of a randomized, placebo-controlled trial. Hepatology 17:383, 1993.
161. Ruiz-Moreno M, Rua MJ, Moraleda G, et al: Treatment with interferon gamma versus interferon alpha and gamma in children with chronic hepatitis B. Pediatrics 90:254, 1992.
162. Lisker-Melman M, Webb D, DiBisceglie AM, et al: Glomerulonephritis caused by chronic hepatitis B virus infection: treatment with recombinant human alpha-interferon. Ann Intern Med 111:479, 1989.
163. Lidman C, Magnius L, Norder H, Weiland O: Interferon alpha-2B treatment in an HIV-infected patient with hepatitis B virus induced nephrotic syndrome. Scand J Infect Dis 25:133, 1993.
164. Wong DKH, Cheung AM, O'Rourke K, et al: Effect of alpha-interferon treatment in patients with hepatitis B e antigen-positive chronic hepatitis B. Ann Intern Med 119:312, 1993.
165. Alter JH. Clinical, virological and epidemiological basis for the treatment of chronic non-A, non-B hepatitis. J Hepatol 11:S19, 1990.
166. Shindo M, DiBisceglie AM, Hoofnagle JH: Long-term follow-up of patients with chronic hepatitis C treated with α-interferon. Hepatology 15:1013, 1992.
167. Viladomiu L, Genesca J, Esteban JI, et al: Interferon-α in acute posttransfusion hepatitis C: a randomized controlled trial. Hepatology 25:767, 1992.

168. Douglas DD, Rakela J, Lin HJ, et al: Randomized controlled trial of recombinant alpha-2α-interferon for chronic hepatitis C. Dig Dis Sci 38:601, 1993.
169. Shibata M, Kumada T, Yamada M, et al: Effects of interferon-α on serum hepatitis C virus in patients with chronic hepatitis C. Dig Dis Sci 38:608, 1993.
170. Iino S, Hino K, Kuroki T, et al: Treatment of chronic hepatitis C with high-dose interferon α-2b. Dig Dis Sci 38:612, 1993.
171. Kleter GEM, Brouwer JT, Heijtink RA, et al: Detection of hepatitis C virus RNA in patients with chronic hepatitis C virus infections during and after therapy with alpha interferon. Antimicrob Agents Chemother 37:595, 1993.
172. Weiland O, Zhang YY, Widell A: Serum HCV RNA levels in patients with chronic hepatitis C given a second course of interferon alpha-2b treatment after relapse following initial treatment. Scand J Infect Dis 25:25, 1993.
173. Lotze MT: AIDS: a surgeon's responsibility. Am Coll Surg Bull 70:6, 1985.
174. Bartlett JG: HIV infection and surgeons. Curr Prob Surg 29:197, 1992.
175. Lane HC, Kovacs JA, Feinberg J, et al: Anti-retroviral effects of interferon-alpha in AIDS-associated Kaposi's sarcoma. Lancet 2:1218, 1988.
176. Miles SA, Wang H, Cortes E, et al: Beta-interferon therapy in patients with poor-prognosis Kaposi sarcoma related to the acquired immunodeficiency syndrome (AIDS). Ann Intern Med 112:582, 1990.
177. Clerici M, Hakim FT, Venzon DJ, et al: Changes in interleukin-2 and interleukin-4 production in asymptomatic, human immunodeficiency virus-seropositive individuals. J Clin Invest 91:759, 1993.
178. Clerici M, Shearer GM: A T_H1–T_H2 switch is a critical step in the etiology of HIV infection. Immunol Today 14:107, 1993.
179. Poli G, Fauci AS: The role of monocyte-macrophages and cytokines in the pathogenesis of HIV infection. Pathobiology 60:246, 1992.
180. Poli G, Fauci AS: Cytokine modulation of HIV expression. Immunology 5:165, 1993.
181. Montaner LJ, Doyle AG, Collin M, et al: Interleukin 13 inhibits human immunodeficiency virus type 1 production in primary blood-derived human macrophages in vitro. J Exp Med 178:743, 1993.
182. Ho M: Interferon as an agent against herpes simplex virus. J Invest Dermatol 95:158S, 1990.
183. Balish MJ, Abrams ME, Pumfery AM, Brandt CR: Enhanced inhibition of herpes simplex virus type 1 growth in human corneal fibroblasts by combinations of interferon-α and -γ. J Infect Dis 166:1401, 1992.
184. Saibara T, Maeda T, Onishi S, Yamamoto Y: Depressed immune functions in the early phase of varicella-zoster virus reactivation. J Med Virol 39:242, 1993.
185. Harms G, Zwingenberger K, Sandkamp B, et al: Immunochemotherapy of visceral leishmaniasis: a pilot trial of sequential treatment with recombinant interferon-γ and pentavalent antimony. J Interferon Res 13:39, 1993.
186. Heinzel FP, Rerko RM, Hatam F, Locksley RM: IL-2 is necessary for the progression of leishmaniasis in susceptible murine hosts. J Immunol 150:3924, 1993.
187. Reed SG, Scott P: T-cell and cytokine responses in leishmaniasis. Curr Opin Immunol 5:524, 1993.
188. Bottasso O, Besuschio S: Lepromatous leprosy treated with recombinant interferon gamma: cutaneous histologic changes. Int J Dermatol 31:813, 1992.
189. Nathan CF, Kaplan G, Levis WR, et al: Local and systemic effects of low doses of recombinant interferon-γ after intradermal injection in patients with lepromatous leprosy. N Engl J Med 315:6, 1986.
190. Nathan C, Squires K, Griffo W, et al: Widespread intradermal accumulation of mononuclear leukocytes in lepromatous leprosy patients treated systemically with recombinant interferon γ. J Exp Med 172:1509, 1990.
191. Sieling PA, Abrams JS, Yamamura M, et al: Immunosuppressive roles for IL-10 and IL-4 in human infection. J Immunol 150:5501, 1993.
192. Browder JF, Araujo OE, Myer NA, Flowers FP: The interferons and their use in condyloma acuminata. Ann Pharmacother 26:42, 1992.
193. Trofatter KF: Interferon treatment of anogenital human papillomavirus-related diseases. Dermatol Clin 9:343, 1991.
194. Kraus SJ, Stone KM: Management of genital infection caused by human papillomavirus. Rev Infect Dis 12:S620, 1990.

Principles of Surgical Treatment

CHAPTER 30

Steve H. Dougherty

Surgical intervention in infections, typically in the form of drainage, debridement, and elimination of ongoing contamination, attempts to achieve two broad goals: eradication of bacterial invaders and other inflammatory stimuli, and dissipation of the host mediator response to such stimuli. Indeed, the host mediator response, especially when manifest as a *systemic inflammatory response*,[1] may be more injurious to the host than the bacterial invaders themselves and may result in multisystem organ failure and death.[2] Even localized inflammation, in spite of its importance in wound healing, can be detrimental to the host. A dramatic example of this is infections associated with foreign bodies where reactive foreign materials, themselves activators of the host defenses, can significantly reduce the number of organisms needed to cause clinical infection.[3] The destructive power of local inflammation can also be appreciated in the process of abscess formation or the generation of pus.

THE PATHOBIOLOGY OF PUS: THE BASIS FOR SURGICAL DRAINAGE

Pus is simply a collection of large numbers of microorganisms, inflammatory cells, and necrotic debris; any local inflammatory stimulus that is sufficiently potent may provoke the generation of pus. Although most pyogenic stimuli are microbiologic and animate, such is not invariably the case. For example, bacteria that have been heat- or antibiotic-killed can still cause pus formation if there are sufficient numbers of them.[4] So, too, can various highly reactive inorganic foreign materials, such as cobalt or copper.[5,6] By activating local host defenses, inflammatory stimuli such as bacteria or foreign bodies trigger the release of lysosomal enzymes, oxygen free radicals, and other inflammatory mediators that are highly tissue-toxic and produce tissue liquefaction and abscess formation.[7–9] Various effects on the complement system and clotting cascade,[3] together with the release of eicosanoids (prostaglandin E_2, thromboxane B_2),[10] cytokines (interleukins),[11] and various acute phase reactants may likewise contribute to tissue damage.

In contrast, where host defenses are deficient, especially in neutropenic states, abscess formation may be blunted or may not occur at all.[12] In such patients—for example, those with tertiary peritonitis, diffuse persistent peritonitis in which well-defined intra-abdominal abscesses do not form—emergence of abscesses may actually signal a resurgence of the host defenses and hence, ironically, the beginning of the patient's recovery. Similarly, patients with severe neutropenia and pneumonia are often unable to produce purulent sputum.[13]

Thus it is primarily the host response to an inflammatory stimulus, rather than the stimulus itself, that is responsible for local tissue destruction and the formation of pus. In order to ameliorate this destructive process, the inflammatory stimulus must be physically eliminated from the focus of inflammation, not just "killed," and the host mediator response must be dissipated. In the case of bacterial abscesses, for example, even "sterile" lesions (those rendered culture-negative with antibiotics) will frequently persist until they are mechanically drained.

In addition to removing dead bacteria and other foreign bodies, surgical drainage or debridement eliminates persisting viable organisms that may be sheltered from antibiotics or from destruction by phagocytes within a fibrin clot or necrotic tissue. By simultaneously removing spilled phagocytic enzymes, activated complement, oxygen free radicals, and probably many other inflammatory mediators, drainage also helps to abolish the vicious cycle of phagocyte chemotaxis, degranulation/oxygen free radical release, and further chemotaxis that causes ongoing tissue destruction. Indeed, through various feedback mechanisms, many inflammatory mediators, such as lysosomal enzymes, do double duty as inflammatory stimuli.[14] Unfortunately, should the host mediator response escalate out of control, it may become "systemic"—autonomous, self-perpetuating, persistent in spite of the eradication of all infected foci—and ultimately lethal.[1,2] This is why early drainage and debridement of surgical infections is so important.

In addition to removing inflammatory stimuli and dissipating the host mediator response, surgical drainage and debridement destroy the bacterial habitat by changing the physiochemical and spatial characteristics of abscesses. In the traditional view, abscesses form to protect the host from disseminated infection. Once an abscess has formed, however, conditions are established which pari passu protect the bacteria from the host. It is not unusual, for example, to find aerobic and anaerobic bacterial concentrations of 10^8 to 10^9 organisms per milliliter of pus obtained from abscesses. Mechanical drainage of such collections probably tips the ecologic balance in favor of the host, and against the bacterial invaders, in many ways including increased oxygen tension, alkaline shifts in pH, alterations in electrolyte concentrations, reduced bacterial inoculum size, evacuation of bacterial metabolic products and complement-poor wound fluid, and perhaps changes in the pressure-volume and surface-to-volume relationships of abscesses. Similarly, drainage of pus may enhance the effectiveness of antibiotics, since many of the latter function relatively poorly under conditions of suppuration, especially anaerobiasis.[15]

APPROACHES TO MANAGEMENT OF SURGICAL INFECTIONS

Treatment of an active focus of bacterial infection, including abscess, can be approached in several ways, including administration of antibiotics, surgical (or radiographically guided percutaneous) drainage of pus, debridement of necrotic tissue, or complete surgical extirpation of the infection.

Antibiotic Cure of Abscesses

Although early cellulitis typically responds quickly to antibiotic therapy without progressing to suppuration, experimental studies have shown that the likelihood of antibiotic cure of an infection without the formation of an abscess diminishes rapidly after the first several hours.[16] As a rule, once an abscess has formed, the infection must be drained before it will resolve. However, abscesses of the liver, kidney, brain, spleen, prostate, pelvis, tubes and ovaries, deep neck spaces, subperiosteal orbit, colon, and perhaps other lesions, as well, have resolved with antibiotic treatment alone. Unfortunately, there are few clinical guidelines for the use of such therapy. In some reports, antibiotics were successful when lesions were diagnosed and treated early in their course (eg, abscesses of the deep neck spaces diagnosed by CAT scan); in other cases, antibiotics without drainage were used for patients who refused surgery. With the exception of amebic liver abscess, actinomycotic abscess, certain brain abscesses, and a few other lesions, however, pus collections, once identified, should be drained. If antibiotic therapy alone is to be used, the ability to demonstrate resolution of the lesion, or the lack thereof, with accurate radiographic imaging techniques assumes particular importance. Serial determination of serum C-reactive protein has also been used to monitor the clinical response of abscesses that were treated without drainage.[17] Of note, even in immunocompromised patients, abscesses of the brain and lung have occasionally been cured using antibiotics alone.[18,19]

In some circumstances, therapy may reasonably consist of antibiotics without drainage if the abscess is likely to drain internally on its own, for example, lung abscess into a bronchus, or appendiceal or diverticular abscesses into the colon. Rarely, even pancreatic abscesses decompress into adjacent bowel or prostatic abscesses decompress into the urethra and resolve. In many reports of abscesses cured by antibiotics, metronidazole, which is especially effective in anaerobic environments, was used, either alone or in combination with other drugs. Other factors that probably favor resolution without surgical drainage include small lesion volume, absence of an associated source of ongoing contamination, and location of the lesion in parenchymal tissues that may concentrate antimicrobial agents (eg, liver, kidney).

Most pus collections, however, will require some sort of therapeutic drainage. Depending on the circumstances, this may include simple needle or catheter aspiration, incision and drainage, incision and curettage with or without primary closure, or complete surgical extirpation.

Needle Aspiration of Pus

In most hospitals, aspiration of pus with needle and syringe is a common procedure. When doubt exists as to the presence or precise location of a pus collection, aspiration may help to establish both the timing for drainage and the surgical approach. If the collection is clinically obvious and not too large, aspiration may also represent definitive therapy. Whenever it is feasible, the use of needle aspiration to search for pus is clearly much safer than blind surgical incision. Aspiration of blood rather than pus, for example, may alert the surgeon to an aneurysm masquerading as an abscess (for a deep pus collection that is suspect, arteriography may be preferable to aspiration).[20,21] On the other hand, if the pus is highly viscous or diffusely dispersed, diagnostic needle aspiration may be misleading. In some necrotizing infections, for example, only open incision is likely to yield an accurate diagnosis (see Chap. 31). Similarly, compared to aspiration of an abscess or an infected body cavity, aspiration of soft tissue cellulitis, even after prior injection of saline, is less likely to yield a microbiologic diagnosis (an exception may be aspiration from the leading edge of an infection that is expanding centrifugally).[22,23]

Recent reports on the use of undirected (nonradiographically guided) therapeutic aspiration have focused mainly on lesions of the head and neck—a region where abscesses are often small, yet close to vital structures, where cosmetic considerations are important, and where incisional drainage may require general anesthesia. Considerable data suggest that outpatient needle aspiration plus oral antibiotics may often be the simplest, most cost-effective therapy for uncomplicated peritonsillar and perhaps other small abscesses of the head and neck (see Chap. 33). Therapeutic arthrocentesis of infected joints remains controversial (see Chap. 46). There are few data that pertain to aspiration of lesions at other sites. In general, for most abscesses larger than a few milliliters, it may be difficult to thoroughly evacuate and irrigate the abscess cavity using only a needle—evacuation and irrigation being crucial if an indwelling drain is not inserted. Likewise, if abscess walls are adherent to surrounding structures, aspiration may fail to adequately collapse the cavity, making recurrence more likely.[24] Additional potential contraindications to aspiration therapy include pus that is too thick to be readily removed, suspicion of an underlying malignancy (eg, in breast abscesses), or the possibility of rupturing a hydatid cyst.

Newer techniques of radiographically guided, percutaneous drainage of deep abscesses are discussed in Chapter 38.

Incisional or Excisional Management of Surgical Infections

Since many pyogenic infections do not present with the classic findings of heat, swelling, pain, redness, and loss of function, a general knowledge of the natural history of lesions occurring at various body sites is important. In perirectal abscess, for example, fluctuance is regularly absent; perianal abscess may cause exquisite tenderness, but no fever. Herpetic infection of paronychial tissues closely mimics bacterial infection, but incision and drainage are of no benefit and may increase morbidity. In contrast, chronic bacterial infections, such as hidradenitis suppurativa or pyoderma fistulans sinifica, which contain woody tissues or thick-walled sinuses, often respond poorly to simple drainage and may require wide excision of the entire process.[25]

The occurrence of certain surgical infections should prompt a search for concurrent underlying diseases. For example, complicated anorectal abscesses may occur in association with Crohn's disease. Anorectal abscess in children may accompany a variety of other problems, including *Enterobius vermicularis* infestation, congenital agranulocytosis, or even chickenpox.[26] Clostridial bacteremia is often associated with underlying hematologic or gastrointestinal malignancy, particularly carcinoma of the colon or rectum.[27] Recurrent staphylococcal abscesses often accompany chronic granulomatous diseases of childhood. Any infection due to an opportunistic pathogen, especially if it occurs in the absence of a known underlying condition, should at least suggest the possibility of acquired immunodeficiency syndrome (AIDS).

When surgical intervention or antibiotic therapy is being considered, it is important to keep in mind that some processes that resemble infections are actually due to noninfectious causes and require little or no operative treatment. For example, purpura fulminans, a symmetrical gangrene of the distal extremities caused by the Shwartzmann and Arthus reactions, can be confused with necrotizing streptococcal fasciitis[28]; so can recluse spider bites. Cutaneous pseudoabscess, an unusual presentation of severe pancreatitis, is actually sterile fat necrosis.[29] Pyoderma gangrenosum, chronic pustules, or erosions resembling pyogenic lesions may be seen in patients with ulcerative colitis. Similarly, certain medications can produce sterile abscess formation at the injection site.[30] Even the systemic inflammatory response and subsequent multisystem organ failure may be triggered by insults other than infection. This systemic inflammatory response sometimes creates quandaries in the critical care unit, for example, when patients with severe acute pancreatitis or trauma appear septic by clinical and physiological measures but are actually not infected at all.[1,2]

When surgical drainage or debridement are being carried out, it is especially important to recognize potential sources of ongoing contamination. Infectious processes associated with foreign bodies or communicating with pilonidal or urachal cysts will seldom completely resolve until the underlying problem is addressed. Undetected branchial cleft cysts, thyroglossal duct cysts, or congenital midline cysts may cause recurrent abscesses of the upper chest or neck, especially in children. Recurrent breast abscess often requires excision of obstructed lactiferous ducts; undetected fistula-in-ano is a common cause of recurrent perirectal or perianal abscess. In patients with Crohn's disease, large, silent abscesses of the thigh, groin, or posterior flank may communicate with an enteric fistula. Similarly, abscess of the medial thigh may sometimes arise from a strangulated femoral hernia. An isolated abscess of the abdominal wall or flank may originate from an underlying perforated carcinoma of the colon, diverticular abscess, or osteomyelitis. Osteomyelitis of the vertebral column or lower ribs sometimes causes retroperitoneal abscess. A perforated sigmoid carcinoma can lead to pelvic, thigh, perirectal, or gluteal abscesses. Bronchopleural or esophagopleural fistulas often seed chronic empyemas.

Since the gastrointestinal tract is a major source of potential contamination during intra-abdominal infection, especially for conditions such as diverticulitis that involve the bowel itself, an understanding of when to divert the fecal stream via colostomy or a more proximally placed stoma is important. For example, colostomy is often necessary for inflammatory or traumatic perforations of the colon, following resection of obstructing lesions, or whenever a primary colonic anastomosis is considered tenuous, as in the presence of generalized peritonitis or host immunodepression. The same may be true of the small bowel, although jejunal and ilial anastomoses are generally considered safer than colonic because of the small intestine's thicker walls and lower concentration of luminal bacteria. Still, in various high-risk circumstances such as severe peritonitis, multiple suture lines, fistulas, or questionable vascular integrity, temporary total diversion of the small intestine (proximal, jejunostomy) may be advisable.[31,32]

In some instances, knowledge of the bacterial flora of a surgical infection can influence overall management quite apart from its impact on antibiotic therapy. For example, enteric organisms recovered from a perianal abscess suggest an associated fistula-in-ano, whereas isolation of predominantly skin flora makes a fistula less likely.[33] Isolation of coliforms from recurrent abscesses of the face or other upper body sites may suggest infection of factitious (self-induced) origin (so does polymicrobial gram-negative bacteremia in otherwise healthy patients). Localized soft tissue infections due to fungi such as *Mucor, Absidia,* or *Rhizopus* occurring in immunocompromised patients are often best managed by total excision (wide debridement). So, too, are fungal abscesses of the brain or lung (excision of fungal lung abscess is controversial).[34,35] Tuberculous cervical abscesses respond better to excision and chemotherapy than to drainage and chemotherapy.[36]

By contrast, some infections require excisional therapy no matter what the cultures show. Mycotic aneurysms, for example, must usually be removed. Necrotizing infections are rarely curable without aggressive surgical debridement. A hemorrhaging lung abscess may require emergency thoracotomy and pulmonary resection.

Incision and Drainage

Ideally, any method of abscess drainage should provide complete evacuation of pus, ease of postoperative wound care, efficient healing, and acceptable cosmetic results. Given the variety of causes, locations, and logistics considerations, however, no single approach is possible. With any technique, an incision adequate to allow complete evacuation, preferably via the shortest feasible route, is crucial. It is also important that septations and loculations within the abscess cavity be broken up, by finger fracture if possible, and that the cavity be thoroughly irrigated. When abscesses are drained by radiographically guided, percutaneous methods, for example, difficulty with recognition and treatment of loculations and septations is one of the commonest causes of failure.[37]

The principal goals of wound management following incision and drainage are to assure that the abscess does not reform and that the cavity heals. Thus wound management should promote resolution of the host inflammatory response (decreased influx of serum proteins, diapedesis of inflammatory cells, etc), coaptation of abscess walls with collapse of dead space, and healing by secondary intention. It is important what sort of cavity remains after the abscess has been evacuated. Deep cavities are usually best managed with drains or loose gauze packs, whereas a superficial defect may require little more than periodic changing of the outer dressing. For most purposes passive drainage is probably as good as suction drainage since abscess cavities are already infected, and retrograde infection via the drain itself is thus not of much concern. Compared to drains, gauze packs are less likely to fall out, they absorb excess fluid, and they may help to debride devitalized surface tissue as they are removed. Packs should be changed frequently (within 48 hours), however, or they may actually impede drainage (this problem has been especially noticeable with packs left in the peritoneal cavity).[38] Packs can usually be discontinued altogether within a few days as the drainage volume decreases. Recently, newer materials such as calcium alginate have been used to pack abscess cavities; calcium alginate aids local hemostasis and is significantly less painful to remove than gauze dressings.[39]

Except perhaps during the initial irrigation and packing of an abscess when topical anti-infectives may help to "cauterize" infected surfaces and kill remaining bacteria, antiseptic irrigation or soaking of dressings with anti-infectives is probably unnecessary; indeed, it may actually damage normal tissue and delay healing. Clean water or saline should suffice. Although bacteremia is probably common following incision and drainage of superficial abscesses, treatment with systemic antibiotics in otherwise healthy patients has never been shown to be of value in the prevention of systemic infections. Macfie and Harvey[40] did show a lower recurrence rate and more rapid healing in drained superficial abscesses when systemic antibiotics were used. Preventive antibiotic therapy may be advisable, however, if the patient is immunocompromised, has valvular heart disease, or if abscess curettage is used. In the presence of systemic toxicity, lymphangitis, or a large surrounding area of cellulitis, a course of antibiotic therapy may be required even if drainage of the liquid central necrotic area is complete.

Mechanical drains are probably used more often than packs to drain abscesses of deep body cavities or solid organs. With either method, however, the ultimate goal is closure of the cavity. For chronically infected wounds or tissue beds, antibiotic suction-irrigation systems are sometimes used. Typically, an antibiotic solution is instilled through one catheter and evacuated through another that is positioned distally or dependently. Such systems have been employed in the management of chronic empyema, osteomyelitis, pyogenic arthritis, pericarditis, peritonitis, infected prosthetic devices or median sternotomy wounds, and, in modified form, even for brain and epidural abscess. Suction-irrigation is particularly effective because it both washes out inflammatory mediators and bacteria and delivers high concentrations of antibiotics to the infected site. In one novel application of this technique, mediastinitis due to a perforated esophagus was managed by having the patient swallow irrigant, which entered the mediastinum through the esophageal defect and was then evacuated by chest tubes.[41] Limitations of suction-irrigation, however, include the tendency of catheters to become occluded after a few days, the possibility of superinfection with resistant organisms, and added requirements for nursing care.

Abscess cavities that are slow to collapse or require periodic reexploration can sometimes be marsupialized—that is, the opening of the abscess made continuous with the outside skin. This prevents premature closure and facilitates surgical access. The Eloesser flap used for chronic empyema is a good example. Marsupialization, or a form of it, has become popular in the treatment of pancreatic abscess or infected pancreatic necrosis. Where there is a large permanent dead space, as may occur after pulmonary resection, a pedicled muscle graft or reconstructive procedure (thoracoplasty) may be required to obliterate the abscess cavity. Experimentally, muscle grafts have been shown to resist bacterial infection; clinically, they provide very effective coverage for chronically infected wounds. Of note, certain sugar-based preparations, including honey, are said to be beneficial for chronically infected wounds and even large abscess cavities, probably by creating an osmotic environment unfavorable for bacteria. Use of platelet-derived growth factor and other enhancers of wound healing are being investigated.[42]

Excision of Abscesses

There is a considerable literature pertaining to the management of soft tissue abscesses by various excisional techniques ranging from curettage to complete extirpation. Practically speaking, abscess excision is probably most useful for lesions that fail to respond to conventional management (antibiotics, drainage, etc) and can be excised—for example, empyema, lung abscess, or abscesses of bone, kidney, spleen, colon (diverticulitis), or prostate. Excision may also be expedient if the surgical approach to the lesion is especially difficult, making subsequent reoperation for further therapy hazardous. Such might be the case for abscesses of the brain or cardiac valve annulus (the issue is controversial for brain abscess). Some abscesses—mycotic aneurysms, myocardial abscess, or lung abscess, for example—may require removal to prevent catastrophic complications. Sometimes even simple cellulitis is a rationale for surgical excision. For example, infections of the gallbladder or appendix are managed by excision (albeit, sometimes deferred) because (1) antibiotic therapy alone may not necessarily cure the infection or prevent serious complications (abscess, peritonitis); (2) excision is relatively safe and, without it, recurrences are common; and (3) the structures involved are nonessential.

In the United Kingdom, curettage and closure of simple soft tissue abscesses have been used since the early 1950s. In the United States, however, the value of this approach has been questioned. Curettage was originally suggested as a technique by which systemic antibiotics could be made available to the abscess cavity. In essence, the approach is intended to create a clean wound—or at least an approximation of such—that heals rapidly by primary intention with little risk of infectious complications. In effect, it represents an attempt to excise abscesses from the inside out. Unfortunately, although curretage and closure may indeed accelerate healing, the reciprocal cost is often an increased number of recurrent abscesses. Curettage without closure appears to ameliorate this problem while still allowing accelerated healing. Curettage still requires general anesthesia. Other limitations include inaccessibility due to the site or size of the abscess, or the presence of adjacent vital structures that could be injured by curettage. For these reasons, curettage and closure of simple soft tissue abscesses have been little used by surgeons in the United States.

Excision of brain abscess, thoracic empyema, and lung abscess and other lesions is discussed in Chapters 34 and 35.

APPROACH TO SURGICAL INFECTIONS IN THE IMMUNOCOMPROMISED HOST

Immunocompromised hosts are a diverse group that includes patients receiving allografts, those receiving chemotherapy or steroids for malignant or autoimmune disease, those at the extremes of age or who are debilitated by uncontrolled infections such as peritonitis, and those with AIDS (see Chap. 51). Other groups, such as patients with diabetes or malnutrition, may be considered immunocompromised as well.

The specific nature of host immune compromise is diverse, with particular defects in host defenses predisposing to specific infectious complications. Patients who are deficient in immunoglobulin production, for example, are more vulnerable to infections with gram-positive cocci, whereas patients with impaired cellular immunity are more susceptible to intracellular pathogens. Patients with severe infections, such as tertiary peritonitis, often have a general or global suppression of their immune defenses, presumably on the basis of the infection itself. Immunocompromised patients often fail to manifest typical signs and symptoms of infection. For example, fever and leukocytosis may be low-grade or absent, especially in the elderly or in patients receiving steroids. Indeed, neutropenia is one of the most common and most important factors predisposing to infection in the immunocompromised host (the major immune defect in patients with AIDS is impaired lymphocyte function, but many develop significant neutropenia as the disease progresses).[43]

Infections in immunocompromised patients may be exotic or commonplace; they may require management with studied conservatism or particularly aggressive operative intervention. Early postoperative infections in renal transplant patients, for example, tend to be of the conventional sort, whereas unconventional infections due to opportunistic organisms such as viruses and fungi occur later (see Chap. 51). Perirectal abscess in neutropenic patients should be diagnosed with caution since the latter generate abscesses poorly; incision and drainage should be deferred unless antibiotic therapy proves inadequate, aspiration demonstrates a drainable fluid collection, or necrotic tissue is obvious. Initial management of neutropenic enterocolitis, the commonest cause of acute abdomen in patients with acute leukemia, should likewise be conservative, employing bowel rest and broad spectrum antibiotics. Acute graft-versus-host disease presenting as an acute abdomen in bone marrow recipients, usually 3 to 4 weeks after transplant, may respond best to increased doses of immunosuppressive agents.

In contrast, *Mucor* infections of the nasal sinuses in diabetic patients are unlikely to be controlled without immediate radical surgical debridement. The same is true of necrotizing streptococcal fasciitis complicating chickenpox in pediatric patients (who are immunosuppressed because of the viral infection) or of opportunistic soft tissue infections due to marine *Vibrio* bacteria.[44] Acute intestinal perforation from cytomegalovirus (CMV) infection, cryptosporidiosis, or candidiasis may require resection of all grossly diseased bowel and diversion by ileostomy or colostomy.

In patients with AIDS, exotic pathogens often cause infections that, save for the pathogen itself, would otherwise be considered conventional: primary peritonitis, cholecystitis, colitis, appendicitis, hepatitis, and pancreatitis due to CMV have all been reported as complications of AIDS. In contrast, conventional pathogens like *Staphylococcus aureus* may cause unusual infections, such as pyomyositis or abscess of the epidural space. In either event, such infections may be the first manifestation of AIDS. Often, of course, both the site of infection and the pathogen are unusual.[45–47] Patients with AIDS can develop infections and other problems that require surgical treatment (see Chap. 53).

Because the microbiology of intra-abdominal infections in immunocompromised patients (*Candida albicans, Enterococcus* species, *Enterobacter* species, and *Staphylococcus epidermidis*) with severe or chronic peritonitis may be inherently different from the flora (*Escherichia coli, Bacteroides fragilis*) of conventional intraperitoneal infections, broadening the spectrum of empiric antimicrobial coverage in such critically ill patients is frequently necessary until culture results are available.[48]

Surgical procedures performed on immunocompromised patients are often done for diagnostic or supportive (tracheostomy, central catheter placement) purposes rather than for therapy.[49] Newer, minimally invasive techniques of inspection and biopsy, such as contrast-enhanced computed tomography (CT) scan, ultrasonography, laparoscopy, or thoracoscopy will probably become increasingly valuable. In one series, simple skin biopsy altered therapy in fully 49 percent of febrile, neutropenic, immunocompromised children.[50] Body fluids and tissue specimens should be studied microbiologically and histologically for conventional bacteria, viruses, acid-fast bacteria, fungi, and protozoa.

Some caveats obtain, however. Although paracentesis and lavage have been particularly helpful in diagnosis of abdominal pain in immunocompromised patients, often providing purulent fluid despite the absence of free air, neutropenic patients may not have a diagnostic number of white blood cells in the peritoneal fluid despite gross peritonitis. Conversely, paracentesis may yield an elevated white blood cell count when the patient has an intestinal lymphoma—but not peritonitis. Similarly, scans using indium-labeled leukocytes can localize intra-abdominal abscesses, but in profoundly neutropenic patients it may be necessary to use labeled donor white blood cells.

REFERENCES

1. American College of Chest Physicians/Society of Critical Care Medicine Consensus Conference: Definitions for sepsis and organ failure and guidelines for the use of innovative therapies in sepsis. Crit Care Med 20:864, 1992.
2. Demling R, LaLonde C, Saldinger P, Knox J: Multiple-organ dysfunction in the surgical patient: pathophysiology, prevention, and treatment. Curr Probl Surg 30:345, 1993.
3. Dougherty SH, Simmons RL: Endogenous factors contributing to prosthetic device infections. Infect Dis Clin North Am 3:199, 1989.
4. DeLong TG, Simmons RL: Comparative effect of various bactericidal agents in vitro on bacterial clearance in vivo. Surg Forum 32:47, 1981.
5. Cohen J: Assay of foreign-body reaction. J Bone Joint Surg 41A:152, 1959.
6. McNamara A, Williams DF: The response to the intramuscular implantation of pure metals. Biomaterials 2:33, 1981.
7. Jackson JH, Cochrane CG: Leukocyte-induced tissue injury. Hematol Oncol Clin North Am 2:317, 1988.
8. Weiss SJ: Tissue destruction by neutrophils. N Engl J Med 320:365, 1989.
9. Ward PA, Kunkel SL: Bacterial virulence and the inflammatory system. Rev Infect Dis 5:S793, 1983.
10. Schultze G, Wagner K, Neumayer HH, et al: Effect of dialyzer membranes on in vitro generation of eicosanoids. Int J Artif Organs 10:275, 1987.
11. Miller KM, Huskey RA, Bigby LF, Anderson JM: Characterization of biomedical polymer-adherent macrophages: interleukin 1 generation and scanning electron microscopy studies. Biomaterials 10:187, 1989.
12. Boddie AW Jr, Bines SD: Management of acute rectal problems in leukemic patients. J Surg Oncol 33:53, 1986.
13. Sickles EA, Greene WH, Wiernik PH: Clinical presentation of infection in granulocytopenic patients. Arch Intern Med 135(5):715, 1975.
14. Dougherty SH, Simmons RL: Infections in bionic man: the pathobiology of infections in prosthetic devices—part I. Curr Probl Surg 19:217, 1982.
15. Dougherty SH, Simmons RL: The biology and practice of surgical drains. Part 1. Curr Probl Surg 29:559, 1992.
16. Burke JF: The effective period of preventive antibiotic action in experimental incisions and dermal lesions. Surgery 50:161, 1961.

17. Mercer LJ, Hajj SN, Ismail MA, Block BS: Use of C-reactive protein to predict the outcome of medical management of tuboovarian abscesses. J Reprod Med 33(Suppl 1):164, 1988.
18. Albrecht H, Stellbrink HJ, Fenske S, et al: *Salmonella typhimurium* lung abscesses in an HIV-infected patient: successful treatment with oral ciprofloxacin. AIDS 6:1400, 1992.
19. Overkamp D, Waldmann B, Lins T, et al: Successful treatment of brain abscess caused by *Nocardia* in an immunocompromised patient after failure of co-trimoxazole. Infection 20:365, 1992.
20. Henry RC: Aneurysm of the internal carotid artery presenting as a peritonsillar abscess. J Laryngol Otol 88:379, 1974.
21. Landreneau RJ, Snyder WH III: Pelvic abscess or pseudoaneurysm: diagnostic and therapeutic dilemma following iliac arterial trauma. Am J Surg 163:197, 1992.
22. Epperly TD: The value of needle aspiration in the management of cellulitis. J Fam Pract 23:337, 1986.
23. Wormser GP, Forseter G, Cooper D, et al: Use of a novel technique of cutaneous lavage for diagnosis of Lyme disease associated with erythema migrans. JAMA 268:1311, 1992.
24. Stroobandt G, Zech F, Thauvoy C, et al: Treatment by aspiration of brain abscesses. Acta Neurochir (Wien) 85:138, 1987.
25. Wittmann DH, Bergstein JM, Georgakas K, et al: Pyoderma fistulans sinifica: misdiagnosis leads to mistreatment (abstract #3). 13th Surgical Infection Society Meeting, April 29–May 1, 1993.
26. Abercrombie JF, George BD: Perianal abscess in children. Ann R Coll Surg Engl 74:385, 1992.
27. Myers G, Ngoi SS, Cennerazzo W, et al: Clostridial septicemia in an urban hospital. Surg Gynecol Obstet 174:291, 1992.
28. Chu DZ, Blaisdell FW: Purpura fulminans. Am J Surg 143:356, 1982.
29. Manji N, Hulyalkar AR, Keroack MA, et al: Cutaneous pseudo abscesses: an unusual presentation of severe pancreatitis. Am J Gastroenterol 83:177, 1988.
30. Starmark JE, Forsman A, Wahlstrom C: Abscesses following prolonged intramuscular administration of perphenazine enantate. Acta Psychiatr Scand 62:154, 1980.
31. Delaney JP, Mulholland MW: The temporary intestinal stoma? Am J Surg 146:668, 1983.
32. Mulholland MW, Delaney JP: Proximal diverting jejunostomy for compromised small bowel. Surgery 93:443, 1983.
33. Eykyn SJ, Grace RH: The relevance of microbiology in the management of anorectal sepsis. Ann R Coll Surg Engl 68:237, 1986.
34. Rosenblum ML, Mampalam TJ, Pons VG: Controversies in the management of brain abscesses. Clin Neurosurg 33:603, 1986.
35. Kosloske AM, Ball WS Jr, Butler C, Musemeche CA: Drainage of pediatric lung abscess by cough, catheter, or complete resection. J Pediatr Surg 21:596, 1986.
36. Cheung WL, Siu KF, Ng A: Tuberculous cervical abscess: comparing the results of total excision against simple incision and drainage. Br J Surg 75:563, 1988.
37. Lang EK, Springer RM, Glorioso LW III, Cammarata CA: Abdominal abscess drainage under radiologic guidance: causes of failure. Radiology 159:329, 1986.
38. Maddaus MA, Simmons RL: Leave the abdomen open for peritonitis: yes, no, maybe? Adv Surg 21:1, 1988.
39. Dawson C, Armstrong MW, Fulford SC, et al: Use of calcium alginate to pack abscess cavities: a controlled clinical trial. J R Coll Surg Edinb 37:177, 1992.
40. Macfie J, Harvey J: The treatment of acute superficial abscesses: a prospective clinical trial. Br J Surg 64:264, 1977.
41. Santos GH, Frater RW: Transesophageal irrigation for the treatment of mediastinitis produced by esophageal rupture. J Thorac Cardiovasc Surg 91:57, 1986.
42. Knighton DR, Ciresi K, Fiegel VD, et al: Stimulation of repair in chronic, nonhealing, cutaneous ulcers using platelet-derived wound healing formula. Surg Gynecol Obstet 170:56, 1990.
43. Bodey GP: Overview of the problem of infections in the immunocompromised host. Am J Med 79:56, 1985.
44. Howard RJ, Lieb S: Soft-tissue infections caused by halophilic marine vibrios. Arch Surg 123:245, 1988.
45. Pirofski L, Casadevall A: Mixed staphylococcal and cryptococcal epidural abscess in a patient with AIDS. Rev Infect Dis 12:964, 1990.
46. Koppel BS, Daras M, Duffy KR: Intramedullary spinal cord abscess. Neurosurgery 26:145, 1990.
47. Fisher EW, Richards A, Anderson G, Albert DM: Laryngeal candidiasis: a cause of airway obstruction in the immunocompromised child. J Laryngol Otol 106:168, 1992.
48. Sawyer RG, Rosenlof LK, Adams RB, et al: Peritonitis into the 1990s: changing pathogens and changing strategies in the critically ill. Am Surg 58:82, 1992.
49. Nugent P, O'Connell TX: The surgeon's role in treating acquired immunodeficiency syndrome. Arch Surg 121:1117, 1986.
50. Allen U, Smith CR, Prober CG: The value of skin biopsies in febrile, neutropenic, immunocompromised children. Am J Dis Child 140:459, 1986.

REGIONAL SURGICAL INFECTIONS

PART VI

Infections of the Skin and Soft Tissues

CHAPTER 31

David H. Ahrenholz, Richard L. Simmons

THE PATHOBIOLOGY OF INFECTIONS OF THE SKIN AND SOFT TISSUES

Anatomy of the Skin, Fasciae, and Muscle

The skin is a two-layered membrane consisting of an outer ectodermal layer, the epidermis, and an inner mesodermal layer, the dermis. The latter is subdivided into two regions, the papillary dermis lying between the epidermal papillae of the skin, and the reticular dermis deep to the papillae. Both consist principally of collagen fibers, although the papillary layer has a finer texture. The epidermis and dermis are firmly cemented together to form a cohesive membrane, which varies in thickness over the surface of the body from 1.5 to 4 mm (see Fig. 31–1). The skin resides on a layer of fatty subcutaneous tissue, the hypodermis or tela subcutanea.

Skin Appendages. Sweat glands, hair follicles, sebaceous glands, apocrine glands, and nails constitute the skin appendages. Because they extend into the hypodermis, infections of these structures can readily spread into adjacent subcutaneous tissue (Fig. 31–2).

Vascular Supply of the Skin. The skin nerves, blood vessels, and lymphatics lie within the dermis, so the superficial layers of the epidermis are relatively isolated from humoral or cellular host defenses. The arterial supply to the skin resides as a flat network near the junction of the superficial fascia and dermis (see Fig. 31–3) originating from branches of larger arteries in the underlying subdermis. Branches pass outward from the deep plexus to form another flat network of small vessels (Fig. 31–3) just below the papillary dermis. From this plexus, arcades of capillaries loop into the papillae and periadnexal dermis. Venules accompany the arteries, forming arteriovenous shunts surrounded by aggregates of smooth muscle cells. These glomus cells regulate skin temperature by altering tissue perfusion.

The lymphatics of the skin follow the arterioles. One plexus resides in the outermost subcutaneous tissue and contains a few valves, while the superficial plexus in the dermis lacks valves. Blind-ended lymphatics in the papillae drain the epidermis. Any infectious focus in the skin can spread circumferentially as erythema, edema, and cellulitis because the superficial blood and lymphatic plexuses lack valves. Thrombosis of the superficial vascular plexus causes foci of cutaneous necrosis, which appear as small ulcers. Deep infections spreading within the fascial cleft between the subcutaneous tissue and the deep fascia (necrotizing

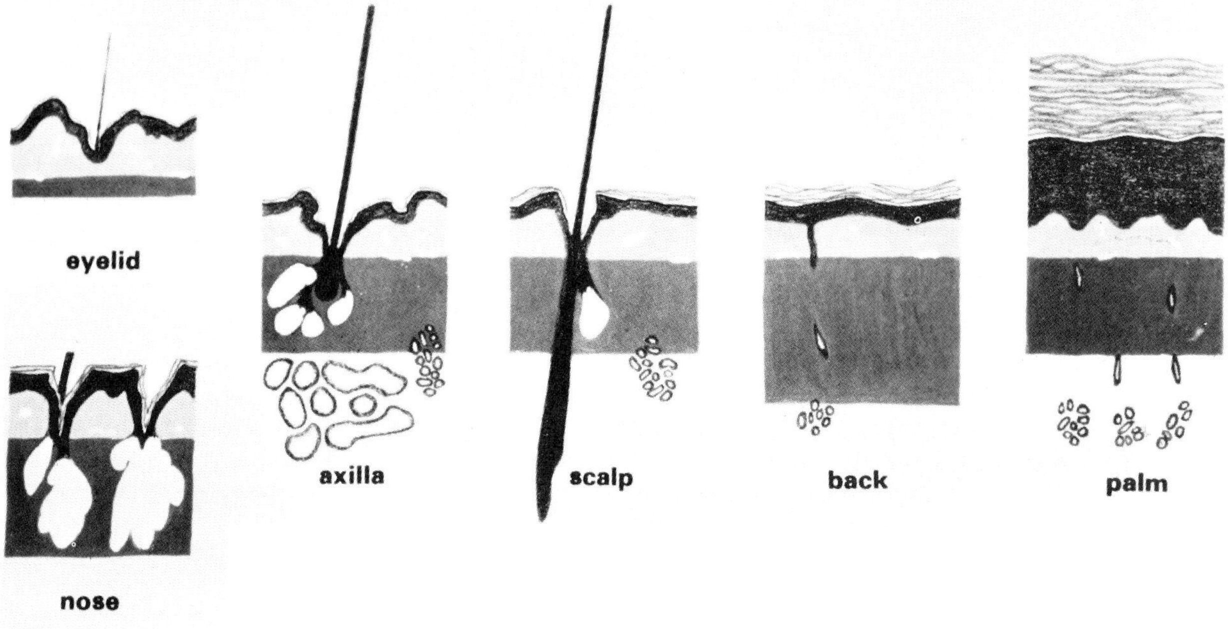

Figure 31–1. Schematic cross-sections of skin in various regions, representing the varying thickness of the epidermis and dermis. The epidermis is thickest on palms and soles. The dermis is thinnest on eyelids and thickest on the back. In many regions the skin appendages reach the subcutaneous tissues. *(From Ackerman AB: Structure and function of the skin. I. Development, morphology and physiology. In Moschella SL, Pillsbury DM, Hurley HJ Jr: Dermatology. Philadelphia, Saunders, 1975, p 1.)*

fasciitis) result in more extensive areas of necrosis only when the infection spreads superficially and causes thrombosis of the deep plexus. Therefore extensive undermining can occur without skin infection if the infection stays in the cleft deep to the subcutaneous tissues where vessels are few.

The Subcutaneous Tissues and Fasciae. All fibrous connective tissue within the body is called fascia except for the specifically organized structures such as tendons, aponeuroses, and ligaments. There are three principal subdivisions of the fascial system: the superficial fascia, the deep fascia, and

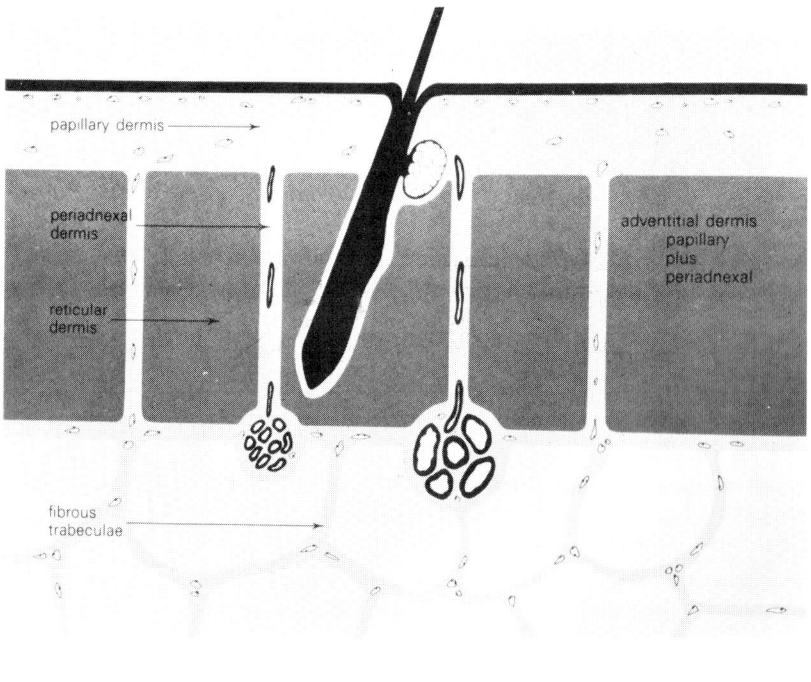

Figure 31–2. The connective tissue of the papillary and periadnexal dermis, which together are called the adventitial dermis, are similar. The fibrous trabeculae of the subcutaneous fat are analogs of the adventitial dermis. *(From Ackerman AB: Structure and function of the skin. I. Development, morphology, and physiology. In Moschella SL, Pillsbury DM, Hurley HJ Jr (eds): Dermatology. Philadelphia, Saunders, 1975, p 1.)*

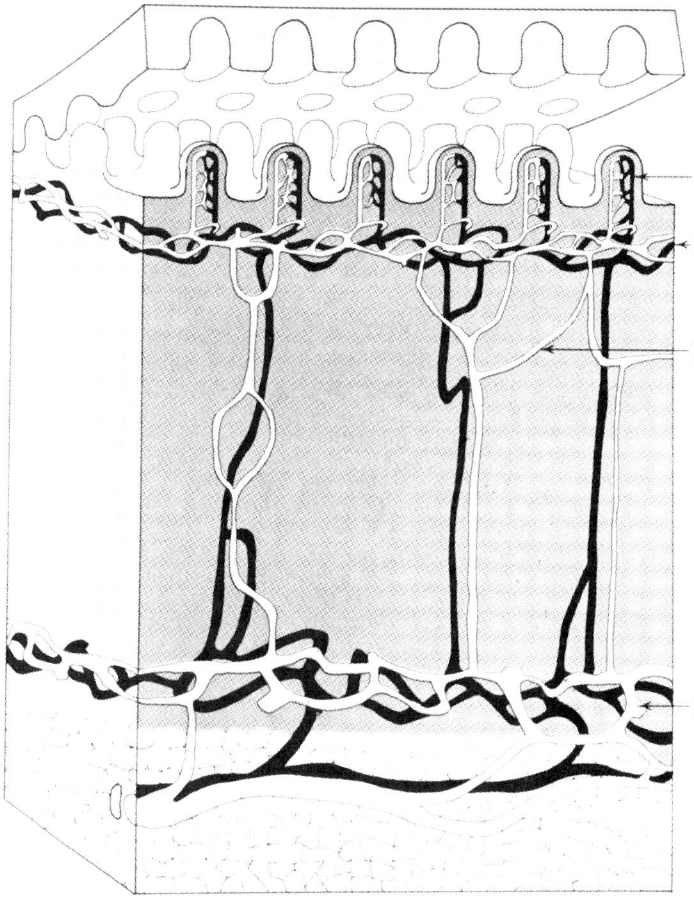

Figure 31–3. The dermal vasculature consists of a three-dimensional network of two plexuses that parallel the skin surface; one in the lower reticular dermis (deep plexus), the other beneath the papillary dermis (superficial plexus). Perpendicularly oriented communicating blood vessels connect the deep and superficial plexuses. The rich capillary supply of the adventitial dermis constitutes a microcirculation, in contrast to the relatively straight, large conduits of the two parallel plexuses and their communicating vessels. *(From Ackerman AB: Structure and function of the skin. I. Development, morphology, and physiology. In Moschella SL, Pillsbury DM, Hurley HJ Jr: Dermatology. Philadelphia, Saunders, 1975, p 1.)*

a subserous fascia. Surgeons generally regard the deep fascia overlying the separating muscle groups as the fascia that deters the spread of infections from superficial layers to the muscular compartments. On the face and scalp, the deep fascia is missing; subcutaneous or submucosal infections meet no deep fascial barrier and readily extend to other tissue planes.

Most soft tissue infections (wound infections, cellulitis, subcutaneous abscesses, lymphangitis, superficial thrombophlebitis) occur within the subdermis or tissue superficial fascia, that is, the subcutaneous layer between the deep fascia and skin. Within this superficial fascia lie the superficial nerves, arteries, veins, lymphatics, as well as mammary glands and muscles of the face.

In most areas, the subcutaneous tissue can be surgically dissected from the deep fascia. These potential spaces are called fascial clefts, and infection can spread readily along these planes. The spread of infection is limited wherever the fascia becomes tightly adherent, that is over bony prominences. Infections of the fascial cleft frequently spare the blood supply of the skin until direct involvement of the superficial fascial vessels occurs. The fascia of the scrotum is tightly adherent to the skin, so infections in this region rapidly cause necrosis of the scrotal skin (Fournier gangrene).

Skeletal Muscle. Striated muscle is composed of long multinucleate fibrillar cells enclosed in an acellular sarcolemma. Bundles of cells are encased in a connective tissue epimysium containing the nerves and vessels. The blood supply is rich—several capillaries may abut on each muscle fiber. Unlike cardiac muscle, which has lymphatics in the endomysium, the lymphatics of skeletal muscle are confined to major connective tissue elements. The low incidence of muscular infection is presumed due to its good blood supply, although some experiments have failed to demonstrate an exceptional resistance to infection.[1]

Microbial Ecology of the Skin

Anatomic and Physiologic Factors. The epidermis is a relatively dry stratified squamous epithelium whose regenerative layers rest on the dermis. The proliferating cells are pushed outward, and cellular degeneration produces the closely packed keratin scales of the stratum corneum. The thick stratum corneum provides the major barrier against infection, since it is virtually impermeable to bacteria, undergoes a constant desquamation, and provides a barrier to fluid loss from the moist tissue below. The normal skin bacteria reside between the desquamating keratinocytes to a depth of two or three cell layers.[2]

The presence of skin appendages increases cutaneous microbial colonization. Eccrine sweat glands (see Fig. 31–2) are found everywhere on the skin in highly variable numbers. The secretory portion lies just beneath the dermis and produces a hypotonic saline solution with small amounts of amino acids, ammonia, urea, and lactic acid, which slightly acidify the skin and have minimal nutrient value for bacteria. Because the eccrine sweat glands have straight ducts and a copious watery secretion, they are rarely the source of primary skin or subcutaneous infections. However, miliaria of the eccrine glands may be clinically misdiagnosed as folliculitis.

Sebaceous glands are found everywhere on the skin except the palms and both surfaces of the feet and discharge their contents into almost every hair follicle on the body. Because the secretory cell dies during secretion, sebaceous glands are called holocrine glands. They produce sebum, a complex mixture of lipids including triglycerides, wax esters, squalene, cholesterol esters, and cholesterol, which are inhibitory to staphylococci, streptococci, and gram-negative organisms but stimulate diphtheroid growth. The diphtheroids, in turn, competitively inhibit the growth of pathogenic organisms. Electron micrographs show the resident bacteria aggregate into microcolonies at the openings of hair follicles, usually adherent to clumps of sebum.[2]

Apocrine secretory glands begin to function under endocrine control at puberty, draining into the hair follicles around the areolae, axillae, and anogenital region. These mesodermal holocrine glands rest in the subcutaneous tissue connected by relatively straight ducts to adjacent hair follicles. Hidradenitis suppurativa is an infection of these apocrine glands. Modified apocrine glands form the ceruminous glands of the ear, Moll glands of the eyelid, and the mammary glands.

Hair follicles are found over most of the skin surface, and bacteria readily colonize their skin openings. The hair can become infected by dermatophytes, and hairy pubic and axillary skin appears more susceptible to many infections.

Other factors affect the skin microflora. At birth, the skin pH is 7 but decreases to 5.5 within the first year of life. Excreted lactate, glutamate, and aspartate acidify the environment; fatty and amino acids contribute little. The temperature is usually about 5C below the internal temperature but varies from region to region. The exposed surface of the skin has a low relative humidity rising to 100 percent only in intertriginous areas.[2]

Many factors limit the normal flora of the skin. A minimal skin flora is maintained by (1) a dry surface, (2) constant desquamation of the superficial keratin layers, (3) the presence of an inhibitory normal bacterial flora, (4) a deficient nutrient supply, (5) an acidic and lipid-rich surface inhibitory to bacteria, and (6) a cool temperature. Changes in these factors increase the bacterial colonization of the skin surface.

Normal Cutaneous Microflora (See Chap. 2). The skin bacterial counts reported by different investigators vary greatly, depending on sampling methods. In 1965, Williamson[3] recorded mean surface bacterial counts of $(2.4 \times 10^6)/cm^2$ in the axillae and $(2 \times 10^5)/cm^2$ on the forehead, while Ulrich[4] reported values of $106/cm^2$ and $348/cm^2$ at the same sites. Most of the reported discrepancies are due to differences in sampling methods. A comparison of aerobic bacterial counts derived by washing techniques is shown in Table 31–1. Counts are dependent on individual hygiene, environmental exposure, endocrine changes, and anatomic site sampled. Typically, the lowest bacterial counts are found on exposed, dry, cool skin surfaces such as the arms and face. Skin folds such as the axillae, perineum, toe webs, and anterior nares have a higher temperature and higher relative humidity, which result in more frequent colonization by all types of bacteria.

Skin has a relatively stable resident flora and a constantly changing transient microbial flora. Transient bacteria collect from the environment, lying free on the skin, and are easily lost with the passage of time. The resident flora are relatively stable in size and composition, consisting mostly of diphtheroids and staphylococci. These organisms reproduce relatively protected within the skin crevices and follicle openings.

Diphtheroids (genus *Corynebacterium*) are gram-positive, nonmotile, catalase-positive, pleomorphic rods. The organisms may be aerobic, microaerophilic, or anaerobic. Aerobes predominate except around sebaceous glands, where anaerobic diphtheroids (especially *C. acnes*) are numerous. Diphtheroids flourish in a lipid environment and break down sebum to produce free fatty acids, which inhibit the growth of other bacteria. Only a few skin diphtheroid species are pathogens, causing

TABLE 31–1. MEAN AND RANGE QUANTITATIVE AEROBIC COUNTS ON SKIN OBTAINED BY SCRUBBING ON 22 HEALTHY INDIVIDUALS

Site	Arithmetic Mean	Geometric Mean	Range
Forehead	1.6×10^5	1.1×10^4	$2.6 \times 10–2.9 \times 10^6$
Sternum	1.5×10^4	2.1×10^3	$6.6 \times 10–1.4 \times 10^5$
Periumbilicus	2.7×10^3	1.4×10^3	$17.9 \times 10–8.0 \times 10^4$
Thigh, upper front	2.3×10^3	7.7×10^2	$9.9 \times 10–2.0 \times 10^4$
Dorsum of foot	8.6×10^2	3.6×10^2	$3.3 \times 10–5.4 \times 10^3$
Back, upper center	1.2×10^4	1.1×10^3	$7–8.2 \times 10^4$
Calf	2.4×10^3	3.1×10^2	$<7–1.5 \times 10^4$
Sole of foot	2.1×10^5	1.6×10^4	$7.2 \times 10–1.6 \times 10^4$
Axilla, lower margin	4.1×10^4	8.7×10^2	$1.3 \times 10–2.8 \times 10^5$
Palm of hand	9.8×10^2	4.4×10^2	$6.6 \times 10–5.6 \times 10^3$

Adapted from Noble WC, Somerville DA (eds): Cutaneous populations. In: Microbiology of Human Skin. London, Saunders, 1974, p 50.

such superficial skin infections as trichomycosis axillaris, erythrasma, pitted keratolysis, and possibly acne. They occasionally produce systemic infection including endocarditis, lymphadenitis, vaginitis, neonatal sepsis, bacteremia, hepatitis, liver abscess, and brain abscess. They are frequent contaminants in blood culture bottles and in mixed infections of the skin and soft tissues but usually play a minor role in the pathogenesis of infection. The bacteria that cause diphtheria may infect the skin, but *C. diphtheriae* is not a member of the normal skin flora.

Micrococcaceae, including the genera *Staphylococcus, Micrococcus,* and *Sarcina,* are the other major components of the human skin flora (see Chap. 2). *Staphylococcus epidermidis* is the most common nondiphtheroid organisms resident on the skin. *Staphylococcus aureus* is not usually a resident organism, although colonization in the nose, axillae, perineum, and toe webs frequently occurs. Nasal carriage is found in 10 to 40 percent of the normal adult population but approaches 100 percent in recently discharged hospital patients. *Staphylococcus aureus* is the most common pathogenic organism found on the skin and the most frequent agent in soft tissue infections. *Staphylococcus epidermidis* and other micrococci are infrequent in soft tissue infections but can cause septicemia or infections of surgical prostheses or of the urinary tract. Streptococci are nonresident on the normal skin.[2]

Of the gram-negative bacilli, only the *Acinetobacter* (*Mima, Herellea*) genus, are part of the normal flora of the axillae, groin, and toe webs. *Proteus* species rarely colonize the skin but are frequently isolated from subcutaneous abscesses of the upper body.[5] The other gram-negative rods are occasionally found in moist areas such as the axillae, groin, and toe webs. On glabrous skin, fecal coliforms disappear rapidly as a result of dessication or good hygiene.

Both the filamentous and yeast forms of fungi are frequently isolated from the skin, but it is difficult to determine whether they are transients acquired from the environment or true inhabitants (Table 31–2). *Pityrosporum orbiculare,* which causes pityriasis vesicolor, is a member of the normal flora in 75 percent of people.

Candida albicans, although frequently found in the vagina and mouth, is a rare cutaneous isolate except in the groin, axillae, and toe webs. These infections are more common in tropical countries. The normal bacterial skin flora inhibit the growth of *C. albicans,* but the use of local antibiotics may permit unrestrained yeast overgrowth. Dermatophytes fre-

TABLE 31–2. YEAST COMMONLY ISOLATED FROM HEALTHY SKIN

Candida parapsilosis
C. guilliermondii
C. pseudotropicalis
C. tropicalis
C. zeylanoides
Debrayomyces hansenii
D. kloeckeri
Torulopsis glabrata
T. famata
Rhodotorula species
Cladosporium species
Trichosporon cutaneum
Cryptococcus species (other than *C. neoformans*)
Saccharomyces species
Geotrichum candidum

From Nobel WC, Somerville DA (eds): The fungal flora. In: Microbiology of Human Skin. London, Saunders, 1974, p 206.

quently colonize the feet and other skin areas but are not always associated with dermatophytic infection.

Viruses are rarely recovered from the skin in the absence of viral disease. Only two skin parasites are commonly found, the mite *Demodex folliculorum* and the flagellate *Trichomonas vaginalis.*[2]

Pathogenesis of Soft Tissue Infections

Experimental Skin Infections. Intact, dry, cornified skin is extremely resistant to infection, and few pathogenic organisms are capable of penetrating and invading intact epidermis. Topical application of even high concentrations of pathogenic bacteria does not initiate an infection.[6] The factors that produce infection include (1) a high concentration of microorganisms; (2) occlusion, which both prevents desquamation and provides a moist environment in which the bacteria can proliferate; (3) nutrients in the area; and (4) sufficient damage to the corneal layer for the organisms to penetrate. Corneal layer damage can be achieved by repeated stripping of the skin with cellophane tape, by plucking hair, by incision, or skin maceration under occlusive dressings. A foreign body within the skin will potentiate most infections and is required for the production of infections from a small inoculum. Experimental folliculitis or impetigo results when *Staphylococcus, Streptococcus,* or *Candida* is applied in combination with these factors. In this sense, skin infections are usually opportunistic, that is, caused by normal skin flora or transient residents that can infect tissue only with impaired local host defenses.

Susceptibility of Soft Tissues to Infection. Subcutaneous and soft tissue infections arise after organisms breach local host defenses, but large numbers of bacteria are necessary to produce suppuration in intact tissue. Roettinger et al[1] found that 3×10^6 *S. aureus* organisms were noninfective when injected into the soft tissues of guinea pigs; 2×10^9 *S. aureus* organisms were required to produce infections consistently. With *Escherichia coli,* 3×10^6 organisms were required to infect more than half the sites. The site of inoculation (tongue, subcutaneous fat, skin, skeletal muscle) did not influence the rate of infection.

The resistance to infection of intact tissue has not been thoroughly studied. Duncan et al[6] noted that the infection rate after exposure of standardized skin abrasions to a mixture of staphylococci and streptococci was dependent on the skin site—15 percent of arm lesions and 38 percent of leg lesions became infected. They hypothesized these differences were due to the decreased cutaneous blood flow to the lower extremity, but such differences are more likely related to the inherent pathogenicity of the local bacteria, the susceptibility of the tissue to trauma, and the size of the inoculum. In people performing manual labor, the hands and arms are the most frequently infected sites, corresponding to the high incidence of trauma.[5] In women, the axillae and submammary regions are frequently infected—minor trauma in both areas results in exposure to a relatively large bacterial inoculum growing in moist skin folds.[5]

Differences in blood supply or tissue P_{O_2} may be an additional factor in regional susceptibility to infection.[6] Ischemic limbs and areas affected by radiation vasculitis and fibrosis are prone to infection. The local injection of epinephrine increases the experimental infection rates for a given bacterial inoculum.[1]

The lymphatic drainage may also affect the infection rate by removing bacteria from sites of inoculation. Delong and Simmons[7] found that bacteria are minimally cleared during the first 6 hours after subcutaneous inoculation, even though lymphatic function is normal. Areas of lymphedema and venous stasis are prone to infection even if the regional nodes are intact.

Role of Trauma in Soft Tissue Infection. Trauma inoculates the bacteria into the soft tissue and simultaneously impairs host defenses. Local tissue injury, edema, and extravasation of blood all contribute to the pathogenesis of soft tissue infections (see Chap. 20).[8]

Foreign Bodies. Foreign bodies have long been recognized to increase the infectivity of small bacterial inocula. Environment contaminants (eg, soil) have also been implicated,[11] and devitalized endogenous tissue may play such a foreign body role. Braided suture materials enhance the development of infection compared with nonfilaments as do surface adhesives such as compound tincture of benzoin, Ace adherent, Vi-drape adhesive, and aerozoin (see Chap. 20).

Not all foreign bodies potentiate infection.[12] Injection of a liquid silicone or a local anesthetic does not stimulate the development of experimental staphylococcal infections.

Epidemiology of Soft Tissue Infections

Most bacterial inocula encounter intact local and systemic defenses. The infection is aborted or limited in extent. A large inoculum or damage to local

TABLE 31–3. COMMONLY REPORTED OCCUPATIONAL INFECTIONS OF THE SKIN AND SOFT TISSUES

Disease	Occupation
Bacteria	
Anthrax	Animal product-associated industries (wool, ivory)
Brucellosis	Meat packers, livestock grazers, veterinarians, contact with domestic animals, especially cattle
Erysipelas	Fishermen, butchers, handlers of raw fish, poultry, and meat products
Glanders	Contact with horses
Tularemia	Hunters, trappers, furriers
Leptospirosis	Farmers, hunters, abattoir workers (domestic animals) and wild animals (squirrels, rats)
Verruca necrogenica (tuberculosis)	Postmortem attendants, pathologists, laundry workers, butchers (butchers' tubercle)
Syphilis	Glassblowers, sharing blowpipes
Trachoma	Sharers of towels
Fungi	
Ringworm	Handlers of horses, cattle, cats, and birds
Sporotrichosis	Gardeners
Viruses	
Orf	Sheep handlers
Epidemic keratoconjunctivitis (shipyard conjunctivitis)	Shipyard workers

Adapted from Hunter D: The Diseases of Occupations. Boston, Little, Brown, 1978.

defenses will permit infection to persist. Few of these minor infections are recorded as occupational diseases. In fact, in California in 1966, only 14,030 occupational dermatoses were due to infections. In four other states, only 9 of 1319 skin illnesses related to occupation were infections. Table 31–3 lists the commonly cited occupational infections of the soft tissues, and Table 31–4 lists those occupations in which the more common pyogenic or more exotic skin infections are seen.

Some rare infections are the result of contact with animal reservoirs of certain microbes. Table 31–5 lists those soft tissue infections in which animal reservoirs are known. Table 31–6 lists those soft tissue infections with known insect vectors. Omitted from this table are the numerous infections caused by the contamination of the traumatic breaks in the skin induced by insect bites themselves or the scratching that frequently ensues.

CLINICAL MANIFESTATIONS AND DIFFERENTIAL DIAGNOSIS OF SOFT TISSUE INFECTIONS

Dermatologists and other clinicians recognize that many soft tissue infections can be diagnosed by the appearance of the cutaneous lesions they produce. The physical characteristics of the lesions immediately indicate the definitive diagnostic maneuver, that is, the need to smear, culture, biopsy, perform serologic studies, special stains, or skin tests, or delay diagnostic maneuvers and await spontaneous

TABLE 31–4. SKIN INFECTIONS ARE MOST LIKELY TO OCCUR IN THE FOLLOWING OCCUPATIONS

Animal handlers (bacteria and fungi)	Felt hat makers
Bakers (fungi)	Fish dressers (erysipeloid)
Barbers and hairdressers	Flour mill workers (fungi)
Bartenders (candidiasis)	Fur processors (zoonoses)
Basket weavers (fungi)	Gardeners (sporotrichosis)
Broom and brush makers (fungi and bacteria)	Janitors
Butchers (zoonoses)	Nurses
Button makers (erysipelas)	Physicians
Canners	Pathologists
Demolition workers	Slaughterhouse and packing house workers
Dairy workers (zoonoses)	Stockyard workers
Dishwashers (candidiasis)	Taxidermists (parasites, zoonoses)
Dock workers	Upholsterers
Embalmers	Veterinarians
Farmers	

Adapted from Pittelkow R: Occupational dermatoses. In Zenz C (ed): Occupations Medicine. Chicago. Year Book Medical Publisher, 1975.

TABLE 31–5. ANIMAL RESERVOIRS FOR INFECTIONS OF THE SKIN AND SOFT TISSUES

Disease	Microbial Organism	Reservoir
Bacteria		
Erysipeloid	*Erysipelothrix insidiosa*	Swine, fish, shellfish, poultry
Anthrax	*Bacillus anthracis*	Sheep, goats, many others
Tularemia	*Francisella tularensis*	Rabbit and other rodents, foxes
Pet bite infection	*Pasturella multocida*	Dogs, cats, many others
Plague	*Yersinia pestis*	Rodents, prairie dogs
Brucellosis	*Brucella* species *B. abortus; B. suis*	Domestic animals, cattle
Rat bite fever	*Streptobacillus moniliformis*	Rodents
Leptospirosis (Weil's disease)	*Leptospira icterohaemorrhagiae*	Domestic animals, wild rodents
Glanders	*Pseudomonas mallei*	Horses
Cat scratch disease	Unknown	Domestic animals
Protozoa		
African trypanosomiasis	*Trypanasoma gambiensis*	
American trypanosomiasis	*T. cruzi*	Dogs, cats, monkeys, pigs, rodents
Leishmaniasis	*Leishmania donovani, L. braziliensis, L. tropica*	Dogs, rodents
Helminths		
Schistosomiasis	*Schistosoma haematobium* *S. mansoni* *S. japonicum*	Snails
Larva migrans	*Ancylostoma braziliensis* *A. caninum* *B. unostomasum phlebotamus*	Dogs, cattle
Trichinosis	*Trichinella spirilis*	Swine
Sparganosis	*Spirometra mansonoides*	Snakes, birds, pigs, frogs, dogs, cats, mammals
Cysticercosis	*Taenia solium*	Swine
Echinococcosis	*E. granulosis*	Dogs, sheep, cattle
	E. multilocularis	Wild animals
Virus		
Cowpox	Pox virus	Cattle
Ecthyma contagiosum	Pox virus	Sheep
Milker's nodules	Paravaccinia	Cattle
Orf	Paravaccinia	Sheep
Vaccinia	Vaccinia	Formerly cattle—now in laboratory

resolution. Many lesions are so common that the diagnosis of rare diseases that mimic them is overlooked. The following discussion presents the characteristic presentations of cutaneous soft tissue infections and the differential diagnostic considerations (see Tables 31–7 to 31–18). The individual diseases are discussed in later sections.

Abbreviated Classification of Soft Tissue Infections

Most soft tissue infections result from traumatic breaks in the skin or adjacent mucosal surfaces, with inoculation of the ambient microbes. The clinical infection produced is determined by the bacterial species introduced and the depth of inoculation (Table 31–7).[13,14] Intracutaneous inocula (level 1) yield pyoderma, impetigo, folliculitis, or erysipelas. These represent a large number of relatively confusing terms for infections that do not require surgical intervention. They will resolve with local care and occasionally antibiotics.

Most surgeons prefer to use a minimal number of terms to describe a clinical infection. Four are especially useful. In the skin, virulent organisms like *Streptococcus pyogenes* produce cellulitis, which manifests as spreading redness and swelling of the dermis and occasionally involves subdermal tissue. These infections are treated with elevation and antibiotics.

Pyogenic organisms like *Staphylococcus aureas*

TABLE 31–6. INSECT VECTORS FOR INFECTIONS OF SKIN AND SOFT TISSUES

Disease	Microbial Organism	Insect Vector
Bacteria		
Bartonellosis	*Bartonella bacilliformis*	Sandfly (*Lutzomyia*)
Plague	*Yersinia pestis*	Flea
Tularemia	*Francisella tularensis*	Deerfly, tick
Rickettsioses	*Rickettsia* species	Tick, mite, louse, flea
Protozoa		
African trypanosomiasis	*Trypanasoma gambiensis*	Tsetse fly
American trypanosomiasis	*T. cruzi*	Kissing bugs (triatomids)
Leishmaniasis (kala-azar)	*Leishmania donovani*	Mosquito (*Phlebotomus*)
Mucocutaneous leishmaniasis	*L. braziliensis*	
Helminths		
Cutaneous loiasis	*Loa loa*	Fly (*Chrysops*)
Onchocerciasis	*Onchocerca volvulus*	Black fly (*Simuliidae*)

in subcutaneous tissue (level 2) produce an abscess, with a fluctuant mass and reddened skin. Without treatment abscesses may spontaneously drain to the surface, but they resolve much quicker with surgical incision. Antibiotics are required if cellulitis is prominent.

Bacteria inoculated into the fascial cleft (level 3) encounter few barriers to rapid lateral spread. Necrotizing fasciitis is the currently accepted generic term for level 3 infections. Even if redness appears in the overlying skin, this infection should not be confused with cellulitis. Surgical debridement of underlying necrotic tissue is necessary after the patient receives fluid resuscitation and appropriate antibiotics.

Muscle fascia is a remarkable barrier to bacterial spread, but once within muscle (level 4), bacteria can cause a variety of serious infections, including streptococcal or staphylococcal myositis or clostridial myonecrosis. Resuscitation, parenteral antibiotics, and extensive debridement or amputation are required for widespread necrosis, but localized abscesses respond to more limited operative intervention.

These terms associate treatment with the level of infection (Table 31–8), but bacteria inoculated at one level may rapidly spread to overlying or subjacent tissue. In describing an infection, it is critical to specify the deepest level involved, so the seriousness of deep infections is appreciated. Thus many older terms have limited usefulness for current infections. Synergistic necrotizing cellulitis is a severe soft tissue infection of diabetics and the elderly, most of whom have muscle necrosis with associated skin necrosis and systemic toxemia (see below). A better term is nonclostridial or enteric myonecrosis, which describes the level 4 infection caused by enteric organisms (see Table 31–7).

In the following section, the variety of terms used to describe the manifestations of skin and soft tissue infections are presented. The term gangrene is specifically avoided in the chapter, because it has

TABLE 31–7. INFECTION SYNDROMES DEFINED BY ORGANISM AND TISSUE LEVEL

Pathogens	Level of Infection: Skin (Level 1)	Subdermis (Level 2)	Fascia (Level 3)	Muscle (Level 4)
Streptococcus pyogenes	Ecthyma contagiosum, erysipelas, cellulitis	Lymphagitis, strep. abscess (rare)	Streptococcal necrotizing fasciitis	Streptococcal myositis
Staphylococcus aureus	Folliculitis, cellulitis (rare)	Abscess	Carbuncle	Pyomyositis
Clostridium perfringens		Clostridial abscess	Clostridial abscess	Clostridial myonecrosis
Combinations				
Staphylococci and Streptococci	?Impetigo	Meleney ulcer	Necrotizing fasciitis	Nonclostridial myonecrosis
Oral flora	Human bite cellulitis	Head and neck abscesses, noma, tropical ulcer	Necrotizing fasciitis	Nonclostridial myonecrosis
Enteric flora	Neutropenic perineal cellulitis	Perineal abscess, diabetic foot infection	Necrotizing fasciitis	Nonclostridial myonecrosis

Adapted from Ahrenholz DH: Necrotizing fasciitis and other infections. In Rippe JM, Irwin RS, Alpert JS, Fink MP (eds): Intensive Care Medicine, 2nd ed. Boston, Little, Brown, 1991, p 1334.

TABLE 31–8. COMMON SOFT TISSUE INFECTIONS AND THEIR TREATMENT

Tissue Level	Term	Common Pathogen	Treatment
Epidermis/dermis (level 1)	Cellulitis	*S. pyogenes*	Antibiotics, heat, elevation
Subcutaneous tissue (level 2)	Abscess	*S. aureus*	Above plus incision and drainage[a]
Fascia (level 3)	Necrotizing fasciitis	Mixed flora	Above plus debridement of necrotic tissue
Muscle (level 4)	Myonecrosis	*C. perfringens*	Above plus radical debridement or amputation; HBO for anaerobic infections

[a] Antibiotics for poorly localised infections only.
Adapted from Ahrenholz DH: Necrotizing fasciitis and other infections. In Rippe JM, Irwin RS, Alpert JS, Fink MP (eds): Intensive Care Medicine, 2nd ed. Boston, Little, Brown, 1991, p 1334.

been used to describe such a wide variety of infectious and noninfectious causes of dermal infarction. Dermal infarction with blackened skin occurs in ischemic dermal necrosis (dry gangrene), embolic dermal infarction (post meningiococcal gangrene), synergistic ulcerating skin lesions (Meleny synergistic gangrene), streptococcal necrotizing fasciitis (streptococcal gangrene), and clostridial myonecrosis (gas gangrene). The term gangrene is associated with such diverse disease states it has become hopelessly confusing to the physician.

Skin Manifestations (Level 1)

Specific terms are used to describe cutaneous diseases. A *macule* is a circumscribed area of abnormal skin color without elevation or depression. The pigment results from melanin or hemosiderin, extravasation of blood, or vascular proliferation or dilation. A *papule* is a solid lesion less than 1 cm in diameter elevated above the surrounding skin. Papules may be the result of epidermal or dermal hyperplasia, local infiltrations, or vegetations. A number of infectious exanthems present as maculopapular eruptions (Table 31–9).[15] Most do not require drainage or debridement. Biopsy may be necessary to differentiate them from similar lesions of a noninfectious origin.

Special forms of maculae include purpura, petechiae, or ecchymosis—all signs of extravasated red cells. Embolic infections (endocarditis, meningococcemia) can present in this way. Infarcts or gangrenous patches are discussed in a subsequent section.

A warty or *verrucous* lesion is a papule composed of multiple, closely packed elevations, which are either dry and keratotic or soft and smooth. Infectious causes include warts, orf, milker's nodules, epidermodysplasia, verruciformis, as well as tuberculosis, leprosy, nocardiosis, and the cutaneous fungi.

A *vesicle* (less than 0.5 cm) or *bulla* (more than 0.5 cm) is a circumscribed elevated lesion containing clear or bloody fluid. Vesicles and bullae arise from a cleavage between skin layers (intra-

TABLE 31–9. DIFFERENTIAL DIAGNOSIS OF GENERALIZED EXANTHEMS

Vesiculopustules	Maculopapules	Urticaria	Petechiae
Drug eruption	Drug eruption	Varicella (urticaria around vesicle)	Drug eruption
Herpes simplex	Secondary syphilis	Coxsackie A5, A9	Bacterial endocarditis
Variola	Scarlet fever	Infectious hepatitis	ECHO 9
Vaccinia	ECHO 9, 16	Mononucleosis	Coxsackie A5, A9
Varicella	Coxsackie A5, A9, A16, B5	*Mycoplasma pneumoniae*	Mononucleosis
Generalized zoster	Reovirus 2	Hepatitis	Rubella
Rickettsialpox	Erythema infectiosum		Thrombocytopenia with many acute infections
Coxsackie A and B	Gianotti-Crosti syndrome		
Reovirus 2	Rubella		
Mycoplasma pneumoniae	Rubeola		
ECHO 4	Hepatitis		
Orf	Infectious mononucleosis		
	Arbovirus (dengue)		
	Rickettsioses		

From Burnett JW, Crutcher WA: Viral and rickettsial infections. In Moschella SL, Pillsbury DM, Hurley HJ Jr (eds): Dermatology, Vol 1. Philadelphia, Saunders, 1975, p 558.

epidermal) or at the epidermal-dermal interface (subepidermal). A subcorneal vesicle characterizes impetigo; intraepidermal vesication may appear as a nodule as in delayed hypersensitivity reactions. Viruses cause degeneration of epidermal cells and produce the vesicles of the viral exanthems, which often have depressed (umbilicated) centers. Trauma from mechanical, thermal, or chemical agents can cause bullae, as can diseases such as pemphigus and pemphigoid.

A *pustule* is a vesicle containing pus or a very superficial abscess of the skin. Not all pustules have an infectious etiology (rosacea, pustular psoriasis). The generalized vesiculopustular exanthems are listed in Table 31–9.

When vesicles or pustules rupture, the exudative lesions produce *crusts* as they dry on the skin surface. The crusts can be serous (yellow), purulent (green or yellow-green), or hemorrhagic (red or brown). *Ecthyma* refers to a shallow ulcerative disease of the epidermis with thick, adherent crusts Table 31–10 lists regional infections that typically present as vesicles, bullae, or crusting lesions.

A *wheal* (hive) is a pale papule—usually sharply circumscribed (eg, a mosquito bite) but sometimes extensive (angioneurotic edema). Wheals simply represent edema of the epidermis and dermis sometimes seen at the edges of erysipelas or cellulitis. Some infections with protozoa or helminths will elicit wheals, for example, Chagas' disease or schistosomiasis.

TABLE 31–10. DIFFERENTIAL DIAGNOSIS OF REGIONAL VESICLES, BULLAE, OR CRUSTS

Bacteria
Impetigo
Bullous impetigo
Folliculitis, furunculosis
Viruses
Herpes simplex
Zoster
Molluscum contageosum (pustular type)
Vesicular stomatitis virus
Kaposi varicelliform eruption
Ecthyma contagiosum (orf)
Cat scratch disease
Fungi
Kerion reactions to dermatophytoses
Vesicular ringworm
Dermatophytid reactions
Parasites
Flea bites
Noninfectious causes
Acne
Pustular psoriasis
Drug sensitivities especially to halides
Erythema multiforme
Pemphigus

Cellulitis is an acute red, tender, swollen area of inflammation within the dermis and spreading to subcutaneous tissues, which is frequently part of any infection of these tissues. Acute lymphangitis can be part of the picture in classic group A streptococcal infections (see subsequent section on lymphangitis). Almost any microbe can be responsible for cellulitis.

Scales are accumulations of desquamated stratum corneum. Any epithelial inflammatory process, including a superficial infection, can induce scaling. Scales can be the only sign of some noninflammatory dermatophytoses.

Subcutaneous Manifestations (Level 2)

A *nodule* is a palpable solid lesion lying principally within the dermis or subcutaneous tissue. Nodules are typical manifestations of granulomatous infections, which sometimes progress to ulceration (*ulceronodular disease*) or even to suppuration or sinus formation. There may be undermining or elevation of the ulcer margin, and the base is clean, covered with a membrane, or thick with granulation tissue. When biopsies are performed, a portion of excised tissue should be homogenized and cultured for fungi as well as aerobic and anaerobic bacteria. Special stains (Giemsa, PAS, mucicarmine, methenamine silver) facilitate the histopathologic diagnosis of fungal or viral infection. The differential diagnoses of nodular and ulceronodular infectious diseases are listed in Table 31–11.

Ulcers are the result of destructive processes that remove the epidermis and varying amounts of underlying tissue. Nodular infectious lesions that ulcerate secondarily are listed in Table 31–11. Table 31–12 lists infections that commonly appear as ulcers without prior nodular lesions. Some are part of a *chancroid complex* in which a primary ulcer is associated with regional adenopathy—the primary chancre of syphilis, primary tuberculosis, and the rare primary cutaneous infections with the dimorphic fungi. In other diseases that present with a chancroid complex, the regional adenopathy predominates and the primary ulcer may be almost invisible, for example, plague, glanders, meliodosis, and rat bite fever. Multiple contiguous ulcers in necrotizing fasciitis suggest the progressive nature of the disease.[16] Most cutaneous ulcers, however, are traumatic lesions that become infected secondarily by ambient bacteria (Table 31–13).

TABLE 31–11. NODULAR AND ULCERONODULAR INFECTIONS OF SKIN AND SUBCUTANEOUS TISSUES

Bacteria
- Pyogenic bacteria
  - Cutaneous abscesses
  - Botryomycosis
  - Hidradenitis suppurativa
  - Acne conglobata
  - Infected epidermal inclusions
    - Sebaceous cyst
    - Pilonidal cyst
- Treponemal infections
  - Benign tertiary syphilis (gumma)
  - Yaws
  - Pinta
- Mycobacterial lesions
  - Leprosy
  - Tuberculosis
    - Lupus vulgaris
    - Tuberculous gumma
- Atypical mycobacteria
  - Swimming pool granuloma
  - Cutaneous atypical mycobacteria
- Sexually transmitted diseases
  - Granuloma inguinale
  - Lymphogranuloma venereum

Fungi
- Inflammatory reactions to dermatophytes
- *Candida* granuloma
- Subcutaneous mycoses
  - Chromoblastomycosis
  - Mycetoma
  - Phaeosporotrichosis
  - Rhinosporidiosis

Fungi (cont.)
- Systemic mycoses
  - Coccidioidomycosis
  - Blastomycosis
  - Paracoccidioidomycosis
  - Histoplasmosis
  - Cryptococcosis
- Sporotrichosis
- Phycomycosis
- Aspergillosis

Viruses
- Warts
- Mollusum contagiosum
- Cowpox
- Milker's nodule

Protozoa and Helminths
- Leishmaniasis
- Cutaneous filarids
  - Onchocerca volvulus
  - Loa loa
  - Dracunculus medinensis

Insect Bites
- Furuncular myiasis
- Trombiculosis

Algae
- Protothecosis

Sporotrichosis causes an unusual form of nodular ulcerative disease. The primary lesion appears as a nodule, ulcer, or infiltrated plaque at the site of entry. Weeks to months later, new nodular-ulcerative lesions appear along lymphatic pathways. Pus may exude when the lesions break down, and the areas can become secondarily infected. The lymphatics between nodules become palpably thickened, but lymph node involvement is unusual. Table 31–14 lists some of the ulceronodular diseases that manifest this clinical *sporotrichoid pattern.*

An *abscess* is a localized accumulation of purulent material situated in the dermis or subcutaneous tissue. The intact skin becomes reddened, tender, and ulcerated. Most abscesses are caused by pyogenic bacteria, but any agent that elicits necrosis and the influx of polymorphonuclear cells can be etiologic. Palpation classically produces fluid shifts within the cavity (fluctuance), but this is an unreliable clinical sign. Rupture or surface necrosis results in purulent drainage. If the abscess is relatively deep in the tissue, the drainage tract from skin to abscess is called a *sinus*. Extensive infections can drain through more than one sinus tract. Table 31–15 lists diseases presenting with abscesses or sinus tracts. Curettings of the tract provide the most reliable culture results.

Cysts are sacs containing liquid or semisolid material and are resilient rather than fluctuant to palpation. Epidermal cysts lined with squamous epithelium and filled with keratinous material are most common. Sebaceous cysts are of pilar origin and can become infected secondarily. A few deep infections appear as cysts—cystic chromoblastomycosis, mycetoma, ecchinococcosis, trichinosis, and cryptococcosis.

Lymphangitis refers to inflammation of lymphatic tissue channels, usually in the subcutaneous tissues, which present on the skin surface. Acute lymphangitis is typically caused by group A streptococci and less commonly by bacterial infections, *S. aureus, Spirillum minus* (rat bite fever), or cer-

TABLE 31–12. PRIMARY INFECTIOUS ULCERS OF THE SKIN WITHOUT PROMINENT UNDERLYING NODULES

Bacteria
- Anthrax
- Diphtheria
- Ecthyma
- Glanders
- Tropical ulcer
- Gangrenous bacterial infections
  - Streptococcal gangrene
  - Necrotizing fasciitis
  - Meleney ulcer
  - Gas gangrene
- Treponemes
  - Primary syphilis
  - Yaws
- Mycobacteria
  - Primary cutaneous tuberculosis
  - Atypical mycobacteria
  - *M. ulcerans*
  - Leprosy
- Chancroid
- Nocardiosis

Fungi
- Primary fungal infections
  - Coccidioidomycosis
  - Blastomycosis
  - Histoplasmosis
- Phycomycosis
- Chromoblastomycosis
- Sporotrichosis

Viruses
- Ulcerated vesicular diseases
  - Herpes simplex
  - Zoster
  - Vaccinia necrosum

Protozoa and Helminths
- Amebiasis
- Leishmaniasis
  - Cutaneous
  - Mucocutaneous
  - Kala-azar
- *Schistosoma cutis*

tain filaria. Chronic lymphangitis leads to a sporotrichoid pattern. Episodes of lymphangitis can produce permanent lymphedema of the distal tissues, making them more susceptible to subsequent infection.

Lymphadenitis occurs when microbial agents reach the lymph nodes and precipitate an inflammatory reaction. Lymphadenitis can be restricted to a solitary node or to a localized group of nodes (regional lymphadenitis), or it can be generalized. Infections that cause regional lymphadenitis are listed in Table 31–16 and those associated with generalized lymphadenitis in Table 31–17. The latter infections rarely come to the attention of the surgeon, since suppuration or an ulceroglandular syndrome is seldom part of the picture. In regional lymphadenitis, the gross features may be those of nonsuppurative, suppurative, or caseous inflammation, depending on the infecting microorganism. Biopsy of nonsuppurative lymphadenitis reveals swelling and hyperplasia of the sinusoidal lining cells and infiltration of leukocytes, which may progress to abscess formation. In granulomatous infections, stellate abscesses become surrounded by palisading epitheloid cells (granulomatous abscess) producing caseous necrosis. Biopsy specimens should be cultured for common and rare etiologic agents and should be stained for fungi, acid-fast organisms, protozoa, and bacteria. The pathologic diagnosis is usually made before isolation in culture of the etiologic agent.

Certain patterns of regional lymphadenopathy suggest the site of inoculation. Pharyngitis and tonsillitis are common precursor diseases of cervical lymphadenitis. Acute regional lymphadenitis caused by pyogenic bacteria is much more common in children than adults and is usually due to *S. aureus* rather than the previously common group A streptococci. Cellulitis and infection of the hand usually produce subpectoral or axillary lymphadenitis and sometimes epitrochlear node swelling. Suppurative iliac lymphadenitis caused by infection of the leg, perineum, or abdominal wall can lead to psoas space abscesses.

Ocular glandular syndromes are caused by conjunctival infection with mycobacteria, tularemia, cat scratch disease, listeriosis, lymphogranuloma, or epidermic keratoconjunctivitis. *Ulceroglandular syndromes* are those in which a small wound of entrance (perhaps an ulcer) is overshadowed by a prominent, sometimes suppurative lymphadenitis, as in tularemia, plague, rat bite fever, and anthrax. Inguinal lymphadenitis (bubo formation) is characteristic of primary infections with syphilis, chancroid, plague, lymphogranuloma venereum, and the primary mycoses. Suppuration is unusual, although the spontaneous rupture of the buboes in lymphogranuloma venereum and chancroid can be mistaken for primary ulcerations.

Manifestations of Deep Infection (Levels 3 and 4)

Deep tissue infections can spread widely along fascial planes with relatively intact overlying skin. Initially, there may be watery drainage from a wound with undermined skin edges. An instrument introduced will pass freely along the fascial cleft. As the

TABLE 31–13. NONINFECTIOUS CAUSES OF LEG ULCERS

Traumatic: Mechanical, physical, chemical, irradiative, heat, cold

Vascular
- Small vessels
  - Vasculitis: allergic and necrotizing angiitis, those associated with connective tissue diseases, malignant atrophic papulosis
  - Embolism: infections (subacute bacterial endocarditis), tumor
  - Livedo reticularis
  - Chronic pernio
  - Hypertensive ischemic leg ulcer
  - Atrophie blanche
  - Raynaud disease
- Large vessels
  - Thromboangiitis obliterans
  - Arteriosclerosis obliterans
  - Chronic venous insufficiency (stasis ulcer)
  - Periarteritis nodosa with or without granuloma
  - Arteriovenous fistula

Hematologic Diseases or States
- Hemoglobinopathies: sickle cell anemia (30 to 50 percent), hereditary spherocytosis, thalassemia (major and minor)
- Dysglobulinemias (hypogammaglobulinemia, cryoglobulinemia, macroglobulinemia)
- Thrombocythemia, polycythemia vera
- Felty syndrome
- Coagulation disorders
- Microthrombotic angiopathy

Metabolic States
- Diabetes mellitus: necrobiosis lipoidica diabeticorum, diabetic dermopathy, peripheral neuropathy
- Porphyria cutanea tarda
- Calcinosis cutis
- Tophaceous gout
- Gaucher disease

Neurologic Diseases
- Tabes dorsalis
- Syringomyelia
- Spina bifida
- Hereditary sensory radicular neuropathy
- Primary amyloidosis (especially familial)
- Congenital indifference to pain

Drug-Induced
- Ergotism
- Halogenoderma
- Barbiturate intoxication
- Methotrexate

Neoplasms
- Epithelioma: melanoma, squamous cell carcinoma, basal cell cancer, complications of Marjolin ulcer
- Cutaneous lymphoma (mycosis fungoides, lymphosarcoma)
- Kaposi sarcoma
- Metastatic carcinoma
- Lymphangioendothelioma and lymphangiosarcoma

Miscellaneous
- Lichen planus
- Pyoderma gangrenosum
- Panniculitides (primary and secondary)
- Epidermolysis bullosa
- Werner syndrome
- Acrodermatitis chronica atrophicans

Adapted from Olsen T: Peripheral vascular diseases, necrotizing vasculitis, and vascular-related diseases. In Moschella SL, Hurley HJ (eds): Dermatology, 2nd ed. Philadelphia, Saunders, 1985, p 1043.

infection spreads, redness and swelling of the overlying skin may mimic cellulitis. Acute streptococcal infection late in the disease course produces bullae of the skin, which become confluent before skin necrosis appears.

Skin necrosis (gangrene) is a late finding in most infections of the fascial cleft, collectively called necrotizing fasciitis. Early diagnosis can only be made operatively, by identifying the separation at the fascial plane of the overlying subcutaneous tissue from muscle fascia. Extensive necrosis occurs late in deep infections caused by streptococcal organisms but is characteristic of mixed infections.

The diagnosis of muscle level infections is even more challenging. Such infections are usually suspected when intense pain, swelling, and watery discharge develop around a postoperative wound or site of penetrating trauma. Radiographs may show gas in the wound associated with myonecrosis. Such gas is not pathognomonic of clostridial myonecrosis (gas gangrene) but may result from perforation of the aerodigestive tract (subcutaneous emphysema) or from anaerobic bacterial metabolism by facultative organisms.[16] The differential diagnosis of tissue gas is listed in Table 31–18.

TABLE 31–14. CAUSES OF A SPOROTRICHLOID PATTERN OF INFECTION

- Sporotrichosis
- Tuberculosis
- Atypical mycobacteria
- Tularemia
- *Scopulariopsis* species
- Mycetomas (*N. braziliensis*)
- Syphilis
- Yaws
- Cutaneous leishmaniasis
- Primary coccidioidomycosis

TABLE 31–15. INFECTIOUS CAUSES OF PERSISTENT DRAINING SINUSES OF SKIN

Bacteria
Pyogenic infection with associated foreign body
Inadequately drained abscess
Carbuncle
Acne conglobata
Infected branchial cleft cyst
Dental sinus
Scrofula or scrofuloderma
Actinomycosis
Nocardiosis
Hidradenitis suppurativa
Necrotizing fasciitis (see Table 31–18)
Clostridial myonecrosis
Infected pilonidal cyst
Fistulas to rectum in Crohn's disease
Enterocutaneous fistulas
Fungi
Kerion
Mycetoma
Cystic chromomycosis
Protozoa
Amebiasis

COMMON PYOGENIC BACTERIAL INFECTIONS

Microbial organisms within a cutaneous lesion are not pathognomonic of infection. Some infections arising in healthy skin and caused by a single virulent species are called primary skin infections (eg, erysipelas, furuncle). The disease is reproduced by inoculation into another animal (Koch's postulates). Primary infection of the skin (level 1) seldom requires surgical therapy.

Bacterial Infections of the Skin and Its Appendages (Level 1)

For the surgeon, it is important to differentiate infections caused by common pyogenic bacteria from the more exotic and rare infections.

Most of the following infections are caused by common pyogenic bacteria and involve the skin (pyoderma) or its appendages.

Impetigo. Impetigo exists in two separate clinical forms: (1) bullous impetigo, consisting of large intraepidermal blebs that rupture leaving thin crusts; and (2) an epidemic form, which progresses from transient vesicles to thick encrustations.[17]

Etiology. The etiology of impetigo has been the subject of much debate. Bullous impetigo is clearly due to *S. aureus,* usually phage type II-71. The more common form of epidemic impetigo is thought to be a primary group A streptococcal infection with rapid *S. aureus* superinfection. Synergistic infections have not been excluded (see Chap. 7).

Epidemiology. Staphylococcus aureus is a frequent contaminant of human skin and is a resident in the anterior nares of many children and about 20 to 30 percent of adults. Impetigo epidemics have been associated with individual nasal or perineal carriers.

Streptococcal pyoderma and impetigo appear primarily in infants and young children during the warm humid months. Predisposing conditions include minor trauma, insect bites, poor hygiene, and preexisting skin disease. Spread within families is common by direct contact with infected material or by insect bites.

Pathogenesis and Pathology. Certain strains of *S. pyogenes* can colonize normal skin, although minor trauma is necessary to initiate infection. The pathogenetic factors of the streptococci are discussed in Chapter 4. The same streptococci causing impetigo can cause erysipelas or wound infections. The initial lesion of impetigo is a vesicle in the superficial epidermis. Acute inflammation with polymorphonuclear cell infiltration follows, and the pustule ruptures leaving an ulcer crater; angiitis, or rarely cellulitis, may follow. Bacteremia is uncommon. Scarring is seldom seen with epidermal lesions alone.

Bullous impetigo produces large superficial skin blebs, which may be extensive in neonates (pemphigus neonatorum). *Staphylococcus aureus,* phage group II, produces an exfoliative toxin—streptococci are rarely found. Cellulitis and lymphangitis are uncommon.

Clinical Manifestations. Impetigo begins as a small red macule, progressing to a vesicle that ruptures leaving a honey-colored crust—the hallmark lesion (Fig. 31–4). Perioral and nasal lesions are most characteristic, but satellite lesions may develop anywhere, occasionally appearing as annular lesions with central healing. The process may last for months, and glomerulonephritis is a feared complication, especially with certain serotypes 12, 4, 2, and 49.

Bullous impetigo presents as vesicles progressing to easily ruptured bullae without erythema (Fig. 31–5).

Diagnosis. Gram stains showing *S. aureus* or streptococcal morphology plus the clinical picture strongly suggest the diagnosis, which is confirmed

TABLE 31–16. INFECTIOUS CAUSES OF REGIONAL LYMPHADENITIS

Disease	Infecting Organism	Regional	Regional with Suppuration (or Caseation)	Inguinal Bubo Formation	Ulcero-glandular
Bacteria					
Pyogenic	Group A strep; *S. aureus*	+	+		
Scarlet fever	Group A strep	+	+		
Diphtheria	*C. diphtheriae*	+			
Fusospirochetal angina	*B. melaninogenicus;* pepto streptococci, etc	+			
Scrofula	*M. tuberculosis*	+	+		
	M. scrofulaceum	+	+		
Syphilis	*T. pallidum*	+			
Chancroid	*H. ducreyi*			+	
Plague	*Y. pestis*	+	+	+	
Tularemia	*F. tularensis*		+		+
Rat bite fever	*Streptobacillus moniliformis* or *Spirillum minus*	+			+
Anthrax	*B. anthracis*	+			+
Melioidosis	*P. pseudomallei*	+	+		
Glanders	*P. mallei*	+	+		
Fungi					
Histoplasmosis	*H. capsulatum*				
	H. capsulatum var. *duboisii*	+			
Paracoccidioidomycosis	*P. brasiliensis*	+			
Rickettsia					
Boutonneuse fever, etc	*R. conori*				+
Scrub typhus	*R. tsutsugamushi*	+			
Rickettsialpox	*R. akari*	+			
Chlamydia					
Lymphogranuloma venereum	*C. trachomatis*			+	
Viruses					
Genital herpes infection	HSV-2	+			
Pharyngoconjunctival fever	Adenovirus (types 3 and 7)	+			
Cat scratch disease	?	+	+		+
Postvaccinial lymphadenitis	*Vaccinia* virus	+			
Protozoa					
African trypanosomiasis	*T. brucei*	+			

Adapted from Swartz MN: Lymphadenitis and lymphangitis. In Mandell GL, Douglas RG Jr, Bennett JE (eds): Principles and Practice of Infectious Diseases, 2nd ed. New York, John Wiley, 1985, p 621.

by isolation of the responsible organism from an unruptured vesicle. Culture of the vesicular fluid or the raw surface is necessary, because many lesions may simulate one phase or another of impetigo or bullous impetigo. Embolic pustular lesions occur in septicemic patients with *Pseudomonas aeruginosa* and *S. aureus,* but these have a characteristic appearance. A variety of serologic tests are available to confirm the diagnosis of staphylococcal or streptococcal infections (see Chap. 4).

Prognosis. Recurrence in the same patient and transmission to family members are common. Most complications with lymphadenitis, soft tissue infection, and cellulitis are self-limited or easily treated. Epidemic nephritis has been found in children following epidemics of impetigo. Although 95 percent of such patients recover, progressive renal failure occasionally follows streptococcal pyoderma.

Treatment. Good hygiene with rupture of vesicles and bullae, and removal of crusts with soap and water, are essential. Washing must be repeated frequently. Topical antibiotic agents are inferior to systemic penicillin, which reduces the incidence of nephritis. Erythromycin has proved useful in mixed

TABLE 31–17. INFECTIOUS CAUSES OF GENERALIZED LYMPHADENITIS

Bacteria
Scarlet fever
Miliary tuberculosis
Brucellosis
Leptospirosis
Syphilis
Melioidosis
Glanders
Fungus
Histoplasmosis
Rickettsia
Scrub typhus
Chlamydia
Lymphogranuloma venerum
Viruses
Measles
Rubella
Infectious mononucleosis
CMV mononucleosis
Dengue fever
West Nile fever
Epidemic (Far Eastern) hemorrhagic fevers
Lassa fever
Protozoa
Kala-azar
African trypanosomiasis
Chagas disease
Toxoplasmosis
Helminths
Filariasis

Adapted from Swartz MN: Lymphadenitis and lymphangitis. In Mandell GL, Douglas RG Jr, Bennett JE (eds): Principles and Practice of Infectious Diseases, 2nd ed. New York, John Wiley, 1985, p 621.

infections with penicillinase-producing staphylococci. Antibiotic sensitivities of staphylococci should be obtained if initial empirical therapy is unsuccessful. Bullous impetigo should be treated with penicillinase-resistant penicillin.

Prevention. Both contamination and minor skin trauma are difficult to control if skin hygiene is neglected. Streptococcal vaccines are not helpful, and elimination of the nasal or perineal staphylococcal reservoir is difficult. Strict skin hygiene and the occasional use of systemic antibiotic chemoprophylaxis (penicillin V) may be useful in limiting spread to contacts while the index case is being treated.

To counter staphylococcal epidemics in newborn nurseries, recolonization with a less virulent strain (strain 502A) has been tried after topical gentamicin or administration of a systemic antistaphylococcal agent.

Ecthyma. Ecthyma is a deeper form of impetigo that begins as a vesicle and progresses to a punched-out ulcer surrounded by a violaceous border covered with a firm eschar (see Fig. 31–4B). The legs of children are most commonly affected, especially in areas of minor trauma, pediculosis, and eczema. Beta-hemolytic streptococci are most often recovered. The crust should be removed and local warm wet compresses applied to remove debris. Antibiotics are the same as for impetigo.

Similar lesions sometimes arise from the hematogenous dissemination of *S. aureus* or *P. aeruginosa* (ecthyma gangrenosa) in patients with seriously compromised defenses such as burn patients. The mortality is greater than 90 percent even with parenteral antibiotics and debridement of infected burn eschar.[18]

Chancriform Pyoderma. This rare disease is of importance only because it resembles a primary syphilitic chancre. Most often, a papulopustule appears on the face near the eyes and progresses to an ulcer 1 to 4 cm in diameter. Regional lymphadenopathy is present, and the disease resolves in 4 to 8 weeks. *Staphylococcus aureus* is found, and the results of serologic tests for syphilis are negative. Antistaphylococcal antibiotics hasten resolution.

Scarlet Fever and the Scalded Skin Syndrome. Scarlet fever is a diffuse erythematous eruption caused by an erythrogenic toxin produced during group A streptococcal pharyngeal soft or tissue infection. Only bacteria infected with a lysogenic bacteriophage produce the toxin. Delayed hypersensitivity to the toxin may also be necessary for the rash, which involves the whole body, blanches on pressure, and gives the skin a sandpaper texture. Immunity to the toxin prevents recurrence. Treatment with penicillin is curative.

Phage group II *S. aureus* produces an exfoliative exotoxin that results in widespread bullae and exfoliation, especially in the newborn-scalded skin syndrome.[17] A toxic epidermal necrolysis (TEN) characterized by superficial epidermal bulla formation without local inflammation results. The infection is elsewhere—not within the affected skin. The diagnosis of a staphylococcal infection may not be evident until sudden fever, skin tenderness, and a scarlatiniform rash appear (staphylococcal scarlet fever). Bullae form and rupture, and a red denuded skin surface results. Toxic shock syndrome is medi-

TABLE 31–18. DIFFERENTIAL DIAGNOSIS OF GAS IN SOFT TISSUE WOUNDS

	Level 3		Level 4				
	Necrotizing Fasciitis[a]	Clostridial Necrotizing Fasciitis	Streptococcal and Staphylococcal Myonecrosis	Nonclostridial Myonecrosis	Clostridial Myonecrosis (Gas Gangrene)	Infected Infarcted Muscle (Vascular Gangrene)	Noninfectious Causes of Gas in Tissues
Predisposing conditions	Diabetes mellitus, abdominal surgery, perineal infection, drug addiction	Local trauma or operation	Local trauma	Diabetes mellitis, local trauma	Local trauma or surgery	Peripheral arterial insufficiency	Blast effects of penetrating trauma; compressed air injuries; entrapment of air under loosely sutured wounds or under ulcers, wound irrigation with hydrogen peroxide; intravenous catheter placement; aerodigestive tract perforation
Swelling	Marked	Moderate	Moderate	Marked	Marked	Moderate or marked	Slight or absent
Skin appearance	Erythematous cellulitis	Minimal discoloration	Erythema	Erythema	Yellow-bronze; dark bullae; green-black patches of necrosis	Discolored or black	Only those due to initiating trauma
Exudate	Seropurulent	Thin, dark	Abundant seropurulent	Serosanguineous	Serosanguineous	0	0
Gas	++	++++	±	++++	++	+++	Variable but present; extends only with aerodigestive tract perforation (eg, subcutaneous emphysema after pneumothorax)
Odor	Foul	Sometimes foul	Slight; "sour"	Foul	Variable; slightly foul or peculiar sweet	Foul	0
Systemic toxicity	Moderate or marked	Minimal	Only late in course	Moderate or marked	Marked	Minimal	0
Muscle involvement	0	0	+++	+++	++++	Infarcted	0

[a] Gas is not associated with streptococcal necrotizing fasciitis.

Modified from Swartz MN: Subcutaneous tissue infections and abscesses. In Mandell GL, Douglas RG Jr, Bennett JE. Principles and Practice of Infectious Diseases, 2nd ed. New York, John Wiley, 1985, p 611.

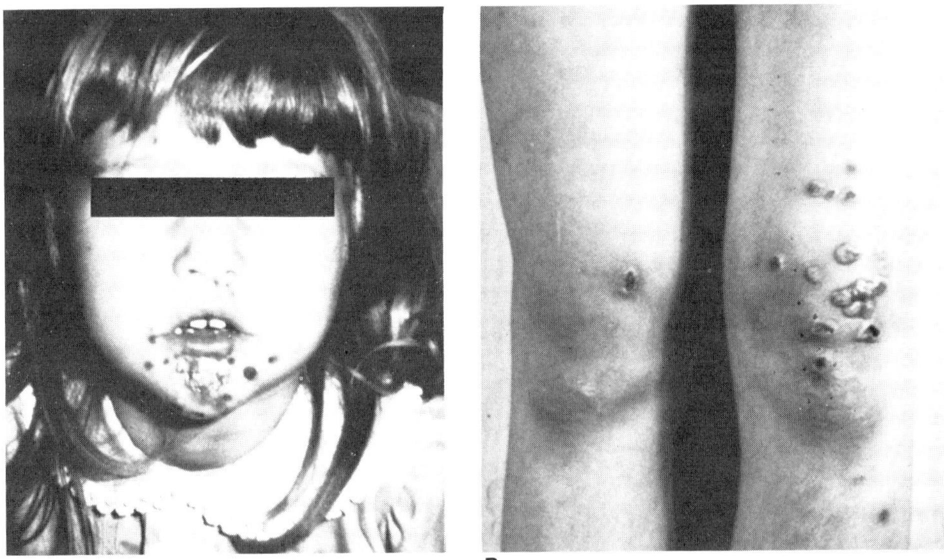

A B

Figure 31–4. Impetigo. **A.** Crusted perioral lesions are characteristic of epidemic impetigo in children. **B.** Ecthyma characterized by punched-out ulcerated nodules is a rare manifestation of streptococcal impetigo. *(Courtesy of Robert W. Goltz, MD, Professor and Head, Department of Dermatology, University of Minnesota, Minneapolis.)*

ated by a staphylococcal toxin, TSST-1 (see Chaps. 3 and 39). A fulminant toxic shock syndrome caused by streptococcal infections of the throat or soft tissue has recently been described.[19] Treatment includes parenteral beta-lactamase-resistant penicillin and fluid resuscitation. For toxic epidermal necrolysis (TEN), the denuded tissue is scrubbed under general anesthesia and covered with pigskin, which markedly lowers the mortality.[20] Steroids are contraindicated for infectious TEN.

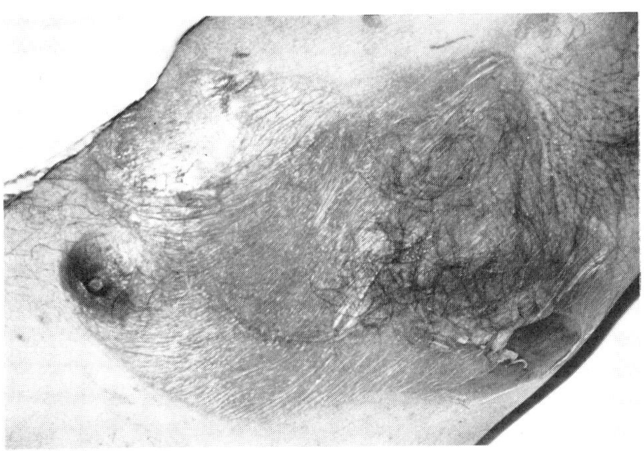

Figure 31–5. Bullous impetigo is caused almost exclusively by staphylococci, usually phage type 71. *(Courtesy of Robert W. Goltz, MD, Professor and Head, Department of Dermatology, University of Minnesota, Minneapolis.)*

Erysipelas

Etiology. This characteristic superficial cellulitis of the skin with extensive lymphatic involvement is almost always due to *Streptococcus pyogenes,* Lancefield group A. Other streptococcal groups (B, C, G in the newborn) and *S. aureus* can also be etiologic agents.

Epidemiology. Infants, children, and the elderly are most commonly affected. Patients with nephrotic syndrome are particularly susceptible. Streptococcal pharyngitis or an infection in the umbilical stump can precede the frank disease. Preexisting lymphatic obstruction or edema from regional nodal dissection or prior episode of lymphangitis are predisposing factors.

Clinical Manifestations. The lesion is painful, indurated, and sharply circumscribed by an advancing border (Fig. 31–6). Fever and leukocytosis are common, but the infection seldom spreads beneath the dermis. A common form involves the bridge of the nose and the cheeks, but the infection can occur anywhere and recurring infections can lead to an elephantiasis-like syndrome with persistent swelling secondary to lymphatic obstruction.

Diagnosis. Diagnosis is based on the typical appearance of the lesion, although other types of cel-

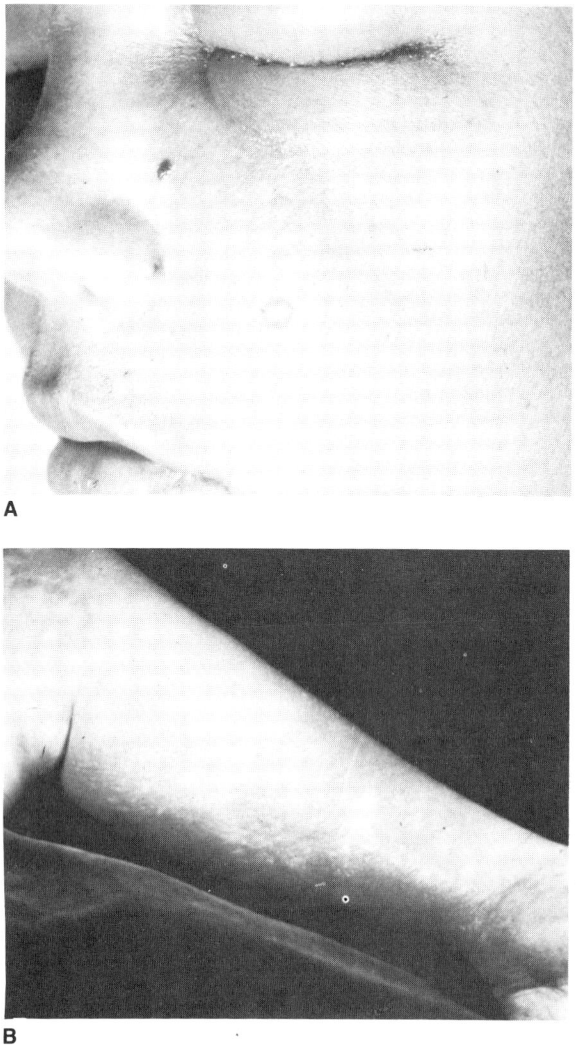

Figure 31–6. Erysipelas edema, a superficial infection, is characterized by induration and a sharply circumscribed border. The most common form extends from the bridge of the nose to the cheeks (A), but infection can occur anywhere (B).

lulitis, dermatitis, or giant urticaria may have a similar appearance. Streptococci can sometimes be aspirated from the edge of the advancing lesion.

Therapy. Therapy should be instituted immediately; parenteral penicillin G (or erythromycin for allergic patients) is usually sufficient.

Erythrasma. This superficial skin disease is caused by *Corynebacterium minutissimum*, a nonmotile gram-positive rod normally found in toe folds, which can induce dry, scaly, slight pink to brown lesions in the groin, pubic, axillary, or intergluteal and inframammary folds. The disease is quite common in patients with diabetes and may coexist with taenia versicolor and cutaneous candidiasis, which generally induces more erythema. The diagnosis is usually made by Wood light—a coral red fluorescence is diagnostic, but the responsible porphyrin pigment can be washed off. Gram stain smears and cultures of scrapings will rule out other or concurrent infections. Surgical incisions through involved areas should be avoided. Treatment with an antibacterial soap is usually effective, but erythromycin used for a week controls more extensive disease.

Erysipeloid. Erysipeloid is an acute slowly developing self-limited infection of the skin, caused by *Erysipelothrix insidiosa* (*rhusiopathiae*), a gram-positive rod that lives in soil and decomposed organic matter. Infection occurs in patients who have handled dead animal matter, meat, fish, or shells. After inoculation into the skin, intense inflammation appears in the dermis. The bacilli are located deep in the corium scattered around the capillaries. A purplish-red nonvesiculated lesion with an irregular raised border is usually seen on the fingers. The lesions itch and burn without lymphangitis or lymphadenitis. Erysipelas, by contrast, typically affects the face and scalp as a bright red, tender lesion that rapidly spreads to produce regional adenopathy and systemic illness. Diagnosis is made by culture of a full-thickness skin biopsy, although aspiration after injection of saline into the periphery of an advancing lesion, or abrasion of the lesion with collection of the exudate may permit adequate culture. It is important to differentiate this organism from the diphtheroids. Erysipeloid may rarely spread to produce a systemic illness with endocarditis and arthritis. The treatment is penicillin or erythromycin.[21]

Folliculitis, Furunculosis, and Carbuncle. *Folliculitis* originates within a hair follicle, usually as a consequence of *S. aureus* infection. When host defenses are impaired, other organisms including normal skin flora may be involved. *Furunculosis* is an infection of several hair follicles within a relatively limited area. A *carbuncle* (boil) is a confluent infection of multiple contiguous follicles in which the infection spreads through the subcutaneous tissue to reach the subcutaneous fascia.

Etiology. Almost all of these infections are due to *S. aureus.* The intrinsic pathogenetic factors associated with this organism are discussed in Chapter

4. *Pseudomonas aeruginosa* folliculitis results from immersion in contaminated swimming pools or whirlpools.[22] *Candida* and gram-negative bacterial folliculitis appear in patients taking antibiotics.[23]

Epidemiology and Pathogenesis. Staphylococcus aureus is frequently found in the anterior nares or perineum, especially in chronic carriers or hospitalized patients.[24] If assiduously sought, it can be found transiently on the skin of most persons. Patients with recurrent folliculitis usually have large numbers of *S. aureus* on their normal skin as well.

Most cases of folliculitis in healthy persons are minor and self-limited. Certain patients, however, seem especially prone to serious or recurrent infections: (1) patients with congenital or acquired hypogammaglobulinemia; (2) patients with diabetes mellitus; (3) patients with cancer or organ transplants receiving immunosuppressive drugs (with adequate skin hygiene, primary bacterial skin infections are uncommon even in these patients); (4) patients with Job syndrome (Hill-Quie syndrome) (this disease consists of eczema, recurrent boils, eosinophilia, and elevated plasma levels of IgE antibodies to staphylococci; influx of neutrophils in this condition may be inhibited by IgE-triggered local histamine release[25]); and (5) chronic granulomatous disease; these patients have a defect of host defenses characterized by recurrent cutaneous and visceral abscesses; their neutrophils lack the ability to kill catalase-positive organisms (see Chap. 13).[26] A number of other conditions sometimes underlie the recurrent appearance of furunculosis: poor hygiene, pediculosis, scabies, excoriations, hyperhidrosis, obesity, hematologic disorders, seborrhea, malnutrition, occupational trauma, exposure of skin to hydrocarbons, and pyogenic infections in family members.

Experimental infection of a hair follicle is difficult. Although the normal skin microflora is concentrated in the sebum within the follicular orifice, the deeper reaches of the hair follicle are sterile. *Staphylococcus epidermidis* and diphtheroids, common in sebum, seldom cause folliculitis. Experimentally, Duncan et al[6] found that local trauma, such as plucking the hair and contaminating the skin with *S. aureus,* produced folliculitis in humans. The trauma to the stratum corneum of hair follicles sustained in shaving results in the frequent appearance of folliculitis of the beard (sycosis barbae). The damaged hair follicle is relatively isolated from host defenses, and edema at the orifice allows contaminated sebaceous secretions to accumulate and suppurate.

Clinical Manifestations. Folliculitis progresses from a small red papule to a vesicle that spontaneously ruptures and resolves with some degree of scarring depending on the depth of destruction (Fig. 31–7). Furunculosis occurs as crops or areas of folliculitis, in traumatized or macerated areas. Certain patients without discernible predisposing causes have repeated episodes of furunculosis over a period of years.

There are superficial and deep forms of folliculitis. Most superficial staphylococcal folliculitis occurs in the scalp, beard, and extremities, especially in macerated areas near wounds and discharges. Elimination of occupational exposure to cutting oils or of occlusive dressings is often curative. Gram-negative folliculitis occurs in acne-prone areas such as the nose in patients treated with antibiotics.[23] *Propionibacterium acnes* scalp infection looks like chronic recurrent folliculitis of the scalp. Cultures are usually sterile, so that Gram stain of purulent smears make the diagnosis. Acne necrotica miliaris is similar but has a necrotic element.

Distinct forms of deep folliculitis have been described. Sycosis barbae (barber's itch) is a pustular folliculitis on the beard area, usually in unshaven parts. Pseudosycosis barbae is a noninfective inflammation caused by ingrown hairs exclusively in shaved areas, especially in black males. Lupoid sycosis is a chronic scarring form of folliculitis. A sty (hordeolum) involves the cilia of the lid margin. Staphylococcal abscess in soft tissue can begin as deep folliculitis.

Perforating folliculitis of the nose begins as a pustule of the nasal vibrissae. In the severe form, it forms an abscess under skin, necessitating surgical drainage and antibiotics.

Carbuncles begin as furuncles on the back of the neck, axilla, or pubic regions (Fig. 31–8). Contiguous spread into adjacent follicles and penetra-

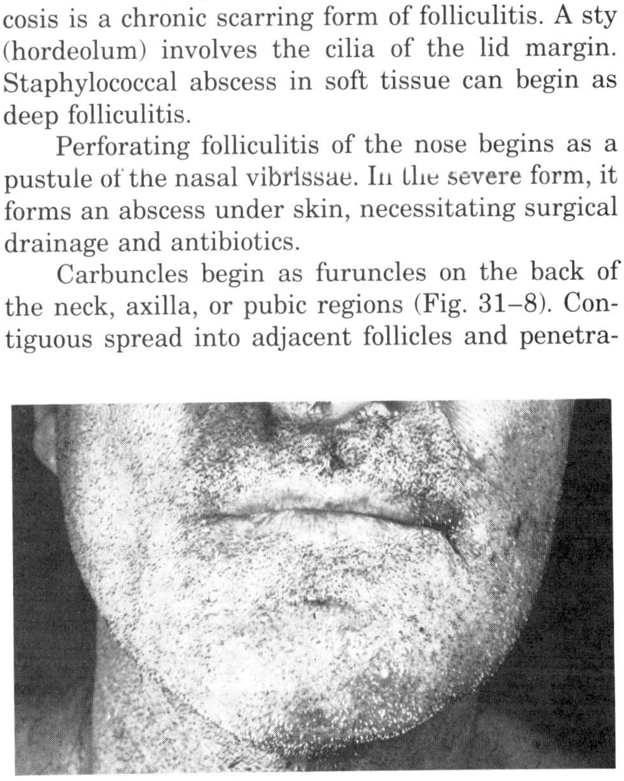

Figure 31–7. Folliculitis of the bearded region.

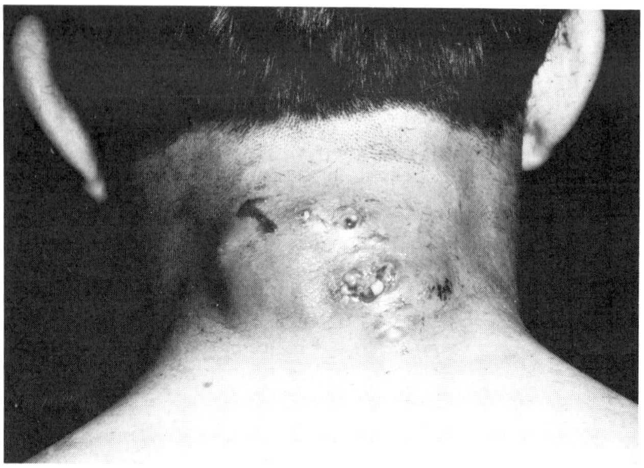

Figure 31–8. The carbuncle in this patient involves the entire back of the neck, with a complex of abscesses with multiple draining sinuses and interconnecting tracts. *(From Armed Forces Institute of Pathology, Neg. No DET B477-4.)*

tion to the subcutaneous space result in an extensive subcutaneous abscess with multiple tracts; a red, painful, tender mass under the skin of the posterior neck with multiple draining sites is diagnostic. Fever and systemic toxicity are common.

Diagnosis. These infections can be diagnosed clinically. Drainage followed by Gram stain will differentiate gram-positive from gram-negative infections.

A variety of other vesicular or pustular diseases may simulate furunculosis (see Table 31–10). Aspiration of the vesicular fluid with Gram stain should rule them out. Rarely, skin infiltration with neoplastic cells mimics furunculosis. Sporotrichosis may resemble furunculosis if the pattern of deep lymphatic infiltration is not recognized.

Treatment. Most small furuncles recede with minimal therapy. Warm skin compresses and good hygiene, such as frequent washing with antiseptic soaps (povidone-iodine), are usually sufficient. Abrasion and maceration should be avoided in order to minimize autoinoculation. Predisposing conditions should be sought and eliminated. Systemic antibiotics are usually not necessary unless lesions are widespread with fever and leukocytosis or there is evidence of impaired host defenses. A penicillinase-resistant penicillin is the preferred choice (erythromycin or clindamycin for the allergic). Incision and drainage are required only for fluctuant or confluent necrotic lesions. After spontaneous or iatrogenic drainage, local antibiotics around the lesion may prevent autoinoculation.

Carbuncles should always be treated with antibiotics in addition to incision and drainage. Extensive incisions and undermining of the flaps are necessary to obtain adequate debridement. Excision to fascia and skin grafting are often required. Carbuncles may recur years after otherwise successful therapy.

Prevention. Staphylococcal skin infections are prevented by good skin hygiene and avoidance of trauma. Plucking eyebrows or upper lip hair should be discouraged. Shaving instruments should be sterilized and replaced when dull. Intranasal antibiotic creams may eliminate the nasal carrier state in certain high-risk patients with recurrent furunculosis. Long-term antibiotic prophylaxis may be required.[27] Predisposing factors should be eradicated. Table 31–19 lists useful advice to patients with recurrent disease. Vaccines or inoculation with less pathogenic *S. aureus* strain 502A is rarely useful.

Acne Vulgaris and Its Variants. Acne vulgaris is a disease of the sebaceous follicles characterized by comedones, papules, pustules, nodules, and cysts. Later, these active lesions are replaced by pits and scars. The primary defect is the plugging of follicles with keratinous debris. If sebum escapes into the tissues, a reaction inflammation occurs in response to free fatty acids released by bacterial lipases. The anaerobic diphtheroid *P. acnes* is an abundant organism in sebaceous glands along with staphylococci and *Pityrosporon* species.[28]

TABLE 31–19. ADVICE FOR PATIENTS WITH RECURRENT FURUNCULOSIS

General skin care: Soap and water should be used to reduce the numbers of *S. aureus* on the body surface and careful handwashing should be performed after contact with lesions. A separate towel and washcloth (carefully washed in hot water before reuse) should be reserved for the patient. Some physicians prefer hexachlorophene, chlorhexidine, or povidone-iodine to soap.

Care of clothing: Sheets and underclothing should be laundered at high temperatures and should be changed daily in problem patients.

Care of dressings: Draining lesions should be covered at all times with sterile dressings to prevent autoinoculation, and the dressings should be wrapped and promptly disposed after removal.

From Swartz MN: Cellulitis and superficial infections. In Mandell GL, Douglas RG Jr, Bennett JE (eds): Principles and Practice of Infectious Diseases, 2nd ed. New York, John Wiley, 1985, p 602.

The diagnosis of acne is seldom confused with true infections. The appearance at adolescence of comedones (blackheads or whiteheads) on the face, back, and shoulders is diagnostic. The inflammatory lesions arise from the closed comedones (whiteheads) and vary from small papules with a red areola to pustules, fluctuant nodules and cysts (Fig. 31–9A). Pits and scars are remnants of prior inflammation deep in the dermis.

The treatment of uncomplicated acne is detailed in dermatology texts. Cleanliness, topical benzoyl peroxide, and topical tretinoin are usually effective. Topical antibiotics (tetracycline, erythromycin, or clindamycin) may be used alone or in combination with the latter. Oral tetracycline or erythromycin is reserved for severe acne vulgaris.[29] Oral tetracycline (500 to 1000 mg/day) will reduce free fatty acid production after several weeks, and treatment is usually continued for months. Tetracycline should not be given to infants with neonatal acne or to pregnant women because of its affinity for mineralized tissue. An increasingly frequent complication is gram-negative folliculitis (*Klebsiella, Enterobacter,* or *Proteus* species). Flare-up of the inflammatory lesions should suggest the diagnosis.

Acne Conglobata. The many forms of inflammatory acne make it an important consideration in the differential diagnosis of folliculitis. Of greatest importance to surgeons is the condition called acne conglobata, an inflammatory disease with comedones, pustules, nodules, and abscesses. Subcutaneous undermining can result in multiple draining sinus tracts. The pus may be foul-smelling and mucopurulent. Healing involves extensive scarring and keloid formation. Adult males rather than adolescents are affected, and the trunk, back, shoulders, and buttocks are most often involved. Hidradenitis suppurativa may be present simultaneously (see Fig. 31–9A). *Staphylococcus aureus* and *Streptococcus pyogenes* group A have both been isolated, but the etiology has not been established.

Systemic antibiotics and topical tretinoin are used initially. If response is inadequate, oral isotrentinoin is usually effective after an initial exacerbation of symptoms.[28] It is both toxic and teratogenic and must be used for short courses only. Intralesional injection of steroids has virtually replaced surgical drainage of inflamed cysts.

Acne Fulminans. Acne fulminans is similar to acne conglobata, but the acute inflammatory ulcers, leukocytosis, and fever affect the backs of adolescent males. Antibiotic therapy must be intensive.

Hidradenitis Suppurativa

Etiology. Hidradenitis suppurativa is a chronic recurrent infection of obstructed apocrine glands in the axillary, perianal, and genital regions. *Staphylococcus aureus* is the most frequent isolate, but *Proteus* species and other enteric gram-negative bacilli and pseudomonads are also found.

Epidemiology. The disease is more common in the axillae of women and the perianal region of men. It never occurs before puberty when these glands begin to function. People with acne and acne conglobata seem especially susceptible.

Pathogenesis. The apocrine glands almost never become infected unless they are first obstructed with keratinous debris. Skin bacteria can then multiply within the gland and produce microabscesses. The gland ruptures and infects adjacent glands, with the surrounding dermal and subcutaneous spaces. Multiple sinus tracts spontaneously drain

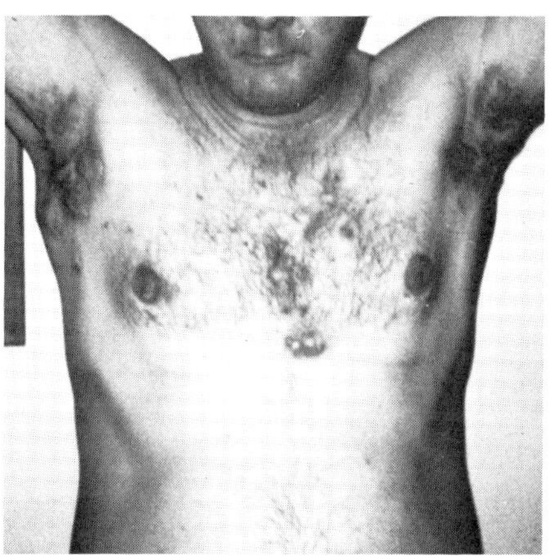

A

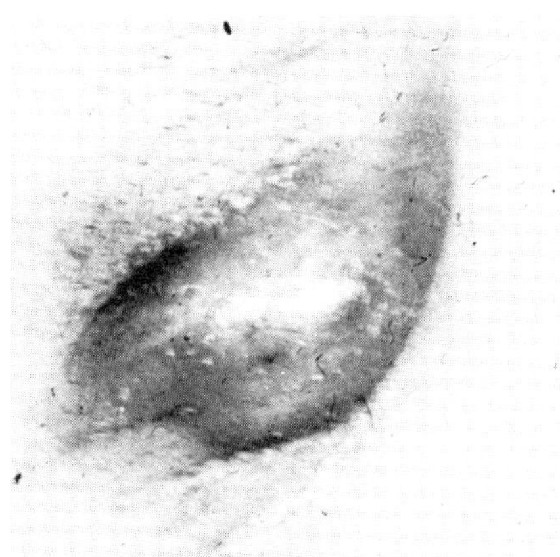

B

Figure 31–9. Hidradenitis suppurativa of the axilla. **A.** Bilateral axillary involvement in an adult male with acne of his face and acne conglobata of his anterior thorax. **B.** A tender, red swelling with multiple sinus tracts. *(Courtesy of Robert W. Goltz MD, Professor and Head, Department of Dermatology, University of Minnesota, Minneapolis.)*

to the skin, giving the appearance of a caruncle.[30] The role of shaving, depilatories, and antiperspirants is unknown.

Clinical Manifestations. A tender red swelling appears in previously healthy persons who may have a history of acne or obesity. If untreated, the boil ruptures and at intervals of weeks to months sequential infections appear. Sinus tracts lead to scarring, which can become so severe that motion of the arm is restricted (see Fig. 31–9). "Bridge" scars spanning old areas of inflammation are characteristic. In the perianal region, scarring can affect the anus and rectum.

Diagnosis. Any abscess in apocrine gland regions should be suspect, but carbuncles, lymphadenitis, or other perineal infections must be excluded. The disease may be confused with tuberculosis and actinomycosis and the sexually transmitted granulomatous diseases.

Treatment. Treatment must vary depending on the stage of disease. Incision and drainage, which may cause sinus formation, should be avoided. In the early stages, antibiotics (penicillinase-resistant penicillin, erythromycin, or clindamycin) should be given until the disease has resolved. Some authorities[30] recommend parenteral therapy followed by oral treatment for 2 weeks. Steroids have also been recommended—either systemically (40 to 60 mg prednisone per day for 7 to 10 days) or intralesionally (5 to 15 mg/ml triamcinalone suspension). Subsequent lesions can be avoided by shaving, depilatories, or deodorants combined with application of an antibiotic ointment in a hydrophilic base (neosporin or gentamicin) and povidone-iodine baths.

Surgical treatment is required in advanced, recurrent, or scarred cases. Piecemeal excisions or repeated incision and drainage is contraindicated. If the process is clearly restricted to one area, it can be excised. In extensive cases, complete full-thickness excision of the entire axillary skin may be required, using skin graft or rotation flaps for closure.[31]

Pyodermas in Immunodepressed Patients—* P. aeruginosa *Pyoderma. Septicemia due to *P. aeruginosa* is common in immunodepressed patients (see subsequent section). They also are susceptible to pyodermas of the nails, toe webs, skin, and external auditory canal.[32]

The bacteriology and pathogenesis of pseudomonal infections are discussed in Chapter 4. Chronically macerated areas of skin such as the toe webs, external auditory canal, paronychial regions of the nails, open wounds, burns, or areas of dermatitis are especially vulnerable.

Several clinical presentations are typical:

1. *Paronychia.* Patients with chronic immersion of hands in water, soaps, and detergents develop painful paronychial lesions with or without characteristic blue-green discoloration of the nails.
2. *Web space infections.* Persistent soreness and scaling of the web tissues occur in patients with hyperhydrosis of the feet or who work in areas of high humidity.
3. *Folliculitis.* Multiple skin pustules occur after immersion in contaminated whirlpool facilities.
4. *External otitis* (see Chap. 33). A swollen, macerated appearance of the external canal without involvement of the drum is characteristic. In diabetic patients, the mortality can be as high as 50 percent.
5. *Superficial pyoderma. Pseudomonas* pyoderma is characterized by irregular, superficial pustular lesions with a greenish-blue purulent exudate (pyocyanin). The pigmented exudate and grapelike odor (trimarethylamine) are distinctive. Mixed infections with other gram-negative rods or with *Candida* may be observed. Some strains produce a fluorescein, which fluoresces yellow-green under a Wood ultraviolet lamp.

Superficial pseudomonal infections are best treated by topical antibiotic therapy (polymyxin B, colistin sulfate) and by drying of the infected area. For local infection, acetic acid, silver nitrate, or gentian violet compresses applied intermittently with long periods of drying are very useful. Paronychia responds to surgical drainage, nail trimming, and 4 percent thymol in chloroform. Acetic acid in 50 percent ethyl alcohol, polymixin (0.1 percent) in acetic acid, or corticosteroids with neomycin are effective for otitis externa. A 5 percent solution of acetic acid used topically is most effective on chronic ulcers.[32] Systemic antibiotics with drainage of the pinna (see Chap. 33) are required for malignant external otitis.

Common Pyogenic Bacterial Infections of the Subcutaneous Tissues (Level 2)

Bacterial soft tissue infections are often part of a continuous spectrum of disease—erysipelas can become subcutaneous cellulitis and thereafter acute streptococcal necrotizing fasciitis. Folliculitis and hidradenitis suppurativa readily become subcutaneous abscesses or a caruncle extending to the fascia. Deeper infections must always be suspected in these patients.

Cellulitis is an acute expanding infection of the skin and superficial subcutaneous tissues characterized by heat, erythema, and edema. It may begin as an erysipelas and advance to necrosis, suppuration, lymphangitis, and lymphadenitis. It is not a single disease entity but a collection of clinical manifestations that can accompany any inflammation of the skin and subcutaneous tissues—both bacterial and nonbacterial. In Tables 31–7 and 31–8, it is listed as a level 1 infection to emphasize the nonsurgical nature of the disease.

Streptococcal Cellulitis

Etiology. Classic cellulitis caused by *S. pyogenes* Lancefield group A (beta-hemolytic streptococcus) appears in unbroken skin, and suppuration is absent. Other gram-positive pyogenic cocci such as *S. aureus, S. pneumoniae,* and many other streptococci (group B in newborns, *S. milleri,* group C, F, G, L) can be involved. Typical cellulitis has been seen with *Erysipelothrix insidiosa* (see erysipeloid section)[21] or mixed gram-negative bacilli.[32] A special form similar to erysipeloid occurs in patients exposed to *Aeromonas hydrophila* during fresh water swimming.[33] *Haemophilus influenzae* can cause cellulitis of the face in children and less often in adults.[32] These special forms are discussed in subsequent sections.

Pathology and Pathogenesis. Cellulitis is a clinical diagnosis characterized by heat, erythema, and edema of the skin surface secondary to local vasodilation and interstitial edema. The skin and superficial subcutaneous tissue are acutely inflamed and infiltrated with polymorphonuclear leukocytes, typically without necrosis or suppuration. Bacteria may be abundant both within and without phagocytes.

The most common predisposing conditions are minor trauma or an underlying skin lesion. Cellulitis may occur as a postoperative wound infection or as a result of perforation of a viscus into the soft tissues, or it may overlay any other suppurative or necrotizing infection of soft tissue or bone. Failure to diagnose the deeper infection increases morbidity and mortality. Up to 5 percent of outpatient burn victims develop cellulitis even if prophylactic antibiotics are used.[34] Cellulitis of an incised wound can be caused by any organism, but most fulminant and rapidly spreading lesions are due to *S. pyogenes.*

Clinical Manifestations. There may be no evidence of previous damage to the skin. Local tenderness, pain, and erythema rapidly progress to a red, swollen lesion associated with malaise, fever, and chills. Unlike erysipelas, the margins are indistinct. The area expands rapidly, and in streptococcal infections, lymphangitis with regional adenopathy and bacteremia is common. Local areas of subcutaneous necrosis, crepitation, and skin breakdown may develop, and abscesses are common sequelae. Crepitus is not seen with streptococcal infections (see Table 31–18). Skin necrosis is diagnostic of severe underlying infection (see subsequent section on streptococcal necrotizing fasciitis).

Diagnosis. Presumptive *S. pyogenes* infections are usually treated with penicillin therapy without laboratory diagnostic studies. A culture obtained by the injection and aspiration of a small volume (0.1 ml) of saline into the advancing edge of the erythematous margin usually is of no diagnostic value because no bacteria are recovered. Treatment failure indicates unsuspected deeper infection or another bacterial etiology.

Any purulent material should be cultured for aerobic and anaerobic organisms, preferably by aspirating pus or obtaining a small tissue biopsy specimen, especially if there is crepitus or a poor response to empiric penicillin treatment (see Table 31–18).

Presumptive Therapy. Early cellulitis is usually of streptococcal origin in the absence of a break in the skin and should be treated with parenteral penicillin G. Erythromycin is used in allergic patients.

Local care of cellulitis includes immobilization and elevation of the infected part to reduce swelling. Warm, moist dressings are useful to reduce local pain, although such treatment probably does not help to localize the infection. Incision and drainage are performed for extension to fascia. Failure to achieve a prompt clinical response to antibiotic therapy is a far more reliable early sign of suppuration. The major mistake is to delay drainage until skin necrosis develops.

Prognosis. Most immunocompetent patients with streptococcal cellulitis treated with parenteral antibiotics are rapidly cured. Rapid progression in areas of local compromise such as chronic edema or ischemia may lead to loss of limb or life. Failure to respond to the presumptive therapy may indicate systemic illnesses, unsuspected foreign bodies, or deep infections with mixed organisms.

Haemophilus Influenzae *Cellulitis*

Etiology. Hemophilus influenzae causes a purple-red cellulitis of the face, neck, or upper extremities of young children. The bacteriology and pathogenic aspects of *H. influenzae* are discussed in Chapter 6.

Pathogenesis. An upper respiratory tract infection precedes most cases of facial cellulitis, and the ear or respiratory tract probably provides the primary septic focus in children. Most adults have bactericidal and anticapsular antibody to *H. influenzae* and are less often afflicted.[35]

Clinical Manifestations. Typically, a young infant or child develops an area of swelling, induration, and purplish discoloration of the face or arm following several days of coryza and fever. The cellulitis can occur in conjunction with otitis media, sinusitis, or epiglottitis and pneumonia. Fever, leukocytosis, and positive blood cultures are common. In children aged 3 to 24 months, this disease must be distinguished from streptococcal, staphylococcal, and pneumococcal cellulitis and erysipelas. Aspiration, Gram stain, and culture of the margin of cellulitis reveal the organisms in about half the cases.

Treatment. Ampicillin (150 to 250 mg/kg per day intravenously in four to six divided doses) is effective in most children. With the recent emergence of R factor-mediated ampicillin-resistant strains, alternative regimens have been recommended, including chloramphenicol (50 to 100 mg/kg daily in children above the age of 3 months) is added for septicemic patients. Cefotaxime and cefatrioxone are useful parenteral antibiotics as well.

Mixed Gram-Negative Cellulitis. Infections caused by mixed facultative and anaerobic organisms are reviewed in Chapter 7. Organisms involved include the enteric pathogens *E. coli, Proteus, Klebsiella, Enterobacter, Serratia,* and *Bacteroides,* usually following contamination of tissue by a break in the skin or bowel mucosa, or oral flora associated with human bite wounds.[36–40] Patients are seen (1) after bowel perforation caused by appendicitis, neoplasm, diverticulitis, or rectal mucosal tear; (2) after colon surgery; (3) with a history of peripheral edema; (4) with vascular insufficiency; or (5) with decubitus, diabetic, or venous insufficiency ulcers. Gas-forming strains of bacteria cause crepitus of soft tissue in patients with poorly controlled diabetes; *Bacteroides* species or anaerobic streptococci are common copathogens (see subsequent sections on deep soft tissue infections).[38–40]

Most of these patients already have level 3 infections beneath the areas of apparent cellulitis and require surgical debridement. Some patients with diabetic foot ulcer or human bite wound may have cellulitis without an underlying purulent or necrotic process. Patients with granulocytopenia or steroid immunosuppression develop mixed bacterial cellulitis of the perineum rather than perineal abscess because neutrophils are required to form pus.[41]

Clinical Manifestations. The typical findings of cellulitis with warmth, redness, and brawny induration are found. Deeper infection is suspected, even in patients with diabetic foot ulcers or human bite wounds, or cancer patients receiving steroids or chemotherapy, unless aspiration for pus is negative. Palpation, aspiration, or imaging studies including ultrasound, computed tomography (CT), or magnetic resonance imaging (MRI) may be required to exclude purulent collections or bowel leak.

Treatment. Immediate treatment with presumptive antibiotics is indicated. Single agents such as cefoxitin, cefotetan, chloramphenicol, ampicillin/sulbactam, or imipenem/cilastatin are effective. The combination of an aminoglycoside with clindamycin, metronidazole, or a semisynthetic penicillin is another option (see Chaps. 7 and 29). Elevation and immobilization are helpful.

Subcutaneous Abscesses. Many infections of the skin and soft tissues present as abscesses in the subcutaneous tissue, especially following foliculitis, cellulitis, or trauma.

Incidence. Localized cutaneous abscesses are a common inducement to visit a physician. At the University of Chicago, approximately 2.5 percent of all adult outpatient visits are for evaluation of such abscesses.[5]

Etiology. The bacteria isolated from 135 subcutaneous abscesses by Meislin et al[5] in otherwise healthy persons are listed in Tables 31–20 and 31–21. *Staphylococcus aureus* is the organism most commonly found, occurring in one-quarter of all abscesses. It is isolated in pure culture 90 percent of the time and accounts for 70 percent of all pure cultures. It is most often found in abscesses of the upper torso and rarely from the perineum, and is almost always resistant to penicillin G.

The majority of subcutaneous abscesses contain mixed bacteria,[5] a finding contrary to tradi-

TABLE 31–20. FREQUENCY OF ISOLATION OF AEROBES FROM 135 OUTPATIENT ABSCESSES

Anatomic Area	*Staphylococcus aureus*	*Staphylococcus epidermidis*	Beta-Hemolytic *Streptococcus* (Group A and B)	Alpha and Nonhemolytic *Streptococcus*	*Corynebacterium* Species (Diphtheroids)	*Proteus mirabilis*	Enterobacteriaceae (Other than *P. mirabilis*)
Head and neck	16[a]	24	4	8	8	12	12
Trunk	18	18	0	9	0	36	0
Axilla	50	9	0	9	5	31	9
Extremity	38	6	6	6	13	6	13
Hand	25	38	38	0	0	13	13
Inguinal	29	0	0	14	0	0	14
Vulvovaginal	8	0	8	21	0	0	8
Buttock	33	0	8	17	25	0	0
Perirectal	0	5	5	48	10	0	10

[a] Numbers indicate percentage of abscesses containing these organisms.
Adapted from Meislin HW, Lerner SA, Graves MH, et al: Ann Intern Med 87:145, 1977.

TABLE 31–21. FREQUENCY OF ISOLATION OF ANAEROBES FROM 135 OUTPATIENT ABSCESSES

Anatomic Area	*Peptococcus* Species	*Peptostreptococcus* Species	*Clostridium* Species	*Eubacterium* Species	*Propionibacterium* Species	*Lactobacillus* Species	*Bacteroides melaninogenicus*	*Bacteroides corrodens*	*Bacteroides fragilis*	Other *Bacteroides* Species	*Fusobacterium* Species
Head and neck	56[a]	0	0	0	28	0	8	8	4	8	0
Trunk	36	9	0	0	36	0	18	9	9	9	9
Axilla	31	9	0	5	14	0	5	0	5	0	0
Extremity	19	6	19[b]	6	0	6	6	13	0	13	0
Hand	13	0	0	0	0	0	0	0	0	0	0
Inguinal	57	57	0	0	0	29	57	29	0	29	14
Vulvo-vaginal	46	62	8	15	8	23	39	31	23	23	46
Buttock	50	25	8	0	0	25	58	33	17	25	25
Perirectal	67	57	10	29	5	14	81	57	47	29	43

[a] Numbers represent percentage of abscesses containing these organisms.
[b] These isolates were all *Clostridium perfringens*.
Adapted from Meislin HW, Lerner SA, Graves MH, et al: Ann Intern Med 87:145, 1977.

tional teaching. The organisms isolated from untreated abscesses depend to a large degree on the site of the infection. Anaerobes are commonly isolated from abscesses of the perineal, inguinal, and buttock region. An average of three to five anaerobic species are found in each abscess. Single species of obligate anaerobic organisms rarely cause suppurative infections. Clostridia species, although common in feces and soil, are only rarely cultured from cutaneous abscesses. The presence of gas within an abscess implies anaerobic metabolism by facultative or anaerobic bacteria. *Bacteroides fragilis* is not found as often as other *Bacteroides* species, although its well-known resistance to penicillin G makes it an important finding in perineal infections (see Table 31–21). Almost all the other anaerobes found in subcutaneous abscesses are sensitive to the penicillins.

Nonperineal infections are most often caused by mixed aerobes (see Table 31–20). *Staphylococcus epidermidis* and enteric gram-negative bacteria were isolated almost exclusively from nonperineal areas. *Proteus mirabilis,* the most common gram-negative aerobe, was more common than all the other Enterobacteriaceae combined. Surprisingly, *Proteus* is rarely isolated from the perineal region and is seen in cutaneous abscesses of the upper torso where it is not a normal inhibitant. *Escherichia coli* is rarely found and only from perineal abscesses.

Culture from subcutaneous abscesses are sterile only if antibiotics have been started or the material has been collected improperly. Truly sterile abscesses most often arise from the injection of foreign material by drug addicts or in psychologically disturbed paramedical personnel (see subsequent section on factitious soft tissue infections).

Pathogenesis and Pathology. Subcutaneous abscesses occur everywhere on the body. Any break in the integrity of the skin permits invasion by the normal flora of the skin and adjacent mucous membranes. The traumatizing instrument is a major source of contamination. Abscesses in the perineum, axilla, and head and neck may arise from infections in apocrine or sebaceous glands. Such abscesses are seen mostly in adults, because these glands become active only after puberty (see preceding section on hidradenitis suppurativa).

Perirectal abscesses commonly arise from anal crypts. Pilonidal abscesses result from secondary infection of pilonidal cysts. Vulvovaginal abscesses usually begin in obstructed Bartholin glands but are rarely due to *Neisseria gonorrhoeae.* Hair follicle infections can extend into the subcutaneous tissues, but infections originating in sweat glands are rare. In general, men present with head and neck, perirectal, and extremity abscesses, while women suffer axillary, vulvovaginal, and perirectal abscesses. The congenital immunodeficiencies and leukocyte abnormalities discussed in Chapters 13–15 should be excluded in infants and children with recurrent abscesses.

Clinical Manifestations. Patients most frequently complain of acute localized pain and swelling around the infected site. Systemic toxicity is unusual, although mild fever and slight tachycardia are common. Induration, redness, lymphedema, lymphangitis, and regional adenopathy may be present. Fluctuance is easy to detect when it overlies firm nonfatty tissue, but it is a late sign of suppuration. It is difficult to estimate the amount of pus in a subcutaneous abscess, especially in the perineum. Needle aspiration through the sterilized skin with recovery of any pus is significant, and incision will almost always reveal more.

Treatment: Superficial Abscesses. The traditional treatment of localized abscesses in the otherwise healthy, nontoxic patient is incision and drainage alone.[41]

INCISION AND DRAINAGE. Drainage of superficial abscesses is readily done in the office or outpatient department. The area is painted with povidone-iodine solution, and a local anesthetic permits incision with a scalpel. Introduction of a gloved finger breaks up all loculations and assures adequate drainage. A dry gauze pack provides hemostasis and is removed the next day, followed by soaks to the affected area. Adequate analgesics are provided.

Usually the incision is made where the abscess points. But midline incisions over the coccyx heal poorly, so a lateral incision is made for infected pilonidal cysts, and infected material is curetted.[42] In many cases this infection resolves with perineal shaving, and careful removal of the ingrown hairs. Radical excision procedures over the sacrum are contraindicated unless a spreading fascial infection is present.

Antibiotics are needed after drainage only if the patient becomes febrile or there are signs of spreading infection. Llera and Levy[43] studied 50 patients undergoing incision and drainage of superficial abscesses and found no decrease in infectious complications in the 27 randomly assigned cephradine versus those receiving no antibiotics.

ALTERNATIVE TREATMENT. Although surgeons are traditionally taught to never primarily close infected wounds, an alternative treatment using incision, curettage, and suture closure of superficial localized abscesses, with or without antibiotic coverage has been used in the United Kingdom. This treatment has not achieved popularity in the United States, and it is contraindicated for deep abscesses, synergistic mixed infections, or patients with constitutional symptoms or impaired host defenses. Jones and Wilson[44] have routinely used intramuscular lincomycin (600 mg) before incision followed by oral clindamycin (150 mg every 6 hours for 4 days). The abscess is incised with the patient under general anesthesia, and the abscess walls are curetted, all clots evacuated, and the cavity obliterated with mattress sutures and a compression dressing. The wound is checked at 5 days and the sutures removed 2 or 3 days later. Primary healing is most successful if skin has not necrosed over the cavity before drainage.

A prospective trial by Macfie and Harvey[41] demonstrated that the mean healing time following incision, currettage, and primary suture with antibiotic treatment was 9 days, but 11.7 percent of patients had recurrences. There were no recurrences in 57 abscesses treated by incision and open drainage with antibiotics, but there was a 7.3 percent recurrence rate after open drainage without antibiotics.

Suture closure without antibiotics may also be successful. Stewart and associates[45] compared incision, curettage, and suture closure to conventional incision, drainage, and dressings in 137 consecutive patients with superficial abscesses. None of the patients received further antibiotics, and all were treated as outpatients. Two of sixty-four patients with primary closure reaccumulated pus and required further treatment. Patients treated with suture closure were off work 4.0 days versus 14.1 days, and time to healing was 7.0 days versus 25.1 days, a remarkable reduction in morbidity.

Treatment: Deep Abscesses. Deep or more extensive abscesses, or infections in compromised hosts, require open drainage and usually antibiotics.

OPERATIVE TREATMENT. In patients with compromised host defenses, deep infections may progress to life-threatening sepsis. Large or extensive abscesses represent failure of local host defenses to limit spread of the process. Drainage in the operating room with the patient under general anesthesia is preferred, since deep infiltration of local anesthetic agents is thought to spread infection to normal tissue. Careful positioning is critical, especially for perirectal abscesses where wide adhesive tape extending from buttock to the table edge can be used to ensure adequate exposure.

The site is scrubbed with povidone-iodine and surgically draped. Bartholin abscesses are incised through the mucosal rather than the cutaneous surface, and all the incisions are placed in the natural skin folds. A small incision permits the surgeon to judge the extent of the cavity with the gloved finger. Probing the wound with instruments is avoided because the abscess walls are easily perforated, contaminating surrounding tissue planes. Adherent necrotic tissue is debrided. Purulent material is obtained for culture and Gram stain. The cavity is irrigated with saline to remove all pus and necrotic debris. Irrigation with antibiotics is probably not necessary, but antiseptics are probably harmful to host tissue.[46]

After debridement, the abscess is loosely packed with a dry gauze pack to obtain hemostasis, and an absorbent dressing is applied. Sanitary napkins work well in the perineal area. After 24 hours the pack is removed and the patient begins warm water soaks or hydrotherapy baths for 20 to 30 minutes three or four times per day. The wound is carefully dried to prevent maceration of the area.

Deep abscess cavities may require daily irrigation or further debridement. Philip[47] has used a Petzer catheter inserted in an abscess cavity and removed after 5 to 10 days. Irrigation of catheters with antibiotics or antiseptics is not necessary in most cases but may have some benefit in deep-seated infections. Irrigation washes out necrotic debris and bacteria, but secondary infections with *Candida, Pseudomonas,* or *Serratia* are common in wounds macerated by prolonged irrigation.

Robson et al[48] suggest that large abscess cavities can be surgically closed when biopsy specimens show fewer than 100,000 organisms per gram of tissue. Other studies are needed, since Schneider et al[49] have shown poor reproducibility of wound biopsy culture counts.

ANTIBIOTICS. Perioperative antibiotics are given to all patients with extensive abscesses, although there is little firm data on which to base this decision. Parenteral antibiotics are indicated in (1) the clinically septic patient with fever and tachycardia; (2) the patient with an abscess in critical areas, that is, mastoid area or central triangle of the face drained by the emissary veins to the cavernous sinus; (3) the patient at risk due to preexisting systemic disease, for example, rheumatic heart disease, Hodgkin's disease, or severe diabetes; and (4) patients receiving immunosuppressive drugs or chemotherapy. Some surgeons prefer to use antibiotics briefly when draining any large multiloculated abscess to treat toxicity secondary to bacteremia induced by surgical trauma. If drainage is adequate, antibiotics need not be administered for the prolonged periods required for systemic infections.

The choice of antibiotic can be based on specific clinical and laboratory findings. For example, infections of the trunk and hands of working persons are frequently caused by *S. aureus* alone; those of the axilla and trunk of women frequently contain *Proteus,* and perineal abscesses contain mixed aerobes and anaerobes (see Tables 31–20 and 31–21). Foul-smelling pus is presumptive evidence of anaerobic infection. A Gram-stained smear of the aspirate will differentiate sterile abscesses, mixed gram-positive and gram-negative abscesses, and abscesses infected with pure *S. aureus* even before operation. For *S. aureus,* a penicillinase-resistant penicillin or cephalosporin is chosen unless methicillin-resistant *Staphylococcus* is suspected[50] and for gram-negative aerobic organisms an aminoglycoside is used. *Bacteroides* infections common in the perineum respond to clindamycin, which is a good choice for staphylococci and anaerobic cocci, which are frequent copathogens.

Page and Freeman[51] obtained the antibiotic sensitivities of aerobes recovered from superficial abscesses in an outpatient clinic. Cloxacillin or clindamycin is effective when *S. aureus* predominates, but an orally administered cephalosporin may be a better choice. For methicillin-resistant *S. aureus* parenteral vancomycin is indicated.[50] For perineal infections in which facultative gram-negative bacilli and anaerobes are both expected, they recommend a combination of ampicillin and clindamycin, which can be given either parenterally or orally. Antibiotics are rarely necessary for more than a few days for a properly drained abscess in an individual with normal host defenses. Arbitrary courses of 7 to 10 days are not necessary. As soon as the wound swelling and purulent drainage resolve (usually 4 to 5 days), antibiotics are discontinued.

In the compromised patient, hospitalization and parenteral administration of antibiotics are indicated; the choices are more varied and the need for prolonged therapy more common. Because staphylococci, gram-negative enteric organisms, and anaerobes are frequently found, we prefer broad spectrum antibiotics (discussed under mixed gram-negative cellulitis), until the pathogens have been isolated and sensitivities determined.

Botryomycosis (Actinophytosis). This rare disease is a small cutaneous or subcutaneous abscess the pus from which appears to contain granules—similar to those seen in mycetoma or actinomycosis. The abscesses are usually single, located in the genital region, and associated with a foreign body. Incision and drainage is curative. The granules consist of clumped *S. aureus* organisms.

Self-Induced Subcutaneous Infections. Self-induced subcutaneous infection is part of a greater problem of factitious illness. Aduan et al[52] describe 32 patients with factitious fever, of whom 11 had recurrent skin infections—three had recurrent polymicrobial bacteremia, and one endocarditis. Most admitted intravenous or subcutaneous inoculation of foreign bodies (dirt, saliva, laboratory bacterial cultures, milk), self-induced excoriation of mucous membranes or skin, as well as thermometer manipulation. Females with medical or paramedical occupations predominated (nurse, student nurse, pharmacist, laboratory technologist, navy corpsman, former medical student). These patients manifested the typical characteristics of Munchausen syndrome. The underlying psychopathology is varied, and the psychodynamics are discussed by Aduan et al.[52]

Numerous cases of similar self-induced infections have been reported. In general, polymicrobial bacteremia in a normal host without underlying malignancy, gastrointestinal tract, biliary tract, or urinary tract obstruction or previous cardiac surgery must be viewed with suspicion. Fortunately, the normal patient usually clears such bacteremia readily and without sequelae. One clue is that patients have bacteremia with multiple organisms. This pattern is so unusual that when it occurs, factitious illnesses should be suspected in patients with subcutaneous infections.

These patients have real illnesses, although they are self-inflicted, and they may confuse the picture with thermometer manipulation and other behaviors. The surgeon seeing patients with recurrent subcutaneous infections should bear this syndrome in mind. The localized infections and episodes of bacteremia are treated as if they were spontaneous. Unfortunately, these patients continue to manipulate and contaminate the wounds, making treatment difficult.

Blunt confrontation of the patient with the factitious nature of his or her disease may precipitate self-destructive behavior or flight. Confrontation, therefore, must not be made until a plan of social-psychiatric care, as described by Wedel,[53] can be arranged.

Infected Bites. Infected bites produce infections caused by the mixed flora of the mouth. A few specific pathogens (*Eikenella corrodens, Pasteurella multocida*) also are encountered.

Infected Human Bites. These injuries can occur in the form of bites or blows to the teeth. The injury itself is usually minor, but subsequent infection can be tragic. The clenched fist injury produces a special wound—the obvious injury to the skin of the knuckle plus a hidden injury to the extensor tendon and the metacarpophalangeal joint capsule. When the fist is opened, the tendons retract so that the deeper parts of the wound are sealed. The anaerobes of the mouth are free to proliferate in the avascular tendon tissues.

Human dental plaque is made up of both aerobic and anaerobic microorganisms. These include *S. aureus,* aerobic and anaerobic streptococci, *Prevotella melaninogenica, Fusobacterium,* spirochetes, viridans streptococci, and *Actinomyces.* All these organisms can be found in human bite infections.[54]

Most human bite infections could be prevented, but patients usually present only after the wound is infected. The principles for prevention of infection in traumatic wounds are discussed in Chapter 24. Devitalized tissue must be excised, foreign particles removed, and blood supply reestablished. Superficial wounds should be left open, unless joints, bone, or tendon is exposed.

If the injury is seen early following wounding, divided tendons, nerves, and blood vessels are repaired—a recommendation that was once controversial.[36] Hospitalization for minor wounds is not required. The part should be splinted at rest and antibiotics administered.[55] Oral penicillins or cephalosporins are highly effective in preventing infection. Tetanus prophylaxis is given, and follow-up examinations are required.

Patients with bite wounds may not comply with antibiotic therapy. Delay in seeking treatment is even more common,[56] and a mixed infection of the soft tissue, tendon, joint, or bone results, presenting as an abscess, cellulitis, lymphangitis, necrotizing fasciitis, osteomyelitis, or septicemia.[55] For localized infections, the extremity is elevated, usually by a sling attached to an intravenous pole. The arm is abducted at the shoulder and held vertically at the elbow to aid lymphatic drainage. A parenteral penicillin or cephalosporin will usually control the infection unless pus is already present in a tendon sheath. Suppuration requires surgical exploration to remove pus and obtain cultures for aerobes and anaerobes.

Eikenella (Bacteroides) corrodens is a frequent pathogen sensitive to penicillin and cefoxitin but resistant to nafcillin, clindamycin, and most aminoglycosides.[56] Seven to ten days of antibiotic therapy may be required, and the overall complication rate is very high. Recurrent infections are usually associated with mixed flora.[57]

Animal Bites. Animal bites should be treated to prevent wound infection, rabies, and tetanus as well as to correct any anatomic injury. Rabies is discussed in Chapter 11, and tetanus is discussed in Chapter 50. Although dog bites are said to be frequently infected, they are less often infected than human bites. Multiple organisms are often isolated,[58] but two specific organisms are of note.

PASTEURELLA MULTOCIDA INFECTIONS. *Pasteurella multocida* is a small, ovoid gram-negative rod (see Chap. 9). The organism is found in the upper respiratory tract of healthy cats, dogs, rats, and mice but can cause hemorrhagic septicemia in these animals. The most common disease in humans is a local infection at the site of an animal bite with redness, swelling, ulceration, and a small amount of seropurulent drainage.[59] A rapidly spreading cellulitis with associated lymphangitis and lymphadenopathy may progress to local necrosis and abscess formation. Fever is usually absent, and leukocytosis is present. The disease must be distinguished from cat scratch disease, ulceroglandular tularemia, and other inoculation infections (see Table 31–5). Isolation of the organism is diagnostic.

Most strains are susceptible to penicillin, which should be administered in doses of 2 to 4 million units intramuscularly daily until the lesion is well healed to avert possible osteomyelitis. Tetracycline is an alternative, except in pregnant women or young children. Abscesses should be surgically drained.

CAPNOCYTOPHAGA CONIMORSUS (DF-E2) INFECTIONS. This thin gram-negative, nonmotile rod can also cause bite wound infections. Usually this is a localized infection characterized by a unique blackened eschar at the injury site, but a fatal overwhelming sepsis syndrome has been described in splenectomized patients.[60] Massive disseminated intravascular coagulation (DIC) is a typical finding. Penicillin, unlike aminoglycosides or methicillin, provides adequate prophylaxis.

RAT BITE FEVER. Rat bite fever, caused by *Streptobacillus moniliformis* or *Spirillum minus*, usually follows the bite or scratch of a rat[61] but may follow ingestion of contaminated food (Haverhill fever was a milk-borne outbreak in 1926). The rat bite has usually healed by the time the systemic illness begins several days later. Fever, chills, headache, and malaise are associated with an erythematous macular or papular rash. A serious arthritis can involve the large joints, and regional adenopathy is common. A small abscess may develop at the bite site. *Spirillum minus* has a lower incidence of arthritis and a slower healing bite wound. The differential diagnosis should include meningococcemia, gonococcemia, viral exanthems, and Rocky Mountain spotted fever. Treatment is penicillin, 600,000 units intramuscularly every 12 hours for 10 to 12 days. Tetracycline and streptomycin are alternatives in the penicillin-allergic patient. Rarely, endocarditis complicates the illness.

CAT SCRATCH DISEASE. This disease is most common in children and adolescents, especially during the winter months. It may arise from a bite or scratch from any pet or from a splinter. After 3 to 30 days, an inflamed papule or pustule appears at the site of inoculation and persists for several weeks (Fig. 31–10). Regional lymphadenopathy, which may suppurate and drain, develops without intervening lymphangitis. Fever and malaise are common, but systemic dissemination is unusual.[62]

The causative organism is unknown, although gram-negative rods are visible on sections of affected lymph nodes.[63,64] Exposure to a pet, the clinical symptoms, and failure to isolate an organism from aspirated pus help establish a presumptive diagnosis. The histologic picture of stellate abscesses surrounded by epithelioid cells is suggestive, and a positive delayed hypersensitivity response to an intradermal skin test (Hanger-Rose test) with an easily prepared antigen is diagnostic. All the causes of a local skin lesion with regional adenopathy must be considered in the differential diagnosis (see Table 31–16).

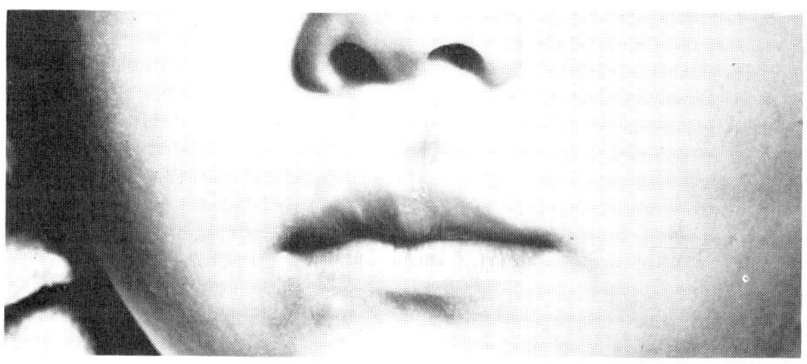

Figure 31–10. Pustule of cat scratch disease at site of inoculation. *(From Armed Forces Institute of Pathology, Neg No. 56-12797.)*

There is no specific treatment, although gentamicin has been administered.[64] The disease is usually self-limited, but adenopathy may persist. Fluctuant nodes are aspirated with an 18-gauge needle, and repeat aspiration may be necessary. Surgical drainage sometimes results in sinus tract formation.

Ulcer Infections

Infections can occur either as a result of inoculation of mixed bacteria into skin and subcutaneous tissue producing an ulcerating primary infection (phagedenic ulcer), or by secondary infection of a chronic open wound caused by systemic illness, local trauma, or tissue ischemia.

Table 31–13 lists the noninfectious causes of skin ulceration. All these ulcers can become secondarily infected and produce cellulitis or subcutaneous abscesses or can progress to the gangrenous infections discussed in a subsequent section.[39,65–67] The secondary infections can be caused by any ambient pathogen, but mixed aerobic and anaerobic infections are most common.

Infections in Malignant Ulcers. Marked bacterial colonization occurs in ulcerated malignant lesions. The ulcers are characteristically grayish with an adherent eschar and a foul smell, yet systemic sepsis is uncommon. In one study of 70 patients, only one blood culture was positive, but an average of four bacterial species were recovered per patient, two-thirds of which were anaerobes (principally *Bacteroides*).[67]

These infections usually respond to antibiotics effective against mixed enteric bacteria. Subsequent resection of the tumor mass prevents recurrence.

Infections in Decubitus Ulcers. Decubitus ulcers are commonly located in proximity to the anus, and anaerobic conditions are present because of tissue necrosis and undermining. In addition, patients with decubitus ulcers are typically debilitated, bedridden, and soiled with feces.

Mitchell[68] reported 24 cases of decubitus ulcers yielding enteric gram-negative facultative organisms, staphylococci, aerobic and anaerobic streptococci, and gram-negative anaerobes—especially *Bacteroides*.

Galpin et al[39] reported 21 patients with systemic sepsis that had begun within a decubitus ulcer with undermined edges. Infection had spread in the fascial cleft beneath apparently normal skin (see subsequent section on necrotizing fasciitis). Ten of the twenty-one patients died in spite of antibiotic treatment and surgical debridement.[39] The undermining and necrosis must be recognized before systemic sepsis supervenes.

Local care includes reducing local pressure, maceration, and fecal contamination. Ulcer excision and primary closure are sometimes effective if thick normal tissue can be used for coverage of bony prominences. Undermined margins of the ulcer suggest a synergistic aerobic and anaerobic infection spreading under apparently normal skin. The presence of multiple contiguous skin ulcers is another clue to the undermining.[39] Osteomyelitis is a common complication and impairs chances of local cure.

Infections of the Diabetic Foot (See Chap. 54)

Pathogenesis. The foot of the diabetic patient is particularly prone to primary soft tissue infections and to ischemic or neuropathic ulceration with secondary infections.[68]

Diabetic patients suffer both large and small vessel disease. Thrombosis of large vessels results in necrosis of a large segment of the leg, which can become secondarily infected. Occlusion of the smaller vessels results in patchy necrotic areas, especially of the toes. Small vessel disease also leads to atrophic skin changes that, after minor trauma, may ulcerate and become infected. An additional type of vascular disease is caused by emboli to the small peripheral vessels from atheromata in the larger vessels.[66]

Although the ischemic changes associated with angiopathy are important, neuropathy is ultimately responsible for most diabetic foot problems that lead to infection. Loss of pain and temperature sensation permits painless trauma of the ischemic foot leading to ulceration. Loss of sensation also produces bone changes such as Charcot's joint or osteolysis, which in turn cause the foot to become deformed. Foot deformities also occur because of muscle atrophy secondary to motor nerve neuropathy. With changes in the configuration of the foot, the gait is altered and new pressure points are created, resulting in ulceration of these points.

Autonomic neuropathy, with an absence of sweating, leads to a dry, cracked skin that may become secondarily infected. Orthostatic hypotension, a complication of autonomic neuropathy, can lead to a decrease in perfusion of these vessels, impairing healing and permitting infection to take hold.

Diabetics are subject to a variety of dermatologic problems that impair local defenses, including eruptive xanthoma, diabetic dermopathy, xanthochromia, necrobiosis lipoidica diabeticorum, bullous diabeticorum, and pruritus. The last three can be associated with cutaneous trauma and ulceration, which subsequently lead to infection.

Diabetics also tend to develop cardiac and renal failure with peripheral edema. This will complicate existing foot problems, impair healing, and increase susceptibility of the foot to infection.

Although the diabetic patient is subject to minor unperceived trauma that leads directly to ulceration of the ischemic foot, the cutaneous fungi and bacteria ultimately lead to infection. There are few differences in the skin flora of diabetics and nondiabetics. Diabetics do not carry pathogenic organisms or yeasts more frequently on the normal skin. Erythrasma, however, occurs more frequently in the diabetic than in normal young adults, and in some studies dermatophytosis of the interdigital areas of the feet is more common in diabetics.

Serious infections are often preceded by minor infections of the toenails, nail beds, and adjacent structures. The fungus invades the distal nail first and disrupts the normal nail-plate—nail bed attachment, permitting air to collect under the nail. As the disease progresses, the fungus invades along the stratum corneum of the nail bed and the excessive horn produced elevates the nail plate. Secondary bacterial invasion by *Pseudomonas* and *Proteus* species is common.

There is little evidence for systemic defects in host defense in the well-controlled diabetic.[69] Hyperglycemia and acidosis do interfere with neutrophil function, but most evidence supports the integrity of host defense—except at the local level, where blood supply and sensation are impaired. It is important to understand the relationship between infection and tissue ischemia in diabetes. Regional infections increase the tissue turgor and metabolic rate of the local tissues. Tissue demand for oxygen is thus increased in the face of relative ischemia. Infection further increases extravascular tissue tension and attracts neutrophils, which release tissue-destructive enzymes. Local thrombosis of small vessels then occurs, perpetuating the vicious cycle.

Etiology. Anaerobic bacteria play an important role in the pathogenesis of diabetic foot infections. Vascular insufficiency creates anaerobic conditions within neuropathic ulcers. Gas in the infected tissues is common. Louie et al[37] cultured the foot ulcers of 20 diabetic patients. Each ulcer yielded an average of 5.8 species per specimen (3.2 aerobes and 2.6 anaerobes). The principal isolates were *Bacteroides* species (17), peptococci (16), *Proteus* species (11), enterococci (9), *S. aureus* (7), clostridia (7), and *E. coli* (6). *Staphylococcus aureus* was found in only 7 of the 20 patients and never in pure culture. Sapico and associates have found similar data.[70] Cultures and sensitivity tests should always be done, preferably utilizing biopsy material, especially if bone is involved. The choice of antibiotics should be broad enough to cover this extensive array of organisms.

Clinical Manifestations. The initial event in diabetic foot infections is a break in the skin followed by penetration of bacteria. These infections begin in subcutaneous tissue (level 2) and readily spread to deeper planes. Certain lesions are typical:

1. The initial break in the skin frequently originates near nails deformed by trauma, fungus infection, or systemic disease in the neuropathic foot. Infections in the nail bed spread on the dorsal and lateral aspects of the toes, blocked from reaching the pad of the toe by fibrous septa that extend from dermis to periosteum. Treatment may require removal of the nail, which must be done cautiously.
2. Toe deformities caused by neurologic imbalances produce characteristic ulcers at the apex of the cock-up deformity or on the callus overlying hammertoes. Infection can spread along the muscles of the great toe to infect the midplantar space.
3. Web infections are particularly hazardous, since they may occur without preexisting anatomic deformity. Infections in the interdigital webs frequently involve the digital arteries and can spread via the lumbrical tendons to deeper structures of the foot.
4. Mal perforans is a chronic indolent ulcer of the sole of the foot, usually over the head of the first, second, and third metatarsal. The tendon, joint, and bone are soon infected because the lesion is painless and the patient does not get off his or her feet.
5. Infections of the middle foot occur only after painless injury by penetrating objects, since the middle foot is not normally subject to pressure. Infection here spreads directly to the central plantar space.
6. Infections of the heel occur over the bony prominences of the calcaneus. When ulceration and necrosis occur in the heel, amputation is required.

Major infections of the foot are of three types (Fig. 31–11): (1) abscesses in the deep spaces of the foot especially in the central plantar space, (2) nonsuppurative phlegmon of the dorsum of the foot, and (3) mal perforans ulcer foot. The deep plantar space may become infected in several ways: direct pentration by foreign bodies in the insensate foot, web space infections extending to the bursa of the lumbrical tendons and following the tendons into the central plantar space, or extension from involvement of the flexor tendon sheath into the central plantar space. Once the infection is established in the plantar space, the characteristic signs of plantar abscess appear—bulging of the areas with loss of the longitudinal arch convexity. The sole of the foot becomes edematous. After a few days, edema of the dorsum of the foot appears, along with fever, malaise, hyperglycemia, and keto-

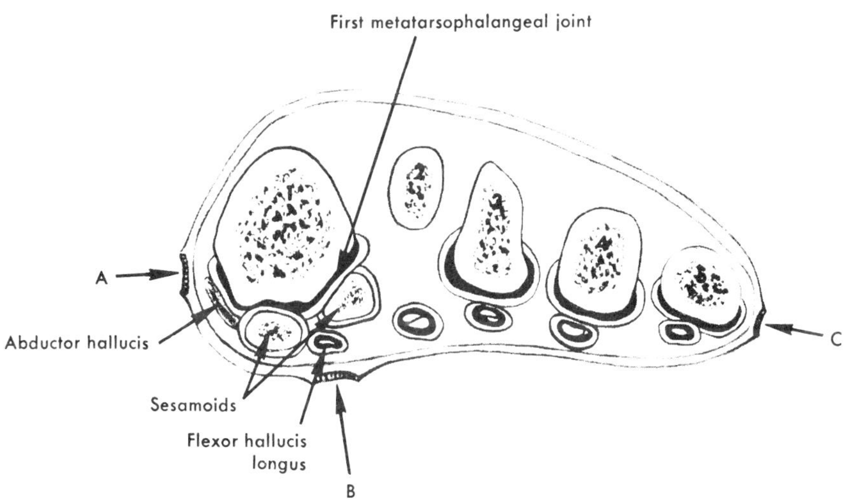

Figure 31–11. Common modes of spread of infection in distal diabetic foot. **A.** Infection from an ulcerated bunion may enter the lateral plantar space or the first metatarsophalangeal joint fairly easily. The joint infection can then penetrate into the central plantar space. **B.** Mal perforans fixes flexor tendons. With progression of infection, the plantar space, or a joint, may be entered. **C.** Ulcerated tailor's bunion finds meager tissue barrier to entry into the fifth metatarsophalangeal joint. *(From O'Neal LW: Surgical pathology of the foot and clinicopathologic correlations. In Levin ME, O'Neal LW (eds): The Diabetic Foot. St Louis, Mosby, 1977, p 108.)*

acidosis. The infection then spreads to the leg along the flexor tendons of the toes. Thrombotic obliteration of small vessels may occur and produce necrosis of the foot. This is first seen in the middle toes, since the plantar digital arteries of the second, third, and fourth toes arise from the plantar arch.

Paronychia or ulcerated calluses on hammertoes produce infections that spread easily to the dorsum of the foot via lymphatics. A dorsal foot phlegmon is produced. In the insensate foot, the infection is aggravated by the dependent position and continued activity. An infective vasculitis then produces necrosis of the skin overlying the phlegmon. Amputation is frequently required.

Osteomyelitis frequently affects the toes and small bones of the feet in diabetic patients. Systemic manifestations are few but pain, swelling, erythema, and indolent ulcers are seen. Both clinically and radiographically, it is difficult to distinguish between osteomyelitis and the osseous lesions of the foot that occur in severe diabetic peripheral neuropathy.[38] MRI scan may be helpful in questionable cases. Most cases of osteomyelitis of the foot and lower leg of these patients begin as chronic perforating ulcers, which may heal and recur repeatedly for years because the predisposing factors resist treatment. In an unhealing ulcer, bacterial invasion may progress at the base of a lesion by spreading along fascia planes or by penetrating fascia and soft tissues to reach the periosteum (see Fig. 31–11).

Treatment. Cellulitis should be treated with broad-spectrum antibiotics (cephamandole, cefoxitin, cefotetan, ampicillin/sulbactam, or gentamicin plus clindamycin), although penicillin is often effective. The foot should be elevated and the diabetes controlled. Abscesses must be drained and necrotic tissue debrided. If the blood supply of the foot is intact or can be restored, the ulcer may heal. Amputation should be avoided because it subjects the opposite foot to further pressure, which can ultimately lead to a second amputation.[66] Many plantar ulcers heal rapidly after metatarsal head resection.[72]

Prevention. Many of the abnormalities in the diabetic foot will ultimately lead to infection as neuropathy progresses and vascular flow is further impaired. Good podiatric treatment and follow-up can minimize many of these problems without reconstructive surgery. Whenever vascular supply is good and healing prompt, correction of the basic deformity should be considered. Ingrown nails, incurving nails, bunions, calluses, and hammertoes do not improve spontaneously. Distal in situ bypass with restoration of tissue perfusion is indicated in selected patients.

Phagedenic Ulcers. Soft tissue inoculation of mixed organisms typically causes cellulitis or abscess, but in some patients the same organisms cause progressive burrowing lesions characterized by a peripheral zone of intense redness and swelling with a central area of leathery skin necrosis. With time the eschar ulcerates, exposing fatty tissue or even fascia. The factors that trigger this unique response are unknown. Collectively, these ulcerating infections have been called phagedenic ulcers. *Mycobacterium ulcerans* causes a similar cutaneous infection (see subsequent section on mycobacterial infections).

Meleney Ulcer. Meleney ulcer (bacterial synergistic gangrene) is an infection primarily of subcutaneous tissue with overlying skin necrosis and rarely spreading along fascial planes. These level 2 infections can be caused by streptococci and staphylococci or mixed enteric organisms (see Table 31–7).

Meleney[73] described the combination of a microaerophilic staphylococcus, found primarily in the periphery of the lesion, and *S. aureus* in the central zone of necrosis (see Chap. 7). The streptococcus is probably *S. evolutus*.[74] Meleney produced the infection experimentally only with the combination of both bacteria, proving the synergistic etiology.[73] More commonly, mixed facultative and anaerobic enteric organisms are isolated from these infections, especially in postoperative wounds or ischemic feet of diabetics.

Meleney ulcer develops most often following abdominal surgery or following a trivial accidental wound in ischemic tissue. The lesion first appears about 2 weeks after wounding, in an area around a suture or wound closure. A purple central area of induration becomes surrounded by a zone of erythema. Pain and tenderness are pronounced. As the lesion progresses, three zones become demarcated: (1) the outer zone is fiery red; (2) the middle zone is purple and tender; and (3) the central portion of the purplish area becomes necrotic, the color changing to a dirty gray-brown or a yellow-green with a typical suede leather appearance.[75] As the lesion spreads outward, the inner margin becomes undermined and ulcerates. Eventually, the center of the lesion becomes a granulating ulcer (Fig. 31–12). The progression is slow but unremitting. The depth is usually limited to the upper third of the subcutaneous fat and rarely extends deep to fascia. Satel-

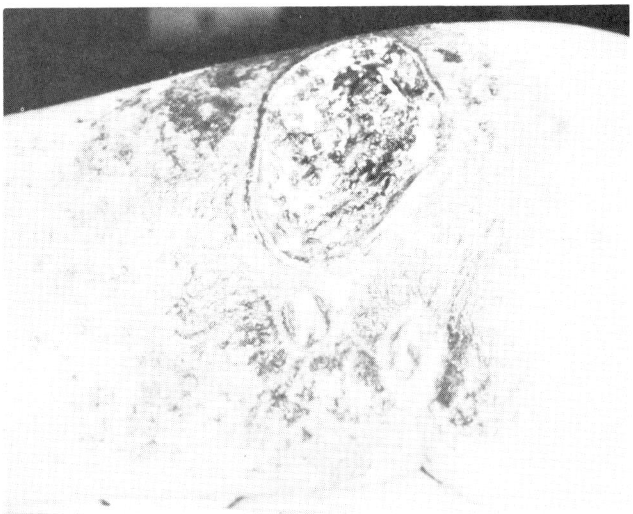

Figure 31–12. Meleney ulcer central necrosis with undermining edges, a purple irregular border, and an outer zone of redness. Satellite lesions surround the ulcer. *(From Baxter CR: Surg Clin North Am 52:1483, 1972.)*

lite lesions may surface as the infection tunnels through the fat. Fever is minimal, but anemia and malnutrition are common.

Antibiotics effective against staphylococci and streptococci, or against mixed enteric bacteria, are indicated, combined with debridement of leathery eschar. Topical silver sulfadiazine or mafenide may also be used.[75] Radical excision is no longer indicated if the tissue is not ischemic. Grainger et al[76] have reported a remarkable response to hyperbaric oxygen therapy in two patients treated concurrently with parenteral antibiotics.

Tropical Ulcer. Tropical ulcer is a similar chronic sloughing ulcer that may take on a more invasive character and that seldom heals spontaneously.[74] The disease is found in all tropical and subtropical regions of Africa, Asia, and the Americas.

Oral flora are found in the wounds. The fusiform bacilli (anerobic gram-negative rods) and a spirochete morphologically identical to *Treponema (Borrelia) vincentii* apparently play a synergistic role (see Chap. 7), but secondary bacterial infection is common.

Tropical ulcer generally affects the ankle and dorsum of the foot.[77] A small painful papule surrounded by a deeply infiltrated dusky red zone soon progresses to a pustule and then to an ulcer, which enlarges in depth and breadth (5 to 10 cm). The margins of the ulcer are flat, and undermining is not prominent, but the base is necrotic, purulent, and foul smelling. The surrounding areas are edematous, but tenderness is minimal. Gradually, the ulcer may extend into deeper structures to destroy muscle, tendon, and periosteum. Untreated lesions commonly reach a diameter of 5 to 10 cm and may persist for years without endangering life.[74]

Fusiform bacilli and spirochetes are abundant in smears from the ulcer base, but secondary colonization of ambient bacteria confuses the picture. Cutaneous diptheria, *M. ulcerans,* and cutaneous leishmaniasis present similar lesions.

Topical therapy, including tyrothricin and combinations of streptomycin, bacitracin, and polymixin, is said to be effective. Systemic penicillin, tetracycline, chloramphenicol, and metronidazole are all very effective.[78] Bed rest, elevation, conservative debridement, plus antibiotic therapy will heal small ulcers and permit skin grafting of larger ones.

Noma. Noma (gangrenous stomatitis, cancrum oris) is a term used to designate all necrotizing infections caused by oral flora involving mucous membranes or mucocutaneous orifices.[74] Although noma occurs most frequently about the mouth, it may also affect the nose, auditory canal, vulva, prepuce, or anus. It is the head and neck equivalent of tropical ulcer.

Fusiform bacilli and spirochetes are found in these lesions. *Prevotella melaninogenica* can be isolated from some specimens, and Emslie[79] has suggested this organism may be a key pathogen in mixed fusospirochete-anaerobic infections.

Children with predisposing systemic disease, malnutrition, poor oral hygeine, measles, smallpox, malaria, and parasitic infections are most often affected. Herpetic gingivostomatitis may trigger acute ulcerative gingivitis and then noma. Adults in concentration camps or with oral carcinomas are occasionally afflicted.[74]

The constitutional symptoms of noma are initially mild, followed by sudden onset of fever, apathy, weakness, and prostration. The odor of the breath or dull red spots on the cheeks may be the first indication of the disease. Inspection of the mouth reveals a dark greenish black area on the gum or buccal mucosa. The surrounding tissues are reddened and swollen to two or three times the normal size. There is an extremely offensive odor. The destructive process progresses with great rapidity, attacking the periosteum and underlying bone. The gums are destroyed, the teeth fall out (Fig. 31–13), and large bony sequestra slough away. In untreated cases, the process may involve the entire mouth and nose, with almost complete destruction of the

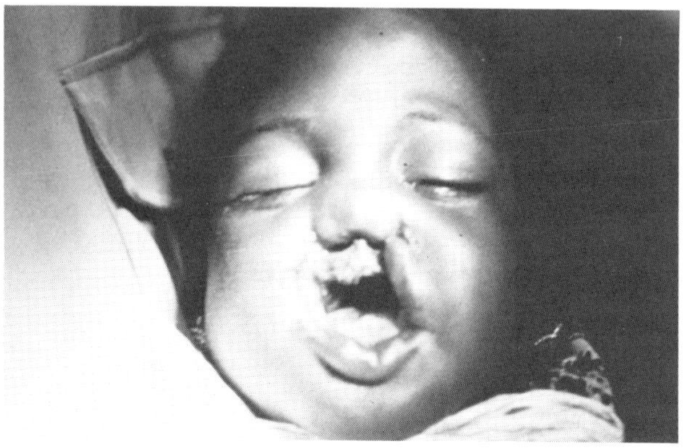

Figure 31–13. Noma (gangrenous stomatitis) of the mouth of an infant. *(From Armed Forces Institute of Pathology, Neg. No. 68-741-3.)*

face before death. The usual duration of the disease without therapy is 5 to 10 days. There is little or no pain, and children sometimes push their fingers through the necrotic areas of the cheek. Hemorrhage is rare because of thrombosis of this area. After treatment, the affected tissue is ultimately sloughed.[74]

Before antimicrobial therapy, the mortality was 70 to 100 percent, and patients who survived had virtually irreparable defects. Intensive penicillin therapy is the best treatment.

BACTERIAL INFECTIONS OF THE FASCIAL CLEFT (LEVEL 3)

The plethora of names applied to necrotizing level 3 infections is of strictly historical significance, because the surgical treatment is the same for each;[14,80] the antibiotic regimens are determined by the infecting organisms. So many terms have been used to describe these infections of the fascia that most surgeons have become hopelessly confused. Necrotizing fasciitis is currently used as the generic term for lack of a better one.

The manifestations depend on the infecting organisms and anatomic location of the infection, modified somewhat by impaired host defenses. There is a variable degree of necrosis of subcutaneous tissues, with hemorrhage, vasculitis, and thrombosis of small arteries and veins and infiltration by polymorphonuclear leukocytes. In clostridial infections, leukocytes are notably absent and gas is abundant. The presence of gas in tissue, previously considered pathognomonic of clostridial infections, implies either mechanically induced air or anaerobic bacterial metabolism that has produced insoluble gases such as hydrogen, nitrogen, and methane (see Table 31–18). Both facultative and obligate anaerobes are capable of such a metabolic activity. These infections occur after inoculation of infecting organisms deep into the tissues. The precipitating event is usually obvious—a crush injury, an operative incision, enterotomy stoma, or a secondarily infected cutaneous ulcer. Perineal fistulas are less visible but common sources of infection. More rarely, rupture of a viscus into the subcutaneous tissues of the abdomen, perineum, or thigh can occur, or infection can begin at a site of an embolic infection in immunodepressed patients.

The extent of skin necrosis is variable. Necrotizing fasciitis from mixed aerobes and anaerobes typically spreads in the fascial cleft between the subcutaneous tissue and deep fascia, sparing the major vessels within the subcutaneous tissue and preserving extensive areas of skin. Debridement can frequently be carried out without removing all the skin. In contrast, streptococcal fasciitis leads to widespread necrosis of all the skin if treatment is delayed.

Streptococcal Necrotizing Fasciitis

Acute streptococcal necrotizing fasciitis, "necrotizing erysipelas," is caused by *S. pyogenes,* Lancefield group A (beta-hemolytic streptococci). Although Meleney first described the condition and its treatment in 1924, the condition was probably the "hospital gangrene" of the Civil War.

Incidence and Epidemiology. Acute streptococcal gangrene is currently a rare disease. Typically, a surgical wound of an extremity is affected, but any region can be infected with or without antecedent trauma.

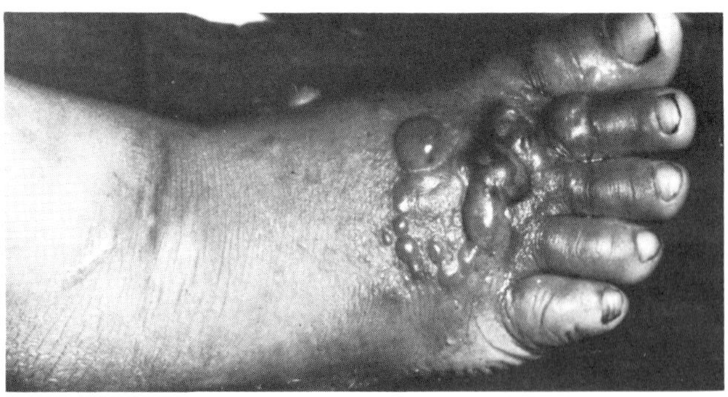

Figure 31–14. Clostridial necrotizing fasciitis of the foot. Bullae, full of black bacteria-laden fluid, are present in the skin. The infection is spreading in the fascial cleft that overlies the tendons of the foot. If tissue gas is absent, it appears clinically identical to some cases of streptococcal necrotizing fascitis. *(From Baxter CR: Surg Clin North Am 52:1483, 1972.)*

Pathogenesis. This is a fulminant form of necrotizing fasciitis that progresses to extensive skin necrosis caused by thrombosis of the blood vessels that supply the skin within the superficial fascia. Destruction of cutaneous nerves may produce local anesthesia. Meleney[81] first believed this disease was an allergic or Shwartzman type of reaction, but it is more likely that the dermal infection is due to a tendency of the streptococcus organism to affect vascular structures of all types (see Chap. 4).

Clinical Manifestations. The clinical course is fulminating. Initially, there is an intense cellulitis around a site of minor trauma or a superficial wound. The affected skin is hot, red, swollen, and extremely painful at first. Fever, chills, tachycardia, and prostration are also present. Within 2 to 4 days, the skin develops dusky, irregular patches and large bullae containing bacteria and a dark exudate (Fig. 31–14). Without treatment, these areas progress to full-thickness cutaneous necrosis and burn-like eschar. Muscle and bone are generally spared. The undermining nature of the infection is recognized by passing a probe without resistance along the fascial plane (Fig. 31–15). Extension through deep fascia can produce myonecrosis and compartmental hypertension. Fasciotomy may be required even if the muscle is not affected. If the untreated patient survives, the slough separates from the underlying tissue in 2 to 3 weeks.

Diagnosis. The differential diagnosis must include clostridial myonecrosis, erysipelas, and cellulitis. The blister fluid will frequently slow gram-positive streptococci on smear. Gas and odor are notably absent. Lymphangitis is uncommon.

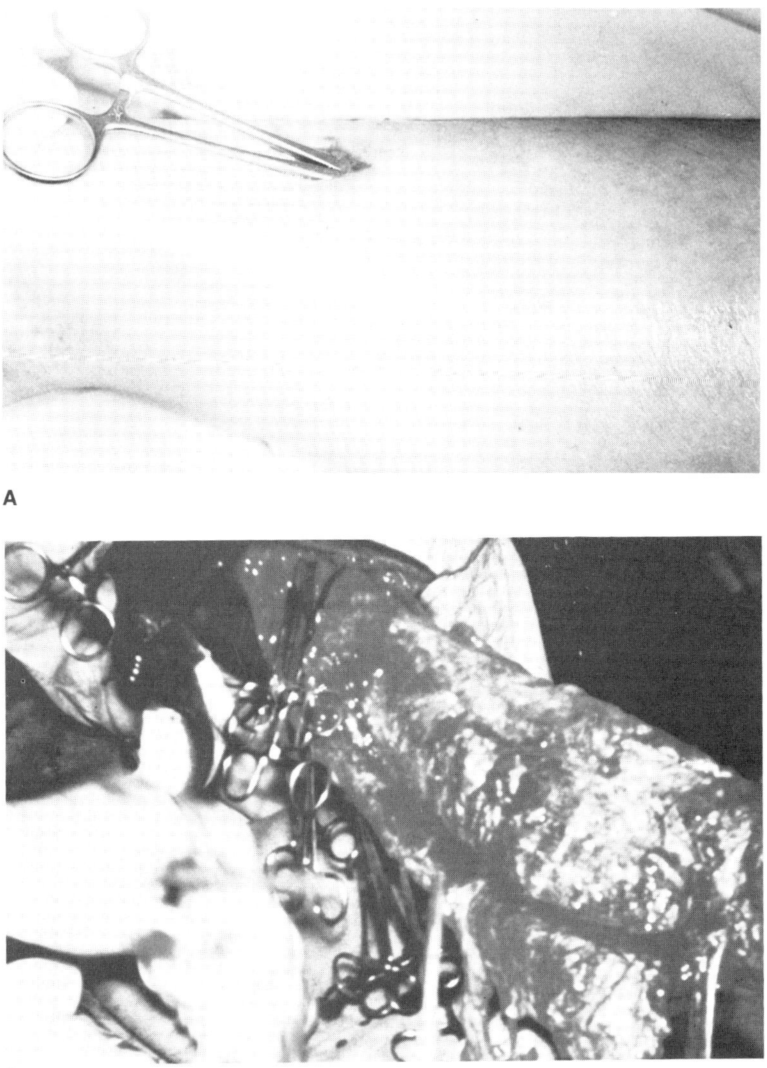

A

B

Figure 31–15. Necrotizing fasciitis. **A.** A probe can be passed along the fascial cleft between the subcutaneous tissue and deep fascia in a patient in whom only a small draining tract is visible. *(From Baxter CR: Surg Clin North Am 52:1483, 1972.)* **B.** Incision reveals extensive necrosis of subcutaneous tissue and fascia. *(Courtesy of P. William Curreri, MD, New York Hospital, Cornell Medical Center, New York.)*

Treatment. High-dose parenteral penicillin G is the treatment of choice, always in conjunction with fluid resuscitation and emergency surgical debridement. An incision along the entire length of the undermined areas should be carried down to the muscles (Fig. 31–14). All the necrotic tissue is excised and undermined, but viable skin is not removed. Some authors spare patent blood vessels to minimize more extensive skin loss.

After incision and debridement through the superficial fascia, the wound is treated by rest, elevation, and frequent dressing changes, which aid in the mechanical debridement. If infection progresses, repeated debridement may be necessary. Skin grafting can be carried out in denuded areas when a granulating base appears. Amputation is especially common in diabetics.

Necrotizing Fasciitis

Definition. Although the term *necrotizing fasciitis* originally described level 3 streptococcal infection,[81] currently it is applied to mixed bacterial infections. Forms of necrotizing fasciitis include streptococcal gangrene, clostridial cellulitis, nonclostridial anaerobic cellulitis, anaerobic cutaneous gangrene, Fournier gangrene, and synergistic necrotizing cellulitis, all having a similar pathogenesis, treatment, and prognosis. Each is an infection of the subcutaneous tissues that spreads in the fascial clefts overlying deep fascia. Skin necrosis results only after the vessels to the skin thrombose. Each of these syndromes was originally described separately, and terminology is hopelessly confusing.

Skin necrosis also occurs with purpura fulminans, triggered by meningococcal septicemia.[82] The patchy areas of necrosis result from disseminated intravascular coagulation and embolic skin infarction. Bacteria are not present in the lesions unless secondary infection occurs. Eschar debridement and skin grafting are indicated.

Etiology. A variety of organisms have been reported as predominant in these infections, including beta-hemolytic streptococcus,[81] often combined with the hemolytic staphylococcus,[83] halophilic marine vibrios,[84] and gram-negative mixed enteric organisms.[85] Rea and Wyrick[85] confirmed that mixtures of bacteria were typical but inadequate collection or laboratory bacteriology techniques frequently failed to document the mixed etiology of this infection.

Current data confirm necrotizing fasciitis is most often a synergistic bacterial surgical infection, produced by the combination of gram-positive cocci and gram-negative bacilli. Both aerobes and anaerobes are typically found. Tables 31–22 and 31–23 list the bacteria cultured from 16 patients with necrotizing fasciitis by Giuliano et al.[83] A total of 75 bacterial species were identified in the 16 patients (Table 31–22). At least one facultative *Streptococcus* was recovered from fifteen patients, a *Bacteroides* species was recovered from ten, and a *Peptostreptococcus* from eight. Giuliano et al[83] concluded

TABLE 31–22. BACTERIA CULTURED FROM NECROTIZING FASCIITIS[a]

Bacteria	Total Number of Isolates
Anaerobic Bacteria (*Gram-Positive*)	
Peptostreptococcus species	8
Peptococcus species	4
Eubacterium species	1
Propionibacterium species	4
Clostridium perfringens	3
Clostridium (not perfringens)	1
Anaerobic Bacteria (*Gram-Negative*)	
Bacteroides (total)	15
B. melaninogenicus	5
B. fragilis	2
B. corrodens	2
B. species	6
Fusobacterium necrophorum	1
Facultative Bacteria	
Streptococcus (total)	22
S. pyogenes (group A)	3
S. agalactiae (group B)	1
Streptococcus (group D) enterococcus	4
S. bovis	2
S. angiosus (group F)	1
Streptococcus, beta-hemolytic (not group A, B, or F)	3
S. intermedius	1
Streptococcus, alpha-hemolytic (not group D)	7
Staphylococcus aureus	0
S. epidermidis	1
Enterobacteriaceae (total)	12
Escherichia coli	4
Citrobacter freundii	1
Klebsiella pneumoniae	2
Enterobacter cloacae	2
Serratia marcescens	2
Proteus mirabilis	1
Aerobic Bacteria	
Pseudomonas aeruginosa	2

[a] All bacteria isolated from each specimen are counted in this table. Individual patient's cultures may contain more than one *Bacteroides,* Enterobacteriaceae, or other group.
From Giuliano A, Lewis F Jr, Hadley K, Blaisdell FW: Am J Surg 134:52, 1977.

TABLE 31–23. BACTERIAL ASSOCIATIONS OBSERVED IN 16 CASES OF NECROTIZING FASCIITIS

	Frequency	All Str, Not Group D	Group D Str	aH Str Not Group D	Group A Str	S	E	B	C	P	PS
Frequency		12	4	6	3	2	9	10	4	4	8
Bacteroides (B)	10	10	4	6	0	0	6	—	2	4	7
Fusobacterium	1	1	1	1	0	0	1	1	1	1	1
Clostridium (C)	4	3	3	1	0	0	4	2	—	0	1
Propionibacterium	4	4	1	3	0	0	2	3	0	2	4
Peptococcus (P)	4	4	1	3	0	0	2	4	0	—	4
Peptostreptococcus (PS)	8	8	2	5	0	0	5	7	1	4	—

When more than one organism of a genus or group is isolated from one specimen, it is counted only once in this table. Str, streptococcus; aH, alpha-hemolytic; S, staphylococcus; E, Enterobacteriaceae.
From Giuliano A, Lewis F Jr, Hadley K, Blaisdell FW: Am J Surg 134:52, 1977.

that there are two types of necrotizing fasciitis. Most commonly, anaerobic bacteria and facultative bacteria (Enterobacteriaceae and streptococci other than group A) act in combination; anaerobes are rarely cultured alone. In the second group, group A *Streptococcus* was isolated alone or in combination with *S. aureus* or *S. epidermidis* representing classic streptococcal gangrene (see preceding section). Howard et al[84] have added marine vibrios as a cause of necrotizing fasciitis.[86]

Giuliano's patients[83] were primarily drug addicts with infections of the upper extremities, trunk, and shoulders, whereas the patients of Stone and Martin[85] were debilitated bedridden patients, frequently with diabetes, with infections of the lower extremities, trunk, and perineal regions. Most had muscle (level 4) involvement. No beta-hemolytic streptococci were found, but there was a higher incidence of facultative gram-negative bacilli (62 percent) and enterococcus (19 percent) in combination with anaerobic *Streptococcus* (51 percent) and *Bacteroides* species (24 percent).

Pathogenesis and Pathology. The infection begins with a break in the skin or mucosa—the subcutaneous or intravenous injection of illicit drugs, an incised wound, an enterostomy, a decubitus ulcer, perineal fistula, or diabetic foot. In neonates with omphalitis, 10 percent may develop necrotizing fasciitis.[87] Diabetes, cardiovascular and renal disease, or starvation or obesity are also risk factors.[85] In drug addicts, extremity infections are usually caused by oral flora rather than the bacteria contaminating the street heroin.[88] In other patients, infections of the trunk, perineum, buttocks, and thighs represent the spread of infection from previously infected sites that had been overlooked or ignored. Phycomycotic gangrene[89] must be considered in all such infections.

Most infections require two or more bacteria to synergistically produce this disease (see Chap. 7). Group A *S. pyogenes* and halophilic *Vibrio* species are capable of producing a necrotizing fasciitis alone.

Clinical Manifestations. The course of necrotizing fasciitis varies. Usually the portal of entry is obvious—the site of trauma, postoperative wound infection, or extension from a previous site of primary infection, ie, perirectal abscess, infected decubitus ulcer, infected diabetic ulcer. It may remain an indolent undermining infection or may become suddenly fulminant and rapidly progress to hypovolemia and death.

In the chronic progressive type, skin redness and swelling predominate. Multiple skin ulcers drain a thin, reddish-brown, foul-smelling fluid characterized as "dishwater pus."[85] Multiple ulcers communicate beneath a superficially normal, but extensively undermined, intervening skin. Crepitance in the soft tissues is frequent, and sensation may range from exquisite local tenderness to anesthesia.

The diagnosis is easily made by passing a probing instrument through the area of necrosis and determining that undermining exists between the subcutaneous tissue and deep fascia (see Fig. 31–15). In simple cellulitis or abscess, such a probing instrument cannot be passed laterally into the fascial cleft.

Frank pus is an unusual finding despite widespread deep necrosis, which is overlooked until the patient is admitted with symptoms and signs of septicemia. At that time, blood cultures are frequently positive. The factors that foster a septicemic rather than an indolent outcome are unknown—but diabetes, anemia, and renal failure are commonly found.

At the other clinical extreme, patients present with extensive areas of cutaneous necrosis with patchy areas of dusky skin progressing to frank eschar formation or bullae (see Fig. 31–14). These patients also demonstrate fever, chills, and shock, but the local process is obvious.

Numerous terms have been applied to these necrotizing infections. Some deserve special comment.

1. *Clostridial necrotizing fasciitis* (*clostridial anaerobic cellulitis*) is a necrotizing clostridial infection of devitalized subcutaneous tissues without involvement of deep fascia or muscle.[80] Gas formation is often extensive. Clostridial species, usually *C. perfringens* or *C. septicum,* can be seen on Gram stain and culture. The infection is usually found at the sites of dirty or inadequately debrided traumatic wounds, especially around the perineum, abdominal wall, buttocks, and lower extremities, that is, areas contaminated with fecal flora. A dark, foul-smelling drainage, often containing fat globules, has been described; frank crepitus seems to extend widely beyond the areas of active infection. X-rays of soft tissue show abundant gas. Sometimes, the clostridia are present in mixed culture with facultative organisms. The operative treatment is identical to necrotizing fasciitis. Adequate surgical treatment of traumatic wounds prevents this disease.
2. *Nonclostridial necrotizing fasciitis* (nonclostridial anaerobic cellulitis, synergistic necrotizing cellulitis) may present an identical clinical picture to clostridial necrotizing fasciitis, with abundant gas formation. Anaerobic organisms predominate. A more virulent form presents with systemic toxicity and bacteremia occurring in patients with diabetes mellitus, obesity, advanced age, and cardiorenal disease.[85] Most infections are located on the lower extremities or near the perineum. Bacteremia and death are common.
3. *Fournier disease* (*Fournier gangrene*)[90] occurs about the male genitals (idiopathic gangrene of the scrotum, streptococcal scrotal gangrene, perineal phlegmon (Fig. 31–16). It involves the scrotum and surrounding perineum, penis, and abdominal wall in patients with diabetes, local trauma, paraphimosis, periurethral extravasation of urine, and perirectal or perineal infections and may follow operation in the area. The rapidly spreading scrotal skin necrosis of the skin is due to interruption of the blood supply by spreading perineal necrotizing fasciitis. The organisms are those seen in necrotizing fasciitis in this region, including facultative enteric organisms (*E. coli, Klebsiella,* enterococci) and anaerobes (*Bacteroides, Fusobacterium,* clostridia, anaerobic peptostreptococci) (see Chap. 49). The prognosis is somewhat better than other forms of perineal necrotizing fasciitis, because rapid necrosis of scrotal skin leads to early diagnosis and treatment.[91]

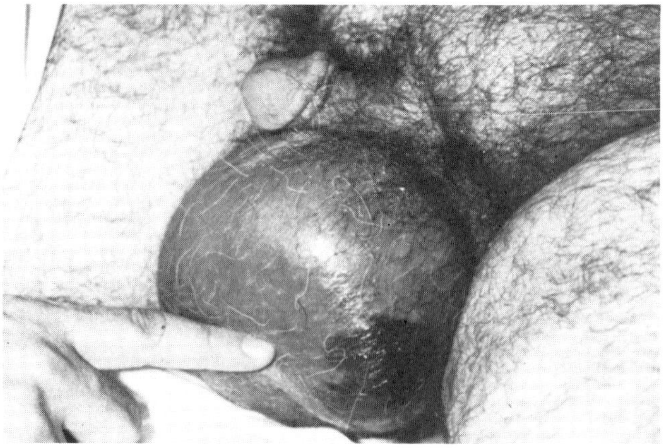

Figure 31–16. Fournier gangrene is necrotizing fasciitis of the scrotum and perineum with a patch of skin necrosis. *(Courtesy of Charles A. Kallick, MD, Cook County Hospital, Chicago.)*

Diagnosis. The diagnosis is usually made on clinical findings (see Table 31–18). The causative agents are readily found on Gram stain of the exudate. Most often mixed gram-positive and gram-negative organisms are found except in patients with streptococcal, clostridial, or *Vibrio* infections. Phycomycotic infections may have a similar presentation, but the diagnosis is confirmed by the histopathologic picture.[89]

Stamenkovic and Lew[92] note the frequent delay in diagnosis and suggest that frozen section examination of tissue biopsy specimens will lead to earlier diagnosis and treatment. Characteristic findings include neutrophil infiltration with fascial necrosis, deep vascular thrombosis, and intact overlying dermis. Mortality was 12.5 percent in patients with diagnosis made within 4 days (usually on the basis of a biopsy) versus 73 percent if the diagnosis was delayed more than 4 days.

Treatment. Infections of the trunk, perineum, perirectal area, buttock, and thigh frequently involve four types of organisms: Enterobacteriaceae, enterococci, anaerobic streptococci, and *Bacteroides*. In these potentially fatal infections, a combination of an aminoglycoside for the Enterobacteriaceae, clindamycin or metronidazole for the anaerobes, and ampicillin for enterococci and peptostreptococci has been standard.[80] Tally and Gorbach[93] note four other classes of antibiotics that may be effective in mixed infections: (1) chloramphenicol, (2) semisynthetic penicillins (carbenicillin, ticarcillin, piperacillin) usually combined with an aminoglycoside, (3) broad spectrum cephalosporins with anaerobic activity (cefoxitin, moxalactam), and (4) imipenem/cilastatin. A more detailed examination of the efficacy of the agents is found in the discussion of peritonitis (see Chap. 38). However, the exceptional beta-lactamase resistance of imipenem and its efficacy in early clinical trials[94] suggest that it may be the agent of choice if only a single agent is used. Chloramphenicol is highly effective but is potentially toxic. Penicillin G in large doses is effective for clostridial or beta-hemolytic streptococcal necrotizing fasciitis.

Blood culture results are frequently positive in patients with necrotizing fasciitis. Antibiotic therapy should be based on the presumptive mixed flora of the wound, since clinical laboratories occasionally fail to recover the anaerobes from a mixed infection.

The primary therapy of necrotizing fasciitis is urgent radical debridement. Bongard et al[95] have used a fluorometric probe after intravenous fluorescein to map the areas of least skin viability in planning debridement incisions. The goal is maximal preservation of viable skin flaps. The incisions should extend to expose normal fascia in all planes. Necrotic soft tissue is resected, but perfused skin flaps are preserved after removal of nonviable fat (see Fig. 31–14). The wounds are packed loosely open with fine mesh gauze, and several small catheters can be placed in the wound for infusion of local antibiotics. Baxter[96] recommends a solution containing 100 mg of neomycin and 100 mg of polymyxin per liter of normal saline. Other authors recommend less toxic agents or none at all.[80]

The fine mesh gauze should be changed frequently during the first days after the operation. In stable patients, hydrotherapy speeds removal of purulent and necrotic material. For toxic patients with ongoing infection, exploration with the patient under general anesthesia every 2 days is often necessary, especially in perineal or truncal infection.

Gozal et al[97] combined radical debridement and parenteral antibiotics with hyperbaric oxygen therapy in 16 patients with only a 12 percent mortality. Riseman et al[98] found the mortality from severe necrotizing fasciitis dropped from 66 percent to 23 percent when HBO therapy was added to broad spectrum antibiotics and aggressive surgical debridement. Although the HBO treated group was sicker on admission, they required fewer additional debridement procedures than the control group (1.2 versus 3.3).

In patients with uncontrolled extremity infection, an amputation may be life-saving. Guillotine amputations have a lower morbidity than primary closure procedures.[99]

Repeated cultures of the wound usually show secondary colonization with *Pseudomonas, Serratia, Candida,* or other opportunists. Mafenide (Sulfamylon) or sliver sulfadiazine can be applied, or, for clean wounds, porcine skin can be used to dress the wound. Later, the remaining skin flaps can be replaced and the open areas covered with meshed, split-thickness autograft. When full thickness of the abdominal wall has been lost, temporary placement of Marlex or Vicryl mesh prevents evisceration until the bowel loops granulate and can be skin grafted.[100] Nonabsorbable mesh left in place has a high incidence of sinus tract formation.

Prognosis. The prognosis is grave and depends in part on the underlying disease, the physiologic condition of the patient, and the organisms in the wound. Mortalities of 8 to 67 percent have been reported with a mean of 35 percent.[14,80] Younger patients, especially drug abusers, have the best prognosis. In the series of Giuliano et al[83] only 2 of 16 patients died.

Early diagnosis and treatment markedly improve the outcome. Sudarsky et al[101] report an overall mortality of 6 percent in 33 patients treated between 1983 and 1987, with no deaths or amputations in patients surgically treated within 48 hours of admission. HBO therapy may also improve survival.[97,98] Infections presenting early with scrotal gangrene (Fournier disease) have a much improved prognosis.[90,91]

A comparison of treatment results between series is possible only with system of risk stratification for these patients. The APACHE (Acute Physiology and Chronic Health Evaluation)[102] and SIS (Surgical Infection Stratification)[103] systems have been proposed to quantitatively evaluate patients with injury or intra-abdominal sepsis (see Chap.

38). Pessa and Howard[104] found that in 33 patients with necrotizing fasciitis, the 11 deaths occurred in patients with significantly higher admission scores in both systems than those of the survivors. Moreover, those patients who died had scores that increased in severity at 3 and 7 days; scores in the survivors were decreased on the same days. The scoring system identify patients at highest risk in whom the most aggressive therapy is indicated.

BACTERIAL INFECTIONS OF MUSCLE (LEVEL 4)

Infections of muscle can present major difficulties in diagnosis, because overlying skin and subcutaneous tissue may obscure the diagnosis. These infections range from relatively limited staphylococcal muscular abscess to life-threatening clostridial myonecrosis[105] (Tables 31–7 and 31–24).

Pyomyositis

Pyomyositis is a primary acute bacterial infection of skeletal muscle, usually due to *S. aureus* in the absence of apparent predisposing conditions.[105] Blood cultures are usually negative, and disseminated staphylococcal sepsis is rare.

Tropical pyomyositis is an endemic disease accounting for 1 to 4 percent of hospital admissions in some tropical areas. In the United States pyomyositis occurs rarely, except in persons who have recently immigrated from the tropics. In some cases, recent trauma to the involved areas suggests that local muscle damage predisposes to infection by transient staphylococcal bacteremia.

Etiology. The disease is usually due to *S. aureus*, with rare cases due to *S. pneumoniae* and *E. coli*. Bacteria can invade muscle either from contiguous sites or hematogenous spread. A fulminant form caused by group A streptococci[106] has been reported with an associated high mortality.

Clinical Manifestations. In the typical case, there is gradual development over several days of localized muscle pain, swelling, and tenderness. Fever generally follows the appearance of local findings, although an acute onset appears in some circumstances.

The muscles of the lower limb and trunk are most frequently affected, and a single muscle group

TABLE 31–24. CLASSIFICATION OF MUSCLE INFECTIONS (LEVEL 4)

Type of Process	Clinical Pattern	Principal Specific Etiologies
Pyogenic and predominantly localized (spreading by contiguity)	Pyomyositis	*S. aureus;* group A streptococcus (rarely);
	Clostridial myonecrosis	*C. perfringens;* occasionally other histotoxic clostridial species
	Nonclostridial myonecrosis (crepitant myositis) anaerobic streptococcal gangrene	*Peptostreptococcus* (plus group A streptococci or *S. aureus*
		Mixed infections: *Bacteroides* and other anaerobic non-spore-forming gram-negative bacilli; *Peptostreptococcus* and various streptococci; *E. coli; Klebsiella; Enterobacter*
	Infected vascular gangrene (infarcted muscle)	Same as for synergistic nonclostridial anaerobic myonecrosis
	Psoas abscess, rectus abscess	Gram-negative bacilli; *S. aureus* mixed infections; *M. tuberculosis*
Nonpyogenic and predominantly generalized	Myalgias	Viral infections (eg, influenza, dengue); infective endocarditis; bacteremias (eg, meningococcemia); rickettsioses (eg, Rocky Mountain spotted fever); toxoplasmosis
	Pleurodynia syndromes	Coxsackievirus B
	Myalgias with eosinophilia	
	Trichinosis	*Trichinella spiralis*
	Cysticercosis (also subcutaneous nodules)	*Taenia solium*
	Muscle degeneration and destruction associated with infections elsewhere	
	Acute rhabdomyolysis	Viral influenza
	Zenker degeneration	*Salmonella typhi*

From Swartz MN: Myositis. In Mandell GL, Douglas RG Jr, Bennett JE (eds): Principles and Practice of Infectious Diseases, 2nd ed. New York, John Wiley, 1985, p 614.

is usually involved. The initial local swelling is diffuse and only moderately tender. Erythema and heat appear only when the infection dissects into the subcutaneous tissues. Leukocytosis and elevation of serum muscle enzyme levels are common. Eosinophilia has been reported but may simply reflect the prevalence of concurrent parasitic infestation in patients from tropical areas.

Treatment. The abscess should be incised and evacuated. Excision is not necessary, but drainage to obtain a clean granulating cavity is essential.

Initial antibiotic therapy should be a beta-lactamase-resistant penicillin or cephalosporin to treat the presumptive *S. aureus,* which should be confirmed by culture results. Failure to improve after drainage and antibiotic therapy suggests the presence of inadequately drained sites.

Infections of Muscle Sheaths

Although experimental studies do not demonstrate that skeletal muscle is more resistant to a standard inoculum of bacteria than fat,[1] infections of viable muscle with pyogenic organisms are rare. Muscle sheaths, on the other hand, can become infected secondary to contiguous infection. Two such sheath infections are relatively common—psoas abscess and rectus sheath abscess.

Psoas Abscess. Psoas abscess is an infection confined within the psoas fascia, usually secondary to contiguous infections. Since the fascial envelope extends into the groin, the infection may point in the inguinal region. The classic cause is pyogenic or tuberculous osteomyelitis, but now it is more commonly the result of the direct extension of intra-abdominal infections, that is, diverticulitis, appendicitis, granulomatous bowel disease, or carcinoma of the colon. A perinephric abscess or secondary infection of a retroperitoneal hematoma is also a predisposing cause. *Staphylococcus aureus* is the most common cause of psoas abscess secondary to vertebral osteomyelitis, and mixed infections arise from perinephric or intraintestinal infections.

The clinical manifestations include fever, lower abdominal back pain, pain referred to the hip or knee, and associated limp. Flexion of the hip may develop from reflex spasm, suggesting septic arthritis of the hip. The psoas sign is evident, that is, pain on passive extension of the hip. Sometimes, a tender mass can be palpated in the groin, and gas may be present on x-rays of the abdomen. Calcification of the psoas abscess suggests a tuberculous etiology. The abscess cavity can be evacuated and drained through the groin or through a flank retroperitoneal approach. Antibiotic therapy and correction of the intraperitoneal source are essential.

Rectus Sheath Abscess. A rectus sheath abscess is usually secondary to a transabdominal operation in which the rectus sheath has been opened by a paramedian or transverse incision. Almost invariably, such infections are the result of extension of intra-abdominal infection or an early manifestation of an enterocutaneous fistula. Contiguous sites of sepsis should always be sought.

Clostridial Myonecrosis (Gas Gangrene)

Clostridial myonecrosis is a rapidly progressive, life-threatening, toxemic infection of skeletal muscles caused by *Clostridium* species (principally *C. perfringens*). It usually follows the contamination of severe crushing muscle injury by soil or feces. It may be part of clostridial necrotizing fasciitis, but in its classic form, muscle is principally involved. Hematogenous spread from a GI malignancy has been documented.[107]

Etiology. Clostridium perfringens is isolated from 80 to 95 percent of the cases.[106] *Clostridium novyi* is found in 10 to 40 percent, *C. septicum* in 5 to 20 percent, and *C. bifermentans, C. histolyticum,* and *C. phallax* have all been implicated. Other aerobes and facultative organisms are also usually isolated. The clinical syndromes produced are all similar. *Clostridium novyi* produce toxemia and massive gelatinous edema with little gas, while *C. septicum* is most often associated with colon carcinoma.[107,108] All *Clostridium* species produce spores that are resistant to physical and chemical agents and persist for long periods in soil.

Epidemiology and Pathogenesis. Clostridium perfringens and other histotoxic clostridial species are the causative organisms. They can be inoculated by trauma, usually associated with muscle injury from blunt trauma or high-velocity wounds. Compound fractures are said to be particularly susceptible because local calcium salts favor clostridial growth. In addition, they are sometimes seen in wounds after large bowel or biliary tract surgery or in the presence of ischemic impairment of a muscular region, especially after amputations of the lower extremity for ischemic gangrene. Cases have followed contaminated injections, especially of vasospastic agents, such as epinephrine. Three factors are usually present in nonhematogenous cases: (1) contamination of wounds with clostridia (eg, fecal contamination), (2) devitalized tissue creating an anaerobic environment, and (3) foreign bodies. Debridement and delayed primary closure of war wounds substantially reduce the incidence. Primary carcinomas of the colon, with or without penetration or perforation, have been associated with hematogenous clostridial myonecrosis caused by *C. septicum*. Immunocompromised patients have a high risk even in the presence of minor trauma.

Clinical Manifestations. The incubation period of clostridial myonecrosis is much shorter than for most pyogenic infections; severe toxemia can occur within 24 hours of wounding. Only group A streptococci or clostridial infections are normally so fulminant. The onset is usually acute—a pain so severe that a vascular catastrophe must be suspected. No other soft tissue infection produces a comparable degree of pain.

The local lesion becomes rapidly edematous, cool, and exquisitely tender. Swollen muscle may herniate through an open wound, and a serosanguineous discharge, which contains numerous gram-positive organisms but few leukocytes, escapes. The wound has a peculiar sweet but foul odor; gas bubbles may be visible in the discharge. Crepitus, if present, is not as prominent as in other anaerobic soft tissue infections. The skin adjacent to the wound is initially swollen and pale, but rapidly takes on a yellowish or bronze discoloration. Tense blebs containing thick, dark fluid develop in the overlying skin, and areas of green-black cutaneous necrosis appear (Fig. 31–17).

Toxemia is usually severe long before cutaneous necrosis appears. Although the systemic signs are nonspecific, they are a prominent part of the clinical picture. The patient is severely ill, pale, sweaty, and apprehensive. Delirium may follow. Tachycardia, hypotension, shock, and renal failure follow in rapid succession. Fever is generally not too high, and hypothermia or jaundice is associated with terminal shock.

Diagnosis. Operative exploration must be profound if one suspects a problem.[109] Bacteremia with *C. perfringens* occurs in only 15 percent of the patients with gas gangrene, but hemolysis, presumably associated with bacteremia, is a common complication, especially after intrauterine infections.

Gram-stained smears of the wound exudate or an aspirate from one of the blebs reveals large gram-positive bacilli with blunt ends but few polymorphonuclear leukocytes. Spores are usually not evident. Other gram-positive and gram-negative bacteria may be present, particularly in grossly contaminated wounds, so that the diagnosis can be overlooked if only bacteriologic diagnosis is sought.

X-rays of the involved areas show extensive and progressive gaseous dissection of muscle and fascial planes in 40 percent of patients.

The diagnosis of crepitant wound infections is outlined in Table 31–18. The degree of toxemia, the rather limited crepitance usually masked by edema, the severe degree of local pain, and the

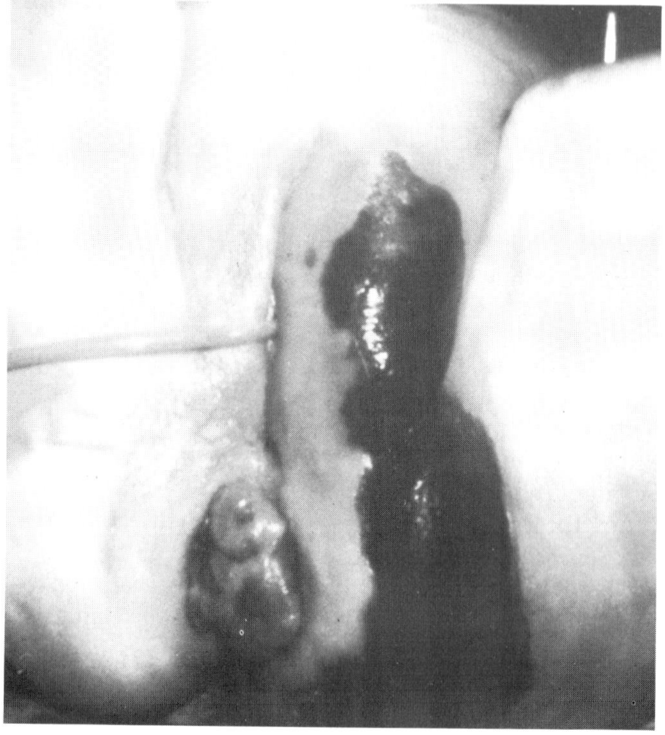

Figure 31–17. Gas gangrene of perianal region and vulva. The lesion is painful, and the skin is bronzed. The central necrotic area overlies a much more extensive area of necrotizing fasciitis and myonecrosis. *(Courtesy of Claude R. Hitchcock, MD, Chief of Surgery, Hennepin County Medical Center, Minneapolis.)*

characteristic skin lesions with bronzing, dark blebs, and gross ischemic necrosis differentiate this disease from nonclostridial level 3 and 4 infections. The absence of leukocytes and the presence of clostridia on smear are helpful diagnostic signs, although clostridia can be part of mixed bacterial necrotizing fasciitis. At exploration, the infected muscle itself may exhibit only pallid edema with an absence of bleeding and failure to contract on electrical stimulation. Later, it becomes discolored to a reddish purple before becoming black and friable.

Treatment. Patients require immediate resuscitation, parenteral antibiotics, and emergency operation to examine the muscles at the site of infection and widely excise the infected tissue. Gram stains of the infected muscle should be carried out during debridement. Only when resected muscle is free of bacteria should debridement be stopped. Some surgeons irrigate the wound in the postoperative period with H_2O_2; others pack the wound with zinc peroxide. All nonviable muscle should be excised and fasciotomies performed to decompress fascial compartments of adjacent uninfected muscle groups. Amputation is a highly effective treatment of distal infections and should be considered in any patient with clostridial myonecrosis who manifests systemic toxicity. The mortality is much higher for truncal and perineal gas gangrene than for limb infections. All wounds should be left to close by secondary infections. Repeated inspection of the wound in the operating room is necessary at frequent intervals after primary debridement to determine if further excision is required. Persistently elevated serum creatine kinase (CK) levels may indicate residual nonviable muscle or progressive infection after primary debridement.[110]

ANTIBIOTIC THERAPY. Antibiotic therapy is essential. Penicillin G is administered intravenously in a dosage of 1 to 2 million units every 2 to 3 hours. Most authorities advocate a second antibiotic (chloramphenicol for mixed infections or an aminoglycoside).[111] Chloramphenicol is a good alternative drug in the penicillin-allergic patient. Clindamycin is superior to penicillin in an experimental dog model.

ANCILLARY SURGICAL THERAPY. Occult malignancy, especially of the GI tract, should be sought if *C. septicum* is recovered.[107,108] If autogenous fecal contamination is responsible for the infection, diversion of the fecal stream will be required. Skin grafting and other reconstructive procedures are almost always required in survivors.

HYPERBARIC OXYGEN THERAPY. Hyperbaric oxygen therapy is indicated as an additive treatment, particularly for patients with diffuse spreading infections.[109,112,113] It may be especially useful in the management of patients with extensive involvement of the trunk or perineum where adequate surgical debridement is difficult. It is not a substitute for debridement and antibiotics.

GENERAL MAINTENANCE. These patients require aggressive fluid resuscitation and management. A Swan-Ganz catheter may be required. Nutritional support is indicated in all patients. Renal failure and secondary organ failure syndromes are common.

ANTITOXIN. A polyvalent gas gangrene antitoxin is no longer available, and its usefulness was controversial. Before the ready availability of penicillin, military surgeons were convinced of its value, although the mechanism of action was unclear.

Prevention. The disease in wartime is more rare than in civilian practice. The military medical policy of wide debridement of all fresh wounds with delayed (4-day) primary closure has effectively reduced the incidence. Prophylactic antibiotics for wounded patients may be useful adjuncts, but excision of all devitalized tissue is the principal prophylactic maneuver. Only 22 cases occurred in 139,000 casualties in Vietnam, where this policy was generally followed. There were 27 cases in Miami in a 10-year period, suggesting that the policy is not followed in civilian practice.[114]

Nonclostridial Myonecrosis

Myonecrosis can be caused by organisms other than *Clostridium*—most prominent among them is the anaerobic *Streptococcus* combined with *S. aureus*.

Anaerobic Streptococcal and Staphylococcal Myonecrosis. This is a rare disease even in wartime. The anaerobic streptococci are usually accompanied by *S. aureus* or group A streptococci (see Table 31–7). The predisposing causes are the same as for clostridial myonecrosis, but the incubation period is longer (3 to 4 days) and the course less fulminating. The wounded area manifests edema and a seropurulent drainage. Pain is not the initial symptom but can become severe. Gas is present but not extensive. The odor may be sour. Toxemia is a later and preterminal sign. When *S. pyogenes* or

S. aureus is present, the wound takes on some of the clinical characteristics of infections with these organisms. Treatment with wide debridement and penicillin is appropriate. Penicillinase-resistant penicillins or cephalosporins should be added for *S. aureus*.

Mixed Enteric Myonecrosis. This muscular infection caused by mixed enteric organisms was originally described by Stone and Martin as synergistic necrotizing cellulitis, and few authors have appreciated the initial statement that "necrosis of muscle and fascia is the rule."[85] This disease has also been called synergistic nonclostridial anaerobic myonecrosis. The elderly, the obese or malnourished, diabetics, and patients with cardiovascular disease or renal failure are at highest risk. The patients are often febrile with marked wound pain and systemic toxicity. Blood cultures are positive in a third of patients.[85]

Antibiotics are the same as used for mixed enteric necrotizing fasciitis. Debrided muscle is gray-green in color and fails to contract with electrocautery stimulation. Truncal involvement is common, precluding definitive amputation. Mortality of 76 percent has been reported.[85]

Infected Vascular Gangrene. Infected vascular gangrene is secondary infection of a dead extremity in which amputation has been delayed. A variety of organisms have been reported, and true clostridial myonecrosis also occurs.

UNUSUAL BACTERIAL INFECTIONS OF THE SKIN NOT USUALLY REQUIRING SURGICAL THERAPY

Cutaneous Anthrax. Anthrax is a zoonotic disease that affects the skin, lungs, and gastrointestinal tract in humans.[115] The cutaneous form accounts for 95 percent of the cases seen in the United States. Meningitis and septicemia are common complications of the pulmonary form with a high mortality.

Etiology. *Bacillus anthracis* is a gram-positive nonmotile encapsulated bacillus producing spores (see Chap. 9).

Epidemiology. The disease is limited to workers in contact with raw wool and hides in agriculture and industry.[116] Consumers are rarely afflicted.

Pathogenesis and Pathology. Anthrax spores are inoculated into skin, eaten, or inhaled. The spores germinate, multiply locally, and produce a toxin that induces regional edema, capillary thrombosis, and tissue necrosis. Pulmonary capillary thrombosis is a major cause of respiratory failure. Gastrointestinal anthrax results in ulceration, edema, and mucosal necrosis with hemorrhagic diarrhea.

Clinical Manifestations. Two to five days after cutaneous inoculation, a small papule appears, which vesiculates. A small ring of vesicles coalesces to form a large vesicle (malignant pustule) with central ulceration and peripheral erythema and edema. In a few days, the clear vesicular fluid becomes black; rupture reveals a depressed ulcer crater with black eschar. Fever, malaise, lymphangitis, and lymphadenopathy may occur, but progression to general toxemia is rare. Usually, the eschar sloughs off and slow healing takes place.

The term malignant edema describes cutaneous anthrax associated with multiple bulli, extensive edema, induration, and systemic toxemia. Meningitis complicating cutaneous anthrax can be fatal.

Diagnosis. The diagnosis is suspected when a nontender, pruritic-papule on an exposed part of the body vesiculates and forms a black depressed eschar. *Bacillus anthracis* can be recovered from vesicular fluid or the ulcer exudate. Staphylococcal skin lesions, tularemia, plague, milker's nodules, and contagious pustular dermatitis (ecthyma contagiosum or orf) are considered in the differential diagnosis. Serologic testing on paired serum specimens confirms the diagnosis. In anthrax meningitis, the organism can be recovered from the cerebrospinal fluid.

Therapy. Cultures should be taken before therapy, since penicillin inhibits bacterial recovery. Parenteral penicillin G is required for severe cases, but oral penicillin G cures the mild cases. Erythromycin, tetracycline, and chloramphenicol are also effective. Antibiotic ointments have no effect.

Prevention. Workers exposed to wool can be immunized. To prevent spread, lesions should be kept covered and soiled dressings incinerated.

Prognosis. Untreated cutaneous anthrax is lethal in 10 to 20 percent of cases; fewer than 1 percent of patients die with effective antimicrobial therapy. Cutaneous lesions progress to a black eschar regardless of therapy. Protective immunity results.

Protective antibody titers are found in some employees of goat hair mills with no history of anthrax, which suggests that subclinical infections occur.[115,116]

Cutaneous Diphtheria. Diphtheria is a systemic illness caused by diphtherial toxin, an extracellular protein elaborated by toxogenic strains of *C. diphtheriae*[101] producing primary pharyngeal infections (see Chap. 9). Cutaneous infection occurs after inoculation into the skin, but without the systemic toxicity and postdiphtheritic complications of myocarditis and polyneuritis.

Etiology and Epidemiology. The characteristics of *C. diphtheriae* and its toxin are discussed in Chapter 9. This organism should be carefully distinguished from other *Corynebacterium* species, including the skin saprophytes. Poor hygiene, especially in tropical areas, predisposes to the cutaneous disease. Patients with cutaneous disease are important reservoirs in epidemics.[117]

Pathogenesis and Pathology. Diphtheria toxin is systemically absorbed from the local site of infection and primarily affects myocardial, renal tubular, and central nervous cells. It is internalized by endocytosis, blocks protein synthesis, and kills affected cells. At the site of local infection, a fibrinopurulent membrane forms without deep tissue erosion.

Clinical Manifestations. Three types of skin disease are described: (1) wound diphtheria—a membrane partially covers the wound, which is surrounded by edema and erythema; (2) primary cutaneous diptheria—a tender pustule ruptures to reveal an oval punched-out ulcer with a gray membrane at the base; the ulcer has edematous, rolled, bluish margins; and (3) superinfection of eczematoid skin. Myocarditis is a rare complication, but neurologic symptoms (blurred vision, diplopia, numbness of the tongue, palatal paralysis, and the Guillain-Barré syndrome) have been described in 3 to 5 percent of patients with cutaneous diphtheria.

Diagnosis. Corynebacterium diphtheriae organisms are visible in methylene blue- or toluidine blue-stained smears of the membrane and are isolated on selective media (Loeffler or tellurite agar). Demonstration of toxin production in vitro confirms the diagnosis.

Treatment. After skin testing and desensitization, diphtheria antitoxin (20,000 to 40,000 units intramuscularly or intravenously) is administered because neurologic complications can occur even in cutaneous disease. Antibiotics (procaine penicillin, 2 million units per day for 7 to 10 days, or erythromycin) and debridement of necrotic tissue may help eliminate the carrier state. Active immunization is also necessary in convalescent patients.[118]

Prevention. Active immunization using toxoid (formalin detoxified diphtheria toxin) prevents the complications of diphtheria but not the infection. Children immunized with diphtheria-pertussis-tetanus (DPT) shots receive the toxoid and immunity lasts only 10 years, so virtually the whole adult population is unprotected. The Schick test uses a minute amount of diphtherial toxin injected intradermally, which causes an inflammatory reaction in 4 to 7 days in the absence of immunity (Schick-positive). The presence of circulating antitoxin blocks the response, indicating immunity (Schick-negative). Reimmunization with highly purified toxoid is advised in combination with tetanus toxoid immunization.

The Treponematoses—Syphilis

Etiology. Treponema pallidum is discussed in Chapter 9. *Treponema pallidum* can produce virtually every manifestation of disease seen in the skin and mucous membranes. In the past, massive textbooks illustrated these presentations. Disease can be acquired by placental transmission from the mother (congenital syphilis), but the infection is usually acquired by sexual activity.[119]

Clinical Manifestations. Approximately 3 weeks after inoculation, primary syphilis produces a chancre, a painless and slightly elevated ucler with a clean base without undermining or raised edges (Fig. 31–18). A nontender, nonfluctuant, rather firm regional lymphadenopathy (bubo) may accompany the chancre (chancre complex). Healing takes 3 to 6 weeks. Secondary bacterial infection or other sexually transmitted disease may produce local pain. Extragenital chancres on the lip, mouth, fingers, breasts, or anus are usually associated with an enlarged unilateral lymph node. Internal chancres in females commonly go unnoticed.

The secondary cutaneous lesions, appearing within a few weeks after the chancre heals, are usually dry, macular, or papular and involve any skin surface. They can mimic any dermatosis, but lesions of the palms and soles suggest the diagnosis. Pustules may occur and lead to surgical consultation; vesicular or bullous lesions are absent. In

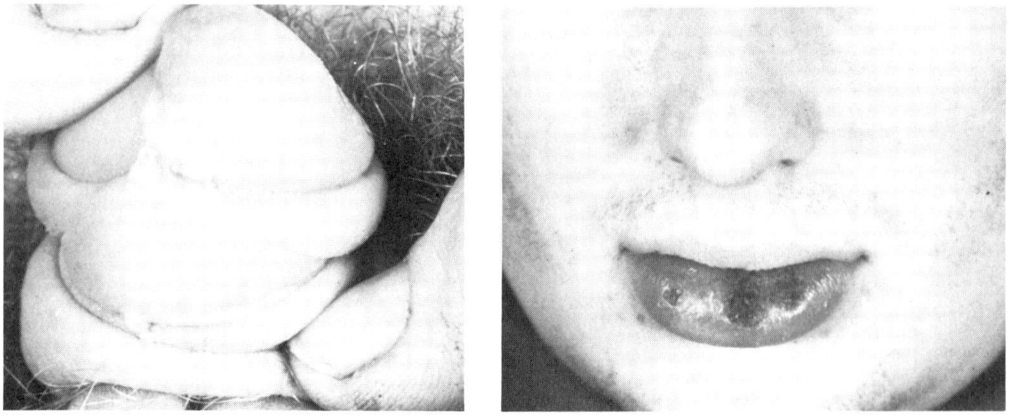

A B

Figure 31–18. A primary syphilis chancre of the **(A)** glans penis and **(B)** lip. *(Courtesy of Robert W. Goltz, MD, Professor and Head, Department of Dermatology, University of Minnesota, Minneapolis.)*

intertriginous areas or on mucous membranes, the papules may coalesce and erode to produce moist gray or red plaques (condyloma lata), which teem with spirochetes. The secondary skin manifestations can be accompanied by low-grade fever, malaise, leukocytosis, laryngitis, arthralgias, and generalized adenopathy. Arthritis, glomerulonephritis, and hepatitis are rare. Relapses can occur, especially within 2 years of the primary infection.

SOFT TISSUE LESIONS IN LATE SYPHILIS. Tertiary syphilis may present as destructive granulomas called gummas (late benign syphilis), most often of subcutaneous tissues but also of bone and other organs. The nodules are usually single but may be grouped or multiple. Breakdown of the skin causes a punched-out lesion with a scalloped border. Coalescence of the lesions produces arsiniform and serpiginous outlines, which are characteristic (Fig. 31–19). The lesions may persist for years, with gradual extension at one border and healing in other areas. Lesions of the mucous membranes of the nose and throat may produce extensive destructive changes, including perforation of the palate (which is pathognomonic in the absence of injury, malignant tumor, or lead poisoning). Treponemes are not demonstrable in the nodules.

Patients with tabes dorsalis or locomotor ataxia may develop indolent pressure ulcers of the toes and feet, or destruction of weight-bearing joints and adjacent bones (Charcot joints), which can become secondarily infected.[119]

Diagnosis. The laboratory diagnosis of syphilis is discussed in Chapter 9. Demonstration of *T. pallidum* in material from a primary or secondary lesion with a dark-field microscope requires skill and experience. The serologic tests for syphilis are obtained and repeated weekly and monthy if they remain negative.

Treatment. Penicillin is the drug of choice in the nonallergic patient for all stages of syphilis. A single intramuscular injection of 2.4 million units of benzathine penicillin G is curative in most cases of primary or secondary syphilis. The gummatous lesions are very susceptible to low-dose penicillin, but other forms of tertiary syphilis should be treated with 2.4 million units of benzathine penicillin per week for 3 weeks (total dose 7.2 million units). Tetracycline, erythromycin, chloramphenicol, and cef-

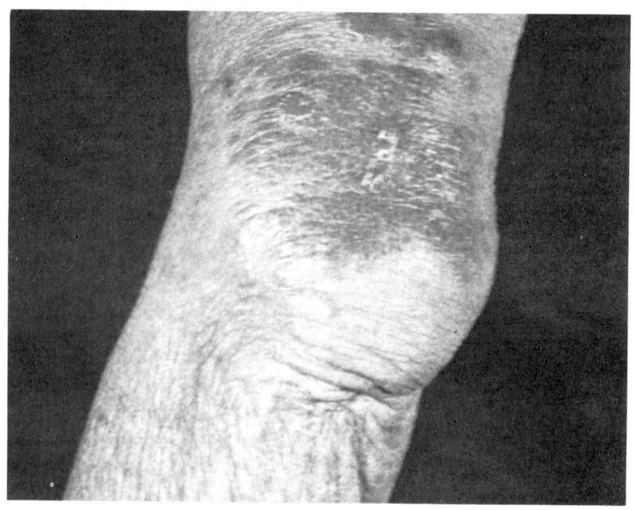

Figure 31–19. Gumma in tertiary syphilis. Several lesions have coalesced, but no ulceration is present. *(Courtesy of Robert W. Goltz, MD, Professor and Head, Department of Dermatology, University of Minnesota, Minneapolis.)*

triaxone are effective alternative drugs. Patients with active neurosyphilis, congenital syphilis, or HIV and syphilis require larger and more prolonged courses of antibiotics.

The Endemic Treponematoses

Yaws, pinta, and bejel are endemic, communicable diseases caused by the treponemes and confined to tropical countries.[120] They are transmitted by nonvenereal contact before puberty, are susceptible to penicillin, and are best controlled by improved hygiene. All yield positive serologic tests for syphilis and have some degree of reciprocal immunity.[119]

Yaws. Yaws (frambesia, pian, buba, bouba) is characterized by early nondestructive skin lesions, a period of latency, and late destructive lesions of skin and bone.

Pathogenesis and Pathology. The organism *Treponema pallidum pertenue* is probably inoculated through traumatic breaks in the skin. Bloodstream invasion rapidly occurs, and the course parallels that of syphilis. The early lesions are not destructive and usually heal. A latent period is followed by granulomatous destructive lesions of bones and skin free of the organism. Hypertrophic periostitis, gummatous periostitis, osteitis, and osteomyelitis affect the bones of limbs, hands, feet, and skull.

Clinical Manifestations. In primary yaws, skin papules appear on exposed skin (usually of the leg), become papillomatous, ulcerate, and heal spontaneously in about 6 months. In secondary yaws, a general eruption of widely dispersed papillomas is accompanied by lymphadenopathy and some malaise. In several months, the eruption heals. Several relapses of secondary lesions may occur over the years and may be accompanied by periostitis, osteitis, and osteomyelitis, particularly involving the shafts of the long bones, fingers, or maxilla.

In tertiary yaws, after an asymptomatic period of 3 or more years, papillomatous lesions of the hands and feet appear, which are now destructive and solitary. Plantar and palmar hyperkeratoses with painful fissures (crab yaws) are the most common late lesions. The late bone lesions of the limbs, hands, and skull may ulcerate through the skin at bony prominences. Impressive destructive ulceration of the nose and palate may occur (gangosa mutilans).

Diagnosis. The diagnosis is difficult in nonendemic areas, yet travel has made the disease worldwide. Dark-field examination of primary or secondary lesions by experts can make the diagnosis. The late lesions are dark-field negative. Serologic syphilis tests are positive.

Prognosis. Yaws may undergo spontaneous resolution, but most cases progress to late lesions with disfigurement, contractures of the hands, and periarticular ulcers. Secondary bacterial infection may cause osteomyelitis. Infection and cure lead to lifelong immunity.

Therapy. A single injection of 600,000 units of procaine penicillin in aluminum monosterate 2 percent (PAM) is curative. Tetracycline and chloramphenicol are also effective.[120]

Surgical Significance. To the surgeon dealing with local manifestations of obscure diseases, the appearance of necrotic ulcerative single lesions may be confusing, especially if secondarily infected. Young adults from endemic areas with lesions not responding to local therapy should be suspect. Surgical therapy should be discontinued and penicillin administered.

Pinta

Etiology. Pinta is caused by the gram-negative spirochete *Treponema carateum.*

Epidemiology. Pinta is chronic, contagious, nonvenereal treponematosis usually affecting adolescents and young adults, limited to tropical Central and South America. Intimate contact with infected persons transmits the disease.[120]

Clinical Manifestations. The changes in pinta are restricted to the skin, especially the epidermis. In the early stages, small erythematous papules gradually enlarge to 1 to 3 cm in diameter, coalesce, and develop satellites, which may persist or disappear. Most characteristic is the variety of colors that may be seen. The early lesions are red and violaceous; later lesions in the face and neck may be blue, brown, slate-gray, or black. Dark blue lesions of the face and neck are said to be striking. The tertiary or late stage results in the development of depigmented areas of the skin. Destructive or necrotic lesions are not seen.[120]

Diagnosis. The diagnosis depends on clinical suspicion and evidence of treponema by dark-field examination of primary and secondary, but not tertiary, lesions. The serologic tests for syphilis are positive. The prognosis of the disease is good, but disfiguring lesions may cause social ostracism.

Therapy. A single dose of long-acting penicillin G, 1.2 million units, is adequate. Tetracyclines and chloramphenicol are also effective. The clinical response may take 6 to 12 months, and repigmentation of tertiary lesions does not occur.[119]

Bejel (Endemic Syphilis). Bejel is a nonvenereal treponematosis acquired in childhood caused by *T. pallidum II endemicum.*[119,120] It is spread predominantly by household contact to prepubertal children among rural populations with poor personal hygiene. The manifestations are those of syphilis. The primary lesion is usually missed, and secondary lesions include mucous membrane patches, anogenital condylomas, and stomatitis of the lateral commissures. The late manifestations are similar to those of venereal syphilis, but the severe cardiovascular and neural lesions are rare. Gummas of the nasopharyngeal area may produce focal disfigurement. Cutaneous gummas often extend laterally, with marked ulceration. The diagnosis is difficult or impossible outside the endemic setting. Serologic test results for syphilis are positive. The optimal treatment is 1.2 million units in a single dose of benzathine penicillin G.

Cutaneous Mycobacterial Infections

Tuberculosis of the Skin. Table 31–25 lists the clinical expressions of cutaneous tuberculosis. Systemic tuberculosis is discussed in Chapter 9. Primary and reactivation infections produce different types of cutaneous responses.

Primary Cutaneous Tuberculosis. The primary inoculation of *M. tuberculosis* into the skin of a previously unsensitized person induces a tuberculous chancre.[144] It is especially common among physicians. A cutaneous inflammatory lesion contains a predominance of polymorphonuclear leukocytes and lymphocytes. Initially, numerous bacilli are seen; later, typical tubercles develop from which acid-fast bacilli are difficult to isolate.

The most common lesion is the chancre, a nodule that evolves into an indolent, firm, nontender, sharply delimited ulcer with regional adenopathy. Other manifestations are the impetiginous lesion, a superficial small ulceration with a loose crust, and the ecthymatous form, with heaped-up margins surrounding a central ulceration. Lymphangitis between the primary chancre and the enlarged node completes the formation of the primary complex. The ulcer slowly involutes and heals with scarring.

Acutely, the acid-fast organisms are easily recovered from currettings or biopsy specimens of the

TABLE 31–25. CLASSIFICATION OF TUBERCULOSIS OF THE SKIN

Types	Mode of Infection or Spread	Bacilli Demonstrable	State of Immunity	Tuberculin Sensitivity	Histologic Caseation
True cutaneous tuberculosis					
Primary Tuberculosis					
Tuberculous chancre	Inoculation	+++	+++	0 (initially)—+ (late)	+++
Miliary	Hematogenous	++	0	0 (terminal anergy)	+++
Secondary Tuberculosis					
Lupus vulgaris	Inoculation	± (with difficulty)	+++	+++	+
Tuberculosis verrucosa cutis	Inoculation	+	+++	+++	++
Scrofuloderma	Local extension	++	+++	+++	+++
Tuberculous gumma	Hematogenous	++	+	+	+++
Tuberculous cutis orificialis	Local extension	++	+	0 (terminal anergy or +++)	+++
Tuberculids					
Papular Forms					
Lupus miliaris disseminatus facei	Hematogenous	0	+++	+++	++
Papulonecrotic tuberculid	Hematogenous	0	+++	+++	+++
Lichen scrofulosorum	Hematogenous	0	+++	+++	0
Nodular					
Erythema induratum	Hematogenous	± (sometimes)	+++	+++	+++

0, absent; +, slight; ++, moderate; +++, considerable.
From Moschella SL: Diseases of the mononuclear phagocytic system (the so-called reticuloendothelial system). In Moschella SL, Hurley HJ (eds): Dermatology, 2nd ed. Philadelphia, Saunders, 1985, p 934.

ulcer and adjacent lymph nodes. The differential diagnosis includes granuloma pyogenicum, luetic chancre, sporotrichosis, subacute tularemia, cat scratch disease, swimming pool granuloma, and epithelioma with metastasis to regional lymph nodes.

Treatment with antituberculous drugs discussed in Chapters 9 and 28 should be effective, although multiply resistant strains are increasingly frequent, especially in AIDS patients.[122] Before the advent of adequate chemotherapy, complete surgical excision of the primary lesion and involved regional lymph nodes was a satisfactory method of treatment. Local excision of fluctuant nodes may still be useful.[121]

Skin Manifestations of Disseminated Primary Tuberculosis. Other forms of tuberculosis of the skin are listed in Table 31–25. Miliary tuberculosis can be primary or secondary. The skin lesion usually consists of malculopapular rash with occasional vesicular changes. Sometimes chronic miliary tuberculosis produces a systemic febrile wasting syndrome, especially in malnourished children. The lesions present as subcutaneous nodules that become fluctuant and drain with undermined ulceration and sinus formation. Histopathologic examination reveals tuberculous granulomata with acid-fast bacilli in the pus (tuberculosis colliquativa).

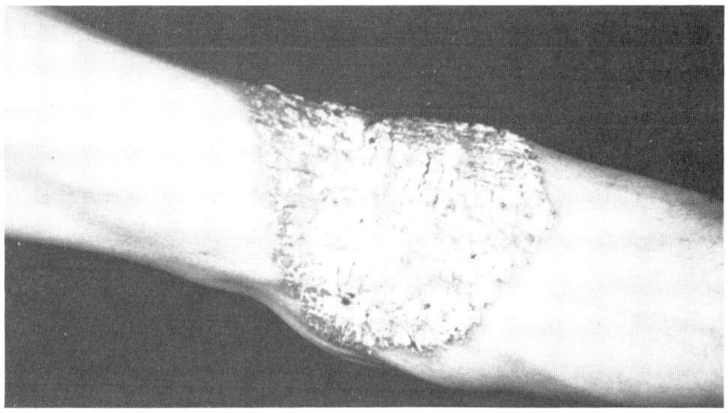

A

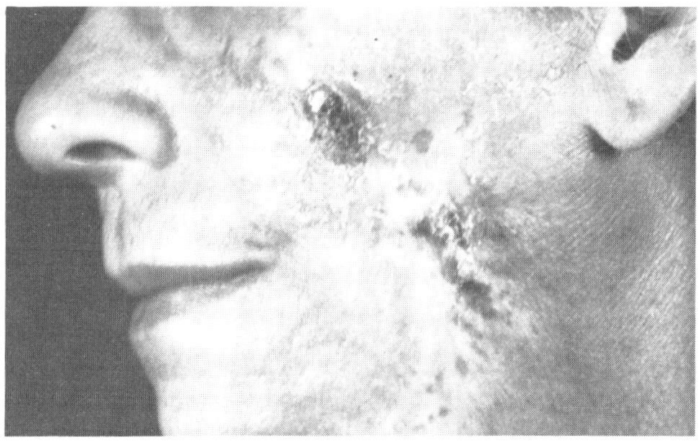

B

Figure 31–20. Tuberculosis of the skin: **(A)** lupus vulgaris, **(B)** lupus vulgaris with carcinoma. *(Courtesy of Robert W. Goltz, MD, Professor and Head, Department of Dermatology, University of Minnesota, Minneapolis.)*

Secondary Tuberculosis

LUPUS VULGARIS. Lupus vulgaris is the most common cutaneous manifestation of tuberculosis and usually affects the face. It may result from inoculation of infected secretions of hematogenous or lymphatic spread.[121] It appears as ulcers, nodules, hypertrophic verrucous or vegetative plaques, sclerotic masses, papillomatous overgrowths, or edematous thickenings (Fig. 31–20). Ulceration secondary to the underlying vegetative lesions can be extensive, and when the lesions resolve, scarring, keloid formation, lymphedema, and functional impairment from contractures remain. The diagnosis depends on biopsy, which reveals typical tuberculoid granulomas, except that caseous necrosis is slight and the tubercle bacilli are difficult to demonstrate on culture (see Table 31–25).

TUBERCULOSIS VERRUCOSA CUTIS. Tuberculosis verrucosa cutis is a warty growth resulting from an inoculation injury in an immune individual.[121] Occupational inoculation of pathologists, surgeons, and morgue attendants leads to verrucoid lesions called verruca necrogenica on exposed areas, particularly fingers and hands. The lesion begins as a deep-seated, dull red papule or pustule, which becomes verrucoid and sometimes crusted with exudate. Although it can be mutilating and destructive, most often the lesion gradually involutes and heals.

Scrofuloderma. Scrofuloderma classically results from the breakdown of cervical nodes with fistula and sinus formation in the overlying skin.[121] The disease formerly predominated in children with bovine tuberculosis with tonsillar involvement and cervical adenitis but is now seen in pulmonary tuberculosis. Painless swellings appear in the neck from a single or a matted group of nodes (Fig. 31–21). Suppuration results in sinus and ulcer formation in the skin. Fungating tumors may result from excessive granulation tissue.

Anorectal Tuberculosis. Tuberculous ischiorectal abscess and fistula in ano are an extension of intestinal tuberculosis.

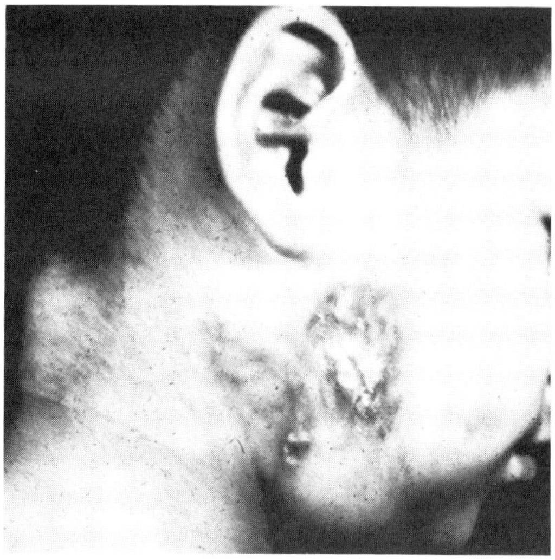

Figure 31–21. Scrofuloderma. *(Courtesy of Robert W. Goltz, MD, Professor and Head, Department of Dermatology, University of Minnesota, Minneapolis.)*

Tuberculids. Tuberculids were once said to be skin lesions resulting from delayed hypersensitivity reactions to tuberculosis elsewhere in the body. Their pathogenesis is currently not clear. The various types are listed in Table 31–25. Although a variety of shapes and forms are observed, the papular or nodular lesions appear in clusters or crops and can undergo spontaneous necrosis and healing. By definition, acid-fast bacteria cannot be isolated.

Atypical Mycobacteria. The pecularities of mycobacteria groups I to IV have been described in Chapter 9, and newer classifications are emerging.[123] These mycobacteria may produce pulmonary disease, cervical adenitis, osteomyelitis, miliary tuberculosis, and skin infections (cutaneous granulomas, ulcers, and abscesses). All infections with groups I to IV mycobacteria produce histologic pictures similar to *M. tuberculosis* except group IV, which does not produce caseating granulomatous disease. PPD skin antigens for each of the major groups are available, but cross-reactivity is common.

Group II mycobacteria, especially *M. scrofulaceum,* usually cause cervical lymphadenitis in children 1 to 3 years of age (Table 31–16). The oropharynx is thought to be the portal of entry when children put foreign bodies in their mouths. The submandibular nodes are involved, rather than the anterior cervical nodes characteristic of scrofula. The disease progresses rapidly and suppurates earlier than tuberculous adenitis. Fever and leukocytosis are absent, the chest roentgenogram is usually negative, and the PPD test results can be negative. Treatment of lymphadenitis is surgical excision. Drug therapy yields equivocal results. Sensitivities are variable *Mycobacterium kansasii* and *M. avium-intracellulare* can both cause lymphadenitis. Although excision may be useful, drug therapy is also important for these organisms.[123] *Mycobacterium avium-intracellulare* causes disseminated disease in AIDS patients, with minimal cutaneous findings.

Group I (*M. kansasii, M. marinum*) and group IV mycobacteria produce a subcutaneous lymphatic sporotrichoid form of infection. The infections listed in Table 31–14 must be excluded.

Most group IV mycobacteria are saprophytes, but *M. fortuitum* and *M. chelonei* can produce deep, painful nodules with indefinite margins that may suppurate, drain, and produce fairly large ulcers after accidental inoculation.[124] *Mycobacterium fortuitum* has been found contaminating Elastoplast dressings and in wound infections.[123] Wide debridement with delayed closure is essential.[125]

Atypical mycobacteria are difficult to eradicate and effective drug combinations have not been defined. They have variable in vitro sensitivity to antituberculous drugs, and usually a combination of two or three drugs is required (see Chap. 9 and Chap. 28). The organisms are rarely susceptible to isoniazid.

SWIMMING POOL GRANULOMA. This is a chronic granulomatous infection at sites of trauma incurred while swimming or cleaning fish tanks. *Mycobacterium marinum* (group I) and perhaps other unclassified mycobacteria are responsible. Histologically, a tuberculoid granulomatous infection is seen with Langhans giant cells but without caseation necrosis. Red papules or pustules that can grow to the size of a pea follow abrasion of elbows (70 percent), knees, dorsa of hands, feet, or nose. Some of the lesions ulcerate and develop brownish crusts. The lesions tend to be solitary but can ascend proximally in a sporotrichoid fashion. Regional lymphangitis and lymphadenopathy have not been described. Healing takes place spontaneously in a few months to several years.

The organisms are susceptible to rifampin and ethambutol but are resistant to streptomycin, isoniazid, and PAS. Surgical excision commonly results in recurrence unless accompanied by chemotherapy. Disinfecting pools and excluding infected individuals from swimming areas are useful preventive measures.

MYCOBACTERIAL PHAGEDENIC ULCERATION. *M. ulcerans* (group III) can lead to inoculation infections of scratches and abrasions in tropical areas of Africa, Australia, and Mexico. The initial papule ulcerates and progresses to a large deep undermined ulcer with a necrotic base. The spreading ulcerative granulomatous process often destroys subcutaneous tissue, including fascia and muscle (Buruli ulcers). The legs are most commonly infected, but lymphadenopathy and systemic illness do not occur. The ulcers are teeming with organisms. Histologically, there is necrosis of the skin and tuberculoid reaction, which differentiate this lesion from mixed bacterial phagedenic ulcers (see preceding section). Spontaneous healing may take place after months. *Mycobacterium ulcerans* is resistant to current antituberculous agents. The only effective therapy presently available is wide surgical excision and skin grafting.

Leprosy. Leprosy (Hansen disease) is a common chronic intracellular nonfatal infectious disease, with many cutaneous manifestations. The diagnosis is made by skin biopsy. Surgical reconstruction of musculoskeletal and cosmetic defects may be required.[126]

Etiology. Mycobacterium leprae is an acid-fast obligate intracellular parasite capable of invading nerves. It fails to grow in culture, but splenectomized mice and rats develop systemic infection following inoculation.

Epidemiology. Leprosy is a common disease in tropical and subtopical regions and is endemic in Texas, Hawaii, California, Louisiana, Puerto Rico, Cuba, Mexico, and Vietnam. Immigration has made it more common in other parts of the United States as well. Transmission is thought to involve human–human contact through breaks in skin, but skin lesions shed relatively few organisms. Nasal secretions and breast milk from infected persons are rich in bacteria. The incubation period is 3 to 5 years.

Pathogenesis and Pathology. Leprosy usually first involves the skin in association with hair follicles and sebaceous glands. It spreads to contiguous skin areas especially along the nerves, dermal appendages, and blood vessels. Lymphohematogenous dissemination occurs early, and spread along the sensory nerves impairs motor fibers within their trunks. The central nervous system is not affected. The granulomatous reaction destroys nerves and dermal appendages, but the epidermis is spared. With progression from the tuberculoid to the lepromatous form, the infiltrating lymphocytes in the granulomas are replaced by foamy histiocytes and bacteria.

Involvement of the lymphoid tissues results in general impairment of cellular immunity with normal or enhanced humoral antibody responses.

Clinical Manifestations. Leprosy produces a progressive spectrum of disease, which progresses from one form to another as the patient's immunologic response changes. Ridley and Joplin[126] have described a spectrum from the most limited form to the most generalized disease as follows: TT—full tuberculoid, BT—borderline tuberculoid, BB—borderline, BL—borderline lepromatous, and LL—full lepromatous. The ends of the spectrum are stable forms of disease; the intermediary stages are clinically unstable.

Indeterminate (borderline) leprosy begins as a flat ill-defined skin lesion on the face and trunk, with minimal sensory changes. There may be a history of contact with a leprosy patient but the diagnosis can only be confirmed by skin biopsy. If punch biopsy specimens are taken at the advancing margin in the early phases, only the acid-last bacilli in nerves suggest the diagnosis. Tuberculoid leprosy occurs when a large erythematous plaque, with clear sharp outer margins, fades to a flattened central zone of rough, anhydrotic, hairless, hypopigmented, and anesthetic skin. This is a response to the development of cell-mediated immunity to the organism.

Lepromatous leprosy (Fig. 31–22), at the other end of the spectrum, appears if effective cell-mcdi ated immunity fails to develop. Diffuse vascular infiltration coarsens the skin. There may be more than 1 billion organisms per gram of tissue with continuous bacteremia and seeding to multiple organs. Symmetrically distributed skin macules, papules, plaques, and nodules (lepromas) are common, with loss of hair (except on the scalp) and edema of the extremities.

The feature common to all forms of leprosy is nerve infection, with denervation of skeletal muscle and characteristic deformities. Ulnar nerve denervation leads to clawing of the fourth and fifth fingers and wasting of intrinsic hand musculature. Posterior tibial denervation causes clawing of the toes and plantar anesthesia. Superficial peroneal nerve denervation leads to footdrop; median nerve destruction produces thenar wasting, loss of thumb opposition, and palmar anesthesia. Wristdrop and

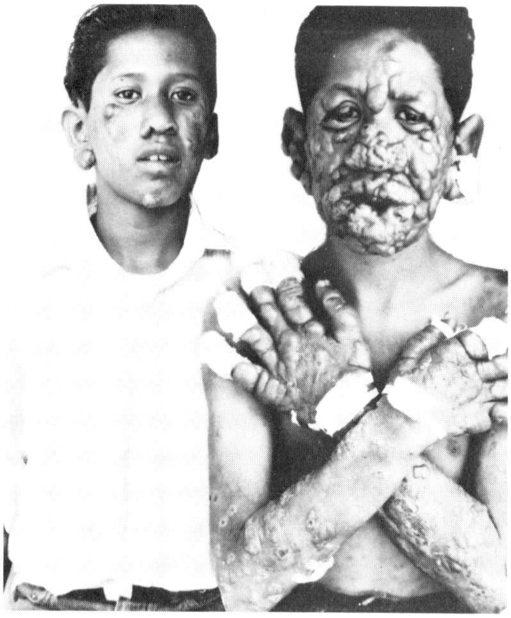

Figure 31–22. Early and late lepromatous leprosy. *(From Armed Forces Institute of Pathology, Neg. No. 75-2479-2.)*

radial nerve destruction occur, and facial nerve involvement produces inability to close the eye, with anesthesia of the cornea and conjunctiva. The anesthetic anterior portion of the eye develops corneal ulceration and blindness. Other deformities develop from destruction of the nasal cartilages with septal perforation. Secondary neuropathic ulcers are common in weight-bearing or easily traumatized areas.

One form of LL leprosy, erythema nodosum leprosum, often leads to diffuse nodular skin lesions during chemotherapy. A high fever, necrosis of the nodules, and neuritis can progress to glomerulonephritis and even death. An Arthus-like reaction is seen in nodule biopsy specimens. Rarely, Lucio phenomenon, erythema necroticans, leads to a necrotizing vasculitis with ulceration and sloughing of large areas of skin.

Diagnosis. The diagnosis depends on properly performed skin biopsies that include both central and peripheral lesions incised deeply enough to include fat. An elliptical excisional biopsy specimen 12 to 15 mm long is better than a punch biopsy specimen. The differential diagnosis includes the entire range of granulomatous skin disease. Acid-fast stains of tissue must be requested in any granulomatous skin biopsy (see Table 31–11).

A lepromin skin test contains a standard suspension of killed leprosy bacilli. A delayed hypersensitivity response is positive. It has no diagnostic value, but in patients with documented leprosy a positive skin test denotes tuberculoid leprosy and a negative result carries a prognosis of lepromatous leprosy if the patient is not treated.

Prognosis. Most indeterminate leprosy is self-limited, but it may evolve into tuberculoid form with severe local damage before infection is arrested. Lepromatous leprosy follows a relentless course to deformity and blindness when neglected. Death is rare except when systemic amyloidosis appears. Tuberculosis or pyogenic infection may also terminate the course.

Therapy. Most *M. leprae* organisms are killed in 3 to 6 months of chemotherapy, but treatment should continue until all *M. leprae* organisms have disappeared from the skin, a matter of at least 5 years with occasional lifelong chemotherapy necessary. Dapsone (DDS, 50 to 100 mg by mouth per day) should cure TT and BT disease. Treatment for BB–LL should combine other drugs (3 to 6 months) with DDS, because resistance develops with DDS monotherapy. Clofazamine (100 mg orally twice weekly) will prevent ENL reactions. Rifampin (600 mg/day) is appropriate for early treatment of BB–LL, since it is bactericidal for *M. leprae*. ENL reactions, if they appear, will require steroids or thalidomide for control. Bullock has summarized the therapeutic approach in detail.[127]

Prevention. BCG immunization may be protective. Prophylactic therapy with DDS may be useful in children.

Surgical Treatment of Leprosy Complications. The surgical complications of untreated or neglected leprosy present special challenges.[128] Orthopedic and plastic procedures may be indicated, including operations for wristdrop, flail foot, tendon transfers in the hand, and sling operations on the eyelids for lagophthalamos. Longitudinal incision of the nerve sheaths is sometimes indicated for relief of severe nerve pain. Plastic operations are useful for deformed noses, gynecomastia, madarosis, sagging face, unsightly earlobes, wasted thumb webs, persistently enlarged and visible great auricular nerves, etc. Orthopedic shoes (molded microcellular rubber insoles on a rigid sole) reduce the risk of plantar ulceration in neuropathic extremities. Adaptive appliances and artificial limbs have been designed to relieve the secondary deformities. Physiotherapy and vocational training are an essential part of the treatment of leprosy.

Glanders

Glanders is a disease of horses, caused by the bacterium *Pseudomonas mallaei,* which is rarely transmitted to humans. The clinical picture takes one of two forms: (1) an acute febrile disseminated infection whose entire course may encompass 10 to 30 days; and (2) an indolent, relapsing, chronic infection of the skin with multiple cutaneous and subcutaneous abscesses and draining sinuses. "Farcy" occurs in horses as nodular subcutaneous abscesses occurring along the course of lymphatics.[118]

Etiology. The pseudomonads are discussed in Chapter 5. Humans are infected by direct contact with horses, but the disease has been nearly eradicated in the United States. The organisms gain entry through abrasions in the skin, via the conjunctivae, by inhalation, or by ingestion.

Clinical Manifestations. In the acute fulminating form, an incubation period of 2 to 5 days is followed by an abrupt febrile illness with headache, malaise, chills, nausea, and vomiting. The more chronic form has similar manifestations over a longer period of time. After several weeks, the typical cutaneous and subcutaneous nodules, abscesses, and draining sinuses develop.

CUTANEOUS LESIONS. In acute glanders, a nodule or cellulitis appears at the site of inoculation. Local swelling and suppuration occur, and the lesion ulcerates. The ulcer is painful and has irregular edges with a gray-yellow base. Nodular ulcerating sores rapidly develop along the lymphatics, forming draining sinuses. Regional adenopathy is present. Widespread dissemination may follow, with multiple nodular necrotic abscesses in subcutaneous tissues and muscle. Lesions frequently coalesce into large necrotic areas. Bacteremic spread produces a generalized eruption or one that is localized to the face and neck consisting of papules, bullae, and pustules in crops. Lesions of the nasal mucosa lead to mucopurulent bloody nasal discharge, and infection may spread to the paranasal sinuses, pharynx, and lungs.

In chronic glanders, cutaneous and subcutaneous nodules appear on the extremities and occasionally on the face. The lesions ulcerate, and draining sinuses develop. Repeated cycles of healing and breakdown may continue for weeks or months. Pneumonia, empyema, meningitis, septic arthritis, and osteomyelitis are common complications. The leukocyte count is usually normal or only slightly elevated. Skin biopsy shows suppurative necrosis containing numerous intracellular and extracellular bacteria. In the chronic form, a granulomatous process with few giant cells suggestive of tuberculosis is seen. The lymphatic nodules resemble lesion of sporotrichosis, but in acute disease, miliary TB, typhoid, staphylococcal mycotic infections, or melioidosis must be excluded.

Treatment. Patients should be isolated. Sulfonamides have been used successfully (sulfadiazine, 100 mg/kg daily in divided doses), and a combination of intramuscular streptomycin with tetracycline has been recommended. Acute glanders formerly had a mortality rate of over 90 percent. Chronic glanders is more successfully treated.[118]

Melioidosis

Melioidosis is caused by the gram-negative bacillus *Pseudomonas pseudomallei,* which, although rare in the United States, is endemic in Southeast Asia[129] (see Chap. 5). Its clinical manifestations are similar to those of glanders, but it is transmitted by contamination of abraded skin with infected soil. Two clinical forms are seen: (1) acute melioidosis with pneumonia or septicemia and (2) chronic melioidosis producing unresolved pneumonia or a cavitary lesion. Both forms can be accompanied by skin lesions with abscesses, sinus development, and localized suppurative infections of bones, joints, liver, spleen.

The acute pneumonic form may appear abruptly with chills, fever, cough, dyspnea, and chest pain, but without skin lesions. The acute septicemic form usually starts with an ulceration at the site of inoculation, lymphangitis, and regional lymphadenitis. Chronic melioidosis may follow the acute disease, usually as an indolent pulmonary infection with multiple superficial abscesses. Late recrudescence of a previous infection may be precipitated by various illnesses, including thermal burns, diabetic ketoacidosis, or pneumonia.[129] The cutaneous manifestations are nonspecific.

In chronic melioidosis, subcutaneous abscesses and draining sinuses from bone or lymph nodes are common features and may occur even in the absence of fever. Sharply circumscribed abscesses are found in many organs and in the subcutaneous tissues.

The disease may imitate typhoid fever, staphylococcal pneumonia, mycotic infections, pulmonary tuberculosis, nocardiosis, fungal infections, and lung abscess.

Treatment. Chloramphenicol is the preferred treatment, with tetracycline and sulfisoxazole as alternatives. Abscesses should be drained.[129]

Bartonellosis (Carrion Disease)

Bartonella bacilliformis, a gram-negative coccobacillus transmitted by sandflies, causes a disease restricted to the valley regions of the Andes Mountains, particularly in Colombia, Ecuador, and Peru.[130] Because the incubation period is 19 to 100 days, visitors have usually returned to their homes before the onset of symptoms, and after the fly bite has been forgotten.

In the first stage, intermittent fever, malaise, myalgias, headache, gastrointestinal irritability, and finally symptoms due to increasingly severe hemolytic anemia appear (Oroya fever). Splenomegaly, pallor, and icterus are characteristic. In the second stage of the disease (verruga peruana) miliary erythematous macules and papules appear on the face and extensor surfaces of the extremities. In addition, subcutaneous nodules 1 to 2 cm in diameter appear in crops on the extremities and may ulcerate and bleed. In the acute phase, the bacilli are easily seen in Giemsa-stained blood smears. Phagocytized *Bartonella* organisms can be seen in the endothelial and histiocytic cells of verrugas if the diagnosis is suspected, but a histopathologic picture resembling a neoplasm has been noted. Blood culture results may be positive even during the cutaneous phase.

Penicillin, streptomycin, tetracycline, and chloramphenicol have all been used successfully. Patients are predisposed to secondary *Salmonella* infections, as are patients with any kind of hemolytic anemia.[130]

Leptospirosis

Leptospirosis is caused by the spirochete *Leptospira interrogans,* which can be cultured on special (Fletcher semisolid) media. The disease is a septicemia derived directly from farm, domestic, or wild animals or indirectly through contaminated water or soil.[131] Organisms enter through a break into the skin, mouth, or conjunctiva, but no local skin lesion appears. After an incubation period of 7 to 14 days, a biphasic infection results, with headache, fever, chills, nausea, vomiting, and myalgias followed by defervescence and a second febrile illness, often with meningitis. Skin lesions are most often produced by *L. icterohaemorrhagiae,* with jaundice, azotemia, and hemorrhagic manifestations in the skin. Surgical implications are negligible. Antibiotics may or may not be useful. Penicillin G and tetracycline are the drugs of choice. In jaundiced patients, the mortality rate may be as high as 40 percent.

Rickettsial Disease

The *Rickettsiae* (discussed in Chap. 9) rarely cause diseases encountered by surgeons. The organisms are transmitted through the skin by arthropod bites and usually produce acute systemic infections of varying severity, characterized by fever, headache, and rash. A surgeon may be asked to treat the primary lesion of scrub typhus or one of the spotted fever groups. The lesion is usually a vesicle that ruptures to form an eschar or, on occasion, a suppurative or necrotic lesion (see Table 6–4). The appearance of the eschar usually precedes the systemic manifestations, so that the diagnosis is not clear. A generalized rash is a common manifestation of the vasculitis associated with systemic rickettsiosis, and diffuse necrosis of the skin caused by ischemic vasculitis can appear.

Tularemia

Human infection with *Francisella tularensis* is discussed in Chapter 9. The ulceroglandular type of tularemia is the most common expression of the disease but oculoglandular, typhoidal, and pulmonary forms are seen.[132]

Inoculation occurs through the bite of infected ticks and flies or contact with infected animals, particularly wild rabbits and hares. Hunters, trappers, and furriers are most often infected. Tick-borne lesions affect the lower extremities; contact-acquired infections affect the upper body.

After an incubation period of 1 to 10 days, fever, sweats, chills, and myalgias are sometimes followed by stupor and coma. Only then does the primary skin lesion develop as a painful papule at the site of entry. The papule enlarges rapidly and undergoes necrosis, producing an indolent ulcer with raised edges and a necrotic base (see Fig. 31–22). The lesion is usually on an exposed extremity, and regional adenopathy develops after the appearance of the chancre-like primary lesion, usually without lymphangitis (see Table 31–16). In a few patients, tender nodules develop along the course of lymphatic channels, similar to sporotrichosis (see Table 31–14). The enlarged nodes may suppurate (Fig. 31–23).

The systemic and febrile infection lasts 2 to 4 weeks with constant bacteremia. In the oculoglan-

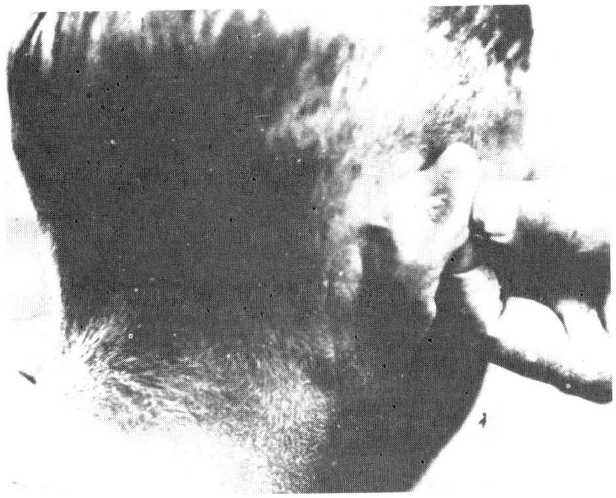

Figure 31–23. Tularemia, caused by a fly bite on the ear, with an enlarged posterior auricular node. *(From Armed Forces Institute of Pathology, Neg. No. 68-5644.)*

dular type, the primary lesion is a purulent conjunctivitis. The constitutional symptoms are so profound that the primary cutaneous lesion and the diagnosis may be missed. However, 90 percent of untreated patients survive, and with treatment, cure is almost universal. The differential diagnosis must include plague, cat scratch disease, melioidosis, and glanders. Since most laboratories are reluctant to isolate the highly contagious organism, serologic diagnosis is preferred. Tularemia agglutination titers become positive in the second week of the illness and remain positive for life. Fluorescent antibody staining may identify the organisms in biopsy specimens or currettings.

An attenuated vaccine administered intradermally by multiple puncture technique is available from the Centers for Disease Control and Prevention, Atlanta, GA. Streptomycin is the drug of choice (15 to 20 mg/kg/day intramuscularly for 7 to 10 days). Tetracycline and chloramphenicol are effective, but relapses occur more frequently. Aspiration or incision and drainage of fluctuant lymph nodes should be delayed until antibiotic therapy is well advanced.

Plague

Plague (*Yersinia pestis*) is an acute, febrile, fatal disease characterized by inflammation of the lymphatics, septicemia, and diffuse hemorrhages into the skin and subcutaneous tissues. Suppurative lymphadenitis with bubo formation is characteristic. Plague occurs worldwide and is endemic in the western United States.

Etiology. *Yersinia pestis* is a short, nonmotile, gram-negative, bipolar-staining, pleomorphic bacillus that is often encapsulated and produces a potent endotoxin. A more complete discussion is available in Chapter 5.

Plague is a disease of rats and other rodents, transmitted incidentally to humans by the bite of a rat flea. It occurs in three forms: bubonic, primary septicemic, and primary pneumonic plague.

Clinical Manifestations. Plague predominates in the bubonic form as an ulceroglandular process with the portal of entry on an extremity. The incubation period is 2 to 10 days. The onset of disease is sudden. The bite mark of the rat flea is inconspicuous, and the hallmark lesion of bubonic plague is the bubo (Fig. 31–24), a large, painful, tender, fixed, matted mass of lymph nodes with overlying skin erythema and a gelatinous consistency. An ulcer resembling the malignant pustule of anthrax may form near the bubo. Complications include septicemia, disseminated intravascular coagulation, pneumonia, and meningitis.[133] The differential diagnosis includes staphylococcal or streptococcal lymphadenitis, tularemia, cat scratch fever, ulceroglandular process, incarcerated hernia, and acute appendicitis (see Table 31–16).

Diagnosis. A Gram stain and culture of material aspirated from affected lymph nodes should be performed on all patients with suspected plague. A fluorescent antibody test, performed by the Centers for Disease Control and Prevention in Fort Collins, CO, is a rapid, specific means of making the diagnosis from various clinical specimens, including bubo aspirates. Acute and convalescent serum specimens

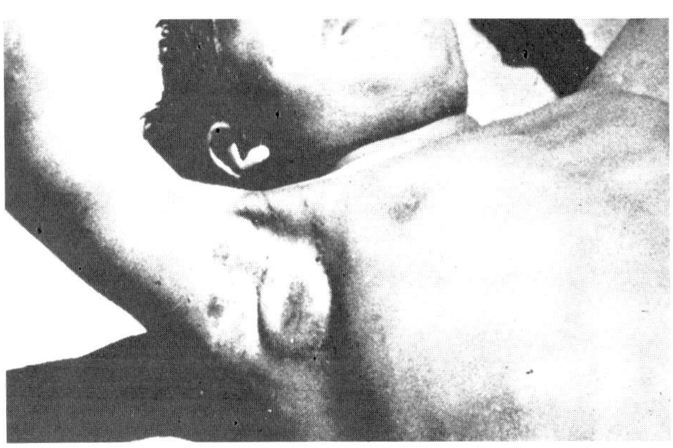

Figure 31–24. The hallmark of plague is an axillary of inguinal bubo. *(From Armed Forces Institute of Pathology, Neg. No. 219 900-7-B.)*

are tested for hemagglutinating antibodies, which appear 8 to 14 days after onset of the disease.

Treatment. The patient is hospitalized and isolated. Streptomycin, 30 mg/kg/day in divided doses, or tetracycline, 30 to 50 mg/kg/day in divided doses, should be given for 10 days.[133] Many patients require aggressive fluid resuscitation. Chloramphenicol is used for meningitis. Plague is an internationally quarantinable disease. Patients should be reported to regional health authorities.

Prevention. Chemoprophylaxis (tetracycline or sulfonamide) is recommended for all contacts with an index case. An effective formalin-killed vaccine is available for persons with high-risk occupations in plague endemic areas.

Nocardia

The etiologic agent and pathogenesis of *Nocardia* infections are discussed in Chapter 6. Soft tissue involvement with *N. asteroides* is usually secondary to hematogenous dissemination from a pulmonary focus in immunodepressed patients. Primary infections of the soft tissues are uncommon. *N. brasiliensis* frequently involves the skin and subcutaneous tissues in tropical regions and is a common cause of mycetoma in tropical regions[134] (see subsequent section on cutaneous fungal infections).

Both *N. asteroides* and *N. brasiliensis* produce suppurative infections of traumatic wounds contaminated with soil organisms. Cellulitis, subcutaneous abscess, pustules, pyoderma, and lymphadenopathy develop. Debridement and drainage may be adequate therapy but should be combined with sulfonamides. Gram stain of purulent drainage shows polymorphonuclear cells and beaded gram-positive branching organisms consistent with *Nocardia*. Rarely, a sulfur granule is seen in a skin biopsy specimen. *Nocardia* takes 2 to 5 days for the colonies to become visible on blood agar plates, and the laboratory diagnosis may be missed unless wound cultures are incubated for at least a week.

Although dissemination of locally inoculated *Nocardia* is rare, undertreatment can result in dissemination of the organism to visceral foci if the more invasive chronic lymphocutaneous infection develops.[134]

Cutaneous manifestations of pulmonary nocardiosis are usually part of a disseminated miliary syndrome with diffuse organ abscesses. Subcutaneous abscesses may be single or multiple, are firm rather than fluctuant, and do not form fistulas. The disease is usually identified at autopsy. Treatment is described in Chapter 6.

Actinomycosis

Actinomycosis is a chronic suppurative infection that forms external sinuses, which discharge characteristic sulfur granules, after endogenous oral commensals invade tissues of the face and neck, lungs, and ileocecal regions. *Actinomyces israelii* is most commonly isolated, but other bacteria are frequently found, especially *Actinobacillus actinomycetemcomitans. Haemophilus* species, *Fusobacterium,* anaerobic and other streptococci, micrococci, staphlococci, and oral *Bacteroides* accompany the cervicofacial, nervous system, and thoracic infections. Coliforms and intestinal anaerobes are often associated with abdominal actinomycosis. The etiologic agent and pathogenesis of these infections are discussed in Chapter 6.

Pathogenesis. The endogenous actinomycoses enter damaged tissues after infection, trauma, or surgical manipulation such as dental extraction. The soft tissues are usually involved before the skin, although mycetoma (see subsequent section) can be caused by the actinomycetes via primary inoculation from contaminated soil. Antecedent disease or operation predisposes to infection, but many infections occur without identifiable trauma.

Clinical Manifestations. The cervicofacial form resembles an acute pyogenic infection along the mandible or even a cold pseudotumor. Spontaneous or operative drainage creates a persistent cutaneous fistula (Fig. 31–25). Adenopathy is not common, although dental roentgenograms may reveal lytic bone lesions. Antibodies may modify this course.

Thoracic infections are the result of aspiration, esophageal injury, or extension into the mediastinal lymph nodes from the neck or the abdomen. Although usually pulmonary disease is manifest, fistulization of the skin and subcutaneous tissues may be the presenting sign (see Fig. 31–24). Disseminated infection may occur from pulmonary disease with subcutaneous abscesses and chronic fistulas. Thoracic antinomycosis is suspected when pulmonary lesions extend directly through the chest wall with bony involvement of vertebra, ribs, or even extension from lobe to lobe within the lung.

Abdominal or pelvic actinomycosis is found after surgery for inflammatory bowel disease or perforation of chronic diverticulitis, duodenal ulcer, or penetrating abdominal trauma. The diagnosis and therapy are discussed in detail in Chapters 6, 33, 35, and 38.

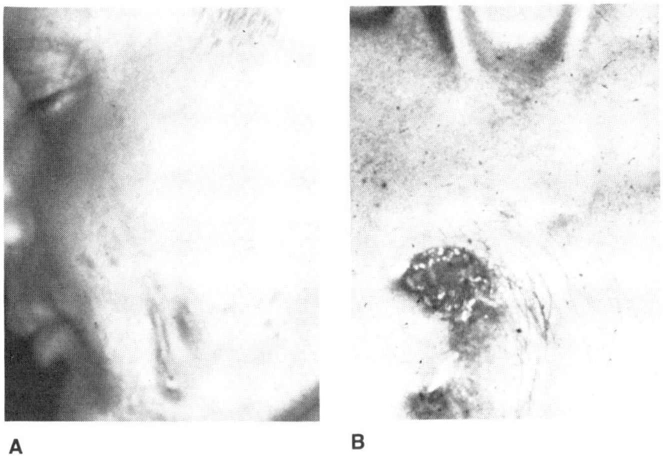

Figure 31–25. Cervicofacial **(A)** and thoracic **(B)** actinomycosis. The findings of a fistula draining an ulceronodular lesion are classic.

Blood-Borne Bacterial Soft Tissue Infections

Many infections cause rash. The following section will briefly discuss infections that metastasize through the bloodstream to the soft tissues.

Meningococcemia. Primary meningococcal suppurative lesions of the soft tissues are rarely seen, but skin lesions are often the most dramatic manifestations of meningococcemia.

Etiology. Neisseria meningitidis is one of the virulent pyogenic cocci discussed in Chapter 4.

Pathogenesis and Pathology. The skin lesions associated with meningococcemia result from damage to small dermal blood vessels.[82] Bacteria become pinocytosed by endothelial cells as well as by polymorphonuclear leukocytes, leading to local endothelial damage, thrombosis, and necrosis of the vessel walls. Edema, infection of overlying skin, and extravasation of red blood cells produce the characteristic progression from macular to hemorrhagic necrotic lesions. The potent endotoxin of *N. meningitidis* may precipitate a dermal Shwartzman reaction. The septic shock syndrome associated with meningococcemia may also be due to the Shwartzman reaction or to endotoxemia.

Most adults possess both IgM and IgG class bactericidal antibodies to *N. meningitidis*. Consequently, most clinical infections occur in children exposed to carriers within the family or in child care centers. Crowding of susceptible individuals, as in military barracks, can also lead to outbreaks of meningococcemia.

Clinical Manifestations. Patients usually become systemically ill, with fever, obtundation, and other manifestations of meningitis. The petechial skin lesions appear on the extremities and trunk. In fulminant meningococcemia, vomiting, stupor, hemorrhagic rash, and hypotension rapidly follow. Survivors develop purpura fulminans (Fig. 31–26). Septic foci in joints, pericardium, endocardium, and lung have been reported. Biopsy reveals organisms in swollen endothelial cells and polymorphonuclear leukocytes in the inflammatory reaction, entrapped by fibrin thrombi within vessels.

Treatment and Prognosis. Meningitis usually responds well to therapy, with recovery in 90 percent of patients, but severe meningococcemia with extensive cutaneous lesions is almost always fatal. Penicillin G (adult dose of 2 million units intravenously every 2 hours) is required. In chronic meningococcemia, lesser doses are effective. Chloramphenicol can be used in penicillin-allergic patients. Some strains are still sulfonamide sensitive. Excision and skin grafting of necrotic areas are indicated in patients who survive septicemia.

Prevention. Chemoprophylaxis is effective in contacts. A single dose of rifampin (600 mg orally for 4 days) is best. Vaccines for groups A and C serotypes have been developed and are useful in certain populations, that is military inductees.

Pseudomonas *Septicemia*

Etiology and Pathogenesis. The bacteriology and pathogenesis of pseudomonad infections are discussed in Chapter 5. *Pseudomonas* septicemia occurs primarily in premature infants, especially those with omphalitis, diarrhea, or urinary tract infection complicating congenital lesions (eg, extrophy of the bladder). Adults who are treated with immunosuppressive drugs or long-term antibiotics,

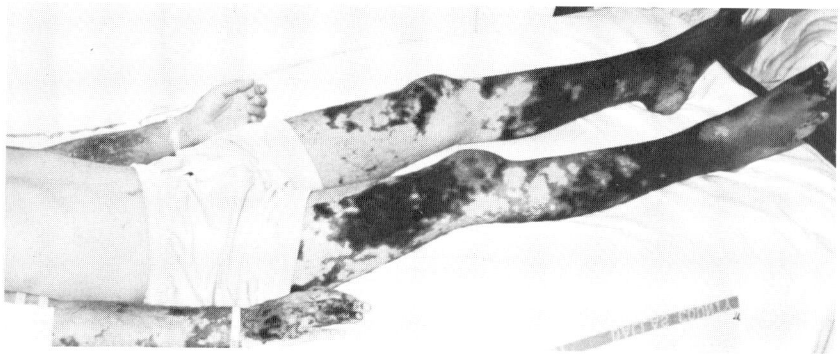

Figure 31–26. The hemorrhagic, advanced stage of meningococcemia. Dry gangrene of the toes and forefeet and full-thickness necrosis of skin are present over 40 percent of the body surface. *(Courtesy of P. William Curreri, MD, New York Hospital, Cornell Medical Center, New York.)*

who are burned, or who require indwelling venous catheters are also susceptible. The distinctive lesion is a necrotizing vasculitis, in which the walls of small arteries and veins are invaded by myriad bacteria. The endothelial surface is intact, and thrombosis is unusual. The occlusion of the vessel by the perivasculitis leads to the formation of cutaneous lesions. The skin is then invaded by bacteria directly. Other organs may be involved in multiple discrete nodular necrotic lesions.

Clinical Manifestation. Sudden worsening of the course of an immunodepressed or burned patient may be the signal that *Pseudomonas* superinfection with bacteremia has occurred. Although hemorrhagic manifestations similar to meningococcemia can occur, *Pseudomonas* usually produces other kinds of skin lesions—vesicles, bullae, macules, papules, or nodular lesions. Several other more deeply situated lesions may prompt surgical consultation in these debilitated patients (see Chap. 42).

The typical lesions are of three types:

1. Round, indurated, ulcerated, painless lesions with central black eschar, surrounded by erythema (necrotic vesicle), are most often found in the anal, genital, or axillary region.
2. Gangrenous cellulitis is a sharply demarcated, superficial, painless, necrotic lesion that may resemble a decubitus ulcer but is not located in a pressure area.
3. *Pseudomonas* abscess (nodular cellulitis) has red, warm nodular lesions situated too deep to feel fluctuant. Incision or aspiration reveals pus, and *P. aeruginosa* can be cultured.

Diagnosis. Aspiration of skin lesions with Gram stain of the smear and culture will reveal the organisms. Blood cultures are frequently positive as well.

Prognosis. Pseudomonas septicemia is frequently the terminal event in a complex illness. Intensive antibiotic therapy can sometimes be effective when combined with elimination of the underlying cause, such as removal of intravascular catheters or excision of infected burn wound eschar.

Treatment. Pseudomonas septicemia will require an aminoglycoside (gentamicin, tobramycin, or amikacin) in combination with ceftazadine or ticarcillin. Aminoglycoside levels should be monitored to assure adequate blood levels, especially in burned children, who may require two to three times the estimated dosage. Blood levels for the betalactam agents are obtained in the sickest patients. The nodular and pustular lesions benefit from incision, drainage, and debridement.

A polyvalent vaccine has been developed against *P. aeruginosa* for use in patients with thermal burns or cystic fibrosis. The results are encouraging in immunocompetent patients but are less impressive in impaired hosts.[32]

Sexually Transmitted Bacteria: Causes of Skin Ulceration

Lymphogranuloma Venereum

Etiology. Lymphogranuloma venereum (LGV) is a venereal disease characterized by suppurative inguinal adenitis. The causative agent is a strain of *Chlamydia trachomatis*. Like all *Chlamydia,* it exists in two forms—the infective nondividing elementary body, which is extracellular, and the intracellular noninfective reticulate body (see Chap. 6).

Incidence and Epidemiology. LGV is endemic in tropical areas of Asia, Africa, and South America, but an increasing number of cases have been found in the United States since the war in Vietnam. It is reported three times as frequently in men as in women and is especially common in patients returning from endemic regions, in male homosexuals, and in the lower socioeconomic classes living in the southeastern United States. Nonsexual transmission has also been reported.[135]

Pathogenesis. After sexual transmission, the extracellular elementary body becomes attached to phagocytes and undergoes endocytosis. It then forms the reticulate body, which grows by binary fission. *Chlamydia* lack the ability to generate energy and must utilize the cell's nucleotide triphosphates. After phagocytosis, the *Chlamydia* can grow within the phagosome without causing lysosomal fusion. Intracellular *C. trachomatis* can then lead to cell death.

Clinical Manifestations. Several days to 3 weeks after exposure, a painless vesicle or papule develops at the site of entry on the penis or vulva. The lesion heals quickly without a scar. In homosexuals, a primary anorectal infection may produce diarrhea, tenesmus, and a rectal discharge.

Two to six weeks after the initial exposure, a painful regional lymphadenopathy develops adjacent to the site of initial infection. For perineal sites, this involves the inguinal and femoral lymph nodes; with anorectal infection, the hypogastric and deep iliac nodes; and with vaginal or cervical infection, the obturator and iliac nodes. The nodes become matted, small abscesses form, coalesce, become necrotic, and ultimately break through the skin to form fistulas. The tracts heal over a period of months, but the scars remain. Systemic manifestations include fever, chills, anorexia, headache, and myalgias. There is a leukocytosis with elevated sedimentation rate and frequently abnormal liver function tests. Approximately 5 percent of men will develop chronic disease, with persistent fistulas or urethral or rectal strictures.

Diagnosis. The diagnosis is established by isolation of the organism from a bubo, although cultures are positive in only about 30 percent of cases. A complement-fixation test with a titer of greater than 1:64 is suggestive. The Frei test, formerly thought to be quite specific, is now rarely used because of low sensitivity and uncertain specificity.

The differential diagnosis includes syphilis, genital herpes, and chancroid. Clinically, LGV presents a more prominent ulcer and greater systemic symptoms than chancroid. Herpes simplex has painful tender vesicles with nonsuppurative regional lymphadenopathy. Syphilis is differentiated from LGV by its positive serologic tests as well as secondary rash and nontender inguinal lymphadenopathy.

Treatment. Fluctuant lymph nodes are aspirated to prevent rupture. Serologic tests exclude syphilis. LGV is sensitive to sulfomanides, 1 g/day for 21 days, or tetracycline, 500 mg/day for 21 days. These help resolve the constitutional symptoms, but the buboes heal slowly. Surgical procedures may be required for strictures, fistulas, or local elephantiasis.

Chancroid

Etiology. Chancroid or soft chancre is a sexually transmitted disease caused by *Haemophilus ducreyi*. These are small pleomorphic gram-negative coccobacilli, which are slow growing and strict parasites. They require hemin and/or nicotinamide adenine dinucleotide (NAD) for growth in culture (see Chap. 9).

Incidence and Epidemiology. Chancroid occurs worldwide, especially where hygiene is poor. It is most common among nonwhite uncircumcised males; only about 10 percent of cases occur in women, who may be asymptomatic carriers.

Clinical Manifestations. After an incubation period of 2 to 5 days, genital or perianal papules, with surrounding erythema, appear. Erosion leads to a soft, undermined, painful, nonindurated ulcer that bleeds easily and may be covered by a necrotic exudate. Multiple ulcerations sometimes appear, which can coalesce and, after superinfection (especially fusospirochetal), destroy the genitalia. Painful, unilateral, inguinal lymphadenitis is characteristic. Like LGV, spontaneous rupture of the abscessed node and fistula formation can occur.

Diagnosis. The differential diagnosis includes primary syphilis, herpes, and lymphogranuloma venereum. The diagnosis is confirmed by the demonstration of *H. ducreyi* on smear and culture of the lesion. The ulcers are cleaned with sterile saline and dried, and exudate from the ulcer border is inoculated into chocolate agar containing Isovitalex and vancomycin. A Gram stain may reveal large numbers of gram-negative coccobacilli usually in chains or "school of fish" patterns. Approximately 10 percent of chancroid patients have primarily syphilis, so dark-field examination to rule out syphilis is required. If these study results are negative, serologic studies for 3 months have been suggested.

Treatment. The treatment of choice is oral sulfisoxazole, 1 g orally every 6 hours for 1 to 2 weeks. Tetracycline has also been successfully used. In Southeast Asia, resistance to these agents has been reported, but kanamycin has been successfully used. Buboes should be aspirated to prevent rupture and fistula formation.[136]

Granuloma Inguinale

Etiology. The causative agent is *Calymmatobacterium (Donovania) granulomatis,* a gram-negative bacterium that usually lives within histiocytes (see Chap. 9). The organisms are encapsulated with small filamentous projections resembling pili.

Incidence and Epidemiology. Granuloma inguinale is common in India, Central Australia, New Guinea, and the Carribean. Fewer than 100 cases are reported annually in the United States. Apparently, it is a mildly contagious sexually transmitted disease that requires repeated exposure for transmission.

Pathology and Clinical Manifestations. The primary genital lesion is a nodule that appears 8 to 80 days after exposure and erodes to form a granulomatous heaped-up ulcer. This progresses slowly, and pathologic examination shows a dense dermal infiltrate of plasma cells and histiocytes, many containing intracellular organisms. The pathognomonic feature is a large infected mononuclear cell, 25 to 90 μm in diameter containing intracytoplasmic cysts filled with deeply staining organisms. The patients have subcutaneous granulomas that resemble buboes. Secondary infection may cause tissue destruction and subsequent scarring. Metastatic spread to bone, joints, and liver may occur.

Diagnosis. The diagnosis is confirmed by a Wright- or Giemsa-stained imprint of fresh granulation tissue. The diagnostic Donovan bodies appear as clusters of blue- or black-staining organisms, which look like safety pins because of chromatin condensation at the poles. Histologic examination of the fixed lesions rarely shows the Donovan bodies.

Treatment. Three-week courses of gentamicin or chloramphenicol are most effective. Tetracycline and ampicillin have been used, but failure rates are high. Clinical response to therapy is indicated by shrinking and decreasing redness of the lesions within 1 week, but medication should be continued until the lesions disappear. The lesions will heal even if drugs are stopped early, but recurrence is frequent.[137]

FUNGAL INFECTIONS

These diseases are of greater interest to dermatologists than surgeons. A few require operation for diagnosis or treatment, and many frequently masquerade as suppurative or malignant lesions.

Superficial Fungal Infections

Dermatophytosis (Tineas, Ringworms). These diseases are caused by the dermatophytes and other fungi that infect the cornified skin—hair and nails. These primary infections are of little importance to the surgeon, but they predispose to deeper local or systemic infections by bacteria or more invasive fungi. The inflammatory manifestations of some can be confused with abscesses and cellulitis.

Etiology. Table 31–26 lists some of the more common dermatophytic fungi and the other species that infect the cornified layers of the skin. Fungi that infect only the hair are omitted. These diseases are usually classified by anatomic region rather than by etiology.

Pathogenesis, Pathology, and General Clinical Manifestations. These fungi invade only dead, cornified layers of the skin, hair, and nails. Only a few organisms are necessary to induce an infection following trauma or occlusion. Dermatophytes grow in filamentous form within the stratum corneum. The downward extension of these hyphae is restricted because certain nutrients, principally iron, are not available in the deeper tissues. Consequently, lateral invasion from the focus of inoculation occurs, leading to the annular pattern seen on the skin surface.

The dermatophytes do not directly damage skin, but a delayed hypersensitivity reaction appears at the borders of the growing fungi after the host becomes sensitized to soluble fungal antigens. The inflammatory response results in a circinate pattern of erythema and edema, followed by exudation. Invasion of hair follicles produces inflamed nodules, deep-seated pustules, and abscesses. The skin becomes inflamed only after cell-mediated immunity to the dermatophyte develops. In its absence, only a dry, erythematous, scaly, pruritic, fissured skin results. Two types of dermatophyte

TABLE 31–26. ETIOLOGIC AGENTS OF THE SUPERFICIAL FUNGUS INFECTIONS OF THE SKIN

	Tinea Capitis	Tinea Barbae	Tinea Cruris	Tinea Pedis	Tinea Unguium	Tinea Versicolor	Tinea Nigra	Tinea Corporis
Dermatophytes								
Microsporum Species								
M. audouinii	Noninflammatory ++++							+
M. canis	++ inflammatory	+ inflammatory						+
M. nanum	+ inflammatory							
M. gypseum	+ inflammatory							+
M. fulvum	+ inflammatory							
Epidermophyton Species								
E. floccosum			++	++	+			+
Trichophyton Species								
T. mentagrophytes	+ inflammatory	+++ inflammatory	+++	+++	+++			+
T. rubrum		+ superficial	+++	++	+++			+
T. tonsurans	+ black dot							+
T. schoenleini	+ favus							
T. concentricum								+
T. furrugineum	+							+
T. violaceum	+ black dot	+ inflammatory			+			+
T. verrucosum	+ inflammatory	+++ inflammatory			+			+
T. megninii	+ inflammatory	+ inflammatory						
T. gallinae	+ favus							
Nondermatophytes								
Pityrosporum orbiculare (*Malassezia furfur*)					+			
Candida Species							+	
Cladosporium Werneckii							+	

+++, very common; +, rare.
Adapted from Jones HE, Harrell ER: Superficial fungus infections of the skin. In Hoeprich PD (ed): Infectious Diseases: A Modern Treatise of Infectious Processes, 2nd ed. Hagerstown, MD, Harper & Row, 1977, p 836.

infection occur: (1) the acute or inflammatory type of infection, associated with cell-mediated immunity to the fungus, which generally heals spontaneously or responds readily to treatment; and (2) the noninflammatory type, which is difficult to eradicate (see Table 31–26).

Hairy regions are particularly favorable for dermatophyte growth, since the hair is composed of nonliving keratin, where the organisms are isolated from cellular defenses. Areas with continuous hair growth, such as the scalp, develop particularly persistent infections.

Clinical Manifestations

TINEA CAPITIS. Ringworm of the scalp ordinarily produces round or oval areas with broken hairs (partial alopecia) in children. The first patch is the largest and the last to disappear. The borders are slightly elevated with central scaling skin, but fungal elements are absent. Itching may be the only symptom. *Microsporum audouini* or *Microsporum canis* fluoresce a bright blue-green under Wood's lamp, but culture is necessary for species identification.

Tinea capitis from *M. audouini* is characteristically noninflammatory, but other forms produce exudative folliculopustules. Permanent alopecia results when severe secondary bacterial infection supervenes. The inflammatory changes (kerions) signal spontaneous cure, although hair regrowth may be slow. Incision and drainage of lesions is almost never necessary.

TINEA BARBAE. Ringworm of the beard presents as a highly inflammatory kerion—a boggy, nodular, exudative circumscribed tumefaction studded with pustules. Suppuration and secondary bacterial invasion are common, but a noninflammatory form also occurs. Differentiation from bacterial folliculitis may be difficult, except that bacterial infections do not produce alopecia.

TINEA PEDIS (ATHLETE'S FOOT). Athlete's foot is the most common type of ringworm. It occurs primarily in young males who wear shoes, and hygienic measures within locker rooms are virtually useless. Three principle forms are described, but gradations occur frequently:

1. The intertriginous form produces maceration, weeping, scaling, and fissuring in the interdigital spaces, with accompanying malodor and pruritus. Scaling differentiates it from the other forms of intertrigo. Warm weather and hyperhidrosis aggravate the condition. Secondary bacterial infection is a serious complication, especially in diabetics.
2. The vesicular form occurs primarily on the instep and may represent a dermatophid (sensitization reaction in the absence of fungi).
3. Squamous ringworm is most frequently caused by *Trichophyton rubrum,* a noninflammatory organism that produces diffuse scaling which makes the foot appear excessively dry.

The first two forms tend to be inflammatory and recurrent. The third is comparatively noninflammatory and extraordinarily persistent.

TINEA CORPORIS. Ringworm of glabrous skin can produce vesicles, scaling, eczematous lesions, or massive granulomas, which may be mistaken for skin cancer. Tropical climates appear to predispose; most lesions remain localized except in patients suffering from systemic diseases such as diabetes and leukemia. The diagnosis requires examination of scrapings from the border of the lesion to exclude a variety of other dermatoses.

TINEA CRURIS. Groin ringworm is extremely common in males and uncommon in females except those wearing tightfitting slacks or panty hose. It is an intertriginous infection starting in the moist crural or perineal folds with extensions onto the thighs. Bilateral involvement produces half-moon-shaped circinate lesions on each upper inner thigh with or without central clearing. Scaling is not a prominent feature. Wood's lamp examination facilitates the diagnosis. Recurrence is due to high environmental temperatures, poor hygiene, and intertriginous moisture.

TINEA UNGUIUM. Superficial fungal infections of the toenails are common in people wearing shoes and may be caused by fungi not classified as dermatophytes. They are frequent in patients with athlete's foot or the chronic squamous type of foot ringworm caused by *T. rubrum*. The distal nail becomes discolored and thickened by subungual hyperkeratosis, which ultimately leads to separation from the nail bed and considerable cosmetic distortion.

TINEA VERSICOLOR. This is an infection of the stratum corneum caused by a nondermatophyte fungus, *Pityrosporon orbiculare* (*P. furfur, Malassezia furfur*). It produces asymptomatic hyperpigmented scaling lesions of no surgical importance.

Diagnosis. Microscopic examination of potassium hydroxide-treated scrapings from the afflicted areas reveals the characteristic hyphal growths. The organisms can be grown in culture if necessary.

Treatment. The details of treatment are best reviewed in dermatology texts. The principles are exemplified in the treatment of athlete's foot. Drying the skin is essential for treatment and prevention. The areas are washed, gently abraded to remove scales and macerated skin, and dried carefully. Continued exposure to the air (eg, going barefoot) is helpful. Dusting powder and cotton inserts are useful if changed before they become wet. Affected nails can be removed, but this will not cure the disease. Prolonged use of topical Whitfield's ointment combined with debridement of infected nails is inexpensive and effective.

Topical application of an azole (miconazole or clotrimazole) as a cream or solution may cure mild cases. Severe cases necessitate the administration of griseofulvin or oral ketoconazole. Tinea versicolor is extirpated with a 1 percent selenium sulfide-based shampoo. Oral griseofulvin is the first-line agent for scalp ringworm.

Superficial Candidiasis. The cutaneous manifestations of candidiasis are commonly seen in dermatologic practice, and as a nosocomial infection in surgical patients whose skin becomes macerated around open wounds or enterostomy sites.

The etiology, pathogenesis, and diagnosis of *Candida* infections are discussed in Chapter 10. The diagnosis of superficial candidiasis is made by microscopic demonstration of the organism in scrapings of the lesion. Cultural isolation of such a common commensal organism from a superficial lesion is not diagnostic. Although superficial candidiasis is not amenable to surgical therapy, extensive mucocutaneous candidiasis frequently precedes or accompanies systemic candidiasis in surgical patients in intensive care units.

Mucocutaneous Candidiasis

THRUSH. Thrush is the most common candidal infection and is frequently seen in patients receiving antibiotics in whom the normal oropharyngeal flora have been altered. Oral nystatin is effective prophylaxis in patients at risk (ie, transplant patients).

The characteristic lesions are white patches on the mucous membranes of the mouth, usually sparing the pharynx. The patches are soft, creamy or crumbly, and poorly adherent, revealing a red base. In extensive cases, the patches may extend into the trachea, upper bronchi, or the esophagus. Perleche (cracks and fissures at the corners of the mouth) may be caused by *C. albicans*. On microscopic examination, the white material is composed of pathognomonic budding cells and filaments.

VULVOVAGINAL CANDIDIASIS. *Candida* is a normal resident of the vagina. Candidiasis occurs more frequently in pregnancy, in diabetes, and in women taking oral contraceptives or antibiotics. A white or yellow curdy discharge containing budding cells and filaments is diagnostic of vaginal candidiasis. The discharge causes itching, redness, and swelling of the vulva (see Chap. 48).

CUTANEOUS CANDIDIASIS. Many varieties of this illness occur:

1. *Candida* intertrigo (diagnosed by the demonstration of large quantities of fungus in scrapings) causes lesions in the groin, axilla, intergluteal cleft, and the inframammary region as a dermatitis. *Candida* intertrigo progresses to a macerated, eroded, red, weeping dermatitis. Debilitated nonambulatory women receiving antibiotics or immunosuppressive therapy are commonly affected.
2. *Candida* paronychia is associated with trauma to the nail or frequent immersion of the hands in water. *Candida albicans* has no keratinolytic enzymes and does not disrupt nail substance but produces nail plate defects by damage to the matrix. The paronychial tissue is swollen and red, but relatively nontender and nonfluctuant although a drop of pus may be expressed from under the nail fold. Several fingers are usually involved. It is unclear whether *C. albicans* is a primary or a secondary invader.
3. Generalized cutaneous candidiasis is a rare generalized eruption.
4. Folliculitis, balanitis, and nodular and granulomatous manifestations are occasionally seen.

CHRONIC MUCOCUTANEOUS CANDIDIASIS. This progressive candidal infection of mucous membranes, skin, and its appendages is usually found in patients with an inability to respond effectively to *Candida* antigens, which are present in high titers. The mucous membranes are covered with thrush, and the skin is covered with candidal paronychia or intertrigo. A generalized hyperkeratotic crusted dermatosis can result in disfiguring granulomas with scarring and loss of hair. Secondary bacterial infection can occur, but candidal dissemination is rare. The disease responds temporarily to systemic amphotericin B but recurs promptly when the drugs are stopped. Ketoconazole controls the disease. Immunostimulation with various experimental preparations (such as levamisole, transfer factor) has been tried. An acquired endocrine (parathyroid, adrenal) disorder has been reported.

Treatment of Superficial Candidiasis. The polyene antibiotics nystatin and amphotericin B are effective, but amphotericin B is rarely required for mucocutaneous candidiasis. Thrush can be prevented by oral nystatin, 500,000 units (5 ml) four times daily. Patients who are immunosuppressed or receiving high-dose antibiotics may require higher doses. Similarly, nystatin can be administered as a vaginal tablet, and the gastrointestinal *C. albicans* can be suppressed by oral nystatin tablets in doses of 1 to 3 million units taken several times a day. Ketoconazole is highly effective for both treatment and prophylaxis.

Candidal intertrigo may resolve rapidly if skin maceration is alleviated. Ointments must be avoided. Amphotericin, miconazole, and clotrimazole creams may be helpful, but nystatin powder is the primary choice.

The Subcutaneous Mycoses and Mycetomas

The subcutaneous mycoses (chromomycosis, sporotrichosis) and the mycetomas are the result of traumatic implantation of the fungus into the skin and subcutaneous tissues. The ensuing disease generally remains localized or slowly spreads to the surrounding tissue. In some diseases, slow extension via lymphatic channels is characteristic (sporotrichosis), but in others, hematogenous or lymphatic dissemination is possible (chromomycosis). The etiologic agents are soil saprophytes, which are quite heterogeneous—their only common feature is the type of local disease produced. Most are sensitive to amphotericin B and the azole antifungals.

Chromomycosis. Chromomycosis includes four clinical entities caused by pigmented fungi: (1) chromoblastomycosis or verrucous dermatitis is the classic form of the disease—a chronic granulomatous infection characterized by warty nodules and plaques that may ulcerate,[138] (2) the brain abscess syndrome (cladosporiosis), (3) a cystic subcutaneous form,[139] and (4) possibly a systemic form.[139]

Etiology. The disease is caused by a wide variety of closely related pigmented fungi, which produce black or brown thick-walled spores in tissue. *Phialophora verrucosa, Fonsecaea pedrosoi, F. compactum, F. dermatitidis,* and *Cladosporium carrioni* are the most common causes of chromoblastomycosis. Other less pathogenic species of these three genera produce cystic chromomycosis, especially *P. gougerotii.*[138]

Epidemiology. Most cases occur in male agricultural workers from humid tropical regions. The spores of soil fungi are implanted by minor trauma to the feet and legs. Children exposed to these conditions rarely develop the disease, suggesting that spores can lie dormant for prolonged periods. The cystic form is the result of mycelial growth in deep puncture wounds.

Pathology. The verrucous lesion shows a pseudoepitheliomatous hyperplasia of the surface epithelium and microabscesses containing neutrophils in the underlying dermis surrounded by epithelioid and giant cell granulomas. Brown yeast cells may be seen in and around the foreign body and Langhans giant cells. Fibrosis may be a feature in chronic cases. The cystic lesion is a mycelial ball surrounded by a thick fibrous capsule.

Clinical Manifestations

CHROMOBLASTOMYCOSIS. This is the classic form of chromomycosis. A small pink scaly papule appears at the site of skin trauma (usually on the foot) and enlarges to a warty tumor, which may persist or spread out to form a plaque. The plaques may be verrucous with central scarring (tuberculoid), extensively scarred with a serpiginous border (syphiloid), scaly (psoriasiform), or indurated with draining sinuses (mycetomatoid). There is no invasion of muscle or bone, but tendon contractures, muscle atrophy, and osteoporosis may occur. Secondary ulceration from trauma or superinfection can lead to lymphedema and elephantiasis. Progress is slow, and satellite lesions along lymphatics may spread to involve a whole limb over 10 to 15 years. Most patients wait to seek medical assistance until they are disabled by lymphedema. Rarely, hematogenous spread and metastases occur to uninvolved areas of the body and the brain. Lymphatic spread is frequent after treatment by cautery and curettage, and biopsies can cause local spread.[138,139]

The differential diagnosis includes blastomycosis, sporotrichosis, mycetoma, tuberculous verrucosa cutis, candidiasis, leishmaniasis, tertiary syphilis, and yaws. The diagnosis of chromomycosis is confirmed by culture of the organisms, by microscopic visualization of the thick-walled dark spores in 20 percent KOH-treated scrapings from the lesions, or by histologic examination of a biopsy specimen showing the granulomatous reaction and spores.[138]

CYSTIC AND NONSPECIFIC CHROMOMYCOSIS (INCLUDING PHAEOSPOROTRICHOSIS). A puncture wound can inoculate the fungi deep into the subcutaneous tissues; single or multiple deep cysts containing masses of brown pigmented fungi of varied morphology result. The clinical designation phaeosporotrichosis is inappropriate, because the disease does not resemble sporotrichosis and the etiologic agents are not related. Phaeomycotic cyst is a better term.

The most common clinical presentation is a cutaneous, subcutaneous, or intramuscular abscess, which evolves into a hard cyst several centimeters in diameter, covered by a raised, thickened epidermis. Occasionally, the cyst may ulcerate and extrude pus containing brown hyphae and sclerotic cells. The regional lymph nodes are not involved, and dissemination is rare. Aspiration of the lesions sometimes results in a chronic fistula.

The differential diagnosis of this form of the disease includes the gumma of tertiary syphilis, sebaceous cyst, foreign body granuloma, tendon sheath ganglion, and sporotrichosis. Demonstration of pigmented fungi in material from lesions and their isolation in culture establish the diagnosis.

Treatment. Traditionally, chromoblastomycosis has been resistant to treatment. In the early verrucous lesion, wide and deep excision and grafting give good results. Curettage and cautery may cause dissemination of infection with lymphatic spread. Systemic amphotericin B is not useful, since fungicidal levels cannot be obtained in vivo. The most promising results have been with the antihelminthic thiabendazole orally (25 mg/kg/day) for 3 to 22 months, or 5-fluorocytosine (100 to 200 mg/kg/day) until healing is complete. Ketoconazole may be combined with 5-FC. Cystic chromomycosis should be excised. Contamination of the surrounding tissue can lead to recurrence.[138]

Sporotrichosis. Sporotrichosis is caused by the fungus *Sporothrix (Sporotrichum) schenckii*. As in all the subcutaneous mycoses, traumatic implantation of the fungus produces a chronic, benign-looking, cutaneous-lymphatic disease. A systemic infection characterized by polyarthritis and pneumonia can occur without the distinctive skin lesions.

Etiology. Sporothrix schenckii is a fungus that grows in tissues as a round or cigarshaped yeast form. Its mycologic properties are discussed in Chapter 10.

Epidemiology. The fungus is found worldwide in soil, decaying vegetation, and gardening supplies and is introduced by accidental cutaneous implantation by a thorn (rose gardener's disease) or other minor trauma. Most cases are reported from Africa, France, Mexico, and the southern United States, especially in persons handling plants.

Pathogenesis and Pathology. After an injury, a small ulcer or subcutaneous nodule appears with erythema and fluctuance. Secondary nodules develop to mark the intermittent course of lymphatic spread. The nodular lesions consist of central necrotic tissue with a few neutrophils, eosinophils, and monocytes surrounded by epithelioid cells and occasional Langhans giant cells. Microabscesses are surrounded by lymphocytes and plasma cells. The asteroid body, amorphous eosinophilic material that radiates from a central fungal cell, is often seen in sporotrichosis as well as coccidioidomycosis and aspergillosis.

Clinical Manifestations. The ulcerating nodular lesions begin in the extremity at a site of injury with centripetal spread marked by multiple subcutaneous nodules along the course of the draining lymphatics (see Fig. 31–27). Little pain or disability results unlike bacterial cellulitis and lymphangitis. A pulmonary form[140] and a disseminated form have also been described. The latter produces multifocal lesions in skin, synovia, or bone especially in metacarpal, phalangeal, or tibial bones.

Diagnosis. Isolation of the fungus is pathognomonic, since it is never a saprophyte in humans. Histologic diagnosis is difficult, since visible fungi

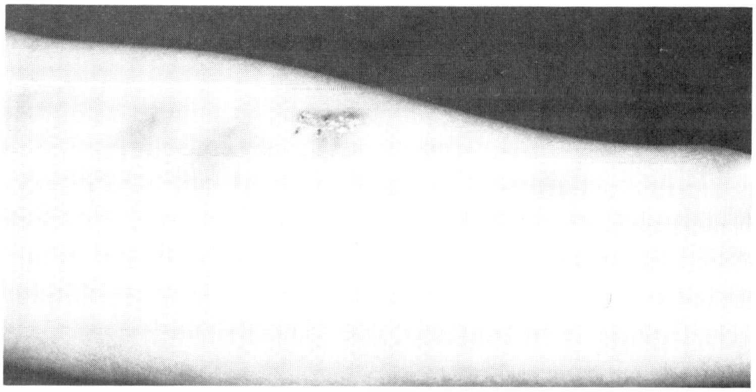

A

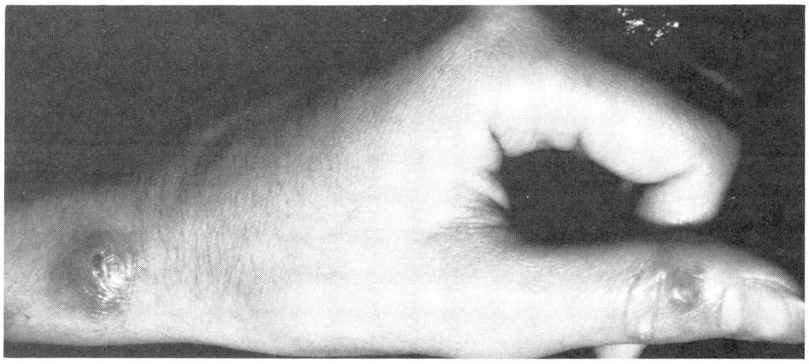

B

Figure 31–27. Sporotrichosis is an ulceronodular lesion with nodules that form along the course of lymphatic vessels. *(Courtesy of Robert W. Goltz, MD, Professor and Head, Department of Dermatology, University of Minnesota, Minneapolis.)*

or asteroid bodies in tissue are rare and secondary bacterial infections are common. Many other chronic granulomatous infections can give an identical clinical picture (see Table 31–14).

Therapy. The cutaneous-lymphatic form responds rapidly to treatment with a saturated solution of potassium iodide (1 g/ml given in a dosage of 9 to 12 g/day in three divided doses). Amphotericin B, to a total dose of 1.5 to 2.5 g, has been employed (see Chap. 10). Mortality and relapses are rare after adequate treatment.

The Mycetomas. A mycetoma is a chronic, granulomatous pseudotumor of the subcutaneous tissues, frequently extending into bone, characterized by abscess formation, sinuses, and fistulas that intermittently drain.[141,142] Fungi and aerobic actinomycetes introduced into the skin by trauma are the causal agents. Although clinically and pathologically identical to mycetomas, cervicofacial actinomycosis caused by anaerobic actinomycetes and botryomycosis caused by some eubacteria are not usually categorized as such (see Table 31–27). The lesions most often occur on the foot as Madura foot, but the disease may occur on any part of the body.

Etiology. The organisms causing mycetomas belong to two groups, fungi and actinomycetes. The mycetomas are consequently divided into two groups, the mycotic mycetomas (eumycetomas or true maduromycoses) and the actinomycotic mycetomas, although the clinical pictures are identical. Almost 90 percent of mycetomas in North and Central America are due to *Nocardia brasiliensis,* but even dermatophytes can cause mycetomas of the scalp and neck. A useful classification is based on the characteristic color of the grossly visible mycetomic grains found in pus or biopsy material (see Table 31–27).

Epidemiology. Mycetomas are common in the tropical and hot temperate zones, especially in tropical North America (Mexico), Central America (except Costa Rica), India, and Africa. They also exist to a lesser extent in the southern United States, southern Europe, and the Near East. Alternating dry and wet seasons favor the disease. Mycetomas develop following a minor injury in mostly barefoot subjects who are in contact with contaminated material (field laborers, farmers, herders, fishermen). Scalp and back mycetomas affect laborers carrying contaminated material on their heads or over the shoulder.

TABLE 31–27. ETIOLOGIC CLASSIFICATION OF MYCETOMAS

Mycotic mycetomas
Caused by eumycetes (branched filaments, 3–4 μm or more in diameter)
Black grain
Madurella mycetomi
M. grisea
Pyrenochaeta romeroi
Phialophora jeanselmei
Leptosphaeria senegalensis
L. tompkinsii
Whitish to yellowish grain
Allescheria boydii-Monosporium apiospermum (*Petriellidium boydii*)
Cephalosporium sp. (*C. recifei, C. falciforme*)
Fusarium sp.
Neotestudina rosatii
Aspergillus nidulans
Actinomycotic mycetomas
Caused by aerobic actinomycetes (branched filaments, 1 μm or less in diameter)
Whitish to yellowish grain
Actinomadura madurae
Streptomyccs somaliensis
Red grain
Actinomadura pelletieri
Small grain (grains invisible to the naked eye)
Nocardia brasiliensis
N. asteroides
N. caviae
Actinomycosis (*Sensu Stricto*)
Caused by anaerobic or microaerophilic actinomycetes (short filaments, 1 μm in diameter)
Yellow grains
Actinomyces israelii
A. bovis
Botryomycosis
Caused by *Eubacteria* (cocci or short rods)
Yellow grains
Actinobacillus lignieresii
Staphylococcus species
Streptococcus species

From Mariat F, Destombes P, Segretain G: Contrib Microbiol Immunol 4:1, 1977.

Pathogenesis and Pathology. A typical mycetoma consists of a large granulomatous tumor with a purulent center surrounded by a thick fibrotic reaction. Communicating, draining sinuses extend along fascial planes and through the skin. The central suppurative zone is in contact with the fungal granules, surrounded by a ring of histiocytes often arranged in palisade fashion and frequently appearing as foreign body giant cells. In a third concentric zone, a subacute nonspecific granuloma is observed containing new capillaries, edema, histiocytes, plasma cells, mast cells, and eosinophils. Lymphocytes are generally localized in a more peripheral zone, sometimes embedded in the fibrotic tissue.

The central grains are an agglomeration of fungal or actinomycotic filaments with a diagnostic shape, composition, and color. Other organisms can cause grain formation, including actinomycosis (*A. israelii*), lumpy jaw (*A. bovis*), botryomycosis (*Staphylococcus* and other bacteria), and cryptic tonsillitis (*Leptothrix*).[141]

Clinical Manifestations. After inoculation, there is a delay before onset of symptoms. The patient first notes a feeling of discomfort at the point of inoculation, accompanied by a small subcutaneous nodule adhering to the skin and sometimes to deeper tissues. The primary lesion subsequently opens to the skin, and grains may be extruded (see Fig. 31–28A). New nodules then form around the initial abscesses. The mycetoma develops slowly, invading along fascial planes, forming fistulas and abscesses in the midst of the inflammatory tumor. Involvement of bone is common. In the foot, for instance, small cavities are formed in the bone, appearing as osseous "geodes," 2 to 10 mm in diameter. The medullary canal and epiphyses can also be invaded. Destruction of bone and the formation of osteophytes can give rise to a complete remodeling or destruction of the bone (see Fig. 31–28B). At this stage of the disease, radiography is of great value, and in some typical cases the diagnosis and prognosis can be made on the basis of x-ray examination.

During the late phase, all the tissues may be involved. When this occurs, secondary bacterial infections supervene, obscuring the diagnosis. Visceral metastases via lymphatics from primary subcutaneous foci can be observed. Pulmonary metastases from primary thoracic mycetomas and abdominal and visceral metastases from mycetomas of the legs, thigh, and perineum have been reported, especially with *Nocardia* and *Actinomadura pelletieri,* perhaps because the small grains of these species can pass easily through the lymphatic vessels.[141,142]

Foot lesions (Madura foot) (see Fig. 31–28B) are most often encountered. The destruction of the metatarsal bones with widespread plantar fibrosis and scarring of tendons gives the foot a characteristic shortened and raised appearance.

Mycetomas develop slowly, spreading over a period of even 25 years or more. Sinuses may heal, only to open again in another area. The patient frequently delays medical therapy because of the absence of pain and the fear of amputation. Although cranial mycetoma can be rapidly fatal, most mycetomas are indolent and compatible with long life.

Diagnosis. Mycetoma must be differentiated from the other diseases that cause persistent draining sinuses (see Table 31–15), including some cancers (sarcoma, Kaposi's disease). The etiologic agent can frequently be identified by the morphology of the grain in tissue sections stained with hematoxylin and eosin. Grains removed from deep biopsy speci-

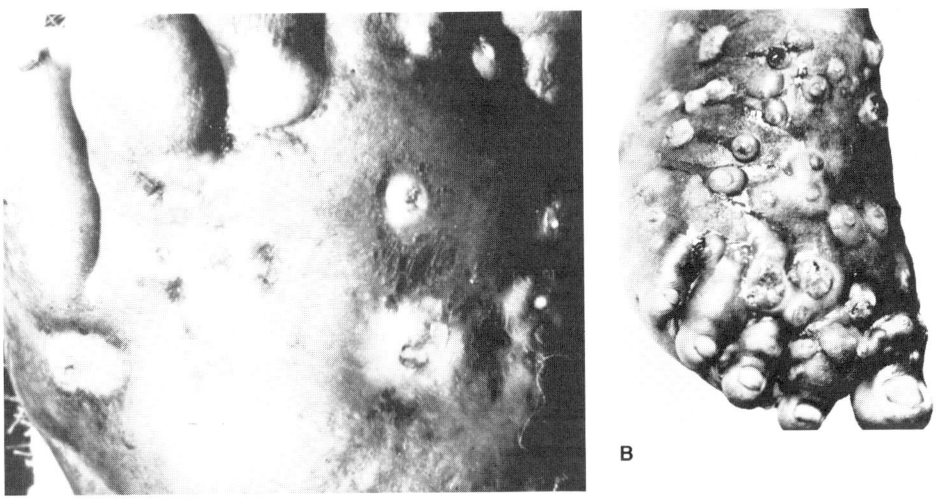

A

B

Figure 31–28. A moderately advanced lesion of mycetoma **(A)** and even later, a Madura foot **(B)**. *(From Armed Forces Institute of Pathology, Neg. No. N-39280 [6490].)*

mens are cultured, but bacterial contamination is common. Serologic tests can also be used.

Treatment. Amputation of the destroyed part is necessary in advanced cases. Chemotherapy includes streptomycin combined with either dapsone or trimethoprime-sulfamethoxazole. Ketoconazole is active against Eumycetes.[142]

Cutaneous and Soft Tissue Infections with Systemic Fungi

The biology, the clinical aspects, and the treatment of systemic infections with *Aspergillus,* the zygomycetes, *Cryptococcus, Histoplasma, Blastomyces, Coccidioides,* and *Paracoccidiodes* have been discussed in Chapter 10. All these fungi can produce both primary and metastatic infection of the skin and soft tissues.

Cutaneous Aspergillosis. Aspergillosis is a disease caused by allergic phenomenon, simple colonization, or true tissue invasion (see Chaps. 10 and 51). A number of *Aspergillus* species have been implicated, but most invasive infections are due to *A. fumigatus.*

Invasive infections are rarely seen in immunocompetent hosts. Immunosuppressed patients sometimes develop necrotic skin ulcers with black eschars at sites of minor trauma, but most infections originate in the lungs. Transpleural extension to bone or soft tissue is rare, as is hematogenous dissemination to soft tissue or bone. Chronic infections of the paranasal sinus may erode into adjacent tissues including the brain. The diagnosis depends on culture isolation and the demonstration of hyphae in tissue specimens. Dissemination from a primary cutaneous infection is unusual.

Cutaneous and wound infections usually begin with blisters or pustules, which progress to hemorrhagic vesicles and progressive skin necrosis, which spreads circumferentially. Smears reveal gram-positive organisms suggesting staphylococci, but histopathologic study demonstrates fungi with broad nonseptate hyphae in the necrotic debris. Drug therapy with amphotericin B is ineffective in the presence of necrotic tissue. Wound infections require wide debridement combined with systemic amphotericin B and topical antifungal therapy to prevent reinfection.

Cutaneous Zygomycosis. Zygomycosis (mucormycosis, phycomycosis) caused by organisms of the genera *Mucor, Absidia,* and *Rhizopus* has been reported mostly in immunosuppressed or debilitated patients (diabetes mellitus, leukemia, lymphoma, renal failure, malnutrition, and malignancy) (see Fig. 31–29A, B). In Uganda, primary subcutaneous infections with zygomycetes are not uncommon even in normal persons, particularly with *Entomophthora* and *Basidiobolus.*[143] The more common

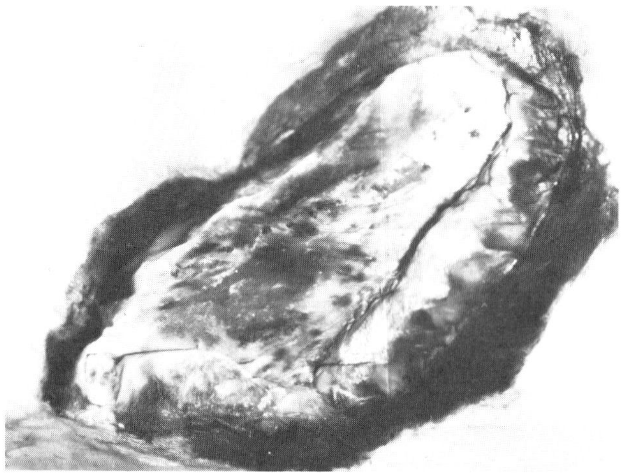

A

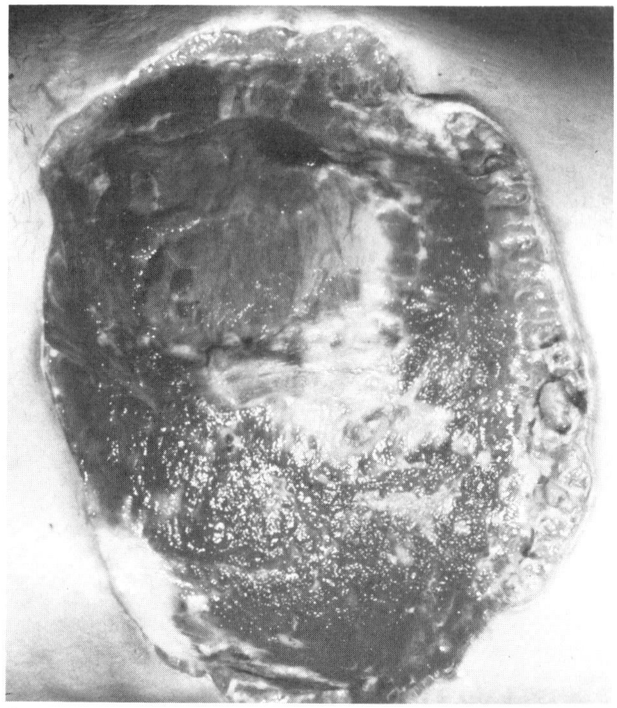

B

Figure 31–29. A. This cutaneous zygomycotic ulcer is surrounded by black necrotic tissue, but debridement must include tissue outside the area of obvious necrosis. **B.** Progressive debridement required to treat this zygomycotic ulcer in the abdominal wall of a renal transplant recipient. There is still a rim of progressive gangrene at the top right of the picture. *(Courtesy of William Sterling, MD, University of New Mexico.)*

rhinocerebral and pulmonary infections in immunosuppressed patients have been discussed in Chapters 10, 33, and 35.

Direct inoculation into the skin accounts for the skin infections, since these fungi are ubiquitous in soil. Burned tissue is susceptible.[144]

It is important to recognize these fungi as a component of mixed necrotizing infections. Diabetic or immunosuppressed patients with recent wounds or operations are usually affected. The lesion begins innocently as a necrotic ulcer or blister in the edge of the wound. Pain is minimal, fever is low grade, and crepitus is absent. The ulcerating lesion progressively expands and invades the skin and soft tissue so that progressive synergistic gangrene or necrotizing fasciitis is suspected. Wide debridement and systemic amphotericin B are required for control.[143,145] Histopathologic examination of the debrided tissue edges is necessary to be assured that debridement is sufficient. Burn wound infections cause a very high mortality.[144]

Cutaneous Coccidioidomycosis

Etiology and Pathogenesis. The diagnosis and treatment of coccidioidomycosis have been discussed in Chapter 10. Extrapulmonary extension from an active, but perhaps asymptomatic, pulmonary focus is more common in blacks and Filipinos; the skin is especially favored. The lesions are granulomas and have few identifying characteristics. Chronic necrotic ulcers or abscesses draining a thick mucoid pus result from necrosis of subcutaneous granulomas. Multiple lesions can fuse, producing extensive ulcerations that ultimately develop veruccous or papillomatous changes. Neoplastic transformation can supervene.

In addition to the systemic cutaneous form, a rare primary cutaneous coccidioidomycosis produces a chancreform syndrome with regional adenopathy. Multiple draining nodules may form along the course of the lymphatics in a sporotrichoid pattern (see Table 31–14). This is a self-limited disease quite different from the localized coccidioidicidal granuloma produced by hematogenous dissemination.

The diagnosis and treatment of disseminated coccidioidomycosis are discussed in Chapter 10. The coccidioidin skin test is diagnostic in limited disease, but patients with disseminated disease become anergic; a rising complement-fixation titer signals progression and dissemination.

The diagnosis is made by demonstrating the characteristic endosporulating spherules on smears of sputum or biopsy specimens or by culture of the fungus. Disseminated disease is treated with amphotericin B, ketoconazole, or itraconazole.

Cutaneous Blastomycosis. The etiology, pathogenesis, diagnosis, and treatment of blastomycosis are discussed in Chapter 10. Forty to 80 percent of the patients with systemic infections will develop skin lesions, which are the initial manifestations 25 to 40 percent of the time. The lesions begin as a papule or nodule, which ulcerates and discharges purulent material. Usually there is a single lesion on the face, wrist, hands, or feet, but any site can be affected (Fig. 31–30). The lesion enlarges eccentrically and clears centrally, leaving a dense scar. Progression is slow but relentless, with an arciform or serpiginous, sharply elevated, verrucous, violaceous border (Fig. 31–30). Miliary abscesses contain organisms and are always found within the abruptly sloping border. Multiple subcutaneous abscesses may be present in disseminated blastomycosis. Accidental inoculation in physicians and laboratory workers leads to a chancreform syndrome with a localized cutaneous plaque and regional adenopathy. The primary lesion heals spontaneously, and the disease involutes.

The diagnosis and treatment of blastomycosis have been discussed in Chapter 10. Biopsy samples should be obtained from the border of the lesions, but the demonstration of round, budding organisms in a potassium hydroxide mount is difficult because

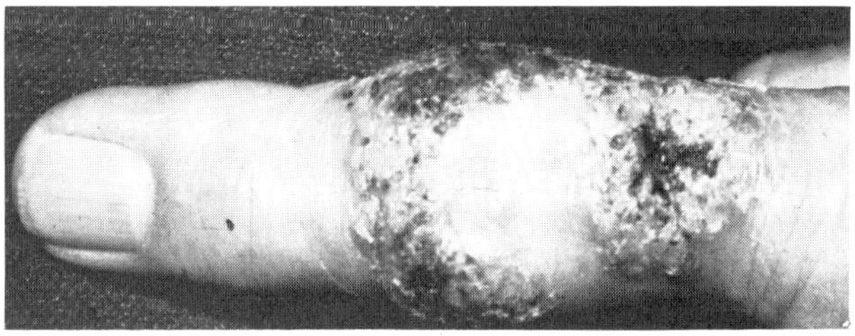

A

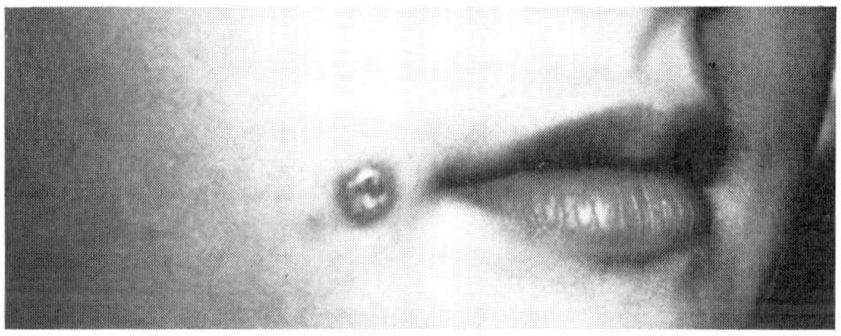

B

Figure 31–30. Cutaneous blastomycosis. **A.** Extensive ulceronodular involvement of the finger. **B.** An early facial lesion. *(Courtesy of Robert W. Goltz, MD, Professor and Head, Department of Dermatology, University of Minnesota, Minneapolis.)*

organisms are sparse. The organism is best cultured by aspirating unruptured subcutaneous nodules. The blastomycin skin reaction has presumptive diagnostic value, and a primary pulmonary source should be sought. Cutaneous blastomycosis must be differentiated from tuberculosis, neoplasm, drug eruptions, syphilis, granuloma inguinale, and other deep-seated fungal infections. Chronic granulomatous pyoderma may be a particular source of confusion.

Treatment with ketoconazole or rarely amphotericin B, has been discussed in Chapter 10. Excision or debridement is usually contraindicated.

Cutaneous Paracoccidioidomycosis. The etiology and pathogenesis of paracoccidioidomycosis have been discussed in Chapter 10. The most common type of disseminated paracoccidioidomycosis is first seen as lymph node enlargement. The skin may be the site of numerous granulomatous ulcerative lesions originating in the mucous membranes of the mouth, tongue, gum, palate, cheek, lips, and occasionally nasal mucosa. A smooth, firm ulcer dotted with punctate hemorrhages rapidly enlarges to produce a hard brawny mass. New ulcers arise in the mouth and also extend rapidly, destroying most of the mucosal surface and spreading out onto the skin around the lips and nose. The lymph nodes of the neck and other sites enlarge massively and necrose to form draining sinuses. Spread to the lung resembles tuberculosis and occurs in over 70 percent of the cases but is seldom seen without associated mucocutaneous and lymphatic involvement. Visceral extension with hepatosplenomegaly is frequently fatal. The thick-walled yeast-like organisms with their diagnostic multiple buds are readily found in biopsy specimens, pus aspirated from lymph nodes, or currettings from mucous membrane lesions (see Chap. 10). Effective antimicrobial agents include sulfonamides, amphotericin B, ketoconazole, or itraconazole.

Lobo Disease (Keloidal Blastomycosis). This chronic localized disease occurs in the northern and Caribbean part of South America and overlaps the endemic area of paracoccidioidomycosis. Lesions may be localized, beginning as intracutaneous nodules that become verrucous and crusted, spreading slowly by peripheral extension or autoinoculation. Lymphatic and visceral involvement is not seen. Excision of localized nodules may be curative. The causative organism *Loboa loboi* is either a variant of paracoccidioidomycosis or a separate species.

Cutaneous Histoplasmosis. Primary histoplasmosis of the skin usually occurs in laboratory or autopsy workers. It produces the typical chancreform syndrome, with a chancre at the site of entry and regional lymphadenopathy. These infections are usually self-limited and seldom result in disseminated disease. Isolated, circumscribed, persistent lesions occasionally occur on the skin and the mucous membranes of the mouth and penis without evidence of disease elsewhere. The lesions are benign expressions of the disease, analogous to the circumscribed pulmonary lesions, and the prognosis is generally good.

Most cutaneous lesions are associated with the progressive form of histoplasmosis. The lesions are not distinctive but usually appear as persistent punched-out or granulomatous ulcers. Other cutaneous manifestations (purpura, crops of papules, chronic abscesses, impetiginous dermatitis, furunculoid and vegetating lesions) are also seen. Lesions of mucous membranes often appear as persistent ulcerative granulomas, which suggest that disseminated disease may arise from the gastrointestinal tract rather than the lung. In immunodepressed patients, either chronic or rapidly progressive disseminated disease can occur.

Diagnosis of the disseminated form, particularly in immunodepressed patients, can be difficult, requiring serologic tests, bone marrow biopsy, and aspiration (see Chap. 10). Amphotericin B or ketoconazole are recommended.

African histoplasmosis, caused by *H. duboisii,* usually presents with multiple subcutaneous and cold osseous abscesses rather than pulmonary disease. Pathologic fractures are common. The endemic area encompasses a wide band that extends across the African continent between the Sahara desert to the north and the Kalahari desert to the south.

Cutaneous Cryptococcosis. Cutaneous lesions are almost always due to hematogenous spread of the organism (*C. neoformans*). Immunosuppressed patients (eg, renal transplant recipients) may have cutaneous lesions but no other symptoms of pulmonary or meningeal disease. Blood and cerebrospinal fluid culture results are frequently positive under these circumstances. The skin lesions can take many forms, including subcutaneous granulomas, papules, nodules, ulcers, or granulating sores. Cutaneous disease should prompt a search for cryptic pulmonary, blood, or meningeal disease. Treatment with amphotericin B and 5-fluorocytosine is effective without excision or debridement.

Cutaneous* Pseudallescheria *Infections. *Pseudallescheria* is a small saprophyte that behaves like *Aspergillus*. Infections of the paranasal sinuses and lung are most common. Like many soil saprophytes (see preceding section on mycetoma), inoculation into the skin will lead to localized granulomatous infection especially in the immunodepressed patient.[146] Surgical debridement combined with amphotericin B or an azole antibiotic is frequently necessary for cure.

Rhinosporidiosis. *Rhinosporidium seeberi,* although never successfully cultured, is thought to be a fungus that forms cysts 10 to 200 μm in diameter in the submucosa of the nose, pharynx, or conjunctiva. Males are more often afflicted. The lesion is painless but enlarges to form a friable pedunculated mass. Excision is curative.

CUTANEOUS ALGAL INFECTIONS

Protothecosis. *Prototheca* organisms are unicellular achloric alga-like organisms, which rarely cause human disease but can enter the body after skin trauma to cause a papulonodular lesion that drains intermittently. Wound infections have been reported. Dissemination in humans is rare. *P. wickerhamii* is the most common isolate. The diagnosis requires histopathologic examination of Gomori methanamine silver- or PAS-stained biopsy specimens. The organisms can be cultured on Sabourand agar. Excision of early lesions may be curative, and response to amphotericin B therapy is reported.

VIRAL DISEASES OF THE SKIN

Surgeons are rarely consulted for viral skin infections, but viral infections increasingly complicate treatment of surgical patients. A few require operation for diagnosis or cure.

Superficial Viral Infections of the Skin

Herpes Simplex. The herpes viruses are discussed as a group in Chapter 11. Their interest for the surgeon resides in their appearance in immunodepressed surgical patients and their occasional tendency to become necrotic and require surgical care.

Etiology. Two types of herpes simplex virus (HSV) are recognized: HSV type 1 is classically associated with nongenital (usually oral) lesions, and type 2 is associated with genital lesions, although changing sexual behavior is altering the sites of infection. The two types can only be distinguished by serologic tests and their effects on cells in tissue culture.

Clinical Manifestations. Cutaneous herpes may present as primary or recurrent disease. Either type 1 or type 2 herpes simplex virus can manifest in any of the clinical forms.

PRIMARY HERPES SIMPLEX INFECTION. Although most primary infections with either virus are subclinical, two classical presentations are described: primary gingivostomatitis (HSV-1) in children aged 2 to 5, and primary vulvovaginitis in adolescents (HSV-2), characterized by a sudden development of painful mucosal lesions, high fever, regional adenopathy, and malaise. The painful vesicles and white plaques appear on the mucosa of mouth, pharynx, gingiva, or vagina, with surrounding erythema and edema (see Fig. 31–31A). Spontaneous resolution takes about 2 weeks, but adenopathy can persist. Recurrence is common with all herpetic lesions.[147]

Primary herpes simplex virus infections can occur in any area as a localized vesicular eruption with regional adenopathy. Primary venereal (usually HSV-2) disease can appear on the penis, vulva, perineum, cervix, or anus (especially in male homosexuals). The exquisitely tender vesicles rupture and ulcerate. An accompanying sacral radiculomeningitis can produce urinary retention and obstipation. Other veneral diseases must be ruled out.

A herpetic whitlow on a finger following slight trauma and contact with an infected patient is an occasional presentation, especially in medical or dental personnel (see Fig. 31–31C). Recurrent herpetic whitlow may be mistaken for bacterial cellulitis because of the surrounding edema and erythema. The grouped, discrete vesicles at the margin of the lesion suggest the diagnosis. Incision and drainage is contraindicated.[147]

Surgical wounds have also been reported as sites of primary herpetic infections. Infection normally subsides but may recur in this site later. Kaposi varicelliform eruption (eczema herpeticum) is a form of primary herpes simplex that can be fatal in infants with eczema and in patients of any age with burns. In eczematous children, fever and umbilicated varicelliform lesions appear over areas of atopic dermatitis. The vesicles, which become hemorrhagic and pustular and may persist for several

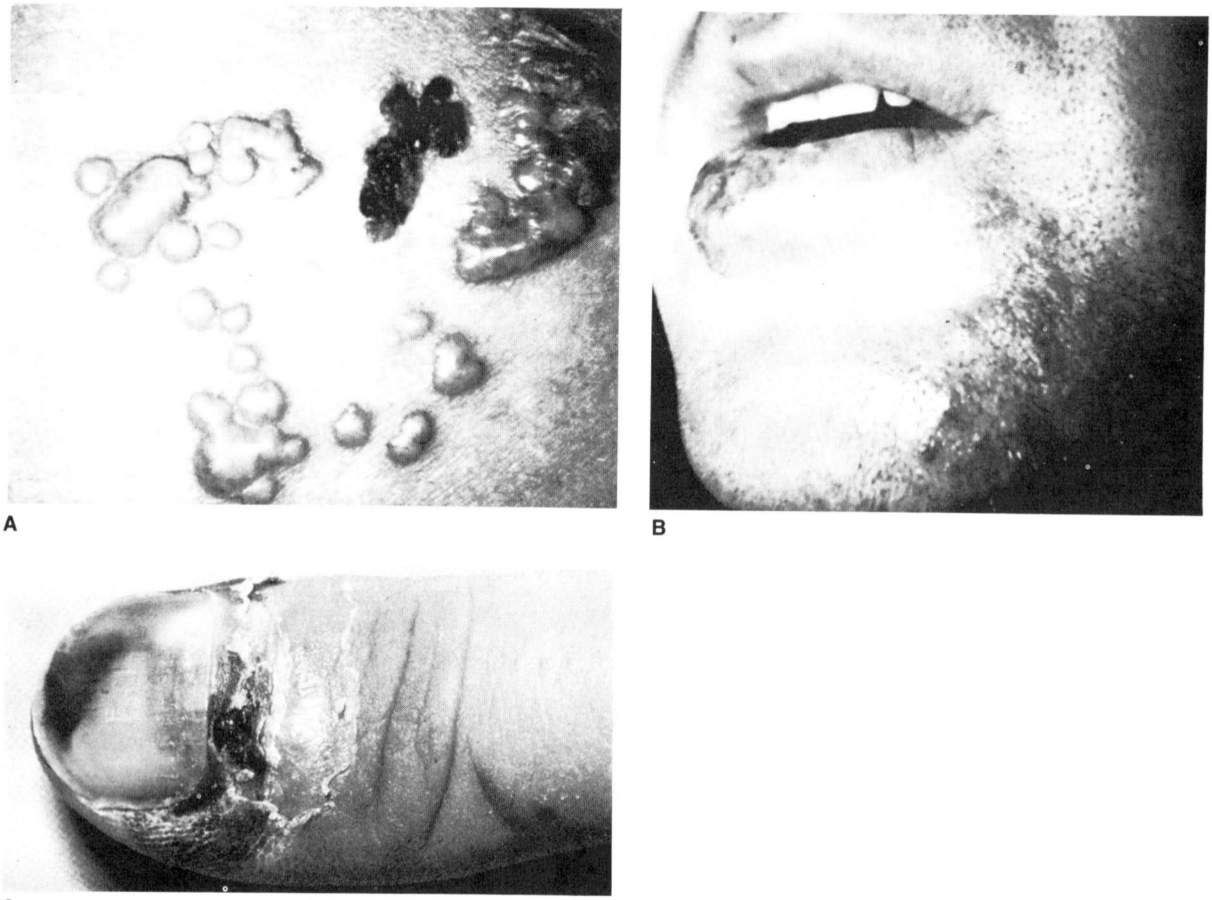

Figure 31–31. **A.** Painful vesicles of primary herpes simplex infection. **B.** Recurrent herpetic lesions of the lips. **C.** Herpetic whitlow in a renal transplant recipient who bites her fingernails.

days to a week, are accompanied by severe adenopathy and local edema. A similar disease occurs in burned patients[148] and may convert second-degree burn areas to third degree; bacterial superinfection is common. Visceral extension has been reported. Because burn patients are already covered with crusts, secondary viral superinfection is difficult to appreciate. The diagnosis is suggested by vesiculation of the margins of the burn wound, followed by an increase in the extent of third-degree burn with patches of bacterial infection and by high fever that does not respond to antibiotics (see Chap. 52). The virus may be cultured from open lesions or seen as viral inclusion bodies on wound biopsy. Surviving patients develop a fourfold or greater rise in herpes neutralizing antibody titers.

RECURRENT HERPES SIMPLEX. Most adults show herpes neutralizing antibodies in their serum, which indicates prior infections. Recurrent lesions often develop after some form of stress such as high fever, prolonged illness, immunosuppression, or exposure to sunlight. The development of painful vesicles grouped on an erythematous base is usually preceded by a local tingling or burning sensation for several hours to days. The lesions usually persist for only a few days without much exudation and are most frequent about the lips, perioral region, or genital region (see Fig. 31–31B). A dangerous form of recurrent herpes affects the eye. The eyelids and palpebral conjunctivae are typically affected, but a dendritic keratitis can develop and progress to include the stroma. Broad spectrum antibiotic ophthalmic solution is critical to prevent bacterial superinfection.

Lesions of the lip, pharynx, and esophagus are sometimes seen in immunodepressed patients. Dissemination of recurrent disease is rare but occasionally occurs without typical cutaneous manifestations in immunosuppressed children. Operative division of the sensory nerve for trigeminal neuralgia is frequently followed by herpetic vesicles, and there is evidence that the herpes virus may remain latent within the trigeminal ganglion.

Diagnosis. The diagnosis of classical primary or secondary infections is simple. Scraping of a vesicle or ulcer with a blade, fixing the smear with alcohol, and staining with Giemsa stain will demonstrate the multinucleate giant cells. This Tzanck preparation is positive for herpes simplex as well as varicella-zoster; by contrast, vaccinia produces intracytoplasmic inclusions. The viruses are rapidly identified by their cytopathogenic effect in tissue culture. Serologic tests are helpful only if a fourfold rise in antibody titer can be demonstrated (see Chap. 11).

Treatment. Acyclovir has been highly effective in clinical trials as an early treatment of primary herpes simplex and varicella zoster, shortening both severity and duration of symptoms.[148,149] Long-term administration reduces genital recurrences. The oral preparation is less effective than the parenteral preparation, but early use even in the immunosuppressed host is highly effective (see Chap. 28).

Varicella-Zoster (Herpes Zoster). The etiology and pathogenesis of varicella-zoster infections have been discussed in Chapter 11.

Varicella. Clinical chickenpox has little surgical significance, although occasional episodes of primary or even secondary disseminated varicella infections occur in immunodepressed children.[150] Superimposed bacterial pyoderma frequently complicates the course of such patients. Bleeding can occur from vesicles in the bladder or nose. Laryngeal edema rarely requires tracheostomy; a fatal purpura fulminans and even intestinal infarction have been reported.[151] Immunosuppressed children who have not had chickenpox should receive zoster immune globulin early after exposure to abort the disease.

Zoster. Shingles is a recrudescence of varicella-zoster virus infection in an "immune" patient. The disease is associated with Hodgkin disease and other lymphomas, radiotherapy, chemotherapy, and organ transplantation, and may signal an occult malignancy. Zoster produces necrotizing ganglionitis of the nerve root and posterior ganglion. Loss of neurofibrils occurs early in affected skin, so that pain and paresthesias precede the cutaneous lesions. Grouped vesicles appear on an erythematous base in a unilateral dermatomal pattern within 1 to 7 days after onset of pain and hyperesthesia (Fig. 31–32A, B). The eruption usually clears in about 2 to 3 weeks, but secondary bacterial infection can prolong the healing time. Regional lymphadenopathy, malaise, and low-grade fever are common, and intractable neuralgia is a feared complication. The most frequently affected dermatomes are thoracic, but any segment can be involved. Herpes zoster affects the eye less often than does herpes simplex. The eye is most in danger when the nasociliary branch of the ophthalmic branch of the trigeminal nerve is affected (see Fig. 31–32A).

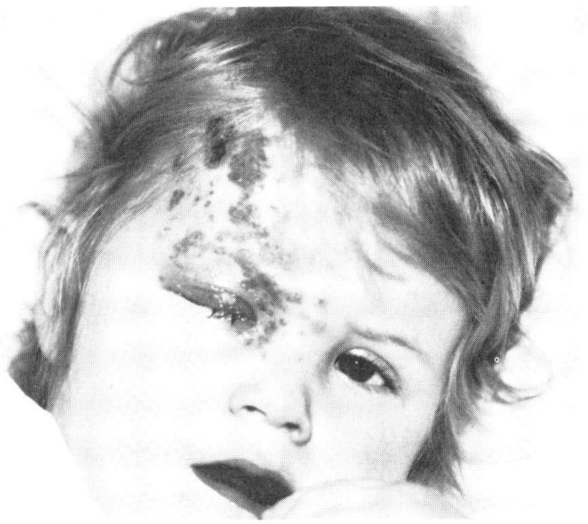

A

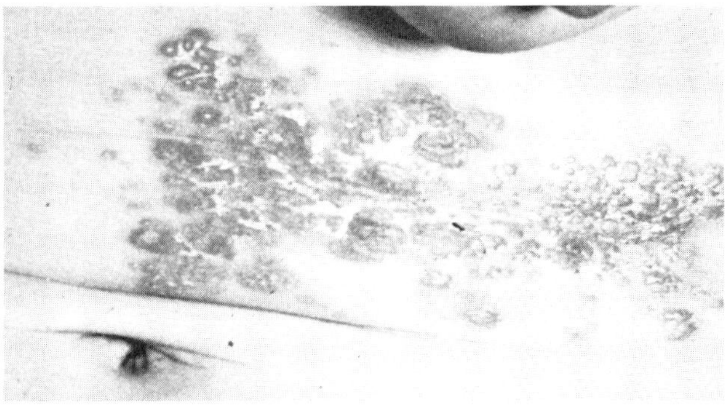

Figure 31–32. A. Zoster on face of a child. **B.** Thoracic zoster in an immunosuppressed adult. *(Courtesy of Robert W. Goltz, MD, Professor and Head, Department of Dermatology, University of Minnesota, Minneapolis.)*

The Ramsay-Hunt syndrome is herpes zoster of the geniculate ganglion, ie, the seventh cranial nerve, which innervates deep facial tissues. Painful vesicles along the uvula, palate, anterior tongue, auricle, and posterior auricular areas may be accompanied by paresis of the face. Glossopharyngeal zoster produces pain in the ear and pharynx with vesiculoulcerative lesions of the soft palate and vesicles of the ear. Vagal zoster may cause paresis of the larynx and pharynx as well as cardiac and epigastric distress. There may be vesicles on the base of the tongue, epiglottis, and arytenoids. Phrenic nerve involvement may paralyze the ipsilateral diaphragm. With thoracic zoster (see Fig. 31–32B), pleural friction rubs may be heard near the involved skin, and at times electrocardiogram changes occur. Lumbosacral involvement mimics renal colic and may result in urinary retention. Generalized zoster is potentially lethal in patients with Hodgkin disease, lymphoma, or leukemia or in severely immunodepressed patients.

The diagnosis depends on finding multinucleate giant cells on a Tzanck preparation and serologic tests.

Vidabarine (adenine arabinoside) is effective in disseminated disease, but its potential toxicity precludes its use in regional zoster.[152] Acyclovir has been highly effective in clinical trials in immunodepressed patients (see Chap. 11 and Chap. 51). The lesions heal faster, fewer new lesions appear, and the pain is reduced. In immunocompromised hosts, acyclovir should be instituted at the first sign of the disease. Intravenous acyclovir should be substituted if progression threatens. An experimental vaccine has been developed for patients at high risk for chickenpox,[153] but its value in the prevention of zoster is unknown.

Warts. Warts, or verrucae, are extremely common viral skin infections characterized by an unpredictable clinical course. Warts are called ectotropic because they affect only the skin and the mucous membranes adjacent to mucocutaneous junctions. Although they are principally an infection of childhood and young adult life, they may be incurable.[154]

Etiology. Warts are caused by DNA human papillomaviruses (HPVs). This conclusion is derived from evidence for their autoinoculation, and transmission from person to person, although the virus has not been cultivated.

Pathogenesis and Pathology. The virus is apparently inoculated through breaks in the skin and stimulates epithelial cell hyperplasia with hyperkeratosis and areas of parakeratosis and papillomatosis. In young verrucae, large vacuolated cells appear in the stratum malpighii and in the granular layer with rounded, deeply basophilic nuclei, which contain aggregates of virus particles on electron microscopy.

Clinical Manifestations. Warts present various morphologic forms. Sessile lesions with a rough gray surface are usually seen on the extremities. Filiform or digitate warts resembling cutaneous horns or nevoid skin tags are commonly encountered on the face and neck. Plantar warts occur where pressure prevents verrucous elevation, especially on the sole where they are often exquisitely painful. The calluslike lesions demonstrate diagnostic obliteration of the skin lines. The wart is usually discernible if the surface of the lesion is shaved off. Plantar warts may be single, multiple, or grouped together in a mosaic fashion. Hyperhidrosis may aid dissemination and seeding of the lesions on the feet. Flat warts, which resemble lightly pigmented nevi, are usually seen in children, especially on the face or forehead.

In moist intertriginous areas, the wart virus causes anogenital warts (condyloma acuminatum), which may be so large and painful that coitus or defecation is avoided (see Fig. 31–33). The lesions are pink or white with a strawberry-like surface and may be sexually transmitted. Differentiation from the highly infectious syphilitic condyloma lata is important. Malignant transformation is commonly reported.[155]

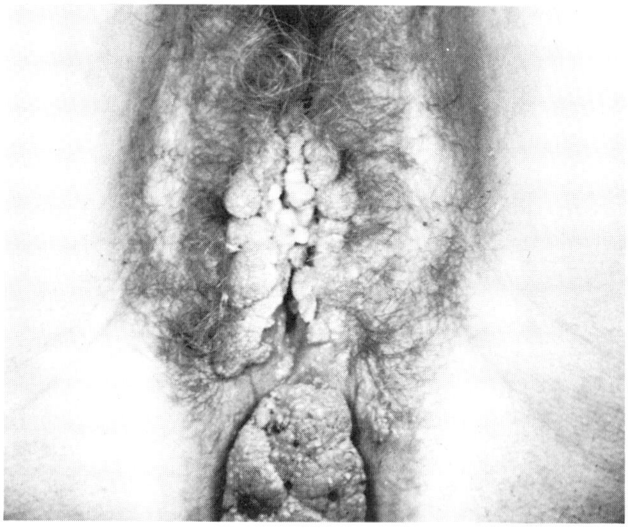

Figure 31–33. Anogenital warts (condylomata acuminatum). *(Courtesy of Robert W. Goltz, MD, Professor and Head, Department of Dermatology, University of Minnesota, Minneapolis.)*

In addition to their varied morphologic pattern, warts have an unpredictable course, undergoing capricious spontaneous disappearance, dissemination, or stubborn persistence. In general, warts disappear with age but commonly recur in immunosuppressed patients.[154]

Treatment. Dermatologists usually treat warts,[154] but surgeons must recognize two principles: (1) the diagnosis must be clear to avoid treating painful calluses or hyperkeratotic pressure points as warts and (2) extensive full-thickness resection is unnecessary because the wart is an entirely intraepidermal tumor.

Scarring from excessive operation may cause a significant permanent disability. The preferred treatment for sessile warts is electrodesiccation or cryosurgery with liquid nitrogen. The top of the wart is shaved, lightly electrocoagulated until it softens, then curretted and the bleeding points cauterized. Undue coagulation of the base of the lesion will retard healing and produce excessive scarring without improving the chances of cure. Cryosurgery is performed cautiously to avoid freezing digital vessels and nerves with consequent permanent paresthesias.

Although most warts need not be removed, periungual warts (those on either the nail fold or under the distal margin of the nail plate) should be removed before the inevitable extension occurs. Local chemotherapy with 10 to 25 percent glutaraldehyde solution, 10 percent formalin ointment, or 0.7 percent cantharidin in acetone, flexible collodion under tape occlusion is preferred to cryosurgery or electrodesiccation. Repeated application of these agents after paring away the white macerated tissue is necessary, but irritant reactions to the medications may limit usefulness.

Plantar warts pose the most serious therapeutic challenge. Irreversible painful scarring on pressure points must be avoided. A wide variety of cauterant chemicals that require repeated application can be used. Repeated nightly applications of 5 to 20 percent formalin solution produce hardening and drying of the skin surface, which may allow the warts to be shelled out. A combination of salicylic acid, lactic acid, and collodion, in a ratio of 1:1:4 (SAL), is useful when only a few warts are being treated. The keratotic surface of the wart is first shaved off, and SAL is self-applied daily for up to 12 weeks.[156]

Podophyllin is effective against warts in moist areas and dry warts after maceration. The wart is trimmed down and a 10 percent solution of podophyllin in benzoin is applied and covered with nonporous adhesive tape to increase maceration. This is repeated at intervals of 48 to 72 hours.

Warts occurring in moist intertriginous areas frequently become numerous and exuberant. A 10 percent solution of podophyllin in benzoin is applied, allowed to dry, and the site powdered with talc. The patient is instructed to wash the area thoroughly in 5 to 6 hours. Sitz baths are helpful in relieving subsequent discomfort. Failure to remove the agent may result in excruciating pain by the following morning. The treatment is repeated every week or two, and scarring is minimal. Sexual partners should be examined and treated to avoid reinfection. Resistant condylomata are excised or electrodesiccated, but excessive scarring can produce strictures in the perianal, periurethral, or vaginal areas. Biopsies will exclude exuberant squamous cell carcinoma.[155]

Molluscum Contagiosum. Molluscum contagiosum is a common pox virus infection of the skin and occasionally causes conjunctivitis in children. Spread occurs by direct contact. Pathologically, the epidermis grows into the dermis to form saccules, which contain clusters of intracytoplasmic virus. Clinically, scattered discrete lesions are found, each a slightly umbilicated, cone-shaped, hard, shiny, pale papule 2 to 5 mm or larger in diameter. Caseous material, which contains the microscopically visible molluscum bodies, can be expressed. In children, the trunk, face, extremities, and conjunctiva are favored sites, but in adults the pubic, genital, and perineal areas are usually affected. Shelling out the inclusions with a currette is curative; light electrocautery or freezing is also effective. The lesions are benign, and wide excision is discouraged.[157]

Viral Exanthems. Many viral illnesses are accompanied by symmetric, erythematous eruptions of the skin (and mucous membranes) called exanthems—measles, atypical measles, rubella, roseola, fifth disease, variola (smallpox), vaccinia, and enteroviral exanthems (see Table 31–9). Rarely is surgical consultation required for either diagnosis or therapy of these diseases, even in immunodepressed patients.

Epidermodysplasia Verruciformis. Epidermodysplasia verruciformis is a rare, probably autosomal recessive condition. Disseminated cutaneous warts appear early in life. The lesions, unlike warts, persist indefinitely and progress to invasive malignancy for which excision is required. Radiotherapy is thought to be contraindicated.

Superficial Viral Infections of the Skin Contracted from Animals

Ecthyma Contagiosum. This pox virus infection produces vesicular and pustular eruptions of the mucocutaneous regions in sheep. Humans are occasionally infected after direct contact with sheep and less often after handling contaminated lumber or clothing. Lesions develop on the hands, to progress from an erythematous macule to a papule and finally an eczematous nodular disease. Lymphadenitis is uncommon. The differential diagnosis includes vaccinia, cutaneous malignancy, verruca, orf, and an infected keratoanthoma. Serologic diagnosis is possible but rarely used.

Milker's Nodules. The paravaccinia virus, a pox virus that infects cow teats or calf muzzles, is sometimes transmitted to the hands of humans. It produces single or multiple firm, nonfixed, sometimes ulcerated and crusted red papules or nodules, 0.5 to 1.5 cm in diameter. The lesions heal in about 6 weeks. Regional adenopathy is common. The virus may be the same as that which causes ecthyma contagiosum. For definitive diagnosis, electron-microscopic examination of crusts from the lesions reveal the cigar-shaped virus, 310 nm long and 140 nm wide, in the cytoplasm of infected cells.

Orf. The paravaccinia virus, which causes contagious pustular dermatitis (orf) in sheep, can spread to persons employed in the wool or meat industries. It is similar in other respects to milker's nodule, which is caused by a similar paravaccinia virus. A self-limited hyperplastic nodular mass results, and electron microscopy reveals long ovoid viral particles.

PROTOZOAN AND HELMINTH INFECTIONS OF THE SKIN AND SOFT TISSUES

The protozoan and helminth infections of interest to surgeons are discussed in Chapter 8. Several of these produce characteristic infections of the skin and soft tissues. Table 8–5 lists the subcutaneous filariads.

Protozoan Infections

Cutaneous Amebiasis. Amebiasis is discussed in Chapter 8; its colonic and hepatic manifestations are discussed in Chapters 43 and 40. Cutaneous amebiasis usually occurs as a direct extension from, or after operation on, diseased viscera. Autoinoculation of the perianal region, buttocks, vulva, and face occurs in patients with colitis. Venereal spread is possible, and penile lesions have been described. The skin lesions spread rapidly and cause death in young patients with dysentery. The lesion consists of a painful ulcerating granuloma (ameboma) containing a purulent exudate with raised erythematous borders and undermined edges. Regional lymphadenopathy is present. The diagnosis is confirmed by finding trophozoites in the fresh material from the edge of the ulcer. Repeated stool examinations should be made even if there is no evidence of dysentery. Both systemic and enteric therapy, as described in Chapter 10, are required. Surgical debridement is contraindicated unless fistulas persist after successful chemotherapy.[158]

Trypanosomiasis. Trypanosomiasis is discussed in Chapter 8. African trypanosomiasis is a systemic infection; the only cutaneous manifestation is a red nodule with lymphangitis and lymphadenopathy at the site of the tsetse fly bite.

American trypanosomiasis (Chagas' disease) caused by *Trypanosoma cruzi* produces a tumor-like edematous mass (Romana sign) at the site of a bite by an infected reduviid bug. The lymphatics and draining lymph nodes become enlarged within 4 to 5 days, followed by hepatosplenomegaly. Myocarditis and meningoencephalitis can be fatal complications of the acute disease. Nifurtimox reduces the duration of acute symptoms but may not eradicate the organisms. The chronic form of disease is characterized by chronic heart failure and megaesophagus and megacolon, without soft tissue manifestations. There is no known treatment for the chronic disease (see Chap. 8).

Leishmaniasis. Infections with *Leishmania* organisms produce either a systemic infection involving the reticuloendothelial system or a localized cutaneous infection without systemic involvement. There are also mucocutaneous infections characterized by cutaneous and metastatic mucous membrane infections. Three species of *Leishmania* have been designated, but they may represent the same organism—*L. donovani* causes kala-azar, *L. braziliensis* causes the mucocutaneous form, and *L. tropica* causes cutaneous leishmaniasis.

Clinical Manifestations

KALA-AZAR. Kala-azar (black death) is a visceral disease that produces fever, emaciation, edema, splenomegaly, and pigmentation of temples and perioral regions.

MUCOCUTANEOUS LEISHMANIASIS (AMERICAN LEISHMANIASIS). Mucocutaneous leishmaniasis is found from Mexico to Argentina, where its vector is the phlebotomus fly. The initial lesion, a hard nodule, appears 2 weeks to 2 months after the fly bite (see Table 31–11). The lesion increases in size (3 to 12 cm), and becomes secondarily infected. A sporotrichoid pattern appears along the lymphatics (see Table 31–14).

The metastatic mucosal involvement is delayed for 3 to 10 years, producing ulcerated granulomatous lesions at the mucocutaneous junctions of the nose or mouth to destroy the nose (Fig. 31–34) or spread to the pharynx, palate, and larynx. Malnutrition and respiratory complications can be fatal.

The diagnosis depends on identification of the organism in smears, cultures, or tissue sections; the leishmanian skin test is almost always diagnostic. Pyoderma, sporotrichosis, syphilis, yaws, chromoblastomycosis, leprosy, and carcinoma must be excluded.

Treatment has traditionally been with the pentavalent antimonials (sodium stibogluconate), but amphotericin B is also effective.[159]

CUTANEOUS LEISHMANIASIS. Oriental sore is a specific granuloma of the skin caused by *L. tropica* in tropical areas of the Eastern Hemisphere. The sand fly (phlebotomus) is the main vector. Most patients are children because the infection produces permanent immunity. A granuloma appears weeks or months after inoculation, grows to 2 cm in size, and ulcerates (see Table 31–11). Secondary bacterial infection is common, but healing is spontaneous. Multiple ulcers are caused by autoinoculation or multiple bites.

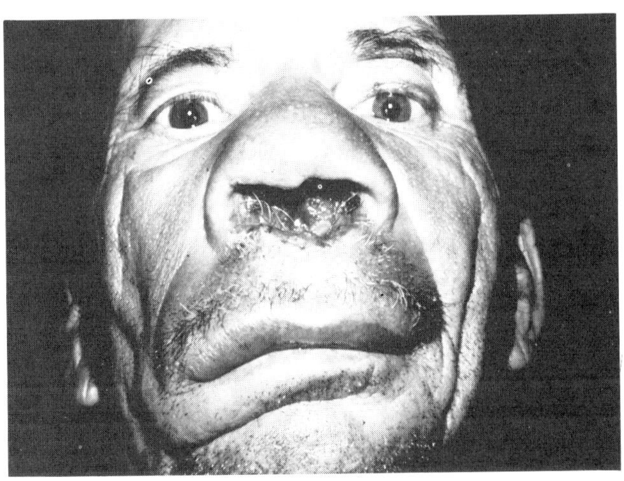

Figure 31–34. Mucocutaneous leishmaniasis of the nose has destroyed the nasal septum and collapsed the nose. *(From Armed Forces Institute of Pathology, Neg. No. 74-8873-1.)*

The diagnosis depends on demonstration of the parasite in stained currettings or aspirates from the ulcer edges. The ulcer surface does not show the parasite.

Surgical excision is not recommended; cryosurgery is useful for some chronic lesions. Pentavalent antimonials such as meglumine antimoniate and sodium stibogluconate are useful for systemic therapy.[159,160]

Helminth Infections

Platyhelminths (Flatworms)

Schistosomiasis. There are several cutaneous lesions associated with schistosomiasis, a parasitic worm that resides in the portal venous system (see Chap. 10). The surgeon is most likely to see the paragenital granulomas that commonly occur in the Middle East where *S. haematobium* is endemic. Granulomatous lesions involve the vaginal area, perineum, and buttocks and are usually associated with extensive communicating fistulas and sinuses. Ectopic cutaneous schistosomiasis produces cutaneous plaques secondary to the hematogenous spread of the worms. Skin or rectal biopsy specimens reveal presence of the ova in both cases. Treatment is described in Chapter 8 (see Table 8–4).

Sparganosis. Sparganosis has a worldwide distribution but occurs mostly in the Orient. The disease is caused by the procercoid larva (sparganum) of *Spirometra mansonides* and *S. mansoni* tapeworms. The definite tapeworm hosts are dogs and cats; people are intermediate hosts after ingesting the ova. The larva penetrates the intestine and develops into a spargoma in the subcutaneous tissue or muscle causing edematous, painful areas. The worm usually dies and produces intense inflammatory tissue destruction and eosinophilia. Incision and drainage with removal of the worm is the preferred therapy. Arsenicals (neoarsphenamine) are said to produce a good response (see Chap. 8).[161]

Cysticercosis. Taenia solium (the pork tapeworm) infects the human intestine after the ingestion of infected incompletely cooked pork. The larval form invades the subcutaneous tissues to produce cysticercosis, manifested by round, rubbery, painless subcutaneous cysts (Fig. 31–35A, B). The diagnosis is made on histopathologic examination of excised cysts. Praziquantel or niclosamide eliminates the adult intestinal worm, but the cysts are usually excised (see Table 8–3).

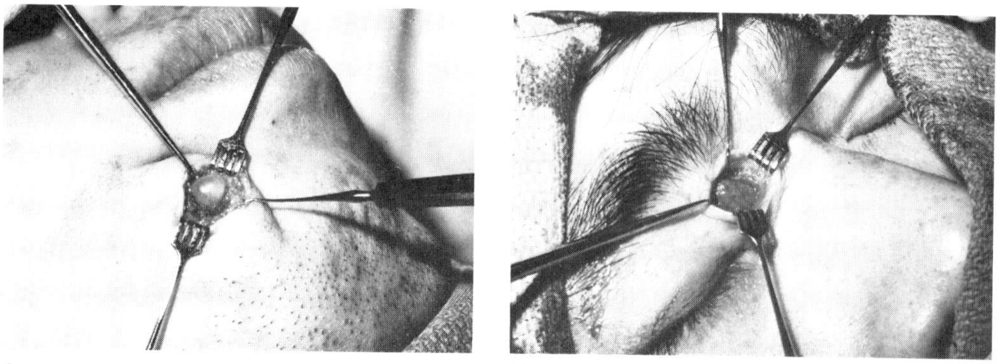

A B

Figure 31–35. Subcutaneous cysticercosis. The larval form of taenia solium (pork tapeworm) in two subcutaneous locations (**A** and **B**) in one patient. *(From Armed Forces Institute of Pathology, Neg. No. 69-2890-3-4.)*

Echinococcosis. The larval form of the dog tapeworms *E. granulosus* and *E. multilocularis* penetrates the intestine and invades various tissues (including liver, lung, and bone) producing soft, painless, fluctuant subcutaneous cysts of various sizes, which calcify or are resorbed. Bouts of urticaria may accompany echinococcosis of various sites. The diagnosis is made on roentgenographic findings of calcified cysts and serologic skin tests. Excision of the intact cysts is diagnostic and therapeutic (see Chap. 8).

Nematodes

Cutaneous Larva Migrans (see Chap. 8, Table 8–5). The surgical significance of cutaneous larva migrans is limited to the need for occasional diagnostic biopsy. Creeping eruption is caused by the infectious larval form of several hookworm species, especially *Ancylostoma braziliense.* The larvae can penetrate the intact skin and migrate beneath the epidermis at 1 to 2 cm per day. The hands, feet, buttocks, and genital areas become marked by serpiginous tracts, 2 to 3 mm wide, with advancing margins and local inflammation caused by a hypersensitivity reaction of the host (Fig. 31–36A, B). Scratching can lead to eczematization or secondary bacterial infection. The diagnosis is suspected by the location and the appearance of the lesions; biopsy at the advancing edge demonstrates the infecting larva. The infection is self-limited but may be chronic—no protective immunity develops.

In the case of autoinfection, systemic thiabendazole by mouth (50 mg/kg body weight per day, in two equal portions, for 2 days, with a maximum daily dose of 3 g) is effective. Adverse reactions to the drug include nausea, vomiting, drowsiness, and hematuria. Local treatment with dry ice or ethyl chloride spray applied to the advancing edge of the burrow blisters the epidermis, and the larva is shed.

Larva currens is caused by the larval form of the human hookworm *Strongyloides stercoralis,* which penetrates the perianal skin. Its migration

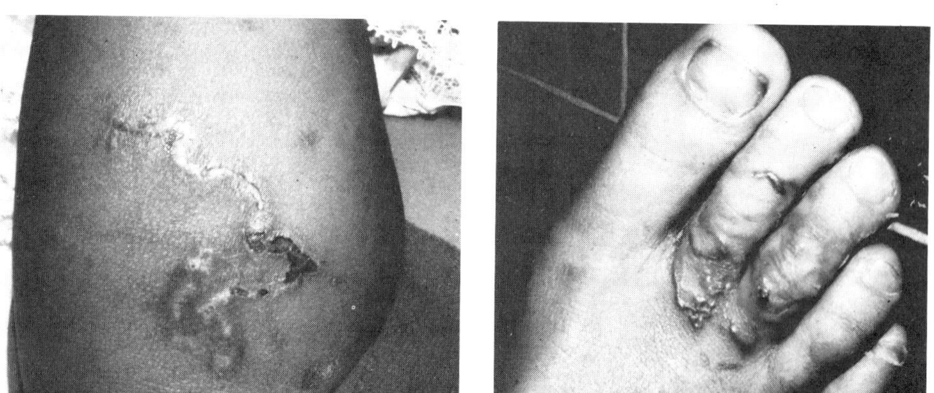

A B

Figure 31–36. Cutaneous larva migrans of the **(A)** arm and **(B)** foot. *(From Armed Forces Institute of Pathology, Neg. Nos. 74-8291-2 and 74-8291-1.)*

is rapid and is accompanied by an intense itching urticarial or papulovesicular rash. The larvae then invade the deeper tissues, and the rash fades. Treatment is identical to larva migrans.[162]

Cutaneous Filariasis. Three tropical species cause the disease: *Dracunculus medinensis* and the true filariae *Onchocerca volvulus* and *Loa loa*. None are endemic to the United States (see Table 8–5).

ONCHOCERCIASIS. *Onchocerca volvulus* is spread by the bite of female black flies, genus *Simulium,* found along the west coast of Africa and from Central America to northern South America. Africans bear lesions on the legs, and in Central America the nodules occur on the head, reflecting the different biting habits of the vectors involved.

The adult worm is long lived (7 to 15 years) but takes a year or so to develop from the larvae injected by the fly. A foreign body granulomatous reaction to the adult worm is produced, which leads to cutaneous nodules. Abscesses may form because the worms occasionally degenerate. The microfilariae released by the adult worm spread out in the tissues, which produce a leathery skin with persistent itching, skin rash, and subcutaneous nodules. When the cornea is involved, blindness may result. The nodules vary greatly in size, from 1 to 8 cm, especially over body prominences (see Fig. 10–17).

The diagnosis depends on the finding of microfilariae in bloodless biopsy specimens of superficial skin taken with a razor blade. The material is teased apart in saline to reveal the swimming microfilariae. The results of a filarial complement-fixation test may be positive. Scabies and superficial mycoses must be ruled out.

Systemic suramin kills adult worms when given as six weekly intravenous injections of 17 mg/kg body weight in each dose. Diethylcarbamazine, or the safer ivemectin, kills microfilariae but not adult worms. Where practical, all nodules should be excised to remove adult worms.

The black fly larvae and pupae are sensitive to DDT in river water; this is the most effective form of control for the insect vector.

LOAIASIS. Infection with *Loa loa* is characterized by transient, inflamed, edematous swellings of the skin called Calabar swellings, thought to be the migration sites of adult worms in the subcutaneous tissue. The erythematous swellings, 5 to 10 cm in size, usually affect the upper limbs. The disease, limited to the west coast of Africa, is transmitted by biting deerflies of the genus *Chrysops*. The swellings result from hypersensitivity to the adult worm or its by-products, and x-rays may reveal calcified worms in tissue. Biopsy is not indicated, and the swellings never suppurate. The worms can be excised. Blood drawn during the day may reveal eosinophilia, sheathed microfilariae, and a positive filarial complement-fixation test. The disease is of little consequence except when the eye, a peripheral nerve, or the central nervous system is involved. Diethylcarbamazine kills both adults and microfilariae.

DRACUNCULIASIS (GUINEA WORM INFECTION). People become infected after ingesting infected water fleas that bear the larvae of the guinea worm *Dracuncula medinensis,* which is endemic in the Middle East, North Africa, and the Caribbean. The larvae invade the intestine and mate. When ready to discharge their larvae, the pregnant female adults migrate to the surface of the skin, possibly selecting regions in humans that are likely to be immersed in cold water. As the adult female worm approaches the skin, a blister is followed by an ulcer several centimeters wide (see Figs. 8–14 and 8–15). The anterior end of the worm then extrudes to discharge the microfilariae. Cellulitis around the ulcer is common, although eosinophils are found locally. The lesion usually occurs on the lower leg but may be found elsewhere including the joints. Observing the protruding worm is diagnostic. The worm may die and calcify in tissues to produce a characteristic roentgenographic picture. Cellulitis and secondary infection often occur if the gravid worm dies in situ or is broken during extraction. Septicemia and tetanus are reported complications.

Gradually winding the worm out of the ulcer by turning on a stick a few centimeters a day can remove the worm intact. Surgical extraction has been practiced. Niridazole has been reported to be lethal to the adult worm in a dose of 25 mg/kg body weight per day by mouth for 7 days; the worm can then be easily withdrawn.[163] Metronidazole resolves inflammation, which facilitates removal of the worm, but it does not kill the worm.

Filariasis. The adult filariae, *Wuchereria bancrofti, Brugia malayi,* and other species of the superfamily Filaroides, live in the lymphatics of the extremities and external genitals proximal to the lymph nodes. Mosquitoes serve as vectors. Elephantiasis takes several years to develop. There are multiple episodes of lymphadenitis or lymphangitis. Ultimately, fribrosis and obstruction of the lymphatics produce thick, dry, course swellings of legs and genitals (Fig. 31–37). The skin may crack, become secondarily infected, and develop chronic ulcers.

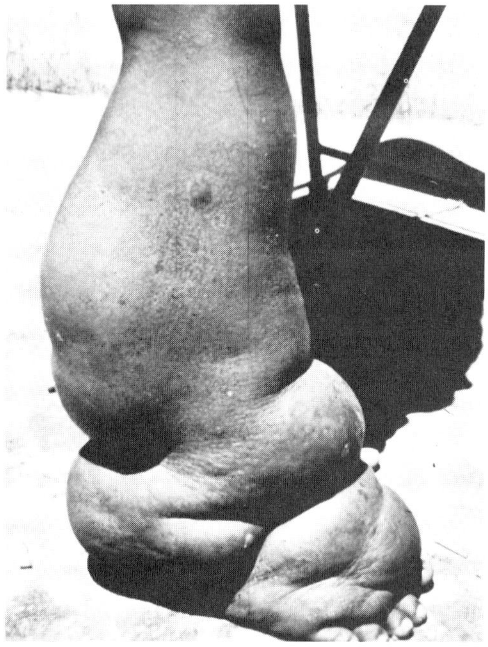

Figure 31–37. Elephantiasis (filariasis) of the leg. *(From Armed Forces Institute of Pathology, Neg. No. 74-6426-2.)*

Early diagnosis in endemic areas can be made by nodal biopsy or an intradermal skin test. During the acute symptomatic phase, the filaria can be seen in thick blood smears.

Treatment of the acute disease with diethylcarbamazine kills the microfilariae, but adult worms are resistant, so recurrence requires treatment. Operation to reduce massive extremity elephantiasis is rarely successful.

REFERENCES

Pathobiology

1. Roettinger W, Edgerton MT, Kurtz LD, et al: Role of inoculation site as a determinant of infection in soft tissue wounds. Am J Surg 126:354, 1973.
2. Noble WC, Somerville DA (eds): Microbiology of Human Skin. Philadelphia, Saunders, 1974.
3. Williamson P: Quantitative estimation of cutaneous flora. In Maibach HI, Hildick-Smith G (eds): Skin Bacteria and their Role in Infection. New York, McGraw-Hill, 1965, p 3.
4. Ulrich JA: Dynamics of bacterial skin populations. In Maibach HI, Hildick-Smith G (eds): Skin Bacteria and Their Role in Infection. New York, McGraw-Hill, 1965, p 219.
5. Meislin HW, Lerner SA, Graves MH, et al: Cutaneous abscesses: Anaerobic and aerobic bacteriology and outpatient management. Ann Intern Med 87:145, 1977.
6. Duncan WC, McBride ME, Knox JM: Experimental production of infections in humans. J Invest Dermatol 54:319, 1970.
7. Delong TG, Simmons RL: Role of the lymphatics in bacterial clearance from early soft tissue infection. Arch Surg 117:123, 1982.
8. Madden JE, Edlich RF, Custer JR, et al: Studies in the management of the contaminated wound: IV. Resistance to infection of surgical wounds made by knife, electrosurgery, and laser. Am J Surg 119:222, 1970.
9. Agarwal DS: Subcutaneous staphylococcal infection in mice: I. The role of cotton-dust in enhancing infection. Br J Exp Pathol 48:436, 1967.
10. Gristina AG, Price JL, Hobgood CD, et al: Bacterial colonization of percutaneous sutures. Surgery 98:12, 1985.
11. Haury BB, Rodeheaver GT, Pettry D, et al: Inhibition of nonspecific defenses by soil infection potentiating factors. Surg Gynecol Obstet 144:19, 1977.
12. Edlich RF, Schmolka IR, Prusak MP, Edgerton MT: The molecular basis for toxicity of surfactants in surgical wounds. I. EO:PO block polymers. J Surg Res 14:277, 1973.

Differential Diagnosis

13. Kolbacha ME, Stankiewicz JA, Clift SE: Severe soft tissue infection of the face and neck: a classification. Laryngoscope 92:1135, 1982.
14. Ahrenholz DH: Necrotizing fasciitis and other infections. In Rippe JM, Irwin RS, Alpert JS, Fink MP (eds): Intensive Care Medicine, 2nd ed. Boston, Little, Brown, 1991, p 1334.
15. Burnett JW, Crutcher WA: Viral and rickettsial infections. In Meschella SL, Pillsbury DM, Hurley HJ Jr (eds): Dermatology, Vol 1. Philadelphia, Saunders, 1975, p 558.
16. Nichols RL, Smith JW: Modern approach to the diagnosis of anaerobic surgical sepsis. Surg Clin North Am 55:21, 1975.

Bacterial Infections of the Skin

17. White A, Brook GF: Furunculosis, pyoderma, and impetigo. In Hoeprich PD (ed): Infectious Diseases, 2nd ed. Hagerstown, Harper & Row, 1977, p 785.
18. Solem LD, Zaske D, Strate RG: Ecthyma gangrenosum: Survival with individualized antibiotic therapy. Arch Surg 114:580, 1979.
19. Wood TF, Potter MA, Jonasson O: Streptococcal toxic shock-like syndrome. The importance of surgical intervention. Ann Surg 217:109, 1993.
20. Heimbach DM, Engrav LH, Marvin JA, et al: Toxic epidermal necrolysis. A step forward in treatment. JAMA 257:2171, 1987.
21. Grieco MH, Sheldon C: Erysipelothrix rhusiopathiae. Ann NY Acad Sci 174:523, 1970.
22. Rinke CM: Hot tub hygiene. JAMA 250:2031, 1983.
23. Leyden JJ, Marples RR, Mills OH, Jr, Kligman AM:

Gram-negative folliculitis—a complication of antibiotic therapy in acne vulgaris. Br J Dermatol 88:533, 1973.
24. Tuazon CU: Skin and skin structure infections in the patient at risk: carrier state of *Staphylococcus aureus*. Am J Med 76(Suppl 5A):166, 1984.
25. Hill HR, Estensen RD, Hogan NA, Quie PG: Severe staphylococcal disease associated with allergic manifestations, hyperimmunoglobulinemia E, and defective neutrophil chemotaxis. J Lab Clin Med 88:796, 1976.
26. Good RA, Quie PG, Windhorst DB, et al: Fatal (chronic) granulomatous diseases of childhood: A hereditary defect of leukocyte function. Semin Hematol 5:215, 1968.
27. Wheat JL, Kohler RB, White A: Prevention of infections of skin and skin structures. Am J Med 76(5A):187, 1984.
28. Leeming JP, Holland KT, Cunliffe WJ: The pathological and ecological significance of microorganisms colonising acne vulgaris comedones. J Med Microbiol 20:11, 1985.
29. Green KE: Contemporary therapy of acne. Postgrad Med 77(6):241, 1985.
30. Hurley HJ Jr: Apocrine glands. In Fitzpatrick TB, Eisen AZ, Wolff K, et al (eds): Dermatology in General Medicine, 2nd ed. New York, McGraw-Hill, 1979, p 473.
31. Broadwater JR, Bryant RL, Petrion RA, et al: Advanced hidradenitis suppurativa. Review of surgical treatment in 23 patients. Am J Surg 144:668, 1982.
32. Weinberg AN, Swartz MN: Gram-negative coccal and bacillary infections. In Fitzpatrick TB, Eisen AZ, Wolff K, et al (eds): Dermatology in General Medicine, 2nd ed. New York, McGraw-Hill, 1979, p 1445.

Infections of the Subcutaneous Tissue

33. Davis WA, Kane J, Garagush V: Human *Aeromonas* infections. Medicine 57:267, 1978.
34. Boss WK, Brand DA, Acampora D, et al: Effectiveness of prophylactic antibiotics in the outpatient treatment of burns. J Trauma 25:224, 1985.
35. Moxon ER: *Haemophilus influenzae*. In Mandel GL, Douglas RG, Bennett JE (eds): Principles and Practice of Infectious Diseases, 3rd ed. New York, Churchill Livingstone, 1990, p 1722.
36. Malinowski RW, Strate RG, Perry JF Jr, Fischer RP: The management of human bite injuries of the hand. J Trauma 19:655, 1979.
37. Louie TJ, Bartlett JG, Tally FP, Gorbach SL: Aerobic and anaerobic bacteria in diabetic foot ulcers. Ann Intern Med 85:461, 1976.
38. Boulton AJM: The diabetic foot. Med Clin North Am 72:1513, 1988.
39. Galpin JE, Chow AW, Bayer AS, Guz LB: Sepsis associated with decubitus ulcer. Am J Med 61:346, 1976.
40. Sickles EA, Green WH, Wiernik PIT: Clinical presentation of infection in granulocytopenic patients. Arch Intern Med 135:715, 1975.
41. Macfie J, Harvey J: The treatment of acute superficial abscesses: A prospective clinical trial. Br J Surg 64:264, 1977.
42. Bascom J: Pilonidal disease: Long-term results of follicle removal. Dis Col Rect 26:800, 1983.
43. Llera JL, Levy RC: Treatment of cutaneous abscess: A double-blind clinical study. Ann Emerg Med 14:15, 1985.
44. Jones NAG, Wilson DH: The treatment of acute abscesses by incision, curettage and primary suture under antibiotic cover. Br J Surg 63:499, 1976.
45. Stewart MP, Laing MR, Krukowski ZH: Treatment of acute abscesses by incision, curettage and primary suture without antibiotics: a controlled clinical trial. Br J Surg 72:66, 1985.
46. Lineaweaver W, Howard R, Soucy D, et al: Topical antimicrobial toxicity. Arch Surg 120:267, 1985.
47. Philip RS: A simplified method for the incision and drainage of abscesses. Am J Surg 135:721, 1978.
48. Robson MC, Shaw RC, Heggers JP: The reclosure of postoperative incisional abscesses based on bacterial quantification of the wound. Ann Surg 171:279, 1970.
49. Schneider M, Vidozola CW, Brooks S: Quantitative assessment of bacterial invasion of chronic ulcers. Am J Surg 145:260, 1983.
50. Sheagren JN: Treatment of skin and skin structure infections in the patient at risk. Am J Med 76(Suppl 5A):180, May 15, 1984.
51. Page RE, Freeman R: Superficial sepsis: The antibiotic choice for blind treatment. Br J Surg 64:261, 1977.
52. Aduan RP, Fauci AS, Dale DC, et al: Factitious fever and self-induced infection: a report of 32 cases and review of the literature. Ann Intern Med 90:230, 1979.
53. Wedel KR: A therapeutic confrontation approach to treating patients with factitious illness. Soc Work 16:69, 1971.
54. Goldstein EJC, Citron DM, Finegold SM: Role of anaerobic bacteria in bite wound infections. Rev Infect Dis 6(Suppl 1):S177, 1984.
55. Goldstein EJC: Infections following human bites. Infect Surg 4:849, 1985.
56. Nunley DL, Saski T, Atkins A, Vetto RM: Hand infections in hospitalized patients. Am J Surg 140:374, 1980.
57. Stromberg BV: Retreatment of previously treated hand infections. J Trauma 25:163, 1985.
58. Weber DJ, Hansen AR: Infections resulting from animal bites. Infect Dis Clin North Am 5(3):663, 1991.
59. Weber DJ, Wolfson JS, Swarz MN: *Pasturella multocida* infections: report of 34 cases and a review of the literature. Medicine (Baltimore) 63:133, 1984.

60. Job L, Horman JT, Grigor JK, Israel E: Dysgonic fermentor-2: a clinico-pathologic review. J Emerg Med 7:185, 1989.
61. Anderson LC, Leary SL, Manning PJ: Rat-bite fever in animal research laboratory personnel. Lab Anim Sci 33:292, 1983.
62. Carithers HA: Cat-scratch disease: an overview based on a study of 1,200 patients. Am J Dis Child 139:1124, 1985.
63. Wear DJ, Margileth AM, Hadfield TL, et al: Cat scratch disease: a bacterial infection. Science 21: 1403, 1983.
64. Bogue CW, Wise JD, Gray GF, et al: Antibiotic therapy for cat-scratch disease? JAMA 262:813, 1989.
65. Manson MH: Pathogenic gas-producing anaerobic bacilli in chronic ulcers. Arch Surg 24:752, 1932.
66. Levin ME, O'Neal LW (eds): The Diabetic Foot, 3rd ed. St Louis, Mosby, 1982.
67. Rotimi VO, Durosinmi-Etti FA: Bacteriology of infected malignant ulcers. J Clin Pathol 37:592, 1984.
68. Mitchell AAB: Incidence and isolation of *Bacteroides* species from clinical material and their sensitivity to antibiotics. J Clin Pathol 26:738, 1973.
69. Gocke TM: Infection complicating diabetes mellitus. In Grieco MH (ed): Infections in the Abnormal Host. New York, Yorke Medical Books, 1980, p 585.
70. Sapico FL, Witte JL, Canawati HN, et al: The infected foot of the diabetic patient: quantitative microbiology and analysis of clinical features. Rev Infect Dis 6(Suppl 1):S171, 1984.
71. Durham JR, Lukens ML, Campanini DS, et al: Impact of magnetic resonance imaging on the management of diabetic foot infections. Am J Surg 162:150, 1991.
72. Griffiths GD, Wieman TJ: Metatarsal head resection for diabetic foot ulcers. Arch Surg 125:832, 1990.
73. Meleney F: Bacterial synergism in disease processes with confirmation of synergistic bacterial etiology of certain type of progressive gangrene of the abdominal wall. Ann Surg 94:961, 1931.
74. Finegold SM (ed): Infections of the skin, soft tissue, and muscle. In: Anaerobic Bacteria in Human Disease. New York, Academic Press, 1977, p 386.
75. Mbonu OO, Nwako FA: Synergistic bacterial gangrene and allied lesions: a unified etiological theory. Int Surg 68:122, 1984.
76. Grainger RW, MacKenzie DA, McLachlin AD: Progressive bacterial synergistic gangrene: chronic undermining ulcer of Meleney. Can J Surg 10:439, 1967.
77. O'Brien JP: Tropical ulcer. In Hunter GW III, Swartzwelder JC, Clyde DF (eds): Tropical Medicine, 5th ed. Philadelphia, Saunders, 1976, p 666.
78. Lindner RR, Adeniyi-Jones C: The effects of metronidazole on tropical ulcers. Trans Soc Trop Med Hyg 62:712, 1968.
79. Emslie RD: Cancrum oris. Dent Pract 13:481, 1963.

Infections of the Fascial Cleft

80. Dellinger EP: Severe necrotizing soft-tissue infections: multiple disease entities requiring a common approach. JAMA 246:1717, 1981.
81. Meleney FL. Hemolytic streptococcus gangrene. Arch Surg 9:317, 1924.
82. Johansen K, Hansen ST: Symmetrical peripheral gangrene (purpura fulminans) complicating pneumococcal sepsis. Am J Surg 165:642, 1993.
83. Giuliano A, Lewis F Jr, Hadley K, Blaisdell FW: Bacteriology of necrotizing fasciitis. Am J Surg 134:52, 1977.
84. Howard RJ, Bennet NT: Infections caused by halophilic marine *Vibrio* bacteria. Ann Surg 217:525, 1993.
85. Stone HH, Martin JD Jr: Synergistic necrotizing cellulitis. Ann Surg 175:702, 1972.
86. Rea WJ, Wyrick WJ Jr: Necrotizing fasciitis. Ann Surg 172:957, 1970.
87. Lally KP, Atkinson JB, Wooley MM, Mahour GH: Necrotizing fasciitis: A serious sequela of omphalitis in the newborn. Ann Surg 199:101, 1984.
88. Moustoukas NM, Nichols RL, Smith JW, et al: Contaminated street heroin: Relationship to clinical infections. Arch Surg 118:746, 1983.
89. Wilson CB, Siber GR, O'Brien TF, Morgan AP: Phycomycotic gangrenous cellulitis. Arch Surg 111:532, 1976.
90. Paty R, Smith AD: Gangrene and Fournier's gangrene. Urol Clin North Am 19(1):149, 1992.
91. Clayton MD, Fowler JE Jr, Sharifi R: Causes, presentation and survival in 57 patients with necrotizing fasciitis of the male genitalia. Surg Gynecol Obstet 170:49, 1990.
92. Stamenkovic I, Lew PD: Early recognition of potentially fatal necrotizing fasciitis: the use of frozen section biopsy. N Engl J Med 310:1686, 1984.
93. Tally FP, Gorbach SL: Therapy of mixed anaerobic-aerobic infections: lessons from studies of intra-abdominal sepsis. Am J Med 78(Suppl 6A):145, June 7, 1985.
94. Solomkin JS, Fant WK, Rivera JO, Alexander JW: Randomized trail of imipenem/cilastatin versus gentamycin and clindamycin in mixed flora infections. Am J Med 78(Suppl 6A):85, June 7, 1985.
95. Bongard FS, Elings VB, Marklson RE: New uses of fluorescence in the surgical management of necrotizing soft tissue infection. Am J Surg 150:281, 1985.
96. Baxter CR: Surgical management of soft tissue infections. Surg Clin North Am 52:1483, 1972.
97. Gozal D, Ziser A, Shupak A, et al: Necrotizing fasciitis. Arch Surg 121:233, 1986.
98. Riseman JA, Zamboni WA, Curtis A, et al: Hyperbaric oxygen therapy for necrotizing fasciitis reduces mortality and the need for debridements. Surgery 108:847, 1990.
99. McIntyre KE, Bailey SA, Malone JM, Goldstone J:

Guillotine amputation in the treatment of nonsalvagable lower-extremity infections. Arch Surg 119:450, 1984.
100. Casali RE, Tucker WE, Petrino RA, et al: Postoperative necrotizing fasciitis of the abdominal wall. Am J Surg 140:787, 1980.
101. Sudarsky LA, Laschinger JC, Coppa GF, Spencer FC: Improved results from a standardized approach in treating patients with necrotizing fasciitis. Ann Surg 206:661, 1987.
102. Knaus WA, Zimmerman JE, Wagner DP, et al: APACHE—acute physiology and chronic health evaluation: a physiologically based classification system. Crit Care Med 9:591, 1981.
103. Meakins JL, Solomkin JS, Allo MD, et al: A proposed classification of intra-abdominal infections. Arch Surg 119:1372, 1984.
104. Pessa ME, Howard RJ: Necrotizing fasciitis. Surg Gynecol Obstet 161:357, 1985.
105. Swartz MN: Myositis. In Mandell GL, Douglas RG Jr, Bennett JE (eds): In Principles and Practice of Infectious Diseases, 3rd ed. New York, Churchill Livingstone, 1990, p 812.
106. Svane S: Peracute spontaneous streptococcal myositis. A report on 2 fatal cases with review of literature. Acta Chir Scand 137:155, 1971.
107. Kudsk KA: Occult gastrointestinal malignancies producing metastatic *Clostridium septicum* infections in diabetic patients. Surgery 112:765, 1992.
108. Pelfrey TM, Turk RP, Peoples JB, Elliot DW: Surgical aspects of *Clostridium septicum* septicemia. Arch Surg 119:546, 1984.
109. Pierce EC: Gas gangrene: A critique of therapy. Surg Rounds 7:17, Aug 1984.
110. Furste W, Lobe TE, Botros NN: Gangrenous soft tissue infections. Infect Surg 4:837, 1985.

Infections of Muscle

111. Burbrick MP, Hitchcock CR: Necrotizing anorectal and perineal infections. Surgery 86:655, 1979.
112. Stevens DL, Bryant AE, Adams K, et al: Evaluation of therapy with hyperbaric oxygen in clostridial myonecrosis. Clin Infect Dis 17:231, 1993.
113. Roding B, Groenveld PHA, Borema I: Ten years of experience in the treatment of gas gangrene with hyperbaric oxygen. Surg Gynecol Obstet 134:579, 1972.
114. Brown PW, Kinman PB: Gas gangrene in a metropolitan community. J Bone Joint Surg 56A:1445, 1974.

Unusual Bacterial Infections of the Skin

115. Brachman PS: Anthrax. In Hoeprich PD (ed): Infectious Diseases, 2nd ed. Hagerstown, Harper & Row, 1977, p 807.
116. Brachman PS, Fekety FR: Industrial anthrax. Ann NY Acad Sci 70:574, 1958.
117. Koopman JS, Campbell J: The role of cutaneous diptheria infection in a diptheria epidemic. J Infect Dis 131:239, 1975.
118. Swartz MN, Weinberg AN: Miscellaneous bacterial infections with cutaneous manifestations. In Fitzpatrick TB, Eisen AZ, Wolff K, et al (eds): Dermatology in General Medicine, 2nd ed. New York, McGraw-Hill, 1979, p 1459.
119. Rhodes AR, Luger AFH: Syphilis and other treponematoses. In Fitzpatrick TB, Eisen AZ, Wolff K, et al (eds): Dermatology in General Medicine, 2nd ed. New York, McGraw-Hill, 1979, p 1677.
120. Demis DJ: Nonsyphilitic treponematoses. In Hoeprich PD (ed): Infectious Diseases, 2nd ed. Hagerstown, Harper & Row, 1977, p 823.
121. Wolff K: Mycobacterial diseases: Tuberculosis. In Fitzpatrick TB, Eisen AZ, Wolff K, et al: Dermatology in General Medicine, 2nd ed. New York, McGraw-Hill, 1979, p 1473.
122. Marwick C: Multidrug-resistant tuberculosis poses challenge. JAMA 267:786, 1992.
123. Johnson RA: Atypical mycobacteria. In Fitzpatrick TB, Eisen AZ, Wolff K, et al: Dermatology in General Medicine, 2nd ed. New York, McGraw-Hill, 1979, p 1505.
124. Wenger JD, Spika JS, Smithwick RW, et al: Outbreak of *Mycobacterium chelonae* infection associated with use of jet injectors. JAMA 264:373, 1990.
125. Rappaport W, Dunington G, Norton L, et al: The surgical management of atypical mycobacterial soft-tissue infections. Surgery 108:36, 1990.
126. Ridley DS, Joplin WH: Classification of leprosy according to immunity: a five-group system. Int J Lepr 34:255, 1966.
127. Bullock WE, Mycobacterium leprae (leprosy). In Mandell GL, Douglas RG Jr, Bennett JE (eds): Principles and Practice of Infectious Diseases, 3rd ed. New York, Churchill Livingstone, 1990, p 1906.
128. Fritschi EP: Reconstructive Surgery in Leprosy. England, Wright, 1971.
129. Sanford JP, Moore WL Jr: Recrudescent melioidosis: a Southeastern Asia legacy. Am Rev Respir Dis 104:452, 1971.
130. Herrer A: Bartonellosis. In Hunter GW III, Swartzwelder JC, Clyde DF (eds): Tropical Medicine, 5th ed. Philadelphia, Saunders, 1976, p 256.
131. Heath CW Jr, Alexander AD, Galton MM: Leptospirosis in the United States: Analysis on 483 cases in man, 1946–61. N Engl J Med 273:857, 915, 1965.
132. Boyce JM: *Francisella tularensis* (tularemia). In Mandel GL, Douglas RG, Bennett JE (eds): Principles and Practice of Infectious Diseases, 3rd ed. New York, Churchill Livingstone, 1990, p 1742.
133. Butler T, Bell WR, Linh NN, et al: *Yersinia pestius* infection in Vietnam: I. Clinical and hematologic aspects. J Infect Dis 129:S78, 1974.
134. Zecler E, Gilboa Y, Elkina L, et al: Lymphocutaneous nocardiosis due to *Nocardia brasiliensis*. Arch Dermatol 113:642, 1977.

135. Richmond SJ, Sparling PF: Genital chlamydial infections. Am J Epidemiol 103:428, 1976.
136. Marmar JL: The management of resistant chancroid in Vietnam. J Urol 107:807, 1972.
137. Hart G: Chancroid, donovanosis, lymphogranuloma venereum. US Department of HEW Publication No. (CDC) 75–8302, 1975.

Fungal Infections of the Soft Tissue

138. Vollum DI: Chromomycosis: a review. Br J Dermatol 96:454, 1977.
139. Carrion AL: Chromoblastomycosis and related infections. New concepts, differential diagnosis, nomenclatorial implications. Int J Dermatol 14:27, 1975.
140. Brook CJ, Ravikrishnan KP, Weg JG: Pulmonary and articular sporotrichosis. Am Rev Respir Dis 116:141, 1977.
141. Mariat F, Destombes P, Segretain G: The mycetomas: clinical features, pathology, etiology and epidemiology. Contrib Microbiol Immunol 4:1, 1977.
142. Emmons CW, Binford CH, Utz JP, Kwon-Chung KJ: The mycetomas. In Medical Mycology, 3rd ed. Philadelphia, Lea & Febiger, 1977, p 437.
143. Gartenberg G, Bottone EJ, Keusch FT, Weitzman I: Hospital-acquired mucormycosis (*Rhizopus rhizopodiformis*) of skin and subcutaneous tissue. Epidemiology, mycology and treatment. Med Intell 299:1115, 1978.
144. Bruck HM, Nash G, Foley FD, Pruitt BA Jr: Opportunistic fungal infection of the burn wound with phycomycetes and *Aspergillus*. Arch Surg 102:476, 1971.
145. Cocanour CS, Miller-Crotchett P, Reed RL, et al: Mucormycosis in trauma patients. J Trauma 32:12, 1992.
146. Halpern AA, Nagel DA, Schurman DJ: *Allescheria boydii* osteomyelitis following multiple steroid injections and surgery. Clin Orthoped 126:232, 1977.

Viral Infections of the Skin

147. Nahmias AJ, Roizman B: Infection with herpes-simplex virus 1 and 2. N Engl J Med 289:667, 719, 781, 1973.
148. Brandt SJ, Tribble CG, Lakeman AD, Hayden FG: Herpes simplex burn wound infections: epidemiology of a case cluster and responses to acyclovir therapy. Surgery 98:338, 1985.
149. Balfour HH: Acyclovir therapy for herpes zoster: advantages and adverse reactions. JAMA 255:387, 1986.
150. Feldhoff CM, Balfour HH Jr, Simmons RL, et al: Varicella in children with renal transplants. J Pediatr 98:25, 1981.
151. Simmons RL, Balfour HH Jr: Complication of disseminated varicella zoster infection (editorial). Surgery 83:486, 1978.
152. Marker SC, Howard RJ, Groth KE, et al: A trial of vidarabine for cytomegalovirus infection in renal transplant patients. Arch Intern Med 140:1441, 1980.
153. Izawa T, Ihara T, Hattori A, et al: Application of live varicella vaccine in children with acute leukemia or other malignant diseases. Pediatrics 60:805, 1977.
154. Pass F: Warts. Biology and current therapy. Minn Med 57:844, 1974.
155. Kovi J, Tillman RL, Lee SM: Malignant transformation and condyloma accuminatum. J Clin Pathol 61:702, 1974.
156. Reichman RC, Bonnez W: Papillomaviruses. In Mandel GL, Douglas RG, Bennett JE (eds): Principles and Practice of Infectious Diseases, 3rd ed. New York, Churchill Livingstone, 1990, p 1191.
157. Hewitt J, Haguenau F: Warts and molluscum contagiosum. In Debre R, Celers J (eds): Clinical Virology. Philadelphia, Saunders, 1970, p 474.

Protozoan and Helminth Infections of the Soft Tissues

158. Sunarwan I: A case of cutaneous amoebiasis. Dermatologica 151:253, 1975.
159. Pearson RD, Sousa A: *Leishmania* species (kala-azar). In Mandell GL, Douglas RG Jr, Bennett JE (eds): Principles and Practice of Infectious Disease, 3rd ed. New York, Churchill Livingstone, 1990, p 2066.
160. Chemotherapy of Parasitic Diseases (Section XI). In Gilman AG, Goodman LS, Gilman A (eds): The Pharmacological Basis of Therapeutics, 6th ed. New York, Macmillan, 1980, p 1013.
161. Taylor RL: Sparganosis in the United States: report of a case. Am J Clin Pathol 66:560, 1976.
162. Katz R, Ziegler J, Blank H: The natural course of creeping eruption and treatment with thiabendazole. Arch Dermatol 91:420, 1965.
163. Muller R: Dracunculus and dracunculiasis. Adv Parasitol 9:73, 1971.

BIBLIOGRAPHY

Ahrenholz DH: Necrotizing fasciitis and other infections. In Rippe JM, Irwin RS, Alpert JS, Fink MP (eds): Intensive Care Medicine, 2nd ed. Boston, Little, Brown, 1991, p 1334.

Finegold SM, George WL: Anaerobic Infections in Humans. New York, Academic Press, 1989.

Maibach H, Aly R (eds): Skin Microbiology: Relevance to Clinical Infection. New York, Springer-Verlag, 1981.

Swartz MN: Skin and soft tissue infections (Section I). In Mandell GL, Douglas RG Jr, Bennett JE (eds): Principles and Practices of Infectious Diseases, 3rd ed. New York, Churchill Livingstone, 1990, p 796.

Yurt RW, Shires GT: Infections related to trauma. In Mandell GL, Douglas RG Jr, Bennett JE (eds): Principles and Practice of Infectious Diseases, 3rd ed. New York, Churchill Livingstone, 1990, p 825.

Infections of the Breast

CHAPTER 32

Gordon Francis Schwartz

Infections of the breast are rarely life threatening, although extremely annoying and uncomfortable. Any soft tissue infection may occur in the breast, and the breast is a relatively common site of infections in women seen by emergency room physicians. Serious infections are usually a product of the breast's unique function of lactation and its anatomic and physiologic development in response to this functional demand.

ANATOMY OF THE BREAST

An understanding of the specific anatomic considerations that may influence the development, containment, or dissemination of infectious processes is necessary as an initial measure.[1] Breast tissue extends from the infraclavicular margin superiorly, the midline medially, down to the sixth or seventh costal cartilage inferiorly, and laterally to the anterior edge of the latissimus dorsi muscle. The breast also extends to a variable degree in a teardrop shape into the axilla as the axillary tail, and even into the hairbearing area. Accessory breast tissue may occur in 2 to 3 percent of individuals (both males and females) along the so-called milk line between the axilla and the groin. If parenchyma is present in the accessory breast tissue, all the diseases that affect the breasts in their usual position are also possible in this ectopic tissue.

The arterial blood supply of the breast originates primarily from perforating branches one through four of the internal mammary artery. In addition, several branches of the axillary artery nourish the breast, the major of these being (1) the highest thoracic artery, above the upper medial border of the pectoralis minor muscle; (2) the pectoral branch of the thoracoacromial artery, which enters the deep surface of the breast; (3) the lateral thoracic artery to the lateral portion of the breast; and (4) the subscapular artery.

The venous drainage of the breast is more important than the arterial supply, not only because of its role as an avenue of dissemination of both infection and cancer, but also because the lymphatic vessels parallel the course of the veins. These venous pathways are divided into several groups. The superficial subcutaneous veins lie below the superficial fascia and may be seen through the intact skin in many patients. These superficial veins usually converge either toward the sternal margin and ultimately empty into the internal mammary veins, or they converge toward the suprasternal notch and empty into the veins of the lower neck (anterior jugular veins). The superficial veins of the breast are often more prominent over an area of disease, whether inflammation, infection, or neoplasm, and differences in the superficial venous pattern between the affected breast and the normal breast may be striking enough to alert the clinician to the possibility of disease. Within the parenchyma of the breast are three groups of veins: the perforating tributaries of the internal mammary veins; the axillary vein, which receives its tributaries in an irregular manner from the deep surface of the chest wall; and the intercostal veins, which communicate with the vertebral veins and empty eventually into the azygos vein and the vena cava. The venous drainage of the breast probably plays an especially important role in dissemination of malignancy to the lungs and bones.

The breast lymphatics begin around the lobules, with collecting channels following mammary ducts centripetally to the areola and its rich subareolar lymphatic plexus. The retroareolar lymphatics and network of cutaneous lymphatics course to the axilla. Details of the lymphatic drainage of the breast have been reviewed elsewhere.[1] In addition to the five identifiable groups of axillary nodes (external mammary, central, scapular, axillary vein, and subclavicular), the internal mammary route of lymphatic drainage of the breast is also important. From the internal mammary nodes, the lymphatic drainage is to the thoracic duct on the left and the lymphatic duct on the right.

The breast is situated between two layers of fascia, the superficial and deep layers of superficial fascia. The superficial layer of fascia is within 2 to 3 mm of the skin, and the deep layer of this (superficial) fascia lies superficial to the fascia and muscles of the chest wall. Between the deep layer of this fascia and the actual muscle fascia is a theoretical space, often called the retromammary bursa, composed of loose areolar tissue. It is this potential space or bursa that allows the breast to move on the chest wall. Projections of the deep layer of fascia traverse the retromammary bursa and pierce the pectoralis fascia, forming the posterior suspensory ligaments of the breast. Small projections of glandular tissue may accompany these fascial projections onto the surface of the pectoralis major muscle.

Throughout the breast parenchyma are Cooper's ligaments, tooth-like projections of areolar tissue that reach superficially to the undersurface of the skin. These ligaments may be seen and palpated through incisions in the breast as fine white strands, invariably accompanied by small blood vessels that perforate the breast. Involvement of Cooper's ligaments by any process that invades or infiltrates them, whether inflammatory or neoplastic, may produce retraction within the breast because the ligaments are shortened by the infiltrative process.

These fascial projections may serve as temporary barriers to the extension of inflammatory processes through the breast and tend to keep the process confined. As the architecture of the breast is maintained, the fluctuance that normally accompanies abscess formation can be masked, and infections may burrow into the parenchyma and be more extensive than the outward appearance of the breast may suggest.

MASTITIS AND BREAST ABSCESS

Lactational Mastitis or Abscess

The most common breast infection, which accompanies pregnancy or nursing, is called lactational mastitis or abscess.[1–6] Although rarely dangerous, impressive symptoms such as malaise and fever may be produced. Abscess is a threat to the breast because, if not treated early, a large portion of mammary parenchyma can be destroyed before the abscess spontaneously drains through the skin.

Etiology. The most common organism associated with lactational mastitis or abscess has been hemolytic, coagulase-positive *Staphylococcus aureus,* reported in from 65 to more than 90 percent of collected series.[4–10] *Staphylococcus epidermidis* and species of *Streptococcus* have also been found. In recent years, lactational abscess has also been associated with other aerobic and anaerobic organisms, such as *Bacteroides.*[7,10–18] If the milk is cultured, the causative organism will sometimes be isolated; if the causative organism comes from the baby's oropharynx, the milk from the contralateral breast may also harbor the same organism without clinical evidence of infection.

Incidence and Epidemiology. The majority of lactational infections occur sporadically after childbirth, but they may also be encountered during pregnancy. Postpartum mastitis strikes fewer than 2 percent of women after delivery, but epidemics affecting up to 10 percent of postpartum women have occurred.[6,10] At one time it was thought that these represented two forms of infection, the epidemic variety being less acute with fewer constitutional symptoms than the sporadic infections, but this arbitrary division is no longer tenable. For some mysterious reason, whether real or because of the manner in which they are reported, about two-thirds of these infections have been associated with first pregnancies. It has also been claimed (although not confirmed) that a woman who has experienced postpartum mastitis once is more likely to develop an infection after subsequent deliveries.

Pathogenesis and Pathology. By definition, lactational infections occur in the breasts of pregnant or lactating women and are related to the physiological phenomena of lactation. During the first trimester of pregnancy the breasts are characterized by ductal spouting and branching, induced by luteal and placental hormones. Near the end of the first trimester there is hypertrophy of the lobular-alveolar units and an actual increase in their number. In the second trimester, secretory activity is initiated and colostrum appears within the alveoli. Enlargement of the breast continues, attributable to alveolar dilation and the accumulation of colostrum, along with increased vascularity. Fat and connective tissue in the breast actually decrease during pregnancy. In the final trimester the secretory cells of the alveoli continue their function as the breast fills with colostrum. The blood supply continues to increase, and flow through the breast by the end of pregnancy may have doubled.

Under the influence of prolactin, after the postpartum withdrawal of placental lactogen and other sex steroids, lactation begins as milk is released into the mammary alveoli and collecting ducts. At the same time, in the first few days after delivery, venous and lymphatic stasis occurs and the breast parenchyma becomes edematous. The composition of colostrum begins to change, and mature milk is available after about 2 weeks. Breast edema, lymphatic stasis, colostrum and milk secretion, and partial ductal obstruction all play a role in the increased susceptibility of the postpartum breast to infection.

Why some women develop lactational infections is poorly understood. It is generally accepted that a cracked or fissured nipple, secondary to continual irritation by the suckling infant, provides a portal of entry for pathogenic organisms from the baby's naso- or oropharynx.[10] This assumes that the infant has been colonized, and the organisms are then passed to the ducts or lymphatics of the nursing mother through the excoriated nipple. For example, there have been rare reports of tuberculous lesions of the nursing breast in nursing women secondary to enteric tuberculosis in the infant.

Many more mothers develop cracked nipples than develop infections of their breasts. Thus it has also been suggested that milk stasis may be a contributing factor, because a missed feeding or weaning has been noted to precipitate infection in some women.

Another unsubstantiated explanation is the altered hormonal status of nursing women. Perhaps the hormonal milieu of the postpartum nursing mother creates a climate that encourages the growth of organisms that might not otherwise be able to establish a foothold. Pregnancy seems to lower resistance to a variety of microbes. Whatever the cause(s), there is no single common denominator to explain the origin of most of these infections, although the introduction of a critical number of bacteria into the dark, warm, nutrient rich environment of the nursing breast would almost seem to invite infection.

Clinical Manifestations. The typical case of lactational mastitis begins in the second to fourth week after delivery.[2,19] The range may be as early as 4 or 5 days after delivery to as late as 1 year.[4] Tenderness is usually the first symptom, accompanied by erythema, usually adjacent to the areolar margin.[20] Induration and edema may follow. General malaise, as with any infectious process, may occur, although at this stage systemic symptoms are not usually present. Fever may occur as the infection continues.

An attempt has been made to quantify the progression of milk stasis through outright abscess on the basis of bacterial counts and leukocyte counts in the mother's milk, along with the clinical findings.[11,12] Milk stasis only may be accompanied by leukocyte counts of less than 1 million per milliliter and bacterial counts of less than 1000 organisms per milliliter of milk, and with counts in this range the process is of short duration without further progression. Inflammation without progression to actual abscess is the most common presentation of lactational mastitis, and in these the bacterial counts remain below 1000 organisms per milliliter of milk, although milk leukocyte counts are more than 1 million per milliliter. Symptoms last typically for 5 or 6 days, and significant improvement is seen with regular emptying of the breast. Clinical infection occurs with bacterial counts of more than 1000 per milliliter of milk and leukocyte counts of more than 1 million per milliliter.

Inflammation without progression to actual abscess is the most common presentation. Symptoms last for 5 to 6 days, and significant improvement is seen with regular emptying of the breast. Of this group of infections, very few will progress to frank abscess if early detection and treatment are instituted. Even prior to the advent of antibiotics, mastitis did not inevitably progress to abscess.

If lactational mastitis does progress without treatment or if it is not detected until later in its course, breast abscess may result. The erythema becomes more pronounced, tenderness and induration increase, and the breast becomes more edematous. Palpation of the breast reveals a mass that is usually exquisitely painful and may be fluctuant. Fever is almost always present, and the systemic signs may be impressive, including malaise, chills, and leukocytosis, as with any acute bacterial infection. Bacteremia is rare.

Diagnosis. The usual surgical dictum of waiting for fluctuance before initiating drainage of an abscess does not apply to the breast. Considerable tissue necrosis may occur within the breast without any palpable evidence of fluctuance; mass and induration may be the only signs. Ancillary diagnostic studies, such as mammography or ultrasonography, are rarely necessary because the diagnosis is clinically evident. Mammography is unpleasant for the nursing patient or for the patient with an abscess, because compression of the breast by the mammographic equipment is necessary to achieve an optimal image. Confirming the presence of mastitis or abscess does not seem to constitute sufficient reason for a woman, especially if she is pregnant, to undergo this examination. The same precautions do not apply for the use of ultrasonography, but its value as a diagnostic aid in mastitis or abscess may be redundant. Champions of ultrasound hail its merits in differentiating a purulent collection that requires drainage from cellulitis that might still respond to antibiotics.[21] Aspiration of a suspected abscess usually will do the same, without the need for the sonogram. Once the clinical diagnosis of abscess has been made, no further confirmatory studies are necessary, and treatment may be instituted forthwith.

Treatment. If treatment begins promptly after mastitis has been diagnosed, further progression may be halted and the process resolved. On the basis of prior data that almost always implicated *Staphylococcus* as the offending organism, treatment with an orally administered synthetic penicillin was the usual recommendation, with erythromycin as an alternative in the allergic patient. Occasional patients may develop significant gastrointestinal symptoms from erythromycin, and in these few patients clindamycin may be a suitable alternative. Cephalosporins have played an increasing role in the initial treatment of these infections as the responsible organisms have become more varied, and currently, one of the orally administered cephalosporins is the initial drug of choice. Even if there is no frank pus present, as is usual in mastitis without abscess, the patient's milk should be cultured. This is even more important now than in past years because the flora responsible for these infections may be unusually resistant to the commonly used antibiotics.[22,23]

If both mother and child are capable of continuing, nursing should not be stopped just because mastitis has occurred, particularly if milk stasis is a factor in the pathogenesis of the infection, because nursing (or at least continuing to empty the breast) may have a beneficial effect.[2,4,12] If nursing must be discontinued, it is probably well to express the milk from the breasts until the infection has resolved. A purulent exudate from the nipple or actual abscess should be justification to stop nursing. Nursing should be stopped altogether if what is considered to be a herpetic lesion of the nipple of the breast develops, even without acute signs of inflammation, because continued nursing may transmit the herpes simplex virus to the infant. Neonatal death from disseminated herpes infections acquired by nursing has been reported.[15,16]

If infection is found early and treatment begins, the erythema, tenderness, and induration diminish within a few days. If the symptoms continue without improvement, an abscess must be suspected.

Occasionally, a suspected breast abscess may be aspirated. If the abscess is small, aspiration with an 18-gauge needle plus vigorous antibiotic therapy may avoid the need for open surgical drainage. If aspiration is attempted, several criteria should be fulfilled. The patient should be examined frequently; if the purulence reaccumulates or if the inflammation does not improve rapidly, open surgical drainage should be performed without delay. The aspirate should be submitted for Gram stain, culture, and sensitivity studies so that the appropriate antibiotic may be selected. When drainage of an abscess is necessary, it is best done in the operating theater with the patient under general anesthesia. Invariably, attempts at drainage in a physician's office with local anesthesia fail, either because the light is poor, the proper instruments and necessary assistants are unavailable, or, more likely, the patient's discomfort precludes adequate exploration, drainage, and irrigation of the wound.

Although many surgical textbooks describe radial incisions in the breast to drain abscesses, supposedly to avoid cutting across ducts, such incisions are perpendicular to the natural skin lines and leave conspicuous scars, especially because these wounds should be left open to heal secondarily (Fig. 32–1). Breast abscesses should be approached through incisions placed in the skin lines, parallel

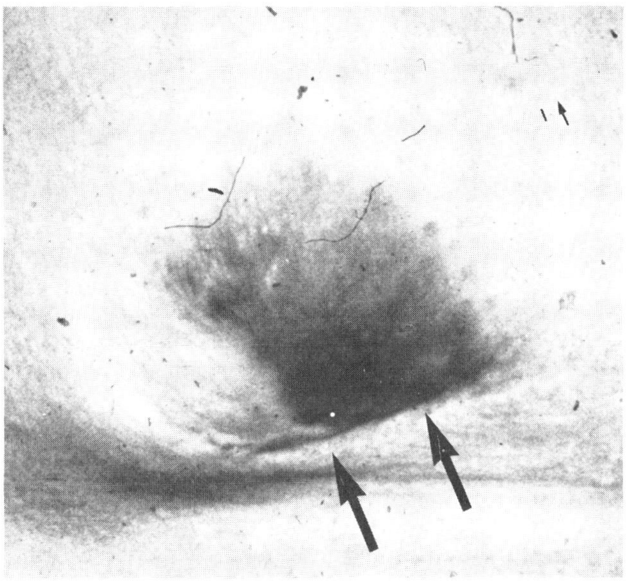

Figure 32–1. Conspicuous scar and deformity of breast after injudicious choice of incision and overzealous excision of inflamed tissues.

to the areolar margin, the same incisions advocated for breast biopsy[1,19,20] (Fig. 32–2). These incisions heal with minimal scarring, even when they are left open. Most breast abscesses occur adjacent to the areolar margin, and therefore a circumareolar incision often may be used, leaving the least conspicuous scar. Finger dissection within the breast may be necessary to fracture the loculations that have formed and to ensure adequate drainage. Although some surgical atlases recommend "counterincisions" to afford dependent drainage, these are rarely necessary and may leave ugly scars. If counterincisions are necessary, they should be placed, when possible, just above (1 to 2 cm) and parallel to the inframammary fold so that the resultant scar will be hidden by the overhanging breast, yet not continually pressed on by the patient's brassiere.

A sample of the wall of the abscess must be examined microscopically each time an abscess of the breast is drained. Carcinoma may mimic an abscess, although the coincidence of lactational abscess and carcinoma is rare. Carcinoma is unusual (although increasing in incidence) in young women, even more rare in the pregnant or lactating patient, but the microscopic examination of all tissues excised at operation is always indicated. A separate specimen should also be submitted to the microbiology laboratory for Gram stain, culture for aerobic and anaerobic organisms, and sensitivity studies, even if previous specimens have been sent.

Copious irrigation of the wound, usually with saline solution mixed with Dakin's solution or peroxide, helps debride the wound. Whether the addition of antibiotic to the saline solution is effective is questionable. Probably it is more important to use a large volume of irrigant. A drain is necessary, to keep the tract open for a minimum of 48 to 72 hours. A latex (Penrose) drain suffices for small abscesses; a packing soaked in Dakin's solution or peroxide is used for larger abscesses. The latex drain can be removed in 2 to 3 days. The packing, when used, is advanced daily until completely removed and is then replaced by a latex drain, which is left in place, changed, and shortened until it is virtually pushed out by the healing wound.

Antibiotics are begun parenterally as soon as the diagnosis is made, prior to drainage, and continued for 7 to 10 days. The oral form may be administered postoperatively when the patient is afebrile or otherwise clinically improved. A cephalosporin is the customary first choice for an antibi-

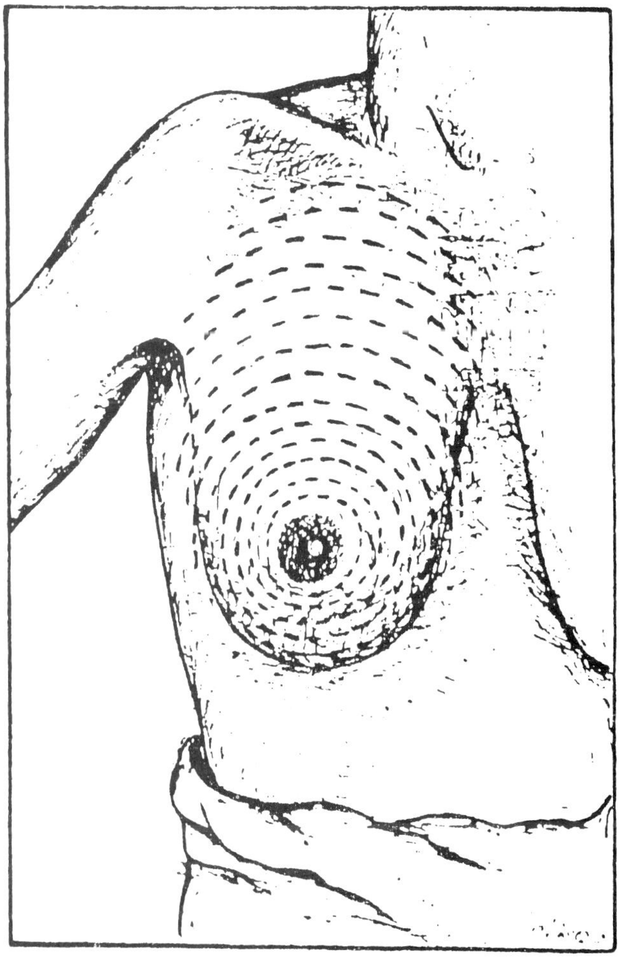

Figure 32–2. Langer's lines in the skin over the breast. *(From Schwartz GF: Surg Clin North Am 53:730, 1973.)*

otic, until the results of Gram stain or culture and sensitivity studies have been reported. The blood supply of the breast is relatively poor, and the antibiotic should be continued until the cellulitis that accompanies the infection has subsided.

Prognosis. Despite the size of the cavity or the depth of the wound, if the drainage incision has been placed in the skin lines, both patient and physician are usually pleased with the final appearance of the healed wound. If the amount of necrosis within the breast is minimal, there is usually neither significant deformity of breast contour nor a large scar.

Prevention. Except for obvious admonitions about personal hygiene, there is no feasible manner in which lactational infections may be completely avoided.

Nonlactational Mastitis and Abscess

The signs and symptoms, diagnosis, and treatment of breast infections in nonpregnant, nonlactating women are similar to those previously described. What is perhaps unusual about these infections is their mysterious origin. As with lactational infections, nonlactational infections occur mainly in young women.[17,20] Almost all are found in premenopausal patients and seem to appear more commonly during the premenstrual phases of the cycle. A history of antecedent factors that predispose to infection is obtained rarely, although embarrassment of the inquiring physician or the patient may cause omission of details about minor trauma to the nipple from "love bites." Any infectious inhabitant of the oropharynx or vagina can cause mastitis by manual or oral stimulation during sexual intercourse or by autoinfection. After the inflammation or infection has begun, the same course of events and treatment pertain for the nonlactating breast as for the patient with a postpartum infection.

Mastitis or abscesses in postmenopausal women often lack overt evidence of acute inflammation.[21] Fever or discomfort is prominent in fewer than 20 percent of patients, and only one-third demonstrate erythema or fluctuance. Leukocytosis is uncommon. Occasionally, fine-needle aspiration may help in the diagnosis.[9] Many postmenopausal patients undergo complete excision of abscesses rather than drainage, because abscesses are not infrequently mistaken for carcinomas (vide infra) because of their indolent characteristics. The organisms are similar to those seen in other infections of the breast, perhaps with an even wider spectrum, but the treatment and outcome are the same.[17,24,25]

Differential Diagnosis. Most important in the nonlactating woman is the differential diagnosis of those conditions of the breast that may mimic infection and that must be excluded, for example, mammary duct ectasia, Mondor's disease, and carcinoma. None of these are infectious in origin but should be discussed in enough detail to facilitate differentiation.

Mammary Duct Ectasia (Plasma Cell Mastitis, Comedomastitis). Mammary duct ectasia is a relative of cystic disease characterized by dilation of the subareolar ducts with contiguous fibrosis and inflammation.[5,26,27] Unlike most breast infections, however, ectasia usually affects the breasts of perimenopausal or postmenopausal women. As the collecting ducts beneath the areola become dilated, they fill with cellular debris. A thick, often blood-stained, toothpaste-like, grumose nipple discharge may occur. If, instead, the process continues peripherally into the breast, the walls of the ducts may become thickened, and the area is infiltrated by lymphocytes and plasma cells. If the intraductal material, a crystalline, lipid substance, ruptures through the duct wall, an intense inflammatory response ensues, with proliferation of giant cells, polymorphonuclear leukocytes, and lymphocytes. The center of the lesion may even break down and cavitate, becoming a sterile abscess filled with this same material. A mass is often palpable. Fibrosis within the breast may produce retraction signs, and the mass may be mistaken for carcinoma.

In some patients with mammary duct ectasia the initial clinical signs may mimic those of infectious mastitis, with erythema, induration, tenderness, and even axillary adenopathy. If the mass is incised, sterile "pus" is obtained. If treated with antibiotics, it resolves, as it does without treatment, in 10 to 14 days. More likely, the ectatic lesion in the breast mimics carcinoma rather than infection, and biopsy is required for diagnosis.

Mondor's Disease (Superficial Phlebitis of the Breast). Mondor's disease, an uncommon lesion that may mimic infection, is named for the French physician who first described it. Usually this phlebitic process involves the thoracoepigastric vein in the lateral half of the breast, and the process may course down across the costal margin onto the abdominal wall (Fig. 32–3).[1] A history of trauma is often noted, and Mondor's disease may follow breast biopsy, usually after about 3 weeks. Pain, tenderness, and erythema overlie a cord-like structure, which may demonstrate retraction along its course. Healing occurs spontaneously in 2 to 3

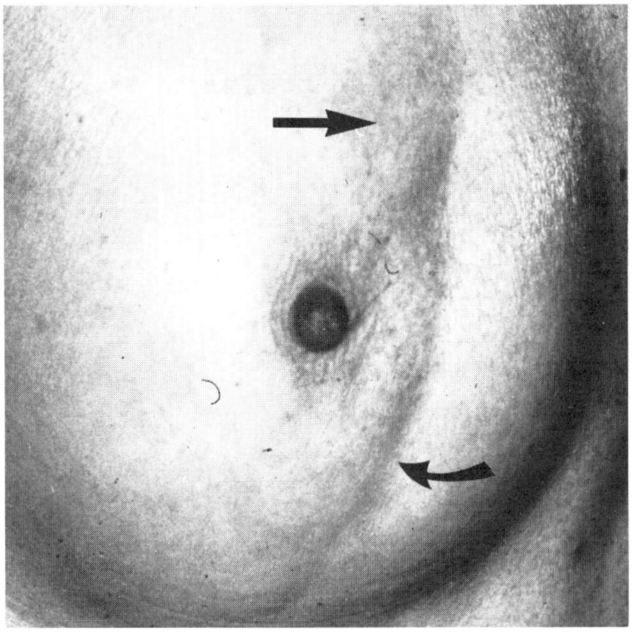

Figure 32–3. Mondor's disease. Upper arrow denotes area of erythema. Lower arrow points to cord-like thrombotic vein, with retraction.

weeks, although it may take as long as 6 to 8 weeks before the cord disappears altogether. Neither biopsy nor treatment is required. Biopsy may be performed if Mondor's disease is not included in the differential diagnosis, but in about one-fourth of reported cases biopsies have been performed unnecessarily.

Carcinoma. Cancer associated with inflammation or infection of the breast is uncommon, and the clinical entity known as inflammatory carcinoma comprises less than 2 percent of all breast cancer. However, the inflammatory type of breast cancer, when it does occur, may resemble an infection, and this diagnosis should be considered when any inflammatory lesion of the breast is encountered.[1]

Inflammatory carcinoma first appears as tenderness or discomfort. Although a mass may be present, it is often overlooked. The hallmark of this, probably the most virulent form of breast cancer, is the apparent inflammatory response of the breast, with actual enlargement of the indurated, edematous breast. There is usually a characteristic pink flush to the skin, but this may be so faint that it is missed. The erythema is most often over the dependent portion of the breast, and the breast itself may be mottled. The reddened skin may feel warm, but there are few, if any, systemic manifestations of inflammation, such as fever or leukocytosis. The majority of patients will have firm, palpable, clinically involved nodes in the axilla, and as many as one-fourth of women with inflammatory carcinoma will have metastatic carcinoma elsewhere, such as the bones, lungs, or liver, at the time of the initial diagnosis. In some ways similar to the evolution of an inflammatory or infectious process, inflammatory carcinoma seems to erupt almost overnight, from almost no apparent findings to its characteristic presentation as global swelling and erythema of the entire breast. Because of the almost universal locally advanced findings at the time of diagnosis, patients with inflammatory carcinoma may erroneously blame their primary care physicians for "delaying" the diagnosis. Malpractice claims by patients with inflammatory carcinoma against their physicians are unfortunately common; ignorance about the explosive nature of this disease, not culpable delay, is responsible for this mistaken inference.

The important differential diagnosis is between inflammatory carcinoma and infection. Many patients with cancer have been given antibiotics mistakenly. Infection or abscess is usually more localized than is inflammatory carcinoma; the latter tends to affect the entire protuberant breast. Mammary duct ectasia must also be considered in the differential diagnosis. Ectasia is also a well-localized rather than a diffuse process, and the inflammatory response it engenders usually resolves within a short period of time.

Advanced breast cancers with ulceration may be accompanied by secondary infection and signs of inflammation. Secondary infections evolve slowly and remain more localized. Redness and edema of the breast associated with ulceration are late signs of advanced localized cancer and customarily are considered clinical signs of "inoperability."

Medullary carcinoma, less often papillary carcinoma, and even comedocarcinoma may undergo central necrosis, which may in turn be followed by erythema and edema of the overlying skin. Only by the microscopic examination of excised tissue can this distinction be made. Carcinoma en cuirasse is a slow process in which the skin of the entire chest wall becomes fibrotic and thickened as the carcinoma advances. Although redness and apparent inflammation may accompany this process, it is usually easy to differentiate from acute inflammation because the evolution of carcinoma en cuirasse is so slow.

Recurrent Subareolar Abscess

Recurrent subareolar abscess is a poorly understood and infrequently recognized chronic infection of the breast. It produces repeated episodes of inflammation and abscess and sometimes has led to total mastectomy in an attempt to control or prevent the infection. This is most unfortunate, because if the diagnosis is made and the appropriate treatment undertaken, mastectomy should never be necessary.

It is possible that the majority of breast abscesses that occur in the periareolar area that are not associated with lactation, or for which a definite portal of entry cannot be established, may be related to this particular lesion. The lesion is usually not diagnosed until after several attempts at cure by incision and drainage.[26,28,29,30] In such abscesses that do not recur, the initial attempt at drainage probably halted the continuing process.

Etiology. The most common infecting organisms are *S. aureus, Proteus, Bacteroides,* and nonhemolytic *Streptococcus.* Recent reports have, however, implicated anaerobic organisms in up to one-half of these patients.[7,17–20] Even corynebacteria have caused recurrent abscesses (and erythrasma, a pruritic superficial skin infection with reddish brown macular lesions).[31,32]

Pathogenesis and Pathology. In normal lactiferous ducts there is an abrupt change from squamous to columnar epithelium 1 to 2 mm beneath the surface of the nipple. Hyperplasia of this squamous epithelium with accumulation of keratin within its lumen of the duct plugs the duct.[33] Dilation and rupture of the proximal duct occur. Bacterial invasion then supervenes, and an abscess is formed, complicated by the keratinized material that acts as an adjuvant foreign body.[5,34] Even if surgical drainage is performed, the suppurative process continues until the squamous epithelium is excised or destroyed. This process may produce a fistula at the edge of the areola, which, if probed, winds its way to the base of the nipple (Figs. 32–4 and 32–5).[33,34] True squamous metaplasia of the nipple ducts may occur, as manifested by transition from squamous to columnar, then back to squamous epithelium deeper in the breast. It has been suggested that this condition must be accompanied by or is a result of inverted nipples, but this does not seem to be substantiated, inasmuch as about half of the patients with these recurring abscesses do not have inverted nipples.[17,35,36]

Diagnosis. If an abscess in the breast seems to be associated with a sinus tract or fistulous opening adjacent to the areolar margin, Gram stained smears and cultures should be performed. If gram-negative bacilli are present, anaerobic cultures should be performed, because *Bacteroides* is a common pathogen in this setting. Clindamycin or metronidazole may be required. Most other infections are caused by staphylococci, and the antibiotic therapy is more straightforward.

The acute abscess must be treated by drainage, as for any breast abscess, but the involved duct(s) must be excised when the infection is quiescent or the abscess will recur. It is sometimes difficult to convince the patient after only the first or second episode that a definitive operation may be neces-

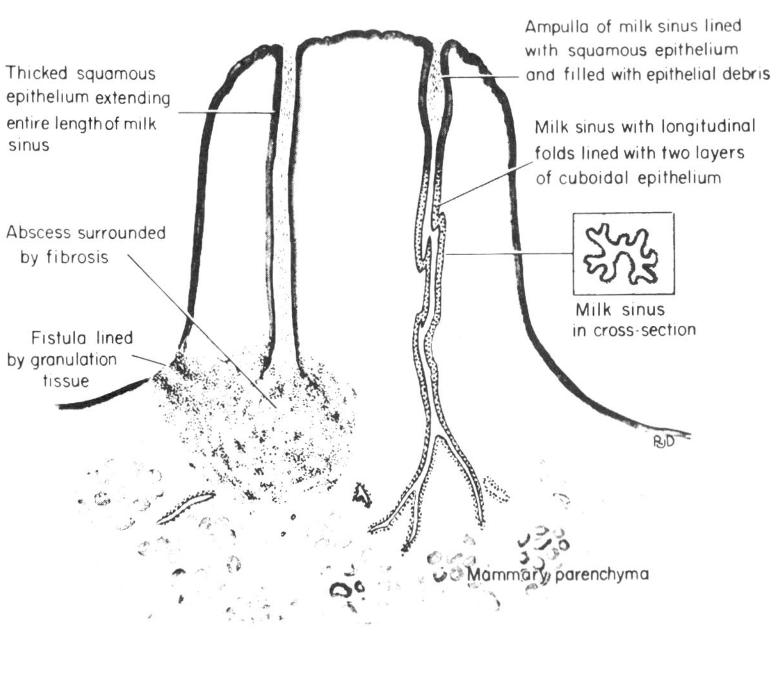

Figure 32–4. Recurring subareolar abscess shown diagrammatically. *(From Haagensen CD: Diseases of the Breast, 3rd ed. Philadelphia, Saunders, 1986.)*

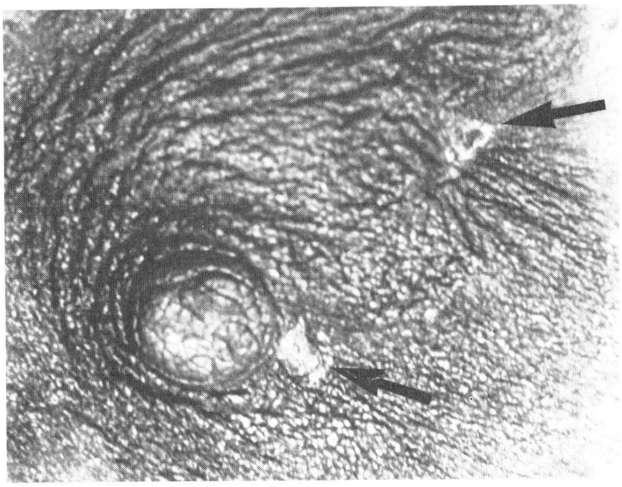

Figure 32–5. Recurring subareolar abscess. Arrows denote openings of sinus tracts beneath nipple-areolar complex.

sary when she is feeling well. After these patients have undergone repeated operations for drainage of recurrent abscesses, however, they are more eager to accept the need for this surgical procedure.

The sinus tract or fistula must be removed in its entirety.[34] This is done by including the opening within a small ellipse of skin at the areolar margin, then dissecting the duct or fistula from the retroareolar area toward the base of the nipple, removing that small aera of nipple where the duct emerges, "coring" it out (Fig. 32–6). The nipple itself may be closed without drainage, although it is usually preferable to leave a sliver of soft latex drain in the circumareolar incision for 24 to 48 hours. This procedure is minimal and is done as the first attempt to eliminate recurrent abscess. In some patients further recurrence may result from the involvement of additional ducts, and in these patients a larger segment of nipple may have to be removed. If recurrence continues despite this treatment, the entire nipple and the underlying major ducts may have to be removed (nipple only, not areola). This will cure the disease without resorting to mastectomy.

In about three-fourths of patients, recurrent abscess will be eradicated by the first *appropriate* surgical attempt; the remainder will need further surgery.

UNCOMMON INFECTIOUS DISEASES OF THE BREAST

Mastitis of the Axillary Tail

The normal extension of the breast into the axilla, known as the axillary tail or tail of Spence, is quite variable and may form a visible mass that enlarges in the premenstrual period or with lactation. If there is no ductal communication between this axillary prolongation of the breast and the remainder of the lactating breast, the tail becomes enlarged, tender, and inflamed and a sterile abscess may form. If this occurs in the primipara, excision of the axillary tissue should be carried out after weaning. Excision may be performed under local anesthesia, and the resultant scar(s) can be hidden inconspicuously in the skin lines of the hair-bearing portion of the underarm.

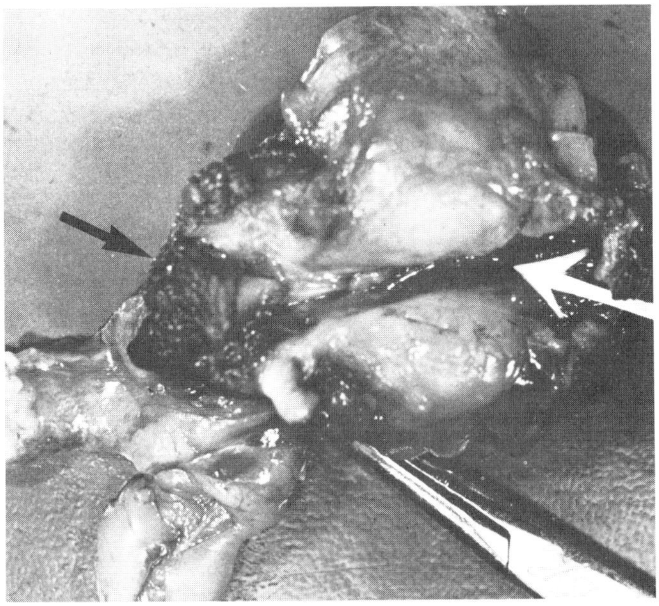

Figure 32–6. Recurring subareolar abscess, gross specimen after excision. White arrow points to squamous lined tract. Black arrow indicates small portion of excised areolar with fistulous opening.

Neonatal Mastitis

About one-third of newborn infants, boys as well as girls, show conspicuous breast enlargement 3 to 4 days after birth, which peaks by 2 or 3 weeks and is gone by 1 month of age. During the time of maximal swelling, a few drops of milky or clear discharge (witch's milk) may escape from the baby's nipple. This is normal; no treatment is indicated.

The only complication of neonatal mastitis is infection, most probably related to the repeated poking and prodding by parents overly concerned about this hypertrophy, especially in infant boys. Organisms may be introduced into the breast. The infection is signaled by erythema, swelling, induration, and pain, and may progress to abscess.[37]

Simultaneous infection of the mother and infant is not rare, and the treatment for both is the same. The organisms implicated in neonatal infections are predominantly *S. aureus,* with reports of gram-negative organisms as well, for example, *Escherichia coli* and even *Salmonella.*[38,39] In cases caused by *Salmonella,* the mastitis is secondary to systemic infection.

If the mastitis in an infant is not cured by antibiotics and requires drainage, it becomes more formidable, not because of the intrinsic danger of the infection but because of the threat of the operative procedure to the breast, especially in an infant girl. Damage to the breast bud from the infection or from the surgical procedure may lead to asymmetry of growth or even failure of the breast to develop at puberty. For this reason, surgical drainage of a breast abscess in the neonate or in any prepubertal girl must be approached with extreme caution.

Prepubertal and Pubertal Mastitis

The prepubertal and pubertal breast, in both boys and girls, may be the site of an inflammatory reaction, manifested by erythema, tenderness, and even the development of a small mass. Such an occurrence is rare, and even fewer progress to form abscesses. The breast is a modified apocrine gland, so it is not unreasonable to imagine that it may become active when the other apocrine glands are stimulated. Treatment of prepubertal and pubertal mastitis is directed at the symptoms, plus the prescription of an appropriate, usually antistaphylococcal, antibiotic.[40]

Inflammatory mastitis also may develop in the adolescent female breast.[41] It is perhaps related to ductal obstruction, because the ducts of the breast are being stimulated by the hormones produced during this time. Treatment is the same as for prepubertal mastitis.

Granulomatous Mastitis

Newly described within the past generation is an inflammatory lesion of the breast that occurs in premenopausal women called granulomatous mastitis.[42,43] A painless mass occurs that resembles carcinoma on clinical examination and thus leads to biopsy.[44] Rather than a central lesion, as with most other inflammatory conditions of the breast, this mass is usually peripheral and confined to the lobular elements of the breast. On microscopic examination, small, sterile abscesses are found within typical granulomatous changes in lobular units, but without accompanying ductal dilation. The initial histologic impression has often been that of mammary duct ectasia, even tuberculous mastitis, but the lack of dilated ducts makes the diagnosis of ectasia untenable, and failure to demonstrate acid-fast organisms makes tuberculosis unlikely.[45,46]

Two different explanations for this lesion have been advanced. The first is akin to the pathogenesis of mammary duct ectasia, a granulomatous response to the contents of ruptured ducts. Another theory is that because the histologic features of this lesion resemble those of cat scratch fever, it may be a response to a similar agent, presumably viral, or it may even represent an unusual autoimmune phenomenon. Treatment is simple excision of the mass, although it has recently been suggested that steroids may be a suitable choice, especially if recurrence is noted after surgical excision.[47] Before steroids are considered, however, it is essential that the usual infectious or neoplastic origins of breast masses have been ruled out by microscopic examination of excised tissue.

Two recent reports have documented three cases of what had been called "granulomatous mastitis" that were thought to be due to histoplasmosis.[48] The etiologic agent was documented in one case by Grocott methenamine silver staining. Whether these are isolated anecdotes or represent the detection of an infectious agent responsible for these enigmatic cases of inflammatory mastitis remains speculative.

Tuberculosis of the Breast

Now a rare lesion of the breast, in the days before specific antituberculous therapy, tuberculous mastitis occasionally accompanied systemic tuberculosis.[49] Even at its peak incidence, tuberculous mastitis may have accounted for only about 2 percent of the breast diseases seen in specialized clinics. Most American physicians, even breast specialists, will never see a tuberculous breast lesion, even though new and aggressive strains of the disease are being seen again among small groups of especially high-risk patients, including the socioeconomically disadvantaged, immigrants from endemic areas, alcohol and drug abusers, and individuals with human immunodeficiency virus (HIV) infections.[50,51] Tuberculosis of the breast was formerly divided arbitrarily into primary (breast only) and secondary (disseminated) forms. In the latter form, the breast was thought to be involved by secondary lymphatic spread of organisms from the axillary nodes or by direct extension from pulmonary intrathoracic lymphatics. In the primary form, a hematogenous source was postulated, with the growth of the bacilli directly in the parenchyma of the breast itself. The most commonly described finding was a painless mass in the breast, progressing to retraction, ulceration, and finally abscess formation.[48] In its early stages, tuberculosis could be easily confused with carcinoma. Axillary nodes were enlarged in a majority (50 to 75 percent) of the cases described. Most patients seemed to be otherwise healthy and did not have the characteristic phthisic appearance associated with this disease. Nipple discharge was rarely present, but if so, if cultured or smeared, the characteristic acid-fast organisms could be demonstrated.[52,53]

Treatment varied, from total mastectomy to antituberculous therapy alone. The most reasonable suggestion would seem to be eradication of the tuberculous focus by local excision of the mass, accompanied by systemic antituberculous therapy.[49] There should be no need for mastectomy unless the lesion is so large that local excision and mastectomy would be virtually synonymous.

Although tuberculous mastitis is rare, at least in Western countries, if a patient with known tuberculosis develops a breast mass, the diagnosis should be considered. At one time it was taught that breast cancer and tuberculosis were mutually exclusive and that the patient with tuberculosis was "immune" to the development of breast cancer. This is untrue. There are case reports of patients with cancer of one breast and tuberculosis of the other, or the two diseases coexisting not only in the same breast but within the same axillary lymph nodes.

Tuberculous mastitis has been reported as a manifestation of HIV infection in a patient suspected of a pyogenic breast abscess.[54] Additionally, the nosocomial transmission of tuberculosis to hospital employees has been associated with the care of patients with (large) tuberculous abscesses.[55] Even these isolated reports emphasize the importance of the prompt identification of the organisms responsible for any breast infection, including mycobacterial smears and cultures in patients thought to be "at risk."

Silicone Mastitis

The general term silicone mastitis describes all those forms of iatrogenic and self-induced infections related to the introduction of liquid silicone or other foreign material into the breast in the attempt to augment its size.[56] These reactions have occurred in response to the implantation or injection of myriad substances into the breast, some of which almost defy the imagination: beeswax, silicone wax, shellac, putty, epoxy resin, and even spun glass.

The characteristic microscopic appearance is a nodal histiocytosis and a local inflammatory reaction to the injected or implanted material. Treatment must include removal of the foreign body, and for this reason total mastectomy has been the unfortunate sequela in some women because the injected substance had permeated the entire breast.

Even the most carefully performed augmentation mammoplasty or reconstruction using an implant can be accompanied by infection of the wound or extrusion of the prosthesis through the skin. With either of these complications it is usually fruitless to attempt to salvage the situation. The prosthesis must be removed and the wound allowed to heal. Later, another attempt at augmentation or reconstruction may be made.

Since April 1992, when the Food and Drug Administration announced that silicone-gel breast implants could not be used for augmentation except through "controlled clinical studies," although women who need them for "breast reconstruction would be assured of access to these studies."[57] their use has been virtually abandoned by most plastic surgeons. Since the "burden of proof of safety rests squarely with the manufacturer,"[57] to most of them, the specter of incurred liability far outweighs the legitimate need of patients whose reconstructions can still be performed using saline filled implants or autogenous flaps.

Toxic Shock Syndrome

Toxic shock syndrome (TSS) is an acute multisystem illness marked by fever, hypotension, rash, and desquamation. Long known as staphylococcal scarlet fever, it reappeared in association with the use of intravaginal tampons in menstruating women.[58] It has been described in virtually every site of staphylococcal infection, including those involving the use of a surgical implant, such as in augmentation mammaplasty, or a tightly placed wound packing.[59–61] It has been even more rarely cited as secondary to breast abscess or postpartum mastitis.[62] The syndrome is caused by toxigenic *S. aureus,* especially those strains that produce toxic shock syndrome toxin 1 (TSST-1) or enterotoxins B or C. Its pathogenesis is discussed in Chapter 4. Recent wounds, including breast biopsies, followed by a systemic illness should be drained and antistaphylococcal antibiotics started. Innocent appearing wounds may contain the bacterium without local signs of infection.

Human Immunodeficiency Virus Infection (HIV/AIDS)

Although not precisely germane to the subject of breast infections, the passage of HIV from mother to infant via nursing should be addressed. Information about the likelihood of an infant being infected from an HIV-positive mother in this manner is sparse.[63,64] Using a decision analysis model, the Centers for Disease Control and Prevention constructed a model suggesting that worldwide infant mortality would be adversely affected by withholding nursing, even if the mother is HIV infected.[65] Nevertheless, in a small number of cases, the seroconversion of infants who nursed from seropositive mothers ranged from 27 to 60 percent.[60,66] Since breast-feeding is so crucial to many societies where HIV infection is encountered in epidemic proportions, recommendations must depend on whether individual or population-based factors are appropriate. In a single case of breast abscess associated with infant HIV-1 infection, it was proposed that the ingestion of inflammatory cells contributed to the transmission of the virus.[60] Therefore it was recommended that HIV-1 infected mothers should discontinue nursing in the presence of mastitis, or when the child reaches an age at which the further benefits of nursing are meager.

Other Infections

The breast has been reported as the locus for many other unusual infectious diseases of bacterial, fungal, or protozoan origin. For example, syphilis of the breast has been described as both primary chancre and secondary gumma, although large clinics may not have a single case in their records.[1]

In areas where the diseases are endemic, hydatid disease, filariasis, leprosy, blastomycosis, sporotrichosis, and actinomycosis of the breast have been reported.[67,68]

Postoperative Wound Infections

Despite the relatively poor blood supply to the breast, operations on the breast are only infrequently accompanied by postoperative wound infections. Breast surgery is considered clean, and prophylactic antibiotics are not indicated. A question often raised is the role of antibiotics in patients with mitral valve prolapse, as this diagnosis has been made more frequently in recent years. We have not recommended the routine use of prophylactic antibiotics in these patients, even though Platt et al.[69] have shown a significant decrease in short- and long-term wound complications after breast biopsy with perioperative prophylaxis. The American Heart Association has not listed breast surgery when recommending the use of prophylactic antibiotics in surgical procedures on patients with varying degrees of risk for endocarditis, including mitral valve prolapse.[70] The recommendations listed only dental, oral and upper respiratory procedures, and gastrointestinal and genitourinary procedures.

Although prophylactic antibiotics may not offer much benefit to breast biopsy or mastectomy, augmentation mammoplasty or reconstruction with a silicone or saline prosthesis, which requires the permanent implantation of a foreign body into the wound, may benefit even though the efficacy of perioperative antibiotic prophylaxis for these procedures has not been established unequivocally.[71,72] The use of silicone breast implants is currently controversial for other reasons, namely, their alleged association with systemic sclerosis and other similar rheumatoid, perhaps autoimmune, syndromes.[73] Parenthetically, even if exonerated fully from these suspicions, the threat of litigation, however unjustified, will certainly influence the enthusiasm with which plastic surgeons approach the use of silicone implants, even for reconstruction in patients who have undergone mastectomy for cancer.

Breast biopsy rarely causes discomfort after the first 24 to 48 hours, so a wound complication should be suspected if pain continues, even if fever, erythema, or fluctuance is absent. Usually some demonstrable serosanguineous or purulent drainage is noted at the incision site, and most often all that is necessary is to open the wound and establish drainage, inserting a small gauze wick or peroxide-soaked packing into the wound to ensure that the wound edges do not seal before effective drainage has been attained. It is customary to initiate a course of antibiotics at the time the wound is opened, usually with a cephalosporin, *while awaiting results of smear and culture.* Most infections would probably respond to drainage alone, but the addition of the appropriate antibiotic may hasten resolution of local cellulitis and any accompanying systemic symptoms. As already noted previously (vide infra), the flora responsible for nonlactational breast abscesses have changed in the past generation, and the same comments pertain to postoperative breast infections.

During major operative procedures on the breast the thin skin flaps created during mastectomy are relatively ischemic and therefore more vulnerable to infection. The likelihood of postoperative wound infection may be minimized by gentle handling of the tissues, sharp dissection with a scalpel rather than with scissors, and wound closure with the finest (00000) sutures. Blunt dissection in the breast or axilla is to be avoided. Even during lengthy operations the blood vessels and other structures that must be secured are small in caliber, even if numerous, and may be tied with the finest synthetic absorbable or nonabsorbable (00000) sutures or clipped. Catgut is especially to be avoided, even though it is absorbable, because of the marked tissue reaction it provokes. Mastectomy flaps may be approximated quite satisfactorily with 00000 sutures of Dexon or Vicryl and 00000 Nylon sutures or staples for the skin. No heavier sutures are required in the breast.

When and if wound infection occurs, the same principles of treatment apply as pertain to other soft tissue infections. Most patients undergoing these operations are otherwise healthy, and their natural defense mechanisms are intact.

The most common organism, even in hospital-acquired infections, is *S. aureus*. These organisms are usually resistant to penicillin (and ampicillin) and require treatment by a synthetic penicillin or one of the cephalosporins. Occasionally, infection by a group A beta-hemolytic *Streptococcus* will occur after mastectomy. This infection is manifested by fever out of proportion to other symptoms and by leukocytosis and wound tenderness, along with considerable erythema in the wound, as well as an exudate. The diagnosis may be made by Gram stained smear of the exudate, which reveals the characteristic gram-positive cocci in chains. Cultures of blood and wound should be followed by high doses of penicillin or erythromycin in the allergic patient.

Other wound infections, such as those caused by gram-negative organisms, anaerobic organisms, or clostridia, are uncommon, although increasing in frequency. The Gram-stained smear and culture should rule these out at the time the infection is recognized and treatment is initiated.

REFERENCES

1. Haagensen CD: Diseases of the Breast, 3rd ed. Philadelphia, Saunders, 1986.
2. Devereux WP: Acute puerperal mastitis: evaluation of its management. Am J Obstet Gynecol 108:78, 1970.
3. Gibberd GF: Sporadic and epidemic puerperal breast infections: a contrast in morbid anatomy and clinical signs. Am J Obstet Gynecol 65:1038, 1953.
4. Marshall BR, Hepper JK, Zirbel CC: Sporadic puerperal mastitis: infection that need not interrupt lactation. JAMA 233:1377, 1975.
5. Sandison AT, Walker JC: Inflammatory mastitis, mammary duct ectasia, and mammillary fistula. Br J Surg 50:57, 1962.
6. Sherman AJ: Puerperal breast abscess: I. Report of an outbreak at Philadelphia General Hospital. Obstet Gynecol 7:268, 1956.
7. Monro JA, Markham NPL: Staphylococcal infection in mothers and infants: maternal breast abscesses and antecedent neonatal sepsis. Lancet 2:186, 1958.
8. Sawyer CD, Walker PH: A bacteriologic and clinical study of breast abscess. Surg Gynecol Obstet 99:368, 1954.
9. Gallblum LI: Subareolar abscess of the breast: diagnosis by fine needle aspiration. Am J Clin Pathol 80:496, 1983.
10. Soltau DHK, Hatcher GW: Some observation on the aetiology of breast abscess in the puerperium. Br Med J 1:1603, 1960.
11. Thomsen AC: Leukocyte counts and microbiologic cultivation in the diagnosis of puerperal mastitis. Am J Obstet Gynecol 146:938, 1983.
12. Thomsen AC: Course and treatment of milk stasis, noninfectious inflammation of the breast and infectious mastitis in nursing women. Am J Obstet Gynecol 149:492, 1984.
13. Ezrati LB: Puerperal mastitis: causes, prevention, management. J Nurs Midwifery 24:3, 1979.
14. Gupta R: Tubercular mastitis. Int Surg 67:422, 1982.
15. Quinn PT: Maternal herpetic breast infection: another hazard of neonatal herpes simplex. Med J Aust 2:411, 1978.
16. Sullivan-Bolyai JZ: Disseminated neonatal herpes simplex virus type I from a maternal breast lesion. Pediatrics 71:455, 1983.
17. Ekland DA, Ziegler MG: Abscess in the nonlactating breast. Arch Surg 107:398, 1973.
18. Leach RD, Phillips I, Eyklyn SJ, Corrin B: Anaerobic subareolar breast abscess. Lancet 1:35, 1979.
19. Newton M, Newton NR: Breast abscess: a result of lactation failure. Surg Gynecol Obstet 901:432, 1973.
20. Knight ICS, Nolan B: Breast abscess. Br Med J 1:1224, 1959.
21. Hayes R, Michell M, Nunnerly HB: Acute inflammation of the breast—the role of breast ultrasound in diagnosis and management. Clin Radiol 44:253, 1991.
22. Kalstone C: Methicillin-resistant staphylococcal mastitis. Am J Obstet Gynecol 161:120, 1989.
23. Rench MA, Baker CJ: Group B streptococcal breast abscess in a mother and mastitis in her infant. Obstet Gynecol 73:875, 1989.

24. Petrek J: Post-menopausal breast abscess. South Med J 75:1198, 1982.
25. Edmiston CE Jr, Walker AP, Krepel CJ, Gohr C: The nonpuerperal breast infection: aerobic and anaerobic microbial recovery from acute and chronic disease. J Infect Dis 162:695, 1990.
26. Abramson DJ: Mammary duct ectasia, mammillary fistula, and subareolar sinuses. Ann Surg 169:217, 1969.
27. Hughes LE: Non-lactational inflammation and duct ectasia. Br Med Bull 47:272, 1991.
28. Zuska JJ, Crile G Jr, Ayres WW: Fistulas of lactiferous ducts. Am J Surg 81:312, 1951.
29. Maier WP: Periareolar abscess in the non-lactating breast. Am J Surg 144:359, 1982.
30. Dixon JM, Thompson AM: Effective management for mammary duct fistula. Br J Surg 78:1185, 1991.
31. Berger SA: Recurrent breast abscesses caused by *Corynebacterium minutissimum.* J Clin Microbiol 20:1219, 1984.
32. Haskell CM: *Corynebacterium parvum* and metastatic breast cancer. Br J Cancer 45:794, 1982.
33. Patey DH, Thackray AC: Pathology and treatment of mammary duct fistula. Lancet 2:871, 1958.
34. Habif DV, Perzin KH, Lipton R, Lattes R: Subareolar abscess associated with squamous metaplasia of lactiferous ducts. Am J Surg 119:523, 1970.
35. Caswell HT, Burnett WE: Chronic recurrent breast abscess due to inversion of the nipple. Surg Gynecol Obstet 102:439, 1956.
36. Caswell HT, Maier WP: Chronic recurrent periareolar abscess secondary to inversion of the nipple. Surg Gynecol Obstet 128:597, 1969.
37. Burry VF, Beezley M: Infant mastitis due to gram-negative organisms. Am J Dis Child 124:736, 1972.
38. Schwarz MD, Rosen RA: Neonatal mastitis due to *Escherichia coli.* Clin Pediatr 13:86, 1974.
39. Stetler H, Martin E, Plotkin S, Katz M: Neonatal mastitis due to *Escherichia coli.* J Pediatr 76:611, 1970.
40. Mayer TC: Treatment of prepubertal mastitis. Lancet 2:721, 1975.
41. Greydanus DE, Parks DS, Farrell EG: Breast disorders in children and adolescents. Pediatr Clin North Am 36:601, 1989.
42. Murthy MSH: Granulomatous mastitis and lipogranuloma of the breast. Am J Clin Pathol 60:432, 1973.
43. Cohen C: Granulomatous mastitis: a review of 5 cases. S Afr Med J 52:14, 1977.
44. Kessler E, Wollock Y: Granulomatous mastitis: a lesion clinically simulating carcinoma. Am J Clin Pathol 58:642, 1972.
45. Alasaratnam TT: Uncommon forms of mastitis. Aust N Z J Surg 51:45, 1981.
46. Galea MH, Robertson JF, Ellis IO, et al: Granulomatous lobular mastitis. Aust N Z J Surg 59:547, 1989.
47. Jorgensen MB, Nielsen DM: Diagnosis and treatment of granulomatous mastitis. Am J Med 93:97, 1992.
48. Houn HY, Granger JK: Granulomatous mastitis secondary to histoplasmosis: report of a case diagnosed by fine-needle aspiration biopsy. Diagnostic Cytopathology 7:282, 1991.
49. Schaefer G: Tuberculosis of the breast: a review with the additional presentation of 10 cases. Am Rev Tuberc 72:810, 1955.
50. Levin AC, Gums JG, Grauer K: Tuberculosis. The primary physician's role in eradication. Postgrad Med 93:46, 1993.
51. Frieden TR, Sterling T, Pablos-Mendez A, et al: The emergence of drug-resistant tuberculosis in New York City. N Engl J Med 328:521, 1993.
52. Alasaratnam TT: Tuberculosis of the breast. Br J Surg 67:125, 1980.
53. Cohen C: Tuberculous mastitis: a review of 34 cases. S Afr Med J 52:12, 1977.
54. Hartstein M, Leaf HL: Tuberculosis of the breast as a presenting manifestation of AIDS. Clin Infect Dis 15:692, 1992.
55. Hutton MD, Stead WW, Cauthen GM, et al: Nosocomial transmission of tuberculosis associated with a draining abscess. J Infect Dis 161:286, 1990.
56. Symmers W St C: Silicone mastitis in "topless" waitresses and some other varieties of foreign-body mastitis. Br Med J 3:19, 1968.
57. Kessler, DA: The basis of the FDA's decision on breast implants. N Engl J Med 326:1713, 1992.
58. Todd J, Fishaut M, Kapral F, Welch T: Toxic-shock syndrome associated with phage-group-1 staphylococci. Lancet 2:1116, 1978.
59. Bartlett P, Reingold A, Graham D, et al: Toxic shock syndrome associated with surgical wound infections. JAMA 247:1448, 1982.
60. Uretsky BF, O'Brien JJ, Courtiss EH, Becker MD: Augmentation mammaplasty associated with a severe systemic illness. Case report. Ann Plast Surg 3:445, 1979.
61. Barnett A, Lavey E, Pearl RM, Vistnes LM: Toxic shock syndrome from an infected breast prosthesis. Ann Plast Surg 10:408, 1983.
62. Demey HE, Hautekeete ML, Buytaert P, Bossaert LL: Mastitis and toxic shock syndrome. Acta Obstet Gynecol Scand 68:87, 1989.
63. Van de Perre P, Simonon A, Msellati P, et al: Postnatal transmission of human immunodeficiency virus type 1 from mother to infant. N Engl J Med 325:595, 1991.
64. Van de Perre P, Hitimana D-G, Simonon A, et al: Postnatal transmission of HIV-1 associated with breast abscess. Lancet 1:1490, 1992.
65. Hu DJ, Heyward WL, Byers RH Jr, et al: HIV infection and breast-feeding: policy implications through a decision analysis model. AIDS 6:1503, 1992.
66. Palasanthiran P, Ziegler JB, Stewart GJ, et al: Breast-feeding during primary maternal human immunodeficiency virus infection and risk of transmission from mother to infant. J Infect Dis 167:441, 1993.

67. Gutierrez Y: Breast nodule produced by *Dirofilaria tenuis*. Am J Surg Pathol 8:463, 1984.
68. Pinto MM, Longstreth GB, Jhoury GM: Fine needle aspiration of *Actinomyces* infection of the breast. A novel presentation of thoracopleural actinomycosis. Acta Cytol 35:409, 1991.
69. Platt R, Zaleznik DF, Hopkins CC, et al. Perioperative antibiotic prophylaxis for herniorrhaphy and breast surgery. N Engl J Med 322:153, 1990.
70. Dajani AS, Bisno AL, Chung KJ, et al: Prevention of bacterial endocarditis: recommendations by the American Heart Association. JAMA 264:2919, 1990.
71. Freedman AM, Jackson IT: Infections in breast implants. Infect Dis Clin North Am 3:275, 1989.
72. LeRoy J, Given KS: Wound infection in breast augmentation: the role of prophylactic perioperative antibiotics. Aesthetic Plast Surg 15:303, 1991.
73. Varga J, Schumacher HR, Jimenez SA: Systemic sclerosis after augmentation mammoplasty with silicone implants. Ann Intern Med 111:377, 1989.

Infections of the Head and Neck

CHAPTER 33

George L. Adams

Although most texts on infectious diseases devote considerable space to viral and bacterial infections of the upper respiratory and aerodigestive tracts, the emphasis in this chapter will be on those situations where surgical intervention is required.

ANATOMIC CHARACTERISTICS OF INFECTIONS OF THE HEAD AND NECK

Infections occurring in the head and neck are unique for several reasons. A rich vascular supply, primarily from divisions of the external carotid artery system, promotes rapid healing after surgery or trauma and permits rapid mobilization of host defenses. Conversely, the coexisting rich venous drainage permits the spread of embolic infection. Retrograde venous flow along the ophthalmic vein to the cavernous sinus and along the mastoid emissary vein to the petrosal vein permits the extension of infection to the meninges and the central nervous system (Fig. 33–1). The predictable pattern of lymphatic channels and lymph nodes provides known routes for the extension of infection.

The mastoids and sinuses are unique air-filled cavities within the head. The sinuses, mastoid cavity, eustachian tube, middle ear, and respiratory portion of the pharynx are lined by respiratory (pseudostratified, columnar, ciliated) epithelium, the condition of which is affected by environmental changes, such as humidity and temperature. The clearance of secretions and contaminants depends on ciliary activity, which in turn is affected by medications, hydration, allergies, and respiratory viral infection. A constantly renewable mucous blanket coats this respiratory epithelium, and it flows continuously toward the pharynx, cleansing the area of foreign material and bacteria. The maxillary sinuses lie in close proximity to the roots of the upper teeth so that dental infections can extend into the sinuses.

The investing fascia of the neck (superficial layer of the deep cervical fascia) acts like a cylinder to surround the important muscles. A separate deeper layer of fascia surrounds the important viscera of the neck, including the pharynx, trachea, and major salivary glands (Fig. 33–2). These fasciae communicate along the region of the carotid sheath. Thus infections are initially confined to specific areas within the neck, but a pathway exists for their spread. These spaces are continuous with similar spaces that extend into the mediastinum.

Developmental Changes

Infections in children can be more serious and have a different clinical course than infections of the

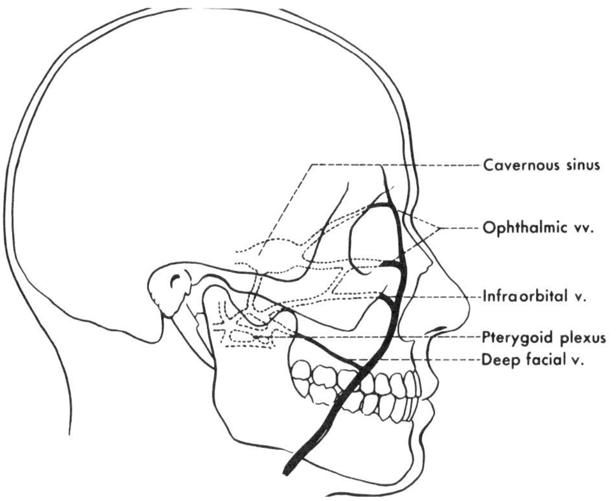

Figure 33–1. Chief connections of the facial vein to the cavernous sinus. *(From Hollinshead HW (ed): The face. In: Anatomy for Surgeons. Volume 1, The Head and Neck, 3rd ed. Hagerstown, MD, Harper & Row, 1982, p 303.)*

same anatomic space with the same organism in an adult. For example, the newborn child has only rudimentary maxillary and ethmoid sinuses, with virtually no development of the frontal sinuses or sphenoid sinus. Thus sinus infections in children are primarily confined to the ethmoid sinuses. Problems in both the frontal and sphenoid sinuses are more likely in the young adult. Although present at birth, the maxillary sinuses continue to increase in size as the contour of the face changes.

The mastoid system is poorly developed in the newborn and develops over the first few years of life. Its development depends on proper eustachian tube function but is affected by structural alterations and defects when present in the child. For example, the eustachian tube of the child lies on a more horizontal plane and is wide and shorter than the adult. Its function is directly dependent on the musculature of the pharynx, primarily of the tensor veli palatini and levator veli palatini. Loss of function in this muscular system, such as occurs in a child with a cleft palate, affects the eustachian tube function, which in turn affects mastoid and middle ear development and physiology.

Structures in the pharynx and nasopharynx also undergo changes related to age. The adenoid mass hypertrophies during early childhood years and can cause nasal and eustachian tube obstruction. Tonsils similarly undergo hypertrophy during this same period and begin to undergo involution in adolescence. Because childhood infections coincide with tonsillar hypertrophy, a causal relationship has been postulated.

The larynx of a newborn, as compared to that of an adult, is disproportionately smaller. Its cartilaginous skeleton is less firm, and the soft tissues are more subject to swelling and edema. The larynx is also located higher in the neck and descends with growth. The disproportionately small size of the upper airway of the child permits airway obstruction to occur with only minimal inflammatory swelling.

The Cartilaginous Support

A large number of appendages and structures in the head and neck are formed from cartilage, rather than bone. Cartilage has no direct blood supply and derives its nutrition entirely from the surrounding perichondrium. Infectious injury to the perichondrium can result in dissolution of the cartilage and loss of its structure. Fibrous tissue, which replaces cartilage, lacks a functional shape. Thus infections that extend into the perichondrium of the ear or nasal septum are not only difficult to control with sys-

Figure 33–2. The deep cervical fascia is itself divided into superficial and deep layers, which encompass trapezius and sternocleidomastoid muscles. The prevertebral layer surrounds the deeper muscles of the neck. The visceral (pretracheal) layer surrounds the trachea, thyroid, and pharyngoesophagus. The visceral and prevertebral layers communicate with the mediastinal fascia. *(From Hollinshead HW (ed): Fascia and fascial spaces. In: Anatomy for Surgeons. Volume 1, The Head and Neck, 3rd ed. Hagerstown, MD, Harper & Row, 1982, p 271.)*

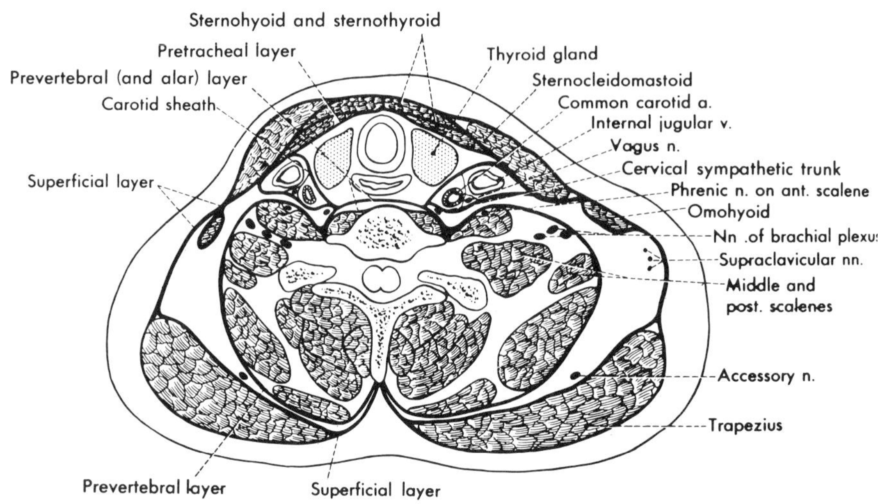

temic antibiotics but leave permanent deformity when they finally resolve. Perichondritis in the larynx, epiglottis, or trachea is uncommon but does occasionally appear after prolonged intubation, trauma, or irradiation. Tracheomalacia with asphyxiation or residual stricture formation are two of the more serious consequences.

INFECTIOUS DISEASES OF THE ORAL CAVITY AND PHARYNX

Most infections of the oral cavity and pharynx can be identified in the course of a routine history and physical examination, with the assistance of appropriate cultures. Certain types of infections have a predilection to extend into the nasopharynx and sinuses, eustachian tube, and mastoid. Treatment and recognition of the pharyngeal problem are therefore important, not only to treat the problem in the oral cavity and pharynx but also to prevent its extension. Patients who have acute infections generally have pain while chewing or swallowing, fever, and cervical lymphadenopathy. Chronic infections may show only erythema, local tenderness, and nontender cervical adenopathy. From many of the acute infections, culture (as taken for suspected beta-hemolytic streptococcal pharyngitis) must be incubated for 24 hours before the organism can be identified. A culture is frequently less informative in the chronic sore throat and chronic oral cavity diseases. If there is a suspicion of infection, a culture should be obtained but a biopsy of the ulceration of whitish plaque tissue may be more revealing. A fungal infection, such as candidiasis, may be present. KOH smear findings along with clinical signs of a thick, whitish exudate may be sufficient to make the diagnosis.

Leukoplakia and Ulcers

White patches and shallow ulcers are common in the mouth and pharynx. Any ulcer that persists for 2 weeks or longer should be evaluated histologically. Other important factors in the patient's history include smoking, denture irritation, alcohol abuse, poor dietary habits, and poor oral hygiene. Medical treatment should include not only the appropriate antibiotics but also instructions on the improvement of oral care, such as sodium chloride and sodium bicarbonate mouthwash, correct care of the teeth, and removal of dentures at night.

Pharyngitis and Tonsillitis

Pharyngitis and tonsillitis are inflammatory diseases of microbial etiology—usually viral or group A streptococci. Both are usually self-limited, but the latter can produce suppurative or nonsuppurative complications.

Viral pharyngitis is most often caused by the adenoviruses (named for adenoid tissue from which they were first isolated) and the coxsackieviruses (types A2, 4, 5, 6, 8, 10), which cause herpangina and acute lymphonodular pharyngitis in children. Herpes simplex virus can cause an ulcerative pharyngitis.

The group A *Streptococcus* is most commonly associated with pharyngitis and rheumatic fever. The streptococci are discussed as a group in Chapter 4. Classically, pharyngitis and rheumatic fever are associated with each other. Glomerulonephritis rarely follows pharyngitis but is most often associated with streptococcal pyoderma.

Viral pharyngitis is a disease of the mucosal cells with superficial necrosis. Extension to the adjacent paranasal sinuses, eustachian tube, and middle ear can lead to obstruction and suppurative complications of these cavities; cervical adenitis and dissemination to lungs are common. Bacteremia can cause metastatic infections.

Tonsillitis

Acute, recurrent, tonsillar pharyngitis occurs in children and particularly young adults. The tonsils become hypertrophic and scarred, and crypt formations associated with chronic sore throat may occur. In others, recurrent episodes of acute tonsillitis with swelling, inflammation, and pain occur. Beta-hemolytic *Streptococcus*, group A, is the most common cause of this infection; however, adenovirus and Epstein-Barr virus (EBV) have also been identified. Acute streptococcal tonsillitis requires treatment with appropriate antibiotics to prevent suppurative complications and rheumatic fever.

The indications for tonsillectomy are still not rigidly established. There is consensus, however, that children younger than 10 who have more than three episodes of culture-documented streptococcal pharyngitis per year for at least 2 years would benefit from tonsillectomy. That benefit is no longer apparent after the children reach age 10.[1,2] Consideration for tonsillectomy and for adenoidectomy should be made separately: they are two distinct operations that do not need to be performed at the same time. There are specific indications for each procedure. Adults require tonsillectomy only after conservative management has failed to eradicate recurrent or chronic tonsillitis. Cultures will reveal mixed aerobic and anaerobic organisms. The most common aerobic organisms include *Hemophilus* species, streptococci, and *Staphylococcus aureus.*

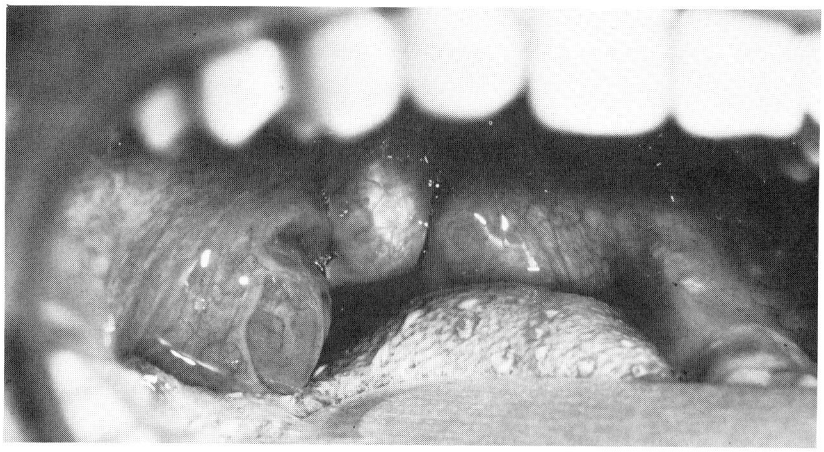

Figure 33–3. Acute right peritonsillar abscess. The tonsil is pushed medially by the abscess. The tonsil may appear enlarged but not infected.

Anaerobic organisms include *Fusobacterium, Bacteroides,* and *Actinomyces* species.[3] The infection resides in the depths of the tonsillar crypts, and penicillin remains the antibiotic of choice.

A child with recurrent episodes of acute otitis media with nasal obstruction from hypertrophied adenoids may benefit from an adenoidectomy. Recurrent streptococcal tonsillitis is an indication for tonsillectomy, not necessarily adenoidectomy. Patients with persistently positive cultures, even after adequate treatment, may have a coexisting infection with a beta-lactamase-producing organism such as *Branhamella catarrhalis.* In this situation, a drug such as clindamycin or amoxicillin-clavulanic acid is effective.

Adults occasionally require tonsillectomy, despite an increased incidence of bleeding and postoperative pain. Current indications include (1) peritonsillar abscess; (2) nasopharyngeal airway obstruction with cor pulmonale; (3) airway obstruction with sleep apnea syndrome, secondary to tonsillar hypertrophy; (4) suspicion of malignancy (lymphoma); (5) repeated documented episodes of beta-hemolytic streptococcal pharyngitis; and (6) chronic tonsillitis.

Peritonsillar Abscess. The most common suppurative complication of acute tonsillitis is the development of a peritonsillar abscess. This usually occurs 3 to 4 days after an acute pharyngitis, even though the tonsillitis may be controlled by antibiotics. Symptoms include trismus, difficulty in swallowing, and pain in the throat. When the patient is coaxed to open the mouth, unilateral pharyngeal swelling is apparent in the region of the soft palate. The tonsil is seen to be pushed toward the midline

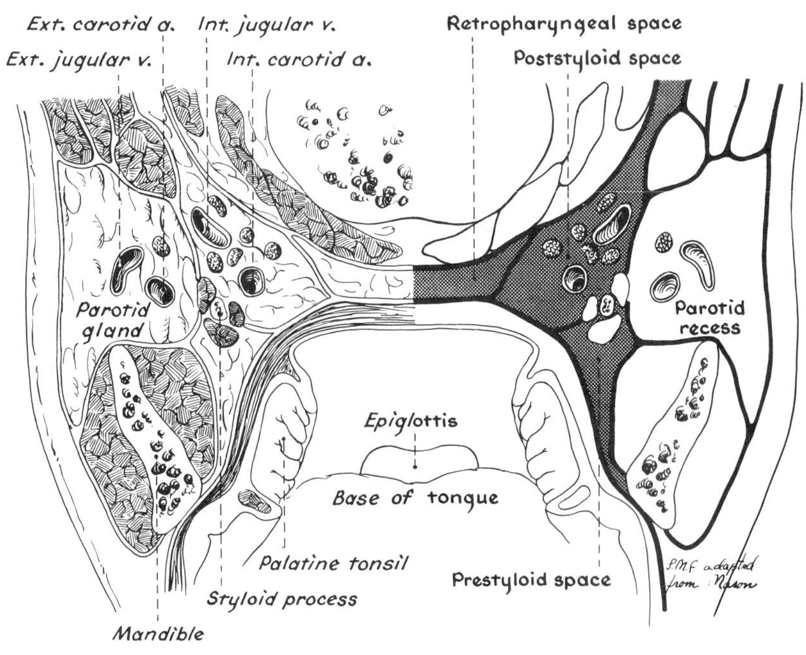

Figure 33–4. Important fascial spaces of the neck: the parapharyngeal (pharyngomaxillary) space is divided into an anterior (prestyloid) and a posterior (poststyloid) space by the styloid process and its attached ligament. *(From Adams G: Special examinations in otolaryngology. In Adams G, Boies LR Jr, Paparella MM (eds): Boies's Fundamentals of Otolaryngology, 5th ed. Philadelphia, Saunders, 1978, p 28.)*

and may no longer be inflamed (see Fig. 33–3). Infection has penetrated the tonsillar capsule and is trapped between the superior pharyngeal constrictor and the tonsil. The possibility of a parapharyngeal space abscess (see Figs. 33–2 and 33–4 to 33–6) occurring as a direct extension of a peritonsillar abscess should always be considered. In fact, a parapharyngeal abscess in a patient who has had a previous tonsillectomy can resemble a peritonsillar abscess. It is important to make this differential diagnosis, because a parapharyngeal abscess is drained through an external or lateral approach to the neck (see Fig. 38–6), but a peritonsillar abscess is drained through an intraoral approach.

Bilateral tonsillectomy immediately for drainage or after a 6-week interval was generally advocated in the past. The reasons for this include a high rate of recurrence of peritonsillar abscess (7 to 25 percent), failure to control the infection with less than adequate drainage, and an 8 percent incidence of bilateral abscesses.

Reports by Herzon[4] and Schechter et al[5] have raised questions about this approach. Both reports advocate use of drainage with a No. 18 spinal needle and 10-ml syringe. After needle aspiration, Herzon advises outpatient therapy with oral antibiotics. Schechter et al still preferred intravenous (IV) antibiotics and hydration. The aspirating needle is inserted into the area of greatest bulging or into three separate areas—superior, central, and inferior—in order to obtain pus for culture. In Schechter's series, 51 percent of the patients were under 25 years of age and 39 percent had a history of previous tonsillar disease. Seventy-two percent of the patient had been on antibiotics before the development of an abscess.

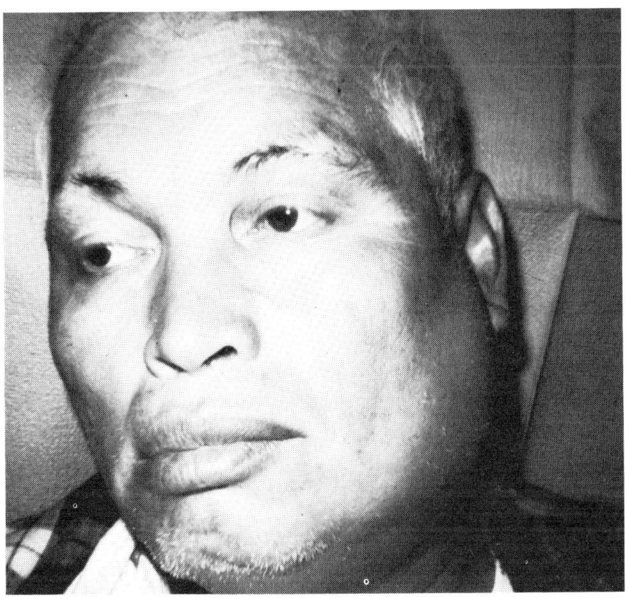

Figure 33–5. Left parapharyngeal space (pharyngomaxillary space) abscess. The left part of the neck and parotid area are diffusely swollen. The angle of the mandible is obliterated.

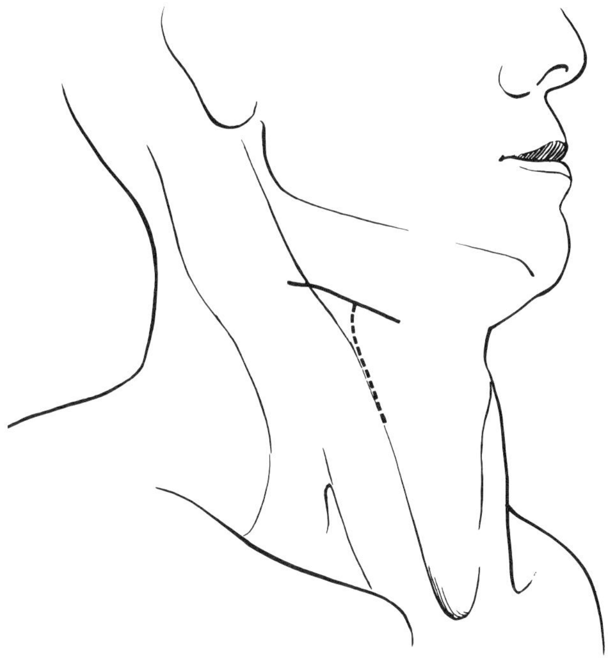

Figure 33–6. Incision described by Mosher to drain a parapharyngeal space abscess. Dotted line indicates possible incision to control extension of infection along the carotid sheath. This same incision can be used to drain infections of the submandibular space and retropharyngeal space.

McCurdy[6] advocates immediate tonsillectomy. It provides improved drainage and requires a shorter hospitalization than an interval tonsillectomy. Patients are given IV penicillin for 12 hours before surgery. Patients allergic to penicillin were given clindamycin. He found no increased blood loss for morbidity in patients having immediate tonsillectomy compared to interval tonsillectomy.

Holt and Tinsley[7] reviewed peritonsillar abscess in children. Thirty-nine percent of these patients had been on an antibiotic before the development of the abscess. Seven percent of their patients developed a recurrent abscess, and 7 percent developed chronic tonsillitis. This compared to an incidence of recurrent abscess of 7 to 16 percent in the literature. They advised surgery for the following circumstances:

1. Previous history of documented recurrent tonsillitis.
2. Obstruction of the airway or abscess in the neck at time of presentation.
3. History of previous peritonsillar abscess.
4. Systemic toxicity at presentation.

These criteria have received general acceptance as indications for tonsillectomy, either immediately or after an interval.

The chemotherapy of peritonsillar abscess is less controversial. The most common organism is *Streptococcus pyogenes,* accounting for about 50 percent of positive cultures. The next most common aerobic organisms recovered include *Streptococcus pneumoniae, Hemophilus influenzae,* and *Staphylococcus aureus.* The most common anaerobic organisms are *Peptostreptococcus* species, *Fusobacterium* species, *Bacteroides* species, and *Peptococcus.* Anaerobic organisms will be recovered more frequently than aerobic organisms, but in approximately 30 percent of patients, no isolate is obtained.

In summary, the preferred treatment for a peritonsillar abscess is as follows:

1. Incision and drainage—either by incision and then spreading the deep tissues with a hemostat, or aspiration with an 18-gauge needle.
2. Oral or intravenous antibiotics, depending on the general status of the patient and need for hydration.
3. Selection of appropriate antibiotics. Penicillin G is the preferred drug: a cephalosporin is an alternative.
4. The decision on tonsillectomy is made on the past history or the severity of systemic manifestations at presentation.

Indications for surgery are a history of repeated acute tonsillitis, chronic tonsillitis, or a previous peritonsillar abscess. An indication for an immediate tonsillectomy would be development of obstruction of the airway or abscess in the neck.

Infectious Mononucleosis. Infectious mononucleosis is an important cause of acute pharyngitis with enlarged tonsils. This infection is probably one of the many diseases caused by the Epstein-Barr virus.[8] The patient has a prodromal syndrome of lethargy and pharyngitis. The tonsils can enlarge and actually obstruct the airway. A membranous exudate is present over the tonsil, and in 30 percent of the cases a culture will reveal an associated group A streptococcus. Cervical adenopathy, particularly of the posterior cervical nodes, becomes evident. The patient may also develop other symptoms, including neurologic disturbances and liver or spleen enlargement. Although enlargement of Waldeyer's ring can cause airway obstruction and cyanosis, tracheostomy is seldom necessary if 40 mg/day of prednisone is used to shrink the lymphoid tissue. The diagnosis is made by examining the peripheral blood smear for atypical lymphocytes and by one of several available heterophile hemagglutination tests (Monospot). If these tests are negative, as they are in 5 to 10 percent of young adults and many infants and children, EBV-specific serologic testing may be necessary.[9] Victims of infectious mononucleosis can be treated at home if their oral intake is satisfactory and their pain is not sufficient to require hospitalization. They should not return to their usual activities for 2 weeks or more, and then only after the disease and particularly spleen enlargement have resolved. There have been reports of splenic rupture when young athletes prematurely return to their sports. Sometimes the tonsils remain hypertrophied after a bout of mononucleosis. If they do not return to normal size in 6 months and symptoms of chronic tonsillitis develop, tonsillectomy is considered.

Dental Infection

The normal oral flora have been discussed in Chapter 2, but individuals actually develop their own normal flora dependent on their general and local dental health, use of antibiotics, and previous irradiation therapy. For example, the oral flora of patients in an intensive care unit will show many gram-negative organisms not ordinarily found in the oral cavity. Sprinkle and Veltri[10] have shown that the oral cavity of a child after repeated episodes of tonsillitis and pharyngitis, and repeated administration of antibiotics, can be restored to a normal flora only after a tonsillectomy. The predominance of anaerobic organisms in the oral cavity reflects the predilection of certain anaerobes for certain microenvironments. For example, some organisms thrive at the junction of the gingiva and teeth, and other species in the gingival-buccal folds. In both these regions the oxygen pressure (Po_2) is usually less than 1 percent. It is important to remember that bacteremia with the potential to seed many metastatic sites (brain, liver, heart valve, prosthesis, etc) is a common consequence of dental procedures. Appropriate chemoprophylaxis is required in all patients at high risk for such complications.

Most of the dental infections discussed in this section are caused by mixed aerobic and anaerobic normal flora of the mouth. Almost all the organisms are sensitive to penicillin. However, penicillin-resistant organisms, especially *Bacteroides fragilis,* are found often enough that culture should be performed in every case not responding promptly to appropriate operative therapy and penicillin.

Gingivitis and Periodontitis. The etiology of these diseases is complex and equivocal. Putative pathogens include spirochetes of the *Treponema* genus (*Treponema denticola*), black-pigmented *Bacteroides* species (formerly called *B. melaninogenicus*), three of which are clearly associated with periodontal disease: *B. gingivalis*—periodontitis, *B. intermedius*—acute necrotizing ulcerative gingivitis (Vincent's angina, trench mouth), and *B. endodalis*—pulpal infections. In Vincent's disease, the gingivae are usually foul smelling and ulcerated. Treatment in severe cases includes a systemic antibiotic, usually penicillin, given for 5 days, and improved oral hygiene, including the use of a peroxide mouthwash. *Bacteroides forsythus* and *Actinobacillus actinomycetemcomitans* may also be implicated—the latter in localized juvenile periodontitis. Precise etiologies of these mixed and synergistic infections are under active investigation. Gingivitis extends to invade the periodontal ligament and acute periodontitis can develop. Besides the gingivae and periodontal ligament, the adjacent alveolar bone becomes infected, with eventual loss of teeth. The complex etiology of periodontal disease contrasts with an apparent clear etiologic role of *Streptococcus mutans* as the cause of dental caries.

Periapical Abscess. Extension of infection up the root canal causes first pulpitis and then a periapical abscess. The patient complains of fever, and percussion of the affected tooth causes pain. In chronic cases, a periodontal pocket develops, which may eventually communicate with the maxillary sinus. Depending on the involved tooth, the apical abscess can perforate either the maxillary or mandibular bone on either the lingual or buccal suture. The abscess with granulation tissue is referred to as a gum boil. The incisor and canine teeth of the mandible are in the middle of the bone and have a thin alveolar plate so that an abscess can perforate either the lingual or buccal alveolar plate. Because the apex of the roots of the second and third mandibular molars extend well below the mylohyoid line, infections from these two teeth may extend directly into the deep neck and into the area of the submandibular lymph node. These two teeth are then most responsible for dental causes of deep neck abscess. Infection of the more anterior mandibular teeth will remain confined by the mylohyoid muscle to the anterior floor of the mouth.

Treatment of acute periapical abscesses requires drainage through a root canal. At a later stage, a root canal filling is made. If the infection has extended through the alveolar plate, this area must also be incised and drained. The decision for a root canal procedure or extraction is up to the dentist. Generally, if a second or third molar is involved and has caused the infection, extraction is preferred, particularly if the molar is dead. The location of the tooth is important in determining whether a root canal drainage should be performed.

Oroantral Fistula. The maxillary premolar and molar teeth are in close proximity to the sinus. In fact, when these teeth are extracted, no effort should be made to prove the depths of the extraction cavity because only a thin membrane of periosteum may be separating the tooth socket from the maxillary antrum. If the membrane is perforated, the hole should be closed and the area cleansed immediately and packed to prevent the formation of an oroantral fistula. If a fistula develops, a palatal buccal flap is devised, the osteitic bone in the area is removed, and the wound is closed primarily. It should be emphasized that if a fistula develops, sinusitis also develops. Establishing better drainage by creating a nasoantral window will enhance clearing of the infection.

Alveolar Osteitis. Alveolar osteitis (dry socket) is a common and feared complication after extraction. Basically, there is a loss of the clot formed at the site of the extraction, and a localized osteitis develops with exposure of the underlying alveolar bone, most commonly after mandibular extractions. A characteristic foul odor develops. Treatment includes cleansing with a warm saline solution to remove the necrotic debris in the socket. Then, some type of antiseptic material is applied to the socket, such as iodoform packing or Eugenol. This treatment may have to be repeated over a period of days. If there is fever with the infection, a systemic antibiotic such as penicillin is used.

Differential Diagnosis of Dental Pain. Sometimes it is difficult to determine whether a patient's pain is secondary to gingivitis, apical abscess, or sinusitis. Approximately 10 to 12 percent of sinusitis is associated with underlying dental disorders. Dental film, such as Panorex, can be helpful in making the differential diagnosis. The most important test for determining pulpitis or periapical abscess is percussion of the suspected teeth. An upright Water's view of the sinuses will aid in determining whether an underlying sinusitis is present. Infection related to the maxillary molars is the most frequent dental cause of sinusitis. In addition, many benign dental tumors appear as bony erosion or an expanding cyst on dental films, Panorex, or maxillary sinus films. Diagnosis includes differentiating cysts from an acute infection. Following extraction, the cyst lining should be removed for histologic diagnosis.

INFECTIOUS DISEASES OF THE MAJOR AND MINOR SALIVARY GLANDS

Anatomic and Physiologic Predisposing Factors

The major and minor salivary glands combine to produce between 1 and 1.5 liters of saliva per day. Saliva is essential for the protection of the teeth and the mucous membrane of the oral cavity and pharynx. Saliva contains enzymes (eg, ptylin, amylase), which help initiate digestion, and certain electrolytes (primarily sodium phosphate, calcium chloride, and bicarbonate and phosphate buffers). IgA that is formed by the plasma cells lining the acini of the parotid gland combines with saliva to form soluble IgA, which inhibits adherence of bacteria to mucosal cells. Ninety percent of saliva is produced by the parotid and submandibular glands. The parotid, a primarily serous salivary gland, emits a thin, watery secretion, the production of which is vastly increased by chewing when stimulated by ascorbic acid. The submandibular glands are mixed serous and mucous glands and produce a more viscous saliva. There is a constant flow of saliva from the submandibular glands, and it too is increased when food is present in the mouth.

The minor salivary glands and sublingual glands produce the remaining 10 percent of saliva. The sublingual glands are primarily mucous glands, located anteriorly in the floor of the mouth, deep to the mylohyoid muscle, just anterior to the submandibular gland. Additional minor salivary glands are located on the lips, buccal mucosa, and along the anterior tonsillar pillar. They are most concentrated at the junction of the hard and soft palate.

The parotid gland is incompletely encapsulated by splitting of superficial layers of the deep cervical fascia. In addition, septa of this fascia extend vertically into the gland, dividing it into many septated smaller sections. The divisions of the facial nerve run through the midportion of the gland, artificially dividing the gland into its more lateral (superficial) lobe and the deep lobe. Approximately 20 lymph nodes are located within the parotid region. These nodes are both extraglandular (lying over the capsular surface of the gland) and deep. The extracapsular nodes receive the lymph from the region of the face, eyelids, scalp, and preauricular areas (such as the tragus). Deep lymph nodes drain the paranasal sinuses, pharynx, and particularly the deeper aspects of the inner ear canal.

The submandibular gland lies inferior to the lower margin of the mandible, but the anteriormost portion of this gland projects medially into the floor of the mouth, through an opening along the lateral border of the mylohyoid muscle. The submandibular duct (Wharton's duct) is 5 to 6 cm long. It passes along the floor of the mouth just deep to the mucosa to enter the oral cavity through a papilla near the lingual frenulum. Thick secretions in this duct are subject to stasis, obstruction, or stone formation.

General Pathogenetic Factors

Infections within the major salivary glands occur as the result of three problems: (1) decreased salivary flow, possibly secondary to drugs, dehydration, or radiation; (2) formation of viscous saliva, caused by abnormal formation of saliva from either generalized systemic disease or drugs; and (3) obstruction to salivary flow by stones in the duct, stricture, or retrograde infection from the oral cavity.

Table 33–1 lists possible effects of systemic medications on the major salivary glands. In addition to the systemic effects, local irritations from dehydration, smoking, oral irritants and astringents, or poor oral hygiene establish an environment in which ascending infection from the mouth is possible. Systemic diseases that cause parotid enlargement and changes in the salivary flow rate include (1) cystic fibrosis, (2) primary aldosteronism,

TABLE 33–1. DRUGS AFFECTING SALIVARY GLANDS

Decreased salivary flow
Parasympathomimeter (atrophic)
Sympathomimeter
Digitalis
Sialadenitis
Heavy metals
Mercury
Bismuth
Enlargement
Iodine
Phenothiazine

(3) Addison's disease, (4) Cushing's disease, (5) cirrhosis, (6) diabetes mellitus, (7) gouty parotitis, and (8) sarcoidosis.

Acute Suppurative Sialoadenitis

Parotitis. Acute suppurative parotitis occurs in the dehydrated postoperative patient, debilitated by disease, with poor oral hygiene. Salivary flow decreases disproportionately with dehydration; even minor degrees of dehydration cause immediate major decrease in salivary flow. Infection usually ascends along the parotid duct. The organism responsible in more than 90 percent of the cases is *S. aureus,* but any organism (*P. aeruginosa,* anaerobes, *Eikenella corrodens, Streptococcus pyogenes*) can also be responsible. Because the parotid is divided by multiple septa, localized fluctuation and suppuration cannot be demonstrated. Instead, diffuse parotid enlargement with tenderness and redness over the involved gland and side of the face are seen. Treatment includes hydration both orally (if possible) and with intravenous fluids, correction of electrolyte disturbances, and administration of intravenous antibiotics, preferably methicillin or cephalosporin derivatives. Improved oral hygiene is also important. Heat applied to the gland (in the form of warm moist packs) may provide some symptomatic relief. If there is no evidence of improvement, some physicians recommend between 400 and 600 rads of cobalt irradiation over a period of 2 to 3 days. This treatment is generally only effective when initiated within the first 48 hours. The radiation decreases the saliva formation and decreases the inflammatory response. If there is no improvement in 4 to 5 days, surgical drainage becomes necessary. A modified Blair or lazy S incision is used. Skin is elevated and a series of incisions are made through the capsule of the parotid gland in multiple areas, being careful to place the incisions parallel to the divisions of the facial nerve. Penrose drains are placed, and the wound is allowed to heal by secondary intention.

Another variant of acute suppurative parotitis—again caused by *S. aureus*—can occur within the first year of life in children. Treatment with systemic antibiotics is usually successful, but failure to respond may necessitate operative drainage as described for the adult.

Submandibular Gland Sialadenitis. Acute infection in the submandibular gland is usually the result of ductal stricture or stone. Antistaphylococcal antibiotics are used before manipulation. Stones felt on bimanual palpation along the course of the duct in the floor of the mouth can be removed by an intraoral incision over the stone. The incision must follow the longitudinal axis of the duct to prevent fistula formation. Stones deep in the hilum of the gland should be removed by a submandibular approach. If there has been an associated, recurrent episode of swelling and a sialadenitis because of the stone, it is worthwhile to remove the entire gland during a quiescent interlude.

Chronic Recurrent Sialadenitis

Chronic sialadenitis is manifested by recurrent acute episodes of sialadenitis, especially of the parotid and submandibular glands. During the quiescent phase, with no evidence of any acute inflammation, sialography may be helpful.

Sialography should demonstrate any area of obstruction in the duct, either extrinsic or intrinsic, stone or stricture. Certain forms of chronic sialadenitis have typical sialographic appearance. Sialectasia shows ectasia of the ductal system similar to the appearance of bronchiectasis on a bronchogram. There may be saccular dilations and areas of obstruction throughout the duct system, primarily in the regions of the small duct lobules. Punctate sialectasis is a term used to describe an end stage of sialadenitis. Spotty collections of contrast throughout the entire glandular system are noted. This appearance is characteristic of Sjögren's disease or benign lymphoepithelial disease. Computed tomography (CT) scan and magnetic resonance imaging (MRI) have reduced the need to perform sialography.

Chronic Nonobstructive Sialadenitis. This disease most commonly affects the parotid gland. Recurrent enlargement and pain are the most frequent symptoms, but there are no calculi. External pressure expresses very viscous saliva from the duct. A sialogram demonstrates tubular changes in the duct, and the x-ray is similar to that seen in tubular bronchiectasis. Treatment involves the use of sialagogues (eg, lemon juice, chewing gum) and increased fluid intake. With increasing symptoms and continuous enlargement that no longer responds to antibiotics and sialogogues, three possible surgical treatments exist. An indirect approach is tympanic neurectomy, that is, sectioning Jacobson's nerve over the promontory of the middle ear. This interrupts the parasympathetic nerve supply to the parotid gland, thus causing a decrease in the salivary flow and atrophy of the glandular tissue. The disadvantage of this technique is the recurrence of saliva flow 18 months later, possibly from alternative neural mechanisms. Another indirect method of treatment is ligation of the parotid duct through an intraoral approach. This surgical treatment requires that a certain amount of parotid function still be present, since the atrophy of the gland depends on the back pressure of the salivary flow to destroy the remaining glandular elements. The third and most effective treatment is total parotidectomy, with preservation of the facial nerve. This resection is performed in a manner similar to the procedure for small benign parotid tumors; however, there is increased risk to the facial nerve. Total rather than superficial parotidectomy is necessary, because the gland is diffusely abnormal with possible small microabscesses and increased fibrosis. Parotidectomy for chronic infection can be technically difficult.

Differential Diagnosis of Salivary Gland Enlargement

It is not always easy to distinguish a chronic inflammation from an underlying parotid tumor because both produce parotid swelling. In addition, cystic masses within the parotid gland, such as a type I or type II pharyngeal cleft cyst, can cause recurrent episodes of parotid swelling. In a type I pharyngeal cleft cyst, there may be cartilaginous duplication of the external ear canal, and the fistulous tract generally exists in the postauricular crease. In a type II pharyngeal cleft cyst, a fistulous tract often enters the upper neck just below the angle of the mandible. Because the tract can pass either medial or lateral to the facial nerve before entering the external ear canal, excision of such a fistulous tract should be performed only after culture, and after antibiotic treatment has removed the acute infection.

A firm nontender mass in the parotid gland that does not fluctuate in size suggests a primary tumor (75 percent are benign pleomorphic adenoma). Fine-needle aspiration (FNA) biopsy can be valuable in this situation. It provides fluid for culture as well as cytology. Failure to make a diagnosis may necessitate a superficial parotidectomy. In children 2 to 10 year of age, atypical mycobacterial infection (*M. avium-intracellulare*) must be included in the differential diagnosis. *Mycobacterium tuberculosis* strain would be more common in adults. Preoperative assessment may include ultrasonic evaluation, CT scan with contrast, or MRI. A properly performed superficial parotidectomy provides a diagnosis and will protect the facial nerve.

INFECTIONS OF THE NOSE AND PARANASAL SINUSES

Serious infections of the nose and paranasal sinuses develop only when the normal physiologic activities of these structures are altered. Normally, the nose acts to cleanse, warm, and humidify inspired air. Most foreign material is deposited on the anterior portion of the middle turbinate. Ciliary activity and the overlying mucous blanket carry the particular debris posteriorly into the nasopharynx. For this to occur normally, the pH of the nose must be neutral. Any of the following events can disrupt these important physiologic activities: (1) an allergic response can cause edema and excess secretion; (2) upper respiratory viral infections severely impair ciliary activity because thick mucus retards ciliary movement; and (3) some medications, both systemic and topical, can interfere with normal ciliary activity (Fig. 33–7). Certain gross anatomic abnormalities—a deviated nasal septum, nasal polyp, tumor, or foreign body—can also obstruct the sinusoidal ostium. Any obstruction, functional or morphologic, impedes the drainage of mucus so that microbial proliferation can occur. The resulting mucosal edema and death of mucosal cells further impede drainage by aggravating the obstruction and abrogating cilial motion. Mucosal regeneration is rapid if obstruction is promptly relieved. If the obstruction is not relieved, the epithelium is permanently damaged: polyps and mucoceles can develop, and chronic sinusitis results. About 10 percent of maxillary sinusitis is associated with preexisting dental infection.

Etiology. The most common bacterial organisms to cause acute sinusitis are pneumococci, strepto-

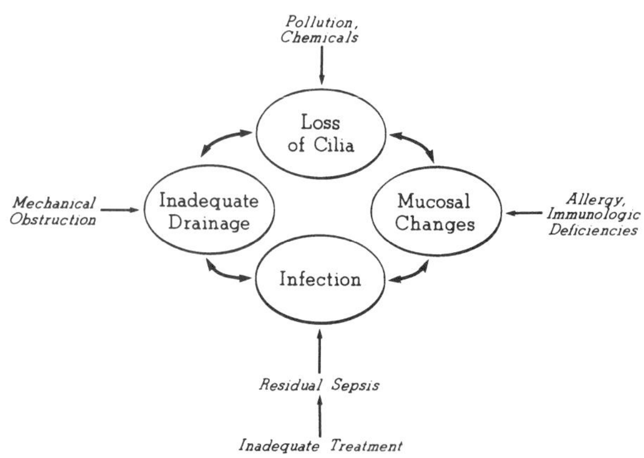

Figure 33–7. Cycle of events leading to chronic sinusitis. *(From Adams GL, Boies LR, Hilger PA (eds): Boies's Fundamentals of Otolaryngology: A Textbook of Ear, Nose, and Throat Diseases, 6th ed. Philadelphia, Saunders, 1989.)*

cocci, staphylococci, and *H. influenzae.* Cultures of the nasal secretions are unreliable in determining the responsible organisms.

Chronic sinusitis and maxillary sinusitis associated with dental infections are more commonly anaerobic because the cavities lose their air content and the increased intrasinusoidal pressure impairs mucosal blood flow. Such infections generally contain large volumes of fetid secretion. Almost all oral, nasal, or pharyngeal anaerobic flora have been found—especially *Peptostreptococcus, Peptococcus, Bacteroides, Veillonella,* and *Actinomyces.* Many anaerobic infections probably result in sterile cultures: bacteria are seen on smear but no growth is found.[11]

General Clinical Manifestations. Pain, headache, fever, and tenderness over the involved area with swelling and redness are common manifestations of acute sinusitis. During chronic infection, the symptoms and signs are much more subtle—congestion, blockage, and chronic nasal discharge. Careful physical examination includes evaluation of the nasal mucosa, search for obstruction by edema or nasal polyps, and examination of nasal secretions. The development of fiberoptic endoscopic sinus scopes facilitates the physician's ability to diagnosis sinus disease (Fig. 33–8). After application of topical decongestant and anesthetic (lidocaine with Neo-Synephrine), the scopes are introduced. The area of the natural ostium, the middle meatus, and the nasopharynx are examined. X-rays of the paranasal sinuses, particularly the upright Water's view of the maxillary and ethmoid sinuses, are helpful. The Caldwell view provides the best information about the frontal sinus. The lateral view is helpful for examination of the ethmoid and frontal sinuses and is essential for evaluation of the sphenoid sinus. Because routine sinus films do not always demonstrate the obstruction or ethmoid sinusitis, a CT scan performed in the coronal plane is required. Decongestant spray is administered 15 minutes prior to scanning to reduce acute edema and better demonstrate structural abnormalities. The coronal CT scan in most circumstances has replaced standard sinus x-rays.

General Aspects of Treatment. Acute sinusitis should respond promptly to medical management. A vasoconstrictor (aqueous 0.25 to 0.50 percent phenylephrine) should be applied as nosedrops every 4 to 6 hours to decrease edema; hot packs or high humidity may provide symptomatic relief. Antibiotics may be necessary especially if fever, pain, and leukocytosis are present. Antibiotics should be continued for 5 days after apparent clinical resolution. In some situations, this may require as much as 2 weeks. The increasing incidence of *H. influenzae* and other penicillin-resistant organisms suggests that amoxicillin plus clavulanic acid be considered as a first line of treatment. The anaerobic organisms in the sinuses are almost always sensitive to these drugs. *Bacteroides fragilis* infections that would be resistant are rare. Rational choice of antibiotic is empirical because reliable noninvasive culture techniques do not exist and nasal cultures are misleading. Aspiration and puncture techniques of obtaining truly diagnostic specimens from each sinus are sometimes necessary and are described in subsequent sections.

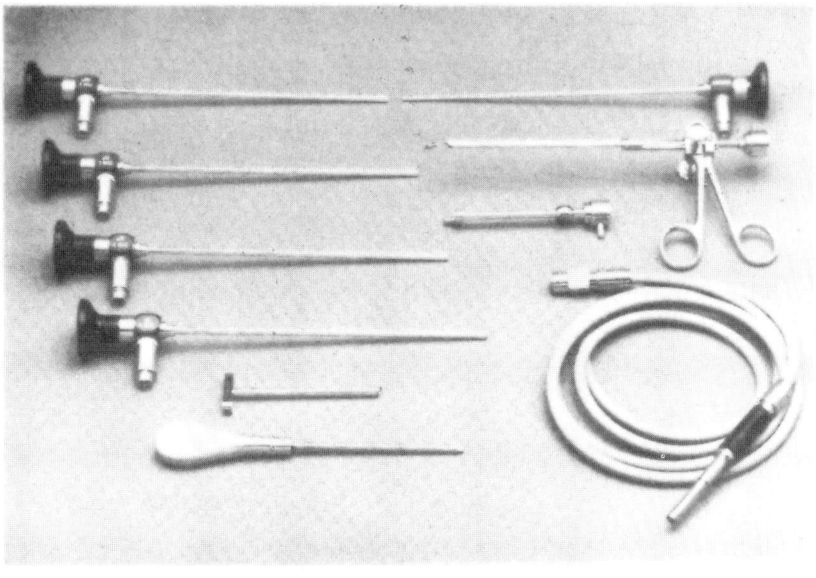

Figure 33–8. Endoscopic sinus surgery instruments. *(From Adams GL, Boies LR, Hilger PA (eds): Boies's Fundamentals of Otolaryngology: A Textbook of Ear, Nose, and Throat Diseases, 6th ed. Philadelphia, Saunders, 1989.)*

During the past 5 years a greater appreciation of sinus and nasal physiology has altered the surgical approach to sinus disease. Development of fiberoptic sinus endoscopy, the coronal CT scan, and recognition that obstruction in the area of the middle meatal complex—that area on the lateral nasal wall above the inferior turbinate into which the frontal and ethmoid sinuses drain—have caused a major difference in surgical approach to sinus disease. Instead of concentrating on the secondary infection that results from obstruction of the maxillary sinus, attention is aimed at the cause within the middle meatal complex by polyps or chronic infection. Alleviation of obstruction in this area is referred to as functional endoscopic sinus surgery. Mucous flow throughout the nose and major sinuses has a specific pattern. Continuously beating ciliary activity pushes the mucous blanket toward the natural sinus ostia. Thus establishing a window into the sinus in an area where gravity drainage could be expected is not felt to be as valuable in standard situations as enlargement of the natural ostium. Credit for appreciation of these techniques is given to Heinz Stanberger, MD, from Graz, Austria, and David Kennedy, MD, from the United States.

Special Forms of Sinusitis

Acute Maxillary Sinusitis. The maxillary sinuses are present at birth and are the most common sinuses to become infected in adults. The maxillary ostium drains into the middle nasal meatus. Infection generally occurs with obstruction of this ostium, whether from a bacterial, viral, or allergic cause. Ten percent result from preexisting dental disease. The coronal CT scan showing an air-fluid level will verify the diagnosis of sinusitis (Fig. 33–9). On the other hand, mucosal thickening of greater than 3 mm can also be considered diagnostic of chronic sinusitis and in the immunocompromised individual, following chemotherapy, AIDS, or a bone marrow transplant, a standard typical fluid level will not be present. (See section on AIDS.) For immunocompromised patients, a much more aggressive approach is initiated from the outset. Sinusitis is a recognized complication of nasal endotracheal intubation, or even nasogastric (NG) tube use, particularly in the intensive care unit (ICU) patient.

In the standard patient, empirical antibiotics and decongestants are selected not on the basis of nasal swab or culture but on recognition that the majority of infections of acute sinusitis are due to *Streptococcus,* pneumococcus, *Staphylococcus,* or *H. influenzae.* In the acute situation, if there is no evidence of improvement after the initiation of 24 to 48 hours of antibiotics, a CT scan is ordered and a culture obtained by placing a trocar into the maxillary sinus. Three options exist. The transnasal technique requires application of a topical anesthetic, such as 4 percent cocaine, to the inferior nasal meatus (Fig. 33–10). With the patient seated, a trocar is pushed through the lateral nasal wall, as high as possible, yet still beneath the inferior turbinate. The trocar is aimed toward the lateral canthus of the eye. With gentle pressure, the trocar passes through the thin bone and enters the maxil-

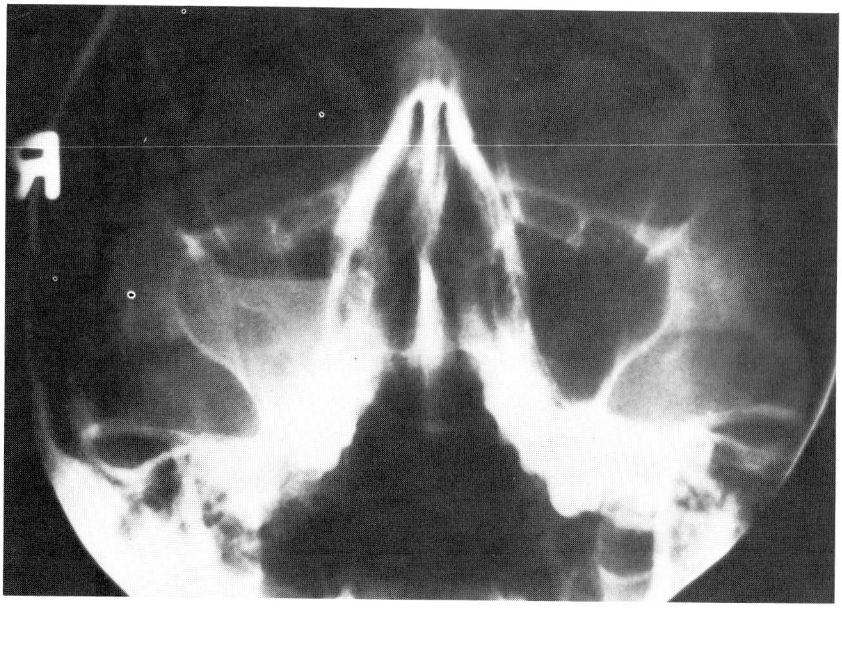

Figure 33–9. Air-fluid level in the right maxillary sinus seen in an upright Water's view of the maxillary sinus.

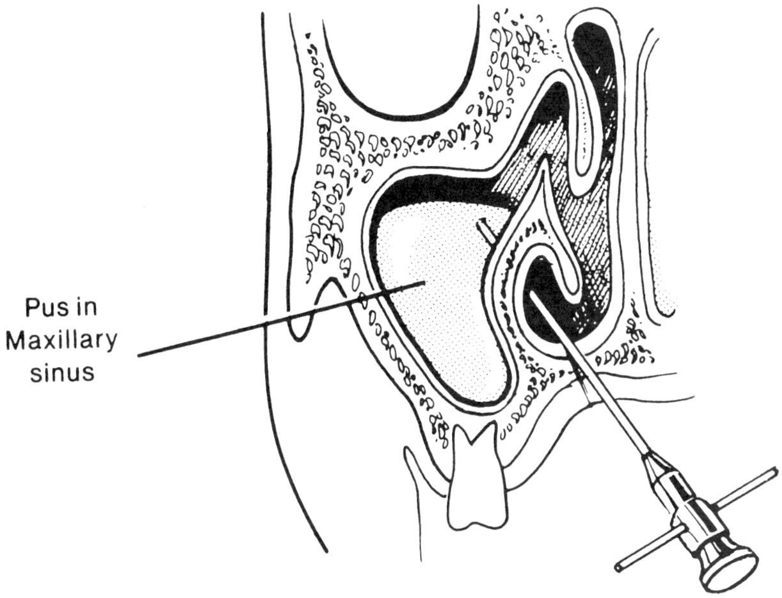

Figure 33–10. Antral irrigation. Purulent secretions in the maxillary sinus can be irrigated by passing a needle through the inferior meatus. *(From Adams GL, Boies LR, Hilger PA (eds): Boies's Fundamentals of Otolaryngology: A Textbook of Ear, Nose, and Throat Diseases, 6th ed. Philadelphia, Saunders, 1989.)*

lary cavity. Aspiration with a syringe will permit removal of purulent material for Gram stain, KOH preparations, and aerobic and anaerobic cultures. An anaerobic infection should be suspected in a chronic infection, dental source, or when purulent foul-smelling material is obtained.

The second antral puncture technique uses cannulation of the natural orifice above the middle meatus. Again, a cocaine topical anesthesia is used, not only for its anesthetic effect but for its vasoconstrictor effect. A specially curve cannula is inserted into the natural ostium, and the sinus is aspirated and culture material obtained.

A third method uses an anterior approach over the canine fossa (Fig. 33–11). Here, injectable local anesthesia (2 percent xylocaine with epinephrine, 1:100,000) is used. By lifting the upper lip, the trocar can be placed directly into the maxillary sinus. The bone is thicker and greater pressure must be applied. This approach can be done using direct visualization, and it can be used in patients with underlying blood dyscrasias. This third technique is preferred because of ease, the ability to directly inject xylocaine with epinephrine, and the ability to apply pressure if bleeding occurs from the site. In the acute phase, aspiration of pus is performed to

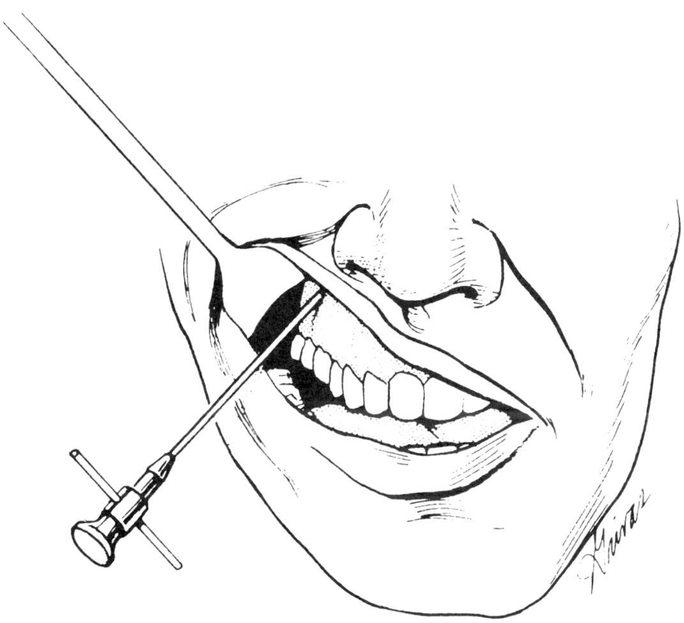

Figure 33–11. Antral irrigation. An alternate method is shown utilizing a needle placed through the canine fossa. *(From Adams GL, Boies LR, Hilger PA (eds): Boies's Fundamentals of Otolaryngology: A Textbook of Ear, Nose, and Throat Diseases, 6th ed. Philadelphia, Saunders, 1989.)*

obtain a Gram stain and culture, but the sinus is not irrigated. The presence of fungal organisms on smear is of concern, but it does not definitely indicate invasive fungal sinusitis. A biopsy procedure in which tissue is obtained is required to demonstrate the invasive nature of fungus and to obtain tissue and specimen for fungal culture.

Chronic Maxillary Sinusitis. Chronic maxillary sinusitis occurs when there is obstruction of the normal drainage through the maxillary ostium. At first, there may be episodes of recurrent acute infections, which resolve with antibiotics and decongestants. Eventually, however, the patient has an almost continuous sinus infection. X-ray studies may no longer reveal a fluid level; instead, an opacified sinus of thickened mucosal lining can be seen. Mucosa thicker than 3 mm is consistent with the diagnosis of chronic sinusitis. Rather than perform repeated antral puncture, with or without repeated lavage of the sinus, a permanent intranasal antrotomy may be established. The preferred technique is to use the endoscopic approach, opening the middle meatal region and enlarging the natural sinus ostia. Further evaluation of the maxillary sinus can be obtained by placing a trocar through the anterior wall of the maxillary sinus sufficiently large to allow passage of a sinus endoscope. Tissue for routine and fungal cultures should be obtained.

The traditional technique for establishing a nasal antral window is a permanent antrostomy beneath the inferior turbinate. It may be considered in patients who have impaired ciliary activity or cystic fibrosis. The mucoperiosteal flap created from the lateral nasal wall is laid into the sinus in an effort to maintain this opening. Even so, at least 30 percent of these openings will close within 1 to 2 years. The incidence of closure is even higher in children.

When the diagnosis of chronic sinusitis is made and a fungal organism is identified, it may be necessary to perform a Caldwell-Luc procedure or radical antrostomy (see Fig. 33–12). In this situation, an opening is created through the anterior wall of the maxillary sinus sufficiently large to allow removal of all diseased maxillary sinus mucoperiosteum (see Fig. 33–13). A large window is then created between the lateral wall of the nose and the

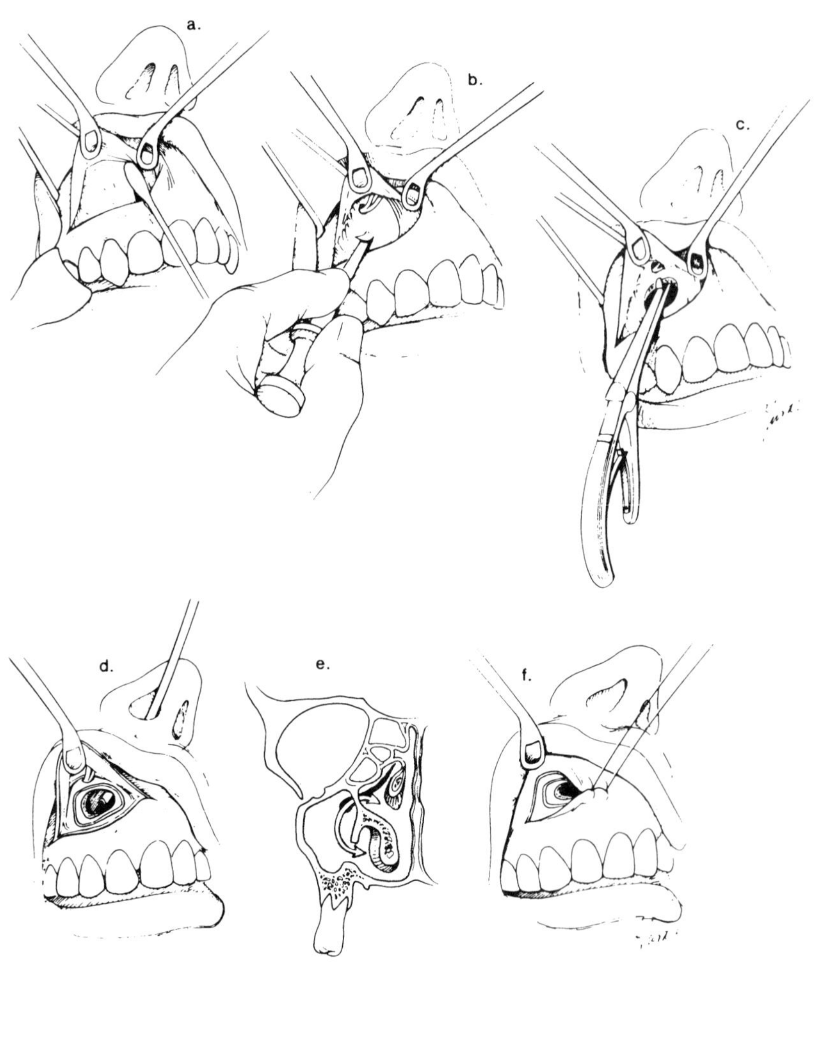

Figure 33–12. Caldwell-Luc procedure. Irreversible maxillary sinus diseases can be treated surgically by **(A)** an incision in the canine fossa and **(B)** removing a portion of the bone of the anterior wall of the sinus. The opening can be enlarged **(C)** with a biting forceps. An opening **(D)** into the inferior meatus similar to a nasoantral window is made to replace the compromised natural ostium. Ventilation and drainage of the sinus can then occur through **(E)** the inferior meatus or the natural ostium if resolution of the sinus disease opens the natural ostium. The operation is completed by **(F)** closure of the oral incision. *(From Adams GL, Boies LR, Hilger PA (eds): Boies's Fundamentals of Otolaryngology: A Textbook of Ear, Nose, and Throat Diseases, 6th ed. Philadelphia, Saunders, 1989.)*

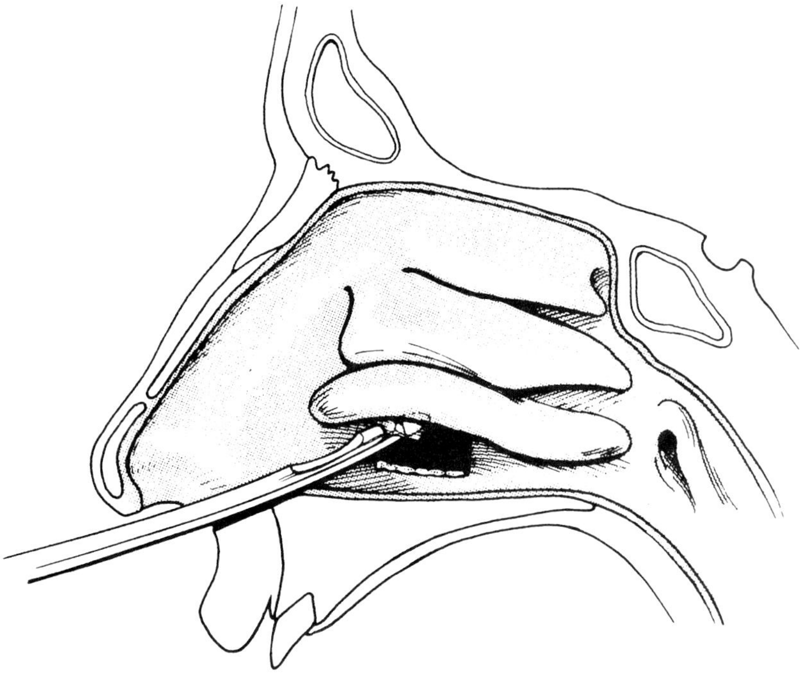

Figure 33–13. Nasoantral window. An opening is made into the maxillary sinus, usually through the inferior meatus as shown. *(From Adams GL, Boies LR, Hilger PA (eds): Boies's Fundamentals of Otolaryngology: A Textbook of Ear, Nose, and Throat Diseases, 6th ed. Philadelphia, Saunders, 1989.)*

medial wall of the maxillary sinus in an effort to allow examination and drainage of the area and make irrigation easier. This procedure is done less often today and is done rarely in children because of the concern over development of the maxillary teeth. A further disadvantage is potential numbness over the cheek due to interference with infraorbital division of the trigeminal nerve.

Acute Frontal Sinusitis. The frontal sinuses are seldom the sites of clinical problems before the teenage years. Acute infection causes fever and severe pain over the sinus and periorbital region. Pressure on the orbital roof will cause exquisite tenderness. Intranasal examination will show congestion, and after application of a topical vasoconstrictor, purulent material can be seen draining from the duct area high in the middle meatus. Infections in this region are more serious than maxillary infections because of the proximity of intracranial structures. In addition, the posterior wall of the frontal sinus is thin and an osteitis of this wall can cause an extradural or subdural abscess.

Hospitalization may be necessary for surveillance. Treatment of acute frontal sinusitis requires systemic antibiotics and topical decongestants. A CT scan is obtained earlier than for other sinus disease because of the propensity to develop intracranial complications. The CT scan may often demonstrate coexisting disease in the ethmoid sinuses and osteomeatal complex area, which may be the cause of the frontal sinusitis. If there is no improvement after 48 hours or if pain and symptoms are becoming worse, an external drainage or trephine procedure is performed (Fig. 33–14). Early intervention is indicated whenever an impending intracranial complication is suspected (Fig. 33–15). An orbital incision is made above the medial canthus just below the brow. The roof of the orbit is exposed, and a drill is used to remove a small amount of bone from the frontal sinus floor. This area is selected because it provides dependent drainage and because the cortical bone in this region is relatively

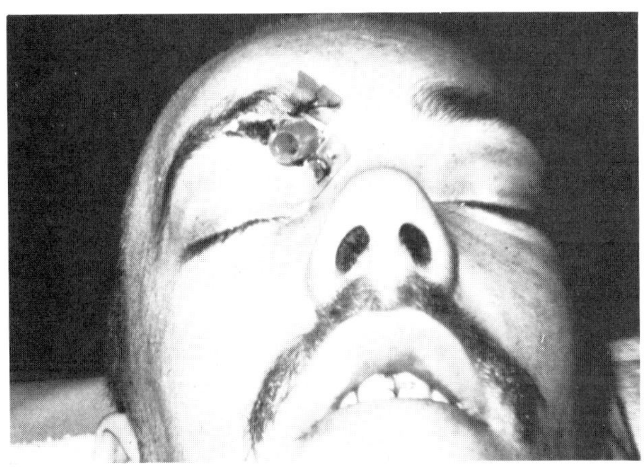

Figure 33–14. Trephine of the frontal sinus for acute suppurative frontal sinusitis. This sinus is entered through the orbital roof. A portion of a No. 24 Silastic chest tube is sewn in place to serve as a drain.

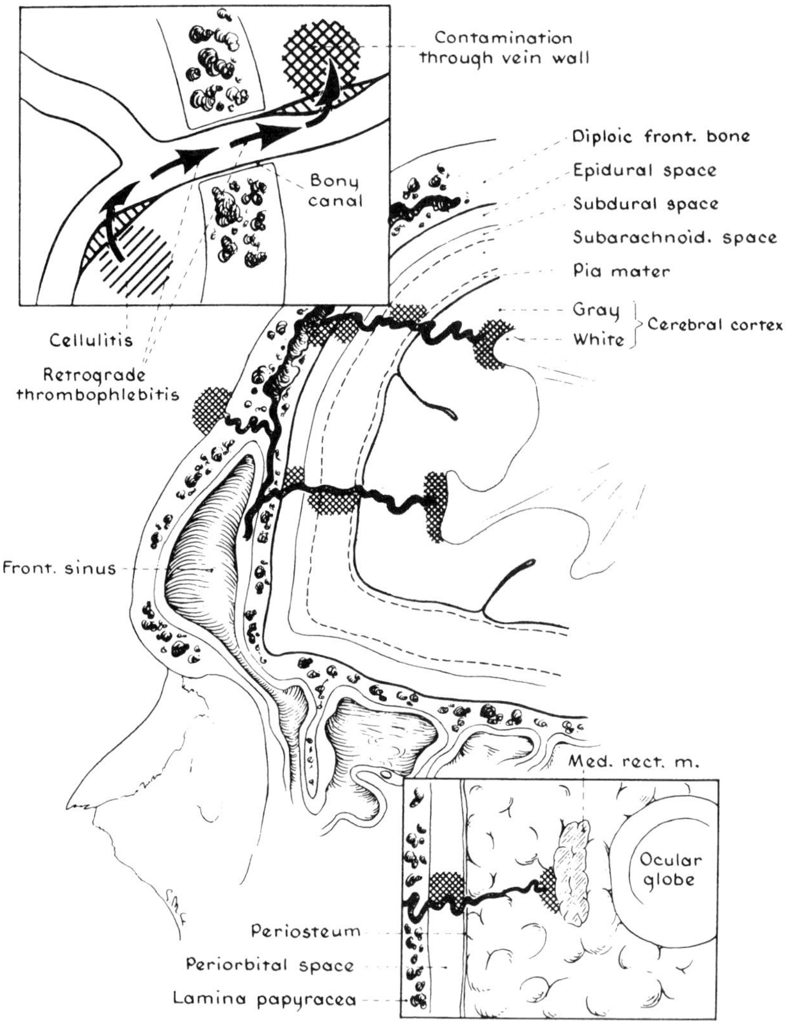

Figure 33–15. Diagrammatic representation of the venous system as the "highway" of extension of suppuration from the sinus mucosa to adjoining structures. Note the depth at which brain abscess develops because of the venous anatomy of the cerebral cortex. *(From Adams GL, Boies LR, Hilger PA (eds): Boies's Fundamentals of Otolaryngology: A Textbook of Ear, Nose, and Throat Diseases, 6th ed. Philadelphia, Saunders, 1989.)*

resistant to osteomyelitis. After obtaining cultures and a Gram stain, a catheter is inserted through the trephine opening and sutured in position. Irrigations with antibiotic solutions or saline are initiated. Once the acute infection has resolved, the nasofrontal duct should again become patent. This can be ascertained by injecting a small amount of dye into the sinus through the tube and checking the nose for the presence of dye. When the duct is patent, the tube is removed. The wound will close spontaneously or with a few sutures or steri-strips. The cosmetic result is acceptable.

Chronic Frontal Sinusitis. Chronic frontal sinusitis may require definitive operation either to establish a drainage path, to replace the occluded nasofrontal duct, or to obliterate the frontal sinus entirely. The Boyden-Sewall procedure establishes a new, larger patent frontal duct, permitting the infection to resolve. Alternatively, since the sinus has little physiologic function, obliteration is a logical alternative. Obliteration requires total removal of all frontal sinus mucosa and plugging the duct through an osteoplastic flap approach.

Ethmoid Sinusitis. The ethmoid sinuses are actually composed of a series of cells (see Fig. 33–16). There are about eight large ethmoid cells, divided into anterior and posterior groups on each side. The anterior group of cells is most closely associated with the anterior portion of the nasal cavity, while the posterior cells extend backward to the region of the sphenoid sinus. They are present at birth, and acute ethmoiditis is most often seen in children or when nasal polyps obstruct the ethmoid ostia. It usually presents as orbital cellulitis. Acute ethmoiditis requires systemic antibiotics and nasal decongestants for treatment.

Chronic ethmoiditis is treated by removing the infected and often polypoid tissue within the ethmoid cells. There are basically three approaches that can be used. The first and perhaps most com-

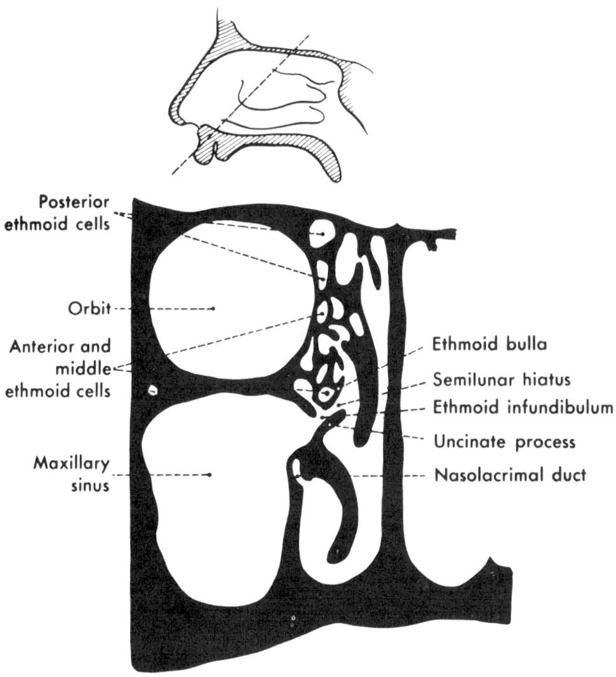

Figure 33–16. The ethmoid air cells, together constituting the ethmoid sinus, are shown in this hypothetical section through the lateral nasal wall. The section represents the slant indicated in the inset. *(From Hollinshead HW (ed): The nose and paranasal sinuses. In: Anatomy for Surgeons, Vol 1, The Head and Neck, 3rd ed. Hagerstown, MD, Harper & Row, 1982, p 235.)*

mon approach is an intranasal ethmoidectomy, which is frequently combined with a nasal polypectomy and can be done under topical anesthesia. Frequently, only the anterior cells can be totally removed with this method. Because of the close association of the ethmoid cells with the optic nerve and the cribriform plate, this technique requires familiarity with the ethmoid anatomy. The roof of the ethmoid cells is higher than the cribriform plate, so that the medial attachment of the middle turbinate is maintained as a landmark to avoid perforating the cribriform plate to prevent a subsequent leak of cerebrospinal fluid. Functional endoscopic sinus surgery (FESS) has become the preferred method for management of both acute and chronic ethmoid disease.

A second approach to the ethmoid cells is the transantral ethmoidectomy. The maxillary sinus is opened via a Caldwell-Luc approach, and the ethmoids are exposed and excised through the medial portion of the maxillary sinus. This approach does not allow access to the more anterior ethmoid cells.

The third approach, external ethmoidectomy (Fig. 33–17), is used for severe or complicated chronic ethmoidal infections. A curvilinear incision is made along the medial canthus and extended along the lateral nasal dorsum. The lacrimal bone, lacrimal sac, and tendon of the superior oblique muscle are identified and preserved. The lamina papyracea of the ethmoid is then perforated and the opening into the ethmoids is enlarged. The anterior ethmoid artery is ligated. Although this approach will leave a scar, it is probably the most effective and safest method of eliminating all chronic diseased tissue in the ethmoid labyrinth.

An external ethmoidectomy is preferred in individuals where the CT scan demonstrates possible

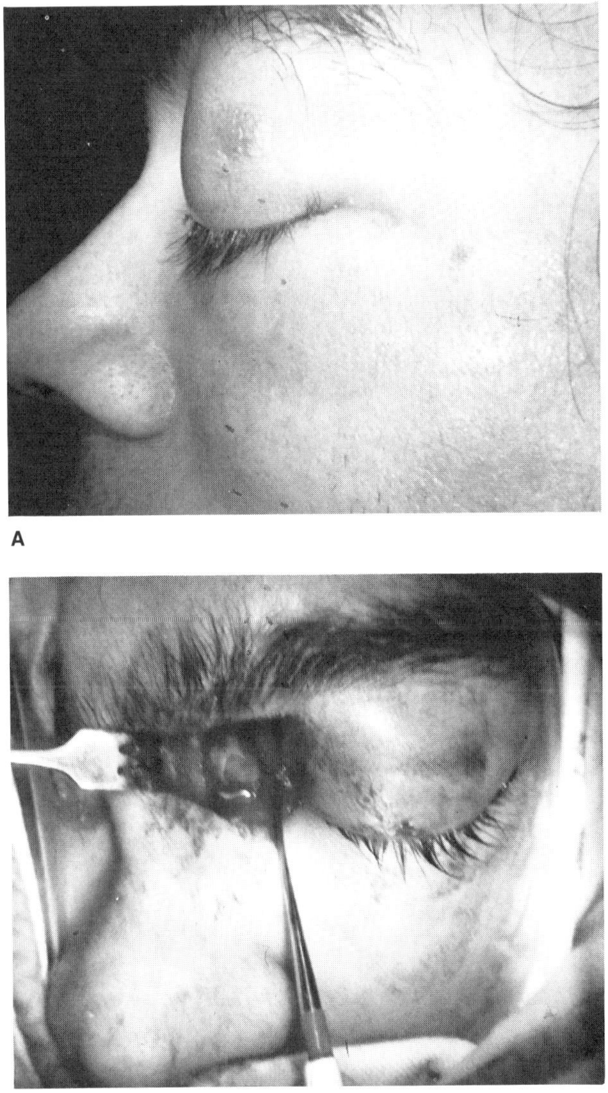

A

B

Figure 33–17. **A.** Acute frontoethmoiditis with extensive edema of the lid. **B.** This patient had rapid deterioration of vision in the left eye. Cavernous sinus thrombosis was suspected but was disproved by venogram. Emergency external ethmoidectomy was performed. Prompt resolution of vision occurred. The responsible organism was *Staphylococcus,* DNase positive.

dehiscence of the lamina papyracea, which divides the contents of the orbit from the ethmoid sinus. In this situation, intranasal ethmoidectomy could result in biopsy or removal of orbital fat with resultant ecchymosis and possible limited extraocular muscle function. For this reason when performing endoscopic sinus surgery, all tissue removed is dropped into a container of saline. Any tissue that remains floating is considered to be orbital fat. Nasal polyps and chronic sinus mucosa will not float.

Sphenoid Sinusitis. The sphenoid sinus is not present at birth and becomes important only in adults. There is close association of the most posterior ethmoid cells to intracranial structures, the optic nerve, ophthalmic division of the fifth nerve, third, fourth, and sixth cranial nerves, and the cavernous sinus. Sphenoid sinusitis is generally associated with infection of all the sinuses. Pain is felt in the midportion of the head or may be referred to the occipital area. Treatment of acute sphenoid infection depends on antibiotics and decongestants. If these modalities are unsuccessful, endoscopic enlargement of the natural ostium allows collection of pus for culture and drainage. Chronic sinusitis may actually require removal of the anterior wall of the sinus, creating a single large cavity opening directly into the posterior nasal cavity and nasopharynx. For complicated cases, the sphenoid sinus is best approached via an external ethmoidectomy because the most posterior ethmoid cells are immediately adjacent to the sphenoid. This protects the orbital contents, optic nerve, and cavernous sinus.

Sinusitis in Children. During the first 2 years of life, the ethmoid sinuses are the only ones that are completely developed and consequently the only ones to become infected. Infection is usually associated with an acute or chronic rhinitis and involves the entire ethmoid labyrinth. A common complication is unilateral or bilateral orbital cellulitis characterized by inflammation and swelling in the periorbital area. Treatment with systemic antibiotics and decongestants is usually sufficient. Surgical drainage is rarely indicated. While viral inflammatory processes may be the inciting cause, secondary bacterial infection follows. The organism responsible is generally of the same group of organisms that causes acute sinusitis in adults. However, in children, *H. influenzae* infection is more frequent.

During the first year of life, the maxillary sinuses are small and only after the second year, when the teeth are developing, do they begin to play a role. Surgical drainage is seldom necessary in children; however, an antral puncture is occasionally required. The Caldwell approach is rarely used in children because the sinus is much smaller and located higher in the maxilla and because the anterior approach threatens the developing teeth. Preferable to repeated antral punctures is placing a catheter into the sinus and taping it to the side of the face. This permits repeated irrigations with either saline or antibiotic solutions.

The frontal sinus develops after 9 years of age and reaches its adult size at approximately 15 years of age. Acute sinusitis in young adults has been associated with swimming and diving. The treatment is similar to that of adults. The technique of endoscopic sinus surgery so successful in adults has been extended to children. Endoscopic removal of polyps, enlarging the natural ostium, and removal of chronically infected anterior ethmoid cells when necessary are performed in children to reduce both ethmoid and maxillary sinus disease.

With recurrent viral rhinitis and sinusitis, the search for the cause of the repeated infections is necessary. Immunologic deficiencies should be considered, but most cases are due to allergy with its attendant nasal polyps, chronic mucoid drainage, and obstruction. When polyps are present in children, the possibility of cystic fibrosis must also be considered, and sweat chloride tests should be performed.

Complications of Sinusitis

Complications of sinusitis occurring with both the acute and chronic forms of the disease can be gradual or sudden in onset. The complications can best be divided into intracranial and extracranial forms.

Extracranial Orbital Complications

Periorbital Cellulitis and Subperiosteal Orbital Abscess. The most common extracranial complications of sinusitis are those that involve the orbit. Extension of infection through the thin lamina papyracea of the ethmoid sinus or from the frontal sinus to the orbit causes first a periorbital cellulitis. When the infection is not controlled, it may advance to form a subperiosteal abscess, accumulating pus between the loosely attached periorbita of the globe and the lamina papyracea. In certain patients, the lamina papyracea is dehiscent. Visual disturbances predominate; ophthalmoplegia of the third nerve leads to diplopia, and increased pressure results in changes in the visual field size and diminished visual acuity. Emergency drainage of the orbit is required along with intravenous antibiotics. An ophthalmologist must measure visual acuity several times a day.

Chandler et al[12] have described the continuum from periorbital cellulitis to intracranial complications such as cavernous sinus thrombosis as a result of paranasal sinus infection. Periorbital cellulitis appears as a redness or inflammation, often bilateral and often in children. There is a high fever, headache, and malaise. It often follows an upper respiratory infection and may occur in individuals with no preceding history of sinus infection. It is by far the most common extracranial complication of sinusitis. Patients who develop complications required a coronal CT scan as well as hospitalization and administration of intravenous antibiotics effective against the same groups of organisms that cause acute sinusitis. Particular care is taken that resistant strains of *H. influenzae* are covered by the antibiotic selection. Vision and extraocular muscle functions are intact at this stage. The majority of infections resolve with antibiotics, but the individual is followed closely every few hours for the development of visual impairment. Failure to show response to antibiotics within 24 to 48 hours, and certainly if there is any worsening of signs, requires repeat of the CT scan to assess for development of a subperiosteal abscess and surgical drainage. An abscess is recognized by CT scan demonstrating inflammation of the periorbita through a dehiscent area in the lamina papyracea. With any of these complications, surgical drainage through an external approach is required. A Penrose drain may be placed for 24 hours and adequate drainage into the nose should be established. Some highly skilled individuals are able to drain this infection through an endoscopic approach.

Orbital Abscess. Extension of the infection through the orbital periosteum into the region posterior to the globe can occur (Fig. 33–18). This space is filled with fat and loose connective tissue. Infection soon leads to fat necrosis. Exophthalmos develops because of increased pressure within the orbit. Increased orbital pressure causes decreased venous drainage and visual loss. The combination of increased venous pressure, inflammation, and possible optic neuritis can lead to blindness.

An orbital abscess can be demonstrated by an orbital axial computed tomography scan. It is essential to differentiate the abscess from a cavernous sinus thrombosis, which may present a clinically similar picture.

The responsible bacterial organisms are *S. pneumoniae* and *S. pyogenes. Hemophilus influenzae* is the most common organism in children. Blood

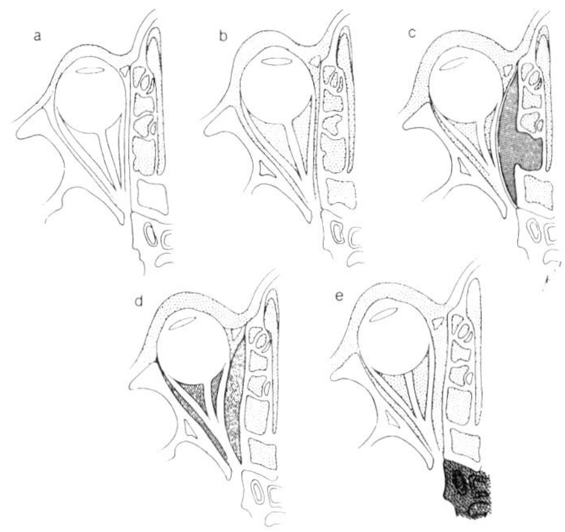

Figure 33–18. Orbital complications of sinus disease. **A.** Ethmoiditis and preseptal celullitis. **B.** Orbital cellulitis. **C.** Subperiosteal abscess. **D.** Orbital abscess. **E.** Cavernous sinus thrombosis. *(From Adams GL, Boies LR, Hilger PA (eds): Boies's Fundamentals of Otolaryngology: A Textbook of Ear, Nose, and Throat Diseases, 6th ed. Philadelphia, Saunders, 1989.)*

cultures may be positive and are more likely than nasal smears to reveal the causative organism. The periorbita should be elevated and the abscess drained under antibiotic coverage. It may be noted at this time that the abscess extends over the roof of the globe yet within the orbit and far more laterally than was recognized. Penrose drains are inserted and gradually advanced daily. Appropriate cultures are obtained. Vision usually returns to normal.

Complications of Frontal Sinusitis

MUCOCELE AND PYOCELE. Complete obstruction of the frontal sinus duct permits development of a cystic lesion, which gradually expands as fluids accumulate within it (see Fig. 33–15). The eye is pushed downward and forward by the enlarging contents of the frontal sinus. The walls of the sinus remain intact but are gradually pushed away over a period of months or years by the enlarging mucocele. The onset has been reported as late as 20 years after trauma to the frontal duct. Infection that develops within the mucocele creates a pyocele. The symptoms of infection, rather than gradual enlargement, predominate. The diagnosis of a frontal sinus mucocele must be considered in evaluation of any patient with a unilateral exophthalmos. Obliteration of the frontal sinus is the best treatment.

FRONTAL BONE OSTEOMYELITIS. Pott's puffy tumor describes a subperiosteal accumulation of pus, which develops from an underlying osteomyelitis of the anterior wall of the frontal sinus. Swelling and edema of the upper eyelid occur, and the eye appears to be pushed downward and forward. The abscess is tender and requires drainage. Usually, a trephine procedure of the frontal sinuses is performed to treat the underlying frontal sinusitis and apparent obstruction of the frontal sinus duct at the same time.

Intracranial Complications of Sinusitis. Symptoms suggesting the development of an intracranial abscess include fever, headache, lethargy, seizure, papilledema, sensory deficit, and cranial nerve paralysis. A CT scan with contrast in actual view is indicated immediately as well as hospitalization for any patient suspected of having intracranial complications.[13,14] Intracranial complications are most often associated with frontal sinusitis and ethmoid sinusitis, but often the patient has a demonstrated pansinusitis, that is, an infection of all sinuses. Frontal lobe abscess and meningitis are the most common intracranial complications.

Epidural Abscess and Meningitis. The intracranial complications of sinusitis occur more as a result of infection in the frontal sinus than the other sinuses. The infection may extend to the meninges directly by osteomyelitis of the posterior wall of the frontal sinus or indirectly by the development of frontal vein phlebitis, extending along the venous drainage and eventually leading to the cavernous or sagittal sinus (see Fig. 33–1). Because veins in this region lack valves, dissemination of the infection by thrombophlebitis is considered a leading cause for development of intracranial complications.

Brain Abscess. When an abscess develops as a complication of sinusitis or mastoiditis, it is usually located directly over the region of the infected sinus or mastoid. Most brain abscesses caused by sinusitis contain anaerobic organisms, particularly anaerobic streptococci, *B. fragilis, Fusobacterium, Veillonella* and other *Bacteroides* species. The most common aerobic organisms are *Staphylococcus aureus* and group A *Streptococcus pyogenes.* Gram-negative aerobes have been identified in infants. At the same time, the cultures from acute and chronic sinusitis demonstrate aerobes—*S. aureus, S. pyogenes, H. influenzae,* and *E. coli.*

Neurosurgical intervention is immediately required. Approaches include both surgical drainage and intravenous antibiotic therapy. The indications for timing and neurosurgical drainage are discussed in Chapter 34. The underlying sinus problem is addressed as previously described.

Cavernous Sinus Thrombosis. The venous drainage from the ethmoid and frontal area extends posteriorly and into a complex of the dural sinuses, referred to as the cavernous sinus (see Fig. 33–1). The veins of the middle one-third of the face have no valves, so the blood can flow in either direction. Through the cavernous sinus pass the optic nerves, the third, fourth, and sixth cranial nerves, and the ophthalmic division of the fifth cranial nerve. Clinical symptoms of a cavernous sinus thrombosis are manifested by loss in visual acuity, headache, fever, meningitis, proptosis, and development of ophthalmoplegia (see Fig. 33–18). Because the cavernous sinuses adjoin each other, the symptoms soon become bilateral, which is the clinical key to the diagnosis. Treatment consists of intravenous penicillin and chloramphenicol. The question of anticoagulation is controversial. Its advantage is possible prevention of an extension of the thrombosis posteriorly to the petrosal veins. The disadvantage of anticoagulation is that thrombi might help to limit the infection to the cavernous sinus. The rarity of this most severe complication with its associated blindness and death has prevented any controlled clinical trials.

Fungal Sinusitis. Fungal infections of the paranasal sinuses present both a chronic indolent infection or an acute fulminant life-threatening infection.[15] This difference is based on the invasiveness of the organism, its tendency toward periocular infiltration, and status of the host.[16]

Fulminant infections are usually due to *Aspergillus* species or the Mucoraceae family (see Chap. 9). Of the five species of *Aspergillus, A. fumigatus* is the most common organism identified in sinus disease. These severe, life-threatening infections occur in immunocompromised patients (individuals with leukemia, diabetes, transplant recipients, especially bone marrow recipients, and individuals receiving chemotherapy).

Sinusitis caused by *Aspergillus* is considered whenever an immunocompromised patient complains of increasing nasal congestion, progressive facial pain, headache, epistaxis, or even change in personality. Physical examination initially reveals only nasal crusts, rhinorrhea, and edema of the skin over the involved sinus. With progressive infection, signs related to the perivascular infiltration with resultant necrosis occur. The turbinate becomes black and black areas develop on the hard palate. Progression leads to orbital complications and chemosis. The CT scan will not show an air-fluid level but indicates only mucosal thickening. This will progress to sinus opacification with areas of hyperattenuation (Fig. 33–19).

Once this diagnosis of invasive aspergillosis is established, immediate aggressive, surgical debridement is mandatory. The invasive nature of the organism must be identified in sinus tissue on hematoxylin-eosin (H&E) stain or preferably methenamine silver stain or periodic acid-Schiff stain. Rapid staining techniques include the white fluorochrome stain and the modified methylene blue stain, which stains the fungal hyphae blue. Presence of a fungus with septate hyphae and dichotomous branching at 45 degrees is strong evidence of invasive *Aspergillus*. There is often not time for further confirming tests and cultures.

In the immunocompromised patient, surgery requires a Caldwell-Luc approach that can be extended to a lateral rhinotomy, medial maxillectomy, or possible septectomy with total ethmoidectomy. Segments of the palate require resection as all involved bone and soft tissue must be excised. Extension into the orbit may require orbital exenteration. Sinus irrigation is begun with amphotericin B (10 to 20 mg/day). The intravenous amphotericin B dose is 0.3 mg/day (total anticipated dose is 2 to 4 g). Rifampin and 5-fluorocytosine may be added. In an effort to obtain better intercellular concentrations, liposomal amphotericin B has become available.[17] These diseases are so rare and survivors so few, that definitive guidelines for therapy cannot be drawn.

Differential diagnosis of *Aspergillus* fungal sinusitis includes *Pseudomonas aeruginosa* sinusitis, which also occurs in immunocompromised patients,[18] noninvasive forms of *Aspergillus,* mucormycosis, and other opportunistic fungi.

Aspergillus is an ubiquitous organism present in soil and water that may be present in the nose and sinuses but may not be invasive. In this situation, it presents with chronic symptoms and oily rhinorrhea. Treatment is still surgical. The sinuses will be filled with thick brown fluid and cheesy material. Removal of all involved mucosa with provision for adequate drainage is all that is necessary. Amphotericin therapy is not indicated.

Rhinocerebral Phycomycosis (Mucormycosis, Zygomycosis). The mucormycoses have been discussed in Chapter 10. This particular form generally begins in the nose and maxillary sinus and has a 50 percent mortality. Most patients are diabetics with ketoacidosis, but cancer patients who are undergoing chemotherapy and debilitated patients with malnutrition are also susceptible. Black crusts, which resemble a recent bloody discharge, initially appear on the turbinates and the nasal

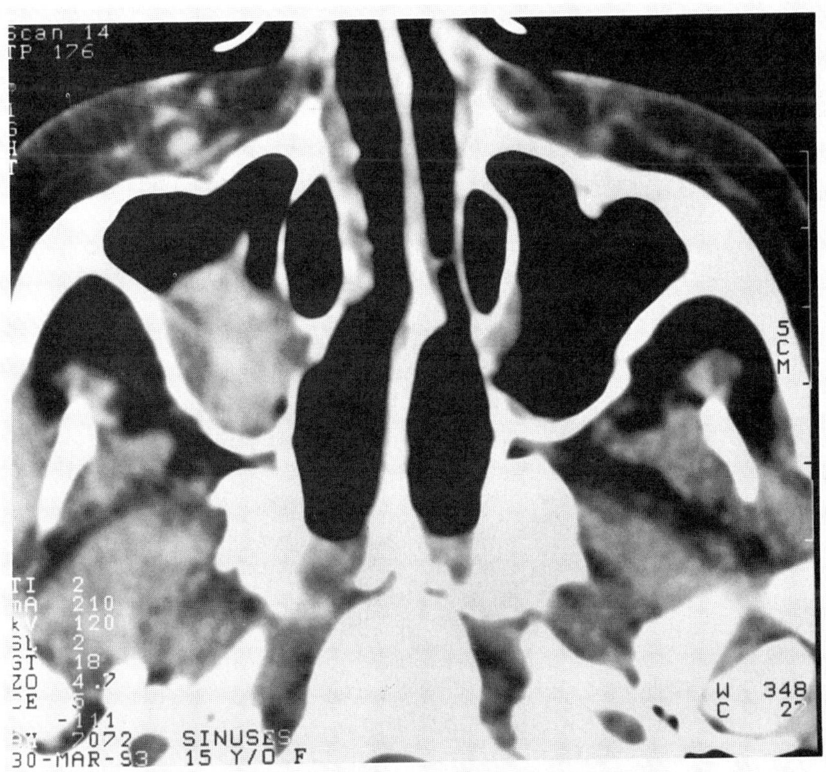

Figure 33–19. Opacification of the right maxillary sinus due to *Aspergillus* infection.

septum. Septal perforation can appear later. An acute maxillary sinusitis develops with facial cellulitis, and the overlying skin of the sinus may become necrotic. The orbit and ethmoid sinus are soon involved, so that proptosis and ophthalmoplegia develop. As the mycotic infection extends directly into this region, blindness ensues with thrombosis of the central retinal artery. Acute infection can extend directly into the brain along venous pathways, for these organisms tend to invade and thrombose vessels. Thus it may extend along the angular vein to the ethmoid vein and then enter the cranium through the superior orbital fissure. Direct extension can occur along the carotid artery or through the cribriform plate. It should be differentiated from cavernous sinus thrombosis by its rapid progression to an orbital apex syndrome and retinal artery occlusion. In cavernous sinus thrombosis, the bacterial infection extends along the vein and the posterior portion of the orbit may be spared, orbital pain is less, and blindness occurs later.

The progression of the disease along the internal carotid artery soon leads to hemiparesis. The fifth and seventh cranial nerves can also be involved. Differential diagnosis includes other problems such as tuberculosis, syphilis, lethal midline granuloma, squamous cell carcinoma, and aspergillosis. The diagnosis is made by biopsy and histologic demonstration of the organism invading the tissue. The presence of the organism in culture is not sufficient to establish its invasive quality.

Treatment requires control of the diabetes, the use of amphotericin B, and surgical debridement of the destroyed tissue. This requires at least a Caldwell-Luc procedure but may require maxillectomy, debridement of the palate, and orbital exenteration.[19] Mortality has been reduced from 80 to 90 percent in the 1950s to 50 percent today. Those patients who survive, however, have severe residual disability. While most fungal infections are caused by these two groups of organisms, there have been reports of severe infections caused by *Bipolaris* species.[20] Infection by this class of organisms is referred to as phycohyphomycosis. It occurs in normally immunocompetent individuals. Treatment requires surgical resection and amphotericin B, but recurrence is possible.

Benign Mucor Sinusitis. While most mucormycosis presents as a fulminating fungal sinus infection, there are now reported cases in which a more benign form of the disease occurs.[21] This infection occurs in individuals with normal immunocompetence and in general good health. It may present with the classic findings of the more common bacterial chronic sinusitis such as headache, nasal obstruction, and a chronic rhinorrhea. A CT scan will demonstrate a mass within the sinus and there may be possible bone destruction. At the time of surgery, tissue specimens will reveal the branching patterns of mucormycosis. There may or may not be invasion of the underlying tissues and usually there is only chronic inflammation of the surrounding mucosa and a large black fungus ball within the sinus. Treatment is the Caldwell-Luc procedure with establishment of a wide drainage window. For sphenoid sinusitis, the anterior wall of the sphenoid sinus is removed. This chronic form of mucormycosis, which may have presented with symptoms of several years duration, requires appropriate surgical management followed by amphotericin B treatment and careful follow-up for persistant disease. The more radical resection reserved for the fulminating type infection is not required.

Facial Cellulitis

Facial cellulitis can develop and spread rapidly over the face from numerous sources. An abscess of the maxillary teeth can cause facial cellulitis and periorbital cellulitis. The symptoms of maxillary sinusitis can include inflammation, swelling, and redness over the cheek.

Cellulitis of the nasal tip is associated with a vestibulitis or inflammation of the vestibule or skin of the nose. There is frequently a history of manipulation of the small vibrissae in the nose. Dryness and cracking of the nasal vestibular skin can contribute to the infection. Cellulitis beginning in the nasal vestibule extends to the tip, causing inflammation. *Staphylococcus aureus* is the pathogen most frequently isolated from the nasal vestibule.

Facial cellulitis can develop after trauma to the region or from manipulation of a furuncle. An abscess can form and can be localized within the cheek. Drainage through a small external incision is preferred. Facial cellulitis should be distinguished from the herpetic lesions seen in varicella-zoster ophthalmicus. In zoster, typical vesiculae develop over the distribution of the sensory divisions of the fifth nerve. Because of possible corneal involvement, ophthalmologic examination is mandatory. The veins in this region permit the infection to extend retrograde toward the cavernous sinus. Thus all areas of cellulitis in the middle one-third of the face are considered potentially serious. Hospitalization and the use of intravenous antibiotics should be considered in every patient with an area of facial or nasal cellulitis. Facial cellulitis in infants and children is often caused by *H. influenzae* and should be treated with ampicillin/clavulenic acid, chloramphenicol, or cefamandole.

INFECTIONS OF THE NECK

Anatomy of the Cervical Fascial Spaces

There are basically four important layers of cervical fascia, which circumferentially divide the neck into compartments (see Fig. 33–2).

The superficial layer is the outermost layer, which completely surrounds the neck like a cylinder. Anteriorly, it lies just beneath the skin and divides to surround the platysma muscle (not shown in Fig. 33–2). The deep cervical fascia is itself divided into a superficial layer and a deep layer. The superficial component of the deep cervical fascia completely encases the neck. Anteriorly, it splits to cover the sternocleidomastoid and trapezius muscles and the parotid and submandibular glands. It is attached firmly to the hyoid bone, which in turn separates it into superior and inferior compartments. Superiorly, it is attached to the lower border of the mandible, and above the parotid it is attached to the zygoma. The deep layer of the deep cervical fascia partially encloses the deep portion of the parotid gland and is attached to the styloid and mastoid processes. A thickening of this layer between the styloid and mandible is called the stylomandibular ligament.

The deepest layer of the deep cervical fascia does not encompass the entire neck; rather it surrounds the muscles associated with the vertebral column, so that it is also called the prevertebral layer. It is important because it extends inferiorly into the mediastinum.

One additional layer of cervical fascia encloses the pharynx, esophagus, larynx, and trachea and thus is referred to as the visceral layer. Anteriorly, where it is closely adherent to the trachea, it is referred to as the pretracheal fascia (see Fig. 33–2). This fascia plane also provides potential access for extension of infection into the mediastinum.

Pharyngomaxillary (Parapharyngeal) Space Infections

The most common potential deep cervical space to become infected is the pharyngomaxillary or parapharyngeal space (see Fig. 33–4). It is a pyramid-shaped space with its base along the base of the skull extending inferiorly to its apex at the hyoid bone. It lies just lateral to the superior constrictor muscle and medial to the parotid gland. It is most often infected as an extension from the pharynx or tonsillar region. Abscesses at the petrous apex, however, can extend into this space. Posteriorly, it is adjacent to the retropharyngeal space, and anteriorly it is closely associated with the submaxillary space (see Fig. 33–4). Infections from the parotid can also extend into the pharyngomaxillary space because the fascia is not complete in the region of the parotid gland. During an infection, the space expands and fills with pus. The close association with the parotid gland causes edema to occur within the gland, and the swelling of the gland then becomes evident in the neck (see Fig. 33–5). Intraoral examination shows the lateral pharyngeal wall in the region of the tonsil to be pushed medially, but the tonsil itself should appear normal.

Because initially a cellulitis infection rather than an abscess is present, intravenous antibiotics are begun. Immediate surgical drainage is indicated if no response to antibiotics is seen or if the infection worsens. The strongest indication for immediate surgical drainage is bleeding from the ear, which suggests that either one of the tributaries of the jugular vein or the branches of the carotid arteries are infected. A CT scan is valuable not only for making this diagnosis but also for demonstrating the extent of involvement.

The external approach to drainage is mandatory. In no case should the abscess be approached intraorally, because a pseudoaneurysm of the carotid artery can rupture and there will be no access to control the hemorrhage. The technique described by Mosher[22] in the 1920s is still the most effective. A transverse incision is made anterior to the sternocleidomastoid muscle two finger-breadths below the margin of the mandible (see Fig. 33–6). The anterior border of the sternocleidomastoid muscle is retracted posteriorly. The fascia overlying the submandibular gland is identified and traced posteriorly and medially, until the space is entered. Next, a finger is passed up and the styloid process palpated. It may be necessary to divide the ligament between the styloid process and the mandible, which is formed by a thickening of the deep cervical fascia. Furthermore, the styloid process itself divides the pharyngeal space into an anterior and posterior compartment. It is almost always the anterior compartment that is infected. This is apparent by the trismus, which develops because of the intimate relationship to the medial pterygoid muscle. The posterior compartment of this space contains primarily the last four cranial nerves, the jugular vein, and the carotid artery. When these structures become infected, the symptoms are usually caused by vascular problems. Soft rubber drains are inserted into the parapharyngeal space and withdrawn gradually over a period of days. Aerobic and anaerobic cultures should be obtained as well as Gram stain. Intravenous antibiotics are continued until the patient's symptoms subside. The wound is approximated and a portion allowed to heal by secondary intention.

Retropharyngeal Space Infections

The retropharyngeal space lies posterior to the superior and middle constrictor muscles of the pharynx (see Fig. 33–4). It is divided into a left and right side by the median raphe. This space is only a potential space. In children under 2 years of age, it contains a few lymph nodes. Suppuration and breakdown of these nodes with adenoid infections in early childhood can result in retropharyngeal space abscesses. In adults, infection of the retropharyngeal space is usually associated with trauma (see Fig. 33–20). This includes instrumentation in the pharynx and particularly traumatic passage of some type of endoscopic equipment. Rarely, tuberculosis will spread into this space from the cervical spine. CT scan and soft tissue lateral x-rays of the neck are very helpful in confirming the diagnosis.

Because the retropharyngeal space can communicate with the prevertebral space, retropharyngeal abscesses can extend into the mediastinum. Immediate drainage with intravenous antibiotic coverage is therefore the best treatment. The preferred approach in children is transpharyngeal with the child in a Rose or head-down position and suction apparatus immediately available to prevent aspiration. A midline incision is then made, the pus is aspirated, and appropriate Gram stains and cultures are obtained (see Fig. 33–21). In certain cases, a chronic lymphadenitis is found in this space rather than a frank abscess. Alternative approaches include a lateral neck incision anterior or posterior to the sternocleidomastoid muscle. The lateral incision is preferred in adults after endoscopic trauma (see Fig. 33–20).

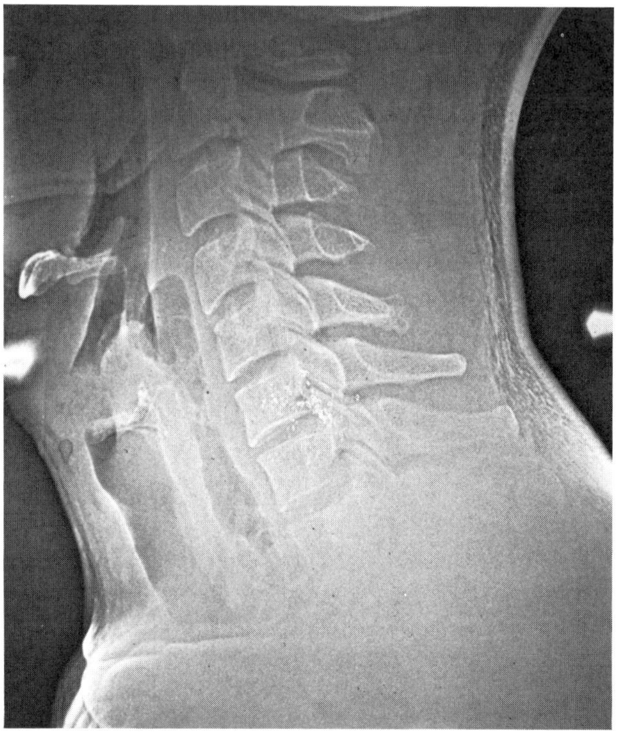

Figure 33–20. Free air in the retropharyngeal space following bullet wound to the neck. A large retropharyngeal space abscess was drained through an external approach.

Suprahyoid Space Infections

The deep cervical fascia attaches firmly to the hyoid bone, thereby confining infection extending from the oral cavity to this suprahyoid space. The anterior belly of the digastric muscle further divides the space into the submental and the submandibular space. Infections from the oral cavity and floor of the mouth, particularly those associated with dental disease or fracture of the mandible, will initially remain between the mucosa of the floor of the mouth and the mylohyoid muscle. As the abscess increases in size and swelling occurs, the tongue is pushed upward and posteriorly so that airway obstruction becomes a threat. Ludwig's angina is a phlegmon of this area characterized by edema rather than suppuration. Incision and release of the tension of the mylohyoid are sometimes necessary to prevent airway obstruction. Tracheostomy should be considered before incision and drainage (Fig. 33–22). The organisms responsible are the aerobic and anaerobic bacteria associated with dental disease and are generally sensitive to penicillin.

Infections in the submandibular space are associated with infections in the gland itself or direct extensions from the floor of the mouth. Another area in which there is a lack of fascial closure and a potential pathway for the rapid spread of infection from the oral cavity to the neck is along the anterior portion of the submandibular gland as it curves around the posterior border of the mylohyoid muscle. Drainage is secured through an incision similar to the one described in Fig. 33–22.

Infections of Masticator Space

The masticator space is formed by the splitting of the superficial layer of the deep cervical fascia to enclose the temporalis, masseter, and medial pterygoid muscles. This space abuts the pharyngomaxillary space, submandibular space, and the parotid

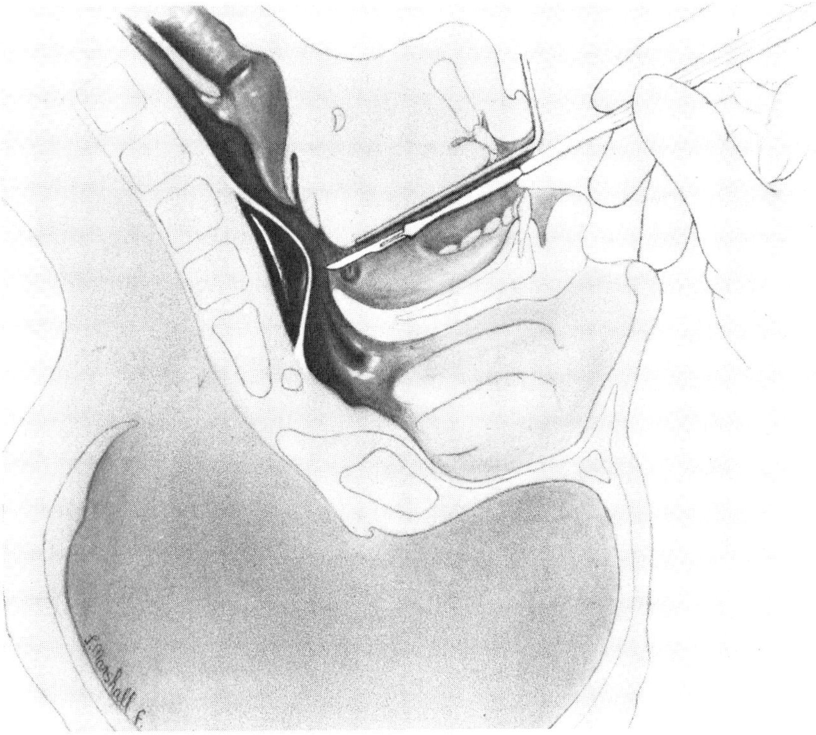

Figure 33–21. Drainage of retropharyngeal space. *(From Adams G: Special examinations in otolaryngology. In Adams G, Boies LR Jr, Paparella MM (eds): Boies's Fundamentals of Otolaryngology, 5th ed. Philadelphia, Saunders, 1978, p 28.)*

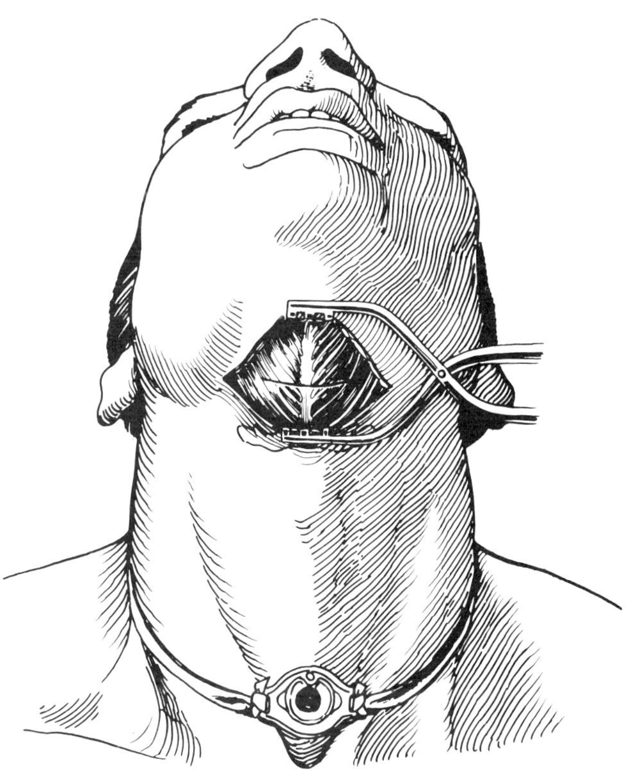

Figure 33–22. Incision and drainage used in Ludwig's angina. The mylohyoid muscle is incised. This patient required a tracheostomy for airway protection before the drainage procedure.

gland. These infections almost always originate in the mandible as a result of dental infection and tend to respond to antibiotic treatment. A 7-day course of antibiotics is generally tried before drainage needs to be considered. When the abscess points into the floor of the mouth or laterally into the gingival sulcus, drainage is indicated. External drainage through the neck is also possible. Should the infection extend upward, a separate incision is made posterolateral to the lateral canthus of the eye above the zygoma. When there is a prolonged indolent infection not responding to the above regimen, actinomycosis or chronic osteomyelitis of the mandible must be considered.

Cervical Necrotizing Fasciitis (Streptococcal Gangrene). Necrotizing fasciitis is a rapidly progressive soft tissue infection of the neck muscles and fascia, which can extend to mediastinitis (see Chap. 31). Although originally described as streptococcal gangrene, it is most often a mixed aerobic-anaerobic bacterial infection consisting of *Staphylococcus aureus,* streptococci, and anaerobic bacteria, which combined have a synergistic effect permitting the infection to spread along the deep layer of the superficial fascia (investing layer). The anaerobic organisms recovered in cervical cases have been normal oral flora plus *Bacteroides* species. A fulminant infection can follow a dental procedure, peritonsillar abscess, relatively minor pharyngitis, or osteoradionecrosis. Patients often have diabetes mellitus, alcoholism, or atherosclerosis.

Initially, the patient is febrile and appears toxic. The skin of the neck is warm and reddened and has firm edema. There is a disproportionate tachycardia. A CT scan will demonstrate definite inflammation of the soft tissue planes of the neck, often bilateral, and with air in the deep tissue. Laboratory tests reveal leukocytosis and anemia. The calcium level is low because of fat necrosis resulting from the binding of calcium by saponification. Initially, this can be confused with cellulitis or erysipelas, but the skin will soon demonstrate areas of necrosis. Initial treatment consists of stabilization of the patient including fluids, blood, and protection of the airway.[22,23] Following are two traditional intravenous antibiotic regimens:

1. Penicillin G, 10 to 20 million units per day, and coverage for *Bacteroides* and *Staphylococcus.*[22]
2. Broad spectrum coverage, including ampicillin, aminoglycosides, and clindamycin (8 g).[24]

The first is only sufficient if group A *S. pyogenes* is the etiologic agent. Polymicrobial flora should be suspected, however. Whichever regimen is initiated, it is changed on the basis of aerobic and anaerobic cultures obtained at the time of surgical debridement. Repeated cultures are necessary.

Upon diagnosis and stabilization of the patient, aggressive surgical intervention is required. Wide skin incisions are made and flaps elevated. Debridement of necrotic muscle, fascia, and fat is necessary. The wound is packed open. If required to protect the airway, a tracheotomy is performed. Failure to see improvement in 24 hours requires a repeat CT scan as it may reveal an area of extension that was not recognized at the initial debridement. Patients often are returned to the operating room two or three times for debridement of necrotic tissue. Mediastinal debridement may be required by midline sternotomy.[25] Additionally, patients will require management of hypotension, hypovolemia, anemia, potential renal failure, and liver and heart failure, as well as respiratory support. Mortality ranges from 10 to 30 percent and is greater in diabetics and elderly people. Hyperbaric oxygen treatment has been advocated but proof is lacking. Often patients are too ill for transfer.

Cervical Adenitis. The lymph nodes of the neck are most easily classified by their relationship to major cervical landmarks: (1) the jugular chain along the jugular vein (subdivided into high, middle, and low); (2) the supraclavicular lymph nodes falling within the triangle formed by the clavicle, anterior sternocleidomastoid muscle, and shoulder; (3) the accessory chain following the accessory nerve and running between the posterior border of the sternocleidomastoid muscle and the anterior margin of the trapezius muscle; (4) the submental nodes in the submental triangle; (5) the submandibular nodes adjacent to the submandibular glands; (6) the parotid nodes next to and within the gland substance; and (7) the retropharyngeal lymph nodes not normally palpable, even when enlarged, which are associated with the posterior lateral aspect of the pharynx.

Tuberculous Cervical Adenitis. The most common form of extrapulmonary tuberculosis is cervical tuberculous lymphadenitis. Any of the mycobacteria discussed in Chapter 9 can be etiologic, but *Mycobacterium tuberculosis* is most common in adults. It has been increasingly common in adults with AIDS. The PPD skin test results are positive. Patients present with solitary, enlarged nontender lymph nodes containing caseating granulomas. After excluding the diagnosis of regional or systemic malignancy, the node should be either excised or have a fine-needle aspiration (FNA). A nonconclusive FNA necessitates a biopsy. The diagnosis is a histologic one, and incisional biopsy may induce a continuously draining fistulous tract. Antituberculosis therapy is described in Chapter 28. It is not known why some individuals develop extrapulmonary tuberculosis. An increased incidence of tuberculosis is reported in individuals with AIDS.

An abscess with caseating granulomas can occur in children caused by atypical mycobacteria. Cervical lymphadenitis can be caused by *M. avium-intracellulare, M. midcrotulaveum,* or *M. scrofulaceum.* Excision of the infected node is usually adequate therapy, and chemotherapy is not required (see Chaps. 9 and 28).

Cat Scratch Disease (Benign Inoculation Lymphoreticulosis). This form of cervical adenitis is diagnosed by history including contact with a cat, and/or regional adenopathy, a site of inoculation, and a positive skin test. It is most likely caused by an unclassified pleomorphic gram-negative bacillus (cat scratch bacillus). Biopsy is not necessary for treatment, but it is necessary to distinguish this from other causes of cervical adenopathy, and excision may be required to eliminate persistent nodes. In one-fourth of the patients, purulent drainage will occur from the node but cultures are usually sterile. This disease is associated with development of acute encephalopathy with neurologic complications similar to those seen in Lyme disease, herpes simplex, and Rocky Mountain spotted fever.[26] The value of antibiotic treatment is not fully documented, but patients have been reported to respond to IV gentamicin sulfate 5 to 7 mg/kg/day. The organism is also sensitive to erythromycin, doxycycline, and many other drugs.

Toxoplasmosis. Cervical lymphadenopathy is the most frequent manifestation of acquired toxoplasmosis. The responsible organism, *Toxoplasma gondii,* is an intracellular parasite in which the final host is the cat. Humans most likely become infected by ingestion of the oocysts after cleaning the litter box of their pet cats and not washing their hands thoroughly afterward. Patients presenting with the cervical form may complain of fatigue, low-grade fever, and muscle weakness. The disease usually runs a benign course with enlarged, mildly tender cervical lymph nodes as the major complaint. However, in extreme cases, the patient becomes acutely ill and can develop splenomegaly, loss of visual acuity, and neurologic symptoms. Diagnosis is made by history of exposure and by indirect fluorescent antibody test. A titer of greater than 1:1024 is considered evidence of recent exposure. Biopsy becomes necessary to distinguish this disease from the similar clinical findings in lymphoma. Histologic examination of the lymph nodes shows a well-preserved node structure with large follicles, which is suggestive, rather than diagnostic, of the disease.

Treatment is unnecessary when cervical lymphadenopathy is the only manifestation of the disease and the fluorescent antibody titer level continues to fall. In the unusual acute form with abdominal and neurologic manifestations, sulfonamide and pyrimethamine are used.

Cervical-Facial Actinomycosis. Actinomycosis is discussed in Chapter 6. The most common presentation of this disease is cervical-facial actinomycosis, or lumpy jaw. This infection usually appears at the angle of the mandible but has also been seen over the lateral part of the neck or even in the midline. The thyroid, deep cervical tissues, and maxillary sinus can all be affected. Acute, painful swelling or swelling and multiple draining fistulas can indicate the infection. Culture can be obtained by biopsy or by direct aspiration of the mass. Yellow particles (sulfur granules), which are actually aggregated bacteria, can sometimes be identified on the dressing. When an abscess suspected of harboring actinomyces is excised, portions should be submitted to both the microbiology and pathology laboratories for evaluation. Gram stains and acid-fast stains should make the diagnosis, since cultures may take 2 weeks for identification.

Actinomycosis responds readily to penicillin (2 to 20 million units per day, intravenous for 2 weeks, followed by oral therapy for 2 months). Tetracycline, clindamycin, and cephalosporins have been used in penicillin-sensitive persons.

Infected Embryologic Deformities

There are three distinct embryologic abnormalities that can present with infection in the neck: (1) cystic hygroma (or lymphangioma), (2) pharyngeal and branchial cleft cysts and fistulas, and (3) thyroglossal duct cysts.

Cystic Hygroma. This diffuse, cystic tumor mass is usually evident within the first 2 years of life. It commonly involves the lower aspects of the neck but can appear anywhere in the cervical region. It is probably an abnormal development of lymph vessels from the jugular lymphatic sacs. Sudden enlargement by infection or hemorrhage into a lymphangioma can cause obstruction of the upper airway. During an acute inflammation, it is better to initially treat the patient with broad spectrum antibiotics until there is resolution of the acute process. Total excision should then be performed to prevent recurrence or further enlargement. The first procedure should be as complete as possible, since all subsequent procedures are more difficult, less likely to remove all lymphangiomatous elements, and more likely to cause damage to underlying cervical structures.

Pharyngeal Cleft Cysts. A pharyngeal cleft cyst can develop from the first, second, or third pharyngeal clefts; the second is most common. During development, both second and third cleft cysts actually develop from the sinus of Hiss. They usually present in childhood as fistulas or masses just posterior to the angle of the mandible along the anterior border of the sternocleidomastoid muscle. Second pharyngeal cleft cysts have a tract leading beneath the digastric muscle above the hypoglossal nerve between the internal and external carotid arteries to the region of the posterior tonsillar pillar. Tracts from the first pharyngeal cleft pass either medial or lateral to the facial nerve and enter the anterior floor of the external ear canal at the junction of the bony and cartilaginous canals. The mass can fluctuate in size, and enlargement can be associated with upper respiratory infection. Acute inflammation should be treated with a broad spectrum antibiotic before resection. The diagnosis can be confirmed and the pathway of the fistulous tract outlined by injection of a radiopaque dye. Treatment is resection. A cyst lying low in the neck may require two transverse or horizontal incisions, which heal with superior cosmetic results, compared to an incision along the anterior border of the sternocleidomastoid muscle. The entire tract should be excised to prevent recurrence. If there is an opening into the pharynx, it should be oversewn, but sometimes the tract is atrophic and does not reach the pharynx.

Thyroglossal Duct Cysts. The thyroid gland originates from the foramen cecum of the tongue and descends through the body of the hyoid bone into the anterior part of the neck. Any residual secretory lining may give rise to a thyroglossal duct cyst, which presents as a midline cystic structure. It can cause respiratory obstruction or a fistula only if infected. The preferred operation (the Sistrunk procedure) removes the cyst and its tract to the base of the tongue including the middle one-third of the hyoid bone. Whenever possible, the acute infection is treated with antibiotics so that surgery can be performed in a quiescent period. Needle aspirations can be useful to help in antibiotic selection.

INFECTIONS OF THE EAR

Infections of the External Ear

Acute External Otitis. Bacterial and fungal infections of the external ear and auricle are common, particularly in summer when external otitis is sometimes called swimmer's ear. Acute external otitis is usually caused by *P. aeruginosa, S. aureus,* or *E. coli,* and the major predisposing factor is persistent moisture from any cause. A low-grade infection ensues and is aggravated by the patient's efforts to scratch or clear the canal. The auricle can become red and tender, and the tenderness can extend into the neck. In advanced cases there is preauricular and occipital adenopathy. Treatment requires cleaning the debris from the canal, insertion of a cotton wick into the canal to enable the medication to penetrate, and the administration of drops into the wick. There are two common types of eardrops available. One type includes topical antibiotics, such as neomycin or colistin, and polymyxin B, combined with a topical steroid. A second contains an acetic acid preparation combined with a steroid in an effort to diminish bacterial growth by lowering the pH of the canal skin.

Chronic External Otitis. This is a superficial infection superimposed on an underlying dermatitis (eczema, psoriasis) and aggravated by the patient's scratching. In long-standing infections, *Aspergillus* and *Candida* superinfection can occur.

Malignant External Otitis. A particular severe form of external otitis caused by *P. aeruginosa* was initially described by Chandler.[27] He noted that external otitis was not limited to the canal in certain elderly diabetic patients but included the surrounding area. Intravenous antibiotics are required because the usual treatment is not effective in these patients. Two regimens include carbenicillin or ticarcillin combined with gentamicin or tobramycin (the two antibiotics should not be mixed) or, most recently, ceftazidine, 2 g every 8 hours (a third-generation cephalosporin effective against *Pseudomonas*). This latter treatment has the advantage of no ototoxicity in patients who may already be hearing impaired.[28,29] Intravenous administration is continued for 2 to 5 weeks. Ciprofloxacin can be substituted in patients who respond well after 2 weeks, but in all cases antibiotics are continued for at least 5 weeks.[30] Debridement of the chronic osteomyelitis in the mastoid and canal may also be necessary, and the surrounding soft tissue beneath the temporal bone may have to be excised in advanced cases. Debridement is never undertaken without prior high-dose combination antibiotic therapy. The advent of current antibiotic regimens has changed this disease from primary surgical debridement to primary medical management.[29–31] When caused by *P. aeruginosa,* the disease has been known to spread along the bony planes of the skull base extend to the contralateral side.

Perichondritis of the Ear. In certain cases, external otitis will extend into the perichondrium of the pinna. The auricle becomes inflamed, swollen, and tender. If the pinna takes on a leathery characteristic, systemic antibiotic treatment is needed in addition to local treatment. The responsible organism is usually *Pseudomonas* and less commonly *Staphylococcus.* This perichondritis can become an actual chondritis. When the blood supply of the perichondrium is interrupted, destruction of the cartilage ensues and resection of cartilage may be needed. Stroud[32] recommends resection of the overlying skin as well as the cartilage.

Various methods have been developed to save as much cartilage as possible and thereby preserve the cosmetic appearance of the auricle (see Fig.

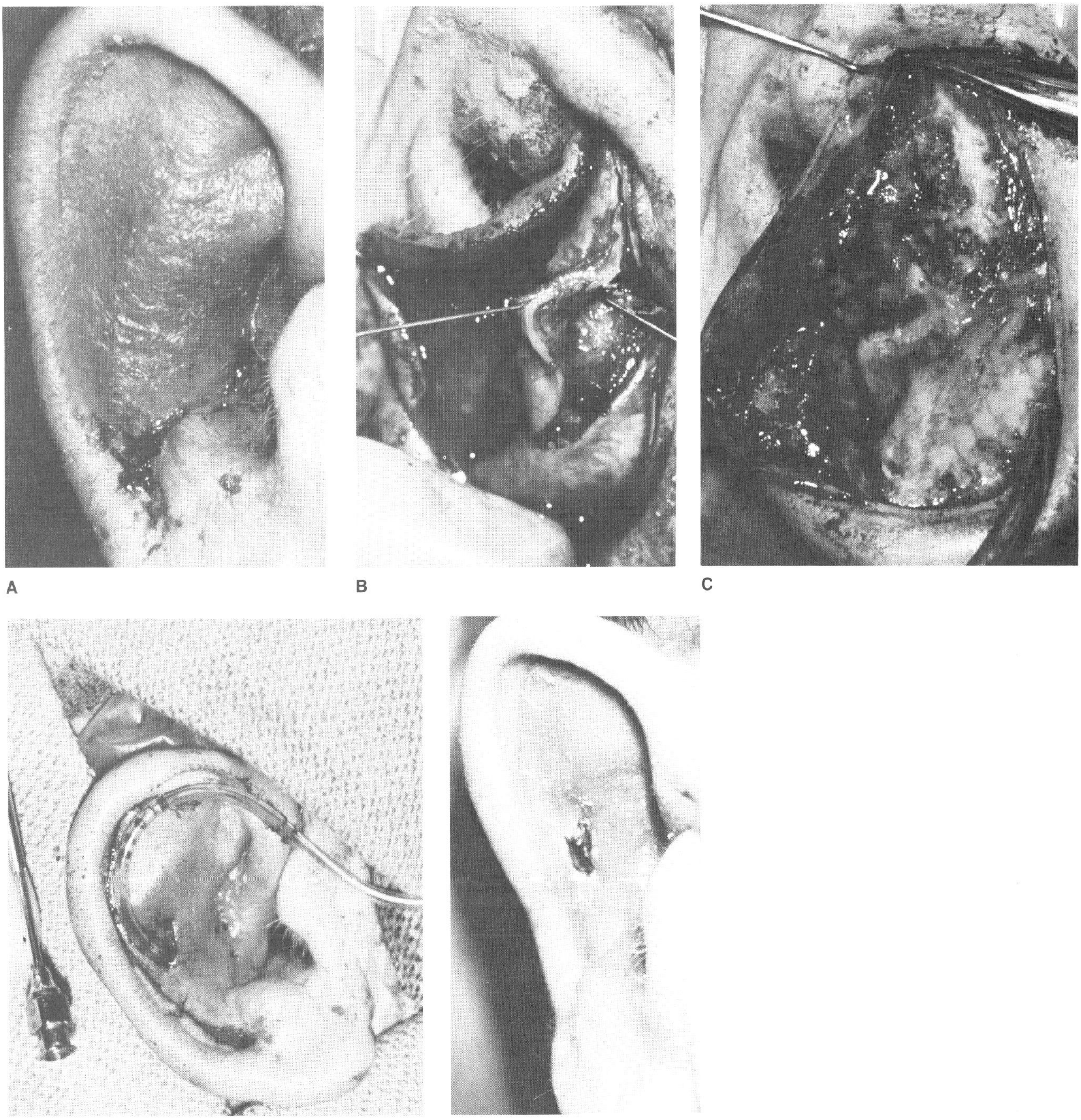

Figure 33–23. **A.** Postoperative acute chondritis of the auricle. **B.** Incision and exposure of infected cartilage. **C.** Removal of all involved cartilage. **D.** Catheter irrigation postoperatively. **E.** Thirteen days after removal of cartilage.

33–23A–E). These methods include debridement of the underlying cartilage and placement of tubes or drains through the auricle, with frequent irrigations with acetic acid or gentamicin solutions. A deformed auricle and a prolonged course of treatment are to be expected.

Viral Infections of the External Ear

Bullous Myringitis. Certain viral infections have a propensity for the external canal, pinna, or tympanic membrane. Bullous myringitis is a viral infection of the tympanic membrane. Because it is preceded by an upper respiratory viral infection and has occasionally been associated with pneumonia, influenza A virus has been incriminated but not definitely established as a cause. The bacterium *Mycoplasma* has also been implicated. Large, painful blebs form on the tympanic membrane and skin of the ear canal. Although some authors have advocated the use of erythromycin, the disease resolves spontaneously in 5 to 7 days. There are usually no adverse long-lasting effects, although some patients have developed sensorineural hearing loss. Secondary bacterial otitis media can develop, requiring systemic antibiotics.

Varicella-Zoster Otitis. The varicella-zoster virus can cause painful vesicles over the distribution of the sensory division of the seventh nerve around the pinna and external canal. The sensory fibers of the seventh nerve supply the posterior superior portion of the external canal and a small area around the conchal region of the auricle. Because the herpetic lesions can occur diffusely over the auricle and the mastoid area, some of the other sensory fibers, such as the second and third cervical divisions of the fifth cranial nerve, must sometimes be affected. Infection of the motor division of the seventh nerve can lead to facial paralysis. The complex of pain, facial palsy, and hearing loss was first described in 1907 by Ramsay Hunt, and the syndrome bears his name. Persistent facial paralysis associated with denervation of the facial muscles has led several authors to advocate immediate facial nerve decompression. Since it is a viral illness, others feel that return of function can be expected. Decompression of the seventh nerve all the way to the internal auditory meatus has been recommended because the viral infection probably infects primarily the seventh nerve medial to the geniculate ganglion. Clinically, it is manifested by decreased tearing on the side of the infection, caused by involvement of the superior petrosal nerve, which supplies the lacrimal glands. Failure of return of function after 4 weeks and evidence on electromyographic or ENOG stimulation of nerve degeneration are indications for decompression of the nerve. Decompression requires microscopic removal of surrounding bone to permit the nerve to swell freely, because its blood supply is diminished by the compression within a confined bony canal. In a few patients with Ramsay Hunt syndrome, there is also involvement of the eighth nerve with decreased sensorineural hearing. The morbidity of such an infection is further aggravated by prolonged neuralgic pain over the distribution of the occipital division of the fifth and seventh nerves. Acute pain can be relieved by analgesics, antivirals, (acyclovir), and systemic steroids. Topical steroids applied to the auricle also provide some relief. Steroids are contraindicated if there is coexisting herpetic involvement of the ophthalmic nerve. Acyclovir if started early might be effective, but oral administration is distinctly inferior to intravenous therapy for most forms of zoster.

Infections of the Middle Ear and Mastoid

Acute Suppurative Otitis Media. Otitis media is most often seen in preschool-age children with eustachian tube dysfunction secondary to infections in the oropharynx, nasopharynx, sinuses, and nose. The infection can initially be caused by a virus, but bacterial infection supervenes, especially with repeated infections. The causative organisms are the pneumococcus, group A *S. pyogenes, B. catarrhalis, S. aureus,* and, in children under 6 years of age, *H. influenzae.* The patient develops fever and otalgia. The tympanic membrane is red and inflamed, and it bulges. Myringotomy was commonly practiced in the past to relieve the pressure and is sometimes still indicated to relieve pain or to obtain an aspirate for culture. Antibiotic treatment usually suffices, however.

Complications of Suppurative Otitis Media

FACIAL NERVE PARALYSIS. When facial nerve paralysis is a complication of acute suppurative otitis media, a wide myringotomy (smile) incision is needed. Cultures should be obtained and intravenous antibiotics started. The facial paralysis usually resolves within 1 to 2 weeks. However, if the paralysis persists or denervation is suspected, a mastoidectomy is urgently indicated. The osteitic bone around the facial nerve is removed only if it is obviously infected. Otherwise, a mastoidectomy with preservation of the posterior canal wall should suffice. The operation also provides an opportunity to rule out any other mastoid or middle ear pathologic condition responsible for paralysis.

ACUTE MASTOIDITIS. Before the advent of penicillin, acute suppurative otitis media led to acute suppurative mastoiditis (see Fig. 33–24). This disease is uncommon today but sometimes occurs in a patient who is undergoing cancer chemotherapy. Myringotomy should be performed with the use of systemic antibiotics. Mastoid decompression is indicated only in cases that do not respond to this conservative regimen, if the pain becomes too severe, or if there is a threat of intracranial complications.

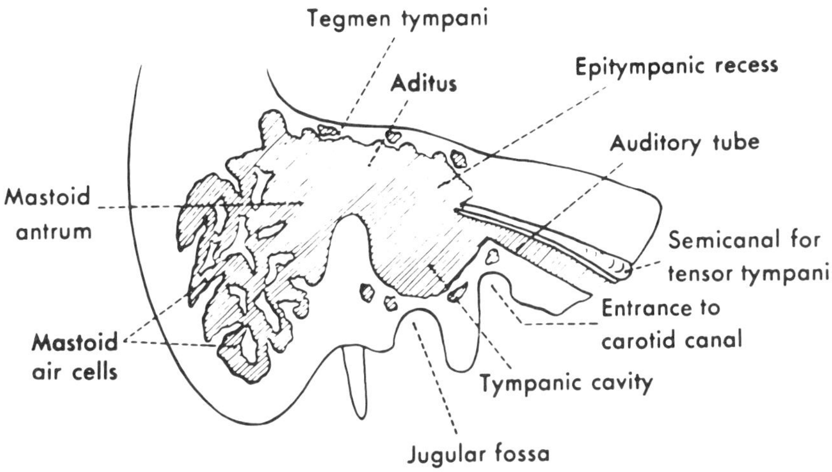

Figure 33–24. Diagram of the middle ear cavity and its connecting air spaces, in a sagittal section. *(From Hollinshead HW (ed): The ear. In: Anatomy for Surgeons. Volume 1, The Head and Neck, 3rd ed. Hagerstown, MD, Harper & Row, 1982, p 167.)*

Acute mastoiditis usually occurs in young children. The onset may be sudden in a well-pneumatized temporal bone. The patient has a fever and appears acutely ill. The tympanic membrane loses the usual landmarks. There is bulging of the posterior and superior canal wall. Subperiosteal swelling, redness, and tenderness to firm palpation can develop in the postauricular area.

Blood cultures and cultures from a myringotomy will identify the organism, most often *H. influenzae* and *S. pneumoniae*. Failure to show improvement after 4 days of antibiotic therapy is sufficient indication for an emergency mastoidectomy (Fig. 33–25).

Development of a subperiosteal abscess is a sign of coalescent mastoiditis. Should the abscess protrude anteriorly, it becomes evident at the zygoma adjacent to the temporalis muscle. Pus that ruptures medial to the cells of the mastoid tip into the digastric groove is called Bezold's abscess. This abscess can extend directly into the retropharyngeal space.

The presence of any of these abscesses is an indication for immediate complete mastoidectomy. It is more difficult to determine whether operation is necessary in "masked" mastoiditis. Antibiotic therapy may be sufficient to eliminate the classic signs of mastoiditis such as pain, fever, and tenderness over the mastoid. However, there may be a recurrence after the antibiotics have been discontinued. Recurrence of pain and drainage along with CT evidence of mastoiditis requires a complete mastoidectomy.

Chronic Otitis Media

Chronic Serous Otitis Media. Far more common in the otologist's practice than the acute form of otitis media are the various forms of chronic otitis media: purulent otitis media, serous otitis media, and mucoid otitis media. Otitis media is the most common cause of hearing loss in school-age children; other symptoms include fullness and pressure in the ear. Sometimes, the onset is gradual, and the teacher is the first to notice hearing loss in a child who is not attentive in class.

Chronic diseases of the middle ear and mastoid are directly related to obstruction of the eustachian (auditory) tube (see Fig. 33–24), which normally opens during swallowing, yawning, or sneezing so that the atmospheric pressure remains equal on both sides of the tympanic membrane. Inflamma-

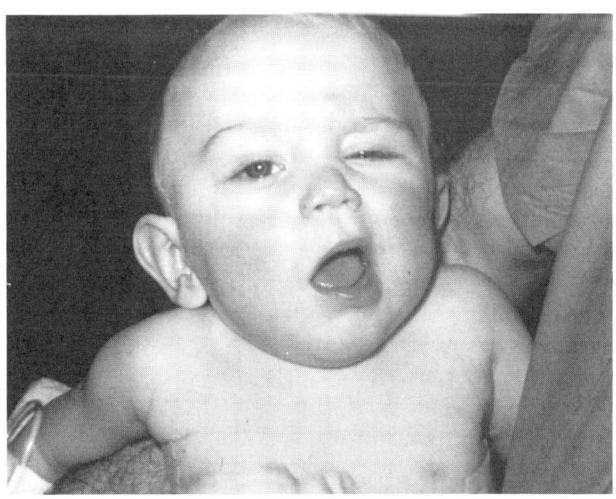

Figure 33–25. Acute suppurative mastoiditis presenting with facial nerve paralysis in a 2-year-old child. Initially, a wide myringotomy was performed with high-dose intravenous antibiotics. Failure to improve in 3 days required an acute mastoidectomy. Granulation tissue and mastoiditis were encountered. The facial nerve was not decompressed. Total recovery of facial nerve function required 6 months.

tion, whether of bacterial, viral, or allergic origin, can induce edema and obstruction of the tube. Air in the mastoid and middle ear is then absorbed, a negative pressure is established within the middle ear cleft, and an effusion forms within the middle ear and mastoid. Return of normal eustachian tube function and patency is essential in the treatment of both acute and chronic diseases of the middle ear and mastoid, although temporary relief can be achieved by myringotomy.

There are many causes of eustachian tube obstruction: allergy, sinusitis, and chronic nasopharyngitis, as well as hypertrophied adenoids. Children with a cleft palate deformity have a much higher incidence of tubal dysfunction and serous otitis media. In adults, there may be other underlying causes, such as tubal blockage caused by a rapid airplane descent, a nasopharyngeal tumor, or previous irradiation to the area. Chronic serous otitis media may also occur after resection of the maxillary and ethmoid sinuses or palate for cancer.

In children with serous otitis media, the middle ear fluid is an exudate not a transudate, and the appearance does not help determine whether bacteria are present. The clear, thin fluid may be just as likely to harbor bacteria as the thick mucoid variety. Changes in the middle ear mucosa also occur in chronic serous otitis media. There are metaplastic changes from low cuboidal epithelium to columnar epithelium with an increased number of goblet cells. In long-standing serous otitis media, fibrosis and diffuse adhesions can occur. In adults, the fluid will not contain pathogenic organisms.

Adenoidectomy is recommended for long-standing cases of chronic otitis media when a conservative medical approach has failed. Medical therapy usually involves systemic and nasal decongestants, and antibiotics when there is a chronic, underlying infection. Adults with serous otitis media require a complete evaluation including examination of the sinuses and nasopharynx.

The most frequently used procedure to keep the pressure across the tympanic membrane equal is myringotomy with insertion of a ventilating tube shaped like a collar button. With relief of the negative pressure in the middle ear, the drumhead returns to its normal position and the fluid resolves. The tube is placed in the anteroinferior or posteroinferior quadrant of the tympanic membrane. It remains in place 3 to 9 months. Myringotomy with tube insertion in children is considered after failure to respond to 2 to 3 months of medical management. Preferred antibiotics include amoxicillin, cefaclor, or a combination of erythromycin ethylsuccinate with sulfisoxazole. A study by Gates et al[33] demonstrates an improved response to treatment when adenoidectomy is performed at the same time as myringotomy. This was true regardless of size of the adenoid bed and suggests that adenoid tissue is more a repository for pathogenic organisms than a cause of mechanical obstruction.

Chronic Otomastoiditis. While acute suppurative otomastoiditis is no longer a common disease, various forms of chronic otomastoiditis are more prevalent today than in the preantibiotic era. Chronic otomastoiditis is generally characterized by a perforated tympanic membrane and intermittent drainage. The aural discharge may occur after upper respiratory infections or after the ear canal has accidently been immersed in water. The organisms associated with this chronic form of disease are entirely different from those seen in the acute phase. They are generally species of *Staphylococcus, P. aeruginosa, Proteus,* and other gram-negative organisms. In addition, anaerobic species including *B. melaninogenicus, B. fragilis,* and peptostreptococci have been found. Treatment of the recurring episodes includes systemic antibiotics and eardrops. Drops containing a combination of neomycin, colistin, or polymyxin B are most often used. X-rays of the mastoid are necessary to determine the extent of the destruction in the bone.

Perforations of the tympanic membrane have been categorized into safe and unsafe. A safe perforation refers to one in the midportion of the tympanic membrane. It usually occurs in the anteroinferior or posteroinferior quadrant. Drainage is associated with an upper respiratory infection that responds to antibiotics and stops after the acute stage is resolved. Unsafe perforations occur in the posterosuperior quadrant of the tympanic membrane and along the margin. Such perforations are usually associated with underlying mastoid disease, especially cholesteatoma. Cholesteatoma is a collection of encapsulated keratinizing squamous epithelium, somewhat like a dermoid cyst that, when entrapped in bone, expands and causes gradual destruction of the surrounding structures. The ossicles, the horizontal semicircular canal, and the facial nerve can be destroyed by a cholesteatoma. Eventually, such destruction can include the tegmen tympani (see Fig. 33–24) and tegmen mastoideum. Such exposure of the dura leads to extracranial and intracranial complications.

The concept of "safe and unsafe" perforations has been challenged. Elevation of the tympanic membrane in a so-called safe perforation has on occasion demonstrated pathologic findings such as granulation tissue mastoiditis. The mastoid cells become filled with chronically infected granulation tissue that is as destructive as cholesteatoma. Topical antibiotic drops with steroids and systemic antibiotics are used to temporarily stop the infection. When these medications are discontinued, drainage and suppuration can recur and surgery becomes necessary.

A third form of chronic otitis media and mastoiditis is known as cholesterin granuloma. This infection is related to chronic granulation tissue mastoiditis and is the result of a breakdown product of cholesterol crystals. CT scanning and MRI have permitted a better assessment of mastoid and middle ear status. It is especially useful when chronic drainage does not respond to conservative treatment and when cholesteatoma is suspected and is mandatory whenever a complaint of chronic otomastoiditis is identified.

TREATMENT OF CHRONIC OTOMASTOIDITIS. The objectives of surgical treatment of otomastoiditis are (1) to remove all infected tissue, (2) to establish a mastoid and middle ear cavity that will no longer be susceptible to repeated infections, and (3) to reestablish the ossicular chain and provide the best hearing possible in an already damaged ear. The operations for establishing an intact tympanic membrane and ossicular chain are referred to as tympanoplasty.

Mastoidectomy can be performed at the time of middle ear exploration. The incision follows the postauricular crease. Fascia may be obtained from the temporalis muscle to be used later as a graft for possible tympanic membrane repair. The muscles and periosteum are elevated from the mastoid bowl. Incisions are made within the external canal so that the auricle may be folded forward. Using a mastoid type of burr, the mastoid cells are carefully exenterated and the antrum of the mastoid cavity is identified. The posterior ear canal wall is preserved if possible, although it is thinned to make certain that all the air cells overlying the facial nerve are also removed. Healthy normal-appearing bone should be identified up to the sigmoid sinus and the sinodural angle, and abnormalities should be looked for in the middle ear. On completion, the ear canal is packed and the postauricular incision is closed, usually without a drain.

A radical mastoidectomy entails complete exenteration of the mastoid cells, middle ear contents, and tympanic membrane, converting it all into one large, clean cavity.

The classic radical mastoidectomy as originally described is now used only for extensive cholesteatoma, for a malignant external otitis, or tumors. Both the posterior canal wall and the lateral attic wall are removed. The floor of the ear canal is lowered to the level of the hypotympanum. The eustachian tube is either plugged with bone chips or muscle or allowed to remain open. Reconstruction of the middle ear space is not possible.

The modified radical mastoidectomy is designed to preserve the middle ear while eradicating all infection from the mastoid process. In contrast to a radical mastoidectomy, a less extensive cholesteatoma has been found. This cholesteatoma needs to be completely exposed and removed. To provide adequate visualization, the entire posterior canal wall may need to be lowered to the level of the facial nerve, thus creating a single cavity between the external ear canal and the mastoid.

When the posterior canal wall is removed, the mastoid bowl can always be checked for recurrence of infection. The disadvantage of such a cavity is a lifelong need to have it cleaned by a physician. Tympanoplasty can be combined with this procedure to reconstruct middle ear structures. When it is felt that all cholesteatoma has been removed, the posterior canal wall can be preserved or reconstructed and the mastoid bowl obliterated.

Intracranial and Extracranial Complications of Middle Ear and Mastoid Disease

Extracranial Complications

Horizontal Canal Fistula. Erosion of the lateral semicircular canal by cholesteatoma can lead to the formation of fistulas between the middle ear and the semicircular canal. Nystagmus, vertigo, and sensorineural hearing loss result. Treatment is by modified radical mastoidectomy with removal of all chronically infected tissue. While the vertigo may eventually subside, no improvement of the hearing loss can be anticipated.

Facial Nerve Paralysis. Infection of the facial nerve can lead to a complete peripheral facial paralysis. In 25 percent of patients, there is an area of dehiscence of the facial nerve close to the region of the oval window without erosion of the bone. When facial paralysis complicates an existing chronic otomastoiditis, immediate mastoidectomy and facial nerve exploration are indicated. Note the difference in management of facial paralysis occurring in this circumstance compared to its occurrence in acute otitis media.

Petrositis. Pneumatization of the petrous portion of the temporal bone is present in 30 percent of adult temporal bones and is usually symmetric. There are two groups of air cells extending to the petrous tip. One group is posterior, passing from the region of the antrum and semicircular canals to the petrous apex. The second group is anterior and inferior, extending from the region of the hypotympanum and the eustachian tube to the petrous tip.

Infection extends from cell to cell within the pneumatized temporal bone. Osteomyelitis can develop if there is incomplete pneumatization of the petrous portion. In addition, the bony labyrinth acts as an obstruction to drainage from the petrous apex into the rest of the mastoid.

Even though the infection in the mastoid can be resolved by antibiotics or operation, an abscess can be overlooked in the petrous tip so that drainage persists after mastoidectomy. Retro-orbital headache and sixth nerve paralysis (Gradenigo's syndrome) is pathognomonic for this condition, which may respond to high-dose intravenous antibiotic therapy. Drainage is required if there is no improvement after 24 hours of intravenous therapy, if symptoms or drainage recur, or if petrositis develops in combination with chronic otomastoiditis. Complete mastoidectomy is first performed, and the anterior and posterior petrous cell tracts are identified. They are used as landmarks and followed to the petrous apex. In the absence of these cell tracts, the method described by Lempert is used. The approach is anterior to the cochlea. The eustachian tube orifice and tensor tympanii muscles are identified, and the carotid artery is followed to the apex. As long as the infection remains within the petrous portion of the temporal bone, no meningeal or spinal fluid abnormalities can be demonstrated. This type of abscess can also rupture into the superior portion of the parapharyngeal space.

Lateral Sinus Thrombosis. Direct extension of infection through the skin layer of cortical bone that overlies the lateral sinus as it makes its sigmoid curve to the jugular vein has been associated with chronic otomastoiditis. In the preantibiotic era, an infected thrombus within the sigmoid sinus was associated with a hectic febrile course, during which septic emboli could pass through the venous drainage system of the brain. The diagnosis is best made by MRI or digital subtraction angiography. Today, this classical picture is unusual and the signs are far more subtle. In fact, thrombosis of the sigmoid sinus may first be recognized at the time of mastoidectomy for chronic otomastoiditis. Removal of the infected clot and packing off of the sinus are necessary. Jugular vein ligation may be required to prevent embolic spread of infected or necrotic tissue. High-dose systemic antibiotics are administered. A lumbar puncture is performed if the preoperative diagnosis is lateral sinus thrombosis. The pressure is measured and compression is applied to each jugular vein in sequence. When compression of one jugular vein causes an elevation in the spinal pressure, the opposite sigmoid sinus is probably blocked by a thrombus. While this test theoretically appears important, it is not dependable.

Suppurative Labyrinthitis. Middle ear infection can cross through the thin round window to include the sensitive membranous labyrinth. The mere presence of a contiguous infection or cholesteatoma can produce vertigo and sensorineural hearing loss and is referred to as serous labyrinthitis. An adjacent infection is sufficient to affect the composition of the perilymph with subsequent deterioration of hearing and balance. Should the infection actually extend into this region, the membranous labyrinth is quickly destroyed. Surgical procedures on the mastoid under this circumstance require opening, draining, and destroying the labyrinth. Fortunately, this complication is rare and such radical treatment is seldom the initial procedure. The surgeon instead removes the infection in the middle ear and mastoid and hopes for a serous labyrinthitis instead. Histopathology reviews in the temporal bone collections have demonstrated total destruction of the membranous labyrinth following infection, deposition of new bone within the otic capsule, and complete calcification of the labyrinthine structures.

Intracranial Complications of Middle Ear and Mastoid Infections. Any of the preceding temporal bone complications of mastoiditis and acute and chronic otitis media can lead to an intracranial complication (see Chap. 34). Pathways of extension include bone erosion of the tegmen of the middle ear or mastoid and thrombophlebitis of the emissary veins draining directly from the mastoid to the dura.

Meningitis. The most common intracranial complication of acute otomastoiditis is meningitis. There is frequently preexisting (acute or chronic) otitis media. Patients develop fever, stiffness of the neck, headache, and eventually nausea with vomiting. Symptoms can progress to coma. Lumbar puncture is essential for diagnosis and to determine the responsible organism, and treatment is by intravenous antibiotics. While waiting for a culture report, the Gram stain of the spinal fluid can be of some help in the selection of the appropriate antibiotics. In addition, it is helpful to differentiate chronic otomastoiditis (associated with cholesteatoma) from the acute meningitis that follows acute otitis media. The organisms most commonly responsible for these different types of infections have been discussed previously. If there is associated chronic otitis media, mastoidectomy to eliminate the source of infection is indicated when the patient is stable and the meningitis has resolved.

Extradural Abscess. The collection of pus over the middle ear or mastoid tegmen, but outside the dura, establishes an extradural abscess. The patient complains of otalgia and severe headache. Typically, there is pulsatile drainage through the tympanic membrane perforation. Such an abscess can be an incidental finding during mastoid operation. Drainage is accomplished through the mastoid with removal of the osteitic bone. Postoperative antibiotics are indicated, and the outlook is usually excellent.

Subdural Abscess (Empyema). The patient becomes acutely ill with headache (first localized, then generalized) and high fever during the course of chronic, purulent otitis media or mastoiditis. Neurologic symptoms progress to include seizure (frequently jacksonian), contralateral hemiplegia, and loss of consciousness. The organism isolated is the same as in the infected ear.

Treatment requires a neurosurgical approach. Drainage is accomplished by either multiple burr holes or craniotomy with placement of drains and irrigation of the subdural space. Multiple brain abscesses may develop. Even today, the mortality rate is 30 percent and patients commonly develop neurologic sequelae (see Chap. 34).

Brain Abscess. Otogenic brain abscess is usually a complication of chronic otitis media or otomastoiditis. Two forms occur: (1) in the temporal lobe of the middle cranial fossa and (2) in the cerebellum (posterior fossa). An abscess in the posterior fossa can result from extension from the sigmoid sinus directly into the cerebellum. An abscess in the temporal lobe can have its origin in the tegmen of the mastoid or middle ear. The course of a cerebellar abscess is more sudden than with an abscess of the middle cranial fossa. A cerebellar abscess is associated with such neurologic signs as ataxia, tremor, and dysdiadochokinesia. Temporal lobe infection can produce headache, seizures, and aphasia. Following control of the abscess, a mastoidectomy may be required to resolve the underlying cause.

Recurrent Bacterial Meningitis. Thirty percent of the cases of meningitis originate in an otogenic or sinus source and all patients require a thorough otolaryngologic examination including CT scan of the mastoids and sinuses. While the mortality rate has decreased because of effective chemotherapy, the morbidity remains high. *Hemophilus influenzae* is the most common cause in children, but *S. pneumoniae* is associated with the highest number of complications in adults. When the ear appears to be the source of trouble, tympanograms and tympanocentesis for bacterial culture are useful.

If the infection appears to arise from a contiguous mastoid bone or paranasal sinus, drainage is required. The operation should usually be limited to drainage, and reconstructive efforts should be avoided. Exenterative procedures should be delayed until recovery from the meningitis. When no immediate source of the infection is evident, patients with recurrent meningitis should be evaluated for a cerebrospinal fluid leak, which in turn might be caused by unrecognized trauma, nasal or ear surgery, or even a congenital bony dehiscence. For example, trauma to the frontal ethmoid region can cause a tear in the dura at the cribriform plate. A complaint of a salty fluid dripping from the nose while in head-down position suggests a leak in the region of the cribriform plate, but similar symptoms can arise from a leak from the middle or posterior cranial fossa into the mastoid or middle ear cavity communicating with the pharynx via the eustachian tube.

There are basically four methods available to identify cerebrospinal fluid (CSF) leaks: (1) CT scan with metrizamide, (2) injection of intrathecal radioactive materials (eg, radioactive albumin), (3) injection of intrathecal dyes, and (4) detection of transferrin in the fluid collections. Pledgets should be placed (1) in the middle meatus in the area of drainage of the nasal frontal duct, (2) high near the cribriform plate, and (3) just below the eustachian tube orifice. Pledgets should be changed at least every 30 minutes, depending on the extent of the leak.

Chemical studies for cerebrospinal fluid rhinorrhea such as glucose determinations can be misleading. Tears and nasal secretions can confuse the results.

During this period, it helps to keep the patient in a sitting position to reduce the cerebrospinal fluid pressure. During the wait, avoid repeated otoscopic examinations to reduce the risk of contamination. When a small CSF leak follows head trauma, it is feasible to wait 3 weeks for spontaneous resolution. Prophylactic systemic antibiotics are not given. After closed head injury, increased CSF pressure with internal hydrocephalus can result. This increased pressure can activate a leak, which closes spontaneously only to reopen. Control of the spinal fluid leakage can be resolved by a shunting procedure, such as a lumbar-peritoneal shunt. Shunts are available with valves that can be opened or closed without additional operations.

To close such leaks, a neurosurgical approach is often more effective than the extracranial route. The brain and underlying dura can be inspected more readily and the fistula can be repaired with a fascia graft. A leak into the sphenoid requires a direct procedure by a transsphenoid approach for effective control and more direct access to the source of the leakage. Rhinorrhea after extensive ethmoid sinus or nasal operation can be repaired by a transnasal-transethmoid approach by developing a regional mucoperiosteal flap by the endoscopic route and thus preserving olfaction. When not successful, frontal craniotomy is needed. A middle fossa craniotomy provides a good access to leaks over the tegmen mastoideum.

Head and Neck Manifestations of Acquired Immunodeficiency Syndrome (AIDS)

The initial manifestations of AIDS is in the head and neck area in 40 percent of patients. Diagnosis is made by history, serum positive for HIV antigen, and T_4 lymphocyte analysis.[34]

The most common oral manifestation of AIDS is oral candidiasis most often caused by *C. albicans.*[35] At some point it is present in 75 percent of AIDS patients. Other oral manifestations include herpetic infection, hairy leukoplakia, gingivitis, oral condylomata, and recurrent aphthous ulcers. Kaposi's sarcoma is a red to bluish appearing flat or raised lesion most often found on the hard palate. Biopsy is required for diagnosis and treatment requires radiation or chemotherapy.

Both acute purulent and serous otitis media are common in AIDS patients. While most often caused by pneumococcus, *E. coli, P. aeruginosa,* or *S. epidermidis,* there are reported cases of extrapulmonary *Pneumocystis carinii* otitis.[36] Diagnosis requires a methenamine silver stain of collected serous fluid. Children who are HIV positive and have a decreased T_4 lymphocyte count have twice the incidence of otitis media as children with a normal T_4 count. Children born to mothers with AIDS who do not seroconvert but develop AIDS have frequent otitis media.[37] In fact, otitis media may be the first infection they develop. Even with myringotomy and PE tube placement, they continue to have recurrent otitis media.

Adult AIDS patients have developed fulminant *Aspergillus* infections of the external canal and mastoid.[38] Invasive canal infections can cause facial nerve paralysis. *Aspergillus fumigatus* mastoiditis can be associated with brain abscess. Patients have survived with radical mastoidectomy and IV amphotericin B (30 mg/day).[39]

Paranasal Sinus Disease. Sinusitis can occur following an upper respiratory infection in AIDS patients. There will be persistent headache, nasal congestion, and fever. Responsible organisms include *S. aureus, S. pneumoniae,* and *P. aeruginosa.* Treatment is primarily medical with amoxicillin and clavulanic acid and decongestants. Worsening of symptoms while on systemic antibiotics requires a limited drainage procedure or irrigation. In an individual who has recurrent maxillary sinusitis, nasoantral windows for permanent drainage are helpful.[40]

Parotid Gland. Large cysts developing in the parotid gland can be an initial manifestation of AIDS.[41,42] The cysts are usually multiple, can be bilateral, and enlarge slowly (Fig. 33–26). They are lined with epithelium and must be differentiated from other lymphoepithelial cysts such as those in Sjögren's syndrome and Warthin's tumor. CT scan

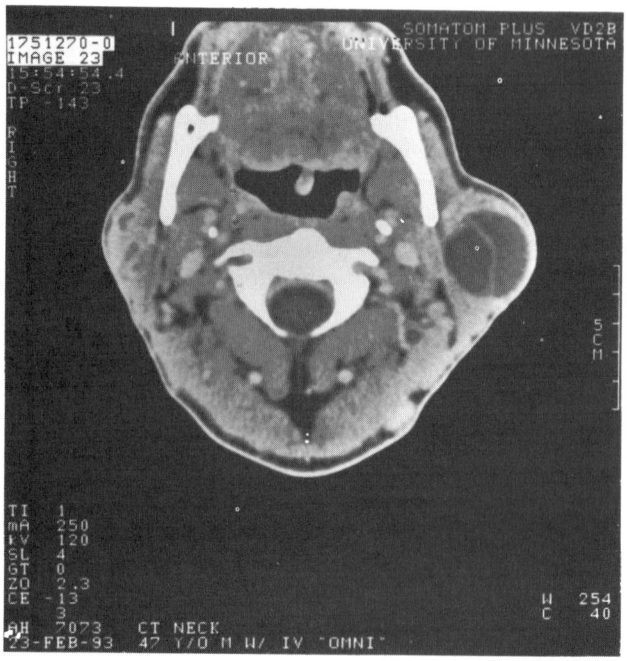

Figure 33–26. Cyst in the left parotid gland.

and FNA are all that are required for diagnosis. If a solid mass is felt in the parotid, biopsy is required for possible lymphoma, tuberculosis, or Kaposi's sarcoma.[43]

Cervical Adenopathy. Cervical lymphadenopathy is common in patients with AIDS-related complex (ARC). The most common site includes the posterior triangle, pre- and postauricular area, and submandibular areas. FNA for cytologic evaluation is necessary to diagnose the presence of carcinoma, lymphoma, Kaposi's sarcoma, or tuberculosis. An open biopsy is necessary when lymphoma is suspected.

INFECTIONS OF THE LARYNX AND TRACHEA

Acute Supraglottitis (Epiglottitis)

Supraglottic laryngitis refers to an acute inflammation of the supraglottic structures, which include the epiglottis, the false cords, and the aryepiglottic folds. It is usually caused by *H. influenzae* type B, but streptococci and staphylococci have also been isolated. Cultures can be obtained from the larynx and blood. Epiglottitis usually occurs in children about 6 years of age, but it has recently shown an increased incidence in adults in their thirties. The onset is marked by severe dysphagia, followed rapidly by refusal to swallow saliva and respiratory distress. The patient can be well in the morning, develop increasing respiratory distress and painful swelling in the afternoon, and be hospitalized and require emergency tracheostomy by dinnertime. The soft and resilient supraglottic tissues in a child permit easy and rapid swelling so that the massive edema of the epiglottis causes airway obstruction. In fact, downward pressure on the posterior tongue can cause the swollen epiglottis to completely obstruct the upper airway. The patient appears acutely ill, with the head extended forward in an effort to maintain an open airway. As it becomes too painful to swallow, the patient will begin to drool. Examination is best performed in the operating room, so that if the swollen epiglottis is seen, an airway can be established. In a patient less severely ill, soft tissue lateral x-ray studies of the neck and chest are obtained. The swollen epiglottis can be seen and the presence of a foreign body or pneumonia ruled out.

Intravenous ampicillin (150 mg/kg/day) was the preferred antibiotic, but because of the 20 percent incidence of resistant strains, the addition of chloramphenicol (100 mg/kg/day) is justifiable in this life-threatening infection. Once the sensitivity is known, ceftriaxone is an alternative. *Hemophilus influenzae* is almost always the cause. The etiology can be confirmed by laryngeal Gram stain and culture or preferably blood culture, because streptococci and staphylococci can cause a similar clinical picture. The major concern, however, is the compromised airway. The current recommendation is examination in the operating room by personnel skilled at bronchoscopy, intubation, and tracheostomy. If the disease is in the advanced stages, it is hazardous to attempt passage of a soft, flexible endotracheal tube through inflamed edematous firm tissues. Under these circumstances in children, a pediatric bronchoscope should be inserted and a tracheostomy performed. With less edema and inflammation, it is possible to insert an endotracheal tube.

The majority of children can be handled by nasotracheal intubation if they are in a pediatric intensive care unit with skilled pediatric intensive care personnel on hand. Otherwise, a tracheostomy is a conservative approach. Establishment of an airway is necessary in a child. The disease has been reported in young adults. Some young adults have been treated in the ICU without a tracheostomy. Steroids have not been demonstrated to be advantageous in the management of epiglottitis.

Acute Laryngotracheobronchitis (Croup)

Acute laryngotracheobronchitis (LTB) should be distinguished from acute supraglottic laryngitis. LTB occurs in a younger age group, generally around 2 years of age. The name croup refers to the typical seal-like barking cough. It is generally caused by parainfluenza virus types I and II and influenza viruses. Respiratory syncitial virus causes about 10 percent of cases. However, superimposed bacterial infections (*Streptococcus, Staphylococcus,* or *H. influenzae*) can occur. The major site of the obstruction is the subglottic area (see Fig. 33–27). It is here that the tissues are most susceptible to swelling and inflammation. Secretions build up within the trachea, and if they become thick the child is unable to raise them.

The child usually has a 2- to 3-day history of an upper respiratory infection with gradually increasing respiratory stridor. As airway obstruction progresses, use of the accessory muscles of respiration become more and more active, and mild cyanosis can appear. There is a low-grade fever and a mild leukocytosis.

When a suspected secondary bacterial infection supervenes, a broad spectrum antibiotic such as ampicillin is generally the antibiotic of choice. With

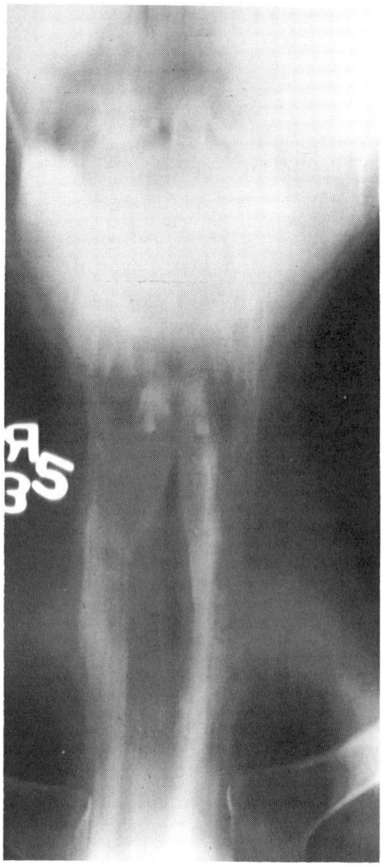

Figure 33–27. Acute laryngotracheobronchitis with subglottic edema.

the compromised airway, these children need high humidity (to liquefy the secretions and avoid the crusting that occurs in the trachea). Aerosolized racemic epinephrine administered by IPPB (0.5 cc in 2.20 percent racemic epinephrine/3 cc normal saline) has been demonstrated to cause relief of laryngeal edema. Steroids have been advocated to reduce the subglottic edema. Dexamethasone is given IV over 1 minute every 4 to 6 hours.

Increasing respiratory distress with a pulse rate greater than 160 and respiratory rate greater than 60 per minute suggest the need for an artificial airway. Arterial blood gases are of little value in determining the need for tracheostomy in upper airway obstruction and can actually be misleading. Both endotracheal intubation and tracheostomy have been used, but the preferred method is tracheostomy. Placing an endotracheal tube through an acutely inflamed subglottic larynx invites complications. Less than 1 percent of children with acute LTB require tracheostomy if proper medical treatment is provided.

Bacterial Tracheitis

Bacterial tracheitis may represent a separate clinical entity, or it may be a complication of acute LTB.[44] It is discussed separately because of its severity, need for antibiotics, and need to establish an artificial airway. In the course of what is felt to be LTB, the child may become acutely more ill, not responsive to racemic epinephrine, and toxic. The white blood cell count is elevated. The child prefers to lie down rather than sit up. This rapid progression in disease is an indication of direct laryngoscopy in the operating room. Endoscopic findings will show subglottic edema and suppurative tracheitis. Cultures are obtained, and in almost all cases *Staphylococcus* is responsible.

An endotracheal tube is inserted or a tracheostomy performed. Antistaphylococcal antibiotics are begun, and the child is kept in the pediatric intensive care unit, where frequent suctioning is required. Crusting may be so extensive that repeated bronchoscopy is necessary for crust removal.

Other Causes of Laryngitis

Diphtheria (see Chap. 9) can create a gray, dirty green membrane with a "mousy" odor over the pharynx. Immunizations have virtually eliminated this disease in the United States. Symptoms include fatigue, mild sore throat, and fever. Death can occur from side effects of the toxin as well as airway obstruction. Treatment includes absolute rest, administration of antitoxin 10,000 units IV, and airway protection including tracheostomy.

Other infections of the larynx include fungal infections (such as *Histoplasma, Blastomyces,* and *Candida* infection) and tuberculosis. Such infections are usually associated with pulmonary involvement with the same organism. Constant cough will cause the infection to spread from the lungs to the larynx. The treatment is the same as required for the pulmonary tissue. Tracheostomy and intubation are not needed in most instances. Other causes of acute laryngeal inflammation can be related to allergic disorders.

Infectious Complications of Tracheostomy

The advent of disposable endotracheal tubes and the increased use of intensive care units for patients who require prolonged intubation have lowered the need for tracheostomy. When an endotracheal tube is in place for prolonged periods (over 72 hours in the adult, or over 2 weeks in the infant), tracheostomy may be necessary. Tracheostomy is frequently necessary preceding an extensive head and neck operation and to maintain an airway after maxillofacial or neck trauma.

Similarly, in the advanced stages of tetanus—Guillain-Barré syndrome (ascending paralysis)—and in other subacute or chronic neurologic disorders, tracheostomy is preferred to prolonged endotracheal intubation, which must later be converted to a tracheostomy.

There are numerous complications associated with tracheostomy. (1) Mediastinal air collections and (2) pneumothorax are most common in children because of the high location of the dome of the pleura. A pneumothorax occurs readily if one deviates even slightly from the midline. Other complications include (3) postoperative bleeding from the tracheostomy site, (4) infection around the tracheostomy tube, (5) dryness of the tracheal mucosa with an associated tracheobronchitis, (6) stenosis developing as the result of localized pressure by the tube or its cuff, (7) difficult decannulation particularly in children, (8) subcutaneous emphysema, (9) erosion of the innominate artery with massive hemorrhage, (10) pneumonia from aspiration, and (11) injury to the recurrent laryngeal nerve.

Infection occurs at the tracheostomy site more frequently when a cuffed tube is used. A patient requires respiratory care because of the loss of ability to cough and clear secretions. Frequent suctioning becomes necessary. Sterile technique is mandatory, and the suction catheter should be placed only 1 to 2 cm beyond the lower tip of the tracheostomy tube. If deeper suctioning is required, it should be performed by a physician. Passing the cannula repeatedly into the major bronchi can cause more irritation and increased secretions. Because the 80 to 90 percent humidity provided by the nose has been bypassed, continuous humidity should be given to the tracheotomy opening. Dry crusts form on the tracheal wall and increase the risk of infection and cannula obstruction. Tracheostomy wounds are left opened to avoid subcutaneous emphysema. Sterile porous dressings are applied to the site and changed frequently. If infection occurs, cultures and Gram stains are indicated. Organisms most frequently encountered are *S. aureus, P. aeruginosa, C. albicans,* and enteric gram-negative rods. Systemic antibiotics should be given, but local care is most important.

Frequent changes of 0.5 percent of acetic acid solution-soaked dressings are useful in reducing *P. aeruginosa* contamination. The tracheostomy tube itself will have to be changed more frequently and careful attention paid to the inner cannula. It will require more frequent cleaning and removal of thick mucus. Disposable inner cannulas are now available.

INFECTIONS ASSOCIATED WITH SURGERY AND RADIATION THERAPY OF THE HEAD AND NECK

Prevention

Tumors of the head and neck are frequently treated by a planned combination of radiation therapy and surgery. When radiation is given first, the surgeon must operate in an irradiated field and complications, although no more frequent, can take longer to resolve. The early effects of radiation include mucositis and skin changes. These effects can be controlled by limiting the radiation field and reducing the daily dosage. Later effects include a proliferative vasculitis with compromise of the blood supply of the treated areas. Ideally, operations should be performed after the early effects have subsided but before the delayed effects of radiation occur. Thus the ideal time for surgery is 4 to 6 weeks after the cessation of radiation. Postoperative radiation therapy is preferred when microscopic cervical metastases are found at operation or when an inadequate margin of normal tissue was resected around the tumor. It has also been used in areas where the overall cure rate for surgery alone is low, such as in the base of the tongue, hypopharynx, or pyriform sinus. The advantage of postoperative radiation therapy is that the tissues are healed before the irradiation is initiated. Although infectious complications occur after operations and radiation therapy, several precautions can decrease their incidence, for example, ensuring that the patient is in the best nutritional status possible, that other diseases such as diabetes are under the best possible control, that preexisting infections have been resolved, and that the operation and all incisions are properly planned.

The blood supply to the neck generally runs in a vertical direction. The poorest blood supply to the neck is across the midline of the neck; therefore the most popular flap design for composite resections or laryngectomy is a half-H or apron flap. The vertical limb of the incision is posterior to the carotid artery and crosses the artery in only one location. If necrosis of the flap should occur, it is unlikely to expose the carotid artery.

In heavily irradiated tissue, such as in a patient who is undergoing a salvage operation when irradiation fails and the oral cavity or pharynx is entered, a controlled fistula pharyngostome should be considered. Closed suction drains are used to decrease fluid accumulation under the flap. The carotid artery can be protected by using muscle flaps or dermal grafts. Heavily irradiated skin may have to be excised and replaced with a deltopectoral flap or pectoralis major myocutaneous flap.

Pharyngocutaneous Fistulas

Pharyngocutaneous fistulas are common complications after ablative head and neck surgery. Cultures of infected wounds are essential because of the variety of organisms responsible. Once thought to be primarily *Staphylococcus,* this organism is now responsible for only 25 percent of infections. Proper local wound care is important. The management of wound infections depends on early recognition and treatment. A patient who develops a low-grade fever and some redness and swelling in the skin flaps should be checked carefully for a fistula. If this occurs, antidiuretic therapy is begun and the flaps must be opened widely and immediately drained. It is important that this be done early to direct the salivary flow away from the carotid artery and from the tracheostomy site or laryngostome if one is present. Antibiotics can be discontinued when the fistula drains only saliva and there is no sign of local or systemic infection. Prolonged use of antibiotics can result in colitis or other complications secondary to *C. difficile* infection.[45] As soon as possible, either horizontal chest flaps or pectoralis major myocutaneous flaps should be rotated to protect the carotid artery.

Osteonecrosis of the Mandible

The blood supply of the mandible can be affected adversely by the combination of operation and radiation. Subsequent bacterial infection leads to a smoldering osteomyelitis (osteonecrosis). Table 33–2 lists the many factors that affect the development of this serious complication. Proliferative vasculitis can actually lead to thrombosis of the vessels and subsequent sclerosis. Sequestra form, which have to be excised. Should an oral cutaneous fistula develop and medical management fail, resection of the involved segment of the mandible is necessary. Before operation, a thorough effort should be made to control the infection with antibiotics against mouth anaerobic flora, such as clindamycin. Frequent oral irrigation and removal of sequestered or exposed bone are required. Particular importance is given to any remaining teeth, and appropriate dental care should be delivered.

Hyperbaric oxygen, delivered at 2 atmospheres pressure for periods of up to 40 hours, has allowed osteonecrosis of the mandible to heal without the need for partial mandibulectomy.

TABLE 33–2. FACTORS INFLUENCING THE DEVELOPMENT OF OSTEORADIONECROSIS

Tumor factors
Tumor overlaying or invading bone (especially floor of mouth)
Large primary tumor
Dental or surgical treatment factors
Elective extractions
Inadequate delay after extractions
Trauma (dentures, surgical salvage)
Patient factors
Poor oral care (poor patient education or poor compliance with instructions)
Poor nutritional status preventing healing
Radiation factors
Salivary suppression
Radical treatment (high dose, high fraction size)
Large volume (decreased collaterals)
Interstitial radiation overlaying bone (especially floor of mouth and base of tongue)
Orthovoltage radiation (should never be used externally, ie, only intraoral treatment acceptable with orthovoltage)

Courtesy of Dr. Robert E. Haselow, Department of Therapeutic Radiology, University of Minnesota.

Osteonecrosis can be prevented by removing any teeth in the potential field of radiation that are not in excellent condition and supported by normal, healthy bone. Patients undergoing radiation therapy should be given fluoride treatments and instructed to practice good oral hygiene. At the time of extraction, the alveolar rim should be smoothed and a primary mucoperiosteal closure obtained. Radiation should not be started after extraction until the bone has healed properly, usually in 10 days.

The development of new infection, particularly *Candida albicans,* must be guarded against by the use of topical antifungal agents (miconazole, nystatin). The saliva flow diminishes after only a few treatments of radiation therapy. The mucosa becomes less able to defend against infection, and a mild mucositis can develop. The use of artificial saliva preparations is often helpful. Patients who begin to lose weight need immediate supplementation with either a nasogastric tube or percutaneous gastrostomy.

Chondritis

High doses of radiation administered to the larynx can result in radionecrosis of the laryngeal cartilage. As the blood supply to the perichondrium diminishes, a chondritis occurs. The thyroid cartilage can become infected and actually dissolve. There is intense pain in the area of skin overlying the cartilages, and fistulas can form. There is swelling, edema, and loss of the normal architectural landmarks of the larynx. Treatment is primarily intensive intravenous antibiotics.[46] Prolonged trials of antibiotic therapy along with wound debridement and cleansing are indicated. Laryngectomy is needed only when complete loss of the skeletal support structures of the larynx or breakdown of overlying skin with fistula formation or intractable pain occurs. Again, hyperbaric oxygen has been helpful.

Wound Infection with Exposure of the Carotid Artery

Pharyngocutaneous or orocutaneous fistulas with breakdown of the cervical flaps in the region of the carotid artery expose the vessel, and infection with oral organisms ensues. This problem usually occurs only when there has been an extensive resection in combination with intensive radiation therapy for advanced disease. Because the normal oral flora have been altered by radiation and operation, the infecting organisms are frequently *Staphylococcus, Pseudomonas,* and other gram-negative organisms. Cultures and Gram stains should be obtained. Intravenous antibiotics are administered, and immediate plans are made for protection of the carotid artery system. The dilemma is complex: the longer the artery remains exposed, the greater the risk of rupture; at the same time, placement of a flap over frank necrosis only hides the impending carotid artery rupture. The vessel must therefore be kept moist with an antibiotic solution or dilute povidone-iodine. The area must be debrided, and a horizontal chest flap or myocutaneous flap can be rotated when the infection is resolved. Cross-matched blood is kept available until healing is assured.

A slight blood loss from an area of eschar over the vessel means rupture is pending (sentinel bleed). There is not time to wait for epithelium to form, and the artery must be ligated in the operating room. If the vessel actually ruptures, pressure is applied over the vessel and a blood transfusion started. Stroke inevitably follows as the vessel is ligated while the patient is in shock, but the incidence can be reduced to less than 30 percent if the blood volume is restored before ligation.

To prevent exposure of the carotid artery should postoperative infection occur, a split-thickness skin graft of 0.013 to 0.014 in. is first elevated from the thigh, and a second graft of 0.013 in. is taken from the underlying dermis. The split-thickness skin graft is then laid back and sutured into position, and the dermal graft is spread over the carotid artery and sutured down to the cervical fascia. An exposed dermal graft will undergo epithelialization. An alternative is to rotate the levator scapula muscle. When the pectoralis major myocutaneous flap is used for oral reconstruction, the muscle segment is used to protect the carotid artery.

INFECTION ASSOCIATED WITH TRAUMA

Trauma to the External Ear

Avulsion. Trauma to the ear varies from a clean laceration to an avulsion of a portion of the auricle to a potentially septic infection (as occurs from a dog or human bite). In the case of a clean laceration or avulsion, all effort is made to protect the cartilage—minimal amounts of tissue are debrided to cover and protect the exposed cartilage and perichondrium. It is even possible to reapproximate an avulsed, clean segment. An antistaphylococcal antibiotic is administered. With a carefully placed external stent, the avulsed segment has a chance to survive. The cartilage is seldom salvageable in cases of avulsion caused by a dog bite. If several hours have elapsed since the injury, it is not worthwhile to attempt reanastomosis of the avulsed segment. Instead, the exposed cartilage can be buried beneath the skin over the mastoid process for later secondary reconstruction. Again, antibiotics are recommended for 5 days. Infection that develops secondarily is treated after appropriate culture and sensitivity studies.

Thermal Injury. Most frostbite injuries are superficial, involving the helix, and should be treated by immediate rapid rewarming with saline-soaked sponges or cotton to a temperature of 38.3C to 42.2C. Broadspectrum antibiotics are administered only to patients in whom a deep injury is suspected. Silver nitrate (0.5 percent) dressings are carefully applied to the auricle. No debridement is undertaken initially. It is important to prevent secondary infection. Large blebs must be neither opened nor aspirated. If they rupture, they must be cleaned daily with antiseptic solutions. When delineation of the devitalized tissues becomes evident, conservative debridement is undertaken.

Burns of the head and neck usually occur in association with other burn injuries and may not be evident initially. More severe injuries will take priority. Again, care should be taken to prevent the spread of infection to the cartilage of the ear. *Pseudomonas aeruginosa* is the most common organism found in this form of smoldering perichondritis. When actual chondritis develops, it is treated like perichondritis, discussed earlier in this chapter.

Traumatic Perforation of the Tympanic Membrane

Perforation of the tympanic membrane can result when foreign objects are introduced into the ear canal and from concussion, such as a slap to the ear. These wounds seldom become infected. Treatment includes protection of the ear from introduction of any foreign material, including water. A baseline audiogram is obtained to rule out damage to the ossicles. The margins of the perforation when examined with the microscope are curled medially under the drumhead and can be retrieved with a microscopic ear instrument. A paper patch is applied to the drumhead to maintain the edges and act as a scaffold. Antibiotics are administered only if infection develops and the ear is kept dry.

Perforations that occur when diving, water skiing, or surfing, however, are almost always associated with an immediate onset of a purulent otitis media. The responsible organisms are initially gram-positive, but soon the gram-negative rods predominate. In addition to systemic antibiotics, a topical antibiotic-steroid eardrop may be helpful. These perforations should not be closed while there is an active infection.

If there is any suspicion that the stapes is dislocated and could be pushed medially into the inner ear, immediate operation is indicated. As a result of such a displacement, the patient has hearing loss as well as vertigo. An emergency stapedectomy may be necessary to save the hearing.

Temporal Bone Fracture

Severe falls and motor vehicle accidents can cause basal skull fractures and associated temporal bone trauma. Three types of temporal bone fractures—longitudinal, transverse, and mixed—can be distinguished by clinical presentation and direction of the fracture on the CT scan.

Otolaryngologic consultation is indicated to assess the extent of injury to the ear and facial nerve, especially if there is bleeding from the external ear canal. A postauricular area of ecchymosis developing over the mastoid region is referred to as Battle's sign and is pathognomonic of temporal bone fracture. Primary care of the patient is by the neurosurgeon who treats the more threatening intracranial injury. It is best to postpone assessment of the extent of ear injury while there is copious bleeding from the ear canal, because attempts to remove the blood clot may introduce pathogenic microbes. The combination of hemorrhage from the ear, hearing loss, and facial nerve paralysis establish the diagnosis of basilar skull fracture. Detailed information about the tympanic membrane in this acute stage is not necessary. The only similar injury that can cause such ear hemorrhage is a direct blow to the symphysis of the mandible, forcing the condyle of the mandible through the anterior aspects of the ear canal, with resultant skin lacerations. Later, when the patient's condition stabilizes and there is no longer active bleeding, crusted blood is removed from the ear canal under aseptic conditions and the extent of the ear injury is determined. A dark blue tympanic membrane indicates that there is a hematoma in the middle ear, and a conductive hearing loss is either because of discontinuity of the ossicles or because this collection of blood prevents ossicular movement. Lacerations of the ear canal usually need no specific treatment and will heal spontaneously. Daily examination of facial nerve function is made. When nerve function is present initially and later decreases, the paralysis will usually recover spontaneously. Facial nerve function that is absent immediately after the trauma is less likely to recover. Such nerve injuries should be explored as soon as the patient's general condition permits. CT scan is valuable in establishing the diagnosis and identifying the site of injury. Testing of facial nerve function provides information on the status of potential facial nerve recovery.

Spinal fluid otorrhea usually ceases spontaneously within 1 week. Failure to stop by conservative treatment requires a combined neurosurgical and otolaryngologic approach to the mastoid region for closure.

Nasal Trauma

Nasal trauma is the most common of all facial injuries. Obvious deformity of the nasal dorsum with deflection to the side and epistaxis bring the patient to the emergency room. In the acute phase when there is significant swelling and the patient is apprehensive, ice packs and analgesics are the best treatment until the swelling subsides. The nasal septum must then be examined because hematomas that develop between the septum and mucoperichrondrium will continue to increase in size, and a complete nasal obstruction will eventually occur. Bilateral nasal packing is inserted and the patient is started on an antistaphylococcal penicillin. An undrained hematoma will lead to abscess, which in turn leads to dissolution of the cartilaginous tissues. Wide drainage with placement of a Penrose drain is required for a septal abscess. In an effort to preserve the physiologic functions and cosmetic appearance of the nose, it will be necessary to replace the missing septal cartilage with autogenous cartilage after the infection is cleared.

Maxillofacial Trauma

Automobile and motorcycle accidents cause the most severe maxillofacial trauma. Although injuries from fist fights and athletic mishaps are more common, they are usually less severe. Any fracture line extending through the tooth-bearing areas of the mandible or maxilla causes an associated laceration of the tightly associated gingiva and must be considered as a compound fracture. Treatment is aimed not only at correcting the fracture but also at prevention of infection and subsequent osteomyelitis.

To prevent large gaps at the fracture sites and avoid exposure of bare bone surfaces, early fragment stabilization is required. This may involve temporary placement of wire ligatures (ivy loops) or the application of portions of arch bars to immobilize the jaw fragments. By stabilizing the mandible, the tongue is also stabilized and the airway protected. Clots of blood and other foreign material need to be removed from the oral cavity.

Loose fragments of bone with attached alveolar mucoperiosteum should not be debrided unless they are definitely dead. Suturing of the mucoperiosteum frequently prevents loss of bone and provides a better opportunity for later reconstruction by the oral surgeon or the prosthodontist.

Tracheostomy and inflated cuffed tracheostomy tubes will keep the severely injured patients from aspirating blood and other foreign materials.

Injury to the maxilla usually exposes the sinus cavity. Fractures through the maxillary and ethmoid sinus cavities tend to develop infection. These sinus cavities need adequate drainage. Obviously, devitalized fragments of bone and soft tissue must be removed. Fractures extending across the frontoethmoid region may displace and obstruct the nasofrontal duct. Such fractures can result in acute frontal or ethmoid sinusitis and can lead to mucocele and pyocele many years (10 to 20) later. For this reason, some physicians advocate the immediate obliteration of the frontal sinus when the duct has been damaged. Others will attempt to reconstruct the duct or perform a trephine to maintain drainage of the sinus while the mucosal reaction subsides and the duct becomes patent again.

Severe epistaxis may be associated with maxillofacial trauma. Anterior packs control some hemorrhages, but, more frequently, when the hemorrhage is severe, a posterior nasal pack is also necessary. The posterior pack is pulled firmly into the posterior choana. This will prevent obstruction of the eustachian tube orifice and resultant otitis media. An antibiotic ointment, such as bacitracin, on the pack reduces the local infection and the associated foul odor. Because obstruction of several sinus ostia occurs when the nasal pack is in position, a systemic antibiotic (such as penicillin) should also be administered. The packs remain in place for 3 to 5 days. Twenty-four hours after removal, antibiotics may be discontinued. Simultaneous occurrence of epistaxis and cerebrospinal fluid otorrhea should be treated with packs to control the hemorrhage, and with systemic antibiotic to prevent meningitis. Persistent cerebrospinal fluid rhinorrhea alone is not a contraindication to reducing a frontoethmoid fracture. In fact, the rhinorrhea may be stopped by reduction of the fracture. When the posterior plate of the frontal sinus is fractured, the cerebrospinal fluid rhinorrhea cannot be expected to stop spontaneously. An open approach can be used to repair the dura and obliterate the sinus. Such procedures are safely undertaken only with simultaneous administration of antibiotics, especially those effective against *S. aureus.*

Blunt Laryngeal Trauma

Blunt injuries to the larynx or trachea will present with subcutaneous emphysema, loss of voice, airway obstruction, and pain and tenderness over the involved cartilage. Flexible fiberoptic endoscopy can be performed in the emergency room and the airway assessed. Tracheostomy is frequently necessary. As soon as the patient's condition permits, within the first 24 to 48 hours if possible, an endoscopic evaluation and open reduction of any fractures of the larynx and trachea should be carried out in the operating room. Delay inevitably results in infection with loss of cartilaginous support. Recurrent laryngeal nerve function should be evaluated. A lateral soft tissue x-ray and esophagogram should be performed to diagnose a ruptured viscus. All wounds of the esophagus, pharynx, and larynx must be drained and systemic antibiotics administered. Severe crush injuries to the larynx and trachea require stenting by either prefashioned endotracheal tubes or Silastic or foam rubber stents. These stents are usually held in position with wire sutures brought out through the neck, tied over a button, and maintained in position for at least 6 to 8 weeks.

In all instances in which massive wounds occur, the patient is treated with an antibiotic that is effective against *S. aureus*. Repeat cultures are performed on any wounds that continue to remain infected, because more resistant and gram-negative organisms show up with time. Tetanus prophylaxis, in the form of tetanus toxoid, is also given to all these trauma patients.

Prophylactic Antibiotics in Head and Neck Surgery. The general principles of prophylaxis should be followed. That is, antibiotic prophylaxis should be directed against the organisms likely to be encountered and should be administered in adequate doses for a brief duration (see Fig. 33–28) (see Chap. 25). Ketcham et al[47] have been acknowledged as authors of the first controlled prospective study to demonstrate the efficacy of prophylactic antibiotics in head and neck cancer surgery. They evaluated the use of chloramphenicol against *Staphylococcus aureus* infections, which was the most common organism associated with wound infection. The antibiotic was started the day prior to surgery and given 2 g every 6 hours for 10 days postoperatively. There were 78 patients in the study, including 20 head and neck patients, before it was discontinued due to the problems in the placebo group. Infection rates were significantly decreased in head and neck cancer surgery and pelvic cancer in the chloramphenicol groups 22 percent (2/9) versus the placebo, 54.5 percent (6/11).

Subsequent prospective studies in head and neck cancer have evaluated drug combinations, duration of administration, and establishment of other risk factors. Most major head and neck cancer surgery involves substantial contamination of the wound with saliva when the upper aerodigestive tract is entered through the neck. The incidence of infection is increased in debilitated patients, alcoholic patients, cases with a long duration, and especially complex cases where a flap closure is required.

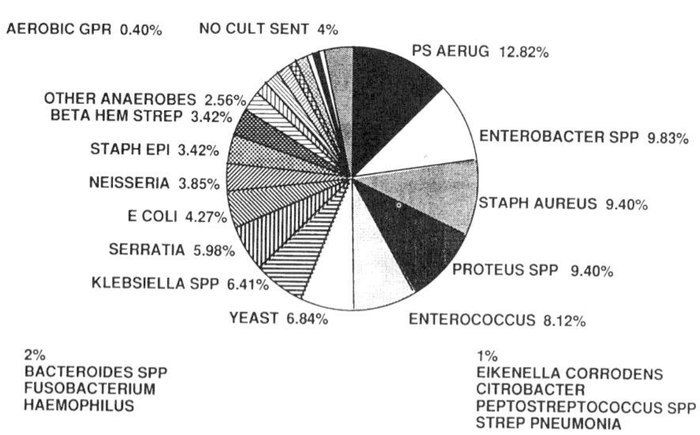

Figure 33–28. Etiologic agents of wound infections of the head and neck during a 15-year period. *(From M. M. Olson and G. L. Adams, unpublished data.)*

In 1972, Becker and Parell[48] studied 55 patients receiving cefazolin 1 g every 2 hours preoperatively and 0.5 g every 6 hours × 4 versus a placebo. Their rate of infection in the cefazolin group was 38 percent (12/32) versus 87 percent (20/23) in the placebo group. Wound infections were due to fistula or abscess formation. *Staphylococcus aureus* was the most common cultured organism, but most infections were mixed aerobic and anaerobic. *Bacteroides fragilis* was not isolated in any of these infections.

Robbins et al[49] at M. D. Anderson Cancer Center studied 330 patients prospectively. They compared cefazolin alone versus cefazolin plus metronidazole. Metronidazole was added in an effort to reduce the incidence of anaerobic infections. The rate of infection in the cefazolin alone group was 9.5 percent versus 18.6 percent in the combination group.

This study additionally demonstrated a direct correlation between wound infection and complexities of this procedure, duration, blood replacement, and tracheostomy. On the other hand, there was no correlation with previous radiation therapy or chemotherapy.

There is general agreement on the benefits of prophylactic antibiotics in clean-contaminated head and neck surgery. Antibiotics have not been demonstrated to be efficacious in clean head and neck surgery. Their use in sinus surgery and nasal septal surgery is still not established. There is consensus that whenever nasal packing is placed for over 24 hours and whenever a posterior nasal pack is required, antibiotic prophylaxis is provided.

Other indications include patients at risk for developing bacterial endocarditis as in aortic valve disease or prosthetic heart valves.

A clear advantage favoring prophylaxis has not been established in patients on steroids, previously irradiated, or diabetic. These groups are at risk for a higher incidence of infection. Malnutrition is associated with poor wound healing and there are studies suggesting preoperative hyperalimentation may decrease postoperative complications.[50]

Other recommended prophylactic antibiotic schedules include ampicillin plus cloxacillin,[51] clindamycin plus amikacin,[52] and gentamicin plus a first-generation cephalosporin. All combinations are active against the normal anaerobes of the mouth and gram-positive facultative bacteria. Current regimens commence 1 hour before surgery and are continued for 24 to 48 hours postoperatively. When an implant is placed (eg, titanium mandible), antibiotics may be continued longer. The highest incidence of postoperative infection occurs in patients undergoing composite resections with flap reconstruction (20 percent).

REFERENCES

1. Mawson SR, Adlington P, Evans M: A controlled study evaluation of adeno-tonsillectomy in children. J Laryngol Otolaryngol 81:777, 1967.
2. McKee WJE: A controlled study of the effects of tonsillectomy and adenoidectomy in children. Br J Prev Med Soc 17:49, 1963.
3. Bieluch VM, Chasin WD, Martin ET, Tally FP: Recurrent tonsillitis: histologic and bacteriologic evaluation. Ann Otol Rhinol Laryngol 98:332, 1989.
4. Herzon FS: Permucosal needle drainage of peritonsillar abscess. Arch Otolaryngol 110:104, 1984.
5. Schechter GL, Sly DE, Roper AL, Jackson RT: The changing face of treatment of peritonsillar abscess. Laryngoscope 92:657, 1982.
6. McCurdy JA; Peritonsillar abscess: a comparison of treatment by immediate tonsillectomy and interval tonsillectomy. Arch Otolaryngol 103:414, 1977.
7. Holt GR, Tinsley PP: Peritonsillar abscess in children. Laryngoscope 91:1226, 1981.
8. Goldstein JC: Grand rounds: Epstein-Barr virus—the ravager. Ann Otol Rhinol Laryngol 87:729, 1978.
9. Tomkinson BE, Sullivan JL: Epstein-Barr virus infection and infectious mononucleosis. In Gorbach SL, Bartlett JG, Blacklow NR (eds): *Infectious Diseases.* Philadelphia, Saunders, 1992.
10. Sprinkle PM, Veltri RW: The tonsil and adenoid dilemma: medical or surgical treatment? Otolaryngol Clin North Am 7:909, 1974.
11. Frederick J, Braude AL: Anaerobic infection of the paranasal sinuses. N Engl J Med 290:135, 1974.
12. Chandler JR, Langenbrunner DJ, Stevens ER: The pathogenesis of orbital complications in acute sinusitis. Laryngoscope 80:1414, 1970.
13. Managlia AJ, Goodwin WJ, Arnold JE, Ganz E: Intracranial abscesses secondary to nasal, sinus, and orbital infections in adults and children. Arch Otolaryngol 115:1424, 1989.
14. Clayman GL, Adams GL, Paugh DR, Koopmann CF: Intracranial complications of paranasal sinusitis: a combined institutional review. Laryngoscope 101: 234, 1991.
15. McGill TJ, Simpson G, Healy GB: Fulminant aspergillosis of the nose and paranasal sinuses: a new clinical entity. Laryngoscope 90:748, 1980.
16. Washburn RG, Kennedy DW, Gebley MG, et al: Chronic fungal sinusitis in apparently normal hosts. Medicine (Baltimore) 67:231, 1988.
17. Fisher EW, Toma A, Fisher PH, Cheesman AD: Rhinocerebral mucormycosis: use of liposomal amphotericin B. J Laryngol Otol 105:575, 1991.
18. Cheung SW, Lee KC, Cha I: Orbitocerebral complications of *Pseudomonas* sinusitis. Laryngoscope 102: 1385, 1992.
19. Ochi JW, Harris JP, Feldman JI, Press GA: Rhinocerebral mucormycosis: results of aggressive surgical debridement and amphotericin B. Laryngoscope 98:1339, 1988.
20. Antoine GA, Raternik MH: *Bipolaris:* a serious new fungal pathogen of the paranasal sinus. Otol Head Neck Surg 100:158, 1989.
21. Henderson LT, Robbins KT, Weitzner S, et al: Benign Mucor colonization (fungus ball) associated with chronic sinusitis. South Med J 81:846, 1988.
22. Mosher HP: President's address: submaxillary fossa approach to deep pus in neck. Trans Am Acad Ophthalmol Otolaryngol 34:19, 1929.
23. Bahna J, Canalis RF: Necrotizing fasciitis (streptococcal gangrene) of the face. Arch Otolaryngol 106:648, 1980.
24. Spankus EM, Flint PW, Smith RJH, Miller RH: Craniocervical necrotizing fasciitis. Otolaryngol Head Neck Surg 92:261, 1984.
25. Lalwani AK, Kaplan MJ: Mediastinal and thoracic complications of necrotizing fasciitis of the head and neck. Head Neck 13:531, 1991.
26. Carithers HA, Margileth AM: Cat-scratch disease. Am J Dis Child 145:98, 1991.
27. Chandler JR: Malignant external otitis: further considerations. Ann Otolaryngol 86:417, 1977.
28. Kimmelman CP, Lucente FE: Use of ceftazidime for malignant external otitis. Ann Otol Rhinol Laryngol 98:721, 1989.
29. Johnson MP, Ramphal R: Malignant external otitis: report on therapy with ceftazidime and review of therapy and prognosis. Rev Infect Dis 12:173, 1990.
30. Lang R, Goshen S, Kitzes-Cohen R, Sade J: Successful treatment of malignant external otitis with oral ciprofloxacin: report of experience with 23 patients. J Infect Dis 161:537, 1991.
31. Kraus DH, Rehm SJ, Kinney SE: The evolving treatment of necrotizing external otitis. Laryngoscope 98:934, 1988.
32. Stroud MH: Treatment of suppurative perichondritis. Laryngoscope 88:176, 1978.
33. Gates FA, Avery CA, Cooper JC, Prihoda TJ: Chronic secretory otitis media: effects of surgical management. Ann Otol Rhinol Laryngol 98(Suppl 138):1, 1989.
34. Lucente FE: Otolaryngologic aspects of acquired immunodeficiency syndrome. Head Clin North Am 75:1389, 1991.
35. Greenspan D, Greenspan JS: Oral manifestations of human immunodeficiency virus infection. Dent Clin North Am 37:21, 1993.
36. Park S, Wunderlich H, Goldenberg RA, Marshall M: *Pneumocystis carinii* infection in the middle ear. Arch Otolaryngol Head Neck Surg 118:269, 1992.
37. Barnett ED, Klein JO, Pelton SI, Luginbuhl LM: Otitis media in children born to human immunodeficiency virus-infected mothers. Pediatr Infect Dis J 11:360, 1992.

38. Hall PH, Farrior JB: *Aspergillus* mastoiditis. Otolaryngol Head Neck Surg 108:167, 1993.
39. Weingarten JS, Crockett DM, Lusk RP: Fulminant aspergillosis: early cutaneous manifestations and the disease process in the immunocompromised host. Otolaryngol Head Neck Surg 97:495, 1987.
40. Rubin JS, Honigberg R: Sinusitis in patients with the acquired immunodeficiency syndrome. Ear Nose Throat J 69:460, 1990.
41. Shugar JMA, Som PM, Ryan JR, et al: Multicentric parotid cysts and cervical adenopathy in AIDS patients. A newly recognized entity: CT and MR manifestations. Laryngoscope 98:772, 1988.
42. Sperling NM, Lin P: Parotid disease associated with human immunodeficiency virus infection. Ear Nose Throat J 69:475, 1990.
43. Huang RD, Pearlman S, Friedman WH, Loree T: Benign cystic vs. solid lesions of the parotid gland in HIV patients. Head Neck 13:522, 1991.
44. Jones R, Santos JI, Overall JC: Bacterial tracheitis. JAMA 242:721, 1979.
45. Griebie M, Adams GL: *Clostridium difficile* colitis following head and neck surgery. Arch Otolaryngol 111:550, 1985.
46. McGovern FH, Fitz-Hugh JS, Constable W: Post radiation perichondritis and cartilage necrosis of the larynx. Laryngoscope 83:808, 1973.
47. Ketcham AS, Bloch JH, Crawford DT, et al: Prophylactic antibiotic therapy in control of staphylococcal infections following cancer surgery. Surg Gynecol Obstet 114:345, 1962.
48. Becker GD, Parell GJ: Cefazolin prophylaxis in head and neck cancer surgery. Ann Otol Rhinol Laryngol 88:183, 1979.
49. Robbins KT, Favrot S, Hanna D, Cole R: Risk of wound infection in patients with head and neck cancer. Head Neck 12:143, 1990.
50. Daley JM, Dudrick SJ, Copeland EM: Parenteral nutrition in patients with head and neck cancer: techniques and results. Otolaryngol Head Neck Surg 88:707, 1980.
51. Dor P, Klastersky J: Prophylactic antibiotics in oral, pharyngeal, and laryngeal surgery for cancer: a double-blind study. Laryngoscope 83:1992, 1973.
52. Gerard M, Meunier F, Dor P, et al: Antimicrobial prophylaxis for major head and neck surgery in cancer patients. Antimicrob Agents Chemother 32:1557, 1988.

Infections of the Nervous System

CHAPTER 34

Perry Black, Michael E. Carey, Thomas M. McCormack

Nervous system infections may be caused by bacteria, viruses, fungi, or parasites, which can cause diffuse or localized disease. This chapter deals primarily with focal infections of the nervous system, which produce a mass of varying size and which may be amenable to surgical intervention. Since primary attention is directed to those lesions with neurosurgical implications, diffuse infections—such as meningitis or encephalitis (other than herpes simplex encephalitis)—are not considered here.

Despite the availability of antibiotic therapy, focal bacterial infections of the central nervous system (CNS) continue to pose a serious problem with disturbingly high mortality and morbidity. Successful management of such infections entails the combination of both surgical decompression of the expanding lesion and carefully selected antibiotic therapy. This is best achieved by a collaborative effort on the part of the neurosurgeon and consultants in infectious disease and clinical microbiology, each contributing the expertise of their respective disciplines.

BRAIN ABSCESS

Pyogenic Brain Abscess

Hematogenous (*metastatic*) brain abscesses occur when bacteria from elsewhere in the body enter the bloodstream and lodge within the brain. Alternatively, brain abscesses may arise from direct brain trauma or from an adjacent inflammation, such as osteomyelitis of the skull, or sinus/mastoid infection. Occasionally, brain abscesses are a sequela of meningitis and occur postoperatively as a complication of craniotomy.

Epidemiology. Cerebral abscess may affect individuals of all ages, with peaks in the preadolescent, young adult, and middle years.[1,2] Males are more frequently involved than females.[3–5] Experience in industrialized countries indicates that an active hospital neurosurgical service may expect to see from four to ten patients each year with pyogenic brain abscess.[6–10] In the United States, the incidence has been estimated to be 1.3 per 100,000 population.[11] The situation in developing countries is quite different. In India,[12–14] pyogenic brain abscess accounts for approximately 8 to 18 percent of all intracranial space-occupying masses, and in the People's Republic of China,[5] a busy neurosurgical service may treat up to 20 brain abscesses a year.

The spectrum of brain infection varies considerably worldwide. Parasitic and tuberculous brain infections are more serious problems than pyogenic abscesses in many countries. Rodriguez et al,[15] in Mexico City, reported that cysticercosis was responsible for 85 percent of all brain infections, while tuberculomas accounted for 11 percent, and pyogenic abscesses for 3 percent. The etiology underlying pyogenic brain abscesses also varies, depending on environmental factors such as trauma[16] or the widespread existence of sinus/mastoid disease.[8] The availability of neurosurgical care and the presence of special units handling many patients with congenital cardiac abnormalities,[17] cystic fibrosis,[18] or immunologic suppression[19] may also alter the underlying etiology.

Etiology. Besides cyanotic heart disease with right-to-left cardiac shunts, pulmonary arteriovenous (A-V) fistulas may lead to brain abscesses because blood circulates from pulmonary arteries to pulmonary veins, bypassing the effective bacterial filtering ability of the pulmonary capillaries.[20,21] In infants and children, cyanotic congenital heart disease is the most common cause of brain abscess (24 percent of cases); other major sources of brain abscesses in children are head trauma, infections of the ear, nose, and throat, and cases of undetermined source.[22,23]

Hereditary hemorrhagic telangiectasia (HHT) is a vascular dysplasia wherein capillaries and small venules are deficient in muscle and elastic tissue. Arterial ectasias and arteriovenous fistulas are also common. More than 200 cases of CNS symptoms associated with HHT have been reported. While many of the CNS complications of this disease are consequent to cerebral arteriovenous malformations (AVMs), CNS infections are likely to occur in association with pulmonary AVMs. Patients with HHT have about 1000 times greater risk of brain abscess than the general population.[24] Brain abscesses have been responsible for about 13 percent of all CNS complications of HHT.[25]

Several reports associate brain abscesses with cystic fibrosis, owing most likely to recurring pulmonary infections seen in this disorder.[18,26,27]

Septic infarction may complicate the clinical course of malignancies, particularly leukemia, carcinoma, and lymphoma.[28] Often patients with systemic malignancies are immunosuppressed either because of the disease or in response to treatment. Thus about 0.5 percent of those dying of systemic cancer will have significant clinical symptoms referable to septic brain infarcts. *Aspergillus* and *Candida* species are the most common causative organisms.

Acquired immunodeficiency syndrome (AIDS) is associated with widespread infections, both systemically and within the CNS. Surprisingly, CNS infections in AIDS are usually caused by protozoa (eg, toxoplasmosis) or fungi rather than the common pyogenic organisms.

Types of Abscess

TRAUMATIC BRAIN ABSCESS. These abscesses may rise from open fractures of the skull, particularly if the dura is torn. Jennett and Miller[29] found an infection rate of 10.6 percent among 359 such fractures, usually occurring from inadequate initial wound care. In other series,[3–7,10,30] the incidence of abscesses consequent to trauma has varied from 3 to 28 percent, possibly to some extent depending on socioeconomic circumstances of various countries and neurosurgical referral patterns. Brain abscess consequent to penetrating missiles incurred in war are a special category. Carey et al[31] reported a 2 percent incidence of such abscesses. Rish et al[32] analyzed Vietnam data and found a 3 percent incidence (37 brain abscesses among 1221 patients with missile wounds to the brain). Many, but not all, of those developing a late brain abscess had associated retained bone fragments. More important than retained bone alone, however, were concomitant orbital facial wounds, wound complications, and multiple operative procedures on the brain.

ABSCESS FROM ADJACENT INFECTION. Chronic infections of the ear, nose, and throat are potential sources of infection that may spread to adjacent brain. In one series, infections of the middle ear and mastoid were the most common source (87 percent), followed by the paranasal sinuses (12 percent) and tonsils (1 percent).[33] In another series, 45 percent of patients with chronic mastoiditis (cholesteatoma) developed intradural sepsis; the bulk of these complications consisted of temporal lobe or cerebellar abscess, and a smaller number were supratentorial or posterior fossa subdural empyemas. Acute mastoiditis was only occasionally (7 percent) associated with intradural infection.[34] Although antibiotics have drastically diminished the incidence of intracranial extension of middle ear/mastoid infection, continued diagnostic vigilance concerning such complications is recommended.[35,36] Bacteria from an adjacent infected paranasal sinus or mastoid may reach the brain by direct extension from the involved sinus through the underlying dura. Bacteria may also reach the brain by local metastatic spread through venous channels that drain the sinus and enter the intracranial compartment as emissary veins. Paranasal sinus infections usually result in frontal lobe abscesses (Fig. 34–1). Mastoid infections may cause temporal lobe or cerebellar abscesses.[37] Temporal lobe abscesses are more common because the roof of the middle ear is thinner than the posterior wall.

Scalp infection, infected subgaleal effusions, or cephalohematomas may also lead to brain abscess with or without associated osteomyelitis. Bacteria from infected bone of the skull (osteomyelitis) may spread directly into the epidural space and reach the subdural compartment and brain by direct extension through the dura. Bacteria from a scalp infection or osteomyelitic bone also may reach the subdural space and brain via emissary veins. Cerebral abscess developing as a late complication of cervical traction occurs rarely; this is thought to occur by penetration of the inner table by the pins of the tongs or halo unit.[38,39]

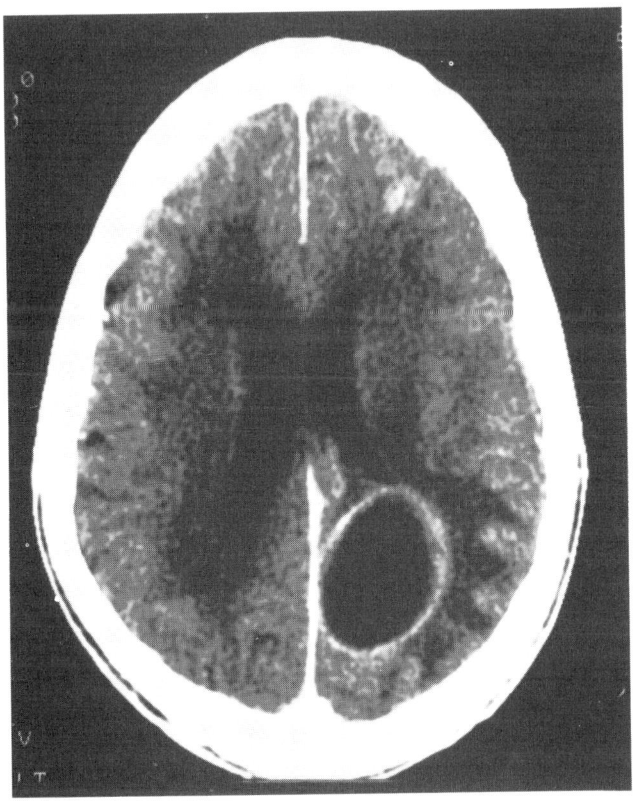

Figure 34–1. Contrast-enhanced axial CT image showing a ring-enhancing mass lesion in the left parieto-occipital lobe with central low density and surrounding vasogenic edema. Note proximity and distortion of left lateral ventricle, predisposing to intraventricular rupture and subsequent ventriculitis. CT-guided stereotaxic biopsy was carried out, with a finding of a bacterial abscess, which was aspirated.

HEMATOGENOUS (METASTATIC) BRAIN ABSCESS. These occur when bacteria from elsewhere in the body colonize the brain. Blood-borne bacteria tend to flow into the middle cerebral artery, so hematogenous abscesses are usually located in the posterior frontal and parietal lobes. Chronic pulmonary infections such as bronchiectasis are an especially common primary source of bacteria, but skin, pelvis, mouth, and long bones are other underlying infective foci. Bacterial endocarditis may also lead to brain abscess, particularly when heart valves are infected with *Staphylococcus aureus* or group D streptococci.[40] In approximately one-fifth of the cases, no apparent source of infection can be found.[2,41]

Metastatic brain abscesses initially occur at the gray-white junction, where blood flow in the brain capillary bed is slowest, but what actually allows a bacterium to adhere to and penetrate a brain capillary is unknown.

About 2 percent of all brain abscesses occur in patients with cyanotic congenital heart disease.[42] Individuals with cardiac venous-to-arterial (V-A) or "right to left" shunts are ten times[17] more likely than normal persons to develop brain abscess because bacteria intermittently present in venous blood may bypass the lungs, enter the arterial system, and pass to the brain. Most cardiac V-A shunts arise as a consequence of Fallot's tetralogy, or dextraposition of the great vessels. Furthermore, patients with cyanosis secondary to V-A shunting are at greater risk of developing brain abscess because the associated elevated hematocrit increases blood viscosity and reduces blood flow. This leads to microinfarction of the brain, which may then become colonized by bacteria. Reduced tissue P_{O_2} concentration in these patients also may enhance bacterial growth within the brain.[17,43] Patients with cyanotic, congenital heart disease also develop strokes from thromboembolic disease. Some authors[44] believe that neurologic signs and symptoms in this population are more commonly caused by brain abscesses rather than vascular occlusion or hemorrhage. They therefore advocate steps to immediately diagnose brain abscess and to begin antibiotic therapy promptly when patients with congenital heart disease develop a "stroke."

The incidence of multiple brain abscesses was found to be 13 percent of cases.[45] In that study, computed tomography (CT) scanning was reported to be vital in the detection of multiple abscesses although it is likely that magnetic resonance imaging (MRI) scanning would be at least equally accurate.

POSTMENINGITIC BRAIN ABSCESS. Considering the frequency of meningitis and the infrequency with which this type of abscess has been reported, this complication of meningitis must be quite rare in the antibiotic era. However, brain abscess may complicate pyogenic meningitis, presumably by direct bacterial colonization of the brain. Neonatal meningitis caused by *Citrobacter* is of particular concern, however, because about 40 percent of these patients develop brain abscess.[46,47] Antecedent brain softening, as from venous infarction, provides an excellent culture medium for bacteria.

Pathology. Initially, a pyogenic brain abscess begins as a focal area of bacteria-laden cerebritis. Host defense mechanisms begin to wall off the infection by capillary proliferation from the surrounding brain. Fibroblasts from the proliferating capillaries lay down collagen fibers to contain the purulent focus. Britt et al[48,49] demonstrated five histologic layers in brain abscess: zone 1, a necrotic center; zone 2, an inflammatory infiltrate mixed with macrophages and fibroblasts surrounding the necrotic center; zone 3, collagenous capsule formation; zone 4, cerebritis with neovascularity and perivascular infiltration of inflammatory cells in the adventitial sheaths of blood vessels surrounding the abscess; and zone 5, reactive astrocytes, gliosis, and cerebral edema. Brain capillaries, from which fibroblasts arise, are more numerous in the cortex and less plentiful in the white matter. Abscess encapsulation is therefore more likely to be complete superficially and deficient in the deeper white matter. Experimental data suggest that hematogenous abscesses are less well encapsulated than abscesses created by direct bacterial implantation, possibly because cerebral ischemia associated with metastatic abscess retards capsule wall formation.[50]

Britt et al[48,49] studied experimental aerobic brain abscess formation and determined four developmental stages: early cerebritis (1 to 3 days), late cerebritis (4 to 9 days); early capsule formation (10 to 13 days), and late capsule formation. Whalen and Hilal's[51] clinical data also indicated that brain abscess encapsulation requires about 2 weeks. Britt et al also studied experimental abscess formation with *Bacteroides,* an anaerobic organism that proved much more virulent than aerobic bacteria. Animals infected with *Bacteroides* did not survive into the late capsule formation stage. Virulent bacterial infections of the brain parenchyma were associated with extensive brain necrosis and edema. Generally, a brain abscess acts as an acute or subacute expanding intracranial mass,[52] often associated with enormous reactive brain swelling. The combination of the abscess mass and swelling may compress vital structures and may cause death by transtentorial herniation. Because of deficient encapsulation in the deep portion of the abscess, it may extend centripetally and rupture into the ventricle,[53] causing fatal ventriculitis/meningitis.

Clinical Manifestations. Brain abscess presents clinically in various ways:[42]

1. The *infectious syndrome*—signs of infection may be local, such as pain, redness, and swelling about an infected frontal sinus. Sometimes only general aspects of infection may be evident, for example, fever, elevated white blood cell (WBC) count, neutrophilia, and increased blood sedimentation rate.
2. The *intracranial hypertension syndrome*—papilledema, nausea, vomiting, and headaches.
3. The *syndrome of focal neurologic signs*—for example, hemiparesis or dysphagia.
4. The *meningeal syndrome*—stiff neck.
5. *Mental disturbances*—especially an alteration in the level of consciousness.

In general, headache is the most common presenting complaint. Fever is present in only half of the patients. Less than half have a focal neurological deficit and nuchal rigidity is uncommon.[1,2] The peripheral white blood cell (WBC) count is normal in 40 percent of the patients. A useful diagnostic feature is the fact that the erythrocyte sedimentation rate (ESR) is usually elevated, except in patients with cyanotic heart disease, in all of whom the ESR is normally low due to their polycythemia.[2,52] Signs and symptoms associated with a brain abscess vary according to the location of the abscess, its size, and whether or not concomitant meningitis is present. Thus the affected individual may have headache, papilledema, and an altered state of consciousness; motor, speech, or visual disturbances; focal or generalized seizures; ataxia; or signs of meningitis.

Brain abscesses are rare in the neonatal period.[54–56] Diagnosis of brain abscess in the neonate is often difficult, because few specific signs or symptoms indicating intracranial infection are present: fever is often absent but vomiting or an enlarging head may be present.[55] Convulsions are the most constant clinical sign in these young patients.[57,58] In the series of Sutton and Ouvrier,[55] the clinical diagnosis of brain abscess was suspected in only 2 of 12 infants. Therefore they recommended that an ultrasound, CT scan, or both be done in all infants presenting with bacterial meningitis.

Diagnostic Studies. When CT scanning is available, this is the primary screening modality for diagnosis of brain abscess. Equally effective, though less widely available, is MRI. Radionuclide (RN) brain scanning is also useful in diagnosis, when CT scanning is not available or is inconclusive. Plain skull films of the head are generally of limited value but may be useful in certain circumstances. Electroencephalography (EEG) may provide evidence of a localized space-occupying mass. Its use has largely been replaced by CT or MRI scanning, when these are available. Lumbar puncture is often contraindicated because of the high risk of cerebral herniation but may be considered with neurosurgical consultation if meningitis must be excluded. Angiography is now used rarely for diagnosis of brain abscess, except when modalities such as CT or MRI are unavailable. Ultrasound may be useful in identifying cerebral shift, especially in young children when the more definitive diagnostic modalities are unavailable.

COMPUTED TOMOGRAPHY SCANNING. CT scanning has revolutionized the diagnosis of brain abscess (see Fig. 34–1). The frequency with which CT identifies brain abscess reflects the prevalence of the disease in the population. Michel et al[59] (France) reported 19 brain abscesses per 8500 scans (0.2 percent), and Danziger et al[6] (South Africa) observed 90 abscesses in 11,300 CT scans (0.8 percent). In addition to promoting early diagnosis, CT scanning allows the clinician to monitor the evolution of the abscess before and after treatment. It has allowed the successful treatment of abscesses in difficult locations, such as the thalamus or brain stem, and multiple brain abscesses.[47,60,61]

One early study[62] indicated that CT scanning had about a 90 percent accuracy in diagnosing brain abscesses, but it was noted that false-negative CT scans were caused by imaging artifacts, failure to give contrast media, and scanning very early in the course of the disease, before encapsulation had occurred. Use of contrast medium for enhancement is mandatory in order to maximize the diagnostic accuracy of the scan. CT scan of brain abscess generally shows a ring-like pattern of smooth, uniform thickness that encloses a hypodense region. The dense ring, in turn, is surrounded by a hypodense area, presumably cerebral edema. Ring enhancement has been attributed to breakdown in the blood-brain barrier (BBB), vascular granulation tissue, or luxury perfusion.[63] Some abscesses appear biloculate or septate on scans.

Ring enhancement on CT scanning may appear within 2 days of the onset of neurologic symptoms. Experimentally,[64,65] a ring pattern consistent with abscess also has been observed in localized cerebritis.[66] Abscess "encapsulation" demonstrated by CT scanning may not correspond to histologic encapsulation; CT ring enhancement was seen with either cerebritis or brain abscess.[67] This observation is of more than theoretical interest for two reasons. First, if a diagnosis of brain abscess was made by CT scan but nothing could be aspirated by needle tapping because the ring-enhancing image was really cerebritis, additional brain damage could result from repeated cannulations in search of the abscess. Second, cerebritis is more amenable to antibiotic treatment than is a brain abscess. Possibly some of the reported cures of brain abscess from antibiotic therapy alone were in reality cures of cerebritis.

Even under experimental conditions, investigators initially had difficulty distinguishing cerebritis from abscess by CT.[65] Clinical and experimental studies have distinguished between cerebritis and frank brain abscess by means of serial CT scans.[64,68] In order to stage the brain abscess by this method, patients were given about 2 ml/kg of contrast medium intravenously. CT scans were then obtained at 5, 10, 20, 30, 45, and 60 minutes after injection. With cerebritis, the ring of enhancement increased for the first 10 to 20 minutes, then plateaued for an hour. The enhancing ring was thick and diffuse when first seen about the periphery of the lesion. With time, the ring tended to migrate toward the center of the lesion, which sometimes did not fill in with contrast. Brain abscesses, on the other hand, showed rapid ring contrast enhancement by 5 to 10 minutes and rapidly faded by 30 minutes. Steroid administration may decrease CT enhancement of brain abscesses in their early stages,[69] but attenuation of CT ring enhancement of a brain abscess with steroid must not be misinterpreted as resolution of infection.[70]

Cystic glioma, tumor metastases, and infarct are common lesions that may mimic abscess on CT scans. Gliomas and metastases tend to have more irregular capsules when enhanced, but, nevertheless, their CT image may be confused with that of an abscess. In one recent analysis,[71] malignant tumor was the initial scan diagnosis in 8 of 26 instances of proved brain abscess. Rapid changes on sequential CT scans favor infection. Providing clinical history to the radiologist may improve the accuracy of CT diagnosis.

CT scanning has proved an effective means for following patient progress after treatment. Some investigators believed that abscess capsule enhancement seen on CT diminished after drainage and that reduced enhancement indicated successful treatment. Conversely, persistent capsule enhancement on follow-up CT studies was thought to indicate that the abscess had refilled or extended.[62] Subsequent studies,[63] however, have indicated that even after complete, successful surgical excision of the abscess, a ring-like zone on contrast enhancement surrounding a low-density zone may be present for some time. Eventually, however, this postexcision ring gradually fades and the excision site is marked only by a region of low cerebral density. Although this persistent ring tends to be more irregular than most abscess capsules, differentiation from recurrent abscess may require considerable clinical acumen plus further sequential CT scans.

MAGNETIC RESONANCE IMAGING. MRI is effective in demonstrating brain abscesses, as well as other infections of the brain.[72] This imaging modality is more sensitive than CT in detecting the sequential changes in the development of a brain abscess.[73] Brant-Zawadzki et al[74] compared MRI and CT imaging of experimental brain abscesses. In the cerebritis stage, CT scans showed ring enhancement corresponding to the inflammatory zone and a surrounding large area of low attenuation. Spin echo MRI showed high intensity in both the dense inflammatory zone and surrounding edematous brain. This high-intensity area on MRI was more extensive than brain changes demonstrated by CT scan. The central core of the abscess was represented on the MRI by a lower intensity area. CT scanning of encapsulated abscesses showed discrete ring enhancement of the capsule, while the spin echo MRI showed a more circumscribed, peripheral, high-intensity area. The authors[74] suggested that MRI is more sensitive than CT in the early detection of cerebritis as well as adjacent cerebral edema. CT and MRI proved equal in detecting the development of central necrosis within an abscess. MRI could differentiate tissue liquefaction from simple edema because edema is seen as an area of high intensity on spin echo images, while liquefaction is shown as a low-intensity region. Capsule staging was better assessed by CT scanning.

Repeated imaging is necessary to follow the course of an abscess; in this regard, an advantage of MRI is the absence of radiation exposure. Gadolinium-DPTA, a paramagnetic contrast agent, enhances MRI imaging as a function of penetration of the BBB.[75]

RADIONUCLIDE SCANS. Radionuclides penetrate the BBB in the presence of inflammation. This alteration allows large molecules tagged with a radioactive moiety to penetrate the BBB and accumulate in the region of a lesion. Isotopic brain scans accurately identify 90 percent of all supratentorial abscesses. Posterior fossa lesions may be missed, however, because of the overlying suboccipital muscles that also take up the isotope. Radioisotope is concentrated in the abscess capsule and surrounding brain.[76] The occasional occurrence of the "ring" or "doughnut" sign may suggest a brain abscess as isotope is taken up by edematous brain and capsule but not by the pus within the abscess. Although RN scans may not distinguish between abscess, cerebritis, or neoplasm, they may delineate early cerebritis and diffuse intracranial infection better than do CT scans,[77] and therefore RN and CT scans may be considered complementary tests.[78] In one series, RN scanning delineated eight of eight brain abscesses whereas CT delineated seven of the eight. Confidence in RN scanning is important because this diagnostic tool may be available in areas where the more expensive CT is not. The use of technetium-99m-DPTA with delayed scans enhances the diagnostic sensitivity of RN scans even further.[79] Thallium localization in an abscess is nonspecific and may be confused with a neoplasm.[80] As an aid in the differential diagnosis between brain abscess and neoplasm, ^{99m}Tc-HMPAO leukocyte scintigraphy and C-reactive protein have been reported to detect brain abscess with high accuracy[81]; any steroids should be stopped for 48 hours before leukocyte scintigraphy but steroids do not interfere with C-reactive protein determination.

SKULL X-RAYS. These are helpful and may show such contiguous sources of infection as osteomyelitis of the skull or sinus/mastoid disease. A shift of the pineal gland indicates an intracranial space-occupying mass. Rarely, gas-forming bacteria within an abscess may cause diagnostic lucencies on skull films.

ELECTROENCEPHALOGRAPHY. This modality may be a useful screen for brain abscess because of the characteristic focal, low-frequency delta wave associated with this lesion. While diagnosis by EEG cannot be expected to be as precise as CT or MRI scanning, EEG is useful in situations when CT or MRI scanning is not available. In one recent series,[82] EEG predicted 11 of 13 abscesses, whereas radioisotopic brain scans localized five of six abscesses and carotid arteriograms localized six of seven lesions. Michel et al[59] compared the efficacy of EEG and CT scans. Among 19 cases, EEG patterns typical of brain abscess were seen in 6 (32 percent), while CT images diagnostic of abscess occurred in 13 (68 percent).

LUMBAR PUNCTURE. This test should not be performed when a brain abscess is suspected because it may lead to transtentorial or tonsillar herniation; furthermore, it rarely provides bacteriologic data since brain abscess only occasionally sheds organisms into the subarachnoid space. Risks of this procedure in the evaluation of brain abscess outweigh its benefits.[2,4,5,52,83]

CEREBRAL ANGIOGRAPHY. Cerebritis results in a characteristic capillary and early venous blush. This angiographic blush is possibly caused by increased cerebral perfusion associated with inflammation, in addition to the accumulation of contrast in dilated capillaries about the involved area. The angiographic diagnosis of brain abscess is made by evidence of a mass lesion and cerebritis. Evidence of leptomeningeal inflammation is indicated by the pooling of contrast within sulci and by halo formation about arterial structures. There is also angiographic staining of neovascular tissue within the abscess (the ring sign).[84,85] Where CT or MRI scanning is not sufficiently diagnostic, arteriography may differentiate tumor from abscess if neovascularity typical of tumor vessels is seen within the mass lesion.

ULTRASOUND. Yang[5] found echoencephalography 87 percent accurate for lateralizing supratentorial abscesses. Occasionally, ultrasound is capable of visualizing an abscess wall. This technique may prove particularly useful for abscess diagnosis in infants with open fontanelles and has been used to guide repeat aspiration in patients with cranial defects.[86]

Organisms Causing Pyogenic Brain Abscess

Streptococci and staphylococci are the most frequent cause of purulent brain abscesses.[1,87–92] In the antibiotic era, more mixed infections caused by gram-positive cocci and gram-negative rods have appeared. *Streptococcus faecalis, Proteus,* and *Bacteroides fragilis* are the organisms most commonly implicated in polymicrobial otogenic abscesses.[93] *Clostridium* is the organism most commonly found in postcraniotomy infection.[93]

Anaerobic bacteria have been increasingly recognized as sources of infection of the CNS, owing to improved methods of isolation and identification. The importance of anaerobic organisms has been recognized since the Heineman and Braude study[94] demonstrating their frequency in brain abscesses. In another study, anaerobic bacteria were isolated from 70 percent of the brain abscesses.[95] Brook[96] confirmed the high incidence of anaerobic organisms in the polymicrobial etiology of intracranial abscess in children. *Bacteroides* species, anaerobic streptococci, and *Fusobacterium,* either singly or in combination, are the most common anaerobes that cause brain abscesses.[48,89,95,97–99] *Bacteroides fragilis* is an obligate anaerobe that tends to produce brain abscesses, especially those following chronic middle ear and mastoid infections. The outer cell wall membrane of *B. fragilis* reacts with serum complement, which completely abolishes polymorphonuclear movement. This may give the bacteria enough time to replicate and overwhelm host defenses. These organisms also produce endotoxins, heparinase, collagenase, and hyaluronidase, which may account for their virulence. Patients with chronic diseases or who are immunosuppressed are more likely to have brain abscesses caused by unusual bacteria, such as *Listeria monocytogenes,* or by fungi. The protozoon *Toxoplasma gondii* is a common cause of CNS infection in patients with AIDS.[100,101]

Antimicrobials. Antimicrobials exert their antibacterial effects in a variety of ways. Some, such as the penicillins,[102] cephalosporins,[103] and vancomycin,[104] inhibit bacterial cell wall synthesis. Others, such as the aminoglycosides (including streptomycin),[105] tetracyclines,[106] chloramphenicol,[106] erythromycin,[107] and rifampin,[108] inhibit RNA synthesis. Chloramphenicol is bacteriostatic because it inhibits microbial protein synthesis by inhibiting peptidyltransferase. This action blocks polypeptide formation at the ribosomal site in the endoplasmic reticulum but does not produce irreversible cell damage. Metronidazole is bactericidal and damages bacterial DNA or other molecules.[109] The sulfonamides[110] inhibit intrabacterial folate synthesis. The polymyxins[111] interact with cell-wall phospholipids and act as cationic detergents or surfactants and increase the permeability of the bacterial cell wall; however, those agents are obsolete today and no longer used.

Penetration of substances across the BBB[112,113] is proportional to their lipid solubility. Antibiotics with greater lipid solubility pass the BBB more readily than do non-lipid-soluble ones. Nonionized molecules pass the BBB more readily than do ionized molecules. Penicillin G is nonlipophilic and is highly ionized at physiologic pH. Hence penicillin and other beta-lactam antibiotics do not cross the normal BBB well. With inflammation, the BBB breaks down, allowing penicillin to enter brain extracellular space.

Antibiotics highly bound to plasma proteins have low effective plasma concentrations, and consequently passage of protein-bound antibiotics across the BBB is poor. High molecular weight and complex antibiotic molecular structure also impede BBB crossover. This latter factor may help explain the poor passage of the aminoglycosides from blood to brain. Even with meningitis, penetration of the aminoglycosides can be achieved only by intrathecal administration.[105] In neonates, however, aminoglycosides do penetrate the cerebrospinal fluid (CSF) in adequate concentration. The above-enumerated factors indicate why antibiotics accumulate poorly in the CNS. Theoretically, active transport mechanisms within the BBB might enhance the passage of some antibiotic molecules from plasma to brain extracellular space.

Clinical data[106] have shown that CSF tetracycline levels are 10 to 20 percent of plasma levels. Under normal conditions, CSF erythromycin is 0 to 2 percent of the plasma level. With meningitis, however, the CSF concentration of this drug may increase to 5 to 10 percent that of plasma. Normally, vancomycin does not cross from plasma to CSF, but in the presence of meningitis, bactericidal levels of the drug may be found in spinal fluid. Despite this fact, up to 3.0 to 5.0 mg of vancomycin may be given intrathecally to combat infection if no response to parenteral administration occurs.[104] Whereas first-generation and most second-generation cephalosporins do not cross the BBB well, cefuroxime, a second-generation cephalosporin, and all third-generation cephalosporins cross the BBB readily.[103] Chloramphenicol is 60 percent protein-bound in plasma. CSF/plasma ratios of the drug vary from 35 to 65 percent regardless of the administration route and the degree of meningeal inflammation. Because the level of protein in CSF is so much lower than that in plasma, chloramphenicol may be relatively more active in CSF than in blood.[114] Most of the organisms involved in brain abscesses are susceptible to chloramphenicol. Phenytoin may increase the effective serum chloramphenicol concentration (even into toxic ranges), whereas phenobarbital may decrease it.[115] The penicillins are bactericidal for most of the common pathogenic bacteria, but some pneumococcal and group B streptococci may be resistant. Metronidazole is soluble in water and is essentially nonionized at physiologic pH. Therefore this molecule rapidly crosses the BBB and cell membranes to achieve anaerobicidal concentrations in the CSF. It is excreted in the urine. A transient opening in the BBB may be induced to allow substances that ordinarily do not pass the barrier into the brain extracellular space.[116] Neuwelt et al[117] increased gentamicin delivery to the brain 30- to 45-fold in rats by giving the drug directly into the carotid artery following BBB opening by mannitol. This approach may have human application.

Human data suggest that penetration of antibiotics into brain abscesses is unpredictable.[89] Fusidic acid has satisfactory abscess accumulation. Chloramphenicol, being a small molecule, penetrates the normal BBB well, but, unfortunately, its uptake into abscess is erratic. Penicillin and ampicillin penetrate abscesses reasonably well, and third-generation cephalosporins penetrate to produce adequate concentrations.

Black et al[118] documented six cases where antibiotics penetrated abscesses in reasonable concentrations, yet the patients continued to deteriorate until surgical treatment was undertaken. They concluded that antibiotics failed once they had reached the contents of the abscess because of poor antibiotic activity within the lesion. They hypothesized that the purulent milieu within the abscess inhibited antibiotic effectiveness.

Experimental evidence suggests that steroid administration in the treatment of experimental brain abscesses retards the passage of some antibiotics through the BBB and into the region of infection. These data suggest that antibiotic dosages should be increased to optimize drug tissue concentrations if steroids are used to treat the edema associated with brain abscesses.

Knowledge of the original infective source is useful when selecting initial antibiotic therapy—even before the organism has been identified—because specific organisms are commonly associated with certain inciting foci. According to de Louvois,[119] abscesses of sinusitic origin are often caused by carboxyphilic streptococci, frequently *Streptococcus milleri,* which are highly sensitive to penicillin. Penicillin (16 to 24 million units/24 h) should therefore be included in the treatment of brain abscesses of sinusitic origin. However, mixed aerobic and anaerobic organisms (such as *Bacteroides*) resistant to penicillin have been cultured from sinus infections.[120] Therefore it may be advisable to treat abscesses of sinusitic origin with metronidazole, in addition to penicillin. Abscesses from mastoid infection are caused by a wide range of aerobic and anaerobic bacteria. Penicillin, chloramphenicol, and metronidazole[98,121,122] or ampicillin, gentamicin, and metronidazole should be started intravenously when treating otogenic brain abscesses because of the high probability of mixed gram-positive, gram-negative aerobic and anaerobic bacteria, including *Bacteroides*. For gram-negative organisms, cefotaxime and ceftriaxone are highly effective. In some cases, clavulanic acid combined with ticarcillin has also been recommended.[123] Post-traumatic abscesses are frequently caused by *Staphylococcus aureus*.[119] Nafcillin would be a good initial antibiotic choice for these abscesses, before specific antibiotic sensitivity testing has been completed. If methicillin resistance is suspected, vancomycin should be used pending sensitivity testing of the isolate.

In rare instances when the organisms are resistant to other antibiotics, quinolones may be effective by virtue of their satisfactory penetration into the CNS. Pefloxacin (not yet available in the United States) and ciprofloxacin are two quinolones that may be considered in these cases.[124] There are, however, no clinical data on the utility of these agents in brain abscess.

DURATION OF ANTIBIOTIC TREATMENT. For aerobic bacterial abscesses, 6 weeks of antibiotic therapy is advisable. For anaerobic abscesses, 8 to 16 weeks of therapy is recommended.[125] The majority of abscesses are mixed aerobic-anaerobic infections; intravenous antibiotic therapy is recommended for 4 to 8 weeks[126]; depending on the response, an additional 4 to 8 weeks of oral therapy may be given. Fungal brain abscesses require antibiotic therapy for months.[126] *Toxoplasma gondii* brain abscess in patients with AIDS is treated indefinitely.[126]

Treatment

SURGICAL TREATMENT OF BRAIN ABSCESSES. Brain abscesses have been treated most commonly by drainage, aspiration, excision, or a combination of these methods. Drainage procedures, wherein a tube is placed into the abscess cavity, were the first to be used systematically.[127] Dandy[128] introduced the technique of abscess aspiration by one or multiple taps through a burr hole, while Vincent et al,[129] in the 1930s, advocated excision via formal craniotomy after encapsulation. Following the introduction of penicillin, LeBeau[130] demonstrated that areas of cerebritis (unencapsulated abscesses) could be excised. Reduction of abscess size by tapping or drainage in the acute phase, followed by excision of the residual capsule, was also advocated at one time.[131] Thorotrast, pantopaque, and micropaque barium have been used in the past to visualize abscess cavities, so that capsule shrinkage after drainage or aspiration could be followed on serial skull films. Such markers should not be used where CT scanning is available for follow-up, because these substances interfere with scan image. One method involves craniotomy, wide abscess incision, and pus drainage under direct vision. With this technique, the empty abscess is irrigated with antibiotic solution and left in situ. In one series, 15 consecutive cures were reported by this technique with little morbidity.[132] However, there would appear to be no particular benefit of this technique over the method of needle aspiration,[2,83] unless a refractory organism is encountered.[133]

The mortality data do not suggest strongly that one treatment type is inherently better than another. In view of the fact that the most immediate threat of brain abscess is its space-occupying mass and reactive brain swelling, the primary role of surgical intervention consists of alleviation of the increased intracranial pressure. This can be achieved by any of the methods in current use. Although the choice is one of controversy at present, the method of choice is probably less important than the relief of increased intracranial pressure (ICP) by any means before irreversible brain damage has occurred.[2,83] While abscess excision may appear logical because the brain infection is totally removed, this form of therapy is usually reserved for patients who have managed to wall off the abscess. Furthermore, patients considered for abscess excision are more often alert and in satisfactory neurological condition, indicating a more optimally functioning brain stem. Brain abscesses containing gas are probably best treated by open craniotomy and excision if it appears that the abscess is related to sinus/mastoid infection or trauma, because the air may result from a dural tear rather than gas-producing bacteria. Not only will the abscess have to be excised but the dural defect will have to be closed.[134] Simpler procedures such as drainage or aspiration are more often used with neurologically compromised patients, or those with surgically inaccessible lesions involving thalamus, basal ganglia, or brain stem. The serious disadvantage of drainage or tapping is that a multiloculated abscess may be incompletely treated. However, CT scanning, perhaps with the use of CT/stereotaxic guidance, should enable targeting of such multifocal lesions for needle aspiration. Furthermore, CT scanning can provide the surgeon with follow-up status of the lesion with repeated aspiration.

It would seem reasonable to suggest therefore that needle aspiration, with CT/stereotaxic guidance, may well become the preferred form of initial management in the future. This may be followed by excision if aspiration should fail. Whatever form of therapy is initially selected, the brain abscess may reaccumulate. It is advisable to observe the patient clinically and obtain repeated follow-up CT brain scans over a period of months and manage the patient accordingly.[135]

The surgical treatment of brain abscesses from cyanotic congenital heart disease has proved especially difficult. Kagawa et al[136] treated 17 patients with this condition by excision following aspiration with no mortality. Despite their success with aspiration followed by excision, they believe that, in the future, simple CT-guided aspiration alone may suffice.

There is no conclusive evidence that there is a difference in postoperative seizure frequency following excision versus tapping or drainage.[137,138] Abscesses in the temporal lobe or in the motor/sensory area of the brain are more susceptible to the development of seizures than lesions involving the frontal or occipital areas.

Although various forms of surgical care may be effective, the mortality is much lower when patients are in satisfactory neurologic condition, as manifested by level of consciousness. Mortality doubles, triples, or quadruples as the level of consciousness decreases, reflecting brain stem compromise from uncal or tonsillar herniation. The obvious conclusion is that for optimal neurologic results a brain abscess must be treated before it has caused irreparable brain stem damage consequent to its mass effect with increased intracranial pressure.

MEDICAL (NONSURGICAL) TREATMENT OF BRAIN ABSCESS. Past experience has indicated that surgery is the appropriate treatment for brain abscess. Nevertheless, in 1971, Heineman, Braude, and Osterholm[139] reported the successful antibiotic treatment of six patients with presumed brain abscess. Each patient had neurologic signs and in some cases EEG findings suggestive of localized intracranial infection. Chow et al[140] reported the successful antibiotic treatment of a patient presumed to have multiple *Listeria monocytogenes* brain abscesses. Traditionalists who believed that pus must be drained or otherwise removed surgically viewed these reports with some skepticism. Because no surgical intervention occurred and no histologic specimen existed, the possibility remained that these medically cured "abscesses" were, in reality, areas of cerebritis, which antibiotics might be expected to penetrate and cure. Furthermore, Black et al[118] did not have good experience with antibiotics alone in the treatment of surgically confirmed brain abscesses: antibiotics penetrated the abscesses adequately, yet viable bacteria were subsequently cultured from them, possibly because pus interfered with antibiotic activity.

The development of CT scanning made earlier diagnosis of brain abscesses more routine, since direct visualization of the lesion was possible. The course of the abscess could be followed while antibiotics were administered, presumably in preparation for surgery. Reports began to appear on occasional abscesses cured by antibiotics alone.[141–148] Computed tomography was used to diagnose and follow the abscesses in most patients, but radionuclide imaging was used once. While these reports appear encouraging, experiments by Enzmann, Britt, and Yeager[64] on dogs correlated CT scans with histologic features and indicated that cerebritis may appear with a peripheral enhancing ring on CT scans and may be confused with a true abscess. Thus some of the medical cures of brain abscess may have been cures of cerebritis instead. This caveat notwithstanding, a growing number of clinical reports have appeared, indicating that some brain abscesses diagnosed and followed by CT may be cured by antibiotics alone. Petit et al[148] reported only 1 death among 14 cases of brain abscess treated with antibiotics alone. Only four of these patients had abscesses larger than 4 cm in diameter. However, medical therapy has succeeded only about 60 percent of the time. Antimicrobials alone are more likely to be successful if the abscess is less than 3 cm in diameter and if antimicrobials are started early.[98,149,150] Leys et al[151] did not find a difference in mortality in medical versus surgical treatment in 56 patients but medically treated patients had fewer sequelae.

Rosenblum et al[149] reported successful treatment in six of ten patients with antibiotics alone and suggested that medical management be undertaken for surgically high-risk patients if they are in good neurologic status. Such patients include those with congenital heart disease, multiple or deep-lying abscesses, as well as those with concurrent meningitis, ependymitis, or hydrocephalus requiring a shunt. A report of 102 patients with brain abscess from 1970 to 1986 suggested that, although medical therapy is appropriate in a few patients, surgery remains the definitive approach for diagnosis and treatment of most brain abscesses.[152] In undertaking the medical treatment of brain abscess, penicillin G and chloramphenicol, with or without gentamicin, are started and periodic CT scans obtained. Alternatively, initial treatment may consist of a combination of metronidazole and cefotaxime (or ceftriaxone or ceftazidime); the combination of metronidazole and cefotaxime covers the common causative organisms in brain abscess and avoids the toxicity of chloramphenicol and gentamicin.[153] After 2 weeks of treatment, the patient is rescanned. Surgery is undertaken if the abscess has enlarged, significant mass effect is present, or if neurologic deterioration has occurred. If the clinical course is stable or improving, antibiotics are continued for an additional 2 weeks. The patient is rescanned weekly, or whenever new symptoms warrant. Surgery is performed if the abscess has not decreased in size after 4 weeks. If the abscess does decrease in size with medical management, antibiotics are continued for 6 to 8 weeks, and CT scans are done up to a year to ensure that the abscess does not recur. Whalen and Hilal[154] presented a series of 20 brain abscesses, 7 of which (35 percent) were cured with antibiotics and without surgery. They considered that two further criteria should be fulfilled when starting and continuing the medical management of brain abscesses: (1) the absence of increased intracranial pressure and (2) a good clinical response to medical treatment within the first week of therapy.

If medical treatment of a brain abscess is to be undertaken, it is recommended that a neurosurgeon be consulted and follow the patient closely in collaboration with a specialist in infectious diseases who is knowledgeable about available antibiotics and their potential for blood-brain barrier and brain abscess penetration. Neurosurgical intervention may have to be considered in the event of clinical deterioration.

Steroids and Brain Abscess. Steroids have been found useful in the treatment of cerebral edema associated with brain tumors.[155,156] Pyogenic brain abscesses are generally associated with significant cerebral edema, and there is a question regarding use of steroids to control the cerebral edema, especially as the mass effect of the swollen, edematous brain may contribute to fatal cerebral herniations. Steroids, however, are known to decrease the immune response consequent to infection and the possibility exists that their use could exacerbate intracranial infections.

Long and Meacham[157] examined the effect of steroid administration upon experimental brain abscess encapsulation. They concluded that dexamethasone may retard but not eliminate abscess capsule formation. Quartey et al[158] also examined the effect of glucocorticoids on experimental brain abscesses histologically and determined that steroids did indeed retard capsule formation, but they noted less edema of the adjacent tissue. Thus steroids showed two opposing effects. Reduction of surrounding edema was beneficial, but retardation of capsule formation was deleterious because viable bacteria remained in the brain. Wallenfang et al[159] used an experimental cat model to physiologically and histologically assess the problem of abscess encapsulation associated brain edema, and the effects of steroid administration. Steroids (0.5 mg dexamethasone/kg) markedly ameliorated brain edema in adjacent and distal brain. Abscess encapsulation was observed, but cats treated with antibiotics and glucocorticoid exhibited a weaker formation of the mesenchymal inflammatory infiltration.[65] Lyons et al[160] studied the effect of short-term, high-dose corticosteroids on CT enhancement of experimental brain abscesses and concluded that the use of high-dose (1.2 mg/kg), short-term (12 hours) corticosteroids did not appear to alter significantly the evolution of intracranial abscess, but, histologically, "some changes" in the amount of collagen deposition were observed. Nevertheless, these investigators could not ascertain whether the high-dose, short-term steroid administration hindered capsule formation. Enzmann et al[69] studied the effect of dexamethasone (1.8 mg/kg) given over 48 hours on the encapsulation of experimental brain abscesses. These authors concluded that a "48 hour course of steroid administration had no noticeable effect on histology of experimental brain abscesses, either in the cerebritis or capsule stage."

In the clinical setting, the use of steroids in the treatment of brain abscess is controversial[161]; some[158] avoid their use for fear of decreasing the inflammatory response and hindering encapsulation, but others believe that steroids are beneficial.[162,163] CT scanning may allow each case to be individualized. If surrounding brain edema is severe and poses a risk of neurologic deterioration, steroids (along with prompt surgical treatment) are recommended because, experimentally, they have been shown to reduce the edema associated with the abscess. It has been suggested that the use of steroids is reasonable in situations where the pathogen is known and specific antibiotic therapy is given concurrently.[2,83] If, on the other hand, the abscess is relatively small (less than 3 cm) and not associated with brain edema, antibiotics may be given alone without steroids.

Current Mortality Associated with Brain Abscess

In the early part of the antibiotic era, the mortality associated with brain abscess remained surprisingly high. In some series, lower mortality was achieved by aggressive diagnosis, timely surgery, close postoperative surveillance, and improved antibiotic usage.[1,164,165] From 1946 to 1977, surgical mortality ranged from 20 to 60 percent. Introduction of CT scanning of the brain in the mid-1970s provided a means of earlier diagnosis; Rosenblum et al[166] attributed 0 percent mortality in their series to this new diagnostic modality. Dohrmann and Elrick[30] observed that the advent of CT scanning had no apparent affect on brain abscess mortality, but Keet[167] documented a decline in mortality from 45 percent in 1952 to 1965 to 17 percent for 1977 to 1986 and attributed this to the use of CT and metronidazole. It would appear that, apart from early diagnosis and possible surgery, *the identification of the offending organism and selection of appropriate antibiotics are of paramount importance in reducing mortality and morbidity.*[2] The information provided by the CT scan regarding the status of the abscess and the surrounding brain does offer the neurosurgeon and other involved clinicians greater latitude in management: to pursue a vigorous course of antibiotic therapy; to tap, drain, or excise the abscess; or to tap and allow further encapsulation before later excision. If CT scanning is not available, clinical judgment plus the relatively accurate diagnostic modalities of EEG, RN scanning, angiography, and ultrasound in infants should permit early diagnosis and decreased mortality.

Sequelae of Management

Gruszkiewicz et al[168] reported a 12 percent incidence of neurologic sequelae among 50 survivors: hemiparesis, seizures, hemianopsia, and aphasia. In the Nielsen et al[169] series, only one-third of 67 patients showed complete neurologic recovery; and Seydoux and Francioli[170] reported 39 cases with 13 percent mortality and 22 percent severe dysfunction. In another series, 15 to 30 percent of survivors had paresis, and 10 to 20 percent had varying degrees of speech and language defects.[171] As expected, parietal abscesses are more prone to be associated with such deficits.[169] Some postabscess disability may be expected in 30 to 50 percent of all patients, whereas total disability occurs in 7 to 17 percent.[137,171] The quality of survival may be poorer in children.[55,171,172] Nielsen et al[169] observed that 29 percent of children but only 9 percent of adults had severe epilepsy, and 33 percent of children but only 13 percent of adults demonstrated intellectual reduction. Hirsch et al,[173] on the other hand, found that almost three-quarters of children who survived their brain abscesses were essentially normal.

Seizures occur in 15 to 55 percent of survivors, but up to 73 percent may report seizures if they are followed up for long periods.[138,174] Frontal and temporal abscesses are more frequently associated with epilepsy.[169] In some series, seizure development was independent of the mode of surgical therapy,[137,171] but in one review,[169] aspiration of the abscess had less of an association with late epilepsy. Aebi et al[175] found this to be true in children as well. Postabscess epilepsy has its peak incidence 4 to 5 years after abscess occurrence and treatment and may lead to death in a small percentage of those who survive their abscess with surgical treatment. Because of this, anticonvulsants should be continued for 5 years after successful brain abscess therapy. Despite a large number of drugs from which to chose, medical control of epilepsy fails in about 25 percent of cases.[169]

With respect to cerebellar abscess, neurologic sequelae following successful treatment may be minimal.[5,37,176]

Actinomycosis. Actinomycosis is a noncontagious, suppurative, bacterial infection characterized by chronic inflammatory induration, sinus tract formation, fever, and leukocytosis.[177–181] *Actinomyces israelii* is responsible for the majority of human actinomycotic infections. Once known as the "ray fungus," *A. israelii* is now recognized as a gram-positive, non-acid-fast anaerobic eubacterium, intermediate between classic bacteria and higher fungi. Unlike *Nocardia, Actinomyces* have not been isolated from the soil. The bacteria reside in natural cavities of humans and animals, particularly in the mouth. The endogenous organism gains entry to the body via breaks in the mucous membranes. Involvement of the CNS (1 to 15 percent of cases) occurs by hematogenous spread from a pulmonary focus or by direct spread from lesions involving the skull, face, and throat, possibly via lymphatics. Actinomycetales *Streptomyces* brain abscesses in AIDS patients have been reported.

Signs and symptoms of an actinomycotic brain abscess depend on location and may include focal neurologic findings as well as increased intracranial pressure. Actinomycotic brain abscess occurs more often than meningitis and subdural empyema caused by that organism. Specific diagnosis can be made by the demonstration of basophilic or amphophilic sulfur granules on microscopic examination of tissue exudates. The organisms are not visible on hematoxylin and eosin sections but may be seen with the Gomori stain. The organisms grow anaerobically.

Surgical aspiration or excision plus penicillin G, 2 to 20 million units/day for 6 to 18 months, forms the basis of treatment. A 28 percent mortality has been reported in cases adequately treated with antibiotics and surgery. Poor prognosis is related to an interval of greater than 2 months before diagnosis and treatment.

Nocardiosis. *Nocardia* are strictly aerobic, gram-positive filamentous bacteria with an unusual propensity to spread from a primary pulmonary focus to the brain.[182–186] The most common species to infect humans is *Nocardia asteroides*. Twenty to 30 percent of patients with *Nocardia* have CNS involvement, which usually occurs as a parenchymal abscess or, uncommonly, as a leptomeningitis. A case of *Nocardia* abscess complicated by a mycotic (infected) cerebral artery aneurysm has been reported. In the United States, 75 percent of nocardial infections occur in immunocompromised persons. The overall mortality of cerebral nocardiosis is 80 percent, largely because this disease occurs in people with serious underlying disease (eg, AIDS, immunosuppression associated with malignancies or following treatment for organ transplantation).

For *Nocardia* brain abscess, surgical aspiration or excision, combined with antimicrobial therapy, forms the basis of treatment. Sulfonamides are the drug of choice; this treatment should be continued for at least 1 year. Good prognostic predictors in cerebral nocardiosis include early diagnosis, appropriate chemotherapy, limited brain involvement, and, most importantly, the absence of serious underlying disease. At least one case of cerebral *Nocardia* brain abscess has been treated successfully medically, using CT to follow abscess resolution.

Multiple Brain Abscesses. Before 1975, the incidence of multiple brain abscesses reported in various series ranged from 4 to 13 percent. Since the advent of CT brain imaging, the reported incidence of multiple brain abscesses has increased to 50 percent. Earlier diagnosis and better antibiotic therapy have improved the prognosis of these lesions.

Rousseaux et al[187] reported on a series of 12 patients who had multiple (two to six) intracranial abscesses whose sizes ranged from 0.5 to 5.0 cm, with an average diameter of 1.7 cm. The causative organism was identified in only three cases. These patients were treated vigorously with intravenous ampicillin, trimethoprim-sulfamethoxazole, and sometimes with an aminoglycoside such as gentamicin, sisomycin, or tobramycin administered intramuscularly. Treatment was continued for about 3 months. The patients were monitored for bone marrow depression, renal toxicity, and cutaneous allergic phenomena. If needed, steroids or mannitol was given initially to combat associated edema. Response to therapy was provided by serial CT scans. In this series, only two patients required surgery and both survived. One patient treated with antibiotics alone eventually died, giving a 10 percent mortality for the ten persons treated without surgery.

During the 3-year interval of their study, only two instances of misdiagnosis by CT were made. In both of those cases, repeated CT scanning and lack of response to treatment indicated that the multiple lesions were tumors. Appropriate surgical therapy was then undertaken.

Boom and Tuazon[188] also have reported the successful antibiotic treatment of seven patients harboring two to ten brain abscesses each. Surgical treatment of these lesions was not considered because of their multiplicity and inaccessibility. A variety of antibiotics were used in these cases: nafcillin, dicloxacillin, chloramphenicol, penicillin G, penicillin V, and rifampin. They used intravenous antimicrobial treatment for about 2 months and then continued oral therapy for several more months. A patient's progress was followed by means of CT scanning.

These investigators concluded that high doses of antibiotics for an extended period may represent an alternative approach in cases of multiple and inaccessible brain abscesses. For this form of therapy to succeed, an early response to antibiotics must occur and follow-up CT scans must be obtained. An early effort at making a microbiologic diagnosis is important to plan optimal antibiotic therapy; CT-guided needle aspiration may be the key to diagnosis. Despite their success in this limited series, the authors reiterated the fact that surgical evacuation of pus remains essential for most brain abscesses.

Subdural Abscess and Empyema. Subdural infection accounts for approximately 10 to 32 percent of all brain abscesses. The incidence of this condition may be higher in developing countries.[3,17,69] Pus in the subdural space can be localized (abscess) or diffuse (empyema). In approximately 50 percent of cases, the subdural pus occurs as an empyema spread widely over a hemisphere (Fig. 34–2). In the remaining half, the pus is loculated as a hemispheral convexity mass (30 percent), in the interhemispheric fissure (10 percent), or in the posterior

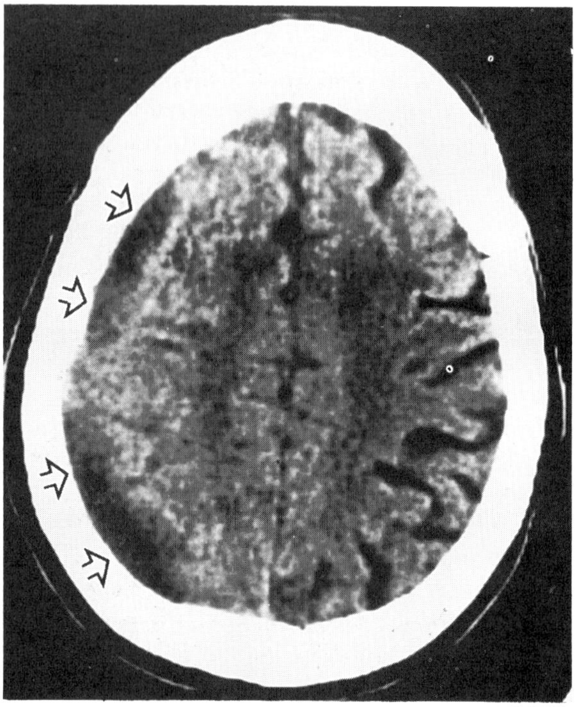

Figure 34–2. CT scan showing right subdural empyema in a 64-year-old woman admitted with sudden onset of generalized seizures. She had low-grade fever, right hemiparesis, and the peripheral white blood cell count was 19,700. With a tentative diagnosis of chronic subdural hematoma, she was taken to the operating room, and burr holes were made; there was an unexpected free flow of grossly purulent material from the subdural space. A craniotomy flap was then turned for removal of a thick yellow membrane on the cortical surface. Microbiologic studies were negative. The patient was placed on broad spectrum antibiotics and she recovered after a prolonged hospital course. There was no antecedent history suggesting source of the infection, although she had a history of chronic obstructive pulmonary disease and an episode of bronchopneumonia 1 month prior to her admission. The subdural collection in this nonenhanced CT scan covers much of the convexity of the right hemispheres (arrows); the cortical markings on that side are diminished. *(From Black P, Carey ME: Focal infections of the central nervous system, skull, and spine. In Grossman RG (ed): Principles of Neurosurgery. New York, Raven Press, 1991, pp 179–221.)*

fossa (10 percent). Acute frontal sinusitis and chronic mastoid infections are the two most common antecedent causes. Chronic otitis media is particularly likely to be the underlying cause of the empyema in developing countries such as India and Sri Lanka.[189] The infecting bacteria may spread in a contiguous fashion from the infected sinus or bone through the adjacent dura and into the subdural space or may spread from the infected sinus to emissary veins that connect with subdural veins. A septic thrombosis forming in a cortical vein creates a nidus of infection that spreads in the subdural compartment in which the pus can spread freely.[134,190,191] Subdural empyema also may occur as a consequence of trauma, cavernous sinus thrombosis, scalp infection, or infected cephalohematoma. In addition, a preexisting subdural hematoma may become infected as a result of concomitant sepsis or, iatrogenically, from needle aspirations. Subdural empyema was reported in 2 percent of patients following the treatment of meningitis.[192] Subdural empyema may complicate a subdural-peritoneal shunt as in the case of perforation of the bowel by the peritoneal end of the shunt catheter.[193] Another unusual source of subdural infection is that associated with the pins penetrating the skull for halo immobilization of the neck.[194]

Bacteriology. In a series of 66 patients with subdural empyema, aerobic or anaerobic streptococci were the infective agents in 37 cases, and staphylococci in six cases.[195] Yoshikawa et al[196] reviewed the bacteriology of subdural empyema and found that the common organisms were aerobic streptococci and staphylococci. *Salmonella* is among the uncommon offending organisms in subdural empyema; in children, *Salmonella* infection of the CNS is more commonly in the form of a subdural empyema, but in adults it is more often in the form of a brain abscess.[197] Twelve percent of cases were caused by anaerobic organisms and 27 percent of the cultures were sterile. If sterile cultures are assumed to be largely composed of inadequately cultured, anaerobic organisms, then about 40 percent of subdural infections may be caused by anaerobes. Khan and Griebel[198] confirm these bacteriologic findings. A higher mortality has been reported in patients with sterile empyema, probably as a result of inadequate therapy.[199] Post-traumatic and postoperative subdural empyemas, however, were caused by *Staphylococcus aureus* or *S. epidermidis.*

Clinical Manifestations. Subdural infection occurs more often in males. Local infection in the region of the affected sinus, scalp, or skull may be evident early, but infection within the subdural space is heralded by intense generalized headache, fever, drowsiness, meningeal signs, and focal neurological findings, such as jacksonian seizures, aphasia, or hemiparesis. Interhemispheric pus often produces a contralateral lower monoparesis, because it involves the medial portion of the motor strip. Evidence of elevated intracranial pressure (drowsiness, papilledema, nausea, vomiting) may also occur. Subdural empyema as a complication of sinusitis may be misdiagnosed as aseptic meningitis or viral encephalitis. Subdural infection is usually less fulminant than bacterial meningitis but more rapidly progressive than a brain abscess. In bacterial meningitis, focal signs are less common, and preceding sinus or mastoid infection need not be present. Clinically, differentiating between subdural infection and brain abscess may be difficult. Subdural abscess and brain abscess may be present concomitantly, but for unknown reasons, this is rare.

Laboratory Findings. Peripheral leukocytosis with a left shift is usual. The ESR is usually elevated. In the series of Khan and Griebel,[198] EEG was performed in 12 of 15 patients with subdural empyema and in 10 there was generalized or unilateral slow-wave activity or unilateral voltage suppression. In a study of EEG in the diagnosis of subdural empyema, the combination of focal theta waves, unilateral depression of cortical activity, and diffuse slowing of background activity has been regarded as being characteristic for subdural empyema and may be more sensitive than CT scanning.[200] Early in the course of the disease, CSF findings may be normal. Later, varying degrees of pleocytosis occur, the protein content increases, and the spinal fluid glucose level remains near normal. The CSF remains sterile unless there is an associated meningitis. Because subdural empyema produces an intracranial mass, there is risk that herniation and death may follow lumbar puncture. Therefore lumbar puncture should generally be deferred in patients with meningitic symptoms and focal neurologic signs until subdural (or brain) abscess has been excluded by CT or MRI scanning or angiography.[2,83,201]

Radiologic Studies. X-rays in cases of subdural empyema often suggest sinus or mastoid infection. Osteomyelitis may be seen about an involved sinus. If osteomyelitis of the cranial vault is the underlying source of subdural infection, it may be evident on skull films. In view of the frequent association of subdural empyema with paranasal sinus disease, plain x-ray studies of the skull and sinuses should be obtained, especially since the initial CT scan may be normal.[202]

Danziger et al[6] analyzed 11,300 CT scans in South Africa and observed 23 (0.2 percent) cases of subdural empyema. On CT scan, a subdural empyema usually appears as a crescentic lesion at the periphery of the brain. Enhancement may demonstrate a rim adjacent to the cortex, and this rim may thicken with time. The ipsilateral ventricle may be displaced. This rim may be thicker with chronic processes. Cerebral edema is not a prominent feature. CT scanning may fail to help in diagnosing subdural empyema, presumably because, at some evolutionary stage in its development, the combination of brain and pus is isodense.[66,203] An illustration of a CT scan showing unilateral subdural empyema is shown in Figure 34–2. The incidence of false-negative CT scans may be reduced by routine use of contrast-enhanced CT in suspected cases and, where feasible, the use of high-resolution scanners.[204]

MRI has been reported as being superior to CT in identifying the presence and extent of subdural empyemas and in distinguishing empyema from chronic subdural hematoma.[205] A similar advantage has been shown in distinguishing *epidural* empyema from *subdural* empyema.[206] Coronal MRI scanning may demonstrate subtemporal extension of the empyema.[73] In some instances, RN scans may reveal the empyema[201,207] and cerebral angiography will also reveal the pus collection.[208] In patients with subdural collections complicating *Hemophilus influenzae* meningitis, CT scanning is not reliable in distinguishing sterile effusions from infected collections (empyema).[209] The accuracy of CT scanning is increased, when combined with examination of *Hemophilus influenzae* capsular antigen; this combination of diagnostic modalities accurately predicts if the subdural collection is infected or is likely to become infected.[209] MRI has been helpful in this differentiation.[210]

In the past, ventriculography was used to diagnose posterior fossa empyema; however, air studies are no longer considered as useful diagnostic modalities when high-resolution CT or MRI scanning is available.

Pathophysiology. Several pathophysiologic processes may be responsible for the rapid clinical deterioration seen in cases of subdural empyema. Bacterial metabolic products or toxins may adversely affect neural-glial function. BBB breakdown may cause cerebral edema. Cortical vein thrombosis may lead to associated cerebral hemisphere infarction, and, finally, the mass of the subdural collection may lead to cerebral herniation.[211]

Treatment. Subdural empyema represents a neurosurgical emergency. Early drainage is essential because antibiotics may not eradicate the infection.[212] The rapid accumulation of subdural pus can dangerously increase intracranial pressure. Once the diagnosis is suspected, large doses of broad spectrum antibiotics should be started (such as a combination of penicillin G, chloramphenicol, and nafcillin) and the patient prepared for operation. Some surgeons drain the pus via multiple burr holes placed over the involved area, while others prefer limited craniectomies or even large craniotomy flaps to expose widely the subdural infection. Bannister et al[195] recommended wide craniotomy; of 66 patients in this series, 14 of 27 patients treated by burr holes died but only 5 of 35 died after craniotomy. Several series have reported that later craniotomy was needed for some patients initially treated by burr holes.[189,201] However, Bok et al[213] have reported that burr holes or a small craniotomy can adequately control the infection. Areas of subdural abscess are copiously irrigated with such antibiotic solutions as bacitracin (or gentamicin). It is crucial that a specimen of the pus be obtained for Gram stain and culture for aerobic, anaerobic, fungal, and mycobacterial organisms to aid in selection of antibiotics.

When an interhemispheric subdural abscess is suspected, the patient's head should be draped so that trephinations or craniectomy can be performed parasagittally from front to back and the entire interhemispheric region may be inspected, drained, and irrigated with antibiotic solution. Any undetected, undrained pus pockets may lead to persistence of the intracranial infection. Posterior fossa subdural empyema is either otogenic in origin or has spread from supratentorial subdural empyema. The diagnosis may be delayed, even with the aid of the new imaging techniques. Posterior fossa craniectomy is recommended as the operation of choice, in preference to posterior fossa burr holes.[214]

In the management of subdural fluid collection in infant *Hemophilus influenzae* meningitis, Curless[215] has reported that subdural taps and systemic antibiotics are usually effective. Another option is burr hole and catheter drainage, along with antibiotic therapy.[216] Although the consensus among most authors favors aggressive surgical evacuation of subdural intracranial empyemas, a minority viewpoint advocates treatment with antibiotics without surgery.[151,217] The latter authors emphasize the use of CT for diagnosis and follow-up during the course of antibiotic treatment.

The primary focus of infection leading to the subdural suppuration also must be vigorously treated. When osteomyelitis of the frontal sinus is present, the infected bone should be removed and the frontal sinus exenterated. If the skull and inner sinus wall appear intact, the involved sinus should be drained. Surgery for sinus, middle ear, or mastoid infection can be performed electively[218] or simultaneously with the evacuation of the subdural empyema. Surgical intervention reduced length of stay and the number of patients requiring reexploration.[219]

Prognosis. Prior to the use of antibiotics, subdural empyema was usually lethal, but mortality has now declined to 10 to 20 percent.[218] In the preantibiotic era, almost all patients died.[220] As with brain abscesses, mortality from subdural empyema increases with neurologic deterioration and for the same reasons.[198,201] Bilateral spread of pus is a common cause of mortality. Early diagnosis and bacteriologic study for selection of proper antibiotics are likely to reduce the mortality. Survivors may be neurologically intact, but focal neurologic deficits, such as hemiparesis or dysphasia, are common. Seizures occur in one-fourth to one-third of survivors but may be controlled by anticonvulsant medication.[198] Calliauw et al[221] followed 18 patients with subdural empyema more than 5 years after successful surgical therapy. None developed seizures after the second year following their empyema. Therefore, anticonvulsants should be given for approximately 2 years after successful treatment of a subdural empyema. A similar experience was reported by Cowie and Williams.[211]

Intracranial Tuberculoma

Tuberculosis of the central nervous system may damage the brain in many ways. A dense basal exudate can form, which may obstruct CSF flow. Extension of this basal exudate into the brain parenchyma itself may cause a border-zone encephalitis. Multiple small foci of ischemia may occur consequent to vasculitis involving many small blood vessels. Infiltration of the meningeal exudate into the walls of larger, basilar blood vessels may cause brain stem infarcts. Intracranial tuberculomas may form, which act as both mass and inflammatory lesions with accompanying edema. The pathologic changes in and around the reactive border zone of tuberculomas has suggested a delayed type of hypersensitivity to tuberculoprotein, which is thought to initiate the "chain of immunologic responses."[222] Occasionally, a more acute form of brain edema develops with a diffuse, perivascular loss of myelin as an allergic hypersensitivity reaction to tuberculoprotein or to the brain's myelin basic protein.[223]

The incidence of focal tuberculous infection of the brain—intracranial tuberculoma—varies according to the prevalence of tuberculosis in the community. While intracranial tuberculosis is extremely common in developing countries, epidemiologic data from developed countries are scarce:

89 tuberculomas were found in 13,000 autopsies (0.68 percent) in Leeds, England (1933),[224] whereas 43 were discovered during 15,000 postmortem exams (0.29 percent) in Los Angeles (1938).[225] Thus physicians in developed countries may fail to recognize the disease because of its rarity. Tuberculosis may be quite prevalent among immigrants from developing areas who come to developed countries.[226] According to reports from countries where intracranial tuberculomas are common, 32 to 50 percent of patients with intracranial tuberculomas are less than 10 years of age and approximately 85 percent are younger than 25.[223,227,228] Tuberculomas may occur anywhere in the brain, but affected children have a high incidence of infratentorial lesions.

Pathology. Grossly, a mature tuberculoma is a well-defined, avascular mass with multiple nodular extensions and a yellowish gritty, caseating central core. In its immature form, the lesion consists of multiple small tubercles with caseating or cystic centers surrounded by edematous brain. More than half are adherent to the dura. Microscopically, the central core of caseous necrosis is surrounded by tuberculous granulation tissue consisting of epithelioid cells, Langhans' giant cells, lymphocytes, polymorphonuclear cells, and plasma cells. Acid-fast bacilli may be seen in either layer. The surrounding brain shows degenerated nerve cells and fibers, swollen astrocytes, and oligodendroglia, as well as thrombosed vessels and multiple microinfarcts. Rarely, frank tuberculous abscess resembling a pyogenic abscess may occur.[229,230] Several cystic tuberculomas resembling gliomas have also been observed.[223,228]

Clinical Manifestations and Diagnosis. Patients with intracranial tuberculomas usually have evidence of the disease elsewhere or have had tuberculosis.[231,232] Fever of a few weeks duration usually precedes the onset of neurologic findings, which will vary according to tuberculoma location. Seizures often occur with supratentorial lesions. Children often evidence a posterior fossa mass: headaches, nausea, vomiting, papilledema, nystagmus, ataxia, and separated cranial sutures or an enlarging head. Unusual presentations of tuberculomas include scalp swelling, or a draining sinus, CSF rhinnorhea, exophthalmos, trigeminal neuralgia, or evidence of pituitary or acoustic nerve "tumors."[223]

Intracranial tuberculomas can be diagnosed with a fair degree of precision by CT, especially in geographic areas where tuberculosis is endemic. The CT scan appearance of an intracranial tuberculoma has been classified as (1) small discs and rings measuring less than 1 cm in diameter with marked contrast enhancement and surrounding low-attenuation edema; (2) large rings but lacking the low central lucency of pyogenic abscesses; a central nidus may be present, the so-called target sign; and (3) large nodular mass, ball-shaped with irregular contours.[233] The lesions may be solitary or multiple. While CT scanning is the ideal diagnostic procedure, it may be unavailable in developing nations where intracranial tuberculomas are most common.[234]

On MRI, tuberculomas have been described as isointensive on T1 and hyperintensive on T2 weighting; marked gadolinium contrast enhancement was seen.[235] When CT or MRI scanning is not available, plain skull x-rays, electroencephalography, RN scans, angiography, and ventriculography are still useful. In general, 2 to 6 percent of intracranial tuberculomas calcify, but, among Eskimos and North American Indians, 60 percent of the lesions show calcification.[223]

Angiographically, a tuberculoma presents as an avascular mass. Vessels in the vicinity may show a reduced caliber, and the midline shift may be small relative to the size of the lesion. Tuberculomas near the surface may occasionally show a blush from meningeal or cortical vessels.

Treatment. Until the advent of CT scanning, surgical resection of intracranial space-occupying lesions caused by tuberculomas was the preferred treatment. Before the development of effective antituberculous chemotherapy, surgical resection of these lesions carried a mortality of up to 85 percent from subsequent tuberculous meningitis.[227] Total excision of the tuberculoma is preferred, but partial excision may be done when large tuberculomas impinge on vital structures, such as the brain stem.[227,228,236] In such cases, a rim of tuberculoma may be left adjacent to the brain.

Following the development of effective drug therapy, operative mortality for intracranial tuberculoma resection fell to about 14 percent, and the incidence of fatal, postoperative tuberculous meningitis was 6 percent. Whereas total excision of the lesion is preferred, partial removal has been advised when large tuberculomas impinge on vital structures.[223,227,228,232] In such cases, it is advisable to treat the residual lesion with antituberculous drugs. Various combinations of rifampin, streptomycin, para-aminosalicyclic acid, and isoniazid are used pre- and postoperatively (see Chap. 24).

Paralleling the development of nonoperative treatment for pyogenic brain abscesses, an initial nonoperative approach for the treatment of intracranial tuberculomas has emerged. This has been possible with the advent of CT and MRI scanning for follow-up. Antituberculous drug therapy alone may be curative, especially for small lesions. A therapeutic trial on antituberculous medication is a reasonable approach. CT-guided biopsy for histology and culture may be carried out for confirmation. Surgical resection may be required to reduce intracranial pressure in the case of large lesions.

In 1983, Harder et al[237] reported on a series of 20 patients with intracranial tuberculomas. Ten patients were treated surgically, whereas ten were treated with antituberculous drugs alone. The progress of the medically treated patients was followed serially by CT scanning. No patients died in either group, but the functional state of those treated medically was significantly better than those who had surgery as their primary therapy.

Tandon and Bhargava[233] reported their experience with 50 patients with intracranial tuberculomas. In these patients, neither vision nor life was threatened by severe intracranial hypertension. All were treated primarily with antituberculous therapy, and serial CT scans were obtained to follow their progress. The authors divided their cases into three groups: (1) lesions larger than 1 cm, (2) multiple ring or disc lesions less than 1 cm in diameter, and (3) solitary ring or disc lesions less than 1 cm in diameter. This study clearly showed that most intracranial tuberculomas resolve under medical management.

In conclusion, it seems that CT scan or CT scan plus angiography can provide a high level of diagnostic confidence with regard to intracranial tuberculomas. If intracranial tuberculoma is suspected, intensive antituberculous therapy is started and continued for 2 weeks. Serial CT scans are obtained to follow the course of treatment, which is continued for at least 12 months.

If the nature of the lesion is in doubt, either a therapeutic trial of antituberculous drugs is initiated or biopsy (stereotaxic or open) is obtained. If there is biopsy confirmation of tuberculoma, it is generally not necessary to excise the lesion, and reliance is placed on antituberculous drugs to optimize long-term neurologic function.

Patients with large tuberculomas, with signs of raised intracranial pressure threatening vision or life, may require surgical excision of the lesion before starting medical treatment. However, if intracranial pressure is not severely elevated, or if visual loss is not threatened, patients suspected of having intracranial tuberculomas can be given a trial of medical therapy. Surgery can be reserved for nonresponders. Papilledema without a serious loss of vision is not considered a contraindication to medical treatment.[238–240]

Steroids may be used when cerebral edema is severe, without fear of exacerbating the intracranial tuberculoma, provided antituberculous therapy is given concurrently. Isoniazid, ethambutol, and rifampin in recommended doses provide adequate coverage.

Intracranial tuberculous lesions may paradoxically enlarge during antituberculous therapy, and resolution of the tuberculous lesion demonstrated on CT scan may take several years. However, long-term therapy may lead to resolution.[241] If CSF pathways are blocked, a shunt procedure may be required.[242]

Herpes Simplex Encephalitis (HSE)

Herpes is probably the most frequent cause of sporadic, viral infection with severe neurologic sequelae in temperate climates, including the United States.[243–246] The occurrence rate is believed to be about two cases per million population per year.[247] The virus infects the nasal mucosa and nasopharynx and penetrates the CNS through the cribriform plate.[248] Pathologically, perivascular lymphocytic infiltration is seen, along with severe necrosis of the medial temporal and orbital frontal lobes. Other areas in the brain are less often involved.[249] Type A Cowdry eosinophilic inclusions are seen in both neurons and glia.[250] Electron microscopy demonstrates herpes virus particles within affected cells.[243] Often, severe temporal lobe swelling accompanies the infection and may cause a significant intracranial mass lesion that may have to be removed surgically.

Clinical Manifestations and Diagnosis. Clinically, HSE is manifested by headache, drowsiness, fever, seizures, and focal neurologic signs. Meningeal signs are not prominent. These nonspecific findings may be seen with many types of encephalitis, but herpes infection is characterized by prominent psychological symptoms early in the disease (global confusion, disorientation, clouding of consciousness, and hallucinations, particularly olfactory and gustatory), because of temporal lobe involvement.[250] Early diagnosis of herpes is paramount because, untreated, the disease has a high mortality and may be associated with severe neurologic sequelae in survivors. EEG usually shows temporal high-voltage sharp waves. RN scanning is characterized by unilateral or bilateral areas of hyperperfusion with focal uptake on the static images. When bilateral, this strongly suggests HSE.[66] After the disease is established, CT scans reveal a low-density area, usually in the medial temporal lobe, unilaterally or bilaterally. There is an irregular pattern of contrast enhancement. These three neurodiagnostic modalities are positive in about 80 percent of cases.[251] MRI scanning is more sensitive than CT in detecting early changes; particularly, petechial hemorrhages, commonly seen pathologically in HSE, may not be detected on CT scanning but are readily seen on MRI scanning, thereby improving diagnostic specificity.[73] Failures probably relate to the stages of the disease at which the tests are performed. Fluorescent antibodies of the herpesvirus antigen and a passive hemagglutinating antibody may be demonstrated in the cerebrospinal fluid. Polymerase chain reaction testing of CSF may also demonstrate the presence of HSV in CSF.[252,253]

Treatment. In the late 1970s, mortality of biopsy-proven HSE was shown to be more than 70 percent[254] and neurologic sequelae were noted to be severe among survivors.[254–257] Adenine arabinoside (Ara-A, vidarabine) was found to be a fairly effective antiviral agent for the treatment of HSE, reducing mortality to about 47 percent[257] (see Chap. 24). After the original report of Whitley et al[257] showing the efficacy of vidarabine, a subsequent study[258] raised questions about the usefulness of this drug, but further uncontrolled studies[251,259] by Whitley's group supported vidarabine, though the mortality of HSE still approximated 50 percent with the use of the drug.

In 1984, Skoldenberg et al[247] studied 51 patients with HSE to compare the effectiveness of vidarabine with acyclovir, a purine nucleoside analog. Acyclovir appeared distinctly more effective than vidarabine, but factors such as level of consciousness, age of patient, and absence of brain biopsies to absolutely prove that each patient had HSE could have affected the results. Subsequent studies indicated the superiority of acyclovir in terms of mortality.[260,261]

Survival was found to be influenced by patient age, level of consciousness, and duration of disease before the start of therapy. Even with statistical adjustments to account for these factors, however, acyclovir was seen to be the superior drug for reducing HSE mortality.

With both drugs, survival and return to normal function have been positively correlated with adequacy of neurologic function. Acyclovir treatment must be started as soon as possible when HSE is suspected. Whitley et al,[257] in particular, believe that brain biopsy is mandatory to confirm the diagnosis. The biopsy can be carried out with CT guidance.[262] Brain biopsy may reveal conditions other than herpes simplex encephalitis, such as tuberculous and cryptococcal meningitis or subdural empyema. The risk to the operating team in obtaining a biopsy in such patients is thought to be minimal.[263] Biopsy is also recommended in infants and children with suspected herpes simplex virus encephalitis.[264] If one suspects HSE, acyclovir should be started even before brain biopsy is obtained. Side effects from acyclovir have, thus far, been minimal, so the drug may safely be continued while awaiting HSE viral cultures. If the herpesvirus is isolated, drug therapy is continued for 10 days. Because acyclovir is nontoxic, one may make a cogent argument for continuing the drug a full 10 days in the face of negative HSE viral cultures because brain biopsy may miss the herpes focus 25 percent of the time.[248]

Despite the safety of antiviral drug therapy, brain biopsy has been recommended in patients with possible HSE.[265,266] These authors state that the rationale is not to confirm HSE but rather to rule out other treatable conditions. Such conditions may be suspected in patients with low CSF glucose, raising suspicion of infections such as tuberculosis, brain abscess, toxoplasmosis, or cryptococcosis. Using decision analysis theory, Soong et al[267] also favor biopsy in selected patients in which HSE is suspected.

Parasitic Abscess

Cysticercosis

Life Cycle. Humans are the definitive hosts for the pork tapeworm, *Taenia solium.* The adult form of the tapeworm lives in the human small intestine. The pig itself becomes infected with the parasite by eating ova or gravid worm segments from human excreta. Once the pig ingests the ova, the surrounding capsule is digested away and contained larvae penetrate the pig's stomach mucosa and are disseminated widely in the animal's body. Humans, after ingesting infested pork, develop a mature tapeworm in the small intestine. Humans can harbor not only the mature tapeworm but may also become infested with the larval form (*Cysticercus cellulosae*). Vomiting or reverse peristalsis delivers proglottids from the small intestine to the stomach.[268–270] In humans, once the larvae penetrate the gastric mucosa, dissemination to the brain is the rule.

Despite these presumed mechanisms of infection, much is unknown about the transmission of the disease. Relative to the probability of fecal-oral contamination, simultaneous infestation with both the adult and larval forms of the parasite is uncommon in those with cysticercosis. Cysticercosis is prevalent in countries where uncooked pork is eaten, but the disease is also endemic in India where eating uncooked or raw pork is very rare.[270]

Incidence. This parasitic infestation is relatively common in economically developing countries such as Mexico, Central and South America, Africa, and India. Although traditionally rare in developed countries,[271] there has been an increasing incidence in children in the United States[272] and in Australia,[273] related to immigrant populations and travelers from endemic areas. The migration of Mexican and Central American people into southern and southwestern states in the United States has made cysticercosis a more common diagnostic consideration in cities such as Los Angeles.[274]

In Mexico and many Central and South American countries, 2 to 5 percent of all pigs slaughtered have evidence of cysticercosis. Among all autopsies performed at the General Hospital in Mexico City, 3.6 percent had evidence of cysticercosis while at the Federal University of Parana, Brazil, 2.2 percent of 7567 brain CT scans showed evidence of cysticercosis. Cerebral cysticercosis recently accounted for 13 to 33 percent of all space-occupying intracranial lesions at the Mexico City General Hospital.[270] By contrast, Courville[275] from the United States found only 22 cases of cysticercosis among 3000 verified brain tumors.

Pathology. Pathologically, the disease may result in (1) meningoencephalitis, (2) granulomatous meningitis, (3) focal granulomas (aseptic abscess), (4) focal cysts, (5) hydrocephalus (communicating or obstructive), (6) ependymitis, or (7) arteritis.[270,276] Living cysts within the brain incite little or no nearby tissue reaction and infested patients may be asymptomatic. When the organisms within the cysts die (after 18 months or so), they cause an intense inflammatory reaction around the cysts. Patients often become symptomatic during this stage, with seizures and focal findings. Finally, dead cysts are reabsorbed and calcification of the lesion occurs; heterotopic bone formation has also been described, presumably secondary to new bone formation around muscle cysticerci.[277] The parasite also may exist in a racemose form about the base of the brain. Some evidence suggests that intraparenchymal brain cysts form if spread to the central nervous system occurs via the carotid artery, whereas the racemose form appears when cerebral spread has occurred via the vertebral artery.

Clinical Manifestations and Diagnosis. Clinical symptomatology depends on the number of cysts, their size, location, and the toxic quality of the parasite. The clinical course of the disease is characterized by remissions and recurrences. Intracranial cysts produce five basic clinical disorders: (1) convulsions, (2) "pseudotumor" from diffuse parenchymal involvement with raised intracranial pressure and small ventricles, (3) intracranial space-occupying lesion (cerebral cysticercosis with focal symptoms), (4) meningoencephalitis, and (5) psychiatric disturbances.[270] Intraventricular cysts occur in 15 to 20 percent of patients with neurocysticercosis. Possibly the larval oncospheres reach the ventricles via the choroid plexus. Intraventricular cysts may lead to positional headaches, rapid deterioration of level of consciousness, and death from acute obstruction of CSF flow. Obstruction to CSF flow by the racemose basal form of the disease is usually more chronic and less catastrophic than obstruction to flow caused by an intraventricular cyst that happens to block the intracerebral CSF pathway.[278]

If the associated basal leptomeningitis is severe and extends to involve the cord, amyotrophy and spastic paresis can also occur. Remote cysts about the chiasm may cause blindness.[279]

Plain x-rays of the skull may reveal evidence of increased intracranial pressure or intracranial calcifications. However, CT and MRI scanning are the best diagnostic modalities. CT scanning is accurate[280] and is particularly useful in detecting parenchymal calcifications within dead larvae.[281] CT can detect intraparenchymatous calcifications and cysts, intraventricular cysts (with the aid of injected contrast media), and hydrocephalus.[282] Cysticercosal calcifications, several millimeters in diameter and scattered through the brain parenchyma, occur in about 65 percent of patients.[283] Calcifications are more common in adults, whereas diffuse homogeneously enhancing lesions are more often seen in children.[284] Cysts occur about 25 percent of the time and these may occur within brain parenchyma or within the ventricles.[283] Over 40 percent will show hydrocephalus by CT, but scanning may not delineate its cause because the intraventricular or subarachnoid parasitic cysts are of CSF density. Furthermore, racemose organisms at the base of the brain will not be delineated by CT scanning. Intraventricular contrast may outline intraventricular cysts, which may change in position.[284] CT scans of the acute parenchymatous form of cysticercosis may reveal (1) diffuse low-density areas within the white matter that enhance with contrast plus compressed but undisplaced ventricles, (2) multiple small low-density areas with discrete rounded central enhancement, or (3) large cystic lesions that "ring enhance." Multiple cystic lesions occur about 85 percent of the time while the lesions are solitary in 15 percent of the cases.[285]

The advent of CT scanning has enabled investigators to follow the natural evolution of intracranial cysticercosis, and intraparenchymal cysts have been observed to disappear spontaneously and be replaced by a small area of calcification.[286] Thus it appears that neural cysticercosis may be well tolerated by some individuals. Spontaneous cyst disappearance makes it somewhat difficult to evaluate drug treatment, which also may cause cyst involution. Contrast enhancement seen about intraventricular cysts indicates the presence of a granular ependymitis with adhesions between the cyst wall and ependyma.[284] When this phenomenon is seen, owing to ependymal inflammation, CSF shunting may be necessary even if the cyst is successfully excised. Before the availability of CT scanning, Skromme-Kadlubik et al[287] tagged anticyst antibodies to indium-113. Intracranial cysticercosal cysts selectively concentrated this isotope and presented increased activity on radioisotope scans.[287]

MRI, especially with the use of intravenous contrast, is also highly accurate in localizing lesions of cerebral cysticercosis.[288] T1 weighted images are effective in early detection of intraventricular lesions.[281]

Peripheral blood smear may show eosinophilia. Spinal fluid glucose is usually low but protein is usually elevated; CSF eosinophilia occurs in about 20 percent of patients.

Indirect hemagglutination tests against cysticercosal antigen may be positive in blood or CSF. CSF complement fixation tests against the parasite generally yield positive results, but the assay can be difficult to perform because no standardized antigens or assay techniques exist. Cysticercosal antigens cross-reacting with echinococcus or schistosomiasis may also be a problem.[289–291] Other tests that have been used to detect cysticercosis include agar gel precipitation, immunoelectrophoresis, counterelectrophoresis, indirect immunofluorescence, blastoid transformation, and skin reaction, each with variable rates of success.[270]

Treatment. Praziquantel is an antihelminthic that is quite effective against cysticercosis. Sotelo et al[292] presented 26 patients treated with this drug. After 3 months all patients had improved clinically and 50 percent were asymptomatic. The drug is tolerated quite well.[293]

Patients receiving praziquantel exhibit side effects owing to the brain's inflammatory reaction to dying and dead parasites. To combat this reaction, some authors have recommended concomitant steroid administration, along with praziquantel. Ciferri[294] compiled four large series of patients with neurocysticercosis treated with praziquantel. Only 11 to 16 percent of patients who received steroids along with praziquantel exhibited adverse reactions, whereas 92 to 100 percent of patients receiving praziquantel alone had adverse reactions from dying parasites. DeGhetaldi et al[295] concluded that praziquantel alone is a remarkably safe drug when administered to healthy volunteers but becomes increasingly hazardous in patients with severe neurocysticercosis. These investigators felt that steroids should be given along with the praziquantel; the benefits of a 1- to 2-month course of steroids to suppress the brain's reaction to dying and dead organisms far outweighed the risks of potential, steroid-induced side effects.

The efficacy of praziquantel may radically alter the indications for surgery in neurocysticercosis. In the past, it was pointed out that up to 90 percent of patients with CT-demonstrated hemisphere lesions have a nonprogressive course not requiring surgery[296] and patients presenting with epilepsy as the only clinical manifestation were often successfully treated with standard antiepileptic drugs alone.[270] One may surmise that patients presenting with a pseudotumor syndrome from miliary cysts, edema, and small ventricles can be treated successfully with praziquantel and steroids.

Should surgery become necessary, the best operative results (75 percent improvement, 24 percent mortality) have been obtained with excision of cysticerci, which form a single, discrete, space-occupying lesion within the brain and produce focal signs. The poorest results (28 percent improvement, 67 percent mortality) have been seen in patients who developed basal leptomeningeal infection.[297] Some authors recommend surgical excision of cysticercosis cysts when they produce focal symptoms and are surgically accessible.[298] In a series of 141 patients with neurocysticercosis, over 50 percent were cured following praziquantel treatment; intraventricular cysts were unaffected by the drug and had to be surgically removed.[299] Intraoperative ultrasound (neurosonography) is helpful in detecting subcortical lesions.[300] Many experienced with cysticercosis cerebri advocate leaving basal cysts in situ. They prefer to deal with the problem of CSF obstruction by communicating the temporal horn with the cisterna ambiens or use of standard CSF shunt.

Spread of the organisms by shunting the CSF is unlikely because cysticercosis cysts are rarely found in the lateral ventricles. Intraventricular cysts are potentially dangerous because they may migrate, plug CSF circulation pathways within the brain, and lead to acute hydrocephalus and abrupt death. They may be removed by a direct surgical approach or stereotaxically.[274] If the cyst is unruptured or has not incited a granular ependymal reaction (determined by enhancement of the cyst on preoperative CT scans), simple cyst removal may suffice. Sometimes, CSF shunts are required even after successful cyst removal if tissue reaction to the parasite obliterates CSF pathways.[274,296] Occasionally, patients with acute obstructive hydrocephalus will require shunting *before* cyst removal in order to reduce intracranial pressure.[278]

Echinococcus Granulosus

Life Cycle and Incidence. Hydatid disease in humans is caused by the larval stage of the tapeworm *Echinococcus granulosus.* The mature worm lives in the intestine of the dog. Ova passed in dogs' feces infect grass eaten by sheep in whose lungs, liver, or other abdominal organs the ova develop into encysted embryos. If a dog eats the offal of infected sheep, the parasite matures in the dog's intestine and its life cycle is repeated. Human infection arises by contamination of food by dust containing viable ova or by oral contamination from the hands after handling infected dogs. Only about 2 percent of those who develop echinococcal disease have CNS involvement.[301] Nevertheless, hydatid cysts account for about 2 to 3 percent of intracranial space-occupying lesions in Ankara, Turkey.[302] Children are affected 2.5 times more frequently than adults. In countries where hydatidosis is common, up to 50 percent of childhood tumors of the CNS turned out to be hydatid cysts.

Pathology. The disease exists in two forms. Intracranially, the discrete and encapsulated hydatid cyst acts as a space-occupying lesion. Because cerebral hydatid cysts are frequently single, surgical therapy is often successful (Fig. 34–3). Most cysts start in the subcortical area and spread deeper into the white matter. The cerebral hemispheres are more often infected than the cerebellum. Intraventricular and even intrasellar cysts have been reported.[303,304] The unencapsulated parasite may invade the bone of the cranium.

Clinical Manifestations and Diagnosis. In children, the peak incidence occurs between ages 5 and 10.

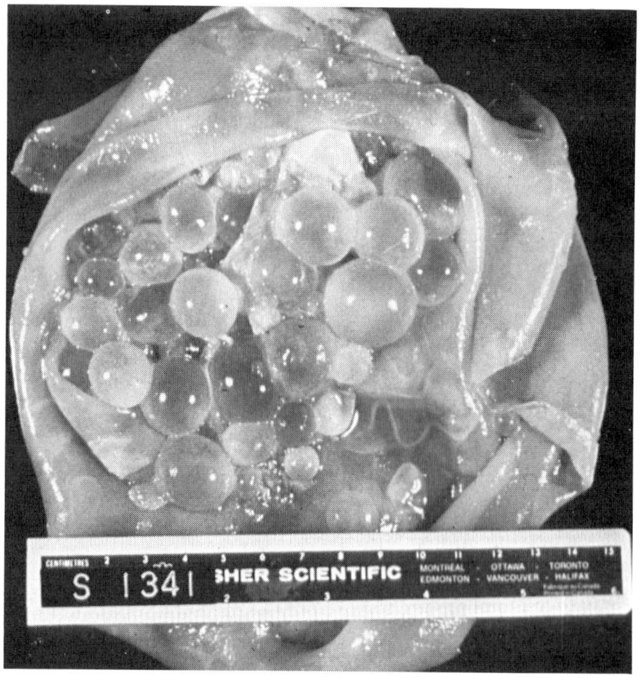

Figure 34–3. Hydatid cysts removed at surgery, unruptured. The outer laminated membrane has been opened, revealing so-called brood capsules contained within. *(Courtesy of George Craven, MD, Department of Neurosurgery, Louisiana State University Medical Center).*

Affected children may have raised intracranial pressure, diminished visual acuity, mental changes, homonymous field cuts, and hemiparesis. Characteristically, however, one is confronted with a child in good general health who lives in an endemic rural area and has elevated intracranial pressure without focal findings.[305] In the adult, the clinical picture is less well defined. Increased intracranial pressure is usually evident, but the differentiation between echinococcal cyst and tumor may be difficult.

Plain x-ray films of the skull in the child may show suture separation or thinning of the cranial vault, whereas RN scans reveal absence of uptake at the cyst site. If angiography is done, it may reveal significant vascular displacement by an avascular mass. CT scanning reveals a cyst, often with nonspecific mass effect.[306] Calcification of the cyst wall may occur, and its presence raises suspicion of echinococcosis cyst. Rarely, there is a fine enhancing rim. The cyst may occur in various sites in the brain, including the aqueduct of Sylvius[307] or the skull.

Treatment. In the presence of increased intracranial pressure, the cyst fluid may be aspirated by puncture via a burr hole and followed by systemic antihelminthic treatment with mebendazole[308] or albendazole.[309] Surgical excision of the encapsulated cyst may be necessary (see Fig. 34–3). The removal can be done by cortical incision, exposure of the cyst, and gentle irrigation between cyst wall and brain. Ozgen et al[310] reported 11 successive cures with surgery.

Cranial hydatid disease also represents an unencapsulated form of the parasite that occurs in either the cranial base or vault. It may result in increased intracranial pressure, focal neurologic disturbances, skull deformity, and cranial nerve palsies. Involved bone of the vault may be widely resected, but this may not be possible with a basal lesion.

Schistosomiasis. Infestation by the trematode worm *Schistosoma* affects an estimated 200 million people worldwide[311] and is endemic in Africa, South America, the Middle East, and the Caribbean. Acute cerebral schistosomiasis can cause a fulminating encephalitis, whereas the chronic form of the disease produces intracranial granulomas with obstruction to cerebrospinal fluid flow, elevated intracranial pressure, and localizing signs. Unfortunately, there are no specific clinical features that are pathognonomic of the disease. Schistosomicidal chemotherapy supplemented with corticosteroids is usually effective.[312]

Toxoplasmosis. *Toxoplasma gondii,* an obligate intracellular protozoon, causes one of the commonest infections in America; from 20 to 70 percent of adults in the United States demonstrate *Toxoplasma* antibodies. In immunocompromised individuals, protozoa invade and destroy cells producing necrotic regions surrounded by an intense mononuclear reaction. Patients may become immunocompromised secondary to AIDS, secondary to treatment for malignancies, or following organ transplantation.[313–316] In the CNS, *T. gondii* infections can be classified into one of three patterns: (1) diffuse encephalopathy with or without seizures, (2) meningoencephalitis, or (3) single or multiple progressive mass lesions. The *T. gondii* trophozoites may be identified by Giemsa-stained preparations of abscess aspirate. Inoculations of purulent material into mice and fluorescent antibody techniques also may enable definite identification of *Toxoplasma* organisms. Pyrimethamine and sulfadiazine (or triple sulfonamides) are the current drugs of choice, and prompt initiation of therapy provides a more favorable outcome. Ultimate prognosis depends on the severity of brain involvement as well as the nature of the underlying systemic disease. In the case of an immunocompromised patient in which the CT scan suggests toxoplasmosis, empirical medical treatment may be started and the patient is followed with serial CT scans. If the lesions clear over the course of a month, this presumes *T. gondii* infection, and brain biopsy may be avoided. (Toxoplasmosis infection is discussed further in this chapter in the section entitled Acquired Immunodeficiency Syndrome (AIDS).)

Paragonimiasis. Paragonimiasis[317] is a parasitic infection caused by the lung fluke *Paragonimus westermani* and related species. The infection is prevalent in the Far East, Southeast Asia, some parts of Africa, and South America. In one endemic area, 24 percent of space-occupying lesions within the brain were caused by *Paragonimus.* It is caused by the ingestion of inadequately cooked crustaceae contaminated with the larval form *Paragonimus,* which migrate from the duodenum to the lungs. Most investigators believe that immature or mature worms follow vascular structures from the chest to the head and enter the brain via foramina at the base of the skull. Entrance through the jugular foramen is highly suspect because most cerebral lesions are posterior, particularly in the occipital, parietal, and temporal lobes. Cerebral paragonimiasis may present as an acute meningoencephalitis, a well-encapsulated granuloma, or a chronic calcified lesion. Seizures, headache, visual disturbances, and hemiparesis are the most common symptoms and signs. Plain x-ray films of the skull may reveal posterior calcifications. CT scanning reveals ring-like or nodular enhancing masses in the early stages.[318,319] Shell-like calcified clusters occur in the chronic form.[320] Cerebrospinal fluid may be normal or abnormal. Occasionally, *Paragonimus* ova may be seen in the CSF. Complement-fixation tests of cerebrospinal fluid against *Paragonimus* antigen are positive in 40 to 80 percent of cases of cerebral infestation. The parasite may also involve the spinal cord. The worms probably migrate into the spinal epidural space directly from the lungs, because an extradural thoracic location is most common.

While medical therapy with praziquantel provides primary treatment, surgery may be performed for intracranial mass lesions that cause increased intracranial pressure. Small cysts may be entirely enucleated. The contents of large cysts are evacuated but the walls are left behind.

Entamoeba Histolytica. Brain abscesses caused by *Entamoeba histolytica*[321–324] usually have a hematogenous origin from *E. histolytica* abscesses of the lung or liver, although at least five cases of direct spread of this organism from bowel to brain have been reported. From 0.7 to 8 percent of hepatic amebiasis will have associated brain involvement. The *E. histolytica* brain abscess is usually solitary and unencapsulated. The abscess progresses rapidly and frequently ends fatally, but several instances have been recorded of survival following aspiration and antiamebic drug therapy.

Trypanosomiasis. A study has suggested that subcurative treatment of systemic trypanosomiasis may permit the parasite to enter the brain and to cause meningoencephalitis.[325] Poisson et al[326] reported the occurrence of pseudotumor associated with *Trypanosoma gambiense.* Clinical signs included progressive hemiplegia and papilledema, although the hemiplegic form has been reported as being unusual.[327] CT scans demonstrated asymmetrical hypodense areas in the white matter, while arteriography showed vascular displacement. Serial CT scanning revealed associated cerebral edema and demyelination. Arsenicals plus corticosteroid treatment led to a rapid clinical improvement in their patient. The differential diagnosis includes tuberculosis, syphilis, and fungal infection.[327]

Fungal Brain Abscess

Fungal infections of the CNS occur sporadically among normal persons (see Chap. 9). More commonly, however, such infections are found in debilitated, diabetic, or immunocompromised individuals (see Chap. 51). Recipients of organ transplants, patients with lymphomas, acute leukemia, and aplastic anemia, and those on cytotoxic chemotherapy are also susceptible, as are those with abnormal immunoglobulins.[328,329] Because of the altered immune response, the host often is unable to confine a fungal brain abscess, and CT scans in such cases often show poorly circumscribed, low-density lesions with little contrast enhancement. These CT characteristics in patients with fungal brain abscesses are often associated with a poor prognosis.[330] Mortality following fungal brain infection is high, not only because of the brain infection itself, but also owing to the underlying disease.

In one neurosurgical series of 78 patients with fungal infections of the CNS, *Coccidioides immitis* and *Cryptococcus neoformans* accounted for two-thirds of the infections; 15 percent were associated with intracranial mass.[331]

Coccidioidomycosis. Coccidioidomycosis[332,333] is caused by a fungus that exists in the mycelial form in hot desert soils and occurs as spherules in the human host. Brain infection usually occurs as a meningitis, which is generally fatal. Hydrocephalus and increased intracranial pressure occur because of obstruction to CSF flow. Shunts are usually required for control of CSF. Until recently, amphotericin B was the only effective treatment, being given either by repeat lumbar injections or via a bubble reservoir under the scalp and connected by a rubber tube placed in the lateral ventricle (Ommaya reservoir). Amphotericin B is toxic in itself and its administration has resulted in significant morbidity. The imidazole antifungal agents, miconazole and ketoconazole, may be effective with less morbidity than amphotericin B. Miconazole is given intraventricularly via an Ommaya reservoir and ketoconazole is taken orally.

Cryptococcosis. CNS cryptococcal infection[334,335] occurs in persons exposed to pigeon and chicken droppings and particularly in debilitated, immunocompromised patients. The organism *Cryptococcus neoformans* reaches the brain or spinal cord by way of the blood and usually produces a meningitis, although space-occupying lesions that require excision have been reported. Currently, 60 percent of cryptococcosis patients who receive amphotericin B are cured. Addition of 5-fluorocytosine may be useful, but this is not well established.

Aspergillosis. Aspergillosis[330,336–344] is caused by a fungus of the genus *Aspergillus.* The infection can involve the meninges, parenchyma, or blood vessels. *Aspergillus fumigatus* is the most common species causing disease in humans. Usually the organism enters the CNS by hematogenous spread from lung or intestine, but occasionally direct penetration occurs from an involved sinus or orbit. Although CNS aspergillosis can occur in otherwise healthy persons, the disease is often associated with drug addiction, AIDS, diabetes mellitus, carcinomatosis, immunosuppression, and other debilitating disorders. Generalized aspergillosis spreads to the CNS about 18 to 50 percent of the time. In the CNS, lesions can be either acute (necrotizing and purulent) or chronic (granulomatous). Fungal arteritis may be caused by extension of the fungus into the walls of cerebral arteries and this may result in cerebral infarction or hemorrhage. In one series of nine fungal brain abscesses among immunocompromised persons, eight were caused by aspergillosis. The clinical findings depend on the site and extent of the lesion. CT scans delineate the extent of neuraxis involvement but are not specific for aspergillosis. Spinal aspergillosis has been reported in normal individuals, the immunocompromised, and following lumbar disc surgery. Although intraventricular and systemic amphotericin B (perhaps in combination with rifampin) can be effective in some cases, the ultimate prognosis is usually guarded because of the underlying systemic disease.

North American Blastomycosis. Blastomycosis[345–351] is a fungal disease caused by *Blastomyces dermatitidis,* a soil saprophyte common in the central part of the United States. The portal of entry into the body is via the lung. Pulmonary blastomycotic lesions may be confused with tuberculosis. Meningitis is the most common form of CNS blastomycosis, but solitary mass lesions in the brain occasionally occur. Clinically, patients may present with headache, coma, confusion, memory loss, aphasia, paresis, increased intracranial pressure, or signs of meningitis. Diagnosis is difficult unless blastomycosis is present elsewhere. Skin testing is of limited value, because blastomycosis antigen cross-reacts with *Histoplasma* and *Coccidioides.* White blood cell count and erythrocyte sedimentation rates are generally normal. CT scanning reveals an isodense or slightly hyperdense solitary mass with contrast enhancement and surrounding edema. The scan appearance may be suspicious for tumor. Definitive diagnosis is based on biopsy and/or culture. Amphotericin B may be curative, but surgical removal of the intracranial lesion may be required.

Phycomycosis (Mucormycosis). Cerebral mucormycosis is an acute, rarely curable fungal disease that affects the nasal sinuses, orbit, and brain.[352–355] The fungus usually becomes pathogenic for humans, in association with predisposing debilitating conditions, such as diabetic acidosis, and altered immune conditions, including use of antibiotics or corticosteroids. Cerebral mucormycosis, however, has been reported following open brain injury alone. Patients with mucormycosis often have proptosis, orbital cellulitis, and total ophthalmoplegia. Central nervous system invasion (acute meningoencephalitis and purulent meningitis) occurs along arteries that transverse the lamina cribrosa. The fungus has a predilection for arterial invasion, which can lead to thrombosis and cerebral infarction, hemorrhage, or dissecting aneurysms.

Paranasal sinus involvement appears as mucosal thickening on CT scans. Bone destruction is occasionally seen. CT scan evidence of intracranial involvement is shown by presence of abscess or infarction. The fungal abscess appears as a low-density mass with variable peripheral enhancement and little surrounding vasogenic edema.

Treatment includes control of the underlying cause, local drainage or debridement of the involved tissue, and use of amphotericin B, both systemically and via local irrigation. Hyperbaric oxygen has been used for treatment of the disease by providing increased oxygen perfusion of tissues distal to occluded arteries. Hyperbaric oxygen may reduce local acidosis and thereby inhibit the growth rate of the fungus.

Histoplasmosis. Histoplasmosis[356] is caused by the dimorphic fungus *Histoplasma capsulatum,* which rarely infects the central nervous system. When the CNS is infected, meningitis usually results, but occasionally parenchymal granulomas occur. Amphotericin B is used for treatment.

Candidiasis. Candidiasis[357–359] is usually a chronic infection caused by various species of the imperfect fungus *Candida.* Central nervous system infection usually follows systemic disease in debilitated persons with diabetes, malignancies, or immunologic problems in those treated with antibiotics, steroids, or immunosuppressive drugs. The usual infection is meningitis, but parenchymal involvement may occur. In infants, *Candida* brain abscess may occur in association with gastrointestinal lesions, postoperatively, or following treatment with antibiotics. *Candida discitis* following bowel surgery in an adult has been reported. Amphotericin B and 5-fluorocytosine are effective drugs, but the ultimate prognosis is often poor because of the underlying disease.

Neurologic Sequelae of Amphotericin. Intrathecal administration of amphotericin B may cause transient or permanent spinal cord dysfunction (myelopathy).[360] Pathologic studies following amphotericin myelopathy in one patient disclosed no evidence of arachnoiditis, suggesting that the dysfunction results from a vascular abnormality (ie, possible transient spasm).

If a patient receiving amphotericin B experiences transient spinal cord symptoms, the amount of drug given intrathecally may be reduced and the injections scheduled farther apart. Alternatively, the drug may be given intraventricularly by means of a reservoir unit. Consideration may be given to changing medication, but when amphotericin B is essential, this may prove difficult. Miconazole may become an alternative to amphotericin B.

Acquired Immunodeficiency Syndrome (AIDS)

The acquired immunodeficiency syndrome (AIDS) and the AIDS-related complex (ARC) have been shown to be caused by the human immunodeficiency virus (HIV). As a result of the immune deficiency, the body is subject to a wide spectrum of opportunistic infections and malignant tumors. In addition, there is increasing evidence that the human immunodeficiency virus type 1 (HIV-1) is neurotropic and can invade the brain directly, although its pathogenesis is not well understood.[361,362]

Since the mortality of AIDS is close to 100 percent, a large literature concerning its protean pathologic manifestations has emerged. The nervous system is significantly involved in the majority (at least 74 percent) of cases.[363–365] A predominant feature is opportunistic infections (crytococcal infection, toxoplasmosis, cytomegalovirus, *Histoplasma* microabscess). Fungal infection, especially by cryptococcus, is the most common cause of meningitis[366]; while toxoplasmosis, a protozoan infection, is the most common cause of abscess formation.[366] Simultaneous infection by more than one microorganism occurs occasionally. Bacterial infections of the CNS are uncommon. HIV encephalitis is common.[364] Primary CNS lymphoma or lymphoma metastatic from extracranial sites occurs in a variable proportion of the cases.[365,367] There are cases where infection and tumor occur in the same patients.[368] Spinal cord involvement occurs with demyelination in the long tracts of posterior columns.[369]

Fifty to 60 percent of patients with AIDS may be expected to develop a neurologic complication.[370] Approximately 10 percent of patients develop intracranial mass lesions, and in about 25 percent of these patients, the lesion is identified before the diagnosis of AIDS is established.[371] The two most common mass lesions are toxoplasmosis abscess and lymphoma. These lesions have neurosurgical implications in terms of the question of biopsy versus medical management.

A large proportion of both the AIDS and non-AIDS population is seropositive for toxoplasmosis, indicating previous subclinical infection. Infection with the protozoon *Toxoplasma gondii,* in patients with AIDS, appears to result from reactivation of prior latent infection.[372] The clinical manifestations of CNS involvement suggest a focal process, especially focal seizures. There may or may not be a focal neurologic abnormality. Lumbar puncture is not helpful, since the CSF may show only a nonspecific lymphocytic pleocytosis. CSF exam, however, is useful in excluding meningitis due to other organisms, including *Cryptococcus neoformans.*[372] On the other hand, clinical judgment needs to dictate whether the risk of the lumbar puncture producing cerebral herniation in the presence of a space-occupying intracranial mass lesion is worth the information concerning the question of meningitis. Measurement of CSF antibody to *T. gondii* is not diagnostically helpful.[372] AIDS patients with toxoplasmosis generally have evidence of past infection (IgG antibody); therefore although serologic testing is of limited value for the diagnosis of toxoplasmosis in AIDS patients, *absence* of the IgG antibody to *T. gondii* tends to exclude that diagnosis.[373]

Both CT and MRI scanning are useful in demonstrating toxoplasmosis in the brain. The lesions may be solitary but are usually multiple. The basal ganglia are the most common site, but the lesions may occur in any portion of the brain including cerebral cortex, cerebellum, and brain stem.[374,375] There is considerable surrounding edema. For CT scanning, double-dose contrast increases the sensitivity of the imaging; ring enhancement is common. Figure 34–4 illustrates CT scanning in a case of toxoplasmosis. MRI may be slightly more sensitive than CT scanning but is not more diagnostically specific than CT.[375] RN brain scintigraphy (isotope brain scan) may also demonstrate localized intracranial infection,[376] although resolution is inferior to that of CT or MRI scanning.

If the diagnostic studies do not reveal a clear-cut diagnosis of toxoplasmosis, then there is a question of carrying out a biopsy for definitive diagnosis. This can be carried out with reasonable safety by CT-guided biopsy technique (under local anesthesia) or by open craniotomy with the aid of ultrasound imaging for localization of the lesion.[372] Another option is that of placing the patient on a trial of the drug combination of pyrimethamine and sulfadiazine. This regimen is highly effective with clinical improvement and shrinkage of the lesions on CT scan within 1 to 2 weeks. Treatment must be continued indefinitely. If there is no improvement within 2 weeks, biopsy may then be considered.[371,372]

In patients with AIDS, primary CNS lymphomas occur in about 2 percent of cases, and, in about one-third, the tumor is the first manifestation of AIDS.[371] The patients may present with confusion, headaches, visual disturbance, memory impairment, and focal neurologic abnormalities such as hemiparesis.[371,377] Seizures occur in about one-third of the patients. CT or MRI scanning reveals mass

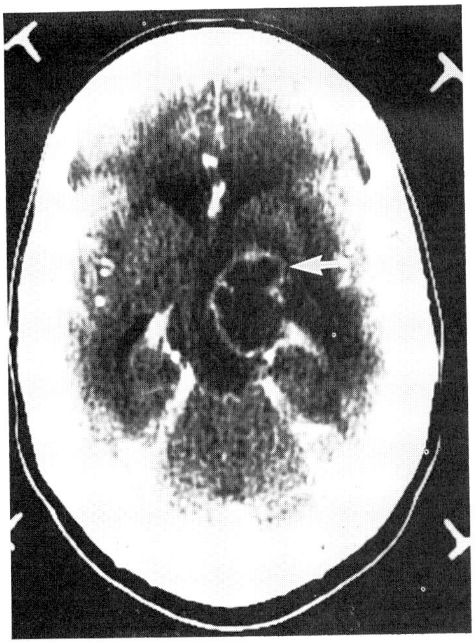

Figure 34–4. CT scan with IV contrast enhancement, showing ring enhancement of lesion in region of thalamus/basal ganglia (arrow). Patient was a 38-year-old woman from Haiti who presented with focal seizures and a rapidly progressive hemiparesis and declining level of consciousness; she was found to be HIV-positive. CT-guided stereotaxic biopsy revealed a toxoplasmosis abscess. She was then treated with pyrimethamine and sulfadiazine, with temporary improvement in her neurologic status, but subsequently she deteriorated and died. *(From Black P, Carey ME: Focal infections of the central nervous system, skull, and spine. In Grossman RG (ed): Principles of Neurosurgery. New York, Raven Press, 1991, pp 179–221.)*

lesions that are multiple in about two-thirds of the cases; the lesions are usually contrast enhancing on CT scanning. MRI is reported as being more sensitive than CT and may show more areas of involvement, but it is not more specific in differentiating the lesion from other AIDS-related diagnostic possibilities.[378]

Other AIDS-related diagnostic possibilities in patients with focal lesions are cerebral toxoplasmosis, progressive multifocal leukoencephalopathy, fungal or bacterial infection, and hemorrhage.[379]

Lumbar puncture for CSF examination may show slight increase in protein and mild lymphocytic pleocytosis.[377] CSF cytology generally does not reveal abnormal cells. Since the CSF findings are nonspecific, the main value of lumbar puncture in diagnosis of CNS lymphoma is to rule out meningitis such as cryptococcus. As mentioned previously, the risk of cerebral herniation has to be considered in the judgment of whether to carry out lumbar puncture in cases where the CT or MRI scan shows significant intracranial mass, and especially if there is a hemispheral shift.

For definitive diagnosis, a CT-guided stereotaxic biopsy may be performed. However, since *Toxoplasma* abscesses are the most common type of cerebral mass lesion in patients with AIDS, and the most amenable to treatment, Rosenblum et al[371] recommend a 3-week antibiotic trial with pyrimethamine and sulfadiazine for any patient with AIDS and intracranial masses. Steroids may also be given briefly if it is necessary to control cerebral edema. Clinical improvement and shrinkage of the lesions confirm toxoplasmosis as a diagnosis. However, if the patient is not likely to survive the 3-week antibiotic trial or if any of the masses fail to respond to the antibiotic treatment, then biopsy is recommended. Furthermore, since toxoplasmosis lesions are usually multiple, a biopsy should probably be performed for solitary mass lesions.

Radiation therapy is the recommended treatment for CNS lymphoma, possibly in conjunction with chemotherapy and steroids.[380] Although the neoplasm responds favorably to radiation therapy, patients usually die of other AIDS complications.

Osteomyelitis of the Skull

The skull is relatively resistant to infection, and its occurrence is associated with one of the following:

1. Infection of an adjacent air sinus, usually the frontal sinus.
2. Head trauma, with scalp laceration and particularly when associated with skull fracture.
3. Postoperatively, following craniotomy.

In one series, there was a 5 percent postoperative infection rate following craniotomy[381] and another series reported a 7 percent incidence of craniotomy infections; in the latter series, bone flap infections represented more than half of all infections after supratentorial craniotomy, while bacterial meningitis accounted for more than half of the infections following suboccipital craniotomy and translabyrinthine operations.[382]

Cranial osteomyelitis may be limited to the skull and may be a low-grade infection, or it may be associated with epidural or subdural empyema, with life-threatening potential. In acute osteomyelitis of the skull, the patient may have fever and localized pain, tenderness, and swelling in the area of the involved bone. On plain x-ray films, localized bone destruction may not become evident until 2 weeks after the onset of the osteomyelitis (Fig. 34–5). Although the area of infected bone may be identified on plain skull films, additional studies,

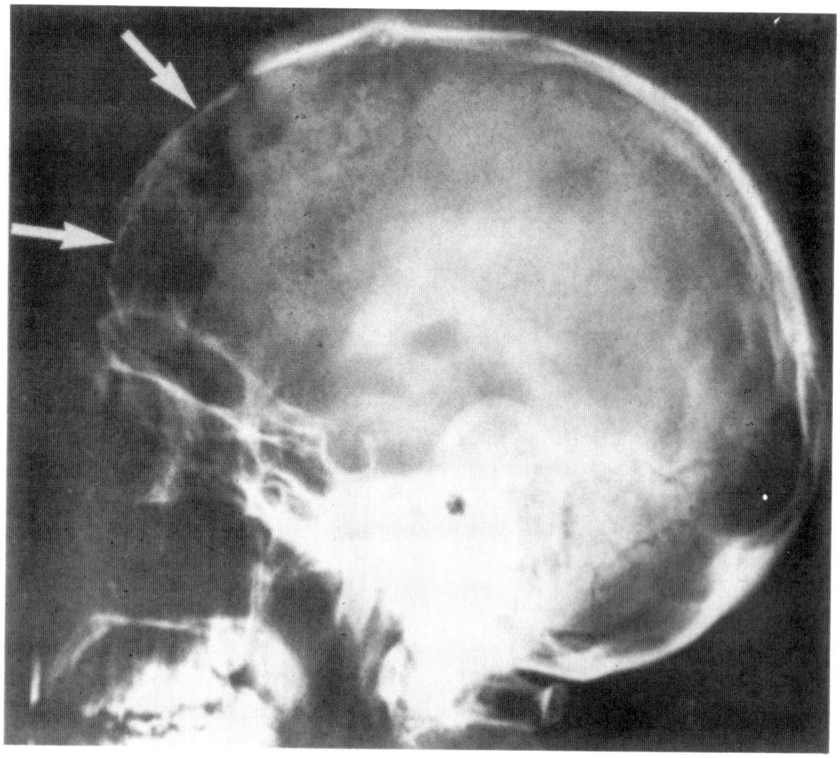

Figure 34–5. Plain skull film showing area of chronic osteomyelitis in the frontal bone (arrows) in a patient who had sustained a depressed skull fracture and frontal paranasal sinus injury.

including isotope bone scan and CT scan of the skull, may be needed to clarify the diagnosis. The offending organism is usually *Staphylococcus*, either *S. aureus* or *S. epidermidis*, or mixed flora.[383]

In acute osteomyelitis, antibiotics are the main treatment. In both the acute and chronic forms, it is important to obtain a culture of the infected area either by needle aspiration or by open operation. Treatment of an infected contiguous source, such as frontal sinusitis, is also necessary. It has been recommended that antibiotics be given intravenously for 1 to 2 weeks, followed by 6 to 12 weeks orally, with intermittent antibiotic serum levels obtained while on oral therapy.[384] Despite the use of antibiotics, chronic osteomyelitis is best treated also with surgical resection (craniectomy) of the involved bone.[383]

SPINAL ABSCESS

Pyogenic Infections

Vertebral Osteomyelitis. Pyogenic vertebral osteomyelitis is commonly associated with antecedent bacterial infection elsewhere in the body. Bacteria from the primary site, such as pelvic or urinary tract infection, spread hematogenously to the vertebral column, either via arteries or via the veins of Batson's plexus.[385–387] A septic embolus produces a localized bone infarction, which results in the development of osteomyelitis.[388] The richly vascularized vertebral body end-plate region is the commonest site of initial infection from hematogenous spread. This disorder occasionally follows penetrating trauma or spinal surgery. *Staphylococcus aureus* is the most common organism responsible for vertebral osteomyelitis, but gram-negative organisms have also been implicated.[386,389–391] *Pseudomonas aeruginosa* is commonly isolated from vertebral osteomyelitis in heroin addicts.[392]

In children, spinal infection usually has an abrupt onset, with malaise, fever, back pain, and spinal tenderness. In adults, however, symptom onset is usually gradual, and up to 3 months may be required to make the diagnosis.[393,394] In both adults and children, diagnosis is commonly delayed, owing to the nonspecificity of the symptoms. For example, spinal pain secondary to vertebral osteomyelitis may be the primary manifestation of infection elsewhere, such as endocarditis.[395,396] Osteomyelitis should be included in the differential diagnosis of persistent or worsening backache in elderly patients with degenerative spinal osteoarthritis.[397] In patients undergoing long-term hemodialysis, however, there are plain x-ray film changes in the spine suggesting osteomyelitis, but which, on investigation, turn out to be "pseudoinfection"; the cause of these changes is not known.[398] The absence of prevertebral soft tissue mass on MRI scanning in hemodialysis patients suggests that the spinal radiographic changes are not due to infection.[399] Osteomyelitis is similarly considered in patients with osteoporosis and vertebral body collapse when there is back pain, fever, and elevated sedimentation rate.[400] Cervical osteomyelitis is considered as a diagnostic possibility months after anterior spine surgery,[401] penetrating wounds of the neck,[402] panfacial trauma,[403] or tracheoesophageal puncture for voice rehabilitation.[404] There is little or no fever and adults usually have no malaise. Back pain is present in about two-thirds of the cases, particularly if the mobile cervical and lumbar areas are affected, rather than the fixed, thoracic spine. Usually on palpation, point tenderness is evident at the involved site. In adults, the leukocyte count is seldom raised but the *ESR is usually elevated.* Some authors[171,405] have noted an association of vertebral osteomyelitis with diabetes, but others have not.[390] The sedimentation rate is said to be the best clue that backache in a diabetic patient is due to something other than benign osteoarthritic changes.[405]

Thoracic and lumbar vertebrae are most frequently involved; the vertebral bodies are more commonly affected than the posterior elements. Generally, more than one spinal level is affected. Pus from an infected vertebra may form a paravertebral abscess or, more importantly, an epidural collection that may compress adjacent neural structures. Collapse of a vertebral body may result in gibbus formation that may impinge on the spinal cord or cauda equina. Either of these mechanisms may lead to paralysis. In one series,[390] 3 of 28 patients with vertebral body infection subsequently developed paralysis.

Plain x-ray findings lag behind signs and symptoms by 2 to 8 weeks.[138] These findings consist of bone rarefication, loss of bony trabeculation close to the cartilaginous plate, and narrowing of the vertebral disc space between involved adjacent vertebrae. An important x-ray observation differentiating osteomyelitis from cancer metastasis is the finding that *the intervertebral disc is commonly destroyed by osteomyelitis, whereas it is generally preserved in metastatic disease.*[406] However, there are exceptions to this rule, so that intact vertebral endplates on MRI scanning do not necessarily exclude osteomyelitis in favor of metastatic disease.[407] Vertebral body collapse is common. In chronic infections, there may be rapid bone regeneration, with the development of dense new bone. RN scanning is sensitive in diagnosing infection in the first several weeks of vertebral osteomyelitis. The combination of an abnormal technetium-99m bone scan and an abnormal gallium-67 scan, showing focal uptake in the spine, is reasonably specific for diagnosis of vertebral osteomyelitis.[408] On the other hand, the finding of indium-111 labeled leukocytes (^{111}In WBCs) is less specific.[409] CT scanning may show bony abnormalities before plain x-ray studies[410] and has the advantage over RN scanning of distinguishing bony from disc space involvement. CT scanning after intravenous contrast injection enhances the rim around an epidural abscess, which adds to the usefulness of this modality.[411] MRI scanning has the same accuracy and sensitivity as RN scanning in detecting osteomyelitis.[406] MRI scans show obliteration of the margin between the disc and the vertebral end-plates[412] (Fig. 34–6). RN scanning is less subject to motion degradation than MRI scanning; if patients cannot tolerate MRI scanning because of claustrophobia, RN scanning can be performed.[406] Myelography with water-soluble contrast followed by CT scanning is useful in outlining epidural abscess, but the value of myelography is declining because of the availability of RN, CT, and MRI scanning.

The responsible organism may be identified by blood culture in cases of acute vertebral osteomyelitis but is usually negative in chronic osteomyelitis.[413] If blood cultures are negative, it is recommended that the organism responsible and its susceptibility to antibiotics be identified. This can be accomplished by percutaneous needle aspiration under fluoroscopic or CT guidance or by open biopsy. Percutaneous CT guidance has been reported as being safe, accurate, and superior to fluoroscopic guidance.[413–416] Both aerobic and anaerobic culture, as well as cultures for tuberculosis and fungi and a search for parasites should be carried out.

Treatment of vertebral osteomyelitis without neurologic deficit consists of bed rest and immobilization, along with antibiotic therapy based on meticulous susceptibility testing of the offending organism(s).[2] Parenteral antibiotics are given for 6 to 8 weeks and oral therapy for an additional 8 weeks.[417] External immobilization may prove a useful adjunct to prevent bony collapse and for patient comfort. Significant paravertebral abscesses may require drainage. A metal stabilization rod may be implanted at the time of surgical drainage for control of pain and to permit postoperative mobilization.[418] Should the spinal cord be compressed by epidural pus or gibbus, decompression of the spinal cord will be necessary either by laminectomy or by an anterior or lateral approach. However, patients with spinal epidural abscess who are in poor medi-

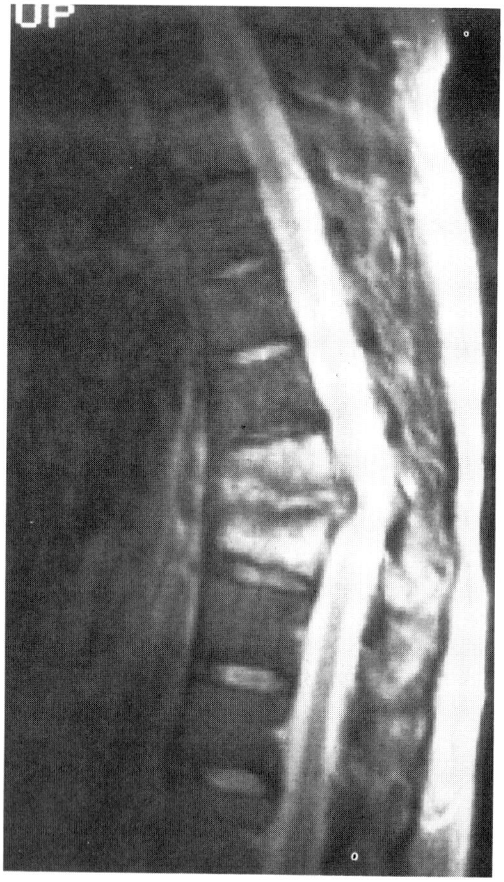

Figure 34–6. MRI scan in 37-year-old patient with history of drug addiction presenting with thoracic spinal pain and rapidly progressive paraparesis. MRI scan suggests osteomyelitis, showing vertebral body collapse, destruction of the endplates, and spinal cord compression. The involved vertebral bodies and intervening disc were resected by a thoracotomy approach and a strut bone graft was placed at the site of the vertebral corpectomies. She had an excellent recovery of neurologic function. The organism proved to be *Staphylococcus,* for which she was placed on an antibiotic regimen. *(From Black P, Carey ME: Focal infections of the central nervous system, skull, and spine. In Grossman RG (ed): Principles of Neurosurgery. New York, Raven Press, 1991, pp 179–221.)*

cal condition or without neurologic deficit may be treated with antibiotics alone without surgery.[417]

Disc Space Infection

Pathophysiology. Infection of the disc space is a relatively uncommon complication following open[419] or percutaneous[420] excision of a herniated disc (usually in the lumbar area)[419] or after lumbar chemonucleolysis.[421] Somewhat more common is the spontaneous development of disc space infection without prior spinal surgery. The latter form is thought to be produced by the hematogenous spread from an infective source elsewhere in the body, although a specific source often remains undetermined. The spontaneous form of disc space infection tends to be more common in children than in adults, which has been attributed to the observation that the disc space early in life is well supplied with blood vessels from the adjacent vertebrae and that these vascular channels gradually disappear by the second or third decade. The normal adult disc is relatively avascular, which probably accounts for the lower frequency of blood-borne infection of the disc in adulthood.

Staphylococcus aureus is nearly always the offending organism in children; this bacterium also predominates in adults, but a wide variety of other organisms may be implicated and hence the importance of isolating the organism, especially in adults, before making a decision regarding selection of antibiotic therapy.

Clinical Manifestations. Discitis can affect the intervertebral disc at any level of the spine but is most common in the lumbar region. Children may be affected from approximately 1 year of age through adolescence. There is a higher incidence of discitis in diabetic adolescents. Children commonly present with low-grade fever, irritability, and malaise. If they are able to describe symptoms, back pain is a prominent complaint and paravertebral muscle spasm is a significant finding on examination. Sometimes the child will present with a limp or will refuse to walk, and the spinal origin of the problem may be missed unless the examiner palpates the spine in search of point tenderness and muscle spasm.

In adults with spontaneous discitis, the onset is generally more insidious, extending over weeks to months before the diagnosis is suspected. Patients complain of well-localized back pain; if the lesion is in the lumbar spine, there is referred pain down one or both legs or to the hip or groin. As in children, there is localized spinal tenderness, paravertebral muscle spasm, and limitation of spinal motion. Neurologic impairment is unusual in children but is more likely in adults, secondary to an extradural inflammatory reaction with spinal cord or nerve root compression. In recent years, it has been observed that intravenous drug users appear to be predisposed to discitis.

Postoperative disc space infection is also difficult to diagnose because patients routinely have back pain and muscle spasm after surgery. However, if the spasm is severe and prolonged (beyond a matter of weeks), disc space infection should be considered, despite the absence of any evidence of wound infection.

Diagnostic Procedures. The white blood cell count in children and adults is often normal or only moderately elevated, but the erythrocyte sedimentation rate is almost uniformly elevated. Blood cultures are positive in about one-quarter of patients with pyogenic infection of the disc space; when positive, the blood culture can be used as a guide for antibiotic therapy and can obviate the need to obtain a culture from the affected disc space.

Plain x-ray films of the involved areas of the spine show localized disc space narrowing as the first radiologic sign, but the films may be normal until several weeks after onset of the symptoms. Narrowing is followed by blurring of the end-plate and irregularity and lytic destruction of the subchondral portion of the vertebral body. In later stages, after many months of healing, there is sclerosis and spontaneous interbody fusion. Laminograms or CT scans are helpful in characterizing the lesion. MRI scanning of disc space infection shows loss of disc height, irregular disc margins, and increased signal from the adjacent vertebral bodies.[422] Differentiating postoperative changes from discitis can be difficult but Boden et al[423] suggest that the combination of enhancing bone marrow, disc space, and posterior annulus fibrosis points to infection over postoperative changes. Radioisotope scanning shows a localized area of increased uptake; spot views using the pinhole collimator provide greater diagnostic detail. The bone scan, however, is of less value in *postoperative* discitis, since increased up take is normally expected following disc surgery. Reliance in the diagnosis of postoperative infection is placed on serial plain x-ray films and CT scans. An experimental study in animals comparing MRI scanning to radioisotope imaging in pyogenic infection of the intervertebral disc revealed that MRI is more sensitive than isotope scanning, particularly in the early stages of the infection.[424] Ultrasonography has also been said to be useful in diagnosis.[425]

Percutaneous needle aspiration of the affected disc space should be seriously considered in an effort to obtain material for culture; identification of the offending organism is crucial in order to select appropriate antibiotics, unless the blood culture has been positive.[2] Disc space culture in children is said to be less vital than in adults, since the organism in children is likely to be *Staphylococcus aureus*. A problem with simple needle aspiration is that the infection is usually not purulent and positive cultures are obtained in no more than one-third of the cases. If no purulent material can be aspirated, 1 to 2 ml of saline may be injected through the needle and the saline reaspirated. An alternative technique that yields positive cultures in about two-thirds of the cases involves use of a trephine biopsy needle, which can be introduced percutaneously under local or general anesthesia or as an open surgical biopsy. This can be done under fluoroscopic or CT guidance. The biopsy/aspiration technique not only provides tissue for histologic examination but also increases the likelihood of obtaining a positive culture. Histologic verification of infection is valuable in patients in whom an organism is not isolated; a further advantage is the occasional finding of an unsuspected tumor. To place the diagnostic procedures in perspective, early radioisotope bone scan and early biopsy of the affected disc are recommended. Where available, the percutaneous nucleotome may be used to obtain specimens for culture and to decompress the affected disc.[426]

Treatment. The key to management is the administration of parenteral antibiotics for 4 to 6 weeks, basing the selection of antibiotic on blood culture or biopsy/aspirate from the affected disc space. Although antibiotics are of proven value for the treatment of vertebral osteomyelitis, there is a question of the effectiveness of antibiotics for disc space infection. At least in the normal, noninfected disc, antibiotics do not penetrate the disc,[427] but it is not clear whether penetration may occur in the presence of discitis. Despite these reservations, the current general consensus favors use of antibiotics in disc space infection. Bed rest is recommended for comfort until the acute symptoms of back pain and spasm subside. Rigid immobilization in a body cast is probably unnecessary. After the initial acute phase, the patient is permitted to ambulate with a simple spinal support for comfort. The erythrocyte sedimentation rate and plain x-ray films of the spine serve to monitor resolution of the infection.[428]

Children tend to recover over the course of a few weeks to several months; the course in adults may be more prolonged. In individuals, usually adults, in whom the symptoms persist and the x-ray films fail to show bone healing, open surgical debridement of the disc can be carried out; a spinal fusion might be added at the time of the disc debridement. Some authors recommend early surgical treatment in some cases, which appears to eradicate the disease.[419] In the unusual circumstance of neurologic impairment secondary to spinal cord or nerve root compression, surgical decompression is mandatory unless there are general medical contraindications. In general, the long-term outlook for most patients with disc space infection is favorable.

Pyogenic Spinal Epidural Abscess. In two U.S. hospitals, the incidence of spinal epidural abscess was between 0.2 and 1.2 per 10,000 admissions, from 1947 to 1974.[429] Acute or chronic forms have been described, depending on whether the clinical course evolved over a few days or several weeks. Pyogenic epidural abscesses may arise hematogenously or by spread from adjacent vertebral osteomyelitis.

Etiology and Pathogenesis. Skin infections are the most common antecedent source.[429–431] *Staphylococcus aureus* has been the most common infecting organism, but streptococci and gram-negative bacteria from preexistent urinary tract infections may also be responsible. Spinal trauma occurring just before the onset of symptoms has been reported in 10 to 40 percent of patients; there is a question whether small, clinically insignificant, traumatic epidural hematomas subsequently become colonized with bacteria.[429,430] Iatrogenic sources include epidural anesthesia, epidural steroid injection, and postsurgical infection.[432–435]

Epidural abscesses can involve any portion of the spine but the thoracic region is most commonly involved. The pus usually lies dorsally, because epidural fat, which is susceptible to bacterial invasion, lies dorsally. The dura is closely approximated to the vertebral bodies anteriorly.[429,430] Anterior epidural abscesses were found in 7 of 39 cases reviewed by Baker et al.[429] In acute hematogenous cases, granulation tissue admixed with pus extends axially over an average of four spinal segments. Chronic epidural abscesses tend to have an even more extensive axial spread than do acute lesions. The dura itself is resistant to bacterial penetration, and spread of infection to the subdural or subarachnoid spaces is rare.

Intuitively, one would imagine that the space-occupying effect of the epidural pus compromises the spinal cord by pressure. Often, however, the neurologic involvement appears out of proportion to any observed pressure effect, and it has been proposed that the neurologic sequelae result from epidural arterial or venous thrombosis, with resultant spinal cord infarction.[436]

Clinical Manifestations. Individuals with acute abscesses are febrile and septic, while those with chronic processes may be afebrile and appear relatively well. Spinal epidural abscesses tend to evolve through four clinical stages: (1) focal spinal pain and tenderness, (2) root pain, (3) paresis, and (4) paralysis.[437] In the acute case, this sequence of events occurs over an average of 7 days, whereas chronic cases may evolve over weeks or months. Once paresis ensues, however, total paralysis generally occurs within 24 hours. *Because the ultimate quality of neurologic recovery varies inversely with the degree and duration of paresis or paralysis, spinal epidural abscess is a true neurosurgical emergency. Immediate operative decompression is mandatory.*

If an individual has the classic clinical syndrome plus evidence of vertebral bone destruction on plain x-ray studies, the diagnosis and approximate locus will be highly suspicious for epidural abscess. In acute cases, however, no osteomyelitis will be evident, and, although the diagnosis may be suspected, the exact locus may be in question. In either case, but particularly in acute cases, imaging by CT scan, MRI, or myelography is indicated in order to delineate the rostral and caudal spread of epidural pus. If myelography is carried out, contrast agent may be injected above or below the suspected site of the lesion, to outline the upper and lower limits of the abscess. Care must be taken when advancing the spinal needle not to introduce bacteria from the epidural to the subarachnoid space. If a spinal puncture is done and spinal fluid examined, the CSF may be turbid or xanthochromic. Pleocytosis may be evident and the protein level elevated. The glucose is often reduced even in the absence of meningitis.

The differential diagnosis of spinal epidural abscess includes meningitis, spinal subdural abscess, acute transverse myelitis, herniated intervertebral disc, vertebral or spinal cord tumors, and vascular lesions.

Treatment. Antibiotics are started when the diagnosis is suspected and while the patient is being prepared for surgery. Since the overwhelming number of cases are due to *Staphylococcus aureus,* empirical therapy is begun with nafcillin, unless an alternative etiology is suggested by history or laboratory findings of an antecedent infection due to another organism (A. Molavi, personal communication). Pyogenic spinal epidural abscess is quite amenable to drainage. The surgical approach depends on the location of the abscess in the spinal canal. At operation, a specimen of pus or granulation tissue is obtained for Gram stain and aerobic and anaerobic culture and sensitivities, as well as fungal and mycobacterial cultures and sensitivities. At surgery, free pus in the epidural space is drained, and the epidural space is irrigated with saline/antibiotic solution. Hulme and Dott[431] recommend excision of chronic granulation tissue, to prevent subsequent dural stricture by scar tissue. In the series of Baker et al,[429] when chronic epidural abscesses were found, the laminectomy wound was closed primarily without difficulty. When acute pyogenic epidural abscess was found, the wound was either packed open for subsequent secondary closure or loosely closed over soft irrigation catheters that could be used to irrigate the epidural space with antibiotic solution in the postoperative phase. Once the specific organism is identified and its sensitivities determined, a specific antimicrobial agent may be selected for further therapy. The role of nonsurgical therapy remains unclear, but if medical treatment is chosen, close neurosurgical observation is desirable.

Acute hematogenous abscesses are not usually associated with vertebral body destruction and spinal instability. If vertebral osteomyelitis coexists with body collapse and gibbus formation has occurred, or if spinal instability is present because of the infection, later stabilization procedures may be necessary.

Prognosis. Before the use of antibiotics, the mortality for epidural abscess ranged from about 30 to 90 percent[430,431]; recent mortality approximates 18 percent.[429,438] In general, the neurologic outcome depends on the degree of cord function remaining prior to drainage and decompression. Patients with no paresis or with weakness less than 36 hours in duration often have excellent neurologic recovery. Those who have been paralyzed for longer than 48 hours generally do not recover neurologic function. Baker et al[429] reported on the outcome (with aggressive diagnosis and surgery) of 32 patients who survived their epidural abscesses: 4 were permanently paralyzed, 5 had paresis, and 23 were neurologically intact.

Spinal Subdural Empyema. Spinal subdural empyema (abscess) is a rare condition. In 1984, Probst and Wicki[439] summarized 14 cases culled from the literature and added 3 of their own. Analysis of these cases led to the conclusion that the origin of the subdural infection was most often hematogenous but that penetration of the dura from a contiguous epidural infection, lumbar puncture, injury, or congenital deformity (eg, dermal sinus tract) could also account for the infection. *Staphylococcus* has been the most common bacterium; diabetes mellitus is a common predisposing cause. Thoracic, thoracolumbar, and lumbar area were all involved with about equal frequency, and several cases occurred where pus extended in the subdural space from cervical to sacral areas.

Pathologically, the inflammation may spread into the subarachnoid space. The arachnoid and dura are thickened. Pus is present subdurally and granulation tissue is fixed not only to the dura but to the spinal cord as well. The more acute the case, the greater the amount of pus; the longer the duration of symptoms, the more likely occurrence of granulation tissue. Infection involves the extra- and intramedullary blood vessels as well. This leads to vascular narrowing and occlusions, particularly venous thrombosis and hemorrhagic infarctions. The nerve roots themselves may be swollen and demyelinated. The white matter of the spinal cord is particularly involved.

Clinically, there is fever and generalized signs of infection. Signs of meningeal irritation may be evident. There may be back pain and spinal cord (myelopathy) or radicular symptoms and signs. The neurologic findings may be secondary to interference with blood supply or due to direct neural compression.

Upon lumbar puncture, frank pus may be returned. Because of compression of the subarachnoid space by the pus, it may be impossible to obtain CSF. When CSF is found, it is often xanthochromic; the cell count is generally elevated. Protein is usually elevated and CSF glucose diminished. Occasionally, however, patients with subdural abscesses have normal CSF.

Plain x-ray studies generally show no bone destruction. Myelography demonstrates an irregular filling defect or a block that may be undifferentiable from epidural abscess. Surgical decompression is essential. Pus, when found, is removed by irrigation. If possible, granulation tissue is removed, but not granulations densely adherent to the spinal cord. Probst and Wicki[439] also recommend early rehabilitation and, of course, treatment of any underlying infection. Of 15 patients who underwent surgery, 6 were cured, 5 improved, and 4 died.

Intramedullary Pyogenic Spinal Cord Abscess. Intramedullary spinal cord abscesses are found in approximately 1 of every 40,000 autopsies. The peak incidence is in the first and third decades; males are more commonly affected than females. The thoracic spinal cord is most commonly involved. Among 55 reported cases, 42 individuals had a single intramedullary abscess, and the remainder had multiple lesions.[440] The predominant organisms were *Staphylococcus* and *Streptococcus.* Antecedent infections of the respiratory tract, spine (including fractures), heart valves, genitourinary tract, soft tissues, and midline spinal skin defects, such as dermoid sinus, had been present in 80 percent of patients. No apparent infected focus could be found in the others. Bacteria can reach the spinal cord by (1) direct implantation secondary to trauma; (2) the bloodstream; or (3) lymphatics from the retropharyngeal space, mediastinum, or abdominal cavity. Such lymphatics course along spinal nerves and communicate with the spinal subarachnoid space and Virchow-Robin spaces. Acute intramedullary abscesses are similar to other CNS abscesses, but they lack the widespread venous infarction seen with epidural abscesses. This may account for their often favorable prognosis.

Clinically, intramedullary abscesses can have acute, subacute, or chronic courses. Neurologic symptoms and signs vary according to abscess location. Acute cases have fever and there may be transverse myelitis. Pain in the neck or back, urinary incontinence, dysesthesias, and monoparesis that progresses to paraparesis or quadraparesis typically occur. Patients with chronic intramedullary abscesses have a stuttering course simulating that of a spinal tumor. Examination of the cerebrospinal fluid is generally unrewarding and may be misleading; pleocytosis may suggest meningitis. Myelography may demonstrate a spinal block and suspicion of an intraspinal mass.

Surgical therapy consists of laminectomy and incision and drainage of the abscess. Occasionally, an intraspinal abscess will masquerade as arachnoiditis, and therefore when localized spinal arachnoiditis is discovered during spinal cord surgery, this should raise suspicion that a spinal cord abscess may be present. As in the case of abscesses in general, antibiotics are started as soon as infection is recognized. When obtained, the pus is Gram-stained and cultured for aerobic, anaerobic, and mycobacteria, as well as fungi, for selection of specific antimicrobial therapy. Postoperatively, patients are followed closely because of a high recurrence rate. Twenty of 55 patients cited above had drainage of the intramedullary abscess: 5 patients died (all before the advent of antibiotics), 6 recovered neurologically, 6 showed some improvement, but 3 remained unchanged.

Spinal Tuberculosis

Tuberculosis may involve the vertebral column, as well as the epidural space, dura, arachnoid, or spinal cord.[228,371,441] Often, the disease is confined to one anatomic area.[442]

Tuberculous Spondylitis (Pott's Paraplegia). Generally, tuberculous spinal infection involves the vertebral body (Pott's tuberculous spondylitis). Tuberculous destruction of the spine, with subsequent spinal cord compression, continues to be a common disease in developing nations. Mathai and Chandy[442] indicated that, in India, 42 percent of their spinal operations for nontraumatic paraplegias were for compression consequent to tuberculous spondylitis. In the United States, this disease is rare. Tuberculous spondylitis most frequently involves the lower thoracic and upper lumbar vertebrae. The disease most commonly affects the vertebral body and is usually limited to one vertebra. Neurologic complications occur in 10 to 25 percent of patients, particularly if the thoracic spine is involved. There are two categories of Pott's paraplegia: early-onset cases, in which the neurologic dysfunction begins within 2 years of the tuberculous spondylitis, and late-onset paraplegia, with the deficit beginning after 2 years. Early cases occur when the disease is active, whereas late cases are associated with a recurrence of the infection following apparent quiescence.

The disease usually starts in the first decade of life but becomes symptomatic and is diagnosed during the third decade. A case of spinal tuberculosis after a closed fracture has been reported[443]; the trauma appeared to predispose the involved vertebrae to hematogenous infection. Though no distinctive pattern of neurologic signs or symptoms exists with Pott's disease,[239] pain and local spine tenderness occur in more than 70 percent of patients. Radicular pain is common. The cause of the cord compression may be epidural abscess, bony compression, or both.

Radiographically, early vertebral body decalcification is seen about the disc with slight diminution of the disc space. Later, frank vertebral erosion and collapse occur and paravertebral or psoas abscess may appear. Sclerotic changes also may be present, because of concomitant bone regeneration and fusion of vertebral bodies. Caseation beneath the anterior spinal ligament causes scalloping of the anterior vertebral border. CT scanning shows the expected vertebral body involvement but, in addition, can depict paraspinal abscess and an epidural tuberculous collection. Contrast enhancement may aid in their delineation. CT is also helpful for guiding aspiration of suspected areas of infection.[444] Myelography often reveals a block at the infection site. Gallium scintigraphy is helpful in identifying bony and paraspinal involvement.[445]

Spinal tuberculosis can be treated medically or surgically. Friedman[444] treated 64 patients with Pott's disease by prolonged administration of antituberculous drugs, bed rest, and spinal bracing. Spinal fusion was not carried out, and laminectomy was reserved for eight patients with paresis. Fifty patients were cured by this approach, but ten others had relapses, and four others died. Hodgson and Stock,[446] on the other hand, advocate operative intervention. The diseased bone is approached anteriorly or laterally and resected. Granulation tissue around the dura is stripped away, and the vertebral bodies are stabilized by strut grafts. They report improved neurologic function even in cases with paralysis. In 1960, they reported the operative results on 35 paralyzed patients. Twenty-six had complete neurologic recovery after operation. Graft complications (slippage, fracture, angulation) occurred in 13 patients and 4 died. Subsequently, Hodgson and colleagues also reported that 19 of 23 paraparetic children made complete neurologic recoveries after decompression and fusion, including 19 of 20 who had been paralyzed.[447] Rajasekaran and Soundarapandian[448] reported long-term follow-up on 81 patients treated for tubercular kyphosis. All were treated by anterior arthrodesis. Fifty-nine percent had good results, all of them had minimal vertebral destruction, limited debridement, small grafts, and lumbar locations as well as good surgical correction of the deformity.[448] Antituberculous drugs are given for at least 18 months after operation. It would appear that Hodgson's patients had more serious bony and neurologic involvement than did Friedman's.

Hsu and Leong[449] reported treatment of 40 patients with tuberculosis of the cervical spine. Forty-three percent of the patients had evidence of cord compression, mainly from pressure by epidural abscess. Surgical therapy was generally by anterior excision of the diseased bone, followed by grafting. In addition, all patients received streptomycin for 3 to 9 months. All patients recovered spinal cord function. Four patients underwent posterior fusion initially, but all eventually required anterior excision and grafting because of progressive kyphosis or persistence of vertebral body infection. Laminectomy is therefore not recommended for Pott's paraplegia because the cord is compressed anteriorly. However, in 10 percent of cases, tuberculous spondylitis involves the neural arch instead of the body. In the latter situation, the spinal cord may be compressed from its dorsal aspect instead of anteriorly. Radiographically, such cases may be mistaken for epidural metastasis. Patients with neural arch involvement invariably have associated dorsally placed epidural abscesses and as such are best treated by laminectomy and antituberculosis therapy.[450]

Tuli[451] reported on the results of aggressive medical and surgical therapy in 200 cases of spinal tuberculosis. Medical treatment for adults consisted of streptomycin, sodium para-aminosalicylate, and isoniazid. Patients were placed on a firm bed or a plaster jacket was used. Gradual mobilization of the patient in a spinal brace was begun after 6 to 9 months. Paravertebral abscesses were aspirated or drained. Decompression of the cord was eventually performed on patients on medical therapy who failed to show progressive recovery of neurologic function. Ninety-four percent of those patients without neurologic deficit recovered without surgery. Thirty-eight percent of those *with* neurologic involvement also recovered without operation. According to Kaufman et al,[452] only 5 to 20 percent of cases of Pott's disease are complicated by neurologic deficit.

The regimen of choice for tuberculosis is a combination of isoniazide, rifampin, and pyrazinamide for 2 months followed by a 4-month or longer course of isoniazide and rifampin.

A 10-year study of 283 cases of spinal tuberculosis in children in Korea showed that antituberculous chemotherapy resulted in satisfactory outcome in 88 percent of the patients.[453] There was no benefit from immobilization either by bed rest or by use of plaster of Paris jacket. Confirming these results, a more recent study from Korea showed that over 80 percent of 265 patients followed for 3 years were successfully managed without surgery.[454]

Intraspinal Tuberculosis. Intramedullary spinal tuberculomas occur much less frequently than does cerebral tuberculosis.[227,228,441] While some intramedullary tuberculomas are primary, others occur in association with cerebral tuberculomas. In addition to paraplegia resulting from the direct effects of infection, tuberculous arachnoiditis and associated vasculitis also may produce neurologic sequelae. Dastur[228] reported that three of six patients in whom spinal tuberculomas were excised made good neurologic recoveries.

Tuberculosis of the coverings of the spinal cord include arachnoiditis, subdural granulomas, and extradural granulomas. Tuberculous arachnoiditis is seen in patients who, in the past, suffered from tuberculous meningitis or pulmonary tuberculosis. Thick, densely organized exudates may encase the entire length of the spinal cord and may cause arteritis and secondary vascular changes leading to transverse myelitis or motor loss. Excision of local arachnoidal granulomas may provide some relief.[223]

Subdural tuberculous granulomas are generally diffuse; the dura is thickened diffusely and the granuloma surrounds the spinal cord. Some authors prefer to relieve the compression surgically while others recommend steroids and antituberculous drugs.

Occasionally, tuberculous epidural granulomas compress the spinal cord but are unassociated with any bony changes. Lacking the usual bone changes associated with tuberculosis, such patients may be misdiagnosed and therefore mismanaged. Myelograms demonstrate a block. These epidural granulomas (tuberculomas) are dorsally placed, and, again, laminectomy and antituberculous drugs are indicated.[450]

Kaufman et al[452] reported seven cases of tuberculous spinal epidural abscess. These patients had back pain for an average of about 3 months. No patient had leukocytosis and only one had a fever greater than 100F. Tuberculous skin tests were positive in only five of the seven. All showed disc space and/or vertebral body involvement. The spinal abscesses contained fibrous granulomas with caseation necrosis. Five of seven patients demonstrated acid-fast bacilli on stain and grew out *Mycobacterium tuberculosis*. All seven underwent surgery, and three died in the postoperative period.

Parasitic Spinal Infection

Spinal Echinococcosis. Hydatid disease due to *Echinococcus granulosus* rarely involves the spine. The echinococcal embryo is carried to a vertebral body, infiltrates, and destroys bone.[455] Thoracic and lumbosacral vertebrae are most commonly involved. The parasite incites little defensive tissue reaction, and adjacent bones such as ribs or pelvis can be invaded. The intervertebral disc is preserved. Spinal cord impingement occurs as the unencapsulated parasite invades the spinal canal or as collapsed bone compresses the cord. Clinical progression of the disease is slow because the parasite enlarges slowly. The common signs and symptoms are pain, motor and sensory deficits, difficulty with bowel and bladder function, paravertebral swelling, and gibbus formation; paraplegia may occur. CT scanning shows bony destruction, extradural isodense mass, and paraspinal extension of the disease.[456]

Spinal decompression by an anterior[457] or posterior laminectomy approach[458] is carried out, depending on location of the neural compression within the spinal canal. Pathologically, the cyst fluid contains the typical hooklet-bearing scolices, and the cyst wall is composed of layers of chitin, typical of echinococcosis. Irrigation of the wound with hypertonic saline for 5 minutes may help destroy the residual organisms. Occasionally, total vertebrectomy is necessary. Mebendazole has been used in conjunction with surgery in the treatment of spinal hydatid disease.[459] Postoperative use of mebendazole has been reported as being effective.[458]

Spinal Schistosomiasis. The infestation can occur as a space-occupying, intramedullary mass, which can extend to involve the cauda equina.[312] It may present clinically as an acute transverse myelitis, causing destruction and atrophy of the cord, or as a progressive neurologic process with slow progressive flaccid paralysis. Males are predominantly affected. In endemic areas, spinal schistosomiasis is considered in patients presenting with spinal cord symptoms. Treatment consists of decompressive spinal surgery and schistosomicidal drugs, which kill the adult female worms and diminish the inflammatory response. Praziquantel and oxaminquine are the current drugs of choice, administered orally, and are relatively safe.[460]

Spinal Cysticercosis. Spinal cysticercosis[461,462] resulting from infestation with the pork tapeworm occurs in only 2 to 5 percent of all cases of neurocysticercosis. Although this form of the disease can occur independently of brain involvement, it usually results from downward spread of intracranial parasites. The cysts may be intramedullary or subdural. Associated arachnoiditis is common. Spinal involvement, though rare, can result in vertebral collapse and spinal cord compression.[463]

***Guinea Worm* (Dracunculus).** Infection with the worm *Dracunculus medinensis* is endemic in Africa and Asia. Rarely, this worm may lodge in the vertebral extradural space causing paraplegia. The associated inflammatory process is of a low-grade, chronic nature but the onset of neurologic symptoms may be sudden and abrupt. Preoperatively, diagnosis is rarely made because the clinical course is indistinguishable from many other extradural spinal infections. Known prior guinea worm infection, peripheral blood eosinophilia, and extraspinal calcified lesions indicating the dead guinea worm may aid diagnosis.[464] The infecting worm causes spinal cord signs, and myelography reveals a block. The worm is discovered in chronic granulation tissue and pus at laminectomy. About half of those operated on improve. Niridazole, specific for guinea worm, has been recommended.[465]

Fungal Spinal Infection

Spinal Blastomycosis. Spinal blastomycosis mainly affects the thoracic and lumbar vertebrae. Clinically and radiologically, blastomycosis may be confused with tuberculosis, and the two diseases may coexist. Accurate tissue or culture diagnosis of the lesion must be made for appropriate treatment with amphotericin B.

Candida. Fungal infection of the spine with *Candida,* although rare, tends to occur in patients after prolonged hospitalization for complex medical problems. Broad spectrum antibiotics and parenteral hyperalimentation have been reported as predisposing factors of *Candida* infection in general.[466] Amphotericin B is effective for treatment of *Candida* vertebral osteomyelitis.[467] Surgical decompression is carried out when there is evidence of spinal cord compression.[468]

Spinal Nocardiosis. Rarely, *Nocardia,* a gram-positive bacteria, spreads hematogenously from the lungs to the vertebral bodies and epidural space and may result in spinal cord involvement. Spinal nocardiosis is treated as any focal spinal infection. A bacteriologic specimen must be obtained for diagnosis. Surgical decompression by an anterior or posterior (laminectomy) approach depends on the site of the infection in the spinal canal.

CONCLUSION

The essential ingredient in management of focal CNS infection is neither medical nor surgical, but rather a combination of antimicrobial administration and judicious surgical intervention. Advances in spinal surgery enable multiple approaches to the spine, which facilitate precise decompression as well as fusion where necessary. The antimicrobial aspects—with the multiplicity of factors of organism identification, antimicrobial susceptibility, and host resistance—afford wide latitude in selection of antimicrobial regimen. Further improvement in therapeutic outcome can be anticipated by meticulous bacteriologic processing and by the application of existing knowledge of antimicrobial therapy.

Many of the conditions involving infection of the nervous system have associated systemic manifestations. Consequently, management of patients with these disorders is best achieved through a multidisciplinary team effort. This is particularly exemplified by AIDS, which consists of a broad spectrum of disorders, so that team management is essential.

Acknowledgments. This chapter represents a revision of previous publications by the authors, particularly the following:

- Black P: Brain abscess. In Kagan BM (ed): *Antimicrobial Therapy,* 2nd ed. Philadelphia, Saunders, 1974, pp 244–252.
- Black P, Carey ME: Focal infections of the central nervous system, skull, and spine. In Grossman RG (ed): *Principles of Neurosurgery.* New York, Raven Press, 1991, pp 179–221.
- Black P, Le Frock JL: Infection of the spine. In Long DM (ed): *Current Therapy in Neurological Surgery.* Philadelphia, BC Decker, 1985, pp 120–124.
- Carey ME: Infectious diseases. In Rosenberg R (ed): *The Clinical Neurosciences, Volume IV: Neurology, Neurosurgery, Neuropathology, Neuroradiology, Neurobiology.* New York, Churchill Livingstone, 1983, pp 1221–1256.
- Carey ME: Infections of the central nervous system. In Howard RJ, Simmons RL (eds): *Surgical Infectious Diseases,* 2nd ed. Norwalk, CT, Appleton & Lange, 1988, pp 469–505.

The assistance of Mary F. McCabe, BA, Research/Editorial Assistant, Department of Neurosurgery, Hahnemann University, and Daniel O. Walsh, MA, in the preparation of the manuscript for this chapter is gratefully acknowledged. John Molavi, MD, Chairman, Division of Infectious Diseases, Hahnemann University Hospital, reviewed those aspects of the manuscript relating to antimicrobial therapy.

REFERENCES

1. Sampson DS, Clark K: A current review of brain abscess. Am J Med 54:201, 1973.
2. Black P, LeFrock JL, Silverberg AL: Management of brain abscess. In Johnson RT (ed): Current Therapy in Neurologic Disease. Philadelphia, BC Decker, 1985, pp 129–133.
3. Alegria C, Lipschitz R, Zwonnikoff G: Intracranial suppuration: a review of 79 cases seen at Baragwanath Hospital over 3 years. S Afr J Surg 20:25, 1982.
4. Nielsen H, Gyldensted C, Harmsen A: Cerebral abscess: aetiology and pathogenesis, symptoms, diagnosis, and treatment; a review of 200 cases from 1935–1976. Acta Neurol Scand 65:609, 1982.
5. Yang SY: Brain abscess: a review of 400 cases. J Neurosurg 55:794, 1981.
6. Danziger A, Price H, Schecter MM: An analysis of 113 intracranial infections. Neuroradiology 19:31, 1980.
7. Dharker SR, Shadangi TN, Vaishya ND, et al: Pyogenic brain abscess: experience with 87 cases. Neurol India 26:126, 1978.
8. Jefferson AA, Keogh AJ: Intracranial abscess: a review of treated patients over 20 years. Q J Med (New Series, XLVI) 183:389, 1977.
9. LeBeau J, Creissard P, Harispe L, et al: Surgical

treatment of brain abscess and subdural empyema. J Neurosurg 38:198, 1973.
10. McClelland CJ, Craig BF, Crockard HA: Brain abscesses in Northern Ireland: a 30 year community review. J Neurol Neurosurg Psychiatry 41:1043, 1978.
11. Nicolosi A, Hauser WA, Musicco M, Kurland LT: Incidence and prognosis of brain abscess in a defined population: Olmstead County, Minnesota, 1935–1981. Neuroepidemiology 10(3):122, 1991.
12. Malik GK, Rastogi GC, Chabra DK, et al: Intracranial space-occupying lesions in children at Lucknow. Indian Pediatr 17:420, 1980.
13. Bhatia R, Tandon PN, Banerji AK: Brain abscess—an analysis of 55 cases. Int Surg 58:565, 1973.
14. Mohanta KD, Rath S: Clinical profile of intracranial space-occupying lesions in children. Indian J Pediatr 48:163, 1981.
15. Rodriguez JC, Gutierrez RA, Valdes OD, Dorfmann JF: The role of computed axial tomography in the diagnosis and treatment of brain inflammatory and parasitic lesions: our experience in Mexico. Neuroradiology 16:458, 1978.
16. Joubert MJ, Stephanov S: Computerized tomography and surgical treatment in intracranial suppuration. Report of thirty consecutive unselected cases of brain abscess and subdural empyema. J Neurosurg 47:73, 1977.
17. Fischbein CA, Rosenthal A, Fischer EG, et al: Risk factors for brain abscess in patients with congenital heart disease. Am J Cardiol 34:97, 1974.
18. Fisher EG, Shwachman H, Wepsic JG: Brain abscess and cystic fibrosis. J Pediatr 95:385, 1979.
19. Hotson JR, Pedley TA: The neurological complications of cardiac transplantation. Brain 99:673, 1976.
20. Feneley MP, Burns MW: Cerebral abscess: manifestation of pulmonary arteriovenous malformations. Aust N Z J Med 13:280, 1983.
21. Ratcliffe PJ, Earl CJ: Recurrent cerebral abscess in association with pulmonary arteriovenous fistulae. J Neurol Neurosurg Psychiatry 45:566, 1982.
22. Jadavji T, Humphreys RP, Prober CG: Brain abscesses in infants and children. Pediatr Infect Dis J 4:394, 1985.
23. Nunez DA: Aetiological role of otolaryngological disease in paediatric intracranial abscess. J R Coll Surg Edinburgh 37(2):80, 1992.
24. Press OW, Ramsey PG: Central nervous system infections associated with hereditary hemorrhagic telangiectasia. Am J Med 77:86, 1984.
25. Sobel D, Normal D: CNS manifestations of hereditary hemorrhagic telangiectasia. AJNR 5:569, 1984.
26. Rabkin CS, Blaser MJ: Brain abscess: a complication of cystic fibrosis in adults (letter). Ann Neurol 15:608, 1984.
27. Kline MW: Brain abscess in a patient with cystic fibrosis. Pediatr Infect Dis J 4:72, 1985.
28. Graus F, Rogers LR, Posner JB: Cerebrovascular complications in patients with cancer. Medicine (Baltimore) 64:16, 1985.
29. Jennett B, Miller JD: Infection after depressed fracture of skull. Implications for management of nonmissile injuries. J Neurosurg 36:333, 1972.
30. Dohrmann PJ, Elrick WL: Observations on brain abscess. Review of 28 cases. Med J Aust 2:81, 1982.
31. Carey ME, Young HF, Rish BL, Mathis JL: Follow-up study of 103 American soldiers who sustained a brain wound in Vietnam. J Neurosurg 41:542, 1974.
32. Rish BL, Caveness WF, Dillon JD, et al: Analysis of brain abscess after penetrating craniocerebral injuries in Vietnam. Neurosurgery 9:535, 1981.
33. Arseni C, Ciurea AV: Cerebral abscesses secondary to otorhinolaryngological infections: a study of 386 cases. Zentralbl Neurochir 49:22, 1988.
34. Mathews TJ, Marus G: Otogenic intradural complications (a review of 37 patients). J Laryngol Otol 102:121, 1988.
35. Gower DJ, McGuirt F, Kelly DL: Intracranial complications of ear disease in a pediatric population with special emphasis on subdural effusion and empyema. South Med J 78:429, 1985.
36. Maksimovic Z, Rukovanjski M: Intracranial complications of cholesteatoma. Acta Otorhinolaryngol Belg 47(1):33, 1993.
37. Morgan H, Wood MW: Cerebellar abscesses: a review of 17 cases. Surg Neurol 3:93, 1975.
38. Celli P, Palatinsky E: Brain abscess as a complication of cranial traction. Surg Neurol 23:594, 1985.
39. Williams FH, Nelms DK, McGaharan KM: Brain abscess: a rare complication of halo usage. Arch Phys Med Rehabil 73(5):490, 1992.
40. Le Cam B, Guivarch G, Boles JM, et al: Neurologic complications in a group of 86 patients with bacterial endocarditis. Eur Heart J 5(Suppl C):97, 1984.
41. Krayenbuhl HA: Abscess of the brain. Clin Neurosurg 14:25,1967.
42. Arseni C, Ciurea AV: Metastatic cerebral abscesses in the frame of cyanogenic congenital cardiopathies. Zentralbl Neurochir 43:271, 1982.
43. Takeshita M, Kagawa M, Yonetani H, et al: Risk factors for brain abscess in patients with congenital cyanotic heart disease. Neurol Med Chir (Tokyo) 32(9):667, 1992.
44. Kurtan R, Griggs RC: Cyanotic congenital heart disease with suspected stroke; should all patients receive antibiotics? Arch Neurol 40:209, 1983.
45. Kratimenos G, Crockard HA: Multiple brain abscess: a review of fourteen cases. Br J Neurosurg 5(2):153, 1991.
46. Curless RG: Neonatal intracranial abscess: two cases caused by *Citrobacter* and a literature review. Ann Neurol 8:269, 1980.
47. Foreman SD, Smith EE, Ryan NJ, Hogan GR: Neonatal *Citrobacter* meningitis: pathogenesis of cerebral abscess formation. Ann Neurol 16:655, 1984.
48. Britt RH, Enzmann DR, Placone RC Jr, et al: Experimental anaerobic brain abscess. Computerized tomographic and neuropathological correlations. J Neurosurg 60:1148, 1984.

49. Britt RH, Enzmann DR, Yeager AS: Neuropathological and computerized tomographic findings in experimental brain abscess. J Neurosurg 55:590, 1981.
50. Wood JH, Lightfoot WE, Ommaya AK: Cerebral abscesses produced by bacterial implantation and septic embolization in primates. J Neurol Neurosurg Psychiatry 42:63, 1979.
51. Whalen MA, Hilal SK: Computed tomography as a guide in the diagnosis and follow-up of brain abscesses. Radiology 135:663, 1980.
52. Carey ME, Chou SN, French LA: Experience with brain abscesses. J Neurosurg 36:1, 1972.
53. Falconer MA, McFarlan AM, Russell DS: Experimental brain abscess in the rabbit. Br J Surg 30:245, 1943.
54. Bhatia R: Brain abscess in children. Indian J Pediatr 50:591, 1983.
55. Sutton DL, Ouvrier RA: Cerebral abscess in the under 6 month age group. Arch Dis Child 58:901, 1983.
56. Tekkok IH, Erbengi A: Management of brain abscess in children: review of 130 cases over a period of 21 years. Childs Nerv Syst 8(7):411, 1992.
57. Pouplard F, Bouderlique C, Berthelot J, et al: Double abscess cerebral de la periode neonatale. Propos d'un cas. Pediatrie 35:619, 1980.
58. Sann L, Lapras C, Duquesnel JC, et al: L'abscess cerebral du nouveau-ne. Pediatrie 35:625, 1980.
59. Michel B, Gastaut JL, Bianchi L: Electroencephalographic cranial computerized tomographic correlations in brain abscess. Electroencephalogr Clin Neurophysiol 46:256, 1979.
60. Ercius MS, Dempsey R, Chandler WF: Successful treatment of solitary thalamic abscess. Case report. J Neurosurg 56:865, 1982.
61. Lunsford LD, Nelson PB: Stereotactic aspiration of a brain abscess using the "therapeutic" CT scanner. A case report. Acta Neurochir (Wien) 62:25, 1982.
62. Claveria LE, du Boulay GH, Moseley IF: Intracranial infections: investigations by computerized axial tomography. Neuroradiology 12:59, 1976.
63. Feely MP, Dempsey PJ: Assessment of the postoperative course of excised brain abscess by computerized tomography. Neurosurgery 5:49, 1979.
64. Enzmann DR, Britt RH, Yeager AS: Experimental brain abscess evolution: computer tomographic and neuropathologic correlation. Radiology 133:113, 1979.
65. Kretzschmar K, Wallenfang T, Bohl J: CT studies of brain abscesses in cats. Neuroradiology 22:93, 1981.
66. Sarwar M, Falkoff G, Naseem M: Radiologic techniques in the diagnosis of CNS infections. Infect Dis Central Nerv Syst 4:41, 1986.
67. Dobkin JF, Healton EB, Dickinson T, Brust JC: Nonspecificity of ring enhancement in "medically cured" brain abscess. Neurology (New York) 34:139, 1984.
68. Britt RH, Enzmann DR: Clinical stages of human brain abscess on serial CT scans after contrast infusion. Computerized tomographic, neuropathological, and clinical correlations. J Neurosurg 59:972, 1983.
69. Enzmann DR, Britt RH, Placone RC Jr, et al: The effect of short-term corticosteroid treatment on the CT appearance of experimental brain abscesses. Radiology 145:79, 1982.
70. Black KL, Farhat SM: Cerebral abscess: loss of computed tomographic enhancement with steroids. Neurosurgery 14:215, 1984.
71. Holtas S, Tornquist C, Cronqvist S: Diagnostic difficulties in computed tomography of brain abscess. J Comput Assist Tomogr 6:683, 1982.
72. Davidson HD, Steiner RE: Magnetic resonance imaging in infections of the central nervous system. AJNR 6:499, 1985.
73. Sze G, Zimmerman RD: The magnetic resonance imaging of infections and inflammatory diseases. Radiol Clin North Am 26:839, 1988.
74. Brant-Zawadzki M, Enzmann DR, Placone RC Jr, et al: NMR imaging of experimental brain abscesses: comparison with CT. AJNR 4:250, 1983.
75. Grossman RI, Wolf G, Biery D, et al: Gadolinium-enhanced nuclear magnetic resonance images of experimental brain abscess. J Comput Assist Tomogr 8:204, 1984.
76. Suwanwela C, Poshyachinda V, Poshyachinda M: Brain scanning in the diagnosis of intracranial abscess. Acta Neurochir (Wien) 25:165, 1971.
77. Lewis SE, Hickey DE, Parkey RW: Radionuclide brain imaging—its role and relation to CT scanning. J Comput Assist Tomogr 2:155, 1978.
78. Masucci EF, Sauerbrunn BJL: The evolution of brain abscess; the complementary roles of radionuclide (RN) and computed tomography (CT) scans. Clin Nucl Med 7:166, 1982.
79. Pinsky S, Yum HY, Patel D, et al: Comparison of radionuclide brainscan and computerized tomography for the detection of intracranial infections. Clin Nucl Med 6:12, 1981.
80. Krishna L, Slizofski WJ, Katsetos CD, et al: Abnormal intracerebral thallium localization in a bacterial brain abscess. J Nucl Med 33(11):2017, 1992.
81. Grimstad IA, Hirschberg H, Rootwelt K: ^{99m}Tc-hexamethylpropyleneamine oxime leukocyte scintigraphy and C-reactive protein levels in the differential diagnosis of brain abscesses. J Neurosurg 77(5):732, 1992.
82. Vignaendra V, Ghee LT, Chawala J: EEG in brain abscess: its value in localization compared to other diagnostic tests. Electroencephalogr Clin Neurophysiol 38:611, 1975.
83. Black P: Brain abscess. In Kagan BM (ed): Antimicrobial Therapy, 2nd ed. Philadelphia, Saunders, 1974, pp 244–252.
84. Raimondi AJ, DiRocco C: Cerebral angiography in meningocerebral inflammatory diseases in infancy and childhood: a study of 35 cases. Neurosurgery 3:37, 1978.
85. Chou SN, Story JSL, French LA, Peterson HO:

Some angiographic features of brain abscess. J Neurosurg 24:693, 1966.
86. Goraj B, Kopytek M: Ultrasound; a method of brain abscess drainage monitoring. Eur J Radiol 12(2):120, 1991.
87. Brook I. Bacteriology of intracranial abscess in children. J Neurosurg 54:484, 1981.
88. Bucy PC: The treatment of brain abscess. Ann Surg 108:961, 1938.
89. de Louvois J, Gortval P, Hurley R: Bacteriology of abscesses of the central nervous system: a multicentre prospective study. Br Med J [Clin Res] 2:981, 1977.
90. Morgan H, Wood MW, Murphey F: Experience with 88 consecutive cases of brain abscesses. J Neurosurg 38:698, 1973.
91. Tutton GK: Cerebral abscess—present position. Ann R Coll Surg Engl 13:281, 1953.
92. VanAlphen HAM, Dreissen JJR: Brain abscess and subdural empyema. J Neurol Neurosurg Psychiatry 39:481, 1976.
93. Ariza J, Casanova A, Fernandez Viladrich P, et al: Etiological agent and primary source of infection in 42 cases of focal intracranial suppuration. J Clin Microbiol 24:899, 1986.
94. Heineman HS, Braude AL: Anaerobic infection of the brain. Observations on eighteen consecutive cases of brain abscess. Am J Med 35:682, 1963.
95. Renu Joshi B: Brain abscesses—a study of the causative organisms with special reference to anaerobes. Indian J Pathol Microbiol 31:44, 1988.
96. Brook I: Aerobic and anaerobic bacteriology of intracranial abscesses. Pediatr Neurol 8(3):210, 1992.
97. Britt RH, Enzmann DR, Remington JS: Intracranial infection in cardiac transplant recipients. Ann Neurol 9:107, 1981.
98. Gillet GR, Garner JE, Bremmer DA: Antimicrobial management of intracranial abscess. Aust N Z J Surg 54:253, 1984.
99. Chandrasekar PH, LeFrock JL: Treatment of anaerobic infections of the central nervous system. Indian J Pathol Microbiol 28:7, 1985.
100. Armstrong D, Wong B: Central nervous system infections in immunocompromised hosts. Annu Rev Med 33:293, 1982.
101. Levy RM, Bredesen DE, Rosenblum ML: Neurological manifestations of the acquired immunodeficiency syndrome (AIDS): experience at UCSF and a review of the literature. J Neurosurg 62:475, 1985.
102. Neu HC: Penicillins. In Mandell GL, Douglas RG Jr, Bennett JE (eds): Principles and Practice of Infectious Diseases, 2nd ed. New York, Wiley, 1985, pp 166–180.
103. Mandell GL. Cephalosporins. In Mandell GL, Douglas RG Jr, Bennett JE (eds): Principles and Practice of Infectious Diseases, 2nd ed. New York, Wiley, 1985, pp 180–187.
104. Fekety R: Vancomycin. In Mandell GL, Douglas RG Jr, Bennett JE (eds): Principles and Practice of Infectious Diseases, 2nd ed. New York, Wiley, 1985, pp 232–235.
105. Lietman PS: Aminoglycosides and spectinomycin: aminocyclitols. In Mandell GL, Douglas RG Jr, Bennett JE (eds): Principles and Practice of Infectious Diseases, 2nd ed. New York, Wiley, 1985, pp 192–206.
106. Standiford HC: Tetracyclines and chloramphenicol. In Mandell GL, Douglas RG Jr, Bennett JE (eds): Principles and Practice of Infectious Diseases, 2nd ed. New York, Wiley, 1985, pp 206–216.
107. Steigbigel NH: Erythromycin, lincomycin, and clindamycin. In Mandell GL, Douglas RG Jr, Bennett JE (eds): Principles and Practice of Infectious Diseases, 2nd ed. New York, Wiley, 1985, pp 224–231.
108. Farr B, Mandell GL: Rifampin. In Mandell GL, Douglas RG Jr, Bennett JE (eds): Principles and Practice of Infectious Diseases, 2nd ed. New York, Wiley, 1985, pp 216–220.
109. Finegold SM: Metronidazole. In Mandell GL, Douglas RG Jr, Bennett JE (eds): Principles and Practice of Infectious Diseases, 2nd ed. New York, Wiley, 1985, pp 220–224.
110. Zinner SH, Mayer KH: Sulfonamides and trimethoprim. In Mandell GL, Douglas RG Jr, Bennett JE (eds): Principles and Practice of Infectious Diseases, 2nd ed. New York, Wiley, 1985, pp 237–244.
111. Fekety R: Polymixins. In Mandell GL, Douglas RG Jr, Bennett JE (eds): Principles and Practice of Infectious Diseases, 2nd ed. New York, Wiley, 1985, pp 235–237.
112. Davson H: The blood-brain barrier. In: Physiology of the Cerebrospinal Fluids. Boston, Little, Brown, 1967, pp 82–103.
113. Norrby R: A review of the penetration of antibiotics into CSF and its clinical significance. Scand J Infect Dis (Suppl) 14:296, 1978.
114. Laferriere CI, Marks MI: Chloramphenicol: properties and clinical use. Pediatr Infect Dis J 1:257, 1982.
115. Krasinski K, Kusmiesz H, Nelson JD: Pharmacologic interactions among chloramphenicol, phenytoin, and phenobarbital. Pediatr Infect Dis J 1:232, 1982.
116. Ohno K, Fredericks WR, Rappoport SI: Osmotic opening of the blood-brain barrier to methotrexate in the rat. Surg Neurol 12:323, 1979.
117. Neuwelt EA, Baker DE, Pagel MA, Blank NK: Cerebrovascular permeability and delivery of gentamicin to normal brain and experimental brain abscess in rats. J Neurosurg 61:430, 1984.
118. Black P, Graybill JR, Carache P: Penetration of brain abscess by systemically administered antibiotics. J Neurosurg 38:705, 1973.
119. de Louvois J: The bacteriology and chemotherapy of brain abscess. J Antimicrob Chemother 4:395, 1978.
120. Grace A, Drake-Lee A: Role of anaerobes in cerebral abscesses of sinus origin. Br Med J 288:758, 1984.
121. Bradley PJ, Shaw MD: Three decades of brain ab-

scess in Merseyside. J R Coll Surg Edinb 28:223, 1983.
122. Ingham HR, Selkon JB, Roxby CM: Bacteriological study of otogenic cerebral abscesses: chemotherapeutic role of metronidazole. Br Med J [Clin Res] 2:991, 1977.
123. Savitz MH, Dickinson T: Drug therapy for intracranial suppuration. Am Fam Physician 37:341, 1988.
124. Norrby SR: 4-Quinolones in the treatment of infections of the central nervous system. Rev Infect Dis 10:S253, 1988.
125. Finegold SM, George WL, Mulligan ME: Anaerobic infections. Part I. Dis Mon 31:1, 1985.
126. Molavi A, Dinubile MJ: Brain abscess. In: Vinken PJ, Bruyn GW, Klawans HL (eds): Handbook of Clinical Neurology, Vol 8(52), Microbial Disease. New York, Elsevier Science Publishers, 1988, pp 143–166.
127. Macewen W. Pyogenic Disease of the Brain and Spinal Cord. Glasgow, Maclehose and Sons, 1893.
128. Dandy WE: Treatment of chronic abscess of the brain by tapping. JAMA 87:1477, 1926.
129. Vincent C, David M, Askenasy H: Sur une methode de traitment des abces subaigus et chroniques des hemispheres cerebraux, large decompression, puis ablation en mass sans drainage, ou ablation en mass sans drainage. J Chir (Paris) 49:1, 1937.
130. LeBeau J: Radical surgery and penicillin in brain abscess. A method of treatment in one stage with special reference to the cure of three thoracogenic cases. J Neurosurg 3:359, 1946.
131. Jooma OV, Pennybacker JB, Tutton GK: Brain abscess: aspiration, drainage, or excision? J Neurol Neurosurg Psychiatry 14:308, 1951.
132. Maurice-Williams RS: Open evacuation of pus: a satisfactory surgical approach to the problem of brain abscess? J Neurol Neurosurg Psychiatry 46:697, 1983.
133. Camarata PJ, Dunn DL, Farney AC, et al: Continual intracavitary administration of amphotericin B as an adjunct in the treatment of *Aspergillus* brain abscess: case report and review of the literature. Neurosurgery 31(3):575, 1992.
134. Young RF, Frazee J: Gas within intracranial abscess cavities: an indication for surgical excision. Ann Neurol 16:35, 1984.
135. Stapleton SR, Bell BA, Uttley D: Stereotactic aspiration of brain abscesses: is this the treatment of choice? Acta Neurochir (Wien) 121(1–2):15, 1993.
136. Kagawa M, Takeshita M, Yato S, Kitamura K: Brain abscess in congenital cyanotic heart disease. J Neurosurg 58:913, 1983.
137. Fischer EG, McLennan JE, Suzuki Y: Cerebral abscess in children. Am J Dis Child 135:746, 1981.
138. Legg NJ, Gupta PC, Scott DF: Epilepsy following cerebral abscess: a clinical and EEG study of 70 patients. Brain 96:259, 1973.
139. Heineman HS, Braude AI, Osterholm JL: Intracranial suppurative disease. Early presumptive diagnosis and successful treatment without surgery. JAMA 218:1542, 1971.
140. Chow AW, Alexander E, Montgomerie JZ, et al: Successful treatment of non-meningitic listerial brain abscess without operation. West J Med 112:167, 1975.
141. Berg B, Franklin G, Cuneo R, et al: Nonsurgical cure of brain abscess: early diagnosis and follow-up with computerized tomography. Ann Neurol 3:474, 1978.
142. Kottas M, Smith LG: A possible new approach to the management of brain abscesses. Infection 6:81, 1978.
143. Rotheram EB, Kessler LA: Use of computerized tomography in nonsurgical management of brain abscess. Arch Neurol 36:25, 1979.
144. Barsoun AH, Lewis HC, Cannillo KL: Nonoperative treatment of multiple brain abscesses. Surg Neurol 16:283, 1981.
145. Kamin M, Biddle D: Conservative management of focal intracerebral infection. Neurology 31:103, 1981.
146. Spirer Z, Jurgenson U, Lazewnick R, Reider-Grossvasser I: Complete recovery from an apparent brain abscess treated without neurosurgery. Clin Pediatr (Phila) 21:106, 1982.
147. Vaquero J, Cabezudo JM, Leunda G: Nonsurgical resolution of a brain-stem abscess. J Neurosurg 53:726, 1980.
148. Petit H, Rousseaux M, Lesoin F, et al: Primaute du traitement medicale des abces cerebraux (19 cas). Rev Neurol (Paris) 139:575, 1983.
149. Rosenblum ML, Hoff JT, Norman D, et al: Nonoperative treatment of brain abscesses in selected high-risk patients. J Neurosurg 52:217, 1980.
150. Mauser HW, van Nieuwenhuizen O, Tummers FC, Willemse J: Conservative and surgical management of focal cerebral infection. Clin Neurol Neurosurg 87:199, 1985.
151. Leys D, Christiaens JL, Derambure P, et al: Management of focal intracranial infections: is medical treatment better than surgery? J Neurol Neurosurg Psychiatry 53(6):472, 1990.
152. Mampalam TJ, Rosenblum ML: Trends in the management of bacterial brain abscesses: a review of 102 cases over 17 years. Neurosurgery 23:451, 1988.
153. Molavi A, Blumberg EA: Infections of the central nervous system. In Schillinger D, Nuss AH (eds): Infections in Emergency Surgery. New York, Churchill Livingstone, 1989, pp 203–270.
154. Whalen MA, Hilal SK: Computed tomography as a guide in the diagnosis and follow-up of brain abscesses. Radiology 135:663, 1980.
155. Galicich JH, French LA: Use of dexamethasone in the treatment of cerebral edema resulting from brain tumors and brain surgery. Am Practit 12:169, 1961.
156. Beks JWF, Walstra GJM: Clinical experiences with

steroids in neurosurgical patients. In Reulen HJ, Schurmann K (eds): Steroids and Brain Edema. New York, Springer-Verlag, 1972, pp 233–238.
157. Long WD, Meacham WF: Experimental method for producing brain abscesses in dogs with evaluation of the effect of dexamethasone and antibiotic therapy on the pathogenesis of intracerebral abscess. Surg Forum 19:437, 1968.
158. Quartey GRC, Johnson JA, Rozdilsky B: Decadron in the treatment of cerebral abscess. An experimental study. J Neurosurg 45:301, 1976.
159. Wallenfang T, Bohl J, Kretzschmar K: Evolution of brain abscess in cats; formation of capsule and resolution of brain edema. Neurosurg Rev 3:101, 1980.
160. Lyons BE, Enzmann DR, Britt RH, et al: Short-term high dose corticosteroids in computed tomographic staging of experimental brain abscess. Neuroradiology 23:279, 1982.
161. Garvey G: Current concepts of bacterial infections of the central nervous system: bacterial meningitis and bacterial brain abscess. J Neurosurg 59:735, 1983.
162. Alderson D, Strong AJ, Ingram HR, Selkon JB: Fifteen-year review of the mortality of brain abscess. Neurosurgery 8:1, 1981.
163. Strong AJ, Ingham HR: Brain abscess. Br J Hosp Med 30:396, 1983.
164. Choudhury AR, Taylor JC, Whitaker R: Primary excision of brain abscess. Br Med J [Clin Res] 2:1119, 1977.
165. Ohaegbulam SC, Saddegi NU: Experience with brain abscess treated by simple aspiration. Surg Neurol 13:289, 1980.
166. Rosenblum ML, Hoff JT, Norman D, et al: Decreased mortality from brain abscesses since advent of computerized tomography. J Neurosurg 49:658, 1978.
167. Keet PC: Cranial intradural abscess management of 641 patients during the 35 years from 1952 to 1986. Br J Neurosurg 4(4):273, 1990.
168. Gruszkiewicz J, Doron Y, Peyser E, et al: Brain abscess and its surgical management. Surg Neurol 18:7, 1982.
169. Nielsen H, Harmsen A, Gyldensted C: Cerebral abscess; a long term follow-up. Acta Neurol Scand 67:330, 1983.
170. Seydoux C, Francioli P: Bacterial brain abscesses: factors influencing mortality and sequelae. Clin Infect Dis 15(3):394, 1992.
171. Carey ME, Chou SN, French LA: Long-term neurological residua in patients surviving brain abscess with surgery. J Neurosurg 34:652, 1971.
172. Krajewski R, Stelmasiak Z: Brain abscess in infants. Childs Nerv Syst 8(5):279, 1992.
173. Hirsch JF, Roux FX, Sainte-Rose C, et al: Brain abscess in childhood: a study of 34 cases treated by puncture and antibiotics. Childs Brain 10:251, 1983.
174. Szenasy J, Nagy A: Epilepsy and brain abscess. Acta Paediatr Acad Sci Hung 20:255, 1979.
175. Aebi C, Kaufmann F, Schaad UB: Brain abscess in childhood–long term experiences. Eur J Pediatr 150(4):282, 1991.
176. Arseni C, Ciurea AV: Cerebellar abscesses; a report on 119 cases. Zentralbl Neurochir 43:359, 1982.
177. Brunon J, Pialat J, Brun Y, et al: Les absces cerebraux actinomyces. Neurochirurgie 26:31, 1980.
178. Causey WA: Actinomycosis. In Vinken PJ, Bruyn GW, Klawans H (eds): Handbook of Clinical Neurology, Vol 35, Part 3, Infections of the Nervous System. New York, Elsevier, 1978, pp 383–393.
179. Louie JA, Kusske JA, Rush JL, Pribram HW: Actinomycotic subdural empyema. J Neurosurg 51:852, 1979.
180. Holtz HA, Lavery DP, Kapila R: Actinomycetales infection in the acquired immunodeficiency syndrome. Ann Intern Med 102:203, 1985.
181. Smego RA: Actinomycosis of the central nervous system. Rev Infect Dis 9:855, 1987.
182. Byrne E, Brophy BP, Perrett LV: Nocardial cerebral abscess: new concepts in diagnosis, management, and prognosis. J Neurol Neurosurg Psychiatry 42:1038, 1979.
183. Causey WA, Lee R: Nocardiosis. In Vinken PJ, Bruyn GW, Klawans H (eds): Handbook of Clinical Neurology, Vol 35, Part 3, Infections of the Nervous System. New York, Elsevier, 1978, pp 517–530.
184. Awad I, Bay J, Petersen JM: Nocardial osteomyelitis of the spine with epidural spinal cord compression—a case report. Neurosurgery 15:254, 1984.
185. Norden CW, Ruben FL, Selker R: Nonsurgical treatment of cerebral nocardiosis. Arch Neurol 40:594, 1983.
186. Hadley MN, Spetzler RF, Martin NA, Johnson PC: Middle cerebral artery aneurysm due to *Nocardia asteroides:* case report of aneurysm excision and extracranial-intracranial bypass. Neurosurgery 22: 923, 1988.
187. Rousseaux M, Lesoin F, Destee A, et al: Developments in the treatment of prognosis of multiple cerebral abscess. Neurosurgery 16:304, 1985.
188. Boom WH, Tuazon CV: Successful treatment of multiple brain abscesses with antibiotics alone. Rev Infect Dis 7:189, 1985.
189. Mahapatra AK, Bahita R, Banerji AK, et al: Subdural empyema in children. Indian Pediatr 21:561, 1984.
190. Schiller F, Cairns H, Russel DS: The treatment of purulent pachymeningitis and subdural suppuration with special reference to penicillin. J Neurol Neurosurg Psychiatry 11:143, 1948.
191. Stern WE, Boldrey E: Subdural purulent collections. Surg Gynecol Obstet 95:623, 1952.
192. Jacobson PL, Farmer TW: Subdural empyema complicating meningitis in infants: improved prognosis. Neurology 31:190, 1981.
193. Dan M, Spiegelmann R: Mixed bacterial subdural empyema complicating subdural peritoneal shunt. Acta Neurochir (Wien) 81:77, 1986.
194. Garfin SR, Botte MJ, Triggs KJ, Nickel VL: Sub-

dural abscess associated with halo-pin traction. J Bone Joint Surg [Am] 70A:1338, 1988.
195. Bannister G, Williams B, Smith S: Treatment of subdural empyema. J Neurosurg 55:82, 1981.
196. Yoshikawa TT, Chow AT, Guze LN: Role of anaerobic bacteria in subdural empyema. Report of 4 cases and review of 327 cases from the English literature. Am J Med 58:99, 1975.
197. Rodriguez RE, Valero V, Watanakunakorn C: *Salmonella* focal intracranial infections: review of the world literature (1884–1984) and report of an unusual case. Rev Infect Dis 8:31, 1986.
198. Khan M, Griebel R: Subdural empyema: a retrospective study of 15 patients. Can J Surg 27:283, 1984.
199. Szuwart U, Bennefeld H: Bacteriological analysis of pyogenic infections of the brain. Neurosurg Rev 13(2):113, 1990.
200. Mauser HW, VanHuffelen AC, Tulleken CAF: The EEG in the diagnosis of subdural empyema. Electroencephalogr Clin Neurophysiol 64:511, 1986.
201. Mauser HW, Tulleken CAF: Subdural empyema. A review of 48 patients. Clin Neurol Neurosurg 86:255, 1984.
202. Hodges J, Anslow P, Gillett G: Subdural empyema—continuing diagnostic problems in the CT scan era. Q J Med 59:387, 1986.
203. Wortzman DJ, Tucker WS, Finlayson DM, et al: Subdural empyema with negative CT scan: a case report. Can J Neurol Sci 7:67, 1980.
204. Weisberg L: Subdural empyema: clinical and computed tomographic correlations. Arch Neurol 43: 497, 1986.
205. Weingarten K, Zimmerman RD, Becker RD, et al: Subdural and epidural empyemas: MR imaging. AJR 152:615, 1988.
206. Tsuchiya K, Makita K, Furui S, et al: Contrast-enhanced magnetic resonance imaging of sub- and epidural empyemas. Neuroradiology 34(6):494, 1992.
207. McKillop JH, Holtzman DS, McDougall IR: Detection of subdural empyema with radionuclides. Clin Nucl Med 5:263, 1980.
208. Luken MG, Whelan MA: Recent diagnostic experience with subdural empyema. J Neurosurg 52:764, 1980.
209. Suchet I, Horowitz T, Kitay S, Cruz RM: The predictive value of computed tomography and *Haemophilus influenzae* capsular antigen in subdural fluid collections. Clin Radiol 39:265, 1988.
210. Ogilvy CS, Chapman PH, McGrail K: Subdural empyema complicating bacterial meningitis in a child: enhancement of membranes with gadolinium on magnetic resonance imaging in a patient without enhancement on computed tomography. Surg Neurol 37(2):138, 1992.
211. Cowie R, Williams B: Late seizures and morbidity after subdural empyema. J Neurosurg 58:569, 1983.
212. Skelton R, Maixner W, Issacs D: Sinusitis-induced subdural empyema. Arch Dis Child 67(12):1478, 1992.
213. Bok AP, Peter JC: Subdural empyema: burr holes or craniotomy? A retrospective computerized tomography-era analysis of treatment in 90 cases. J Neurosurg 78(4):574, 1993.
214. Morgan DW, Williams B: Posterior fossa subdural empyema. Brain 108:983, 1985.
215. Curless RG: Subdural empyema in infant meningitis: diagnosis, therapy, and prognosis. Childs Nerv Syst 1:211, 1985.
216. Pattisapu JV, Parent AD: Subdural empyemas in children. Pediatr Neurosci 13:251, 1987.
217. Leys D, Destee A, Petit H, Warot P: Management of subdural intracranial empyemas should not always require surgery. J Neurol Neurosurg Psychiatry 49:635, 1986.
218. Kubic CS, Adams RD: Subdural empyema. Brain 66:18, 1943.
219. Hoyt DJ, Fisher SR: Otolaryngologic management of patients with subdural empyema. Laryngoscope 101(1 Pt 1):20, 1991.
220. Silverberg AL, DiNubile MJ: Subdural empyema and cranial epidural abscess. Symp Infect Central Nerv Syst 69:361, 1985.
221. Calliauw L, dePraetere P, Verbeke L: Postoperative epilepsy in subdural suppurations. Acta Neurochir (Wien) 71:217, 1984.
222. Dastur DK, Dave UP: Fine structure of cellular and vascular reaction in brain tuberculomas: a model for phagocytosis in the CNS. Pathol Res Pract 181:721, 1986.
223. Dastur DK: Neurosurgically relevant aspects of pathology and pathogenesis of intracranial and intraspinal tuberculosis. Neurosurg Rev 6:103, 1983.
224. Garland HG, Armitage J: Intracranial tuberculomata. J Pathol Bacteriol 37:461, 1933.
225. Evans HS, Courville CB: Calcification and ossification in tuberculoma of the brain. Review of the literature and report of three cases. Arch Surg 36:637, 1938.
226. Lees AJ, MacLeod AF, Marshall J: Cerebral tuberculomas developing during treatment of tuberculous meningitis. Lancet 1:1208, 1980.
227. Arseni C: Two hundred and one cases of intracranial tuberculoma treated surgically. J Neurol Neurosurg Psychiatry 21:308, 1958.
228. Dastur HM: A tuberculoma review with some personal experiences. Part I—Brain. Part II—Spinal cord and its coverings. Neurol India 20:111, 1972.
229. Rab SM, Bhatti IH, Ghani A, Khan A: Tuberculous brain abscess. J Neurosurg 43:490, 1975.
230. Whitener DR: Tuberculous brain abscess. Report of a case and review of the literature. Arch Neurol 35:148, 1978.
231. Rammurthi B, Varadarajan MG: Diagnosis of tuberculomas of the brain. Clinical and radiological correlation. J Neurosurg 18:1, 1961.
232. Sinh G, Pandya SK, Dastur DK: Pathogenesis of un-

usual intracranial tuberculomas and tuberculous space-occupying lesions. J Neurosurg 29:149, 1968.
233. Tandon PN, Bhargava S: Effect of medical treatment of intracranial tuberculoma—a CT study. Tubercle 66:85, 1985.
234. Danesi MA, Arigbabu SO, Mordi PN, Ojikutu NA: Intracranial tuberculoma in Lagos, Nigeria. Trop Geogr Med 37:279, 1985.
235. Shen WC, Cheng TY, Lee SK, et al: Disseminated tuberculomas in spinal cord and brain demonstrated by MRI with gadolinium-DTPA. Neuroradiology 35(3):213, 1993.
236. Obrador S: Intracranial tuberculomas—a review of 47 cases. Neurochirurgia (Stuttg) 1:150, 1958/59.
237. Harder E, Al-Kawi MZ, Carney P: Intracranial tuberculoma: conservative management. Am J Med 74:570, 1983.
238. Traub M, Colchester ACF, Kingsley DPE, Swash M: Tuberculosis of the central nervous system. Q J Med (New Series L111) 209:81, 1984.
239. Rossi LN, Duzioni N, Terzi F: Intracranial tuberculomas in a child: regression on the CT scan under conservative therapy. Neuropediatrics 16:228, 1985.
240. Tang LM, Swash M: Tuberculosis of the nervous system: a modern problem (editorial). J R Soc Med 78:429, 1985.
241. Nazaki H, Takashima S, Ishihara T, Aoyagi T: Paradoxical expansion of intracranial tuberculomas during chemotherapy. Rinsho Shinkeigaku 32(1):91, 1992.
242. Dastur HM: Diagnosis and neurosurgical treatment of tuberculous disease of the CNS. Neurosurg Rev 6:111, 1983.
243. Baringer JR: Human herpes simplex virus infections. Adv Neurol 6:41, 1974.
244. Boyle RS, Landry PJ: Herpes simplex encephalitis. Aust N Z J Med 7:408, 1977.
245. Johnson KP, Rosenthal MS, Lerner PI: Herpes simplex encephalitis: the course in 5 vitrologically proven cases. Arch Neurol 27:103, 1972.
246. Johnson RT: Treatment of herpes simplex virus encephalitis. Arch Neurol 27:97, 1972.
247. Skoldenberg B, Forsgren M, Alestig K, et al: Acyclovir versus vidarabine in herpes simplex encephalitis. Lancet 2:707, 1984.
248. Thong YH: Chemotherapy for herpes simplex encephalitis. Med J Aust 1:388, 1981.
249. Fieldman RA, Shende MC: Herpes simplex virus encephalitis simulating a frontoparietal convexity neoplasm. Surg Neurol 3:329, 1975.
250. Drachman DA, Adams RD: Herpes simplex and acute inclusion-body encephalitis. Arch Neurol 7:45, 1962.
251. Whitley RJ, Soong S-J, Linneman C, et al: Herpes simplex encephalitis; clinical assessment. JAMA 247:317, 1982.
252. Puchhammer-Stockl E, Popow-Kraupp T, Heinz FX, et al: Establishment of PCR for the early diagnosis of herpes simplex encephalitis. J Med Virol 32(2):77, 1990.
253. Aurelius E, Johansson B, Skoldenberg B, Forsgren M: Encephalitis in immunocompetent patients due to herpes simplex virus type 1 or 2 as determined by type-specific polymerase chain reaction and antibody assays of cerebrospinal fluid. J Med Virol 39(3):179, 1993.
254. Maxwell GM, Thong YH, Manson JI, Robertson CF: Herpes simplex encephalitis: treatment with adenine arabinoside and cytosine arabinoside. Med J Aust 1:181, 1978.
255. Higazi I: Tuberculoma of the brain. A clinical and angiographic study. J Neurosurg 20:378, 1963.
256. Taber LH, Greenberg SB, Perez FI, Couch RB: Herpes simplex encephalitis treated with vidarabine (adenine arabinoside). Arch Neurol 34:608, 1977.
257. Whitley RJ, Soong SJ, Dolin R et al: Adenine arabinoside therapy of biopsy-proven herpes simplex encephalitis (National Institute of Allergy and Infectious Disease Collaborative Antiviral Study). N Engl J Med 297:289, 1977.
258. Wenman WM, Brunton JL, Lank BA, Ronald AR: Herpes simplex encephalitis: poor outcome despite adenine arabinoside therapy. Can Med Assoc J 126:819, 1982.
259. Whitley RJ, Soong SJ, Hirsch MS, et al: Herpes simplex encephalitis, vidarabine therapy, and diagnostic problems. N Engl J Med 304:313, 1981.
260. Skoldenburg B: Herpes simplex encephalitis. Scand J Infect Dis Suppl 80:40, 1991.
261. Whitley RJ: Herpes simplex virus infections of the central nervous system. Encephalitis and neonatal herpes. Drugs 42(3):406, 1991.
262. Lunsford LD, Martinez AJ, Latchaw RE, Pazin GJ: Rapid and accurate diagnosis of herpes simplex encephalitis with computed tomography stereotaxic biopsy. Surg Neurol 21:249, 1984.
263. Schlitt MJ, Morawetz RB, Bonnin JM, et al: Brain biopsy for encephalitis. Clin Neurosurg 3:591, 1986.
264. Kohl S, James AR: Herpes simplex virus encephalitis during childhood: importance of brain biopsy diagnosis. J Pediatr 107:212, 1985.
265. Sawyer J, Ellner J, Ransohoff DF: To biopsy or not to biopsy in suspected herpes simplex encephalitis: a quantitative analysis. Med Decis Making 8:95, 1988.
266. Fishman MA: Brain biopsy in herpes simplex encephalitis. Acta Paediatr Jpn 34(3):344, 1992.
267. Soong SJ, Watson NE, Caddell GR, et al: Use of brain biopsy for diagnostic evaluation of patients with suspected herpes simplex encephalitis: a statistical model and its clinical implications. NIAID Collaborative Antiviral Study Group. J Infect Dis 163(1):17, 1991.
268. Dixon HHF, Lipscomb FM: Cysticercosis: an analysis of follow-up of 450 cases. Med Res Counc Spec Rep Ser (Lond) 299:1, 1966.
269. Trelles JO, Trelles L: Cysticercosis of the nervous system. In Vinken PJ, Bruyn GW, Klawans H (eds): Handbook of Clinical Neurology, Vol 35, Part 3. In-

fections of the Nervous System. New York, Elsevier, 1978, pp 291–320.
270. Tandon PN: Cerebral cysticercosis. Neurosurg Rev 6:119, 1983.
271. Whittle IR, Dorsch NW: Neurocysticercosis in Australia. Med J Aust 2:156, 1981.
272. Mitchell WG, Crawford TO: Intraparenchymal cerebral cysticercosis in children: diagnosis and treatment. Pediatrics 82:76, 1988.
273. Pascoe M, Saines N, Lyall I, Nolan C: Cerebral cysticercosis: a case report with particular reference to recent advances in diagnosis and treatment. Aust N Z J Med 17:55, 1987.
274. Appuzo MLJ, Dobkin WR, Zee CS, et al: Surgical considerations in treatment of intraventricular cysticercosis. J Neurosurg 60:400, 1984.
275. Courville CB: Intracranial tumors. Notes upon a series of 3,000 verified cases with some current observations pertaining to their mortality. Bull Los Angeles Neurol Soc (Suppl 2) 32:1, 1967.
276. Stern WE: Neurosurgical considerations of cysticercosis of the central nervous system. J Neurosurg 55:382, 1981.
277. Spencer RF, Ganpath V: Heterotopic bone formation following cerebral cysticercosis. S Afr Med J 74:35, 1988.
278. Estanol B, Kleriga E, Lyo M, et al: Mechanisms of hydrocephalus in cerebral cysticercosis: implications for therapy. Neurosurgery 13:119, 1983.
279. DeVilliers JC: Cysticercosis of the nervous system. S Afr Med J 63:769, 1983.
280. Rodriquez-Carbajal J, Boleaga-Duran B, Dorfsman J: The role of computed tomography (CT) in the diagnosis of neurocysticercosis. Childs Nerve Syst 3:199, 1987.
281. Zee CS, Segall HD, Boswell W, et al: MR imaging of neurocysticercosis. J Comput Assist Tomogr 12:927, 1988.
282. Minguetti G, Ferreira MV: Computed tomography in neurocysticercosis. J Neurol Neurosurg Psychiatry 46:936, 1983.
283. Mazer S, Antoniuk A, Ditzel LFS, Araujo JC: The computed tomographic spectrum of cerebral cysticercosis. Comput Radiol 7:373, 1983.
284. Byrd SE, Locke GE, Biggers S, Peroy AK: The computed tomographic appearance of cerebral cysticercosis in adults and children. Radiology 144:819, 1982.
285. Rodriguez-Carbajal J, Salgado P, Gutierrez-Alvarado R, et al: The acute encephalitic phase of neurocysticercosis. Computed tomographic manifestations. AJNR 4:51, 1983.
286. Miller B, Grinnell V, Goldberg MA, Heiner D: Spontaneous radiographic disappearance of cerebral cysticercosis: three cases. Neurology 33:1377, 1983.
287. Skromme-Kadlubik G, Celis C, Ferez A: Cysticercosis of the nervous system. Diagnosed by means of specific radiommunoscan. Ann Neurol 2:343, 1977.
288. Hesselink JR, Healy ME, Press GA, Brahme FJ: Benefits of Gd-DTPA for MR imaging of intracranial abnormalities. J Comput Assist Tomogr 12:266, 1988.
289. Dawood AA, Moosa A: Cerebral cysticercosis in children. J Trop Pediatr 30:136, 1984.
290. Thomson AJ, DeVilliers JC, Moosa A, Vandellen J: Cerebral cysticercosis in children in South Africa. Ann Trop Paediatr 4:67, 1984.
291. Nash TE, Neva FA: Recent advances in the diagnosis and treatment of cerebral cysticercosis. N Engl J Med 311:1492, 1984.
292. Sotelo J, Escobedo F, Rodriquez-Carbajal J, et al: Therapy of parenchymal brain cysticercosis with praziquantel. N Engl J Med 310:1001, 1984.
293. Lawner PM: Medical management of neurocysticercosis with praziquantel. Bull Clin Neurosci 48:102, 1983.
294. Ciferri F: Praziquantel for cysticercosis of the brain parenchyma (letter). N Engl J Med 311:733, 1984.
295. DeGhetaldi LD, Norman RM, Douville AW: Praziquantel for cysticercosis of the brain parenchyma (letter). N Engl J Med 311:732, 1984.
296. McCormick GF, Zee CS, Heiden J: Cysticercosis cerebri: review of 127 cases. Arch Neurol 39:534, 1982.
297. Stepian L. Cerebral cysticercosis in Poland: clinical symptoms and operative results in 132 cases. J Neurosurg 19:505, 1962.
298. Ramina R, Arruda WD, Parolin MKF, Prestes ACF: When and on what to operate in multiple cerebral cysticercosis cysts? J Neurol Neurosurg Psychiatry 51:1006, 1988.
299. Robles C, Sedano AM, Vargas-Tentori N, Galindo-Virgen S: Long-term results of praziquantel therapy in neurocysticercosis. J Neurosurg 66:359, 1987.
300. Rosner NH, Doris PE, Singh RR: Cerebral cysticercosis. Demonstration by intraoperative neurosonography. J Ultrasound Med 6:623, 1987.
301. Arana-Iniquez R: Echinococcus. In Vinken PJ, Bruyn GE, Klawans H (eds): Handbook of Clinical Neurology, Vol 35, Part 3. Infections of the Nervous System. New York, Elsevier, 1978, pp 175–208.
302. Kaya U, Ozden B, Turker K, Tarcan B: Intracranial hydatid cysts: study of 17 cases. J Neurosurg 42:580, 1975.
303. Rahimizadeh A, Hadadian K: Hydatid cyst of the fourth ventricle. Neurosurgery 14:787, 1984.
304. Ozgen T, Bertan V, Kansu T, Akalin S: Intrasellar hydatid cyst. J Neurosurg 60:647, 1984.
305. Anderson ME, Bickerstaff ER, Hamilton JG: Cerebral hydatid disease in Britain. J Neurol Neurosurg Psychiatry 38:1104, 1975.
306. Gomori JM, Cohen D, Eyd A, Pomeranz S: Water lily sign in CT of cerebral hydatid disease: a case report. Neuroradiology 30:358, 1988.
307. Gokalp HZ, Erdogan A: Hydatid cyst of the aqueduct of Sylvius. Case report. Clin Neurol Neurosurg 90:83, 1988.
308. Braunsdorf EW, Schmidt D, Rautenberg M: Cere-

bral manifestation of hydatid disease in a child. Childs Nerv Syst 4:249, 1988.

309. Todorov T, Vutova K, Petkov D, Balkanski G: Albendazole treatment of multiple cerebral hydatid cysts: case report. Trans R Soc Trop Med Hyg 82:150, 1988.
310. Ozgen T, Erbengi A, Bertan V, et al: The use of computerized tomography in the diagnosis of cerebral hydatid cysts. J Neurosurg 50:339, 1979.
311. Bird AV: Schistosomiasis of the central nervous system. In Vinken PJ, Bruyn GW, Klawans HL (eds): Handbook of Clinical Neurology, Vol 35, Part 3. Infections of the Nervous System. New York, Elsevier, 1978, pp 231–241.
312. Scrimgeour EM, Gajdusek DC: Involvement of the central nervous system in *Schistosoma mansoni* and *S. haematobium* infection. Brain 108:1023, 1985.
313. Britton CB, Miller JR: Neurologic complications in acquired immunodeficiency syndrome (AIDS). In Johnson KP (ed): Neurologic Clinics, Vol 2, No 2. Philadelphia, Saunders, 1984, pp 315–339.
314. Levy RM, Pons VG, Rosenblum ML: Central nervous system mass lesions in the acquired immunodeficiency syndrome (AIDS). J Neurosurg 61:9, 1984.
315. Resnick L, DiMarzo-Veronese F, Schupbach J, et al: Intra-blood-brain-barrier synthesis of HTLV-III from specific IgG in patients with neurologic symptoms associated with AIDS or AIDS-related complex. N Engl J Med 313:1498, 1985.
316. McLeod R, Berry PF, Marchall WH Jr, et al: Toxoplasmosis presenting as brain abscess: diagnosis by computerized tomography and cytology of aspirated purulent material. Am J Med 67:711, 1979.
317. Oh SJ: Paragonimiasis in the central nervous system. In Vinken JP, Bruyn GW, Klawans H (eds): Handbook of Clinical Neurology, Vol 35, Part 3. Infections of the Nervous System. New York, Elsevier, 1978, pp 243–266.
318. Lee SH, Rao KCVG: Paragonimiasis. In Cranial Computed Tomography. New York, McGraw-Hill, 1983, pp 540–542.
319. Udaka F, Okuda B, Okada M, et al: CT findings of cerebral paragonimiasis in the chronic state. Neuroradiology 30:31, 1988.
320. Yoshida M, Moritaka K, Kuga A, Anegawa S: CT findings of cerebral paragonimiasis in the chronic state. J Comput Assist Tomogr 6:195, 1982.
321. Mousa AH: Amebiasis in the tropics. J Egypt Public Health Assoc 48:148, 1983.
322. Rananavare MM: Evolution of amoebic lesions. Indian J Pathol Bacteriol 12:101, 1969.
323. Reddy DR, Rao JJ, Krishna RV: Amoebic brain abscess. J Indian Med Assoc 63:61, 1974.
324. Banerjee AK, Bhatnagar RK, Bhusnurmath SR: Secondary cerebral amebiasis. Trop Geogr Med 35:333, 1983.
325. Schmidt H, Bafort JM: African trypanosomiasis: treatment-induced invasion of brain and encephalitis. Am J Trop Med Hyg 34:64, 1985.
326. Poisson M, Bleibel JM, Regnier A, et al: Formes pseudo-tumorales de la trypanosomiase africaine a *Trypanosoma gambiense*. Etude clinique et tomoden. Sem Hop Paris 56:1979, 1980.
327. Sonan T, Giordano C, Boa F, Dumas M: Hemiplegic forms of human African trypanosomiasis. Bull Soc Pathol Exot Filiales 81:459, 1988.
328. Armstrong D, Wong B: Central nervous system infections in immunocompromised hosts. Annu Rev Med 33:293, 1982.
329. Britt RH, Enzmann DR, Remington JS: Intracranial infection in cardiac transplant recipients. Ann Neurol 9:107, 1981.
330. Enzmann DR, Brant-Zawadzki M, Britt RH: CT of central nervous system infections in immunocompromised patients. AJR 135:263, 1980.
331. Young RF, Gade G, Grinnell V: Surgical treatment for fungal infections in the central nervous system. J Neurosurg 63:371, 1985.
332. Goldstein E, Lawrence R: Coccidioidomycosis of the central nervous system. In Vinken PJ, Bruyn GW, Klawans H (eds): Handbook of Clinical Neurology, Vol 35, Part 3. Infections of the Nervous System. New York, Elsevier, 1978, pp 443–457.
333. Harrison HR, Galgiani JN, Reynolds AF, et al: Amphotericin B and imidazole therapy for coccidiodal meningitis in children. Pediatr Infect Dis 2:216, 1983.
334. Roberts M, Rinaudo PA, Tilton RC, et al: Treatment of multiple intracerebral cryptococcal granulomas with 5-fluorocytosine. Case report. J Neurosurg 37:229, 1972.
335. Weenink HR, Bruyn G, Klawans H: Cryptococcus of the central nervous system. In Vinken PJ, Bruyn GW, Klawans H (eds): Handbook of Clinical Neurology, Vol 35, Part 3. Infections of the Nervous System. New York, Elsevier, 1978, pp 459–502.
336. Bhalla D, Kumar S, Pal DN, et al: Aspergilloma of the frontal lobe. Acta Neurochir (Wien) 55:135, 1980.
337. Byrd B, Weiner MH, McGee ZA: *Aspergillus* spinal epidural abscess. JAMA 248:3138, 1982.
338. Fisher BD, Armstrong D, Yu B, Gold JWM: Invasive aspergillosis: progress in early diagnosis and treatment. Am J Med 71:571, 1981.
339. Mawk JR, Erickson DL, Chou SN, Seljeskog EL: *Aspergillus* infections of the lumbar disc spaces. J Neurosurg 58:270, 1983.
340. Savaria-Gomez J: Aspergillosis of the central nervous system. In Vinken PJ, Bruyn GW, Klawans H (eds): Handbook of Clinical Neurology, Vol 35, Part 3. Infections of the Nervous System. New York, Elsevier, 1978, pp 395–400.
341. Nov AA, Cromwell LD: Computed tomography of neuraxis aspergillosis. J Comput Assist Tomogr 8:413, 1984.
342. Weiland D, Ferguson RM, Peterson PK, et al: Aspergillosis in 25 renal transplant patients. Epidemiology, clinical presentation, diagnosis, and management. Ann Surg 98:622, 1983.

343. McKee DF, Barr WM, Bryan CS, Lunceford EM: Primary aspergillosis of the spine mimicking Pott's paraplegia. J Bone Joint Surg [Am] 66A:1481, 1984.
344. Corvisier N, Gray F, Gherardi R, et al: Aspergillosis of ethmoid sinus and optic nerve, with arteritis and rupture of the internal carotid artery. Surg Neurol 28:311, 1987.
345. Leers WD: North American blastomycosis. In Vinken PJ, Bruyn GW, Klawans H (eds): Handbook of Clinical Neurology, Vol 35, Part 3. Infections of the Nervous System. New York, Elsevier, 1978, pp 401–411.
346. Titrud LA: Blastomycosis of the cervical spine. Minn Med 58:729, 1975.
347. Kravitz GR, Davies SF, Eckman MR, Sarosi GA: Chronic blastomycotic meningitis. Am J Med 71:501, 1981.
348. Bell RM, Starshak RJ, Sty JR, Harb JM: Solitary intracranial blastomycotic abscess. Wis Med J 82:23, 1983.
349. Osmund JD, Schweitzer G, Dunbar JM, Villet W: Blastomycosis of the spine with paraplegia. S Afr Med J 45:431, 1971.
350. Detrisac DA, Harding WG, Greiner AL, et al: Vertebral North American blastomycosis. Surg Neurol 13:311, 1980.
351. Roos KL, Bryan JP, Maggio WW, et al: Intracranial blastomycoma. Medicine (Baltimore) 66:224, 1987.
352. Dhermy P: Phycomycosis (mucormycosis). In Vinken PJ, Bruyn GW, Klawans H (eds): Handbook of Clinical Neurology, Vol 35, Part 3. Infections of the Nervous System. New York, Elsevier, 1978, pp 541–555.
353. Ignelzi RJ, VanderArk GD: Cerebral mucormycosis following open head trauma. J Neurosurg 42:593, 1975.
354. Price JC, Stevens DL: Hyperbaric oxygen in the treatment of rhinocerebral mycormycosis. Laryngoscope 90:737, 1980.
355. Gamba JL, Woodruff WW, Djang WT, Yeates AE: Craniofacial mucormycosis: assessment with CT. Radiology 160:207, 1986.
356. Lawrence RM, Goldstein E: Histoplasmosis. In Vinken PJ, Bruyn GW, Klawans H (eds): Handbook of Clinical Neurology, Vol 35, Part 3. Infections of the Nervous System. New York, Elsevier, 1978, pp 503–515.
357. Tveten L: Candidiasis. In Vinken PJ, Bruyn GW, Klawans H (eds): Handbook of Clinical Neurology, Vol 35, Part 3. Infections of the Nervous System. New York, Elsevier, 1978, pp 413–442.
358. Haruda F, Bergman MA, Headings D: Unrecognized *Candida* brain abscess in infancy: two cases and a review of the literature. Johns Hopkins Med J 147:182, 1980.
359. Hayes WS, Berg RA, Dorfman HD, Freedman MT: Case report 291. Diagnosis: *Candida discitis* vertebral osteomyelitis at L1–L2 from hematogenous spread. Skeletal Radiol 12:284, 1984.
360. Carnevale NT, Galgiani JN, Stevens DA, et al: Amphotericin-B-induced myelopathy. Arch Intern Med 140:1189, 1980.
361. Price RW, Brew B, Sidtis J, et al: The brain in AIDS: central nervous system HIV-1 infection and AIDS dementia complex. Science 239:586, 1988.
362. Johnson RT, McArthur JC, Narayan O: The neurobiology of human immunodeficiency virus infections. FASEB J 2:2970, 1988.
363. Gray F, Gherardi R, Scarvilli F: The neuropathology of the acquired immune deficiency syndrome (AIDS). A review. Brain 111:245, 1988.
364. Lantos PL, McLaughlin JE, Schoitz CL, et al: Neuropathology of the brain in HIV infection. Lancet 1(8633):309, 1989.
365. Anders KH, Guerra WF, Tomiyasu U, et al: The neuropathology of AIDS: UCLA experience and review. Am J Pathol 124:537, 1986.
366. Gonzales MF, Davis RL: Neuropathology of acquired immunodeficiency syndrome. Neuropathol Appl Neurobiol 14:345, 1988.
367. Loureiro C, Gill PS, Meyer PR, et al: Autopsy findings in AIDS-related lymphoma. Cancer 62:735, 1988.
368. Michalany J, Mattos ALA, Michalany NS, et al: Acquired immune deficiency syndrome (AIDS) in Brazil. Necropsy findings. Ann Pathol 7:15, 1987.
369. Rhodes RH: Histopathology of the central nervous system in the acquired immunodeficiency syndrome. Hum Pathol 18:636, 1987.
370. McArthur JH, Palenicek JG, Bowersox LL: Human immunodeficiency virus and the nervous system. Nurs Clin North Am 23:823, 1988.
371. Rosenblum ML, Levy RM, Bredesen DE: Neurosurgical implications of the acquired immunodeficiency syndrome (AIDS). Clin Neurosurg 34:419, 1988.
372. Mills J: *Pneumocystis carinii* and *Toxoplasma gondii* infections in patients with AIDS. Rev Infect Dis 8:1001, 1986.
373. Luft BJ, Brooks RG, Conley FK, et al: Toxoplasmic encephalitis in patients with acquired immune deficiency syndrome. JAMA 252:913, 1984.
374. Olsen WL: Neuroradiologic abnormalities in AIDS. Curr Probl Diagn Radiol 17:89, 1988.
375. Post MJD, Sheldon JJ, Hensley GT, et al: Central nervous system disease in acquired immunodeficiency syndrome: prospective correlation using CT, MR imaging, and pathologic studies. Radiology 158: 141, 1986.
376. Shih WJ, Domstad PA, DeLand FH: Opportunistic intracranial infection in AIDS detection by technetium-99m DTPA brain scintigraphy. J Nucl Med 27:498, 1986.
377. Levy RE, Bredesen DE: Central nervous system dysfunction in acquired immunodeficiency syndrome. J Acquir Immune Defic Syndr 1:41, 1988.
378. Ramsey RG, Geremia GK: CNS complications of AIDS: CT and MR findings. AJNR 151:449, 1988.
379. Snider WD, Simpson DM, Nielsen S, et al: Neurological complications of acquired immune deficiency

syndrome: analysis of 50 patients. Ann Neurol 14:403, 1983.
380. Levy RM, Bredesen DE, Rosenblum ML: Neurologic manifestations of the acquired immunodeficiency syndrome (AIDS): experience at UCSF and review of the literature. J Neurosurg 62:475, 1985.
381. Balch RE: Wound infections complicating neurosurgical procedures. J Neurosurg 26:41, 1967.
382. Blomstedt GC: Infections in neurosurgery: a retrospective study of 1143 patients and 1517 operations. Acta Neurochir (Wien) 78:81, 1985.
383. Bullitt E, Lehman RAW: Osteomyelitis of the skull. Surg Neurol 11:163, 1979.
384. Haines SJ, Shou SN: Infections of the scalp and osteomyelitis of the skull. In Wilkins RH, Rengechary SS (eds): Neurosurgery, Vol 3. New York, McGraw-Hill, 1985, pp 1964–1967.
385. Batson OV: The function of the vertebral veins and their role in the spread of metastases. Ann Surg 112:138, 1940.
386. Waldvogel FA, Medoff F, Swartz NM: Osteomyelitis: a review of clinical features, therapeutic considerations, and unusual aspects. N Engl J Med 282:316, 1970.
387. Wiley AM, Trueta J: The vascular anatomy of the spine and its relationship to pyogenic vertebral osteomyelitis. J Bone Joint Surg [Br] 41B:796, 1959.
388. Ratcliffe JF: Anatomic basis for the pathogenesis and radiologic features of vertebral osteomyelitis and its differentiation from childhood discitis. Acta Radiol Diagn 26:137, 1985.
389. Collert S: Osteomyelitis of the spine. Acta Orthop Scand 48:283, 1977.
390. Griffiths HED, Jones DM: Pyogenic infection of the spine: a review of 28 cases. J Bone Joint Surg [Br] 53B:383, 1971.
391. Verner EF, Musher DM: Spinal epidural abscess. Med Clin North Am 69:375, 1985.
392. Jabbari B, Pierce JF: Spinal cord compression due to pseudomonas in a heroin addict. Case report. Neurology 27:1034, 1977.
393. Stern WE, Balch RE: Surgical aspects of nonspecific inflammatory and suppurative disease of the vertebral column. Am J Surg 112:314, 1966.
394. Stone DB, Bonfiglio M: Pyogenic vertebral osteomyelitis. A diagnostic pitfall for the internist. Arch Intern Med 112:491, 1963.
395. Demers C, Tremblay M, Lacourciere Y: Acute vertebral osteomyelitis complicating *Streptococcus sanguis* endocarditis. Ann Rheum Dis 47:333, 1988.
396. Ullman RF, Strampfer MJ, Cunha BA: *Streptococcus mutans* vertebral osteomyelitis. Heart Lung 17:319, 1988.
397. Thompson D, Bannister P, Murphy P: Vertebral osteomyelitis in the elderly. Br Med J [Clin Res] 296:1309, 1988.
398. Williams JL, Moller GA, O'Rourke TL: Pseudoinfections of the intervertebral disc and adjacent vertebrae. AJR 103:611, 1968.
399. Rafto SE, Dalinka MK, Schiebler ML, et al: Spondyloarthropathy of the cervical spine in long-term hemodialysis. Radiology 166:201, 1988.
400. McHenry MC, Duchesneau PM, Keys TF, et al: Vertebral osteomyelitis presenting as spinal cord compression fracture. Arch Intern Med 148:417, 1988.
401. Kuriloff DB, Blaugrund S, Ryan J, O'Leary P: Delayed neck infection following anterior spine surgery. Laryngoscope 97:1094, 1987.
402. Craig JB: Cervical spine osteomyelitis with delayed onset tetraparesis after penetrating wounds of the neck. S Afr Med J 69:197, 1986.
403. Maher DP, Rappaport NH, Kopaniky DR: *Pseudomonas* cervical osteomyelitis in a polytrauma patient. J Trauma 27:1301, 1987.
404. Andrews JC, Mickel RA, Hanson DG, et al: Major complications following tracheoesophageal puncture for voice rehabilitation. Laryngoscope 97:562, 1987.
405. Baldwin N, Scott AR, Heller SR, et al: Vertebral and paravertebral sepsis in diabetes: an easily missed cause of backache. Diabetic Med 2:395, 1985.
406. Modic MT, Feiglin DH, Piraino DW, et al: Vertebral osteomyelitis: assessment using MR. Radiology 157:157, 1985.
407. Michael AS, Mikheal MA: Spinal osteomyelitis: unusual findings on magnetic resonance imaging. Comput Med Imaging Graph 12:329, 1988.
408. Adatepe MH, Powell OM, Isaacs GH, et al: Hematogenous pyogenic vertebral osteomyelitis: diagnostic value of radionuclide bone imaging. J Nucl Med 27:1680, 1986.
409. Fernandez-Ulloa M, Vasavada PJ, Hanslits ML, et al: Diagnosis of vertebral osteomyelitis: clinical, radiological, and scintigraphic features. Orthopedics 8:1144, 1985.
410. Brant-Zawadzki M, Burke VD, Jeffrey RB: CT in the evaluation of spine infection. Spine 8:358, 1983.
411. Whelan MA, Schonfeld S, Post JD, et al: Computed tomography of nontuberculous spinal infection. J Comput Assist Tomogr 9:280, 1985.
412. Hyman RA, Gorey MT: Imaging strategies for MR of the spine. Radiol Clin North Am 26:505, 1988.
413. Hoffer FA, Strand RD, Gebhardt MC: Percutaneous biopsy of pyogenic infection of the spine in children. J Pediatr Orthop 8:442, 1988.
414. Kattapuram SV, Rosenthal DI: Percutaneous biopsy of the cervical spine using CT guidance. AJR 149:539, 1987.
415. Cotty PH, Fouquet B, Pleskof L, et al: Vertebral osteomyelitis: value of percutaneous biopsy. J Neuroradiol 15:13, 1988.
416. Frager DH, Goldman MJ, Seimon LP: Computed tomography guidance for skeletal biopsy. Skeletal Radiol 16:644, 1987.
417. Leys D, Lesoin F, Viaud C: Decreased morbidity from acute bacterial spinal epidural abscesses using computed tomography and nonsurgical treatment in selected patients. Ann Neurol 17:350, 1985.
418. Redfern RM, Miles J, Banks AJ, Dervin E: Stabilisation of the infected spine. J Neurol Neurosurg Psychiatry 51:803, 1988.

419. Fernand R, Lee CK: Postlaminectomy disc space infection. Clin Orthop 209:215, 1986.
420. Blankstein A, Rubinstein E, Ezra E, et al: Disc space infection and vertebral osteomyelitis as a complication of percutaneous lateral discectomy. Clin Orthop 225:234, 1987.
421. Zeiger HE, Zampella EJ: Intervertebral disc infection after lumbar chemonucleolysis: report of a case. Neurosurgery 18:616, 1986.
422. Heller RM, Szalay EA, Green NE, et al: Disc space infection in children: magnetic resonance imaging. Radiol Clin North Am 26:207, 1988.
423. Boden SD, Davis DO, Dina TS, et al: Postoperative discitis: distinguishing early MR-imaging findings from normal postoperative disk space changes. Radiology 184(3):765, 1992.
424. Szypryt EP, Hardy JG, Hinton CE, et al: A comparison between magnetic resonance imaging and scintigraphic bone imaging in the diagnosis of disc space infection in an animal model. Spine 13:1042, 1988.
425. Rubaltelli L, DeGerone E, Caterino G: Echographic evaluation of tubercular abscesses in lumbar spondylitis. J Ultrasound Med 9(2):67, 1990.
426. Yu WY, Siu C, Wing PC, et al: Percutaneous suction aspiration for osteomyelitis. Report of two cases. Spine 16(2):198, 1991.
427. Gibson MJ, Karpinski MRK, Slack RCB, et al: The penetration of antibiotics into the normal intervertebral disc. J Bone Joint Surg [Br] 69B:784, 1987.
428. Borner M, Follath F: Antibiotic therapy and long-term course in spondylodiscitis. Schweitz Med Wochenschr 119:19, 1987.
429. Baker AS, Ojemann RG, Swartz MN, Richardson EP: Spinal epidural abscess. N Engl J Med 293:463, 1975.
430. Heusner AP: Nontuberculous spinal epidural infections. N Engl J Med 239:845, 1948.
431. Hulme A, Dott NM: Spinal epidural abscess. Br Med J [Clin Res] 1:64, 1958.
432. Ericsson M, Algers G, Schliamser SE: Spinal epidural abscess in adults: review and report of iatrogenic cases. Scand J Infect Dis 22(3):249, 1990.
433. Lynch J, Zech D: Spondylitis without epidural abscess formation following short-term use of an epidural catheter. Acta Anaesthesiol Scand 34(2):167, 1990.
434. Reynolds PC, Hahn MB: Early diagnosis of a spinal epidural abscess. Reg Anesth 16(1):57, 1991.
435. Sonden B: Epidural abscess—a rare but severe complication after epidural anesthesia. Lakartidningen 88(26–27):2401, 1991.
436. Browder J, Meyers R: Pyogenic infections of the spinal epidural space; a consideration of anatomic and physiologic pathology. Surgery 10:296, 1941.
437. Wheeler D, Keiser P, Rigamonti D, Keay S: Medical management of spinal epidural abscesses: case report and review. Clin Infect Dis 15(1):22, 1992.
438. Redekop GJ, Del Maestro RF: Diagnosis and management of spinal epidural abscess. Can J Neurol Sci 19(2):180, 1992.
439. Probst CH, Wicki G: Spinale subdurale empyema und abszesse. Schweiz Arch Neurol Neurochir Psychiatr 134(1):53, 1984.
440. Menezes AH, Graf CJ, Perrett GE: Spinal cord abscess: a review. Surg Neurol 8:461, 1977.
441. Kocen RS, Parsons M: Neurological complications of tuberculosis: some unusual manifestations. Q J Med 39:17, 1970.
442. Mathai KV, Chandy J: Tuberculous infections of the nervous system. In Ojemann RG, Shillito J (eds): Clinical Neurosurgery, Vol 14. Baltimore, Williams & Wilkins, 1967, pp 145–177.
443. Govender S, Charles RW, Ballaram RS, Achary DM: Vertebral osteomyelitis after a closed fracture of the spine. S Afr Med J 73:124, 1988.
444. Friedman B: Chemotherapy of tuberculosis of the spine. J Bone Joint Surg [Am] 48A:451, 1966.
445. Lisbona R, Derbekyan V, Novales-Diaz J, Veksler A: Gallium-67 scintigraphy in tuberculous and nontuberculous infectious spondylitis. J Nucl Med 34(5):853, 1993.
446. Hodgson AR, Stock FE: Anterior spine fusion for the treatment of tuberculosis of the spine. The operative findings and results of treatment in the first 100 cases. J Bone Joint Surg [Am] 42A:295, 1960.
447. Bailey HL, Gabriel M, Hodgson AR, et al: Tuberculosis of the spine in children. Operative findings and results in one hundred consecutive patients treated by removal of the lesion and anterior grafting. J Bone Joint Surg [Am] 54A:1633, 1972.
448. Rajasekaran S, Soundarapandian S: Progression of kyphosis in tuberculosis of the spine treated by anterior arthrodesis. J Bone Joint Surg [Am] 71(9):1314, 1989.
449. Hsu LCS, Leong JCY: Tuberculosis of the lower cervical spine (C2 to C7). A report on 40 cases. J Bone and Joint Surg [Br] 66B:1, 1984.
450. Babhulkar SS, Tayade WB, Babhulkar SK: Atypical spinal tuberculosis. J Bone and Joint Surg [Br] 66B:239, 1984.
451. Tuli SM: Results of treatment of spinal tuberculosis by "middle-path" regime. J Bone Joint Surg [Br] 57B:13, 1975.
452. Kaufman DM, Kaplan JG, Litman N: Infectious agents in spinal epidural abscesses. Neurology 30:844, 1980.
453. Medical Research Council: A 10-year assessment of controlled trials of inpatient and outpatient treatment of plaster-of-paris jackets for tuberculosis of the spine in children on standard chemotherapy. J Bone Joint Surg [Br] 67B:103, 1985.
454. Anonymous: Controlled trial of short-course regimens of chemotherapy in the ambulatory treatment of spinal tuberculosis. Results at three years of a study in Korea. Twelfth report of the Medical Research Council Working Party on Tubercu-

losis of the Spine. J Bone Joint Surg [Br] 75(2):240, 1993.

455. Perani D, Scotti G, Scialfa G, D'Angelo V: Hydatid disease of spine: a case report. J Neurosurg Sci 27:55, 1983.
456. Claudon M, Bracard S, Plenat F, et al: Spinal involvement in alveolar echinococcosis: assessment of two cases. Radiology 162:571, 1987.
457. Charles RW, Govender S, Naidoo KS: Echinococcal infection of the spine with neural involvement. Spine 13:47, 1988.
458. Tavoulari-Chrysophaki KG, Emmanouilidou AJ: Primary diagnosis of intraspinal echinococcosis by cytologic examination of cyst fluid. Acta Cytol 33:138, 1989.
459. Fiennes AG, Thomas DG: Combined medical and surgical treatment of spinal hydatid disease: a case report. J Neurol Neurosurg Psychiatry 45:927, 1982.
460. Efthimiou J, Denning D: Spinal cord disease due to *Schistosoma mansoni* successfully treated with oxaminquine. Br Med J 288:1343, 1984.
461. Roy RN, Bhattacharya MB, Chatterjee BP, et al: Spinal cysticerosis. Surg Neurol 6:129, 1976.
462. de Villiers JC: Cysticercosis of the nervous system. S Afr Med J 63:769, 1983.
463. Vlok GJ, Wells MC: Vertebral cysticercosis: a case report. S Afr Med J 73:730, 1988.
464. Khwaja MS, Dossetor FB, Lawrie JH: Extradural guinea-worm abscess: report of two cases. J Neurosurg 43:627, 1975.
465. Adeloye A: Extradural compression by guinea worm (letter). Surg Neurol 19:482, 1983.
466. Dupont B, Drauhet E: Cutaneous, ocular, and osteoarticular candidiasis in heroin addicts: new clinical and therapeutic aspects in 38 patients. J Infect Dis 152:577, 1985.
467. Friedman BC, Simon GL: *Candida* vertebral osteomyelitis: report of three cases and a review of the literature. Diagn Microbiol Infect Dis 8:31, 1987.
468. Kashimoto T, Kitagawa H, Kachi H: *Candida tropicalis* vertebral osteomyelitis and discitis. Spine 11:57, 1986.

Thoracic Surgical Infections

CHAPTER 35

Stewart M. Scott, Gulshan K. Sethi, Timothy Takaro, Thomas J. Enright

Infections of the chest can be divided into four regions: (1) the chest wall, (2) pleural spaces, (3) lungs and airways, and (4) the mediastinum. In each area, both primary and postoperative infections are considered.

These divisions are somewhat artificial, because infections in one area commonly involve neighboring areas. For example, pneumonias or lung abscesses are a major cause of pleural empyema. In turn, a loculated empyema may burrow through the chest, simulating an abscess of the chest wall (empyema necessitatis). Chronic mediastinal infections may result from primary lung infections, such as histoplasmosis or tuberculosis, and acute mediastinal infections that result from perforations of the esophagus or bronchopleural fistulas quickly cause infections of the pleural cavities.

The mouth and nasopharynx are normally host to many microorganisms and, being in continuity with the upper and lower airways of the lungs, provide natural and major portals of entry into this region. The result can be aspiration pneumonitis, lung abscess, or a communicable infectious disease transmitted by droplet from patient to patient, as in tuberculosis. Noncommunicable diseases may also result from inhaled or aspirated endogenous or exogenous agents, such as bacteria, viruses, fungi, protozoa, or gastric contents. Pathogenic organisms can also enter the thoracic contents through the bloodstream or lymphatics, via the fascial spaces from the neck, or from beneath the diaphragm.

Disturbances of normal physiologic pressure differentials may also cause serious consequences. For instance, if the normally negative intrapleural pressure is lost, the potential pleural space becomes an actual space, with partial or complete collapse of the lung and an invitation for intrapleural infection. Abnormal mediastinal masses, unusual enlargement or infection of mediastinal lymph nodes, and intense fibrous tissue inflammatory mediastinal reaction can produce a variety of clinical syndromes (superior vena caval syndrome, middle lobe syndrome) or abnormal fistulous communications between organs and adjoining spaces.

Pathogenetic factors are discussed regionally. It is enough to point out that the congenital anatomic disorders (tracheoesophageal fistulas, pulmonary sequestration, mediastinal cysts of almost any variety), acquired conditions [trauma, airway or esophageal obstruction, operative procedures, ischemia (pulmonary thromboembolic disease)], or compromised host defense mechanisms all play important roles in surgical infections of the chest.

Fortunately, this region lends itself to examination by the traditional methods of physical examination, by x-ray methods including angiography, computed tomography (CT) scanning, and magnetic resonance imaging (MRI) and by techniques involving radionuclides.

The increased use of corticosteroids, drugs to treat cancer, and drugs to control rejection of transplanted organs, along with the emergence of acquired immunodeficiency syndrome (AIDS) has changed the spectrum of thoracic infections. Many viruses, bacteria, fungi, and protozoa that once rarely caused human infections now are being encountered as opportunistic organisms and many newly identified microorganisms are emerging as potential pathogens.

INFECTIONS OF THE CHEST WALL

The thorax constitutes approximately 20 percent of the total body surface. Only those infections specific to the chest wall and that may require special considerations in management are discussed here. Infections of the skin and subcutaneous tissue are discussed in Chapter 31.

Abscess of the Chest Wall

Etiology and Pathogenesis. An abscess of the chest wall may arise as a primary infection or as a complication of septicemia. However, an abscess can result from an intrathoracic infection that penetrates the thoracic wall.[1,2] Thus abscesses may be associated with osteomyelitis of the ribs or sternum or with costal chondritis of pyogenic, mycobacterial, or fungal origin. Actinomycosis, discussed in detail later, is the most common granulomatous infection of the chest wall and is characterized by chronically draining sinuses, the discharge typically containing sulfur granules. Uncommon now, an undrained empyema may erode through the chest wall and present as a subcutaneous abscess. This so-called empyema necessitatis may drain spontaneously, forming an intermittently draining sinus. Occasionally, radionecrosis and infected skin ulcers may follow mastectomy and radiation therapy. Though uncommon, it may penetrate through the necrotic chest wall and cause empyema or pericardial abscess.[1]

SUBSCAPULAR AND SUBPECTORAL ABSCESSES. Subscapular and subpectoral abscesses are two specific, but uncommon, infections peculiar to the chest wall. A subscapular abscess may arise from an infected posterolateral thoracotomy incision and was formerly a common complication of Schede's thoracoplasty performed for the treatment of chronic empyema. A subpectoral abscess can occur from a suppurative lymphadenitis that involves the lymph nodes underlying the axillary portion of the pectoralis muscle after infection of the upper extremity or upper chest wall.[2]

Clinical Manifestations. Acute pyogenic abscesses of the chest wall may cause chills, fever, severe local pain, and tenderness. Leukocytosis is usually present. Empyema necessitatis caused by tuberculosis produces a cold abscess without signs of local inflammation.

Treatment. Pyogenic abscess of the chest wall requires surgical drainage, as with any soft tissue infection, combined with the use of antibiotics. In patients with radionecrosis of the chest wall after mastectomy, resection of the chest wall and reconstruction with myocutaneous flaps offer good palliation and can significantly improve the quality of life. The treatment of the underlying cause (actinomycotic infections, empyema necessitatis) is discussed in subsequent sections.

Infections of the Costal Cartilages: Costal Chondritis

Pathogenesis. Costal cartilage, being composed of hyaline cartilage devoid of blood vessels, derives its nutrition by diffusion from the perichondrium. Because of this avascularity, costal cartilage, especially if it has been exposed, injured, or denuded of perichondrium, is especially vulnerable to infection. The cartilage then acts as a foreign body, with the development of chronic infection and draining sinuses. Healing often occurs only after the infected cartilage has completely been removed.

Incidence and Etiology. Costal chondritis arises most often after operation and trauma, especially as a consequence of infected median sternotomy wounds. In former times, blood-borne infection or that arising from adjacent structures by way of the regional lymphatics occurred. Now, all those pyogenic microbacterial and fungal organisms that infect the sternum are found.[3–5] Costochondritis may occur after radical mastectomy, especially if it is associated with infection or radiation therapy.

Clinical Manifestations. The clinical manifestations of costal chondritis vary with the offending organisms. With pyogenic infections the area over the infected cartilage can develop signs of acute inflammation, including erythema, swelling, and tenderness, and there may be systemic signs of sepsis. Infections caused by mycobacteria, fungi, or bacteria of low virulence may produce minimal local, and often no, systemic symptoms. Only local tenderness followed by spontaneous drainage may occur. Occasionally, it has been mistaken for a neoplasm. Infections of the costal arch on one side may extend to the opposite side either through the involvement of the xiphisternum or as a result of secondary osteomyelitis of the sternum. Thoracic x-rays are usually not helpful but occasionally show evidence of associated bony destruction. Computed tomography may confirm the site and degree of tissue destruction. The diagnosis is usually confirmed at operation. Incision of pyogenic infections may release copious amounts of pus and liquefied cartilage. With *Candida* infections, the cartilage may be partly liquefied and replaced with pink, poorly vascularized, loose granulation tissue. Smears with Gram stain and acid-fast stain should suggest the appropriate diagnosis.

Treatment. Infections of costal cartilage are notoriously chronic but can be controlled by early and adequate therapy. Appropriate antibiotics should be administered, and complete excision of the involved soft tissues and cartilage should be performed promptly. Here, anatomic considerations become important. The first four and sometimes five costal cartilages are individually attached to the sternum and can be completely resected separately. The sixth and seventh costal cartilages and sometimes the fifth are joined not only to the sternum but to each other and to the eighth, ninth, and tenth costal cartilages, the lowermost four forming one side of the costal arch. Complete excision of this large cartilaginous plate is undesirable because it compromises chest wall stability. Therefore, as a first step, that portion of cartilage that is infected and a substantial segment of adjacent normal cartilage may be excised subperichondrially and the denuded ends of the cartilage covered by preserved perichondrium. Other tissues, such as muscle, if available, may also be used to cover the cartilage. If the infection persists, complete excision of the costal arch is necessary. Wound coverage should be individualized, and primary skin coverage is desirable. The older concept of mandatory open drainage has been changed by availability of more effective antimicrobial drugs and tube suction drainage. Adjacent tissues should be mobilized to completely cover the bone and cartilage. If the wound is left open primarily or occurs as a breakdown of primary closure, it should be irrigated with antimicrobial solutions. Wray et al[5] found that 0.25 percent acetic acid irrigation was better than antibiotics, amphotericin B, or local packing with iodoform gauze, especially with chondritis caused by *Candida albicans.*

Prevention. Postoperative costochondritis can be prevented by proper precautions in draining intrathoracic or upper abdominal infections, as well as in closing the sternum. Wire sutures should not be placed through the costal cartilages. Chest tubes should be placed adjacent to ribs rather than cartilages. When an empyema or pulmonary abscess is drained, a portion of a rib rather than cartilage should be excised. If an infection lies beneath one of the upper four cartilages the entire cartilage should be removed and the denuded rib ends covered by perichondrium and muscles.

Infections of Sternum and Ribs: Median Sternotomy Wound Infections

Osteomyelitis of the sternum and ribs as a result of blood-borne infection is rare, is often difficult to eradicate, is usually associated with severe morbidity, and does not differ significantly from osteomyelitis in any other part of the skeletal system (see Chap. 46). Sternal osteomyelitis occurs most commonly after median sternotomy, an incision used in the majority of cardiac operations. Postoperative infection is a dreaded complication because anterior mediastinitis with extension to the aortic and cardiac suture lines, prosthetic grafts, and intracardiac prostheses can occur.

Incidence. The incidence of wound infections after median sternotomy has been reported as low as 0.16 percent and as high as 6 percent.[6–15] In the experience of most surgeons it will occur in 1 or 2 percent of patients, depending on the number of high-risk patients being operated. In a review by Grossi et al,[7] sternal wound infection occurred in 0.97 percent of 7949 patients undergoing median sternotomy. Sethi et al,[9] reporting on 1150 VA cooperative study patients, found an incidence of sternal wound infection of 2.2 percent in patients having an internal mammary artery bypass graft and 2.0 percent for patients having a saphenous vein bypass graft. Mediastinitis occurred in 0.8 percent of the patients in each group.

Etiology. A wide spectrum of microbial organisms may be involved either singly or in combination. Staphylococci and gram-negative enteric bacilli alone or in combination with other organisms are most commonly reported.[7] Methicillin-resistant *Staphylococcus aureus* (MRSA) is being cultured with increasing frequency.[13] Occasionally, sternal and secondary mediastinal infections caused by *My-*

cobacterium fortuitum[11,12] and *Candida*[7] have been reported. Smears, Gram stains, KOH preparations, and acid-fast stains, as well as culture, are indicated if proper therapy for the unusual organism is to be chosen.

Pathogenesis. As in all wound infections, sternal infections and associated mediastinitis apparently occur more frequently in association with chronic debilitation and malnutrition, use of corticosteroids, and prolonged operative time. External cardiac massage and prolonged mechanical ventilation postoperatively predispose to sternal instability and infection. Opinions differ regarding the significance of the technique of dividing and reapproximating the sternum, reoperation for bleeding, low cardiac output syndrome, and other factors. Grossi et al[7] identified as significant risk factors postoperative bleeding requiring reexploration, low cardiac output requiring circulatory support, ventilatory support for more than 24 hours, and severe infections caused by the same organisms at other sites such as lung or urinary tract. Repeat sternotomy was not a risk factor in their experience nor was using the internal mammary artery (2.9 percent infection versus 1.4 percent for saphenous vein). Cosgrove et al[8] studied the incidence of sternal wound infection in computer-matched patients. No infection occurred in patients receiving only saphenous vein bypass grafts. One infection (0.3 percent) occurred in the group of 335 patients receiving a single internal mammary artery (IMA) graft and eight of 338 patients (2.4 percent) developed sternal wound infection after bilateral IMA grafts. These differences were not statistically significant but both age over 60 years and diabetes mellitus were significant risk factors. Diabetic patients undergoing bilateral IMA grafting had a 16.7 percent incidence of sternal wound infection compared to 0.7 percent in nondiabetic patients undergoing bilateral IMA grafting.

The incidence of sternal wound infection associated with heart and lung transplantation is not appreciably different from that observed in the general cardiac surgical population even though transplant patients receive drugs to control rejection. Mediastinitis, which occurred in 12 of 420 heart transplant patients (2.8 percent) reported by Karwande et al[15] was 2.7 times more likely to occur in patients with ischemic cardiomyopathy than in other transplant patients.

Clinical Manifestations and Diagnosis. The diagnosis of sternal wound infection and underlying anterior mediastinitis is not difficult if the patient has persistent, unexplained fever, drainage through the incision, and dehiscence of the sternum early in the postoperative period. When the infection is indolent, however, the diagnosis can be extremely difficult. Cellulitis that involves the incision or local tenderness over the sternum and costal cartilages, along with unexplained fever, should raise suspicion. Thoracic x-ray studies may show air under the sternum. Computed tomography may show evidence of undrained pus collection and extent and depth of wound infection. Aspiration of the sternal wound and the anterior mediastinal space may be necessary to prove the diagnosis. A radioactive gallium scan will occasionally help detect a mediastinal abscess. With sternal wound infections caused by atypical myobacteria, patients generally do not appear ill. There may be no or minimal elevation of temperature and only slight redness and moderate tenderness in the area of the incision. The watery drainage from the wound may not appear until several weeks after operation.

Treatment. Systemic antibiotic administration is essential, especially if intracardiac prosthetic grafts or valves have been used. If Gram stain of purulent material reveals gram-positive cocci, antistaphylococcal therapy should be started. Culture and sensitivity tests should be performed and antibiotics chosen accordingly.

Conventional treatment of wound infection, such as opening of the wound and maintenance of wide-open drainage, may not be feasible because the heart, mediastinum, or pleural cavities may be exposed. Fortunately, it may not always be necessary. Selection of the appropriate therapy depends on the time of appearance and duration of the wound infection and its possible association with an anterior mediastinitis. Superficial wound infections may be managed by debridement, local wound packing, and antibiotics. Major infections, with sternal instability, osteomyelitis of the sternum, or obvious mediastinal involvement, require a more aggressive approach.

For infections of limited extent and short duration, prompt reopening of the entire sternotomy, removal of sutures, and debridement of mediastinum, sternum, and subcutaneous tissues should be carried out.[7,16,17] Two chest tubes are placed under the sternum, one for irrigation and the other for drainage. If the pleural cavity has been opened, an additional tube is inserted into the pleural cavity. The sternal edges are reapproximated with multiple wire sutures, and the subcutaneous tissues are packed with gauze soaked with povidone-iodine. Continuous irrigation with antibiotic solution is initiated and continued for 10 to 14 days (Fig. 35–1). Neomycin-bacitracin solutions (1 g neomycin, 50,000

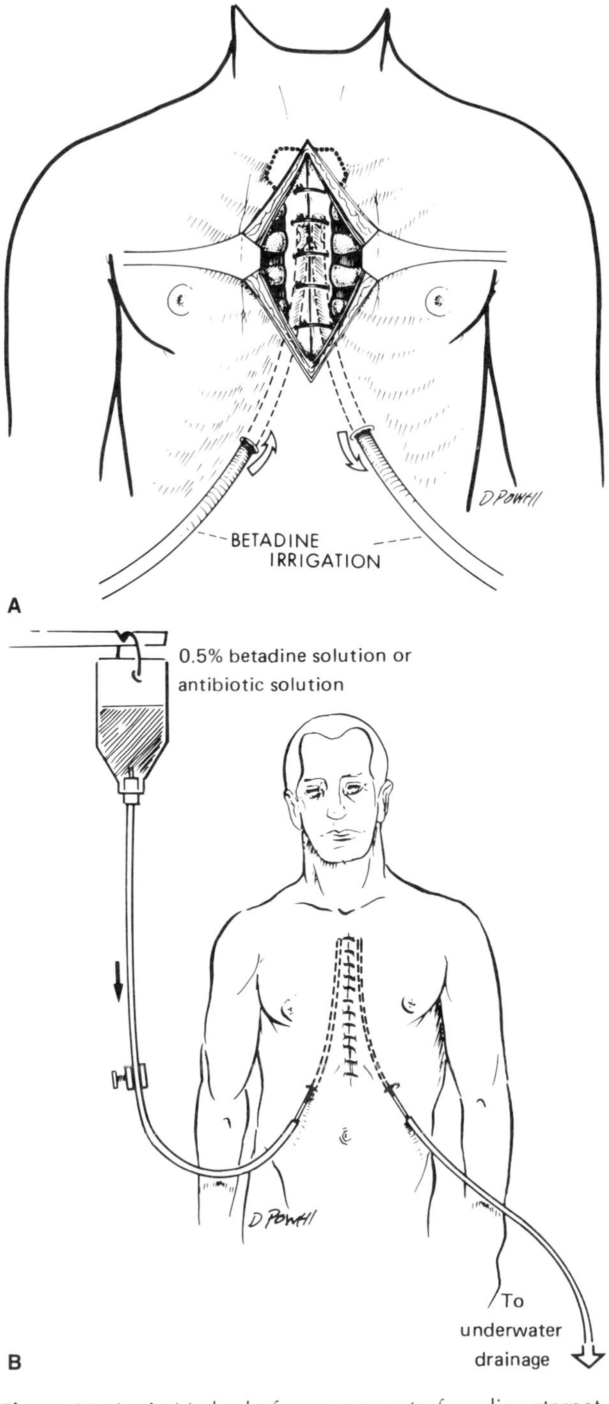

Figure 35–1. A. Method of management of median sternotomy wound infection. The subcutaneous tissues, sternum, and mediastinal tissues are thoroughly debrided. The necrotic tissues are cultured and antibiotic sensitivities performed. The entire wound is irrigated with copious amounts of Betadine or antibiotic solution. Two chest tubes are placed under the sternum, and the sternum is approximated with interrupted wires. Fascia, subcutaneous tissues, and skin are approximated. If the pleural cavity is entered, it is drained by a separate chest tube. **B.** Continuous irrigation with 0.5 percent povidone-iodine (50 to 100 ml/h) or antibiotic solution is begun immediately after the operation and continued for 7 to 10 days. Care is taken to ensure that appropriate amounts of solution are retrieved by the drainage tube each hour.

units of bacitracin in normal saline solution, 50 to 100 ml/h) have been suggested,[7,16] but the toxic effects of neomycin require caution. Equally effective results should be obtainable by using solutions that contain other antibiotics selected on the basis of bacterial sensitivity. We, and others,[17] use an irrigant of 0.5 percent povidone-iodine solution, which is both bactericidal and fungicidal but also has some toxic effect on tissue. Its short-term use until the wound surface is granulating is not dangerous. If antibiotic irrigants are chosen, frequent cultures of the irrigant effluent should be taken to see if overgrowth with fungi or other organisms has occurred. If so, the addition of antifungal therapy is required. It is recommended by Grossi et al,[7] that irrigations be continued for 4 or 5 days after daily cultures of effluent are negative. Adequate dosages of appropriate systemic antibiotics should also be administered, and repeated blood cultures should be obtained to detect the occurrence of endocarditis.

Healing of the sternum in an afebrile patient is successful in up to 90 percent of patients.[7,16,17] If the infection continues or appears late (more than 4 to 6 weeks postoperatively) or the osteomyelitis is complicated by adjacent costal chondritis, a more radical procedure is necessary to eradicate the infection. The wound should be opened in its entire length, and radical debridement of the mediastinum, including the edges of sternum and other involved tissues, should be performed. Local antibiotic irrigation and frequent dressing changes are necessary for a prolonged period. If the combination of thorough surgical debridement and antimicrobial therapy should fail to eliminate the infection, then a more aggressive approach such as complete excision of the sternum and of the neighboring cartilages, and coverage of the exposed mediastinum with an omentum flap may be necessary.[18] An alternate and probably superior procedure is direct closure of the wound with viable muscle flaps to obliterate the dead space.[14,19–22] In these instances, it is imperative that the wound be adequately drained and that there be no residual loculated area of infection, as indicated by persistent febrile course. The infected cartilages and sternum should be debrided back to healthy tissues and bleeding bone. The wound is then covered with the appropriate muscle flap constructed from either the pectoralis major or rectus abdominis muscle (Fig. 35–2). The effectiveness of this procedure in reducing morbidity and mortality has prompted many surgeons to combine debridement with muscle flap construction in a single stage.[22] It is of utmost importance that positive nitrogen balance be maintained with dietary supplements by either enteral or intravenous hyperalimentation. Meanwhile, the patient should

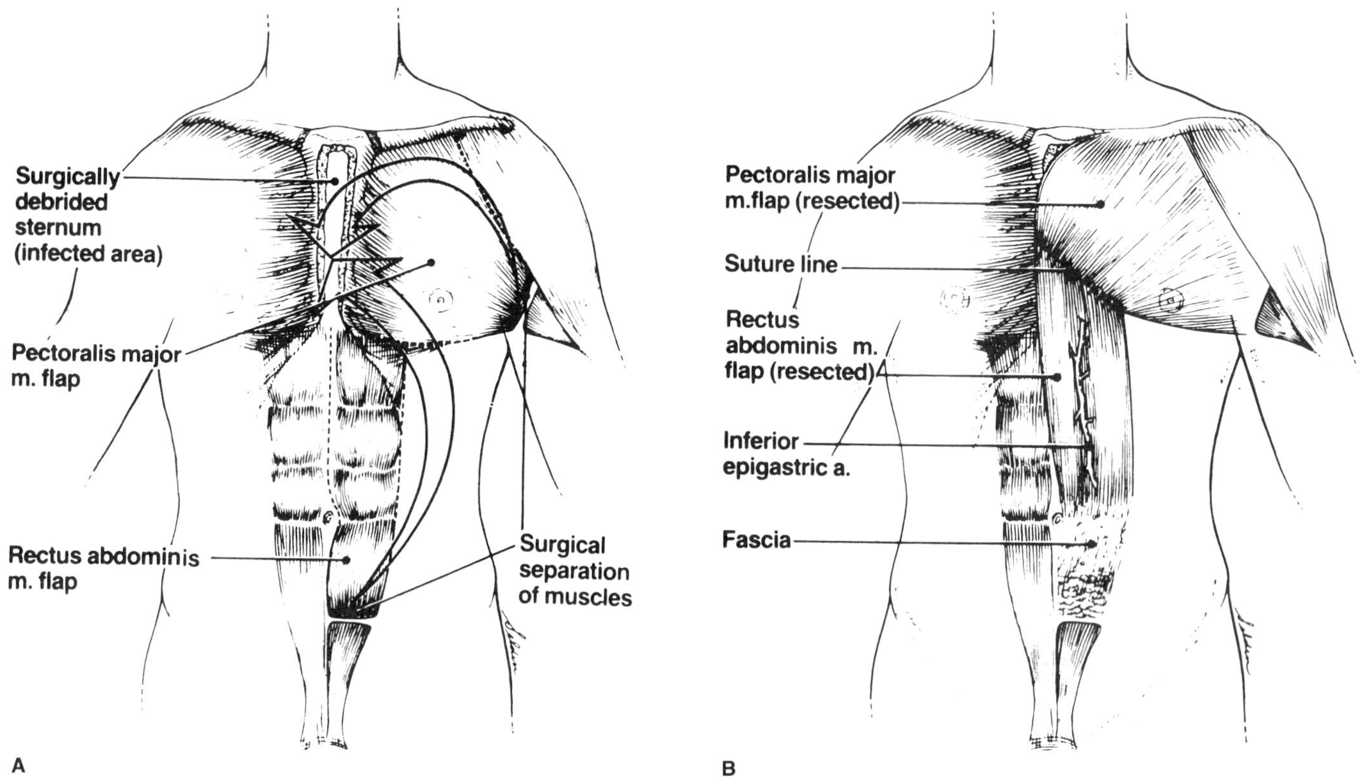

Figure 35–2. A. Surgically debrided sternum and mediastinum with planned muscle flaps. **B.** Rectus muscle inserted into wound. *(From Acinapura AJ, Godfrey N, Romita M, et al: J Cardiovasc Surg 26:443, 1985.)*

receive sufficient concentrations of appropriate antibiotics.

Prevention. A review of the predisposing factors suggests that several measures can be taken to avoid median sternotomy wound infections. First, adequate preoperative and intraoperative skin preparation must be used. Patients should receive 0.5 percent povidone-iodine whirlpool baths for 15 minutes, twice a day for 1 or 2 days prior to operation. Shaving is done approximately 18 hours before operation, and abrasion of the skin must be avoided. Many authorities think that shaving should be postponed until immediately prior to operation (see Chap. 24). At operation the skin is thoroughly scrubbed for 10 minutes with povidone-iodine soap, and the povidone-iodine scrub solution is applied over the skin. Disposable plastic drapes in which the povidone-iodine is already incorporated can be used.

Wound infections can also be avoided by the prophylactic use of antibiotics. The principles of their use are discussed extensively in Chapter 28. It is only necessary to reiterate here that the agent chosen should achieve therapeutic blood and tissue concentrations during the operation. Many cephalosporins are excreted rapidly so that tissue levels may be low unless the drug is administered frequently.

Intraoperative preventive measures include avoidance of excessive tissue damage and prolonged operative time. Accurate midline incision and sternal divisions with the high-speed oscillating saw avoid injury to the cartilage and damage to the sternal periosteum. The use of bone wax to control the bleeding from sternal marrow should be avoided. This would reduce the amount of foreign material left behind (a possible factor in one serious epidemic). Meticulous hemostasis and early detection and correction of coagulation abnormalities are necessary to reduce postoperative bleeding. If reexploration of the mediastinum is necessary, the patient must be returned to the sterile operating room. A second antibiotic to cover gram-negative organisms should be added at this time. It is important to place tubes in the mediastinum and pleural cavity to avoid cardiac tamponade and mediastinal hematoma. Complete closure of the pericardium is usually easily accomplished in patients who are undergoing operations for congenital heart disease and valvular disease. However, it may produce compression or kinking of bypass conduits in patients undergoing aortocoronary bypass grafting. We attempt to close the pericardium with interrupted nonabsorbable sutures in all patients except those undergoing aortocoronary bypass procedures. In these patients the thymus tissue and mediastinal pleurae are approximated.

Interrupted wire sutures in adults and nonabsorbable sutures in infants and small children should be placed either through the bone or parasternally, not through the costal cartilages. Occasionally, a figure-of-eight suture technique or other modification of the interrupted technique may be necessary for firm closure. Basically, stable closure of the sternum is essential: instability of the chest wall repair is an important predisposing factor to sternal dehiscence and secondary infection.[6] Where clustering of cases of mediastinitis occurs, an epidemiologic investigation may be necessary to identify a carrier or other cause of perioperative infection.[13,14]

Postoperatively, if prolonged mechanical ventilation becomes necessary, it should be given through a nasotracheal tube to avoid the use of tracheostomy, at least until the tissue planes have become obliterated. All precautions should be taken to avoid pulmonary and systemic infections.

Prognosis. The reported mortality rates for patients with sternal wound infections range from 8.4 to 28.6 percent.[7,8] Early and aggressive use of pectoral muscle flaps has done much to improve the prognosis for the patients. Muscle flaps constructed during a second operation following drainage and debridement[18,21] or in a single-stage operation[22] have not only lowered mortality rates but have markedly reduced hospital lengths of stay. Patients undergoing cardiac transplantation,[15] patients with concomitant cytomegaloviral[23] infection, and patients with mycobacterial infection[12] have a poorer prognosis.

Infections Involving Implanted Prosthesis

Pacemakers. Infections have been reported in 0 to 19 percent of patients following pacemaker implantation. However, infection probably is becoming less frequent as pacemakers are being made smaller and techniques for implantation are being improved. The erosion and necrosis of overlying skin associated with the older, larger pacemakers is unlikely to occur now except possibly in very thin or very young patients.[24] The organisms most often identified with pacemaker infections are *Staphylococcus epidermidis* and *Staphylococcus aureus.* Other organisms reported include *Klebsiella, Escherichia coli, Pseudomonas, Serratia, Enterobacter, Proteus, Aspergillus, Candida,* and *Mycobacterium avium.*[25]

Treatment. Conservative management with local irrigation and systemic antibiotics has a high failure rate and is rarely indicated. An infected pulse generator should be explanted, the pacemaker pocket should be surgically debrided, and any systemic infection present should be appropriately treated.[26] Temporary pacing may be necessary before a new pacemaker can be implanted in the opposite side remote from the infection. The pacemaker lead must be removed if it is infected or if septicemia is present (see Chap. 36). Echocardiography must be done to detect vegetations, infected thrombi, or endocarditis. Leads with bulbous, tine, or screw-type tips may become entrapped, making their removal difficult and dangerous. Prolonged traction is sometimes successful. The wide variety of extraction devices that have been used serves to illustrate the difficulties encountered. A contaminated lead may sometimes be safely abandoned in a high-risk patient. An infected lead may require thoracotomy and cardiopulmonary bypass for its safe removal.[25]

Vascular Prosthetic Grafts. Infections of vascular prosthetic grafts are discussed in detail in Chapter 37. Since vascular procedures involving the axillary artery are being performed with increasing frequency, axilloaxillary and axillofemoral bypass grafts are special cases that involve the thoracic wall. Infections of these grafts are common, unfortunately, because the patients who require them are old and debilitated and already have systemic infections in preexisting prosthetic grafts. In a patient with a thin layer of subcutaneous tissue, the constant pressure and pulsations of the arterial prosthesis, especially over the costal arch, may cause necrosis and erosion of the overlying skin and result in graft infection. Local signs of acute infection include warmth, erythema, swelling, local tenderness, and, ultimately, drainage of pus from the wound. Exposure of a graft in the wound is evidence enough for the presumptive diagnosis. Systemic signs, such as fever, night sweats, and tachycardia, may also occur.

The principles of treatment of all infected vascular prostheses are discussed in Chapter 37. Only total graft excision results in resolution of infection, though appropriate parenteral antibiotics must be used. The arterial reconstruction should be performed via a noncontaminated route and delayed if possible.

Miscellaneous Infections of the Chest Wall

Two other conditions that produce nonsuppurative inflammatory swelling of the chest wall should be noted. Both are usually self-limiting and may be confused with infections of the chest wall.

Mondor's syndrome is a superficial phlebitis of the thoracoepigastric vein and its branches. It is characterized by the presence of a subcutaneous cord, with variable inflammatory signs. The condition does not require specific therapy, and complete resolution can be expected within weeks or months.

Tietze's syndrome is a painful, nonsuppurative swelling of one or more costal cartilages, usually the second. Adults of either sex may be affected. The clinical picture may be suggestive of chondritis or cartilaginous tumor. The symptoms are usually self-limiting, but recurrences may occur. Appropriate specific treatment has not been defined.

Infections of the Pleural Cavities (Empyema)

Purulent collections in the pleural cavities are among the oldest conditions that surgeons have been called on to treat, judging from the Hippocratic literature. "Pus in the chest" is no less important today to the thoracic surgeon, although the clinical circumstances that cause it are considerably different from those of ancient times. Since the availability of antibiotics, the incidence of empyemas has dropped sharply, and the causative organisms have changed.

In this section, pleural empyemas are discussed in general terms. It must be recognized, however, that there are important differences between empyemas of pyogenic origin and those caused by actinomycotic, fungal, or protozoan organisms and that empyemas of aerobic, anaerobic, and postoperative origin also differ.

Etiology and Pathogenesis. Pleural empyemas are not ordinarily primary infections. They usually occur in response to a primary infection elsewhere, most commonly pneumonia. This, however, may not be apparent when the empyema is fully developed. Probably the most common pathogenetic mechanism is rupture of a necrotic subpleural lung abscess or pneumonitis into the pleural cavity, although spread from lymphatic and hematogenous sources may also occur. The primary pneumonic process or abscess may, in turn, be the result of a variety of conditions, including bronchial obstruction (tumor, foreign body), bronchial infection (bronchiectasis), or emphysema (ruptured infected bleb). The mediastinum, subdiaphragmatic areas, chest wall, and dorsal spine can also be the sites of the primary infections that lead to an empyema (Fig. 35–3).

Such conditions as esophageal perforation, bronchopleural fistula, ruptured infected mediastinal lymph node, or subphrenic or intrahepatic abscess, including amebic abscess, have all been recognized as causes of empyema, as have external sources such as trauma, needle aspiration, and thoracotomy tubes.[27] Infection of the pleural cavity (empyema) occurs if a hemothorax or a residual air space becomes infected after thoracotomy or if the pleural cavity is significantly contaminated during pulmonary resection or esophageal surgery (see Fig. 35–3). Thirty-three percent of empyemas occur after surgery, and another 10 percent are iatrogenic, occurring after thoracentesis, thoracostomy, or some other invasive procedure.[28]

Post-traumatic empyema is a serious problem in wartime. The incidence was 6 percent during the war in Vietnam.[29] Bacterial contamination of the pleural space can readily occur from penetrating injuries of the thorax, but infection is uncommon unless foreign material, such as clothing or organic matter, is retained in the pleural cavity. Air in the pleural space, especially in combination with hemothorax, doubles the likelihood of an empyema.

ETIOLOGIC AGENTS. In the preantibiotic era, empyema was usually produced by pneumococci or streptococci. As effective antibiotics against these organisms became available, the incidence of empyema dropped significantly. In the late 1950s, however, pleuropulmonary infections caused by *Staphylococcus aureus,* resistant to all available antibiotics, increased for a time, especially in the young.[30] In the Johns Hopkins Hospital from 1955 to 1958, *Staphylococcus* caused 92 percent of empyemas in children younger than 2 years.[30] In the 1980s and 1990s, staphylococcal pneumonia and empyema have been uncommon in children. *Streptococcus pneumoniae, Hemophilus influenzae,* and mixed aerobic/anaerobic organisms predominate in pediatric infections.[31]

Half or more infections are polymicrobial. With the use of anaerobic culture techniques, anaerobes and microaerophilic organisms have been identified with increasing frequency in empyema fluids.[32] Anaerobes are particularly common in empyemas arising from aspiration pneumonitis or in association with subdiaphragmatic infections. Table 35–1 lists the organisms identified from 83 patients with em-

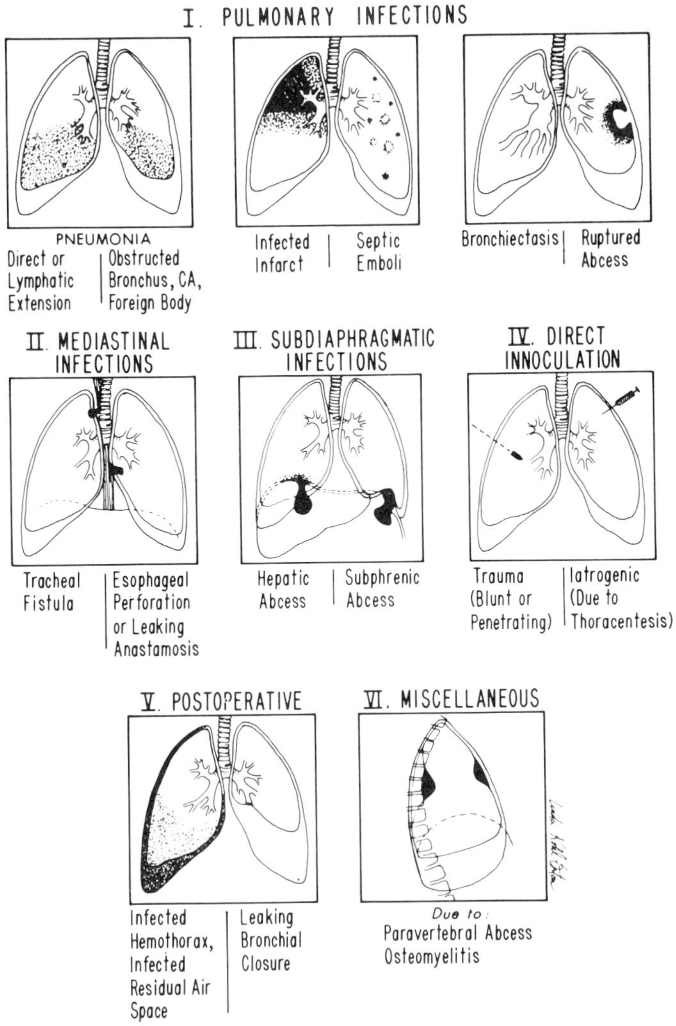

Figure 35–3. Etiology of thoracic empyema. *(Adapted from Snider GL, Saleh SS: Dis Chest 54:410, 1968.)*

pyema in a laboratory with a strong interest in anaerobic bacteria. Tuberculous empyema is now rare. Amebic empyema and actinomycotic and nocardial empyemas also occur and are referred to in later sections.

Pathology. Empyemas may be encapsulated and localized to various regions of the pleural cavity, such as an interlobular location or a mediastinal or intrapulmonary region. They may also involve the entire pleural space. At first, during the exudative stage, the fluid is thin and has a low cell content, and the visceral pleura is still elastic, so that the lung can be reexpanded. When increasing numbers of polymorphonuclear leukocytes and fibrin deposition begin to appear, the fibrinopurulent stage has been reached, and the visceral and parietal pleural surfaces begin to adhere. Finally, when the exudate has thickened so that more than 75 percent of an empyema fluid sediments on standing and fibroblasts have invaded the fibrinous layer over the pleural membranes, it is called an organizing empyema. Recognition of these distinctions in the natural course of pneumococcal and streptococcal empyemas by Graham and Bell in 1918 led to the use of closed drainage.[33] These three stages correspond only roughly with temporal conceptions of acute, subacute, and chronic empyema. Initially, all empyemas are acute, and chronicity develops if they are inadequately treated or if the primary condition is not controlled.

Empyema necessitatis (Fig. 35–4) is an encapsulated empyema that has burrowed through the chest wall into the subcutaneous tissues. It is still occasionally seen after pneumonectomy. A bronchopleural fistula occasionally can be the result of a neglected empyema rupturing through a fresh or old bronchial closure or into the lung. The reverse is usually the case: the diseased lung or the bronchopleural fistula gives rise to the empyema.

Clinical Manifestations. The symptoms and signs of the empyema may be continuous with those of the primary infection. Pleuritic pain and persis-

TABLE 35–1. BACTERIOLOGY OF LUNG ABSCESS (45 CASES) AND EMPYEMA (83 CASES)[a]

Bacteriologic Results	Lung Abscess	Empyema
Only anaerobes recovered	26/45 (58%)	29/83 (35%)
Anaerobes and aerobes recovered concurrently	19/45 (42%)	34/83 (41%)
Anaerobic isolates		
Fusobacterium nucleatum	19 (3)[b]	16/3
F. necrophorum	1	
Bacteroides melaninogenicus	18 (1)	13
B. fragilis	9	13 (1)
B. oralis	5	8
B. corrodens	2	
Unidentified gram-negative bacilli	4	3
Peptostreptococcus	14 (4)	12
Peptococcus	14 (1)	14 (1)
Microaerophilic streptococcus	6 (3)	15 (5)
Veillonella	4	6
Eubacterium lentum	4	
Eubacterium species	3	5 (1)
Catalase-negative, non-spore-forming gram-positive bacilli	3	9
Propionibacterium species	6	4
Clostridium species	2 (1)	13 (1)
Aerobic and facultative isolates		
Staphylococcus aureus	6	17 (6)
Streptococcus faecalis	3	5
Streptococcus pneumoniae	2	5 (2)
Streptococcus pyogenes	1	4
Klebsiella pneumoniae	3	6 (1)
Escherichia coli	6	11
Proteus mirabilis	2	2
Hemophilus influenzae	1	1
Pseudomonas aeruginosa	3	10 (2)

[a] Data from Wadsworth and Sepulveda Veterans Hospitals.
[b] Numbers in parentheses are numbers recovered in pure culture.
From Finegold SM: Anaerobic Bacteria in Human Disease. New York, Academic Press, 1977.

tence of fever in spite of adequate chemotherapy, especially when the pneumonic process has largely subsided, suggest the diagnosis. The patient looks toxic and has chills and fever. The physical findings of empyema are typical of pleural effusion and include diminished movement of the affected hemithorax, impaired note on percussion, and reduced breath sounds and tactile and vocal resonance over the involved area. A large empyema may displace the mediastinum to the contralateral side and produce significant cardiopulmonary dysfunction on a mechanical basis alone.

Anemia, dyspnea, lassitude, debility, and clubbing of the fingers may develop in the chronic stages. The signs of empyema necessitatis have been described. If the pus takes another route and erodes into a bronchus, forming a bronchopleural fistula, sudden emptying of a large empyema into a bronchus may flood the bronchial tree and even drown the patient. Should this situation be suspected, the patient must be instructed to lie on the affected side to prevent leakage of empyema contents into the bronchus until the empyema can be definitely drained. Figures 35–5 and 35–6 are representative of the many appearances empyema may have.

In chronic empyema, movement of the involved hemithorax can be severely restricted. If fibrothorax occurs, the trachea may be displaced toward the affected side, and the size of the involved hemithorax can decrease significantly. Amyloidosis may ultimately develop after a long-standing chronic empyema.

Diagnosis. In the preantibiotic era, thoracentesis, with the aspiration of purulent fluid from the pleural space, established the diagnosis unequivocally. Today, a patient may have clear pleural fluid, and organisms may not even be cultured from aspirates by conventional techniques. Yet a pleural infection that is masked by antibiotics or caused by anaerobic organisms can be present. Even though the patient is usually febrile, the pleural infection may

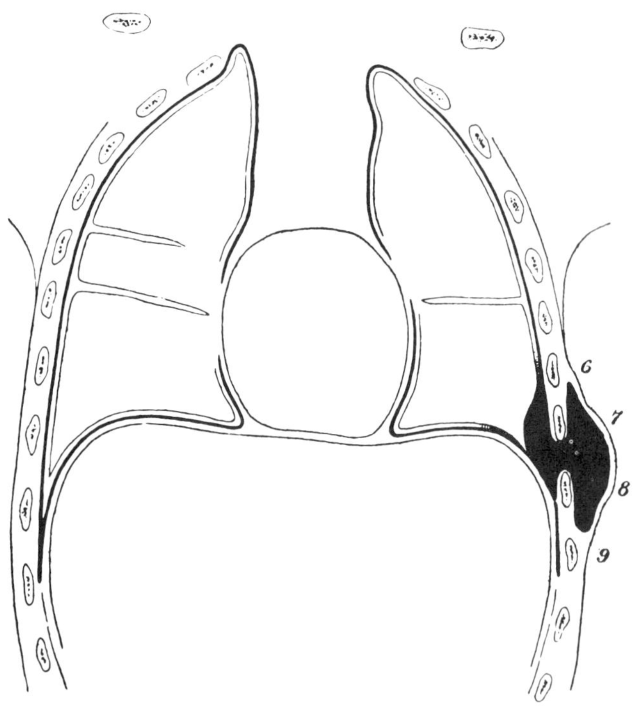

Figure 35–4. Diagram of empyema necessitatis showing its characteristic components: encapsulated pleural empyema, the narrow opening between the ribs through which the empyema has burrowed, and the externally presenting collection of pus in the subcutaneous tissues. *(From Ashurst APC: Int Clin 4:173, 1916.)*

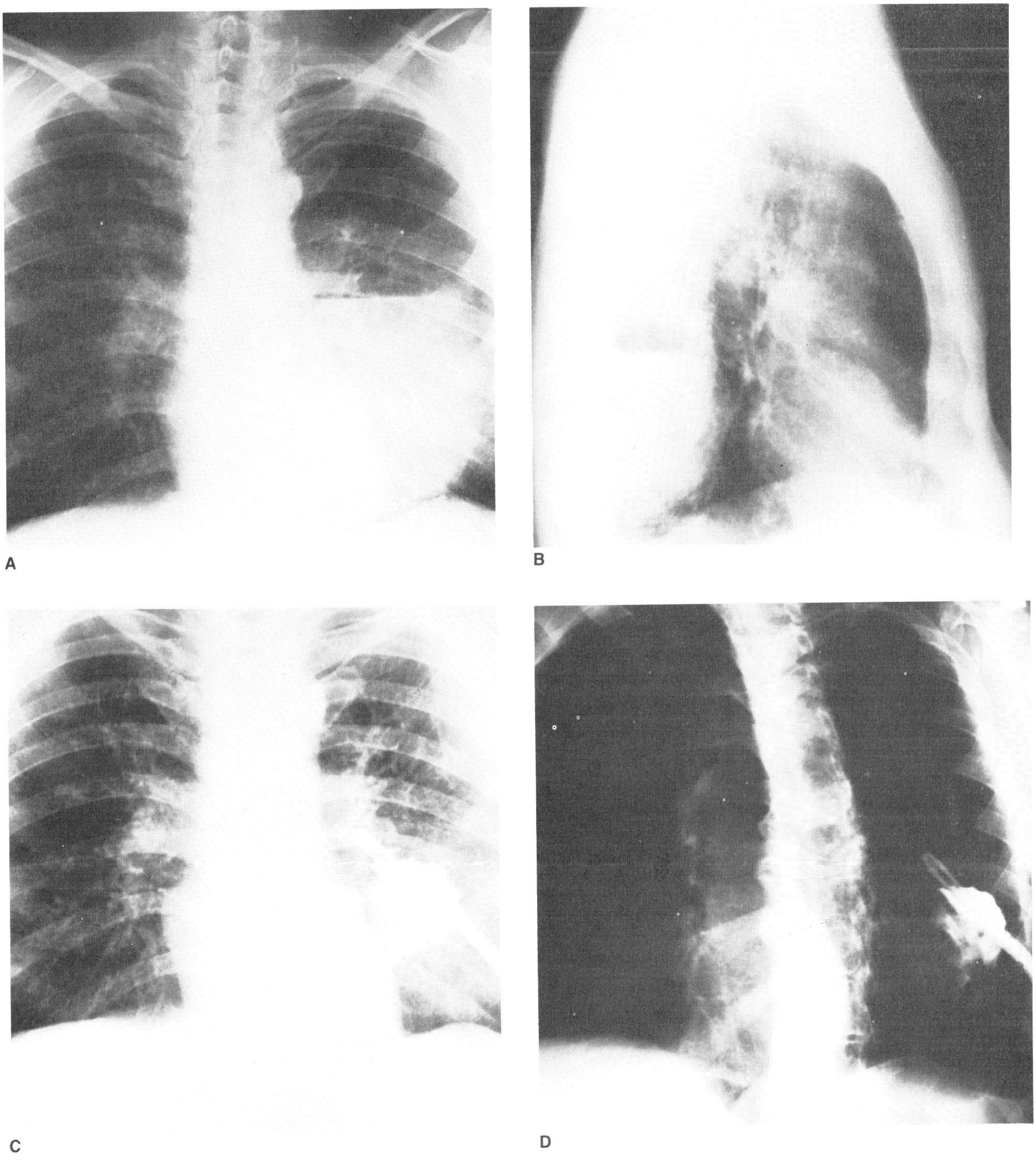

Figure 35–5. Postpneumonic empyema for which rib resection and open drainage were carried out. *Streptococcus pneumoniae* was cultured from aspirate. Posteroanterior **(A)** and lateral **(B)** views showing posterior location of empyema cavity containing air-fluid level. **C, D.** Sinograms 5 weeks after open drainage show residual space. A wide-bore tube was left in place until the space was completely obliterated 6 weeks later. *(From Takaro T, Scott SM, Bridgman AH, et al: Curr Probl Surg 14:6, 1977.)*

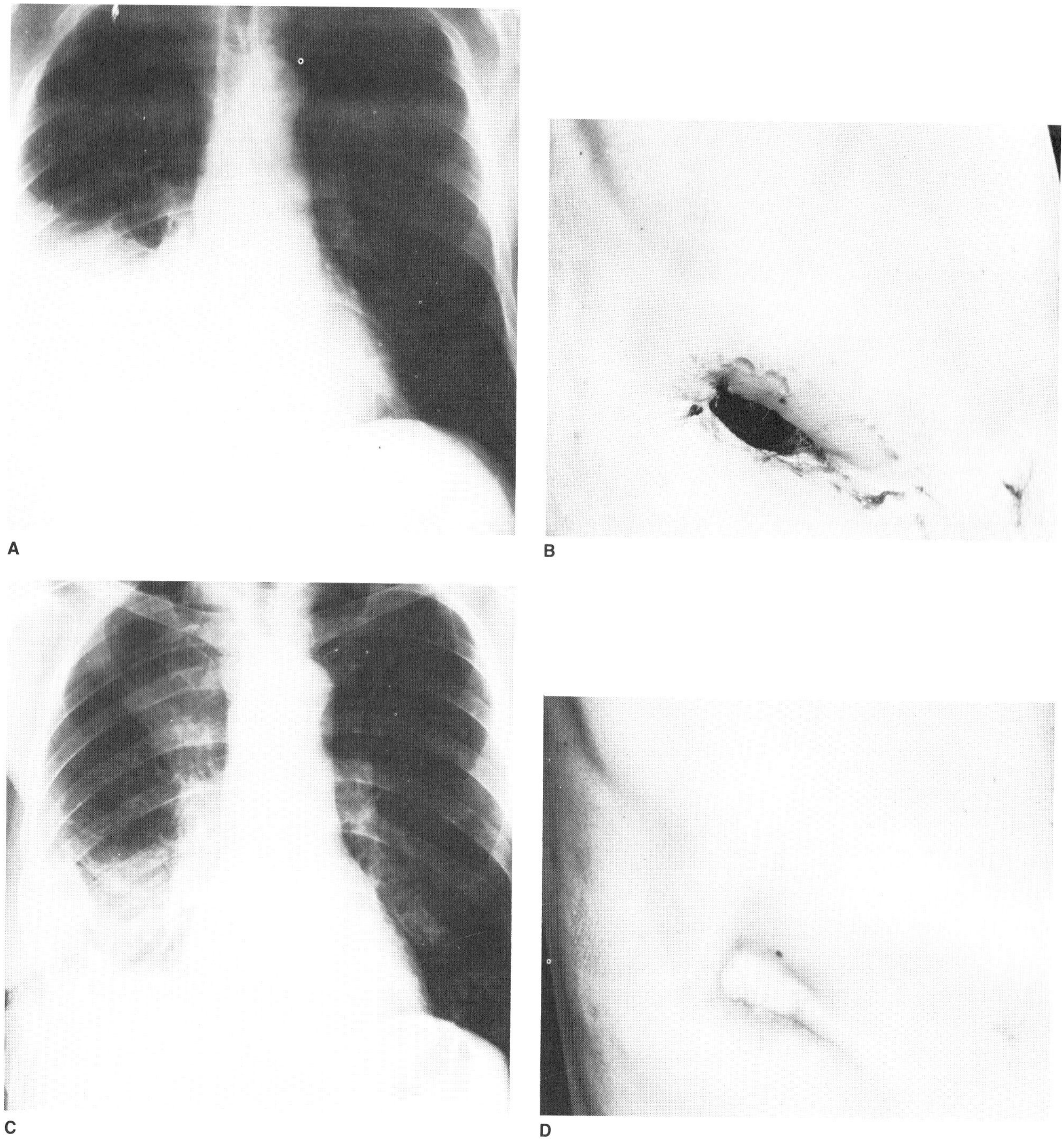

Figure 35–6. Management of chronic empyema of 3 months duration, using a modified Eloesser pedicled skin flap (see Fig. 35–7). Cultures of material from the empyema space grew a mixture of aerobic and anaerobic bacteria. **A.** X-ray on admission. **B.** Appearance of chest wall 3 weeks after resection of segments of the eighth and ninth ribs and establishment of the flap. X-ray **(C)** and chest wall **(D)** 4 months after drainage procedure. *(From Takaro T, Scott SM, Bridgman AH, et al: Curr Probl Surg 14:6, 1977.)*

not become clinically evident until the antibiotics have been discontinued.

Aspirated material is sent to the laboratory for bacteriologic examination, including Gram stain, culture, and antibiotic sensitivity testing. The use of anaerobic culture techniques is essential. The possibility that the empyema may be the result of tuberculosis, actinomycosis, or fungal infections should be considered if response to therapy is slow, if the patient has chronic empyema or a draining sinus, or if the pus contains sulfur granules (the hallmark of an actinomycotic infection). In cases of amebic empyema, the characteristic anchovy sauce type of pus can be aspirated from the pleural cavity. This fluid and stools should be examined for *Entamoeba histolytica* and serologic procedures carried out (see Chap. 8). A hepatic source must be sought and eliminated.

Occasionally, bronchoscopy may be necessary to exclude the possibility of an intrabronchial tumor, an inhaled foreign body, or a bronchopleural fistula. The presence of a bronchial fistula can be confirmed by injecting 1 percent methylene blue into the empyema cavity and observing the expectorated material for blue dye.

Treatment. "It is sad to think of the number of lives which are sacrificed annually by the failure to recognize that empyema should be treated as an ordinary abscess, by free incision" (Osler, 1892).[34]

There are three major objectives in the treatment of an empyema. The first is control of the etiologic agent, usually by specific antimicrobial therapy. The second is evacuation of the contents of the empyema. The third, intimately related to the second, is restoration of normal lung function by reexpansion of the underlying lung.

Thoracentesis or needle aspiration of an empyema is nearly always the primary step. This single maneuver can establish the diagnosis, obtain material for identification of the etiologic agent, and, at least in the exudative stage, evacuate the contents of the empyema space. Mandal and Thadepalli[35] report success with thoracentesis alone for 25 percent of 112 patients with primary parapneumonic empyema. Both ultrasound and CT scan are extremely helpful in locating empyemas and directing needles and catheters into the space for drainage.[36,37]

TUBE THORACOTOMY. Even in the exudative stage of an empyema, it is often wise to insert an intercostal tube for continuous closed drainage, especially when complete evacuation of the empyema space is unlikely to be achieved safely by needle aspiration alone. Thoracotomy tube drainage is especially important if systemic toxicity has not been controlled adequately. A pleural fluid pH less than 7.2 indicates an infection that requires chest tube drainage.[38] A chest tube, if adequate in size and properly positioned, will ensure achieving the twin objectives of complete evacuation of the empyema space and reexpansion of the lung, provided the closed drainage procedure is carried out in the exudative or fibrinopurulent stages (see Fig. 35–5).

The course of disease is followed by the clinical response of the patient and by frequent x-rays of the chest. Fluid should be cultured frequently, and the antibiotic treatment should be modified as indicated. After 2 to 3 weeks, the tube may be converted to open drainage if it seems necessary. Before conversion to open drainage, however, the fibrinopurulent stage of empyema must have been reached, so that the lung does not collapse. The size of a residual cavity can be assessed by injecting saline solution into the cavity. The tube can be removed safely when the volume of the cavity is less than 10 ml (see Fig. 35–5). Tube thoracostomy is usually inadequate for postoperative empyema.

OPEN DRAINAGE. While many patients with postpneumonic empyema do respond to thoracentesis or tube thoracostomy (64 percent in the Mandal and Thadepalli series),[35] more aggressive therapy is usually needed for patients with empyema following surgery or trauma. Immunosuppressed patients and substance abusers have a high failure rate with chest tube drainage.

Open drainage should be instituted if there are multiple pus pockets, if the pus is very thick and contains fibrin flakes, if the empyema is first seen in the organizing stage, or if it appears to be inadequately drained. Persistence with closed intercostal drainage for adults is a common error.

Chronic empyema can result from inadequate or delayed earlier drainage procedures, some underlying primary condition such as a bronchopleural fistula, or esophagopleural fistula. A full investigation into the possible causes for the chronicity should always be made.

Because of prolonged infection, patients with chronic empyema often have anemia, depleted plasma proteins, and low blood volume. These should be corrected by blood transfusions and by a high-vitamin, high-protein diet. A positive nitrogen balance is essential for control of chronic infection and healing of fistulas or wounds. Appropriate and adequate antibiotic coverage is necessary before, during, and after operations.

RIB RESECTION. The mainstay of management for chronic empyema should be adequate open drainage at the most dependent part of the cavity. This can be accomplished by resecting a short 5-cm section of the most dependent rib overlying the empyema cavity. This technique allows the surgeon to explore the cavity, break up any loculations with a finger, clean away fibrin and debris, and establish drainage with a large bore tube.[39]

LIMITED THORACOTOMY. A small thoracotomy with chest tubes can be used to accomplish the same as a rib resection procedure. Should decortication be necessary, the thoracotomy can be extended. Braimbridge[40] has advocated the use of a laparoscope to debride an empyema cavity and avoid open drainage in noncompliant patients.

ELOESSER FLAP. Open drainage can be modified by creation of an Eloesser flap or one of its modifications. This procedure is especially valuable in the treatment of postpneumonectomy empyema or for a large secondarily infected tuberculous empyema. It is also useful in the management of empyema where the tube drainage would be uncomfortable, such as high in the axilla or in the paravertebral area. Its virtue is to maintain the drainage indefinitely, preventing premature closure (Figs. 35–6 and 35–7).

Sterilization of an empyema cavity, as described by Stafford and Clagett,[41] is especially useful when empyema develops after pneumonectomy. A window is created by suturing the subcutaneous tissues to the pleura after rib resection. The empyema cavity is irrigated daily with half-strength Dakin's solution for 6 to 8 weeks. After the pleural cavity has diminished in size and become lined with clean, healthy granulation tissue, the sinus tract or window is excised, the cavity is irrigated with saline solution and filled with 0.25 percent neomycin solution, and the chest wall is closed in layers. The dangers of systemic neomycin administration must be recalled and literal application of this technique avoided.

A modification of this method, which is more convenient for the patient and avoids a two-stage procedure, is advocated by Provan[42] and by Karkola et al.[43] Intrapleural antibiotic irrigation using two thoracostomy tubes, one near the apex of the space to instill the solutions and the other for drainage, has been applied successfully even when an open bronchopleural or esophagopleural fistula is present. The problem of bronchial aspiration is circumvented by careful positioning of the patient until the fistula is closed.

DECORTICATION. Occasionally, in chronic empyema, the thick peel that forms over the visceral pleura may trap enough underlying lung to produce respiratory embarrassment. This peel may also prevent healing of the empyema, because with the rigid thickened lining, the cavity cannot close. Decortication to remove the thick pleural peel may improve function and encourage healing.

In certain other circumstances, decortication can be more efficient than open drainage. For example, in the management of an infected hemothorax, the intrinsically normal lung becomes imprisoned by its nonelastic, fibrinopurulent investment. With few exceptions, however, decortication is not generally advocated as primary treatment for most types of empyema.

Occasionally, a relatively small empyema cavity may be excised en masse (empyemectomy) without opening it, thus avoiding spillage of its contents into the uninvolved pleural space. This might be especially applicable in cases where the empyema pocket has never been subjected to open drainage or

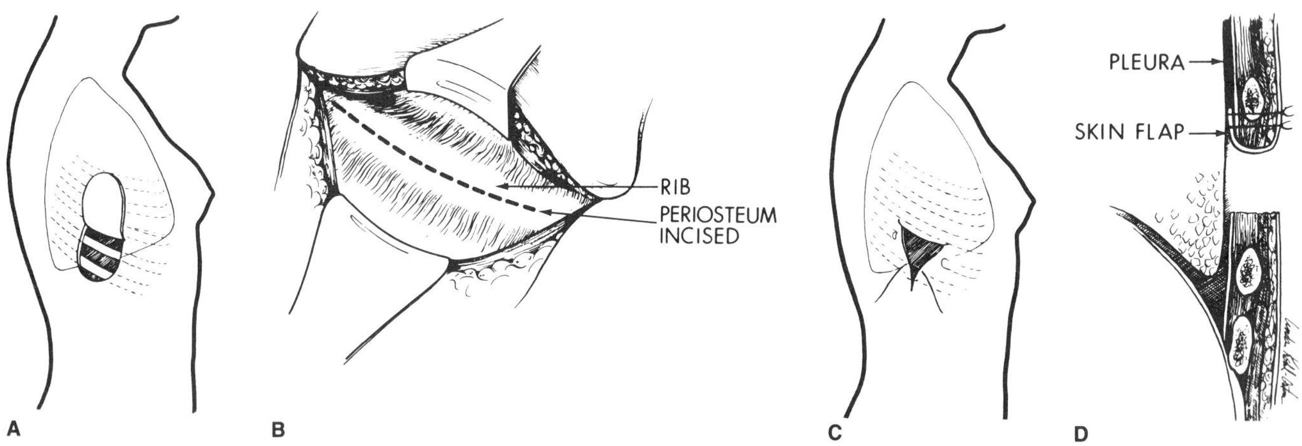

Figure 35–7. Eloesser flap drainage procedure. **A.** Full-thickness skin flap is elevated. We sometimes resect portions of two ribs rather than one. **B.** Preparation for subperiosteal resection of rib. **C.** Completed operation, showing skin flap inverted and sutured to parietal pleura at superior edge of thoracotomy wound. In most instances, fewer sutures than shown would be used inferiorly, to avoid diminishing the opening. **D.** Cross-section of thoracic wall, showing relationship of inverted skin flap to the parietal pleura. *(Adapted from Eloesser L: Ann Thorac Surg 8:355, 1969.)*

where the chronic encapsulation is either obviously infected or of unknown origin.

THORACOPLASTY. To obliterate a large (especially an apical) empyema cavity or close a coexistent bronchopleural or esophagopleural fistula, it is sometimes necessary to collapse the chest wall.[44] The procedures available include the conventional thoracoplasty, the classic Schede's thoracoplasty, and modifications of these (Fig. 35–8).

Additional special procedures may be necessary when an empyema is present along with a chronic bronchopleural or esophagopleural fistula. The empyema cavity is obliterated, if possible, by a pedicled flap (fashioned from the serratus anterior, latissimus dorsi, pectoralis major, or subscapularis muscles, from intercostal muscle bundles or omentum). The muscle flap is brought down (or in) to fill the empyema space and to seal the fistula.[45–47] Some tailoring of the chest wall may be necessary to permit these muscle flaps to reach their objectives (Fig. 35–9).

INFECTIONS OF THE LUNGS AND AIRWAYS

Lung Defense Mechanisms Against Infection

The defense mechanisms of the lung have been reviewed extensively by Newhouse et al.[48,49] Mucociliary functions have been described in detail by Thompson et al.[50] The majority of potentially harmful particles and microbes in inhaled air are eliminated before reaching the alveoli. In fact, the normal lung is sterile from the first bronchial division to the terminal lung segments.

Inhaled particles can be deposited in the respiratory tract as a result of impaction, sedimentation, brownian motion, turbulent diffusion, and even electrostatic forces. Whether the particle is retained depends on how it was inhaled (through the nose or the mouth), its size, shape, and density, and the air flow velocity and aerodynamic characteristics of the airway. For example, large particles are eliminated as the air passes the nasal vibrissae. Particles larger than 10 μm encounter the moist surface of the nasal septum and turbinates[51] and impact on the posterior wall of the pharynx, where the tonsils and adenoids are conveniently located. The few particles larger than 10 to 15 μm that remain will impact at the carina or within one or two bronchial divisions.

Because of the rapid increase in the cross-sectional area of the bronchial tree beyond the tenth bronchial division, air flow rates fall rapidly. Beyond this division, particles 0.2 to 5 μm in size sediment by gravity. The majority of bacteria thus sediment to the distal bronchial walls in these areas of stagnant air flow.

Particles of 0.1 μm and smaller are deposited mainly as the result of brownian motion because of their constant bombardment by gas molecules. Particles between 0.5 and 0.1 μm are least affected by inertial, gravitational, and brownian forces, and only about 20 percent are retained in the lung.[52]

Despite these defenses, some large, irregular particles, such as asbestos fibers, are capable of reaching the lung periphery because their aerodynamic characteristics prevent their retention in the upper airways. Similar factors may govern other particles.

Airway Reflexes. Two airway reflexes exist: bronchoconstriction and cough. Stimuli of various types can produce vagally mediated reflex contraction of the airway smooth muscle and mucosal edema in both the upper and lower respiratory tract. Such stimuli, including mechanical irritation of the nose, trachea, or larynx, inhalation of irritant gases, some droplet aerosols, and chemically inert dusts can produce bronchoconstriction or trigger the cough reflex.[48,49] Bronchoconstriction is characterized by a concurrent reduction in airway caliber without decreasing the number of ventilated pulmonary units. The protection resides in the prevention of the deep penetration by mechanical or chemical irritants.

The cough reflex helps remove excess secretions and foreign bodies in the trachea or major bronchi. The reflex begins with a deep inspiration, after which expiration is initiated against a closed glottis with an elevation of intrapleural pressure to well over 100 mm Hg. When the glottis is suddenly opened, the pressure within the trachea and major bronchi falls to a much lower level, resulting in a high transbronchial pressure and rapid reduction in bronchial caliber. Two effects then result: (1) secretions retained on the walls of the bronchus occupy a larger proportion of the cross-sectional area of the narrowed lumen and can temporarily occlude it, and (2) the flow rates throughout the bronchial tree are greatly augmented. The resulting high air flow velocity propels the mucous plug toward the mouth. Compression from the high intrathoracic pressures may also produce a milking action, which clears mucus into larger airways for subsequent expulsion. Cough is an effective means of expelling foreign bodies and secretions, but chronic bronchitis, emphysema, or cystic fibrosis can retard the

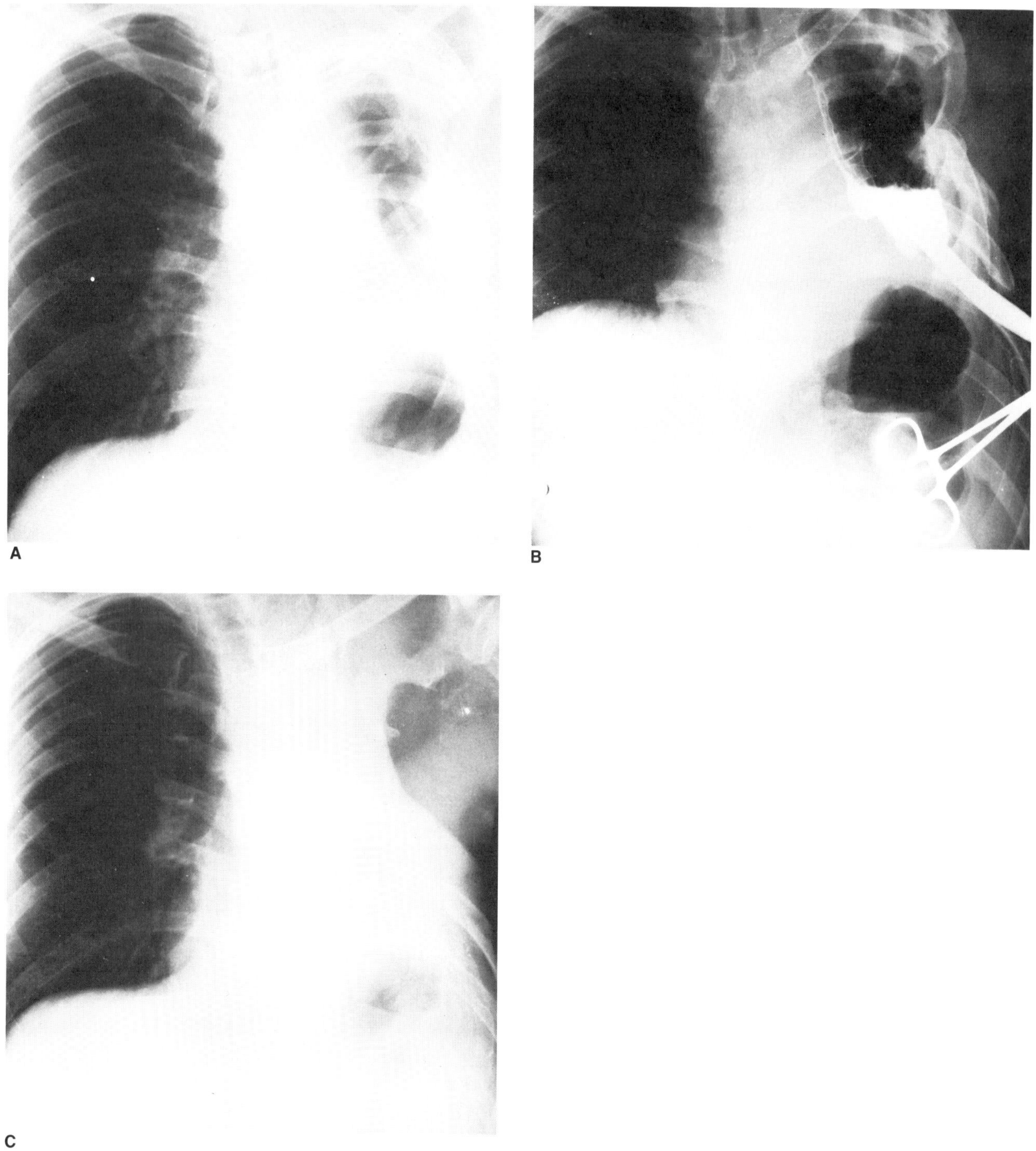

Figure 35–8. Management of intractable, chronically draining empyema space, using a modified Schede's thoracoplasty, in young Vietnam veteran who had emergency pneumonectomy 4 years before admission. This was followed by empyema, with several previous unsuccessful attempts elsewhere to reduce or to sterilize the empyema space. Bronchoscopy and bronchography showed a healed left bronchial stump. Mixed flora (*Pseudomonas, Enterobacter* species, and enterococci) were cultured from purulent contents of the empyema space. The large space was completely unroofed of its calcific external wall after resection of portions of six ribs. The wound was packed and only partially closed, leaving a large opening for drainage and changes of dressing. Healing was uneventful and was essentially complete in approximately 3 months. **A.** X-ray after previous rib resections and attempts to sterilize empyema space. **B.** Sinogram outlining extent of space. **C.** Appearance 1 year postoperatively. *(From Takaro T, Scott SM, Bridgman AH, et al: Curr Probl Surg 14:6, 1977.)*

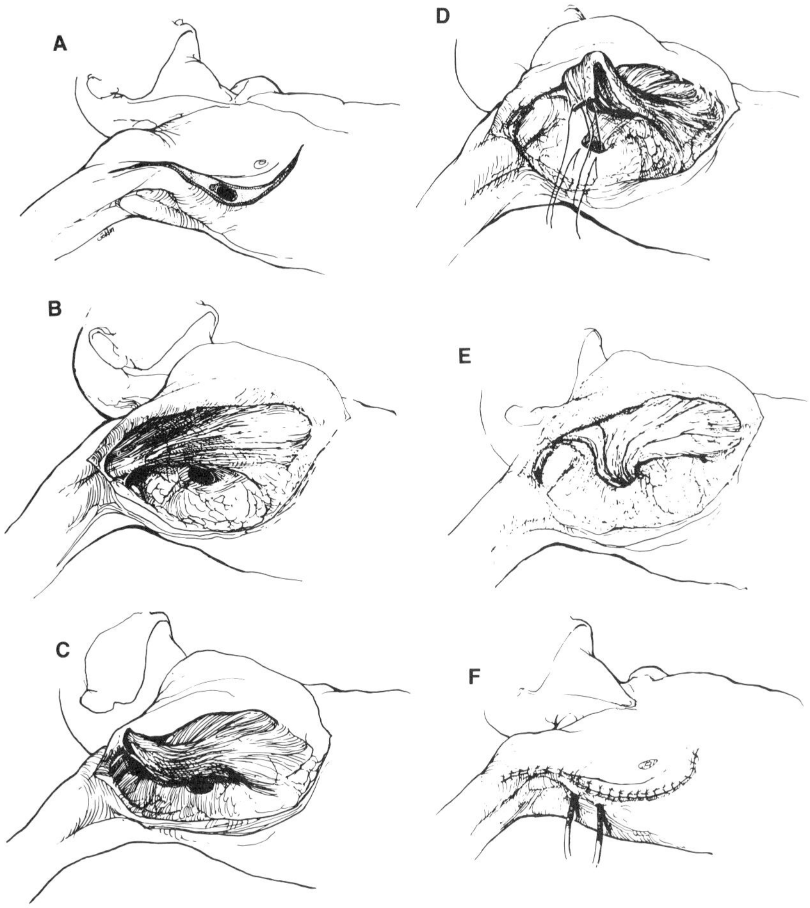

Figure 35–9. Steps in closure of a bronchopleural fistula using a pedicled muscle graft. **A.** Incision extends along border of pectoralis major muscle into axilla and includes fistulous tract. **B.** Pectoralis major muscle is dissected to its insertion on the humerus. **C.** The muscle is detached from its insertion and is unfolded to provide an adequate graft. **D.** It is then sutured into the space and stump with absorbable sutures. **E.** The muscle is shown sutured in place. **F.** The wound is closed, with subcutaneous drainage only. *(From Barker WL, Faber LP, Ostermiller WE, Jr, et al: J Thorac Cardiovasc Surg 62:393, 1971.)*

cough mechanism, and an inefficient cough can cause retrograde movement of secretions to the lung periphery or aspiration from one lung into the other.

Tracheobronchial Secretions and Mucociliary Transport. The respiratory airways from distal nasopharynx to terminal bronchioles are lined by mucus-covered, ciliated epithelium that removes deposited particles by means of mucociliary transport mechanisms. The larger particles that impact or sediment on the mucosa are swept upward by this mechanism, to be swallowed or spit out. The smaller particles that sediment in regions distal to the terminal bronchioles are not handled in this way.

Structure of Mucociliary Transport System. The mucociliary transport system has two components. The respiratory epithelium is lined by cells, each of which bears approximately 200 cilia. Airway secretions are produced by both mucosal goblet cells and submucosal mucus-secreting glands. The resulting mucous blanket consists of two layers: (1) a 5-μm high-shear periciliary fluid that has the physical characteristics of a sol that bathes the cilia from the surface of the epithelial cell to their apex, and (2) above this level, a 2-μm lower-shear gel with greater viscoelasticity. Effective airway clearance depends on maintenance of this viscoelasticity, which can be altered by proteases, lysozymes, and DNA from lysed inflammatory cells and bacteria.

The gel layer is impermeable to water and may protect the subjacent epithelium and periciliary fluid from dehydration, ionic disequilibrium, and penetration of toxic substances. The gel layer also probably provides an important barrier to biologic agents because it contains secretory IgA and a number of nonspecific soluble factors that can act as defenses.

Airway secretions contain a variety of antimicrobials, antioxidants, and antiproteases. Among the antimicrobial substances are lactoferrin and transferrin, which are iron-binding proteins. Lysozyme, secretory IgA, IgG, complement, defensins, and free fatty acids are also present.

Oxidant-mediated epithelial cell injury is protected by the presence in mucin of a number of antioxidants including lactoferrin, vitamin E, catalase, and others.

Proteolytic injury is caused by proteases from inflammatory cells. Antiproteases are present in airway secretions, the most abundant of which is alpha-1-protease inhibitor (alpha-1-antitrypsin). Alpha-1-antitrypsin can inhibit bacterial enzymes as well as collagenase, plasmin, thrombin, and proteases and elastase derived from lysosomes of neutrophils.[53,54] In addition, alpha-1-antitrypsin is probably identical to the chemotactic factor inactivator present in normal serum, and Ward and Talamo[53] have suggested that a deficiency in alpha-1-antitrypsin may permit neutrophils to damage the lung. In fact, emphysema is one consequence of congenital alpha-1-protease inhibitor.

Cilia and Mucociliary Transport. Cilia do not beat in synchrony but sequentially, in metachronal waves. The mucous blanket appears to provide a mechanical linkage between cilia, and a neuroidal pacemaker network has been hypothesized to explain the coordinated movement. The cilia beat at a frequency of between 1000 and 1500 cycles per minute. The tip of the cilium is in contact with the undersurface of the mucous gel only during the maximum velocity of the effector stroke.[55] Cilial motion is generated by peptids known as dynein arms through a complex transfer of high-energy phosphate bonds from adenosine triphosphate (ATP).

There is a progressive increase in the velocity of the mucous blanket toward the upper airways. Particles in the proximal bronchi are cleared with a half-time of about 30 minutes, whereas particles on the distal mucosa are removed with half-times up to several hours. All material deposited on the normal ciliated epithelium is removed in less than 24 hours.[56]

Ciliary movement is influenced by many physical and chemical stimuli. Autorhythmicity of cilia may be controlled by physiologic amines, such as serotonin, that might act as local pacemaker substances. Oxygen appears to be essential for ciliary motion. A number of agents appear to be toxic to cilia. High concentrations of carbon dioxide and oxygen, cigarette smoke, pentobarbital, atropine, and alcohol are toxic to cilia. Viruses damage mucociliary clearance, and *Mycoplasma pneumoniae* infection can slow tracheobronchial clearance for as long as 1 year.

Phagocytic Defenses (Alveolar Macrophages)

Although the major clearance mechanism of the lung consists of the mucociliary transport system, alveolar macrophages are responsible for the physical removal of inhaled particles. Alveolar macrophages can be specifically or nonspecifically activated during infections.[57] Activated macrophages have a higher lysosomal enzyme level, are more phagocytic, and possess more bactericidal activity than do nonactivated cells.[57] Once activated, macrophages display a nonantigen-specific capacity to ingest and kill apparently irrelevant organisms. It should be emphasized, however, that specific inactivation of bacteria by activated macrophages is nearly always quantitatively greater than nonspecific activation. The primary bactericidal activity in the resting lung is dependent on this macrophage system.

Immunologic Defenses

Alveolar macrophages interact with IgG, IgA, and IgE through cell surface receptors to stimulate phagocytosis and the secretion of a growing list of macrophage products. The lungs are not generally regarded as lymphoid organs, but submucosal lymphoid deposits respond to both systemic and aerosolized antigens. Local mucosal presentation of antigen is a more efficient mode of obtaining local immunity.

It is now known that secretory IgA antibody acts as a primary defense mechanism at all mucosal surfaces (see Chaps. 12 and 15). IgA antibody present in nasal and upper respiratory tract secretions is better correlated with resistance to viral or bacterial infection than in serum antibody.[58]

IgA in bronchial mucus is in the secretory form, consisting of a dimer IgA together with two additional nonimmunoglobulin moieties, known as secretory component and J chain. IgA-containing cells predominate at lymphoid sites in the lamina propria, and relatively few cells containing IgM or IgG are normally found at these sites. Although normally only a few IgE-containing cells are found in these mucosal tissues, the relative number of such cells is greater in the respiratory tract and associated lymphoid tissue. In chronic respiratory tract disease, the number of cells that produce IgA and IgE tends to rise at a rate disproportionate to that in other classes.

Evidence indicates a predominantly IgG response in the lower respiratory tract to several antigens.[59] IgA-containing cells predominate in the upper and middle portions of the tract but are rarely, if ever, seen around bronchioles, even in infection.

IgA appears, at first glance, to be an ineffectual antibody. It cannot fix complement and therefore cannot serve to lyse microorganisms. It cannot opsonize microbes for phagocytosis by neutrophils or macrophages. More likely, IgA acts to neutralize toxins or viruses and to prevent bacterial colonization of mucosal surfaces, because bacteria sensitized with IgA appear unable to adhere to mucous membranes.

Patients with IgA deficiency do, on the average, have more respiratory tract infections, but some deficient patients are normal. These people appear capable of replacing the IgA with IgM.

Special Procedures in Diagnosis of Pulmonary Infections

Special techniques are available to aid in diagnosing pulmonary infiltrates. These techniques are especially helpful for diagnosing pulmonary infiltrates in immunologically compromised hosts. Pulmonary lesions in these patients—cancer patients receiving chemotherapy or radiation, patients receiving immunosuppressive drugs, patients with congenital immunodeficiency disorders, lymphoproliferative disorders, or AIDS—are frequently caused by organisms that do not result in sputum production or are difficult or impossible to culture. To diagnose these infections tissue specimens are frequently required. Rapid diagnosis is necessary so that specific therapy can be instituted.

Sputum examination is helpful when the sputum is copious or can be induced. It is not helpful in the diagnosis of viral infections or *Pneumocystis carinii*. Because sputum is always contaminated with oral bacteria, culture results are unreliable. This is especially true if one is looking for anaerobic bacteria. Oral contamination can be avoided by transtracheal needle aspiration but in compromised patients with low platelet counts there is a danger of bleeding. Bronchoalveolar lavage (BAL) with 100 ml of sterile saline is the method of choice for diagnosing opportunistic infections in immunocompromised hosts.[60] *Pneumocystis carinii* can be identified in 50 percent of specimens. Lavage is helpful in identifying cellular contents of the lung, diagnosing malignancies, and evaluating interstitial disease.

Bronchoscopy with the rigid bronchoscope has long been used for diagnosis and therapy to culture and wash out thickened bronchial secretions. This technique has some of the same drawbacks as sputum collection, because the bronchoscope must be passed through the mouth and can become contaminated by oral bacteria. Bronchoscopy with a flexible bronchoscope has largely replaced the rigid bronchoscope for diagnosis. The flexible bronchoscope can be directed into the subsegmental bronchi of the affected pulmonary segments to collect secretions from the specific location affected. Any obstruction, such as that due to tumor, can be visualized and a biopsy specimen obtained. Biopsy of the lung can also be accomplished through the bronchoscope by penetrating the bronchus with the biopsy forceps to obtain lung tissue. Viral infections and *P. carinii* can be diagnosed in this manner. Hanson et al[61] reported 62 percent accuracy in the diagnosis of infectious lung disease in 37 patients with transbronchial biopsy through the flexible fiberoptic bronchoscope. Hemorrhage (more than 100 ml) occurred in 26 percent of the patients and pneumothorax in 19 percent. However, Anderson[62] reported only a 1 percent incidence of bleeding and a 12 percent incidence of pneumothorax. Low platelet levels in many of these patients increases the risk of hemorrhage that cannot be directly controlled. However, in patients with proved pulmonary tuberculosis, transbronchial biopsy for culture was only 18 percent accurate.[63] Special sheathed catheters have been developed to try to circumvent contamination with oral bacteria. A sheathed catheter is passed through the flexible bronchoscope into the bronchus. A gelatin plug at the end is then punched out by the culture tip, and cultures are obtained. The sheathed catheters may provide more reliable culture results. One drawback to the use of flexible bronchoscopy is that these patients frequently have severe hypoxia, and the bronchoscope can occupy a substantial portion of the airway, especially in children. Supplementary oxygen cannot be given, as it can with the rigid bronchoscope.

The lack of reliability of cultures and risk of uncontrolled hemorrhage in many of these severely immunocompromised hosts have led to more direct sampling of lung tissue. In general, three methods are used: percutaneous needle biopsy, thoracoscopic biopsy, and open lung biopsy.

Needle biopsy can be performed under fluoroscopic control[64,65] and computed tomography[66] to ensure that the diseased portion of the lung has been entered. This technique can be helpful for diffuse pulmonary infiltrates as well as for solid tumors.[67] Several biopsy needles are available. Trephine air drill biopsy was able to provide the diagnosis in 82 percent of immunocompromised patients with diffuse lung disease.[67] Hemorrhage occurred in 18 percent (3 of 17) of the patients. One patient required transfusion, and 60 percent (10 of 17) developed a pneumothorax; 8 of the 10 patients required a chest tube. This technique has the advantage of being performed with local anesthesia in the cooperative patient. Aspiration of diffuse pulmonary infiltrates with a thin needle does not yield reliable results.

Thoracoscopy was introduced in 1921, at which time it was used primarily for dividing pleural adhesions to produce pulmonary collapse in tuberculosis therapy.[68] Recent introduction of video-assisted thoracoscopy has made this procedure an extremely effective diagnostic tool and in many instances a reliable approach for surgical procedures.[69] The visualization afforded by videothoracoscopy is often better than that provided by a thoracotomy. Procedures reported to have been done in this way with no operative mortality include lobectomy, wedge resection, lung biopsy, pleural biopsy, pleurodesis, decortication, mediastinal biopsy, pericardiectomy, sympathectomy, and pleural irrigation for empyema.[69–71] For most patients, postoperative pain with thoracoscopy is much less than that experienced with a thoracotomy, especially if a chest tube is not used. Hospital stay for thoracoscopy is as little as 3 or 4 days.

The technique of video-assisted thoracoscopy requires using a double-lumen endotracheal tube and general anesthesia. The patient is placed on an operating table in the standard lateral position for a posterolateral thoracotomy and draped widely to allow for multiple ports. A 1- to 2-cm incision is made in the midaxillary line over the sixth or seventh intercostal space. Through this incision the surgeon can explore the chest with his/her finger to detect a lesion and to ascertain if the pneumothorax is complete. A 10- to 12-mm trocar is inserted through this opening, through which the thoracoscope is passed. After exploration with the video camera, additional ports for instruments are made at sites most convenient for the procedure anticipated. For procedures not associated with bleeding or air leak, no chest tube is required.

Open lung biopsy for diffuse pulmonary infiltrates can be done safely in both adult and pediatric patients through a small anterior thoracotomy.[72] Leight and Michaelis[73] obtained diseased tissue in 100 percent of 42 consecutive open lung biopsies. A specific diagnosis was made in 30 patients (74 percent). Delayed pneumothorax occurred in three patients and wound dehiscence in one patient. In cooperative patients, open lung biopsy can be performed under local anesthetic.[74]

Noninvasive aids for diagnosing lung infections include computed tomography (CT) scan, magnetic resonance imaging (MRI), positron emission tomography (PET), lung scans, and gallium-67 scans. New immunochemical techniques have been developed to improve cytologic screening (DNA probes, immunofluorescent antibodies) and shorten the time required to identify organisms in culture.[75]

Viral Infections

Viral infections may be encountered by the thoracic surgeon performing lung biopsy or seen as complications in immunocompromised surgical patients. The most frequent virus occurring in patients following heart and lung transplantation is the cytomegalovirus (CMV) (see Chap. 51).[76] This virus has long been observed in patients after extracorporeal circulation but only recently has it been shown that patients with CMV at the time of cardiac surgery have greater morbidity than patients who are CMV-negative at the time of surgery.[77] Pneumonitis occurs in patients with CMV and low CD4 counts. While there is a case on record of cytomegaloviral infection presenting as a solitary pulmonary nodule,[78] ordinarily the disease occurs as diffuse interstitial pneumonitis, suggestive of pulmonary edema, or as bilateral nodular infiltrates. Fever and leukopenia are present.

Other viral infections causing pneumonitis or esophagitis are herpes simplex, herpes zoster-varicella, Epstein-Barr virus (EBV).

Bacterial Infections

Postoperative Lung Complications. Although many postoperative complications that involve the lungs are associated with infection, the infection is often overshadowed by other clinical problems, such as mechanical airway obstruction, pleural space problems, respiratory insufficiency, or graft rejection. Nevertheless, postoperative lung complications will be discussed briefly, chiefly in relation to the element of lung infection.

Definition. Pulmonary complications associated with lung infection include retained secretions, localized pneumonitis, atelectasis, pneumonia, lung abscess, and adult respiratory distress syndrome from sepsis or other causes. Any of these can be exacerbated by previous conditions, most notably chronic obstructive pulmonary disease, and by operations on any of the thoracic contents, the chest, or the abdominal wall.

Pathogenesis. Retention of pulmonary secretions, the most common complication, results from aspiration of saline solution or gastric juice into the airways or ineffective cough and hampered ventilation. If the atelectasis is unrelieved, infection will occur.

Aspiration pneumonia results from the inhalation of oronasopharyngeal secretions laden with microorganisms or gastric contents of high acidity, with the development of either a bacterial or a chemical pneumonia. It can also lead to lung abscess. Sepsis is the most commonly identified factor in adult respiratory distress syndrome in the absence of preexisting pulmonary dysfunction. The pathogenesis of this complex state is unclear, but circulating endotoxins from gram-negative organisms are involved. Other factors are recumbency, pulmonary or peritoneal infection, aspiration, fluid overload, fat or particulate microaggregate embolism, oxygen toxicity, and left ventricular failure. Neutrophils that aggregate within the lung and attach to endothelial cell surfaces are activated by endotoxins and complement. Activation results in release of oxygen free radicals and proteases, which are damaging to the lung.

Clinical Manifestations. The symptoms and signs of retained secretions are easily recognized. Pneumonitis and atelectasis may be heralded by low-grade fever, rales, or rhonchi, with x-ray evidence of patchy areas of pneumonitis. Aspiration pneumonia may be difficult to distinguish from atelectasis if it is localized to one lobe or lung. Under some circumstances, it may resemble pulmonary edema. Adult respiratory distress syndrome associated with sepsis usually begins with symptoms and signs of respiratory insufficiency, which may at first be mild. As it progresses, it is characterized by fever, hypotension, hyperventilation, oliguria, arterial hypoxemia, and hypocarbia. Blood cultures are usually positive. In the patient with full-blown adult respiratory distress syndrome, the symptoms and signs are more severe and less responsive to elevated inspired oxygen concentrations.

Treatment and Prevention. For retained secretions, a methodical progression of measures should be used. First, the patient should be encouraged to cough effectively and repeatedly with the aid of analgesics and physical support. If this is ineffective in eliminating secretions, transnasal aspiration of the trachea and main bronchi should be done, using a sterile catheter. Hypoxia can be avoided by hyperoxygenating the lungs before suctioning and keeping the active suctioning brief.

The next step should be bedside bronchoscopy using the fiberoptic bronchoscope if secretions are thin. Otherwise, the rigid bronchoscope should be used. If bronchoscopy is unsuccessful, endotracheal intubation and mechanical ventilation should follow. Tracheostomy allows ready and repeated access to the lower respiratory tract and should be resorted to if secretions cannot be managed through the endotracheal tube or if prolonged mechanical ventilation is anticipated.

For pneumonitis and atelectasis, essentially the same measures are used, but with increased vigor. Appropriate antibiotic should be administered, as determined by culturing material aspirated from the lower respiratory tract for both aerobic and anaerobic organisms.

Aspiration pneumonia will also require close monitoring of blood gases, elevated levels of inspired concentrations of humidified oxygen, and, possibly, assisted ventilation.

By far the best course, for both patient and surgeon, is prevention. Careful assessment of the patient's respiratory reserve prior to operation and individualized preparation are vital, especially for patients with chronic obstructive lung disease. Smoking must be stopped, tracheobronchial secretions must be reduced or eliminated, and localized infection must be brought under control or eliminated.

Chest physiotherapy instituted prior to operation appears to be helpful, although proof of this is lacking. All measures to prevent aspiration of gastric contents during the induction of anesthesia, the course of the operation, and the postoperative period are essential. Prompt postoperative institution of a coughing regimen and of transnasal endotracheal aspiration for retained secretions is mandatory.

The prevention and management of postoperative lung infections will probably occupy more time and cause more concern to the surgeon than any other condition described in this chapter.

The mortality rate for adult respiratory distress syndrome is 60 percent. The treatment is primarily antibiotics, oxygen, and ventilator support. Monoclonal antibodies that bind endotoxin and tumor necrosis factor alpha (TNF-α) are under investigation as are interleukin 1 receptor blockers and prostaglandin E_1. Scavengers for free radicals such as N-acetylcysteine and ibuprofen may be helpful.[79]

Lung Abscess

Definition. Not all localized collections of "pus in the lung" qualify for our definition of lung abscess. A lung abscess is a localized area of suppuration in the lung followed by central necrosis of tissue and (usually) cavitation. A lung abscess, by this definition, excludes collections of pus in preexisting cavities or potential spaces. For the purposes of clarity therefore, encysted and interlobar empyemas and infected pulmonary or bronchial cysts are not considered in this section, although they can be construed by some as abscesses in the lung.

Historical Note. Putrid lung abscess has been recognized for centuries, but treatment was always relatively ineffective. Incision and drainage, although described more than a century and a half ago,[80] were rarely performed, even though the beneficial effects of providing prompt egress for collections of pus were understood. Usually, the diagnosis of lung abscess was delayed, and patients were in a debilitated and toxic state by the time surgical drainage was performed, with understandably discouraging results. In 1942, however, a series of early, open drainage procedures was reported in 122 patients with putrid lung abscesses, with only 3 percent mortality.[81] It was this unprecedented success that led to the need for greater precision in the diagnosis and topographic localization of lung abscesses on the chest wall based on segmental bronchial anatomy. Lord Brock[82] provided the groundwork for the evolution of appropriate treatment, and the principles he emphasized remain valid. In the two-stage procedure of drainage, adherence of the visceral pleura to the parietal pleura was either identified as having already occurred or was deliberately provoked by packing the rib bed with gauze after segmental rib resection. In the second stage, drainage of the lung abscess was carried out through the prepared area, thereby avoiding contamination of the pleural space and resulting empyema. Later, resective procedures for chronic lung abscesses were introduced, almost completely displacing the two-stage procedure.

The most important advance in managing lung abscesses, however, was the introduction of antibiotics in the late 1940s. As a result, far fewer pneumonias developed into abscesses. Even when an abscess developed, effective antibiotic treatment controlled most acute lung abscesses. Surgical treatment declined in popularity, and open drainage became rare.

Over the years, however, the microbes that cause lung abscesses have changed as a result of the extensive use of antibiotics and other agents, including antineoplastic drugs, corticosteroids, and immunosuppressive drugs. Opportunistic organisms have replaced primary pathogens as the cause of lung abscesses, so that as the incidence of primary lung abscesses has decreased, the incidence of opportunistic lung abscesses has increased.

Pathogenesis. Primary lung abscesses usually occur in patients with dental or oral infections during a period of decreased consciousness, which is usually accompanied by suppression of the normally protective cough reflexes, as in alcoholism, anesthesia, neurologic disorders, and submersion. Other causes of aspiration include drug ingestion or addiction, diabetic coma, and esophageal disorders. Infectious debris slips by gravity into the airway or is inhaled by the obtunded patient, preferentially into one of the three segmental bronchi most directly in line with the upper airways. Approximately three-quarters of primary lung abscesses occur in three lung segments: the superior segments of the lower lobes of both lungs and the posterior segment of the right upper lobe (Fig. 35–10). Such is not the case for opportunistic lung abscesses, which can occur in all segments with approximately equal frequency, although the right lung is more commonly involved than the left. The old adage that primary aspiration lung abscess almost never occurs in edentulous patients has repeatedly been shown to be incorrect.[83]

The aspirated material causes bronchial occlusion and produces atelectasis of the lung tissue supplied by the blocked bronchus. This area may become infected by the organism carried down with the aspirate, producing a suppurative pneumonia. If the infection progresses, an area of focal necrosis and liquefaction can be produced.

This propensity of anaerobic bacteria to cause tissue necrosis and abscess formation has been related to their production of short-chain fatty acids, which protect the bacteria from phagocytosis (and cause the putrid discharge), to their polysaccharide capsule, and to an antigen-specific T cell lymphokine that regulates abscess formation.[83–85]

The pathogenesis of opportunistic lung abscesses is not as readily understood. These abscesses occur in patients who are either very young or very old and who have serious, associated conditions ranging from prematurity to incurable malignancy. In these patients, lung abscesses occur as

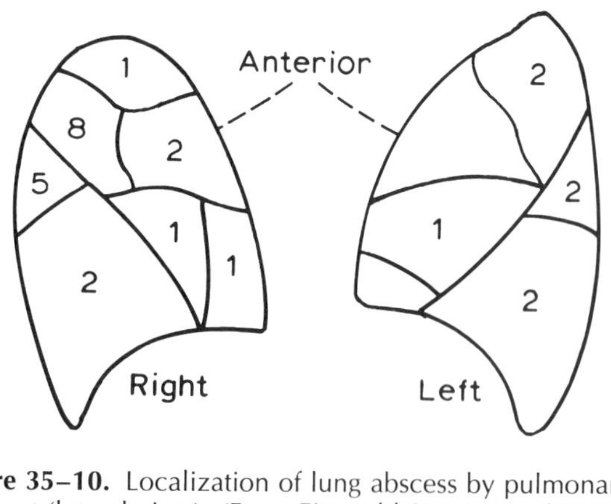

Figure 35–10. Localization of lung abscess by pulmonary segment (lateral view). *(From Finegold SM: Anaerobic Bacteria in Human Disease. New York, Academic Press, 1977.)*

a complication of a systemic disease. Prematurity, bronchopneumonia, congenital defects that require surgical treatment, the postoperative state itself, the presence of other infections, blood dyscrasias, and systemic diseases are all common predisposing conditions in early infancy. Systemic diseases, malignancies (especially of the lung and oropharynx), prolonged use of corticosteroids, immunosuppressive or radiation therapy, and, again, the postoperative period constitute the common conditions of the older age group in which opportunistic lung abscesses are seen. Such conditions often cause multiple (rather than single) abscesses, the majority of which are acquired in the hospital.

Etiology. The most common organisms responsible for primary aspiration lung abscesses are anaerobic bacteria (see Table 35–1). The fusobacteria, *Bacteroides* species, peptostreptococci, and peptococci are most commonly seen.[83] Aerobic bacteria (*Streptococcus pneumoniae, S. aureus,* beta-hemolytic streptococci, *Klebsiella* species, *Pseudomonas aeruginosa, Escherichia coli*) are less commonly true etiologic agents but are often implicated because they are cultured from expectorated sputum by simple aerobic cultural techniques. Bartlett et al[86] have demonstrated the need for anaerobic cultural methods, preferably using percutaneous transtracheal aspiration, if accurate bacteriologic studies uncontaminated with nasopharyngeal flora are to be obtained. These are not without hazard, and alternative methods using protected brush catheters in association with fiberoptic bronchoscopy have been introduced.[87] In common practice, the organisms often cannot be isolated because antibiotic therapy has already been started. Often, however, the technique for obtaining material for study is self-defeating because the bacteriostatic additives in injectable saline solutions that are used to obtain lung washings are the bacterial suppressive action of local anesthetic agents used at bronchoscopy or bronchography have inhibited bacterial growth.[87–89]

The types of bacteria isolated in opportunistic lung abscesses differ from those that cause aspiration disease. Although *S. aureus* is still a common causative organism, alpha-hemolytic streptococci, *Neisseria catarrhalis, S. pneumoniae, Pseudomonas, Proteus, E. coli,* and *Klebsiella* all appear. Occasionally, after prolonged antibiotic treatment, rather unusual bacteria and fungi are all that remain to be cultured from the sputum.

Clinical Manifestations. The typical onset of lung abscess is insidious, with cough and fever, sometimes in association with chest pain. Hemoptysis often signals the evacuation of the necrotic contents of the abscess cavity, after which purulent and sometimes foul-smelling sputum is produced. The color (green, brown, gray, or yellow) is usually not helpful, although the production of anchovy- or chocolate- colored sputum should suggest amebic abscess. After the contents of the abscess are evacuated, clinical evidence of toxicity subsides.

The early physical signs of lung abscess are similar to those of localized pneumonia or consolidation. Later, the signs of cavitation may be elicited, as well as those of a pleural effusion, if empyema supervenes. Clubbing of the digits occurs only in patients with long-standing infection.[90]

Sometimes, severe toxemia, dyspnea, cyanosis, and septic shock overshadow symptoms and signs of staphylococcal pneumonia or lung abscess in infants or children, especially if rupture of the abscess and pyopneumothorax have occurred.

THORACIC X-RAY STUDIES. Initially, an area of nonspecific, dense pneumonic consolidation may be seen. After evacuation of the necrotic center through a connecting bronchus, a typical air-fluid level is observed on films taken with the patient in the upright position or in the lateral decubitus position if the patient is too ill to sit up (Fig. 35–11). In time, the cavity may shrink and disappear, but occasionally a cavity will assume a cyst-like appearance. Atelectasis, pneumothorax, pleural thickening, or effusion may confuse the typical picture. For example, complete or partial opacification of an entire hemithorax is occasionally seen in infants with staphylococcal pneumonias, because of their predilection to develop into infected, thin-walled pneumoceles associated with pleural effusion, empyema, or pyopneumothorax. Even such extensive x-ray changes can disappear rather dramatically after appropriate therapy.

Diagnosis. A significant infection in a dependent pulmonary segment in combination with known orogingival or dental disease and a probable history of obtunded consciousness should suggest the possibility of a lung abscess. This diagnosis is strongly supported by the presence of purulent sputum and even more strongly if a fluid level can be identified in a characteristic lesion on the thoracic x-ray taken in the upright position. Any pneumonia can rapidly lead to lung abscess in immunocompromised patients.

DIFFERENTIAL DIAGNOSIS. Many conditions can be mistaken for lung abscess, especially on x-ray ex-

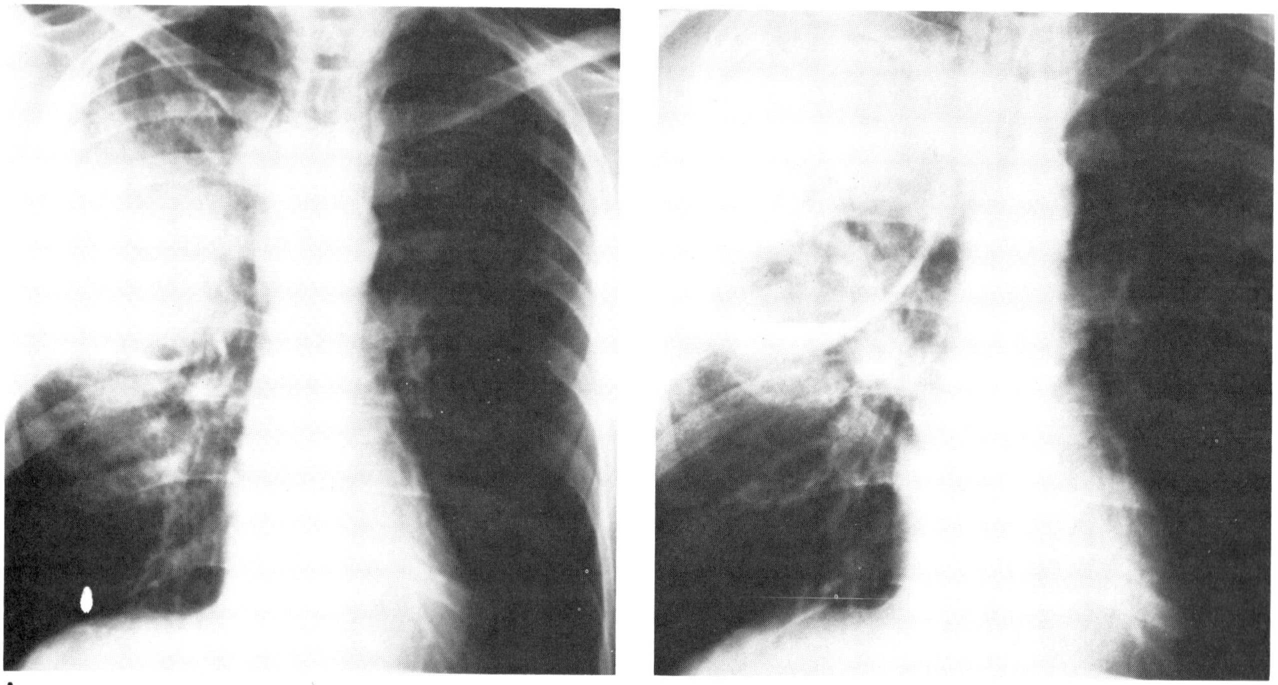

A B

Figure 35–11. Evolution of a lung abscess. This 50-year-old alcoholic man had a febrile illness and the pneumonic lesions seen in **A.** Note small area of cavitation near the base. The patient received high doses of penicillin. Over the course of 3 days, he began to cough up quantities of yellow-green odorous material. **B.** The thoracic x-ray 3 days later shows a large cystic lesion with a fluid level. It is probable that a small lung abscess ruptured into and was loculated by the interlobar fissure, forming an interlobar empyema. With continued therapy the process resolved, leaving only a thickened pleura and moderate reduction in lung volume.

aminations. These include lung tumors, tuberculosis, fungal infections of the lung, actinomycosis, bronchiectasis, pneumonia, aseptic necrosis of a tumor, and secondary infection of cysts or bullae.

Bacteriologic examination of the sputum for fungi and tubercle bacilli, sputum cytology, chest tomography, bronchoscopy, and bronchography may be needed in the differential diagnosis of atypical cases. The radiographic appearance of a carcinoma that has excavated can sometimes be confusing. The irregular lobulated contour containing an irregular central cavity with a thickened wall is helpful. A bronchogenic carcinoma should also be suspected if the lesion responds poorly to antibiotic therapy. An encysted subacute or chronic pleural or interlobar empyema may appear as a well-defined shadow that closely resembles an abscess. On a lateral x-ray examination, however, the empyema shadow is usually oval and interlobar or subpleural. Computer tomography may be helpful in delineating the abscess.[91,92] Tuberculous or fungal cavities do not usually appear with a fluid level or in the clinical setting described. Bacteriologic and mycologic studies are obviously essential for differential diagnosis.

Cysts of the lung are spherical (often without a clear-cut outline) and thin-walled, with little or no inflammation surrounding them. Infected, hydatid cysts are a problem only in endemic areas—Utah, Canada, and Alaska. It may be difficult to differentiate an abscess from a hydatid cyst after the cyst has ruptured and becomes secondarily infected, because then it has become a chronic lung abscess. A positive reaction to a Casoni skin test (not completely reliable) or eosinophilia and the occurrence of urticaria are helpful in diagnosing echinococcosis.

Treatment

MEDICAL TREATMENT. Prolonged antimicrobial therapy is the best treatment for primary aspiration lung abscess. If all primary lung abscesses were appropriately treated, there would be little place for operation in this disease.[86] Appropriate management includes an attempt to obtain secretions from the lower respiratory tract either by percutaneous transtracheal aspiration or by fiberoptic bronchoscopy and special brush catheters for bacteriologic studies.[87]

An effective regimen is penicillin G, 5 to 20 million units per day, either orally (the lower dose) or intravenously (the higher dose).[93] Because penicillin-resistant strains of anaerobic organisms have emerged, clindamycin 600 mg IV every 6 hours is slightly more effective and is considered by many to be the treatment of choice.[83] Metronidazole (Flagyl), which is not active against aerobic or microaerophilic organisms, is effective against anaerobic bacteria, especially in combination with penicillin. Four weeks of treatment have been recommended,[93] but the parenteral administration need be continued only until the patient's fever and toxicity have subsided and x-ray evidence of improvement is seen. After this, antibiotics are given orally, and treatment is continued until cavitation disappears and clinical cure is attained. Oral antibiotics may be required for 3 to 20 weeks, but with this treatment, operation for primary lung abscess is almost never required. Kanamycin may be the best drug for *Klebsiella* infection. Combinations of drugs may be needed in drug-resistant cases.

Bronchoscopy is often appropriate, to look for foreign bodies, to rule out endobronchial tumor, and to aid in evacuating abscesses. If bronchoscopic manipulation to achieve transbronchial drainage of large abscesses is required, great care should be exercised to avoid spillage of pus into the opposite lung. Drowning has been reported in these circumstances. The refinement of transbronchoscopic drainage by catheterization of the appropriate bronchus by an arteriographic catheter (through a rigid bronchoscope, with or without fluoroscopic guidance) is more helpful than the flexible fiberoptic bronchoscope (Fig. 35–12). Physical measures, including postural drainage and percussion of the thorax, may be helpful, but proof of this is lacking.

SURGICAL TREATMENT. Operations are reserved for the complications of lung abscess, including chronicity, serious hemoptysis, the development of bronchopleural fistula, and empyema. Operation should not often be required but is occasionally useful in neglected or inadequately treated patients, in older people with suspected malignancy, and for giant abscesses where the risk of contralateral aspiration is great.

Pulmonary resection (usually lobectomy) should be used if a large (6 cm or more) or smaller, thick-walled, residual cavity remains after 8 weeks of intensive antibiotic therapy, especially if there are continuing or recurring symptoms. Patients with sizable hemoptysis are at risk not so much because of the threat of exsanguination as because of

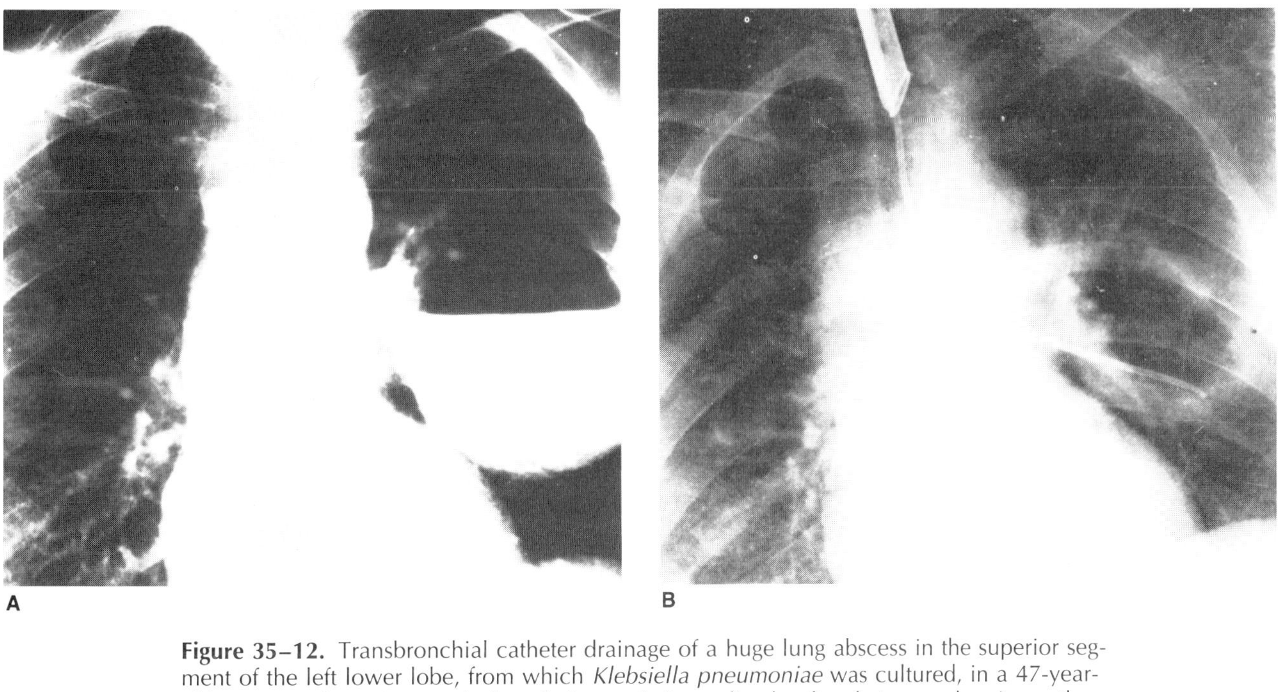

A B

Figure 35–12. Transbronchial catheter drainage of a huge lung abscess in the superior segment of the left lower lobe, from which *Klebsiella pneumoniae* was cultured, in a 47-year-old man. **A.** Thoracic x-ray before drainage. **B.** Immediately after drainage, showing catheter in the cavity. A Cordis right coronary angiographic catheter was used. The procedure was repeated 3 days later, again with evacuation of pus. The patient was ultimately discharged with a thin-walled, 2-cm cavity in the left lower lobe. *(From Connors JP, Roper CL, Ferguson TB, et al: Ann Thorac Surg 19:254, 1975.)*

the hazard of asphyxiation and may require emergency operation.[94] Radiologic features that can be seen in patients with severe hemoptysis include (1) alternate emptying and refilling of the abscess cavity in serial chest films (the emptying may correlate with an episode of hemoptysis, the refilling with periods of minimal or no hemoptysis), (2) an air-fluid level with differences in the radiolucency of the fluid phase and changes in location in the abscess cavity on changes in position, and (3) a persistent density with patchy radiolucencies. The persistent density may indicate an abscess cavity filled with blood clots.[94]

Special care is necessary when operating on patients with lung abscesses because of the possibility of flooding the airways with blood or pus. Appropriate anesthetic and operative techniques must be used to prevent this material from entering the uninvolved portions of the lung. These techniques include the use of a tracheal divider or placing the patient in the prone or supine position to prevent contralateral lung contamination and airway obstruction. The involved bronchus should be clamped as soon as possible after the chest is opened. A long, cuffed endotracheal tube passed into the main bronchus on the nonoperative side and blockage of a draining bronchus with a Fogarty-type catheter during bronchoscopy prior to intubation are less satisfactory methods but are sometimes necessary. Empyemas must be drained, and a pulmonary abscess that ruptures into the pleural cavity can be treated as an empyema. Closed-tubed thoracostomy drainage of a lung abscess is generally contraindicated because a large bronchopleural fistula may result. Nevertheless, giant or neglected abscesses can sometimes be rapidly cured with simultaneous closure of the abscess and the fistula by closed drainage. Aspiration is thereby avoided. This is particularly useful in seriously ill patients who would not be expected to tolerate a formal thoracotomy. When patients with life-threatening hemoptysis cannot safely undergo major thoracic operations because of severe respiratory insufficiency, bilateral disease, inability to locate the site of bleeding, or because the patient refuses operation, nonsurgical treatment must be used. Several radiologists have reported successful control of pulmonary hemorrhage by embolizing the bronchial and nonbronchial arteries.[95]

OPPORTUNISTIC ABSCESSES. Because of effective antibiotic therapy, the mortality rate in primary lung abscesses has declined from approximately 25 percent to less than 5 percent. Unfortunately, this is not true of opportunistic lung abscesses. Opportunistic lung abscesses require more aggressive diagnostic and therapeutic measures. Invasive diagnostic methods, such as percutaneous transtracheal aspiration and even direct needle aspiration of the lung, may be justified to determine the etiologic agent because specific therapy may be necessary.

Occasionally, percutaneous transthoracic drainage can cause dramatic decompression of an abscess cavity, which can result in its obliteration and subsequent healing. Newson et al[96] successfully treated opportunistic abscesses in desperately ill patients by inserting a plastic intravenous catheter directly into the abscess cavity, aspirating the pus, and instilling antibiotics. The mortality rate continues to be high, however (75 to 90 percent), in immunocompromised patients who have lung abscesses.

Prevention. Lung abscesses can be prevented in some circumstances. Whenever possible, tonsillectomy, tooth extraction, and operations on paranasal sinuses should be performed with the patient under local rather than general anesthesia. If a foreign body is inhaled, it should promptly be removed by bronchoscopy. All acute lung infections should be treated promptly with appropriate antimicrobial drugs. Prevention of aspiration during the postanesthetic state, and during any state of altered consciousness, will prevent aspiration pneumonitis and abscess formation. Finally, maintenance of good oral hygiene would probably reduce the risk of putrid lung abscesses.

Hematogenous Lung Abscesses and Septic Pulmonary Infarcts. Hematogenous lung abscesses are not considered here. They are usually associated with bacteremia, are almost always multiple, and do not usually require operative intervention. Vidal et al[97] have suggested surgical intervention for lung abscesses secondary to pulmonary infarction in patients who respond poorly to medical treatment. McMillan et al[98] reported that of 12 patients (many heroin addicts) with septic embolism and infected infarcts who required thoracotomy, only one died.

Bronchiectasis. To Laennec and his pupils belongs the credit for the earliest descriptions of bronchiectasis, although the term was not introduced until 1846 (by Hasse). Not much could be done about this "loathsome disease" for a century after its recognition, but in 1922 Sicard and Forestier introduced bronchography, which permitted visualization, localization, and assessment of its severity.[99] Drainage procedures similar to those used for empyema or lung abscess were predictably accompanied by disastrous results. Surgical treatment of bronchiectasis became firmly established only after Kent and Blades[100] pioneered lung resection using individual ligation of the lobar hilar structures. The frequency of the disease has declined since the introduction of effective antibiotics.

Pathogenesis

ACQUIRED BRONCHIECTASIS. Infection and bronchial obstruction are the two major factors contributing to the development of acquired bronchiectasis. Infection may be associated with abnormal host defense, the most common being panhypogammaglobulinemia. The decline in the incidence of bronchiectasis in children is probably the result of the control of pertussis, measles, influenza, and bronchopneumonia by immunization and antibiotics.

Causes of bronchial obstruction include aspiration of foreign bodies, retained mucopurulent secretions, bronchial tumors, and external bronchial compression by enlarged peribronchial lymph nodes associated with chronic lung infections (tuberculosis, histoplasmosis, and coccidioidomycosis).

Middle lobe syndrome refers to the particular susceptibility of this lobe to bronchiectasis. Two factors appear to be involved in its susceptibility: the acute angle at which the middle lobe bronchus arises from the bronchus intermedius, making it more susceptible to compression, and the poor collateral ventilation of the middle lobe, which leads to atelectasis and pneumonitis when the proximal bronchus becomes obstructed.[101]

Because bronchiectasis is frequently preceded by pneumonitis but not bronchial obstruction, the traction theory for the origin of bronchiectasis has evolved. According to this hypothesis, after pneumonia, scarring and contracture of the tissue that surrounds the entrapped bronchi occur. Traction on the external circumference of the bronchi causes dilation. The distal branches of the segmental bronchi, having the least cartilaginous support, then become dilated. The bronchial dilation that follows the healing of a tuberculous infection or a chronic lung abscess can leave a residual bronchiectatic segmental or subsegmental bronchus.

CONGENITAL BRONCHIECTASIS. The strongest evidence for a congenital link in the cause of bronchiectasis is found in Kartagener's syndrome, a triad of conditions including situs inversus, pansinusitis, and bronchiectasis.[102] Whereas bronchiectasis at one time affected about 0.5 percent of the general population, it has been identified in 20 to 25 percent of patients with situs inversus and dextrocardia. A genetic abnormality, carried as an autosomal recessive trait, has been suggested, but such a relationship was not identified in the 1972 series from the Mayo Clinic.[102] Ultrastructural studies of a genetic disorder associated with the dynein arms of cilia or with a lack of radial spokes suggest abnormalities of mucociliary transport as a factor in the pathogenesis of some forms of bronchiectasis. Homozygous alpha-1-antitrypsin deficiency, a condition that is associated with pulmonary emphysema, is occasionally accompanied by bronchiectasis.[103]

Bronchiectasis is also seen in children with cystic fibrosis. These patients with tenacious bronchial secretions, abnormal bronchial mucosa, and impaired ciliary function ultimately die of complications of diffuse pulmonary disease. Adult cystic fibrosis with bronchiectasis and *Pseudomonas* colonization has become increasingly common.

Pathology. Bronchiectasis is most frequently located in the basal segments of the lower lobes. Although the superior segments are usually free of disease, the lingula may be involved in patients with left lower lobe bronchiectasis, and the right middle lobe may be bronchiectactic in patients with right lower lobe disease.

The bronchi are dilated, and if secondary infection is present, they can be filled with mucopurulent secretions. The bronchial wall is partially destroyed and replaced with fibrous tissue. Both acute and chronic inflammatory changes may be present. The bronchial arteries are hypertrophied, and enlarged anastomoses between the bronchial and pulmonary arteries can be found. These anastomoses can cause significant arteriovenous shunting. Severe hemoptysis may be a consequence of this rich network of high-pressure vessels.

Etiology. Infection is secondary to obstruction in bronchiectasis, and the infecting organisms are frequently mixed. When anaerobes are found, *Bacteroides, Fusobacterium,* and anaerobic streptococci are most frequently cultured. *Pseudomonas aeruginosa,* a common colonizer in cystic fibrosis, is known to elaborate a variety of substances that damage bronchi and may play a significant role in the development of bronchiectasis.[104]

Clinical Manifestations. Cough, production of mucopurulent sputum, fever, and pleuritic pain occur intermittently when secondary infection supervenes. Much of the time the patient may be asymptomatic. Recurrent episodes of bronchopneumonia are often accompanied by pleuritic pain and an increase in copious, foul-smelling sputum so severe that the social consequences exceed the threat to health. Patients with upper lobe bronchiectasis may have no symptoms. Chronic or recurring hemoptysis, rather than productive cough, may be the primary symptom. Hemoptysis occurs in 41 percent of patients with localized disease and in 66 percent of patients with diffuse disease.[105] Bronchiectasis is the most common cause of hemoptysis in children. Malnutrition and pulmonary insufficiency can develop when the disease is advanced. The classic physical findings of cyanosis, digital clubbing, and weight loss are rarely seen.

Percussion may reveal localized dullness. Moist, bubbling rales may be heard on auscultation over the affected areas, and coarse expiratory rhonchi are present during acute exacerbations.

Diagnosis. The diagnosis of bronchiectasis should be suspected in a patient with frequent respiratory tract infections, chronic productive cough, and hemoptysis. Because of the impact of antibiotics on the natural course of this disease, its symptoms are likely to be subtle. Thoracic x-ray studies may demonstrate only nonspecific findings, such as atelectasis, fibrosis, and pleural thickening. In severe cases, dilated bronchi partially filled with purulent secretions may be identified by the presence of multiple air-fluid levels.

Computed tomography has largely replaced bronchography for diagnosing bronchiectasis because it is noninvasive (Fig. 35–13). High-resolution CT scans are convenient for both patient and physician but are often unable to resolve motion artifacts or inspissated mucus, or to distinguish bronchiectasis from other chronic lung disease with cystic abnormalities.[106]

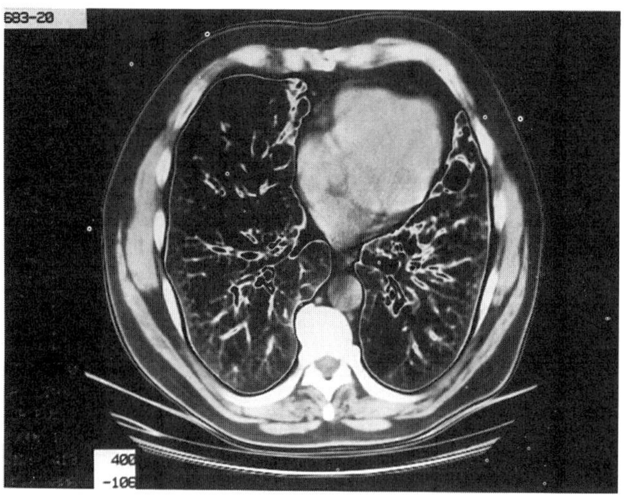

Figure 35–13. CT scan showing saccular bronchiectasis in the right middle lobe and in the lingula of the left lung. Note the dilated thin-wall bronchi.

The only definitive method of diagnosing bronchiectasis is by bronchography. This is ordinarily performed only if operation is contemplated. It is also used occasionally to help exclude a tumor, foreign body, or a rare congenital abnormality. It is best performed after appropriate treatment of acute infection and after special efforts, such as postural drainage, have been made to evacuate secretions. The bronchi must be relatively free of secretions if a technically good bronchogram is to be obtained (Fig. 35–14).

Bronchoscopic examination may be performed at the same time as bronchography and may provide additional information, such as the specific segments that are the sources of purulent secretions and the visualization of bronchostenosis, foreign body, or neoplasm. Bacteriologic study of secretions obtained directly through the bronchoscope, uncontaminated with nasopharyngeal secretions (or local anesthetic agents), can give a more accurate diagnosis, so that more specific antibiotic therapy can be used. Finally, removal of thick purulent secretions is, in itself, therapeutic.

The differentiation between acute or chronic purulent bronchitis that causes cylindrical bronchiectasis, which may be reversible by vigorous antibiotic treatment, and true nonreversible bronchiectasis can be difficult to determine during bronchoscopy. Chronic bronchitis may be the cause of secondary infection in bronchiectasis. The bronchographic appearance of cylindrical ectasia, with bronchi of uniform caliber crowded together and with rather diffuse involvement of both lungs, is more suggestive of chronic bronchitis or reversible bronchiectasis than of true surgical bronchiectasis.

Treatment. Control of infection and relief of bronchial obstruction are the two most important measures in the treatment of bronchiectasis. The most common secondary infecting organisms are *Hemophilus influenzae,* a variety of streptococci, *S. aureus, K. pneumoniae, E. coli,* fusiform bacilli, and Vincent's spirochetes. When the patient's sputum is purulent, appropriate antibiotics should be given. Broad spectrum antibiotics that have been effective are tetracycline, oxytetracycline, and ampicillin. Ampicillin combined with cloxacillin or benzylpenicillin is effective against *S. aureus*. Vigorous antibiotic treatment and pulmonary toilet will reverse

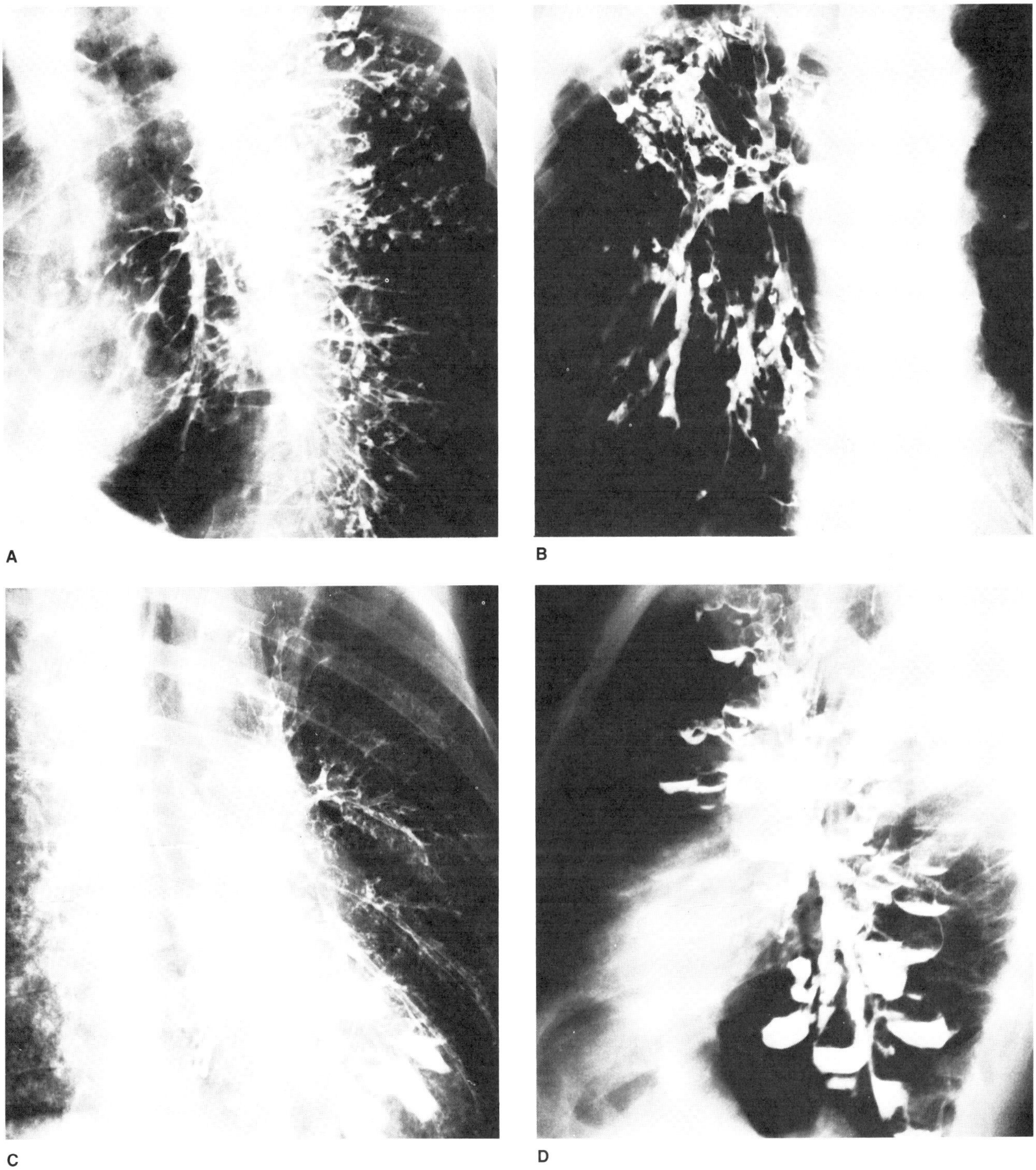

Figure 35–14. Varieties of bronchiectasis revealed during bronchography. **A.** Bronchiolectasis, generalized involvement of very small bronchi, best seen in upper lung field. This is not a surgical condition. **B.** Marked distortion of bronchi following tuberculous infection, right upper lobe. This is also not usually a surgical condition per se. **C.** Localized postpneumonic saccular bronchiectasis, basal segments, left lower lobe. This patient was treated successfully by resection of the basal segments of the left lower lobe. **D.** Saccular bronchiectasis involving the entire left lung. The right lung was normal. This patient was treated successfully by left pneumonectomy. *(From Takaro T, Scott SM, Bridgman AH, et al: Curr Probl Surg 14:6, 1977.)*

many of the bronchoscopic and bronchographic findings of chronic bronchitis and cylindrical bronchiectasis.

Coughing, endotracheal suction, and postural drainage are all effective in removing bronchial secretions. Postural drainage requires training and conscientious performance to be effective. In addition to the use of postural drainage to remove bronchial secretions, cough can be enhanced with the use of bronchodilators and humidifiers. Isoproterenol, epinephrine, and phenylephrine are useful bronchodilators and can be used in nebulizers. Endotracheal aspiration of secretions is used when coughing and postural drainage are ineffective.

Should symptoms remain or recur after an adequate trial of medical therapy, operation should be considered. These symptoms would include continuing episodes of pneumonitis, continuing production of 30 to 60 ml of purulent sputum daily, or frequent episodes of hemoptysis. The patient's general condition and pulmonary reserve, in particular, must be considered.

The best results can be anticipated in patients with limited or localized disease, especially those with unilateral disease restricted to the basal segments.[107] Eighty percent of patients with localized disease were relieved of all symptoms by operation. Only 36 percent with diffuse or multisegmental disease were rendered asymptomatic, although 50 percent were improved.[105] With bilateral disease the side with the greater degree of involvement should be resected first. A maximum amount of pulmonary tissue should be conserved. Resection of the opposite lung will not always be necessary.[105]

Operative mortality for pulmonary resection for bronchiectasis is now less than 1 percent, and the incidence of bronchopleural fistula and empyema has been between 3 and 5 percent.[108]

Prognosis. Bronchiectasis is no longer of considerable prominence in thoracic surgery. Prior to the advent of the antibiotic era, the average life expectancy of patients with bronchiectasis was less than 10 years.[99] Most patients now have a nearly normal life span.[109]

Pulmonary Tuberculosis

Definition and Etiology. Lung disease caused by mammalian tubercle bacilli (*Mycobacterium tuberculosis* and *M. bovis*) is designated pulmonary tuberculosis. Nontuberculous mycobacterial lung infection is caused by mycobacteria other than mammalian tubercle bacilli (*Mycobacterium* types I through IV). The bacteriologic characteristics of these organisms are described more completely in Chapter 9.

Thoracic surgeons once called pulmonary tuberculosis the "king of diseases," a title earned eight centuries ago. Surgeons formerly devised a number of ingenious operations to collapse the portions of the lungs occupied by cavities, such as artificial pneumothorax and pneumoperitoneum, extrapleural thoracoplasty, and plombage operations. When antimicrobial agents became available, pulmonary resection became the operation of choice, but with the advent of effective antimicrobial therapy, surgery for tuberculosis is now rarely needed.[110]

Incidence. The decline in deaths from tuberculosis (from 63 to just 2 per 100,000 over a 45-year span) and the decrease in active cases (from 77 to 9.4 per 100,000) are two of the more remarkable developments of this century.[111] Most of the decline in mortality occurred prior to the advent of antituberculous agents. Thus the initial decline is attributable to improvements in public health. The more recent decline was associated with the discovery of effective chemotherapy. However, the disease has not disappeared. In fact, after a century of decline it may be reemerging. In the United States in 1985 there were only 2200 new cases of pulmonary tuberculosis. In 1991 there were 26,283 cases reported and one-third of those observed in New York City were resistant to one or more drugs.[112,113] In the developing world (as of 1990), tuberculosis accounts for 18.5 percent of adult deaths.[112]

Pathogenesis. The pathogenesis of tuberculosis is discussed in Chapter 9. Typically, inhalation of tubercle bacilli leads to peripheral, pulmonary, necrotizing pneumonitis and hilar lymph node involvement, which is sometimes very prominent, especially in children. This comprises the primary Ghon complex, which nearly always heals. In a minority of cases, a caseous necrotic focus will excavate and empty its liquefied contents into a bronchus to produce cavitation and signal reinfection. There may then be either intrabronchial, lymphatic, or hematogenous spread of disease, or it may regress, fibrose, and calcify. A tuberculoma is formed when the contents of a caseating focus become inspissated. Bronchiectasis or atelectasis may result from partial or complete bronchial obstruction due to intrinsic disease (endobronchial disease with ulceration and scarring) or from extrinsic obstruction due to enlarged hilar lymph nodes. Rupture of a caseous subpleural focus into the pleural cavity may produce a tuberculous effusion or empyema. Tuberculosis of the larynx, mediastinal, supraclavicular, and cervical lymph nodes, pericardium, and chest wall may all occur. Extrathoracic hematogenous spread to any of the organs of the body, especially meninges, bones, joints, or peritoneal cavity, was common in earlier years and may again become common should tuberculosis reemerge when AIDS and overpopulation strain the resources of public health organizations.

Clinical Manifestations. The onset of pulmonary tuberculosis can be insidious, with vague complaints of anorexia, fatigue, weight loss, and low-grade fever. A more acute onset includes fever, cough, aching, sweating, and hemoptysis. Chest pain is usually caused by tuberculous pleurisy. Physical signs are not often helpful but should be sought in cases of pleural effusion, atelectasis, bronchiectasis, consolidation, or appreciable cavitation. Hoarseness may indicate laryngitis.

Thoracic x-ray studies can vary in appearance, depending on the extent and type of disease. Tuberculosis can mimic almost any other pulmonary disease on x-ray examination. The lesions of surgical interest are the open cavity, the tuberculoma, bronchiectasis, and various combinations of atelectatic or destroyed lobes or lungs that can mimic bronchogenic carcinoma.

A number of x-ray patterns may be identified in patients with postprimary tuberculosis:

1. Local exudative lesions represent alveolar consolidation, which may be patchy or confluent. The lymphatic drainage markings radiating toward the hilus are accentuated.
2. Local fibroproductive lesions are defined more sharply, although their size and shape may vary. Fibrosis and contracture are evidenced by a decrease in lung volume, and retraction of the hilus and trachea toward the lesion is common.
3. Cavitary lesions have moderately thick walls, but, with healing, these tend to become quite thin, the inner surface linings are smooth, and air-fluid levels are seen (see Fig. 35–15). The cavities may disappear following adequate therapy, but some persist as open negative cavities. Computed tomography scans may be necessary to verify the persistence of some cavities after therapy.

The x-ray manifestations of pulmonary disease due to mycobacteria other than *M. tuberculosis* cannot be differentiated from those due to *M. tuberculosis*. Some features are more characteristic, however. There is a greater tendency for cavitation with multiple thin-walled cavities than with infection with the tubercle bacillus, and exudative lesions are uncommon, as are hematogenous dissemination and pleural effusion.

Diagnosis. The diagnosis of tuberculosis is solely dependent on identification of the infecting organisms or the histologic features and demonstration of the organism in the lung. A negative skin test result excludes the diagnosis unless miliary tuberculosis is present or an immunosuppressed patient is being examined. The principal differential diagnosis is cancer, but any chronic pulmonary infection can have a similar presentation.

Treatment. The contemporary treatment of tuberculosis by chemotherapeutic agents has been summarized by Van Scoy and Wilkowske.[114] The need for therapy and the duration of treatment depend on the category of disease.

The universally recognized first-line drugs are isoniazid, ethambutol, streptomycin, pyrazinamide, and rifampin, and all are associated with some degree of toxicity (see Chap. 9). There are also several second-line drugs, which are generally less effective and more toxic. Uncomplicated pulmonary tuberculosis is treated with isoniazid, rifampin, and pyrazinamide for 2 months followed by isoniazid and rifampin for 4 more months. Pyrazinamide is bactericidal for actively dividing organisms. For prophylaxis, isoniazid is given for 6 to 12 months unless contacts are isoniazid-resistant.

Certain principles in the use of drug therapy in pulmonary tuberculosis must be adhered to: (1) never use a single drug when there is clinical evidence of disease, (2) a failing regimen (ie, continued sputum positivity) indicates drug resistance, (3) never add only a single drug to a failing regimen, and (4) add two drugs to which sensitivity has been demonstrated.

Surgical treatment should strongly be considered under the following circumstances:[115]

1. The persistence of cavitary disease, bronchial disease, or granulomatous nodular disease, with sputum smears and cultures that remain positive for *M. tuberculosis* for 3 to 6 months when appropriate antimicrobial therapy with at least two drugs is being used.
2. The persistence of significant (larger than 2 cm in diameter) nodular disease or a destroyed lobe or lung even without positive sputum cultures. The rationale here is that the antimicrobial agents penetrate dense

fibrous tissue in insufficient concentration to adequately sterilize the lesion.

3. The presence of thick-walled cavities even when sputum cultures are negative (ie, open negative cavities in patients who cannot be relied on to continue long-term antimicrobial therapy—18 months).
4. Lesions suspected of being bronchogenic carcinoma. Carcinomas can occur in an area previously damaged by tuberculous infection (scar carcinoma). A tuberculoma can usually be resected when carcinoma is suspected even without drug coverage (Fig. 35–15).
5. Significant hemoptysis or hemorrhage if the source can be located and is resectable (bronchiectasis, broncholithiasis, mycetoma in a tuberculous cavity).[116]
6. A lobe or lung trapped by a tuberculous empyema that is unexpandable even after decortication.

Operation is rarely required for childhood tuberculosis. Purulent tuberculous empyema is seldom encountered, but when it is, decortication may be necessary, with or without resection of a portion of the underlying diseased lung.

The complications of operations for tuberculosis include the usual problems that follow major thoracotomy and lung resection, especially persistent pleural air space, bronchopleural fistula, empyema, or spread of tuberculosis.[117] Before operation patients should be given a drug to which their bacilli are sensitive, because the complication rate is high if the organisms are resistant. Ideally, at least one primary drug to which the organisms are sensitive should be used. When upper lobectomy plus resection of the superior segment of the lower lobe is required, a prior concomitant posterolateral thoracoplasty involving the upper three to five ribs can prevent the development of a significant space problem, empyema, or bronchopleural fistula.[118] If these complications develop, they should be managed like pleural empyemas. The problem of the long-term effects of thoracoplasty on cardiorespiratory function following pneumonectomy has been reviewed.

The operative management of massive hemoptysis (200 to 300 ml in 24 hours) requires special attention. Success with this difficult problem requires locating the source of hemorrhage by bronchoscopy during active bleeding, the use of double-lumen endotracheal dividers, and judicious selection of patients.[110] Bronchial arterial embolization might be considered in inoperable candidates.[95]

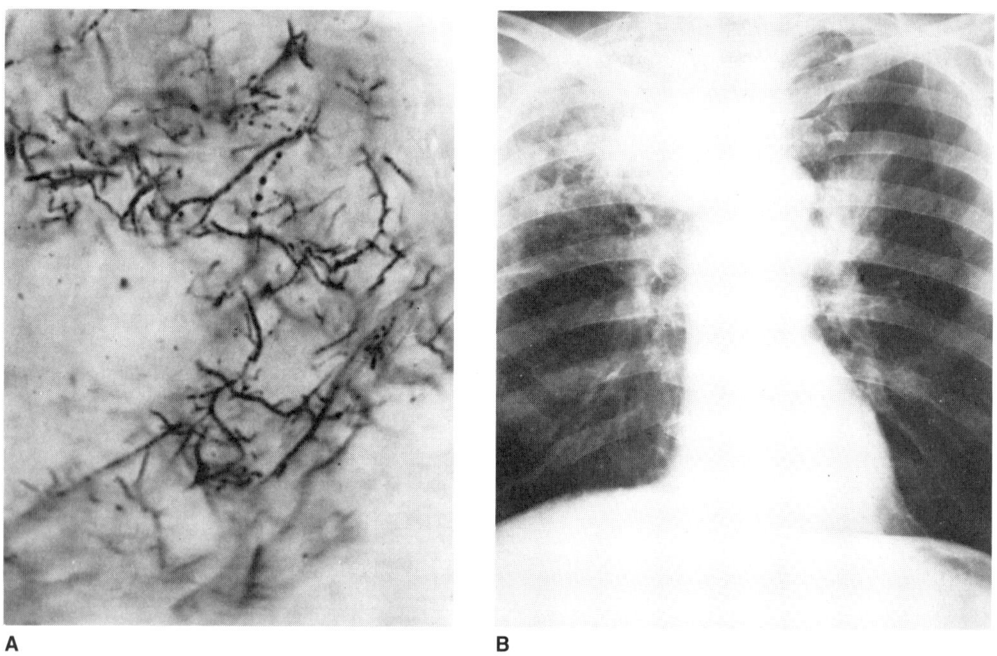

A B

Figure 35–15. A. *Nocardia asteroides.* These organisms have been mistaken for tubercle bacilli because of acid-fast staining characteristics. Gram. ×1000. **B.** X-ray of thorax shows pneumonic lesion of nocardiosis, right lung, and left parahilar infiltrate. *Nocardia asteroides* was cultured from the sputum. The patient received a course of sulfadiazine and recovered. *(From Takaro T: Thoracic Actinomycetic and Mycotic Infections: In Goldsmith EI (ed): Practice of Surgery. New York, Harper & Row, 1978.)*

When operating on a drug-resistant, sputum-positive patient, Pomerantz et al[119] recommend reinforcing the bronchial closure with a muscle flap constructed from latissimus dorsi, serratus anterior, or intercostal muscle. They also recommend 3 months of preoperative drug therapy.

In general, the long-term prognosis has been excellent: 90 to 96 percent of patients who have had operations are free of disease at 5 years.[120] Even in developing countries, excellent results are obtained.

Nontuberculous Mycobacterial Lung Infections

Etiology. The microbiologic characteristics of mycobacteria are discussed in Chapter 9. The causative organisms in human disease are largely confined to *Mycobacterium kansasii, M. avium-intracellulare, M. xenopi, M. fortuitum-chelonei,* and *M. scrofulaceum* (see Table 9–2).[121]

Pathogenesis. The pathogenesis of these diseases is obscure. The disease is not transmitted by droplet infection from person to person but appears instead to be acquired from natural sources in the environment. The majority of cases are reported in adult men with preexisting pulmonary lesions (pneumoconiosis, previous tuberculosis, chronic bronchitis, bronchiectasis, chronic obstructive lung disease, and chronic aspiration pneumonitis) or immunologic deficiency disease. Disseminated disease due to *M. avium-intracellulare* occurs in 40 percent of AIDS patients. Cases do occur, however, in men and women without apparent lung disease or immunologic deficiency states. Malignant disease is a recognized risk factor.

Clinical Manifestations and Diagnosis. Symptoms are insidious, often overshadowed by preexisting chronic lung disease, and include persistent and productive cough, weakness, dyspnea, and weight loss. Occasionally, hemoptysis and chest pain are present. Cervical lymphadenitis may be observed in children.

Diagnosis may be difficult, because symptomatically, radiographically, and histologically, nontuberculous lung infections caused by *Mycobacteria* cannot reliably be distinguished from pulmonary tuberculosis. Skin tests may be helpful, but extensive cross-reactions may interfere with proper interpretation. Ultimately, the diagnosis depends on microbiologic evidence—the characteristic appearance of *M. kansasii* on smears—and on cultures of material obtained by sputum collection, transtracheal aspiration, or bronchoscopy. Other clinical syndromes include lymphadenitis, skin lesions, infections of the bones and joint, and urologic infections. Cases of disseminated disease have also been reported.

Treatment. A combined medical-surgical approach is favored.[119,122] For *M. kansasii* infection, isoniazid, ethambutol, and rifampin should be used for a minimum of 24 months. In most instances this will result in cure. For *M. avium-intracellulare* infection, which responds less readily to drug therapy, four drugs are recommended.[123] This expensive, uncomfortable, intensive treatment may also be toxic and can be modified by subsequent drug susceptibility studies and by the course of the disease.

Operation is reserved for medical treatment failures and should be used without inordinate delay. If the residual disease is localized enough to be resectable after 6 to 8 months of appropriate drug treatment, it should be excised. This will rarely be necessary with *M. kansasii* infection but will be required in an appreciable percentage of *M. avium-intracellulare* infections. Even with adjunctive surgical treatment the relapse and late mortality rates can be high. However, the overall late results in surgically treated patients are distinctly better than in those patients in whom operation is not carried out.[122,124,125]

Melioidosis

Incidence and Epidemiology. Melioidosis is a glanders-like infection of humans and animals that occurs endemically in Southeast Asia. Natural immunity is probably attained in the indigenous population, but military personnel during the Vietnam war acquired the disease in skin abrasions, in burns, and by ingestion or inhalation.[126]

Etiology. The organism responsible is *Pseudomonas pseudomallei,* a gram-negative bacillus that is ordinarily a saprophyte in damp tropical soils. Although the organism grows readily on standard culture media, it probably is not often recognized.[127] A characteristic wrinkling of the colonies occurs at about 72 hours and can be hastened by culturing at room temperature.

Clinical Manifestations. This rare disease occurs in several forms: (1) asymptomatic cases identified only by positive serologic findings, (2) acute localized suppuration, (3) acute pulmonary infection (the most common form), (4) acute septicemia (a highly lethal form), (5) chronic suppuration in which abscesses may be found in any organ, and (6) recrudescent infection in which any of the preceding overt forms may occur months or years after exposure. The outcome is fatal in more than 50 percent of cases, even with vigorous and appropriate therapy.[128]

Clinically, the disease resembles either pulmonary tuberculosis or chronic fungal infection. Many of the cases seen at large military medical centers were initially diagnosed as pulmonary tuberculosis. The full spectrum of x-ray findings—infiltration, cavitation, pleural effusion, empyema—can be seen. Hemagglutination, direct agglutination, and complement fixation tests are aids in diagnosis if a fourfold or greater rise in titer occurs in paired sera.[128]

Treatment. Antibiotics found to be effective in vitro, usually tetracycline, should be used for a minimum of 30 days. Other antibiotics might have to be used, singly or in a variety of combinations, including novobiocin, chloramphenicol, trimethoprim, sulfadiazine, and kanamycin.[128]

If pulmonary lesions remain after 6 months of antibiotic therapy, an operation is probably indicated. Ideally, sputum cultures should be negative at the time of operation, but this is not likely. Lobectomy, rather than segmental resection, is the best operation to avoid the development of bronchopleural fistula.[129] Good results can be expected.

INFECTIONS WITH THE ACTINOMYCETES

Actinomyces and *Nocardia* morphologically resemble fungi because they form hyphae with true branching and are spore producing, but they are true bacteria. Their microbiologic and pathologic characteristics are discussed in Chapters 6 and 9. This distinction is clinically important because these two diseases do not respond to the major antimycotic agent, amphotericin B, but do respond to antibacterial agents, such as penicillin and sulfonamides.

Actinomycosis

Definition. Actinomycosis is a chronic infection caused by the anaerobic Actinomycetaceae *Actinomyces israelii*. The disease is characterized by suppuration, with the formation of abscess and sinuses, in association with dense scarring. Characteristic yellow-brown granules, sulfur granules, are sometimes seen in material draining from abscesses or sinuses. Such material must be cultured under anaerobic conditions.[130]

Actinomyces israelii is a normal inhabitant of the oral cavity. Therefore the diagnosis can only be confirmed if the organism is recovered from closed tissue spaces, from draining sinuses or abscesses, or is shown to be invasive in histopathologic sections.

Clinical Syndromes. Three clinical forms of actinomycosis are recognized: cervicofacial (see Chap. 33), thoracic, and abdominal (see Chap. 38).

Thoracic actinomycosis can develop as an extension of the cervicofacial variety or even by extension from a subphrenic collection. Most commonly it results from bronchopulmonary invasion from aspirated material. It appears first as a pneumonic suppurative process, which may be associated with an abscess, similar to suppurative pneumonia caused by other agents. Hemoptysis may occur. The infection may be so indolent that symptoms are few until pleural or chest wall involvement becomes apparent. Thus, although empyema and chronically draining chest wall sinuses are characteristic, they are usually late stages of an insidious pulmonary process in the form of a nonspecific-appearing pulmonary infiltration, consolidation, or hilar mass sometimes strongly suggestive of bronchogenic carcinoma.[131,132] Colonization of an existing cavity may also occur resulting in a "fungus ball."[133]

X-ray signs that are helpful clinical clues for actinomycosis are pleural fluid with chest wall involvement including ribs and periosteum, penetration of interlobar fissures, and vertebral destruction. The infection rarely extends into the pericardium.

Treatment. Penicillin should be used in high doses for a prolonged period: a treatment of 20 million units of penicillin daily for 1 to 3 months is recommended. The prognosis after effective treatment is good.

Operations are sometimes indicated to remove a destroyed lobe, to drain an empyema, or to excise a sinus, but drug therapy is usually curative.[134] Suspicion of bronchogenic carcinoma is the most common indication for operation. Adequate and prolonged drug therapy to prevent reactivation of disease or development of empyema is important during and after thoracotomy.

The main problem with actinomycosis appears to be diagnosis rather than treatment: the correct diagnosis was made in fewer than 10 percent of patients in one series.[135]

Nocardiosis

The microbiology and pathogenesis of nocardiosis are discussed in Chapter 9. Nocardiosis is a chronic infection usually caused by *Nocardia asteroides* (but also by several other species) and characterized by primary pulmonary involvement, with secondary hematogenous dissemination to other organs, especially the central nervous system.[136] The diagnosis is very difficult to make, but infection may be fatal unless adequate specific antimicrobial therapy is used. In most recent reports, nocardiosis is seen as an opportunistic infection in patients with disordered immune systems associated with malignancy, organ transplantation, or immunosuppressive therapy.[136–138] It is infrequent in AIDS patients.[139]

Pathogenesis and Pathology. *Nocardia* is aerobic and widely disseminated in soil, grains, grasses, and several species of animals.

The organism apparently enters via the respiratory tract and produces a necrotizing pneumonitis, progressing to abscess formation. Encapsulation is incomplete, so that spread to adjacent pulmonary tissue, pleura, and chest wall, as well as dissemination, is common. All organs may be involved, and brain abscesses are especially common. The histopathologic appearance is not diagnostic, although clumps of organisms may be seen and mistaken for *M. tuberculosis* (see Fig. 35–15).

Clinical Manifestations. Classic nocardiosis, like actinomycosis, is characterized by fever, a necrotizing pneumonia productive of thick, purulent sputum, and chronic or subacute progression to involvement of the chest wall, with subcutaneous abscesses and draining sinuses. The exudate rarely will contain sulfur granules similar to those observed in actinomycosis. Most commonly, however, an immunosuppressed patient will have nonspecific flu-like symptoms of cough, malaise, fever, weakness, night sweats, weight loss, and, occasionally, hemoptysis and pleuritic chest pain. On thoracic x-ray studies, a variety of presentations, including solitary nodules, nonspecific infiltrates, or cavitary disease, may be seen, and confusion with tuberculosis is common (see Fig. 35–15). Localized pneumonic or infiltrative lesions may suggest bronchogenic carcinoma. In the clearly opportunistic form of the disease, the progress to cavitation and dissemination can be accelerated. The most frequent site of extrapulmonary spread is to the brain.

Diagnosis. Diagnosis is difficult and is frequently made at autopsy. A chronically ill or immunologically depressed patient with a subacute pulmonary infection (perhaps with evidence of nonspecific central nervous system involvement) is suggestive. The isolation of *Nocardia* from sputum, transtracheal aspiration, bronchoscopic washings, sinus drainage, or lung biopsy is diagnostic because the organism is not a respiratory tract saprophyte. The diagnosis can be missed in the laboratory if the technicians are not informed of the possibility of nocardiosis.

Nocardia grows so slowly that the cultures are frequently discarded. Antibiotics in fungal media suppress its growth. Overgrowth by oropharyngeal or sinus tract bacteria can obscure it, and histopathologic evidence is inconclusive because hematoxylin and eosin stain does not stain it. The Gram stain, methenamine silver stain, and acid-fast stain do. Serologic tests are useless. Because the differential diagnosis includes most of the fungi for which treatment is amphotericin B, empiric treatment is not attempted. Diagnosis of chronic pneumonias in compromised patients requires direct lung biopsy and culture of the specimen. When skin lesions are present, the organisms can usually be found.[136] Identification is simple if the diagnosis of nocardiosis is considered.

Treatment. Sulfadiazine, 4 to 8 g daily, or sulfisoxazole (Gantrisin) in divided doses totaling 12 g daily is recommended for subacute and chronic infections. A minimum of 2 to 3 months of therapy is usually necessary, but treatment may have to be prolonged up to 6 to 8 months.[136] Minocycline HCl and the combination of trimethoprim and sulfamethoxazole have been effective drug therapies.[140,141] Cefotaxime, imipenem, and amikacin may be considered for the sulfonamide-sensitive patient.[136]

The drainage of abscesses may be necessary, but pulmonary resection is rarely indicated. Sulfonamide coverage of any operation is recommended even though resection has been done safely without drug coverage.

Pulmonary Mycoses

The microbiologic characteristics of the fungi and the diagnostic problems that they present are discussed elsewhere (see Chaps. 10 and 51). This section focuses on the clinical problems of thoracic mycotic infections. Surgeons encounter these infections when biopsy of the lung is required to achieve a diagnosis and when treatment is necessary for residual disease in immunosuppressed patients.

Pulmonary infections caused by *Histoplasma capsulatum, Blastomyces dermatitidis, Coccidioides immitis, Paracoccidioides brasiliensis,* and *Cryptococcus neoformans* are common, especially in endemic areas. The patients are usually asymptomatic and the disease is self-limited. Except for *Cryptococcus,* which is a pandemic yeast, they are dimorphic, endemic fungi and all are resistant to destruction by phagocytes, which is why they are pathogenic. They occur in soil, infect by inhalation, and cause disseminated disease in patients with defective cell-mediated immunity (eg, patients with AIDS).[142]

Opportunistic fungi are those that because they are destroyed by neutrophils, do not cause disease in normal hosts. Infection occurs in patients with neutropenia or depressed phagacytic function, which is frequently caused by corticosteroid treatment and cancer chemotherapy. The most common fungal infections in cancer patients are aspergillosis and candidiasis but other fungi may be present such as Zygomycetes, *Fusarium* species, and *Torulopsis glabrata*.[143]

Transplant patients who receive drugs that suppress cell-mediated immunity are especially prone to pulmonary infections. When infection is due to a fungus the mortality rate is high. Infections frequently observed in organ and bone marrow transplant patients are aspergillosis, histoplasmosis, coccidioidomycosis, cryptococcosis, candidiasis, pseudallescheriasis, and zygomycosis.[144]

Histoplasmosis. Histoplasmosis can be an acute or chronic infectious disease caused by *Histoplama capsulatum,* which is endemic to North American. (see Fig. 35–16).

Pathology. The tiny spores of *H. capsulatum* when inhaled into alveoli transform at body temperature into yeast. The yeast are phagocytized by macrophages but remain viable until immunity develops in about 2 weeks. The early lesion in the lung is pneumonitis with necrosis (rarely cavitation) and an inflammatory response in the adjacent lymph nodes.[145] Both become calcified similar to the Ghon complex of primary pulmonary tuberculosis. Multiple, dense pulmonary infiltrations or calcifications are characteristic of histoplasmosis as healing occurs. In chronic progressive histoplasmosis, which develops in lungs that have previously been damaged, there may be granulomatous infiltration, caseation, cavitation, and fibrosis as well as centrilobular or bullous emphysema. Nodular histoplasmosis, often solitary but sometimes multiple, is characterized by concentric deposition of dense collagen, in the center of which can be found (using Grocott's stain) the stained shells or capsules of dead yeast cells. In addition, benign progressive multinodular histoplasmosis has been reported.[146]

Clinical Manifestations. The acute pulmonic form of histoplasmosis may be mild and the symptoms confused with those of an ordinary respiratory tract infection, or the disease may go undetected. Rarely, a more violent reaction is seen, with fever, prostration, weakness, and chest pains lasting from weeks to months. Diffuse nodular densities may be noted on the chest x-ray films, which may subsequently either disappear completely or calcify (Fig. 35–17).

There may be no symptoms at all with chronic granulomatous histoplasmosis. The disease is often discovered on a routine chest x-ray examination.

Chronic cavitary histoplasmosis resembles chronic pulmonary tuberculosis both symptomatically and radiographically. Pulmonary fibrosis can occur after healing has taken place. Areas of emphysema are common and may give rise to pulmonary insufficiency and cor pulmonale.

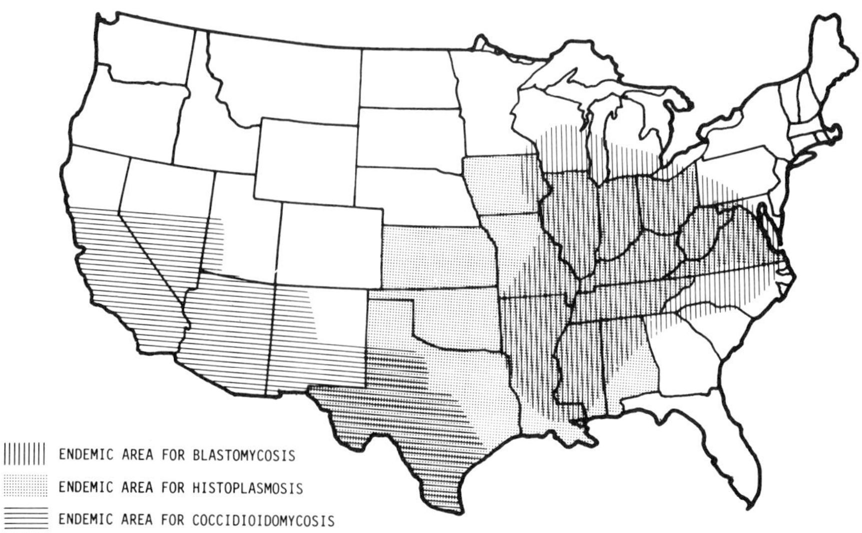

Figure 35–16. Map showing approximate areas in the United States recognized as endemic for North American blastomycosis, histoplasmosis, and coccidioidomycosis. *(From Takaro T: Thoracic Actinomycetic and Mycotic Infections: In Goldsmith EI (ed): Practice of Surgery. New York, Harper & Row, 1978.)*

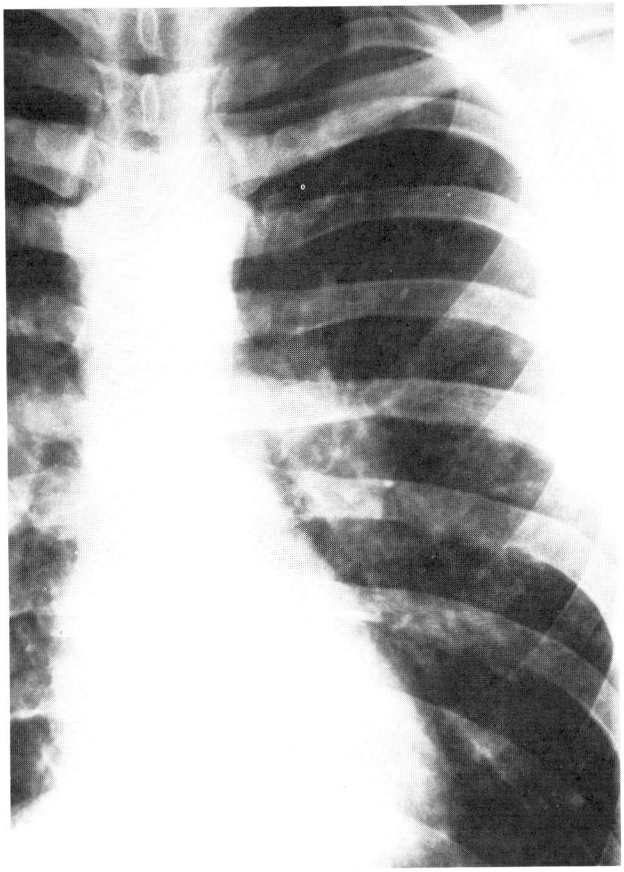

Figure 35–17. Acute histoplasmosis. Thoracic x-ray of a 26-year-old male construction worker with a febrile illness of 10 days duration, accompanied by malaise and weight loss. Note fine nodular infiltrates, especially on the left. Histoplasmin skin test was strongly positive. Mediastinal lymph node biopsy showed a granuloma with central necrosis. In this area, on Gomori silver methenamine stains, innumerable small oval yeast cells were seen. The patient made an uneventful recovery without specific therapy, and the fine nodular infiltrates cleared.

Mediastinal involvement occurs in response to *H. capsulatum* antigen and may be manifest as large mediastinal granulomas or as mediastinal fibrosis.

Progressive disseminated histoplasmosis occurs in infants as a fulminating disease, in elderly adults as a subacute illness, and in immunocompromised patients causing various and often mild pulmonary symptoms.

Diagnosis. Skin tests, serologic tests, and complement fixation are of limited value (see Chap. 10), especially in endemic areas.[147]

A definitive diagnosis depends on the demonstration of *H. capsulatum* in sputum cultures or histologic evidence of organisms compatible with *H. capsulatum* in sputum or tissue. The organism may be recovered from bone marrow, blood, lymph node, or lung tissue. Bronchoalveolar lavage, puffy coat examination, blood cultures, and bone marrow biopsy may be required to diagnose progressive disseminated disease.

Treatment. Acute histoplasmosis rarely requires treatment but should a life-threatening infection develop the patient should receive amphotericin B until symptoms subside.

Chronic cavitary histoplasmosis should be treated with ketoconazol 400 mg/day for 6 months. Itraconazole if available is equally effective and less toxic. Pulmonary resection has no advantage since it does not lower the relapse or death rate. If resectional surgery is undertaken it should be accompanied by amphotericin B or ketoconazole.[148]

All patients with progressive disseminated histoplasmosis should be treated with amphotericin B (40 mg/kg or 2 g total). AIDS patients require continuing therapy to avoid relapse.[149]

The role of surgery is primarily diagnostic, particularly when a solitary nodule is present in a patient at risk for cancer. The complications of chronic fibrosing mediastinitis caused by histoplasmosis may require surgical relief.

North American Blastomycosis

North American blastomycosis is a suppurative and granulomatous infectious disease caused by *Blastomyces dermatitidis,* which attacks primarily the lungs, skin, bone, and genitourinary tract.[150] The microbiologic, epidemiologic, and pathogenetic aspects of this fungus are discussed in Chapter 10. The endemic areas of the United States are shown in Figure 35–16.

Pathology. North American blastomycosis characteristically induces a granulomatous and pyogenic reaction, with microabscesses and giant cells and, occasionally, caseation, cavitation, and fibrosis. Special stains reveal the round, thick-walled yeast cell, measuring 5 to 20 μm in diameter, with a single budding cell. Endogenous reinfection, as in pulmonary tuberculosis, has been documented.[151]

Clinical Manifestations. As in histoplasmosis and coccidioidomycosis, the acute pulmonary infection may be mild or asymptomatic. If clinically evident, a bilateral basilar pneumonia is seen, which usually resolves spontaneously, though progression can occur (see Chap. 10). Some patients present with fever, productive cough, and toxic symptoms.

Chronic pulmonary blastomycosis is characterized by cough (usually productive only of mucoid sputum), chest pain, and occasional hemoptysis, though fever, malaise, weight loss, weakness, and other nonspecific symptoms may be the only complaints. Physical signs are not characteristic or particularly helpful.

Concomitant involvement of distant sites, especially bone, prostate, epididymis, and skin, is frequent. The skin is involved in two-thirds of the cases as papules or papulopustules, which enlarge slowly, ulcerate, and exhibit elevated, cyanotic edges with peripheral microabscesses (see Chap. 31). The organisms are found in the edges. The lesions may appear anywhere, both on exposed and unexposed portions of the skin, and are characterized by chronicity. Healing may occur, leaving a soft noncontracting scar.

THORACIC X-RAY STUDIES. Consolidation is characteristic of acute disease. Chronic blastomycosis is seen most commonly with fibronodular lesions with or without cavitation (reminiscent of pulmonary tuberculosis), but consolidation, mass lesions, diffuse patterns, pleural involvement, and hilar lymphadenopathy are also observed. Bronchogenic carcinoma is always in the differential diagnosis.

Diagnosis. A definitive diagnosis requires positive identification of the organism. This can be by culture of the sputum or aspirate, or biopsy specimens of skin or bone. Culture requires several weeks, which may be too long a wait for severely ill patients. The examination of bronchial washings or sputum by cytologic techniques (Papanicolaou) for *B. dermatitidis* has been helpful.[152] Lung biopsy may be necessary to make the diagnosis but, unfortunately, is occasionally followed by dissemination of the disease. The major differential diagnostic problem in the endemic areas of blastomycosis is bronchogenic carcinoma.[153] A preoperative diagnosis is important to avoid an unnecessary radical resection. Serologic and intracutaneous diagnostic tests cannot be relied on for a definitive diagnosis (see Chap. 10).

Treatment. Blastomycosis should be treated whenever the definitive diagnosis can be made. Patients with mild or moderate disease should receive ketoconazole, 400 mg/day for 6 months. Severely ill patients should receive amphotericin B, 40 mg/day (total dose 2 g).[154]

Surgery is indicated if bronchogenic carcinoma is suspected after efforts have been made, especially in endemic areas, to rule out North American blastomycosis. Drug treatment should follow operation if the diagnosis is made at operation, unless the pulmonary lesion has been macroscopically excised at surgery.[155] Cavitary lesions should be resected if they persist after adequate drug therapy because viable organisms usually persist in unresolved cavities even if they cannot be recovered in the sputum. Pulmonary blastomycosis is a serious disease, with a 5-year mortality rate of approximately 20 percent.

Coccidioidomycosis

Coccidioidomycosis is a suppurative and granulomatous infectious disease whose etiologic agent, *Coccidioides immitis,* is inhaled from spore-laden dust. The microbiologic, pathogenetic features of this disease, as well as its generalized form, are reviewed in Chapter 10. The endemic area is shown in Figure 35–16.

Pathology. The gross lesions resemble those of pulmonary tuberculosis. The primary complex is composed of a parenchymal pneumonitis with regional lymph node involvement. This phase may not be detected clinically. Reinfection, which may be the result of reactivation of the primary complex, produces caseous nodules, effusions, pneumonic areas, cavities, and calcified, fibrotic, and ossified areas (Fig. 35–18). Dissemination can occur (see Chap. 10).

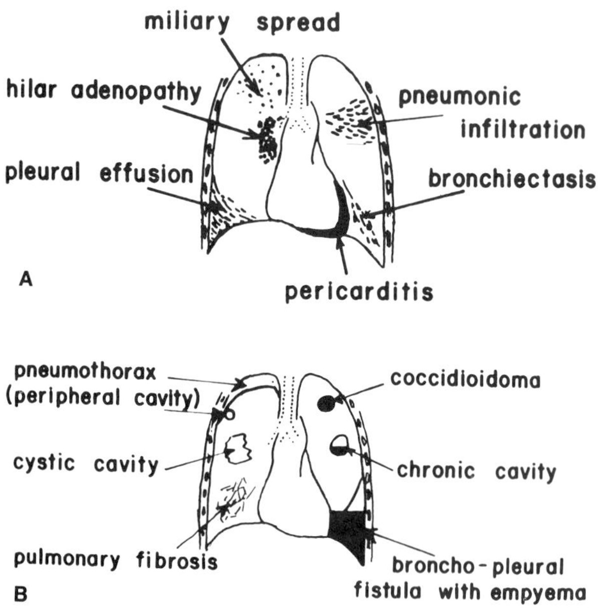

Figure 35–18. Varieties of pulmonary manifestations of coccidioidomycosis. **A.** Acute stage. **B.** Chronic stage. *(From Paulson GA: Pulmonary surgery in coccoidioidal infections: In Ajello L (ed): Coccidioidomycosis. Tucson, University of Arizona Press, 1967.)*

The histologic lesions of coccidioidomycosis are those of granuloma formation with suppuration. With special stains, large (15 to 80 μm) spherules, packed with tiny endospores when mature, or the endospores themselves can be seen. Rarely, a mycetoma or fungus ball,[155,156] as seen in aspergillosis, is observed.

Clinical Manifestations. Most cases of primary infection are asymptomatic. However, about 25 percent of patients have symptoms, especially Filipinos, blacks, diabetics, and pregnant women. Coccidioidomycosis begins with nonspecific respiratory tract symptoms or a flu-like illness with malaise, headaches, and fever. There may be pleuritic pain and cough productive of mucoid or, rarely, bloody sputum. Erythema multiforme, erythema nodosum, or less specific morbilliform rashes are observed occasionally, especially in female patients. Mild arthritic manifestations that commonly pass under the name of desert rheumatism are also sometimes seen. The x-ray findings are nonspecific. In the acute stage, miliary lesions, pneumonic infiltrates, hilar adenopathy, or pleural and pericardial effusions can be observed. With chronic coccidioidomycosis, solitary nodules or coin lesions representing coccidioidal granulomas, chronic, thin-walled cavities sometimes with a fluid level, pneumothorax, fibrosis, or empyema can be seen.

Diagnosis. A positive culture of sputum (or other body fluid or tissue) is necessary for a definitive diagnosis. In acute coccidioidal pleural effusion, cultures of pleural biopsy specimens can be more rewarding than cultures of the fluid.[157] The details of skin tests and serologic tests are discussed in Chapter 2. Strongly suggestive evidence of coccidioidomycosis is provided by a recent conversion of the coccidioidin skin test to positive or by positive serology. Serologic tests are available; early coccidioidal infection is usually detected by immunodiffusion assay for IgM antibodies. Rising serial complement fixation tests mean severe disease or even dissemination, and a falling titer usually indicates regression or improvement.

Treatment. Amphotericin B is time tested, but fluconazole may prove to be useful. Ketoconazole is suppressive but not curative and is not recommended. Treatment should be restricted to those patients with (1) severe acute pulmonary disease; (2) disseminated disease; (3) threatened dissemination, that is, a persistently high (greater than 1:64) complement fixation test titer; (4) cavitary disease with positive sputum cultures; (5) progressive chronic pulmonary lesions; (6) prophylaxis during pulmonary resection or excision or drainage of abscesses, sinus tracts, lymph nodes, or necrotic bone; and (7) prophylaxis in patients with active coccidioidomycosis, during corticosteroid therapy for whatever reason, during pregnancy, or in the diabetic patient.[158] Patients with AIDS require in addition long-term suppressive therapy.

The indications for resective surgery for coccidioidomycosis include localized granulomatous lesions and cavitary disease (Fig. 35–19). Whereas the majority of undiagnosed solitary pulmonary nodules occurring in patients in the endemic area prove to be coccidioidomas, 26 to 35 percent are found to be malignant.[159] Therefore, even in the endemic area, a coccidioidal granuloma must be resected if the diagnosis cannot be proved, especially if the patient is 35 to 40 years of age or older with a history of cigarette smoking.

Known coccidioidal granulomas do not require resection. Localized resection in more than 700 cases collected by Marks et al[160] was accompanied by a complication rate of approximately 10 percent, many of them minor air leaks or small bronchopleural fistulas.

For cavitary lesions, the indications for thoracotomy are clearer. They include persisting cavities 2 cm or greater in diameter despite drug therapy, those that are enlarging, thick-walled, or ruptured, those associated with severe or recurrent hemoptysis, those occurring in diabetic or pregnant patients, and those coexisting with pulmonary tuberculosis.[160,161] Therapy with amphotericin B is recommended by some, but it is not clear that the use of this drug has resulted in significantly fewer complications of bronchopleural fistula, empyema, and recurrent cavitation.[162]

Paracoccidioidomycosis (South American Blastomycosis)

This is a chronic granulomatous infection that involves the skin, mucous membranes, lymph nodes, and visceral organs (including the lungs), caused by *Paracoccidioides brasiliensis* (see Chap. 10),[163] which is endemic to Central and South America.

Cavitary pulmonary disease occurs in about one-third of patients, and bilateral disseminated and polymorphic lung lesions seem to be the rule.[163,164] Surgery is indicated only for diagnostic biopsy. The disease is fatal unless treated. Amphotericin B can be curative. Ketoconazole or itraconazole for 6 to 12 months is the treatment of choice.

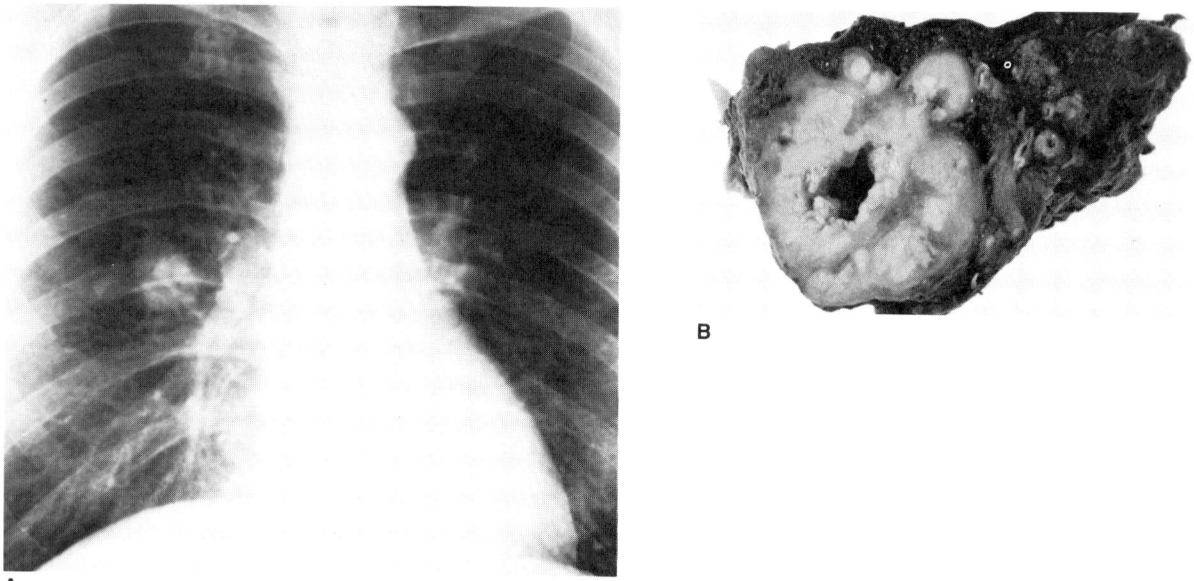

B

A

Figure 35–19. Coccidioidal granuloma. **A.** Thoracic x-ray of a 45-year-old asymptomatic male chronic smoker from Texas who was refused a job as a foodhandler because of this dense, irregularly shaped nodule in the superior segment of the right lower lobe. All diagnostic studies proved negative or normal. **B.** Chronic granuloma containing central cavitation found in resected segment. A small satellite nodule was also resected. Fungal stains showed typical spherules packed with endospores. *(From Takaro T: Lung Infections and Diffuse Interstitial Diseases of the Lungs: In Sabiston D, Spencer F (eds): Gibbon's Surgery of the Chest. Philadelphia, Saunders, 1983.)*

Cryptococcosis

Definition. Cryptococcosis is a subacute or chronic infection caused by a yeast, *Cryptococcus neoformans* (formerly known as *Torula histolytica*), that primarily attacks the bronchopulmonary tree but also has a special predilection for the central nervous system.[165] Though meningitis is the most feared clinical manifestation, benign bronchopulmonary forms are more common. The number of patients with opportunistic infections with *C. neoformans* has increased.[166] Most patients with cryptococcal infection have AIDS. The microbiologic, epidemiologic, and pathogenetic aspects of the fungus and its systemic diseases are discussed in Chapter 10.

Pathology. The respiratory tract is the portal of entry, and a primary complex (a pulmonary granuloma) with hilar node involvement, as in pulmonary tuberculosis, is characteristic.[167,168] However, there is little acute inflammatory response. The lesions are often solid, and the cut surface may be shiny, as in a mucoid carcinoma. Central necrosis, cavitation, and calcification are uncommon. The organisms can easily be identified in properly stained tissue. Pleural effusions and empyemas occur,[169] and dissemination to parts of the body other than the central nervous system is also described.

Clinical Manifestations. Pulmonary symptoms are nonspecific, insidious, and frequently absent. Cough, bloody sputum, low-grade fever, weakness, and lethargy are sometimes seen. Spontaneous remission sometimes occurs. Inasmuch as it is often an opportunistic infection, the manifestations of the primary disease may overshadow those of cryptococcosis, and the diagnosis may become apparent only if abnormalities on thoracic x-ray studies call attention to the lungs or symptoms referable to the central nervous system suggest meningitis. The x-ray features are not sufficiently characteristic to be of diagnostic help. Infiltrative, mass, nodular, cavitary, and diffuse miliary lesions have all been described.[165] Pleural effusion is unusual but is becoming recognized more frequently.[169] Cavities are rare.

Diagnosis. Cryptococcus may be isolated from sputum, bronchial washings, bronchial brushing, or percutaneous needle aspiration, as well as from cerebrospinal fluid, where it should always be sought (India ink preparation). Often the diagnosis is made from a resected lung specimen or at autopsy. No specific skin test for cryptococcosis is available.

Cryptococcal antigen in the cerebral spinal fluid is useful in diagnosing cryptococcal meningitis. The antigen is also usually present in the serum of AIDS patients and patients with disseminated disease.

Treatment. Amphotericin B and 5-fluorocytosine are effective singly or in combination to treat all proved disease.[148] In the unusual event that the diagnosis of pulmonary cryptococcosis has been firmly established prior to operation and pulmonary resection is being considered, drug therapy should be tried.

If the diagnosis is made only after thoracotomy (the usual situation), fungal therapy may not be necessary but is recommended in at-risk patients to prevent subsequent meningitis.

Fluconazole, 200 to 400 mg/day, is effective for pneumonia when given for 6 months and can be used for suppressive treatment of AIDS patients and other immunosuppressed patients.[148]

Sporotrichosis

The dimorphic mold, *Sporotrichum schenckii,* discussed in detail in Chapter 10, usually causes a cutaneous and lymphatic disease but rarely pulmonary disease.[170]

Clinical Manifestation. Pulmonary sporotrichosis is reported so rarely that it is hazardous to make generalizations. When recognized, however, the symptoms resemble pulmonary tuberculosis, and the course is slow. Localized cavitary disease is most common,[171,172] but a variety of clinical patterns, including hilar lymphadenopathy, pleural effusion, lobular consolidation, fibrosis, and multiple nodules, has been reported.[173–175] Many patients with pulmonary disease work with plants and plant products. Such occupations put persons in contact with the plant and soil fungus.

Diagnosis. Although the organism is a saprophyte, it is not commensal of humans. The diagnosis is made on the basis of its culture and identification from the resected specimens, sputum, or bronchial brushings. The preculture diagnosis is usually tuberculosis, sarcoidosis, or opportunistic fungus. Biopsy diagnosis may be difficult because the organism is sparse in tissue. The pathogenicity for animals can be established by inoculation. The serum agglutinins for *Sporotrichum* should be 1:50 or greater.

Treatment. Combined lung resection of localized cavitary disease, together with potassium iodide, amphotericin B, or both, is probably the best treatment, although there are few patient data available. A saturated solution of potassium iodide is given in a dosage of 9 to 12 g/day. Amphotericin B (see Table 10–2) should be used as well for pulmonary disease.[148]

Pulmonary Mycoses Caused by Opportunistic Fungi

Aspergillosis. In recent years, aspergillosis has become the third most common systemic fungal infection (after histoplasmosis and coccidioidomycosis) and one with the most rapidly rising incidence.[176] The usually saprophytic *Aspergillus fumigatus* (or some other member of the species) can cause three distinctly different clinical syndromes: aspergillus bronchitis (an allergic disease), aspergilloma (fungus ball), or invasive, necrotizing aspergillus infection.[177] The organisms and all three types of disease are discussed in Chapter 10.

Pathology. In pathologic materials, the coarse, fragmented, septate, branching hyphae are found, either as short strands or ball-like clusters, which can be identified only by isolation in culture.

Most of the surgically resected lesions of aspergillosis are aspergillomas.[178,179] A fungus ball is actually a matted sphere of hyphae, fibrin, and inflammatory cells, which appears grossly as a round or oval, friable, gray, red, brown, or yellow necrotic-looking mass. It is ordinarily found lying in an upper lobe cavity, the wall of which is often smooth and may be thick or thin, with relatively little evidence of inflammatory reaction. There usually is evidence, however, of previous chronic lung disease in this area, for example, tuberculosis, sarcoidosis,[180] histoplasmosis, bronchiectasis, bronchogenic cyst, chronic lung abscess, or cavitating carcinoma, but sometimes there is no obvious evidence of preexisting pulmonary damage (Fig. 35–20). A true necrotizing pneumonia with abscess formation is found in immunologically compromised patients.

Clinical Manifestations. Aspergillomas occupying preexisting cavities usually produce no symptoms. Sometimes, cough with bloody or blood-streaked sputum is seen. An aspergilloma can be identified as a mass shifting within a cavity or cyst on changes in position of the patient. Thus, in an x-ray film of the thorax exposed in the upright position, a crescentic radiolucency above a rounded radiopaque lesion is suggestive of aspergilloma (see Fig. 35–20).

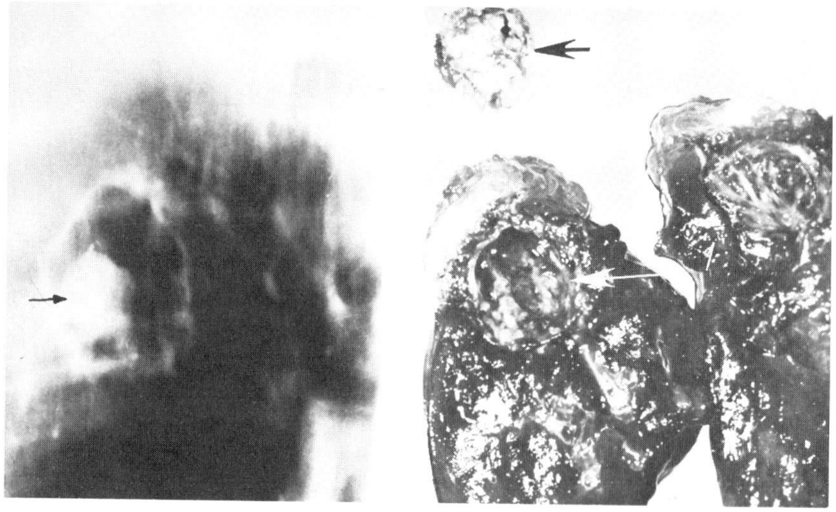

Figure 35–20. Aspergillosis. **A.** Tomogram showing cavitary lesion, right upper lung field, containing a fungous ball or aspergilloma (*arrow*), lying free in a cavitary lesion. The ball characteristically will alter its location in the cavity as the patient changes position. **B.** Resected specimen of a right upper lobe, showing smooth-lined chronic cavity (*white arrow*) from which fungus ball (*black arrow*) was lifted out. *(**A.** From Aslam: Aslam PA, Larkin J, Eastridge CE, et al. Chest 57:94, 1970. **B.** From Takaro T: Thoracic Actinomycetic and Mycotic Infections: In Goldsmith EI (ed): Practice of Surgery. New York, Harper & Row, 1978.)*

Initial symptoms of invasive *Aspergillus* pneumonias include chronic fever, cough, and sputum, which may progress to involve the pleura. Multiple abscesses can be seen within the lung and in other tissues, especially the brain.

Aspergillus pericarditis in the immunocompromised patient has also been reported.[181]

Diagnosis. The finding of *Aspergillus* cells in the sputum alone does not justify the diagnosis of aspergillosis. If the clinical picture of aspergilloma is present and sputum cultures are positive for *Aspergillus,* the diagnosis is probable.

Transtracheal aspirates or direct lung aspirates by thin-walled 18-gauge needles may provide a definitive diagnosis and are especially useful in immunosuppressed patients.

Treatment. Medical treatment of aspergilloma has generally been unsatisfactory.[182] Amphotericin B is the most satisfactory treatment and may be curative even in immunodeficient patients. Diiodohydroxyquinoline and rifampin have been reported to be helpful in combination with amphotericin B.[183] Persistent, long-term, high-dose therapy may be required. The indications for resection of an aspergilloma are not clear. Severe hemoptysis is an obvious indication, but routine surgical excision probably is not indicated. The reported complication rates are high.[184]

In difficult situations, where resection is indicated but cannot be carried out safely, cavernostomy or the endobronchial or endocavitary instillation of sodium iodide or amphotericin B has occasionally been helpful.[185,186]

Aspergillus empyema, or pleural aspergillosis, has been treated by intrapleural amphotericin B or nystatin and by pleural drainage, pleurectomy, thoracoplasty, and repair of bronchopleural fistulas.[187]

Mucormycosis (Phycomycosis). Mucormycosis (phycomycosis, zygomycosis) is a rare fungal infection caused by genera belonging to the class Zygomycetes, discussed in Chapter 10. Disease-causing organisms in this group include species of *Absidia, Rhizopus, Mucor, Mortierella,* and *Basidiobolus.*[130] Many of these organisms are saprophytic, occurring as molds on manure and foods and producing spores that can be inhaled. Characteristically, direct blood vessel invasion, thrombosis, and infarction of invaded organs occur, with tissue destruction and cavitation in patients with compromised host defenses.

Clinical Manifestations. As noted in Chapter 10, mucormycosis is usually rapidly fatal, occurring especially in acidotic diabetes, in patients with lymphomas or leukemias, or in persons receiving intensive or prolonged antimetabolite, antibiotic, or steroid therapy. Extensive necrosis of areas around the face (paranasal sinuses, orbit, mucous membranes) and the brain may be seen, in addition to cutaneous and subcutaneous infection. Pulmonary mucormycosis usually develops rapidly as a nonspecific bronchitis and pneumonia. Signs and symptoms of thrombosis and infarction manifested by severe chest pain, pleural friction rub, and bloody sputum appear. Massive fatal pulmonary hemorrhage has been reported.[188] Two fatal cases of necrotizing chest wall infections followed aortocoronary bypass surgery in which Elastoplast dressings were used.[189] Kidney transplant patients usually develop a necrotizing pneumonia with abscess formation.

Diagnosis. Biopsy is essential, because the diagnosis depends on the identification of wide (6 to 50 μm), nonseptate, branching hyphae in and around thrombosed vessels, especially well seen with hematoxylin and eosin stain. Culture permits identification of the particular species but does not alter therapy.

Treatment. Most patients die.[190,191] Drug therapy with amphotericin B plus excision and drainage are necessary in debilitated, desperately ill patients.[192] Transthoracic drainage of a necrotic lobe was lifesaving in one patient (R. L. Simmons, personal communication), and success following lung resections is reported.[193,194] Control of diabetes is obviously essential, but control of the other predisposing conditions may be impossible.

Pseudoallescheriasis (Monosporosis)

Pseudoallescheria boydii is an inhabitant of soil that appears to act as a secondary invader of previously damaged lung tissue, such as a tuberculous cavity, a cyst, or a bronchial saccule.[195] A fungus ball is sometimes formed. Amphotericin B has not been effective. Localized resections have been performed in ten patients, with two deaths.[196] Conservative management is recommended for asymptomatic patients without cavitary disease or bronchiectasis. Resection is advocated for good risk patients with localized cavitary disease or to help make a definitive diagnosis when bronchogenic carcinoma is suspected. Cardiac valve prostheses infected with *P. boydii* have been reported in two patients.[197]

Emerging Fungal Infections. A consequence of modern chemotherapy for cancer, transplantation, and the increasing incidence of AIDS is the emergence of disease due to organisms not previously known to cause human infection. Hyalohyphomycosis is an infection by any one of the many colorless, septate filamentous fungi and includes *Fusarium, Penicillium,* and *Cephalosporium.* Phaehyphomycosis is infection caused by pigmented septate filamentous molds such as *Alternaria* and *Bipolaris.*[130]

Candidiasis

Although *Candida* species commonly affect mucous and cutaneous surfaces, deep or systemic infections of the lungs and other tissues also occur. *Candida albicans* and other fungi of this genus—*guilliermondi, stellatoidea, krusei, tropicalis, parapsilosis,* and *glabrata*—can all cause disease. Microbiologic and pathogenic features are discussed in Chapter 10.

Clinical Manifestations and Diagnosis. Invasive candidiasis is an opportunistic infection rarely seen except in the presence of intensive or prolonged antibiotic therapy, especially with multiple drugs or immunosuppressive or cytotoxic therapy.[198] Debility, senescence, prematurity, starvation, prolonged shock, multiple operations, multiple or mixed infections, bone marrow depression by lymphomas or antitumor drugs, radiation therapy, disseminated malignancies, and antibiotic or steroid therapy render the patient susceptible. Under these conditions, normal bacterial flora of patients may be suppressed, allowing an overgrowth of the often-present saprophytic species of *Candida.*

Invasion can take place through the skin, the bloodstream (via needles or catheters used for intravenous therapy), the lungs, or the gastrointestinal tract. *Candida* pneumonia, abscess, septicemia, and generalized infection may result, frequently with a fatal outcome.[199] Even tracheal obstruction associated with a *Candida* fungus ball has been reported.[200] *Candida* species in the sputum are of no diagnostic or prognostic importance, so the diagnosis depends on finding *Candida* in bronchial or lung biopsy tissue, the bloodstream, or evidence of *Candida* ophthalmitis. Candiduria frequently accompanies candidiasis but is not diagnostic. Biopsy proof of tissue invasion in immunosuppressed or otherwise compromised patients who have symptoms and signs of pneumonia or septicemia requires that drug therapy be given promptly.[201] On the other hand, Rosenbaum et al[202] suggest that some forms of *Candida* pneumonia are self-limited and require no treatment.

Treatment. The combination of amphotericin B and 5-fluorocytosine is the most promising regimen available.[199]

Prevention. Prophylactic nystatin and amphotericin B therapy by mouth have been shown to suppress gastrointestinal *Candida* and reduce the infection rate in debilitated patients who are taking antibiotics.[203,204]

PROTOZOAN INFECTIONS

Thoracic Amebiasis

Thoracic complications of amebiasis are rare. They occur secondary to amebic hepatic abscess, usually on the right. The liver abscess (see Chap. 40) may erode or rupture through the diaphragm without the formation of a subphrenic abscess. The second abscess, in the superadjacent, right lower, or middle lobe of the lung, or an empyema may lead to a hepaticobronchial fistula.[205]

In 90 percent of cases, pathologic changes are confined to the right lower hemithorax. Chest pain, fever, cough, and the expectoration of material variously described as resembling chocolate or anchovy sauce or catsup are characteristic. The liver is tender and enlarged. A history of dysentery or diarrhea may be suggestive.

X-ray findings include moderate fixation, elevation, or localized bulge of the right side of the diaphragm, pleural effusion, pneumonic consolidation, or abscess formation, usually in the right lower lung field.

Entamoeba histolytica organisms are reported in pus, sputum, or aspirated material only in about one-fourth of patients. In many patients, a presumptive diagnosis must be made, which is supported by the finding of *E. histolytica* in stools and by positive results of a serologic test for the organism.

Although right pleuropulmonary amebiasis is typical, extension of a hepatic amebic abscess into the left lung has been reported.[206] Abdominal symptoms and physical manifestations of amebiasis may be minimal. The diagnosis can therefore be confused with tuberculosis, pneumonia, or lung abscess.

Therapy should be directed toward cure of the liver abscess.[207,208] Aspiration and drug therapy are described in Chapter 40. Thoracic procedures are rarely indicated.

Pneumocystis Carinii Pneumonia

This is an opportunistic infection in the form of a diffuse interstitial pneumonitis, which occurs in congenitally immunodeficient and pharmacologically immunosuppressed patients (see Chap. 51). It was first recognized in epidemic form during World War II in people of central Europe whose nutritional status was presumably at a low level.[209] Today it is epidemic in HIV-infected patients and is the initial infection in 65 percent of these patients.[210]

Etiology. Pneumocystis carinii is so named for its discoverer, Carini. This organism occurs in thick-walled or thin-walled cystic forms, 5 to 12 μm in diameter. It has a double-walled outer membrane and within are three to eight intracystic bodies. The organism stains with silver methenamine (Gomori) stains. Although classified as protozoan, recently demonstrated RNA sequences suggest it may be a fungus.[211]

Clinical Manifestations. The disease almost invariably occurs in patients with impaired cellular immunity.[209] Renewed interest in this disease emerged in the early 1980s when it was recognized with increasing frequency in patients with AIDS.[212]

The peculiar combination in patients at risk, often infants or children, of dyspnea, tachypnea, dry nonproductive cough, fever, flaring of the nasal alae, intercostal retraction and sometimes cyanosis with minimal auscultatory signs, and the x-ray findings of unilateral or bilateral diffuse (ground-glass) infiltrates, or localized areas of pneumonitis or consolidation, should lead to a suspicion of *P. carinii* pneumonia. An air bronchogram silhouetted against a ground-glass infiltrate is a typical radiographic appearance. Marked hypoxemia and hypocapnia characterize this clinical picture.

Diagnosis. The diagnosis depends on the demonstration of organisms in sputum, bronchial brushings, bronchoalveolar washings, or lung tissue. Because the diagnosis can be made practically 100 percent of the time by bronchoalveolar lavage and transbronchial lung biopsy, thoracotomy or thoracoscopy is seldom necessary.[213] The morbidity and mortality of open biopsy in desperately ill hypoxemic patients cannot be underestimated. Both percutaneous needle aspiration and transbronchoscopic lung biopsy can be followed by pneumothorax and hemorrhage. Touch preparations of biopsy material stained with silver methenamine are used to identify the organisms. Inasmuch as multiple coexistent infections may be present, bacterial and fungal cultures and histopathologic examinations should also be performed.

Treatment. The need for precise diagnosis derives from the toxicity of the only treatment formerly available, pentamidine isethionate. Currently, trimethoprim-sulfamethoxazole appears to be an excellent alternative as does the antiprotozoan agent, atovaquone.[214] If all attempts at diagnosis short of open lung biopsy have failed, empirical therapy can be carried out and open lung biopsy reserved for those patients who do not respond to the drugs.[214] Because of severe hypoxemia, supplemental oxygen therapy is often necessary. Patients with AIDS and *Pneumocystis* pneumonia require a longer duration of treatment and have higher relapse rates than other adults with known causes of immunosuppression.[215,216] With progression, lung compliance is seriously reduced, and the use of respirator support becomes essential.

Prognosis. Untreated, *P. carinii* pneumonia is often fatal. In patients treated early and adequately, 65 to 75 percent survive. Prognosis is best for those with arterial Po_2 greater than 70 mm Hg and an arterial-alveolar gradient less than 35 mm Hg.[217]

Prevention. Trimethoprim-sulfamethoxazole has been shown to be an effective prophylactic agent in high-risk patients, that is, children with acute leukemia, patients who have received transplants, and patients with AIDS.

PULMONARY ECHINOCOCCOSIS: HYDATID DISEASE OF THE LUNG

Etiology. Pulmonary echinococcus disease is caused by the larval form of the small tapeworm, *Echinococcus granulosus,* or, rarely, *Echinococcus multilocularis.*

Pathology. The cyst itself consists of a germinal layer and cyst fluid containing brood capsules and scoleces. A succession of acellular, white, hyaline layers are laid down outside the cyst, which is thus enclosed by a laminated cyst membrane. As the cyst enlarges, it usually reaches the pleural surface. Compression of the surrounding lung produces a thin fibrous layer of atelectatic lung around the hydatid, variously called capsule, adventitia, or pericyst.

The cyst may remain dormant for many years. However, it poses a hazard to the patient because it may rupture at any time, resulting in formation of daughter cysts or, uncommonly, in death due to asphyxiation or to a hypersensitivity reaction to the contents of the cyst. In any event, a ruptured cyst may become infected, forming a chronic lung abscess or a localized bronchiectactic area. One report describes an infected hepatic hydatid cyst that eroded into the right pleural space. The empyema was treated successfully only after resection of the cyst.

Clinical Manifestations and Diagnosis. Symptoms are minimal unless there is significant compression of an airway or a mediastinal structure (eg, esophagus, great veins) or unless the cyst ruptures. At such time there may be dramatic expectoration of cyst fluid, followed by an allergic rash and sometimes fever. If secondary infection occurs, the symptoms of lung abscess or bronchiectasis predominate.

The diagnosis is suggested most commonly by the characteristic x-ray film appearance of round or oval radiopaque shadows of a very homogeneous water-like density, with clear-cut borders and little or no evidence of reaction around them (Fig. 35–21), usually located in the middle or lower lung fields. When air enters the perivesicular space, a characteristic thin crescentic shadow is seen, which is quite unlike the semilunar shadow seen with aspergillomas. The most unusual and unique x-ray sign, the water lily sign, consists of a lenticular shadow rising from a fluid level in a cyst. This is seen after rupture of the cyst and partial evacuation of its contents, with the torn vesicular or germinal layer floating on the surface of the retained fluid.[218] The Casoni skin test for *Echinococcus* disease is not completely reliable.

Treatment. The diagnosis of such a lesion in an area where pastoral as opposed to sylvatic echinococcosis is found, that is, where sheep and cattle are raised, is an indication for excision. Operations that conserve pulmonary parenchyma are advocated wherever possible. There are surprisingly vehement differences of opinion about the appropriate procedure for cystectomy. Peschiera,[218] who reports a large series of cases from Peru, is certain that the best method is partial aspiration of the cyst at open thoracotomy first, with instillation of formalin into the cyst. After that, the cyst is opened and removed together with the adventitial pericyst formed by the patient's own lung. On the other hand, others favor simple enucleation of the intact cyst, especially if it is not under tension (Fig. 35–22). First, the nonadherent cleavage plane between cyst and pericyst is widely opened. Then the anesthetist is requested to inflate the lung. This allows the fragile intact cyst to roll out or to be extruded into a waiting spoon, hand, or basin without the need to grasp or touch the cyst. Sometimes 10 ml of 10 percent sodium chloride solution is instilled into the cyst as a preliminary maneuver.[219] The remaining space in the lung parenchyma in both methods is obliterated after careful control of small and large bronchial fistulas with or without removal of the fibrous pericyst. If lung tissue has been destroyed by prolonged

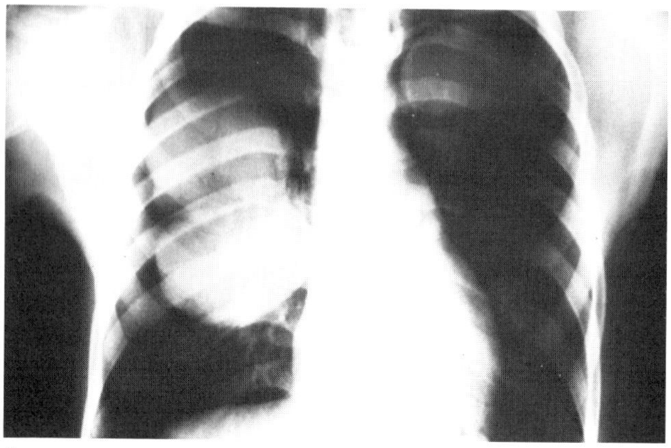

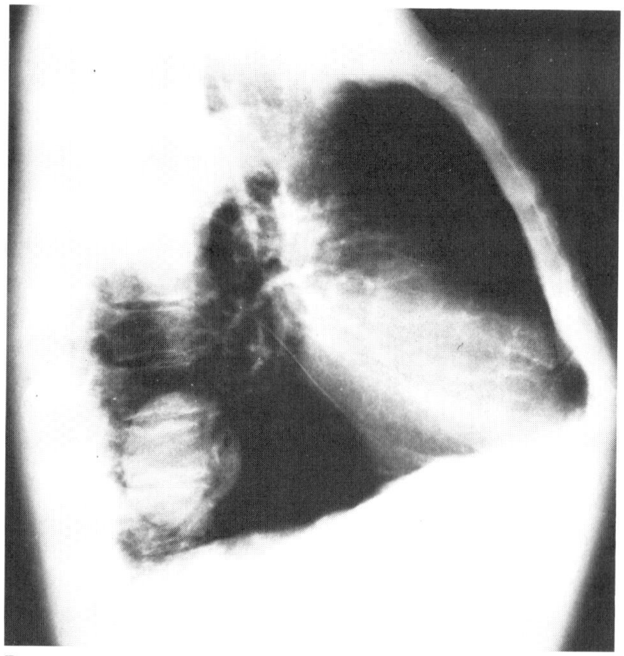

Figure 35–21. Thoracic x-rays showing *Echinococcus* cysts. **A.** Multiple and bilateral cysts. In both x-rays, the characteristic appearance of large, rounded shadows of homogeneous density with clear-cut borders is well shown. **B.** Solitary cyst lying posteriorly behind the heart. *(**A.** From Wolcott MW, Harris SH, Briggs JN, et al: J Thorac Cardiovasc Surg 62:465, 1971. **B.** From Lichter I: Thorax 27:529, 1972.)*

compression or infection, segmental resection or lobectomy may be necessary after removal of the cyst. Nonoperative treatment with mebendazole or albendazole is recommended for the asymptomatic patient with the less common sylvatic or forest type of echinococcosis, which is observed in Alaska and Northern Canada where moose and caribou are hunted, as opposed to the more common and more serious pastoral disease in which operation is clearly indicated.[220,221]

Whatever operation is performed, it must be done carefully so that contents of the cyst are not spilled, which will lead to anaphylaxis and formation of daughter cysts. The instillation of a 10 percent povidone-iodine solution or 10 percent sodium chloride solution has been recommended to sterilize the cyst prior to attempts at excision (T. Hau, personal communication).

INFECTIONS OF THE MEDIASTINUM

Infections of the mediastinum are uncommon but serious. They are often iatrogenic and pose many management problems. The mediastinum extends from the thoracic inlet to the diaphragm and partitions the two pleural cavities. It is bounded anteriorly by the sternum and posteriorly by the thoracic vertebrae. Because of the many structures within this portion of the thoracic cavity, it is usually subdivided for easier description. The superior mediastinum lies above a plane that extends between the lower manubrium and the fourth thoracic vertebra. It contains the thymus gland, trachea, esophagus, and the aortic arch, and it is in direct continuity with the neck and its fascial planes. The inferior mediastinum is separated into anterior, middle, and posterior compartments. The anterior mediastinum contains only lymph nodes and connective tissue. The middle mediastinum contains, in addition to these, the trachea, mainstem bronchi, the heart and pericardium, and the ascending aorta. The posterior mediastinum contains the esophagus, vagus nerves, descending thoracic aorta, azygos veins, and the thoracic duct.

Infections of the mediastinum may result either from disease or from injury primarily affecting mediastinal structures or by extension of infection from adjacent regions, such as the neck, the pleural cavities, the lungs, or the abdominal cavity. Metastatic infections of the mediastinum by way of the bloodstream are rare.

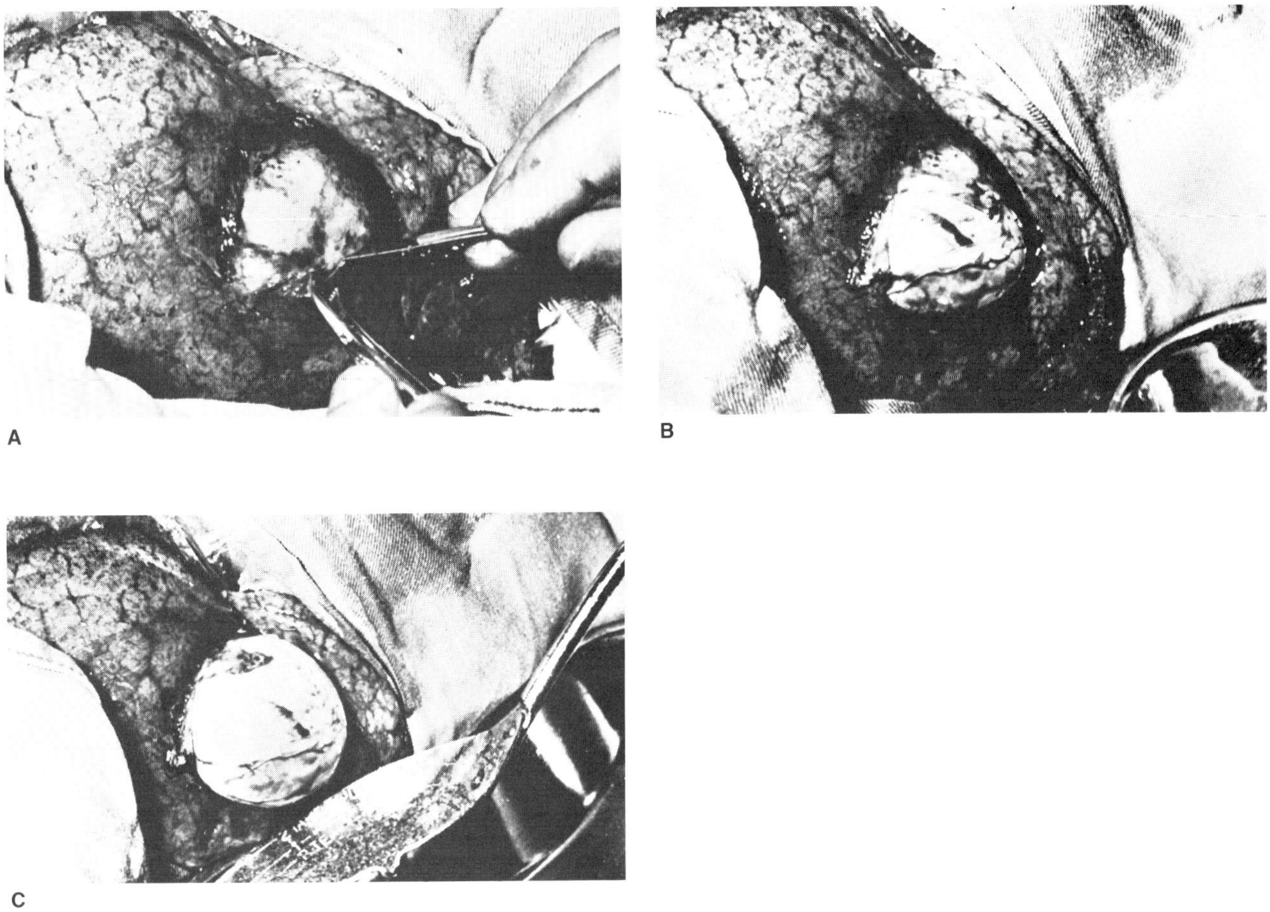

Figure 35–22. Excision of *Echinococcus* cyst. **A.** Adventitia of subpleural cyst is carefully incised. **B.** Opening is widened promptly so cyst does not extrude through too small an opening and rupture. **C.** Anesthetist inflates lung, extruding cyst gradually into spoon or basin. Cyst must not be grasped or touched for fear of rupturing it. *(From Lichter I: Thorax 27:529, 1972.)*

Three fascial spaces in the neck—the pretracheal, the retrovisceral, and the perivascular—communicate with the mediastinum and thus provide ready avenues for the spread of infections into this vital area (see Chap. 33). The pretracheal space is formed from the pretracheal fascia and its fusion with the buccopharyngeal fascia and the carotid sheaths. It extends from the thyroid cartilage to the anterior mediastinum, where the pretracheal fascia blends into the pericardium. The retrovisceral space lies between the esophagus and the prevertebral fascia. It extends from the base of the skull to the posterior mediastinum. The perivascular space, containing carotid arteries, jugular vein, and vagus nerve, extends into the mediastinum along with these structures (Fig. 35–23).

Negative intrathoracic pressures may cause infection in these classic cervical fascial spaces to spread to the mediastinum, but the infectious process may not be contained or confined to these spaces.[222] Likewise, positive pressures relative to intrathoracic pressures may cause the fluid contents of a ruptured trachea, bronchus, or esophagus to be introduced into the mediastinum.

Retroperitoneal infections may extend into the mediastinum through the various openings in the diaphragm. However, this is rarely a cause of mediastinitis since the advent of antibiotic therapy.

Acute Infections of the Superior Mediastinum

Pathogenesis. Acute mediastinitis involving the superior mediastinum is rarely a primary infection. It occurs most commonly by extension from the cervical region, including the oropharyngeal area, via the fascial planes or the lymphatics. Currently, esophageal perforation due to instrumentation is

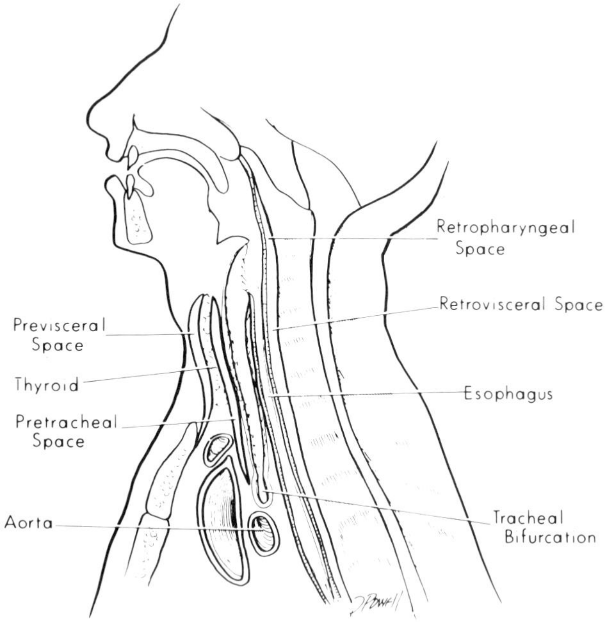

Figure 35–23. Three fascial planes along which infections may extend from the neck into the mediastinum are illustrated in this diagram. These are the previsceral space, the pretracheal space, and the retropharyngeal or retrovisceral space. Infections due to retropharyngeal abscesses or to perforations of the cervical esophagus usually extend along the retrovisceral space. *(Adapted from Pearse HE Jr: Ann Surg 108:508, 1938.)*

the most common cause,[223] but extensions of retropharyngeal abscess can also occur.[224] Surprisingly, mediastinitis due to tracheostomy, a common operative procedure invariably contaminated with microbes, is quite rare.

Retropharyngeal abscesses may extend into the retrovisceral space and from there into the mediastinum. Since 1960 there have been 43 reports of acute mediastinitis arising from retropharyngeal infections secondary to dental caries.[225] The associated mortality of 36 percent is attributed at least in part to delay in treatment and inadequate cervical drainage. When spread of infection from the root space of a tooth occurs, it is usually controllable with antibiotics. Rarely, it may extend from the mandible either into the pterygomandibular or infratemporal spaces or to the area above or below the mylohyoid muscle (Ludwig's angina). Once the retropharyngeal tissues become infected, an abscess may form, which can then spread along the retrovisceral, pretracheal, or perivascular spaces into the mediastinum (see Fig. 35–23) (see Chap. 33).

Retropharyngeal spread and mediasatinitis may occur in patients with cellulitis of the head and neck[226] and cellulitis of the face.[227] Mediastinal radiographic changes and presumed mediastinitis have been observed after sclerotherapy for esophageal varices.[228] Suppurative mediastinitis from an infected subclavian catheter is a reported complication of long-term parenteral nutrition.[229]

Mediastinal infections caused by esophageal perforation are always serious, and the mortality is high unless the perforation is recognized early and promptly treated. It is usually the result of perforation of the cervical esophagus with a rigid esophagoscope, often because of pressure of the posterior esophageal wall against a cervical vertebral spur.

Etiology. Infections caused by dental abscesses are usually mixed infections, because of the synergistic effects of anaerobic streptococci and *Bacteroides,* which together can cause a necrotizing inflammation.[225] Routine culture results may be reported as negative unless anaerobic organisms are suspected and anaerobic culture techniques are used.[230] However, gram-negative, pleomorphic rods on a smear may suggest *Bacteroides,* and because gas-forming organisms may be present, air in the retropharyngeal space may be seen on x-ray films.[231]

Infections due to esophageal perforation contain oral flora (ie, mixed organisms), principally gram-positive aerobes and anaerobes at first. Later, the flora resemble that recovered from retropharyngeal infections, as anaerobes proliferate.

Clinical Manifestations. Pain is the most prominent symptom of cervical esophageal rupture. It occurs suddenly and is usually localized near the site of perforation. Occasionally, it is referred to the chest. Pain occurring with swallowing and cervical flexion are also common manifestations. There may be fever and localized cervical tenderness. Crepitation is usually present, and there may be radiographic evidence of cervical emphysema. A lateral view of the cervical spine will show anterior displacement of the trachea and an air-fluid level if a retrovisceral abscess has formed. Computed tomography (CT) may be even more helpful in the early identification of these signs of mediastinitis and in determining the adequacy of surgical treatment. Contrast studies using a thin opaque material will usually demonstrate an esophageal leak.

Treatment

RETROPHARYNGEAL AND DENTAL ORIGIN. The treatment of mediastinitis caused by cervical and dental infections consists of surgical drainage and antibiotics. *Staphylococcus aureus, Streptococcus,* and *Bacteroides,* the most common infecting organisms, are usually sensitive to clindamycin and chloramphenicol.

Cervical abscesses should be drained widely. A lateral incision along the posterior border of the sternocleidomastoid muscle can be extended to inspect and drain the pretracheal, perivascular, or retrovisceral spaces. Adequate drainage of the superior mediastinum can be obtained by this approach (Fig. 35–24). If the infection has spread to the inferior mediastinum, transthoracic or subxiphoid drainage is necessary. Wheatley et al[225] recommend aggressive treatment with subxiphoid drainage, tracheostomy, and broad spectrum aerobic and anaerobic antibiotics. Their recommenda-

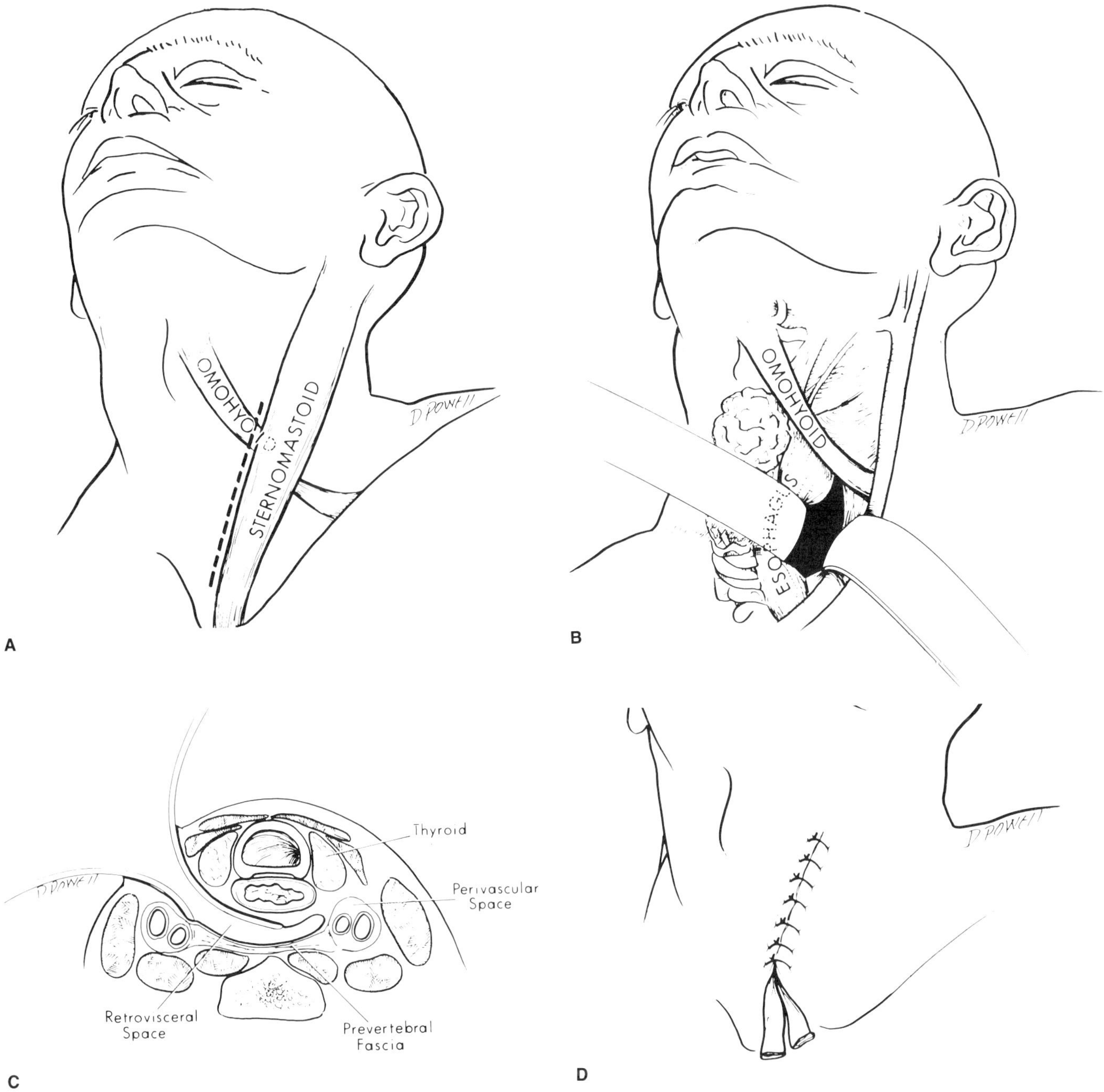

Figure 35–24. Cervical approach for draining the fascial planes of the neck and the upper mediastinum to the level of the fourth thoracic vertebra. **A.** Line of skin incision along anterior border of the sternomastoid muscle. **B.** Exposure of the retrovisceral space. **C.** Cross-sectional view of the approach to the retrovisceral space and the adjacent perivascular spaces. **D.** Rubber drains inserted into the dependent portion of the retrovisceral space. *(Adapted from Payne WS, Larson RH: Surg Clin North Am 49:999, 1969.)*

tions are supported by the high mortality (40 percent) of descending necrotizing mediastinitis treated otherwise.

ESOPHAGEAL PERFORATION DUE TO INSTRUMENTATION. The treatment of cervical esophageal perforation is surgical drainage of the retrovisceral space, as described previously. This procedure is prophylactic and will prevent abscess formation and the spread of infection to the mediastinum if the esophageal perforation is recognized early. If treatment is delayed, both cervical suppuration and superior mediastinitis may be adequately drained through the cervical approach. The wound should be cultured for both aerobic and anaerobic organisms, and appropriate antibiotics should be instituted. Penicillin G is usually found to be an excellent first-choice antibiotic unless a preexisting infection with a penicillin-resistant organism is present, since most oral flora are sensitive. If treated within 24 hours, 90 percent of patients will survive.[232]

Anterior Mediastinitis

One of the most frequent causes of mediastinitis is infection following median sternotomy. The cause and management of this condition are described in the section on chest wall infections.

Rarely, mediastinitis may develop in the postoperative period in the absence of sternal dehiscence or sternal wound infection. If the patient has only fever and leukocytosis, the diagnosis may be difficult to establish. If the chest x-ray shows a pleural effusion, increasing substernal opacification, or mediastinal widening, and the patient does not respond to antibiotic treatment, mediastinal exploration and drainage may be required, as described previously. A CT scan is especially helpful and can be used to demonstrate imperfect sternal closures when sternal dehiscence and sternal clicks are absent, and when retrosternal air-fluid, hematoma, or abscess are present.[233]

The presence of foreign material, such as Teflon pledgets, Dacron grafts, and epicardial pacemaker electrodes, poses a special problem. All foreign material should be removed when possible. Engleman et al[234] reported healing of mediastinitis following ventricular aneurysmectomy only after they removed the Teflon-felt used to buttress the ventricular suture line. Moseley et al,[235] however, reported success in sterilizing an infected Hancock prosthesis used to repair a truncus arteriosus. Only rarely does a chronic abscess develop from an acute infection unless a foreign body is present. The complications of mediastinitis may take a long time to become evident, as illustrated by one patient with postoperative sternal dehiscence, in whom a large mycotic aortic aneurysm developed at the site of aortic cannulation 2 years after aortocoronary arterial bypass surgery.[236]

Infections of the Middle Mediastinum

The pathogenesis and treatment of cardiac and pericardial infections are discussed in Chapter 36.

Mediastinal Granulomas and Chronic Fibrosing Mediastinitis. These are probably different stages of the same disease. They are most frequently located in the right paratracheal region and are due to histoplasmosis, tuberculosis, or, more rarely, to sarcoidosis, nocardiosis, actinomycosis, *aspergillosis,* or syphilis.[237,238] In the granulomatous phase, the large yellow and white masses of lymph nodes are often cystic and filled with caseous material. Microscopically, various stages of caseating granuloma are seen, and with Gomori methenamine silver nitrate stain, the yeast-like structures of *Histoplasma* are sometimes found. Cultures for *Histoplasma* and *Mycobacterium* are almost always negative.

Most patients are asymptomatic, but occasionally they may have symptoms caused by encroachment on important structures traversing the mediastinum, such as the superior vena cava, pulmonary veins, esophagus, trachea, or a bronchus.[239-242] Such encroachment may produce severe symptoms, depending on the structure that is compromised. They may include cough, hemoptysis, or the expectoration of broncholiths. Productive cough and wheezing may result if bronchiectasis develops. When the middle lobe alone is involved, the so-called middle lobe syndrome may be recognized on thoracic x-ray films or on bronchography. The formation of an esophageal traction diverticulum may follow the development of an abscess in a mediastinal node, with erosion into the esophageal wall. Fistula formation between the trachea and esophagus, with harassing cough on taking fluids, may be another complication.[243]

Treatment. Fibrosis of the mediastinum can produce superior vena caval obstruction and thus the superior vena caval syndrome, significant airway obstruction, or pulmonary hypertension primarily caused by pulmonary venous obstruction.[244,245] When the pericardium is involved, a granulomatous pericarditis can result. Constrictive pericarditis, however, is rare.[246]

Because of the seriousness of some of the complications of healed mediastinal granulomas and chronic mediastinitis—such as middle lobe syndrome, superior vena caval syndrome, broncholithiasis, esophagotracheal fistula, and pericarditis—appropriate corrective or extirpative surgical therapy may be required, depending on the severity of the symptom and the feasibility of relieving it surgically.[243,247,248] Some lesions may be difficult to manage by operation. Therefore early resection of asymptomatic mediastinal granulomas to forestall such more intractable problems has been recommended and is probably appropriate.[249,250] If complement fixation titer for *Histoplasma* is elevated, a prolonged course of ketoconazole may be effective, at least in treating superior vena caval obstruction without surgery.[251] CT scanning is useful in demonstrating the relative size and location of calcified mediastinal masses, and MRI may be used to demonstrate obstruction of mediastinal vascular structures without the need of intravascular contrast material.[250,252]

Posterior Mediastinitis

Posterior mediastinitis is largely caused by esophageal perforation. Other causes, such as paravertebral abscess, are much less common.

Esophageal Perforation (see also Chap. 42)

Pathogenesis. After the cricopharyngeal area, the second most common site of instrumental perforation of the esophagus is the lower third of the esophagus where it narrows just above the diaphragm. Less commonly, the midesophagus, weakened by tumor or fresh caustic burn, can be perforated. Introduction of the flexible fiberoptic esophagoscope has greatly reduced the incidence of instrumental perforations.

Other causes of esophageal perforation include ingestion of foreign bodies, penetrating injuries, blunt trauma, caustic burns, and anastomotic leak after esophageal resection. Belsey and Hiebert[253] reported a 12 percent incidence in their series, and Payne and Larson[223] stated that 50 percent of the deaths that occur after esophageal surgery are the result of an anastomotic leak. Improved operative techniques (eg, the right-sided approach to esophageal resection and possibly automatic stapling devices) may help to reduce the incidence of this dreaded complication.

Perforation of the esophagus from either blunt or penetrating injury when in association with multiple injuries can obscure the diagnosis. The ingestion of foreign bodies is an infrequent cause of esophageal perforation, but, when it occurs, the foreign body must be removed by endoscopy or at operation.

Postemetic esophageal tear, Boerhaave's syndrome, has a 20 percent or more mortality as a result of the severe necrotizing mediastinitis.[254]

Clinical Manifestations. Symptoms of esophageal perforation include substernal or epigastric pain, fever, dysphagia, and shortness of breath. Sometimes, the pleura is involved, and there may be signs of pleural effusion or pneumothorax. X-ray signs include widening of the mediastinum or emphysema, pleural effusion, and pneumothorax. A mediastinal air-fluid level may be present.

Boerhaave's syndrome resembles an acute abdominal crisis (eg, perforated peptic ulcer, a spontaneous pneumothorax) or a myocardial infarction but not a ruptured esophagus. Subcutaneous and mediastinal emphysema are early signs of a ruptured esophagus, and the diagnosis can be confirmed by x-ray studies by having the patient swallow a thin aqueous contrast medium to demonstrate extravasation.

The diagnosis of an anastomotic leak is not always clear. There may be an insidious onset of symptoms, with low-grade fever and leukocytosis. If chest tubes are still in place, the instillation of methylene blue into the esophagus and its identification in drainage fluid confirms the presence of a leak between the esophagus and the pleural space. A swallow of thin radiopaque contrast medium also may demonstrate either an anastomotic fistula or a paraesophageal abscess. Rarely will the disruption of an anastomosis be manifest as an acute catastrophic event with chest pain and hypotension. If this occurs, pleural drainage must be maintained, oral intake stopped, antibiotic coverage given, and appropriate fluid and volume replacement provided.

Pain is the most prominent symptom of an esophageal perforation caused by a foreign body. Fever and leukocytosis will also occur in time. If the foreign body is radiopaque, an x-ray film may be diagnostic, or a rent in the esophagus may be found at the time esophagoscopy is performed for removal of the foreign body.

Treatment. The best results in managing acute perforation of the distal esophagus whether the result of instrumental perforation or postemetic rupture have been obtained with early suture repair and drainage of the mediastinum. Attar et al[232] reported 3 deaths (17 percent) in 17 patients treated by primary repair and drainage within 24 hours of perforation. When repair of the esophagus is reinforced with autogenous tissue, either pleura or muscle, the results have been better. The incidence of fistula in 99 patients undergoing reinforced repair of esophageal perforation was 13 percent and the mortality was 6 percent.[232]

When the diagnosis of esophageal perforation is delayed beyond 24 hours, the results of treatment are not satisfactory. The mortality for delayed treatment of both cervical and thoracic esophageal perforations was 45 percent in 33 patients reported by Attar et al.[232]

In some instances, esophagectomy is the procedure of choice. Orringer and Stirling[255] reported 3 deaths in 24 patients and Attar et al[232] reported 2 deaths in 9 patients treated by esophagectomy.

Apparently, if the injury is recognized promptly (within 20 hours), oral intake is immediately stopped, and nasogastric and intrapleural drainages are initiated, together with the administration of antibiotics and steroids, some patients will do well without direct reparative surgery. In any event, after 20 to 24 hours, direct suture repair often fails. Unfortunately, late recognition of perforation is associated with a higher mortality rate for both nonoperative and direct reparative modes of treatment.

If a patient should survive beyond 1 month without surgery, an excisable fibrous tract may form, and then the fistula can be closed. The problem of esophagopleural fistula is discussed briefly in the section dealing with empyemas.

Postoperative esophagopleural fistula formations can usually be managed with intrapleural drains and without direct operative repair. If, however, reflux from the stomach or jejunum cannot be controlled or the breakdown of the anastomosis is so large that salivary flow is profuse, diversion of the refluxing intestine or of the proximal esophagus will be necessary.

Paravertebral Abscess. Although uncommon, a paravertebral abscess may develop from pyogenic osteomyelitis of the spine. The diagnosis is characteristically delayed by the obscure symptoms, which are usually limited to back pain, muscle spasm, and fever. X-ray studies of the chest may reveal vertebral destruction and a paravertebral abscess. A gallium-67 scan has been reported to be helpful in identifying pyogenic osteomyelitis.[256] *Staphylococcus aureus* is most frequently isolated. However, when there has been a history of antecedent urinary tract infection, gram-negative organisms are usually present. Identification of the organism is not always possible, and nonoperative treatment is generally successful.

Tuberculosis was another well-known cause of vertebral osteomyelitis and paravertebral abscess in earlier years. These abscesses developed from the upper thoracic vertebrae and either remained localized or extended inferiorly. When they extended along the psoas muscle, a cold abscess appeared in the abdominal wall or upper thigh. In addition to back pain, symptoms were those related to the presence of tuberculosis: fever, cough, and malaise. A chest x-ray examination often revealed a sharp convex shadow between the vertebrae and the esophagus. Posterior mediastinal abscesses were and still may be drained by excising short segments of one or more posterior ribs and entering the abscess extrapleurally (Fig. 35–25).

Echinococcus *Mediastinal Cysts.* Hydatid cysts due to *E. granulosus* occur anywhere in the human body, although the liver is the most common organ affected. Occasionally, the primary site of the disease will be the mediastinum, usually the posterior mediastinum where rib and vertebral body erosion sometimes occurs. They may cause compression of the spinal cord, superior vena cava, or branches of the aortic arch. When the anterior mediastinum is involved, hydatid cysts may cause tracheal compression or produce a Horner's syndrome. Myocardial disease is discussed in Chapter 36.

Anthrax. Anthrax is discussed in Chapter 9. Anthrax spores inhaled into the lungs may become phagocytosed and transported to mediastinal lymph nodes. Spores germinate there and cause a host reaction, which in turn results in an acute hemorrhagic mediastinitis. *Bacillus anthracis* is sensitive to both penicillin and streptomycin.

Infections of the Esophagus

Candida *Esophagitis.* Infections of the esophagus are extremely rare, and most are of no surgical significance. However, esophagitis due to *Candida* is not only the most common fungus infection of the esophagus, but it is the most frequent of all forms of esophagitis. Esophageal candidiasis is seen in debilitated patients receiving cancer chemotherapy and antibiotics, in patients with diabetes mellitus and primary parathyroidism, in patients with AIDS, and in patients immunosuppressed for tissue and organ transplantation.[257–259]

Candida albicans is the usual organism, although *C. krusei, C. tropicalis,* and *Torulopsis glabrata* are sometimes present. The disease may be acute or chronic. Symptoms include dysphagia and odynophagia, and esophagitis can occur without the

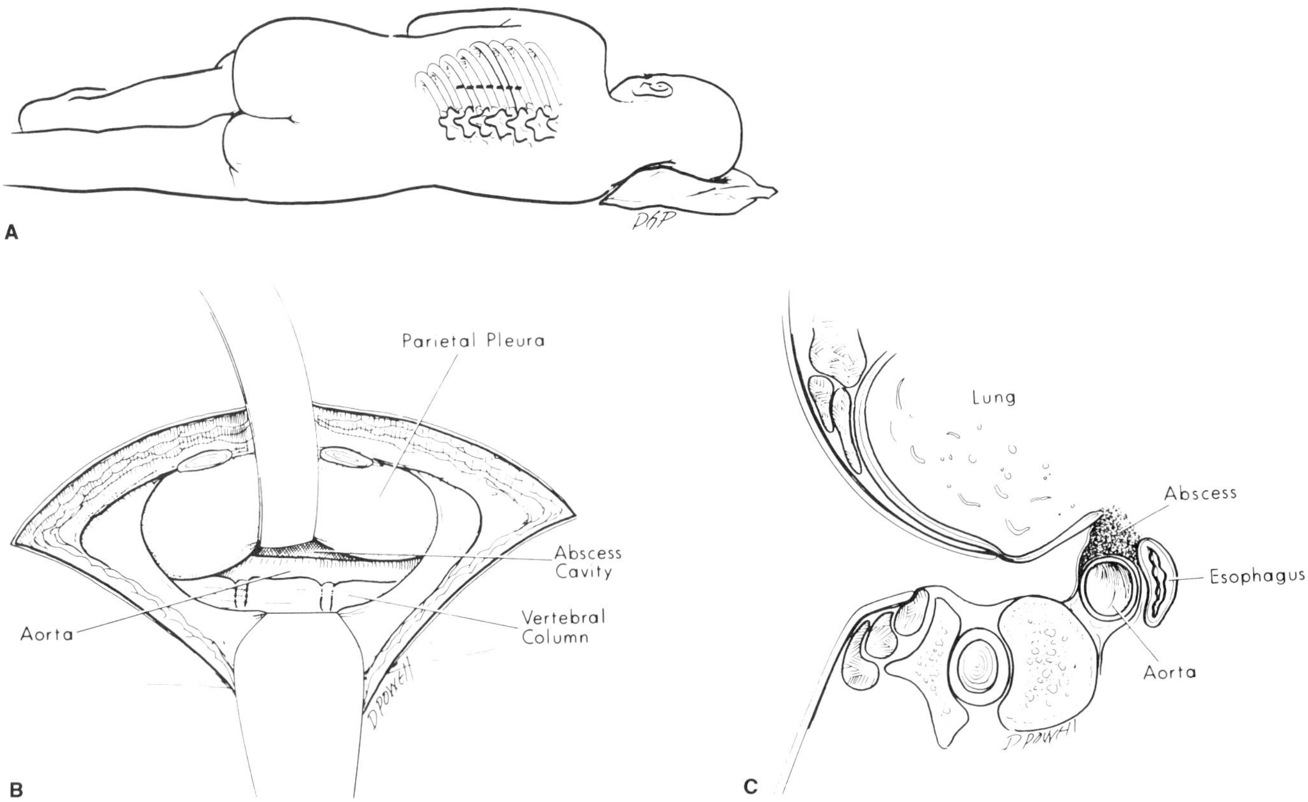

Figure 35–25. Drainage of posterior mediastinum. **A.** Skin incision lateral and parallel to vertebral bodies. **B.** Parietal pleura is retracted laterally to expose abscess cavity. **C.** Cross-section showing exposure of abscess cavity. *(Adapted from Seybold WD, Johnson MA III, Leary WV, et al: Surg Clin North Am 30:1155, 1950.)*

presence of thrush in the mouth. The esophagus develops a green or white pseudomembrane. The mucosa under the membrane is red and necrotic. These areas may become scarred and strictured. A double-contrast esophagogram often shows changes, especially in the lower two-thirds of the esophagus.[260] There may be spasm and lack of peristalsis, and the mucosa is irregular or sometimes ulcerated. Orringer and Sloan[261] reported three patients with esophageal stricture caused by monilial esophagitis and reviewed the literature.

Candida esophagitis in the nonimmunocompromised patient usually responds to nystatin taken as an oral suspension, 400,000 units every 2 hours while awake. The severely debilitated patient may require much greater concentrations of nystatin. For the immunocompromised patients and patients unresponsive to nystatin, flucytosine 150 mg/kg/day in four divided doses, ketoconazole 100 to 400 mg/day, and topical miconazole are effective against *Candida*.[261,262] For systemic candidiasis, intravenous amphotericin B is most effective. Once a fibrous stricture develops, antifungal drugs are of little value. Chronic esophageal dilation may be necessary and occasionally esophageal bypass surgery.

Viral Esophagitis. Herpetic esophagitis is an occasional complication of surgery in immunocompromised patients. It may or may not be associated with herpetic gingivostomatitis. In transplant patients, reactivation of the disease usually occurs in the first 4 weeks post-transplant and is characterized by dysphagia. Herpetic vesicles are seen on the pharynx and can be visualized by esophagoscopy. Esophagrams show discrete, widely separated ulcers and plaque-like defects with ulceration.[263] Superinfection with *Candida* can be prevented by nystatin. Most often the disease resolves spontaneously without stricture.

Cytomegalovirus esophagitis occurs in patients with AIDS and transplants and may complicate the course of the immunodepressed surgical patient.[264] The radiographic appearance may be that of a large flat ulcer.[260] The most effective drug is ganciclovir.[264]

REFERENCES

Infections of the Chest Wall

1. McKenna RJ, McMurtrey MJ, Larson DL, Mountain CF: A perspective on chest wall resection in patients with breast cancer. Ann Thorac Surg 38:482, 1984.
2. Bryant LR, Morgan C Jr: Chest wall, pleura, lung and mediastinum. In Schwartz SI, Shires GT, Spencer FC, Storer EH (eds): Principles of Surgery, 4th ed. New York, McGraw-Hill, 1984, pp 603–732.
3. Williams CD, Cunningham JN, Falk EA, et al: Chronic infection of the costal cartilages after thoracic surgical procedures. J Thorac Cardiovasc Surg 66:592, 1973.
4. Reckler JM, Flemma RJ, Pruitt BA Jr: Costal chondritis: an unusual complication in the burned patient. J Trauma 13:76, 1973.

Sternal Wound Infections

5. Wray TM, Bryant RE, Killen DA: Sternal osteomyelitis and costochondritis after median sternotomy. J Thorac Cardiovasc Surg 65:227, 1973.
6. Stoney WS, Alford WC Jr, Burrus GR, et al: Median sternotomy dehiscence. Ann Thorac Surg 26:421, 1978.
7. Grossi EA, Culliford AT, Krieger KH, et al: A survey of 77 major infectious complications of median sternotomy: a review of 7,949 consecutive operative procedures. Ann Thorac Surg 40:214, 1985.
8. Cosgrove DM, Lytle BW, Loop FD, et al: Does bilateral internal mammary artery grafting increase surgical risk? J Thorac Cardiovasc Surg 95:850, 1988.
9. Sethi GK, Copeland JG, Moritz T, et al: Comparison of postoperative complications between saphenous vein and IMA grafts to left anterior descending coronary artery. Ann Thorac Surg 51:733, 1991.
10. Sarr MG, Gott VL, Townsend TR: Mediastinal infection after cardiac surgery. Ann Thorac Surg 38:415, 1984.
11. Kuritsky JL, Bullen MG, Broome CV, et al: Sternal wound infections and endocarditis due to organisms of *Mycobacterium fortuitum* complex. Ann Intern Med 98:938, 1983.
12. Sethi GK, Simons WJ, Scott SM: *Mycobacterium fortuitum* infections of the mediastinum. J Cardiovasc Surg 26:307, 1985.
13. Gaynes R, Marosok R, Mowry-Hanley J, et al: Mediastinitis following coronary artery bypass surgery: a 3-year review. J Infect Dis 163:117, 1991.
14. Ehrenkranz NJ, Pfaff SJ: Mediastinitis complicating cardiac operations: evidence of postoperative causation. Rev Infect Dis 13:803, 1991.
15. Karwande SV, Renlund DG, Olsen SL, et al: Mediastinitis in heart transplantation. Ann Thorac Surg 54:1039, 1992.
16. Bryant LR, Spencer FC, Trinkle JK: Treatment of median sternotomy infection by mediastinal irrigation with an antibiotic solution. Ann Surg 169:914, 1969.
17. Thurer RJ, Bognolo D, Vargas A, et al: The management of mediastinal infection following cardiac surgery: an experience utilizing continuous irrigation with povidone-iodine. Cardiovasc Surg 68:962, 1974.
18. Arnold PG: Reconstruction of sternum and anterior chest wall. Clin Plast Surg 8:389, 1981.
19. Jurkiewicz MJ, Bostywick J, Hester TR, et al: Infected median sternotomy wound. Ann Surg 191:738, 1980.
20. Acinapura AJ, Godfrey N, Romita M, et al: Surgical management of infected median sternotomy: closed irrigation vs muscle flaps. J Cardiovasc Surg 26: 443, 1985.
21. Nahai F, Morales L Jr, Bone DK, et al: Pectoralis major muscle turnover flaps for closure of the infected sternotomy wound with preservation of form and function. Plast Reconstr Surg 70:471, 1982.
22. Jeevanandam V, Smith CR, Rose EA, et al: Single-stage management of sternal wound infections. J Thorac Cardiovasc Surg 99:256, 1990.
23. Domart Y, Trouillet JL, Fagon JY, et al: Incidence and morbidity of cytomegaloviral infection in patients with mediastinitis following cardiac surgery. Chest 97:18, 1990.

Pacemaker Infections

24. Siddons H, Nowak K: Surgical complications of implanting pacemakers. Br J Surg 62:929, 1975.
25. Brodman R, Frame R, Andrews C, et al: Removal of infected transvenous leads requiring cardiopulmonary bypass or inflow occlusion. J Thorac Cardiovasc Surg 103:649, 1992.
26. Meyers MR, Parsonnet V, Bernstein AD: Extraction of implanted transvenous pacing leads: a review of a persistent clinical problem. Am Heart J 121:881, 1991.

Empyema

27. Scott S: The pleura and empyema. In Sabiston DC Jr (ed): Textbook of Surgery. Philadelphia, Saunders, 1991, p 1718.
28. Lemmer JH, Botham MJ, Orringer MB: Modern management of adult thoracic empyema. J Thorac Cardiovasc Surg 90:849, 1985.
29. Patterson LT, Schmitt HJ Jr, Armstrong RG: Intermediate care of war wounds of the chest. J Thorac Cardiovasc Surg 55:16, 1968.
30. Ravitch MM, Fein R: The changing picture of pneumonia and empyema in infants and children: a review of the experience at the Harriet Lane Home from 1934 through 1958. JAMA 175:1039, 1961.
31. Kosloske AM, Cartwright KC: The controversial role of decortication in the management of pediatric empyema. J Thorac Cardiovasc Surg 96:166, 1988.
32. Bartlett JG, Finegold SM: Anaerobic infections of the lung and pleural space. Am Rev Respir Dis 110:56, 1974.

33. Recollections: Evarts A. Graham. Ann Thorac Surg 9:272, 1970.
34. Hood M: Discussion of ref. 28. J Thorac Cardiovasc Surg 90:854, 1985.
35. Mandal AK, Thadepalli H: Treatment of spontaneous bacterial empyema thoracis. J Thorac Cardiovasc Surg 94:414, 1987.
36. VanSonnenberg E, Nakamoto SK, Mueller PR, et al: CT and ultrasound-guided catheter drainage of empyemas after chest-tube failure. Radiology 151:349, 1984.
37. Mace AH, Elyaderani MK: Ultrasonography in the diagnosis and management of empyema of the thorax. South Med J 77:294, 1984.
38. Van Way C III, Narrod J, Hopeman A: The role of early limited thoracotomy in the treatment of empyema. J Thorac Cardiovasc Surg 96:436, 1988.
39. Hood RM: Surgical Diseases of the Pleura and Chest Wall. Philadelphia, Saunders, 1985, p 96.
40. Braimbridge M: Discussion of ref. 28. J Thorac Cardiovasc Surg 90:853, 1985.
41. Stafford EG, Clagett OT: Postpneumonectomy empyema: neomycin instillation and definitive closure. J Thorac Cardiovasc Surg 63:771, 1972.
42. Provan JL: The management of postpneumonectomy empyema. J Thorac Cardiovasc Surg 61:107, 1971.
43. Karkola P, Kairaluoma MI, Larmi TK: Postpneumonectomy empyema in pulmonary carcinoma patients: treatment with antibiotic irrigation and closed-chest drainage. J Thorac Cardiovasc Surg 72:319, 1976.
44. Pairolero PC, Trastek VF: Surgical management of chronic empyema: the role of thoracoplasty. Ann Thorac Surg 50:689, 1990.
45. Hankins JR, Miller JE, McLaughlin JS: The use of chest wall muscle flaps to close bronchopleural fistulas; experience with 21 patients. Ann Thorac Surg 25:491, 1978.
46. Virkkula L: Treatment of bronchopleural fistula. Ann Thorac Surg 25:489, 1978.
47. Miller JI: Empyema thoracis. Ann Thorac Surg 50:343, 1990.

Pulmonary Defense Mechanisms

48. Newhouse M, Sanchis J, Bienenstock J: Lung defense mechanisms. N Engl J Med 295:990, 1976.
49. Newhouse M, Sanchis J, Bienenstock J: Lung defense mechanisms. N Engl J Med 295:1045, 1976.
50. Thompson AB, Schultz HD, Sisson JH, et al: Airway mucociliary clearance. In Bone RC (ed): Pulmonary and Critical Care Medicine. St Louis, Mosby Year Book, 1993, Chap 1, p 1.
51. Proctor DF, Wagner HN: Mucociliary particle clearance in the human nose. In Davis CN (ed): Inhaled Particles and Vapours, II. London, Pergamon, 1967, p 25.
52. Muir DCF, Davies CN: The deposition of 0.5μ diameter aerosols in the lungs of man. Ann Occup Hyg 10:161, 1967.
53. Ward PA, Talamo RC: Deficiency of the chemotactic factor inactivator in human sera with α_1-antitrypsin deficiency. J Clin Invest 52:516, 1973.
54. Catz EG, Speir WA Jr: α_1-Antitrypsin deficiency. South Med J 77:479, 1984.
55. Hilding AC: Experimental studies on some little understood aspects of the physiology of the respiratory tract and their clinical importance. Trans Am Acad Ophthalmol Otolaryngol 65:475, 1961.
56. Sanchis J, Dolovich M, Rossman C, et al: Pulmonary mucociliary clearance in cystic fibrosis. N Engl J Med 288:651, 1973.
57. Mackaness GB: The monocyte in cellular immunity. Semin Hematol 7:172, 1970.
58. Waldman RH, Mann JJ, Small PA Jr: Immunization against influenza: prevention of illness in man by aerolized inactivated vaccine. JAMA 207:520, 1969.
59. Hand WL, Cantey JR: Antibacterial mechanisms of the lower respiratory tract. I. Immunoglobulin synthesis and secretion. J Clin Invest 53:354, 1974.

Diagnosis of Pulmonary Infections

60. Daniele RP, Elias JA, Epstein PE, Rossman MD: Bronchoalveolar lavage: role in the pathogenesis, diagnosis, and management of interstitial lung disease. Ann Intern Med 102:93, 1985.
61. Hanson RR, Zavala DC, Rhodes ML, et al: Transbronchial biopsy via flexible fiberoptic bronchoscope: results in 164 patients. Am Rev Respir Dis 114:67, 1976.
62. Anderson HA: Transbronchoscopic lung biopsy for diffuse pulmonary disease: results in 939 patients. Chest 73:734, 1978.
63. Stenson W, Aranda C, Bevelaqua FA: Transbronchial biopsy culture in pulmonary tuberculosis. Chest 83:883, 1983.
64. Stevens GM, Jackman RJ: Outpatient needle biopsy of the lung: its safety and utility. Radiology 151:301, 1984.
65. Khouri NF, Stitik FP, Erozan YS, et al: Transthoracic needle aspiration biopsy of benign and malignant lung lesions. AJR 144:281, 1985.
66. Gatenby RA, Mulhern CB Jr, Broder GJ, Moldofsky PJ: Computed-tomographic-guided biopsy of small apical and peripheral upper-lobe lung masses. Radiology 150:591, 1984.
67. Cunningham JH, Zavala DC, Corry RJ, Keim LW: Trephine air drill, bronchial brush, and fiberoptic transbronchial lung biopsies in immunosuppressed patients. Am Rev Respir Dis 115:213, 1977.
68. Jacobeus HC: The practical importance of thoracoscopy in surgery of the chest. Surg Gynecol Obstet 34:289, 1922.
69. Mack MJ, Aronoff RJ, Acuff TE, et al: Present role of thoracoscopy in the diagnosis and treatment of diseases of the chest. Ann Thorac Surg 54:403, 1992.
70. Lewis RJ, Sisler CE, Caccavale RJ: Imaged thoracic

lobectomy: should it be done? Ann Thorac Surg 54:80, 1992.
71. Donnelly RJ, Page RD, Cowen ME: Endoscopy assisted microthoracotomy: initial experience. Thorax 47:490, 1992.
72. Cheson BD, Samlowski WE, Tang TT, Spruance SL: Value of open-lung biopsy in 87 immunocompromised patients with pulmonary infiltrates. Cancer 55:453, 1985.
73. Leight GS Jr, Michaelis LL: Open lung biopsy for the diagnosis of acute, diffuse pulmonary infiltrates in the immunosuppressed patient. Chest 73:499, 1978.
74. Thompson DT: Lung biopsy with local anesthesia: report on 100 cases with the use of a recently introduced technique. J Thorac Cardiovasc Surg 75:429, 1978.
75. Marty JJ, Mehta AC: Pulmonary cytology. In Bone RC (ed): Pulmonary and Critical Care Medicine. St Louis, Mosby Year Book, 1993, Chap 3, p 1.

Viral Infections

76. Bahnson HT, Hardesty RL, Griffith BP, et al: Management of complications in transplantation: heart-lung. In Waldhausen JA, Orringer MB (eds): Complications in Cardiothoracic Surgery. St Louis, Mosby Year Book, 1991, p 425.
77. Vander Salm TJ: Cytomegalovirus: more dangerous to the cardiac surgical patient than we thought? Chest 97:3, 1990.
78. Ravin CE, Smith GW, Ahern MJ, et al: Cytomegaloviral infection presenting as a solitary pulmonary nodule. Chest 71:220, 1977.

Bacterial Infections

79. Bone RC: The adult respiratory distress syndrome. In Bone RC (ed): Pulmonary and Critical Care Medicine. St Louis, Mosby Year Book, 1993, Chap R3.
80. Hochberg LA: Thoracic Surgery before the Twentieth Century. New York, Vantage Press, 1960.
81. Neuhof H, Touroff ASW: Acute putrid abscess of the lung: hyperacute variety. J Thorac Surg 12:98, 1942.
82. Brock RC: Lung Abscess. Oxford, Blackwell, 1952.
83. Bartlett JG: Anaerobic bacteria (aspiration pneumonitis and lung abscess). In Bone RC (ed): Pulmonary and Critical Care Medicine. St Louis, Mosby Year Book, 1993, Chap 4, p 1.
84. Eftimiadi C, Tonetti M, Cavallero A, et al: Short-chain fatty acids produced by anaerobic bacteria inhibit phagocytosis by human lung phagocytes. J Infect Dis 161:138, 1990.
85. Crabb JH, Finberg R, Onderdonk AB, et al: T cell regulation of *Bacteroides fragilis*-induced intraabdominal abscesses. Rev Infect Dis 12:S178, 1990.
86. Bartlett JG, Rosenblatt JE, Finegold SM: Percutaneous transtracheal aspiration in the diagnosis of anaerobic pulmonary infection. Ann Intern Med 79:535, 1973.
87. Wimberley NW, Bass JB Jr, Boyd BW, et al: Use of bronchoscopic protected catheter brush for the diagnosis of pulmonary infections. Chest 81:556, 1982.
88. Conte BA, Laforet EG: The role of the topical anesthetic agent in modifying bacteriologic data obtained by bronchoscopy. N Engl J Med 267:957, 1962.
89. Davidson M, Tempest B, Palmer DL: Bacteriologic diagnosis of acute pneumonia: comparison of sputum, transtracheal aspirates, and lung aspirates. JAMA 235:158, 1976.
90. Schweppe HI, Knowles JH, Kane L: Lung abscess: an analysis of the Massachusetts General Hospital cases from 1943 through 1956. N Engl J Med 265:1039, 1961.
91. Stark DD, Federle MP, Goodman PC, et al: Differentiating lung abscess and empyema: radiography and computed tomography. Am J Roentgenol 141:163, 1983.
92. Williford ME, Godwin JD: Computed tomography of lung abscess and empyema. Radiol Clin North Am 21:575, 1983.
93. Weiss W, Cherniack NS: Acute nonspecific lung abscess: a controlled study comparing orally and parenterally administered penicillin G. Chest 66:348, 1974.
94. Thoms NW, Wilson RF, Puro HE, Arbulu A: Life-threatening hemoptysis in primary lung abscess. Ann Thorac Surg 14:347, 1972.
95. Harley JD, Killien FC, Peck AG: Massive hemoptysis controlled by transcatheter embolization of the bronchial arteries. Am J Roentgenol 128:302, 1977.
96. Newson SWB, Milstein BB, Stark JE: Local chemotherapy for *Pseudomonas* lung abscess. Lancet 2:530, 1974.
97. Vidal E, LeVeen HH, Yarnoz M, Piccone VA Jr: Lung abscess secondary to pulmonary infarction. Ann Thorac Surg 11:577, 1971.
98. McMillan JC, Milstein SH, Samson PC: Clinical spectrum of septic pulmonary embolism and infarction. J Thorac Cardiovasc Surg 75:670, 1978.
99. Ochsner A: Bronchiectasis: a disappearing pulmonary lesion. NY State J Med 75:1683, 1975.
100. Kent EM, Blades B: Surgical anatomy of pulmonary lobes. J Thorac Surg 12:18, 1942.
101. Bradham RR, Sealy WC, Young WG Jr: Chronic middle lobe infection: factors responsible for its development. Ann Thorac Surg 2:612, 1966.
102. Miller RD, Divertie MB: Kartagener's syndrome. Chest 62:130, 1972.
103. Longstreth GF, Weitzman SA, Browning RJ, Lieberman J: Bronchiectasis and homozygous alpha$_1$-antitrypsin deficiency. Chest 67:233, 1975.
104. Nagaki M, Shimura S, Tanno Y, et al: Role of chronic *Pseudomonas aeruginosa* infection in the development of bronchiectasis. Chest 102:1464, 1992.
105. Sealy WC, Bradham RR, Young WG Jr: The surgical treatment of multisegmental and localized bronchiectasis. Surg Gynecol Obstet 123:80, 1966.

106. McGuinness G, Naidich DP, Leitman BS, McCauley DI: Bronchiectasis: CT evaluation. AJR 160:253, 1993.
107. Ripe E: Bronchiectasis. I. A follow-up study after surgical treatment. Scand J Respir Dis 52:96, 1971.
108. Sanderson JM, Kennedy MCS, Johnson MF, Manley DCE: Bronchiectasis: results of surgical and conservative management. A review of 393 cases. Thorax 29:407, 1974.
109. Barker AF, Bardana EJ Jr: Bronchiectasis: update of an orphan disease. Am Rev Respir Dis 137:969, 1988.
110. McLaughlin JS, Hankins JR: Current aspects of surgery for pulmonary tuberculosis. Ann Thorac Surg 17:513, 1974.
111. Centers for Disease Control: Tuberculosis—United States 1984. MMWR Morb Mortal Wkly Rep 34:300, 1985.
112. Bloom BR, Murray CJL: Tuberculosis: commentary on a reemergent killer. Science 257:1055, 1992.
113. Goble M, Iseman MD, Madsen LA, et al: Treatment of 171 patients with pulmonary tuberculosis resistant to isoniazid and rifampin. N Engl J Med 328:527, 1993.
114. Van Scoy RE, Wilkowske CJ: Antituberculous agents. Mayo Clin Proc 67:179, 1992.
115. Harrison LH: Current aspects of the surgical management of tuberculosis. Surg Clin North Am 60:883, 1980.
116. Butz RO, Zvetina JR, Leininger BJ: Ten-year experience with mycetomas in patients with pulmonary tuberculosis. Chest 87:356, 1985.
117. Sethi GK, Takaro T: Management of complications following pulmonary resection for infections of mycobacterial, actinomycetic, and fungal origins. In Cordell AR, Ellison RG (eds): Complications of Intrathoracic Surgery. Boston, Little, Brown, 1979.
118. Tamimi TM, Hankins JR, Miller JE, et al: The value of thoracoplasty before extensive unilateral resection for pulmonary tuberculosis. Am Surg 42:71, 1976.
119. Pomerantz M, Madsen L, Goble M, Iseman M: Surgical management of resistant mycobacterial tuberculosis and other mycobacterial pulmonary infections. Ann Thorac Surg 52:1108, 1991.
120. Johnson G Jr, Peters RM: Pulmonary resection for tuberculosis: life table analysis of results. Ann Thorac Surg 1:634, 1965.

Opportunistic Infections

121. Simor AE, Salit IE, Vellend H: The role of *Mycobacterium xenopi* in human disease. Am Rev Respir Dis 129:435, 1984.
122. Banks J, Hunter AM, Campbell IA, et al: Pulmonary infection with *Mycobacterium xenopi:* review of treatment and response. Thorax 39:376, 1984.
123. Cotton P: Medicine's arsenal in battling "dominant dozen," other AIDS-associated opportunistic infections. JAMA 266:1476, 1991.
124. Moran JF, Alexander LG, Stab EW, et al: Long-term results of pulmonary resection for atypical mycobacterial disease. Ann Thorac Surg 35:597, 1983.
125. Corpe RF: Surgical management of pulmonary disease due to *Mycobacterium avium-intracellulare.* Rev Infect Dis 3:1064, 1981.
126. Spencer H: Pathology of the Lung: Excluding Pulmonary Tuberculosis, Vol 1, 3rd ed. Oxford, Pergamon, 1977, pp 258–261.
127. Everett ED, Nelson RA: Pulmonary melioidosis: observations in thirty-nine cases. Am Rev Respir Dis 112:331, 1975.
128. Sanford JP: *Pseudomonas* species (including melioidosis and glanders). In Mandell GL, Douglas RG Jr, Bennett JE (eds): Principles and Practice of Infectious Diseases. New York, Churchill Livingstone, 1989.
129. Zajtchuk R, Guiton CR, Sadler TR, et al: Surgical treatment of pulmonary melioidosis. J Thorac Cardiovasc Surg 66:838, 1973.
130. Rippon JW: Medical Mycology. The Pathogenic Fungi and the Pathogenic Actinomycetes. Philadelphia, Saunders, 1988.
131. Harrison RN, Thomas DJB: Acute actinomycetic empyema. Thorax 12:406, 1979.
132. Merdler C, Greif J, Burke M, et al: Primary actinomycotic empyema. South Med J 76:411, 1983.
133. Severo LC, Kaemmerer A, Camargo JJ, et al: Actinomycotic intracavitary lung colonization. Mycopathologia 108:1, 1989.
134. Jensen BM, Kruse-Andersen S, Andersen K: Thoracic actinomycosis. Scand J Thorac Cardiovasc Surg 23:181, 1989.
135. Weese WC, Smith IM: A study of 57 cases of actinomycosis over a 36-year period: a diagnostic "failure" with good prognosis after treatment. Arch Intern Med 135:1562, 1975.
136. Caputo GM, Aber RC: Pneumonia due to higher bacteria (*Nocardia* and *Actinomyces* species). In Bone RC (ed): Pulmonary and Critical Care. St Louis, Mosby Year Book, 1993, Chap 7, p 1.
137. Beaman BL, Burnside J, Edwards B, Causey W: Nocardial infections in the United States, 1972–1974. J Infect Dis 134:286, 1976.
138. Curry WA: Human nocardiosis: a clinical review with selected case reports. Arch Intern Med 140:818, 1980.
139. Rodriquez JL, Barrio JL, Pitchenik AE: Pulmonary nocardiosis in the acquired immunodeficiency syndrome. Diagnosis with bronchoalveolar lavage and treatment with non-sulphur containing drugs. Chest 90:912, 1986.
140. Petersen EA, Nash ML, Mammana RB, Copeland JG: Minocycline treatment of pulmonary nocardiosis. JAMA 250:930, 1983.
141. Smego RA Jr, Moeller MB, Gallis HA: Trimethoprim-sulfamethoxazole therapy for *Nocardia* infections. Arch Intern Med 143:711, 1983.

Fungal Infections of the Lung

142. Diamond RD: The growing problem of mycosis in patients infected with the human immunodeficiency virus. Rev Infect Dis 13:480, 1991.
143. Anaissie EJ, Bodey GP: Fungal infections in patients with cancer. Pharmacotherapy 10:164S, 1990.
144. Peterson PK: Pulmonary mycoses in organ transplant recipients. In Sarosi GA, Davies SF (eds): Fungal Diseases of the Lung. New York, Grune & Stratton, 1986, p 299.
145. Chick EW, Dillon ML, Tahanasab A: Acute cavitary histoplasmosis. Chest 71:674, 1977.
146. Palayew MJ, Frank H: Benign progressive multinodular pulmonary histoplasmosis: a radiological and clinical entity. Radiology 111:311, 1974.
147. Davies SF, Sarosi GA: Pulmonary mycoses. In Bone RC (ed): Pulmonary and Critical Care Medicine. St Louis, Mosby Year Book, 1993, Chap 6, p 1.
148. Terrell CL, Hughes CE: Antifungal agents used for deep-seated mycotic infections. Mayo Clin Proc 67:69, 1992.
149. Sarosi GA, Johnson PC: Progressive disseminated histoplasmosis in the acquired immunodeficiency syndrome: a model for disseminated disease. Semin Respir Infect 5:146, 1990.
150. Davies SF, Sarosi GA: Blastomycosis. Eur J Clin Microbiol Infect Dis 8:474, 1989.
151. Laskey W, Sarosi GA: Endogenous reinfection in blastomycosis. Am Rev Respir Dis 115:266, 1977.
152. Sanders JS, Sarosi GA, Nollet DJ, Thompson JI: Exfoliative cytology in the rapid diagnosis of pulmonary blastomycosis. Chest 72:193, 1977.
153. Poe RH, Vassallo CL, Plessinger VA, Witt RL: Pulmonary blastomycosis versus carcinoma: a challenging differential. Am J Med Sci 263:145, 1972.
154. Bradsher RW: Blastomycosis: fungal infections of the lung update: 1989. Semin Respir Infect 5:105, 1990.
155. Edson RS, Keys TF: Treatment of primary pulmonary blastomycosis: results of long term follow-up. Mayo Clin Proc 56:683, 1981.
156. Thadepalli H, Salem FA, Mandall AK, et al: Pulmonary mycetoma due to *Coccidioides immitis.* Chest 71:429, 1977.
157. Lonky SA, Catanzaro A, Moser KM, Einstein H: Acute coccidioidal pleural effusion. Am Rev Respir Dis 114:681, 1976.
158. Baker EJ, Hawkins JA, Waskow EA: Surgery for coccidioidomycosis in 52 diabetic patients, with special reference to related immunologic factors. J Thorac Cardiovasc 75:680, 1978.
159. Read TC: Coin lesion, pulmonary, in the Southwest (solitary pulmonary nodules). Ariz Med 29:775, 1972.
160. Marks TS, Spence WF, Baisch BF: Limited resection for pulmonary coccidioidomycosis. In Ajello L (ed): Coccidioidomycosis. Tuscon, University of Arizona Press, 1967, p 73.
161. Cunningham RT, Einstein H: Coccidioidal pulmonary cavities with rupture. J Thorac Cardiovasc Surg 84:172, 1982.
162. Ampel NM, Wieden MA, Galgiani JN: Coccidioidomycosis: clinical update. Rev Infect Dis 11:897, 1989.
163. Bouza E, Winston DJ, Rhodes J, Hewitt WL: Paracoccidioidomycosis (South American blastomycosis) in the United States. Chest 72:100, 1977.
164. Restrepo A, Robledo M, Giraldo R, et al: The gamut of paracoccidioidomycosis. Am J Med 61:33, 1976.
165. Perfect JR: Cryptococcosis. Infect Dis Clin North Am 3:77, 1989.
166. Khoury MB, Godwin JD, Ravin CE, et al: Thoracic cryptococcosis: immunologic competence and radiographic appearance. Am J Roentgenol 142:893, 1984.
167. Salyer WR, Salyer DC, Baker RD: Primary complex of *Cryptococcus* and pulmonary lymph nodes. J Infect Dis 130:74, 1974.
168. Baker RD: The primary pulmonary lymph node complex of cryptococcosis. Am J Clin Pathol 65:83, 1976.
169. Salyer WR, Salyer DC: Pleural involvement in cryptococcosis. Chest 66:139, 1974.
170. Rohatgi PK: Pulmonary sporotrichosis. South Med J 73:1611, 1980.
171. Scott SM, Peasley ED, Crymes TP: Pulmonary sporotrichosis: a report of two cases with cavitation. N Engl J Med 265:453, 1961.
172. Jay SJ, Platt MR, Reynolds RC: Primary pulmonary sporotrichosis. Am Rev Respir Dis 115:1051, 1977.
173. England DM, Hochholzer L: Primary pulmonary sporotrichosis: report of 8 cases with clinicopathologic review. Am J Surg Pathol 9:193, 1985.
174. Haponik EF, Hill MK, Graighead CC: Case report: pulmonary sporotrichosis with massive hemoptysis. Am J Med Sci 297:251, 1989.
175. Fields CL, Ossorio MA, Roy TM: Empyema associated with pulmonary sporotrichosis. South Med J 82:910, 1989.
176. Fraser DW, Ward J, Ajello L, et al: Aspergillosis and other systemic mycoses: the growing problem. JAMA 242:163, 1979.
177. Pennington JE: *Aspergillus* lung disease. Med Clin North Am 64:475, 1980.
178. Battaglini JW, Murray GF, Keagy BA, et al: Surgical management of symptomatic pulmonary aspergilloma. Ann Thorac Surg 39:512, 1985.
179. Daly RC, Pairolero PC, Piehler JM, et al: Pulmonary aspergilloma. Results of surgical treatment. J Thorac Cardiovasc Surg 92:981, 1986.
180. Wollschlager C, Khan F: Aspergillomas complicating sarcoidosis: prospective study in 100 patients. Chest 86:585, 1984.
181. Walsh TJ, Bulkley BH: *Aspergillus* pericarditis: clinical and pathologic features in the immunocompromised patient. Cancer 49:48, 1982.
182. Denning DW, Stevens DA: Antifungal and surgical

treatment of invasive aspergillosis: review of 2,121 published cases. Rev Infect Dis 12:1147, 1990.
183. Horsfield K, Nicholls A, Cumming G, et al: Treatment of pulmonary aspergillosis with di-iodohydroxyquinoline. Thorax 32:250, 1977.
184. Faulkner SL, Vernon R, Brown PP, et al: Hemoptysis and pulmonary aspergilloma: operative versus nonoperative treatment. Ann Thorac Surg 25:389, 1978.
185. Eguchi S, Endo S, Sakashita I, et al: Surgery in the treatment of pulmonary aspergillosis. Br J Dis Chest 65:111, 1971.
186. Bennett MR, Weinbaum DL, Fiehler PC: Chronic necrotizing pulmonary aspergillosis treated by endobronchial amphotericin B. South Med J 83:829, 1990.
187. Parry MF, Coughlin FR, Zambetti FX: *Aspergillus* empyema. Chest 81:768, 1982.
188. Murray HW: Pulmonary mucormycosis with massive fatal hemoptysis. Chest 68:65, 1975.
189. Gartenberg G, Bottone EJ, Keusch GT, Weitzman I: Hospital-acquired mucormycosis (*Rhizopus rhizopodiformis*) of skin and subcutaneous tissue. N Engl J Med 299:1115, 1978.
190. Record NB Jr, Ginder DR: Pulmonary phycomycosis without obvious predisposing factors. JAMA 235: 1256, 1976.
191. Murray HW: Pulmonary mucormycosis: one hundred years later. Chest 72:1, 1977.
192. Hauch TW: Pulmonary mucormycosis: another cure. Chest 72:92, 1977.
193. Gribetz AR, Chuang MT, Burrows L, Teirstein AS: *Rhizopus* lung abscess in renal transplant patient successfully treated by lobectomy. Chest 77:102, 1980.
194. Wright RN, Saxena A, Robin A, et al: Pulmonary mucormycosis (phycomycetes) successfully treated by resection. Ann Thorac Surg 29:166, 1980.
195. Travis LB, Roberts GD, Wilson WR: Clinical significance of *Pseudallescheria boydii:* a review of 10 years' experience. Mayo Clin Proc 60:531, 1985.
196. Jung JY, Salas R, Almond CH, et al: The role of surgery in the management of pulmonary monosporosis: a collective review. J Thorac Cardiovasc Surg 73:139, 1977.
197. Gordon G, Axelrod JL: Case report: prosthetic valve endocarditis caused by *Pseudallescheria boydii* and *Clostridium limosum.* Mycopathologia 89:129, 1985.
198. Armstrong D: Candida species. In Sarosi GA, Davies SF (eds): Fungal Disease of the Lung. Orlando, FL, Grune & Stratton, 1986, pp 167–174.
199. Schiffman RL, Johnson TS, Weinberger SE, et al: *Candida* lung abscess: successful treatment with amphotercin B and 5-flucytosine. Am Rev Respir Dis 125:766, 1982.
200. Spear RK, Walker PD, Lampton LM: Tracheal obstruction associated with a fungus ball. Chest 70:662, 1976.
201. Haron E, Vartivarian S, Anaissie E, et al: Primary *Candida* pneumonia. Medicine (Baltimore) 72:137, 1993.
202. Rosenbaum RB, Barber JV, Stevens DA: *Candida albicans* pneumonia. Diagnosis by pulmonary aspiration, recovery without treatment. Am Rev Respir Dis 109:373, 1974.
203. Carpentieri U, Haggard ME, Lockhart LH, et al: Clinical experience in prevention of candidiasis by nystatin in children with acute lymphocytic leukemia. J Pediatr 92:593, 1978.
204. Ezdinli EZ, O'Sullivan DD, Wasser LP, et al: Oral amphotericin for candidiasis in patients with hematologic neoplasms. JAMA 242:258, 1979.

Protozoan and Helminth Infections

205. Rodriguez C: Pulmonary and pleural amebiasis. In Shields TW (ed): General Thoracic Surgery. Philadelphia, Lea & Febiger, 1972, p 650.
206. Furst SR: Pleuropulmonary amebiasis. Chest 100:293, 1991.
207. Metronidazole (Flagyl) for amebiasis. Med Lett Drugs Ther 14:39, 1972.
208. Adeyemo AO, Aderounmu A: Intrathoracic complications of amebic liver abscess. J R Soc Med 77:17, 1984.
209. Burke BA, Good RA: *Pneumocystis carinii* infection. Medicine (Baltimore) 52:23, 1973.
210. Watts JC, Chandler FW: Evolving concepts of infection by *Pneumocystis carinii.* Pathol Annu 26:93, 1991.
211. Edman JC, Kovacs JA, Masur H, et al: Ribosomal RNA sequence shows *Pneumocystis carinii* to be a member of the fungi. Nature 334:519, 1988.
212. Murray JF, Felton CP, Garay SM, et al: Pulmonary complications of the acquired immunodeficiency syndrome (Report of a National Heart, Lung, and Blood Institute Workshop). N Engl J Med 310:1682, 1984.
213. Ognibene FP, Shelhamer J, Gill V, et al: The diagnosis of *Pneumocystis carinii* pneumonia in patients with the acquired immunodeficiency syndrome using subsegmental bronchoalveolar lavage. Am Rev Respir Dis 129:929, 1984.
214. Nicolau DP, Ross JW, Nightingale CH, Quiniliani R: Focus on atovaquone. Hosp Formul 28:341, 1993.
215. Delorenzo LJ, Maguire GP, Wormser GP, et al: Persistence of *Pneumocystis carinii* pneumonia in acquired immunodeficiency syndrome. Chest 88:79, 1985.
216. Small CB, Harris CA, Friedland GH, Klein RS: The treatment of *Pneumocystis carinii* pneumonia in the immunodeficiency syndrome. Arch Intern Med 145:837, 1985.
217. Zurlo JJ: Respiratory infections and acquired immunodeficiency syndrome (AIDS). In Bone RC (ed): Pulmonary and Critical Care Medicine. St Louis, Mosby Year Book, 1993, Chap 3, p 1.
218. Peschiera CA: Hydatid cysts of the lung. In Steele J

(ed): The Treatment of Mycotic and Parasitic Diseases of the Chest. Springfield, IL, CC Thomas, 1964, p 201.
219. Xanthakis D, Efthimiadis M, Papadakis G, et al: Hydatid disease of the chest: report of 91 patients surgically treated. Thorax 27:517, 1972.
220. Pinch LW, Wilson JF: Nonsurgical management of cystic hydatid disease in Alaska: a review of 30 cases of *Echinococcus granulosus* infection treated without operation. Ann Surg 178:45, 1973.
221. Pinch LW, Wilson JF: Nonsurgical management of cystic hydatid disease in Alaska: a review of 30 cases of *Echinococcus granulosus* infection treated without operation. Ann Surg 178:45, 1973.

Mediastinitis

222. Pearse HE Jr: Mediastinitis following cervical suppuration. Ann Surg 108:588, 1938.
223. Payne WS, Larson RH: Acute mediastinitis. Surg Clin North Am 49:999, 1969.
224. Moncada R, Warpeha R, Pickleman J, et al: Mediastinitis from odontogenic and deep cervical infection: anatomic pathways of propagation. Chest 73:497, 1978.
225. Wheatley MJ, Stirling MC, Kirsh MM, et al: Descending necrotizing mediastinitis: transcervical drainage is not enough. Ann Thorac Surg 49:780, 1990.
226. Perfect JR: Mediastinitis complicating cellulitis of the head and neck. South Med J 73:1378, 1980.
227. Calandra GB, MacKowiak PA: Retropharyngeal abscess, mediastinitis, and pleural effusion complicating streptococcal facial erysipelas. South Med J 74:1031, 1981.
228. Saks BJ, Kilby AE, Dietrich PA, et al: Pleural and mediastinal changes following endoscopic injection sclerotherapy of esophageal varices. Radiology 149:639, 1983.
229. Fallon WF Jr, Golocovsky M, Paul BK, Champion HR: Suppurative mediastinitis as a complication of long-term total parenteral nutrition therapy via subclavian vein. Clin Care Med 9:558, 1981.
230. Sprinkle PM, Veltri RW, Kantor LM: Abscesses of the head and neck. Laryngoscope 84:1142, 1974.
231. Janecka IP, Rankow RM: Fatal mediastinitis following retropharyngeal abscess. Arch Otolaryngol 93: 630, 1971.
232. Attar S, Hankins JR, Suter CM, et al: Esophageal perforation: a therapeutic challenge. Ann Thorac Surg 50:45, 1990.
233. Kay HR, Goodman LR, Teplick SK, Mundth ED: Use of computed tomography to assess mediastinal complications after median sternotomy. Ann Thorac Surg 36:706, 1983.
234. Engelman RM, Saxena A, Levitsky S: Delayed mediastinal infection after ventricular aneurysm resection. Ann Thorac Surg 25:470, 1978.
235. Moseley PW, Ochsner JL, Mills NL, Chapman J: Management of an infected Hancock prosthesis after repair of truncus arteriosus. J Thorac Cardiovasc Surg 73:306, 1977.
236. Crosby IK, Tegtmeyer C: Mycotic aneurysm of the ascending aorta following coronary revascularization. Ann Thorac Surg 25:474, 1979.
237. Prager RL, Burney P, Waterhouse G, Bender HW Jr: Pulmonary mediastinal and cardiac presentations of histoplasmosis. Ann Thorac Surg 30:385, 1980.
238. Ahmad M, Weinstein AJ, Hughes JA, Cosgrove DE: Granulomatous mediastinitis due to *Aspergillus flavus* in a nonimmunosuppressed patient. Am J Med 70:887, 1981.
239. Katzenstein ALA, Mazur MT: Pulmonary infarct: an unusual manifestation of fibrosing mediastinitis. Chest 77:521, 1980.
240. Mendelson EB, Mintzer RA, Hidvegi DF: Venoocclusive pulmonary infarct: an unusual complication of fibrosing mediastinitis. AJR 141:175, 1983.
241. James EC, Harris SS, Dillenburg CJ: Tracheal stenosis: an unusual presenting complication of idiopathic fibrosing mediastinitis. J Thorac Cardiovasc Surg 80:410, 1980.
242. Chipps BE, Shinnar S, Pickard LR, et al: Spontaneous resolution of multilobar atelectasis secondary to fibrinous mediastinitis. J Pediatr 100:935, 1982.
243. Hutchin P, Lindskog GE: Acquired esophagobronchial fistula of infectious origin. J Thorac Cardiovasc Surg 48:1, 1964.
244. Fairbank JT, Tampas JP, Longstreth G: Superior vena caval obstruction in histoplasmosis. Am J Roentgenol Radium Ther Nucl Med 115:488, 1972.
245. Greenwood MF, Holland P: Tracheal obstruction secondary to *Histoplasma* mediastinal granuloma. Chest 62:642, 1972.
246. Picardi JL, Kauffman CA, Schwarz J, et al: Pericarditis caused by *Histoplasma capsulatum*. Am J Cardiol 37:82, 1976.
247. Pate JW, Hammon J: Superior vena cava syndrome due to histoplasmosis in children. Ann Surg 161: 778, 1965.
248. Rosenbaum AE, Schweepe HI Jr, Rabin ER: Constrictive pericarditis, pneumopericardium, and aortic aneurysm due to *Histoplasma capsulatum*. N Engl J Med 270:935, 1964.
249. Zajtchuk R, Strevey TE, Heydorn WH, Tresure RL: Mediastinal histoplasmosis: surgical considerations. J Thorac Cardiovasc Surg 66:300, 1973.
250. Weinstein JB, Aronberg DJ, Sagel SS: CT of fibrosing mediastinitis: findings and their utility. AJR 141:247, 1983.
251. Urschel HC Jr, Razzuk MA, Netto GS, et al: Sclerosing mediastinitis: improved management with histoplasmosis titre and ketoconazole. Ann Thorac Surg 50:215, 1990.
252. Farmer DW, Moore E, Amparo E, et al: Calcific fibrosing mediastinitis: demonstration of pulmonary vascular obstruction by magnetic resonance imaging. AJR 143:1189, 1984.
253. Belsey R, Hiebert CA: An exclusive right thoracic

approach for cancer of the middle third of the esophagus. Ann Thorac Surg 18:1, 1974.
254. Lyons WS, Seremetis MG, deGuzman VC, Peabody JW Jr: Ruptures and perforations of the esophagus: the case for conservative supportative management. Ann Thorac Surg 25:346, 1978.
255. Orringer MB, Stirling MC: Esophagectomy for esophageal disruption. Ann Thorac Surg 49:35, 1990.
256. Goldberg M, Balthazar E, Nichols R: Subacute pyogenic osteomyelitis of the thoracic spine diagnosed by gallium scan: case report. Ill Med J 148:62, 1975.
257. Pass HI, Macher AM, Shelhammer JH, et al: Thoracic manifestations of the acquired immune deficiency syndrome. J Thorac Cardiovasc Surg 88:654, 1984.
258. McDonald GB, Sharma P, Hackman RC, et al: Esophageal infections in immunosuppressed patients after marrow transplantation. Gastroenterology 88:1111, 1985.
259. Jones JM, Glass NR, Belzer FO: Fatal *Candida* esophagitis in two diabetics after renal transplantation. Arch Surg 117:499, 1982.
260. Levine MS: Radiology of esophagitis: a pattern approach. Radiology 179:1, 1991.
261. Orringer MB, Sloan H: Monilial esophagitis: an increasingly frequent cause of esophageal stenosis? Ann Thorac Surg 26:364, 1978.
262. Hawkins C, Armstrong D: Fungal infections in the immunocompromised host. Clin Haematol 13:599, 1984.
263. Levine MS, Laufer I, Kressel HY, Friedman HM: Herpes esophagitis. AJR 136:863, 1981.
264. Goff JS: Infectious causes of esophagitis. Annu Rev Med 39:163, 1988.

BIBLIOGRAPHY

Bone RC: Pulmonary and Critical Care Medicine. St Louis, Mosby Year Book, 1993.
Hood MR: Surgical Diseases of the Pleura and Chest Wall. Philadelphia, Saunders, 1986.
Rippon JW: Medical Mycology. Philadelphia, Saunders, 1988.
Sabiston DC, Spencer FC: Surgery of the Chest. Philadelphia, Saunders, 1990.
Sarosi GA, Davies SF: Fungal Diseases of the Lung. New York, Raven Press, 1993.
Shields TW: Mediastinal Surgery. Philadelphia, Lea & Febiger, 1991.

Infections of the Heart

CHAPTER 36

Raymond A. Amoury

CARDIAC DEFENSES AGAINST INFECTION

Several anatomic and physiologic characteristics of the heart serve to prevent infection. The most important are the combined effects of the rapid flow of blood through the heart, which normally washes out any organism before it can proliferate, and the smooth endothelial surface, to which bacteria cannot adhere. When the endothelium is damaged, platelets and fibrin form a thrombotic vegetation to which bacteria can adhere. In addition, the slower turbulent flow that results impairs washout and permits proliferation in situ.

Similar protective factors are at work within the myocardium itself. The coronary arteries supply a rich capillary bed. Myocardial contraction eliminates stasis from this vascular network. Any organism that enters the coronary circulation is rapidly washed out. The rich lymphatic supply of the myocardium has a similar function. Miller et al[1] found that dogs with impaired cardiac lymph drainage are more prone to develop acute endocarditis and myocarditis following intravenous injection of staphylococci than are dogs with normal lymphatics. For these reasons, myocardial infection is rarely seen even after myocardial infarction, unless endocarditis is also present. Of minor importance is the action of the pulmonary vascular bed to filter microbes from the circulation before they reach the coronary vessels.

Certain other characteristics of the heart serve to localize or restrict infections when they occur. The pericardial sac is the best example, but several other factors are at work as well. The thick, fibrous, and elastic subendocardial tissues appear to act as a natural barrier against the spread of endocardial infection to the myocardium.[2] The trabeculae carneae tend to entrap foreign bodies (eg, cardiac pacing wires), which tend to become infected.[3] The sinuses of Valsalva are obviously sites of turbulent blood flow and are well-recognized sites of infection.[4]

INFECTIONS OF THE MYOCARDIUM

Myocarditis and Myocardial Abscess

Myocardial Infection in Patients with Coronary Artery Disease. Infection is a rare complication of coronary artery disease, even with advanced ischemia and myocardial necrosis. The same may be said for patients with hypertension, left ventricular hypertrophy, and secondary ischemia. In fact, isolated abscesses of the myocardium seldom occur except in association with endocarditis. Gopalakrishna et al[2] reported a case of myocardial abscess that developed within a myocardial infarction. The infection was caused by group F streptococci, which had metastasized from a metatarsal osteomyelitis. They found 11 other cases in the English literature due to *Staphylococcus aureus* (four cases), *Escherichia coli* (two cases), *Clostridium perfringens* (two cases), *Streptococcus pneumoniae* (one case), beta-hemolytic *Streptococcus pyogenes* (one case), and *Bacteroides* (one case). A primary distant focus of infection was recognized as the source in six cases.

The mechanism of abscess formation within a myocardial infarction is uncertain, but it does not appear to be the result of septic embolization to a major coronary artery, because the artery is usually occluded by a bland thrombus. In addition, the artery walls show no evidence of arteritis. Bacteria probably penetrate the infarct via surrounding collaterals.[2]

Myocardial Infection in Patients with Septicemia. Interstitial myocarditis, myocardial abscess, and mural endocarditis limited to nonvalvular endothelium without valvular lesions or vegetations and with patent coronary arteries are extremely rare. Milstoc and Berger[3] have described a case caused by coagulase-negative *S. aureus.* The sequence of events is presumed to be septicemia, usually from an obvious site, with production of a focus of interstitial myocarditis and subsequent formation of an abscess. The abscess and surrounding interstitial myocardial process then extend to and disrupt the endothelial surface with deposition of a mass of fibrin, bacteria, and blood elements on the endocardial surface.

Myocardial Infection in Patients with Bacterial Endocarditis. Most myocardial abscesses appear in the upper interventricular septum of patients with aortic (or, less often, mitral) endocarditis.[4] The organisms are those that infect the valve. The diagnosis of myocardial abscess is seldom made during the patient's life but should be suspected when a patient with aortic or mitral endocarditis develops conduction disturbances resulting from septal involvement. Echocardiography can be used to support the diagnosis if septal thickening is found. The use of gallium-67 citrate imaging can be helpful when all other diagnostic maneuvers fail. Drainage and valvular replacement have been effective.[4]

Echinococcus *Infection of the Myocardium.* *Echinococcus* is an uncommon cause of infection of the heart and is treatable only by operation. The diagnosis should be considered in patients with cardiac symptoms who have been in an endemic area.[5]

Epidemiology, Incidence, and Pathogenesis. The epidemiology of echinococcosis is discussed in Chapter 12. Echinococcosis is endemic in sheep-raising countries. Humans are accidental hosts after ingesting ova on contaminated vegetables or after handling dogs that shed ova in their feces. In 1977 Shakibi et al[6] reported on the surgical treatment of echinococcal cysts of the heart in two patients and reviewed the world's literature.

Less than 2 percent of the patients with echinococcosis have cardiac involvement, because the larvae must first escape the hepatic and pulmonary filters to reach the coronary arteries. The left ventricular wall and the interventricular septum are most frequently infected, perhaps because of their more extensive blood supply. In a report of 842 cases of thoracic hydatid cysts only two cases involved the heart.[7]

Clinical Manifestations. Most patients with *Echinococcus* disease of the heart are asymptomatic, and the diagnosis is first made by x-ray studies. When symptoms occur, they are generally caused by the enlarging cyst or its rupture. Arrhythmias can result from interference with the conduction system of the interventricular septum. In some cases, heart murmurs are caused by papillary muscle dysfunction that causes valvular insufficiency. A pulmonary systolic ejection murmur can result from the establishment of flow gradients between the right ventricular chamber and pulmonary artery, because of the projection of a cyst into the right ventricular outflow tract. Precordial pain appears to be related to episodes of partial cyst rupture into the pericardium, causing pericarditis, which in turn causes either severe fibrosis (constrictive pericarditis) or pericardial effusion with tamponade. Rupture into a chamber is even more common, as there is no overlying pericardium to reinforce the cyst wall. Rupture into the left ventricle results in systemic emboli, which, if not fatal, can produce metastatic lesions or infarcts. Acute and chronic cor pulmonale and metastatic pulmonary echinococcosis can follow rupture into the right ventricle.

Diagnosis. The most important historic point in the diagnosis is previous hydatid disease in other organs (liver or lung). The Casoni intradermal test and the less specific complement fixation test results are corroborative when positive but do not rule out the diagnosis when they are negative. In Qian's[7] series the Casoni test yielded false-positive results in as many as 37.5 percent of cases. The author used simultaneous, multiple tests including an enzyme-linked immunosorbent peroxidase assay with a 94 percent sensitivity.[7] Eosinophilia is found in less than 25 percent of the patients and may indicate recent infection or rupture. Absence of eosinophilia may indicate death or degeneration of the cyst. Electrocardiographic abnormalities have been noted with hydatid cysts and help to distinguish them from ventricular aneurysms.

X-ray findings are not diagnostic but vary with the stage of the disease. Plain films in various projections help locate the cysts and fluoroscopy reveals an absence of paradoxical pulsation, but the most specific finding is the appearance of a calcification within a mass or in its periphery. Such peripheral calcification, if constrictive pericarditis is not present, indicates *Echinococcus* disease of the heart.

Angiocardiography is the most informative of the radiologic studies because it indicates the degree of penetration of a cyst into a cardiac chamber and differentiates a cyst from a ventricular aneurysm. Coronary arteriography shows displacement of vessels by a cyst and its lack of vascularization. The differential diagnosis includes mediastinal and cardiac tumors, pericardial cysts, and ventricular aneurysms. In those rare cases where the cyst presents with atrioventricular conduction disturbances, echocardiograph localization of a mass in the interventricular septum may be adequate and has been reported in a patient in whom atrioventricular conduction was restored after removal of a hydatid cyst of the interventricular septum.[8]

Treatment. Excision is the only effective treatment for cardiac echinococcosis. If the cyst is accessible, it can be aspirated and any remaining viable scoleces can be killed by the instillation of 2 percent formalin, ether, or, preferably, concentrated (30 percent) sodium chloride to prevent dissemination if the contents are spilled. The cyst can then be opened to remove its germinative lining.

When a cyst projects into a cardiac chamber with danger of rupture, a cardiopulmonary bypass is recommended for greater mobilization of the heart and adequate control should an intracavitary cyst rupture or a ventricle be perforated. In addition, bypass allows for resection of the heart wall if necessary, as in treating an aneurysm of the ventricle. A one-stage operation for treatment of cardiac and pulmonary echinococcosis has been described.[9]

Trypanosoma cruzi *Infection of the Myocardium.* Myocarditis in Chagas' disease is caused by *T. cruzi* and can result in severe cardiomyopathy. Dynamic cardiomyoplasty using latissimus dorsi has been reported as a palliative procedure in such patients, as cardiac transplantation has resulted in a high incidence of recurrence of *T. cruzi* infection.[10]

Myocardial Infections in the Immunologically Compromised Patient. Many factors can alter host resistance to make a patient abnormally susceptible to myocardial infections (see Chap. 51). For example, myocardial abscesses occurred in 67 percent of patients with *Aspergillus* endocarditis.[11] Candidal myocardial infections have been reported in patients treated with steroids, in leukemia patients treated with chemotherapeutic drugs, and in patients with burns. Most of these patients have small, diffuse abscesses that are not amenable to drainage (Fig. 36–1). Myocardial abscess in the interventricular septum has been reported in a hemophiliac with AIDS-related complex. This was successfully treated with debridement and patch repair with autologous pericardium.[12]

Myocardial Infections Caused by Trauma. Nonpenetrating chest trauma can cause cardiac contusion and, occasionally, valvular injury, such as

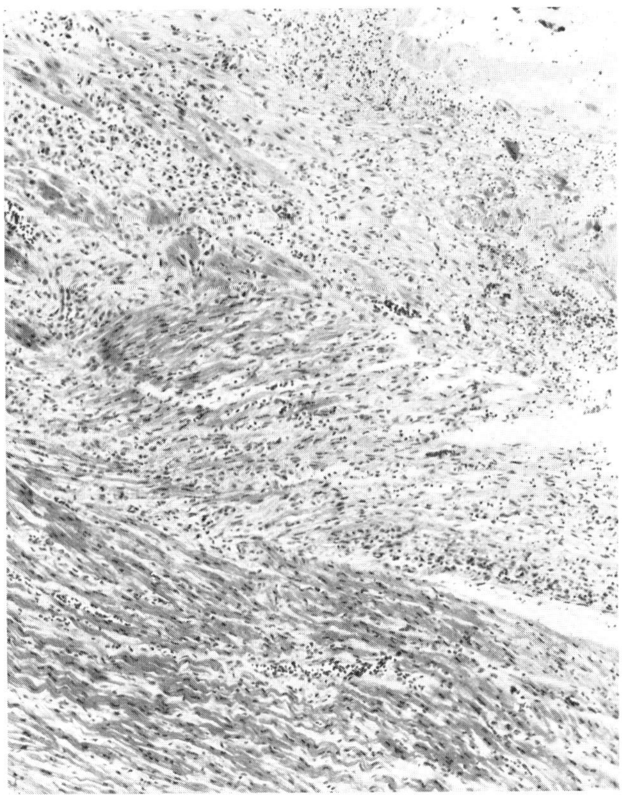

Figure 36–1. Microabscesses in the myocardium of a severely burned child. Multifocal abscesses were present at postmortem examination. She died as a consequence of *Staphylococcus aureus* (coagulase-positive) sepsis.

aortic insufficiency. Infection of a traumatically damaged valve is rare.[13] Penetrating wounds of the heart can cause both pericarditis and endocarditis. Enders et al[14] emphasize that both wound infection and intracardiac infection are less common than expected. *Pseudomonas aeruginosa* and *S. aureus* have been reported as etiologic agents.[15] Projectiles embedded in the heart for a long time may also be sites for infection.[16]

INFECTIVE ENDOCARDITIS

Infective endocarditis (IE) is the most important infection of the heart. This subject has been reviewed in detail in monographs edited by Kaye,[17] Kaplan and Taranta,[18] Rahimtoola,[19] and Bisno[20] and, most recently, in the comprehensive text also edited by Kaye.[21] This section discusses only infections of the native endocardium. Subsequent sections deal with prosthetic valve endocarditis.

Classification, Incidence, and Underlying Heart Disease. The established classification of endocarditis into acute and subacute forms has given way to a classification based on the identity of the causative microorganism and underlying anatomy, because both clinical features and treatment vary according to the organism.[17,21,22] The incidence of infectious endocarditis ranges from 0.3 to 3 per 1000 hospital admissions. More than one-half of the patients are older than 50. Because endocarditis is found at areas of turbulence, such as at damaged or deformed valves, and at sites of high pressure, cardiac conditions associated with turbulence predispose to these infections. Several factors predispose to infective endocarditis (Table 36–1).

RHEUMATIC HEART DISEASE. Nearly 50 percent of the patients with endocarditis have had rheumatic heart disease, but the incidence is falling. Earlier reports implicated rheumatic carditis in one-third of pediatric patients with endocarditis in contrast to more recent series where 1.5 to 10 percent occur on valves damaged by rheumatic valvulitis.[22] The mitral valve is most frequently deformed by the rheumatic process and is the most common site for endocarditis. The aortic valve is next most commonly deformed, and it is infected alone or in combination (usually with the mitral valve) in over half the patients. Infection of the tricuspid valve occurs in less than 10 percent of patients with rheumatic heart disease and is usually accompanied by infection of the aortic or mitral heart valve.

TABLE 36–1. FACTORS PREDISPOSING TO THE DEVELOPMENT OF INFECTIVE ENDOCARDITIS

- CARDIAC
  - Congenital lesions
    - Ventricular septal defect
    - Tetralogy of Fallot
    - Aortic stenosis
    - Pulmonic stenosis
    - Complex cyanotic anomalies
    - Patent ductus arteriosus
    - Systemic to pulmonary artery shunts
  - Lesions of obscure etiology
    - Mitral valve prolapse
    - Idiopathic hypertrophic subaortic stenosis
    - Bicuspid aortic valve
    - Myxomatous degeneration of cardiac valves
  - Acquired lesions
    - Rheumatic valvular disease
    - Degenerative cardiac lesions
      - Arteriosclerotic valvular disease associated with valvular insufficiency
      - Calcific aortic stenosis
      - Calcific mitral stenosis
      - Traumatic valvular lesions
  - Patients with prosthetic cardiac valves
  - Patients with pacemakers
- NONCARDIAC
  - Compromised hosts
  - Patients with intravenous devices
    - For hyperalimentation
    - For prolonged administration of medications
    - For cancer chemotherapy
  - Drug addiction: "mainliners"

From Arbulu A, Asfaw I: Infective endocarditis. In Bave AE, Geha AS, Hammond GL, et al (eds): Glenn's Thoracic and Cardiovascular Surgery, 5th ed. Norwalk, CT, Appleton & Lange, 1991, p 1647.

CONGENITAL HEART DISEASE. Approximately one-fifth of the patients with IE have congenital heart lesions. Patent ductus arteriosus, ventricular septal defects, bicuspid aortic valve, coarctation of the aorta, pulmonic stenosis, and tetralogy of Fallot are the most commonly associated lesions. In children, IE accounts for 0.24 to 0.55 per 1000 hospital admissions.[23]

NO APPARENT HEART DISEASE. Certain organisms can attack normal valves and cause endocarditis in patients without underlying heart disease. As many as 50 percent or more of the patients with endocarditis caused by *S. aureus, Streptococcus pneumoniae,* group A beta-hemolytic *Streptococcus,* and *Enterococcus* species may have no underlying heart disease. Opportunistic infections also occur on normal valves in patients with defects in host defenses, in those receiving antibiotic therapy, and in drug addicts. In addition, patients having prolonged use of central venous or umbilical catheters may also develop infectious endocarditis. High-risk neonates and older infants may even develop endocarditis without catheter exposure.[24] In one case this occurred on a normal mitral valve and was secondary to sepsis. Debridement of the vegetations and closure of a perforation of the posterior leaflet resulted in a good outcome.[25] Invasive monitoring and nutritional support using intravascular catheters are also risk factors for endocarditis.[27–29] A rare case of nonbacterial thrombotic endocarditis has been reported with the use of a peritoneovenous shunt in a patient with ascites.[26]

DEGENERATIVE HEART DISEASE. Degenerative or atherosclerotic lesions seldom predispose to infection, but the incidence appears to be increasing in the older population, especially in men with calcific aortic stenosis. Rare cases of endocarditis in patients with coronary artery disease have been reported.

ARTERIOVENOUS FISTULAS. Peripheral arteriovenous fistulas have been created in animals to produce endocarditis, and this association has been found in humans with acquired arteriovenous fistulas. Patients with hemodialysis shunts in place can also develop endocarditis, and Quintiliani and Ganguli[30] reported a rare association of splenic arteriovenous fistula with bacterial endarteritis and endocarditis caused by coagulase-negative *Staphylococcus.* Coronary arteriovenous fistulas are rare lesions and are seldom complicated by bacterial endarteritis.

OTHER PREDISPOSING LESIONS AND CONDITIONS. Subaortic stenosis was a major cause of endocarditis in the preantibiotic era, and acute endocarditis is occasionally seen in patients with idiopathic hypertrophic subaortic stenosis.[31,32] Mitral involvement can also occur. Mitral valve prolapse syndrome is a recently defined lesion that predisposes to IE[33,34] and now appears to be the most common lesion predisposing to IE in adults. The incidence of risks of IE have been summarized.[22] Syphilitic aortitis is seldom found in patients with endocarditis and does not appear to increase a patient's susceptibility.

A rare cause of IE is infection in a cardiac tumor. Flynn et al[35] reviewed the literature and reported a *Veillonella* infection in a right atrial myxoma with survival following resection. Diabetes mellitus may increase the susceptibility of patients to IE with accelerated atherosclerosis and occurrence of calcific nodular valve lesions, in addition to soft tissue and urinary tract infections, which can serve as sources of bacteremia.[22] The uncommon occurrence of IE in pregnancy has also been summarized[22] with dental procedures being more common portals of entry for bacteria than vaginal delivery or cesarean section. Predisposing factors noted included premature labor, premature rupture of membranes, prolonged third stage of labor, and manual removal of the placenta.[22]

Pathology of Infective Endocarditis. The pathology of IE must include the pathologic alterations in the heart and in other organs.

CARDIAC PATHOLOGY. Vegetations are classically found on the valves of patients with IE (Fig. 36–2). These lesions vary in number, size, color, and consistency and tend to localize on the atrial surfaces of the atrioventricular valves and on the ventricular surfaces of the semilunar valves. Histologically, the vegetation consists of an amorphous mass of fibrin, leukocytes, and masses of red blood cell debris and bacteria. These may be suppurative, or show destruction of the underlying valve, or both. Granulation tissue is seen at the base of the lesion, with a nonspecific inflammatory response. The bacteria may be difficult to identify or may be seen at the surface or in the interior of the vegetation. If antibiotic therapy is successful, fibrosis, hyalinization,

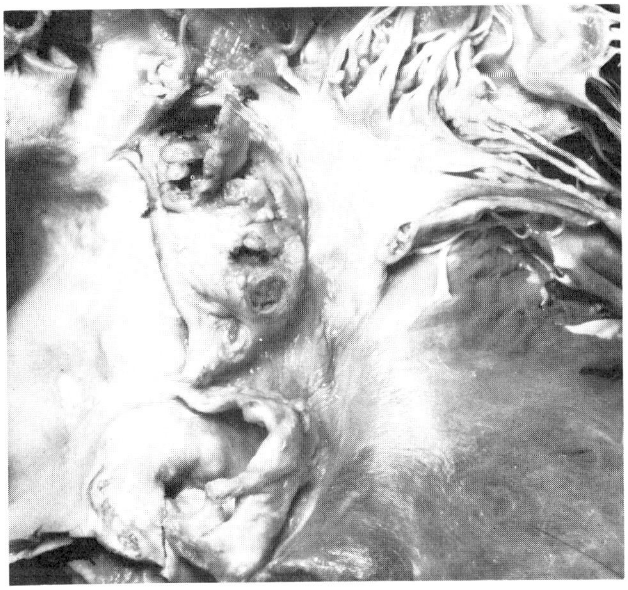

Figure 36–2. Aortic valve showing background of rheumatic fibrosis and retraction of one cusp. Other two cusps show numerous vegetations from bacterial endocarditis caused by beta-hemolytic *Streptococcus. (Courtesy of Jesse E. Edwards, MD, Department of Pathology, United Hospitals, Inc., Miller Division, St. Paul, Minnesota).*

and calcification of the vegetation occur with reendothelialization. Outpouchings, or aneurysms, of portions of a valve can develop in an area of valvulitis from scarring and altered hydrodynamics. Other destructive effects produced by vegetations are perforation, erosive aneurysms of the sinus of Valsalva, ruptures of papillary muscles or of chordea tendineae, and abscesses of the valve ring at times with fistula formation and rupture of the interventricular septum[36,37] (Fig. 36–3). Mural thrombi in the atria or ventricles can occur at sites of turbulence (eg, ventricular septal defects, stenotic or regurgitant valves) but mural endocardial infection is rare in the absence of concomitant valve infection.[38]

Myocarditis is an important complication of endocarditis and is recognized with increased frequency. Its pathogenesis is unclear, but ischemic damage secondary to coronary artery occlusion by emboli, damage as a result of microbial toxins, invasion of the myocardium by microorganisms, and activity of immune complexes resulting in a vasculitis of arterioles and capillaries have all been suggested as causes. Myocardial abscesses containing bacteria have been found in about one-fifth of cases. Involvement of the pericardium is uncommon.[38] In acute IE, pericarditis is usually due to extension from an aortic or other ring abscess, from an infected aneurysm of the ascending aorta, or from a myocardial abscess. Noninfective pericarditis may occur with rheumatic carditis and in immune complex related diseases.[38]

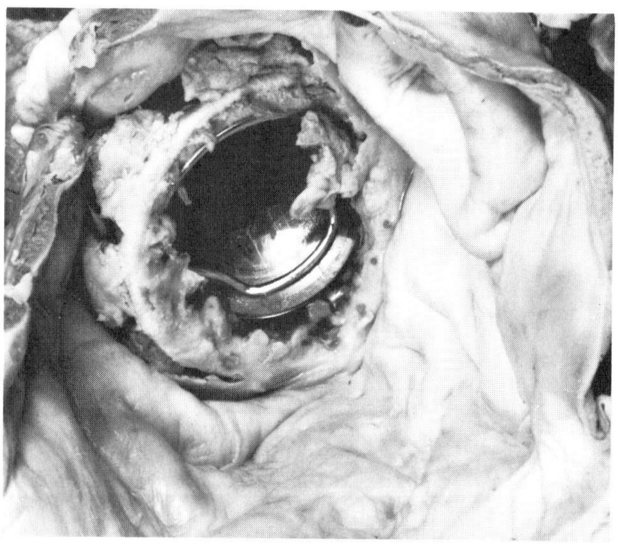

Figure 36–3. Interior of left atrium and view of Bjork-Shiley prosthesis from above. Vegetations and dehiscence of prosthetic valve seat are the result of bacterial infection. *(Courtesy of Jesse E. Edwards, MD, Department of Pathology, United Hospitals, Inc., Miller Division, St. Paul, Minnesota.)*

PATHOGENESIS OF THE CARDIAC LESIONS. The characteristic lesion in IE is an infected thrombus or vegetation on the endocardial surface, usually along the closing edges of the valve leaflets or cusps. There seem to be two mechanisms by which valves can become infected. The first is embolization of microorganisms to the valvular interstitium. This mechanism is unlikely because valves are vascularized only at their proximal parts, which are rarely colonized early in the disease. The more likely mechanism is infection of the endocardium by implantation of microorganisms on the endocardial surfaces of the valve.

The primary valvular lesion appears to be the result of platelet aggregation induced by contact with a foreign surface, that is, the endocardial surface previously damaged by disease or hemodynamic alteration. A nonbacterial thrombus composed largely of platelets becomes adherent to the site of endothelial damage.[37–39] Such sterile thrombi are found in patients with rheumatic heart disease, as well as in patients with malignant and wasting disease and with connective tissue disorders, such as systemic lupus erythematosus (SLE). They serve as predisposing sites for bacterial endocarditis in rheumatic heart disease, but for obscure reasons are often harmless in the other conditions. Subsequent bacteremia can result in colonization of the platelet fibrin mass with the establishment of infection. Although nonbacterial thrombotic endocarditis (NBTE) is generally seen in adults over 50 years of age, it has been found in neonates and in patients with collagen diseases such as SLE, burns, septicemia, disseminated intravascular coagulation (DIC), and in association with intracardiac catheters. It has been speculated that a hypercoagulable state may be promoted by intravascular mucin produced by adenocarcinomas. In SLE, direct endothelial cell injury from the deposition of circulating immune complexes add to a hypercoagulable state to produce NBTE. In patients with DIC the fibrinolytic activity of normal endothelial cells is lost and localized areas of thrombosis can occur.[39]

Nonbacterial and bacterial endocarditis share the same location and frequency of involvement. For example, in both acute rheumatic fever and bacterial endocarditis the atrial surface of the mitral valve and the ventricular surface of the aortic valve are most frequently involved, followed by the aortic, the tricuspid, and, rarely, the pulmonic valves.

Platelet aggregation can be induced by a variety of stimuli in addition to thrombin, epinephrine, and adenosine diphosphate.[38] Clawson[40] has pointed out that some common bacterial pathogens, such as staphylococci and streptococci, may themselves act to stimulate platelet aggregation. This results in the incorporation of the bacteria into the aggregate. The location of large numbers of bacteria deep within the sanctuary of a platelet-fibrin mass provides a mechanical barrier to their elimination by phagocytes and probably to penetration by antibiotics and antibodies. Clawson has reviewed other interactions between platelets and bacteria.[40] Once the sterile thrombus is in place, bacteremia from any source can infect the damaged valve—a local infection in the skin, infected thrombi within the bloodstream, and direct inoculation of bacteria into the circulation. Most cases of clinical endocarditis, however, appear to arise from transient bacteremia, which occurs in normal individuals without a septic focus. Manipulation of contaminated mucosal surfaces can produce transient bacteremia. For example, people develop bacteremia after brushing their teeth or using an oral irrigation apparatus (Table 36–2). Tooth extraction causes a mixed bacteremia, with viridans streptococci and *Bacteroides melaninogenicus* as the predominant organisms in a majority of patients. The frequency of bacteremia from these sources is related to the degree of periodontal disease and the degree of trauma inflicted during the procedure, with infection being the more important factor. In addition, sigmoidoscopy and barium enema can both induce bacteremia, as do transurethral prostatic resection, cystoscopy, urethral dilatation and catheterization, abortion, delivery, and instrumentation of the female reproductive tract.[41] The properties of certain bacteria that enable them to adhere to endothelium are discussed in a subsequent section.

TABLE 36–2. INCIDENCE OF BACTEREMIA AFTER VARIOUS PROCEDURES

Procedure/Manipulation	Percentage of Positive Blood Cultures
• DENTAL	
Dental extraction	18–85
Periodontal surgery	32–88
Chewing candy or paraffin	17–51
Tooth brushing	0–26
Oral irrigation device	27–50
• UPPER AIRWAY	
Bronchoscopy (rigid scope)	15
Tonsillectomy	28–38
Nasotracheal suctioning/intubation	16
• GASTROINTESTINAL	
Upper GI endoscopy	8–12
Sigmoidoscopy/colonoscopy	0–9.5
Barium enema	11
Percutaneous needle biopsy of liver	3–13
• UROLOGIC	
Urethral dilatation	18–33
Urethral catheterization	8
Cystoscopy	0–17
Transurethral prostatic resection	12–46
• OBSTETRIC/GYNECOLOGIC	
Normal vaginal delivery	0–11
Punch biopsy cervix	0
Removal/insertion of IUD	0

From Scheld WM, Sande MA: Endocarditis and intravascular infections. In Mandell G, Douglas RG, Bennett JE (eds): Principles and Practice of Infectious Diseases, 3rd ed. New York, Churchill Livingstone, 1990, p 673.

Valve dysfunction can result from either obstruction or destruction of the valve. As a result of continued deposition of platelets and fibrin, the vegetation can grow and obstruct the orifice. This is especially likely in fungal endocarditis but has also been reported with staphylococcal endocarditis of the mitral valve.[42] In other instances, especially in *S. aureus* endocarditis, destruction of tissue with resulting valvular insufficiency can be the result. In still other cases, healing with scar formation can produce valvular insufficiency or stenosis. Infection can also extend into the myocardium from the periphery of a valve, as into the mitral annulus or along the sinus of Valsalva into the aortic ring, and produce burrowing abscesses. Septic emboli from infected, necrotic, calcified vegetations can produce infarcts in the lung, heart, brain, kidneys, spleen, liver, and extremities. Metastatic abscesses may develop especially when *S. aureus* endocarditis is the source of the emboli. Septic embolization to the vasa vasorum or direct bacterial invasion of the arterial wall can predispose to the formation of mycotic aneurysms in the sinus of Valsalva and the aorta and its branches with the potential for rupture.

EXPERIMENTAL ENDOCARDITIS. Some experimental models of endocarditis have shed light on the pathogenesis of the disease. For example, endocarditis occurs naturally in the opossum, in which the stress of captivity appears to predispose to the infection. As in humans, the infection is caused by viridans streptococci, and the mitral and aortic valves are primarily involved. Bacterial inoculation consistently produces the disease in this species. Experimental endocarditis can be produced in many other animals; transarterial trauma to the aortic and mitral valves, high altitude, hypothermia, polycythemia, and administration of vasoactive substances all predispose to valvulitis and vegetations.

Lillehei et al[43] created arteriovenous (AV) fistulas in dogs as a method of producing endocardial changes and increasing the likelihood of valve deformities and endocarditis. The shunt must be large enough to increase cardiac output; the number and dimension of the fistulas required varied inversely with the age of the animal; younger animals required significantly more peripheral shunt flow to produce endocarditis. These investigators concluded that any condition that increased cardiac output could cause endocardial damage, leading to a nonbacterial thrombotic endocarditis that subsequently became infected.

Experimental endocarditis can be achieved in rabbits or rats by positioning a polyethylene catheter within the heart. Catheters cause endothelial cell damage by direct contact with valve surfaces and by causing flow disturbances. In this manner, the catheter induces vegetations, which can then become infected. If the catheter is removed long enough (before microbial inoculation) for the valve to reendothelialize, susceptibility to colonization is reduced.[44] The level of metabolic activity of bacterial colonies in these vegetations was determined using tritiated L-alanine. The colonies in the periphery of the vegetation are the most active, whereas those in the interior are less active. Because some antibiotics depend on cell wall synthesis and cell division for their bactericidal action, the interior organisms may be difficult to eradicate. Hooke and Sande[45] prevented development of thrombotic vegetations by anticoagulation, but this did not prevent valvular colonization. The authors suggested that the fibrin vegetation actually retarded the disease by containing the bacteria. In the treated animals, the absence of vegetations allowed for more rapid eradication of infection, suggesting that rapid bacterial division on the outside of the vegetation makes them more susceptible to penicillin. These studies have definite correlates in clinical disease, especially in prosthetic valve infections.

A number of investigators have studied the possible role of cardiac lymphatic obstruction in the pathogenesis of cardiac disease, but the exact role in endocarditis is not yet clear. Symbas et al[46] studied the susceptibility to endocarditis in three groups of dogs. In six dogs no surgical procedure was done; in six dogs the cardiac lymphatics were interrupted; and in six animals two AV fistulas were created. Five million *S. aureus* organisms were injected intravenously three times at 3-day intervals. None of the control dogs developed endocarditis, and only one dog in the group with interrupted cardiac lymphatics developed chronic myocarditis without endocarditis. In the group with AV fistulas, three out of the six dogs developed endocarditis with gram-negative rods but not with the injected staphylococci.

Animal models of endocarditis provide important data in planning prophylactic and therapeutic antimicrobial regimens. For example, bacteriostatic drugs were of no value in experimental streptococcal endocarditis even when used on a sensitive organism for a prolonged period; bactericidal regimens were necessary. Multiple factors are involved in models using viridans streptococci, *Staphylococcus aureus, Streptococcus faecalis, Pseudomonas, Candida,* and *Aspergillus.*[47] These studies indicate that effective prophylaxis is dependent on use of a microbicidal regimen that will achieve high blood levels for 6 hours or more after an episode of bacteremia.

Noncardiac Pathologic Features Associated with Infective Endocarditis

KIDNEY. Diffuse glomerulonephritis (GN) is characterized by hypercellularity in all glomeruli with two variants described with IE. Acute proliferative GN resembles poststreptococcal GN with swollen endothelial cells and neutrophils in glomeruli in contrast to the membranoproliferative variant that shows mesangial widening.[38]

Diffuse GN may be a reaction to circulating antigen-antibody complexes. This concept is supported by electron microscopic studies showing dense, subepithelial deposits in the glomeruli of patients with endocarditis and nephritis, as well as deposits of immune globulins in glomerular basement membranes. Chronicity of infection may be important, as it is necessary for the organism or its antigens to stimulate antibody production and also to supply antigen for the formation of soluble complexes. The site of deposition in the glomeruli appears to depend on the size of the complex. In this way, small complexes formed under conditions of antigen excess are found in a subepithelial locus and are associated with diffuse proliferation. Large antigen-antibody complexes formed under conditions of antibody excess are deposited on the inside of the glomerular basement membrane and are accompanied by focal nephritis.

Other renal lesions include interstitial nephritis, petechiae, and emboli from infected cardiac vegetations, which can cause mycotic aneurysms, arteritis, and renal abscesses. Embolic (or focal) GN is characterized by discrete deposits of fibrin, sclerosis, and infarcts in scattered glomeruli. Focal GN may also show the granular deposits of immunoglobulin, especially IgG and complement (C_1) with immunoflorescence.[38]

SKIN. Petechiae and subungual splinter hemorrhages may be caused by emboli or hypersensitivity vasculitis. Osler nodes are the painful, erythematous elevations found in the digital pads, and these may be caused by hypersensitivity vasculitis, probably secondary to immune complex deposition. Janeway nodes are painless hemorrhagic lesions that occur on the palms, soles, or tips of the digits. They are necrotic and contain polymorphonuclear leukocytes and bacteria.[37]

SPLEEN. Splenomegaly is frequently found. Microscopically, there is hyperplasia of lymphoid follicles and often considerable proliferation of reticuloendothelial cells, probably resulting from chronic stimulation of the reticuloendothelial system from prolonged bacteremia and circulating immune complexes.[38] Splenic infarcts are noted in about one-third of patients coming to autopsy.

CENTRAL NERVOUS SYSTEM AND EYE. Mycotic aneurysms, embolic infarcts, and arteritis are all common. Additional findings include intracerebral and subarachnoid hemorrhage and encephalomalacia. Meningitis is uncommon. In the eye, petechial hemorrhages in the conjunctiva and retina are common, as are flame-shaped retinal hemorrhages.[37] White spots, or cotton-wool exudates, are also seen and histologically represent small infarcts in the nerve fiber layer of the retina, while the white-centered petechial hemorrhages (so-called Roth spots) are due to extravasated red blood cells with small collections of leukocytes. They also occur in other conditions.

IMMUNOLOGIC PHENOMENA. A number of immunologic phenomena accompany endocarditis. Circulating antibodies against the pathogen appear. Hypergammaglobulinemia is associated with an increase in the plasma cells of the bone marrow. Approximately half the patients have positive serum tests for rheumatoid factor within 6 weeks. Complement levels may be low in patients in whom immune complex GN develops. Circulating cryoglobulins may appear and cause vascular occlusions in the digits of some patients. Hyperstimulation of the macrophage system is manifested by histiocytes in the peripheral blood. The role, if any, of each of these findings in the pathogenesis of the clinical manifestations of IE is, as yet, not clear.[41]

Etiology of Infective Endocarditis

COMMON INFECTIOUS AGENTS. Although almost any bacteria are capable of producing bacterial endocarditis, streptococci and staphylococci account for 90 to 95 percent of cases in which an infecting organism can be identified (Table 36–3).

TABLE 36–3. FREQUENCY OF VARIOUS ORGANISMS CAUSING INFECTIVE ENDOCARDITIS[a]

Organism	NVE (%)	IV Drug Abusers (%)	Early PVE (%)	Late PVE (%)
Streptococci	65	15	10	35
Viridans, alpha-hemolytic	35	5	<5	25
S. bovis (group D)	15	<5	<5	<5
S. faecalis (group D)	10	8	<5	<5
Other streptococci	<5	<5	<5	<5
Staphylococci	25	50	50	30
Coagulase-positive	23	50	20	10
Coagulase-negative	<5	<5	30	20
Gram-negative aerobic bacilli	<5	5	20	15
Fungi	<5	5	10	5
Miscellaneous bacteria	<5	5	5	5
Diphtheroids, propionibacteria	<1	<5	5	<5
Other anaerobes	<1	<1	<1	<1
Rickettsia	<1	<1	<1	<1
Chlamydia	<1	<1	<1	<1
Polymicrobial infection	<1	5	5	5
Culture-negative endocarditis	5–10	5	<5	<5

[a] These are representative figures collated from the literature; wide local variations in frequency are to be expected. NVE, native valve endocarditis; PVE, prosthetic valve endocarditis.

From Durack DT: Infective and noninfective endocarditis. In Hurst JW, Logue RB, Rackley CE, et al (eds): The Heart, Arteries and Veins, 6th ed. New York, McGraw-Hill, 1986, p 1130.

STREPTOCOCCI. Streptococci are the causative microorganisms in 60 to 80 percent of blood culture-positive cases of IE[48,49] The viridans streptococci account for more than one-half of cases of streptococcal endocarditis. The viridans streptococci (*S. mitior, S. sanguis, S. milleri, S. salivarius,* and *S. mutans*) are alpha-hemolytic and generally not typeable in the Lancefield system. *Streptococcus bovis* normally inhabits the gastrointestinal tract of humans. It is a group D streptococcus and is an important cause of IE. *Streptococcus bovis* bacteremia has been associated with carcinoma of the colon and other gastrointestinal lesions and can occur in patients without gastrointestinal symptoms. This suggests that the lower gastrointestinal tract should be evaluated when *S. bovis* is isolated from blood cultures.[48,49] Enterococci cause between 10 and 20 percent of the cases, but the relative incidence is increasing. Enterococci were previously classified as Lancefield's group D. They are now established as a separate genus. They are normally found in the gastrointestinal and genital tracts and may show alpha-, beta-, or gamma-hemolysis on blood agar. Microaerophilic and anaerobic streptococci, nonhemolytic streptococci, group A beta-hemolytic streptococci, and streptococci of other groups account for the rest. Group B streptococcal sepsis is a serious problem in neonates but it is an uncommon cause of endocarditis. Group C streptococcal endocarditis is rare, with 16 cases reported.[50] Almost all cases of anaerobic endocarditis are due to streptococci.[51]

The biology and taxonomy of the streptococci are discussed in Chapter 4. The dextran-forming strains were more often found in endocardial infection than the nondextran-producing strains, although the role of dextran is not completely known. Dextran-like polysaccharides (eg, glucan) may be important in adherence of these bacteria to both teeth and endocardial tissue. In a rabbit model, Dall et al[52] have shown that treatment of dextran-producing streptococcal endocarditis with dextranase and penicillin resulted in higher rates of sterilization compared to penicillin alone.[52] Theoretically, dextranase hydrolyzes the dextran glycocalyx, reduces adherence, and renders the streptococci more susceptible to penicillin. The potential for developing a hypersensitivity reaction to the enzyme precludes its use clinically.

Striking differences in adherence of bacteria to endocardial tissue can be observed. Enterococci are most adherent, followed by staphylococci and viridans streptococci. *Pseudomonas aeruginosa* and *E. coli* are much less adherent. This may be related to fibronectin, which is secreted by endothelial cells, platelets, and fibroblasts. It occurs in thrombotic lesions in response to vascular injury. Gram-negative organisms do not bind to fibronectin but *S. aureus,* viridans streptococci, *S. pneumoniae,* other streptococci, and *Candida* species have fibronectin receptors, which appear to be lipoteichoic acid on some streptococci. Organisms may become coated with soluble fibronectin and attach to normal heart valves, collagen, or fibrin. The roles of fibronectin, tissue thromboplastin, thrombospondin, and slime have been summarized by Livornese and Korzeniowski.[39] The ability to adhere to valvular endothelium may be an essential characteristic of the bacteria that cause human endocarditis. An intriguing hypothesis has been raised by studies of endothelial cell monolayers, which have shown that vascular endothelium can phagocytize *S. aureus* and *Candida.*[53,54] Theoretically, these organisms can make contact with an intact valve and, following phagocytosis, can multiply intracellularly and destroy the endothelial cell, causing destruction of the endothelial surface and induction of platelet and fibrin deposition.[39]

STAPHYLOCOCCI. Staphylococci are the causative microorganisms in 10 to 30 percent of cases with positive blood cultures. The biology of the staphylococci is discussed in Chapter 4. Coagulase-positive staphylococci are isolated much more frequently than coagulase-negative staphylococci, especially in patients with the acute form of bacterial endocarditis. Coagulase-positive staphylococci can attack either normal or previously damaged heart valves and cause rapid destruction of valve substance with a fulminant and often fatal course. Death can occur within days from overwhelming bacteremia and within weeks from heart failure. Multifocal abscesses also occur from septic emboli and infarcts.

Coagulase-negative staphylococci account for only 1 to 3 percent of blood culture-positive endocarditis and are seen in patients with more subacute disease. These organisms usually attack heart valves with preexisting abnormalities or damage, without causing rapid destruction. The adherence properties of *S. epidermidis* may be related to the production of slime. This extracellular mucoid substance may also play a role in cerebrospinal fluid shunt infections. In the rat, Baddour et al[55] found slime-positive strains of *S. epidermidis* to produce endocarditis much more consistently than when the animals were challenged with slime-negative inocula of these organisms. The role of slime production in IE is unclear as is its correlation with pathogenicity.[52]

The incidence of coagulase-positive staphylococcal endocarditis is increasing in drug addicts and patients with endocarditis following prosthetic valve replacement. In the latter group, coagulase-negative staphylococci are also a major cause of endocarditis.[56]

UNCOMMON INFECTIOUS AGENTS. Table 36–4 lists the less common and rare organisms associated with endocarditis. Almost all species of bacteria have been reported. Pneumococci have become uncommon causes of infective endocarditis (5 percent of cases) since effective therapy of pneumonia and otitis media became available. Once established, pneumococci can attack normal or previously damaged valves and can cause rapid destruction. The gonococcus can attack and destroy either normal or previously damaged heart valves and was once a common cause of right heart endocarditis. It is now seldom seen.

Aside from the anaerobic streptococci, the most common anaerobes causing endocarditis are *Bacteroides* and *Actinomyces*.[51]

MIXED INFECTIONS. Two or more organisms are seldom involved simultaneously except in *Candida* infections, in which bacteria such as *S. aureus* may coexist with and probably precede the *Candida* infection. Prolonged antibiotic treatment of bacterial endocarditis can predispose to fungal superinfection.

FUNGI. Fungal endocarditis is uncommon (see Table 36–4), occurring principally in (1) narcotics addicts; (2) patients receiving intravenous hyperalimentation; (3) patients receiving steroids, cytotoxic agents, and broad spectrum antibiotics; and (4) patients with infected intracardiac prostheses.[56] *Candida, Aspergillus,* and *Histoplasma* species are the most common causes of fungal endocarditis, with *Candida* leading in overall frequency. *Candida albicans* is the most common candidal organism isolated, but *C. tropicalis, C. krusei, C. parapsilosis,* and other candidal species have also been found.

TABLE 36–4. UNCOMMON AND RARE ORGANISMS IN ENDOCARDITIS

• PYOGENIC COCCI	• OTHER RARE CAUSES
S. pneumoniae	Meningococci
N. gonorrhoeae	*Coxiella burnetii*
	Diphtheroids
• GRAM-NEGATIVE BACILLAE	*Spirillum minus*
Salmonella	*Listeria*
Streptobacillus moniliformis	Micrococci
Serratia marcescens	Propionibacterium
Bacteroides	
Hemophilus	• FUNGI
Brucella	*Candida* } Most common
Yersenia	*Aspergillus* } Most common
Cardiobacterium	*Histoplasma* } Most common
Actinobacillus	*Blastomyces*
Citrobacter	*Cryptococcus*
Chlamydia	*Mucor*
• PARASITES	*Torulopsis*

CELL WALL-DEFICIENT FORMS. These forms are usually isolated using hypertonic media when routine blood cultures are sterile. They are induced by antibiotics, and their presence does not necessarily implicate them in the pathologic process. Their persistence during therapy and subsequent reversion to the parent form may explain some relapses. The failure of penicillin as the sole therapy against enterococcal endocarditis is illustrative. In this situation, cell wall-deficient forms may be induced by penicillin. Successful therapy requires the addition of an aminoglycoside that is active against these bacterial forms. The frequency of cell wall-deficient bacteria in endocarditis is unknown and their virulence in causing IE uncertain. For example, in experimentally produced NBTE in rabbits, single intravenous injections of streptococci, staphylococci, *Proteus mirabilis,* or *Candida albicans* all led to the development of IE. However, no infection occurred after injection of L-forms of *S. faecalis* or coxsackie B-4 virus.[57]

COXIELLA BURNETII. The cause of Q fever has been found also to cause endocarditis in patients with underlying heart disease. *Coxiella burnetii* is the only established cause of rickettsial endocarditis and affects prosthetic heart valves, as well as native valves. Blood cultures are usually negative, and although the course of the disease is characteristic of IE, antibiotic therapy is usually unsuccessful, and valve replacement plus antimicrobial therapy is often required. It is possible to isolate the organism by inoculating the patient's blood into guinea pigs; however, a rise in titer of complement-fixing antibody to *C. burnetii* is usually necessary to make the diagnosis[58] (see Chap. 9).

VIRUS INFECTIONS. These can cause valve lesions in animals, but there is no evidence that viral infections can cause a clinical syndrome resembling bacterial or fungal endocarditis.

Clinical Manifestations Infective endocarditis is capable of multiple organ system involvement, and clinical manifestations can therefore show marked variability. Variations in the patient's course will also depend on the offending organism. Endocarditis caused by viridans-type streptococci has an insidious onset, with nonspecific complaints such as fever and malaise, which may persist for weeks. Acute endocarditis caused by *S. aureus* has a more fulminant course with high fever, congestive heart failure, and emboli as possible complications. In short, the clinical diagnosis is unreliable—only persistently negative blood cultures exclude the diagnosis.

Fever is virtually always found. It is usually remitting and seldom exceeds 39C unless the infection is staphylococcal, pneumococcal, or gonococcal in origin.

A cardiac murmur is present in almost all patients but may be absent in those with acute endocarditis and in drug addicts in whom tricuspid valve involvement may not be accompanied by a murmur. Changing murmurs—once thought to be characteristic of the disease—are not common. An aortic diastolic murmur is significant and can be seen in some patients with staphylococcal endocarditis.

Splenomegaly is a frequent finding. A number of cutaneous signs can be seen. Osler nodes and Janeway nodes have been discussed in preceding sections. Petechiae are found in 20 to 40 percent of patients and are thought to represent blood extravasated from superficial capillaries damaged by vasculitis.[38]

Neurologic complications occur in 20 to 40 percent of patients and represent a major symptom in one-half of them. Manifestations are varied and include major cerebral emboli and mycotic aneurysms. Cerebral emboli most frequently involve the middle cerebral artery and its branches and can cause hemiplegia, cortical sensory loss, aphasia, ataxia, and confusion. Mycotic aneurysms can result from septic emboli. These lesions occur at bifurcations of small arteries and are most often seen with viridans streptococcal infections. Mycotic aneurysms are small and seldom cause space-occupying neurologic signs. Rupture is a grave threat, and subarachnoid, cortical, or intraventricular hemorrhage can be disastrous.

An acute brain syndrome ranging from mild personality change to frank psychosis has been reported in patients even without focal neurologic findings. Cerebrospinal fluid analysis shows increased numbers of cells, increased protein, and a normal glucose concentration. *Staphylococcus aureus* is usually the causative organism and can occasionally produce acute purulent meningitis. Meningoencephalitis should be considered when signs and symptoms of toxic encephalopathy and meningitis are found in the same patient. Small, multifocal brain abscesses can also result from an embolic shower in staphylococcal endocarditis. They are usually too scattered and minute for surgical treatment and respond to antibiotics in most cases.[38]

The renal changes have been noted in preceding sections. Microscopic hematuria is found in approximately one-half of patients. Reversible renal failure is more typical of subacute or chronic endocarditis. Renal infarction is usually associated with staphylococcal endocarditis.

Laboratory Findings in Infective Endocarditis

HEMATOLOGY. Normochromic, normocytic anemia is found in nearly all patients. The low reticulocyte count, low serum iron, and reduced percent saturation of iron-binding capacity are found in spite of adequate iron stores in the bone marrow. These findings are seen in many chronic infections and are attributed to decreased erythrocyte production in the marrow caused by slow release of iron from tissue macrophages.[41]

Except for patients with acute endocarditis, normal white blood cell counts and normal differential counts or a mild shift to the left are seen. Leukopenia and thrombocytopenia are found in a minority of patients.[58]

Large mononuclear cells of the monocyte-macrophage lineage have been found in the marrow and in capillary blood; the ear lobe is a good source. Ingested organisms can sometimes be seen in these phagocytic cells, but more often they contain vacuoles and cellular debris.[58]

Powers and Mandell[59] have described a technique for the preparation of a concentrated monolayer of neutrophils and monocytes using a drop of venous blood. There is good correlation between the finding of bacteria within leukocytes, a clinical diagnosis of endocarditis, and the presence of positive blood cultures. A positive result may be considered as a strong indication to start therapy.

Erythrocyte sedimentation rates are consistently elevated. Although the test is nonspecific, a normal value is presumptive evidence against the diagnosis unless the patient is in congestive heart failure.

URINE. Microscopic hematuria, proteinuria, red blood cell casts, and white blood cell casts may all be found. Proteinuria is seen more commonly than hematuria.[58]

TEICHOIC ACID ANTIBODIES. The presence of precipitating antibodies to teichoic acid may be useful in the diagnosis of serious staphylococcal infections (see Chap. 4). Positive reactions are found in over three-fourths of patients with staphylococcal endocarditis,[58] and the technique may be of value in patients with negative blood cultures. Other special tests may be required when the ubiquitous *S. epidermidis* is isolated in order to demonstrate that the bacteria in each culture are the same organisms and therefore the tissue pathogen rather than contaminated cultures containing different *S. epidermidis* strains. Two such tests rely on the uniqueness of electrophoretic patterns of plasmid DNA[60] and endonuclease digests of chromosomal DNA.[61] Thus confirmation of an identical coagulase-negative organism isolated from the blood of a patient with fever and a previously damaged valve or an intracardiac prosthesis, central venous line, or transvenous cardiac pacemaker strongly suggests endocarditis.

IMMUNOFLUORESCENT ANTIBODIES. Skin immunofluorescence in deposits of immunoglobulin and complement has been demonstrated in punch biopsies from patients with IE as compared with bacteremic patients.[62]

Diagnosis

BLOOD CULTURES. The most important test result in establishing a diagnosis of IE is a positive blood culture (Table 36–5). Because the bacteremia of endocarditis is usually continuous, timing of venipuncture is not critical. Two or three separate sets of blood cultures should be collected within a 24-hour period. Skin preparation and collection of separate sets are most important, as some organisms found in the skin can cause endocarditis. In similar fashion, too large a volume of blood contaminated during a single venipuncture can result in a false-positive diagnosis. An adequate volume in adults is approximately 20 ml drawn at each venipuncture and inoculated in equal parts into two 100-ml vacuum blood culture bottles. One bottle should be used for anaerobic culture and the other vented transiently to allow for recovery of both anaerobic and aerobic organisms. Werner et al[63] report that the first blood culture was positive in 96 percent of the cases of streptococcal endocarditis, and one of the first two blood cultures was positive in 89 percent of the cases. In endocarditis caused by microorganisms other than streptococci, the first blood culture was positive in all cases. The incidence of positive results was slightly reduced when the patient had received an antimicrobial agent within 2 weeks. Endocarditis can be caused by a number of microorganisms that are difficult to culture using routine techniques. In some cases of "culture-negative" endocarditis, the patient may be infected with fastidious gram-negative rods of the oropharyngeal flora such as in the HACEK (*Hemophilus-Actinobacillus-Cardiobacterium-Eikenella-Kingella*) group, nutritionally deficient-streptococci, bacterial L-forms (cell wall-deficient organisms), species of *Brucella* and *Neisseria, Legionella, Corynebacterium,* anaerobic bacteria, mycobacteria, *Nocardia,* rickettsial species, chlamydial species, fungi, and possibly viruses. Serologic studies are needed to diagnose IE caused by *Chlamydia* species, *Coxiella burnetii,* and, in some cases, *Brucella.* Fungal endocarditis may be more difficult to diagnose as blood cultures are often negative for growth of *Candida* species and especially for *Aspergillus* species, and in cases of *Histoplasma* endocarditis. Serologic tests for fungal endocarditis have still to be developed.[64] Although the yield is low, evaluation of the buffy-coat smear has been used for the rapid detection of bacteria before blood cultures become positive. Gram-positive cocci are more likely to be present in large enough numbers to give a positive smear. The prognosis is grave, however, as the concentration of organisms required for a positive buffy-coat smear is so great that death usually follows.[65]

TABLE 36–5. CRITERIA FOR DIAGNOSIS OF INFECTIVE ENDOCARDITIS

At least one of the following:

1. Histopathologic evidence of infective endocarditis

or

2. Multiple positive blood cultures in the absence of another known primary source of bacteremia together with at least two of the following signs or symptoms of infective endocarditis: fever, new or changing murmur, newly developed splenomegaly, hypersensitivity, or microvascular phenomena (eg, Janeway lesions, Osler nodes, Roth spots)

or

3. Intermittently positive blood cultures, or negative blood cultures when cultures were first obtained only after empiric antimicrobial therapy, with at least three signs or symptoms of infective endocarditis (as stated above)

From Steckelberg JM, Murphy JG, Ballard D, et al: Ann Intern Med 114:635, 1991.

ECHOCARDIOGRAPHY. Localization of the valvular site may be helpful in planning surgical therapy. Obtaining quantitative cultures of blood proximal and distal to a valve is dangerous, because vegetations can be dislodged. The best current procedure is echocardiography. Vegetations are best seen on aortic and mitral valves, but even there they must be large. Thomson et al[66] reviewed the ultrasound characteristics of vegetations on the aortic, mitral, and tricuspid valves in a total of 17 patients. Echocardiography correctly identified the abnormality in 11 valves. They found eight valves with false-negative results and indicated that a negative echocardiogram does not exclude IE. The echocardiographic criteria for diagnosis of IE are noted in Table 36–6. In a recent review of imaging, Sokil[67] emphasizes the use of two-dimensional echocardiography especially with Doppler, including pulsed and wave flow mapping in assessing valve function and detecting vegetations. The latter can remain morphologically stable for many months after bacteriologic cure; however, a change in morphology can occur after a clinically evident embolic event. Transesophageal echocardiography (TEE) allows for increased accuracy when evaluating native valves as well as prosthetic valves for endocarditis as the position of the sensor near the heart results in more precise imaging. Cardiac catheterization is generally unnecessary in the diagnosis of IE. Computed tomography (CT) is of limited use because of cardiac motion; however, magnetic resonance imaging (MRI) can be helpful in detecting valvular regurgitation. Riba et al[68] demonstrated in rabbits that platelets labeled with indium-111 resulted in cardiac imaging sensitive enough to detect endocardial lesions. The clinical utility of this test has not been proved.

Treatment

MEDICAL MANAGEMENT. The therapy for IE has been extensively reviewed.[69] In theory, bactericidal therapy is best determined on the basis of in vitro sensitivity studies and is administered parenterally for the most consistent results. The duration of therapy is determined by the organism. Serum bactericidal activity should be monitored. Levison[70] has detailed various in vitro assays used in the management of IE including pharmacokinetics of antimicrobial agents, use of broth dilution, and diffusion methods of determining minimal inhibiting concentrations (MICs) and minimal bactericidal concentrations (MBCs). Treatment with the selected agent should not be shortened or interrupted without good reason such as a documented hypersensitivity reaction. A variety of regimens against specific organisms have been tabulated by Baldassarre and Kaye.[69] This includes susceptibilities of both common and less common organisms encountered, presence or absence of cardiac prostheses, and regimens used in patients sensitive to penicillin.[69]

TABLE 36–6. ECHOCARDIOGRAPHIC CRITERIA FOR DIAGNOSIS OF INFECTIVE ENDOCARDITIS

- AORTIC VALVE
  - Shaggy nonuniform thickening in systole and/or diastole with unrestricted leaflet motion
  - Shaggy echoes moving longitudinally across the aortic valve
- MITRAL VALVE
  - Thick shaggy echoes from either leaflet, with unrestricted leaflet motion either attached to or moving behind the leaflets
  - Systolic flutter of the prolapsing segments of the mitral valve
- TRICUSPID VALVE
  - Shaggy thickening of the anterior leaflet with a mass of echoes behind the anterior leaflet

From Thomson KR, Nanda NC, Gramiak R: Radiology *125:473, 1977.*

STREPTOCOCCAL ENDOCARDITIS. Hook and Guerrant[71] have advocated determining the minimal inhibitory concentration of penicillin G for an isolate, and base their therapy on whether or not a strain of streptococci is inhibited at an arbitrary level of 0.1 μg/ml of penicillin G. Streptococci (usually viridans streptococci) are best treated with penicillin alone or in combination with streptomycin. Almost all patients respond, but bacteriologic cure is not achieved in all and relapses have occurred. Penicillin G (1.2 million units intramuscularly every 6 hours, or 20 million units a day by constant infusion) should be given for 4 weeks, plus streptomycin (0.5 g intramuscularly every 12 hours) for 2 weeks. The efficacy of shorter term therapy has been reported by Wilson and Geraci.[72]

In patients with hypersensitivity to penicillin, cefazolin should be substituted at a dose of 1 to 2 g every 6 hours. For organisms resistant to cephalosporins as well as penicillin, vancomycin (0.5 g every 6 hours for 4 weeks with streptomycin for the first 2 weeks) should be used intravenously.

In view of the in vitro synergism between streptomycin and penicillin against most enterococci, both drugs are used for 6 weeks. The dose schedule for streptomycin for adults is 1 g every 12 hours intramuscularly for 2 weeks, then 0.5 g every 12 hours for an additional 4 weeks. Penicillin G is given by constant intravenous infusion 20 million units daily for 6 weeks. Ampicillin (6 to 12 g/day) may be substituted for penicillin, and gentamicin (3 to 5 mg/kg/day divided into three doses) may be substituted for streptomycin.

In patients in whom disturbances of vestibular function occur, streptomycin may need to be stopped after 4 weeks. Aminoglycoside levels should be measured periodically, since the pharmacokinetics of these drugs is variable and doses may need readjustment frequently even in the absence of obvious renal function impairment. Cephalosporins have no place in the treatment of enterococcal endocarditis, because enterococci are generally resistant.

Clinical and therapeutic aspects of streptococcal endocarditis including the viridans and beta-hemolytic streptococci[48,73] and enterococci[74] have been detailed.

STAPHYLOCOCCAL ENDOCARDITIS. Only penicillinase-resistant penicillins are reliable and must be used for 4 to 6 weeks. Methicillin, nafcillin, oxacillin, or the cephalosporins can be used to treat staphylococcal endocarditis. Some physicians add gentamicin or tobramycin to these regimens. The presentation and antimicrobial and surgical management of patients with native valve and prosthetic valve endocarditis due to coagulase-positive and coagulase-negative staphylococci have recently been reviewed by Karchmer.[75]

PNEUMOCOCCAL, GONOCOCCAL, AND MENINGOCOCCAL ENDOCARDITIS. Endocarditis caused by these organisms usually responds to high doses of penicillin G (20 million units/day) given continuously by the intravenous route for 4 weeks.

ENDOCARDITIS CAUSED BY GRAM-NEGATIVE ORGANISMS. Therapy should be based on the results of in vitro sensitivity tests. A cephalosporin with or without an aminoglycoside is frequently selected. Penicillin G or ampicillin with an aminoglycoside (for Enterobacteriaceae such as *E. coli, Proteus mirabilis,* or *Salmonella*), cephalosporins (for *E. coli, P. mirabilis,* or *Klebsiella* species), and extended spectrum penicillin (or piperacillin or ticarcillin) and an aminoglycoside plus valve replacement (for *Serratia marcescens*) are commonly used. Carbenicillin is used for *Enterobacter* species, *Proteus* species other than *P. mirabilis,* or *Pseudomonas aeruginosa.*[76] Other antipseudomonal drugs are also used for *P. aeruginosa.* Bodey[77] has reviewed the beta-lactam antibiotics including the penicillins, the monobactams, and the carbapenems. These agents act by inhibiting cell wall synthesis. Experience in patients with endocarditis is limited, and their use should be determined by organism sensitivity and resistance to other antibiotics. The epidemiology, clinical features, and management of patients with endocarditis due to gram-negative bacteria including Enterobacteriaceae, *Pseudomonas* species, *Neisseria* species, the HACEK (*Hemophilus* species, *Actinobacillus actinomycetemcomitans, Cardiobacterium hominis, Eikenella corrodens,* and *Kingella* species) organisms, and *Brucella* have recently been reviewed by Hessen and Abrutyn.[76]

The use of quinolones in endocarditis patients is limited. Neu[78] outlined the broad spectrum of organisms that can be treated with these agents and noted successful treatment of *S. aureus* endocarditis in drug addicts as well as *Pseudomonas* endocarditis using oral ciprofloxacin and rifampin for staphylococcal infections and ciprofloxacin in combination with an antipseudomonal penicillin for *Pseudomonas* endocarditis.

ENDOCARDITIS CAUSED BY ANAEROBES. Anaerobic organisms are uncommon causes of endocarditis. Penicillin G is the treatment of choice for most anaerobes, but *Bacteroides fragilis* strains are highly resistant. Most strains of *B. fragilis* are sensitive in vitro to clindamycin and chloramphenicol, but the prognosis is grave. Both are bacteriostatic rather than bactericidal. Metronidazole may prove more effective.

FUNGAL ENDOCARDITIS. Fungal endocarditis remains a challenging problem because the drug of choice, amphotericin B, is highly toxic. Amphotericin B in combination with flucytosine may be more effective. In general, however, surgical intervention in addition to antifungal therapy is necessary for cure in most cases (see subsequent section).

ENDOCARDITIS WITH NEGATIVE CULTURE. The management of the uncommon patient with typical findings of endocarditis and negative blood cultures is empirical. Most clinicians treat such patients as they would those with enterococcal endocarditis unless the course is fulminant, in which case they are treated as if they had staphylococcal endocarditis. Organisms that may be implicated include fungi, anaerobes, diphtheroids, cell wall-defective bacteria, and *C. burnetii.*

Most patients with IE will be cured of their disease by appropriate antibiotic therapy alone and have a 5-year survival rate of 50 to 85 percent.[79] The mortality in viridans-type streptococcal endocarditis is about 10 to 15 percent and is due to damage that had occurred by the time therapy was initiated. Some patients will require surgical intervention to control the infection or the hemodynamic consequences of infection.

SURGICAL MANAGEMENT OF INFECTIVE ENDOCARDITIS. In 1964, Yeh et al[80] first demonstrated the feasibility of valve replacement with a prosthesis in six patients with endocarditis of the aortic valve who had been successfully treated with antibiotics before operation. The following year Wallace et al[81] accomplished valve replacement successfully in a patient with active infection. Since that time, an increasing number of cases of surgically treated endocarditis have been reported,[82–89] and IE has become a well-recognized indication for cardiac surgery when congestive failure persists or worsens in spite of aggressive medical management.[85–89]

In their detailed review of 293 cases of left-sided endocarditis, Jung et al[83] found the mean age of the surgical patient to be 30 to 40 years, with men predominating approximately 3 : 1. A history of a preexisting congenital or acquired heart disease can be elicited in 60 percent of patients. Where identified, streptococci (mostly of the viridans type) were the commonest infecting organisms, followed by staphylococci and pneumococci.

INDICATIONS FOR OPERATION. The most common indication for surgical intervention is congestive heart failure with hemodynamic deterioration caused by destruction of heart valves and their supporting structures (Table 36–7).[83] It is the only indication in 84 percent of the patients and is combined with embolization or resistant organisms in 12 percent. Resistant infection with repeated septic embolization or drug toxicity constitutes the indication in the remaining 4 percent. Despite the fact that the mitral valve is the most common valve infection, the aortic valve is replaced in 71 percent, the mitral valve in 19 percent, and both valves in 10 percent of the patients.[83] This experience reflects the devastating consequences of aortic insufficiency as compared with mitral insufficiency.

TABLE 36–7. INDICATIONS FOR SURGICAL INTERVENTION

- MAJOR CRITERIA
  - Progressive heart failure
  - Significant heart failure: fails to improve after "simple" medical treatment
  - Major embolism
  - Persistent bacteremia despite appropriate antibiotics
  - Fungal endocarditis
  - Patients with intravascular devices
  - Patients developing heart block
  - Prosthetic valve dehiscence or obstruction
  - Relapse of infection following adequate medical treatment
- MINOR CRITERIA
  - Congestive heart failure resolved with medical treatment
  - Simple "minor" embolism
  - Large left-sided or right-sided vegetation (seen on echocardiogram)
  - Early mitral valve closure or flail valve leaflets
  - Prosthetic valve endocarditis caused by other than highly penicillin-resistant streptococci
  - Gram-negative rod tricuspid endocarditis
  - Persistent fever without other identifiable cause
  - New regurgitant murmurs in aortic prosthetic endocarditis
  - Lack of appropriate cell wall antibiotic

From Arbulu A, Asfaw I: Infective endocarditis. In Baue AE, Geha AS, Hammond GL, et al (eds): Glenn's Thoracic and Cardiovascular Surgery, 5th ed. Norwalk, CT, Appleton & Lange, 1991, p 1647.

Septic cerebral emboli complicate the courses of 20 to 40 percent of patients with left-sided endocarditis.[88] In 106 patients who underwent valve replacement at the University of Illinois Hospital, Ting et al[88] found that 45 had cerebral septic infarctions. Hospital mortality among the 106 patients was 9 percent. There was a 16 percent mortality (7/45) in the patients with septic cerebral emboli. The authors concluded that in the absence of a hemorrhagic infarct, valve replacement can be performed with minimal risk of a perioperative stroke.[88]

Valves demonstrate the usual vegetations, disruption of leaflets and supporting structures, perforations, and tears of valve cusps.[80–89] Abscesses of the annulus, which sometimes extend into the interventricular septum or myocardium, mycotic aneurysm of the sinuses of Valsalva, or fistulous connections between cardiac chambers or into the pulmonary artery are also found. A rare indication for operative correction has been reported by Bove and associates[90] in a patient with streptococcal endocarditis and complete endocardial cushion defect.

OPERATIVE CORRECTION. The operative procedure consists of valve replacement in the great majority of patients. In some of the earlier cases, aortic and mitral cusp replacement and valvuloplasty were generally unsuccessful. Successful mitral valvuloplasty has now been reported in one case[91] and repair of the mitral valve apparatus is described using a variety of techniques in 22 patients.[92] In cases of aortic valve IE, the situation may be complicated by aortic root abscesses, fistulas, and, in some cases, annulus destruction. Complex repairs include excision of the valve, debridement of infected material, and translocation of an aortic prosthesis to the supravalvular aorta with relocation of the coronary artery using vein grafts or direct anastomosis into an aortic conduit using Danielson's technique.[87,93] Replacement with a mechanical versus a bioprosthesis remains controversial. Cryopreserved homografts have been unsuccessful,[94] as have other bioprosthetic valves.[95] Operative techniques in infective endocarditis have been reviewed by Lau et al.[96]

RESULTS OF SURGICAL TREATMENT. Patients with *active* disease are at high risk. The early mortality was 30 percent and the late mortality 7 percent.[83] For inactive patients whose indications were hemodynamic or embolic, the early and late mortality figures were 12 percent and 11 percent, respectively. The early mortality rates were comparable (approximately 20 percent) in patients undergoing aortic, mitral, or aortic and mitral replacement. The most significant factor affecting mortality rate was the degree of cardiac decompensation present at the time of operation. Procedures carried out because of severe congestive heart failure carried a mortality of 34 percent, in contrast to elective operations where the mortality rate was 15 percent.

One of the potential dangers of valve replacement in endocarditis is infection of the prosthetic valve. Only 12 of 293 patients with IE developed infection of the prosthesis, and only 5 of 162 operated on during the active phase developed infection by the original organism. One patient developed infection by a different organism. Of six additional patients who developed infection of the prosthesis, three were in the inactive stage and the stage was not specified in three other patients.[83] All the patients with infected prostheses died. Lewis et al[97] noted only one case of reinfection in 86 patients undergoing natural valve replacement for IE in the active phase. It appears that the procedure is safer than delaying the operation in patients with uncontrolled heart failure. Bacteria have usually been eliminated from the circulation and the infected valve within days of starting effective antibiotic treatment unless the organisms are drug-resistant or inaccessible, as in a bulky vegetation or nidus of calcification. In the case of organisms that are inaccessible, operative excision and debridement may actually be essential to eliminate the infection. Jung et al[83] feel that this explains why the variable duration of antibiotic therapy preoperatively has no bearing on the mortality rate or rate of recurrence of infection on the implanted prosthesis. If one can assume that patients reported in most surgical series would succumb to their disease without operative intervention, a combined early (22 percent) and late (9 percent) mortality rate of 31 percent, though high, is better than a 100 percent mortality. It is probable that the results could be improved if the operation were undertaken before irreversible congestive heart failure and such anatomic complications as aortic root abscesses, sinus of Valsalva aneurysms, and fistulas occur. The emphasis on earlier operation is clearly seen in the series of Boyd et al.[84] In their 45 patients with primary endocarditis, survival was improved when the operation was carried out promptly in those with both controlled and uncontrolled infection. Dreyfus et al[87] felt that a successful outcome in the operative treatment of IE was improved if patients had received antibiotic treatment for at least 1 week before operation; however, improved results were obtained in the Al Jubair et al[89] series of 65 patients who underwent operation within 3 days of starting antibiotic therapy. Cukingnan et al[98] found a probability of survival at 5 years for all patients with active endocarditis to be 53 percent with no significant difference in survival curves in subgroups with natural valve endocarditis.

Valve replacement is almost always necessary for fungal and *Pseudomonas* endocarditis, which rarely respond to chemotherapy alone. If the tricuspid valve is infected (see subsequent section on drug addiction), excision of the valve without immediate replacement is in order.

Prophylaxis. According to Korzeniowski and Kaye[22] there is no definitive evidence that antimicrobial prophylaxis is effective in preventing IE. Only half of patients will have a previously recognized cardiac lesion and an apparent portal of entry (excluding drug abusers) is demonstrated in patients with IE less than 25 percent of the time. Theoretically, fewer than 10 percent of cases of IE are preventable using antibiotic prophylaxis. Nevertheless, penicillin at 6-hour intervals for 48 hours may be effective. Patients who are allergic to penicillin should receive 2 g cefazolin plus an aminoglycoside, or 1 g vancomycin intravenously. The best regimen for preventing enterococcal endocarditis is ampicillin plus gentamicin. No firm dosage schedules have been established, but 2 g ampicillin followed by 0.5 g every 6 hours plus 3 to 5 mg/kg gentamicin in three divided doses for a total of 48 hours given simultaneously should be adequate. The prophylactic doses of penicillin used to prevent group A streptococcal infection and recurrent rheumatic fever will not prevent bacterial endocarditis.[22] Korzeniowski and Kaye[22] have tabulated procedures where prophylaxis is both indicated and not indicated along with a number of specific regimens tailored to specific risk groups and specific procedures.

Infective Endocarditis in Drug Addicts

Infective endocarditis in drug addicts is an entity of increasing concern. Bacteremia obviously arises by injection of unsterile material and the use of unclean needles, syringes, and other paraphernalia. Most often, endogenous skin or oral bacteria are inoculated. In addition to direct intravenous inoculation, bacteria may enter the circulation from foci of phlebitis or through regional lymphatic absorption from areas of bacterial cellulitis.

Preexisting heart disease is present in only about 20 percent of narcotic addicts presenting with their initial episode of endocarditis, in sharp contrast to the 60 percent of nonaddicts with endocarditis. The mechanism of endocarditis beginning on normal structures is uncertain. Repeated intravenous injections of foreign material may traumatize the endocardial surfaces, causing roughened areas that serve as sites for aggregation of platelets and development of platelet thrombi. Highly contaminated systemic venous flow could explain the frequency of right heart endocarditis in drug abusers. The tricuspid valve is infected in 55 percent of 270 cases, the aortic valve in 35 percent, the mitral valve in 30 percent, and the pulmonary valve in only 2 percent of these patients.[99]

Etiology. The microbiology of infective endocarditis in drug addicts is different from that in nonaddicts. *Staphylococcus aureus* is the most common pathogen (45 to 56 percent). Aerobic gram-negative bacilli account for approximately 15 percent, fungi (usually *Candida*) for 11 percent, streptococci for 10 percent, and enterococci for 8 percent. Enterococcal endocarditis may occur more frequently in some series.[99] *Pseudomonas* is identified in one-third of the gram-negative bacillary infections and often involves the tricuspid valve. Borow et al[100] caution that transient *Pseudomonas* bacteremia in an addict may mimic right-sided endocarditis and may actually require a much shorter course of therapy. It may be that virulent organisms (eg, staphylococci) are necessary to initiate endocardial infection in addicts without preexisting heart disease, but once valvular damage has occurred, the addict becomes susceptible to infection with less virulent organisms.

Clinical Manifestations. The patients are generally young adult men with symptoms of acute onset and short duration. Fever is present in 90 percent, with pleuritic chest pain, increased sputum production, or hemoptysis occurring in about 30 percent. Exertional dyspnea, orthopnea, and paroxysmal nocturnal dyspnea occur in 15 percent and are manifestations of heart failure. The other manifestations and complications of endocarditis are those noted previously in nonaddicts. Pulmonary complications often dominate the clinical picture caused by emboli from the right heart.

Three specific syndromes have been identified[99]:

1. Staphylococcal endocarditis. Valve destruction occurs early, and septic pulmonary emboli with pulmonary infiltrates are common. Although right-sided involvement predominates, either or both sides of the heart may be involved. The mortality increases with aortic or mitral valve involvement over that from isolated tricuspid valve involvement because of the hemodynamic derangements of valvular insufficiency of the left side of the heart.
2. Gram-negative bacillary endocarditis. The most commonly involved organisms are of the *Klebsiella-Enterobacter* group, *E. coli,* and *Pseudomonas. Serratia marcescens* and *Herellea vaginicola* have also been found. Infection of both sides of the heart can result from gram-negative bacteria, although left-sided endocarditis predominates and is associated with a mortality of approximately 90 percent. This is caused in part by the relative resistance of these bacteria to antibiotics, *Pseudomonas* being especially difficult to treat. In view of this, Meyerowitz et al[101] have recommended early operation for left-sided *Pseudomonas* endocarditis in drug addicts.[101] They characterized these infections as aggressive with early invasion of the myocardium that requires wide debridement of the annulus to remove any vegetations or intramyocardial abscess wall. In mitral infections they recommend removing a second rim of the annulus for separate culture at the time of mitral valve replacement to demonstrate if valve resection has eliminated all the infected tissue. If early reinfection of the prosthesis occurs, it should be removed and replaced with another prosthesis.
3. *Candida* endocarditis. These very serious infections are often superimposed on a previous episode of bacterial endocarditis. A mixed fungal and bacterial infection was present in four of the five addicts with *Candida* endocarditis reported earlier by Harris et al.[102] The clinical course is less acute, and the left side of the heart is most often involved. Large vegetations occur in fungal endocarditis, and those in the left heart may embolize to other organs and to large peripheral arteries (eg, the aortic or femoral

bifurcations). The prognosis in fungal endocarditis is dismal.[99]

Treatment. The treatment is the same in addicts as in nonaddicts, with the exception of the addict with (bacterial or fungal) tricuspid endocarditis caused by resistant organisms. In these circumstances, the best results are achieved when the tricuspid valve has been excised without replacement. Four of the five patients so treated by Arbulu et al[103] were alive and free of infection and hemodynamic problems from 7 to 17 months after operation. Based on this experience, Arbulu et al[104] expanded their series to 55 patients over a 20-year period, with an overall mortality rate of 29 percent. Six (11 percent) required prosthetic valve placement. Stern et al[105] have used immediate replacement of the tricuspid valve with porcine bioprostheses in ten addicts with tricuspid endocarditis. All left the hospital free of infection and heart failure. Three returned to intravenous drug abuse and died. A reparative approach including valvuloplasty and annuloplasty has also been used in 12 patients (six heroin addicts), which resulted in improved hemodynamics, low recurrence of tricuspid endocarditis, and a favorable long-term outlook without need of prosthetic valve replacement.[106] As noted above, left-sided *Pseudomonas* endocarditis requires aggressive therapy that is the same for addicts as for nonaddicts.[101]

Prognosis. Reinfection of addicts with successfully treated endocarditis is a common problem. Some[18] have suggested remedies such as antibiotic prophylaxis and improved personal hygiene. Obviously, the surgeon will require professional social and psychologic assistance in the rehabilitation of these patients. Hiratzka and associates[107] have reviewed their operative experience with IE in 18 drug users compared with 14 nondrug users. They found a 30-day mortality rate of 6 percent in drug users and 7 percent in nonusers. This was in contrast to a higher late mortality rate in drug users of 39 percent versus 7 percent in nonusers. Persistent infection with the same organism occurred in 2 of 18 users, whereas late reinfection with a different organism occurred in 4 of the 18 drug users and 1 of the 14 nonusers.[107] The subject of IE in intravenous drug users has recently been thoroughly reviewed.[108]

Infective Endocarditis and the Acquired Immunodeficiency Syndrome (AIDS)

In patients with human immunodeficiency virus (HIV) infection, with or without AIDS, structural heart disease is uncommon.[38] Left ventricular dilatation and hypokinetic function have been observed using echocardiography.[109] Pericarditis, myocarditis, and nonbacterial thrombotic endocarditis are more commonly seen than IE.[110–112] Cammarosano and Lewis[111] described autopsy findings in 41 patients with AIDS. In ten there were significant cardiac changes. Metastatic Karposi's sarcoma was found in the epicardium or myocardium in four patients while NBTE while embolization was found in three and *Cryptococcus neoformans* endocarditis was found in one patient. Niedt and Schinella[112] did a clinicopathologic study of 56 autopsies on patients with AIDS and found lipochrome deposition in the heart. They, however, noted necrotizing arteritis in three cases with cytomegalovirus.[112]

Many HIV victims are intravenous drug abusers. Consequently, their clinical presentation is that of intravenous drug abusers with IE. They show a prevalence for right-sided valve lesions and are at increased risk for fungal endocarditis (*Candida, Cryptococcus, Aspergillus*). Intravenous drug abusers with AIDS are more profoundly immunocompromised than those without AIDS. They frequently have coexisting *Pneumocystis* or other forms of pneumonia and have a more fulminant course with IE than drug abusers without AIDS.[38] Successful valve replacement has been reported in four intravenous drug abusers infected with HIV but without AIDS. Three survived. There was no apparent downhill acceleration in their immune function as a consequence of anesthesia and operation.[113]

Pacemaker Endocarditis

Permanent cardiac pacemakers have revolutionized the management of patients with cardiac arrhythmias. As with any procedure involving the implantation of foreign bodies, pacemaker infection is a threat that may involve the pacing system at any point outside the heart or within the endocardium. The infections of the subcutaneous pacemaker pocket are discussed in Chapter 35. This section focuses on infections within the heart.

Incidence. Intravascular infection is an uncommon complication. Schwartz and Pervez[114] reported the first case of acute bacterial endocarditis in a patient with a permanent transvenous pacemaker. In 1972, Imparato and Kim[115] reviewed the complications found in 200 patients with permanent cardiac pacemakers. Six patients (5 percent) developed skin erosions caused by the hardware, and all but one developed secondary infection of the pacemaker pockets and catheter tracts. In none of the five could the electrodes be extracted at the time of removal of the pacemakers from their infected pockets (trapped endocardial electrode). In three cases, the trapped electrodes were severed distal to the infected pacemaker pockets and left within their venous tracts. This resulted in the delayed appearance of septicemia in one patient, persistent septicemia in another, and migration of the electrode in the third. The rate can be reduced. Conklin et al[116] reported an infection rate on all pacemaker procedures of 0.13 percent (1 of 726), but these results are unusual. Grogler et al[117] reported a 3.2 percent incidence of infection of generator pocket infections in 1376 pacemaker operations and a 1.9 percent incidence of infected electrode channels. In most cases, infection could be directly related to operation, but a few appeared months to years after implantation.

Pathogenesis and Bacteriology of Pacemaker Endocarditis. Endocardial electrodes can become infected by one of two major mechanisms. In the more frequent type, the infected pacemaker generator (and site) acts as a foreign body that allows a direct extension of organisms along pacemaker wires with or without systemic bacteremia. Cultures most often reveal *S. aureus* followed by *S. epidermidis* and *Klebsiella*. Other organisms that have rarely been encountered include *E. coli, Candida, Serratia, Flavobacterium,* and other Enterobacteriaceae. The less frequent type is caused by metastatic implantation of bacteria from a distant site. As expected, any microorganism can be involved.[118] Diagnosis of pacemaker-induced endocarditis depends on clinical suspicion, positive blood cultures and possible verification using two-dimensional echocardiography (sector scanning) to detect right atrial vegetations.[119]

Treatment. High doses of antibiotic drugs should be used in all cases of prosthetic endocarditis. The surgical treatment of the infected pacemaker generator and external wires has been discussed in Chapter 35. The standard treatment is removal of all infected foreign bodies including extrathoracic electrode segments, drainage, and antibiotics. Sterile electrode tracts seldom need to be disturbed. The in situ management of the infected pulse generator has been reported by Dargan and Norman[120] and is described in Chapter 35. Successful in situ treatment of a pacemaker infection has been reported using an omental pedicle graft spread over the pacemaker with closure of the pocket around a drain. This was especially beneficial in a report of a neonate with congenital heart block who had a limited number of sites to replace an infected pacemaker.[121] Salvage of exposed and infected pulse generators by relocation to deeper subfascial sites has been reported.[122] When infection has spread from the pulse generator or external wires into the heart or has involved the endocardial electrode by metastatic spread from a distant focus, all foreign material must be removed. Removal of the electrode is usually accomplished by graded traction on the electrode. The wire is tensed until the tugging caused by ventricular motion is felt. The wire is then taped to the chest and the procedure repeated as slack is developed in the wire and the electrode wire is removed completely.[115] Obviously, a new pacemaker system must be in place before removal is attempted.

Salvage and reuse of an infected pacemaker system have been reported using explanation, gas sterilization, and reimplantation of the pulse generator with subsequent replacement of epicardial or endocardial leads.[123]

The most difficult problem is the trapped electrode. Retention is due to ensheathment of the larger tip of the electrode by fibrous tissue, which prevents its easy withdrawal through the fibrous ring just proximal to it. Trapped electrodes have sometimes required thoracotomy, cardiopulmonary bypass, and cardiotomy for removal.[124] In elderly and high-risk patients a technique has been described for surgical extraction of permanent pacing leads and electrodes using a limited right extrapleural thoracotomy, purse-string right atriotomy, and a snare to engage the lead under fluoroscopic control. Cardiopulmonary bypass must be available should an atrial or ventricular tear occur, or should it be necessary to open the heart to dissect trapped electrodes free of encasing fibrous tissue.[125]

Prophylaxis of Pacemaker Infections. Hartstein et al[126] retrospectively analyzed 298 pacemaker procedures. There was no significant difference in infection rate between the group given prophylactic antibiotics and the group given no or inadequate prophylactic antibiotics. Prospective studies have not been completed. The authors[126] concluded that drains should be avoided in battery pack plus pacing wire procedures. Conklin et al[116] noted that the one infection in their series resulted from repeated efforts to aspirate a pouch hematoma. They recommend that a pouch hematoma be treated by prompt operation, evacuation of the hematoma, and primary closure of the pouch.

Although late intracardiac infections are unusual, chemoprophylaxis with antibiotics (see preceding section on prophylaxis of endocarditis) should be carried out in patients with intravascular pacemakers whenever bacteremia-inducing procedures are contemplated (see Table 36–2).

INFECTIONS AFTER HEART SURGERY

Chest wall wound infections have been discussed in Chapter 35. The following sections discuss intracardiac infections after heart surgery.

Endocarditis in the Absence of an Intracardiac Prosthesis

Incidence and Consequences. There is limited information regarding the incidence of endocarditis after cardiac surgery in the absence of an intracardiac prosthesis. An incidence of 2 percent was once estimated. Geraci et al[127] reported on the experience of the Mayo Clinic from 1946 through 1962 with bacterial endocarditis and endarteritis after approximately 4300 cardiac or large vessel operations, excluding coarctation of the aorta and lesions distal to this site. There were 24 patients (0.5 percent) with bacterial or fungal endocarditis, 12 of whom had undergone intracardiac operations. Four had congenital aortic stenosis, four had mitral stenosis, and four had atrial septal defects (with associated pulmonic stenosis and patent ductus arteriorsus in one patient each). Seven patients died.[127]

Pathogenesis. Experience is so limited that the pathogenetic factors are not clear. Cardiopulmonary bypass probably plays an important role in many cases of postoperative endocarditis (see subsequent section), as must preexisting infection, suture material, and extracardiac foreign bodies. Damaged valves and suture lines are most often affected. Late infections have involved Teflon-reinforced, ventricular suture lines.[128] The role of sepsis and additional factors, such as operative contamination and intravascular catheters, in postoperative endocarditis is better documented in patients with prosthetic valve endocarditis and is discussed in that section.

Etiology. Staphylococcus aureus is responsible for more than half of the cases, with *S. epidermidis, Streptococcus pyogenes* (group A), *P. aeruginosa,* and other gram-negative rods responsible for the rest.[127,128] Fungi are rare etiologic agents: *C. albicans,*[128] *Mucor,* and *Histoplasma*[127] have been cultured from suture lines and damaged valves.

Pathology. The pathologic changes of postoperative endocarditis in the absence of an intracardiac prosthesis are similar to those previously described for endocarditis when the valves are affected. Most of the nonvalvular infections involve cardiotomy and aortotomy suture lines. The highest incidence of fatal infections have followed operations for aortic stenosis—aortic suture line separation, mycotic aneurysm formation, and aortic valve cusp infection have all been noted. Mitral (and sometimes aortic) vegetations were a dominant feature in heart infections after mitral commissurotomy, and myocardial abscess and atrial thrombi were also seen.[127,128]

Clinical Manifestations. The clinical diagnosis of postoperative endocarditis in the absence of an intracardiac prosthesis can be elusive. Embolic signs and splenomegaly were each noted in four instances.[127] The appearance of new or changing murmurs is not as striking as in patients with infected intracardiac prostheses. Persistent early or late unexplained fever is often the only sign. When combined with positive blood cultures, intracardiac infection should be suspected. X-ray studies and lung scans can be useful in detecting pulmonary emboli and infarcts, and ultrasound studies can at times document intracardiac vegetations as well as pericarditis with effusion. Angiocardiography is useful in suture line disruption and where an exact assessment of a residual defect is important before reoperation.[127]

Treatment

MEDICAL THERAPY. The patient should be started on a bactericidal antibiotic regimen, giving adequate doses for a sufficiently long period and regulating the course of treatment by determination of bactericidal levels of antibiotics in the patient's serum. Most of the patients described by Geraci et al[127] who were cured with antibiotic therapy alone had undergone repair of an atrial septal defect with silk suture or commissurotomy for valve stenosis. The diagnosis of bacterial endocarditis in patients successfully treated can never be proved, but three patients with similar signs clearly received inadequate courses of antibiotic therapy and died of their infections, as did four patients treated aggressively with antibiotic therapy.[127]

In some patients, infection cannot be eradicated but can be suppressed by indefinite antibiotic administration. This approach is more commonly required in patients with infected prostheses.

SURGICAL TREATMENT. In hemodynamically stable patients, surgical treatment should be considered only after an adequate trial of effective bactericidal antibiotic therapy for 4 or more weeks. Those in whom relapse occurs after therapy or where bacteremia is not controlled are candidates for reoperation.

The first report of endocarditis following direct repair of ventricular septal defect was that of Mandel et al[129] in 1958. The patient died of a coagulase-positive staphylococcal infection on the intact line of closure of this defect, which was covered with granulations containing gram-positive cocci. In 1960 Teitel and Florman[130] described a patient with *Pseudomonas aeruginosa* endocarditis on a silk suture after repair of an atrial septal defect. There was no other foreign material in the heart and the patient recovered after the removal of the suture.

In 1961, Kelsch and Thomson[131] reported cure of a patient with postoperative endocarditis by removing the infected silk sutures used to close a ventricular septal defect. Hemodynamic instability requires urgent operations as in native endocarditis.

Prevention

TECHNICAL ASPECTS. The principles of bacterial control in the operating room, patient preparation, and operative technique are the same as in patients in whom prostheses are inserted (this is discussed in a subsequent section on technical aspects of prophylaxis of infection during implantation of a prosthesis).

ANTIBIOTIC PROPHYLAXIS. Prophylactic antibiotics are usually used in patients undergoing open heart surgery but for shorter times than in patients who require valve replacement. With current methods of prophylaxis, the rate of postoperative endocardial infection is low in the absence of an intracardiac prosthesis. Most trials reflecting the beneficial effects of antibiotic prophylaxis have been performed during the implantation of intracardiac prostheses.

Endocarditis in the Presence of an Intracardiac Interventricular Prosthetic Patch

Incidence and Consequences. Postoperative endocarditis is a rare event in the many patients who have undergone closure of a ventricular septal defect (VSD) using a patch of prosthetic material. Thirteen cases had been reported[132–137] with Nakayama et al[138] subsequently adding two patients with probable infected VSD repairs, and Jackson and Hicks[139] reporting a unique case from our institution. Nakayama et al[138] emphasized the management of the peripheral arterial embolic complications of bacterial endocarditis, while Jackson and Hicks[139] detailed successful management of a vancomycin-tolerant *S. aureus* infection by removal and replacement of an infected VSD patch, and the addition of trimethoprim-sulfamethaxazole to the vancomycin regimen. Seven of the patients died after receiving multiple (often massive) courses of antibiotics in an effort to eradicate their infections. In general, where information was available, patches had partially detached from the interventricular septum.

Organisms were seen on histologic examination of fibrin and granulation tissues in five cases at the site of the patch and recurrent ventricular septal defect. In one patient the patch had detached completely and embolized to the abdominal aorta.[137] There was no apparent predilection to infection with any type of patch material. In five survivors infection was of late onset with *Micrococcus* species alone or in association with other gram-positive cocci in three cases (*S. aureus* isolated in two of these cases).[138,139] Only one of the survivors required cardiac reoperation.[139] In general, the hemodynamic sequelae of these infections are not as severe as in prosthetic valve infections.

It is not clear whether bacterial infection at the site of a VSD patch precedes or follows its partial detachment. It is probable that either or both mechanisms are responsible in a given case. Thus the patch and suture material could serve as a nidus for infection with its subsequent partial detachment, or partial detachment could set the stage for turbulence, formation of thrombotic vegetations, and secondary infection. In patients with mixed bacterial and fungal infection, *S. epidermidis* and *E. coli* infections were thought to have preceded superimposed *Aspergillus* and *Candida* infections.[134] Use of multiple and prolonged courses of antibiotics were considered important predisposing factors to these mixed and fatal infections.[56,134]

In spite of the right-sided localization of the endocarditis, peripheral venous blood cultures were, for the most part, commonly positive, and peripheral systemic manifestations, such as splenomegaly and petechial hemorrhages, were seen in the majority of cases where data were available. Obviously, emboli from these right-sided lesions went preferentially to the lungs rather than to the systemic circulation.

Echocardiography can be helpful in establishing the anatomy of the septum and in detecting thrombotic vegetations. This can be important in documenting an intracardiac focus of infection as the source of bacteremia in those patients who survive without cardiac reoperation.[140]

Prosthetic Valve Endocarditis

In the 1960s postoperative endocarditis became more frequent, especially in patients with acquired heart disease and in those in whom intracardiac prostheses were used. In 1966 Amoury et al[134] reported an early experience with 13 instances of postoperative endocarditis following a total of 568 open heart operations. In this group, 357 patients required intracardiac prostheses, with 223 intracardiac patches and 134 patients receiving 154 valve prostheses. Endocarditis was most common after aortic valve replacement, less common after intracardiac patch prosthesis, and least common when no prosthesis was used. Other studies in the 1960s confirmed these findings.[141] Although the incidence has been further reduced, prosthetic valve endocarditis (PVE) is still a major complication, with serious consequences.

Epidemiology and Incidence. To more accurately assess the incidence of PVE, it is necessary to define the diagnostic criteria. Wilson[142] considers PVE to be present if two of three criteria are fulfilled: (1) at least two positive blood cultures contain the same microbial species; (2) surgical or autopsy specimens show evidence of bacterial endocarditis; and (3) at least two of the following clinical signs are found—fever, appearance of a new regugitant murmur, newly developed splenomegaly, and signs of peripheral emboli.

The disease can be further divided into early onset PVE, appearing within 2 months of operation, and late onset PVE. Wilson[142] found PVE in 45 of 4586 patients (0.98 percent) given 4706 prosthetic valves. Early onset PVE occurred in 16 (0.35 percent) and late onset PVE in 29 (0.63 percent). In patients with early onset PVE, the mean time from operation to onset of symptoms was 17 days (range 1 to 45 days). In the late onset group the mean delay was 26 months (range 72 days to 10 years). The aortic valve was involved more frequently than the mitral valve. All age groups were equally susceptible. A wound infection was the portal of entry in 5 of the 16 early cases (31 percent), but no obvious portal was present in the rest. In the late onset group five of the patients with endocarditis caused by viridans streptococci had either antecedent trauma, surgical procedures, or dental work. Two of three patients with late onset PVE caused by group D streptococci had prior or concomitant urinary tract infection with the same organism. None of the remaining 22 patients with late onset PVE had an obvious portal of entry.

Both early and late onset PVE may follow contamination of prostheses in the perioperative period, and considerable attention has been focused on this period in a patient's course. Ankeney and Parker[143] studied 383 open heart operations during which 1555 intraoperative blood cultures were secured. *Staphylococcus epidermidis* grew in 7.5 percent of these samples and diphtheroids in 9.8 percent. The greatest number of positive cultures were in specimens taken from the recently assembled and primed pump and from the suction line during bypass when the pump and blood are most exposed to the operating room air.

In similar studies of 400 patients, Yeh et al[141] obtained positive cultures from the primed oxygenator preoperatively in 37: *Staphylococcus* (7), *Streptococcus* (2), diphtheroids (7), *Alcaligenes* (20), and *Paracolobactrum* (1). Nineteen had positive blood cultures from the pump equipment after bypass: *Staphylococcus* (2), diphtheroids (6), *Alcaligenes* (5), and *Proteus, Mima, Bacillus, Aerobacter, Pseudomonas,* and unidentified gram-negative rods (1 each). Only two developed bacterial endocarditis due to the same organism (diphtheroid and *Pseudomonas maltophilia*) found in the pump equipment. Of these 400 patients,[141] 32 had positive blood cultures at some time after cardiopulmonary bypass, and 18 of these were considered to have PVE.

Another source of potential contamination that has received increasing attention in patients undergoing sternotomy and open heart operations are glove punctures and tears. These obviously expose the extracorporeal circuit, the patient, the operators, and, more importantly, an implanted cardiac prosthesis to organisms from the skin of the hands of the operating team. Conversely, of course, the operating team is exposed to the patient's blood with the potential risk of exposure to hepatitis B, hepatitis C, and HIV. Wong et al[144] examined the incidence of glove punctures during cardiac operations in 48 adult patients. Out of a total of 514 gloves tested there were 162 gloves (31.5 percent) that had one or more punctures. Only 20 glove punctures were recognized by the operating team in contrast to 185 glove punctures detected only by testing. The most important finding from the study was that 61 percent of gloves worn by scrub nurses had one or more punctures compared to 23.6 percent of surgeons.

In view of the accumulated data, and in spite of the numerous potential sources of intraoperative contamination, most infections arise postoperatively rather than intraoperatively. Contamination most often arises from arterial and venous cannulations, cannulation of the heart, tracheostomy, endotracheal intubation, and bladder catheterization.

Etiology (Bacteriology). A variety of organisms have been reported in patients with PVE (Tables 36–8 and 36–9). Both gram-positive and gram-negative organisms are found. Staphylococci and streptococci are the most frequently encountered gram-positive organisms in almost all series, but almost any pathogen or saprophyte can be encountered. Table 36–9 cites case reports of the rarely encountered bacteria that cause PVE.[145–171] Mixed infections are uncommon—most involve *Staphylococcus* and another bacterium or a fungus. The special characteristics of fungal infections are described in a subsequent section.

Pathology of Prosthetic Valve Endocarditis. The pathologic findings seen in endocarditis after valve replacement have been extensively documented.[172] Thrombotic vegetations on prostheses of various types, separation of sutures anchoring prostheses, pseudoaneurysm and mycotic aneurysms of the ascending aorta, microabscesses in the myocardium, and abscess of the aortic valve ring are frequently noted (see Fig. 36–3). There are no pathologic alterations distinctive for a given organism.[134] Thrombi are typically located at the junction of the struts and the metallic rings of the prosthesis, with extension up the struts. Ring abscesses are frequently present and most often involve the entire valve annulus and spread to adjacent structures in more than half the cases. For example, aortic ring abscesses frequently burrow through the ascending aorta into the periaortic space, through the atrial septum into the right atrium, into the left atrium, through the ventricular septum into the right ventricle, or into the anterobasal left ventricular wall. The ring abscess of infected mitral prostheses can burrow through the atrial wall into the pericardial space. These features are apparently the result of the rolling motion of the rigid frame of the valve prosthesis. The more severe changes around the aortic valve may be caused by the greater turbulence across the aortic prosthesis than around the mitral valve.[172]

TABLE 36–8. SUMMARY OF MICROORGANISMS ISOLATED FROM BLOOD CULTURES OR PROSTHESES IN FOUR STUDIES CONTAINING 260 PATIENTS WITH 262 EPISODES OF PVE (1962 TO 1982)

	Number of Isolates[a]					
Microorganisms	Early	Percentage of Early Total	Late	Percentage of Late Total	Total	Percentage of Total
Gram-positive						
Coagulase-negative staphylococci	34	43	51	28	85	32
Staphylococcus aureus	12	15	14	8	26	10
Enterococci	1	1	15	8	17	6
Nonenterococcal streptococci	3	3	48	27	50	19
Diphtheroids	10	13	5	3	15	6
Listeria	1	1	1	0.5	2	1
Gram-negative						
Gram-negative bacilli	8	10	13	7	21	8
Gram-negative coccobacilli[b]	0	0	9	5	9	3
Neisseria	0	0	1	0.5	1	1
Fungi[c]	6	8	9	5	15	6
Polymicrobial	3	3	4	2	7	3
Culture negative or not done	3	3	11	6	14	5
Total number of isolates (% of total)	81(31)		181(69)		262(100)	

[a] *Early* and *late* are defined as PVE occurring at less than 60 and at 60 or more days postvalve implantation, respectively.
[b] Includes *Actinobacillus, Cardiobacterium,* and *Hemophilus.*
[c] Includes *Candida, Aspergillus,* and *Scopulariopsis.*
From Heimberger TS, Duma RJ: Infect Dis Clin North Am 3:221, 1989.

TABLE 36–9. PROSTHETIC VALVE ENDOCARDITIS: UNCOMMON BACTERIA

Microorganism	Reference
Neisseria perflava	
N. meningitidis	145, 146
Hemophilus aphorphilus	147
Actinobacillus actinomycetemcomitans	148
Actinobacillus	149
Mima polymorpha (*Acinetobacter*)	150
Pseudomonas maltophilia	151
Nocardia asteroides	153
Brucella melitensis	154, 155
Listeria monocytogenes	156, 157
Diphtheroids	107, 149, 158
Corynebacterium diphtheriae	98, 149
Bacillus cereus	108, 159
Cardiobacterium hominis	160, 161, 162
Mycobacterium fortuitum (group IV)	163, 164
M. chelonei (group IV)	114, 115, 165, 166, 167
M. gordonae (group II)	117, 168
Acid-fast, not identifiable	169
Rickettsia burnetti	119, 120, 170, 171

Several important clinical events can clearly be related to the pathologic findings. The appearance of an aortic diastolic murmur probably coincides with the formation of a discrete paravalvular leak and aortic insufficiency. An alternate explanation could be the interposition of a tail of thrombus onto the rim of the cage, thereby preventing complete seating of the ball during ventricular diastole.[134,172] The appearance of abnormal rhythms and defects in impulse propagation are probably the result of extension of the infection into the interventricular septum. Complete heart block frequently means that an abscess involves the AV node or bundle of His. Left bundle branch block does not correlate with infection of the conduction system. In such patients idiopathic atrophy and fibrosis of the proximal portion of the left bundle are found. The principal causes of death are congestive heart failure (85 percent), central nervous system embolus, and generalized infection.

Aortic valves are more commonly infected than mitral valves. Infected aortic prostheses tend to become detached more often than mitral, and infected mitral prostheses tend to become obstructed by vegetations more often than aortic.

Pathogenesis. From the foregoing, the pathogenesis of PVE can be deduced and the major factors summarized. Transient bouts of bacteremia from contaminated intravascular catheters or procedures (dental, rectal, gynecologic) serve as microbial sources (see Table 36–2). The bacteria lodge in areas of turbulence, stasis, and microthromboses. Such disturbances are seen wherever significant pressure gradients exist across a defect or a valve. High-velocity flow through a narrow orifice produces diminished lateral pressure locally and determines the sites of endocardial bacterial lesions. The use of metal frame prostheses within the heart introduces a well-defined area of rigidity, producing local turbulence, and often a small gradient.

The cloth fixation ring and sutures provide an inert foreign body anchored in the turbulent stream. Barney et al[173] found that 100 percent of dogs inoculated intravenously with a predetermined dose of *S. mitis* developed endocarditis if a prosthesis was inserted or if an aortic valve had been damaged. No infection occurred in a similarly exposed control group and in a group with right ventriculotomies.

The changes in systemic host defense caused by pump oxygenators should also be noted, although their contribution to PVE is probably minor. The bactericidal activity in the sera of patients after open heart surgery using standard nonmembrane oxygenators is depressed, and transient defects in the phagocytic functions of leukocytes concurrently appear. Jacob and his colleagues[174] have shown that exposure of blood to cellophane membranes activates the complement cascade in the fluid phase. Circulating leukocytes become aggregated and embolize to capillary beds, especially in the lung. There, activation of the oxidative and enzymatic digestive processes may take place. This scenario, for which there is convincing experimental and clinical evidence, would account for both the humoral and transient cellular antimicrobial defects after cardiopulmonary bypass.

The further effects of cardiopulmonary bypass on platelets may have an indirect bearing on infection by predisposing to abnormal hematomas and sternal instability. Blood collections are easily infected.

The extracardiac effects of extracorporeal circulation may be important here. Intestinal necrosis is a rare but grave complication after open heart surgery, as is necrotizing enterocolitis.[175] These clear-cut episodes of loss of intestinal viability testify to the possibility that transient compromise of the gastrointestinal barrier may occur during bypass, which may permit endogenous intestinal organisms to seed the bloodstream.

Experimental Studies in the Pathogenesis of PVE

THE ROLE OF PREEXISTING THROMBOSIS. The experimental production of infective endocarditis has been discussed in a previous section. The same basic designs have been applied to PVE, and these methods have been reviewed by Archer.[176] In small animals, the most consistent model of endocarditis has resulted from passage of a polyethylene catheter into either side of the heart. This abrades the ventricular endocardium and produces the sterile vegetations characteristic of nonbacterial thrombotic endocarditis. Such lesions can consistently be colonized with inoculated bacteria. These thrombi resemble the thrombi often found on the struts of prosthetic valves.

Archer[176] studied colonization of catheter-induced vegetations by intravenously inoculated *S. aureus, S. faecalis,* and *P. aeruginosa.* He showed that gram-negative bacteria adhere to or multiply in endocardial vegetations at a slower rate than gram-positive bacteria and that most bacteria adhere passively to nonbacterial thrombotic endocarditis lesions without prior interaction with other blood elements. The latter observations stand in contrast to other studies, which suggest that bacteria agglutinate platelets during the production of vegetations. It is likely that turbulent flow around natural valves or prostheses and the inherent characteristics of individual organisms are the most important factors determining the deposition of microorganisms on natural and prosthetic valves. Archer[176] also made the important observation that tightly interwoven fibrin acts as a barrier to the effective migration of phagocytes. He found that, although fibrin is loose at the surface of a vegetation, it is packed tightly in the region just below the surface and contains colonies of bacteria in areas that are devoid of phagocytes. Bacterial agglutination of platelets is necessary for bacteria to localize on vegetations. Bacterial infection of a sterile platelet-fibrin thrombus may occur after organisms are caught on the surface of a platelet-fibrin lattice and are buried by accretion of platelets and fibrin from the circulation. Multiplication occurs in the depths of this lattice unimpeded by phagocytes.

ROLE OF BACTEREMIA. A somewhat different view, which assigns bacteria a primary role in thrombus formation, should be noted. Jones et al[177] related the frequency of massive thrombus accumulation on prosthetic heart valves in dogs to the common occurrence of bacteremia in these animals. If the dogs could be rendered free of bacteremic episodes by means of an elemental diet, preoperative gut decontamination, and systemic antibiotics, the valves remained free of thrombus.

ROLE OF CLOTH COVERING TO THE PROSTHESIS. Prostheses with the base and struts entirely covered with thin, porous fabric have been designed to minimize thromboembolism, though totally cloth-covered valves remain susceptible to infection with large inocula of *S. aureaus.* Prophylactic antibiotics prevented PVE in a comparative study by Detmer et al.[178]

ROLE OF BACTERIAL INOCULUM SIZE. A calf model for prosthetic tricuspid valve endocarditis using *S. aureus* of varying inoculum sizes was developed by Grogan et al.[179] They determined that the dose required to colonize an endothelialized tricuspid prosthesis was 10^7 to 10^8 *S. aureus* organisms. Smaller inoculum sizes did not produce PVE in the late onset period in the calves tested. In contrast, early onset PVE was produced in three of four calves within 7 days after direct inoculation of 10^2 to 10^3 *S. aureus* into the prosthetic valve sewing ring with the heart open. The authors also examined simultaneous cultures from the right atrium, right ventricle, and aorta and demonstrated a 1000- to 10,000-fold decrease in bacterial titers across the combined pulmonary and systemic capillary beds. The bacterial titer of jugular vein blood was low, whereas the right atrial and right ventricular titers were 10,000 times greater. Corresponding aortic cultures varied in titer.

Clinical Manifestations. The diagnosis of PVE is more difficult to establish in patients in the postoperative setting than in unoperated patients. Although the same symptoms and signs are found (Table 36–10), they require cautious interpretation, as they can all occur in the absence of bacteremia after cardiopulmonary bypass. In general, patients with early onset PVE have shaking chills and splenomegaly. Changing murmurs usually appear at the same time as the first positive blood culture, both in the early and late cases, but in some patients changing murmurs are not noted until more than 1 month after the first positive blood culture. Embolic accidents can occur at any time.

Although the single consistent finding in all patients is still fever, a febrile response occurs commonly in patients after bypass in the absence of infection. For example, in infants, overheating by the environment is a common artifact. More detailed investigation must be instituted for daily unex-

TABLE 36–10. CLINICAL MANIFESTATION OF PROSTHETIC VALVE ENDOCARDITIS

Symptom/Sign	Early PVE (%)	Late PVE (%)
Fever	95–100	95–100
New/changing murmur	50–70	40–60
Congestive heart failure	30–100	30
Shock	33	0–10
Conduction abnormality	15–20	5–10
Splenomegaly	20–30	15–40
Emboli	5–30	10–40
Petechiae	30–60	40–50
Osler's nodes, Janeway lesions, Roth spots	5	15
Anemia	75	75
Leukocytosis	40	30–50
Hematuria		65

From Douglas JL, Cobbs CG: Prosthetic Valve Endocarditis. In Kaye D (ed): Infective Endocarditis, 2nd ed. New York, Raven Press, 1992, p 375.

plained temperature elevations above 38.4C, which persist postoperatively beyond 10 to 14 days. Evaluation should be particularly thorough in patients who demonstrate the triad of fever, splenomegaly, and a change in heart sounds.

The most significant change in heart sounds is usually the appearance of an aortic diastolic murmur. Dysfunction of a prosthetic mitral valve is indicated by the progression of a systolic murmur, and thrombosis of a mitral prosthesis can be heralded by the disappearance of the characteristic clicking sound. Cheng et al[180] state that this change should arouse immediate suspicion of massive thrombosis of the prosthesis. They reported a patient with an infected mitral prosthesis where the infection provided a nidus for progressive, fatal thrombosis.

Laboratory Examination in the Diagnosis of PVE

HEMATOLOGIC FINDINGS. Anemia is uncommon, and leukocytosis is mild. Differential counts generally show predominance of neutrophils, and atypical lymphocytes are rarely noted. Erythrocyte sedimentation rates are consistently elevated. Leukocytosis in the diagnosis of infection after cardiac valve surgery has previously been emphasized, but only one-third of the patients with PVE have leukocytosis.[56]

URINARY FINDINGS. Microscopic hematuria and variable degrees of proteinuria are present in the majority of the patients. The degree of hematuria is not impressive, nor is the associated microscopic pyuria. Urine cultures are usually sterile.[56]

X-Ray Studies and Other Special Diagnostic Examinations in PVE

X-RAY STUDIES. Stinson et al[181] reviewed some of the radiologic signs in endocarditis after prosthetic valve replacement. They noted that loosening of a prosthesis may occur with or without infection, but that extensive disruption of a suture line with gross valve movement is more likely caused by a destructive infectious process. The authors described the double-exposure appearance of a disrupted prosthesis on prolonged exposure x-ray studies and distinguished between the gross angulation of a loose mitral prosthesis and the slight angulation that occurs with normal mitral valve action. In contrast, an aortic prosthesis normally moves very little during the cardiac cycle, and minor degrees of tilt on prolonged exposure may be significant. Gross angulation usually signifies detachment of most of the suture line. Fluoroscopy characteristically shows a rapid tilt or "flip" as the base of a partially detached prosthesis changes its axis during systole.

Cinefluoroscopy allows more deliberate examination, and, if there is still doubt, appropriate contrast studies are done using a cine or multiple frame technique. Cinefluoroscopy is especially valuable in assessing valve dysfunction secondary to endocardial infection. Unstable and "rocking" valves can be seen in patients with PVE. In addition, valve dehiscence, abnormal excursion of poppets, and incomplete seating of poppets through tissue ingrowth and obstruction can be detected fluoroscopically.[67] Although cineangiography is not helpful in demonstrating vegetations, contrast injections can define the presence and location of aortic root abscesses.[67]

The diagnostic features of malfunction of mitral valve prostheses has been outlined. Cine studies or rapid frame exposures usually clarify valve motion and angulation. As in aortic valve dysfunction, cardiac catheterization and cineangiography should be done promptly when noninvasive studies are inconclusive.

The clinical examination and x-ray studies are not only useful in a diagnostic sense, but they can also have therapeutic implications, for example, by dictating the removal of an unstable valve before the hemodynamic alterations are too advanced.

ECHOCARDIOGRAPHY. The use of echocardiography in the diagnosis of infective endocarditis on natural valves is well established.[66] The use of echocardiography for the detection of valve vegetations in the diagnosis of PVE has increased of late. Bioprostheses, such as porcine heterograft valves, are better studied by echocardiographic examination than mechanical prostheses, which are so echodense that echocardiographic assessment is difficult and vegetations are hard to detect. Doppler color-flow mapping may be useful in an indirect sense by showing abnormal jets of valvular regurgitation. Cardiac catheterization is generally unnecessary in documenting complications of PVE.[67]

ISOTOPE SCANNING. The experimental imaging of infective endocarditis with indium-111 labeled blood cellular components has been noted. Riba et al[68] demonstrated in rabbits that indium-111 labeled platelets (but not leukocytes) resulted in cardiac imaging that was sensitive enough to detect endocarditis. Isotope angiocardiography has been used clinically in detecting a malfunctioning tricuspid valve prosthesis by Malcolm et al.[182] They used technetium-99 pertechnetate and isotopically outlined a large right atrium with a striking hold-up of isotope in the great veins and right atrium. Isotope scanning may be a useful noninvasive adjunct in the diagnosis of PVE where infection has caused valve dysfunction. The technique would be more valuable in right-sided prostheses, where imaging and activity-time curves for intravenously administered isotope are maximal before forward flow and dilution.[182]

Diagnosis. The definitive diagnosis is established only by a positive venous blood culture. This is the most critical examination performed in both the diagnostic evaluation and subsequent assessment of patients developing intracardiac infections postoperatively. If the patient is receiving antibiotics, therapy is discontinued for 2 days. Venous samples from different sites are taken daily for 3 consecutive days and each specimen is inoculated into one or more flasks. The venipuncture site must be well prepared, and sterile gloves must be worn. The cultures should then be incubated in aerobic and anaerobic media for 3 weeks. Penicillinase should be added to the culture media. If the cultures remain sterile, bacterial endocarditis is highly unlikely. When indicated, the specimens should also be studied for fungi, which, like the bacteria, usually show growth within 10 days. Antibiotic therapy can be resumed while awaiting the results.

Single isolated positive cultures should not be disregarded as contaminants. If the culture results are equivocal, a series of cultures should be repeated before either embarking on a prolonged course of therapy or discarding the diagnosis. The diagnosis of endocarditis is more certain if a large proportion of separately drawn blood cultures and inoculated flasks show growth of the same organism.

In a few cases it may be difficult to identify the site of infection in a patient with sustained bacteremia when there is no clinical or x-ray evidence of valve dysfunction. Bach et al[183] localized infection in an aortic bypass graft, which extended from the thoracic to the abdominal aorta, using intra-arterial catheters and quantitative bacterial counts on blood samples taken upstream and downstream from the graft. The same principle can be applied to those rare patients with intracardiac prostheses and bacteremia in whom there is no definite evidence of endocarditis and no other obvious extracardiac source for bacteremia.

Treatment. The management of patients with PVE can be divided into three areas: (1) general care, (2) antimicrobial therapy, and (3) surgical considerations.[184]

GENERAL CARE. Special attention should be directed to the organ systems most commonly affected in PVE. The major complications of PVE have been noted in the preceding sections and include congestive heart failure, arrhythmias, myocardial infarction secondary to coronary artery emboli, and myocardial abscess. Standard parameters that merit serial studies include repeated physical examinations, electrocardiograms, and x-ray studies of the chest. Other tests that may be useful in specific cases include fluoroscopy, echocardiography, and cardiac catheterization for hemodynamic studies and at times for quantitative cultures to assist in localization of a focus of infection.

Careful repeated evaluation of renal function is also indicated to adjust antibiotic dosage. Diminished renal function significantly alters the pharmacokinetics of most antibiotics, and antibiotic dosages should be reviewed daily in any patient who is uremic. Acute tubular impairment in PVE can be caused by aminoglycoside toxicity, and prerenal azotemia can be caused by cardiac failure as well as the glomerulonephritis seen as part of the vasculitis of PVE. The central nervous system, the skin, and the reticuloendothelial system should also be evaluated and followed.

ANTIMICROBIAL THERAPY. After a microbiologic diagnosis is established by means of blood cultures, therapy can be initiated. If the illness is more acute, therapy can be started after the collection of three blood cultures several hours apart. Initial therapy, when possible, should include two drugs with synergistic bactericidal activity against the suspected or identified pathogen (see Tables 36–8 and 36–11).

The principles outlined in the sections of infective endocarditis also apply to the patient with PVE. Samples of organisms isolated from the blood cultures should be saved until treatment has been completed, so that susceptibility testing can be performed. Serum bactericidal activity and direct measurement of blood antibiotic concentrations should be done to study the adequacy of drug dosage. Se-

TABLE 36–11. GUIDE TO ANTIMICROBIAL THERAPY OF PVE IN ADULTS

Microorganism	Recommended Antibiotic Regimen	Minimum Duration of Therapy (wk)	Alternative Antibiotic Regimen for Penicillin-Allergic Patient
• GRAM POSITIVE			
Nonenterococcal streptococci			
Penicillin-susceptible (MIC < 0.2 μg/ml)	Aqueous penicillin G[a] or aqueous penicillin G[a] plus streptomycin[d] or gentamicin[e]	6 4–6 (penicillin) 2 (aminoglycoside)	Vancomycin[b] or cephalothin[c] or Cephalothin[c] plus streptomycin[d] or gentamicin[e]
Penicillin-resistant (MIC > 0.2 μg/ml but <0.5 μg/ml) Nutritionally deficient variants	Aqueous penicillin G[a] plus gentamicin[e]	6	Vancomycin[b] or Cephalothin[c] plus streptomycin[d] or gentamicin[e]
Enterococci[f]	Penicillin G[a] or Ampicillin[g] plus gentamicin[e] or streptomycin[d]	6	Vancomycin[b] plus gentamicin[e]
Staphylococci[h]			
Coagulase positive, methicillin-sensitive	Nafcillin[i] or oxacillin plus/minus gentamicin[e]	6–8 (nafcillin) 2 (aminoglycoside)	Cephalothin[c] plus/minus gentamicin[e] or Vancomycin[b]
Coagulase positive, methicillin-resistant	Vancomycin[b] plus/minus gentamicin[e]	6–8 (vancomycin) 2 (aminoglycoside)	None
Coagulase negative	Vancomycin[b] plus rifampin[j] plus/minus gentamicin[e]	6–8 (vancomycin) 2 (aminoglycoside)	
Diphtheroids Gentamicin-susceptible	Aqueous penicillin G[a] plus gentamicin[e] or Vancomycin[b] plus/minus gentamicin[e]	6 6–8	Vancomycin[b]
Gentamicin-resistant	Vancomycin[b]	6–8	
• GRAM NEGATIVE			
Gram-negative bacilli	Third-generation cephalosporins, carbapenems, monobactams or broad spectrum penicillins (eg, piperacillin) plus an aminoglycoside until organism speciated and MIC and MBC studies are performed[b]	6	
Gram-negative coccobacilli	Ampicillin[g] plus streptomycin[d] or third generation cephalosporin[l]	6	

Includes *Hemophilus* species, *Actinobacillus actinomycetemcomitans* and *Cardiobacterium hominis.* All of the following doses are for adults with normal renal function:

[a] Aqueous penicillin G, 20 million units IV daily given in divided doses every 4 hours.
[b] Vancomycin, 0.5 g IV every 6 hours or 1.0 g IV every 12 hours.
[c] Cephalothin, 2 g IV every 4 hours (or equivalent first-generation cephalosporin).
[d] Streptomycin, 0.5 g IM every 12 hours.
[e] Gentamicin, 1 mg/kg IV every 8 hours maintenance. Aminoglycoside levels should be monitored to avoid renal dysfunction and ototoxicity.
[f] Aqueous penicillin G, 20–30 million units IV daily given in divided doses every 4 hours.
[g] Ampicillin, 12–15 g daily, in divided doses, every 4 hours for non-beta-lactamase-producing organisms.
[h] Isolates should be tested for susceptibility to aminoglycosides to aid in selection of the best agent. If the organism is resistant to all aminoglycosides, these agents should not be used or should be discontinued.
[i] Nafcillin, 2.0 g IV every 4 hours.
[j] Rifampin, 300 mg orally every 8 hours.
[k] Maximum allowable doses of third-generation cephalosporins, monobactams, carbapenems, and broad spectrum penicillins should be used.
[l] If a beta-lactamase-positive microorganism is isolated, a beta-lactamase-resistant third-generation beta-lactam should be used.

From Heimberger TS, Duma RJ: Infect Dis Clin North Am 3:221, 1989.

rum levels should be assessed at standardized times after administration. Synergism assays of the bactericidal activity of cell wall active agents such as penicillins and aminoglycosides can be carried out. As noted, this is especially important in patients with changing renal function.

Prolonged parenteral therapy with appropriate doses of antibacterial drugs is the most dependable approach. Oral antibiotics have not gained wide acceptance for the treatment of patients with PVE. Gardner et al[184] note that the average duration of parenteral therapy was 5 weeks. Patients infected with staphylococci or gram-negative bacilli were usually treated longer, whereas patients infected with viridans streptococci or nongroup D streptococci often received shorter treatment courses.

SURGICAL CONSIDERATIONS. The management of most patients with PVE hinges on antimicrobial therapy. Over the past three decades[134,185,186] it has become apparent that reoperation and replacement of the prosthesis must be carried out for patients with congestive heart failure, valve dysfunction, and multiple septic emboli or when medical therapy fails.[134,185,186] Using these common criteria, however,[187] the mortality for patients with PVE averages 56 percent.

In view of these poor results, Gardner et al[184] reexamined the concept of prompt valve replacement versus medical treatment alone. The obvious goal is to excise the diseased prosthesis before the infection spreads into critical structures (ie, septic emboli, interventricular septum, myocardial abscesses) or produces congestive heart failure. Arguments against prompt valve replacement include the risks of persistent or recurrent infection that could necessitate a second reoperation. One of the consequences of recommending early operations is that valve replacement will be done in some patients who could have been cured with antibiotics alone. In rebuttal, Gardner et al[184] argue that the operative mortality in cardiac surgery is correlated chiefly with a degree of congestive heart failure at the time of operation and that a policy of prompt valve replacement would probably lower the operative mortality to that seen in elective valve replacement (less than 10 percent).

Prognosis. Patients with an early onset of PVE had a high mortality (76 percent) and were infected chiefly by staphylococci, gram-negative bacilli, or *Candida* (Table 36–12). Patients with late onset PVE had a lower mortality (44 percent) and were more commonly infected with streptococci.

Twenty-two percent of patients were treated by valve replacement. The indications for surgery were (1) significant valvular leak and congestive heart failure (64 percent), (2) persistent or recurrent bacteremia (35 percent), and (3) peripheral emboli (22 percent). Several of the patients had more than one indication for operation. The overall mortality was 61 percent (63 of 103 cases) for patients treated with antibiotics alone and 39 percent (12 of 32 cases) for patients treated by valve replacement plus antibiotics. Gardner et al[184] emphasize that patients who died shortly after diagnosis were frequently too ill to benefit from any therapy, and that this group unfairly prejudiced the treatment results. Consequently, they analyzed a subgroup of patients who survived at least 1 week after the diagnosis of PVE.

Gardner et al[184] concluded that the result of therapy with antimicrobial drugs alone approaches the success rate of valve replacement only for patients with late onset infection caused by highly sensitive organisms, such as the viridans strepto-

TABLE 36–12. SUMMARY OF MORTALITY RATES OF PVE WITH RESPECT TO VALVE POSITION AND EARLY VERSUS LATE ONSET IN THREE STUDIES CONTAINING 144 PATIENTS (1962 TO 1982) WITH AN OVERALL MORTALITY RATE OF 53 PERCENT[a]

Reference Number	Total Number of Patients with PVE	Number of Deaths/Number of Patients with PVE				Number of Deaths/Number of Patients with PVE			
		Aortic Valve	%	*Mitral Valve*	%	*Early*[b]	%	*Late*[b]	%
1	48	25/33	76	8/15	53	12/16	75	21/32	66
2	45	18/34	53	7/11	64	14/16	88	11/29	38
3	51	13/38	34	5/13	38	5/9	56	13/42	31
Total	144	56/105	53	20/39	51	31/41	76	45/103	44

[a] References 187, 211, and 247.
[b] *Early* and *late* are defined as PVE occurring less than 60 and at 60 days or more postvalve implantation, respectively.
From Heimberger TS, Duma RJ: Infect Dis Clin North Am 3:221, 1989.

cocci, who do not have valve dysfunction, congestive heart failure, multiple septic emboli, or refractory infection. They suggest that the more liberal indications for surgery might yield a greater salvage.[184] Douglas and Cobbs[186] have recently reviewed the management of PVE and concisely summarized antimicrobial therapy. Cowgill et al[188] reviewed several major series and stated relative and absolute indications for surgical intervention by valve replacement. Absolute indications are (1) congestive heart failure, moderate to severe due to valve dysfunction; (2) refractory sepsis despite optimal antibiotic treatment; (3) fungal PVE; (4) valve obstruction; (5) unstable prostheses as evidenced by fluoroscopy; and (6) new onset heart block. Relative indications include the following: (1) mild congestive heart failure due to valve dysfunction; (2) nonstreptococcal organism; (3) embolism; (4) vegetation as evidenced by echocardiography; (5) perivalvular leak; (6) relapse following completion of therapy; (7) early onset PVE; and (8) culture-negative PVE despite empirical therapy. In general, Cowgill et al[188] felt that medical therapy is most likely to succeed for penicillin-sensitive streptococcal PVE, mitral rather than aortic PVE, and tissue as opposed to mechanical prostheses.

Baumgartner et al[189] reviewed 75 patients with PVE who underwent valve replacement. The patients were divided into two groups. The "healed" group included 12 patients who had completed a planned course of antibiotic therapy before operation, while in the second group of 63 patients with "active" PVE, operation was performed before completion of therapy. Staphylococcal organisms were the causative agents in seven patients (43 percent) with early PVE. Staphylococcal and streptococcal organisms accounted for late PVE in 58 patients (47 percent). The operative mortality for all patients with PVE was 23 percent (25 percent for "active" PVE, 8 percent for "healed" PVE). The authors found no correlation between duration of preoperative antibiotic therapy and operative outcome. Recurrent or residual endocarditis occurred in seven patients (15 percent) with "active" PVE. In their review of 116 patients with PVE, Calderwood et al[190] found an in-hospital mortality rate of 23 percent. Coagulase-negative staphylococci were the most common infecting organisms in those patients who developed PVE in their 12 months following operation. Eleven of 89 survivors (12 percent) had relapse of PVE during the follow-up interval. Nine relapses occurred in the 56 survivors of medical therapy (16 percent) compared with two of 33 patients (6 percent) following medical-surgical therapy. The latter difference was not statistically significant. The authors felt the beneficial role of operation in these patients was confirmed by the higher risk of relapse for patients with coagulase-negative staphylococcal PVE treated medically (27 percent) than for those treated surgically (5 percent). Complex surgical procedures are sometimes required to replace prosthetic valves especially when there has been destruction of the annulus and/or in the case of valve ring abscesses. Reconstructive techniques used in 23 patients have been reported by Rocchiccioli et al.[191] Standard valve replacements were attempted in nine patients but two showed rapid dehiscence and required complex procedures at reoperation. All were hospital survivors. The 14 other surgically treated patients had almost complete destruction of annular roots and required complex reconstruction. There were five postoperative deaths but nine patients survived with no further evidence of infection with a near follow-up of almost 3 years.[191]

Antibiotic Prophylaxis in Patients with Prosthetic Intracardiac Devices

A patient with a prosthetic intracardiac device has a chance of contracting endocarditis when undergoing dental or other procedures long after complete recovery has taken place (see Table 36–2). Bacteremia can even result from gingival ulcers caused by ill-fitting dentures, and late endocarditis may result from this mechanism. A vigorous prophylactic antibiotic program should be begun in patients with prosthetic cardiac valves who are about to undergo dental or other procedures. The prophylactic program must be more intensive than the prophylactic penicillin regimen recommended for patients with rheumatic heart disease who are candidates for surgical procedures. It includes the use of broad spectrum antibiotics for 2 days before a dental procedure to reduce the number of organisms in the mouth. On the day before, the day of, and for 3 to 5 days following the procedure, parenteral procaine penicillin (600,000 units every 6 hours) and gentamicin (1.5 mg/kg every 8 hours) or streptomycin (0.5 g every 12 hours) are given. Gentamicin is generally preferred because intravenous dosing assures one of adequate blood and tissue antibiotic concentrations. Methicillin (5 g) is given intravenously during the day of operation and oxacillin (4 g orally) for 3 to 5 days after the procedure.

In pediatric patients prophylaxis may be administered or continued after the induction of anesthesia, when intravenous access is established, sparing the patient the discomfort and apprehension of a needle stick. Drug selection and duration depend on the procedure (eg, dental, oral, respiratory) where penicillin or ampicillin (1.0 to 2.0 g) plus gentamicin (1.5 mg/kg) can be used a half-hour before the procedure and repeated 8 to 12 hours later. For genitourinary and gastrointestinal procedures, ampicillin is generally selected. In penicillin-sensitive patients vancomycin or a cephalosporin is commonly substituted, although erythromycin could be used.

In a concise summary, Dajani et al[192] have tabulated conditions and operative procedures where endocarditis prophylaxis is both recommended and not recommended. They have also recommended standard and alternate prophylactic regimens for patients with preexisting heart disease and in patients following insertion of prosthetic heart valves and correlated these regimens for patients having dental, oral, and upper respiratory procedures as well as genitourinary and gastrointestinal procedures.

Fungal Prosthetic Valve Endocarditis. Although intracardiac fungal infection is uncommon after open heart surgery, the diagnosis should be considered in those patients suspected of having endocarditis in whom routine blood cultures are sterile. Characteristically, *Aspergillus* and *Candida* vegetations are found impairing the function of the prosthetic valve and widespread septic emboli are present. McLeod and Remington[193] surveyed more than 300 cases of fungal endocarditis from the literature. More than half occurred on prosthetic valves. Many of the case reports contained only partial information, and their analysis was based only on those cases in which a specific factor was mentioned. Their tabulated information is most useful, and the percentages stated in their tables refer solely to the percentage of patients in whom a specific parameter was defined.

Etiology. Table 36–13 lists the valves involved by various fungi in 170 cases of endocarditis that occurred after cardiac surgery.[193] Obviously, *Aspergillus* and *Candida* species predominate. Table 36–14[194–203] lists the more unusual fungal prosthetic valve infections.

Incidence. Fungal PVE is uncommon; its incidence relative to bacterial PVE is shown in Table 36–8. McLeod and Remington[193] found no apparent preferential predisposition of any specific type of valve for fungi and no predilection of any specific fungus for a particular valve.

Pathogenesis. Fungi are everywhere. They can be found in ventilating systems near and in the operating room and recovery rooms. Operating room equipment and anesthesia equipment are both contaminated, as are occasional homograft valves, porcine heterograft valves, and suture material. Fungi

TABLE 36–13. VALVES INVOLVED BY VARIOUS FUNGI IN 170 CASES OF FUNGAL ENDOCARDITIS OCCURRING AFTER CARDIAC SURGERY

Fungus	Total	No Implant	Prosthesis[a]	Homograft	Heterograft	Fascia lata	Other Cardiac Surgery
Aspergillus	43	4	28(30)	3	0	5	3
Candida albicans	65	11	34(36)	16	1	0	3
Candida (non-*albicans*)	32	10	15(26)	4	0	0	3
Candida (species not specified)	15	0	9	4	1	0	1
Coprinus species	1	0	1	0	0	0	0
Cryptococcus neoformans	1	0	1	0	0	0	0
Curvularia geniculata	1	0	0	1	0	0	0
Histoplasma capsulatum	2	2	0	0	0	0	0
Paecilomyces varioti	2	0	1	1	0	0	0
Penicillium species	3	0	3	0	0	0	0
Phialophora	2	0	1	0	1	0	0
Phycomyces	1	0	1	0	0	0	0
Saccharomyces cerevisiae	2	0	2	0	0	0	0
Torulopsis glabrata	1	0	0(1)	0	0	0	0
Total	171	27	112	29	3	5	10

[a] Figures in parentheses include cases in which infection recurred on prosthesis after fungal infection on a different valve.
From McLeod R, Remington JS: Postoperative fungal endocarditis. In Duma RJ (ed): Infections of Prosthetic Heart Valves and Vascular Grafts. Baltimore, University Park Press, 1977, p 171.

TABLE 36–14. PROSTHETIC VALVE ENDOCARDITIS: UNCOMMON FUNGAL INFECTIONS

Microorganisms	Reference
Paecilomyces varioti	194, 195, 196
Histoplasma capsulatum	197, 198
Curvularia geniculata	199
Mucor species	200
Penicillium chrysogenum	201
Penicillium species	202
Petriellidium boydii (*Allescheria boydii*)	203

may also be introduced into the circulation by trauma to the trachea or colonization of the lower airways during intubation and mechanical ventilation. Other wound infections and intravenous catheters and solutions are well-known sources. The turbulence and jet effects, which produce endocardial surface trauma and thereby predispose to platelet deposition and adherence of organisms, have been stressed by Robboy and Kaiser.[204] They found four lethal cases in which the fungi had implanted on patches of neoendocardium consisting of platelets, fibrin, and fibroblasts that developed as ingrowths of host endocardium onto the sewing cloth rather than on the metallic parts of the valve.

Concomitant bacterial and fungal infections have been reported in a number of cases. In fact, antibiotics had been administered before the development of fungal endocarditis in 68 percent of McLeod and Remington's cases.[193] Intravenous catheters had been used in 43 percent. The same bacteria that occur as common causes of bacterial endocarditis also occur in conjunction with fungal endocarditis. These are organisms that have a greater ability to adhere to heart valves in vitro, and the adherence properties of bacteria may well be related to fungal implantation on a valve. In addition, staphylococci grow better in vitro in the presence of *C. albicans* than in pure culture.[193]

ROLE OF ANTIBIOTICS IN PREDISPOSING TO FUNGAL INFECTION. The role of antibiotics in predisposing to fungal infection has received considerable attention (see Chaps. 10 and 46). Antibiotics may predispose to fungal infection by eliminating intestinal bacteria that normally compete for nutrients and produce antifungal agents, thereby allowing fungal overgrowth, which in turn leads to fungemia. In addition, antibiotics are thought to interfere directly with cellular fungicidal mechanisms. Cooper et al[205] found that antibiotics were necessary in dog models to produce *C. guilliermondi* endocarditis.

Pathology. One of the most characteristic features of fungal endocarditis is the large, bulky vegetations (2 to 8 cm in largest diameter). Fungal vegetations can produce aortic insufficiency by valvular destruction, interference with valve closure by a vegetation, and destruction of paravalvular tissue and secondary paravalvular leaks. Fungal vegetation in a prosthetic valve may also prevent proper seating of the ball or disc in the metallic ring and thereby lead to regurgitation. In addition, stenosis of a valve orifice may be caused by vegetations interfering with flow across the valve.

The vegetations histologically reveal debris, fibrin, and large colonies of organisms with either yeast or hyphal forms, or both. Organisms are present both on the surface and within the vegetation. In addition, histiocytes, lymphocytes, and neutrophils are seen within vegetations and at their periphery. Patches of neoendocardium, which appear to have developed as ingrowths of host endocardium onto the sewing ring of artificial valves, are involved with foci of infection.

Nonvalvular cardiac involvement in fungal endocarditis includes myocardial abscesses, fistulas, coronary emboli and infarction, aneurysms of the atrioventricular valve ring, and destruction and perforation of the interventricular septum and papillary muscles. In addition, myocarditis and pericarditis have also been seen. The pathologic findings of fatal fungal pericarditis have been detailed in two patients following aorta-coronary bypass operations.[206] Both were immunosuppressed with glucocorticoids used to reduce cerebral edema following cardiac arrests. In the first case both *Candida* and *Aspergillus* were present and the bypasses were all invaded by *A. fumigatus* (which can cause necrosis of blood vessels) and this produced extensive myocardial infarctions. In the second case *C. albicans* was involved, and the coronary vessels remained patent. Both patients had *S. epidermidis* infection and were on broad spectrum antibiotics.[206]

Hepatic involvement most frequently consists of chronic passive congestion or small hepatic abscesses. Enlarged spleens are commonly found and show congestion and at times splenic infarcts and abscesses. Renal abnormalities are present in the majority of patients, with infarction, abscesses, and fungal pyelonephritis. Focal glomerulitis as seen in bacterial endocarditis has also been noted.

Emboli can occur to almost any site within the body, most commonly the kidney, the central nervous system, the lower extremities, and the spleen.

Cerebral emboli have been associated with mycotic aneurysms. As stated earlier, *Aspergillus* is an especially virulent embolic agent in that it invades and causes necrosis of walls of small- to medium-sized arteries and veins. Although the prognosis with embolism is grave, a patient with a saddle embolus secondary to *Candida* endocarditis was salvaged by first excising an infected mitral valve (site of a previous mitral commissurotomy and replacement with a mechanical prosthesis). This was followed by resection of the aortic bifurcation (with its contained saddle embolus) and reconstruction with a Y-graft 2 weeks later.[207]

Clinical Manifestations. McLeod and Remington[193] note that an antemortem diagnosis of fungal endocarditis is made in approximately one-half of the reported cases.

Special attention should be paid to intravenous drug abusers, patients who have received antibiotics, those in whom intravenous catheters have been used for any length of time, and patients with infected catheter sites. Fungal endocarditis should also be suspected in patients with disseminated fungal disease. These historical features can be deceptive in that they may antedate an obvious illness by months and at times even years. Fungal endocarditis should also be suspected in patients who have persistent fever even after therapy for proven bacterial endocarditis, and those in whom endocarditis is suspected but where blood culture results are repeatedly negative. Moyer and Edwards[208] have recently reviewed fungal endocarditis. The most common clinical features are the same as those seen in bacterial PVE, except that embolic phenomena are more prevalent.[193,208] Seventy-two percent of the patients with fungal PVE had emboli, in contrast to 27 percent of those with bacterial endocarditis.[209]

Laboratory Findings. The laboratory and electrocardiographic findings in fungal endocarditis are the same as in all endocarditis. X-ray studies may be useful. Lesions in the lungs secondary to septic pulmonary emboli include consolidations, streaks in the parenchyma, pleural effusions, or at times nodular densities. Areas of increased lucency secondary to pulmonary ischemia may at times be seen. McLeod and Remington[193] note that the inflammatory response is deficient in leukopenic patients, and pulmonary findings may be much less impressive even during an active fungal infection. Arteriograms may demonstrate bulky emboli in the lungs. Abnormal echoes may be produced by the large vegetations, which modify the motions of prosthetic devices.

SEROLOGIC STUDIES. Serologic studies in the diagnosis of fungal disease are discussed in Chapter 10. McLeod and Remington[193] note that among the more promising methods of detecting candidiasis are those that detect precipitating antibodies, such as those against mannan (a surface polysaccharide of *Candida*), or detection of actual antigenemia. None are diagnostic because false-positive reactions are too common. Podzorski et al[210] have suggested a special role for fungal mannan in the pathogenesis of candidiasis. They proposed that catabolites of fungal mannan significantly suppress cell-mediated immunity to candidiasis and may perpetuate infecton.

CULTURES. All thromboemboli should be cultured for fungi. Histologic examination of tissue can also be very helpful in identifying fungal elements and is independent of cultures that may be sterile. Bone marrow cultures may also be useful.

McLeod and Remington[193] tabulated the results of blood cultures in fungal endocarditis (Table 36–15). Blood cultures were frequently positive in *Candida* endocarditis (64 to 93 percent), but they were seldom positive in endocarditis caused by *Aspergillus*. Several reasons have been proposed for the negative blood cultures: (1) differences in growth characteristics of certain fungi; (2) low numbers of organisms because fungi grow in mycelial masses rather than as separate organisms—it may be necessary to culture larger volumes of blood than usually necessary for bacterial endocarditis; (3) fungi may be trapped in capillary beds, and arterial cultures may be more useful than venous blood cultures in some cases; (4) the possible emergence of L-forms in patients with fungal endocarditis has also been postulated; in patients with negative cultures, hypertonic media should be used to pick up possible L-form transformation[193]; and (5) fungi may not cloud the culture medium as bacteria do, so that the cultures are erroneously discarded.

Blood cultures should be examined by Gram stain even when the culture medium appears to be negative. Therefore variations in media may be helpful in achieving growth of some of the fungi.[193]

Treatment and Prognosis. The results of therapy are dismal; only 16 percent of patients with *Candida* infections and 5 percent of those with *Aspergillus* survive.[193]

Patients with fungal PVE seldom survived when given amphotericin B (22 percent) alone,

TABLE 36–15. DATA ON BLOOD CULTURES, SEROLOGY, AND SURVIVAL IN PATIENTS WITH ENDOCARDITIS CAUSED BY DIFFERENT FUNGI

Fungus	Total Cases Reported	Percentage with Positive Blood Cultures	Percentage with Positive Serology	Percentage Surviving
Aspergillus	43	13 (4/30)		5
Candida albicans	65	81 (47/58)	100 (9/9)	18
Candida (non-*albicans*)	32	93 (26/28)	100 (4/4)	14
Candida (species not specified)	15	64 (7/11)	100 (2/2)	13
Coprinius species	1	0 (0/1)		0
Cryptococcus neoformans	1	100 (1/1)	0 (0/0)	0
Curvularia geniculata	1	0 (0/1)		0
Histoplasma capsulatum	2	0 (0/2)	0 (0/0)	0
Paecilomyces varioti	2	50 (1/2)		0
Penicillium species	3	0 (0/2)		0
Phialophora	2	50 (1/2)		0
Phycomyces	1	0 (0/0)		0
Saccharomyces cerevisiae	2	100 (2/2)		50
Torulopsis glabrata	1	0 (0/0)		0

Figures outside parentheses: percentage of patients with the parameter. Numerators of figures inside parentheses: patients with the parameter. Denominators of figures inside parentheses: those patients in whom it was possible to define this parameter from the data presented.
From McLeod R, Remington JS: Postoperative fungal endocarditis. In Duma RJ (ed): Infections of Prosthetic Heart Valves and Vascular Grafts. Baltimore, University Park Press, 1977, p 163.

whereas 11 of 22 who received both amphotericin B and operation survived. In brief, drugs alone are not adequate therapy for fungal prosthetic valve endocarditis. Replacement of the valve is necessary in the vast majority of cases. Delay is rarely justified. Preoperative amphotericin B does not improve the outcome, but intravenous doses of the drug should be started on the day of operation, to be continued for long periods. Local irrigations of the endocardium with a 1 percent solution of amphotericin B may be helpful.[193]

In their review, Moyer and Edwards[208] outline therapy. The drugs useful for fungal PVE are those useful for fungal infections in general—amphotericin B and 5-fluorocytosine. The efficacy of the triazoles such as fluronazole and itraconazole is uncertain[208] (see Chap. 28). The combinations of amphotericin B and 5-fluorocytosine are additive or synergistic. Synergy of a combination of amphotericin B and rifampin has been noted against *C. albicans* and combinations have been fungicidal against *Histoplasma*. Rifampin and low-dose amphotericin B have been used successfully in inhibiting growth of *Saccharomyces*.

PVE Involving Tissue Valves. The use of tissue valves has increased in the past decade because the incidence of thromboembolism is reduced when compared with mechanical prostheses. Various tissue substitutes have been employed and the experiences with prosthetic valve endocarditis documented.[211]

Aortic Homograft Valves. In 1962, Ross[212] carried out the first clinical placement of an aortic valve homograft in the subcoronary position. In an earlier series, the homografts were sterilized and preserved in 4 percent formaldehyde solution buffered to a pH of 5.6. Acute bacterial endocarditis (*S. aureus*) was one of the most important postoperative complications and accounted for one of five deaths. Gonzalez-Lavin et al[213] reported on 259 patients who had undergone aortic valve replacement with preserved homograft valves. Most valves showed fragmentation of collagen fibers, resulting in diminution in tensile strength.

Although the incidence of endocarditis was not increased by the use of preserved aortic homografts, graft failure requiring reoperation was too common. Sometimes, endocarditis appeared to precede valve failure. Sterilization of homograft valves by either irradiation or beta-propiolactone solution produced acellularity with a loss of fibrillar structure, separation of collagen fibers, and disruption of elastic fibers. The changes were accentuated in most cusps removed for dysfunction. The most pronounced changes were found in cusps that had been affected by a previous episode of bacterial endocarditis. These valves had thickening, fibrosis, and areas of calcification. These findings encouraged the search for other tissue valve prostheses.

Porcine Aortic Xenograft (Hancock) Valves. In view of the shortcomings already noted in some types of tissue valves, the use of xenografts has gained in popularity. Porcine aortic xenografts have been studied extensively and closely resemble their human counterparts. Buch et al[214] emphasized the method of preservation of valves. Formaldehyde preservation of porcine aortic xenografts failed to provide stable collagen cross-linking, resulting in tissue disruption. Glutaraldehyde preservation, in contrast, improves collagen polymerization and is not appreciably biodegraded. In 1975, Buch et al[214] reported on 120 patients who underwent mitral valve replacement with a Hancock "stabilized glutaraldehyde process: porcine aortic xenograft." Enterococcal endocarditis developed in only one patient, 20 months after surgery, and responded to ampicillin and probenicid therapy. Further experience has suggested to Magilligan et al[215] that the Hancock porcine xenograft is (1) as susceptible to infection as are rigid prostheses, (2) relatively resistant to early postoperative bacteremia, (3) easier to sterilize than rigid prostheses, and (4) more durable than other tissue valves in the face of PVE.[215]

The Hancock porcine valve continues to gain acceptance in many centers, but some later failures may be caused by low-grade infections due to atypical mycobacteria.[164–169] Some fastidious atypical mycobacteria can be cultured only after prolonged incubation in special media and have been found in 8 of 24 Hancock valves.[167] Whether this organism is *Mycobacterium avium-intracellulare,* which commonly infects pigs, or some other atypical mycobacterium is unknown. Currently, glutaraldehyde stabilization of the collagen matrix of the valve is an effective sterilizing agent as well. Valves are not released to users until a quarantine period has passed and control cultures have been proved to be sterile.[167–169] Rossiter et al[211] in 1978 undertook an extensive study comparing heterograft tissue valves and mechanical valves. Pathologic changes of infective endocarditis as seen in Hancock bioprostheses have been detailed by Bartolotti et al[216] in nine patients. The offending organisms were gram-negative bacteria in three patients (*Klebsiella pneumoniae, Enterobacter cloacae,* and *Serratia marcescens*), gram-positive in two (*S. aureus* and viridans streptococci), and fungi in four (*Candida* species in three and *Aspergillus* in one). In most cases there were friable vegetations on the porcine valve cusps, which were the source of septic emboli in five cases. Calcification and valve dysfunction remain risks in porcine xenograft prostheses.

Norenberg et al[163] found half the cases of bacterial PVE were caused by opportunistic bacteria, and 13 to 20 percent were caused by fungi. Unusual organisms have especially been noted in tissue valves (see Tables 36–9, 36–13, and 36–14).

Valved Extracardiac Conduits. Infection has been noted in the valved, extracardiac conduits used in the Rastelli procedure to establish continuity between the right ventricle and pulmonary arteries, thereby allowing total correction of such anomalies as transposition of the great vessels, truncus arteriosus, pulmonary atresia with ventricular septal defect, and double outlet right ventricle. Surgical pathology seen in 39 children referred to Mayo Clinic for replacement of porcine-valved Hancock extracardiac Dacron conduits has been detailed by Edwards et al.[217] Successful management has been described in one case of a presumed staphylococcal infection of a conduit-aortic homograft by replacement with a Hancock conduit,[218] and in another case by debridement and continuous irrigation of a staphylococcal infection that was sterilized with the prosthesis being left in place.[219] Shea et al[220] reported for the first time an infection involving a ventricular apical to descending aorta conduit. It was polymicrobial and fatal.

Antibiotic Prophylaxis for Patients Having Heart Surgery

Antibiotic prophylaxis should be given for 72 hours or less (see Chap. 25). Various antibiotics have been used either singly or in combination with satisfactory results.

In this regard the value of prophylactic antibiotics has been shown by Fong et al[221] in patients undergoing coronary artery bypass procedures in a double-blind, randomized trial using an antistaphylococcal penicillin (methicillin) or a cephalosporin for 3 days. Hillis et al[222] concluded that no more than 2 days of antibiotic prophylaxis was necessary for patients undergoing coronary bypass grafting. Cephalosporins have been used increasingly for prophylaxis because they are effective against most strains of *S. aureus* and *S. epidermidis.* This is especially important in the case of *S. epidermidis* where a number of strains are resistant to semisynthetic penicillins. The pharmacokinetics of the cephalosporins have been studied in some detail and penetration characteristics have been evaluated for some of these drugs.

Akl and Richardson[223] further studied cephalosporin kinetics by determining serum cefazolin levels during cardiopulmonary bypass. They found that one dose given intramuscularly before operation resulted in adequate and stable serum cefazolin levels in patients undergoing cardiopulmonary bypass for up to 3 hours, and possibly longer.

INFECTION OF ARTIFICIAL HEARTS

There is limited experience with totally implanted mechanical hearts; however, infections, complications, and postmortem microbiologic and ultrastructural findings have been described in 1988 in three related reports.[224–226] In the first report of four of the longest term recipients of the Jarvik-7 artificial heart, the major limiting factor was infection arising from the device lines, with spread to the mediastinal periprosthetic space. Infections were due to coagulase-negative staphylococci, *Staphylococcus aureus, P. aeruginosa,* and other *Pseudomonas* species. Intravascular line sepsis with *Candida* also occurred. Intensive antimicrobial treatment to eradicate or suppress the infections resulted in multiresistant strains of bacteria. Thrombi infected with coagulase-negative staphylococci were found in both the right and left atria and in the prosthetic ventricles. The authors concluded that prolonged use of the device beyond 30 days should be reserved for patients for whom no other form of life support is available.[225]

The postmortem microbiologic findings in two patients showed a variety of organisms including three distinct species of *Pseudomonas* in one patient. In one case thrombi were observed at the site of atrial anastomoses; a thrombus from the mitral valve was infected with cultures positive for *P. aeruginosa* and *Bacteroides fragilis*. The latter anaerobe is highly unusual in a heart infection.[224] In the third related article the authors[226] examine biomaterial-centered sepsis and the total artificial heart (TAH). This ultrastructural study identifies a failure of true tissue integration and diffuse, adhesive bacterial colonization of the several biomaterial surfaces of a total artificial heart. The surfaces of a TAH are not well integrated into host tissues and both transmission and scanning electromicrographs show a failure of true tissue integration and diffuse, adhesive, polymicrobial colonization.[226] It is obvious that further investigation is needed to overcome these major obstacles.

INFECTION FOLLOWING HEART TRANSPLANTATION

Infection and rejection are the two most serious complications following heart and heart and lung transplants, and will be dealt with very briefly here are there appear to be few infections of the heart itself following orthotopic transplantation (see Chap. 51). Greene et al[227] undertook an exploratory analysis of time-dependent risk for infection, rejection, and death after cardiac transplantation in 95 patients from Johns Hopkins Medical Institutions. The rates of rejection and infection as episodes per patient were determined within each of ten intervals following transplantation. A total of 19 deaths, 281 rejection episodes, and 180 distinct infections were available for analysis. The hazard function for rejection appeared biphasic with a rapidly decelerating early phase during the first year followed by a constant late phase. This was followed by an approximately 2-year risk of infection after operation and, finally, a late constant phase.[227]

Several reports have been published indicating the appearance of legionnaires' disease,[228] *Pneumocystis carinii,*[229] and aspergillosis in a cardiac recipient.[230] The radiographic appearance of infection and acute rejection of the lung after heart and lung transplant has been well described by Millet et al.[231] Mediastinitis is also a serious recognized complication and has been reported by Karwande et al.[232] Mediastinitis developed in 12 of 420 cardiac transplant patients. Computed tomographic scanning was a valuable method in the diagnosis of mediastinitis. Debridement and muscle-flap coverage were successful in 4 of 12 patients.

It is of interest that there have apparently been only two reports of intracardiac infection following transplantation. The first was in a "hybrid" heart, where a left ventricular bypass procedure was done with a cardiac allograft.[233] Prosthesis endocarditis finally necessitated removal of an aortic prosthesis and partial resection of the infected (*S. aureus*) recipient left ventricle, which was excluded from the circulation. The patient continued to survive 3 years after cardiac allograft.[233]

The apparently single case of endocarditis occurring in an orthotopically transplanted heart was reported by Khoo et al.[234] The patient presented with an abscess in his sternotomy 33 months after orthotopic cardiac transplantation. Blood cultures grew *S. aureus* and he died 34 days after the onset of his illness. Postmortem examination showed acute bacterial endocarditis with dense colonies of gram-positive cocci on the structurally normal leaflets of the mitral valve and microabscesses in the myocardium of the transplanted heart.

It is appropriate to note here that the shortage of donor organs has led to the use of potentially infected donor hearts for cardiac transplantation in 16 patients reported by Lammermeier et al.[235] There were three early and six late deaths. The authors noted surprisingly few infectious complications in this group of recipients and felt that this practice should be considered when other options are not available. The interior of the donor hearts should be structurally normal and the leaflets, cusps, and endocardium may be resistant to the many factors that predispose to endocarditis in spite of host defenses hampered by immunosuppression, catheters, and other conduits for bacterial and fungal entrance and the many other sources of bacteremia and fungemia that occur in these postoperative patients.

POSTOPERATIVE SYNDROMES

Three identifiable postoperative syndromes have been described earlier in patients after cardiac surgery, with and without the use of extracorporeal circulation: the postpericardiotomy, postperfusion, and postcardiotomy syndromes.[236]

Postpericardiotomy Syndrome

The postpericardiotomy syndrome is delayed in onset and follows trauma, myocardial infarction, or a variety of cardiac surgical procedures. Fever and chest pain are the predominant symptoms, with evidence of pericarditis confirmed by physical examination, electrocardiogram, x-ray studies, or echocardiography. The incidence can be as high as 30 percent. Heart-reactive antibodies have been found in many patients, particularly in association with serologic evidence of infection with coxsackie B1-B6 or cytomegalovirus (CMV). Engle et al[237,238] suggest that a recent viral illness or reactivation of a latent illness may trigger the immunologic response that constitutes the postpericardiotomy syndromes.

The syndrome is usually mild and self-limited, although pericardial tamponade has been reported. Rest, fluid restriction, and diuretics are commonly recommended. Systemic steroids are effective in patients with severe or prolonged symptoms.

A prospective study was carried out in children by Webber et al[239] on autoantibody production after cardiopulmonary bypass. The authors attempted to relate antibody production to the postcardiotomy syndrome. Although many of the patients produced autoantibodies, no association was found between these antibodies, which included anticardiolipin antibodies, and the occurrence of the postpericardiotomy syndrome.

In a study using electrophoresis of myocardial proteins and the Western blot technique of detecting anti-heart antibodies, Akl et al[240] followed the formation of anti-heart antibodies for the first 9 months after cardiac surgery and attempted to correlate these findings with the development of the postpericardiotomy syndrome. They found that only 25 percent (9/36) of patients showed any increase in the preexisting levels of anti-heart antibodies or developed anti-heart antibodies with new reactivities. None of the patients developed specific manifestations of the postpericardiotomy syndrome.[240] By contrast, the authors noted (in a prior study) that a high incidence of anti-heart antibodies formed after cardiac transplantation and concluded that this was due to a humoral immune response to the presence of alloantigens on the grafted heart rather than as a result of the surgical procedure, as shown by the low incidence of increase of anti-heart antibodies where the patients underwent nontransplant heart operations.[240]

Postperfusion Syndrome

The postperfusion syndrome consists of fever, an atypical lymphocytosis, and splenomegaly appearing most commonly 2 to 6 weeks after an episode of extracorporeal circulation. Pericarditis and pleurisy are not dominant findings. Rising titers of antibodies to cytomegalovirus (CMV) during the course of the syndrome, and isolation of the virus from body fluids have implicated this virus as the causative agent.[241] Identification of the parainfluenza virus in tissue cultures from patients with a similar disorder suggested that multiple viruses or virus strains may be producing different clinical varieties of the syndrome in various parts of the world. Because the CMV resides in the leukocyte fractions of fresh blood, primary CMV infections could be acquired. Other evidence suggests that latent CMV may become reactivated by alterations in host defense induced by extracorporeal circulation (see Chap. 11).[237,238] This syndrome is benign and usually mildly symptomatic. The importance of correct diagnosis lies in differentiating more serious causes of fever such as bacterial endocarditis and hepatitis.

Postcardiotomy Syndrome

The postcardiotomy syndrome exhibits features of both postpericardiotomy and the postperfusion syndromes. Kirsh et al[236] characterized it by the onset of prolonged fever, tachycardia, and mucosal lesions within a few days after operation. Recurrent fever, pleuropericardial friction rub, hepatomegaly, and splenomegaly develop 3 to 6 weeks later. The course is benign, and only supportive treatment is necessary.

Postcardiac Injury Syndrome. A relatively new entity has now been proposed by Khan[242] termed the postcardiac injury syndrome (PCIS).[242] This encompasses the postmyocardial infarction syndrome (PMIS) and the postcardiotomy syndrome (PCS)[243] and post-trauma syndrome. It encompasses these entities, which share many common features in spite of different etiologic mechanisms. Postcardiac injury syndrome is characterized by fever, pleuropericardial pain, pericarditis, and pulmonary involvement with pleural effusions with or without lung infiltrates. Viruses may play a role. The course is usually benign but rare complications include tamponade, constriction, anemia, and coronary bypass occlusion. As noted previously, anti-inflammatory agents may be useful in managing these patients.

Fever After Heart Surgery. Undiagnosed febrile illnesses are common after open heart surgery and may or may not conform to the clinical syndromes discussed. Freeman et al[244] found a fourfold or greater rise in complement-fixing antibody titer to CMV in three (4 percent), and to *M. pneumoniae* in 14 (19 percent) of 74 patients. There was no serologic evidence of infection with influenza A and B, mumps, the psittacosis-lymphogranuloma venereum group of agents, *Chlamydia*, or *Coxiella burnetii*. Caul and co-workers[241] found complement-fixing antibodies to cytomegalovirus in 21 of 55 cardiac surgical patients. There was no correlation between CMV infection and age, sex, blood group, or season. All the patients received fresh blood, but none of those receiving less than 5 pints became infected. The authors speculated, as have others, on whether some of these infections are caused by fresh blood used in extracorporeal circuits.

Burch and Colcolough[243] have suggested that some viruses, especially the coxsackie B group, are capable of infecting the heart and remaining dormant for long periods of time to be activated when conditions are suitable. They found a number of instances in which viral antigen was detected within the myocardium and valves of experimental animals many months after the initial infection. They felt that some instances of chronic valvular and myocardial disease, thought previously to be rheumatic in origin, might have been caused by viruses. In addition, these findings make it conceivable that the postperfusion and perhaps the postpericardiotomy, postcardiotomy, and postcardiac injury syndromes may result from activation of a dormant cardiac virus after the trauma of operation, transfused blood, and extracorporeal circulation.

Hornick[245] also emphasizes that, in addition to bacterial contamination of parenteral solutions, other agents may also be transfused with debilitating effects (ie, CMV, hepatitis viruses, Epstein-Barr virus). These agents can both induce infection and depress host defenses so that superinfection can occur.

Obviously, not all febrile illnesses are infective in origin. The role of transfused blood per se and altered host immunologic reactivity has been investigated by Roses et al.[246] They studied the etiology of postoperative fevers in 97 patients after cardiac surgical procedures. Of this group, 26 had unexplained fevers, whereas only six of all the patients had a postpericardiotomy syndrome. The pathogenetic mechanisms have included exacerbation of rheumatic fever, inflammatory response to blood in the pericardial cavity, autoimmune responses to traumatized cardiac tissue, and reaction of the patient to leukocytes in transfused blood. Atypical lymphocytes occurred almost twice as frequently in patients with prolonged fevers after the first postoperative week, in whom no specific etiology could be defined, compared with subjects who were afebrile after the first postoperative week. This group also received more units of transfused blood during operation. There was no correlation, however, between such cellular activation and the appearance of lymphocytotoxic antibodies against a standard reference panel of lymphocytes obtained from 30 normal donors of different HLA phenotypes. This suggested that the atypical lymphocytes reflected a cellular rather than a serologic immune response to massive blood transfusions.

REFERENCES

Myocardial Infections

1. Miller AJ, Pick R, Kline IK, Katz LN: The susceptibility of dogs with chronic impairment of cardiac lymph flow to staphylococcal valvular endocarditis. Circulation 30:417, 1964.
2. Gopalakrishna KV, Kwon KH, Shah A: Metastatic myocardial abscess due to group F streptococci. Am J Med Sci 274:329, 1977.
3. Milstoc M, Berger AR: True bacterial mural endocarditis. Chest 59:103, 1971.

4. Mildvan D, Goldberg E, Berger M, et al: Diagnosis and successful management of septal myocardial abscess: a complication of bacterial endocarditis. Am J Med Sci 274:311, 1977.
5. Tellez G, Nojek C, Juffe A, et al: Cardiac echinococcosis: report of three cases and review of the literature. Ann Thorac Surg 21:425, 1976.
6. Shakibi JG, Safavion MH, Azar H, Siassi B: Surgical treatment of echinococcal cysts of the heart: report of two cases and review of the world literature. J Thorac Cardiovasc Surg 74:941, 1977.
7. Qian Z: Thoracic hydatid cysts: a report of 842 cases treated over a thirty-year period. Ann Thorac Surg 46:342, 1988.
8. Ottino G, Villani M, DePaulis R, et al: Restoration of atrioventricular conduction after surgical removal of a hydatid cyst of the interventricular septum. J Thorac Cardiovasc Surg 93:144, 1987.
9. Aris A, Leon C, Bonnin JO, et al: One-stage surgical treatment of cardiac and pulmonary echinococcosis. Ann Thorac Surg 31:564, 1981.
10. Rossi MA, Braile DM, Souza DRS, et al: Dynamic cardiomyoplasty in chronic Chagas' heart disease: clinicopathological data. Ann Thorac Surg 51:649, 1991.
11. Woods GL, Wood RP, Shaw BW Jr: *Aspergillus* endocarditis in patients without prior cardiovascular surgery: report of a case in a liver transplant recipient and review. Rev Infect Dis 11:263, 1989.
12. Egan TM, Maitland A, Sinave C, et al: Myocardial abscess in a patient with AIDS-related complex: pericardial patch repair. Ann Thorac Surg 49:481, 1990.
13. Morgan MG, Glasser SP, Sanusi ID: Bacterial endocarditis: occurrence on a traumatically ruptured aortic valve. JAMA 233:810, 1975.
14. Enders GC, Graeber GM, Poirier RA: Wounds traversing two or more cardiac chambers. Case presentation of two survivors and review of the literature. J Thorac Cardiovasc Surg 76:83, 1978.
15. Pate JW, Richardson RL: Penetrating wounds of cardiac valves. JAMA 207:309, 1969.
16. Symbas PN, DiOrio DA, Tyras DH, et al: Penetrating cardiac wounds: significant residual and delayed sequelae. J Thorac Cardiovasc Surg 66:526, 1973.

Infective Endocarditis

17. Kaye D (ed): Infective Endocarditis. Baltimore, University Park Press, 1976.
18. Kaplan EL, Taranta AV (eds): Infective Endocarditis. Dallas, American Heart Association, 1977.
19. Rahimtoola SH (ed): Infective Endocarditis. New York, Grune & Stratton, 1978.
20. Bisno AL (ed): Treatment of Infective Endocarditis. New York, Grune & Stratton, 1981.
21. Kaye D (ed): Infective Endocarditis, 2nd ed. New York, Raven Press, 1992.
22. Korzeniowski OM, Kaye D: Infective endocarditis. In Braunwald E (ed): Heart Disease, 4th ed. Philadelphia, Saunders, 1992, p 1078.
23. Rosenthal A, Nadas AS: Infective endocarditis in infancy and childhood. In Rahimtoola SH (ed): Infective Endocarditis. New York, Grune & Stratton, 1978, p 149.
24. Oelberg DG, Fisher DJ, Gross DM, et al: Endocarditis in high-risk neonates. Pediatrics 71:392, 1983.
25. Hartyanszky IL, Lozsadi K, Huttl T: Successful surgical management of mitral valve endocarditis in a 13-month-old child. J Thorac Cardiovasc Surg 96:831, 1988.
26. Kaplansky M, Reyes CV: Nonbacterial thrombotic endocarditis associated with the use of a peritoneovenous shunt. Tex Heart Inst J 14:215, 1987.
27. Powell DC, Bivins BA, Bell RM, et al: Bacterial endocarditis in the critically ill surgical patient. Arch Surg 116:311, 1981.
28. Michel L, Marsh HM, McMichen JC, et al: Infection of pulmonary artery catheters in critically ill patients. JAMA 245:1032, 1981.
29. Gutti JE, Reichek N, Mullen JL: Endocarditis complicating home hyperalimentation. Arch Surg 116:933, 1981.
30. Quintiliani R, Ganguli P: Splenic arteriovenous fistula with bacterial endoarteritis and endocarditis. JAMA 214:727, 1970.
31. Nagle JP: Idiopathic hypertrophic subaortic stenosis and bacterial endocarditis. JAMA 200:163, 1967.
32. Frank S, Braunwald E: Idiopathic hypertrophic subaortic stenosis. Clinical analysis of 126 patients with emphasis on the natural history. Circulation 37:759, 1968.
33. Weinstein AJ, McHenry MC: Bacterial endocarditis in a patient with mitral valve prolapse. Arch Intern Med 139:1191, 1979.
34. Cheitlin MD, Byrd RC: The click-murmur syndrome. A clinical problem in diagnosis and treatment. JAMA 245:1357, 1981.
35. Flynn W, Garcia-Rinaldi R, Roehm JOF Jr, Crawford ES: Surgical treatment of infected right atrial myxoma. Ann Thorac Surg 27:242, 1978.
36. Roberts WC: Characteristics and consequences of infective endocarditis (active or healed or both). In Rahimtoola SH (ed): Infective Endocarditis. New York, Grune & Stratton, 1978, p 55.
37. Krause JR, Levison SP: Pathology of infective endocarditis. In Kaye D (ed): Infective Endocarditis. Baltimore, University Park Press, 1976, p 55.
38. McFarland MM: Pathology of infective endocarditis. In Kaye D (ed): Infective Endocarditis, New York, Raven Press, 1992, p 57.
39. Livornese LL Jr, Korzeniowski OM: Pathogenesis of infective endocarditis. In Kaye D (ed): Infective Endocarditis, 2nd ed. New York, Raven Press, 1992, p 19.
40. Clawson CC: Role of platelets in the pathogenesis of endocarditis. In Kaplan EL, Taranta AV (eds): Infective Endocarditis. Dallas, American Heart Association, 1977, p 24.
41. Levison ME: Pathogenesis of infective endocarditis.

In Kaye D (ed): Infective Endocarditis. Baltimore, University Park Press, 1976, p 29.
42. Reeve R, Reeve JS, Matula G, Lawson W: Mitral obstruction by vegetations of staphylococcal endocarditis. JAMA 228:75, 1974.
43. Lillehei CW, Bobb JR, Visscher MB: The occurrence of endocarditis with valvular deformities in dogs with arteriovenous fistulas. Ann Surg 132:577, 1950.
44. Sande MA: Experimental endocarditis. In Kaye D (ed): Infective Endocarditis. Baltimore, University Park Press, 1976, p 11.
45. Hook EW, Sande MA: Role of the vegetation in experimental streptococcus viridans endocarditis. Infect Immun 10:1433, 1974.
46. Symbas PN, Cooper T, Gantner GE Jr, Willman VL: Lymphatic drainage of the heart: effects of experimental interruption of lymphatic vessels. Surg Forum 14:254, 1963.
47. Sande MA: Antibiotic therapy of experimental endocarditis. In Kaplan EL, Taranta AV (eds): Infective Endocarditis. Dallas, American Heart Association, 1977, p 33.
48. Roberts RB: Streptococcal endocarditis. The viridans and beta-hemolytic streptococci. In Kaye D (ed): Infective Endocarditis, 2nd ed. New York, Raven Press, 1992, p 191.
49. Tunkel AR, Mandell GL: Infecting microorganisms. In Kaye D (ed): Infective Endocarditis, 2nd ed. New York, Raven Press, 1992, p 85.
50. Goldberg P, Shulman ST, Yogeo R: Group C streptococcal endocarditis. Pediatrics 75:114, 1985.
51. Finegold SM: Cardiovascular infections. In Finegold SM (ed): Anaerobic Bacteria in Human Disease. New York, Academic Press, 1977, p 182.
52. Dall L, Barnes WG, Lane JW, Mills J: Enzymatic modification of the glycocalyx in the treatment of experimental endocarditis due to viridans streptococci. J Infect Dis 156(5):736, 1987.
53. Hammill RJ, Vann JM, Proctor RA: Phagocytosis of *Staphylococcus aureus* by cultured bovine aortic endothelial cells: model for post-adherence events in endovascular infections. Infect Immun 54:833, 1986.
54. Rotrosen D, Edwards JE Jr, Gibson TR, et al: Adherence of *Candida* to cultured vascular endothelial cells: mechanisms of attachment and endothelial penetration. J Infect Dis 152:1264, 1985.
55. Baddour LM, Christensen GD, Hester MG, Bisno AL: Production of experimental endocarditis by coagulase-negative staphylococci: variability in species virulence. J Infect Dis 150:721, 1984.
56. Amoury RA: Infection following cardiopulmonary bypass. In Norman JC (ed): Cardiac Surgery. New York, Appleton-Century-Crofts, 1972.
57. Tunkel AR, Scheld WM: Experimental models of endocarditis. In Kaye D (ed): Infective Endocarditis, 2nd ed. New York, Raven Press, 1992, p 37.
58. Mandell GL: The laboratory in diagnosis and management. In Kaye D (ed): Infective Endocarditis. Baltimore, University Park Press, 1976, p 155.
59. Powers DL, Mandell GL: Intraleukocytic bacteria in endocarditis patients. JAMA 227:312, 1974.
60. Archer GL, Karchmer AW, Vishniavsky N, Johnston JL: Plasmid-pattern analysis for the differentiation of infecting from noninfecting *Staphylococcus epidermidis*. J Infect Dis 149:913, 1984.
61. Goering RV, Duensing TD: Rapid field inversion gel electrophoresis in combination with an rRNA gene probe in the epidemiological evaluation of staphylococci. J Clin Microbiol 28:426, 1990.
62. Lowenstein MB, Urman JD, Abeles M, Weinstein A: Skin immunofluorescence in infective endocarditis. JAMA 238:1163, 1977.
63. Werner AS, Cobbs CG, Kaye D, Hook EW: Studies on the bacteremia of bacterial endocarditis. JAMA 202:199, 1967.
64. Kaye KM, Kaye D: Laboratory findings including blood cultures. In Kaye D (ed): Infective Endocarditis, 2nd ed. New York, Raven Press, 1992, p 117.
65. Reik H, Rubin SJ: Evaluation of the buffy-coat smear for rapid detection of bacteremia. JAMA 245:375, 1981.
66. Thomson KR, Nanda NC, Gramiak R: The reliability of echocardiography in the diagnosis of infective endocarditis. Radiology 125:473, 1977.
67. Sokil AB: Cardiac imaging in infective endocarditis. In Kaye D (ed): Infective Endocarditis, 2nd ed. New York, Raven Press, 1992, p 125.
68. Riba AL, Thakur ML, Gottschalk A, et al: Imaging experimental infective endocarditis with indium-111 labeled blood cellular components. Circulation 59:336, 1979.
69. Baldassarre JS, Kaye D: Principles and overview of antibiotic therapy. In Kaye D (ed): Infective Endocarditis, 2nd ed. New York, Raven Press, 1992, p 169.
70. Levison M: In vitro assays. In Kaye D (ed): Infective Endocarditis, 2nd ed. New York, Raven Press, 1992, p 151.
71. Hook EW, Guerrant RL: Therapy of infective endocarditis. In Kaye D (ed): Infective Endocarditis. Baltimore, University Park Press, 1976, p 167.
72. Wilson WR, Geraci JE: Antimicrobial therapy for penicillin-sensitive streptococcal endocarditis: two week regimens. In Bisno AL (ed): Treatment of Infective Endocarditis. New York, Grune & Stratton, 1981, p 61.
73. Bush LM, Johnson CC: Clinical syndrome and diagnosis. In Kaye D (ed): Infective Endocarditis, 2nd ed. New York, Raven Press, 1992, p 99.
74. Eliopoulos GM: Enterococcal endocarditis. In Kaye D (ed): Infective Endocarditis, 2nd ed. New York, Raven Press, 1992, p 209.
75. Karchmer AW: Staphylococcal endocarditis. In Kaye D (ed): Infective Endocarditis, 2nd ed. New York, Raven Press, 1992, p 225.
76. Hessen MT, Abrutyn E: Gram-negative bacterial endocarditis. In Kaye D (ed): Infective Endocarditis, 2nd ed. New York, Raven Press, 1992, p 251.

77. Bodey GP: Penicillin, monobactums, and carbapenems. Tex Heart Inst J 17:315, 1990.
78. Neu HC: Use of fluoroquinolone antimicrobial agents by cardiovascular and cardiopulmonary surgeons. Tex Heart Inst J 17:12, 1990.
79. Lerner PI, Weinstein L: Infective endocarditis in the antibiotic era. N Engl J Med 274:199, 259, 323, 388, 1966.
80. Yeh TJ, Hall DP, Ellison RG: Surgical treatment of aortic valve perforation due to bacterial endocarditis. A report of six cases. Am Surg 30:766, 1964.
81. Wallace AG, Young WG Jr, Osterhout S: Treatment of acute bacterial endocarditis by valve excision and replacement. Circulation 31:450, 1965.
82. Manhas Dr, Hessel EA II, Winterschied LC, et al: Open heart surgery in infective endocarditis. Circulation 41:841, 1979.
83. Jung JY, Saab SB, Almond CH: The case for early surgical treatment of left-sided primary infective endocarditis. J Thorac Cardiovasc Surg 70:509, 1975.
84. Boyd AD, Spencer FC, Isom OW, et al: Infective endocarditis. An analysis of 54 surgically treated patients. J Thorac Cardiovasc Surg 73:23, 1977.
85. David TE, Bos J, Christakis GT, et al: Heart valve operations in patients with active infective endocarditis. Ann Thorac Surg 49:701, 1990.
86. Attum AA, Masri Z, Yared SF, et al: Infective endocarditis: diagnosis, treatment, and mortality as related to surgical timing and infectious organism. Tex Heart Inst J 14:401, 1987.
87. Dreyfus G, Serraf A, Jebara YA, et al: Valve repair in acute endocarditis. Ann Thorac Surg 49:706, 1990.
88. Ting W, Silverman N, Levitsky S: Valve replacement in patients with endocarditis and cerebral septic emboli. Ann Thorac Surg 51:18, 1991.
89. Al Jubair K, Al Fagih MR, Ashmeg A, et al: Cardiac operations during active endocarditis. J Thorac Cardiovasc Surg 104:487, 1992.
90. Bove EL, Kavey REW, Sondheimer HM, Parker FB Jr: Subacute bacterial endocarditis and complete endocardial cushion defect. Ann Thorac Surg 34:466, 1982.
91. Fleisher AG, David I, Mogtader A, Hutchinson JE III: Mitral valvuloplasty and repair for infective endocarditis. J Thorac Cardiovasc Surg 93:311, 1987.
92. Hendren WG, Morris AS, Rosenkranz ER, et al: Mitral valve repair for bacterial endocarditis. J Thorac Cardiovasc Surg 103:124, 1992.
93. Danielson GK, Titus JL, DuShane JW: Successful treatment of aortic valve endocarditis and aortic root abscesses by insertion of prosthetic valve in ascending aorta and placement of bypass grafts to coronary arteries. J Thorac Cardiovasc Surg 67:443, 1974.
94. Tuna IC, Orszulak TA, Schaff HV, Danielson GK: Results of homograft aortic valve replacement for active endocarditis. Ann Thorac Surg 49:619, 1990.
95. Cooley DA: Surgical considerations in infective endocarditis. Tex Heart Inst J 16:263, 1989.
96. Lau JM, Guinn GA, Beall AC Jr, et al: Operative techniques in infectious endocarditis. Ann Thorac Surg 32:351, 1981.
97. Lewis BS, Agathangelow NE, Colsen PR, et al: Cardiac operation during active infective endocarditis. J Thorac Cardiovasc Surg 84:579, 1982.
98. Cukingnan RA Jr, Carey JS, Witting JH, Cimochowski GE: Early valve replacement in active infective endocarditis. Results and late survival. J Thorac Cardiovasc Surg 85:163, 1983.
99. Cannon NJ, Cobbs CG: Infective endocarditis in drug addicts. In Kaye D (ed): Infective Endocarditis. Baltimore, University Park Press, 1976, p 111.
100. Borow KM, Alpert JS, Pennington J: Transient *Pseudomonas* bacteremia in a heroin addict. JAMA 240:560, 1978.
101. Meyerowitz PD, Gardner P, Campbell C, et al: Earlier operation for left-sided *Pseudomonas* endocarditis in drug addicts. J Thorac Cardiovasc Surg 77:577, 1979.
102. Harris PD, Yeoh CB, Breault J, et al: Fungal endocarditis secondary to drug addiction. J Thorac Cardiovasc Surg 63:980, 1972.
103. Arbulu A, Thomas NW, Wilson RF: Valvulectomy without prosthetic replacement. J Thorac Cardiovasc Surg 64:103, 1972.
104. Arbulu A, Holmes RJ, Asfaw I: Tricuspid valvulectomy without replacement. J Thorac Cardiovasc Surg 102:917, 1991.
105. Stern HJ, Sisto DA, Strom JA, et al: Immediate tricuspid valve replacement for endocarditis: indications and results. J Thorac Cardiovasc Surg 91:163, 1986.
106. Yee ES, Ullyot DJ: Reparative approach for right-sided endocarditis. J Thorac Cardiovasc Surg 96:133, 1988.
107. Hiratzka LF, Nelson RJ, Oliver CB, Jengo JA: Operative experience with infective endocarditis. Drug users compared with nondrug users. J Thorac Cardiovasc Surg 77:355, 1979.
108. Sande MA, Lee BL, Mills J, Chambers HF III: Endocarditis in intravenous drug users. In Kaye D (ed): Infective Endocarditis, 2nd ed. New York, Raven Press, 1992, p 345.
109. Levy WS, Simon GL, Rios JC, Ross AM: Prevalence of cardiac abnormalities in human immunodeficiency virus infection. Am J Cardiol 63:86, 1989.
110. Francis CK: Cardiac involvement in AIDS. Curr Probl Cardiol 15:571, 1990.
111. Cammarosano C, Lewis W: Cardiac lesions in acquired immune deficiency syndrome (AIDS). J Am Coll Cardiol 5:703, 1985.
112. Niedt GW, Schinella R: Acquired immunodeficiency syndrome: clinicopathologic study of 56 autopsies. Arch Pathol Lab Med 109:727, 1985.
113. Brau N, Esposito RA, Simberkoff MS: Cardiac valve replacement in patients infected with the human immunodeficiency virus. Ann Thorac Surg 54:552, 1992.

114. Schwartz IS, Pervez N: Bacterial endocarditis associated with a permanent transvenous cardiac pacemaker. JAMA 218:736, 1971.
115. Imparato AM, Kim GE: Electrode complications in patients with permanent cardiac pacemakers. Ten years experience. Arch Surg 105:705, 1972.
116. Conklin EF, Giannelli S Jr, Nealon TF Jr: Four hundred consecutive patients with permanent transvenous pacemakers. J Thorac Cardiovasc Surg 69:1, 1975.
117. Grogler FM, Frank G, Greven G, et al: Complications of permanent transvenous cardiac pacing. J Thorac Cardiovasc Surg 69:895, 1975.
118. Charez CM, Conn JH: Septicemia secondary to impacted infected pacemaker wire. J Thorac Cardiovasc Surg 73:796, 1977.
119. Eichhorn EJ, Winters WL Jr, Crawford S, et al: Bacterial endocarditis and right atrial vegetation. Detection by two-dimensional echocardiography. JAMA 246:2724, 1981.
120. Dargan EL, Norman JC: Conservative management of infected pacemaker pulse generator sites. Ann Thorac Surg 12:297, 1971.
121. Brunswick RA, Moynihan PC, Webb WR: Treatment of pacemaker infection in the neonate. J Thorac Cardiovasc Surg 80:123, 1980.
122. Garcia-Rinaldi R, Revuelta JM, Bonnington L, Soltero-Harrington L: The exposed cardiac pacemaker. Treatment by subfascial pocket relocation. J Thorac Cardiovasc Surg 89:136, 1985.
123. Mansour KA, Kauten JR, Hatcher CR Jr: Management of the infected pacemaker: explantation, sterilization and reimplantation. Ann Thorac Surg 40:617, 1985.
124. Hong-Barco P, O'Toole J, Gerber ML, et al: Endocarditis due to six entrapped pacemaker leads and concomitant recurrent coronary arteriosclerosis. Ann Thorac Surg 46:97, 1988.
125. Byrd CL, Schwartz SJ, Sivina M, et al: Technique for the surgical extraction of permanent pacing leads and electrodes. J Thorac Cardiovasc Surg 89:142, 1985.
126. Hartstein AI, Jackson J, Gilbert DN: Prophylactic antibiotics and the insertion of permanent transvenous cardiac pacemakers. J Thorac Cardiovasc Surg 75:219, 1978.
127. Geraci JE, Dale AJD McGoon DC: Bacterial endocarditis and endoarteritis following cardiac operations. Wis Med J 62:302, 1963.
128. Looser KG, Allmendinger PD, Takata H, et al: Infection of cardiac suture line after ventricular aneurysmectomy. J Thorac Cardiovasc Surg 72:280, 1976.
129. Mandel W, Hoffman MS, Heitzman GH, Kass I: Endocarditis following ventricular septal defect repair. Calif Med 88:248, 1958.
130. Teitel M, Florman AL: Postoperative endocarditis due to *Pseudomonas aeruginosa.* JAMA 172:329, 1960.
131. Kelsch JV, Thomson NB Jr: Bacterial endocarditis complicating repair of a ventricular septal defect. Report of a case cured after removal of silk sutures. N Engl J Med 265:1245, 1961.
132. Linde LM, Heins HL: Bacterial endocarditis following surgery for congenital heart disease. N Engl J Med 263:65, 1960.
133. Lord JW Jr, Imparato AM, Hackel A, Doyle EF: Endocarditis complicating open heart surgery. Circulation 23:489, 1961.
134. Amoury RA, Bowman FO Jr, Malm JR: Endocarditis associated with intracardiac prostheses. Diagnosis, management, and prophylaxis. J Thorac Cardiovasc Surg 51:36, 1966.
135. Fraser RS, Rossall RE, Dvorkin J: Bacterial endocarditis after open heart surgery. Can Med Assoc J 96:1551, 1967.
136. Stanton RE, Lindesmith GC, Meyer BW: *Escherichia coli* endocarditis after repair of ventricular septal defects. N Engl J Med 279:737, 1968.
137. Gersony WM, White NR: "Patch embolization" following repair of ventricular septal defect. A complication of bacterial endocarditis. Am J Cardiol 26:315, 1970.
138. Nakayama DK, O'Neill JA Jr, Wagner H, et al: Management of vascular complications of bacterial endocarditis. J Pediatr Surg 21:636, 1986.
139. Jackson MA, Hicks RA: Vancomycin failure in staphylococcal endocarditis. Pediatr Infect Dis J 6:750, 1987.
140. Younkin SW, Brandriss MW, Steigbigel RT: Well-tolerated bacteremia of five years' duration. JAMA 248:2310, 1982.
141. Yeh TJ, Anabtawi IN, Cornett VE, et al: Bacterial endocarditis following open-heart surgery. Ann Thorac Surg 3:29, 1967.
142. Wilson WR: Prosthetic valve endocarditis: incidence, anatomic location, cause, morbidity, and mortality. In Duma RJ (ed): Infections of Prosthetic Heart Valves and Vascular Grafts. Baltimore, University Park Press, 1977, p 3.
143. Ankeney JL, Parker RF: Staphylococcal endocarditis following open heart surgery related to positive intraoperative blood cultures. In Brewer LA (ed): Prosthetic Heart Valves. Springfield, IL, CC Thomas, 1969, p 719.
144. Wong PS, Young VK, Youkana A, Wright JE: Surgical glove punctures during cardiac operations. Ann Thorac Surg 56:108, 1993.
145. Levin S, Balagtas R, Susmano A, et al: Meningococcus endocarditis at the site of Starr-Edwards mitral prosthesis. Arch Intern Med 129:963, 1972.
146. Jephcott AE, Hardesty CA: Meningococcal septicemia in a patient with a prosthetic valve. A successfully treated case. Br J Clin Pract 30:180, 185, 1976.
147. Goldsweig HG, Matsen JM, Castaneda AR: *Hemophilus aphrophilus* endocarditis in a patient with a mitral valve prosthesis: case report and review of the literature. J Thorac Cardiovasc Surg 63:408, 1972.
148. Stauffer JD, Goldman MJ: Bacterial endocarditis due to *Actinobacillus actinomycetemcomitans* in a

patient with a prosthetic aortic valve. Calif Med 117:59, 1972.
149. Juffe A, Miranda AL, Rufilanchas JJ, et al: Prosthetic valve endocarditis by opportunistic pathogens. Arch Surg 112:151, 1977.
150. Buchanan TM: *Mima polymorpha* endocarditis: a patient with two artificial heart valves. South Med J 65:693, 1972.
151. Fischer JJ: *Pseudomonas maltophilia* endocarditis after replacement of the mitral valve: a case study. J Infect Dis 128:S771, 1973.
152. Dismukes WE, Karchmer AW: The diagnosis of infected prosthetic heart valves: bacteremia versus endocarditis. In Duma RJ (ed): Infections of Prosthetic Heart Valves and Vascular Grafts. Baltimore, University Park Press, 1977, p 61.
153. Vlachakis ND, Gazez PC, Hairston P: Nocardial endocarditis following mitral valve replacement. Chest 63:276, 1973.
154. O'Meara D, Eykyn S, Jenkins BS, et al: *Brucella melitensis* endocarditis: successful treatment of an infected prosthetic mitral valve. Thorax 29:377, 1974.
155. Ehrenhaft JL: Discussion of Kaiser GC, Willman VL, Thurmann M, Hanlon CR: Valve replacement in cases of aortic insufficiency due to active endocarditis. J Thorac Cardiovasc Surg 54:491, 1967.
156. Weinstein GS, Nichols NJ, Rogers MR, et al: Endocarditis of aortic valvular prosthesis due to *Listeria monocytogenes*. Chest 69:807, 1976.
157. Saravolatz LD, Burch KH, Madhavan T, Quinn EL: Listerial prosthetic valve endocarditis: successful medical therapy. JAMA 240:2186, 1978.
158. Jackson G, Saunders K: Prosthetic valve diphtheroids endocarditis treated with sodium fusidate and erythromycin. Br Heart J 35:931, 1973.
159. Block CS, Levy NL, Fritz VU: *Bacillus cereus* endocarditis: a case report. SAfr Med J 53:556, 1978.
160. Tuazon CU, Murray HW, Levy C, et al: Serious infections from *Bacillus* sp. JAMA 241:1137, 1979.
161. Geraci JE, Greipp PR, Wilkowske CJ, et al: *Cardiobacterium hominis* endocarditis, four cases with clinical and laboratory observations. Mayo Clin Proc 53:49, 1978.
162. Spernoga JF, Laskowski L, Marr JJ, Burmeister RW: *Cardiobacterium hominis* endocarditis. South Med J 72:85, 1979.
163. Norenberg RG, Sethi GK, Scott SM, Takaro T: Opportunistic endocarditis following open heart surgery. Ann Thorac Surg 19:592, 1975.
164. Robicsek F, Daugherty HK, Cook JW, et al: *Mycobacterium fortuitum* epidemics after open-heart surgery. J Thorac Cardiovasc Surg 75:91, 1978.
165. Altmann G, Horowitz A, Kaplinsky N: Prosthetic valve endocarditis due to *Mycobacterium chelonei*. J Clin Microbiol 1:531, 1975.
166. Repath F, Seabury JH, Sanders CV, Dumer J: Prosthetic valve endocarditis due to *Mycobacterium chelonei*. South Med J 69:1244, 1976.
167. Tyras DH, Kaiser GC, Barner HB, et al: Atypical mycobacteria and the xenograft valve. J Thorac Cardiovasc Surg 75:331, 1978.
168. Lohr DC, Goeken JA, Doty DB, Donta ST: *Mycobacterium gordonae* infection of a prosthetic aortic valve. JAMA 231:1528, 1978.
169. O'Rourke MF, Shanahan MX, Harkness JL: Endocarditis with an acid-fast organism after porcine heart-valve replacement. Lancet 2:686, 1978.
170. Kristinsson A, Bentall HH: Medical and surgical treatment of Q-fever endocarditis. Lancet 2:693, 1967.
171. Morgans CM, Cartwright RY: Case of Q-fever endocarditis at site of aortic valve prosthesis. Br Heart J 31:520, 1969.
172. Arnett EN, Roberts WC: Clinicopathology of prosthetic valve endocarditis. In Duma RJ (ed): Infections of Prosthetic Heart Valves and Vascular Grafts. Baltimore, University Park Press, 1977, p 17.
173. Barney JD, Williams GR, Cayler GG, Bracken EG: Influence of intracardiac prosthetic materials on susceptibility to bacterial endocarditis. Circulation 26:684, 1962.
174. Jacob HS, Craddock PR, Hammerschmidt DE, Moldow CF: Complement-induced granulocyte aggregation: an unsuspected mechanism of disease. N Engl J Med 302:789, 1980.
175. Amoury RA: Necrotizing enterocolitis. In Holder TM, Ashcraft KW (eds): Pediatric Surgery, 2nd ed. Philadelphia, Saunders, 1992, p 341.
176. Archer GL: Experimental endocarditis. In Duma RJ (ed): Infections of Prosthetic Heart Valves and Vascular Grafts. Baltimore, University Park Press, 1977, p 43.
177. Jones RD, Akao M, Cross FS: Bacteremia and thrombus accumulation on prosthetic heart valves in the dog. J Surg Res 9:293, 1969.
178. Detmer DE, Morrow AG, Marsh HH III, Braunwald NS: Experimental endocarditis following cardiac valve replacement. J Thorac Cardiovasc Surg 60:46, 1970.
179. Grogan EL, Sande MA, Clark RE, Nolan SP: Experimental endocarditis in calf after tricuspid valve replacement. Ann Thorac Surg 30:64, 1980.
180. Cheng TO, Kinhal V, Tice DA: Fatal thrombosis of the Starr-Edwards mitral valve prosthesis associated with bacterial endocarditis. Diagnostic significance of a disappearing prosthetic click. Chest 57:151, 1970.
181. Stinson EB, Castellino RA, Shumway NE: Radiologic signs in endocarditis following prosthetic valve replacement. J Thorac Cardiovasc Surg 56:554, 1968.
182. Malcolm AD, Ahuja SP, Chamberlain MJ: Malfunction of tricuspid valve prosthesis shown by isotope angiocardiography. J Thorac Cardiovasc Surg 71:134, 1976.
183. Bach MC, Lewin EB, Sheaff ET, et al: Localization of endovascular infection by selective catheterization with serial cultures. J Thorac Cardiovasc Surg 69:377, 1975.

184. Gardner P, Saffle JR, Schoenbaum SC: Management of prosthetic valve endocarditis. In Duma RJ (ed): Infections of Prosthetic Heart Valves and Vascular Grafts. Baltimore, University Park Press, 1977, p 123.
185. Killen DA, Collins HA, Koenig MG, Goodman JS: Prosthetic cardiac valves and bacterial endocarditis. Ann Thorac Surg 9:238, 1970.
186. Douglas JL, Cobbs CG: Prosthetic valve endocarditis. In Kaye D (ed): Infective Endocarditis, 2nd ed. New York, Raven Press, 1992, p 375.
187. Wilson WR, Jaumin PM, Danielson GK, et al: Prosthetic valve endocarditis. Ann Intern Med 82:751, 1975.
188. Cowgill LD, Addonizio VP, Hopemen AR, Harken AH: A practical approach to prosthetic valve endocarditis. Ann Thorac Surg 43:450, 1987.
189. Baumgartner WA, Miller DC, Reitz BA, et al: Surgical treatment of prosthetic valve endocarditis. Ann Thorac Surg 35:87, 1983.
190. Calderwood SB, Gwinski LA, Karchmer AW, et al: Prosthetic valve endocarditis. Analysis of factors affecting outcome of therapy. J Thorac Cardiovasc Surg 92:776, 1986.
191. Rocchiccioli C, Chastre J, Lecompte Y, et al: Prosthetic valve endocarditis. The case for prompt surgical management. J Thorac Cardiovasc Surg 92:784, 1986.
192. Dejani AS, Brisno AL, Chung KJ, et al: Prevention of bacterial endocarditis. Recommendations by the American Heart Association. JAMA 264:2919, 1990.
193. McLeod R, Remington JS: Postoperative fungal endocarditis. In Duma RJ (ed): Infections of Prosthetic Heart Valves and Vascular Grafts. Baltimore, University Park Press, 1977, p 163.
194. Uys CJ, Don PA, Schrire V, Barnard CN: Endocarditis following cardiac surgery due to the fungus *Paecilomyces.* S Afr Med J 37:1276, 1963.
195. Silver MD, Tuffnell PG, Bigelow WG: Endocarditis caused by *Paecilomyces varioti* affecting an aortic valve allograft. J Thorac Cardiovasc Surg 61:278, 1971.
196. McClellan JR, Hamilton JD, Alexander JA, et al: *Paecilomyces varioti* endocarditis on a prosthetic aortic valve. J Thorac Cardiovasc Surg 71:472, 1976.
197. Weaver DK, Batsakis JG, Nishiyama OH: *Histoplasma* endocarditis. Arch Surg 96:158, 1968.
198. Alexander WJ, Mowry RW, Cobbs CG, Dismukes WE: Prosthetic valve endocarditis caused by *Histoplasma capsulatum.* JAMA 242:1399, 1979.
199. Kaufman SN: *Curvularia* endocarditis following cardiac surgery. Am J Clin Pathol 56:466, 1971.
200. Khicha GJ, Berroya RB, Escano SB Jr, Lee CS: Mucormycosis in a mitral prosthesis. J Thorac Cardiovasc Surg 63:903, 1972.
201. Upshaw CB Jr: *Penicillium* endocarditis of aortic valve prosthesis. J Thorac Cardiovasc Surg 68:428, 1974.
202. Hall WJ III: *Penicillium* endocarditis following open heart surgery and prosthetic valve insertion. Am Heart J 87:501, 1974.
203. Roberts FJ, Allen P, Maybee TK: *Petriellidium boydii (Allescheria boydii)* endocarditis associated with porcine valve replacement. Can Med Assoc J 117:1251, 1977.
204. Robboy SJ, Kaiser J: Pathogenesis of fungal infection of heart valve prostheses. Hum Pathol 6:711, 1975.
205. Cooper T, Morrow A, Roberts W, Herman L: Postoperative endocarditis due to *Candida:* clinical observations in the experimental production of the lesion. Surgery 50:341, 1961.
206. Carrel TP, Schaffner A, Schmid ER, et al: Fatal fungal pericarditis after cardiac surgery immunosuppression. J Thorac Cardiovasc Surg 101:161, 1991.
207. Kawamoto T, Nakano S, Matsuda H, et al: *Candida* endocarditis with saddle embolism: a successful surgical intervention. Ann Thorac Surg 48:723, 1989.
208. Moyer DV, Edwards JE Jr: Fungal endocarditis. In Kaye D (ed): Infective Endocarditis, 2nd ed. New York, Raven Press, 1992, p 299.
209. Utley J, Mills J, Hutchinson J, et al: Valve replacement for bacterial and fungal endocarditis. A comparative study. Circulation 48(Suppl 3):42, 1973.
210. Podzorski RP, Herron MJ, Fast DJ, Nelson RD: Pathogenesis of candidiasis. Immunosuppression by cell wall mannan metabolites. Arch Surg 124:1290, 1989.
211. Rossiter SJ, Stinson EB, Oyer PE, et al: Prosthetic valve endocarditis: comparison of heterograft tissue valves and mechanical valves. J Thorac Cardiovasc Surg 76:795, 1978.
212. Ross DN: Homograft replacement of the aortic valve. Lancet 2:487, 1962.
213. Gonzalez-Lavin L, Al-Janabi N, Ross DN: Long-term results after aortic valve replacement with preserved aortic homografts. Ann Thorac Surg 13:594, 1972.
214. Buch WS, Pipkin RD, Hancock WD, Fogarty TJ: Mitral valve replacement with a Hancock stabilized glutaraldehyde valve. Arch Surg 110:1408, 1975.
215. Magilligan DJ Jr, Quinn EL, Davila JC: Bacteremia, endocarditis, and the Hancock valve. Ann Thorac Surg 24:508, 1977.
216. Bartollotti V, Thiene G, Milano A, et al: Pathological study of infective endocarditis on Hancock porcine bioprostheses. J Thorac Cardiovasc Surg 81:934, 1981.
217. Edwards WD, Agarwal KC, Feldt RH, et al: Surgical pathology of obstructed, right-sided, porcine-valved extracardiac conduits. Arch Pathol Lab Med 107:400, 1983.
218. Thompson J, Dirksen TH, Nube M, Brom AG: Prosthesis endocarditis—treatment of a case occurring five years after a Rastelli-Ross operation. J Thorac Cardiovasc Surg 72:28, 1976.
219. Moseley PW, Ochsner JL, Mills NL, Chapman J: Management of an infected Hancock prosthesis after repair of truncus arteriosus. J Thorac Cardiovasc Surg 73:306, 1977.

220. Shea PM, Folkerth TL, Vieweg WVR, et al: Endocarditis involving a left ventricular apicoaortic valve-bearing conduit. South Med J 72:882, 1979.
221. Fong IW, Baker CB, McKee DC: The value of prophylactic antibiotics in aorta-coronary bypass operations. J Thorac Cardiovasc Surg 78:908, 1979.
222. Hillis DJ, Rosenfeldt FL, Spicer WJ, Sterling GR: Antibiotic prophylaxis for coronary bypass grafting. J Thorac Cardiovasc Surg 86:217, 1983.
223. Akl BF, Richardson G: Serum cefazolin levels during cardiopulmonary bypass. Ann Thorac Surg 29:109, 1980.
224. Dobbins JJ, Johnson GS, Kunin CM, DeVries WC: Postmortem microbiological findings of two total artificial heart recipients. JAMA 259:865, 1988.
225. Kunin CM, Dobbins JJ, Meio JC, et al: Infectious complications in four long-term recipients of the Jarvik-7 artificial heart. JAMA 259:860, 1988.
226. Gristina AG, Dobbins JJ, Giammara B, et al: Biomaterial-centered sepsis and the total artificial heart. Microbial adhesion vs. tissue integration. JAMA 259:870, 1988.
227. Greene PS, Cameron DE, Augustine S, et al: Exploratory analysis of time-dependent risk for infection, rejection, and death after cardiac transplantation. Ann Thorac Surg 47:650, 1989.
228. Fuller J, Levinson MM, Kline JR, Copeland J: Legionnaires' disease after heart transplantation. Ann Thorac Surg 39:308, 1985.
229. Saigenji H, Kaneko M, Rhenmen B, et al: *Pneumocystis carinii* pneumonia after heart transplantation. Ann Thorac Surg 52:107, 1991.
230. McCalmont TH, Silverman JF, Geisinger KR: Cytologic diagnosis of aspergillosis in cardiac transplantation. Arch Surg 126:394, 1991.
231. Millet B, Higenbottam TW, Flower CDR, et al: The radiographic appearances of infection and acute rejection of the lung after heart-lung transplantation. Am Rev Respir Dis 140:62, 1989.
232. Karwande SV, Renlund DG, Olsen SL, et al: Mediastinitis in heart transplantation. Ann Thorac Surg 54:1039, 1992.
233. Losman JG, Curcio A, Barnard C: Normal cardiac function with a hybrid heart. Ann Thorac Surg 26:177, 1978.
234. Khoo DE, Zebro TJ, English TAH: Bacterial endocarditis in a transplanted heart. Pathol Res Pract 185:445, 1989.
235. Lammermeier DE, Sweeney MS, Haupt HE, et al: Use of potentially infected donor hearts for cardiac transplantation. Ann Thorac Surg 50:222, 1990.
236. Kirsh MM, McIntosh A, Kahn DR, Sloan H: Postpericardiotomy syndrome. Ann Thorac Surg 9:158, 1970.
237. Engle MA, Klein AA, Hepner S, Ehlers KH: The postpericardiotomy syndromes. Cardiovasc Clin North Am 2:11, 1976.
238. Engle MA, Ehlers KH, O'Loughlin JE Jr, et al: The postpericardiotomy syndrome: iatrogenic illness with immunologic and virologic components. In Engle MA (ed): Pediatric Cardiovascular Disease. Philadelphia, FA Davis, 1981, p 381.
239. Webber SA, Wilson NJ, Fung MY, et al: Autoantibody production after cardiopulmonary bypass with special reference to postpericardiotomy syndrome. J Pediatr 121:744, 1992.
240. Akl ES, Latif, Dunn MJ, et al: Antiheart antibodies following open heart surgery: incidence and correlation with postpericardiotomy syndrome. Eur J Cardiothorac Surg 6:503, 1992.
241. Caul WO, Clarke SKR, Mott MG, et al: Cytomegalovirus infections after open-heart surgery. Lancet 1:777, 1971.
242. Khan AH: The postcardiac injury syndromes. Clin Cardiol 15:67, 1992.
243. Burch GE, Colcolough HL: Postcardiotomy and postinfarction syndromes—a theory. Am Heart J 80:290, 1970.
244. Freeman R, King B, Hambling MH: Infective complications of open-heart surgery and the monitoring of infections by the NBI test. Thorax 28:617, 1973.
245. Hornick RB: Source of contamination in open-heart surgery. In Duma RJ (ed): Infections of Prosthetic Heart Valves and Vascular Grafts. Baltimore, University Park Press, 1977, p 81.
246. Roses DF, Rose MR, Rappaport FT: Febrile responses associated with cardiac surgery: relationships to the postcardiotomy syndrome and to altered host immunologic reactivity. J Thorac Surg 67:251, 1974.
247. Masur H: Prosthetic valve endocarditis. J Thorac Cardiovasc Surg 80:31, 1980.

BIBLIOGRAPHY

Bisno AL (ed): Treatment of Infective Endocarditis. New York, Grune & Stratton, 1981.

Brewer LA (ed): Prosthetic Heart Valves. Springfield IL, CC Thomas, 1969.

Duma RJ (ed): Infections of Prosthetic Heart Valves and Vascular Grafts. Baltimore, University Park Press, 1977.

Kaplan EL, Taranta AV (eds): Infective Endocarditis. Dallas, American Heart Association, 1977.

Kaye D (ed): Infective Endocarditis, 2nd ed. New York, Raven Press, 1992.

Rahimtoola SH (ed): Infective Endocarditis. New York, Grune & Stratton, 1978.

Vascular Infections

CHAPTER 37

Hugh A. Gelabert, Wesley S. Moore

ARTERIAL INFECTION

Despite almost 50 years of "modern" antibiotic era, infections of the vascular tree remain among the more difficult infectious problems. These infections are frequently difficult to diagnose. Once they present in an obvious manner, they are frequently well advanced. Once diagnosed they are difficult to clear, and the relapse rate is considerable. Finally, they are dangerous infections frequently causing loss of limb and life. The most complete classification of spontaneous arterial infections, which stresses both the arterial pathology and the infectious etiology, is the system suggested by Wilson et al[1] (Table 37–1).

Incidence of Arterial Infection. Historically, the most common cause of arterial infection was hematogenous seeding of an artery from an endocardial infection. The antibiotic era has decreased the incidence of arterial infection caused by endocardial infection. In 1923, Stengel and Wolferth[2] reported that bacterial endocarditis was the source of 86 percent of arterial infections. Pneumonia and osteomyelitis were the next most common causes of arterial infection.[1,3] Aortic infections were much more common than visceral or peripheral arterial infections in most early series.[1,4] Ninety-five percent of arterial infections with aneurysm formation were etiologically related to endocarditis as recently as 1949.[1] In 1951, penicillin treatment of bacterial endocarditis lowered the rate of arterial infection caused by septic emboli from 80 to 47 percent.[5] Because bacterial endocarditis and mycotic aneurysms are not reportable diseases, the exact incidence is unknown. Wilson et al[1] estimate the incidence of bacterial endocarditis at 1 in 1000 to 6000 hospital admissions but suggest that the actual incidence may be much higher. Pelletier and Petersdorf[3] recently reported that 18 percent of 125 patients with bacterial endocarditis had mycotic aneurysms and that 13 percent died of aneurysm rupture.

Infected atherosclerotic aneurysms are reported with increasing frequency. An autopsy series by Sommerville et al[6] of 20,201 cadavers suggests an incidence of over 3 percent (6 of 170) with infected atherosclerotic abdominal aortic aneurysms. Essentially all types of soft tissue and organ infections have been associated with infected atherosclerotic aneurysms, but the primary source of infection is unknown in one-third to one-half of the cases. The true incidence of infected atherosclerotic aneurysms may be higher, but most vascular surgeons do not culture abdominal aortic aneurysms at the time of operation. The reported data suggest the laminated clot from clinically uninfected infrarenal abdominal aortic aneurysms with culture organisms in 13 percent (28 of 210) of cases.[7] The significance of this observation in

TABLE 37–1. DIFFERENTIAL FEATURES OF SPONTANEOUS ARTERIAL INFECTIONS

Feature	Mycotic Aneurysm	Infected Aneurysm	Microbial Arteritis	Traumatic Infected Pseudoaneurysm
Etiology	Endocarditis	Bacteremia	Bacteremia	Trauma, narcotic addiction
Sex	F > M	M	M	M or F
Age	30–50	Over 50	Over 50	Under 30
Incidence	Rare	Unusual	Common	Common
Number	Multiple	Single	Single	Multiple
Site	Visceral, intracranial, aorta, and peripheral arteries	Distal aorta	Aortoiliac, superficial femoral arteries; congenital or traumatic vascular defects	Femoral, carotid, or sites of injection
Bacteriology	Gram-positive cocci	*Staphylococcus, Escherichia coli*	*Salmonella* species	Polymicrobial flora
Mortality	Moderate (25%)	High (90%)	High (75%)	Low (10%)

From Wilson SE, Van Wagenen P, Passaro E Jr: Curr Probl Surg 15:1, 1978.

the pathophysiology of infected aortic aneurysms is unknown.

Microbial arteritis,[1] the invasion of preexisting arterial lesions during noncardiac bacteremia, is probably more common than is suspected. Its recognition is probably obscured since many early arterial infections may be sterilized by antibiotic therapy. Preexisting arterial lesions include congenital cardiovascular abnormalities, atherosclerotic vascular disease, hypertensive vascular disease, and prior traumatic vascular insult. MacBeth et al[7] have recently published data concerning arterial wall microbiology in elective clean vascular reconstructive procedures. They documented an overall 43 percent (38 of 88) incidence of positive arterial cultures and there were no significant differences in the incidence of positive arterial cultures in three different anatomic areas: neck, abdomen, and extremity. The significance of this observation with respect to arterial infection awaits further study. The differentiating feature between microbial arteritis and mycotic aneurysms is that the source of arterial infection in microbial arteritis is noncardiac.

We have reported a surprisingly high incidence of bacteremia with clinical diagnostic tests or invasive procedures that involve mucous membrane trauma. The incidence of bacteremia ranged from 8 percent for hemodialysis to 60 to 90 percent for dental extractions. Bacteremias have been documented in healthy individuals without mucous membrane trauma, but the incidence is probably less than 1 percent. In healthy persons with mucous membrane trauma, bacteremia is usually of no consequence. However, patients with vascular lesions, either intrinsic (eg, rheumatic heart disease, atherosclerotic vascular disease) or extrinsic (eg, vascular surgery, vascular trauma) are at increased risk for arterial or valvular infection (5 to 15 percent).[8] The exact incidence of microbial arteritis, however, is unknown. The potential for arterial infection to occur must be considered in any patient with congenital or acquired cardiovascular disease, or prior cardiovascular surgery, who has sustained a clinically significant episode of either bacteremia or septicemia.[9]

False aneurysms differ from true arterial aneurysms in that the wall of the false aneurysm is made of compressed periarterial fibrous tissue and clot rather than of adventitia, media, and intima. Increases in numbers of invasive diagnostic tests, vascular operations, and traumatic injuries have increased the incidence of infected arterial false aneurysms in recent years. The poor prognosis associated with any untreated infected aneurysm demands that any patient with bacteremia or septicemia and a history of vascular surgery or vascular trauma must be evaluated closely.

Secondary arterial infections are those that result from the extension of sepsis from an infection located adjacent to an artery. Common infectious sites include periarterial abscess, lymphangitis with lymph node involvement, osteomyelitis, phlebitis, and infected pseudocysts. Common clinical scenarios include pancreatitis, appendicitis, and pneumonia. These infections may occur after vascular surgery when a prosthetic graft has been implanted. Although the reported incidence of secondary or contiguous arterial infections caused by periarterial infections is low,[10] these infections must be suspected in patients with a history of arterial trauma or surgery who have evidence of a systemic infection. Host immunocompetence is an important factor with this type of arterial infection. Kyriakides et al[11] and Walsh et al[12] noted an increased incidence of arterial infections caused by periarterial infections in immunosuppressed renal transplant patients. Contiguous arterial infections in nonimmunosuppressed hosts have also been documented after gastrointestinal procedures. Kerr and Tilney[13] noted an external iliac arterial infection that resulted from a pelvic abscess after a routine colonic resection. Although any artery theoretically can be infected through extension of a perivascular infection, infections of the thoracic and abdominal aortas are most common.[1] Although the incidence of contiguous arterial infection is unknown, this diagnosis must be considered when there is an abscess or inflammatory process adjacent to an artery.

The invasion of preexisting arterial lesions during endocardially induced bacteremia, the creation of iatrogenic arterial injuries that subsequently become infected, and secondary septic pulmonary parenchymal abscess and pulmonary arterial mycotic aneurysms are almost entirely diseases of the 20th century. These infections result most often from iatrogenic, diagnostic, or operative intervention or intravenous drug abuse. Intravenous drug addiction is currently the leading cause of septic emboli in the arterial tree.[1] Septic emboli to the pulmonary artery or lung parenchyma may also result from septic thrombophlebitis of the arm, pelvis, or leg. Most often, septic thrombophlebitis also is associated with either iatrogenic procedures or intravascular drug abuse. Griffith et al[14] have reported that the incidence of infected arterial emboli is approximately 2 to 3 percent of all arterial emboli. The diagnosis of septic arterial emboli or secondary pulmonary or parenchymal infection should be suggested in patients with a recent history of intravenous drug abuse or iatrogenic arterial manipulation.

The last type of arterial infection to be considered results from arterial erosion into the gastrointestinal tract: the aortoenteric fistula. This infection may not be diagnosed prior to death and is almost always fatal unless it is treated appropriately. The abdominal aorta is most commonly involved. A typical example is an aortoenteric fistula with erosion into the duodenum caused by an untreated expanding abdominal aneurysm. The incidence of these lesions is extremely low. The significance of the lesion is that expanding major arterial aneurysms, in proximity to the gastrointestinal tract, have a substantial risk for erosion with rapid hemorrhage and subsequent death.

Location. Although spontaneous infections have the potential to occur in any artery, large or medium sized, large arterial degenerative changes predispose the thoracic and abdominal aorta and its major branches to arterial infection (Fig. 37–1).[1,2,4] An obvious exception to this rule is the significant number of peripheral arterial infections associated with arterial trauma, operations, invasive diagnostic tests, and intravenous drug abuse (Fig. 37–2).[15] Overall, arterial infections usually involve the aorta, the visceral arteries, and the peripheral arteries in decreasing frequency. Distal extremity vessels and intracranial vessels are not as commonly involved—the significant exception being intracranial fungal infections secondary to fungal endocarditis.[15] Arterial infections caused by bacterial endocarditis usually involve visceral, peripheral, or intracranial vessels. Arterial infections that result from noncardiac-related bacterial invasion usually involve the aorta and its major branches or the extremity vessels.

Pathogenesis. The cause of arterial infections depends on the size of the artery. In small arteries,

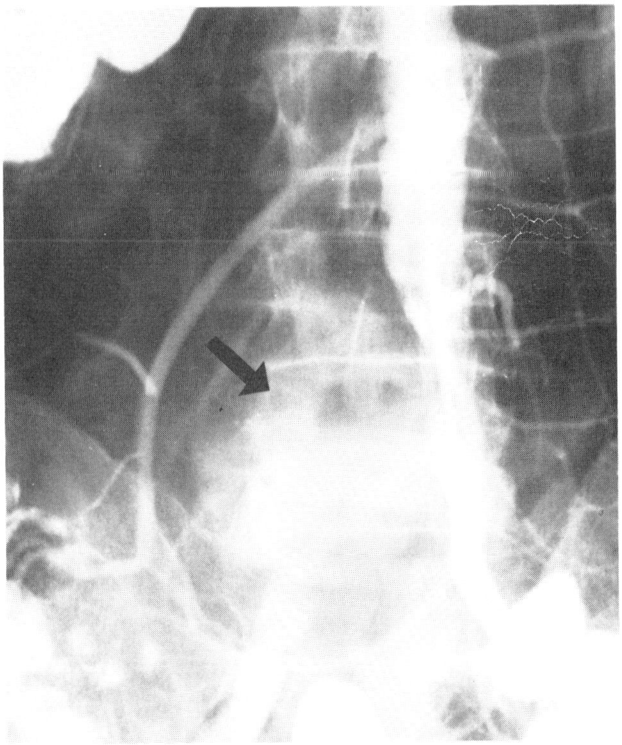

Figure 37–1. *Salmonella* arteritis of the aortoiliac bifurcation resulting in rupture and pseudoaneurysm formation (arrow). *(From Wilson SE, Van Wagenen P, Passaro E Jr: Curr Probl Surg 15:1, 1978.)*

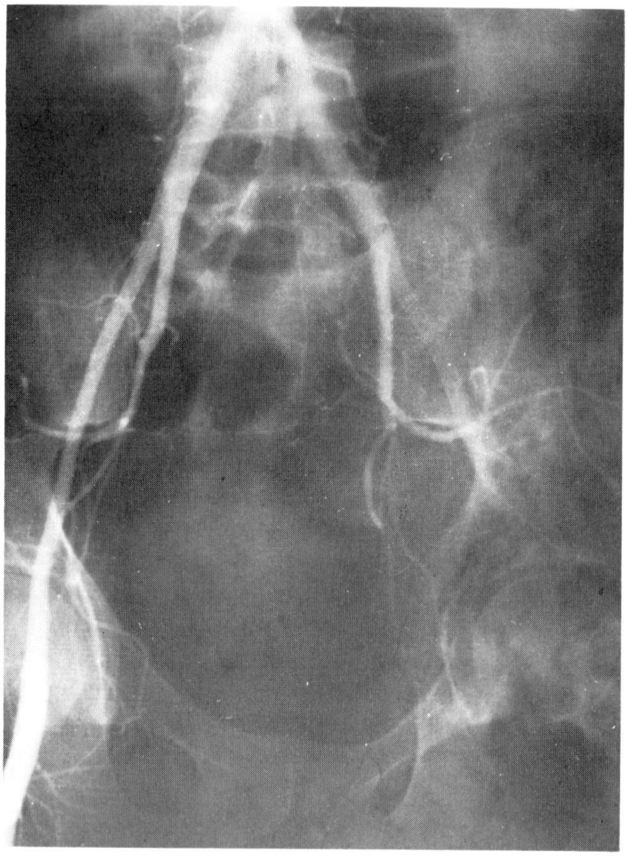

Figure 37–2. Arteriogram in heroin addict with mycotic aneurysm of common femoral artery that caused thrombosis of vessel. Abundant gas production in soft tissue of thigh resulted from anaerobic peptostreptococcal infection. *(From Anderson CB, Butcher HR, Ballinger WF: Arch Surg 109:712, 1974.)*

which are predisposed to degenerative changes, bacteria or septic emboli probably lodge in the vessel wall and lead to locally invasive intimal infections. This results in a transmural arteritis and subsequent aneurysm formation from arterial wall degeneration. In large arteries, however, bacteremia or emboli may lodge in areas of intimal or medial disease on the luminal side of the artery, or they may lodge in the vasa vasorum, with secondary ischemic degeneration of the media. This medial degeneration is followed by aneurysmal degeneration of the arterial wall. Arterial bifurcations, congenital cardiovascular abnormalities, areas of localized cardiovascular trauma, and primary noninfected arterial aneurysms all predispose to arterial infection.

In the embolic type of arterial infection, there is usually an identifiable source of infection such as bacterial endocarditis.[1,2,15] Arterial infection may also occur as a direct result of inoculation at the time of vascular trauma or operation. Examples of this latter etiology include intravenous drug abuse,[16] brachial arterial infection after coronary catheterization, and infection after vascular surgery.[1,8] Finally, arterial infection may occur as a direct extension (contiguous arterial infection) from a perivascular infection, such as thoracic tuberculous aortitis adjacent to tuberculous mediastinal lymph nodes, arterial infection from contiguous periarterial abscesses,[10] or erosion into the superior mesenteric artery or aorta by a pancreatic pseudocyst.[1,13] As noted earlier, host immunocompetence and host debilitation are important in the pathogenesis of arterial infections.[11,12]

Systemic diseases that are associated with medial degeneration or obliterative endarteritis of the vasa vasorum, such as Marfan's syndrome and Behçet's disease,[17] have been associated with an increased incidence of arterial aneurysm formation and subsequent infection. Arteries affected by such diseases are at increased risk of infection from bacteremia or emboli. These lesions can therefore be loosely grouped in the category of predisposing lesions. Discussion of the arteritides and subsequent secondary arterial infection has purposely been excluded from this discussion. Rosenberg et al[18] provide an excellent review of noninfective arterial inflammatory diseases.

Microbiology. The bacteriology of spontaneous arterial infections is essentially that of bacterial endocarditis. Historically, hemolytic streptococci, *Streptococcus pneumoniae,* and *Hemophilus* were the most common organisms. More recently, an increasing incidence of *Salmonella* species and staphylococci have been reported. Other organisms include enterococci, gonococci, diphtheroids, *Serratia, Escherichia coli, Yersinia, Pseudomonas, Klebsiella, Proteus, Citrobacter, Campylobacter* species, *Arizona hinshawii, Brucella suis,* and anaerobic organisms, including *Clostridium, Peptostreptococcus,* and *Bacteroides.* MacBeth et al[7] have called attention to both the high incidence (45 percent; 35 of 77) of positive arterial cultures in clean elective vascular cases and the fact that *S. epidermidis* was the organism in 71 percent (27 of 38) of the positive cultures. The implications of these data for the occurrence of microbial arteritis or graft infection are unknown and require further analysis. Mycobacterial infections have been reported throughout the entire history of spontaneous arterial infections. Arterial infections caused by endocardial emboli tend to be of primarily gram-positive cocci, whereas infections in preexisting arterial lesions caused by nonendocardial bacteremia are more commonly the result of *Salmonella* and a variety of gram-negative rods. Arterial infections that result from perivascular spread are most commonly associated with *Salmonella,* staphylococci, mycobacteria, and fungi. The bacteriology of arterial infection is reviewed in detail by Wilson et al.[1]

The morbidity and mortality of arterial infections are related to the infecting bacteria. Gram-negative infections result in a much higher morbidity and mortality than do gram-positive infections.[1,4] Of special note are arterial infections caused by *Salmonella* species (see Fig. 37–1). Three types of arterial lesions have been noted with *Salmonella:* (1) focal arteritis with saccular aneurysm formation and rupture, (2) diffuse suppurative arteritis with development of a fusiform aneurysm and rupture, and (3) secondary infection complicating degenerative arterial lesions such as atherosclerotic plaques. Unlike other bacterial arterial infections that require 6 to 12 weeks of antibiotic therapy, *Salmonella* infections require at least 6 months of oral therapy after acute intravenous therapy is concluded.[1]

Almost all reports of fungal arterial infections have been associated with fungal endocarditis[18] or cardiovascular trauma. These include intravenous drug abuse, arterial surgery, and invasive diagnostic procedures.[16] Fortunately, fungal endocarditis or arteritis is a rare disease. It is most commonly seen in debilitated or immunosuppressed patients.[19] The most commonly reported fungal organisms include *Candida, Histoplasma, Rhodotorula, Aspergillus,* and *Blastomyces.* Prognosis for either fungal endocarditis or fungal mycotic aneurysms, even with excision and intensive antifungal treatment, is often poor.

Viral arterial infections have not been documented in humans. Herpesvirus and measles virus, however, have caused arterial lesions that are similar to immunologic connective tissue disorders demonstrated in animals.[20]

Manifestations. The signs and symptoms of arterial infections depend on the infectious etiology and the location of the arterial infection. The relationship between bacterial endocarditis and arterial infection is dependent on the timing, duration, and treatment of the endocardial disease. Patients are usually in the second to fourth decades of life. The signs and symptoms of mycotic aneurysms are those of bacterial endocarditis: fever, weight loss, cardiac murmur, peripheral embolization (petechiae, rose spots, splinter hemorrhages), neurologic symptoms (central nervous system emboli), or organ failure.

As the incidence of endocarditis-related infections has decreased, noncardiac-induced arterial infections have become much more common. These infections may be characterized by their nonspecific clinical presentations. They most commonly present with symptoms resembling any systemic infection. Many are asymptomatic until they reach an advanced stage. Sommerville et al[6] emphasized the difficulty of distinguishing patients with infected abdominal aortic aneurysms from those with noninfected aneurysms. Acute vascular insufficiency in the setting of systemic infection should be considered a symptom of an infected arterial emboli.

Most commonly, physical examination will serve to reveal the presence of an arterial infection only when the affected arteries are in close proximity to the overlying skin. Thus femoral, popliteal, and brachial artery infections may be revealed by a rapidly expanding pulsatile mass, skin erythema, or tenderness. Deeper arterial beds such as the iliac and aorta may escape detection on physical examination until late in the course of the disease. Accordingly, the identification of an arterial infection frequently relies on the recognition of the combination of predisposing factors (arterial trauma, vascular surgery, arterial punctures) and the subtle nonspecific signs of a low-grade systemic infection.

At best, clinical laboratory testing may identify the presence of bacteremia or leukocytosis. Otherwise, laboratory testing is frequently not helpful in conclusively making the diagnosis of an arterial infection. Blood cultures may at times suggest the possibility of an arterial infection when the identified organism is *Salmonella.* Overall, positive blood cultures, have not proved useful as a diagnostic test in the absence of an arterial or graft enteric fistula.[1,21]

The role of plain x-ray studies is limited in the evaluation of patients suspected of harboring an arterial infection. X-ray studies may reveal vascular calcifications that suggest aneurysm formation. Additionally, they may demonstrate bone destruction caused by osteomyelitis. This information is insufficient to secure the diagnosis of an arterial infection; further testing is invariably required. Accordingly, such x-ray studies are frequently omitted.

Arteriography plays a central role in the diagnosis of arterial infections by identifying the location of the arterial defect, suggesting its etiology, and providing information required to plan the repair of the lesion. Once an arterial infection is suspected, arteriography is the next step in establishing a diagnosis and commencing treatment. The etiology may be suggested by the location and shape of the aneurysm. Saccular aneurysms that extrude from the side of a major artery are considered infectious in origin until proven otherwise. Finally, arteriograms may differentiate between arterial embolization with arterial occlusion or thrombosis caused by contiguous infection.

Ultrasonography is of limited value in the diagnosis of either aneurysms or arterial occlusion. While duplex scanning may reveal the presence of atherosclerotic plaques, arterial occlusions, and aneurysms, it is subject to many limitations that render it less than ideal for the diagnosis of an arterial infection. Additionally, there is not sufficient experience with duplex data to reliably detect these lesions.

Computer-assisted tomography (CAT) scanning has found increasing favor among vascular surgeons as a means of evaluating the presence of abdominal and thoracic arterial aneurysms. In addition to identifying the presence of aneurysms, CAT scans may provide sufficient detail to suggest that the aneurysm may be infectious. A saccular para-aortic aneurysm would thus be suspected of being septic. CAT scans may detect fluid surrounding a prosthetic graft or the extension of an inflammatory mass between the aorta and adjacent bowel. Such signs are strongly suggestive of vascular infections.

There are several reports that suggest that radionuclear scans are valuable in both diagnosis and localization of mycotic and infected aneurysms.[22,23] In addition, radiologic or radionuclear evidence of an infection adjacent to a major vessel in a patient with signs of a systemic infection suggests an arterial infection.

The sudden onset of bacteremia, localized pain, localized murmur or bruit, or pulsatile mass in the area of a suspected abscess indicates an arterial infection.[21] It is difficult to diagnose abdominal, thoracic, and intracranial arterial infections without arteriography or CAT scans. Most particularly, we cannot overemphasize the difficulty in diagnosing visceral arterial aneurysms without using arteriography. Typically, physical examination and routine laboratory evaluations in a patient with an infected visceral arterial aneurysm will reveal fever, abdominal pain, and signs of systemic illness. Although some visceral aneurysms, such as those involving the proper hepatic artery, may be associated with specific symptom complexes (signs of cholecystitis, hepatitis, or hematobilia), they are not, by themselves, diagnostic in any individual patient. The high morbidity and mortality of untreated infected visceral arterial aneurysms can only be reduced through a high degree of suspicion and angiography.

Treatment and Results. The management of arterial infections is a combination of antibiotic therapy and operation. However, successful treatment is also related to their location.

Large doses of culture-specific antibiotics are commenced preoperatively and continue through the operation and at least 6 to 8 weeks postoperatively or longer, depending on the aneurysm and the organism.[1,4] Adequate serum antibiotic levels must be checked and maintained during all phases of therapy. There is evidence to suggest that levels of antibiotics vary in human aortic tissues with the different classes of antibiotics.[24] Bactericidal, rather than bacteriostatic, drugs should be used. Antibiotic pharmacokinetics are important in establishing effective treatment schedules. Without operative treatment, infected arterial lesions may continue to enlarge and either rupture or remain a reservoir for continued bacteremic infection in spite of antibiotic therapy. Sterilization of a preexisting endocarditis is especially important to minimize the risk of contaminating newly implanted vascular prostheses.

Surgical treatment should include excision of the infected artery and surrounding tissue, exclusion from the arterial circulation if excision is not possible, and vascular reconstruction, if required, through uninfected tissues. Simple ligation and excision are the best treatment if the arterial infection involves a noncritical artery or as immediate treatment if the arterial infection involves a critical artery but the collateral flow is acceptable. Reconstruction should be performed as needed but as late as possible (preferably 3 to 6 months) after the primary operation. In many cases, immediate arterial reconstruction is required. The principles of arterial reconstruction in infected fields are discussed in a later portion of this chapter. However, there are two basic rules: (1) prosthetic grafts must be routed outside any potentially infected area to avoid recurrent graft infection and (2) arterial continuity through an infected area can only be assured with fresh autogenous tissue grafts.[1,7]

Management of aortic or other large retroperitoneal arterial vascular infections is possible only with total excision of the involved arterial segment and surrounding tissue. We prefer to use a monofilament suture for oversewing the proximal and distal portions of the remaining artery. If possible, we use a two-layer closure, employing a continuous suture reinforced with interrupted sutures. The area should be retroperitonealized, if possible, and drained, using retroperitoneal flank drains. Copious amounts of intraoperative local antibiotic irrigation should be used. A closed-system antibiotic irrigation during the postoperative period, much like the closed systems used for open fractures, can be employed.

Successful management of visceral arterial infections is difficult because they involve end-organ vessels with poor collateral supply. In addition, extensive dissection may injure the surrounding structures. Techniques used for management of infected visceral arterial aneurysms include endoaneurysmorrhaphy, ligation and excision, and excision with primary grafting. All the various vascular techniques attempt to minimize dissection because the aneurysm in usually densely adherent to surrounding structures as a result of the inflammatory process. Because it is not usually possible to route a visceral graft through an uninfected area, it is best to use fresh autogenous arteries or veins for reconstruction of infected visceral arterial lesions. It must be emphasized that drainage of infected vascular lesions must be thorough and that any revascularization procedures must be performed through clean tissue planes, if possible.

Infected peripheral arterial lesions are usually the easiest lesions to diagnose and treat because of the ease of both examination and operative access, the amount of potential collateralization, and the presence of noninfected tissue compartments that can be used for extra-anatomic vascular reconstruction. Regardless of the location of the vessel, the presence of a perivascular abscess or infection is an absolute indication for surgical drainage.

Several types of arterial lesions, especially atherosclerotic abdominal aneurysms, are often not recognized as being infected prior to operation. All atherosclerotic abdominal aneurysms or questionable and unusual arterial lesions should have their wall or intraluminal contents cultured and Gram stained. If an infection is suspected, based on operative findings or Gram stain, excision of the lesion and management as previously described are mandatory. If the cultures return to positive during the postoperative period, antibiotic therapy should be continued with culture-specific antibiotics. Unfortunately, objective criteria for determining the duration of antibiotic therapy have not been established. We recommend 4 to 6 weeks of treatment based on the current recommendations for treatment of active endocarditis.

Excised specimens also should always be cultured, not only because blood cultures will not always be positive but because cardiovascular infections may be polymicrobial, and adequate adjunctive antibiotic therapy depends on identification of specific organisms. The increased appearance of antibiotic-resistant organisms in arterial infections emphasizes the need for accurate culture information.

The relatively poor long-term results in management of arterial lesions in critical arteries strongly suggest that both postoperative arteriography and long-term follow-up with noninvasive tests, such as CAT scan, are mandatory. In addition, strong consideration should be given for extended oral antibiotic coverage (6 to 12 months) after the completion of acute surgical antibiotic therapy, although the data to support such an approach are not yet available.

Fungal organisms, *Candida* species in particular, tend to preferentially embolize to both intracranial and extremity vessels. The tendency for these fungal lesions to embolize is related to the poor adherence of fungal vegetation to the vascular surfaces. Surgeons should be aggressive in exploring arteries suspected of being occluded by fungal emboli, especially those suspected of being infected with *Candida* because embolectomy can be performed safely, even in the most debilitated patient.

INFECTIONS IN VEINS

Unlike arteries, veins are rarely infected unless a foreign body lies in the venous system. The most notable exception to such a general statement is the occurrence of pyelophlebitis with appendicitis, necrotic bowel, abdominal abscesses, and other types of abdominal sepsis.[25] The intrinsic venous resistance to bacteremia-induced infection is probably related to the lack of degenerative changes in the venous system, which predispose veins to bacterial seeding and subsequent infection. The low incidence of venous infection in postphlebitic limbs or in venous segments that have sustained trauma suggests that venous injury alone is not a predisposing lesion. The best hypotheses to explain the low incidence of spontaneous venous infection (without the introduction of extrinsic organisms into the venous system) include (1) the lack of predisposing lesions in the venous system; (2) differences in flow and pulsatility compared with the arterial system; and (3) differences in morphology of the veins, such as the lack of a vasa vasorum, as seen in large- and medium-sized arteries.

Venous infections are almost always associated with direct microbial inoculation. For this reason the subsequent sections on venous infection emphasize postinfusion phlebitis and suppurative phlebitis. Nonsuppurative venous inflammatory diseases have been reviewed by Abruzzo.[26]

Umbilical Arterial and Venous Catheters

The increased use of both umbilical arterial and venous catheters in neonatal units has brought with it a host of complications, including vascular thrombosis, organ infarction, and visceral ischemia.[27] Balagtas et al[28] reviewed the infectious risks of umbilical venous catheterization in 86 newborn infants. They reported that 52 percent of all umbilical venous catheters were colonized with bacteria within 48 hours of insertion (primarily with staphylococci and coliform organisms). Most importantly, they found that the incidence of catheter colonization was not related to the duration of catheterization.[28] A prospective study by Anagnostakis et al[27] of 65 newborn infants with umbilical venous catheters revealed that 53 percent of the umbilical cord stumps were contaminated prior to catheter placement, even though the stump was cleaned before catheterization, and that 62 percent of the umbilical venous catheters were colonized at the time of removal. In addition to the high rate of catheter bacterial colonization, both studies documented an 8 to 10 percent incidence of catheter-related bacteremia and sepsis.[27,28] Balagtas et al[28] showed that, although prophylactic antibiotics (penicillin and kanamycin) did not decrease the overall incidence of catheter colonization, the antibiotics significantly decreased the incidence of bacteremia. Most studies (except Balagtas et al[28]) suggest that prophylactic antibiotics did not significantly change the risk of sepsis, the incidence of positive umbilical catheter blood cultures, or the incidence of catheter bacterial colonization.[27] This is consistent with studies of other intravascular catheters.[29–31] Everyone agrees that umbilical arterial and venous catheters should be removed as rapidly as possible.[27]

Peripheral Catheter-Related Phlebitis

Nosocomial venous infusion infections are discussed in Chapter 22. True suppurative phlebitis is much less common, but the true incidence is difficult to determine the reported incidence of postinfusion or suppurative phlebitis ranges from 0.2 to 15 percent.[29] This variation is related to (1) the type of catheter used, because steel scalp venous needles are associated with a lower incidence of infection than are plastic catheters[29]; (2) techniques of venipuncture and catheter care and maintenance; and (3) the high incidence of inflammatory but nonsuppurative phlebitis seen with all types of venous catheters.

Intravenous catheter tips often show positive cultures without the occurrence of local suppurative phlebitis. The incidence of culture-positive intravenous catheter tips in some studies is as high as 47 percent, although the incidence of suppurative phlebitis can range from 5 to 16 percent. This apparent discrepancy suggests that there are errors in culture technique (which can introduce nonpathogenic bacteria onto the catheter) or differences in the parameters of the clinical diagnosis of suppurative phlebitis versus nonsuppurative postinfusion phlebitis. This also suggests that there are two etiologies—irritation and infection—important to the pathogenesis of true suppurative phlebitis. The histopathologic changes noted in postinfusion phlebitis strongly support irritation as one of the important etiologic factors. Early phlebitis demonstrates endothelial swelling and increased numbers of neutrophils (PMNs) in the media of the vein. As the degree of the phlebitis becomes more severe, endothelial cell loss increases, and increased numbers of PMNs are noted in the media. In addition, there is pyknosis of many medial muscle cells. Finally, in the most severe form, phlebitic veins demonstrate wall necrosis. These changes are noted with and without bacteria, and it is therefore difficult to suggest that the changes are caused only by localized infection or irritation. There is little question, however, that infection is involved in the pathophysiology of suppurative phlebitis (pus in vein lumen). The most common organisms are skin organisms, *Staphylococcus aureus* and streptococci, although almost all major groups of gram-positive and gram-negative organisms have been reported, as well as yeasts and fungi.[30]

Cannula-related sepsis is a risk with intravenous therapy, and the risk is higher with plastic indwelling catheters than with steel scalp venous needles (see Chap. 26). Although there are no comparable double-blind studies, the incidence of cannula-related sepsis for scalp venous needles and for plastic catheters would appear to be less than 0.5 percent and over 5 percent, respectively. Postinfusion phlebitis or catheter-related infections, excluding true suppurative phlebitis, usually respond to treatment after the catheter is removed. True suppurative phlebitis, however, is lethal unless the involved venous segment is excised.[26,28,29,32] Suppurative phlebitis is seen most commonly with leg intravenous catheters[29] and with prolonged intravenous cannulation with plastic catheters (longer than 48 hours).[26,28,29] In addition, there is an increased risk of suppurative phlebitis in burn patients,[29] debilitated or immunosuppressed patients, and patients with cancer.[29]

The clinical sign of inflammation and unexplained fever in a patient with no obvious source of infection suggest intravenous catheter-related infection. The local signs of inflammation and infection are often absent, however, in patients with cancer, burns, immunoincompetence, or severe debilitation. If suppurative phlebitis is suspected, exploratory venotomy is indicated.

Infections with Central Venous Catheters

All of our previous statements regarding infections related to peripheral intravenous cannulation also apply to central venous catheters; however, a few specific points deserve emphasis. The techniques of insertion and intravenous catheter care are extremely critical to both catheter patency and catheter-related infections, especially in immunologically compromised patients. Properly inserted and maintained central venous catheters can be used for total parenteral nutrition for extended times without the occurrence of catheter-related sepsis. These same lines cannot be used, however, for administration of medication, for central venous pressure measurements, or for routine intravenous administration, without a high risk of catheter-related sepsis after 48 to 72 hours (see Chap. 26).

The risk of central venous catheter-related infection varies with the infection status of the patient. In a review of 130 consecutive percutaneous subclavian catheters, Mogensen et al[30] noted no catheter-related infections in 64 noninfected patients and both a 10 percent (9 of 66) incidence of catheter-related sepsis and a 25 percent (17 of 66) incidence of positive catheter cultures in patients with previous septic foci. In the 17 patients with positive catheter cultures, 14 had positive cultures of catheter contents, and 9 had positive blood cultures drawn from other venipuncture sources. In addition, in the group with previous septic foci, the incidence of catheter-related sepsis varied directly with the duration of catheter placement.[30]

In addition to improper catheter insertion, improper catheter maintenance, or errors in the use of a hyperalimentation line, an often overlooked and not unusual source of sepsis is the contamination of the intravenous solution itself.

Deep Venous Thrombosis and Infection

In the absence of iatrogenic or penetrating traumatic injury, the incidence of suppurative phlebitis with spontaneous deep venous thrombosis is exceedingly low. Septic deep venous thrombosis occurs most commonly after intravenous drug abuse, pelvic or urologic surgery, and peripheral arterial or venous surgery. Traumatic septic deep venous thrombosis is most often related to intravenous drug abuse and, much less commonly, to severe crushing injuries of the lower extremities. There has always been a suspicion that spontaneous deep venous thrombosis was caused by infection, especially with L-forms (wall-deficient bacteria). Nicolaides et al[33] reviewed 420 surgery patients screened by iodine-125 fibrinogen for deep venous thrombosis. They found a statistically significant increase of deep venous thrombosis with postoperative infection and with the perioperative use of antibiotics in the absence of postoperative infection. Although there is little question that the incidence of deep venous thrombosis is increased with operation, it is difficult, at best, to suggest that the Nicolaides study conclusively proves an infectious cause of deep venous thrombosis. The bulk of data suggests that deep venous thrombosis is related to local vascular trauma, local hypercoagulation, stasis, and possibly hypofibrinolysis of the venous endothelium. There are no conclusive data to suggest a primary infection in most cases of deep venous thrombosis.

INFECTION IN IRRADIATED ARTERIES AND VEINS

Radiation probably induces vascular damage by obliterating small nutrient wall vessels, such as the vasa vasorum, that supply the media of small, medium, and large arteries. Obliteration of these nutrient vessels causes tissue (media) hypoxemia and subsequent wall degeneration. Radiation treatment can cause both arterial aneurysm formation and atherosclerosis with stenosis and occlusion. The type of arterial injury caused by a specific form of radiation therapy is unpredictable. The predilection of irradiation to disproportionately injure small nutrient vessels probably accounts for the lesser incidence of recognized radiation-associated venous injury because there are few nutrient vessels in most veins. Any histopathologic changes caused by radiation might predispose the artery or vein to an increased risk of infection (both cardiac and noncardiac bacteremia and septicemia). The relative resistance of the venous system to infection from bacteremia accounts for the low incidence of irradiation-related venous infections. Svanberg et al[34] demonstrated decreased endothelial fibrinolytic activator activity in irradiated vessels compared with nonradiated control vessels and a decreased rate of endothelial fibrinolytic activity in irradiated vessels with passage of time after radiation therapy. Intravascular thrombosis is probably an important predisposing lesion for arterial and venous infection with respect to a bacteremic challenge, especially in a debilitated, immunosuppressed, or cancer patient (Fig. 37–3). The relationships between the vascular changes, the venous and arterial endothelial fibrinolytic activity, and the subsequent vascular thrombosis and infection are unknown.

There is no question that the loss of endothelial fibrinolytic activator activity denotes biochemical, if not histologic, injury and that decreased endothelial fibrinolysis is associated with an increased incidence of local vascular thrombus formation or vessel thrombosis. It is attractive to hypothesize that radiation-induced changes in endothelial fibrinolytic activity may be associated with either an increased incidence of arterial and venous infection or a decreased resistance of irradiated arteries and veins to infection from bacteremic challenge.

It is recognized that irradiated tissues have severely decreased resistance to infection, and it is reasonably safe to predict that there should be an increased incidence of contiguous arterial infection in those patients who have had local irradiation over the artery in question. However, there is only the common clinical observation that carotid arterial rupture after combined excision and radiation therapy for head and neck cancer is much more frequent than that following either treatment alone.

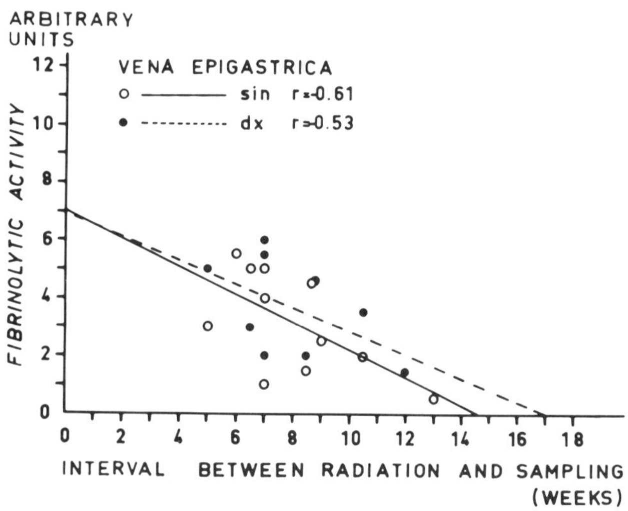

Figure 37–3. Comparison between fibrinolytic activity in superficial veins and interval between radiation and sampling. *(From Svanberg L, Åstedt B, Kullander S: Acta Obstet Gynecol Scand 55:49, 1976.)*

INFECTION IN VASCULAR GRAFTS

Infection that involves a vascular graft is a rare but disastrous complication. Morbidity and mortality from graft infection have been extremely high because of the critical location of the graft as well as the necessity to remove the graft material, particularly in the instance of a prosthetic graft, after infection has been established. The incidence, natural history, and management are influenced by the type of material used for grafting, the location of the graft, and the functional distribution of the arterial blood supply for which the graft was intended.

Historic Perspective. The first reported clinical series of infected prosthetic grafts appeared in the late 1950s. Schramel and Creech[35] collected six cases of infected prostheses. Of four grafts located in the femoral or femoropopliteal regions, three were treated by excision, resulting in two major amputations—one hip disarticulation and one high above-knee amputation. Two grafts were in the aortic or iliofemoral region, and both were treated by excision. One patient had above-knee amputation, and the other died from continued sepsis.

Harrison[36] used dogs to compare the effect of infection on aortic homografts with experimental infection in Teflon prostheses. Two groups were employed: in the first group, grafts were implanted in an infected wound, and in the second group, the grafts were placed in a contaminated wound. In the first group, 5 of 11 dogs died from disruption of an infected homograft, and 5 of 10 dogs experienced complications of infection in a Teflon prosthesis, but only two disrupted. In the second group of implants, in contaminated wounds, six of nine dogs developed infection in a homograft, and five of the six dogs died from disruption. Seven out of eleven Teflon grafts became infected, and there were three deaths from disruption. The authors concluded that the only difference between the behavior of Teflon and homografts in the presence of infection or contamination was the incidence and mode of death. The Teflon graft harbored sepsis, whereas the homograft promptly disrupted, leading to exsanguination.

Humphries et al[37] reported a clinical series of 11 infected homografts collected in 525 arterial reconstructive procedures, an incidence of 2 percent. All of these 11 homografts ruptured from lysis of the grafts, presumably the result of the proteolytic effect of the infection. Prompted by a clinical experience of having an aortic homograft lyse and exsanguinate following resection and replacement of a mycotic aortic aneurysm, Foster et al[38] carried out a similar study to compare the effect of infection on Teflon grafts and homografts. They observed that all the homografts that became infected disrupted and exsanguinated, whereas the plastic prostheses remained intact. They cautioned, however, that the plastic prostheses appeared to continue to harbor infection.

Following these initial clinical and experimental reports, many case reports were published that confirmed the serious nature of infection that complicates vascular grafts. This led the way toward an in-depth search for the etiology, methods of management, and prevention of graft infection.

Incidence. The incidence of graft infection is difficult to quantitate for several reasons. First, the actual number of graft infections is low, and, second, graft infections do not necessarily appear in the immediate postoperative course. They may be delayed for months or even years before they become clinically manifest. There are a number of factors that appear to affect the reported incidence of graft infection in the various series. These factors include the type of graft (autogenous versus prosthetic) and the type of fabric employed in the construction of the prosthetic material. Live autogenous grafts appear to be far more resistant to infection and therefore have a lower incidence of infection in contrast to a foreign body implant.[39–41] In addition, the type of fabric used for the prosthetic graft will have a major effect on the healing properties of the graft. Late infections are considerably fewer in grafts that have a more complete healing response than in those that are more inert to tissue ingrowth.[42] The location of the graft appears to have a major effect on the likelihood of subsequent infection. Infection is also influenced by the appropriate use of antibiotic prophylaxis.[43,44] In analyzing various series, it is important to evaluate the number of operations per year, the number of grafts at risk in a given time interval, and the relative proportion of types of operative procedures and locations when comparing the incidence of graft infection from one series to another.

The overall incidence of graft infection ranges from 1.34 to 6 percent.[45–48] The larger, current series gives the best idea of the problem. In 1972, Szilagyi et al,[49] in a detailed review, evaluated their experience between the years 1952 and 1971, which included 3347 arterial reconstructive procedures. Of the 2145 prosthetic grafts, 40 became infected, an incidence of 1.9 percent. Of the 445 vein grafts, two (0.4 percent) became infected. There was one (0.2 percent) arterial infection in 492 endarterectomies, and 265 reconstructions were performed with arterial allografts, in which there was one (0.4 percent) infection. These authors also analyzed the incidence of infection by the site of insertion and noted that the incidence of infection in aortoiliac grafts was 0.7 percent; in aortofemoral grafts, 1.6 percent; in femorofemoral grafts, 0.9 percent; and in femoropopliteal grafts, 3.0 percent.[49] In 1974, Goldstone and Moore[43] reviewed 566 prosthetic graft implantations performed between 1959 and 1973. Fourteen infections were reported, for an overall incidence of 2.5 percent. These data were broken down into two time intervals, corresponding to a change in the regimen used for antibiotic prophylaxis. Between 1959 and 1965, antibiotics were used in an inconsistent fashion, usually beginning antibiotic treatment in the postoperative period. Nine of the 222 grafts inserted during this interval became infected, for an overall infection rate of 4 percent. Between 1966 and 1973, modern methods of antibiotic prophylaxis, which included preoperative, intraoperative, and postoperative administration of antibiotic medication, were instituted. There were 341 grafts placed during this second period, of which five became infected, for an overall incidence of 1.5 percent. An analysis of the incidence of graft infection as a function of location is shown in Table 37–2, which also compares the incidence of graft infection in the two periods analyzed. Lorentzen et al[47] recently reviewed 2411 consecutive prosthetic graft implantations over a 4-year period (1978 to 1981) and reported 62 (1.6 percent) graft infections. They also noted that graft infection occurred only when the groin had been incised and that 48 percent (30) of patients with graft infection had wound complications in the groin.

Pathogenesis. There are many causes of graft infection. Some have been proved either by clinical observation or by experimental means, and others

TABLE 37–2. INCIDENCE OF GRAFT INFECTION AS A FUNCTION OF GRAFT LOCATION AND ERA OF IMPLANTATION

Anatomic Location	Infection Rate *1959–1965* (%)	*1966–1973* (%)	*1959–1973* (%)
Aortoiliac	1.3	1.2	1.2
Aortofemoral	5.7	1.2	3.0
Axillofemoral	8.0	3.1	5.3
Femorofemoral			7.7
Femoropopliteal			2.3

Adapted from Goldstone J, Moore WS: Am J Surg 128:225, 1974.

represent hypothetical ways in which a prosthesis can become contaminated.[7,42,50–53]

TRAUMATIC WOUNDS. Arterial trauma from war or civilian injuries represents an obvious source of bacterial contamination. Such infections may compromise a vascular repair by producing a combination of wound and graft sepsis. Because every traumatic wound is contaminated to some degree, the arterial repair should preferentially employ autogenous tissues. In those instances in which prosthetic grafts have been implanted directly in contaminated or infected wounds, the incidence of subsequent infectious complications is extremely high. Contaminated wounds represent a major cause of vascular graft sepsis. A noteworthy exception is the experience reported by the Baylor group. They have been able to successfully use prosthetic grafts for arterial reconstruction in contaminated extremity and abdominal injuries.[54]

IMPROPER STERILIZATION OF GRAFT OR SURGICAL INSTRUMENTS. This mechanism probably represents an infrequent, but self-evident, source of contamination of a vascular graft.

BREAK IN STERILE TECHNIQUE. Strict aseptic technique must be followed throughout the procedure. In patients with distal extremity infections, the use of double gloves when draping, careful isolation of the infected focus, and moisture-resistant drapes are all important adjuncts in the prevention of wound or prosthetic graft infections.

SKIN CONTACT. Because the skin cannot be sterilized, large exposed areas of skin continue to harbor organisms on the surface. A prosthetic graft, if allowed to come in contact with the skin, can pick up skin organisms. Skin contact with a graft may occur most commonly in relatively superficial grafting sites, such as the femoral, popliteal, and axillary arteries. This may partially account for the relatively higher incidence of graft infection when prostheses are implanted in these locations. In addition to the skin surface as a source of organisms, the cut edges of skin represent another source of skin contact and transfer of organisms.

SURGICAL TECHNIQUE. It is almost redundant to stress the importance of surgical technique in the prevention of graft infection. Lorentzen et al[47] noted that in 50 of 62 patients with graft infections the most important predisposing or precipitating factor was unsatisfactory surgical technique. In that series, poor surgical technique, including such factors as skin necrosis, hematoma, lymphocele, reoperation because of hemorrhage or thrombosis, and prolonged ileus, constituted 75 percent of the total number of predisposing factors.[47]

INFECTED LYMPH GLANDS OR LYMPHATICS. Lymph glands or lymphatics may be a source of organisms, particularly when there is infection present in the extremity. Incisions to expose arteries that must pass through lymph glands or lymphatic channels will spill contaminated lymph and may represent a major source of contamination of prostheses. Femoral incisions represent the most obvious source for this mode of contamination. Rubin et al[53] have presented data suggesting that lymphatics probably contribute to the development of acute graft infection in two ways. First, by absorbing bacteria and transporting them into the systemic circulation, thus allowing hematogenous contamination of a graft. Or second, by directly bathing the implanted graft with bacteria when lymphatics are disrupted in the course of surgery. These data suggest that careful isolation, transection, and ligation of inguinal lymphatics at the time of arterial reconstruction might minimize acute graft sepsis.

INTESTINAL TRANSUDATE. It is common practice to place the loops of small bowel in a sack when preparing the exposure of the abdominal aorta. There have been reports that the liquid that collects in the plastic bag is contaminated with bacteria. Return of this liquid to the abdominal cavity may bathe the prosthesis and increase the likelihood of graft infection. Other reports, however, have failed to confirm bacterial contamination in this fluid, which may reflect a beneficial effect of prophylactic antibiotics.

INFECTED ARTERIAL OR ANEURYSM CONTENT. On occasion, an abdominal or peripheral aneurysm may be infected prior to repair. The prosthetic graft will inevitably be contaminated. There is also evidence that bacteria are always present in the laminated thrombus lining an abdominal aortic aneurysm. MacBeth et al[7] reported that 3 of 11 (27 percent) aortic aneurysm clot cultures grew bacteria. Previous reports in the literature document a total of 28 positive cultures (13.3 percent) out of 210 aortic aneurysm contents cultures.[53–57] The relationship between infected aneurysm contents and subsequent graft infection is uncertain.

As noted in the section on arterial infections, MacBeth et al[7] reported that 43 percent (38/88) of arterial cultures in clean elective vascular reconstructive procedures grew organisms. In addition, when they reviewed their incidence of graft infection (3/335), graft infections only occurred in patients with positive arterial cultures. If bacterial colonization of the arterial wall is a factor in the pathogenesis of graft infection, however, other factors also must be involved, since the incidence of prosthetic infection is so much lower (0.9 percent) than the incidence of positive arterial cultures (43 percent).[7]

FALSE ANEURYSMS. Although most investigators believe that the majority of arterial prosthetic false aneurysms are caused by technical errors, Bandyk[58] has reported a surprisingly high incidence of positive cultures of *S. epidermidis* in clinically noninfected false aneurysms. However, whether such culture data support a clinical diagnosis of graft infection requires further study.

COMBINED OPERATIONS. The performance of another operation at the time of vascular repair may also be a source of bacterial contamination of the arterial graft. This is particularly true with appendectomy, cholecystectomy, and colectomy. A clean vascular surgical procedure should never be intentionally combined with a contaminated or clean contaminated operation.

TRANSIENT BACTEREMIA. External contamination of the prosthetic graft is most common, but internal contamination during transient bacteremia also occurs. Bacteria in the arterial blood may deposit on the luminal surface of the graft and ultimately lead to a prosthetic infection. Sources of transient bacteremia in the perioperative period include Foley catheters, endotracheal tubes, secondary infections such as pneumonia or urinary tract infection, and, in general, any vigorous mucous membrane manipulation. Transient bacteremia may also be a cause of late graft infection in those instances where the lining of the graft is incomplete. We strongly recommend the use of antibiotic prophylaxis in those patients undergoing mucous membrane manipulation (dental surgery, cystoscopy, proctoscopy) with vascular prostheses in place.

Etiology. It is possible for any organism to infect a graft, and there is a wide spectrum of organisms reported to have infected prostheses. These include such unlikely organisms as *Mycobacterium tuberculosis* and *Histoplasma capsulatum*. It was previously believed that most graft infections were caused by *S. aureus* and fewer to gram-negative organisms. Table 37–3 lists the organisms found in prosthetic graft infections in several recent series.[7,43,46,49,50,52,59] Multiple organisms are frequently found; however, recent reports by Bandyk et al[59] and MacBeth et al[7] have pointed out that

TABLE 37–3. SPECTRUM OF ORGANISMS INFECTING VASCULAR GRAFTS

	Percentage of Patients with Cultured Organisms					
Organism	*Conn et al*[46]	*Szilagyi et al*[49]	*Liekweg and Greenfield*[52]	*MacBeth et al*[7]	*Goldstone and Moore*[43]	*Bandyk*[58]
Aerobacter	10.25	—	—		—	
Bacteroides	—	2.5	0.6		—	
Corynebacterium	—	2.5	0.6		—	
Escherichia coli	10.25	22.5	13.4		15.0	
Enterococcus	10.25	—	1.8		—	
Enterobacter	2.5	—	—		—	
Klebsiella	7.5	—	5.4	21		
Proteus	13.0	7.5	4.8			
Providencia	—	—	—		4.0	
Pseudomonas	13.0	2.5	6.1	29	7.0	
Salmonella	—	—	1.2		—	
Serratia marcescens	10.25	—	—		—	
Staphylococcus, coagulase negative	—	15.0	—	27	—	60
Staphylococcus albus	2.5	—	3.6		26.0	
Staphylococcus aureus	18.0	32.5	50.0	9	41.0	
Streptococcus	2.5	5.0	8.5		—	
Unknown	—	10.0	16.0		7.0	
Total infections	39	40	188	22	27	30

there appears to be a change in the recent microbiology of prosthetic infection and that most graft infections are now primarily caused by *S. epidermidis*.

Each of the groups[7,43,46,49,50,52,59] also analyzed the type and frequency of infection as a function of the interval between operation and clinical presentation and of the location of the clinical infection. They noted that the median interval between graft implantation and the appearance of infection was 3.5 months. Table 37–4 identifies the infecting organism and frequency of those infections that occurred earlier and later than 3.5 months, as a function of location.

Exposure of the graft to skin bacteria in a superficial subcutaneous site like the groin is the most important factor in graft infection. The low-virulence skin organism *S. epidermidis* is most often found late after grafting, and it is conceivable that a dormant period intervenes between contamination and clinical infection. The increased risk of graft infection when the graft extends below the inguinal ligament should encourage a greater degree of care when extending prosthetic reconstruction in that area. Finally, the frequency of *Staphylococcus* species as the infecting organisms should direct one to antibiotic prophylaxis that includes *Staphylococcus* species in its bactericidal spectrum.[7,43,59] Although there are recent reports calling increased attention to *S. epidermidis* as an important pathogen in prosthetic infection,[5,7] objective evidence to support a change in antibiotic prophylaxis away from cephalosporins is not yet available.[60]

Clinical Manifestations. Infection in a vascular graft may have a wide spectrum of clinical manifestations. The clinical appearance of a graft infection is dependent on three major factors: the duration between implantation and appearance of sepsis, the type of graft material involved in the infectious process, and the location of the vascular conduit.

TABLE 37–4. SPECTRUM AND LOCATION OF INFECTIONS WITHIN OR AFTER 3.5 MONTHS OF OPERATION

	Within 3.5 Months		After 3.5 Months	
Organism	*Groin*	*Elsewhere*	*Groin*	*Elsewhere*
Escherichia coli	0	2	1	1
Providencia	—	—	0	1
Pseudomonas	1	1	—	—
Staphylococcus albus	—	—	7	0
Staphylococcus aureus	9	0	1	1
Unknown	—	—	2	0

From Goldstone J, Moore WS: Am J Surg 128:225, 1974.

ACUTE GRAFT INFECTION. Acute vascular graft infections usually occur as a consequence of a postoperative wound infection. Therefore acute graft infections are most often limited to those reconstructive procedures that come in close proximity to the skin (femoral, popliteal, axillary, carotid-subclavian anastomoses). The initial manifestations of sepsis include the characteristics of a wound infection: fever, leukocytosis, redness, induration, and abscess formation. The specific manifestations of acute sepsis around the vascular conduit depend on the type of material used for the vascular graft.

LATE GRAFT INFECTION. Most graft infections appear months to years after a vascular reconstructive procedure. The signs of sepsis may be quite subtle. Patients are frequently afebrile, and the white blood cell count is often normal. One consistent although nonspecific laboratory finding, both clinically and experimentally, has been an elevated erythrocyte sedimentation rate. Specific manifestations of infection often depend on the type of graft material and the location of implantation.

Manifestations of Sepsis as a Function of the Graft Material

PLASTIC PROSTHESES. Dacron is a textile, that is, a multifibered foreign body. Once infecting organisms contaminate a dacron prosthesis, they continue to be harbored in the graft fabric. Systemic antibiotic therapy alone will not succeed in eradicating contaminating organisms from the prosthesis. Expanded PTFE is not a textile but its surface interstices are also difficult to sterilize. In some instances, however, PTFE grafts can be preserved.

Infections in any plastic prosthesis can manifest itself in several ways including anastomotic breakdown with formation of a false aneurysm, graft thrombosis, a purulent draining sinus, wound breakdown with exteriorization of the prosthesis, systemic sepsis, and septic emboli.

Table 37–5 lists the modes of onset and clinical manifestations of graft infections in an older[45] and more recent[41] series. The clinical manifestations can be divided into two general patterns. In the first, the diagnosis is readily evident. There is persistent purulent wound drainage, wound abscess, or exteriorization of the graft. In the second, the diagnosis is subtle—persistent low-grade fever, sys-

TABLE 37–5. PRESENTING CLINICAL MANIFESTATIONS OF PROSTHETIC GRAFT SEPSIS

Complications	Number	
	Fry and Lindenauer[45]	*Goldstone and Moore*[43]
Graft occlusion	4	8
Localized infection and draining sinus	3	14
False aneurysm	1	13
Local hemorrhage	1	7
Systemic sepsis or shock	2	5
Persistent pelvic abscess	1	—
Septic emboli	—	2
Total	12	49

temic sepsis, septic embolization, graft thrombosis, ureteral obstruction, an abdominal mass, a false aneurysm, and gastrointestinal hemorrhage.

Liekweg and Greenfield[52] analyzed the mode of presentation of 164 cases from the literature as a function of anatomic location (Table 37–6).

PRESERVED HOMOGRAFTS. Freeze-dried preserved homografts were introduced by Gross et al[61] in 1949 and represented a major breakthrough in the availability of materials for grafting of large vessels. Sepsis complicating the use of this material, however, is particularly disastrous. Because the material is nonviable, sepsis results in rapid proteolytic digestion of the graft material, which promptly leads to disruption and massive hemorrhage. Early experimental studies by Foster et al[38] confirmed this observation and indicated that plastic prostheses, although continuing to harbor infection as a foreign body, at least remain intact, thus preventing disruption and hemorrhage from the body of the graft. The various manifestations of sepsis in preserved homografts are again dependent on the location of the homografts, but, ultimately, hemorrhage is the final common pathway. Freeze-dried preserved arterial homografts are not in clinical use at the present time. However, a new material has been introduced to the market and is currently being employed for vascular reconstruction and dialysis access. This is the tanned, externally supported umbilical vein. This material is not viable and possesses the identical characteristics of freeze-dried preserved homografts when their clinical use is complicated by sepsis.

BOVINE XENOGRAFTS. Carotid arteries, obtained from cows and processed by digestion and tanning to yield a collagen tube, were formerly used for dialysis access procedures. When sepsis complicated a bovine xenograft disruption and hemorrhage ensued.

FRESH AUTOGENOUS GRAFTS. Fresh autogenous artery and vein grafts have been used for a variety of vascular grafting operations. Specifically, the autogenous saphenous vein has been used for femoropopliteal replacement, patch angioplasty, coronary bypass, and extrathoracic cerebrovascular bypass procedures. Fresh autogenous arteries (eg, hypogastric, external iliac, reconstituted thrombectomized superficial femoral) have been used as renal arterial replacements or as replacements in septic fields as a vascular replacement material. These conduits tend to be quite resistant to the immediate complications of sepsis, provided there is prompt treatment of the surrounding septic processes, including drainage, irrigation, and antibiotic therapy. However, if the surrounding sepsis is profound and is not treated in time, infection will lead to proteolytic disruption of the autogenous vascular material, with breakdown and hemorrhage.

Sepsis as a Function of Graft Location. Sepsis as a function of graft location will produce not only the evidence of the systemic problem but also features

TABLE 37–6. CLINICAL MANIFESTATION OF PROSTHETIC GRAFT INFECTION AS A FUNCTION OF LOCATION

Mode	Aortoiliac (%)	Aortofemoral (%)	Iliofemoral (%)	Femoropopliteal (%)
Wound purulence	10.4	43.6	42.8	74.5
Sepsis	24.1	18.2	7.1	0.0
False Aneurysm	10.4	9.1	14.2	9.1
Hemorrhage	20.8	7.2	7.1	7.2
Sinus tract	6.9	9.1	21.4	7.2
Upper gastrointestinal bleeding	27.5	18.2	0.0	0.0
Graft occlusion	0.0	9.1	7.1	1.8

Adapted from Liekweg WG Jr, Greenfield LJ: Surgery 81:335, 1977.

that are unique to the organ being supplied or organs adjacent to the infected graft. For example, infection in an abdominal graft can produce a fistula into adjacent duodenum, small bowel, or large intestine. Thus the first presenting manifestation of graft sepsis may be massive upper or lower gastrointestinal bleeding. It is well to remember this fact when any patient with a history of vascular replacement in the abdomen presents with gastrointestinal bleeding. Under such circumstances, gastrointestinal bleeding is graft sepsis until proved otherwise.[62] It is dangerous to attribute bleeding to another lesion even if changes such as gastritis or duodenal ulceration are relatively easy to demonstrate.

As long as the sepsis is confined to the shaft of the prosthetic graft, it may remain relatively quiet for some time. If the shaft is superficial to the skin surface, the infection may ultimately become visible as an abscess or a draining sinus. Once the infection extends to the anastomosis between the plastic prosthesis and host artery, the inflammatory process ultimately destroys the host tissue at the junction and leads to the formation of a septic false aneurysm. If the anastomosis is relatively close to the skin surface, the presence of a false aneurysm will easily be appreciated on physical examination. If the anastomosis is within the abdomen or chest cavity, the false aneurysm may not be obvious until it produces a mass effect, obstructing an adjacent organ, or produces exsanguinating hemorrhage. The specific manifestations as a function of the type of reconstructive procedure as documented by Liekweg and Greenfield[52] are summarized in Table 37–6.

Natural History, Morbidity, and Mortality. Uncontrolled infection involving a tissue graft (fresh autograft, preserved homograft, heterograft) results in proteolytic digestion of the graft, disruption, and exsanguinating hemorrhage. A prosthetic graft infection has a slower and more insidious natural history. The foreign material continues to harbor infecting organisms, but the rate at which infection spreads along the course of the prosthesis to involve the anastomoses is quite variable. If the organism is of low virulence, such as *S. epididmidis,* the infection may remain quiescent for years. If the infecting exudate has egress, as through an exposed graft or a draining sinus, the progression of the infection to the anastomotic areas may be quite delayed. On the other hand, if the infecting organisms are virulent or if the infection remains confined to a closed space, the infection will progress rapidly along the length of the graft to ultimately involve the anastomosis. Once the anastomosis is involved, anastomotic disruption occurs, resulting in the development of pseudoaneurysms and, ultimately, exsanguinating hemorrhage.

The morbidity and mortality associated with graft infection are great even when a management program is appropriately instituted. Bouhoutsos et al[50] reported their experience with 14 infected grafts, seven aortofemoral or iliofemoral and seven femoropopliteal grafts. Three patients died in the aortofemoral series, in spite of treatment (mortality, 29 percent). Two major lower extremity amputations were required in the femoropopliteal group (amputation rate of 28.6 percent). Fry and Lindenauer,[45] reporting their experience with 12 infected grafts, had 9 deaths (mortality rate of 75 percent) in spite of a vigorous attempt at surgical management. Conn et al[46] in their series of 22 graft infections had a 40.9 percent mortality rate and a 27 percent lower extremity amputation rate. Goldstone and Moore,[43] reporting on 27 patients with graft infection, had 10 deaths (a mortality rate of 37 percent), and another 6 patients underwent major lower extremity amputation (an amputation rate of 22 percent). The mortality rate of infrainguinal prosthetic graft infections is relatively low compared with infections involving aortic grafts; however, the amputation rate is high. In a recent review of 3731 infrainguinal graft infections, Durham et al[63] reported a 9.1 percent mortality and a 69.7 percent amputation rate. Szilagyi et al[49] and Liekweg et al[64] have looked at mortality and amputation as a function of the graft location (Table 37–7).

TABLE 37–7. MORBIDITY AND MORTALITY OF INFECTED GRAFTS AS A FUNCTION OF LOCATION

	Szilagyl et al[49]		Liekweg and Greenfield[52]	
Anatomic Location	*Mortality (%)*	*Amputation (%)*	*Mortality (%)*	*Amputation (%)*
Aortoiliac	40.0	0.0	58.6	34.5
Aortofemoral	52.6	10.5	43.5	13.0
Femoropopliteal	0.0	50.0	9.9	32.7
Total grafts	34		153	

When a graft infection presents primarily with bleeding into the gastrointestinal tract, the prognosis is usually grave in spite of aggressive management. Elliot et al[62] report a mortality rate of 73.7 percent despite aggressive management in 19 patients with aortic or paraprosthetic enteric fistulas. However, Perdue et al[65] more recently reported a salvage rate of 86 percent (five of six aortoduodenal fistulas) with aggressive early surgical intervention.

Diagnosis

HISTORY. Anyone with a vascular graft in place, particularly a plastic prosthesis, is a candidate for infection, regardless of length of time between implantation and subsequent presentation of the clinical problem. In evaluating a patient with suspected graft infection, the following points are of value:

1. The surgeon's operative report. The report from the original implantation should carefully be reviewed to elicit any potential intraoperative problems that may have predisposed to graft infection. These would include an inadvertent enterotomy, grafting in the presence of a coexistent septic problem (eg, infected, gangrenous extremity; intra-abdominal sepsis; trauma), combined operations, such as simultaneous appendectomy, cholecystectomy, or colectomy, or failure to reretroperitonealize the graft.
2. A history of postoperative wound complications. This may suggest continued wound sepsis.
3. A history of repeated redo operations. Recurrent false aneurysms or graft thrombosis may have been signs of a subtle graft infection that was not obvious at the time of initial repair.[58,66] Also, each time a graft is reexposed de novo contamination is possible.
4. A history of infection or potential bacteremic exposure. An acute urinary tract infection, pulmonary infection, or mucous membrane manipulation or instrumentation, such as dental extraction or endoscopy, may have provided an opportunity for introduction of bacteria into the bloodstream.
5. A patient with a history of intra-abdominal vascular grafting who has gastrointestinal bleeding. Such a patient must be considered as a candidate for graft infection and paraprosthetic-enteric fistula until proved otherwise.

PHYSICAL EXAMINATION. In performing a physical examination on a patient with suspected graft sepsis, the examiner must keep in mind the specific manifestations that graft sepsis may demonstrate. These include absence of pulsation associated with a graft limb thrombosis, a palpable pulsatile mass suggesting a false aneurysm at one of the anastomoses, a draining sinus through one of the incision sites, abscess formation along the course of the graft or in the area of a healed incision, exposed graft, fever, wound erythema, and petechiae over the skin in the distribution of blood flow from a prosthetic graft, indicating the possible presence of septic emboli.

LABORATORY STUDIES. Routine laboratory studies should be performed to identify nonspecific inflammation or infection. These include a white blood cell and differential blood count, erythrocyte sedimentation rate, and blood cultures. It should be noted that some less virulent forms of graft infection may be present with a normal white blood cell count, as well as a normal differential. The erythrocyte sedimentation rate has been uniquely sensitive in suggesting possible sepsis; however, this test is quite nonspecific. Finally, blood cultures may be helpful, if positive. However, many patients with graft infection will have negative blood cultures.

SPECIAL STUDIES. Special diagnostic studies are often helpful in establishing the presence of graft sepsis.

ARTERIOGRAPHY. An arteriogram may reveal irregularity in the area of an anastomosis, a false aneurysm, or graft thrombosis, all of which may be indirect evidence of sepsis. It can be difficult to interpret a single arteriogram when looking for evidence of graft infection, and therefore comparison with previous studies may be helpful. In instances of gastrointestinal bleeding, the arteriogram sometimes reveals the arterioenteric fistula.

SINOGRAM. If the patient has a draining sinus, the insertion of a small catheter and the careful injection of contrast material is often helpful in making the diagnosis of periprosthetic infection.[11] If the sinogram demonstrates a tract around the graft, as evidenced by the appearance of corrugations corresponding to the prosthesis, the diagnosis of graft sepsis is confirmed. It should be noted, however, that sinogram catheter manipulation may induce bacteremia.

ASPIRATION. A careful attempt at needle aspiration of the perigraft space under sterile conditions can be helpful if there is a fluid collection around the graft. The fluid obtained should be cultured, and a positive culture confirms graft sepsis. CAT scanning may be a useful adjunct for needle aspiration of a deep lying graft.

ENDOSCOPY OR BARIUM STUDIES. Upper gastrointestinal barium studies or endoscopy are generally useful only for delineation of prosthetic erosion or fistula, or documentation of the presence or absence of bleeding from other sources of upper gastrointestinal hemorrhage such as peptic ulcer disease.

ULTRASONOGRAPHY, GALLIUM, AND INDIUM WHITE BLOOD CELL SCANNING. Gooding et al[67] have documented the role of ultrasonography in delineating pseudoaneurysms, perigraft fluid collections, and graft infections in aortobifemoral grafts. However, a negative ultrasound does not rule out a graft infection and the accuracy of ultrasound varies with the experience of the radiologist. If positive, gallium scanning may be useful in the diagnosis of graft infection.[68] Once again, however, a negative scan does not rule out a graft infection. In spite of initial promising results, the diagnostic value of indium white blood cell scanning is unclear.[69]

CAT SCAN. Although CAT scanning is being used with increasing frequency to diagnose abdominal and inguinal graft infection,[70] the interpretation of postoperative tomographic scans has been limited because of the absence of studies documenting the normal appearance of routine uncomplicated aortic grafts. Quarfordt et al[71] presented tomographic scan data on 29 uncomplicated patients (17 aortoiliac, and 12 aneurysmal disease) who were studied on a mean of 7, 48, and 102 days after surgery. That study provides important baseline data for the use of CAT scans in the postoperative period.

Treatment. The management of a vascular graft infection depends on several factors: the type of material involved, the location, the patency of the prosthesis, the extent to which the graft is involved in the septic process, and the effect of the graft infection on the patient.

GENERAL PRINCIPLES. If the infection involves an autograft or homograft artery or vein, it may be possible to manage the patient by conservative means. Drainage, debridement, and intensive antibiotic therapy with careful observation are appropriate. If a preserved tissue graft, such as a freeze-dried homograft or a preserved allograft, becomes infected, removal of the graft is usually required. The same is true of a synthetic prosthesis, which must be removed to eradicate the septic problem.

The general principles for management of an infected plastic prosthesis or a preserved tissue graft would observe the following sequence:

1. *Remove the infected graft.* Only by removing the entire graft will total control of the septic process be assured, because any portion of the foreign body left behind may continue to harbor infection.
2. *Debride all infected arterial tissue.* Failure to debride all infected arterial tissue is a significant error since this tissue will frequently proceed to disintegrate in the face of the infectious process and lead to exsanguination. In the course of removing the infected graft, the adjacent arterial segments should be debrided to the point where the artery appears normal: there should be no edema, no inflammation, and the tissue should have a normal tensile strength. Although some surgeons have advocated intraoperative histologic assessment, most experienced surgeons believe that the distinction between healthy and diseased artery may safely be made on the basis of intraoperative examination.
3. *Close involved arteries with monofilament suture.* The use of a braided, polyfilament suture in the face of infected tissue presents the potential risk of suture line infection. The braided sutures are more likely to provide bacteria with a suitable environment in which they may proliferate. Accordingly, monofilament suture is recommended for closure of any open vessels in the operative field.
4. *Repair blood vessel defects with autogenous tissue.* In the instance of an end-to-side anastomosis, closing the arteriotomy simply without compromising apparent flow through the artery is ideal. If a considerable circumference of the artery has been effaced or destroyed by the septic process, it may be necessary to close the arteriotomy site with a patch to maintain flow through the parent or recipient vessel. The ideal material would be fresh autogenous vein. It should be recognized that there is some risk in such a repair since the infectious process, if not well controlled, may destroy the patch or parent artery.

5. *Debridement, irrigation, and drainage.* Once the graft has been removed, any septic tissue or exudate must carefully be debrided, the wound generously irrigated with antibiotic solution, and drainage provided. Debridement of the infected and inflamed retroperitoneal and periarterial tissue is a very important element in controlling an arterial infection since these tissues may serve to perpetuate the infection. For retroperitoneal infections, closed drains are used routinely when gross purulence is encountered. Infections involving superficial arteries such as the femoral or popliteal vessels may be managed by open packing to allow the formation of granulation tissue and secondary wound closure.
6. *Long-term antibiotics.* The principal cause of management failure in the surgical treatment of graft sepsis is persistent sepsis in the periarterial tissues or continued sepsis in the arterial wall proper. Arterial and graft cultures from the site of prosthetic graft infection have both prognostic and therapeutic implications. MacBeth et al[7] reported 8 of 14 arterial disruptions when both artery and graft cultures were positive; none of the eight arteries disrupted when only the graft was contaminated. Massive doses of antibiotics to which the organisms are sensitive will help to eradicate the problem of arterial contamination even after graft removal. Treatment with intravenous therapy during the 2 weeks following graft excision should be followed by 3 to 6 months of oral antibiotics.
7. *Extra-anatomic revascularization.* If the patient has an organ or an extremity that is dependent on blood flow through the graft, blood flow must be reestablished or the organ or extremity will be sacrificed. In the case of a peripheral vascular graft, it is our practice to remove the infected graft first and then evaluate the circulation to the extremity. If collateral circulation is adequate to maintain viability of the limb, immediate revascularization is withheld because of the increased risk of contamination of the new graft. However, if the extremity is clearly nonviable after graft removal, extra-anatomic revascularization is attempted.

It should be noted that many other authors recommend revascularization before removal of the infected prosthesis, and we have adopted this approach when managing aortic prosthetic infections. A review by Trout et al[72] strongly suggests that remote bypass with a prosthetic graft should precede removal of an infected graft or surgery for a graft enteric erosion fistula. Based on a literature review of aortic prosthetic infections and graft enteric erosions or fistulas, that study reported decreased mortality rates from 71 percent (10 of 14) to 20 percent (6 of 23) and from 53 percent (40 of 115) to 17 percent (5 of 29), respectively, if remote bypass was performed first. Lower extremity ischemia for the period required to revascularize distal tissues is obviously a major stress in the already infected patient.

Specific Problems

AORTOENTERIC FISTULA. After appropriate blood replacement, a rapid exploration should be carried out. The fistula site is usually obvious because the bowel is adherent to the phlegmon. If the fistula is between the proximal anastomosis and the duodenum, proximal control of the aorta is best obtained immediately below the diaphragm. The iliac arteries distal to the iliac anastomoses are then mobilized and controlled. As with elective arterial reconstruction, heparinization prior to clamping the arteries is recommended. Careful dissection can now be carried out between the graft and the duodenum. Once the duodenum is disconnected, nonviable tissue is debrided and the bowel is oversewn transversely. The graft is excised from the distal anastomoses, debridement is carried out, and the arteriotomy sites are closed with monofilament suture, providing an adequate cuff of both proximal and distal artery. If possible, specimens of residual artery and resected graft should be obtained for culture and sensitivity testing. It is desirable to interpose tissue between the aortic closure and the duodenal closure. This is best accomplished by developing an omental pedicle to place over the aortic stump. After closure of the arteriotomies, the proximal and distal clamps are removed. The perigraft tissues are carefully debrided and generously irrigated with antibiotic solution. Closed suction drains are placed, and the abdomen is closed. The drapes are then removed, and the extremities are carefully evaluated for evidence of capillary blood flow to the toes. If the extremities are obviously ischemic, the patient is reprepped and redraped, and an axillary-bifemoral bypass is performed. High-dose antibiotic therapy is administered in the postoperative period and should be continued for up to 3 months. Antibiotic therapy is based on the assumption that polymicrobial intestinal flora are always present in this circumstance.

AORTOFEMORAL GRAFT SEPSIS. The management of infection of an aortofemoral bypass graft depends on the extent to which the graft is involved in the infectious process. It is possible for the infection to be confined to the distal end of one femoral limb, leaving the proximal graft and opposite femoral limb sterile. It is also possible for the entire prosthesis to be infected, which necessitates the complete removal of the bifurcation graft. The initial surgical maneuver is to establish the extent of the septic process. If the patient has localized sepsis at one groin, the approach we recommend is a suprainguinal, retroperitoneal exploration of the proximal limb of that graft. If that portion of the graft demonstrates a good fibrous tissue incorporation of the prosthesis, and no evidence of perigraft exudate is present, the graft limb is divided near the bifurcation, a segment of graft is removed and cultured, and the proximal and distal portions of the excised segment are oversewn. The objective of this maneuver is to disconnect the proximal sterile portion of the graft from the distal infected portion and to allow an interposition of viable soft tissue between the divided segments of the graft. At a second procedure, the femoral incision is reopened, the infected limb of the graft is disconnected from the femoral artery, and the femoral arteriotomy is oversewn. The distal portion of the graft is then pulled out from the retroperitoneal tunnel, thus leaving the proximal graft and opposite graft limb functioning with flow to the opposite extremity. With good blood flow to the opposite extremity, ligation of one side of the bifurcation graft will usually not jeopardize the viability of the extremity on that side. There is often sufficient cross-pelvic collateral flow to support the disconnected leg. The femoral wound on the infected side is usually packed open and allowed to close secondarily. A drain is placed in the retroperitoneal tunnel to ensure good drainage of the contaminated tunnel site. Topical antibiotic irrigation is carried out, as well as long-term administration of systemic antibiotics. If the graft culture returns positive in spite of the benign clinical appearance of the incorporated graft, long-term antibiotic therapy is indicated. Unless there are clinical findings to suggest graft infection of the residual graft limb, we would not recommend total excision of the graft based on culture data alone. However, careful patient follow-up is appropriate and CAT scans may be a useful long-term diagnostic tool.

If both graft limbs are involved, or if the body of the graft is involved, removal of the entire graft is required. Following graft removal, if the extremities appear nonviable, an extra-anatomic bypass is necessary. If the superficial femoral arteries are open, an axillary bypass skirting wide of the contaminated femoral wound can be carried down and anastomosed to the midsuperficial femoral artery. If the superficial femoral arteries are occluded, an axillary-to-popliteal bypass can be performed. Many authorities would, if possible, perform the revascularization procedure before removal of the graft in order to preserve continuous perfusion of the lower extremities.

When sepsis is confined to one femoral site, an alternative mode of grafting is possible. A new graft limb is anastomosed to the proximal aortic graft and brought through the obturator foramen to the superficial femoral artery. This is a more extensive operative method of circumventing the contaminated femoral site and is therefore less desirable.

FEMOROPOPLITEAL GRAFT SEPSIS. Infection of a femoropopliteal bypass graft presents itself in two principal manners. It may occur acutely when an autogenous bypass graft becomes infected in the course of an acute wound infection. The second presentation is that of a late graft infection, usually associated with the use of prosthetic grafts. If an autogenous tissue graft is infected, open drainage and irrigation will usually clear the sepsis and allow wound closure. When a prosthetic graft is involved, the entire graft must be removed. If the viability of the extremity is compromised, reconstruction is best carried out with an autogenous saphenous vein. When a vein is not available, an endarterectomized superficial femoral artery may be used.

SEPSIS IN A DIALYSIS ACCESS ARTERIOVENOUS FISTULA. Because of its subcutaneous location, the response to therapy of an infection in a dialysis access graft may easily be observed. This had led to a more conservative approach to the management of this problem. Dialysis graft infections are initially treated with intravenous antibiotics. If a discrete area of fluctuance develops, it is incised and drained. The infected graft is removed and a new graft is implanted through a new tunnel, which circumvents the area of sepsis. Such management has the advantage of preserving the arterial and venous anastomosis as well as preserving the dialysis site. Frequently, the septic portion of the graft is localized and so limited that the remaining graft may be used even as the new segment is incorporating.

New Concepts in the Management of Graft Sepsis

FRESH TISSUE GRAFT REPLACEMENT. In 1961, Moore et al[39] experimentally demonstrated that fresh autogenous veins could be placed in infected fields and would function as vascular conduits while allowing eradication of the local infection. In a clinical study, Wylie[40] demonstrated that autogenous arterial grafts could be placed in an infected field and function while the systemic sepsis was clearing. While this is an exciting concept, the availability of autogenous arteries is limited, and the portion of autogenous artery removed must be replaced with a plastic graft to maintain arterial continuity. Theoretically, this is a disadvantage, because the graft replacing the donor autogenous artery may become secondarily infected.

Fresh arterial allografts were experimentally used in the management of arterial infection by Moore et al[41] in 1975. They demonstrated that fresh allograft arteries could be implanted in infected fields, would permit infection to be cleared, and would function as a viable conduit. The fresh allograft did as well as the fresh autograft control.

Unfortunately, however, clinically satisfactory methods for arterial allograft preservation and storage have not been developed to the point of allowing widespread clinical use. Preliminary reports on detergent extracted arterial homografts are promising, but such grafts are not yet available for clinical evaluation.[73]

A recent clinical report by Kieffer et al[74] has detailed the use of fresh allografts obtained in the course of cadaveric organ procurement. Because of limitation of donors and the emergent nature of most operations, no attempt was made to match tissue or even blood types. They successfully treated 43 patients with infected aortic prostheses with a combination of immediate or delayed in situ aortic reconstruction using fresh cadaveric aortic allografts. In the course of their experience, four patients suffered allograft complications: one occlusion, one graft enteric fistula, and two ruptures (one fatal). With a mean follow-up period of 13.8 months, they concluded that allograft replacement represented a major advance in the management of infected aortic prostheses.[74]

LOCAL ANTIBIOTIC IRRIGATION. There are occasional reports documenting the success of topical irrigation of an exposed graft with antibiotic solution, which permits the development of granulation tissue and closure of the septic wound site. The only cases that were successful, however, were those in which only a segment of the shaft of the graft was exposed. In no instance was this method successful if an anastomotic site was exposed.[63,75,76]

LOCAL EXCISION, DRAINAGE, AND SUPPRESSIVE ANTIBIOTIC THERAPY. On occasion, when the total excision of an infected graft is impossible, due either to the critical location or to systemic illness, another approach has been used with some success. Local excision of the obviously infected portion of the graft, particularly that involving a distal femoral anastomosis, is carried out. The wound is generously irrigated with antibiotic solution. The proximal septic process can frequently be controlled by the permanent systemic administration of antibiotics. Thus the high-risk patient is permitted to live out his or her abbreviated remaining life span.

This approach has recently been modified in some patients with localized graft infections of limited extent. Calligaro and associates[77] reported a series of 42 patients with either peripheral graft infections or infected femoral portions of aortic grafts. They preserved these grafts by judicious debridement of infected tissues, use of open wound packing, use of muscle flap coverage, and prolonged administration of antibiotics. Four patients (10 percent) died; nine graft were ultimately lost; and one limb was amputated. Overall, the graft salvage was 28 of 42 grafts (67 percent).[77] In a similar effort, Miller[78] reported partial replacement of 42 infected arterial grafts by replacing the involved portion of the grafts with a segment of PTFE, which was routed to a clean site. Additional adjuncts included debridement of the infected site, as well as parenteral antibiotics. Only 3 of 42 patients died and 6 of 42 limbs were amputated. The author concluded that partial graft replacement was an effective and simpler method of managing limited graft infections.

These reports emphasize the variety of approaches that have been employed to individualize the management of prosthetic graft infections as well as the complexity of these problems. It should be noted that even in the best of hands these problems are frequently devastating and have a high chance of resulting in loss of limb and life.

Antibiotic-Bonded Grafts

Clarke and Morgraf[79] first reported studies on antibiotic graft bonding. In that study, a silver-allantoin-heparin combination was bonded to Dacron and decreased the sepsis rate from 100 percent (5 of 5) to 15 percent (1 of 7) in a canine vena cava model. McDivitt[80] reported a decrease in topical *E. coli* sepsis from 100 percent (5 of 5) to 11 percent (2 of 19) with heat and pressure bonding of tetracycline to Dacron in a canine model. Moore et al[81] have more recently reported the resistance of Dacron-collagen-aminoglycoside bonded aortic grafts in dogs to *S. aureus* infusions, where antibiotic-bonded grafts had an 8 percent (2 of 17) infection rate compared with 100 percent (13 of 13) of untreated grafts. Finally, both Prahlad et al[82] and Greco et al[60] have reported similar data using noncovalent antibiotic bonding to PTFE grafts. Most importantly, however, Greco et al[60] demonstrated that surfactant-treated PTFE grafts could absorb parenterally administered penicillin G in clinically significant concentrations compared with control grafts. This later study clearly suggests that prosthetic graft infections might be prevented or treated by antibiotic-bonded grafts.

More recently, we have reported our experience using a rifampicin-impregnated collagen coated Dacron graft for in situ repair of prosthetic aortic graft infections.[83] By administration of parenteral antibiotics for a period of 2 weeks along with debridement and the use of the rifampicin-bonded graft, the incidence of reinfection of the in situ replacement graft was lowered from 100 percent to about 20 percent. One remarkable insight gained from this experiment was confirmation of the importance of long-term antibiotic therapy. After 2 weeks of parenteral antibiotics, the incidence of positive tissue cultures from the retroperitoneum was remarkably lower than when shorter periods of antibiotic administration were employed. Comparison of the cultures of grafts and the perigraft tissues revealed that while infection appeared to have been cleared from the graft, it persisted in the adjacent tissues, thus supporting the concept of prolonged administration of antibiotics in the management of graft infections.

Prevention of Graft Sepsis. Obviously, the best method of managing graft sepsis is prevention. Recognition of the causative factors in prosthetic sepsis is helpful in designing a program to reduce the incidence and thus help prevent this dreaded complication.

ANTIBIOTIC PROPHYLAXIS. Experimental reports and a recent, controlled, clinical trial have demonstrated that the perioperative use of systemic and topical prophylactic antibiotics is effective in reducing the incidence of graft infection.[43,44,84–86] Antibiotic prophylaxis should ensure bactericidal tissue levels during the entire operation (see Chap. 25). Because the most common organism associated with graft sepsis is *Staphylococcus,* prophylactic antibiotics should be selected with this organism in mind. Our drugs of choice are cephalosporins, which are bactericidal not only for *Staphylococcus* but also for several gram-negative organisms that have been identified as causes of graft sepsis. During the course of operation, another dose of prophylactic antibiotic is administered, and postoperative antibiotic prophylaxis is continued until all the lines, such as Foley catheter, nasogastric tube, and arterial and venous cannulas, are out of the patient—usually 2 to 3 days.

PREVENTION OF INTRAOPERATIVE GRAFT CONTAMINATION. The skin is a potential source of organisms that may contaminate a graft. Every attempt should be made to avoid bringing the graft in contact with the skin. This is best accomplished by the use of plastic adhesive drapes that will cover the large exposed area of skin often present during vascular surgical procedures. Plastic drapes are far superior to cloth drapes, because cloth drapes become moistened and permit the migration of contaminated fluids through the cloth surface. One other source of skin contamination not often recognized is the cut edge of skin. This is particularly important in superficial grafting sites such as femoral or popliteal wounds. Bringing a graft into contact with the cut edge of skin is as bad as allowing direct surface skin contact with the prosthesis. Skin edge contact can be avoided by appropriate wound edge draping with antibiotic-moistened sponges and by keeping this potential source of contamination in mind when handling a graft in a superficial site.

Another source of intraoperative contamination is the contaminated lymphatic, particularly in femoral incisions.[53] In making a femoral incision, it is important to avoid incising directly through lymph nodes and lymphatics, particularly in patients who have gangrenous changes of the extremity, because there may well be bacterial contamination of lymphatic channels or the lymph nodes themselves. Transected lymphatic channels or nodes should be ligated and excised.[53]

Particular care should be paid to the closure of superficial grafting sites, because wound sepsis, if it occurs, offers a major risk for extension and graft contamination. We advocate closing wounds in several layers and using subcuticular rather than transcutaneous sutures, particularly in incisions over the femoral artery.

Another way to help maintain the sterility of the operative field and the graft during placement is to practice generous irrigation of the graft and wound with antibiotic solutions during the entire operative procedure. Experimental data have demonstrated that topical wound irrigation will significantly reduce the risk of graft sepsis.[81,85,86]

LATE ANTIBIOTIC PROPHYLAXIS. Prosthetic vascular grafts will inevitably have incomplete healing of their linings, and these raw spots are always susceptible to implantation from circulating bacteria.[42] Patients should be instructed to inform their other physicians of the presence of the vascular graft and the need for using prophylactic antibiotic therapy when undergoing such procedures as dental extraction, mucous membrane manipulation, or endoscopy. Patients with prosthetic grafts should also be more concerned about superficial infection and the prompt treatment of systemic infection by antibiotic therapy.

REFERENCES

1. Wilson SE, Van Wagenen P, Passaro E Jr: Arterial infection. Curr Probl Surg 15(9):1, 1978.
2. Stengel A, Wolferth CC: Mycotic (bacterial) aneurysms of intravascular origin. Arch Intern Med 31:527, 1923.
3. Pelletier LL Jr, Petersdorf R: Infective endocarditis. In Harrison T (ed): Harrison's Principles of Internal Medicine, Vol 1, 8th ed. New York, McGraw-Hill, 1977, p 797.
4. Jarrett F, Darling RC, Mundth ED, Austen WG: The management of infected arterial aneurysms. J Cardiovasc Surg 18:361, 1977.
5. Cates J, Christie R: Subacute bacterial endocarditis: a review of 442 patients treated in 14 centers appointed by the Penicillin Trials Committee of the Medical Research Council. Q J Med 20:93, 1951.
6. Sommerville RL, Allen EV, Edwards IE: Bland and infected arteriosclerotic abdominal aortic aneurysms—a clinicopathologic study. Medicine (Baltimore) 38:207, 1959.
7. MacBeth GA, Rubin JR, McIntyre RE, et al: The relevance of arterial wall microbiology to the treatment of prosthetic graft infection: graft infection vs arterial infection. J Vasc Surg 1:750, 1984.
8. Moore WS, Malone JM: The use of prophylactic antibiotics in vascular surgery. J Surg Pract 6:24, 1977.
9. Sullivan JJ Jr, Mangiardi JL: Surgical management of mycotic aneurysms. Ann Surg 148:119, 1958.
10. Shapiro SL: Carotid artery erosion secondary to pharyngeal infection. Eye Ear Nose Throat Mon 52:513, 1974.
11. Kyriakides GK, Simmons RL, Najarian JS: Mycotic aneurysms in transplant patients. Arch Surg 111:472, 1976.
12. Walsh TJ, Zachary JB, Hutchins GM, Sterioff S: Mycotic aneurysm with recurrent sepsis implicating post-transplant nephrectomy. Johns Hopkins Med J 141:85, 1977.
13. Kerr AL, Tilney NL: Mycotic aneurysm from unrecognized colonic sepsis. J R Coll Surg Edinb 22:271. 1977.
14. Griffith G, Maull K, Sachatello C: Septic pulmonary embolization. Surg Gynecol Obstet 144:1, 1977.
15. Bennett DE, Cherry JK: Bacterial infection of the aortic aneurysms: a clinicopathologic study. Am J Surg 113:321, 1967.
16. Yellin AE: Ruptured mycotic aneurysm: a complication of parenteral drug abuse. Arch Surg 112:981, 1977.
17. Jenkins A, MacPherson A, Nolan B, Housley E: Peripheral aneurysms in Behçet's disease. Br J Surg 63:199, 1976.
18. Rosenberg TF, Medsger TA Jr, DeCicco FA, Fireman P: Allergic granulomatous angiitis (Churg-Strauss syndrome). J Allergy Clin Immunol 55:56, 1975.
19. Collins CR Jr, Rich NM, Hobson RW, et al: Multiple mycotic aneurysms due to *Candida* endocarditis. Am J Surg 186:136, 1977.
20. Smith KO, Cehle WD, Sanrord BA: Evidence for chronic viral infections in human arteries. Proc Soc Exp Biol Med 147:357, 1974.
21. Gladstone JL, Friedman SA, Cerruti MM, Jomain SL: Treatment of *Candida* endocarditis and arteritis. J Thorac Cardiovasc Surg 71:835, 1976.
22. Michal JA III, Coleman RE: Localization of gallium 67 citrate in a mycotic aneurysm. Am J Roentgenol 129:1111, 1977.
23. Sukerkar AN, Dulay CC, Anandappa E, Asokan S: Mycotic aneurysm of the hepatic artery: case diagnosed with radionuclide imaging and ultrasound. Radiology 124:444, 1977.
24. Mutch D, Richards C, Brown RD, Mulder DS: Bioactive antibiotic levels in human aorta. Surgery 92:1068, 1982.
25. Liebman PR, Patten MT, Manny J, et al: Hepatic-portal venous gas ill adults: etiology, pathophysiology, and clinical significance. Am Surg 187:281, 1978.
26. Abruzzo JL: The spectrum of systemic vasculitis. J Med Soc NJ 74:227, 1977.
27. Anagnostakis D, Kamba A, Petrochilou V, et al: Risk of infection associated with umbilical vein catheterization: a prospective study in 74 newborn infants. J Pediatr 86:759, 1975.
28. Balagtas RC, Bell CE, Edwards LD, Levin S: Risk of local and systemic infections associated with umbilical vein catheterization: a prospective study in 86 newborn patients. Pediatrics 48:359, 1971.

29. Maki DG, Drinka PJ, Davis TE: Suppurative phlebitis of an arm vein from a "scalp-vein needle." N Engl J Med 292:1116, 1975.
30. Mogensen JV, Frederiksen W, Jensen JK: Subclavian vein catheterization and infection: a bacteriological study of 130 catheter insertions. Scand J Infect Dis 4:31, 1972.
31. Rubio T, Riley HD Jr: Serious systemic infection associated with the use of indwelling intravenous catheters. South Med J 66:633, 1973.
32. Stein JM, Pruitt BA Jr: Suppurative thrombophlebitis: a lethal iatrogenic disease. N Engl J Med 282:1452, 1970.
33. Nicolaides AN, Kakkar W, Field ES, et al: Prostatectomy and deep vein thrombosis. Br J Surg 59:487, 1972.
34. Svanberg L, Astedt B, Kullander S: On radiation-decreased fibrinolytic activity of vessel walls. Acta Obstet Gynecol Scand 55:49, 1976.
35. Schramel RJ, Creech O Jr: Effects of infection and exposure on synthetic arterial prostheses. Arch Surg 78:271, 1959.
36. Harrison JH: Influence of infection on homografts and synthetic (Teflon) grafts: a comparative study in experimental animals. Arch Surg 76:67, 1958.
37. Humphries AW, Hawk WA, DeWolfe VG, LeFevre FA: Clinicopathologic observations on the fate of arterial freeze-dried homografts. Surgery 45:59, 1959.
38. Foster IH, Berzins T, Scott HW Jr: An experimental study of arterial replacement in the presence of bacterial infection. Surg Gynecol Obstet 108:141, 1959.
39. Moore WS, Blaisdell FW, Cardner M, Hall AD: Effect of infection on autogenous vein arterial substitutes. Surg Forum 13:235, 1962.
40. Wylie EJ: Vascular replacement with arterial autografts. Surgery 57:14, 1965.
41. Moore WS, Swanson RJ, Campagna G, Bean B: The use of fresh tissue arterial substitutes in infected fields. J Surg Res 18:229, 1975.
42. Roon A, Malone JM, Moore WS, et al: Bacteremic infectability: a function of vascular graft material and design. J Surg Res 22:489, 1977.
43. Goldstone J, Moore WS: Infection in vascular prostheses: clinical manifestations and surgical management. Am J Surg 128:225, 1974.
44. Kaiser AB, Clayson KR, Mulherin JL Jr, et al: Antibiotic prophylaxis in vascular surgery. Ann Surg 188:283, 1978.
45. Fry WJ, Lindenauer SM: Infection complicating the use of plastic arterial implants. Arch Surg 95:600, 1967.
46. Conn JH, Hardy JD, Chavez CM, Fain WR: Infected arterial grafts: experience in 22 cases with emphasis on unusual bacteria and techniques. Ann Surg 171:704, 1970.
47. Lorentzen JE, Nielson OM, Arendrop H, et al: Vascular infection: an analysis of 62 graft infections in 2411 consecutively implanted synthetic vascular grafts. Surgery 98:81, 1985.
48. Bunt TJ: Synthetic vascular graft infections. I. Graft infections. Surgery 93:733, 1983.
49. Szilagyi DE, Smith RF, Elliott JP, Vrandecic MP: Infection in arterial reconstruction with synthetic grafts. Ann Surg 176:321, 1972.
50. Bouhoutsos J, Chavatzas D, Martin P, Morris T: Infected synthetic arterial grafts. Br J Surg 61:108, 1974.
51. Fry WJ: Vascular prosthesis infections. Surg Clin North Am 52:1419, 1972.
52. Liekweg WC Jr, Greenfield LJ: Vascular prosthetic infections: collected experience and results of treatment. Surgery 81:335, 1977.
53. Rubin JR, Malone JM, Goldstone J: The role of the lymphatic system in acute arterial prosthetic graft infections. J Vasc Surg 2:92, 1985.
54. Vaughan CD, Mattox RL, Feliciano DV, et al: Surgical experience with polytetrafluoroethylene (PTFE) as a replacement graft for traumatized vessels. J Trauma 19:403, 1979.
55. Ernst CB, Campbell HC, Daugherty ME, et al: Incidence and significance of intraoperative bacterial cultures during abdominal aortic aneurysmectomy. Ann Surg 185:626, 1977.
56. Williams RD, Fisher FW: Aneurysm contents as a source of graft infection. Arch Surg 112:415, 1977.
57. McAuley CE, Steed DL, Webster MW: Bacterial presence in aortic thrombosis at elective aneurysm resection: is it clinically significant? Am J Surg 147:322, 1984.
58. Bandyk D: Vascular graft infection epidemiology, bacteriology, and pathogenesis. In Bernhard VM, Towne J (eds): Complications in Vascular Surgery. New York, Grune & Stratton, 1985, p 471.
59. Bandyk DF, Berni CA, Thiele BI, Towne J: Aortofemoral graft infection due to *Staphylococcus epidermidis.* Arch Surg 119:102, 1984.
60. Greco RS, Trooskin SZ, Donetz AP, Harvey RA: The application of antibiotic bonding to the treatment of established vascular prosthetic infection. Arch Surg 120:71, 1985.
61. Gross RE, Bill AH Jr, Peirce EC: Methods for preservation and transplantation of arterial grafts: observations on arterial grafts in dogs. Report of transplantation of preserved arterial grafts in 9 human cases. Surg Gynecol Obstet 88:689, 1949.
62. Elliott JP Jr, Smith RF, Szilagyi DE: Proceedings: aortoenteric and paraprosthetic-enteric fistulas. Problems of diagnosis and management. Arch Surg 108:479, 1974.
63. Durham JR, Rubin JR, Malone JM: Management of infected infrainguinal bypass grafts. In Bergan JJ, Yao JS (eds): Reoperative Arterial Surgery. New York, Grune & Stratton, 1985.
64. Liekweg WC Jr, Levinson SA, Greenfield LJ: Infection of vascular grafts: incidence, anatomic location,

etiologic agents, morbidity, and mortality. In Duma RJ (ed): Infections of Prosthetic Heart Valves and Vascular Grafts. Baltimore, University Park Press, 1977, p 239.
65. Perdue CD, Smith RC, Ansley JD, Constantino MJ: Impending aortoenteric hemorrhage: the effect of early recognition on improved outcome. Ann Surg 192:237, 1980.
66. Santiani U: False aneurysms following arterial reconstruction. Surg Gynecol Obstet 152:357, 1981.
67. Gooding GHW, Effney DJ, Goldstone J: The aortofemoral graft: detection and identification of healing complications by ultrasonography. Surgery 89:94, 1981.
68. Causey DA, Fajman WA, Perdue GD, et al: Gallium scintigraphy in postoperative synthetic graft infections. Am J Radiol 134: 1041, 1980.
69. Brunner MC, Mitchell RS, Baldwin JC, et al: Prosthetic graft infection: limitations of indium white cell scanning. J Vasc Surg 3:42, 1986.
70. Haaqa JR, Baldwin CN, Reich NE, et al: CT detection of infected synthetic grafts: preliminary report of a new sign. Am J Roentgenol 131:317, 1978.
71. Quarfordt PC, Reilly LM, Mark AS, et al: Computerized tomographic assessment of graft incorporation after aortic reconstruction. Am J Surg 150:227, 1985.
72. Trout HH, Rozloff, L, Giordano JH: Priority of revascularization in patients with graft enteric fistulas, infected arteries, or infected arterial prostheses. Ann Surg 199:669, 1984.
73. Malone SM, Brendel K, Duhamel RC, Reinert RL: Detergent extracted small-diameter vascular prostheses. J Vasc Surg 1:181, 1984.
74. Kieffer E, Bahnini A, Kosas F, et al: In situ allograft replacement of infected infrarenal aortic prosthetic graft infections: results in forty-three patients. J Vasc Surg 17:349, 1993.
75. Colden CT, Lovett WL, Harrah JD, et al: The treatment of extruded and infected permanent cardiac pulse generators: application of a technique of closed irrigation. Surgery 74:575, 1973.
76. Popovsky J, Singer S: Infected prosthetic grafts. Arch Surg 115:203, 1980.
77. Calligaro KD, Veith FJ, Schwartz ML, et al: Are gram-negative bacteria a contraindication to selective preservation of infected prosthetic arterial grafts? J Vasc Surg 16:337, 1992.
78. Miller JH: Partial replacement of an infected arterial graft by a new prosthetic polytetrafluoroethylene segment: a new therapeutic option. J Vasc Surg 17:546, 1993.
79. Clark RE, Morgraf HW: Antibacterial vascular grafts with improved thromboresistance. Arch Surg 109: 159, 1974.
80. McDivitt NB: Commentary to Moore WS, et al: Development of an infection-resistant vascular prosthesis. Arch Surg 116:1403, 1981.
81. Moore WS, Chvopil M, Seiffert C, Keown K: Development of an infection-resistant vascular prosthesis. Arch Surg 116:1403, 1981.
82. Prahlad A, Harvey RA, Greco RS: Diffusion of antibiotics from a polytetrafluoroethylene-benzalkonium surface. Am Surg 47:515, 1981.
83. Colburn MD, Moore WS, Chvapil M, et al: Use of an antibiotic-bonded graft for in-situ reconstruction following prosthetic graft infections. J Vasc Surg 16:651, 1992.
84. Parsa F, Gordon HE, Wilson SE: Intraoperative antibiotics in the prevention of experimental Dacron graft infection. Vasc Surg 10:64, 1976.
85. Pitt HA, Postier RC, MacGowan WAL, et al: Prophylactic antibiotics in vascular surgery: topical, systemic, or both? Ann Surg 192:356, 1980.
86. Lord JW Jr, Rossi C, Daliana M: Intraoperative antibiotic wound lavage: an attempt to eliminate post operative infection in arterial and clean general surgical procedures. Ann Surg 185:634, 1977.

Peritonitis and Other Intra-abdominal Infections

CHAPTER 38

A. B. Nathens, David H. Ahrenholz, Richard L. Simmons, Ori Rotstein

ANATOMY AND PHYSIOLOGY OF THE PERITONEAL CAVITY

Anatomy

The peritoneum is the largest serous membrane in the body. In the male, it consists of a closed sac, a part of which lines the abdominal wall, while the remainder is reflected over the contained viscera. In contrast, in the female, the lateral ends of the uterine tubes open into the peritoneal cavity. That part of the serous membrane which lines the abdominal wall is referred to as the parietal peritoneum, while that which is reflected over the contained viscera constitutes the visceral portion of the peritoneum. The peritoneal surface consists of a single layer of flat mesothelial cells that reside on a basement membrane, which in turn overlies a bed of connective tissue consisting of adipose cells, macrophages, fibroblasts, lymphocytes, a few mast cells, and collagen and elastic fibers.[1] Reepithelialization of peritoneal defects after injury occurs over the entire surface of the injured site simultaneously; thus large areas of injury reepithelialize as rapidly as a smaller wound.[2] Peritoneal reepithelialization is modulated by macrophages recruited into the peritoneal cavity after injury.[3,4]

The cavity defined by the peritoneal surface represents the largest preformed extravascular space in the body, but normally the viscera are in contact along their serosal surfaces. The peritoneal cavity is divided into greater and lesser sacs, which communicate through the foramen of Winslow. In health, the space contains less than 50 ml of clear yellow fluid with a specific gravity of less than 1.016 and less than 3 g/dl protein. Solute concentrations are nearly identical to those in plasma. The normal fluid contains fewer than 300 cells/mm^3, 50 percent of which are macrophages, 40 percent lymphocytes, and the remainder, eosinophils, mast cells, and an occasional mesothelial cell.[5,6] Peritoneal fluid has minimal antibacterial activity, mostly related to the presence of complement.[7] Macrophage colony-stimulating factor (M-CSF) has been documented in peritoneal fluid and presumably contributes to the differentiation of blood monocytes from peritoneal macrophages.[8]

Fluid Exchange

The surface of peritoneum approximates that of the total cutaneous surface (1.7 m^2). Most of this membrane behaves as a passive, semipermeable barrier to the diffusion of water and low molecular weight solutes, making peritoneal dialysis an effective treatment for chronic renal failure. Studies of dialysis patients have shown that the functional exchange surface of the peritoneal cavity is approximately 1 m^2.[9] The efficiency of fluid exchange is proportional to the membrane surface area and is increased by alterations in local splanchnic blood flow or peritoneal membrane permeability.[10,11] During peritoneal dialysis, hyperosmolar solutions can induce a net flow of 300 to 500 ml of water per hour into the peritoneal space.[9] Peritonitis due to bacteria, chemical irritants, or enzymes can similarly induce exudation of fluid, potentially resulting in hypovolemia in the affected patient.

Particulate and Microbial Absorption

Although the entire peritoneal surface participates in fluid and low molecular weight solute exchange, particulate matter is absorbed specifically by the diaphragmatic lymphatics.[12–14] In most areas, the mesothelial cells lining the peritoneal cavity form a carpet of closely packed, flattened cells covered with numerous microvilli that minimize shear between adjacent viscera[15,16] (Fig. 38–1). On the inferior surface of the diaphragm, however, special lymphatic collecting vessels (lacunae) under the mesothelial basement membrane open into the peritoneal cavity by small pores (stomata) (Figs. 38–1 and 38–2).[13] Fluid flows rapidly through the stomata into the la-

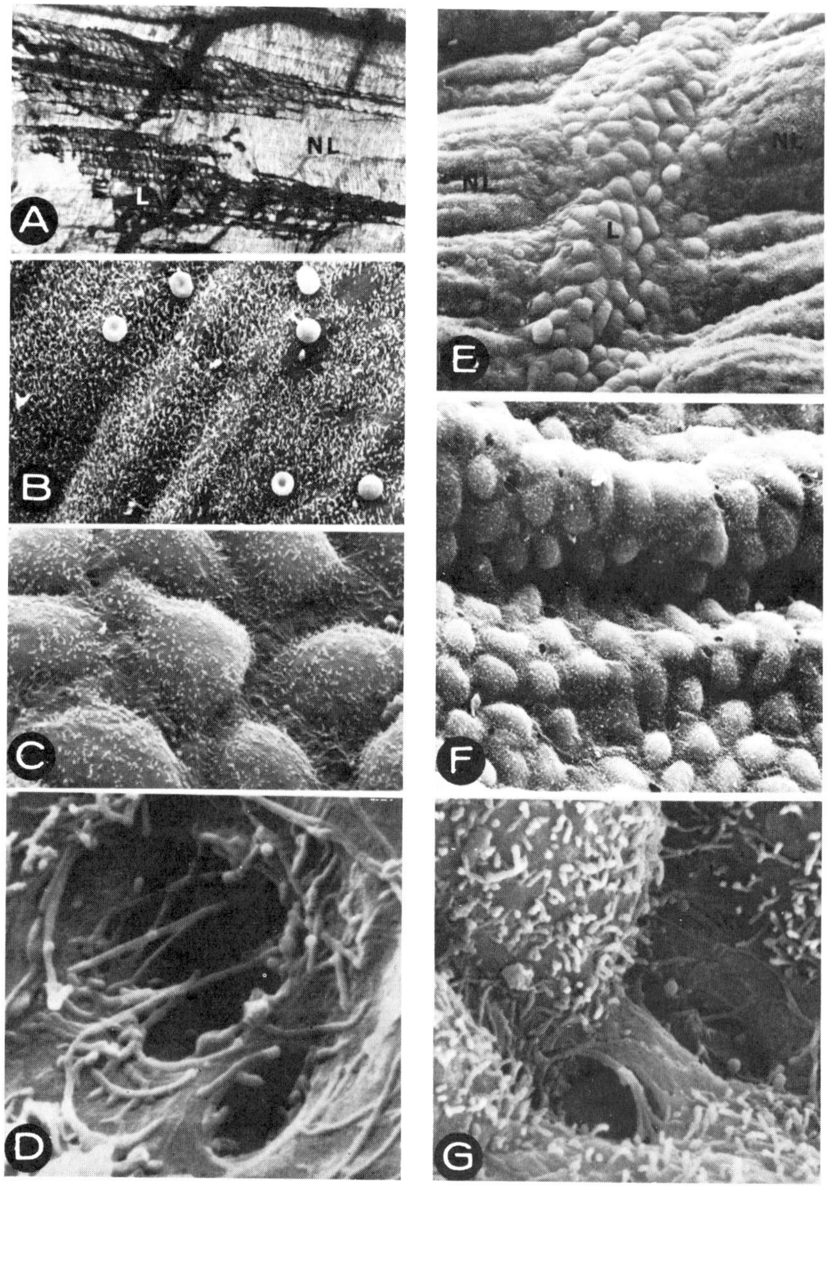

Figure 38–1. The topography of the peritoneal surface by light and scanning electron microscopy (SEM). **A.** Low-power photomicrograph of the peritoneal surface of the diaphragm showing the lacunar areas labeled with India ink. Lacunar areas (L) are sharply delineated from nonlacunar areas (NL). ×8. **B.** Higher power of a nonlacunar area. The mesothelial cells lining the surface are flat, and they have many microvilli. Boundaries between individual cells are not seen. ×713. **C.** Mesothelial cells of a lacunar area. Each cell is distinctly outlined. Many interdigitating processess and a few small stomata between them are seen at the border of each cell. ×1800. **D.** High-power micrograph of a complex stoma. The upper portion of the stoma overlies a deep pit and is encircled at its rim by several cell processes. The lower portion of the stoma is smaller, and the surface of another cell can be seen beneath its opening. ×12,300. **E.** Peritoneal surface of the diaphragm observed with the SEM. The mesothelial cells over nonlacunar areas are flattened, and individual cells cannot be distinguished. The mesothelial cells overlying a lacunar area protrude toward the lumen of the peritoneal cavity and have distinct boundaries. A muscular contraction, probably due to the action of the fixative, caused folding of the surface of the diaphragm. ×360. **F.** High power of a lacunar area. The mesothelial cells lie on ridges over the lacuna. The nucleus of each individual cell is represented by a round swelling in the center of each cell. Numerous stomata can be seen between adjacent cells. ×680. **G.** A stoma between two adjacent mesothelial cells is shown. Processes extend between the cells and bridge the opening of the stoma. Underneath the opening is seen the surface of another cell. ×6888. *(From Tsilibary EC, Wissig SL: Am J Anat 149:127, 1977.)*

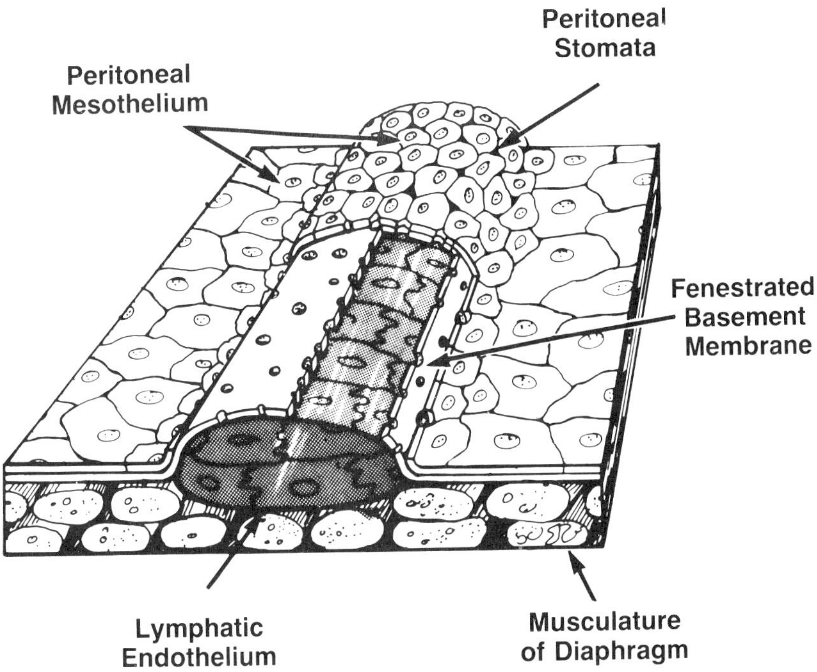

Figure 38–2. Schematic view of lymphatic lacunae on the peritoneal surface of the diaphragm. The mesothelial cells are flattened and polygonal everywhere but over the lymphatics, where they are smaller, with stomata between the cells. These stomata correspond to fenestrations of the underlying basement membrane. The lymphatic endothelium lines the lymphatic lacuna and probably communicates with the peritoneal cavity through the stomata. *(Adapted from Allen L: Anat Rec 67:89, 1936.)*

cunae with relaxation of the diaphragm during expiration. Contraction of the diaphragm during inspiration empties the lymphatics into efferent ducts, aided by the simultaneous drop in endothoracic pressure. One-way valves in the thoracic lymphatics prevent reverse flow. In most animals, the chief route of drainage of the diaphragmatic lymphatics is by the right thoracic duct. The drainage route for the human diaphragmatic lymphatics is uncertain, but at autopsy the anterior mediastinal lymphatics of patients dying of peritonitis contain bacteria, even though the remainder of the thoracic cavity is sterile.[17]

The size of the stomata (8 to 12 μm) determines the minimum size of particles that are readily absorbed from the peritoneal cavity. Only a few polystyrene beads 20 μm in diameter can be absorbed but 10-μm sized beads pass through easily.[13] Thus bacteria measuring 0.5 to 2.0 μm in diameter pass readily through the much larger stomata. Bacteria are not absorbed to any extent from nondiaphragmatic peritoneal surfaces.

The removal of fluid by the diaphragmatic lymphatics creates a cephalad flow of peritoneal fluid (Fig. 38–3). Autio[18] found that contrast material injected into the ileocecal region after routine appendectomy or cholecystectomy rapidly accumulated in the pelvis and, to a lesser degree, in the right paracolic and subhepatic areas. Lesser amounts accumulated along the left paracolic gutter and into the left subphrenic space. When contrast medium was injected into the right infrahepatic space near the duodenum, the dye spread to the right suprahepatic space, the left infrahepatic space, the right paracolic gutter, and the pelvis. These patterns correspond to the sites where abscesses form after peritonitis in humans (see Fig. 38–3B).

HOST RESPONSE TO PERITONEAL INJURY

Local Response

Bacterial contamination of the peritoneal cavity initiates a complex series of events that result in the eradication of all particulate matter and microorganisms. The three major defense mechanisms responsible include (1) mechanical clearance of bacteria via the diaphragmatic lymphatics, (2) phagocytosis and destruction of suspended or adherent bacteria by phagocytic cells, and (3) sequestration and localization of bacteria by a fibrinous inflammatory exudate.[19]

Mechanical Clearance. The early mechanical clearance of bacteria via the diaphragmatic lymphatics begins almost immediately upon bacterial spillage. Bacteria appear in the mediastinal lymphatics within 6 minutes of inoculation, and in the bloodstream within 12 minutes.[20] Bacterial removal by this method serves to clear approximately 80

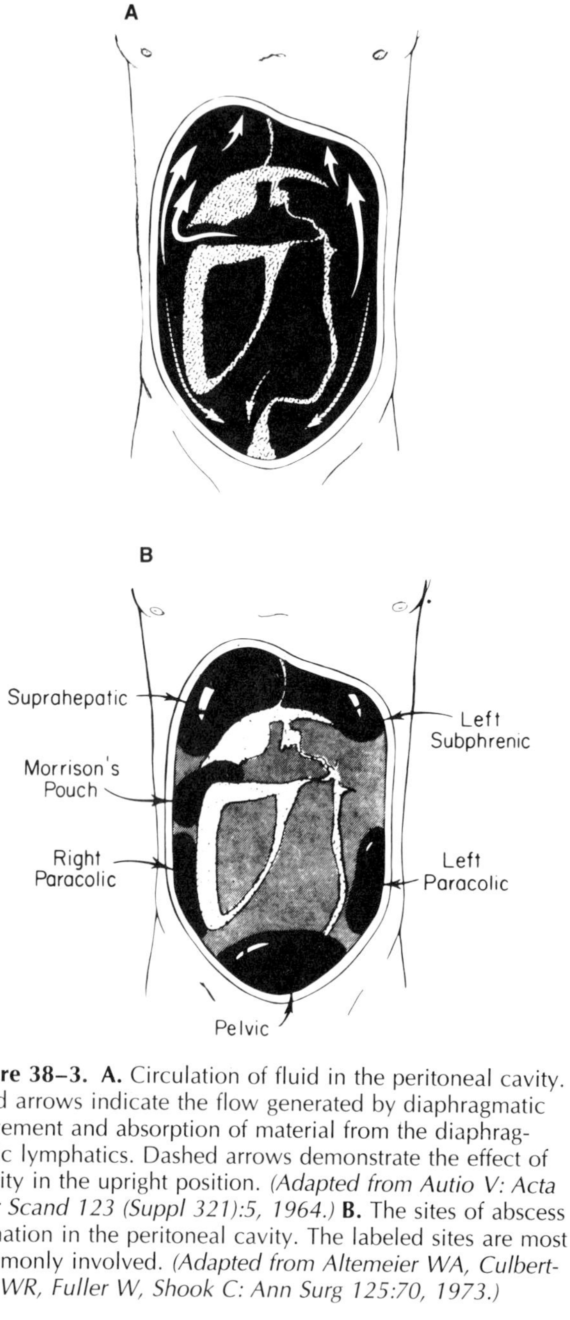

Figure 38–3. **A.** Circulation of fluid in the peritoneal cavity. Solid arrows indicate the flow generated by diaphragmatic movement and absorption of material from the diaphragmatic lymphatics. Dashed arrows demonstrate the effect of gravity in the upright position. *(Adapted from Autio V: Acta Chir Scand 123 (Suppl 321):5, 1964.)* **B.** The sites of abscess formation in the peritoneal cavity. The labeled sites are most commonly involved. *(Adapted from Altemeier WA, Culbertson WR, Fuller W, Shook C: Ann Surg 125:70, 1973.)*

percent of the bacteria initially inoculated into the peritoneal cavity within 30 minutes. Multiple factors affect the clearance of particulate matter. Hypoventilation induced by general anesthetics, analgesics, or impaired diaphragmatic function alters the normal diaphragmatic pumping action. Mechanical ventilation, especially with positive end expiratory pressure (PEEP), impairs clearance via its effect on intrathoracic pressure.[21] Laparotomy with manipulation of the viscera leading to ileus causes a delay in clearance time as a result of impaired intraperitoneal circulation of bacteria.[22] In 1944, Steinberg[20] demonstrated that absorption of bacteria from the peritoneal cavity was delayed by the upright position and accelerated by the head-down position. As early as 1900, Fowler[23] used the semiupright position in patients with peritonitis to prevent the rapid absorption of toxins from the peritoneal cavity. Although early mechanical clearance via diaphragmatic lymphatics reduces bacterial numbers in the peritoneal cavity, the result is bacteremia, which if massive can result in an overwhelming systemic response in the form of sepsis.

Phagocytosis. The initial peritoneal response to bacterial contamination is characterized by hyperemia, exudation of fluid into the peritoneal cavity, and a marked influx of phagocytic cells. During the first hour after contamination, resident peritoneal macrophages are the predominant phagocytic cells, while over the next 2 to 6 hours, there is a massive influx of neutrophils.[24] The mediators of this response are many and include cytokines, growth factors, arachidonic acid metabolites such as prostaglandins and leukotrienes, as well as products of both the complement and coagulation cascades (see Chap. 16).

The early local inflammatory response is mediated by numerous proinflammatory cytokines, the sources of which are both resident peritoneal macrophages and possibly peritoneal mesothelial cells. The former produce interleukin 1 (IL-1) and tumor necrosis factor (TNF) in response to lipopolysaccharide derived from gram-negative enteric bacteria. Peritoneal mesothelial cells are capable of producing granulocyte colony-stimulating factor (G-CSF), M-CSF, IL-1, IL-6, and IL-8 in response to lipopolysaccharide or TNF.[8] G-CSF induces neutrophil maturation and release from bone marrow, whereas IL-8 acts as a potent activator and chemoattractant for polymorphonuclear leukocytes. M-CSF induces blood monocytes to differentiate into peritoneal macrophages. IL-1 increases the influx of neutrophils into the peritoneum by augmenting neutrophil-endothelium interactions and transendothelial migration of neutrophils and stimulates macrophage procoagulant activity. Both TNF and IL-1 prime neutrophils for phagocytosis and microbicidal killing. IL-6 is important in initiating the acute phase response and priming other inflammatory cells.[25–28]

Activation of the complement cascade results in the formation of C3a and C5a, both of which are potent chemoattractants. Degranulation of peritoneal mast cells releases vasoactive substances with a resultant outpouring of fluid rich in complement and serum opsonins that bind to bacteria. Recent studies have also documented a central role for mast cells in recruiting neutrophils into the peritoneal cavity during peritoneal inflammation. C3b plays a vital role in opsonization of bacteria, which are then removed by lymphatics or engulfed in situ by the phagocytic cells. Cyclooxygenase products modulate the immune response and alter vascular permeability. The increase in vascular permeability brings with it a large fluid influx into the peritoneal cavity, which may impair bacterial opsonization by diluting opsonins and may impair phagocytosis by altering the neutrophil's ability to reach the bacterium.[29] In addition, fluid sequestration in the peritoneal cavity may contribute to the development of hypovolemic shock.

Sequestration and Localization of Bacteria. Fibrin deposition appears to play an important role in localizing infection, not only by incorporating large numbers of bacteria within its interstices, but also by causing loops of intestine to adhere to each other and the omentum. This process creates a physical barrier against both local and systemic dissemination of bacteria.[30,31] The exudation of protein-rich fluid containing fibrinogen into the peritoneal cavity underlies fibrin deposition. The conversion of fibrinogen to fibrin is promoted by the release of tissue thromboplastin from both mesothelial cells and stimulated peritoneal macrophages in response to stimulation by both aerobic and anaerobic bacteria.[32] The gram-negative anaerobe *Bacteroides fragilis,* a common isolate from intra-abdominal abscesses, promotes fibrin deposition by inducing procoagulant activity in macrophages via the production of tissue factor.[33] This mechanism may represent the critical initiating event involved in abscess formation by this common anaerobe. Furthermore, a plasminogen activator, which is responsible for the activation of fibrinolytic enzymes and is normally present in the mesothelial and submesothelial cell membranes, disappears in the presence of bacterial infection.[34]

Systemic Response

The systemic response to intra-abdominal infection involves two phases. Initially, massive fluid losses associated with third space fluid shifts result in the classic picture of hypovolemia. It appears that acute generalized peritonitis has the same hemodynamic effect as a 50 percent or greater body surface burn and therefore requires aggressive fluid resuscitation. Following resuscitation, the patients exhibit features associated with a systemic inflammatory response. The patient is febrile unless elderly or immunocompromised. Hemodynamic parameters reflect a hyperdynamic circulation, with tachycardia, low systemic vascular resistance, high cardiac output, and a narrowed arteriovenous O_2 difference. Hyperglycemia and nitrogen wasting reflect the hypermetabolic state associated with sepsis. The later stages of this systemic inflammatory response are manifested by remote organ dysfunction, culminating in the multiple organ dysfunction syndrome with its high associated mortality.

There are many lines of evidence to suggest that the morbidity and mortality associated with intra-abdominal infection are related to the magnitude of the host's systemic inflammatory response.[35] Intravenous infusion of TNF into both humans and experimental animals mimics the hemodynamic alterations that follow the administration of bacterial endotoxin. Both TNF and IL-1 cause fever and neutrophilia and IL-6 initiates the acute-phase protein response characteristic of infection.[36–38] The central role of these cytokines in mediating the septic response is illustrated by the ability of antibodies, directed against either TNF or endotoxin, or receptor antagonists such as IL-1RA (IL-1 receptor antagonist) to abrogate components of this response.[39–43] Teleologically, cytokines must play a vital role in the host's immune response as they are products of some of the most highly conserved genes in mammalian evolution.

PERITONITIS

Peritonitis is defined as inflammation of the peritoneum and may be the result of a microbial stimulus or any of a number of noninfective stimuli. *Primary* peritonitis refers to inflammation of the peritoneal cavity without a documented source of contamination from the gastrointestinal tract. *Secondary* peritonitis occurs as a result of contamination of the peritoneal cavity following perforation of a hollow viscus or transmural necrosis of the gastrointestinal tract. Complicated primary or secondary peritonitis has recently been described conceptually as *tertiary* peritonitis.

Secondary Bacterial Peritonitis

Etiology and Incidence. When Kirschner[44] reviewed 1626 cases of peritonitis treated between 1895 to 1925, he found the vast majority to be due to appendicitis. Presently, the most common causes of secondary bacterial peritonitis include perforation of the colon due to either diverticulitis, carcinoma or volvulus, perforated appendicitis, postoperative peritonitis occurring as a result of anastomotic disruption, and perforated gastric or duodenal ulcer[45] (Table 38–1). Microorganisms may contaminate the peritoneal cavity due to one or more of a combination of processes such as trauma, neoplasia, and vascular or inflammatory diseases.

Bacteriology. The spectrum of microorganisms inoculating the peritoneum after perforation of the gastrointestinal tract depends on the level of perforation.[46] Normally, the stomach and duodenum are sterile, and consequently perforation of these organs initially causes a sterile, chemical peritonitis. The relative achlorhydria associated with gastric ulcers or the use of antacids or H_2 receptor antagonists permits gastric colonization with gram-positive oral anaerobes, *Candida* species, and facultative gram-negative bacilli resulting in greater contamination at the time of perforation.[47] By contrast, the terminal ileum and the colon contain more than 500 different species of bacteria at a concentration of up to 10^{12} bacteria/g, with an anaerobe/aerobe ratio of 100:1.[48] The spectrum of peritoneal isolates at the time of laparotomy reflects this phenomenon (Table 38–2). However, while larger numbers of bacteria are spilled into the peritoneum, early events cause a marked simplification of the flora.

Most commonly, the resultant infection is polymicrobial, containing a mixture of aerobic and anaerobic bacteria. In a recent study of 339 peritoneal culture specimens in patients with peritonitis, 76 percent contained mixed aerobic and anaerobic bacteria, with the most frequent combination being *Escherichia coli* and *B. fragilis.* Anaerobic organisms were present alone in only 13 percent and aerobic in only 11 percent of specimens.[49] Polymicrobial infections are present in 59 to 67 percent of patients, with an average of 2.9 to 3.9 isolates/patient at the time of initial laparotomy.[49–52] The predominant gram-positive organisms are nonenterococcal streptococci and enterococci.[45,53,54]

TABLE 38–1. SOURCE OF PERITONITIS BY SITE OF ANATOMIC ORIGIN

Origin of Peritonitis by Anatomic Origin	Kirschner 1926	Solomkin et al 1990
Stomach and duodenum	11%	11%
Small bowel	12%	7%
Large bowel		25%
Appendix	58%	24%
Pancreas and biliary tract	2%	11%
Postoperative	N/A	20%
Other	17%	2%

Adapted from Kirschner M: Arch Klin Chir *142:253, 1926; and Solomkin JS, Dellinger EP, Christou NV, et al:* Ann Surg *212:581, 1990.*

Bacterial Synergy. Bacterial synergy is defined as the cooperative interaction of two or more bacterial species to produce a result not achieved by the individual bacteria acting alone.[55] Several experimental studies suggest that synergistic interactions occur between aerobic and anaerobic organisms (see Chap. 7). The classic studies of Weinstein et al[56] established the role of the various components of the infecting inoculum in the pathogenesis of intra-abdominal infection. In these investigations, gelatin capsules containing a mixture of cecal contents and barium sulfate were implanted into the pelvic region of rats. The animals demonstrated a biphasic response to sepsis in the peritoneal cavity. The first phase, the peritonitis phase, was characterized by diffuse peritoneal inflammation and was associated with a significant mortality (43 percent). Surviving animals entered a second phase characterized by the presence of intra-abdominal abscesses.[56] Despite the complex cecal inoculum, the peritonitis phase demonstrated a predominance of *E. coli,* enterococci, *B. fragilis,* and *Fusobacterium* species, while anaerobes predominated during the abscess stage.[57]

Onderdonk et al[58] extended these studies by incorporating known quantities of bacteria within gelatin capsules. Pure cultures of *B. fragilis, Fusobacterium varium, E. coli,* or enterococci did not induce intra-abdominal abscesses, nor did combinations of the two aerobes or the two anaerobes. By contrast, a mixed anaerobe-aerobe inoculum consistently produced intraperitoneal abscesses. Subsequently, Onderdonk concluded that early mortality was due to *E. coli* and late abscess formation due to the presence of both an aerobe and anaerobe. Gentamicin, an aminoglycoside with gram-negative coverage, prevented early deaths but had no effect on subsequent abscess formation. Clindamycin, a potent antianaerobe, did not prevent early deaths but provided protection against abscess formation. Rotstein et al[59–61] extended the concept of synergism beyond late abscess formation when it was demonstrated that the presence of *B. fragilis* increased the lethality in an *E. coli* fibrin clot model of peritonitis.

Several hypotheses have been proposed to explain microbial synergy. It may occur as a result of some combination of mutual protection from phagocytosis and intracellular killing, production of essential growth factors, or lowering of the oxidation-reduction potential.[62–64] The principles of aerobic-

TABLE 38–2. PERITONEAL ISOLATES AT LAPAROTOMY

Organism	Solomkin et al*	Mosdell et al†	Organism	Solomkin et al	Mosdell et al
Gram-negative aerobic and facultative anaerobes			Gram-positive aerobic and facultative anaerobes		
Escherichia coli	56.8	68.4	Nonenterococcal streptococci	35.8	25.9
Enterobacter species	13.5	6.1	Enterococci	23.5	10.5
Klebsiella species	15.4	17	*Staphylococcus aureus* or *S. epidermidis*	10.5	10.5
Pseudomonas aeruginosa	14.8	19.1			
Proteus species	6.2	2.7	Anaerobic organisms		
Serratia marcescens	1.2	4.1	*Bacteroides fragilis*	22.8	44.5
Morganella species	1.2	—	Other *Bacteroides*	21	—
Citrobacter species	3.1	3.4	*Clostridium* species	17.9	5.8
Others	3.7	7.5	Peptococci/streptococci	7.4	16
			Fusobacterium species	6.2	5.1
Yeast			*Lactobacillus* species	5.6	—
Candida species	18.6	4.1	*Eubacterium* species	4.3	—
			Others	12.4	3.7

* Percent of patients
† Percent of abscesses
Adapted from Solomkin JS, Dellinger EP, Christou NV, et al: Ann Surg 212:581, 1990; and Mosdell DM, Morris DM, Voltura A, et al: Ann Surg 214:543, 1991.

anaerobic synergism provide the rationale for the current antimicrobial regimes in intra-abdominal infection.

The concept of bacterial synergism is not unique to intra-abdominal infection and is noted in many other surgical infections such as necrotizing soft tissue infection, Meleny synergistic gangrene, and gynecologic infections. The mechanisms of bacterial synergy are discussed in Chapter 7.

Adjuvant Substances. The mixed bacterial inoculum released into the peritoneal cavity following gastrointestinal perforation is invariably accompanied by other substances that serve to promote local infection. Common adjuvants include blood, fluid, bile, feces, fiber, gastric mucin, barium, and foreign bodies. The mechanisms underlying this effect vary but are generally related to the ability of the adjuvant material to promote bacterial growth and/or impair local host defenses.

Blood is an extremely potent adjuvant for intra-abdominal infection. Several of its components contribute to this effect. Hemoglobin reduces the median lethal dose of *E. coli* in the peritoneal cavity of the rat by 10^5.[65] The effect is related to the ability of hemoglobin to enhance bacterial proliferation, increase virulence, and impair host defenses. Iron is an essential growth factor for several bacteria, including *E. coli.*[66] In vitro studies using an iron-depleted medium demonstrate that the addition of iron enhances *E. coli* growth.[67] Additionally, culture filtrates of *E. coli* grown in hemoglobin markedly reduce neutrophil migration and microbicidal activity.[65]

Platelets and fibrin also contribute to the pathogenesis of intra-abdominal infection. Platelets impair clearance of bacteria from the peritoneal cavity, presumably by physically occluding diaphragmatic lymphatics.[68] Products of platelet degranulation may also contribute by altering resident macrophage function. Although advantageous in terms of preventing dissemination of contamination within the peritoneal cavity and limiting systemic bacteremia,[31] fibrin deposition has several adverse effects on the local response to infection. Polymerizing fibrin mesh sequesters large numbers of bacteria within its interstices, allowing microorganisms to proliferate in an environment inaccessible to local host defense mechanisms.[30] Furthermore, fibrin impairs phagocytosis by limiting migration of phagocytic cells[69] and coating microorganisms, reducing efficient opsonization.[70] In addition, microbicidal killing is reduced in the presence of fibrin.[71] Ahrenholz et al[72] inoculated the peritoneal cavity of rats with *E. coli* in saline or enmeshed within a fibrin clot. Injection of *E. coli* resulted in a high early mortality rate but no abscesses in survivors. In contrast, enmeshing similar numbers of bacteria within a fibrin matrix abrogated early mortality[72] but induced late abscess formation. These studies demonstrate the paradox of bacterial sequestration by fibrin.

Intraperitoneal fluid also appears to promote local infection. A sublethal inoculum of *E. coli* becomes lethal when injected in direct proportion to the volume of saline infused.[29] This effect is attributed to the dilution of opsonic proteins such as complement and immunoglobulins. In addition, macrophages require a surface to trap and ingest bacteria and thus, when in suspension, are incapable of doing so.

Intraperitoneal instillation of bile in an *E. coli* peritonitis model increases mortality.[73] Several mechanisms have been implicated, including impaired phagocytosis,[74] altered neutrophil microbicidal activity, and migration,[75,76] as well as impaired bacterial clearance via the diaphragmatic lymphatics.[77] Feces, fiber, and mucin activate the complement cascade and thus deplete and compete for local opsonins.[78] Barium impairs neutrophil function both directly and indirectly by inducing an intense fibrinous reaction.[79] Foreign bodies including drains, suture material, hemostatic agents such as Gelfoam and Oxycel, and even missile fragments[80] clearly potentiate infection. The interaction between neutrophils and foreign bodies causes premature degranulation and release of toxic oxygen radicals by the neutrophils, thereby rendering these cells functionally incapacitated when subsequently stimulated.[81,82] A similar activation state has been demonstrated for peritoneal macrophages.

Although the mechanisms of action of all intraperitoneal adjuvants are not known, meticulous hemostasis, copious lavage to remove all types of adjuvant substances from the peritoneal cavity, and aspiration of all excess irrigant may reduce the incidence of recurrent intra-abdominal infection after operation.

Clinical Manifestations. Textbook descriptions of secondary bacterial peritonitis tend to equate it with the acute abdomen. In fact, the manifestations are variable depending on the specific disease, its location in relation to the other viscera and serosal surfaces, and host factors such as immunosuppression or recent operation. Visceral perforation is a frequent cause of secondary bacterial peritonitis. The resulting rapid contamination of the peritoneal cavity often produces the classic acute abdomen. Pain is of recent onset and may be sudden or appear over several hours. Whereas the pain at onset could be localized, generalized pain develops rapidly. Movement, coughing, or jarring the bed aggravates the symptoms. In diffuse peritonitis, tenderness is found over the entire abdomen and rebound tenderness is diffuse and severe. Although conventional wisdom professes the value of rebound tenderness, its specificity is probably no higher than 50 percent[83] and likely reflects only a more dramatic way of demonstrating tenderness and guarding. At first, the patient lies still, with shallow respirations and voluntary muscular guarding of the abdomen. As the parietal peritoneum becomes inflamed, rigidity ensues due to reflex muscular spasm. Anorexia, nausea, and vomiting are present from the onset, but the patient is thirsty, and urine output is low. Ileus results in abdominal distention and hyperresonance, and bowel sounds are usually diminished or absent.

Fever and tachycardia are almost always present, except in patients who are in some way immunocompromised. The patient is initially alert and irritable but, without treatment, gradually becomes obtunded. The patient normally dies of dehydration and hypovolemic shock, not sepsis. If a patient is being carefully monitored and fluid resuscitation is appropriate, the development of a hyperdynamic circulation, with a concurrent drop in arteriovenous oxygen extraction, hyperglycemia, and acidosis, may be detected before any other symptoms appear. Hypotension is more common in the elderly and young, both of whom frequently have more subtle localizing signs. Septic shock is usually a late event except in the case of a ruptured abscess.

Peritonitis developing from a prior site of visceral inflammation, such as appendicitis, diverticulitis, or tubo-ovarian abscess, usually has a less dramatic presentation unless an abscess suddenly ruptures to effect contamination of the entire peritoneal surface. Patients usually first note a dull aching pain in the abdomen. This centrally perceived sensation is generally slow in onset, dull, and poorly localized. Unlike cutaneous pain, visceral pain is elicited either by distention, inflammation, or ischemia, stimulating the sensory neurons within the visceral peritoneum. Rectal or vaginal exam may reveal tenderness or fluctuance of a pelvic abscess. Once the parietal peritoneum of the anterior abdominal wall is affected, the distribution of pain fibers permits the perception of localization pain. If the abscess remains deep in the pelvis or under the diaphragm, abdominal tenderness may be difficult to elicit.

Similarly, postoperative patients with peritonitis have unreliable signs of developing intraperitoneal infection. Incisional pain, postoperative analgesics, or respiratory complications may mask the intraperitoneal irritation. Fever and ileus are such common nonspecific signs in postoperative patients that their significance tends to be ignored. Even when sepsis becomes obvious, other sources of infection must be ruled out.

Patients who are immunocompromised have little in the way of abdominal findings. Patients receiving steroids, with underlying malignancy, chronic renal failure, diabetes, or other chronic illness, may also present difficult diagnostic challenges. Some patients, especially those who have had an operation in the immediate past, may present with multiple organ system failure as the only indication of continuing intra-abdominal sepsis—usually an abscess rather than peritonitis (see the section on abdominal abscess in this chapter).

Laboratory Studies. A leukocytosis exceeding 11,000/mm^3, with a shift to immature neutrophil forms, is one of the hallmarks of peritonitis. Leukopenia is compatible with overwhelming sepsis. Biochemical data reflect the degree of dehydration, with elevated blood urea nitrogen and a metabolic acidosis. Microscopic hematuria and pyuria occur with inflammation adjacent to the urinary tract, but the presence of bacteria, white blood cell casts, and large numbers of erythrocytes in the urine should suggest a urinary tract source of the pain. Amylase levels are usually normal unless pancreatitis, a proximal gastrointestinal tract perforation, or bowel infarction are responsible for the peritoneal inflammation.

Blood cultures are positive in 24 to 30 percent of patients with peritonitis. The most common microbes recovered are *E. coli, B. fragilis,* or *Enterococcus.*[19,45] A polymicrobial bacteremia, especially with *E. coli* and *Enterococcus*, frequently reflects the presence of intra-abdominal infection.[84] Similarly, any patient presenting with an anaerobic bacteremia should have intra-abdominal infection considered as a possible source of sepsis.[85]

Imaging Studies. Plain films of the abdomen and an upright chest x-ray should be considered routine in the elucidation of the cause of abdominal pain. The chest x-ray will frequently reveal free air below the diaphragm in the case of a perforated viscus or, alternatively, may reveal a nongastrointestinal etiology of upper abdominal pain, such as pneumonia. Positioning patients in the left lateral decubitus position may heighten the sensitivity for detecting free intraperitoneal air.[86] This position has several advantages in that it allows free air to accumulate between the abdominal wall and liver, thereby eliminating confusing shadows caused by an irregular diaphragm, gastric bubble, and intraluminal bowel gas. Additionally, it allows escape of air through the foramen of Winslow, thereby permitting visualization of retroperitoneal air. Pneumoperitoneum is seen in only 55 to 69 percent of gastroduodenal perforation, 30 to 41 percent of small bowel perforations and 37 to 46 percent of colonic perforations, suggesting that lack of free air does not rule out hollow viscus perforation.[87,88] Free air is seen for up to 3 weeks following laparotomy,[89] making its value in the postoperative patient somewhat questionable. However, an increase in the amount of air on sequential films may be indicative of anastomotic dehiscence. If clinical presentation is not consistent with the radiologic findings, films can be supplemented with injection of a water-soluble contrast agent.

Supine, decubitus, and upright abdominal films may also contribute to diagnosis by providing evidence of mechanical intestinal obstruction, volvulus, intussusception, and occasionally mass effects due to abscesses or neoplastic processes. More commonly, mild distention of the small and large intestine with air-fluid levels and bowel loops separated by intraperitoneal fluid are found. Gas seen in unusual places is usually indicative of an underlying pathologic process. Gas within the biliary tree or gallbladder suggests a fistulous communication, emphysematous cholecystitis, or cholangitis. Gas within the mesenteric venous system, portal vein, or hepatic venous system suggests an advanced gastrointestinal inflammatory or ischemic process. Rarely, pneumatosis intestinalis or retroperitoneal air may be seen following endoscopy. Extraluminal gas with a fluid level or gas bubbles is suggestive of an abscess in which the infecting organisms are undergoing anaerobic metabolism.

Ultrasonography may provide supportive evidence of an intra-abdominal inflammatory process. Less than 100 ml of peritoneal fluid can be visualized. Alterations in the configuration of bowel acoustic patterns or altered peristaltic activity provides further support. Real-time ultrasonography is now the most commonly used imaging study in the assessment of patients with right upper quadrant peritonitis. The caliber of both the intrahepatic and extrahepatic biliary tree, the presence of biliary calculi, the morphologic features of the gallbladder wall, and the presence or absence of an ultrasonographic Murphy's sign can be documented.

Ultrasonography may be useful in equivocal cases of appendicitis,[90,91] with a specificity and sensitivity on the order of 90 and 80 percent, respectively. Typical sonographic findings include the presence of a periappendiceal phlegmon or thick-walled dilated appendix with tenderness on graded compression. It is perhaps especially valuable in females with middle to lower abdominal pain within the reproductive age group by providing evidence of appendicitis while ruling out the presence of tuboovarian disease.[92] In a similar manner, ultrasonography can provide evidence of diverticulitis by virtue of the presence of a diverticular phlegmon, colonic wall thickening, or tenderness with graded compression.[93,94] The widespread availability, coupled with accuracy and noninvasiveness, has resulted in the use of ultrasonography as an adjunct to the physical exam, with some centers providing sonography equipment for use by surgeons in the emergency department.

The use of computed tomography (CT) has had a significant impact on the diagnosis of equivocal cases of peritonitis. Unlike ultrasonography, imaging is not affected by overlying gas, bone, or adipose tissue. The two significant advantages over conventional radiography include the appreciation of intra-abdominal pathology in three dimensions and the excellent contrast discrimination between different tissues. CT is invaluable in detecting minute quantities of intraperitoneal fluid, a significant clue to peritoneal inflammation. In one prospective study, CT provided a diagnosis in 95 percent of cases and altered the primary therapeutic strategy in 30 percent of patients.[95] Federle et al[96] demonstrated an 85 percent sensitivity for the CT diagnosis of bowel infarction, although other studies have been less optimistic.[97] The most reliable criteria of infarction were the presence of portal or mesenteric venous gas, intramural gas in the presence of a thickened bowel wall, or focal bowel dilatation.[96] CT is the procedure of choice for imaging the retroperitoneum and is useful for the diagnosis and grading of the severity of pancreatitis by demonstrating the extent of peripancreatic edema, as well as the presence or absence of associated fluid collections. Furthermore, it is invaluable in the detection of fluid collections as the result of complicated appendicitis or diverticulitis.

Adjunctive Diagnostic Modalities. Although the diagnosis of secondary peritonitis is most often based on clinical parameters, occasionally adjunctive techniques are required in an attempt to elucidate the presence or absence of peritoneal inflammation requiring laparotomy. History and physical examination may be unreliable as a result of altered mentation due to head injury, dementia, or encephalopathy. Paralysis, either iatrogenic or occurring as the result of spinal cord injury, may make the diagnosis of peritonitis difficult. Both diagnostic peritoneal lavage and diagnostic laparoscopy may be useful in selected patients.

DIAGNOSTIC PERITONEAL LAVAGE. Diagnostic peritoneal lavage may be useful in the diagnosis of intra-abdominal infection.[98–100] The presence of gross pus, turbid fluid, bile, or a positive Gram stain suggest intra-abdominal pathology. When the aspirate is grossly negative, microscopic examination of the effluent is necessary. Early studies used the traditional criterion of 500 WBC/mm^3 after a 1-liter saline lavage to denote a positive lavage.[99] Recent studies have suggested that the presence of as few[101] as 200 WBC/mm^3 or 250 to 500 WBC/mm^3 with less than 75 percent neutrophils[100] be considered positive. False negatives may occur in well-localized inflammatory processes, as well as immunocompromised patients unable to mount a significant white blood cell response.

DIAGNOSTIC LAPAROSCOPY. As a result of its efficacy in the treatment of both acute and chronic cholecystitis, the laparoscope has become an important addition to the armamentarium of the general surgeon.[102] The benefits of laparoscopy in the evaluation of acute abdominal pain are only now being appreciated. Negative laparotomy rates of 25 percent[103] using the traditional clinical examination and laboratory studies have dramatically been reduced when diagnostic laparoscopy is performed prior to laparotomy. In one series, laparotomy was avoided in 55 percent of patients.[104] Patterson-Brown et al[105] have demonstrated that selective laparoscopy performed in patients for whom the need for operation was uncertain reported a reduction in error rate from 19 to 0 percent. Unnecessary appendectomies were reduced from 22 to 8 percent.[106] The most common indication for laparoscopy is lower abdominal or pelvic pain in young women, especially in the right iliac fossa. There are proponents for universal use of laparoscopy in this subgroup of patients in an attempt to reduce the rate of unnecessary laparotomy.[107–109] The normal appendix can be visualized with laparoscopy in more than 75 percent of patients.[107,110] The other advantage of laparoscopy is its capacity for therapeutic intervention. Furthermore, laparoscopy has been used in the diagnosis and treatment of numerous other conditions traditionally considered to be an indication for laparotomy, such as mesenteric infarction[104,111] and perforated peptic ulcer.[112,113]

Management. The management of a patient with peritonitis involves three phases: (1) a preoperative phase, in which fluid resuscitation and initiation of antibiotic therapy are paramount; (2) operative intervention to achieve control of the peritoneal contamination and effect peritoneal toilet; and (3) the postoperative phase in which the patient requires ongoing resuscitation and antibiotics as well as frequent reassessment to provide early recognition of complications.

PREOPERATIVE. The main objectives in preparing patients with secondary peritonitis for operation are fluid resuscitation and the initiation of antibiotic therapy. Fluid resuscitation entails both the administration of fluids and the monitoring of fluid status. All patients with peritonitis have some degree of hypovolemia and thus adequate volumes of fluid should be administered to restore and maintain tissue perfusion. Adequacy of resuscitation may be assessed by monitoring blood pressure, central venous pressure, and urine output. In the elderly or critically ill patient, resuscitative measures must be directed by invasive monitoring techniques such as arterial cannulation for continuous and repeated evaluations of blood pressure and arterial blood gases. Central venous pressure monitoring, preferably with a Swan–Ganz catheter to measure pulmonary and left atrial pressures, may be necessary. Measurement of urine output with an indwelling catheter remains an excellent measure of end-organ perfusion.

The systemic inflammatory response characteristic of the septic state results in increased permeability of the pulmonary vasculature and transudation of fluid into the alveoli. The severity ranges from mild hypoxemia to the clinical and radiologic equivalent of the adult respiratory distress syndrome (ARDS). Additionally, reflex abdominal rigidity and diaphragmatic spasm may impair ventilation. Furthermore, patients may present in septic shock if the process is advanced. Therapy must be directed appropriately and at times may require mechanical ventilation and inotropic support in the intensive care unit in preparation for urgent laparotomy.

Ileus of varying degrees occurs in most cases of diffuse peritonitis. Air swallowing and intestinal contents distend the bowel, further impairing diaphragmatic excursion. Preoperative nasogastric intubation may decompress the bowel, reducing vomiting and the discomfort associated with abdominal distention.

As a general principle, sedatives and analgesics are withheld in patients with suspected peritonitis until the decision is made to perform a laparotomy. This allows for repeated and systematic clinical evaluation during the period of observation.

ANTIBIOTIC THERAPY OF INTRA-ABDOMINAL INFECTION. A recent position paper from the Antimicrobial Agents Committee of the Surgical Infection Society has helped clarify the use of antibiotics in intra-abdominal infection.[114] Excluded from consideration were disease processes in which contamination has occurred but infection is not established, or conditions in which a localized infectious process is dealt with entirely by excision. The common feature of these diagnoses is the minimal degree of peritoneal soiling at the time of laparotomy (Table 38–3). In these cases, antibiotic therapy is considered prophylactic and prolonged therapy is not indicated. A preoperative dose of antibiotics followed by two doses within 24 hours is sufficient.

Two cardinal principles underlie the use of antimicrobial agents in established intra-abdominal infection. The first principle is the initiation of antibiotic therapy at the time the clinical diagnosis of peritonitis is made—thus prior to laparotomy and certainly before culture data are available. Secondly, antimicrobial therapy should include an agent or a combination of agents with activity against both aerobic and anaerobic bacteria. Evidence from in vitro data, numerous animal studies, and clinical trials has led to the general acceptance of the requirement for the use of *empiric therapy* directed against *E. coli* and other common members of the family Enterobacteriaceae, in addition to *B. fragilis*. In the past, dual-agent therapy with an aminoglycoside and antianaerobe such as metronidazole or clindamycin was considered the gold standard. The development of second- and third-generation cephalosporins, the carbapenems, and monobactam agents have resulted in the availability of several single-agent or combination regimens of equal or improved efficacy.

Decisions regarding a particular regimen are based on consideration of both efficacy and toxicity profiles in each particular patient. Most patients acquiring secondary peritonitis outside the hospital may be treated adequately with a single broad spectrum agent (Table 38–4). Peritoneal isolates in such patients do not usually demonstrate significant antimicrobial resistance. Single-agent therapy using second-generation cephalosporins possessing

TABLE 38–3. CONDITIONS IN WHICH ANTIMICROBIAL THERAPY IS CONSIDERED PROPHYLACTIC

Intra-abdominal Pathology
Early acute appendicitis
Acute suppurative appendicitis
Simple acute cholecystitis
Gastroduodenal ulcer perforation
Traumatic enteric perforations
Simple dead bowel

Adapted from Bohnen JMA, Solomkin JS, Dellinger EP, et al: Arch Surg 127:83, 1992.

TABLE 38–4. ANTIBIOTIC THERAPY IN SECONDARY PERITONITIS

Single Agents	Combinations
Community-acquired infections of mild to moderate severity	
Cefoxitin	Antianaerobe plus aminoglycoside
Cefotetan	Antianaerobe plus third-generation cepholosporin
Cefmetazole	
Ticarcillin-clavulinic acid	Clindamycin plus aztreonam
Severe infections	
Imipenem-cilastin	

Adapted from Bohnen JMA, Solomkin JS, Dellinger EP, et al: Arch Surg 127:83, 1992.

anaerobic coverage such as cefoxitin, cefotetan, or cefmetazole or the use of ticarcillin with a beta-lactamase inhibitor in the form of ticarcillin-clavulanic acid are of documented efficacy in patients with community-acquired peritonitis of mild to moderate severity.[114]

Patients in whom intra-abdominal infection develops within the hospital environment or who are immunocompromised, debilitated, critically ill, or otherwise at risk for resistant organisms require special consideration. In these patients, the use of imipenem-cilastin is of documented efficacy as demonstrated by Solomkin et al[45] and Hackford et al.[50] Dual-agent regimens in these patients include the use of an antianaerobe (clindamycin or metronidazole) in combination with a third-generation cephalosporin such as cefotaxime and ceftizoxime. Alternatively, the use of the monobactam aztreonam in addition to clindamycin is useful.[115,116] In this latter regimen, metronidazole should not be substituted for clindamycin, in order to ensure some degree of gram-positive coverage.

The classic dual-agent regimen of an aminoglycoside and an antianaerobe has fallen into disfavor due to problems with both the toxicity profile and efficacy of aminoglycosides. The relative risk of aminoglycoside-induced nephrotoxicity has been estimated at approximately 8 to 18 percent. High-risk groups include the elderly, patients with preexisting renal disease or liver disease, and patients with recent episodes of hypotension.[117] The efficacy of aminoglycosides is reduced significantly by frequent underdosing and consequently an inability to maintain therapeutic levels. Solomkin et al[45] documented an average of 3.8 to 4.6 days to reach therapeutic levels in patients treated with aminoglycosides for intra-abdominal infection. The efficacy of aminoglycoside therapy is dependent on the rapid achievement of peak serum levels, which are four to eight times the anticipated minimum inhibitory concentration. Current recommendations for aminoglycosides include initial dosing at 2 mg/kg for gentamicin, tobramycin, and netilmicin and 20 mg/kg for amikacin, with an initial dosing interval of 12 hours.[118] Peak and trough levels should be obtained on the first or second dose providing for an early change in either dose or interval. The septic, hyperdynamic patient with normal renal function and expanded extracellular fluid volume (hence a greater volume of distribution) may require up to five times the daily recommended dose to achieve therapeutic levels.[119,120] Additionally, recent evidence suggests that the activity of gentamicin may be reduced in the local environment of an intra-abdominal abscess. The activity of gentamicin is reduced 16- to 32-fold by lowering pH from physiologic ranges to levels typically found within an abscess. Furthermore, hypoxia may interfere with oxygen-dependent transport of the drug across bacterial membranes.[121,122]

Inadequate or inappropriate use of empiric antibiotic therapy results in poor outcome with regard to length of hospital stay, wound infections, postoperative abscesses, and rate of reoperation.[53] There is no beneficial effect even when antibiotics are subsequently changed on the basis of culture results to include the use of appropriate agents.[53] As a result, the use of intraoperative cultures to guide therapy has come into question. Dougherty et al[123] demonstrated that bacterial cultures appeared to have influenced antibiotic therapy in less than 7 percent of patients and were most useful in guiding therapy only after the onset of postoperative infections. Clearly, they remain valuable in detecting the presence of organisms which may have potentially devastating effects, such as *Clostridium perfringens,* as well as to allow for epidemiologic tracking of organisms and resistance patterns.

The guidelines for determining the duration of antibiotic therapy in patients after operative management have been well delineated by retrospective analyses of outcome in patients following discontinuation of antibiotics. If a patient is afebrile, has a normal leukocyte count, and has a band count of less than 3 percent, the chance of recurrent sepsis following discontinuation of antibiotic therapy is virtually zero.[124] The probability of recurrent infection if the temperature or leukocyte count is elevated ranges from 33 to 55 percent.[125] Using these criteria, antibiotics may be discontinued as early as the fourth postoperative day. If persistent leukocytosis or fever is present by postoperative days 7 to 10, a diligent course should be initiated to locate the source of persistent sepsis.

CANDIDA AND *ENTEROCOCCI*. The significance of peritoneal isolates containing either Enterococci or *Candida* species is controversial. Enterococci are resistant to many of the antibiotic regimens used for intra-abdominal infection, including most beta-lactams.[126] Antibiotics with activity against enterococci, such as ampicillin and vancomycin, are not bactericidal against most strains, requiring the addition of an aminoglycoside to induce a synergistic effect.[127] Experimental and clinical evidence suggest that polymicrobial intra-abdominal infections do not require the addition of antienterococcal coverage on an empiric basis. Furthermore, it is not necessary to add antienterococcal coverage if initial intraperitoneal cultures reveal Enterococci and the patient is doing well. Enterococcal bacteremia in the context of intra-abdominal infections is quite rare, attesting to the low virulence of this organism. Therapy is indicated in situations where the patient is immunocompromised or the isolate occurs on the background of previous antibiotic therapy or postoperative peritonitis. This is especially true in patients with valvular heart disease or a prosthetic heart valve.[128] There is no doubt about the need for antienterococcal therapy when enterococcal bacteremia is documented,[129] although its efficacy in reducing mortality is questionable.[130,131]

Isolation of *Candida* from peritoneal fluid occurs frequently following proximal gastrointestinal tract perforation, reflecting its predominance in this part of the gut. When isolated at the first laparotomy for community-acquired intra-abdominal sepsis, antifungal therapy is not warranted. However, if *Candida* is isolated at subsequent laparotomies for complicated intra-abdominal infection, antifungal therapy should be implemented. Additionally, in the patient immunocompromised as a result of immunosuppressive drug regimens or by virtue of being critically ill, antifungal therapy is necessary.[114] Recent experimental evidence suggests that *C. albicans* and *E. coli* may act synergistically to increase mortality when present as copathogens.[132] Solomkin et al[133] demonstrated an improvement in mortality associated with antifungal therapy in patients in whom amphotericin B therapy was initiated after isolation of *Candida* from the peritoneal cavity, but before the onset of candidemia and multiple organ failure. Sawyer and Dunn[134] recommend a minimum 7- to 10-day course of amphotericin B at a dose of 0.3 to 0.5 mg/kg/day when the presence of *Candida* is limited to the peritoneal cavity.

OPERATIVE INTERVENTION. Presently, aggressive operative management of secondary peritonitis is the treatment of choice. Surgical management of secondary peritonitis involves three fundamental principles: (1) elimination of the source of contamination, (2) reduction of bacterial contamination, and (3) prevention of recurrent infection.

ELIMINATION OF THE SOURCE OF CONTAMINATION. The operative technique used to control contamination depends on the location and nature of the pathology in the gastrointestinal tract. In general, peritoneal contamination is controlled by closing, excluding, or resecting the perforated viscus. Perforation of the duodenum due to peptic ulcer disease may be patched safely with a piece of omentum, while a perforated gastric ulcer is either included in a distal gastric resection with a subsequent gastroduodenal or gastrojejunal anastomosis or locally excised with primary closure.

Peritoneal soiling as a result of perforation of the small bowel is dealt with by resection followed by primary anastomosis. If peritoneal contamination is particularly extensive or if there is concern about the viability of the intestine, resection plus proximal and distal enterostomy may be necessary. This holds true for proximal colonic perforation as well. Appendicitis is treated with resection (ie, appendectomy).

Considerable controversy exists over the management of perforation of the left colon, usually occurring as a result of diverticulitis or sigmoid carcinoma. Control of peritoneal contamination is usually accomplished by resecting the perforated segment and exteriorizing the proximal end as an end colostomy, and dealing with the distal end by creating a mucous fistula or oversewing it. Restoration of intestinal continuity is performed 2 to 3 months later, once the acute inflammatory process has settled.

It was previously thought that primary anastomosis in the setting of peritonitis is at high risk for dehiscence and should be avoided. Recent evidence suggests that it is not the presence of peritonitis that places the anastomosis at risk, but the proximal fecal loading associated with an unprepared bowel.[135–138] Anastomotic dehiscence may occur as a result of the mechanical disruption associated with a fecal bolus or due to the development of a local inflammatory process at the site of anastomosis, resulting in altered collagen metabolism. Preliminary trials suggest that the use of an intracolonic bypass device consisting of a soft, pliable tube anastomosed to the submucosa of the proximal colon may protect the anastomosis from the effects of fecal loading, providing for a safe primary anastomosis. The device is expelled 10 to 14 days postoperatively. Ravo et al[139] demonstrated the efficacy of such a device in 28 patients with left colonic perforations of various etiologies with no mortality and no evidence of anastomotic leaks. More recently, Rosati et al[140] reported similar encouraging results, with an anastomotic leak rate of only 8.7 percent. Although promising, patient selection no doubt plays a role in outcome. Further testing in clinical trials is necessary to define those patients most likely to benefit.

REDUCTION OF BACTERIAL CONTAMINATION. The second major goal of operative management of peritonitis is to reduce the bacterial inoculum. At operation, gross purulent exudates should be aspirated, and loculations in the pelvis, paracolic gutters, and subphrenic regions should be gently opened and debrided. If present, an attempt should be made to remove particulate debris, such as fecal matter or barium sulfate.

Although intraoperative peritoneal lavage with saline or antibiotic-saline combinations has become a standard procedure during surgery for peritonitis, there is no evidence that it reduces mortality or the incidence of intra-abdominal septic complications in patients receiving broad spectrum perioperative systemic antibiotics. A recent prospective study by Schein et al[141] documented no improvement in either surgical complications or mortality using saline lavage with or without the addition of chloramphenicol. The use of peritoneal lavage with or without antibiotics may have deleterious effects on local host defenses. Saline itself acts as an adjuvant by impairing phagocytosis and leukocyte migration.[29] Antibiotics or antiseptics in the lavage fluid may impair neutrophil chemotaxis[142] and microbicidal killing.[143] Furthermore, irrigation with antibiotics may increase adhesion formation.[144] As a result of the undocumented beneficial effects of intraoperative peritoneal lavage, it is recommended that peritoneal toilet be limited to thorough cleansing with suction and moist swabs.[145]

The concept of radical peritoneal debridement as advocated by Hudspeth[146] involves complete exploration of the peritoneal cavity using a vertical midline incision from xiphoid to pubis. All loculations and abscess cavities are identified and eliminated. The bowel is decompressed with a long intestinal tube and all fibrinous deposits are debrided from both the parietal and visceral peritoneal surfaces. Initial results in an uncontrolled trial were excellent.[146] However, a subsequent study in which this technique was compared to standard methods demonstrated no advantage and suggested a possible deleterious effect, probably due to excessive bleeding caused in mechanical debridement.[147]

PREVENTION OF RECURRENT INFECTION. Several techniques have been utilized to prevent recurrent infection within the peritoneal cavity. The use of drains, continuous postoperative peritoneal lavage, and relaparotomy have all been used to achieve this end. As demonstrated by Kirschner[44] in 1926, it is impossible to drain the free peritoneal cavity in patients with diffuse peritonitis. Drains left in situ are not innocuous. Visceral or vascular erosion with fistulization or bleeding may occur, with potentially disastrous consequences. Drains may also act as adjuvants by providing a site for bacterial adherence and subsequent biofilm formation.[148] Finally, drains may provide a tract for the retrograde spread of infection into otherwise sterile tissue.[149] Haller et al[150] demonstrated that children with Penrose drains placed during operations for free peritonitis secondary to perforated appendicitis averaged 3.7 more hospital days than those without drains. For these reasons, the use of drains is ill-advised unless their purpose is to evacuate a well-defined abscess cavity, establish a controlled fistula, or effect continuous postoperative peritoneal lavage.

The concept of continuous postoperative peritoneal lavage has received much attention as a means of reducing postoperative sepsis.[151–154] At the time of initial surgery, peritoneal drains are left in situ and lavage is begun in the immediate postoperative period. Lavage is performed with large exchange volumes (more than 2 liters) during each 3-hour cycle to ensure dispersion of fluid throughout the peritoneum and to prevent loculations. Broad spectrum antimicrobials as well as low-dose heparin are usually included in the lavage fluid. Lavage is continued for 48 to 72 hours, or until the effluent is clear.

Studies of this technique are difficult to evaluate because of poor experimental design. Washington et al[151] demonstrated a reduction in postoperative abscess formation in patients who underwent postoperative lavage with a mixture of cefamandole, erythromycin, and heparin. However, the control group was not randomly selected and received no lavage at all. Thus, considering the number of variables, one could not attribute improved outcome to antibiotic lavage alone. A prospective randomized controlled study demonstrated that postoperative lavage containing neither antibiotics nor heparin did not benefit patients who were not already receiving broad spectrum systemic therapy.[152] However, the control group of patients had a trivial rate of infection, thereby making evaluation of the technique difficult. This technique is extremely labor intensive, necessitates intensive care monitoring, and is potentially complicated by the development of enteric fistulas from erosion of the cannula. A well-performed, prospective randomized trial of postoperative peritoneal lavage in high-risk patients would better define the efficacy of this technique.

The two surgical approches to prevention of recurrent intra-abdominal infection are scheduled relaparotomy and open management. Planned relaparotomy, or etappenlavage as it is known in the German literature, is the practice of performing repeat operations at fixed intervals (usually 24 to 72 hours) regardless of the patient's clinical condition. In this way, the development of new collections is prevented before their deleterious systemic effects are manifest. The difficulties arising from frequent exploration, with its forceful, repeated closure of the abdominal wall, have resulted in the development of the open abdomen approach, or laparostomy. Reported benefits of this technique include the conceptual advantage of treating the entire peritoneal cavity as one large collection, with its exposure allowing for drainage. Other possible advantages include improved ventilation[155] and renal perfusion.[156] Classically, the open abdomen approach involves leaving the fascia opened with saline gauze packing. Complications of this technique include evisceration, massive fluid losses, spontaneous fistulas, and contamination of the open wound. In addition, it is now realized that an open abdomen does not obviate the need for repeat abdominal exploration.

As a result of the disadvantages associated with the above techniques, a compromise has been employed using a semiopen technique with various temporary abdominal closure methods. The use of a Marlex or Dexon mesh with or without an insewn zipper provides ready access to the peritoneal cavity. In addition, the mesh prevents evisceration in the early postoperative period, reduces the risk of spontaneous fistulization, allows for drainage of fluid and pus through its interstices, and may function as an exit site for a stoma or drain. In this technique, the zipper is opened and the entire abdomen is manually explored. Adhesions between loops of bowel are lysed, while fibrinous exudates and fluid and necrotic debris are debrided. Repeat laparotomies are performed daily to ensure prompt treatment of new septic foci and early recognition of enteric fistulas. Once clinical evidence of sepsis subsides and the peritoneal cavity appears clean as determined by the presence of healthy granulation tissue, the explorations are discontinued. Nonabsorbable mesh (Marlex) may be removed at 7 to 9 days, once adhesions eliminate the possibility of evisceration. The resultant defect is either closed with a split-thickness skin graft or allowed to heal by secondary intention. The probability of late hernia formation is high.[157]

Reports evaluating this technique have been quite favorable. Objective interpretation is difficult due to the heterogeneity of the patient populations with regard to severity of illness and underlying disease processes. Two studies used the APACHE II stratification system to define the severity of illness, thereby permitting comparison of outcome to an accepted standard.[158,159] In one, the technique was applied to patients with diffuse, nonlocalizing peritonitis.[158] The mortality in patients receiving a mesh at the time of reoperation for postoperative peritonitis was one-third the rate predicted on the basis of APACHE II scores. Evaluation of the subgroups of APACHE II scores indicated that critically ill patients with scores higher than 25 had a mortality of 100 percent, whereas those with low scores already had a low mortality that was independent of treatment. These data suggest that patients with midrange APACHE II scores are the ones who may derive the greatest benefit from this approach, a finding confirmed by Garcia-Sabrido et al.[159] However, based on a compilation of 642 patients from 22 series, Schein et al[145] concluded that there was insufficient evidence to recommend that either open management or planned relaparotomy improves outcome in postoperative peritonitis. Enteric fistulas are a significant complication associated with the open abdomen approach despite the use of mesh. Mastboom et al[160] demonstrated a fistula rate of 13 percent in patients treated with such an approach with 14 patients developing 53 small bowel perforations attributable to the use of mesh.

ABDOMINAL CLOSURE. The approaches described above are reserved for those patients with severe intra-abdominal infection. In the majority of patients, abdominal wall closure is accomplished with a single fascial layer of either interrupted or running monofilament suture. In the elderly, malnourished, or immunocompromised patient, full-thickness abdominal wall retention sutures are used in addition to fascial closure. Care should be taken not to tie these sutures too tightly, as abdominal distention and abdominal wall swelling may cause pressure necrosis at suture insertion sites, leading to stitch abscesses and spreading cellulitis.

The risk of wound infection associated with diffuse peritonitis exceeds 20 percent, and therefore wounds should be managed by delayed primary closure of the skin and subcutaneous tissues.[161] The wound is loosely packed with saline-soaked gauze during operation, and the gauze is changed every 8 hours for 3 to 4 days. If the wound appears clean with a granulating base, skin edges can be apposed with skin tapes or fine sutures. If any question exists about the wound, it should be left open and allowed to close secondarily.

Prognosis. The ultimate outcome of an episode of secondary peritonitis is determined by many factors, some of which are controlled directly by the surgeon. These include the correct choice and timing of antibiotics, as well as nutritional and hemodynamic support. Technical factors, such as a poor anastomoses or the performance of an anastomosis in a contaminated field, are potentially catastrophic errors. Most important is the delay in operative intervention, with a significant rise in mortality when intervention is delayed more than 24 hours after presentation.[162] Delay in diagnosis is probably the most significant contributing factor to the high mortality associated with postoperative peritonitis, ranging from 50 to 60 percent.[162,163] The unreliability of the physical examination in patients during the postoperative period combined with overreliance on diagnostic imaging studies likely contribute to the delay.[162,164]

Patient-specific factors contributing to an unfavorable prognosis include advanced age and poor nutritional status. Chronic disease states such as cardiac disease,[163] malignancy, and the use of corticosteroids[165] adversely affect outcome. Nonspecific impairment of immune function as measured by the delayed type hypersensitivity (DTH) reaction to common recall antigens is predictive of both septic complications and mortality.[166,167] Outcome may also be correlated with the anatomical origin of peritoneal contamination. Bohnen and colleagues[165] documented a mortality rate of 10 percent in patients with appendicitis and perforated duodenal ulcers, in contrast to a mortality rate of 50 percent when contamination arose from other sites. Similar low rates associated with appendicitis have been documented by other investigators.[168]

The morbidity and mortality of intra-abdominal infection vary widely among studies. Studies examining the efficacy of antibiotics in intra-abdominal infection tend to include patients within a defined age limit, with normal organ function, and with minimally deranged physiologic parameters. As a result, these studies show a very favorable outcome for intra-abdominal infection, with a mortality in the range of 3 to 5 percent. Conversely, studies specifically designed to investigate mortality associated with intra-abdominal infection have yielded rates exceeding 20 percent. This discrepancy is consistent with the fact that peritonitis is not a homogeneous disease, but rather one that poses a high risk of complications for some patients and a low risk for others. The ability to stratify patients into these risk groups is of paramount importance. It allows prediction of those patients at high risk toward whom new and innovative therapies should be directed. Additionally, stratification of patients into risk groups enhances our ability to interpret the results of studies examining new treatments.

A surgical infection stratification system has been developed for patients with intra-abdominal infection.[168] In a five-center study, 178 patients with established intra-abdominal infection were found to have an overall mortality of 24 percent. Multivariate analysis has determined that the Acute Physiology Score (APS), malnutrition, and age were the most reliable predictors of outcome. The APS represents the degree of deviation from normal of 33 routinely measured laboratory tests or physical findings. A discriminant function based on these parameters could predict survival with 84 percent accuracy. Presently, the APACHE II system is used most commonly and has been found to accurately predict outcome in most patients.[165] However, in a group of critically ill patients, Cerra found that the APACHE II score tended to underestimate the risk of multiple organ failure and mortality.[298] Poenaru and Christou[167] demonstrated the improvement of the predictive value of the APACHE II system when DTH scores were added to the discriminant analysis, reflecting the importance of host immune function in prognosis.

Tertiary Peritonitis

The term tertiary peritonitis has been proposed to describe persistence or recurrence of peritonitis in the critically ill patient despite adequate surgical and antibiotic therapy of primary or secondary peritonitis.[170,171] In most patients, the combination of appropriate antibiotic therapy, timely surgical intervention, and normal host defense mechanisms results in complete resolution of the infection and subsequent recovery. Even when infection persists, localization of the process with subsequent abscess formation limits the magnitude of the systemic response and permits straightforward management by means of either percutaneous drainage or directed surgical drainage.

The developments of critical care units, broad spectrum antibiotics, and nutritional support have produced a subset of patients who are able to survive their initial operative intervention, but whose postoperative course is characterized by a prolonged ICU stay, multiple laparotomies, and organ dysfunction—the syndrome of tertiary peritonitis. Mortality has been documented as high as 64 percent despite aggressive surgical and antibiotic therapy.[171] At laparotomy, poorly defined, serosanguinous collections are often found, rather than discrete purulent abscesses. This likely represents an inability on the part of the host to localize an infectious process, reflecting global immune dysfunction. Additional support for this hypothesis is provided by the flora associated with tertiary peritonitis. Peritoneal cultures yield organisms markedly different than community-acquired, secondary peritonitis. Potentially pathogenic organisms traditionally thought to be of low virulence such as *Enterococcus, Candida, Staphylococcus epidermidis,* and *Pseudomonas aeruginosa* predominate.[171,172] Their presence may reflect either selection by antibiotic pressures or markers of the impaired systemic and local host defenses of the multiple organ dysfunction syndrome.

Early studies of multiple organ failure in patients with peritonitis demonstrated a strong association between organ failure and the presence of uncontrolled residual infection in the peritoneal cavity.[173–175] This resulted in a trend toward exploratory or "blind" laparotomy in patients with organ dysfunction and was extended to patients without recent gastrointestinal tract manipulation and negative imaging studies. However, subsequent studies documented the rarity of intra-abdominal infection in the majority of such cases. At present, the practice of directed exploration is advocated in which laparotomy is performed only if supported by findings on physical exam, imaging studies, or blood cultures.[176,177] However, in the presence of advanced organ dysfunction, definitive management of an intra-abdominal source of infection rarely succeeds in altering outcome.[178]

Primary Peritonitis

Primary peritonitis refers to infection of the peritoneal cavity in the absence of a documented source of contamination from the gastrointestinal tract. On the basis of the pathophysiology and microbiology, four variants of primary peritonitis are recognized.

Primary Peritonitis in Childhood. In 1581, Fernel described a 7-year-old girl who developed painless diarrhea and died. At autopsy, the abdomen was distended with putrid purulent peritoneal fluid. This probably represents the first description of primary peritonitis. Due to the widespread use of antibiotics, primary peritonitis is declining in frequency. It once accounted for 10 percent of all abdominal emergencies in children, with 75 percent of the cases occurring in children less than 5 years old.[179] More recently, McDougal et al[180] found that primary peritonitis accounted for 2.1 percent of all pediatric abdominal emergencies, 17.6 percent of diffuse peritonitis in infants, and 13.4 percent of diffuse peritonitis in children. Primary peritonitis in children follows a bimodal age distribution.[179,181] In infants, it occurs within the first 2 months of life, and females predominate. In childhood, the peak incidence is from 5 to 9 years of age (mean 8.5), and a more equal distribution of males and females is seen.[182] Children with nephrotic syndrome or cirrhosis appear to be at particularly high risk.[180,183,184]

The most common isolates include gram-positive cocci, such as *Streptococcus pneumoniae* and group A streptococci,[180,185] except for cirrhotics, in whom gram-negative organisms are present in half.[184] Several sources for these organisms are possible. The pneumococcus commonly colonizes the genital tract of infant females, and retrograde ascent of the fallopian tubes may result in intraperitoneal contamination. Additionally, pneumococcal bacteremia is characteristic of pneumococcal respiratory tract infections, so that hematogenous seeding of the peritoneal cavity is possible. Contiguous spread is possible, as primary peritonitis is often associated with lower lobe pneumonia in adults.[186] Beale and Hackett[187] documented reflux of urine into the uterus of a child; this may aid the spread of bacteria to the peritoneal cavity and would account for the high incidence of prior or concurrent urinary tract infections in girls who develop primary peritonitis.[180]

The clinical presentation mimics that of secondary bacterial peritonitis with presenting signs and symptoms consisting of fever, nausea, vomiting, and abdominal pain. Abdominal examination reveals diffuse tenderness, rebound tenderness, guarding, and absence of bowel sounds. Children presenting with evidence of peritonitis usually undergo laparotomy with a provisional diagnosis of acute appendicitis, unless evidence of underlying renal disease is noted. The diagnosis is made after a negative laparotomy, when gram-positive organisms are cultured from the peritoneal swabs. Antibiotic therapy is directed against the offending organism. In most cases parenteral penicillin G is adequate. Any child with gram-positive primary peritonitis should be evaluated for occult renal disease. Fifty percent of patients in one series had nephrotic syndrome that was not suspected until peritonitis developed.[184]

Peritonitis Associated with Urogenital Infection. The association between ascending genital tract infections and intra-abdominal infection was first noted in the 1930s, at which time *Neisseria gonorrhea* was implicated. Presently, *Chlamydia trachomatis* is recognized as the major etiologic agent. The most common form of peritonitis involves a localized inflammatory process involving Glisson's capsule and adjacent peritoneum, referred to as perihepatitis, or Fitz-Hugh-Curtis syndrome. Other variants are rare and include periappendicitis[188] and perisplenitis.[189] Diffuse chlamydial peritonitis presenting as generalized abdominal pain has been described and may be complicated by chronic ascites.[190,191] Contamination of the peritoneal cavity most likely occurs following involvement of the endometrium and fallopian tubes. The resulting ascending infection reaches the peritoneal cavity and likely continues cephalad along the paracolic gutters. A report of gonococcal perihepatitis in a male suggests that hematogenous spread is possible.[192]

The acute presentation classically begins with sudden pleuritic pain in the right upper quadrant, often associated with nausea and anorexia. The pain may be referred to the right shoulder as a result of diaphragmatic irritation. Chills, fever, sweats, and headache occur less often. The liver is often tender, with evidence of guarding. A friction rub is noted in only 15 percent of patients.[193] The diagnosis should be considered in young, sexually active women. Accompanying symptoms of pelvic inflammatory disease may be mild or absent[194,195]; therefore examination of the cervix for discharge and cervical swabs are necessary to confirm the diagnosis. Chlamydial antibody titers are usually elevated, often higher than 1:1000.[193] Definitive diagnosis is made by laparoscopy, at which time the typical "violin string" adhesions between the liver capsule and adjacent structures are seen. The treatment regimen is similar to that of pelvic inflammatory disease. Outpatient therapy consists of a single intramuscular dose of ceftriaxone, followed by doxycycline orally for 14 days. Inpatients receive cefoxitin and doxycycline intravenously until improvement occurs, followed by oral doxycycline to complete a 14-day course.[193]

Primary Peritonitis and the Immunocompromised Host. Patients immunosuppressed for any variety of reasons may develop primary peritonitis. Patients with systemic lupus erythematosus on steroids may develop infection, usually with encapsulated bacteria.[196] This presents a diagnostic problem, as 10 to 37 percent of patients will manifest abdominal pain as a part of their symptomatology—the majority of which represent other peritoneal inflammatory syndromes, such as serositis, vasculitis, or pancreatitis.[197] Additionally, patients who receive immunosuppression following transplantation or chemotherapy for neoplasia may develop spontaneous peritonitis. Patients with the acquired immunodeficiency syndrome may develop primary peritonitis as a result of cytomegalovirus (CMV) infection or a variety of other opportunistic pathogens.[198]

Spontaneous Bacterial Peritonitis in Cirrhotics. The most frequent form of primary peritonitis is that which occurs in cirrhotic patients with ascites. Routine admission paracentesis documented an incidence as high as 27 percent in this patient population.[199] Furthermore, it accounts for 30 percent of all infections in cirrhotic patients.[200,201] The low protein content of cirrhotic ascites predisposes to infection as a result of its low opsonic activity. Immunoglobulin and complement levels are significantly reduced as compared to normal ascitic fluid.[202] Patients at highest risk are those with ascitic fluid protein concentrations of less than 1 g/dl.[203] Additionally, patients with advanced liver disease have impaired reticuloendothelial function, resulting in impaired clearance of otherwise innocuous spontaneous bacteremia.[204]

Hematogenous seeding of the ascitic fluid is the most likely mechanism by which the peritoneal fluid becomes infected, although bacterial translocation through the intact gut or lymphatogenous spread has not been excluded.[205] The infection is monomicrobial in 90 percent of cases. The most common isolates are *E. coli, Streptococcus* species, and *Klebsiella* species. Anaerobes are rare, reflecting the hostile environment created by the relatively high Po_2 of ascitic fluid.[206,207] Characteristic of spontaneous bacterial peritonitis are the low concentrations of organisms encountered in the peritoneal fluid. As few as 1 to 2 organisms/ml have been documented.[208]

Clinical presentation is variable and symptoms are often subtle. Patients may have a low-grade fever with minimal or no tenderness. Frequently, the presenting symptoms are the result of hepatic decompensation. A known cirrhotic presenting with worsening encephalopathy, hepatorenal syndrome, or increasing ascites should undergo diagnostic paracentesis to rule out the diagnosis of spontaneous bacterial peritonitis. Coagulopathy is not a contraindication to the procedure.[208] Paracentesis of ascitic fluid is clearly the most valuable diagnostic tool. Fluid should be examined for the cell count and differential, pH, lactate, glucose, LDH, protein, Gram stain, and culture. Due to the relatively few organisms present, ascitic fluid is most accurately cultured by inoculating 10 to 20 ml into aerobic and anaerobic blood culture bottles at the bedside.[209] To obviate the 24- to 72-hour delay in obtaining a diagnosis, a few rapid tests are used to guide the initiation of therapy. In many studies, an elevated neutrophil count (greater than 250/mm^3), a reduced pH (less than 7.35), and an elevated lactate level (greater than 32 mg/dl) have been found to be highly predictive of the presence of peritonitis.[210,211] Recently, it has been demonstrated that evaluation of the neutrophil count is the most valuable test for the detection of peritonitis, and that elevation of this count is an indication for therapy despite the presence of negative cultures.[212] There is evidence that the clinical course and outcome of culture-negative neutrocytic ascites is identical to that of the culture-positive cohorts, suggesting that these are the same disease process.[213]

Of critical importance in the cirrhotic patient is the differentiation of primary versus secondary peritonitis. A negative laparotomy in a patient with end-stage liver disease carries with it a mortality of 80 percent.[214] It is difficult to distinguish these entities on the basis of clinical findings, as a patient with 10 to 20 liters of ascites rarely exhibits the classic signs of peritonitis. Additionally, an elevated neutrophil count does not differentiate primary from secondary peritonitis. Peritonitis associated with perforation may be identifiable on the basis of the initial ascitic fluid analysis of neutrocytic ascites (PMN > 250/mm^3) and is characterized by a typical pattern of biochemical tests, fulfilling at least two of the following criteria: ascitic fluid total protein greater than 1 g/dl, glucose less than 50 mg/dl, and lactate dehydrogenase greater than the upper limit of normal for serum.[215] If these criteria are positive, additional investigation with plain radiographs and water-soluble contrast studies should be performed to rule out gastrointestinal tract perforation. Ultrasound or CT scans may be useful to rule out the presence of localized or loculated infection. If such investigations are negative and the suspicion of secondary peritonitis remains, a repeat paracentesis should be performed 48 hours after the initiation of antibiotic therapy.[216] In primary peritonitis, the neutrophil count falls rapidly, whereas in secondary peritonitis, it remains stable or rises.[217] Indications for laparotomy include a fluid aspirate positive for gross feces or bile, radiologic investigation suggestive of a perforated viscus, cultures revealing mixed aerobic/anaerobic flora, or failure to improve on medical management.

Empiric antibiotic therapy should be initiated once neutrocytic ascites is documented. The antimicrobial of choice is parenterally administered cefotaxime.[218] The broad spectrum of this antibiotic includes activity against over 90 percent of the causative organisms and attains ascitic fluid concentrations over 20 times higher than the minimal inhibitory concentration for most sensitive strains.[219] The use of cefotaxime has supplanted conventional therapy with ampicillin and an aminoglycoside as a result of the high incidence of nephrotoxicity in this patient population.[218] A 5-day course of therapy is adequate, as longer courses provide no benefit with regard to mortality, cure rate, or recurrence rate.[220] Hospital mortality for cirrhotic patients in whom spontaneous bacterial peritonitis develops is approximately 50 percent, reflecting the severity of the underlying liver disease. Infection-related mortality is thought to be less than 30 percent and is improving as a result of earlier and improved treatment regimens.[208,221] Survivors of the initial episode have a high rate of recurrence, approaching 69 percent at one year, and have a significantly lower survival than comparable cirrhotic patients in whom spontaneous bacterial peritonitis does not develop.[222] Selective intestinal decontamination using oral norfloxacin, to reduce the level of gram-negative aerobes in the gut, lowered the probability of recurrence from 68 to 20 percent at 1 year.[223] Overall mortality was not altered, suggesting that spontaneous bacterial peritonitis is a predictor of poor outcome as a result of progressive liver failure, rather than an independent cause of increased mortality.

Unusual Forms of Primary Peritonitis

Tuberculous Peritonitis. In the United States, conditions are suitable for a major increase in the morbidity and mortality from tuberculosis. Since 1984, the expected continued decline in tuberculosis-associated morbidity has not occurred. In fact, in 1986, the morbidity began to increase.[224] Contributing factors are the mass migration from countries in which tuberculosis is endemic, coupled with the emergence of a new and highly susceptible group of immunocompromised patients in the form of AIDS. Additional factors are the increase in the population of persons who are elderly or socioeconomically deprived, both of which are considered high-risk groups.[225,226] Tuberculous peritonitis occurs in 2 percent of all patients with tuberculosis and in 30 to 67 percent of patients with abdominal tuberculosis.[224,227] The disease has a female preponderance and is most commonly seen in the third to fourth decade of life.[227]

Etiology. The microbiologic characteristics of *Mycobacterium tuberculosis* are discussed elsewhere in this textbook (see Chap. 9). Other forms of mycobacteria, such as *Mycobacterium avium-intracellulare,* are rarely implicated in peritonitis.

Pathogenesis. There are several ways in which tuberculous peritonitis may develop.[228] Most commonly, hematogenous spread occurs from a primary extraperitoneal focus, such as the lung.[229] Direct contamination from an infected mesenteric lymph node or tuberculous enteritis may occur. Similarly, contamination may follow the onset of tuberculous salpingitis in females. Only rarely is reactivation of latent peritoneal tuberculosis responsible.

Clinical Manifestations. The disease is insidious in onset, with symptoms developing over a 1- to 3-month period. In a series of 145 patients,[227] the most common symptoms included increasing abdominal girth secondary to ascites (73 percent), fever and night sweats (54 percent), anorexia (47 percent), weight loss (44 percent), and abdominal pain (35 percent). On physical exam, ascites was present in 95 percent of patients. In the remainder, the abdomen may have a "doughy" feel related to adherent loops of bowel, enlarged nodes, and a thickened omentum. Positive PPD skin tests are found in almost 60 percent of patients. Laboratory abnormalities include an elevated ESR and a normochromic, normocytic anemia. The leukocyte count is variable. An abnormal chest x-ray is present in 40 percent of patients, and sputum is positive for acid-fast bacilli in under 20 percent of cases.

Diagnosis. Tuberculous peritonitis should be suspected in patients presenting with the insidious onset of symptoms described above. A history of exposure to tuberculosis, a positive PPD test, and an abnormal chest X-ray study are helpful but, if normal, do not preclude the diagnosis. Paracentesis rarely yields visible organisms, but if a liter of ascites fluid is cultured, the organism will be recovered in 80 percent of cases.[230] Ascitic fluid characteristically has a high protein content (2.5 g/dl), low glucose level (less than 30 mg/dl), and a leukocyte count greater than 200/mm^3, with a predominance of lymphocytes.[226] Several investigators have demonstrated that the level of adenosine deaminase (ADA) in ascitic fluid correlates well with the presence of tuberculous peritonitis. An elevated level of ADA (greater than 32.2 U/liter) has a diagnostic sensitivity of 94 to 100 percent and specificity of over 95 percent.[225,231]

Ultrasound or computed tomography may reveal evidence of free or loculated fluid, an ileocecal mass, or retroperitoneal lymph node enlargement. More subtle signs include mesenteric thickening, adherent loops of bowel, and omental thickening.[232] The signs are relatively nonspecific and are as equally likely to represent a neoplastic process.

Diagnosis is made by laparoscopy. Characteristic findings include a thickened peritoneum with miliary yellow-white tubercles. Occasionally, only scattered erythematous patches are seen. Rarely, a fibroadhesive peritonitis occurs, resulting in thick adhesions and rendering laparoscopic examination difficult and uninformative. In this situation, open peritoneal biopsy is indicated.[233] In most cases, diagnosis can be made on the gross findings supplemented with a directed laparoscopic peritoneal biopsy. Pathologic examination reveals caseating granulomas in 82 to 100 percent of patients.

Treatment. Chemotherapeutic agents may be initiated on the basis of the gross appearance at laparoscopy, pending histology and culture results.[234] In general, extrapulmonary tuberculosis should be managed with drug regimens adequate for pulmonary tuberculosis (see Chap. 28). Specific 6- and 9-month regimens have been used successfully. The 6-month regimen is particularly useful for patients who must be under surveillance during therapy and involves triple-agent therapy with isoniazid, rifampin, and pyrazinamide.[235] The most common reason for therapeutic failure is noncompliance; however, the possibility of drug resistance should always be considered. Mortality is less than 7 percent in most series.[230]

Actinomycosis. Actinomycosis is a chronic, suppurative infection characterized by formation of multiple abscesses, draining sinuses, and abundant granulation tissue. The three major clinical presentations include involvement of the cervicofacial, thoracic, and abdominopelvic regions.[236] Males are affected two to three times more frequently than females. The disease occurs most often in middle-aged individuals and less commonly in adolescents and children.[237] Actinomycosis is encountered worldwide but is unusual in the United States.

Etiology. The *Actinomyces* organisms are gram-positive, non-spore-forming microaerophilic or obligate anaerobic bacteria. Their fastidious growth and microscopic appearance resemble that of many fungi, and they were considered as such until the 1950s.[238] *Actinomyces israelii* is usually responsible for the disease in humans.

Pathogenesis. *Actinomyces* organisms are part of the normal commensal flora of the oral cavity and tonsillar crypts. They are swallowed and reach the distal bowel. Abdominal actinomycosis is most commonly discovered after appendectomy or drainage of a periappendiceal abscess, although the disease has been described in association with diverticular disease[239,240] and intrauterine devices.[241] The stomach, liver, gallbladder, pancreas, small bowel, anorectal region, pelvis, abdominal wall, and other sites can also be involved.[237] Usually, a single organ is affected, and disseminated intra-abdominal actinomycosis is uncommon.

Actinomyces israelii probably cannot invade the intact mucous membrane, but disruption of gastrointestinal mucosa by recent disease or trauma allows the organisms to penetrate into adjacent tissue. Immunocompromised states, such as those caused by corticosteroids or diabetes, may be contributory.[242] Other pathogenic bacteria are virtually always associated with actinomycotic abscesses, and a synergistic interaction between *Actinomyces* and other microorganisms has been postulated. Coliforms and anaerobic, gram-negative bacilli are commonly found in abdominal actinomycosis. The hallmark of actinomycosis is a localized suppurative mass that forms an abscess and spreads by direct extension without regard for tissue planes, often ending in a draining sinus tract.

Clinical Manifestations. Abdominal actinomycosis is one of the great imitators in medicine. Actinomycosis generally presents as a chronic, localized inflammatory process associated with fever and leukocytosis. The diagnosis is often not suspected in the absence of a draining sinus. There is usually a latent interval of days to weeks between the onset of symptoms and presentation with a persistent, draining sinus.

In the early stages, abdominal actinomycosis may be indistinguishable from other inflammatory processes including appendicitis, Crohn's disease, diverticulitis, and pelvic inflammatory disease. The majority of patients have had an episode of acute abdominal inflammation in the recent past. Constitutional symptoms such as malaise, fever, chills, anorexia, and weight loss are not uncommon. The most characteristic physical signs are a palpable mass or a visible sinus tract or fistula. The mass may be confused with a neoplastic process.

Diagnosis. A preoperative diagnosis of actinomycosis is difficult. As an initial diagnosis, this disease is suspected in less than 10 percent of cases.[239] Laboratory tests are not helpful in differentiating other inflammatory or neoplastic processes. Contrast studies are usually nonspecific and may demonstrate fistulas or a mass effect. Computed tomography may demonstrate abdominal masses crossing fascial planes and involving multiple anatomic compartments, a finding not inconsistent with neoplastic disease.[239,243] The diagnosis is made by histologic examination of pus or curettings obtained from the fistula tract. Sulfur granules, 1 to 2 mm in size, are seen in more than 60 percent of cases.[244] Microscopic examination shows a zone of granulation tissue surrounding one or more oval eosinophilic granules. Beaded or filamentous, non-acid-fast bacilli radiate from this granule. The sulfur granules represent colonies of *Actinomyces,* but *Nocardia* species and some fungal infections may have a similar appearance. Cultures are more specific, although bacteriologic confirmation of the diagnosis occurs in less than 50 percent of the cases because of failure to obtain anaerobic cultures or overgrowth of other bacteria.[245]

Treatment. Operative management is required for localized abscesses and for excision of fistula and sinus tracts, after which the diagnosis is usually made. Percutaneous drainage of periappendiceal actinomycosis has been described.[246] The antibiotic of choice is penicillin given parenterally for at least several weeks, with duration depending on the extent of disease and clinical response. This is followed up by a regimen of oral penicillin for 3 to 12 months, with follow-up to document clinical and radiologic cure. Cure is achieved in 88 to 96 percent of cases, and mortality is low.[247]

Amebic Peritonitis. Amebic peritonitis is unusual in the United States, although numerous cases were reported in individuals returning from Vietnam (see Chap. 8). The asymptomatic carrier state in the United States may reach 5 percent[248] and amebic dysentery may be misdiagnosed as ulcerative or granulomatous colitis. Progression to toxic megacolon is common. Three or 4 percent of patients with amebic dysentery present with profound shock associated with perforation of the colon or small bowel. The mortality of mixed amebic and fecal peritonitis is 75 to 100 percent but can be lowered by early operation. Chronic cases, with formation of pericecal ameboma, have been reported.[249] Patients treated by simple appendectomy often develop fecal fistulas, which fail to heal until appropriate antiamebic therapy is begun.

Hepatic abscesses are a common manifestation of amebic infection. Abscesses of the left lobe or the inferior surface of the liver can rupture into the peritoneal cavity, although most amebic abscesses of the liver are situated on the superior hepatic surface and tend to perforate into the pleural space (see Chap. 40). Amebic peritonitis occurs in 6 to 9 percent of patients with hepatic abscesses[250] and rupture may be preceded by increasing right upper quadrant pain. These patients present with abdominal distention and fever and may deteriorate quite rapidly, but a rigid abdomen is not always present.

In the United States, most of these patients are male, have emigrated from or have recently traveled to Latin America, or have served in Vietnam. The organisms may be overlooked in Gram-stain specimens of peritoneal exudates and are best seen in fixed specimens stained with iron-hematoxylin. Shaggy perforations of the cecum or ruptured liver abscesses discovered at laparotomy suggest the diagnosis, and the microbiology laboratory should be notified. Serologic test results, so valuable for the diagnosis of hepatic abscesses, are almost always negative in acute peritonitis secondary to amebic bowel perforation (see Chap. 43).

In the United States, the diagnosis is usually made at laparotomy as the disease is uncommon and is rarely considered preoperatively. The trophozoites are best seen on biopsy of the liver abscess or cecal wall. For cecal perforation, resection with exteriorization of the bowel ends is indicated because suture closure or primary anastomosis usually fails.[248] Drains usually result in formation of sinus tracts. Antimicrobial therapy should be directed against both amebae and the polymicrobial bacterial flora associated with perforation of the colon. Systemic amebicide treatment with metronidazole is indicated. Eradication of the amebic reservoir (see Chap. 8) requires both intestinal and extraintestinal amebicidal drugs.

Other Granulomatous Infections. Almost any disseminated fungal disease (see Chap. 10) or parasite (see Chap. 8) can reach the peritoneal cavity to produce a granulomatous intra-abdominal infection. *Pityrosporum, Nocardia,* and *Strongyloides* have been occasional causes of peritoneal infection by invasion of the bowel wall and perforation or, more rarely, by hematogenous dissemination.

PERITONITIS ASSOCIATED WITH PROSTHETIC DEVICES

Peritonitis as a Result of Peritoneal Dialysis

In the United States, approximately 13 percent of the total 100,000 patients receiving dialysis treatment use continuous ambulatory peritoneal dialysis (CAPD).[251] Peritonitis related to CAPD is a common clinical problem and is the most significant complication associated with this form of dialysis. The incidence of peritonitis was much higher in the early 1980s, but more experience and general improvements in cuffed catheter design (eg, the Tenckhoff catheter) have decreased the rate to about 1.3 episodes per patient per year.[252] However, there are those patients who, as a result of poor compliance with aseptic techniques or individual susceptibility to infection, get three or more episodes of peritonitis per year. Over 60 percent of patients develop peritonitis during the first year of dialysis, reflecting the breaches in aseptic technique that occur during the early months of CAPD.[253]

Etiology. CAPD peritonitis is usually caused by normal skin commensals, most commonly *Staphylococcus* and *Streptococcus* species[253] (Table 38–5).

TABLE 38–5. MICROBIOLOGY OF CAPD PERITONITIS

Organism	%
• GRAM POSITIVE	
Staphylococcus (coagulase negative)	30–45%
Staphylococcus aureus	10–20%
Streptococcus species	10–15%
Enterococci	3–5%
Diptheroids	1–2%
• GRAM-NEGATIVE	
Escherichia coli	8–12%
Pseudomonas aeruginosa	5–8%
Enterobacter	2–3%
Acinobacter	2–3%
Klebsiella	2–3%
Proteus	2–3%
• FUNGI	
Candida species	5–15%

Adapted from Saklayen MG: Med Clin North Am 74:997, 1990.

Gram-negative organisms such as *E. coli, Enterobacter,* and *Klebsiella* are less frequent and account for approximately 20 percent of all cases. *Pseudomonas aeruginosa* occurs in 5 to 8 percent of episodes. Fungal organisms constitute 5 to 15 percent of all cases, with *Candida* species predominating.[253]

In the great majority of patients, CAPD peritonitis is a monomicrobial infection. If a polymicrobial infection is documented, or the peritoneal cultures show evidence of anaerobes such as *Bacteroides fragilis,* the presence of hollow viscus perforation must be considered. Cultures fail to grow any organisms in 3 to 30 percent of patients and probably reflect the variability in culture techniques in different microbiology laboratories.[253,254]

Pathogenesis. There are several potential portals of entry by which bacteria can gain access to the peritoneal cavity. Bacteria may penetrate via (1) an intraluminal route, by contamination of lines, connectors, or fluid; (2) a periluminal route (the use of a Dacron cuff on the catheter to permit tissue ingrowth and stabilize the catheter has markedly decreased infection rates); (3) a transmural route, by infection from the intestinal lumen, which may occur through the intestinal wall without obvious perforation[255] or at the site of preexisting diverticular disease[256]; (4) a hematogenous route; or (5) an ascending vaginal infection. The peritoneal cavity is usually able to clear small inocula of bacteria efficiently. However, the presence of a foreign body in the peritoneal cavity in combination with large fluid volumes may impair local host defenses and thereby permit small numbers of bacteria to establish infection. Chronic fibrin deposition on the catheter has also been postulated as an important factor leading to recurrent infection. Bacteria within the mesh are protected from the action of antibiotics and may act as a nidus for persistent infection.

Clinical Manifestations. The manifestations of peritonitis in patients on peritoneal dialysis are variable and may include mild abdominal pain, low-grade fever, and mild abdominal tenderness. Occasionally, patients are asymptomatic and their disease is manifested by the development of cloudy dialysis fluid, a feature occurring in 98 percent of cases.[257] If the dialysate fluid is clear, diagnosis of CAPD peritonitis should be suspect even in the presence of abdominal pain or fever. A cloudy dialysate fluid in the absence of symptoms requires a diagnostic workup for peritonitis.[253] The symptomatology depends on the virulence of the infecting organism and the time course of infection.

Diagnosis. Evaluation of suspected CAPD peritonitis includes obtaining peritoneal fluid for cell count, Gram stain, and culture. Criteria for the diagnosis of peritonitis include at least two of the following conditions: (1) presence of organisms on Gram stain or culture of the dialysate; (2) cloudy dialysis fluid with a WBC count greater than 100/mm^3, of which more than 50 percent are neutrophils; and (3) signs and symptoms of peritoneal inflammation.[258] A Gram stain is useful in predicting the type of organisms in only 30 to 40 percent of episodes.[253] It allows for early detection of fungal peritonitis and prompt institution of antimycotic agents. A high WBC count with a preponderance of mononuclear cells implies the possibility of tuberculous peritonitis and warrants further diagnostic evaluation.[259] The presence of pneumoperitoneum on chest x-ray examination in a patient on CAPD does not necessarily imply a perforated viscus. The finding is relatively common, occurring in 27 percent of patients on peritoneal dialysis.[260]

Treatment. After dialysate has been collected for diagnostic studies, three quick exchanges of peritoneal dialysis are performed, which serve to reduce the degree of abdominal discomfort. Once the cell count documents the presence of peritonitis, empiric antibiotic therapy is initiated. The use of a first-generation cephalosporin such as cefazolin or cephalothin in combination with an aminoglycoside has proved effective in most patients. In centers where a high incidence of methicillin-resistant *Staphylococcus aureus* has been demonstrated, vancomycin is preferred over the cephalosporins.[252] Antibiotics should be adjusted appropriately once culture results become available. If cultures are negative and the patient shows evidence of clinical improvement, the antibiotics should be continued.

Intraperitoneal administration of antibiotics is preferred in CAPD peritonitis. This method facilitates self-administration by the patient, permits a high level of antibiotics within the peritoneal cavity, and allows enough of the antibiotic to be absorbed to achieve bactericidal serum levels. An initial loading dose of 500 mg/liter of cephalosporin and 1.5 to 2.0 mg/kg of any of the aminoglycosides results in adequate serum levels.

Maintenance doses of 125 to 250 mg/liter of cephalosporin and 4 to 8 mg/liter of aminoglycoside are then continued for 7 days after the last positive culture has been obtained.[252] Serum levels of the aminoglycoside should be monitored and the dose adjusted appropriately.

Pseudomonas aeruginosa may pose a difficult management problem. Clinical experience has demonstrated that *Pseudomonas* peritonitis in CAPD patients is very difficult to treat and antibiotic treatment without catheter removal has a high probability of failure.[252] Once *P. aeruginosa* has been identified, an antipseudomonal aminoglycoside administered intraperitoneally should be continued. A second antipseudomonal antibiotic, either piperacillin or ceftazidime, should be added. If the former is chosen, it should be administered intravenously, as the ureidopenicillins inactivate the aminoglycosides when in solution.[252]

If cultures reveal the presence of fungal peritonitis, then catheter removal is recommended. Amphotericin B has very low efficacy when used intraperitoneally because of the low pH of the dialysate. Additionally, it causes severe peritoneal irritation. Complete eradication with antifungal therapy alone is rare and probably relates to adherence of fungi to the peritoneal dialysis catheter. Following catheter removal, 10 days of systemic amphotericin therapy is indicated.[252]

Adjuvant Therapy. Adjuvant therapy including heparin at 500 to 2000 U/liter is frequently used until the dialysate effluent clears. This usually occurs within 2 to 3 days. Heparin reduces fibrin formation, which tends to occlude the catheter. Additionally, it may prevent the development of fibrinous adhesions, which reduce the surface area for peritoneal exchange and provide sanctuary for organisms. Urokinase has been used in the early phase of treatment with varying rates of success.[261,262]

Treatment Failure. Within 48 hours of initiating therapy, most patients with CAPD peritonitis demonstrate considerable clinical improvement. The remainder show evidence of response by 48 to 96 hours. Those patients not improving by this time are considered treatment failures,[252] and reevaluation with repeat cell count, Gram stain, and cultures is necessary. Consideration should be given to the possibility of secondary bacterial peritonitis or the presence of unusual organisms, such as mycobacteria, fungi, or fastidious organisms.

In addition, reassessment of the antimicrobial regimen is required. If *Staphylococcus aureus* has been isolated, then the cephalosporin should be discontinued and vancomycin added. Addition of oral rifampin, 600 mg/day, is recommended.[252] The possibility of an exit site infection should be considered. A similar regimen should be employed for *Staphylococcus epidermidis* that fails to respond to a first-generation cephalosporin. If *Enterococcus* has been isolated, and the patient failed on ampicillin or vancomycin alone, then an aminoglycoside should be added.

The presence of anaerobic bacteria or gram-negative organisms not responding to the appropriate antibiotic regimen requires removal of the catheter, followed by 5 to 7 days of intravenous antibiotic therapy. A diligent search for intra-abdominal pathology should be undertaken, including contrast studies of the gastrointestinal tract, computed tomography, and, rarely, exploratory laparotomy.

Relapsing Peritonitis

Peritonitis recurring within 4 weeks of completing antibiotic therapy and where the same organisms are recovered is referred to as relapsing peritonitis.[252] Relapsing infections with staphylococci should be treated with vancomycin and rifampin as described previously for approximately 4 weeks. If no response is noted after 96 hours, the catheter should be removed. Additionally, a second relapse is an indication for catheter removal. Relapsing peritonitis caused by gram-negative organisms should raise suspicion of an underlying intra-abdominal abscess, and appropriate imaging studies should be undertaken. In the absence of intra-abdominal pathology, a repeat trial of antibiotic therapy with an aminoglycoside is warranted.

Conventionally, catheter removal is followed by interim hemodialysis for 2 to 3 weeks. Recently, there is evidence that immediate replacement with a permanent catheter is possible with minimal septic morbidity.[262,263] This may preserve the peritoneal cavity for dialysis by preventing the formation of adhesions. It also reduces the morbidity related to the initiation of temporary hemodialysis.

The significance of exit site and tunnel infections lies in their propensity to contaminate the peritoneal cavity. These infections usually cause only mild local symptoms or may be asymptomatic. Exit site infections produce local inflammation and a purulent discharge. Tunnel infections are difficult to diagnose, particularly if there is no accompanying exit site infection. In about 50 percent of patients, these infections can be managed by daily cleansing of the exit site with a disinfectant, together with oral administration of antibiotics. Catheter removal is indicated when there is a persistently infected exit site or tunnel tract. The catheter may be replaced at a new site as a one-stage procedure.

The management of patients whose peritoneal fluid cultures reveal multiple enteric organisms deserves consideration. Organisms appearing during the first 24 to 48 hours after percutaneous insertion of a temporary catheter suggest perforation of a hollow viscus. Laparotomy should be performed for closure of the perforated segment of bowel and for reinsertion of the catheter. In long-term dialysis patients, the most likely disease processes are perforated diverticulitis, perforated ulcers, or appendicitis. Water-soluble contrast studies of the gastrointestinal tract may help confirm the diagnosis and the need for operation. If the contrast examination is normal and the patient demonstrates clinical improvement on antibiotics with negative dialysate cultures, conservative management may be continued. In a series of ten patients treated in this manner, four patients had persistent abdominal pain, all of whom demonstrated intra-abdominal pathology requiring surgical intervention at the time of laparotomy.[264] The remaining six patients responded to antibiotic therapy and did not require laparotomy, suggesting that local host defenses cleared a predominantly localized process.

Two other forms of peritonitis have been associated with CAPD. Eosinophilic peritonitis may present within a few days of placement of the Tenckhoff catheter. The peritoneal fluid is cloudy, with an abundance of eosinophils. The disease is self-limited and is thought to occur as a result of an allergic reaction to the catheter tubing.[265]

Sclerosing encapsulating peritonitis is a significant complication of recurrent peritoneal dialysis cannula infections. It is characterized clinically by a progression from nausea, vomiting, abdominal pain, and impaired ultrafiltration during CAPD, to complete small bowel obstruction.[266] Pathologically, sclerosing encapsulating peritonitis appears to be an inflammatory process that transforms the peritoneum into thick fibrous tissue, resulting in dense adhesions. The small bowel is often encased by a thick grayish white membrane similar in appearance to a cocoon.[267] This inflammatory response has been associated with recurrent CAPD peritonitis, the use of acetate or antiseptics in the dialysate, and possibly concomitant use of beta-blockers.[268] Others have implicated the silicone catheter itself in the pathogenesis of sclerosing encapsulating peritonitis.[269] If left untreated, mortality is high as a result of complications related to the development of recurrent small bowel obstruction and necrosis, enterocutaneous fistulas, and malnutrition. Surgical treatment consists of meticulous lysis of the extensive fibrinous peritoneal reaction. The surgeon should be prepared for a difficult and tedious operative procedure.

Peritonitis Associated with Peritoneovenous Shunt

Patients with chronic liver disease and intractable ascites may require a peritoneovenous shunt as a palliative procedure. These patients are a high-risk group for infectious complications as a result of preexisting protein-calorie malnutrition and impaired cell-mediated immunity. In one recent series, 21 percent of 85 peritoneovenous shunt insertions were followed by major infection.[270] More recently, Hillaire et al[271] documented a 14 percent risk of spontaneous bacterial peritonitis within the first 10 postoperative months. The mortality in these patients was over 60 percent.[271] When shunt infection occurs, systemic antibiotic therapy and shunt removal are almost always required.[272]

Infections Associated with Ventriculoperitoneal Shunts

The diagnosis and treatment of infected ventriculoperitoneal shunts are discussed in detail in Chapter 34. Ventriculoperitoneal shunts drain cerebrospinal fluid from the obstructed ventricles to the peritoneal cavity. Shunt infection rates as high as 20 percent have been reported.[273] The patients usually present with septicemia, headache, neck stiffness, and evidence of increased intracranial pressure.

Acute abdominal infection is rare with ventriculoperitoneal shunts,[273,274] but primary shunt infection can lead to seeding of the peritoneal cavity. Usually, central nervous system symptoms are minimal compared with the abdominal findings. Children usually have a history of several days of anorexia, fever, abdominal pain, nausea, and vomiting. A leukocytosis is characteristic. All patients with a shunt and abdominal pain should have a percutaneous puncture of the shunt. Analysis of the fluid usually shows decreased glucose, and recovery of organisms is diagnostic.

Staphylococcus aureus and *S. epidermidis* are the most common pathogens. Gram-positive organisms suggest primary shunt infection, but gram-negative organisms may indicate an ascending infection from primary or secondary peritonitis. The recommended treatment is high-dose intravenous and intraventricular antibiotics for 2 weeks, followed by shunt replacement and an additional 2 weeks of antibiotics.[274]

DISEASES MIMICKING BACTERIAL PERITONITIS

Other noninfectious diseases can present with acute abdominal pain and may mimic peritonitis. Periodic peritonitis (Mediterranean fever, periodic polyserositis), porphyria, sickle cell crises, and diabetic ketoacidosis can all mimic an acute abdominal catastrophe, but laparotomy fails to demonstrate pathologic findings.

INTRA-ABDOMINAL ABSCESSES

Abscesses are well-defined collections of pus that are walled off from the rest of the peritoneal cavity by inflammatory adhesions, loops of intestine and their mesentery, the greater omentum, and other abdominal viscera. Abscesses represent the successful result of normal host defense mechanisms in the peritoneal cavity. Complete resolution of the abscess by host defenses, however, is frustrated by the ability of the contents of the abscess center to locally impair host cell function.

Abscesses may occur in the peritoneal cavity, either within or outside abdominal viscera, as well as in the retroperitoneum. Nonvisceral abscesses arise in two settings: (1) following resolution of diffuse peritonitis in which a loculated area of infection persists and evolves into an abscess and (2) following a perforation of a viscus or an anastomotic breakdown that is successfully walled off by peritoneal defense mechanisms. Visceral abscesses are most commonly due to hematogenous or lymphatic spread of bacteria to the organ. Retroperitoneal abscesses may originate through several mechanisms, including perforation of the gastrointestinal tract into the retroperitoneum or hematogenous or lymphatic spread of bacteria to retroperitoneal organs, as occurs in the setting of pancreatitis.

Abscesses most commonly arise following an abdominal operation. Such postoperative abscesses account for 46 to 74 percent of all cases.[275,276] Most (over 30 percent) postoperative abscesses are due to a documented anastomotic leak. The predominance of these abscesses occur after colorectal surgery[277] (Table 38–6), reflecting the large bacterial inoculum from a leak in the distal gut. Diverticular disease, appendicitis, inflammatory bowel disease, and perforated colonic carcinomas account for the remainder. The incidence is changing, with a notable decrease in the number of patients presenting with appendiceal abscess and an increase in those patients with diverticular abscesses.

TABLE 38–6. INCIDENCE OF POSTOPERATIVE ABSCESS FORMATION IN RELATION TO SITE OF INITIAL OPERATION

Site of Initial Operation	Incidence of Postoperative Abscess (%)
Colorectal	30
Urologic	19
Gastric	15
Pancreatic/biliary	15
Small bowel	5
Appendiceal	5
Esophageal	4
Splenic	3
Gynecologic	2

Adapted from Olson MM, Allen MO: Arch Surg 124:356. 1989.

Anatomy of Abscess Formation

Intraperitoneal Spaces. The posterior peritoneal reflections and mesenteric attachments of the intra-abdominal viscera divide the intraperitoneal space into anatomic areas where abscesses can form (Figs. 38–3, 38–4, and 38–5).[278] The transverse mesocolon divides the peritoneal cavity posteriorly into an upper and lower space. The greater omentum lies immediately adjacent to the anterior abdominal wall and functionally completes the division. The lower peritoneal space is, in turn, divided into right upper and left lower portions by the diagonal origin of the small bowel mesentery.

The intraperitoneal circulation described previously follows the pattern shown in Figure 38–4.[278,279] The most dependent recess is the pelvis, where the pouch of Douglas lies between the rectum and the body of the uterus, and the perirectal and perivesical fossae lie lateral to the rectum and bladder. The peritoneal circulation favors unilateral spread of exudate because the phrenocolic ligament, which spans the diaphragm, spleen, and splenic flexure of the colon, interrupts the flow into the left subphrenic space during respiration (see Fig. 38–4).[279] Left subphrenic abscesses are therefore commonly associated with retrogastric (lesser sac) lesions. Bilateral subphrenic abscesses are uncommon since the right and left subhepatic spaces are separated by the falciform ligament. The left subhepatic space is divided by the gastrohepatic omentum into an anterior space and a lesser sac (see Figs. 38–4 and 38–5). Abscesses can form in any of these areas.

The lesser sac communicates with the general peritoneal cavity via the foramen of Winslow between the free border of the gastrohepatic omentum

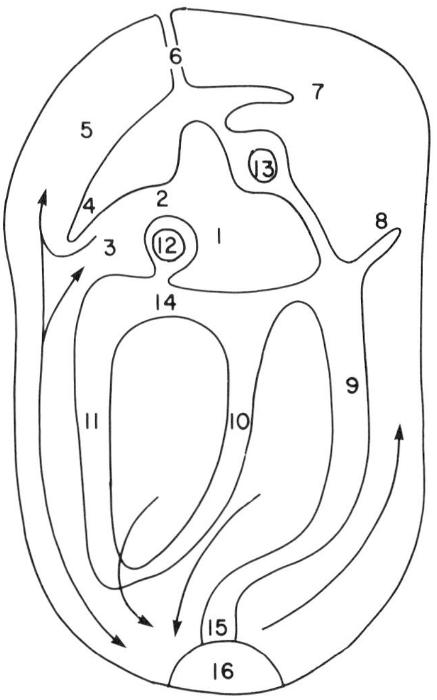

Figure 38–4. Schematic diagram of the posterior peritoneal reflections and recesses of the peritoneal cavity. *1.* Lesser sac. *2.* Foramen of Winslow. *3.* Morison's pouch. *4.* Right triangular ligament. *5.* Right subphrenic space. *6.* Falciform ligament. *7.* Left subphrenic space. *8.* Phrenicolic ligament. *9.* Bare area of the descending colon. *10.* Root of the small bowel mesentery. *11.* Bare area of ascending colon. *12.* Duodenum. *13.* Esophagus. *14.* Root of the transverse mesocolon. *15.* Bare area of rectum. *16.* Bladder. *(From Levison ME: In Mandell GL, Douglas RG Jr, Bernett JE (eds): Principles and Practice of Infectious Diseases, Vol 1. New York, Wiley, 1979, p 609.)*

and the posterior parietal peritoneum. The opening is small, so visceral perforations elsewhere in the peritoneal cavity rarely produce suppuration of the lesser sac.

Primary lesser sac abscesses can spread downward via the foramen of Winslow, across the hepatic flexure of the colon into the right gutter, and then upward into the subphrenic space. The movement of water-soluble contrast material selectively injected into various intraperitoneal spaces is depicted in Figure 38–4.[279] The mobility of the small bowel tends to limit the accumulation of fluid in the central portion of the peritoneal cavity under normal circumstances. However, truly massive abscesses (horseshoe abscesses) may extend down one gutter to the pelvis and up the opposite side.[280] Pelvic abscesses occur below the brim of the true pelvis.

Retroperitoneal Spaces. There is a potential space between the peritoneum and the transversalis fascia that extends from the diaphragm superiorly to the brim of the true pelvis inferiorly and to the lateral borders of the quadratus lumborum muscles.[280,281] The retroperitoneal space extends across the midline, but most infections are unilateral.

The renal fascia surrounding the kidneys and enclosing the great vessels separates the retroperitoneal space into anterior and posterior compartments (see Fig. 38–5). The anterior retroperitoneal

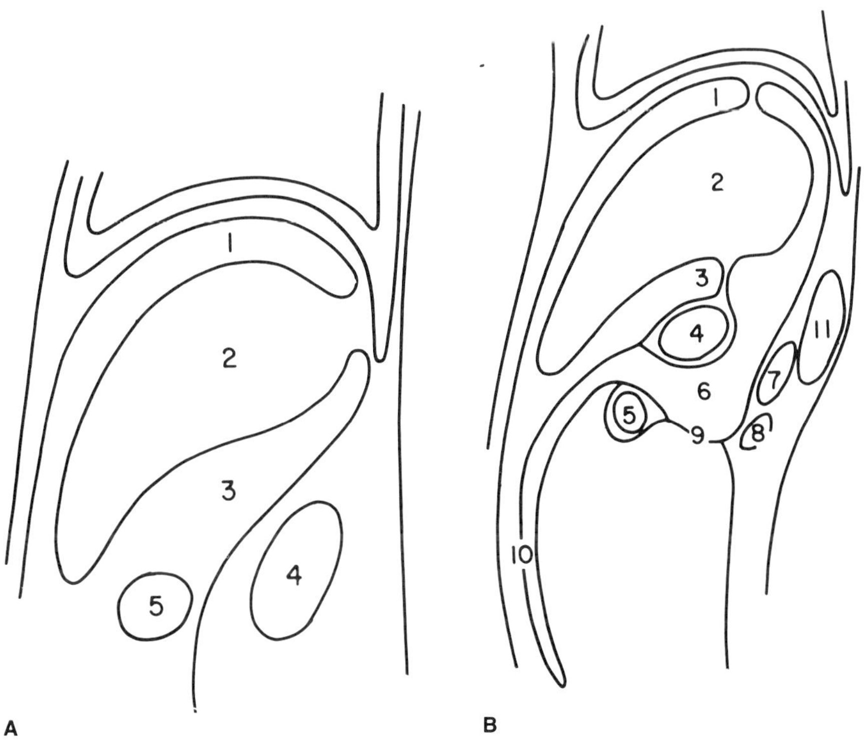

Figure 38–5. Schema of a sagittal section of the peritoneal cavity. **A.** Right upper quadrant. *1.* Subphrenic space. *2.* Liver. *3.* Subhepatic space. *4.* Right kidney. *5.* Transverse colon. **B.** Left upper quadrant. *1.* Subphrenic space. *2.* Liver, left lobe. *3.* Subhepatic space. *4.* Stomach. *5.* Transverse colon. *6.* Lesser sac. *7.* Pancreas. *8.* Duodenum. *9.* Transverse mesocolon. *10.* Omentum. *11.* Left kidney. *(From Levison ME: In Mandell GL, Douglas RG Jr, Bernett JF (eds): Principles and Practice of Infectious Diseases, Vol 1. New York, Wiley, 1979, p 609.)*

space is bordered by the posterior peritoneum and the anterior portion of the renal fascia (Fig. 38–6).[282] The posterior peritoneal space is subdivided into superior and inferior divisions by the posterior leaf of the renal fascia. The renal compartment of the posterior retroperitoneal space is closed superiorly and open inferiorly, favoring the downward spread of infection.

The retrofascial space is posterior to the transversalis fascia and encloses the dorsal spine and muscles. It is not strictly a part of the retroperitoneal space but is included in most studies because its position is truly retroperitoneal.

The anterior retroperitoneal space contains the esophagus, duodenum, pancreas, bile duct, portal and splenic veins, appendix, ascending and descending colon, and rectosigmoid. The posterior (perinephric) space contains the kidneys, ureters, gonadal vessels, aorta, inferior cava, and lymph nodes. The retrofascial (ileopsoas) space encloses the twelfth rib, spine, and paraspinous muscles. Rarely, an extraperitoneal perforation of a viscus such as a perforated colonic diverticulum or carcinoma may tract down along the psoas in association with the femoral neurovascular complex and produce an abscess in the thigh.

Microbiology. The bacteria that cause intra-abdominal abscesses are similar to those that cause secondary bacterial peritonitis and thus represent a mix of anaerobic and aerobic gut flora (Table 38–7). In the postoperative patient, resistant gram-negative organisms may be present, due to the use of empiric broad spectrum antibiotics in the preoperative setting. Additionally, such organisms may develop when antibiotics are used empirically for postoperative febrile episodes in attempt to "treat the fever" rather than drain the abscess.

Clinical Manifestations. Diffuse generalized peritonitis usually produces such intense abdominal symptoms that the diagnosis is obvious, but intra-abdominal abscesses frequently have less impressive findings. Enteroparietal abscesses produce pain, tenderness, and a palpable, diffuse abdominal mass. Interloop, intramesenteric, and subphrenic abscesses are more cryptic because the visceral peritoneum is innervated by splanchnic rather than somatic pain fibers, and no mass can be palpated. Additionally, patients with subphrenic abscesses may have hiccups, cough, tachypnea, or jaundice.[283] Nonspecific thoracic manifestations include pleural effusions, elevation of the diaphragm, and decreased basilar breath sounds.[284,285] Retroperitoneal abscesses may only produce lumbar or ileopsoas muscle spasm. Chronic psoas abscesses may present with an irritable hip and back pain with a flexion deformity of the hip and wasting of the

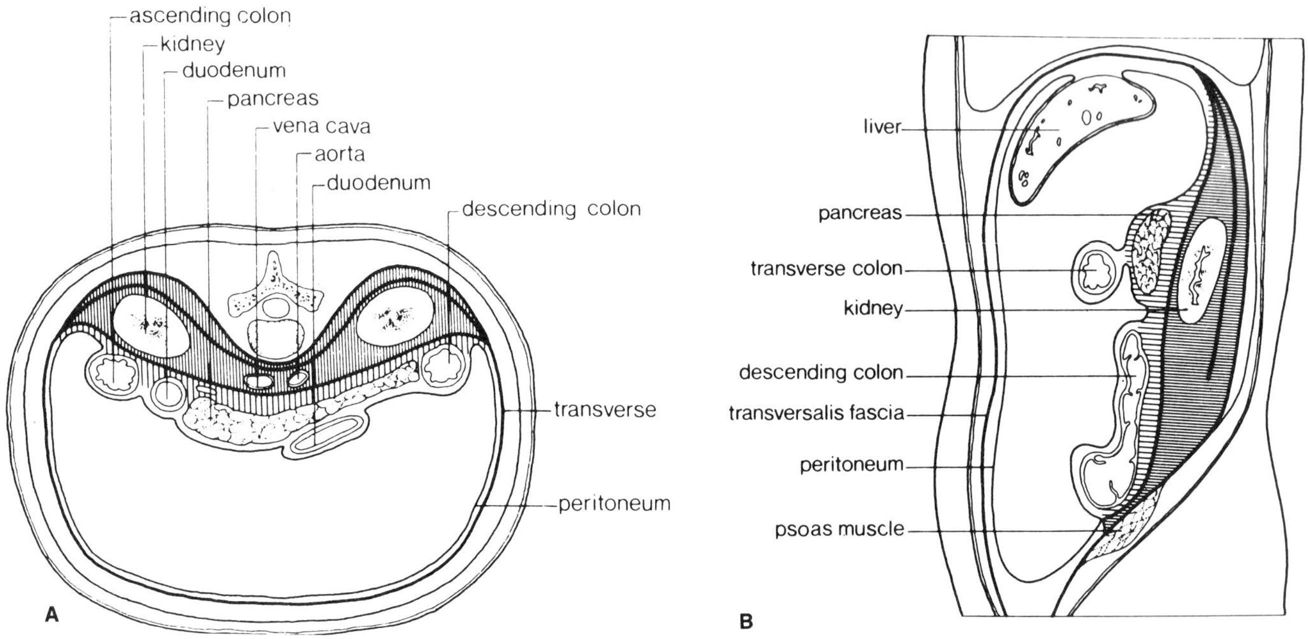

Figure 38–6. Details of the retroperitoneal space. **A.** Cross section. **B.** Sagittal section. Note the anterior compartment and the perinephric-perivascular posterior compartment. The retroperitoneal muscles are not strictly considered part of the retroperitoneum. *(From Goris RJA, Lubbers EJC, Oostveen HW, van den Dries ACP: In de Boer HHM (ed): Intraabdominal Sepsis. Utrecht, Bunge Scientific Publishers, 1979, p 47.)*

TABLE 38–7. MICROBIOLOGIC FLORA OF INTRA-ABDOMINAL ABSCESSES

Organisms	Olson et al 1989	Olak et al 1986
Aerobes only	58%	75%
Anaerobes only	9%	—
Mixed aerobic/anaerobic	33%	24%
Escherichia coli	38%	46%
Enterococcus	38%	25%
Bacteroides	31%	17%
Klebsiella	19%	39%
Pseudomonas	17%	9.3%
Candida species	14.7%	9.3%
Enterobacter	12.5%	9.3%
Serratia	11.3%	—
Proteus	8%	3.7%
Clostridium	10.2%	7.4%
Staphylococcus epidermidis	4.6%	13%
S. aureus	1.1%	5.6%

Adapted from Olson MM, Allen MO: Arch Surg 124:356, 1989; and Olak J, Christou NV, Stein LA, et al: Arch Surg 121:141, 1986.

quadriceps femoris.[286] Pelvic abscesses can be palpated on rectal examination but usually give few symptoms. Occasionally, diarrhea may be the presenting symptom due to irritability of the sigmoid colon as a result of the adjacent abscess.

Constitutional symptoms such as anorexia and malaise are frequent. Systemic signs of inflammation such as fevers and chills are often present. Laboratory investigation adds little to confirm the diagnosis. Leukocytosis with a left shift may be noted.

In the postoperative patient, the abdominal symptoms are masked by incisional pain, postoperative analgesics, and the reluctance of the surgeon to admit the possibility of a complication. Physical examination is notoriously unreliable in this period—all patients are distended and tender. Additionally, the clinical findings associated with an intra-abdominal abscess may be masked by the administration of antibiotics to the patient. The median time from initial operation to clinical presentation in a series of 114 abscesses was 8 days.[277] In this same series, the median time from presentation of abscess symptoms to drainage was 4 days. As noted previously, in the face of antibiotic therapy, the presence of a fever and/or a leukocytosis with more than a 3 percent band count is highly indicative of persistent sepsis and should direct the physician to more intensive radiologic investigation.[124,125] At times, the first sign of postoperative abscess formation may be progressive organ dysfunction leading to multiple organ failure.[174]

Diagnosis. Diagnosis is based on clinical suspicion of an abscess and radiologic confirmation. Conventional plain film radiographs of the abdomen may reveal loculated extraluminal gas collections or mottled soft tissue masses, either of which is indicative of abscess formation. More subtle signs include the presence of a localized ileus, or obliteration of the psoas shadow or flank stripes. Chest x-ray examinations may document the presence of a pleural effusion or atelectasis, suggesting the presence of a subphrenic collection.[287]

The availability of modern imaging techniques such as ultrasonography and computed tomography has revolutionized both the diagnosis and treatment of intra-abdominal abscesses. Ultrasonography (US) is rapid and noninvasive and does not expose the patient to further irradiation. The availability of mobile machines permits bedside and intraoperative examination. The test can be completed and interpreted within an hour. The disadvantages of the system are that it requires an intact abdominal wall overlying the abscess. Thus it is difficult to study patients with drains, open wounds, or stomas because of the lack of acoustic windows. The presence of an intestinal ileus usually reduces the sensitivity of an ultrasound examination, as its images may be obscured by gas. These problems are particularly relevant in the postoperative critically ill patient with an ileus and multiple operative interventions. Additionally, the examination is extremely operator dependent and requires interpretation. Reports of the sensitivity and specificity of US in detection of intra-abdominal abscesses usually are in the range of 80 to 90 percent, depending on the site of the abscess and skill of the operator.[288,289] The use of endoluminal probes allows transvaginal or transrectal visualization and drainage of deep pelvic abscesses, an advantage not offered by other techniques.[290,291]

Computed tomography (CT) has several advantages over the use of US and proves to be the most accurate technique available for the diagnosis of intra-abdominal abscesses.[288,292] Knochel et al[288] documented a sensitivity of 97.5 percent and specificity of 85 percent. Its advantages include higher resolution, little need for operator skill in interpretation, and an ability to see deep to bone and gas-filled structures without the need for an intact abdominal wall. It has proved excellent in visualizing the retroperitoneum, a distinct disadvantage noted with US. Optimal detection by CT scan depends on the administration of intravenous contrast material and gastrointestinal contrast to opacify bowel. Gastrointestinal contrast improves the differentiation of fluid-filled bowel from an abscess. However, interloop abscesses, which represent approximately 4 percent of all abscesses, remain poorly visualized on CT scan.[293]

Radionuclide scanning techniques using either gallium-67 citrate or indium-111 have been used in the diagnosis of intra-abdominal abscesses. Gallium has an affinity for iron-binding proteins present on leukocytes and on bacterial surfaces and thus is concentrated at sites of infection.[294] The detection of an abscess is based on increased uptake outside expected sites. However, gallium is excreted in the colon and accumulates in the stool. Frequently, an enema is necessary to clear radiolabeled stool before scanning to allow for proper interpretation of the study. Other disadvantages of this technique include the false-positive imaging of neoplasms and the 24- to 72-hour delay required between injection of the radionuclide and the scanning procedure.

In a white blood cell scan, indium-111 in the form of the chelate indium-111 oxyquinoline is used to label leukocytes drawn from the patient.[288,295] After labeling, the cells are reinjected into the patient, and the patient is scanned with a gamma camera. A major shortcoming associated with this technique is the significant number of false-negative results in patients with chronic infections, which are less likely to lead to accumulation of acute inflammatory cells.[288] Neither indium-111 nor gallium-67 scans are effective in the early postoperative period. Peritoneal inflammation at this time will attract the isotopes, and all sites at which dissection has occurred will show isotope localization. Patients more than 2 weeks postoperatively, when acute inflammation has quiesced, may benefit from these scanning techniques.[296]

Treatment. The three basic principles guiding the management of intra-abdominal abscesses include (1) supportive care, (2) antibiotic administration, and (3) drainage—percutaneous or operative.

SUPPORTIVE CARE. Patients with intra-abdominal abscess show a spectrum of clinical presentations, ranging from relatively well with low-grade fever to those with septic shock. In general, these patients have intravascular volume depletion that calls for fluid resuscitation and monitoring. The intensity of resuscitation and monitoring depends on the status of the patient. Vital signs, urine output, and mental status should be monitored hourly if necessary. In the critically ill individual, Swan–Ganz catheterization and invasive arterial monitoring are essential to direct initial resuscitation, particularly if administration of inotropic agents is necessary.

Hypoxemia may be present for several reasons. Atelectasis, basilar pneumonia, and pleural effusions may exist secondary to abdominal distention and elevation of the diaphragm or a subdiaphragmatic inflammatory process. If the process is advanced, early signs of organ dysfunction may develop in the form of the adult respiratory distress syndrome or renal dysfunction, both of which may cause significant management problems. Intubation and mechanical ventilation may be required to maintain adequate oxygenation.

Nutritional support is important to prevent further debilitation. Patients in whom abscesses develop in the postoperative period are already at a nutritional disadvantage because they have usually spent 7 to 10 days without adequate caloric intake. The marked catabolic response associated with sepsis further aggravates this problem. If tolerated, the enteral route is preferred.[297,298]

ANTIBIOTICS. Antibiotic therapy should be directed against the microorganisms most likely to be recovered from the abscess, which almost always include a combination of aerobic and anaerobic bacteria. As for secondary peritonitis, administration of antibiotic combinations or single agents that are active against both aerobes and anaerobes is necessary to achieve optimal coverage.

General supportive management and antibiotic therapy serve primarily as adjuncts to drainage of the abscess cavity. Antibiotics are unlikely to be effective for numerous reasons, including poor penetration of antibiotics into the abscess center, inactivation of antibiotics in the microenvironment of infection, and inactivity of the drug against a large bacterial inoculum[299] (Table 38–8). Drainage of an abscess usually reverses these adverse effects and increases the efficacy of the antibiotics.

DRAINAGE

PERCUTANEOUS DRAINAGE. Over the last 10 years, there has been an increasing trend toward percutaneous drainage of intra-abdominal abscesses. The original criteria for percutaneous abscess drainage were limited to well-defined, uniloculated collections without evidence of enteral communication and required a drainage route not traversing uncontaminated viscera.[300] The increasing experience of invasive radiologists and improved imaging techniques have recently permitted a liberalization of the indications for percutaneous abscess drainage. Percutaneous drainage has now become the treatment of choice in the majority of cases. The best results have been achieved for single well-defined

TABLE 38–8. ADVERSE EFFECTS OF THE MICROENVIRONMENT OF ABSCESSES ON HOST IMMUNE FUNCTION

Factor	Effect
Hypoxia	Impaired neutrophil migration and killing, reduced aminoglycoside activity
Low pH	Impaired neutrophil migration and killing, reduced aminoglycoside activity
Large numbers of stationary phase bacteria	Reduced antibiotic efficacy due to inoculum effect and absence of bacterial proliferation
High concentration of bacterial by-products, components, and toxins	Impaired phagocytic cell function, local tissue damage, complement depletion
Necrotic debris	Neutrophil deactivation, complement depletion
Fibrin	Reduced access of cells to bacteria, impaired microbicidal killing

Adapted from Rotstein OD, Brisseau GF: The microenvironment of infection. In Fry DE (ed): Surgical Infection. Boston, Little, Brown (in press).

abscesses without evidence of enteric connection, with no adjacent tumor and no tissue necrosis, defined as *simple abscesses.* Multiple or multiloculated abscesses, those that form a fistula to surrounding organs or bowel, and abscesses containing viscous fluid, debris, or necrotic material are defined as *complex.*[301] These were formerly thought to be absolute contraindications to catheter drainage, but successful percutaneous management of even these entities is being regularly reported.[302–304]

Percutaneous abscess drainage was initially performed as a two-stage procedure by first locating the abscess with US or CT scan and then transferring the patient to a fluoroscopy suite for catheter insertion. Presently, guidance has become a one-stage procedure performed entirely with CT scan or US, reducing the need to move the patient with the inherent risk of guidewire displacement. Intravenous antibiotics are administered prior to the procedure. Percutaneous drainage is accomplished by a modified Seldinger technique. A fine needle (22 or 20 gauge) is guided into the collection initially both for localization and for aspiration of a sample of fluid. Following this, a guidewire is placed through the needle into the cavity and then an 8.3F-14F catheter is placed into the cavity over the guidewire, and the latter is then removed. There are very little data to support the notion that larger tubes (more than 14F) lead to more effective drainage. The principal determinant of efficacy is the presence of multiple large side holes that do not become plugged with the abscess contents.[305]

Once in place, catheters are either placed to gravity drainage or to low suction. Saline irrigation on a daily basis should be used to maintain catheter patency. Weekly sinograms and/or imaging with CT or US are useful for follow-up of cavity size as well as to determine whether any enteral communication exists. Criteria for removal of the percutaneous catheter are (1) clinical resolution of sepsis as determined by defervescence, normalization of leukocyte count, and return of appetite, (2) the purulent drainage changes to small amounts of clear, serous fluid; and (3) radiologic evidence of resolution of abscess on sinogram or CT scan.[25] At this point, the catheter can be withdrawn slowly over 1 or 2 days.

A poor clinical response indicates ineffective drainage due to either inadequate catheter size or position, an undrained area of contiguous abscess, a large enteric communication, or the presence of a second abscess. If the patient has not improved markedly by 48 hours after initial percutaneous drainage, another CT scan should be performed. Any residual abscesses can then be percutaneously drained or the catheter repositioned as necessary. However, if there is residual infection that cannot be adequately drained, or if no residual collections are found, then consideration should be given to performing a formal laparotomy. The surgeon must be wary of unwarranted delay of surgical drainage despite failed attempts at percutaneous drainage. If an attempt at percutaneous drainage is unsuccessful, there is little to be gained by temporizing.

Successful percutaneous abscess drainage has been redefined and is divided into two categories.[306] *Curative success* refers to complete cure with drainage such that no further operative or percutaneous management is necessary. *Palliative success* implies the use of percutaneous drainage in cases where cure is impossible such as an unresectable, infected tumor mass or, more frequently, as a temporizing measure to stabilize the patient prior to definitive operative management. Flancbaum et al[302] described a series of 14 patients, all of whom had intra-abdominal abscesses as a result of a perforated viscus who were treated initially with percutaneous abscess drainage, thus obviating the first stage of the traditional two-stage surgical approach. For treatment of peridiverticular abscess, the need for two- or three-stage surgical procedures can be reduced or eliminated. Bowel resection and primary anastomosis can be accomplished at operation in an elective setting after percutaneous abscess drainage in 66 to 74 percent of patients.[307,308]

With an overall success rate of 81 to 89 percent, percutaneous abscess drainage compares favorably to most surgical series and is somewhat dependent on the type, location, and etiology of the abscess(es).[301,309–313] Simple abscesses are successfully drained in 82 to 95 percent of cases, whereas complex collections are associated with a 45 to 69 percent success rate. There is an increased risk of failure when the collection occurs as a result of hematoma, foreign body, fungal infections, or necrotic tissue.[301,306] Malangoni et al[314] noted that complex abscesses were treated successfully more often by operative than by percutaneous methods, in contrast to the equivalent results achieved with simple collections. Complications occur in 5 to 10 percent of cases and include systemic sepsis, soft tissue infection of the abdominal wall, hemorrhage, diffuse contamination of the peritoneal or thoracic cavity, pneumothorax, and fistula formation.[301,310]

OPERATIVE DRAINAGE. Prior to the advent of percutaneous drainage, the controversy regarding extraserous versus transperitoneal drainage of intra-abdominal abscesses engendered much debate. Advocates of the extraserous approach cited a reduction in peritoneal contamination, fistula rate, and hemorrhagic complications.[315] Those favoring transperitoneal drainage have noted the high rate of multiple abscesses in patients and the increased mortality rate associated with inadequate drainage of these missed abscesses.[312,316,317] Furthermore, the transperitoneal approach allows for identification and management of the inciting cause of the abscess.

This debate is now moot. Improved imaging modalities such as computed tomography and ultrasound have reduced the likelihood of missing abscesses to under 5 percent.[288,292] Percutaneous drainage is analogous to a nonoperative extraserosal approach without the disadvantage of missing a second potentially drainable collection. Presently, the controversy revolves around percutaneous drainage and transperitoneal drainage. Clearly, operative drainage should be undertaken when an abscess is inaccessibly deep and the radiologist feels there is no safe route to drain it percutaneously. Ill-defined or multiple abscesses often require full exploration to ensure adequate drainage of all collections and control of the inciting process. Additionally, failure of the patient to improve after percutaneous drainage may reflect the presence of an infected phlegmon, which may not be adequately evacuated using percutaneous methods.[318] Finally, fluid collections developing in the early postoperative period (less than 72 hours) are usually not amenable to percutaneous treatment, since the collection is rarely localized. This frequently represents an anastomotic dehiscence, which requires surgical intervention to deal with the bowel as well as the extensive dissemination of intestinal contents.

Prognosis. The mortality rate attributable to intra-abdominal abscesses is difficult to discern due to the degree of heterogeneity in these patients. Furthermore, the literature does not differentiate the prognoses from abscesses versus peritonitis. In a series of 143 patients over a 5-year period, Fry et al[312] reported a mortality of 32 percent. Determinants of death were the presence of organ failure, lesser sac or subphrenic abscesses, positive blood cultures, recurrent or multiple abscesses, and age over 50. In this series, abscesses occurring as a result of appendicitis or perforated ulcers were excluded. Fry attributed the deaths to inadequate drainage and failure of host defense mechanisms. Olson and Allen[277] documented that persistent abscesses were present in 41 percent of patients at autopsy, again implicating inadequate drainage as a contributing factor to mortality.

Deveney et al[275] compared the mortality in two series of patients. Thirty-one patients treated for intra-abdominal abscesses between 1973 and 1978 before the use of computed tomography, ultrasonography, and percutaneous drainage were compared to 66 patients treated between 1981 and 1986, when these modalities were available. Mortality was less in the second group of patients (21 versus 39 percent). This decreased mortality was accompanied by a greater proportion of patients with predrainage localization, successful initial drainage, and a decreased incidence of predrainage organ failure. There was no difference in mortality in those patients in the latter group treated with percutaneous drainage or laparotomy, suggesting that the reduction in mortality was entirely attributable to earlier and more precise localization rather than to the particular drainage technique used.[275]

INTRA-ABDOMINAL FISTULA

It is important to distinguish between intra-abdominal infections that are fed by continuous contamination in the form of a fistula, and those that result from a single episode of contamination. A fistula is an abnormal communication between two epithelialized surfaces. The tract may be lined by epithelium but usually consists of granulation tissue. Fistulas are frequently found in association with intra-abdominal infection and, as an ongoing source of peritoneal contamination, may result in recurrent or persistent abscess formation.

Intestinal fistulas can be *internal* or *external* (enterocutaneous). Internal fistulas connect two organs of the same or different systems, whereas external fistulas connect the gut, directly or indirectly, with the body surface. External fistulas are further described according to their output. A *high-output* fistula discharges more than 500 ml/day as effluent, whereas a *low-output* fistula discharges a smaller volume. *End fistulas* are those arising from a hollow viscus where there is no further gastrointestinal tract continuity, effectively forming an ostomy. *Lateral fistulas* are those originating in partial defects of the gastrointestinal tract.

Etiology. Fistulas are either congenital or acquired. A patent vitellointestinal duct is an example of the former. Its presence is marked by persistent drainage rather than intra-abdominal infection and, as such, will not be discussed further. The vast majority of fistulas occur as the result of acquired conditions, either due to spontaneous disease processes or iatrogenic injury on the part of the surgeon[319] (Table 38–9). Regardless of the etiology, fistulas arise by one or more of several mechanisms[319]: (1) penetrating trauma, including operation with simultaneous perforation of intestine and an adjacent structure; (2) inflammatory adherence with degeneration of the common wall; (3) perforation of the gastrointestinal tract with abscess formation that subsequently perforates adjacent structures; or (4) an abscess outside the gastrointestinal tract that perforates into the intestine.

Any intrinsic intestinal parasites that elicit necrosis or granulomatous host reactions can lead to fistula formation. Table 38–10 lists some of these rare infectious causes that will require special treatment.[319] Many are not considered preoperatively and the diagnosis is usually made after resection or biopsy of the fistula tract.

Spontaneous Fistula

Not uncommonly, fistulas occur as a result of subacute perforation of the gastrointestinal tract. Host defenses localize the perforation, with the formation of an abscess. The abscess then spontaneously drains externally, as occurs with a colovaginal or colovesical fistula due to a paracolic abscess secondary to diverticulitis. Alternatively, the fistula may not be discovered until the abscess is evacuated and the cavity continues to drain gastrointestinal contents.

Fistulas occurring as a result of Crohn's disease are very common. The transmural penetration of the fissures characteristic of the disease results in localized perforations of the bowel wall and ab-

TABLE 38–9. FISTULAS: ETIOLOGY AND CLASSIFICATION

- I. Congenital
- II. Acquired
  - Spontaneous
    - Infectious
      - Intrinsic
      - Extrinsic
    - Inflammatory
      - Inflammatory bowel disease
    - Neoplastic
      - Benign
      - Malignant
    - Traumatic
      - Blunt
      - Penetrating
      - Foreign body
        - Cholelithiasis\choledocholithiasis
      - Irradiation
  - Iatrogenic
    - Intentional
      - Enteroenterostomy, gastroenterostomy
    - Unintentional
      - Inadvertent enterotomy
      - Serosal tear
      - Technically poor anastomosis
        - Impaired vascular supply
        - Tension
      - Suture line defects
      - Drains

Adapted from Webster MW Jr, Cary LC: Curr Probl Surg 13:5, 1976; and Rubelowsky J, Machiedo GW: Surg Clin North Am 71:147, 1991.

TABLE 38–10. RARE PRIMARY INFECTIOUS ETIOLOGIES OF INTRA-ABDOMINAL FISTULAS

Site	Infectious Etiology
Enterocutaneous	Tuberculosis, amebiasis, actinomycosis
Enteroenteric	Tuberculosis, typhoid, syphilis
Enterorespiratory	Tuberculosis, histoplasmosis, actinomycosis, nonspecific adenitis, syphilis, aortic aneurysm, gumma
Biliorespiratory and biliopericardial	Amebiasis, echinococcosis
Nephro or ureteroenteric	Tuberculosis, echinococcosis, bilharziasis
Enteropericardial	Tuberculous adenitis

Adapted from Webster MW Jr, Carey LC: Curr Probl Surg 13:5, 1976.

scess formation. As shown previously, it is the spontaneous or induced drainage of these abscesses that leads to the formation of fistulas.

Malignancy may result in the formation of fistulas following direct invasion into adjacent viscera. Common examples of this type of fistula are the gastrocolic fistula produced by extension of a carcinoma of the stomach and colovesical fistula from extension of a sigmoid carcinoma. Alternatively, malignant perforation of the gastrointestinal tract may occur, leading to subsequent abscess and fistula formation.

Foreign bodies, such as a gallstone, may induce the formation of a fistula as a result of pressure necrosis and perforation into an adjacent hollow viscus. The chronic inflammatory process associated with cholelithiasis facilitates this process, resulting in either a cholecystoduodenal or cholecystocholedochal fistula.

Radiation enteritis is strongly associated with the formation of fistulas. Spontaneous fistula may develop in up to 6 percent of patients after radiotherapy.[320] Over 30 percent of such patients develop enterocutaneous fistula postlaparotomy.[321]

Iatrogenic Fistula

Gastrointestinal fistulas occur most commonly as a result of technical errors due to careless dissection of adhesions leading to unrecognized enterotomies, devascularization of the gut wall, or anastomotic leakage. Additionally, poor placement of drains may impair healing of enterotomy sites or erode into normal bowel. When the intestinal breakdown is so sudden that no preexisting peritoneal inflammation has taken place, diffuse peritonitis will result. However, the inflammatory process and perforation usually occur over several days, and an abscess develops. A fistula forms once the collection either spontaneously drains through the wound or is identified as a postoperative complication and is then drained.

The risk of postoperative fistula formation is related to both site-specific and patient-specific factors. These factors will be outlined below.

Esophageal Surgery. The well-developed defense mechanisms of the peritoneal cavity make intraperitoneal sites rather resistant to anastomotic breakdown. The esophagus is prone to anastomotic dehiscence because of its extraperitoneal location, the absence of a well-developed seromuscular layer to hold sutures, and tension across the anastomosis. Presternal esophagogastrostomies have a higher incidence of fistula formation compared to retrosternal anastomoses. End-to-side esophagogastrostomy and esophagojejunostomy have lower leakage rates than end-to-end anastomosis, probably because tension is less frequent with the end-to-side anastomoses. Colon interposition for total esophageal replacement is frequently followed by an anastomotic leak in the neck.[322]

Gastric Surgery. Gastrostomy sites frequently (6 to 10 percent) become persistent fistulas after removal of the gastrostomy tube.[319] Anastomotic leakage is common acutely after gastric bypass for obesity because swallowed air can readily distend the partially devascularized proximal gastric pouch and rupture a suture line if the nasogastric tube fails to function. Gastrojejunostomy with or without antrectomy has a low anastomotic leak rate.[323]

The blown duodenal stump is a feared complication after gastrectomy and Billroth II reconstruction, since one-half of the deaths after gastrectomy are caused by this complication.[324] Suture line failures account for the majority of these fistulas, and the operative report usually notes that stump closure was difficult. The incidence of leak is decreasing, however. Soeters et al[323] reported that only 0.6 percent of 280 gastrectomy patients operated on between 1960 and 1975 developed fistulas.

Duodenal Fistula. The lateral duodenal fistula arising with the duodenum in continuity (ie, after blunt trauma or unrecognized operative duodenal perforation) has traditionally been considered a more serious complication.[325] Rarely, perforation of a duodenal diverticulum may be the cause. These fistulas have a serious prognosis because all the gastric and duodenal contents exit into the fistula site, whereas only biliary and pancreatic secretions are lost to the skin surface from the end fistula after a Billroth II reconstruction.

Small Bowel Fistula. Fistulas from the small bowel are typically iatrogenic, but the incidence is increased by intrinsic bowel disease, such as Crohn's disease, or radiation injury. Early suture closure of traumatic small bowel perforation rarely results in a fistula. Proximal small bowel fistulas typically have a high output and may present very difficult management problems.

Colonic Surgery. Colonic anastomotic leaks are decreasing in frequency. Intraperitoneal anastomoses have a lower fistula rate than do extraperitoneal anastomoses. A rate as high as 50 percent has been reported in low anterior anastomoses studied routinely with radiocontrast enemas in the early postoperative period.[326] Clinical leakage rates after such anastomoses are much lower (10 to 30 percent). The use of the automatic circumferential stapling device for the creation of low anterior anastomoses has further reduced the fistula rate (1.1 percent).[327]

Patient-Specific Factors. Any factor that adversely affects wound healing, such as chronic corticosteroid use, malnutrition, vitamin deficiency, or diabetes mellitus, can increase the risk of fistula formation. Local factors that impair wound healing, such as an impaired blood supply due to atherosclerosis, radiation fibrosis, or hypovolemic shock, also markedly increase the risk of fistulas. Hermreck and Crawford[328] found that anastomotic leak occurred in 80 percent of patients who developed a period of shock after esophageal surgery versus an 8 percent leak rate in patients not experiencing shock.

Clinical Manifestations. Table 38–11 lists the clinical problems created by gastrointestinal fistulas. The septic problems will be emphasized, since these may be life-threatening, and the other problems frequently persist even after the infectious element is controlled. Acute acquired fistulas due to operative or accidental trauma present with the general symptoms and signs of a cryptic intra-abdominal abscess. Fever, leukocytosis, prolonged ileus, and poorly localized abdominal pain are characteristic.[329] Signs consistent with partial intestinal obstruction are common. Steadily increasing drainage from a drain site may be found, but more often a wound infection is opened only to subsequently drain enteric contents. Occasionally, patients will rapidly improve after drainage is established, but, more often, the patient continues to look and feel ill. This correlates with the degree of pooling within the abscess cavity. The most proximal small bowel fistulas are usually the most symptomatic because of the corrosive nature of pancreatic-duodenal contents. Activated pancreatic exocrine secretions can digest both the external skin and peritoneal surfaces. Acute internal fistulas will resemble abscesses unless by chance they decompress themselves into adjacent organs.[330] If enteroenteric or biliary enteric fistulas result, the diagnosis may be delayed until symptoms of malabsorption appear. Spontaneous drainage of intra-abdominal contents into the bronchial tree, renal pelvis, or bladder may occasionally be life-threatening.

TABLE 38–11. COMPLICATIONS AND CLINICAL MANIFESTATIONS OF ENTEROCUTANEOUS FISTULAS

• NUTRITIONAL	• SEPTIC
Dehydration	Peritonitis
Electrolye disturbances	Abscess
Malnutrition	Systemic sepsis
Vitamin deficiencies	Multiple organ dysfunction
Trace element deficiencies	
• TPN RELATED (CHRONIC)	• LOCAL
Catheter-related sepsis	Bleeding
TPN cholestasis	Skin excoriation
Venous thrombosis	Wound dehiscence

Diagnosis. The diagnosis of enterocutaneous fistulas is usually readily apparent when enteric contents appear at the skin surface. Sinograms and enteric contrast studies usually are successful in outlining the tract, diagnosing abscesses that lie along it, and establishing their origin. The oral administration of methylene blue or powdered charcoal may document a fistula in doubtful cases, whereas water-soluble contrast materials available sometimes fail to detail all anatomic defects. Chemical analysis of the drainage fluid is sometimes valuable in determining its source (eg, amylase, bilirubin, creatinine).

Certain points regarding the diagnostic approach to fistulas are to be emphasized. The information obtained will determine whether conservative or urgent surgical management is required. Investigation should be centered on determining the origin of the fistula as well as the presence or absence of distal obstruction. Furthermore, information regarding the condition of the bowel around and distal to the fistula is important. The noninvasive methods previously described for the diagnosis of intra-abdominal abscesses can all be useful. Because complete distal obstruction or anastomotic dehiscence virtually precludes spontaneous closure, early surgical intervention must be undertaken when investigations document their presence.

Treatment. The therapeutic approach to an intestinal fistula is outlined in the following points.[329] The urgency of any intervention is dictated by the problems that threaten the patient.

1. Correct the fluid and electrolyte imbalances. These are especially troublesome in upper intestinal fistulas from which fluid losses can be enormous.
2. Control infection by early adequate drainage of the tract and of any abscess cavities. Reber et al[331] found that 81 percent of 186 fistula patients were septic on admission.

Furthermore, intra-abdominal infection is the principal cause of mortality in these patients.

3. Provide adequate nutrition. Total parenteral nutrition has revolutionized the therapy of enteric fistulas.[329,331–333] Adequate calories must be administered with sufficient amino acids, free fatty acids, vitamins, and trace elements. Enteral alimentation, either proximal to a colonic fistula or distal to an esophageal or gastric fistula, may be possible and preferable to parenteral alimentation.[320]
4. Repeat the contrast studies at intervals to document healing and identify those patients requiring surgical correction.
5. Control skin excoriation, especially in patients with proximal gastrointestinal tract fistulas. Skin problems may be especially troublesome while awaiting spontaneous closure. Karaya gum, Stomadhesive, and fitted acrylic appliances all offer improved care in this area.
6. Reduce the volume of secretions entering the fistula from the bowel and avoid pooling within the tract. Both somatostatin[334,335] and cimetidine[331] have been shown to be effective in this regard.

Early Management of Enteric Fistulas

MANAGEMENT OF LOCAL INFECTION. The therapeutic goal of early management is to convert the fistula from the state of a partially drained abscess cavity into a narrow linear tract as rapidly as possible. As soon as an enteric fistula is recognized, oral intake is stopped. The majority of fistulas occur in the postoperative patient when ileus is still present. Therefore nasogastric decompression is usually indicated as soon as the intestinal leak is suspected, to prevent further distention of anastomoses and to minimize the output of enteric contents.

The failure to treat the intra-abdominal infection associated with fistulas is the leading cause of morbidity and mortality, accounting for over 70 percent of all deaths.[336,337] Athanassiades et al[338] found severe intraperitoneal infection in 35 of 70 fistula patients. In 21 patients, clinical signs of sepsis preceded the appearance of the fistula, but in 14 patients sepsis appeared after the fistula presented. Pooled secretions within the abdominal cavity must be continuously and efficiently evacuated along with loculated intraperitoneal abscesses. Percutaneous drainage permits early abscess drainage and may obviate the need for operative intervention.[304]

Antibiotic therapy should be directed toward the polymicrobial enteric flora. Proximal small bowel fistulas typically have low numbers of bacteria per milliliter of fluid, but because of their large fluid volume and high content of digestive enzymes, pooling of the secretions causes autodigestion of peritoneal surfaces. Distal fistulas have a less caustic output but so many pathogenic bacteria that abscesses are inevitable if adequate drainage is not immediately established. Over a period of time, the septic focus is localized and a fibrous tract relatively resistant to bacterial invasion is formed. Only at that time do antibiotics become unnecessary.

NUTRITIONAL SUPPORT. The combination of limited oral intake, an accelerated catabolic state due to sepsis, and excessive losses of gastrointestinal tract secretions leads to profound malnutrition. Prior to 1960, nutritional problems were the major cause of death in patients with intestinal fistulas. Chapman et al[339] reported a mortality rate of 57 and 65 percent in patients with high-output duodenal fistula and jejunal and ileal fistulas, respectively. However, in those patients receiving adequate nutritional support, the mortality was only 18 percent.[339] Recent series document lower mortality rates in the range of 7 to 37 percent.[335,336,340] Improvements in mortality and spontaneous closure rate over this time have been attributed to improvements in nutritional support.

Most patients with enterocutaneous fistulas will require total parenteral nutrition for several weeks, so careful attention should be paid to free fatty acid, vitamin, and trace element requirements.[333] Some authors feel that high-dose vitamin C administration augments wound healing.[329] Zinc deficiency is an occasional finding in patients with enterocutaneous fistulas.[329] Symptoms respond dramatically to the addition of zinc to the hyperalimentation solution. Several patients have developed hypocalcemia with tetany due to unsuspected magnesium deficiency. The hypocalcemia is refractory to calcium supplementation until adequate magnesium levels are obtained. Severe hypophosphatemia also can occur.

Recently, the importance of enteral nutrition in reducing septic complications and improving the immune status of critically ill patients has gained increased recognition.[297,298] In a large series of 335 patients, Levy et al[320] have documented that up to 85 percent of patients with high-output enterocutaneous fistulas can be supported on enteral therapy alone, with similar mortality rates to those on parenteral nutrition. In patients with proximal enteric fistulas, enteral nutrition is possible once access to the distal tract of the fistula is obtained. This can be accomplished via a gastrostomy or jejunostomy and the use of viscous or elemental feedings to assure nutrient absorption and slowing of intestinal transit time.[320]

It is sometimes possible to collect the drainage from duodenal or high jejunal fistulas for reinfusion into a distal limb of small bowel.[324] Although this is applicable only in selected patients, a reduced complication rate for fluid, electrolyte, and protein losses justifies its use when possible.

WOUND MANAGEMENT. As soon as a fistula is recognized, urgent attempts must be made to protect the skin. The proximal, high-output fistulas are especially difficult management problems because of the resulting skin excoriation. Ideally, the patient with enterocutaneous fistula should be positioned so that gravity can continuously assist the drainage of enteric contents. A circle bed or a Stryker frame is useful for this purpose. Unfortunately, the awkward positions that result are uncomfortable. An alternative choice, which has the additional advantage of protecting the skin from the digestive enzymes, is suction drainage of the cavity. Sump tubes offer the most efficient fluid removal. Hard plastic tubes that are capable of eroding into the bowel or slipping into the bowel should be avoided. On the other hand, pliable drainage tubes (eg, Jackson-Pratt drains) are relatively difficult to position unless they are placed at operation. One option is a large-diameter, soft latex tube with a smaller intraluminal sump tube introduced into the fistula at bedside and placed to achieve low continuous suction. Persistence of a well-drained fistula in the absence of distal obstruction or malignancy, however, may be due to the drain itself. When the tract is long and fibrous, most drains can be removed, allowing spontaneous closure of the fistula.

Stomadhesive pads are useful in protecting the skin and allowing healing of the excoriated areas. A ring of Stomadhesive or similar material around the mouth of the fistula forms a watertight seal when used in conjunction with karaya paste. A disposable drainage bag can be placed on top of the Stomadhesive to collect the effluent from the fistula. Additionally, the use of Stomadhesive allows for excellent fixation of a sump drain. Custom silicone castings of the abdominal wall defect have been used in management of enterocutaneous fistulas that were so irregular that conventional stoma appliances could not be used. Silicone castings of the abdominal wall are made after occluding the fistula with a disposable syringe. After the casting hardens, the syringe is removed and karaya paste is applied to the undersurface of the casting. A conventional stoma appliance is applied to the surface of the casting. Such castings allow patients to be ambulatory, and, in one series, five of the six patients so treated were discontinued from total parenteral nutrition and treated as outpatients.[333] Although none had spontaneous closure of the fistula, their direct hospital costs were reduced and adequate nutrition was maintained during this period.

Several investigators propose that acidification of the output prevents activation of the proteolytic pancreatic enzymes responsible for digestion of the abdominal wall.[341] Lactic acid solution (0.45 percent) has been dripped into the wound and aspirated continuously in an attempt to flush away the highly caustic material.[341] Similarly, adherent ion-exchange resin pads with an acidic pH have been applied around fistula tracts in an attempt to prevent activation of these enzymes.

CONSERVATIVE VERSUS OPERATIVE MANAGEMENT. Once resuscitation, intra-abdominal infection, and nutritional support are dealt with, consideration must be given to the timing and need for fistula repair. If the investigations outlined above indicate the fistula communicates with the bowel and the bowel is in continuity without distal obstruction or evidence of active disease, then it is reasonable to attempt conservative management. The latter consists of nutritional support, wound management, and frequent clinical and radiologic reassessment to detect complications. Evidence of peritonitis or ongoing local or generalized sepsis suggests the need for urgent intervention. At surgery, no attempt should be made to perform a primary closure or anastomosis, since this will rarely heal. Rather, stomata or attempts at defunctioning should be undertaken. If the underlying bowel from which the fistula originates is abnormal as a result of inflammatory bowel disease, irradiation, malignancy, or primary infection such as tuberculosis or actinomycosis, then surgical management is indicated. Timing of the procedure will depend on the chronicity and nature of the underlying disease process. A very short fistula tract (less than 2.0 cm) rarely closes spontaneously as a result of epithelialization of the tract.[342] The longer and more narrow the tract, the higher the resistance to flow and the greater the likelihood that conservative management will be successful. A foreign body, such as a drain or prosthesis, precludes spontaneous closure. The factors affecting spontaneous closure and the closure rate are outlined in Table 38–12.[331]

TABLE 38–12. FACTORS AFFECTING SPONTANEOUS FISTULA CLOSURE

Factor	Closure Rate (%)
Local infection	Virtually 0
Complete anastomotic dehiscence	Virtually 0
Retained foreign body	Virtually 0
Epithelialization of tract	Virtually 0
Distal obstruction	Virtually 0
Crohn's disease	8
Irradition of small bowel	14
Tract <2 cm	17
Malignancy	26
Closure rate with none of these factors	32

Adapted from Reber H, Roberts C, Way LW, et al: Ann Surg 188:460, 1978.

Overall, a 30 to 38 percent rate of spontaneous closure has been demonstrated in many large studies.[320,337]

Somatostatin, a gastrointestinal hormone with pronounced inhibitory effects on gastrointestinal, pancreatic, and biliary secretions, has proved effective in the management of enterocutaneous fistulas. Spiliotis et al[334] have demonstrated a reduction in the time to achieve a 50 percent drop in fistula output from 6 days to 3 days in patients receiving somatostatin. Additionally, the time to spontaneous closure was reduced to 18 days from 27 days in controls. The disadvantages associated with somatostatin include its short half-life and a high incidence of glucose intolerance. A somatostatin analog has been developed, which has shown similar promise without troublesome side effects.[335]

Several reports have indicated that over 90 percent of fistulas will spontaneously close within 4 to 6 weeks of initial presentation in the setting of optimal management.[331,343] After this time period, some future requirement for surgery should be considered. Patient factors as well as local factors will help dictate the optimal timing for surgical intervention.

Table 38–13 relates the spontaneous enterocutaneous fistula closure rate with the site of enteric origin. Small bowel fistulas close spontaneously far less often than do esophageal, gastric, or colocutaneous fistulas. Two important factors influencing spontaneous closure are malnutrition and underlying sepsis, both of which can be dealt with during this period of conservative therapy.[337] Additionally, early operation in the presence of malnutrition may be detrimental, and as demonstrated by MacFayden et al,[344] this period of nutritional support improves the outcome in patients eventually going on to operative repair.

Operative Management of Specific Fistulas

SPECIFIC MANAGEMENT PROBLEMS IN ENTERIC FISTULAS. In general, resection with primary anastomosis is the therapy of choice for management of an enterocutaneous fistula. Local conditions such as extensive adhesions, carcinomatosis, or severe radiation changes in the bowel may preclude resection and make bypass or exclusion more attractive alternatives. Specific levels of fistula formation cause different problems that require brief consideration.

ESOPHAGEAL FISTULAS. After total esophagectomy, fistulization at the proximal suture line of the interposed bowel in the neck is a rather common occurrence.[322] Generalized necrosis of the bowel must be ruled out, since this is a surgical emergency. Saliva is relatively nontoxic if adequately drained, so drainage and maintenance of nutrition usually result in a spontaneous closure of these fistulas unless there is intestinal discontinuity.

Esophagogastrostomy and esophagojejunostomy leakage within the chest represent somewhat more formidable problems. After a Roux-en-Y anastomosis, there is no pancreatic or biliary flow through the anastomosis and only saliva passes into the mediastinum. Leakage is usually manifested by a pleural effusion and sepsis. Penicillin plus an aminoglycoside should be used for early antibiotic therapy, as the hospitalized patient most often has altered oral flora. Placement of a chest tube transpleurally to lie near the site of leakage will be adequate therapy only if the pleural cavity is drained and the reexpanded lung contacts the site of leak, allowing it to seal. If the fistula persists, thoracotomy with suture closure of the leak, decor-

TABLE 38–13. SPONTANEOUS CLOSURE RATE BY SITE OF FISTULA

Origin of Fistula	Spontaneous Closure (%)
Esophagus	82
Stomach	43
Duodenum (end)	50
Duodenum (lateral)	27
Jejunum	21
Ileum	19
Pancreas	67
Bile ducts	60
Cecum/appendix	44
Colon	30
Rectum	30

Adapted from Reber H, Roberts C, Way LW, et al: Ann Surg 188:460, 1978.

tication of the pleura, drainage of pleural loculations, and reexpansion of the lung may be required to seal the fistula. Diverting cervical esophagostomy may be necessary.[328]

A more complicated situation is produced if the esophagus has been anastomosed to the side of a jejunal loop or a partially obstructed stomach. In these cases, an enteropleural or gastropleural fistula is created, which will continue to contaminate the pleura with feculent flora. Consistent patient survival will only be achieved by taking down the anastomosis and diverting salivary flow.[345]

Esophageal perforation can result from esophagoscopy or bouginage. If the perforation is recognized early, successful primary suture can be undertaken. In contrast, postemetic rupture has a poor prognosis because the rupture usually forces a large quantity of contaminated gastric contents into the mediastinum. Early primary suture repair is indicated but usually fails if extensive mediastinitis is present. Buttressing the closure with the stomach fundus may reinforce the repair. The mediastinum must be drained into the pleura, and a drainage tube can be left near the suture line in the event that it fails. Esophageal diversion and drainage rather than operative closure have been advocated for late cases because of the high failure rate of closure.[346]

Postoperatively, the patient must be maintained on parenteral feeding or enteral feeding via a feeding jejunostomy. The saliva must be aspirated via a tube placed just above the leak. Constant aspiration of the stomach via a gastrostomy may be required to prevent regurgitation of gastric contents. If the fistula volume remains large, cervical esophagogastrostomy or a bowel interposition procedure is necessary. This has been advocated as a primary procedure in cases of severe mediastinitis with esophageal necrosis.

GASTROCUTANEOUS FISTULAS. Gastrocutaneous fistulas most frequently result after removal of a temporary gastrostomy.[319] Most other gastrocutaneous fistulas appear when an inflammatory or neoplastic process binds the gastric wall to the anterior abdominal wall or after gastric surgery, especially if distal obstruction is present. A short tract without associated extensive abscess formation usually occurs. Excision of the mucosa-lined tract is curative in the absence of obstruction.

Gastrojejunocutaneous fistulas may follow an anastomotic disruption or as a late complication of a perforated anastomotic ulcer.[330] If this fistula occurs acutely as the result of an anastomotic disruption, an associated abscess is common. Drainage of the abscess, antibiotic therapy, gastric decompression, and adequate nutrition should lead to fistula closure. By contrast, the formation of a gastrojejunocutaneous or gastrojejunocolonic fistula due to a perforated anastomotic ulcer is usually an indolent process with penetration of the ulcer into the abdominal wall or colon. This is rarely associated with abscess formation and usually requires operative intervention after the patient's condition is optimized. An adequate ulcer operation consisting of reresection of the stomach and reconstruction of the gastrojejunostomy with or without repeat vagotomy is indicated. Primary colonic anastomosis is appropriate if the colon has been prepared preoperatively.

DUODENOCUTANEOUS FISTULAS. There are two types of duodenocutaneous fistulas: (1) an end duodenal fistula, which usually results from a blown duodenal stump closure following gastrectomy and gastrojejunostomy (Billroth II reconstruction); and (2) a lateral duodenal fistula, which follows the inadvertent or planned duodenotomy. All such fistulas present difficult management problems because of the high enzyme content of the effluent and thus require excellent stoma care.

Prevention may be the best therapy, since placement of an end or lateral duodenostomy tube routinely for difficult duodenal stump closure nearly eliminates this complication.[324] Anderson et al[325] noted that placement of a periduodenal drain at operation reduces the mortality if a leak later occurs.

The most frequent cause of an end duodenal fistula is the breakdown of the duodenal suture line following closure of the duodenal stump after gastrectomy. A subhepatic abscess is an almost constant feature of such fistulas. Percutaneous drainage will often serve to treat local infection and heal the fistula, provided no distal obstruction is present. The response to conservative therapy should be followed for 1 to 2 weeks. If the patient remains stable and effluent volume is on the decline, then further nonoperative management is warranted. Garden et al[347] demonstrated spontaneous closure in 12 out of 13 patients with end duodenal fistulas. Despite a mean output of 1130 cc/day, the mean time to spontaneous closure was only 28 days.

In the presence of afferent limb or anastomotic obstruction, surgical intervention will likely be necessary. Anatomical definition of the underlying process should be discerned preoperatively by endoscopy, gastrointestinal contrast studies, and fistulograms. Patients should be prepared preoperatively with nutritional support and prophylactic antibiotics.

Lateral duodenal fistulas have a higher mortality and may persist chronically. With the lateral fistula even control of secretions and local infection may be difficult. Diverticulization of the duodenum requires closure of the duodenal perforation, accompanied by antrectomy, vagotomy, duodenostomy, and Billroth II gastrojejunostomy, with conversion of the lateral duodenal fistula to an end duodenal fistula. Other methods include effecting pyloric exclusion and gastrojejunostomy or using a serosal patch of jejunum to seal the defect in the duodenum.

JEJUNAL AND ILEAL FISTULAS. Operation to relieve intestinal obstruction secondary to extensive adhesions is the usual cause.[323,338] Inadvertent and unrecognized enterotomies lead to spillage of enteric contents. In the postoperative period, these patients often present with peritonitis, abscess formation, or bilious drainage through the abdominal wound. The latter two can usually be managed by effecting drainage percutaneously, while the former requires reoperation. At relaparotomy, the enterotomy should be exteriorized and distal obstruction addressed. For fistulas managed percutaneously, a search for distal obstruction should be performed with a view to subsequent correction if obstruction exists.

Leaking intraperitoneal ileocolonic anastomoses often close spontaneously on a low residue diet once local infection is controlled by percutaneous or surgical intervention. An exception is ileocolonic anastomotic failure because of intrinsic disease, such as residual Crohn's disease. In these cases, control of local infection with percutaneous drainage followed by delayed surgical intervention is the treatment of choice.

ENTEROENTERIC FISTULAS. In contrast to all the enterocutaneous fistulas, enteroenteric fistulas rarely cause gross intraperitoneal soiling. They usually represent spontaneous internal drainage of a localized abscess or perforation of a local inflammatory process. As a result, the patients have fewer septic episodes and frequently will appear chronically ill rather than acutely ill. Enteroenteric fistulas, however, seldom close spontaneously and usually require segmental resection of the diseased bowel. Many of the patients require intensive nutritional therapy because of chronic malnutrition but seldom present with fluid and electrolyte problems, skin excoriation, or sepsis. In this respect, they represent much less complex clinical management problems.

CECAL OR APPENDICEAL FISTULAS. Cecal fistula after drainage of a perforated appendix is seldom a major problem if the infection is adequately controlled. The fistula behaves much like a cecostomy and usually closes spontaneously. The persistence of such fistulas may indicate the presence of distal obstruction and should be regarded as an indication for investigation of the large bowel.[348]

COLONIC FISTULAS. Colonic fistulas may occur as a result of an anastomotic leak or due to a primary disease processes, most commonly diverticulitis or malignancy. External fistulas are seldom problematic and tend to have a low output with little metabolic sequelae. The majority of such fistulas follow operation on the large bowel, such as resection and anastomosis or closure of colostomy. Rarely, a spontaneous fistula may form as a result of a carcinoma eroding through the anterior abdominal wall or a large diverticular abscess pointing and discharging externally. Management principles are the same as most other fistulas, with an emphasis on dealing with the underlying infection. A liquid or low residue diet will reduce the volume of output while maintaining nutrition. In the absence of distal obstruction, underlying colonic disease, or an associated abscess cavity, the fistulas will likely close with conservative management. If the fistula does not close with such therapy and there is no evidence of residual local infection, then primary anastomosis is safe, providing an adequate mechanical bowel preparation is possible.

Coloenteric fistulas result when a loop of small bowel becomes part of a large inflammatory or malignant process. The manifestations are variable, depending on the location of the fistula in the small and large bowel. Diarrhea, with significant metabolic and nutritional derangements, may occur. Such fistulas rarely close spontaneously. Operative management includes en bloc resection of the inflammatory mass. Primary anastomosis of the small bowel is almost always performed unless the patient is very high risk with a significant amount of peritoneal contamination. Similarly, a primary colonic anastomosis is possible in the absence of localized infection or a compromised patient.

Colovesical fistulas are usually complications of inflammatory and neoplastic diseases of the colon and bladder. Diverticulitis is the most common cause, accounting for approximately 75 percent of all cases.[349,350] The remainder occur as a result of carcinoma of the colon or bladder and Crohn's disease. Rarely, a colovesical fistula occurs as a result of anastomotic dehiscence. Presenting symptoms include dysuria and recurrent urinary tract infections in over 90 percent of patients. Fecaluria and pneumaturia are also common and are features in 75 percent of patients.[350] Other manifestations include systemic sepsis and passage of urine per rectum. Men are more frequently affected, as interposition of the uterus between the sigmoid colon and the bladder is protective. A previous hysterectomy is noted in over 50 percent of women so presenting.[349] Diagnostic tests include a barium enema, which provides evidence of colonic disease and may demonstrate the fistula in 25 percent of cases. This may be followed by sigmoidoscopy to obtain a pathologic diagnosis. Cystoscopy is most sensitive, providing evidence of the fistulous opening or localized inflammation and bullous edema of the bladder mucosa in the region of the dome.[349,350] The majority of such fistulas do not close spontaneously. Most can be managed by resection and primary anastomosis of the affected colon and bladder repair.

Colovaginal fistulas are rare and are most often the result of diverticulitis. Occasionally, anastomotic disruption of a low colonic anastomosis with drainage into the vagina or inadvertent incorporation of the vagina in the anastomosis is causative.[351,352] Patients may present with flatus and feces per vagina, and the fistula may be visualized with colposcopy or vaginography and barium enema. As shown previously, most cases require operative management, in which case a one-stage repair is possible.[353,354]

SPECIAL PROBLEMS. Internal fistulas to the respiratory tract or pleural cavity will require tube or open thoracostomy drainage of the empyema to evacuate enteral or biliary secretions so that they cannot contaminate the bronchial tree.[355] Associated pneumonia and lung abscess will require the approaches described elsewhere in this text. In the case of esophagopleural fistulas, however, it is important to recognize that failure to achieve rapid and complete pleural drainage with tube thoracostomy may be the result of pleural adhesions or restrictive fibrosis of the lung. In either case, open thoracotomy is necessary with proper placement of drainage tubes and decortication of the pleural surface to permit full expansion of the lung and obliteration of the abscess cavity. Prompt recognition of this problem is required to permit healing.

The special problems of fistulas to the pericardium are those of acute pericarditis, namely, tamponade and adequate drainage of a purulent pericarditis.

Prognosis. Recent reports demonstrate mortality rates that vary between 7 and 37 percent,[335,336,340] reflecting the heterogeneity of this patient population. Sitges-Serra et al[356] proposed a classification of postoperative enterocutaneous fistulas to achieve improved stratification into more homogeneous groups. They divided patients into three groups: group I, esophageal, gastric, small bowel fistulas (low- or high-output); group 2, fistulas draining through a large abdominal wall defect; and group 3, appendiceal and colonic fistulas. The mortality rates in these groups were 18, 60, and 0 percent, respectively. Schein and Decker[336] modified this classification and stratified fistulas into four types, again with an emphasis on a large abdominal wall defect associated with a high mortality (Table 38–14).

Numerous studies have documented that prognosis is directly related to how rapidly infection is controlled. Athanassiades et al[338] reported twice the number of fistula-related deaths in septic versus nonseptic fistula patients. Soeters et al[323] found that if sepsis was controlled, the mortality was 0 as compared to 81 percent in those patients with uncontrolled sepsis. Schein and Decker[336] identified infection or multiple organ failure as the cause of death in 72 percent of patients.

Other factors that may be of prognostic significance include fistula output of more than 1500 ml/day[320] and poor nutritional status.[337] Altomare et al[340] used logistic regression analysis to determine factors correlating with mortality. Only the APACHE II score and serum albumin were predictive of mortality, reflecting the importance of nutritional status in affecting outcome.

Enterocutaneous fistulas remain a feared complication for the general surgeon because of their

TABLE 38–14. MORTALITY IN RELATION TO SITE OF FISTULA

Type	Site	Mortality
I	Esophagus/gastroduodenal	17%
II	Small bowel	33%
III	Large bowel	20%
IV	All sites associated with abdominal wall defect >20 cm^2	60%

Adapted from Schein M, Decker GA: Am J Surg 161:435, 1991.

extreme morbidity and frequent iatrogenic etiology. Early control of sepsis and careful attention to nutritional status will decrease the early mortality of this problem. These fistulas represent one end of the spectrum of intraperitoneal sepsis where a perforated viscus continues to pour contaminated material into and through the peritoneal cavity. Control of peritoneal infection requires removal of the bacteria and agents that potentiate their virulence, administration of appropriate antimicrobial chemotherapeutic agents, prevention of ongoing or recurrent contamination, nutritional and hemodynamic support, and careful observation for indicators of recurrent infection. These general principles are applicable to all types of intraperitoneal infections.

REFERENCES

1. Allen L: The peritoneal stomata. Anat Rec 67:89, 1936.
2. Raferty AT: Regeneration of parietal and visceral peritoneum. Br J Surg 60:293, 1973.
3. Rodgers KE, Dizerega GS: Modulation of peritoneal re-epithelialization by postsurgical macrophages. J Surg Res 53:542, 1992.
4. Fukasawa M, Campeau JD, Yanagihara DL, et al: Regulation of proliferation of peritoneal tissue repair cells by peritoneal macrophages. J Surg Res 49:81, 1990.
5. Dixon CF, Rixford EL: Cytologic response to peritoneal irritation in man: a protective mechanism. Am J Surg 25:504, 1934.
6. Golden GT, Shaw A: Primary peritonitis. Surg Gynecol Obstet 135:513, 1972.
7. Bercovici B, Miller MJ, Sacks TG: Antimicrobial activity of human peritoneal fluid. Surg Gynecol Obstet 141:885, 1975.
8. Lanfrancone L, Boraschi D, Ghiara P, et al: Human peritoneal mesothelial cells produce many cytokines (granulocyte colony-stimulating factor [CSF], granulocyte-monocyte-CSF, macrophage-CSF, interleukin-1 [IL-1], and IL-6) and are activated and stimulated to grow by IL-1. Blood 80:2835, 1992.
9. Henderson LW, Nolph KD: Altered permeability of the peritoneal membrane after using hypertonic peritoneal dialysis fluid. J Clin Invest 48:992, 1969.
10. Henderson LW: The problem of peritoneal membrane area and permeability. Kidney Int 3:409, 1973.
11. Gutman RA, Nixon WP, McRae RL, et al: Effect of intraperitoneal and intravenous vasoactive amines on peritoneal dialysis: study in anephric dogs. Trans Am Soc Artif Intern Organs 22:570, 1976.
12. MacCallum WG: On the mechanism of absorption of granular materials from the peritoneum. Bull Johns Hopkins Hosp 14:105, 1903.
13. Allen L, Weatherford T: Role of fenestrated basement membrane in lymphatic absorption from the peritoneal cavity. Am J Physiol 197:551, 1956.
14. Richardson JD, DeCamp MM, Garrison RN, et al: Pulmonary infection complicating intra-abdominal sepsis: clinical and experimental observations. Ann Surg 195:732, 1982.
15. Tsilibary EC, Wissig SL: Absorption from the peritoneal cavity: SEM study of the mesothelium covering the peritoneal surface of the muscular portion of the diaphragm. Am J Anat 149:127, 1977.
16. Janik JS, Apkarian R, Nagarah HS, et al: An ultrastructural study of enteric serosa after surgical management. Surg Gynecol Obstet 154:491, 1982.
17. Yoffey JM, Courtice FC: Lymphatics, Lymph and Lymphoid Tissue. Cambridge, MA, Howard Press, 1956.
18. Autio V: The spread of intraperitoneal infection: studies with roentgen contrast medium. Acta Chir Scand 123 (Suppl 321):5, 1964.
19. Hau T, Arenholz DH, Simmons RL: Secondary bacterial peritonitis: the biologic basis of treatment. Curr Probl Surg 16:1, 1979.
20. Steinberg B: Infections of the Peritoneum. New York, Hoeber, 1944.
21. Last M, Kurtz L, Stein TA, et al: Effect of PEEP on the rate of thoracic duct flow and bacterial clearance from the peritoneal cavity. Am J Surg 145:126, 1983.
22. Higgins GM, Beaver MG, Lemon WS: Phrenic neurectomy and peritoneal absorption. Am J Anat 45:137, 1930.
23. Fowler GR: Diffuse septic peritonitis, with special reference to a new method of treatment, namely, the elevated head and trunk posture to facilitate drainage into the pelvis. With a report of nine consecutive cases of recovery. Med Rec 57:617, 1900.
24. Dunn DL, Barke RA, Ewald DC, Simmons RL: Macrophages and translymphatic absorption represent the first line of defense in the peritoneal cavity. Arch Surg 122:105, 1987.
25. Rotstein OD: Peritonitis and intra-abdominal abscesses. In Wilmore DW, Brennan MF, Harken AH, et al (eds): Scientific American: Care of the Surgical Patient. New York, Scientific American, 1992, pp 1–24.
26. Ford-Hutchinson AW: Leukotriene B4 in inflammation. CRC Rev Immunol 10:1, 1990.
27. West MA: Mechanisms of Leukocyte Activation: Current Topics in Membranes and Transport. New York, Academic Press, 1990.
28. Mason MJ, van Epps DE: In vivo neutrophil emigration in response to interleukin-1 and tumor necrosis factor alpha. J Leukoc Biol 45:62, 1989.
29. Dunn DL, Barke RA, Ahrenholz DH, et al: The adjuvant effect of peritoneal fluid in experimental peritonitis: mechanism and clinical implications. Ann Surg 199:37, 1984.
30. Dunn DL, Simmons RL: Fibrin in peritonitis: III.

The mechanism of bacterial trapping by polymerizing fibrin. Surgery 92:513, 1982.
31. Zinsser HH, Pryde AW: Experimental study of physical factors, including fibrin formation, influencing the spread of fluids and small particles within and from the peritoneal cavity of the dog. Surgery 130:818, 1952.
32. Sinclair SB, Rotstein OD, Levy GA: Disparate mechanisms of induction of procoagulant activity by live and inactivated bacteria and viruses. Infect Immun 58:1821, 1990.
33. Rosenthal GA, Levy G, Rotstein OD: Induction of macrophage procoagulant activity by *Bacteroides fragilis*. Infect Immun 57:338, 1989.
34. Hau T, Payne WD, Simmons RL: Fibrinolytic activity of the peritoneum during experimental peritonitis. Surg Gynecol Obstet 148:415, 1979.
35. Marshall JC, Sweeney D: Microbial infection and the septic response in critical surgical illness. Arch Surg 125:17, 1990.
36. St. John RC, Dorinsky PM: Immunologic therapy for ARDS, septic shock and multiple-organ failure. Chest 103:932, 1993.
37. Pinsky MR, Vincent JL, Alegre M, et al: Serum cytokine levels in human septic shock. Chest 103:565, 1993.
38. Giroir BP: Mediators of septic shock: new approaches for interrupting the endogenous inflammatory cascade. Crit Care Med 21:780, 1993.
39. Vincent J-L, Bakker J, Marecaux G, et al: Administration of anti-TNF antibody improves left ventricular function in septic shock patients. Chest 101:810, 1992.
40. Fisher CJ, Opal SM, Dhainaut JF, et al: Influence of anti-tumor necrosis factor monoclonal antibody on cytokine levels in patients with sepsis. Crit Care Med 21:318, 1993.
41. Wortel CH, von der Mohlen MAM, van Deventer SJH, et al: Effectiveness of a human monoclonal anti-endotoxin antibody (HA-1A) in gram negative sepsis: relationship to endotoxin and cytokine levels. J Infect Dis 166:1367, 1992.
42. Granowitz EV, Porat R, Mier JW, et al: Pharmacokinetics, safety and immunomodulatory effects of human recombinant interleukin-1 receptor antagonist in healthy humans. Cytokine 4:353, 1992.
43. Van Dissel JT, Van Furth R, Compier BA, et al: Survival in selected patients with gram-negative sepsis after adjunctive therapy with HA-1A. Lancet 341:959, 1993.
44. Kirschner M: Die Behandlung der akuten eitrigen freien Bauchfellentzundung. Arch Klin Chir 142: 253, 1926.
45. Solomkin JS, Dellinger EP, Christou NV, Busuttil RW: Results of a multicenter trial comparing imipenem/cilastin to tobramycin/clindamycin for intraabdominal infections. Ann Surg 212:581, 1990.
46. Poenaru D, De Santis M, Christou NV: Imipenem versus tobramycin—antianaerobe antibiotic therapy in intra-abdominal infections. Can J Surg 33:415, 1990.
47. Ruddell WSJ, Axon ATR, Findlay JM, et al: Effect of cimetidine on the gastric bacterial flora. Lancet 1:672, 1980.
48. Stone HH, Kolb LD, Geheber CE: Incidence and significance of intraperitoneal anaerobic bacteria. Ann Surg 181:705, 1975.
49. Brook I: A 12 year study of aerobic and anaerobic bacteria in intra-abdominal and postsurgical abdominal wound infections. Surg Gynecol Obstet 169:387, 1989.
50. Hackford AW, Tally FP, Reinhold RB, et al: Prospective study comparing imipenem-cilastin with clindamycin and gentamicin for the treatment of serious surgical infections. Arch Surg 123:322, 1988.
51. Gonzenbach HR, Simmen HP, Amgwerd R: Imipenem (N-F-Thienamycin) versus netilmicin plus clindamycin. Ann Surg 205:271, 1986.
52. Walker AP, Nichols RL, Wilson RF, et al: Efficacy of a beta-lactamase inhibitor combination for serious intra-abdominal infections. Ann Surg 217:115, 1993.
53. Mosdell DM, Morris DM, Voltura A, et al: Antibiotic treatment for surgical peritonitis. Ann Surg 214: 543, 1991.
54. Schaberg DR, Culver DH, Gaynes RP: Major trends in the microbial etiology of nosocomial infection. Am J Med 91(3B):72S, 1991.
55. Bjornson HS: Bacterial synergy, virulence factors, and host defense mechanisms in the pathogenesis of intraabdominal infections. In Simmons RL (ed): Topics in Intraabdominal Surgical Infection. Norwalk, CT, Appleton-Century-Crofts, 1982, pp 65–78.
56. Weinstein WM, Onderdonk AB, Bartlett JG, Gorbach SL: Experimental intra-abdominal abscesses in rats: development of an experimental model. Infect Immun 10:1250, 1974.
57. Onderdonk AB, Weinstein WM, Sullivan NM, et al: Experimental intra-abdominal abscesses in rats: quantitative bacteriology of infected animals. Infect Immun 10:1256, 1974.
58. Onderdonk A, Bartlett J, Louie T, et al: Microbial synergy in experimental intra-abdominal abscesses. Infect Immun 13:22, 1976.
59. Rotstein OD, Kao J: The spectrum of *Escherichia coli–Bacteroides fragilis* pathogenic synergy in an intraabdominal infection model. Can J Microbiol 34:352, 1988.
60. Rotstein OD, Pruett TL, Simmons RL: Lethal microbial synergism in intra-abdominal infections. Arch Surg 120:146, 1985.
61. Rotstein OD, Pruett TL, Wells CL, Simmons RL: The role of *Bacteroides* encapsulation in the lethal synergy between *Escherichia coli* and *Bacteroides* species studies in a rat fibrin clot peritonitis model. J Infect 15:135, 1987.
62. Tofte RW, Peterson PK, Schemling D, et al: Opsonization of four *Bacteroides* species: role of the classi-

cal complement pathway and immunoglobulin. Infect Immun 27:784, 1980.
63. Rotstein OD, Pruett TL, Fiegel VD: Succinic acid, a metabolic by-product of *Bacteroides* species, inhibits polymorphonuclear leukocyte function. Infect Immun 48:402, 1985.
64. Lev M, Krudell KC, Milford AF: Succinate as a growth factor for *Bacteroides melananinogenicus.* J Bacteriol 108:175, 1971.
65. Pruett TL, Rotstein OD, Fiegel VD, et al: Mechanism of the adjuvant effect of hemoglobin in experimental peritonitis: VIII. A leukotoxin is produced by *Escherichia coli* metabolism in hemoglobin. Surgery 96:375, 1984.
66. Ward CG: Influence of iron on infection. Am J Surg 151:291, 1986.
67. Bullen JJ: The significance of iron in infection. Rev Infect Dis 3:1127, 1981.
68. Dumont AE, Maas WK, Iliescu H, et al: Increased survival from peritonitis after blockade of transdiaphragmatic absorption of bacteria. Surg Gynecol Obstet 162:248, 1986.
69. Rotstein OD, Pruett TL, Simmons RL: Fibrin in peritonitis V. Fibrin inhibits phagocytic killing of *E. coli* by human polymorphonuclear leukocytes. Ann Surg 203:413, 1986.
70. Whitnack E, Beachey EH: Inhibition of complement-mediated opsonization and phagocytosis of *Streptococcus pyogenes* by D fragments of fibrinogen and fibrin bound to cell surface M protein. J Exp Med 162:1983, 1985.
71. Kazura JW, Wenger JD, Salata RA, et al: Modulation of polymorphonuclear leukocyte microbicidal activity and oxidative metabolism by fibrinogen degradation products D and E. J Clin Invest 83:1916, 1989.
72. Ahrenholz DH, Simmons RL: Fibrin in peritonitis. I. Beneficial and adverse effects of fibrin in experimental *E. coli* peritonitis. Surgery 88:41, 1980.
73. Andersson R, Tranberg KG, Bengmark S: Bile peritonitis in acute cholecystitis. Hepatopancreatobiliary Surg 2:7, 1990.
74. Andersson R, Tranberg KG, Alwmark A, Bengmark S: Factors influencing the outcome of *E. coli* peritonitis in rats. Acta Chir Scand 155:155, 1989.
75. Cho J, Rotstein OD, Pruett TL: The adjuvant effect of bile salts in experimental peritonitis. Surg Forum 35:231, 1984.
76. Iwanaga M, Nakagawara A, Matsuo S, et al: Impaired polymorphonuclear leukocyte function in biliary atresia: role of bilirubin and bile acids. J Pediatr Surg 22:967, 1987.
77. Andersson R, Willen R, Massa G, et al: Effect of bile on peritoneal morphology in *E. coli* peritonitis. Scand J Gastroenterol 25:405, 1990.
78. Finlay-Jones JJ, Kenny PA, Nulsen MF, et al: Pathogenesis of intraabdominal abscess formation: abscess-potentiating agents and inhibition of complement-dependent opsonization of abscess inducing bacteria. J Infect Dis 164:1173, 1991.
79. Yamamura M, Nishi M, Furubayashi H, et al: Barium peritonitis. Report of a case and review of the literature. Dis Colon Rectum 28:347, 1985.
80. Poret HA, Fabian TC, Croce MA, et al: Analysis of septic morbidity following gunshot wounds to the colon: the missile is an adjuvant for abscess. J Trauma 31:1088, 1991.
81. Zimmerli W, Waldvogel FA, Vaudaus P, et al: Pathogenesis of foreign body infection: description and characteristics of an animal model. J Infect Dis 146:487, 1982.
82. Zimmerli W, Lew PD, Waldvogel FA: Pathogenesis of foreign body infection: evidence for a local granulocyte defect. J Clin Invest 73:1191, 1984.
83. Liddington MI, Thomson WH: Rebound tenderness test. Br J Surg 78:795, 1991.
84. Ing AF, Mclean APH, Meakins JL: Multiple-organism bacteremia in the surgical intensive care unit: a sign of intraperitoneal sepsis. Surgery 90:779, 1981.
85. Fry DE, Garrison RN, Polk HC Jr: Clinical implications in *Bacteroides* bacteremia. Surg Gynecol Obstet 149:189, 1979.
86. Miller R, Becher G, Slabough R: Detection of pneumoperitoneum: optimal body position and respiratory phase. Am J Roentgenol 135:487, 1980.
87. Winek TG, Mosely S, Grout G, Luallin D: Pneumoperitoneum and its association with ruptured abdominal viscus. Arch Surg 123:709, 1988.
88. Roh J, Thompson J, Harsed R, et al: Value of pneumoperitoneum in diagnosis of visceral perforation. Am J Surg 146:830, 1983.
89. Harrison I, Litwer H: Studies of the incidence and duration of postoperative pneumoperitoneum. Ann Surg 145:591, 1957.
90. Sim KT, Picone S, Crade M, Sweeney JP: Ultrasound with graded compression in the evaluation of acute appendicitis. J Natl Med Assoc 81:954, 1989.
91. Abu-Yousef MM, Bleicher JJ, Maher JW, et al: High resolution sonography of acute appendicitis. Am J Roentgenol 149:53, 1987.
92. McGrath FP, Keeling F: The role of early sonography in the management of the acute abdomen. Clin Radiol 44:172, 1991.
93. Schwerk WB, Schwarz S, Rothmund M: Sonography in acute colonic diverticulitis. Dis Colon Rectum 35:1077, 1992.
94. Verbanck J, Lambrecht S, Rutgeerts L, et al: Can sonography diagnose acute colonic diverticulitis in patients with acute intestinal inflammation? A prospective study. J Clin Ultrasound 17:661, 1989.
95. Taourel P, Baron MP, Pradel J, et al: Acute abdomen of unknown origin: impact of CT on diagnosis and management. Gastrointest Radiol 17:287, 1992.
96. Federle MP, Chun G, Jeffery RB, et al: Computed tomographic findings in bowel infarction. J Radiol 142:91, 1984.
97. Smerud MJ, Johnson CD, Stephens DH: Diagnosis of bowel infarction: a comparison of plain films and CT scans in 23 cases. Am J Roentgenol 154:99, 1990.

98. Lobbato V, Cioroiu M, LaRaja RD, et al: Peritoneal lavage as an aid to diagnosis of peritonitis in debilitated and elderly patients. Am Surg 51:508, 1985.
99. Richardson JD, Flint LM, Polk HC Jr: Peritoneal lavage: a useful diagnostic adjunct for peritonitis. Surgery 94:826, 1983.
100. Alverdy JC, Saunders J, Chamerlin WH, Moss GS: Diagnostic peritoneal lavage in intra-abdominal sepsis. Am Surg 54:456, 1988.
101. Larson FA, Haller CC, Delcore R, Thomas JH: Diagnostic peritoneal lavage in acute peritonitis. Am J Surg 164:449, 1992.
102. Zucker KA, Bailey RW, Flowers J: Laparoscopic management of acute and chronic cholecystitis. Surg Clin North Am 72:1045, 1992.
103. Adams JD, Chan M, Clifford PC, et al: Computer aided diagnosis of acute abdominal pain: a multicenter study. BMJ 293:800, 1986.
104. Nagy AG, James D. Diagnostic laparoscopy. Am J Surg 157:490, 1989.
105. Paterson-Brown S, Eckersley JRT, Sim AJWS, Dudley HAF: Laparoscopy as an adjunct to decision making in the acute abdomen. Br J Surg 73:1022, 1986.
106. Paterson-Brown S, Thompson JN, Eckersley JRT, Ponting GA: Which patient with suspected appendicitis should undergo laparoscopy? BMJ 296:1363, 1988.
107. Spirtos NM, Eisenkop SM, Spirtos TW, et al: Laparoscopy—a diagnostic aid in cases of suspected appendicitis. Its use in women of reproductive age. Am J Obstet Gynecol 156:90, 1987.
108. Foster HM: Which patients should undergo laparoscopy? BMJ 297:489, 1988.
109. Paterson-Brown S: Emergency laparoscopic surgery. Br J Surg 80:279, 1993.
110. Paterson-Brown S, Olufunwa SA, Galazka N, Simmons SC: Visualization of the normal appendix at laparoscopy. J R Coll Surg Edinb 31:106, 1986.
111. Iberti TJ, Salky BA, Onofrey D: Use of bedside laparoscopy to identify intestinal ischemia in postoperative cases of aortic reconstruction. Surgery 105:686, 1989.
112. Mouret P, Francois Y, Vignal J, et al: Laparoscopic treatment of perforated peptic ulcer. Br J Surg 77:1006, 1990.
113. Nathanson LK, Easter DW, Cuschierei A: Laparoscopic repair/peritoneal toilet of perforated duodenal ulcer. Surg Endosc 4:232, 1990.
114. Bohnen JMA, Solomkin JS, Dellinger EP, et al: Guidelines for clinical care: anti-infective agents for intraabdominal infection. Arch Surg 127:83, 1992.
115. Berne TV, Appleman MD, Chenella FC, et al: Surgically treated gangrenous or perforated appendicitis: a comparison of aztreonam and clindamycin versus gentamicin and clindamycin. Ann Surg 205:133, 1987.
116. Birolini D, Moraes MF, de Souza OS: Aztreonam plus clindamycin versus tobramycin plus clindamycin for the treatment of intraabdominal infections. Rev Infect Dis 7:S724, 1985.
117. Smith CR, Moore RD, Lietman PS: Studies of risk factors for aminoglycoside nephrotoxicity. Am J Kidney Dis 8:308, 1986.
118. Ho JL, Barza M: Role of aminoglycoside antibiotics in the treatment of intra-abdominal infection. Antimicrob Agents Chemother 31:485, 1987.
119. Fry DE, Pitcher DE: Antibiotic pharmacokinetics in surgery. Arch Surg 125:1490, 1990.
120. Niemiec PWJR, Allo MD, Miller CF: Effect of altered volume of distribution on aminoglycoside levels in patients in surgical intensive care. Arch Surg 122:207, 1987.
121. Bryant RE: Effect of the suppurative environment on antibiotic activity. In Root RK, Sande MA (eds): New Dimensions in Antimicrobial Therapy. New York, Churchill Livingstone, 1984, pp 313–337.
122. Jackson GG: Gentamicin. Practioner 198:855, 1967.
123. Dougherty SH, Saltzstein EC, Peacock JB, et al: Perforated or gangrenous appendicitis treated with aminoglycosides. Arch Surg 124:1280, 1989.
124. Stone HH, Bourneuf AA, Stinson LD: Reliability of criteria for predicting persistent or recurrent sepsis. Arch Surg 120:17, 1985.
125. Lennard ES, Dellinger EP, Wertz MJ: Implications of leukocytosis and fever at conclusion of antibiotic therapy for intraabdominal sepsis. Ann Surg 195:19, 1982.
126. Hoffman SA, Moellering RC Jr: The enterococcus: "putting the bug in our ears." Ann Intern Med 106:757, 1987.
127. Moellering RC Jr, Wennersten CBG, Weinberg AN: Studies on antibiotic synergism against enterococci: II. Effect of various antibiotics on the uptake of ^{14}C-labelled streptomycin by enterococci. J Clin Invest 50:2580, 1971.
128. Maki DG, Agger WA: Enterococcal bacteremia: clinical features, the risk of endocarditis, and management. Medicine (Baltimore) 67:248, 1988.
129. Barie PS, Christou NV, Dellinger EP, et al: Pathogenicity of the enterococcus in surgical infections. Ann Surg 212:155, 1990.
130. Barrall DT, Kenney PR, Slotman GJ, Burchard KW: Enterococcal bacteremia in surgical patients. Arch Surg 120:57, 1985.
131. Garrison RN, Fry DE, Berberich S, Polk HC: Enterococcal bacteremia. Ann Surg 196:43, 1982.
132. Burd RS, Raymond CS, Dunn DL: Endotoxin promotes synergistic lethality during concurrent *Escherichia coli* and *Candida albicans* infection. J Surg Res 52:537, 1992.
133. Solomkin JS, Flohr AB, Quie PG, Simmons RL: The role of *Candida* in intraperitoneal infections. Surgery 88:524, 1980.
134. Sawyer MD, Dunn DL: Antimicrobial therapy of intra-abdominal sepsis. Infect Dis Clin North Am 6:545, 1992.
135. Ravo B, Metwally N, Yeh J, et al: Effect of fecal loading with/without peritonitis on the healing of a

colonic anastomosis: an experimental study. Eur Surg Res 23:100, 1991.

136. Ravo B, Metwally N, Castera P, et al: The importance of intraluminal fecal contact and peritonitis in colonic anastomotic leakages: an experimental study. Dis Colon Rectum 31:868, 1988.
137. Irvin TT, Goligher JC: Aetiology of disruption of intestinal anastomoses. Br J Surg 60:461, 1973.
138. Smith SR, Connolly JC, Golmere OJ: The effect of fecal loading on colonic anastomotic healing. Br J Surg 70:49, 1983.
139. Ravo B, Mishrick A, Addei K, et al: The treatment of perforated diverticulitis by one stage intracolonic bypass procedure. Surgery 102:771, 1987.
140. Rosati C, Smith L, Deitel M, et al: Primary colorectal anastomosis with the intracolonic bypass tube. Surgery 112:618, 1992.
141. Schein M, Gecelter G, Freinkel W, et al: Peritoneal lavage in abdominal sepsis. A controlled clinical study. Arch Surg 125:1132, 1990.
142. Majeski JA, McClellan MA, Alexander JW: Evaluation of leukocyte chemotactic response in the presence of antibiotics. Surg Forum 16:83, 1975.
143. Hansbrough JF, Zapata-Sirvent RL, Cooper ML: Effects of topical antimicrobial agents on the human neutrophil respiratory burst. Arch Surg 126:603, 1991.
144. Rappaport WD, Holcomb M, Valente J, Chvapil M: Antibiotic irrigation and the formation of intraabdominal adhesions. Am J Surg 158:435, 1989.
145. Schein M, Hirshberg A, Hashmonai M: Current surgical management of severe intraabdominal infection. Surgery 112:489, 1992.
146. Hudspeth AS: Radical debridement in the treatment of advanced generalized bacterial peritonitis. Arch Surg 110:1233, 1975.
147. Polk HC, Fry DE: Radical peritoneal debridement for established peritonitis: the result of a prospective randomized clinical trial. Ann Surg 192:350, 1980.
148. Costerton JW, Irwin RT, Cheung K-J: The bacterial glycocalyx in nature and disease. Am Rev Microbiol 35:299, 1981.
149. Cerise EJ, Pierce WA, Diamond DL: Abdominal drains: their role as a source of infection following splenectomy. Ann Surg 171:764, 1970.
150. Haller JD, Shaker IJ, Donahoo JS: Peritoneal drainage versus non-drainage for generalized peritonitis from ruptured appendix in children. Ann Surg 177:595, 1973.
151. Washington BC, Villalba MR, Lauter CB: Cefamandole-erythromycin-heparin peritoneal irrigation: an adjunct to the surgical treatment of diffuse bacterial peritonitis. Surgery 94:576, 1983.
152. Hallerback B, Andersson C, Englund N, et al: A prospective randomized study of continuous peritoneal lavage postoperatively in the treatment of purulent peritonitis. Surg Gynecol Obstet 163:433, 1986.
153. Stephen M, Lowenthal J: Continuing peritoneal lavage in high risk peritonitis. Surgery 85:603, 1979.
154. Leiboff AR, Soroff HS: The treatment of generalized peritonitis by closed postoperative peritoneal lavage: a critical review of the literature. Arch Surg 122:1005, 1987.
155. Richardson JD, Trinkle JK: Hemodynamic and respiratory alteration with increased intraabdominal pressure. J Surg Res 20:401, 1976.
156. Caldwell CB, Riccotta JJ: Evaluation of intraabdominal and renal hemodynamics. Curr Surg 43:495, 1986.
157. Ivatury RR, Nallathambi M, Rao PM, et al: Open management of the septic abdomen: therapeutic and prognostic considerations based on APACHE II. Crit Care Med 17:511, 1989.
158. Walsh GL, Chiasson P, Hedderich G: The open abdomen. The marlex mesh and zipper technique: a method of managing intraabdominal infection. Surg Clin North Am 68:25, 1988.
159. Garcia-Sabrido JL, Tallado JM, Christou NV, et al: Treatment of severe intra-abdominal sepsis and/or necrotic foci by an "open-abdomen" approach. Arch Surg 123:152, 1988.
160. Mastboom WJB, Kuypers HHC, Schoots FJ, Wobbes T: Small bowel perforations complicating the open treatment of generalized peritonitis. Arch Surg 124:689, 1989.
161. Bernard HR, Cole WR: Wound infections following potentially contaminated operations. JAMA 184: 290, 1963.
162. Bohnen J, Boulanger M, Meakins JL, Mclean APH: Prognosis in generalized peritonitis. Arch Surg 118:285, 1983.
163. Christou NV, Barie PS, Dellinger EP, et al: Surgical Infection Society intra-abdominal infection study. Prospective evaluation of management techniques and outcome. Arch Surg 128:193, 1993.
164. Pitcher WD, Musher DM: Critical importance of early diagnosis and treatment of intraabdominal infection. Arch Surg 117:328, 1982.
165. Bohnen JMA, Mustard RA, Oxholm SE, Schouten D: APACHE II score and abdominal sepsis. Arch Surg 123:225, 1988.
166. Maclean LD, Meakins JL, Taguchi K, et al: Host resistance in sepsis and trauma. Ann Surg 182:207, 1975.
167. Poenaru D, Christou NV: Clinical outcome of seriously ill surgical patients with intra-abdominal infection depends on both physiologic (APACHE II score) and immunologic (DTH score) alterations. Ann Surg 113:130, 1991.
168. Dellinger EP, Wertz MJ, Meakins JL, et al: Surgical infection stratification system for intra-abdominal infection. Arch Surg 120:21, 1985.
169. Cerra FB, Negru F, Abrams J: APACHE II score does not predict multiple organ failure or mortality in postoperative surgical patients. Arch Surg 125:519, 1990.
170. Rotstein OD, Meakins JL: Diagnostic and therapeu-

tic challenges of intraabdominal infections. World J Surg 14:159, 1990.
171. Nathens AB,. Rotstein OD, Marshall JC: Tertiary peritonitis: clinical features of a complex nosocomial infection. Crit Care Med 21(Suppl):S129, 1993.
172. Rotstein OD, Pruett TL, Simmons RL: Microbiologic features and treatment of persistent peritonitis in patients in the intensive care unit. Can J Surg 29:247, 1986.
173. Ferraris VA: Exploratory laparotomy for potential abdominal sepsis in patients with multiple organ failure. Arch Surg 118:1130, 1983.
174. Polk HC, Shields CL: Remote organ failure: a valid sign of occult intraabdominal infection. Surgery 81:310, 1977.
175. Hinsdale JG, Jaffe BM: Re-operation for intra-abdominal sepsis. Ann Surg 199:31, 1984.
176. Sinanan M, Maier RV, Carrico J: Laparotomy for intra-abdominal sepsis in patients in an intensive care unit. Arch Surg 119:652, 1984.
177. Bunt TJ: Non-directed relaparotomy for intra-abdominal sepsis. A futile procedure. Am Surg 52:294, 1986.
178. Norton LW: Does drainage of intraabdominal pus reverse multiple organ failure? Am J Surg 149:347, 1985.
179. Fowler R: Primary peritonitis: changing aspects 1956–1970. Aust Paediatr J 7:73, 1971.
180. McDougal WS, Izant RJ Jr, Zollinger RM Jr: Primary peritonitis in infancy and childhood. Ann Surg 181:310, 1975.
181. Armitage TG, Williamson RC: Primary peritonitis in children and adults. Postgrad Med J 59:21, 1983.
182. Nohr CW, Marshall DG: Primary peritonitis in children. Can J Surg 27:179, 1984.
183. Wilfert CM, Katz SL: Etiology of bacterial sepsis in nephrotic children 1963–1967. Pediatrics 42:840, 1968.
184. Speck WT, Dresdale SS, Mcmillan RW: Primary peritonitis and the nephrotic syndrome. Am J Surg 127:267, 1974.
185. Harken AH, Shochat SJ: Gram-positive peritonitis in children. Am J Surg 125:769, 1973.
186. Golden GT, Shaw A: Primary peritonitis. Surg Gynecol Obstet 135:513, 1972.
187. Beale G, Hackett AH: A case of uterine reflux of urine in a girl and its suggested role in primary peritonitis. N Z Med J 69:158, 1969.
188. Mardh PA, Wolner-Hanssen P: Periappendicitis and chlamydial salpingitis. Surg Gynecol Obstet 160: 304, 1985.
189. Gatt D, Jantet G: Perisplenitis and perinephritis in the Curtis-Fitz-Hugh syndrome. Br J Surg 74:110, 1987.
190. Haight JB, Ockner SA: Chlamydial trachomatis perihepatitis with ascites. Am J Gastroenterol 83:323, 1988.
191. Marbet UA, Stalder GA, Vogtlin J, et al: Diffuse peritonitis and chronic ascites due to infection with *Chlamydia trachomatis* in patients without liver disease: new presentation of the Fitz-Hugh-Curtis syndrome. BMJ (Clin Res) 293:5, 1986.
192. Kimball MW, Knee S: Gonococcal perihepatitis in a male. N Engl J Med 282:1080, 1970.
193. Baumgardner DJ: Abdominal pain: *Chlamydia* as culprit. Postgrad Med 85:281, 1989.
194. Wolner-Hanssen P, Westrom L, Mardh PA: Chlamydial perihepatitis. Scand J Infect Dis Suppl 32:77, 1982.
195. Baumgardner DJ, McCanse DE: Peritonitis and small bowel obstruction. IMJ 171:75, 1987.
196. Lipsky PE, Hardin JA, Schour L, Plotz PH: Spontaneous peritonitis and systemic lupus erythematosus. Importance of accurate diagnosis of gram-positive bacterial infections. JAMA 232:939, 1975.
197. Pollak VE, Grove WJ, Kark RM, et al: Systemic lupus erythematosus simulating acute surgical conditions of the abdomen. N Engl J Med 259:258, 1958.
198. Wilcox CM, Forsmark CE, Darragh TM, et al: Cytomegalovirus peritonitis in a patient with the acquired immunodeficiency syndrome. Dig Dis Sci 37:1288, 1992.
199. Pinzello G, Simonetti RG, Craxi A, et al: Spontaneous bacterial peritonitis: a prospective investigation in predominantly nonalcoholic cirrhotic patients. Hepatology 3:545, 1983.
200. Hoefs JC, Runyon BA: Spontaneous bacterial peritonitis. Dis Mon 31:1, 1985.
201. Wyke RJ: Problems of bacterial infection in patients with liver disease. Gut 28:623, 1987.
202. Akalin HE, Laleli Y, Telatar H: Bactericidal and opsonic activity of ascitic fluid from cirrhotic and noncirrhotic patients. J Infect Dis 147:1011, 1983.
203. Andreu M, Sola R, Sitges-Serra A, et al: Risk factors for spontaneous bacterial peritonitis in cirrhotic patients with ascites. Gastroenterology 104:1133, 1993.
204. Rimola A, Soto R, Bory F, et al: Reticuloendothelial system phagocytic activity in cirrhosis and its relation to bacterial infections and prognosis. Hepatology 4:53, 1984.
205. Hallak A: Spontaneous bacterial peritonitis. Am J Gastroenterol 84:345, 1989.
206. Targan SR, Chow AW, Guze LB: Role of anaerobic bacteria in spontaneous peritonitis of cirrhosis. Report of two cases and review of the literature. Am J Med 62:397, 1977.
207. Sheckman P, Onderdonk AB, Bartlett JG: Anaerobes in spontaneous peritonitis. Lancet 2:1223, 1977.
208. Runyon BA: Spontaneous bacterial peritonitis: an explosion of information. Hepatology 8:171, 1988.
209. Runyon BA, Canawati HN, Akriviadis EA: Optimization of ascitic fluid culture technique. Gastroenterology 95:1351, 1988.
210. Garcia-Tsao G, Conn HO, Lerner E: The diagnosis of bacterial peritonitis: comparison of pH, lactate concentration, and leukocyte count. Hepatology 5: 91, 1985.

211. Yang C-Y, Liaw Y-F, Chu C-M, et al: White count, pH, and lactate in ascites in the diagnosis of spontaneous bacterial peritonitis. Hepatology 5:85, 1985.
212. Hoefs JC: Diagnostic paracentesis: a potent clinical tool. Gastroenterology 98:230, 1990.
213. Terg R, Levi D, Lopez P, et al: Analysis of clinical course and prognosis of culture-positive spontaneous bacterial peritonitis and neutrocytic ascites. Evidence of the same disease. Dig Dis Sci 37:1499, 1992.
214. Garrison RN, Cryer HM, Howard DA, Polk H: Clarification of risk factors for abdominal operations in patients with hepatic cirrhosis. Ann Surg 199:648, 1984.
215. Runyon BA, Hoefs JC: Ascitic fluid analysis in the differentiation of spontaneous bacterial peritonitis from gastrointestinal tract perforation into ascitic fluid. Hepatology 4:447, 1984.
216. Akriviadis EA, Runyon BA: Utility of an algorithm in differentiating spontaneous from secondary bacterial peritonitis. Gastroenterology 98:127, 1990.
217. Runyon BA, Hoefs JC: Spontaneous vs. secondary bacterial peritonitis: differentiation by response of ascitic fluid neutrophil count to antimicrobial therapy. Arch Intern Med 146:1563, 1986.
218. Felisart J, Rimola A, Arroyo V, et al: Cefotaxime is more effective than is ampicillin-tobramycin in cirrhotics with severe infections. Hepatology 5:457, 1985.
219. Runyon BA, Akriviadis EA, Sattler FR, Cohen J: Ascitic fluid and serum cefotaxime and desacetyl cefotaxime levels in patients treated for bacterial peritonitis. Dig Dis Sci 36:1782, 1991.
220. Runyon BA, McHutchison JG, Antillon MR, et al: Short-course versus long-course antibiotic treatment of spontaneous bacterial peritonitis. Gastroenterology 100:1737, 1991.
221. Runyon BA, McHutchison JG, Antillon MR, et al: Short-course versus long-course antibiotic treatment of spontaneous bacterial peritonitis. A randomized controlled study of 100 patients. Gastroenterology 100:1737, 1991.
222. Tito L, Rimola A, Llach J, et al: Recurrence of spontaneous bacterial peritonitis in cirrhosis: frequency and predictive factors. Hepatology 8:27, 1988.
223. Gines P, Rimola A, Planas R, et al: Norfloxacin prevents spontaneous bacterial peritonitis recurrence in cirrhosis: results of a double-blind, placebo-controlled trial. Hepatology 12:716, 1990.
224. Rieder HL, Cauthen GM, Kelly GD, et al: Tuberculosis in the United States. JAMA 262:385, 1989.
225. Lingenfelser T, Zak J, Marks IN, et al: Abdominal tuberculosis: still a potentially lethal disease. Am J Gastroenterol 88:744, 1993.
226. Jayanthi V, Probert CS, Sher KS, et al: The renaissance of abdominal tuberculosis. Dig Dis 11:36, 1993.
227. Manohar A, Simjee AE, Haffejee AA, Pettengell KE: Symptoms and investigative findings in 145 patients with tuberculous peritonitis diagnosed by peritoneoscopy and biopsy over a five year period. Gut 31:1130, 1990.
228. Dineen P, Homan WP, Grafe WR: Tuberculous peritonitis: 43 years' experience in diagnosis and treatment. Ann Surg 184:717, 1976.
229. Lougheed JC, Saporta J, Holmes J: Treatment and current status of tuberculous peritonitis. Am Surg 29:850, 1963.
230. Singh MM, Bhargava AN, Jain KP: Tuberculous peritonitis. An evaluation of pathogenetic mechanisms, diagnostic procedures and therapeutic measures. N Engl J Med 281:1091, 1969.
231. Voigt MD, Kalvaria I, Trey C, et al: Diagnostic value of ascites adenosine deaminase in tuberculous peritonitis. Lancet 1:751, 1989.
232. Ramaiya LI, Walter DF: Sonographic features of tuberculous peritonitis. Abdominal Imaging 18:23, 1993.
233. Mimica M: Usefulness and limitations of laparoscopy in the diagnosis of tuberculous peritonitis. Endoscopy 24:588, 1992.
234. Bhargava DK, Shriniwas, Chopra P, et al: Peritoneal tuberculosis: laparoscopic patterns and its diagnostic accuracy. Am J Gastroenterol 87:109, 1992.
235. Van Scoy RE, Wilkowske CJ: Antituberculous agents. Mayo Clin Proc 67:179, 1992.
236. Cope VZ: Visceral actinomycosis. BMJ 2:1311, 1949.
237. Berardi RS: Abdominal actinomycosis. Surg Gynecol Obstet 149:257, 1979.
238. Burden P: Actinomycosis. J Infect 19:95, 1989.
239. Harris LA, DeCosse JJ, Dannenberg A: Abdominal actinomycosis: evaluation by computed tomography. Am J Gastroenterol 84:198, 1989.
240. Manoussakis CA, Triantafillidis JK, Dadioti P, et al: The role of computed tomography in the assessment of patients with abdominal actinomycosis. Am J Gastroenterol 85:213, 1990.
241. Schiffer MA, Elquezabel A, Sultana M: Actinomycosis infections associated with intrauterine contraceptive devices. Obstet Gynecol 45:67, 1975.
242. Evans TN, Fitzgerald EJ: Abdominal actinomycosis. Br J Clin Pract 44:499, 1990.
243. Allen HA, Scatarige JC, Kim MH: Actinomycosis: CT findings in six patients. Am J Roentgenol 149:1255, 1987.
244. Brown JR: Visceral actinomycosis. Hum Pathol 4:319, 1973.
245. Wyngaarden JB, Smith LH: In: Cecil's Textbook of Medicine. Philadelphia, Saunders, 1988, pp 1673–1674.
246. Goldwag S, Abbitt PL, Watts B: Case report: percutaneous drainage of periappendiceal actinomycosis. Clin Radiol 44:422, 1991.
247. Putman HC Jr, Dockerty MB, Waugh JM: Abdominal actinomycosis: analysis of 122 cases. Surgery 28:781, 1950.
248. Brooke MM: Epidemiology of amebiasis in the US. JAMA 188:519, 1964.

249. Judy KL: Amebiasis presenting as an acute abdomen. Am J Surg 127:275, 1974.
250. DeBakey ME, Oschner A: Hepatic amebiasis: 20 year experience and analysis of 263 cases. Int Abstr Surg 92:209, 1951.
251. Health Care Financing Research Report: End-Stage Renal Disease, 1988. Washington, DC, Government Printing Office, 1989.
252. Keane WF, Everett ED, Fine RN, et al: CAPD related peritonitis management and antibiotic therapy recommendations. Peritoneal Dial Bull 7:55, 1987.
253. Saklayen MG: CAPD peritonitis. Incidence, pathogens, diagnosis, and management. Med Clin North Am 74:997, 1990.
254. Vas SI: Microbiologic aspects of chronic ambulatory peritoneal dialysis. Kidney Int 23:83, 1983.
255. Wells CL, Rotstein OD, Pruett TL: Intestinal bacteria translocate into experimental intraabdominal abscesses. Arch Surg 121:102, 1986.
256. Wu G, Khanna R, Vas SI, et al: Is extensive diverticulosis of the colon a contraindication to CAPD. Peritoneal Dialysis Bull 3:180, 1983.
257. Peterson PK, Matzke GR, Keane WF: Current concepts in the management of peritonitis in continuous ambulatory peritoneal dialysis patients. Rev Infect Dis 9:604, 1987.
258. Vas SI: Peritonitis during CAPD: a mixed bag. Peritoneal Dialysis Bull 1:47, 1981.
259. Ludlam H, Jayre D, Philips I: *Mycobacterium* tuberculosis as a cause of peritonitis in a patient undergoing continuous ambulatory peritoneal dialysis. J Infect 12:75, 1986.
260. Svetilas C, Tannenberg A: Pneumoperitoneum with peritoneal dialysis. Lancet 1:910, 1971.
261. Pickering SJ, Bowley JA, Fleming SJ, et al: Urokinase for recurrent CAPD peritonitis. Lancet 1:1258, 1987.
262. Williams AJ, Boletis I, Johnson BF, et al: Tenckhoff catheter replacement or intraperitoneal urokinase: a randomized trial in the management of recurrent continuous ambulatory peritoneal dialysis. Peritoneal Dialysis Int 9:65, 1989.
263. Paterson AD, Bishop MC, Morgan AG, et al: Removal and replacement of Tenckhoff catheter at a single operation: successful treatment of resistant peritonitis in continuous ambulatory peritoneal dialysis. Lancet 2:1245, 1986.
264. Spence PA, Mathews RE, Khanna R, et al: Indications for operation where peritonitis occurs in patients on chronic ambulatory peritoneal dialysis. Surg Gynecol Obstet 161:450, 1985.
265. Digenis GE, Khanna K, Pantalony D: Eosinophilia after implantation of the peritoneal catheter. Peritoneal Dialysis Bull 2:98, 1982.
266. Kittur DS, Korpe SW, Raytch RE, Smith GW: Surgical aspects of sclerosing encapsulating peritonitis. Arch Surg 125:1626, 1990.
267. Tsunoda T, Mochinaga N, Eto T, et al: Sclerosing encapsulating peritonitis combined with peritoneal encapsulation. Arch Surg 128:353, 1993.
268. Slingeneyer A: Preliminary report on cooperative international study on sclerosing encapsulating peritonitis. Contrib Nephrol 57:239, 1987.
269. Chefjec G, Stanley MM, Greenlee HB, Reinhardt GF: Diffuse peritoneal fibromatosis in cirrhotics following LeVeen peritoneovenous shunt insertion. Gastroenterology, 77:A7, 1979.
270. Prokesch RC, Rimland D: Infectious complications of the peritoneovenous shunt. Am J Gastroenterol 78:235, 1983.
271. Hillaire S, Labianca M, Borgonovo G, et al: Peritoneovenous shunting of intractable ascites in patients with cirrhosis: improving results and predictive factors of failure. Surgery 113:373, 1993.
272. Greig PD, Langer B: Peritoneovenous shunts for intractable ascites. In Sabiston DC (ed): Textbook of Surgery. Philadelphia, Saunders, 1991, pp 1030–1035.
273. Hubschmann OR, Countee RW: Acute abdomen in children with infected ventriculoperitoneal shunts. Arch Surg 115:305, 1980.
274. Reynolds M, Sherman JO, Melone DG: Ventriculoperitoneal shunt infection masquerading as an acute abdomen. J Pediatr Surg 18:951, 1983.
275. Deveney CW, Lurie K, Deveney KE: Improved treatment of intra-abdominal abscess. Arch Surg 123:1126, 1988.
276. Olak J, Christou NV, Stein LA, et al: Operative vs percutaneous drainage of intra-abdominal abscesses. Comparison of morbidity and mortality. Arch Surg 121:141, 1986.
277. Olson MM, Allen MO: Nosocomial abscess. Results of an eight-year prospective study of 32,284 operations. Arch Surg 124:356, 1989.
278. Altemeier WA, Culbertson WR, Fullen WD, Shook CD: Intra-abdominal abscesses. Am J Surg 125:70, 1973.
279. Mitchell GAG: The spread of acute intraperitoneal effusions. Br J Surg 28:291, 1941.
280. Altemeier WA, Culbertson WR, Fidler JP: Giant horseshoe intraabdominal abscess. Ann Surg 181: 716, 1975.
281. Patterson HC: Left subphrenic abscesses. Am Surg 43:430, 1977.
282. Goris RJA, Lubbers EJC, Oostveen HW, van den Dries ACP: Retroperitoneal infection. In de Boer HHM (ed): Intra-abdominal Sepsis. Utrecht, Bunge Scientific Publishers, 1979, p 47.
283. Sherman NJ, Davis JR, Jesseph JE: Subphrenic abscess. A continuing hazard. Am J Surg 117:117, 1969.
284. Carter R, Brewer LA: Subphrenic abscess: a thoracoabdominal clinical complex. Am J Surg 108:165, 1964.
285. Boyd DP: The intrathoracic complications of subphrenic abscess. J Thorac Cardiovasc Surg 38:771, 1959.
286. Durning P, Schofield PF: Diagnosis and manage-

ment of psoas abscess in Crohn's disease. J R Soc Med 77:33, 1984.
287. DeCosse JJ, Poulin TL, Fox PS, Condon RE: Subphrenic abscess. Surg Gynecol Obstet 138:841, 1974.
288. Knochel JO, Koehler PR, Lee TG: Diagnosis of abdominal abscesses with computed tomography, ultrasound, and In-111 leukocyte scans. Radiology 137:427, 1980.
289. Taylor KJW, Wasson JFM, De Graaf C, et al: Accuracy of grey-scale ultrasound diagnosis of abdominal and pelvic abscesses in 220 patients. Lancet 1:83, 1978.
290. vanSonnenberg E, D'Agostino HB, Casola G, et al: US-guided transvaginal drainage of pelvic abscesses and fluid collections. Radiology 181:53, 1991.
291. Bennett JD, Kozak RI, Taylor BM, Jory TA: Deep pelvic abscesses: transrectal drainage with radiologic guidance. Radiology 185:825, 1992.
292. Dobrin PB, Gully PH, Greenlee HB, et al: Radiologic diagnosis of an intraabdominal abscess. Do multiple tests help? Arch Surg 121:41, 1986.
293. Baker ME, Blinder RA, Rice RP: Diagnostic imaging of abdominal fluid collections and abscesses. CRC Crit Rev Diagn Imaging 25:233, 1986.
294. Hoffer P. Gallium mechanisms. J Nucl Med 21:282, 1980.
295. Dutcher JP, Schiffer CA, Johnston GS: Rapid migration of 111-indium labelled granulocytes to sites of infection. N Engl J Med 304:586, 1981.
296. Fry DE, Clevenger FW: Reoperation for intra-abdominal abscess. Surg Clin North Am 71:159, 1991.
297. Moore F, Feliciano D, Andrassy R, et al: Early enteral feeding, compared with parenteral, reduces postoperative septic complications: the results of a meta-analysis. Ann Surg 216:172, 1992.
298. Cerra F: Nutrient modulation of inflammatory and immune function. Am J Surg 161:230, 1991.
299. Rotstein OD, Brisseau GF: The microenvironment of infection. In Fry DE (ed): Surgical Infection. Boston, Little, Brown (in press).
300. Hau T, Haaga JR, Aeder MI: Pathophysiology, diagnosis, and treatment of abdominal abscesses. Curr Probl Surg 21:1, 1984.
301. Gerzof SG, Johnson WC, Robbins AH, Nabseth DC: Expanded criteria for percutaneous abscess drainage. Arch Surg 120:227, 1985.
302. Flancbaum L, Nosher JL, Brolin RE: Percutaneous catheter drainage of abdominal abscesses associated with perforated viscus. Am Surg 56:52, 1990.
303. Lambiase RE, Cronan JJ, Dorfman GS, et al: Postoperative abscesses with enteric communication: percutaneous treatment. Radiology 171:497, 1989.
304. Papanicolaou N, Mueller PR, Ferucci JT Jr, et al: Abscess-fistula association: radiological recognition and percutaneous management. Am J Roentgenol 143:811, 1984.
305. Gobien RP, Stanley JH, Schabel SI, et al: The effect of drainage tube size on adequacy of percutaneous abscess drainage. Cardiovas Int Radiol 8:100, 1985.
306. Pruett TL, Rotstein OD, Crass J, et al: Percutaneous aspiration and drainage for suspected intra-abdominal infection. Surgery 96:731, 1984.
307. Stabile BE, Puccio E, van Sonnenberg E, Neff CC: Preoperative percutaneous drainage of diverticular abscesses. Am J Surg 159:99, 1990.
308. Mueller PR, Saini S, Wittenburg J, et al: Sigmoid diverticular abscesses: percutaneous drainage as an adjunct to surgical resection in 24 cases. Radiology 164:321, 1987.
309. Hemming A, Davis NL, Robins RE: Surgical versus percutaneous drainage of intra-abdominal abscesses. Am J Surg 161:593, 1991.
310. Haaga JR. Imaging intraabdominal abscesses and nonoperative drainage procedures. World J Surg 14:204, 1990.
311. Goletti O, Lippolis PV, Chiarugi M, et al: Percutaneous ultrasound-guided drainage of intra-abdominal abscesses. Br J Surg 80:336, 1993.
312. Fry DE, Garrison N, Heitsch RC, et al: Determinants of death in patients with intraabdominal abscess. Surgery 88:517, 1980.
313. Brolin RE, Nosher JL, Leiman S: Percutaneous catheter versus open surgical drainage in the treatment of abdominal abscesses. Am Surg 150:102, 1984.
314. Malangoni MA, Shumate CR, Thomas HA, Richardson JD: Factors influencing the treatment of intra-abdominal abscesses. Am J Surg 159:167, 1990.
315. Stone HH, Mullins RJ, Dunlop WE, Strom PR: Extraperitoneal versus transperitoneal drainage of the intra-abdominal abscess. Surg Gynecol Obstet 159:549, 1984.
316. Halasz NA: Subphrenic abscess myths and facts. JAMA 214:724, 1970.
317. Surakiatchanukul S, Ram MD: Current patterns of subphrenic abscess. Am J Surg 125:718, 1973.
318. Pruett TL, Simmons RL: Status of percutaneous catheter drainage of abscesses. Surg Clin North Am 68:89, 1988.
319. Webster MW Jr, Cary LC: Fistulae of the intestinal tract. Curr Probl Surg 13:5, 1976.
320. Levy E, Frileux P, Cugnenc PH, et al: High-output external fistulae of the small bowel: management with continuous enteral nutrition. Br J Surg 76:676, 1989.
321. Mortensen E, Nilsson T, Vesterhauge S: Treatment of intestinal injuries following irradiation. Dis Colon Rectum 17:638, 1974.
322. Yamato T, Hamanaka Y, Hirata S, Sakai K: Esophagoplasty with an autogenous tube gastric flap. Am J Surg 137:597, 1979.
323. Soeters PB, Ebeid AM, Fischer JE: Review of 404 patients with gastrointestinal fistulas. Impact of parenteral nutrition. Ann Surg 190:189, 1979.
324. Welch CE, Rodkey GV: A method of management of the duodenal stump after gastrectomy. Surg Gynecol Obstet 98:376, 1954.

325. Anderson GW, Goss JC, Lawrence GH: External duodenal fistula. Am Surg 43:666, 1977.
326. Sharefkin J, Joffe N, Silen W, Fromm D: Anastomotic dehiscence after low anterior resection of the rectum. Am J Surg 135:519, 1978.
327. Chassin JL, Rifkind KM, Sussman B, et al: The stapled gastrointestinal tract anastomosis: incidence of postoperative complications compared with the sutured anastomosis. Ann Surg 188:689, 1978.
328. Hermreck AS, Crawford DG: The esophageal anastomotic leak. Am J Surg 132:794, 1976.
329. Fischer JE: The management of high-output intestinal fistulas. Adv Surg 9:139, 1975.
330. Miller HI, Dorn BC: Postoperative gastrointestinal fistulas. Am J Surg 116:382, 1968.
331. Reber H, Roberts C, Way LW, Dunphy JE: Management of external gastrointestinal fistulas. Ann Surg 188:460, 1978.
332. Thomas RJS, Rosalion A: The use of parenteral nutrition in the management of external gastrointestinal tract fistulae. Aust N Z J Med 48:535, 1978.
333. Freund H, Anner C, Saltz NJ: Management of gastrointestinal fistulas with total parenteral nutrition. Int Surg 61:273, 1976.
334. Spiliotis J, Vagenas K, Panagopoulos K, Kalfarentzos F: Treatment of enterocutaneous fistulas with TPN and somatostatin, compared with patients who received TPN only. Br J Clin Pract 44:616, 1990.
335. Nubiola P, Badia JM, Martinez-Rodenas F, et al: Treatment of 27 postoperative enterocutaneous fistulas with the long half life somatostatin analogue SMS 201-995. Ann Surg 210:56, 1989.
336. Schein M, Decker GA: Postoperative external alimentary tract fistulas. Am J Surg 161:435, 1991.
337. Prickett D, Montgomery R, Cheadle WG: External fistulas arising from the digestive tract. South Med J 84:736, 1991.
338. Athanassiades S, Notis P, Tountas C: Fistulas of the gastrointestinal tract. Experience with 81 cases. Am J Surg 130:26, 1975.
339. Chapman R, Foran R, Dunphy JE: Management of intestinal fistulas. Am J Surg 108:157, 1964.
340. Altomare DF, Serio G, Pannarale OC, et al: Prediction of mortality by logistic regression analysis in patients with postoperative enterocutaneous fistulae. Br J Surg 77:450, 1990.
341. Hollender LF, Otteni F: Treatment of postoperative external fistulas of the small intestine. Surg Annu 7:295, 1975.
342. Rubelowsky J, Machiedo GW: Reoperative versus conservative management for gastrointestinal fistulas. Surg Clin North Am 71:147, 1991.
343. Monod-Broca P: Treatment of intestinal fistulas. Br J Surg 65:685, 1977.
344. MacFayden BV, Dudrick SJ, Ruberg RL: Management of gastrointestinal fistulae with parenteral hyperalimentation. Surgery 74:100, 1973.
345. Meijer WS, Schmitz PIM, Jeekel J: Meta-analysis of randomized controlled clinical trials of antibiotic prophylaxis in biliary tract surgery. Br J Surg 77:283, 1990.
346. Patton AS, Lawson DW, Shannon JM, et al: Reevaluation of the Boerhaave syndrome. A review of fourteen cases. Am J Surg 137:560, 1979.
347. Garden OJ, Dykes EH, Carter DC: Surgical and nutritional management of postoperative duodenal fistulas. Dig Dis Sci 33:30, 1988.
348. Ellis H, Irving M: Gastrointestinal and biliary fistulae. In Schwartz S, Ellis H (eds): Maingot's Abdominal Operations. Norwalk, CT, Appleton & Lange, 1989, pp 315–334.
349. Rao PN, Knox R, Barnard RJ, Schofield PF: Management of colovesical fistula. Br J Surg 74:362, 1987.
350. Mileski WJ, Joehl RJ, Rege RV, Nahrwold DL: One-stage resection and anastomosis in the management of colovesical fistula. Am J Surg 153:75, 1987.
351. Bard V, Cohen Z, Ross T: An unusual intraoperative complication of stapled colorectal anastomosis: report of a case and review of the literature. Can J Surg 36:165, 1993.
352. Fleshner PR, Schoetz DJ Jr, Roberts PL, et al: Anastomotic-vaginal fistula after colorectal surgery. Dis Colon Rectum 35:938, 1992.
353. Grissom R, Snyder TE: Colovaginal fistula secondary to diverticular disease. Dis Colon Rectum 34:1043, 1991.
354. Colonna JO, Kang J, Giuliano AE, Hiatt JR: One-stage repair of colovaginal fistula complicating acute diverticulitis. Am Surg 56:788, 1990.
355. Rotstein OD, Pruett TL, Simmons RL: Gastropleural fistula: report of three cases and review of the literature. Am J Surg 150:392, 1985.
356. Sitges-Serra A, Jaurrieta E, Sitges-Creus A: Management of postoperative enterocutaneous fistulas: the roles of parenteral nutrition and surgery. Br J Surg 69:147, 1982.

Biliary Tract Infections

CHAPTER 39

Pamela A. Lipsett, Henry A. Pitt

Infections of the biliary tract are one of the most common intra-abdominal infectious problems. Although the biliary tree is normally sterile, the high incidences of gallstones in Western countries and of intrahepatic stones in Asia frequently create situations that result in biliary tract infections. The widespread availability of nonoperative biliary interventions has also increased the infectious complications in patients with malignant biliary tract obstruction. This chapter will review the anatomy, physiology, and bacteriology of the biliary tract, the common gallbladder, and bile duct infections, cholecystitis and cholangitis, as well as rare infections such as cholangiohepatitis and those seen in patients with acquired immune deficiency syndrome.

ANATOMY, PHYSIOLOGY, AND BACTERIOLOGY

Anatomy

The biliary tree begins at the bile canaliculi within the hepatic parenchyma. Multiple branches of the tree pass more centrally toward the right and left hepatic ducts. Most patients have a hepatic duct bifurcation although a small percentage have three ducts that come together to form the common hepatic duct (CHD). The right hepatic duct leads relatively directly into the CHD, whereas the left hepatic duct usually enters the CHD at a greater angle. This anatomic difference may explain, in part, why intrahepatic stones and associated "oriental cholangiohepatitis" occurs more commonly on the left.

At the point where the cystic duct enters the biliary tree, the CHD becomes the common bile duct (CBD). This point of entrance is quite variable, and a relatively low entrance of a relatively large cystic duct may predispose to common duct stones[1] and therefore to cholangitis. Rarely, the cystic duct may enter the right hepatic duct. The length and diameter of the cystic duct are also quite variable, and this duct is unique in that the valves of Heister participate in the two-way flow of bile. Increased resistance to flow through the cystic duct may predispose to gallstone formation[2] and therefore also to acute cholecystitis.

The gallbladder is a very compliant structure that stores bile between meals and empties approximately three-quarters of its contents in response to ingested food. The gallbladder's tip is called the fundus, and the body and neck are the structures that lead into the cystic duct. Hartmann's pouch lies adjacent to the gallbladder's neck. Obstruction of the cystic duct by a gallstone is the most frequent cause of acute cholecystitis. Rarely, a large stone impacted in Hartmann's pouch or in the cystic duct may obstruct the common hepatic duct—the Mirrizi syndrome—resulting in obstructive jaundice and cholangitis.

The common bile duct enters the duodenum near the junction of the second and third portions. The sphincter of Oddi is a complex structure at the lower end of the bile duct, which regulates the flow of bile and pancreatic juice. This sphincter is a one-way valve that normally prevents the regurgitation of duodenal juice and bacteria from entering the biliary system. However, dysfunction or stenosis of the sphincter of Oddi may result in reflux of duodenal contents or bile stasis. In this setting, bacterial colonization may occur, and primary common duct stones may form. If a common duct stone obstructs the distal bile duct or lodges in the sphincter of Oddi, cholangitis will result.

The arterial blood flow to the biliary system comes from various branches of the hepatic artery. Within the wall of the common duct, two main arteries run in the three and nine o'clock positions. The main arterial supply to the gallbladder is the cystic artery, which usually arises from the right hepatic artery. With respect to biliary infections, however, the venous and lymphatic anatomy may be more relevant. Venous drainage of the gallbladder is primarily through small veins that enter the liver directly. A venous plexus from the extrahepatic bile ducts drains into the portal vein. Within the liver, however, the bile canaliculi communicate with the hepatic venules through the space of Disse. This pathway is one route by which bacteria may gain access to the systemic circulation in patients with cholangitis.

With increased biliary pressures, both cholangiovenous and cholangiolymphatic reflux may occur. Within the liver lymphatic channels drain to the lymphatic nodes in the porta hepatis. Lymphatic drainage of the gallbladder is toward the cystic duct lymph nodes. The extrahepatic biliary lymphatics also drain toward the cystic duct nodes as well as those surrounding the bile duct. All these nodes drain toward the celiac nodes. Lymph flow then extends through central channels to the thoracic duct. Through this lymphatic route bacteria may also gain access to the systemic circulation.

Physiology

The liver normally produces between 500 and 1000 ml of bile each day. Two of the major components of bile, water and bile salts, are very efficiently conserved by the body.[3] Water in bile excreted by the liver is absorbed both in the gallbladder and in the intestinal tract. The gallbladder is actually one of the most efficient absorptive surfaces in the body. As a result, gallbladder bile is very concentrated when compared to hepatic bile (Table 39–1). Bile salts are almost all reabsorbed by the ileum, creating an efficient enterohepatic circulation (EHC). As a result of gallbladder concentration and the EHC, approximately 90 percent of the bile salt pool resides in the gallbladder in the fasting state.

TABLE 39–1. COMPOSITION OF HEPATIC AND GALLBLADDER BILE

Characteristics	Hepatic	Gallbladder
Na (mEq/liter)	160	270
K (mEq/liter)	5	10
Cl (mEq/liter)	90	15
HCO_3 (mEq/liter)	45	10
Plt	7.8	7.2
Bilirubin (mEq/liter)	1.5	15
Cholesterol	4	18
Phospholipids (mEq/liter)	8	40
Bile acids (mEq/liter)	50	150

Adapted from Klein AS, Lillemoe KD, Yeo CJ, Pitt HA: Liver, biliary tract, and pancreas. In O'Leary JP (ed): The Physiologic Basis of Surgery. Baltimore, Williams & Wilkins, 1993.

In response to a meal the gallbladder empties the majority of its contents into the duodenum within 1 hour.[3] In the fasting state small amounts of hepatic bile are continuously delivered to the duodenum by the sphincter of Oddi. In addition, in coordination with phase III of the migrating myoelectric complex, the gallbladder empties approximately 15 percent of its contents on a regular basis during fasts. Thus bile flow is a dynamic process and is relatively rapid considering the small volume of the ductal system. This constant clearing process is one of the factors that keeps the bile sterile.

Bile has many components including water, biliary lipids, and proteins.[3] The three major classes of lipid are cholesterol, phospholipids, and bile salts. While the milieu of bile may be a nutrient source for certain organisms like the coliforms, high concentrations of bile salts tend to inhibit bacterial growth. Bile salts are relatively more potent inhibitors of anaerobic than of aerobic organisms. This fact may explain why anaerobic infections of the biliary tract are less common than in other abdominal infections. Bile also has very high levels of the immunoglobulins, IgA, IgG, and IgM. These immunoglobulins also play an important role in maintaining a sterile biliary tree.

Bacteriology

Cultures of the normal gallbladder and bile duct bile are usually sterile.[4] The pathway by which bacteria infect the biliary tree has not been firmly established.[5] Possibilities include ascending infection from the duodenum, lymphatic spread, and vascular dissemination from portal venous or hepatic arterial flow. Although the spread of organisms from the duodenum seems logical, no convincing evidence suggests that this factor is important in patients having a normal sphincter mechanism.[6] Dineen[7] has demonstrated that lymphatic flow is caudad from the liver into the periduodenal area. In addition, Dineen has demonstrated that portal vein bacteremia is the most efficient way to deliver bacteria into bile and that biliary obstruction further increases the concentration of bacteria in bile after portal venous bacteremia. Patients with oriental cholangiohepatitis and ulcerative colitis have been shown to have portal venous bacteremia.[7]

Under normal circumstances portal venous bacteremia is effectively cleared by the hepatic reticuloendothelial system. These bacteria are excreted into the bile, which is then innocently secreted back into the small intestine. Thus diseases that influence the reticuloendothelial system and normal bile flow will increase the likelihood of clinical biliary tract infection. Hepatic arterial bacteremia certainly can cause biliary tract disease such as hepatic abscesses, but this mechanism is uncommon except in situations where bacteremia is sustained, such as bacterial endocarditis.

When bacteria do gain access to the biliary tree, the organisms most likely to be isolated are gut-derived aerobes. In most analyses of biliary bacteriology the three most common organisms are the gram-negatives *Escherichia coli* and *Klebsiella* and the gram-positive *Enterococcus.*[4,6] Other gram-negative aerobes such as *Pseudomonas* and *Enterobacter* species are more likely to appear after the biliary tree has been manipulated. Anaerobes are isolated from bile less commonly. Anaerobes are more common in elderly patients and in those with complex biliary problems and severe forms of cholecystitis and cholangitis. When anaerobes are present, *Bacteroides fragilis* and *Clostridium perfringens* are the most common species. Yeast, especially *Candida albicans,* may also be a common isolate in patients who have been treated with antibiotics.

The precise role of bacteria in the formation of gallstones has been debated. Most authorities now believe that bacteria are not important in the pathogenesis of cholesterol or black pigment gallstones.[8] However, brown pigment stones are thought to be caused by bacteria, especially gram-negative rods. Brown pigment stones occur most commonly as primary common duct stones in Western countries and intrahepatic stones in the Orient. Kaufman et al[8] have demonstrated gram-negative bacteria and their casts within brown pigment stones (see Fig. 39–1). Maki[9] suggested that beta-glucaronidase produced by gram-negative organisms hydrolyses bilirubin glucuronide into free bilirubin and glucuronic acid. The free bilirubin carboxyl group has a high affinity for calcium and forms calcium bilirubinate, which then complexes with varying additional biliary proteins and small amounts of cholesterol to form stones. As mentioned above, not all gallstones are formed via an infectious pathogenic mechanism. Gender, pregnancy, diet, obesity, rapid weight loss, and gallbladder stasis clearly are important factors in noninfectious gallstone formation (see Table 39–2).[10]

Antibiotic Excretion

A great deal has been written about the importance of antibacterial concentrations of antimicrobial agents in the biliary tree. Some of the newer broad spectrum penicillins and cephalosporins produce

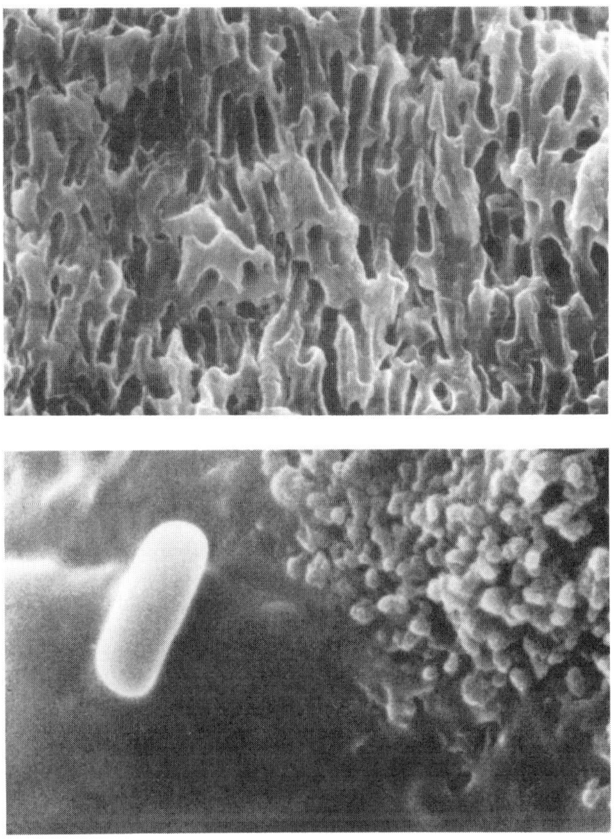

Figure 39–1. A. Electron micrograph of gallstone demonstrating casts from gram-negative rods within the gallstone substance. ×7500. *(From Kaufman HW, Magnuson TH, Lillemoe KD, Pitt HA: Ann Surg 209:584, 1989.)* **B.** Further magnification of additional area of the same gallstone as part **A** with an actual gram-negative rod. ×24,000.

TABLE 39–2. RISK FACTORS FOR GALLSTONES

Female gender
Pregnancy
Diet
Obesity
Rapid weight loss
Cirrhosis
Hemolytic anemia
Sickle cell disease
Hereditary spherocytosis
Crohn's disease, ileal disease
Ulcerative colitis
Intestinal bypass surgery
Genetic factors
Pima Indian
Vagotomy

very high concentrations in bile (see Chap. 24). However, when the cystic duct or the common bile duct is obstructed, even agents that normally achieve very high biliary levels are poorly concentrated. Moreover, gentamicin, an aminoglycoside not concentrated in bile, has proved efficient in reducing wound sepsis and treating bacteremia in patients with biliary tract infections.[11] Keighley and associates[11] have clearly demonstrated that biliary concentration of antibiotics are not as important as antibacterial spectrum, particularly in patients with biliary obstruction. Thus specific antibiotics for treating biliary infections should be selected on the basis of their antibacterial spectrum rather than on their biliary excretion.[12–15]

GALLBLADDER INFECTIONS

As with cholangitis, infections of the gallbladder may present with a wide spectrum of disease. Most patients who develop gallbladder infections have gallstones. However, only approximately 15 percent of patients with cholesterol or black pigment gallstones and chronic cholecystitis have bacteria in their gallbladders at the time of cholecystectomy.[8,16] The likelihood of isolating bacteria increases in patients with acute cholecystitis, especially as the disease progresses. At the far end of this spectrum of cholecystitis are patients with empyema of the gallbladder or emphysematous cholecystitis where the infection may be life-threatening. Before discussing these severe infections, the role of antibiotic prophylaxis will be addressed.

Antibiotic Prophylaxis

The development of a wound infection following biliary tract surgery depends on the bacteriologic status of the bile and the degree of wound contamination during the operation. A myriad of prospective, randomized trials of antibiotics for prophylaxis have been carried out for open cholecystectomy and other common open biliary tract procedures. Good data are not yet available on the role of prophylactic antibiotics for patients undergoing laparoscopic cholecystectomy. However, the principles learned with open procedures should be applicable to the laparoscopic operations.

Previously, antibiotic prophylaxis was recommended for patients at "high risk" of having bactibilia.[12,17] These risk factors were (1) age greater than 70 years, (2) recent cholangitis, (3) prior biliary tract surgery, (4) jaundice, (5) acute cholecystitis within 1 month, (6) choledocholithiasis, and (7) gallbladder empyema.[18] Several authorities[19,20] have championed the use of intraoperative Gram stains to guide the use of antibiotics in the operating room. Accuracy rates coincided with subsequent cultures greater than 75 percent of the time, and advocates of this approach suggested that antibiotics be used when bacteria were seen in Gram stains.

A recent meta-analysis of greater than 1400 patients involved in randomized trials confirmed the benefit of prophylaxis in all patients undergoing open cholecystectomy.[23] In this meta-analysis a first-generation cephalosporin was as efficacious and more cost effective than second- or third-generation cephalosporins. Moreover, in several studies one dose of a preoperative antibiotic was as effective as a 5-day course. These principles should also apply to patients undergoing laparoscopic cholecystectomy even though the wound infection rate may be lower than with the open technique. Whether more broad spectrum antibiotics are indicated for prophylaxis in patients undergoing more complicated biliary tract surgery remains a matter of debate as this question has not been addressed in proper randomized trial.

Acute Cholecystitis

Acute cholecystitis is an inflammatory process of the gallbladder that occurs when the cystic duct becomes obstructed. In more than 90 percent of cases, acute cholecystitis is caused by gallstones.[15] Other unusual etiologies of cholecystitis include cholangiocarcinoma and primary gallbladder cancer. In a small minority of patients acute cholecystitis occurs in the absence of gallstones or cancer, and these patients often represent a more difficult diagnostic dilemma.[16]

Pathogenesis. In acute cholecystitis, gallbladder bile infection is a secondary, rather than a primary, event. With cystic duct obstruction, bile remains static, while the gallbladder continues to secrete fluid, electrolytes, and proteins. As a result, the gallbladder swells and becomes tense, inflamed, and edematous. As the inflammatory process spreads within the gallbladder, the surrounding portal structures become involved. Frequently, the omentum will travel to the right upper quadrant to attempt to "police" the inflammatory process. Failure to relieve the cystic duct obstruction either spontaneously or by invasive measures results in a further increase in intraluminal pressure within the gallbladder. As the intraluminal pressure exceeds capillary blood flow, vascular compromise ensues, gangrene of the gallbladder wall develops, and perforation with bile peritonitis can develop (Fig. 39–2).

The gallbladder fundus is the most frequent area of perforation because the gallbladder wall blood supply in this area is the poorest.[18] Because bile flow is an important mechanism for the clearance of the small numbers of bacteria that may enter the biliary system, gallbladder obstruction and stasis eventually lead to bacterial proliferation. However, in most cases the inflammatory process is primary and bacterial infection is secondary.

Gallstones are found with increased frequency in certain patient populations and may be related to other disease processes[10] (see Table 39–2). Patients with cirrhosis, chronic hemolytic anemias, such as sickle cell disease and hereditary spherocytosis, Crohn's disease, ulcerative colitis, prior intestinal bypass surgery, and rapid weight loss are all at increased risk for developing gallstones. Therefore each of these groups of patients are also at increased risk for acute cholecystitis.

Acute cholecystitis is a very rare event in patients without gallstones; most of these patients who develop acute acalculous cholecystitis have other major illnesses and are frequently found in an intensive care unit. These patients may be recovering from prior surgery,[21–23] extensive burns,[24] or major trauma.[25–27] Risk factors seemingly associated with this disease include parenteral nutrition,[28,29] mechanical ventilation,[22,26] multiple blood transfusions,[25] high doses of narcotics,[27] antibiotic administration,[30] and hypotension[26] (Table 39–3). In these patients a combination of gallbladder stasis and perhaps ischemia may be important pathogentic factors. Additionally, patients with the acquired immune deficiency syndrome (AIDS) are at special risk for acalculous biliary tract disease, and these patients will be discussed separately.[31–34]

Clinical Features. Abdominal pain is the most prominent clinical feature of acute cholecystitis (Table 39–4). Typically, the onset of pain occurs several hours after a fatty late night meal. The pain is usually located at the right subcostal margin but may occur in the epigastrium and may radiate to the tip of the right scapula as the peritoneum becomes inflamed. The pain is usually not colicky but is constant, severe, and usually associated with

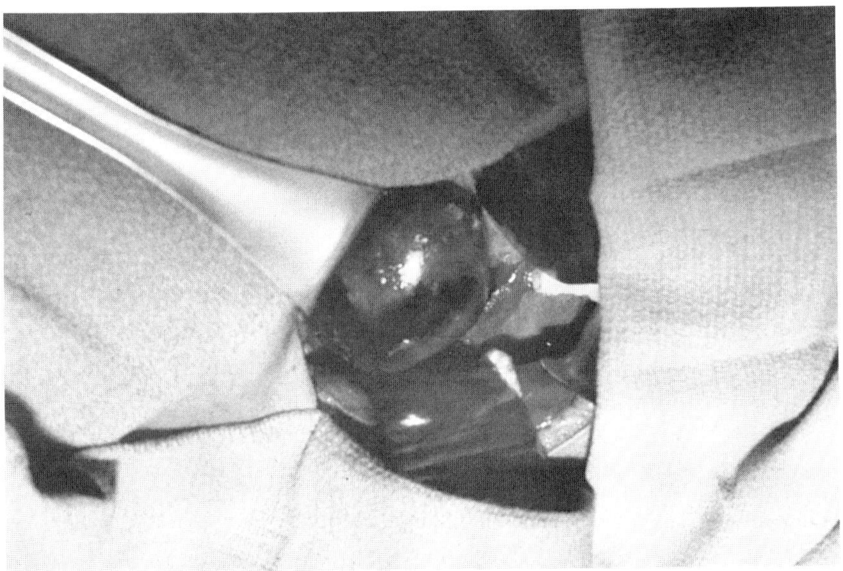

Figure 39–2. Intraoperative photograph of a gallbladder with acute cholecystitis and focal gangrene of the gallbladder wall at the fundus.

TABLE 39–3. RISK FACTORS FOR ACALCULOUS CHOLECYSTITIS

Acquired immune deficiency	Medical illnesses (severe)
Antibiotics	Narcotics (high dose)
Blood transfusions (multiple)	Postoperative state
Burns	Total parenteral nutrition
Hypotension	Trauma
Mechanical ventilation	Vasculitis

nausea. As the disease progresses, vomiting may occur but is usually not profuse. As the inflammatory process continues, fever may develop.

The clinical examination includes muscular guarding and tenderness in the right subcostal area. Point tenderness over the gallbladder that halts the patient's inspiratory effort is a positive Murphy's sign. In up to one-quarter of cases the gallbladder will be palpable; and as it distends, it moves laterally and inferiorly. A rigid abdomen in a patient with acute cholecystitis suggests that a complication such as gangrene and/or rupture of the gallbladder has developed.

Diagnosis. In patients with known gallstones the diagnosis is usually straightforward. The laboratory evaluation usually demonstrates a slight elevation of the white blood cell (WBC) count (10,000 to 15,000 cells/mm^3) and liver function tests. The bilirubin may be mildly elevated (2 to 3 mg/dl) as the inflammatory process continues. Plain radiographs of the abdomen usually are nonspecific, but in 10 to 15 percent of patients, radiopaque gallstones may be demonstrated. In a small minority of cases the gallbladder itself can be calcified (poreclin) or gas can be seen within the gallbladder, its wall or within the biliary tree. In the acute setting oral cholecystograms are of no value because of problems with vomiting, ileus, altered liver function, and the time involved. Intravenous cholangiography is no longer performed because of low accuracy and concerns about allergic reactions.

Depending on the availability of each test in a specific center, both ultrasonography and biliary scintigraphy are helpful in establishing this diagnosis. The ultrasonography reveals calculous disease, a distended gallbladder often with an edematous wall (Halo sign), and pericholecystic fluid (Fig. 39–3). Sonographic tenderness also can be demonstrated over the gallbladder. Biliary scintigraphy depends on the hepatic uptake of the tracer and biliary secretion. If the cystic duct is patent and the gallbladder can accommodate fluid, the tracer will enter the gallbladder, and additional tracer will be excreted into the duodenum (Fig. 39–4). Both of these studies are sensitive and specific when uti-

TABLE 39–4. CLINICAL FEATURES OF ACUTE CHOLECYSTITIS

• PRESENTATION	
Age	40–50s
Female/male	3:2
Fever	90%
Chills	50%
Nausea	70%
RUQ pain	95%
RUQ tenderness	95%
Palpable mass RUQ	25%
Jaundice	30%
• LABORATORY FINDINGS	
WBC > 10,000	70%
WBC > 20,000	5%
Bilirubin > 1.5	30%
Bilirubin > 5.0	5%
Alkaline phosphatase ↑	40%
SGOT/SGPT ↑	50%
Amylase ↑	15%

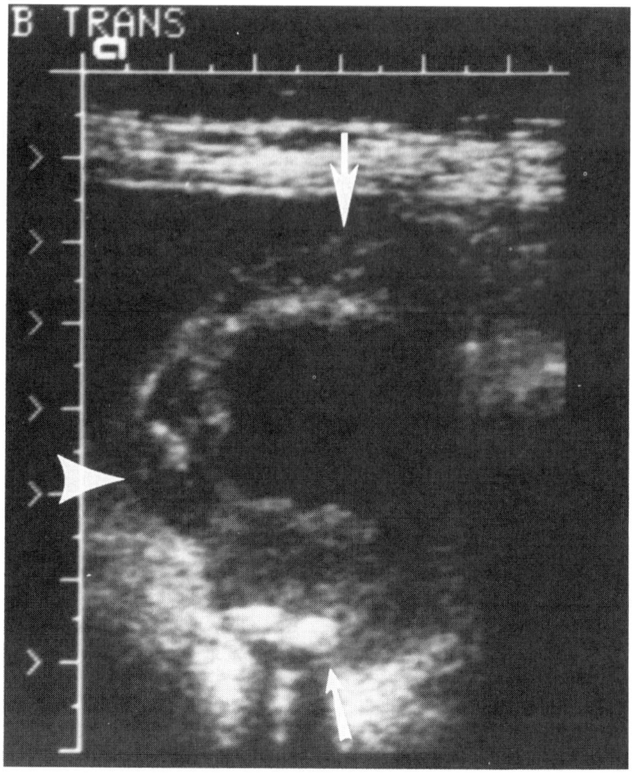

Figure 39–3. Transverse section of a right upper quadrant ultrasound demonstrating gallstones (small arrow), a thickened gallbladder wall with a halo sign (top arrow), and a focal collection of air within the gallbladder wall suggesting impending perforation (curved arrow).

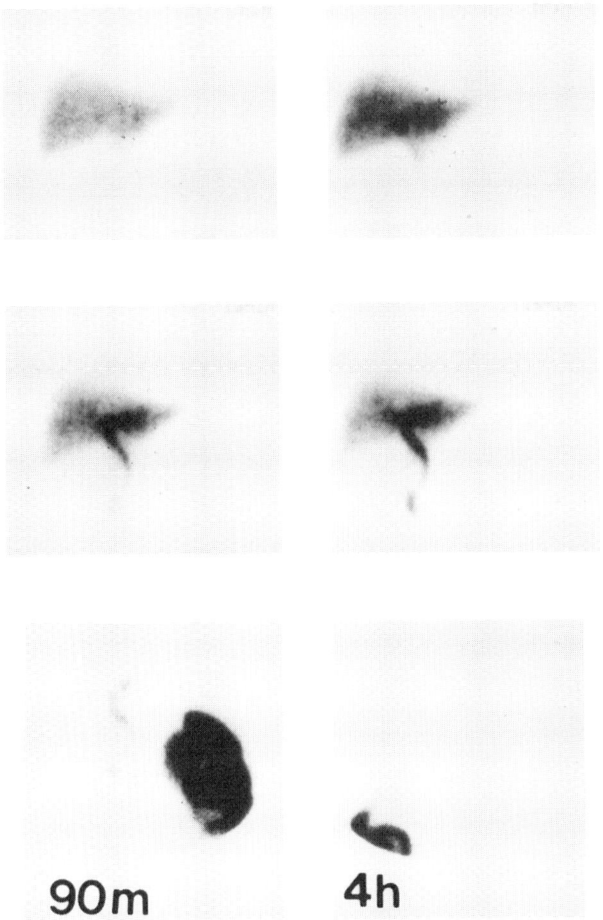

Figure 39–4. A. Technetium hepatobiliary scan of a middle-aged woman with fever, right upper quadrant pain, and nausea demonstrating uptake in the liver at 2 (a) and 5 (b) minutes and biliary secretion by 10 (c) and 15 (d) minutes. **B.** After 90 minutes there has been flow into the duodenum and small bowel without filling the gallbladder. By 4 hours the contrast is in the right lower quadrant. The gallbladder never filled, suggesting acute cholecystitis as the diagnosis.

lized with the appropriate patient population.[35] However, comparative studies suggest that scintigraphy is more accurate because some patients with acute cholecystitis have enough intestinal and colonic gas due to ileus to prevent full evaluation of the gallbladder.

Microbiology. Thompson and colleagues[36] reported that 42 percent, and Lee et al[14] found that 63 percent of patients with acute cholecystitis had positive gallbladder bile cultures (Table 39–5). Both the gallbladder bile and the gallbladder wall contained the same microorganisms. *Escherichia coli, Klebsiella,* and *Enterobacter* species were the most common gram-negative organisms, while *Enterococcus* and other *Streptococcus* species were common gram-positive organisms. Anaerobes were isolated in only 11 percent of patients, and fungi were rarely seen.[14] Thus the bacteriology is similar whether acute or chronic cholecystitis is present. The gram-negative coliforms account for approximately two-thirds of the isolated organisms; the gram-positive enterococci are present in 20 to 30 percent of the patients; and anaerobes are rarely found. While the organisms are the same, patients with acute cholecystitis generally have more bacteria (10^6 to 10^9 versus 10^5) and are more likely to have positive cultures (40 to 60 percent versus 15 to 30 percent) than patients with chronic cholecystitis.

Treatment. Many cases of acute cholecystitis resolve spontaneously, and the disease continues to the chronic phase. Much debate has occurred with respect to the merits of early (within 1 to 2 days of symptom onset) versus late (after more than 6 weeks) operative intervention. On the basis of four randomized trials, the balance of opinion supports early cholecystectomy.[17,37] Early operative intervention has the benefit of shortened hospitalization and sooner return to work without increased morbidity or mortality. Early cholecystectomy may also abort the development of complications of acute cholecystitis (empyema and perforation). Moreover, the dissection if done within the first 3 days of the disease process is often easier.

In the vast majority of patients with acute cholecystitis the treatment of choice is cholecystectomy. Even with acute inflammation, many of these cholecystectomies may be completed by the laparoscopic technique. However, the surgeon should have a low threshold for converting to an open procedure in these patients. Open cholecystostomy is rarely indicated as it may not be an adequate operation to resolve the septic process in patients with empyema or gangrene of the gallbladder. Subtotal cholecys-

TABLE 39–5. ANTIBIOTIC CHOICE IN ACUTE CHOLECYSTITIS

Infecting Organism[a]	Percentage of Patients Positive
Escherichia coli	48
Klebsiella species	22
Enterococcus/Streptococcus species	25
Enterobacter species	4
Proteus species	2
Clostridium species	5
Bacteriodes species	1
Other	6

[a] Note many patients have mixed infections.

tectomy may be a reasonable compromise when the inflammatory process in the porta hepatis makes identification of the common duct essentially impossible. Another option to be considered in carefully selected severely ill patients is percutaneous cholecystostomy. However, if sepsis or organ failure continues, cholecystectomy may be the more conservative approach.

If there is suspicion of significant gallbladder pathology requiring admission, the patient should be kept without oral alimentation and hydrated intravenously. Parenteral antibiotics should be utilized as the disease progresses and the possibility of infection increases with the majority of patients demonstrating bactibilia at the time of operation. In most patients with acute cholecystitis antibiotics can be discontinued in 2 to 3 days after cholecystectomy. However, in patients in whom a complication of cholecystitis such as empyema, perforation, emphysematous cholecystitis, or gangrene has developed, antibiotics should be administered for a longer period of at least 5 to 7 days. As a general guideline, antibiotics may be stopped when the patient remains afebrile and the WBC count returns to normal.

The antibiotics selected for these patients should offer coverage against the aerobic enteric gram-negative rods, which comprise the majority of bacteria found in acute cholecystitis. Although some authors have suggested that intraoperative Gram stains should guide the decision whether or not to utilize antibacterial agents, most authorities recommend preoperative coverage in all patients.[19] Operative bile cultures can be utilized to modify antibiotic therapy if necessary, and the presence of gram-positive rods suggesting *Clostridium* species may be an indication for high-dose penicillin therapy.[38] Many antibacterial agents have proved efficacious for the treatment of acute cholecystitis.[14,19,34,39–43] Examples of appropriate agents and their bacterial coverage are presented in Table 39–6.

Outcome. Although the morbidity and mortality for acute cholecystitis exceed that of chronic cholecystitis, most patients will do well when the disease is promptly recognized and treated. Septic complications following acute cholecystitis are much more likely when the disease has failed to resolve spontaneously or treatment has been delayed. While earlier reports suggested that the mortality was as high as 5 percent in these patients, recent reports[44] suggest that mortality is less than 1 percent for patients with acute cholecystitis.

TABLE 39–6. ANTIBIOTIC CHOICE IN ACUTE CHOLECYSTITIS

Antibiotic for uncomplicated cholecystitis (2–5 days)
Penicillins
Ampicillin
Ureidopenicillins (pipercillin, mezlocillin)
Combinations (ampicillin/sulbactam, ticarcillin/clavulanic acid)
Cephalosporins
First-generation (cefazolin)
Second-generation (cefotetan, cefoxitin)
Third-generation (ceftriaxone, cefotaxime, cefoperazone)
Antibiotics for complicated cholecystities (5–7 days)
Ampicillin + aminoglycoside
Pipercillin/mezlocillin
Combination penicillins (ampicillin/sulbactam, ticarcillin/clavulanic acid)
Second-generation cephalosporin ± ampicillin
Third-generation cephalosporin ± ampicillin
Monobactam (imipenem)
Fluoroquinolone (ciprofloxacin, perfloxacin)

Hydrops

Hydrops develops when the gallbladder mucosal lining continues to secrete mucus in the face of complete obstruction of the cystic duct. Clinically, patients present with some degree of right upper quadrant pain and a smooth, nontender mass in the right upper quadrant. These patients usually have "white bile" because all the bilirubin pigment has been absorbed. This viscous white bile is normally sterile. If bacteria are present within the gallbladder, hydrops will progress to an empyema of gallbladder. The treatment of hydrops of the gallbladder is cholecystectomy. Antibiotics are probably indicated for perioperative prophylaxis only and may be discontinued if operative cultures are sterile.

Empyema

If the cystic duct remains obstructed as infection is established, the purulent process may progress within the gallbladder. The gallbladder becomes greatly distended and tense. The combination of infection and increased gallbladder wall pressure once again enhance the chance of gallbladder wall necrosis and perforation.[45]

Because empyema of the gallbladder is a complication of acute cholecystitis, the initial 48 hours of symptomatology of an empyema are indistinguishable from acute cholecystitis. However, after 48 hours when most patients with acute cholecystitis feel symptomatically improved, patients who are developing an empyema have a more severe clinical course. Fever is often significant (38.7C to 40C), as is abdominal pain and tenderness. A tender right upper quadrant mass is often palpable. Generalized peritonitis with a rigid abdomen is unusual but often indicates that perforation of the gallbladder has occurred. In elderly or immunosuppressed patients, the magnitude of abdominal signs may be less than anticipated. In any patient undergoing medical treatment for acute cholecystitis with continued signs of systemic toxicity, empyema of the gallbladder should be considered.

The diagnosis is established on the basis of the history and physical examination. Typically, the laboratory values reveal a significantly elevated WBC count often above 20,000 cells/mm^3. Liver function tests are often mildly abnormal, much as in acute cholecystitis. As with uncomplicated acute cholecystitis, cholescintigraphy will indicate cystic duct obstruction and ultrasonography will usually indicate gallstones and a fluid-filled, swollen gallbladder.

Early operative intervention is the treatment of choice for empyema of the gallbladder. After intravenous hydration, stabilization, and parenteral antibiotics, cholecystectomy should be performed. Although occasionally cholecystostomy or drainage is used as a temporizing measure in the critically ill patient, frequently the gallbladder wall is necrotic and thus warrants excision. While the incidence of anaerobes is low in patients with uncomplicated acute cholecystitis, up to 45 percent of patients with empyema of the gallbladder will have a polymicrobial infection that includes anaerobes.[45] Thus antibiotics with anaerobic coverage are indicated in patients suspected or found to have empyema of the gallbladder. Both the morbidity and mortality are increased in this small subset of patients. Therefore removal of the gallbladder may be life-saving even in patients with significant associated diseases.

Emphysematous Cholecystitis

Emphysematous cholecystitis is synonymous with acute gaseous cholecystitis, aerocholecystitis, pneumocholecystitis, and gas gangrene of the gallbladder. Emphysematous cholecystitis is an uncommon and very serious variant of acute cholecystitis.[45] This disease is characterized and diagnosed by the presence of gas on a plain radiograph, ultrasound, or computed tomography (CT) scan in the gallbladder lumen, in the gallbladder wall, or in the biliary ducts, which is caused by gas-forming microbes (Fig. 39–5). Other causes for air to be observed in the gallbladder or bile ducts include a biliary-enteric surgical anastomosis, a spontaneous internal biliary fistula, a traumatic biliary fistula, an incompetent sphincter of Oddi, and percutaneous endoscopic intervention.

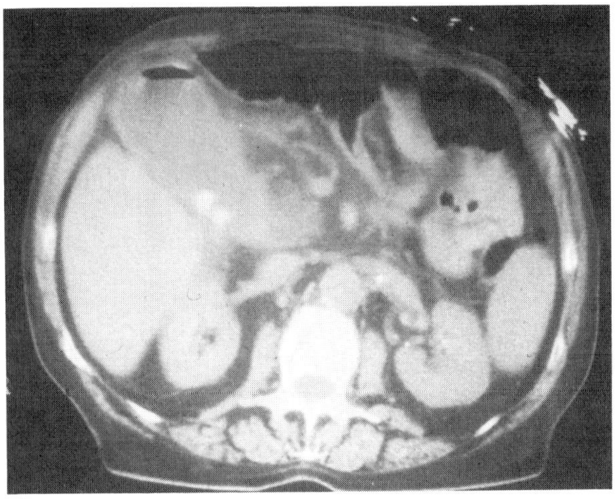

Figure 39–5. CT scan from an elderly man who was toxic and jaundiced. Abdominal film was normal. Air is seen within the gallbladder lumen and gallstones are seen in the neck of the gallbladder. Intraoperative cultures from the gallbladder demonstrated both *Clostridium welchii* and toxigenic *E. coli.*

In emphysematous cholecystitis, gas is produced by facultative and anaerobic bacteria. *Clostridium perfringens* is the most common offending organism although *Escherichia coli, Klebsiella,* and anaerobic streptococci have been implicated.[44–47] Men are much more likely to have this disease and diabetes is associated in 30 to 50 percent of patients[48] (Table 39–7). The features that differentiate patients with emphysematous cholecystitis from patients with uncomplicated acute cholecystitis are presented in Table 39–8. The diagnosis of emphysematous cholecystitis must be established early to prevent the high mortality associated with

TABLE 39–7. DIAGNOSTIC POSSIBILITIES OF AIR IN THE RUQ ON PLAIN FILM

Emphysematous cholecystitis
Enteric biliary anastomosis
Incompetent sphincter of Oddi
Spontaneous internal biliary fistula
Traumatic biliary fistula
Cholangitis
Liver abscess
Mesenteric infarct

TABLE 39–8. DIFFERENTIAL FEATURES IN ACUTE AND EMPHYSEMATOUS CHOLECYSTITIS

Feature	Acute	Emphysematous
Diabetes	10%	30%
No gallstones	10%	50%
Gallbladder perforation	4%	20%
Mortality	4%	15%
Clostridium species	<5%	~50%

this disease. Thus plain films are suggested in any ill patient with acute cholecystitis in search for gas in the gallbladder or bile ducts (see Fig. 39–5). If gas is identified, early operative intervention is warranted. Broad spectrum antibiotics should include coverage for *Clostridium* species and facultative coliforms. Thus high-dose penicillin should be part of the antibiotic regimen. As with empyema of the gallbladder, cholecystectomy is the treatment of choice for patients with emphysematous cholecystitis.

ACUTE CHOLANGITIS

Cholangitis is an infection of the biliary ductal system. Charcot was the first to clinically recognize cholangitis and describe the triad of fever, jaundice, and right upper quadrant pain in 1877.[49] He postulated that "stagnant bile" was often seen in association with an obstruction. In the 1940s the importance of bacteria in the pathogenesis of cholangitis was appreciated, and systemic antibiotics were utilized for treatment.

Reynolds and Dargan[50] added to Charcot's triad with two additional signs of sepsis: shock and mental obtundation. During the 1960s and 1970s, the term *suppurative cholangitis* was used to describe this toxic form of cholangitis. However, not all patients with this severe form of cholangitis have pus in their bile ducts, and not all patients with pus in their bile ducts have septic shock. Therefore, in recent years, we and others have preferred the use of the term *toxic cholangitis* to describe the patients at the most severe end of this clinical spectrum.[51]

Etiology. The most common causes of biliary obstruction are choledocholithiasis, benign strictures, obstructed anastomotic strictures, and malignant strictures. Analysis of the literature[37,52,53] and our own data suggest that the etiology of cholangitis has changed in recent years (Table 39–9). While Pitt and Longmire[52,53] reported that 80 percent of cholangitis was secondary to stone disease, choledocholithiasis has been much less common in recent patients at The Johns Hopkins Hospital. On the other hand, malignant strictures and sclerosing cholangitis are increasingly the cause of cholangitis at tertiary referral centers. Many factors are undoubtedly responsible for these etiologic changes at our institution and probably reflect a combination of the tertiary nature of our practice and the increased use of biliary stents, both endoscopic endoprostheses and transhepatic stents.

Pathophysiology. Clinical cholangitis results from a combination of two factors: significant bacterial concentration in the bile and biliary obstruction (Fig. 39–6). With increased intraductal pressure, reflux of bacteria into hepatic veins and perihepatic lymphatics occurs and results in bacteremia.[54] Biliary obstruction is critical in this process as both biliary stagnation with bacterial proliferation and increased intraductal pressures occur.[54,55] Gallstones and parasites can act as foreign bodies, which can cause both obstruction and act as a nidus for bacterial overgrowth.

Normal biliary pressures range from 7 to 14 cm H_2O.[56] When bile flow is partially or completely obstructed, pressures may increase from 15 to 30 cm H_2O.[56] Jacobsson et al[54] have demonstrated that with biliary pressures just greater than the secretory pressure of the liver (15 cm H_2O) approximately 10 percent of radiolabeled bacteria reflux

TABLE 39–9. CHANGING ETIOLOGY OF CHOLANGITIS AT THE JOHNS HOPKINS HOSPITAL

	Percentage of Patients			
Etiology	*1952–1974 (N = 76)*	*1976–1978 (N = 40)*	*1983–1985 (N = 48)*	*1986–1989 (N = 96)*
Choledocholithiasis	70	70	32	28
Benign strictures	13	18	14	12
Malignant strictures	17	10	30	57
Sclerosing cholangitis	0	3	24	3

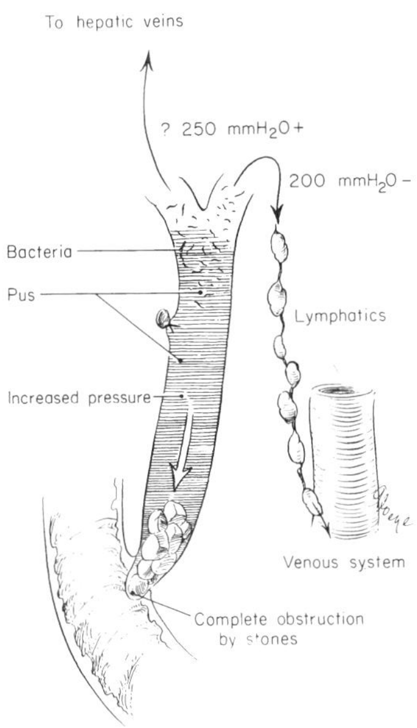

Figure 39–6. Schematic representing the contributing pathogenic factors in acute cholangitis. Both obstruction and infection are necessary to cause cholangitis. *(From Pitt HA, Longmire WP Jr: Suppurrative cholangitis. In Hardy JM (ed): Critical Illness, 2nd ed. Philadelphia, Saunders, 1980, p 380).*

into the bloodstream although the majority of these bacteria are destroyed in the liver.

Fever and chills associated with cholangitis are the result of a systemic bacteremia and the inflammatory mediators produced by cholangiovenous or cholangiolymphatic reflux of bacteria.[38,54,57,58] As noted previously, cultures of the normal gallbladder and biliary tree are usually sterile. However, in the presence of stones in the gallbladder[39,55] and common bile duct,[6,13,17,59] the incidence of positive cultures ranges from 15 to 50 percent and 60 to 90 percent, respectively. With complete ductal obstruction, as is usually present with malignancy, only 25 to 40 percent of bile cultures are positive prior to biliary manipulation.[39,60] The organisms most commonly cultured from bile are *Escherichia coli, Klebsiella pneumonia,* and enterococci. Anaerobes such as *Bacteroides fragilis* have been isolated in 25 to 30 percent of patients with choledocholithiasis and cholangitis.[14,17,59]

Clinical Manifestations. A wide spectrum of disease is often seen in patients with acute cholangitis. Some patients may have a self-limited illness and never seek medical attention, while others present with a life-threatening illness consisting of mental confusion, hypotension, fever, jaundice, and abdominal pain. These latter patients have *toxic* cholangitis and were first described by Reynolds and Dargan.[50]

Although gallstones are more common in women than men, cholangitis is observed with equal frequency in males and females. In a recent series from Johns Hopkins, University of California, Los Angeles (UCLA), and the Olive View Medical Center in Los Angeles, the mean age of presentation was 51 years and did not vary depending on the benign or malignant nature of the obstruction.[39] Fever is the most common presenting symptom in patients with cholangitis. However, the presenting symptoms have changed as the etiology of cholangitis has changed at our institution (Table 39–10).[39,61] Jaundice was previously a common physical finding occurring in 79 to 90 percent of patients with cholangitis at Johns Hopkins. However, only two-thirds of patients now are clinically jaundiced. This finding may be explained by the increased numbers of patients with malignant obstruction and indwelling stents.

Abdominal pain is common but is usually mild (see Table 39–10). Because abdominal pain is now less common in patients with cholangitis, Charcot's triad of fever, jaundice, and abdominal pain is even less common than previously.[39] The severe toxic form of cholangitis is still consistently present in 4 to 5 percent of all patients. Physical findings, similar to disease severity, are somewhat variable. Jaundice and mild to moderate right upper abdominal tenderness are seen in as many as two-thirds of patients. However, severe tenderness on physical examination should prompt consideration of an alternative diagnosis such as acute cholecystitis.

Diagnosis. The diagnosis of acute cholangitis should be considered in all patients who present with any of the triad symptoms of fever, jaundice, or abdominal pain. The presence of known choledocholithiasis, a history of biliary surgery, or an indwelling biliary catheter should increase clinical suspicion.

TABLE 39–10. CLINICAL PRESENTATION OF CHOLANGITIS AT THE JOHNS HOPKINS HOSPITAL

	Percentage of Patients		
Symptom	*1952–1974* (*N* = 76)	*1976–1978* (*N* = 40)	*1983–1985* (*N* = 48)
Fever	65	98	92
Jaundice	79	90	67
Abdominal pain	79	78	42
Chills	79	63	65
Shock	5	5	4

Most patients will have abnormal laboratory findings, which include leukocytosis, hyperbilirubinemia, and elevations of both alkaline phosphatase and the liver transaminase values.[14,38] Saharia and Cameron[57] noted that 79 percent of patients had a WBC count greater than 10,000 cells/mm^3. Thompson et al[38] have found the mean WBC count in patients with cholangitis to be 13,600 cells/mm^3 while others have demonstrated a mean WBC count as high as 19,000 cells/mm^3. A small minority of patients will present with leukopenia, often a manifestation of overwhelming gram-negative sepsis.

Most patients with cholangitis have abnormalities of liver function tests. Thompson and associates[38] have noted a correlation between the etiology of the obstruction and the pattern and degree of liver function test abnormalities. As expected, patients with malignant obstruction had higher elevations of alkaline phosphatase (531 versus 278 IU, $p < 0.02$) when compared with patients who had a benign obstruction causing cholangitis. In contrast, patients with benign obstruction more frequently had higher elevations of liver transaminases, usually secondary to acute obstruction with stone disease. Although liver function abnormalities are usually present in patients with acute cholangitis, their presence is nondiagnostic and systemic sepsis, hepatitis, and other causes must also be considered in the differential diagnosis. However, entirely normal liver function tests are unusual in patients with this cholangitis.

As many as one-third of patients may have an elevated serum amylase, which often indicates that a benign condition such as choledocholithiasis is present.[52] The tumor marker CA19-9 may be markedly elevated in patients with benign biliary obstruction and acute cholangitis. Albert et al[62] have demonstrated that therapy and resolution of the acute disease process will allow the CA19-9 level to return to normal.

In most cases plain radiographs of the abdomen are of little diagnostic value in patients with acute cholangitis. In a small percentage of cases radiopaque gallstones may be seen and, even more uncommonly, pneumobilia may be noted.[61] Nuclear medicine scans are helpful in the diagnosis of acute cholecystitis but not acute cholangitis. Ultrasonography and CT scans will not establish the diagnosis of acute cholangitis but may well note dilated ducts or an etiologic factor such as gallstones, a pancreatic mass, or a liver abscess (Fig. 39–7).

Cholangiography is usually required prior to or as a part of therapy. Direct cholangiography tests via either the endoscopic retrograde (ERC) route or via the percutaneous transhepatic (PTC) route are equally informative. In general, the endoscopic route is preferred if common duct stones or a periampullary tumor is expected, whereas the percutaneous route[63] has advantages if a perihilar obstruction is suspected. Cholangitis can occur as the result of either procedure, but generally a low incidence of 3 to 7 percent can be expected.[57,67]

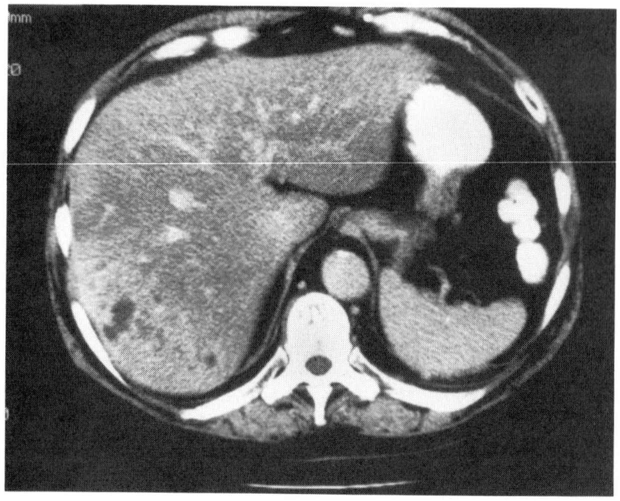

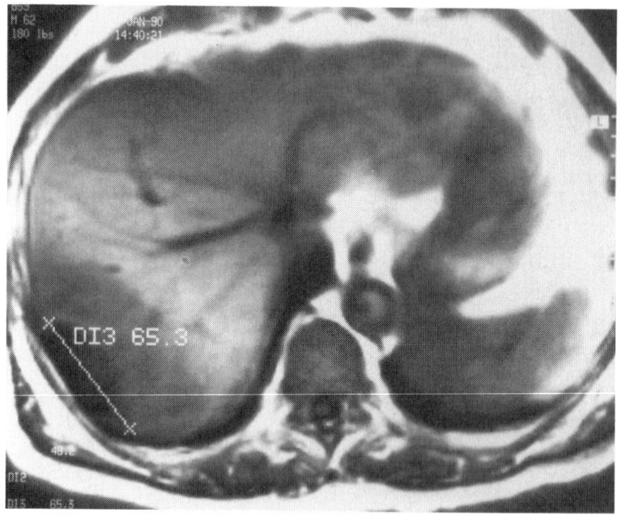

Figure 39–7. A. Computed tomography scan from a patient with an obstructed biliary enteric anastomosis demonstrating a small peripheral liver abscess in the posterior aspect of the right hepatic lobe. *(From Pitt HA, Couse NF: Biliary sepsis and toxic cholangitis. In Moody FG (ed): Surgical Treatment of Digestive Diseases, 2nd ed. Chicago, Year Book Medical Publishers, 1990, p 32.)* **B.** Corresponding magnetic resonance image demonstrating the same area as seen above.

Microbiology. As previously discussed, the combination of biliary obstruction and bactibilia cause bacteremia. High fever, chills, and, particularly, hypotension signify that bacteremia is likely in patients with acute cholangitis. In one of the early series from Johns Hopkins, 50 of 78 patients with acute cholangitis had blood drawn shortly after admission, and 20 patients (26 percent) had bacteremia.[61] *Escherichia coli* and *Klebsiella* species accounted for 17 of the 20 cases. In the most recent series, 21 percent of patients had bacteremia, but *E. coli* and *Klebsiella* species represented a smaller proportion of the organisms that were isolated.[38]

In most series mutliple organisms are present in the biliary tree.[14,39,52,61,62] Along with the changing etiology and presentation of patients with cholangitis, biliary bacteriology has changed significantly at Johns Hopkins (Table 39–11). Previously, the common enteric coliforms, *E. coli* and *Klebsiella* species, and the gram-positive enterococci predominated. In more recent years as more patients with malignant obstruction and indwelling tubes are experiencing cholangitis, additional, more resistant, organisms are now common.[38] *Enterobacter* and *Pseudomonas* species are now common gram-negatives isolated from the infected biliary tract. Anaerobes such as *Bacteroides* species continue to play a small but significant role in severe biliary infections.[14,38]

Treatment. Patients with acute cholangitis represent a wide spectrum of illness. A small number of patients with mild intermittent fevers may be managed with oral antibiotics as outpatients. However, the majority require admission, intravenous hydration, and intravenous antibiotics. A small number of patients will require critical care management with invasive monitoring devices and cardiopulmonary support. Adequate, but careful, hydration is important as these patients are particularly prone to renal insufficiency. If pressors are required, low-dose dopamine should be employed to help preserve renal blood flow.

ANTIBIOTIC THERAPY. All patients with acute cholangitis require antibiotic therapy. However, no general consensus exists about specific antibiotic regimens. For severe cholangitis, antibiotic selection should include adequate gram-negative anaerobic and, probably, enterococcal coverage. Aminoglycosides provide excellent coverage for most gram-negative organisms, but a narrow therapeutic-toxic window makes their use somewhat unpopular in jaundiced patients who are prone to renal compromise.[11,12,38] In the critically ill patients with a large volume of distribution, aminoglycosides are most typically underdosed and may not provide optimal bactericidal coverage if given as the standard 2-mg/kg dose. Large doses (4 mg/kg) at 24-hour intervals have rapid bactericidal effect with minimal toxicity.[64] In addition, the judicious use of antibiotic levels with rapid results reporting can allow both safe and efficacious use of aminoglycosides as alternative coverage for gram-negative organisms found in the biliary tree.[65]

Third-generation cephalosporins, ureidopenicillins, monobactams, and fluroquinolones offer excellent options for treatment. Ureidopenicillins, such as pipercillin, offer the advantage of additional coverage of the enterococci and provide reasonable anaerobic coverage.[38] This spectrum is also true of the monobactams, but the intravenous fluroquinolone, ciprofloxacin, does not cover anaerobes, and an additional agent for anaerobes such as metronidazole should be added. Some third-generation cephalosporins provide some anaerobic coverage, but no currently available third-generation cephalosporin provides adequate enterococcal coverage.

A randomized study of 46 patients with cholangitis from the Mayo Clinic demonstrated that mezlocillin, a ureidopenicillin, compared favorably with an ampicillin/gentamicin combination.[66] Twenty of 24 patients (83 percent) were cured with mezlocillin therapy compared with only 9 of 22 patients (41 percent) treated with ampicillin and gentamicin. In

TABLE 39–11. ACUTE CHOLANGITIS BILIARY BACTERIOLOGY AT THE JOHNS HOPKINS

	Percentage of Patients		
Bile Culture	*1976–1978* (*N* = 40)	*1983–1985* (*N* = 48)	*1986–1989* (*N* = 96)
Escherichia coli	55	55	39
Klebsiella species	41	32	54
Enterococcus	41	55	34
Bacteroides species	28	9	15
Enterobacter species	0	33	34
Pseudomonas species	0	23	24

addition, fewer toxic or adverse events were seen with mezlocillin treatment.

In a recent study from Johns Hopkins, the Olive View Medical Center, and UCLA, 96 patients were treated with either pipercillin or ampicillin and tobramycin.[38] No significant differences were seen between the treatment groups, but the outcome of therapy was released to the type of obstruction (malignant versus benign) (Fig. 39–8). Thus, in this study, pipercillin was an effective single-agent therapy for the treatment of acute cholangitis.

BILIARY DECOMPRESSION. The majority of patients who present with acute cholangitis will respond to supportive therapy with intravenous hydration and antibiotics and will not require urgent biliary decompression. However, approximately 15 percent of patients with cholangitis present with septic shock and will require urgent decompression of the biliary tree. In an effort to identify these high-risk patients with acute cholangitis, Gigot et al[67] found seven independent risk factors that predicted mortality: (1) acute renal failure, (2) liver abscess, (3) cirrhosis, (4) high malignant strictures, (5) percutaneous transhepatic cholangiography, (6) female gender, and (7) age. When given proportional weight, a score of 0 to 27 could be obtained with 7 being the cutoff point. Mortality was 1.8 percent in patients with less than 7 points while those with over 7 points had a mortality of 49 percent. Although these data have not been tested prospectively and utilized for management decision-making, the group of patients with significant risk seem well suited for consideration of biliary decompression.

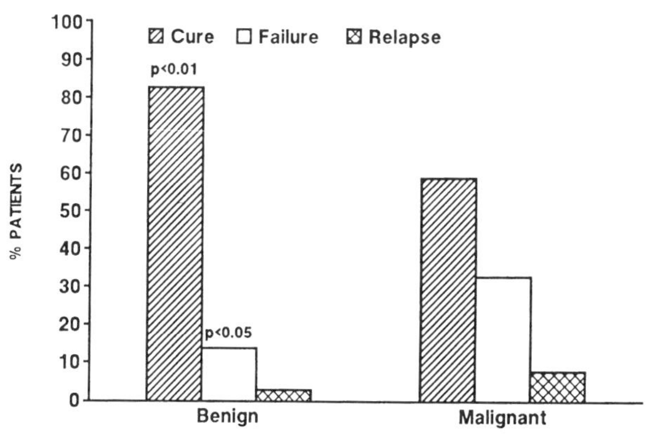

Figure 39–8. Response rates (cure, failure, or relapse) of 96 patients treated for acute cholangitis. Rather than antibiotic treatment (pipercillin versus ampicillin-tobramycin), etiology of the obstruction (benign versus malignant) appeared to significantly predict response to therapy, with the outcome significantly worse when malignant obstruction was present. *(From Thompson JE Jr, Pitt HA, Doty JE, et al: Surg Gynecol Obstet 171:275, 1990.)*

Certainly, clinical deterioration or failure to demonstrate objective clinical improvement within the first 24 hours warrants urgent biliary decompression.

Percutaneous transhepatic biliary drainage (PTD) is an established technique for decompressing a dilated biliary tree in patients who have obstructive jaundice.[68–70] The ability to perform PTD alleviates the need for general anesthesia and the stress of a complicated operative procedure. In the setting of septic shock, a catheter should be placed to establish biliary drainage without the need for extensive cholangiography. Pessa et al[70] reported 42 patients with urgent biliary drainage prior to definitive therapy with a 7 percent morbidity and a 5 percent mortality. The two deaths in this series occurred in patients who underwent drainage while in septic shock. If the patient has had a previous biliary enteric anastomosis or is known to have a perihilar obstruction, percutaneous transhepatic drainage is the preferred route of biliary decompression.

In patients with acute cholangitis secondary to choledocholithiasis, endoscopic treatment with papillotomy alone or with placement of an endoscopic endoprosthesis may be the treatment of choice. Lai and colleagues[71] randomized 82 patients with toxic cholangitis to receive either urgent surgical decompression or endoscopic treatment. Patients undergoing operative treatment were significantly more likely to develop respiratory failure and require ventilatory support (Table 39–12). Moreover, the mortality in this series was significantly less in patients undergoing endoscopic versus operative drainage. If endoscopic expertise is available, this report suggests that emergency endoscopic drainage should be offered to patients with severe cholangitis secondary to choledocholithiasis.

If the expertise for percutaneous or endoscopic drainage is not available, operative decompression will be necessary as a life-saving measure for patients with toxic cholangitis. Timely intervention is essential in the successful management of these patients. Biliary decompression is warranted even in patients with persistent hypotension. Lai et al[71,72] demonstrated that, in 30 patients with persistent shock, outcome was not different from patients who had been successfully resuscitated preoperatively. The extent of surgical intervention should be guided by the hemodynamic status of the patient intraoperatively. In any unstable patient, choledochoscopy and cholangiography should not be performed. Exploration and drainage alone were performed in 24 of 44 patients in Lai's series. Since common duct obstruction is an etiologic factor in

TABLE 39–12. OUTCOME OF ENDOSCOPIC VERSUS SURGICAL DECOMPRESSION FOR TOXIC CHOLANGITIS

Measurement	Endoscopic Papillotomy Nasobiliary Drainage[a]	Surgical Decompression
Number of patients	41	41
Ventilatory support	29%	63%
Morbidity	34%	66%
Mortality	10%	32%

[a] $p < 0.03$ versus papillotomy.
Adapted from Lai ECS, Mokf PT, Tan ESY, et al: N Engl J Med 326:1582, 1992.

acute cholangitis, cholecystectomy alone is not adequate therapy for this disease. In general, choledochotomy with placement of a T-tube will be necessary if an emergent procedure is indicated. More definitive procedures can be performed when the patient has adequately stabilized.

Outcome. As might be anticipated, patients with toxic cholangitis are at considerable risk for developing organ system failure. In patients with ongoing sepsis, inflammatory mediators and endogenous hormones contribute to reduced systemic vascular resistance, altered permeability, and relative hypovolemia, which all contribute to reduced renal blood flow and an increased risk of acute renal failure. Thus adequate volume replacement is essential for successful outcome. In patients with underlying hepatic or renal failure, circulating endotoxin may also contribute to additional morbidity. Preventative therapy with oral bile acids, lactulose, or internal biliary drainage is directed toward the prevention of absorption of endotoxin through the mucosa of the small bowel into the portal bloodstream.[73,74]

In addition to underlying risk factors, the development of a liver abscess considerably increases morbidity and mortality.[75] The etiology of the biliary obstruction and number of hepatic abscesses are of prognostic importance. In patients with toxic cholangitis who fail to respond to initial management, a liver abscess should be considered. In patients with biliary obstruction and multiple small abscesses, biliary drainage may be adequate. However, with larger collections separate drainage of the abscess will usually be required. Percutaneous abscess drainage is often sufficient, but open surgical drainage may be required if sepsis persists or treatment of the underlying cause is necessary.

In most series approximately 5 percent of patients presenting with acute cholangitis do not survive. The highest mortality is in patients with toxic cholangitis who comprise about 10 to 15 percent of all patients. In addition to the prognostic factors identified by Gigot and colleagues,[67] Lai et al,[72] Little,[76] and numerous others have documented additional risk factors for mortality. Concomitant medical disease, renal failure, and low albumin are important additional risk factors. These factors are also considered in more general prognostic scores such as the Acute Physiology and Chronic Health Score (APACHE). This score is a measure of illness and prognosis on admission to the intensive care unit irrespective of the particular underlying disease process.

Nonetheless, the etiology of biliary obstruction causing acute cholangitis does predict outcome. For example, Thompson et al[38] demonstrated that rather than a particular antibiotic therapy, benign or malignant obstruction predicted initial cure rate (59 versus 83 percent). The mortality in this series was 5 percent with many of the patients who died having had liver and/or renal failure. Thus recognition of high-risk patients by identifying risk factors in the history, clinical presentation, and laboratory evaluation should indicate which septic patients require urgent biliary decompression. With this information, mortality should be kept to a minimum.

RARE INFECTIONS

Acute cholecystitis and acute cholangitis are by far the most common biliary tract infections. In the West gallstones in the gallbladder or common bile duct are the usual cause, and common gut-derived bacteria are responsible for the infectious process. However, a number of other unusual infectious agents may cause infections of the biliary tract that are rarely observed in Western cultures. The rare infections that will be discussed in this section include oriental cholangiohepatitis, bile peritonitis, *Salmonella* cholecystitis, and AIDS-related infections.

Oriental Cholangiohepatitis

Oriental cholangiohepatitis or recurrent pyogenic cholangitis is prevalent in East Asians but now occurs throughout the world due to the ease of travel. As the name implies, recurrent pyogenic cholangitis is a clinical syndrome characterized by repeated infections of the biliary system by pus-forming bacteria. Oriental cholangiohepatitis is usually caused by intrahepatic stones and/or strictures and may be associated with parasites such as *Ascaris* or *Clonorchis.* In contrast to Western calculous disease, cholangiohepatitis is equally common in males and females and generally occurs in young or people in lower socioeconomic groups and in rural areas.[77,78]

The clinical diagnosis is similar to acute cholangitis with fever, pain, and jaundice. The physical examination reveals a febrile, jaundiced patient with mild right upper quadrant or epigastric pain; a right upper quadrant scar from previous surgery is often present. Initial conservative management with intravenous fluids and antibiotics should be utilized, but this patient population is twice as likely to fail conservative therapy and require biliary decompression than a typical Western patient with acute cholangitis.[78,79]

Repeated episodes of infection result in ductal change, primarily stricture formation. Typically, these changes are seen in the larger ducts, especially at the origin of the left hepatic duct. In the smaller intrahepatic ducts, a combination of strictures and proximal dilatation may be seen. Stones are commonly found within the intrahepatic biliary tree and often are numerous. However, in most cases the gallbladder is normal, even with severe intra- and extrahepatic disease. The stones in these patients are brown pigment, irregular in shape and size, usually brown externally and yellow or light brown internally, and are soft, usually crumbling into an amorphous mass with minimal pressure. Typically, these stones are culture positive, and a nidus of a dead parasite or a clump of bacteria may be seen deep within these stones.

Due to the diffuse nature of this disease and the repeated attacks, parenchymal liver disease may result. Frequently, the left lobe of the liver is most involved, atrophies, and becomes a mass of intrahepatic stones in dilated ducts.[78] Bile cultures most commonly show a mixture of bowel organisms. Although anaerobes are often isolated, they are rarely an independent pathogen. *Clonorchis sinensis* and *Ascaris lumbricoides* are also commonly found in this patient population, but an etiologic role is unclear because the incidence of infestation is similar in other surgical patients without cholangiohepatitis. Moreover, in the Philippines clonorchiasis is absent, but cholangiohepatitis is prevalent.[78,79]

Complications during an acute attack of cholangiohepatitis are common and include liver abscesses, acute pancreatitis, and empyema of the gallbladder.[78] In Asia, many patients are initially managed conservatively without emergent investigations. Once the disease is quiescent, ultrasonography usually provides adequate information about the intrahepatic biliary tree as CT scans are generally unavailable in many Asian countries. Cholangiography again is essential, and ERCP may be utilized when extrahepatic disease is primarily suspected (Fig. 39–9). However, PTC provides more precise localization if ultrasonography suggests intrahepatic disease. Both methods may provide drainage of the biliary tree, but caution should be exercised when utilizing endoscopic drainage

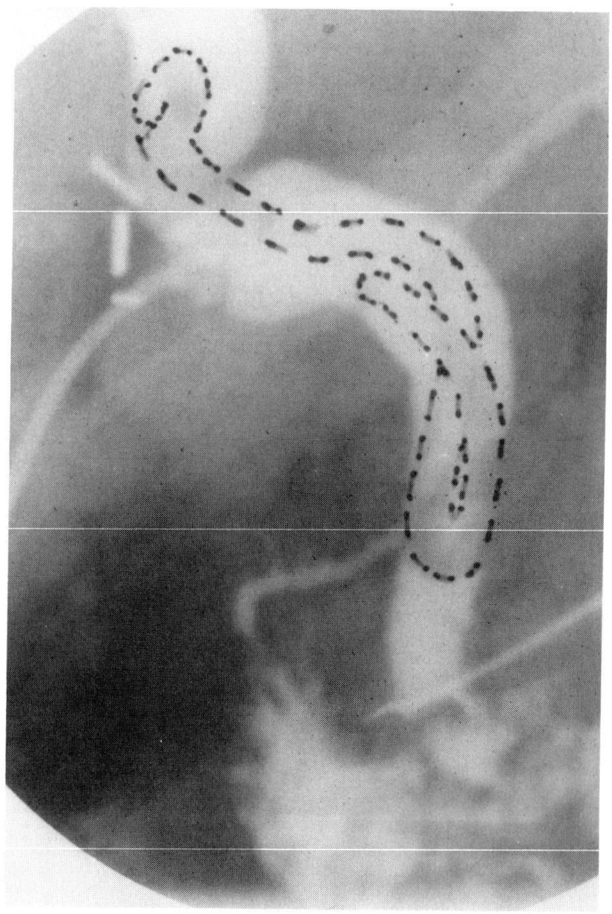

Figure 39–9. Intraoperative cholangiogram demonstrates dilated extrahepatic biliary tree in an Asian patient with cholangiohepatitis. Dots outline the presence of *Ascaris* adult worm causing biliary obstruction.

through a small catheter for treatment of an acute attack. As previously described, this infected bile is thick, usually contains significant debris, and is likely to occlude a small-diameter catheter.

If the patient deteriorates after 24 hours of conservative management despite supportive care, biliary drainage is essential. Although endoscopic and transhepatic drainage certainly can be used initially if available, the bulk of management in many Asian countries is operative intervention. Choledochotomy and removal of stones, mud, and debris with insertion of a large T-tube are typical. Emergent measures do not treat strictures or other pathology, and definitive care can be performed when the patient has stabilized. Definitive management depends on the extent of the intrahepatic disease and the degree of hepatic fibrosis. Often the bulk of disease is located in the left lobe or even in the lateral segments (II and III). If significant focal cirrhosis is also present, hepatic resection may be indicated. However, if the disease is bilateral or only minimal fibrosis is present, definitive surgery should include a cleanout of intrahepatic ducts, dilatation and transhepatic stenting of strictures, and access to the biliary tree for postoperative percutaneous choledochoscopy. We prefer access via transhepatic stents whereas others recommend placement of a portion of a Roux-en-Y hepaticojejunostomy in a subcutaneous or subfascial position.

Salmonella Infections

Salmonella infections are important public health problems throughout the world.[80] The incidence of *Salmonella* biliary tract infections in the United States is expected to increase as immigrants, foreign travel, and patients with AIDS increase.[81,82] Salmonellosis can cause many diseases, including (1) gastroenteritis, (2) enteric fever (typhoid and paratyphoid), (3) bacteremia, (4) acute cholecystitis, and (5) a chronic carrier state. These last two varieties, which apply to the biliary tract, will be discussed in more detail.

Acute cholecystitis associated with *Salmonella typhi* and gallstones is not rare. The bacteria accumulate in the gallbladder during a systemic infection and can proliferate, causing typical acute cholecystitis. The most common predisposing conditions associated with *Salmonella* hepatobiliary infections include anatomical abnormalities of the biliary tree, sickle cell disease, a history of previous typhoid fever, ethanol abuse, and gastric achlorhydria.[83] Acalculous cholecystitis has occasionally been reported in *Salmonella typhi*[84] and other *Salmonella* stereotypes.[85] As with other forms of acute cholecystitis, the mainstay of treatment is cholecystectomy.

Occasionally, the chronic *Salmonella* carrier state may be prolonged when *Salmonella* bacteria are associated with gallstones. Under these circumstances, the biliary tree may harbor significant numbers of bacteria (more than 10^9), which are then excreted into the stool, prolonging the carrier state. Usually, prolonged antibiotic treatment of the carrier state is not successful in the presence of gallstones. Thus in patients whose livelihood depends on a free bacterial state, a cholecystectomy may be indicated even in the absence of biliary symptoms. With both acute cholecystitis and the chronic carrier situation, perioperative ceftriaxone is the antibiotic treatment of choice.

Bile Peritonitis

Bile peritonitis can result from any perforation of a bile-containing structure. If the bile is sterile, a chemical peritonitis develops. Among the constituents of bile, the detergent bile salts are the most toxic to peritoneal surfaces. However, severity of bile peritonitis depends entirely on the underlying pathology and whether the bile is initially infected. If bile peritonitis is associated with perforation from infected gangrenous cholecystitis or an empyema, a highly virulent peritonitis will result. The signs, symptoms, severity, and treatment are also related to the extent to which bile permeates the peritoneal cavity.

When the gallbladder or biliary tree perforates, the omentum may very efficiently wall off the process, and the result is a localized abscess rather than bile peritonitis. Alternatively, the leaking bile may remain in the right upper quadrant extending around the liver in the subhepatic and subphrenic spaces as a biloma without free communication with the entire peritoneum. These patients may present with fever, chills, localized pain and tenderness, and/or signs of diaphragmatic irritation. Often, initial management of these patients will include percutaneous drainage of the infected biloma as well as the biliary tract. Definitive surgical treatment of the underlying biliary pathology may usually be delayed until often the infectious process has resolved. With more generalized peritoneal spillage of infected bile, a much lower threshold for operative intervention should be adopted. In this setting, debridement and lavage of peritoneal surfaces are indicated, and cholecystectomy should be performed if the gallbladder is the source of bile spillage. However, if the source of infected bile is the biliary tree, external drainage may be life-saving, and definitive repair may be more likely to succeed at a later date.

AIDS Infections

Most patients who are infected with human immunodeficiency virus (HIV) and who have abdominal pain do not have a pathologic process that will require surgical intervention (see Chap. 53). However, among the increasing number of surgical procedures being performed in this patient population, biliary tract disease accounts for over one-third of the cases. Calculous disease resulting in acute or chronic cholecystitis accounts for a minority of cases in this patient population. Acalculous acute cholecystitis with typical symptoms and signs has been more commonly the rule. The etiology of the cystic duct obstruction in some cases has been Kaposi's sarcoma or obstructing lymph nodes from lymphoma or *Mycobacterium avium-intracellulare* intra-abdominal disease. In addition to the typical biliary tract organisms seen in acute cholecystitis, fungi are more common, and cytomegalovirus has also been implicated as the cause of cholecystitis.

Cholangitis has also been reported in patients with AIDS.[34] While the etiology of the bile duct obstruction has been atypical, the presenting symptoms, usually fever, jaundice, and abdominal pain, are common. *Cryptosporidium* has been isolated in the bile of this patient group and is extremely difficult to eradicate.[33,86] Cytomegalovirus and *Cryptosporidium* have both been implicated in patients who are HIV-positive and have a sclerosing cholangitis type of illness. In these patients, appropriate titers and cultures and biopsies should be performed so that specific therapy can be undertaken. The decision as to whether endoscopic, percutaneous, or surgical treatment of cholangitis should be undertaken must be individualized on the basis of the exact etiology, extent, and site(s) of biliary obstruction and the stage of the immune deficiency process.

CONCLUSIONS

Biliary tract infections are very common and are usually associated with gallstones either in the gallbladder, common bile duct, or, in the Orient, in intrahepatic ducts. While management usually includes the use of systemic antibiotics, definitive treatment often requires removal of the gallbladder or decompression of the biliary tree. In recent years, the introduction of nonoperative biliary manipulations has provided alternatives to surgery as a mode for biliary decompression. However, this advance has also resulted in an increased incidence of cholangitis in patients with indwelling tubes for palliation of biliary and pancreatic malignancies. This trend has been accompanied by a broader spectrum of bacterial infections with the emergence of resistant organisms and yeast as more common biliary tract pathogens. The possibility of parasitic infection must also be considered in patients from the Orient; and viral, parasitic, and mycobacterial infections of the biliary tree should be considered in patients who are immunocomprised.

REFERENCES

1. Bornman PC, Kottler RE, Terblanche J, et al: Does low entry of the cystic duct predispose to stones in the common bile duct? Br Med J 297:31, 1988.
2. Pitt HA, Roslyn JJ, Kuchenbecker SL, et al: The role of cystic duct resistance in the pathogenesis of cholesterol gallstones. J Surg Res 30:508, 1981.
3. Klein AS, Lillemoe KD, Yeo CJ, Pitt HA: Liver, biliary tract, and pancreas. In O'Leary JP (ed): The Physiologic Basis of Surgery. Baltimore, Williams & Wikins, 1993, pp 255–292.
4. Csendes A, Fernandez M, Uribe P: Bacteriology of the gallbladder bile in normal subjects. Am J Surg 129:629, 1975.
5. Scott AJ, Kahn GA: Origin of bacteria in the bile duct. Lancet 2:790, 1967.
6. Edlund YA, Mollstedt BO, Ouchterlong X: Bacteriologic investigation of the biliary system and liver in biliary tract disease correlated to clinical data and microstructure of the gallbladder and liver. Acta Chir Scand 116:461, 1959.
7. Dineen P: The importance of the route of infection in experimental biliary obstruction. Surg Gynecol Obstet 119:1001, 1964.
8. Kaufman HW, Magnuson TH, Lillemoe KD, Pitt HA: The role of bacteria in gallbladder and common duct stone formation. Ann Surg 209:584, 1989.
9. Maki T: Pathogenesis of calcium bilirubinate gallstone: role of *E. coli,* beta-glucuronidase and coagulation by inorganic ions, polyelectrolytes, and agitation. Ann Surg 164:90, 1966.
10. Strasberg SM, Clavien PA, Harvey PRC: Pathogenesis of cholesterol gallstones. HPB Surg 3:79, 1991.
11. Keighley MR, Baddeley RM, Burdon DW, et al: A controlled trial of parenteral prophylactic gentamicin therapy in biliary surgery. Br J Surg 62:275, 1975.
12. Keighley MR, Drysdale BB, Quorashi AH: Antibiotic treatment of biliary sepsis. Clin North Am 55:1379, 1975.
13. Pitt HA, Postier RG, Cameron JL: Consequences of preoperative cholangitis and its treatment on the outcome of surgery for choledocholithiasis. Surgery 94:447, 1983.
14. Lee W, Chang KJ, Lee CS, Chen KM: Surgery in cholangitis: bacteriology and choice of antibiotic. Hepatogastroenterology 39:347, 1992.
15. MacLean LD, Goldstein M, MacDonald JE, Demers

R: Results of cholecystectomy in 1000 consecutive patients. Carr Surg 18:459, 1975.
16. Babb RR: Acute acalculous cholecystitis. J Clin Gastroenterol 15:238, 1992.
17. Keighley MR, Flinn R, Alexander-Williams J: Multivariate analysis of clinical and operative findings associated with biliary sepsis. Br J Surg 63:528, 1976.
18. Ahmad MM, Macon WL: Gangrene of the gallbladder. Am Surg 49:155, 1983.
19. Keighley MRB, McLeish AR, Bishop HM, et al: Identification of the presence and type of biliary microfluid by immediate gram stains. Surgery 81:469, 1977.
20. McLersh AR, Keighley MRB, Bishop HM, et al: Selecting patients requiring antibiotics in biliary surgery by immediate gram stains of bile at operation. Surgery 81:473, 1977.
21. Glenn F: Acute acalculous cholecystitis. Ann Surg 189:458, 1979.
22. Howard RJ: Acute acalculous cholecystitis. Am J Surg 141:194, 1981.
23. Meijer WS, Schmitz PIM, Jeekel J: Meta-analysis of randomized, controlled clinical trials of antibiotic prophylaxis in biliary tract surgery. Br J Surg 70:283, 1990.
24. Munster AM, Goodwin MN, Bruitt BA: Acalculous cholecystitis in burned patients. Am J Surg 122:591, 1971.
25. Lindberg EF, Griman GLB, Smith L: Acalculous cholecystitis in Vietnam casualties. Ann Surg 171:152, 1970.
26. Stevens PE, Harrison NA, Ramford DJ: Acute acalculous cholecystitis in acute renal failure. Intensive Care Med 14:411, 1988.
27. Flanchaum LF, Majerus TC, Cox EF: Acute post traumatic acalculous cholecystitis. Am J Surg 150:252, 1985.
28. Peterson SR, Sheldon GF: Acute acalculous cholecystitis. Am J Surg 138:814, 1979.
29. Roslyn JJ, Pitt HA, Mann LL, et al: Gallbladder disease in patients on long-term parenteral nutrition. Gastroenterology 84:148, 1983.
30. Parry SW, Pelias ME, Browder W: Acalculous hypersensitivity cholecystitis: hypothesis of a new clinicopathologic entity. Surgery 104:911, 1988.
31. Savocd PE, Longo WE, Zucker KA, et al: The increasing prevalence of acalculous cholecystitis in outpatient results of a 7 year study. Ann Surg 211:433, 1990.
32. Kavin W, Jonas RB, Chowdhurg L, Kabin S: Acalculous cholecystitis and cytomegalovirus infection in the acquired immunodeficiency syndrome. Ann Intern Med 104:53, 1986.
33. Hinnart K, Schwartz A, Rotterdam H, Rudski C: Cytomegaloviral and cryptosporidial cholecystitis in two patients with acquired immunodeficiency syndrome. Am J Surg Pathol 13:57, 1989.
34. Iannuzzi C, Belghiti J, Erlinger S, et al: Cholangitis associated with cholecystitis in patients with acquired immunodeficiency syndrome. Arch Surg 125:1211, 1990.
35. Szlabick RE, Catto JA, Fink-Bennett D, Vantura V: Hepatobiliary scanning in the diagnosis of acute cholecystitis. Arch Surg 115:540, 1980.
36. Thompson JE Jr, Bennion RS, Doty JE, et al: Predictive factors for bactibilia in acute cholecystitis: indications for therapy. Arch Surgery 125:261, 1990.
37. Järvinen HJ, Hästacka J: Early cholecystectomy for acute cholecystitis. Ann Surg 191:501, 1980.
38. Thompson JE Jr, Pitt HA, Doty JE, et al: Broad spectrum penicillin as adequate therapy for acute cholangitis. Surg Gynecol Obstet 171:275, 1990.
39. Muller EL, Pitt HA, Thompson JE Jr, et al: Antibiotics in infections of the biliary tract. Surg Gynecol Obstet 165:285, 1987.
40. Pitt HA, Postier RG, Gadacz TR, Cameron JL: The role of topical antibiotics in "high-risk" biliary surgery. Surgery 91:518, 1982.
41. Sarr MG, Parikh KH, Saref H, et al: Topical antibiotics in high risk biliary surgical patients: a prospective randomized study. Am Surg 155:337, 1989.
42. Kanter MA, Gellhoed GW: Biliary antibiotics: clinical utility in biliary surgery. South Med 80:1007, 1987.
43. Dooley JS, Hamilton-Miller JMT, Brumfitt W, Sherlock S: Antibiotics in the treatment of biliary infection. Gut 25:988, 1984.
44. Roslyn JJ: Current status of cholecystectomy. In Pitt HA (ed): Diseases of the Liver, Biliary Tract and Pancreas. Chicago, American College of Surgeons, 1990 pp 107–110.
45. Doty JE, Pitt HA: Management of empyema of the gallbladder. Infect Surg 5:271, 1986.
46. Lorenz RW, Steffen HM: Emphysematous cholecystitis: diagnostic problems and differential diagnosis of gallbladder gas accumulations. Hepatogastroenterology 37:103(SII), 1990.
47. Sawyer RB, Kennedy TJ, List JE, et al: Acute emphysematous cholecystitis. Arch Surg 86:484, 1963.
48. Mentzer RM, Golden GI, Chandler JG, Horsley JS: A comparative appraisal of emphysematous cholecystitis. Am J Surg 129:10, 1975.
49. Charcot JM: Lecons surles maladies du fore des voices biliares et des veins Paris. Faculte de Medicine de Paris, Bourneville et Sevestre, 1877.
50. Reynolds BM, Dargan EL: Acute obstructive cholangitis: a distinct clinical syndrome. Ann Surg 150:299, 1959.
51. Lipsett PA, Pitt HA: Acute cholangitis. Surg Clin North Am 70:1297, 1990.
52. Pitt HA, Couse NF: Biliary sepsis and toxic cholangitis. In Moody FG (ed): Surgical Treatment of Digestive Disease, 2nd ed. Chicago, Year Book Medical Publishers, 1990, pp 332–350.
53. Pitt HA, Longmire WP Jr: Supprative cholangitis. In Hardy JM (ed): Critical Surgical Illness, 2nd ed. Philadelphia, Saunders, 1980, p 380.
54. Jacobsson K, Ellander J, Rosengren B: Cholangiovenous reflux. Acta Chir Scand 123:316, 1962.
55. Flemma RJ, Flint LM, Osterhout S, Shingleton WW:

Bacteriologic studies of biliary infection. Ann Surg 166:563, 1967.
56. Mallet-Guy P: Value of preoperative manometric and roentgenographic examination in the diagnosis of pathologic changes and functional disturbances of the biliary tract. Surg Gynecol Obstet 94:385, 1952.
57. Huang T, Bass JA, Williams RD: The significance of biliary pressure in cholangitis. Arch Surg 98:629, 1969.
58. Stewart L, Pellegrini CA, Way LW: Cholangiovenous reflux pathways as defined by corrosion casting and scanning electron microscopy. Am Surg 155:23, 1988.
59. Pitt HA, Postier RG, Cameron JL: Biliary bacteria: significance and alterations after antibiotic therapy. Arch Surg 117:445, 1982.
60. O'Connor MJ, Schwartz ML, McQuarrie DG, Sumner HW: Cholangitis due to malignant obstruction to biliary outflow. Ann Surg 193:341, 1981.
61. Saharia PC, Cameron JL: Clinical management of cholangitis. Surg Gynecol Obstet 142:369, 1976.
62. Albert MA, Steinberg WM, Henry JP: Elevated serum levels of tumor marker CA19-9 in acute cholangitis. Dig Dis Sci 33:1223, 1988.
63. Okuda K, Tunikawa K, Emara T, et al: Nonsurgical percutaneous transhepatic cholangiography: diagnostic significance in medical problems of the liver. Am J Dig Dis 19:21, 1974.
64. Parker SE, Davey PG: Practicalities of once daily aminoglycoside dosing. J Antimicrob Chemother 31:4, 1993.
65. Miyagawa CI: Aminoglycosides in the intensive care units: an old drug in a dynamic environment. New Horizons 1:172, 1993.
66. Gerecht WB, Henry NK, Hoffman WW, et al: Prospective randomized comparison of mezlocillin therapy alone with combined ampicillin and gentamicin therapy for patients with cholangitis. Arch Intern Med 149:1279, 1989.
67. Gigot JF, Leese T, Dereme T, et al: Acute cholangitis: multivariate analysis of risk factors. Ann Surg 209:435, 1989.
68. Gould RJ, Vogelzang RL, Neiman HL, et al: Percutaneous biliary drainage as an initial therapy in sepsis of the biliary tree. Surg Gynecol Obstet 160:523, 1985.
69. Kadir S, Baassiri A, Barth RH, et al: Percutaneous biliary drainage in the management of biliary sepsis. Am J Roentgenol 138:25, 1982.
70. Pessa ME, Hawkins IF, Vogel SB: The treatment of acute cholangitis: percutaneous transhepatic biliary drainage before definitive therapy. Ann Surg 205: 389, 1987.
71. Lai ECS, Mokf PT, Tan ESY, et al: Endoscopic biliary drainage for severe acute cholangitis. N Engl J Med 326:1582, 1992.
72. Lai EC, Tam PC, Patterson I, et al: Emergency surgery for severe acute cholangitis: the high risk patients. Am Surg 211:55, 1990.
73. Pain ME, Cahill CJ, Barley ME: Perioperative complications in obstructive jaundice therapeutic considerations. Br J Surg 73:775, 1985.
74. Dawson JL: Postoperative renal function in obstructive jaundice: effect of mannitol diuresis. Br Med J 1:82, 1965.
75. Oschner A, DeBarkey M, Murray S: Pyogenic abscess of the liver. II: An analysis of 47 cases with review of the literature. Am J Surg 40:292, 1938.
76. Little JM: A prospective evaluation of computerized estimates of the risk of management of obstructive jaundice. Surgery 102:474, 1987.
77. Choi TK, Wong J, Ong GB: The surgical management of primary intrahepatic stones. Br J Surg 69:86, 1982.
78. Wong J, Choi TK: Recurrent pyogenic cholangitis. Dig Surg 3:265, 1986.
79. Fan ST, Lai ECS, Mok FPT, et al: Acute cholangitis secondary to hepatolithiasis. Arch Surg 126:1027, 1991.
80. Centers for Disease Control: Update: milk-borne salmonellosis. MMWR Morb Mortal Wkly Rep 34:215, 1985.
81. Claser JB, Morton-Kute L, Berger SR: Recurrent *Salmonella typhimurium* bacteremia associated with AIDS. Ann Intern Med 102:189, 1985.
82. Jacobs SL, Gold JW, Murray HW, et al: *Salmonella* infections in patients with AIDS. Ann Intern Med 102:186, 1985.
83. Cohen JI, Bartlett JA, Corey JR: Extra intestinal manifestations of *Salmonella* infections. Medicine (Baltimore) 66:349, 1987.
84. Alvalos ME, Cerulli MA, Lee RS: Acalculous acute cholecystitis due to *Salmonella typhi*. Dig Dis Sci 37:1772, 1992.
85. James RA, Morris G, Winter R, Keston-Jones RM: Acalculous cholecystitis due to *Salmonella vircow*. Br J Clin Pract 44:767, 1990.
86. Teixidor HS, Godwin TA, Ramrez EA: Cryptosporidiosis of the biliary tract in AIDS. Radiology 180:51, 1991.

Infections of the Liver and Spleen

CHAPTER 40

Toni Hau

The structure and function of the liver and the spleen can be altered during many systemic infections, and some infections can involve these organs diffusely (Table 40–1). Many cases of hepatitis lead to cirrhosis with associated portal hypertension, intestinal varices, hemorrhage, and hypersplenism, all of which may become surgical problems, the treatment of which lie outside the scope of this book. In addition, patients with cirrhosis are prone to develop sepsis and primary peritonitis (see Chap. 38), and infections of the biliary tract can lead to liver infection (see Chap. 38). This chapter is limited to discussions of infections and infestations of the liver and the spleen whose treatment or diagnosis frequently require surgical consultation.

The liver and the spleen are the major reservoirs of the fixed macrophage population in the body. As blood passes through both organs, it is in intimate and prolonged contact with sinusoidal macrophages, one of whose functions is to clear the filtered blood of microorganisms. The liver filters the portal blood so that pathogenic or opportunistic microbes that escape the gut are usually trapped by the Kupffer cells. Both the liver and the spleen clear the arterial blood of circulating organisms.[1]

INFECTIONS OF THE LIVER

Despite continuous exposure to microbial organisms and their toxins, the liver of humans, unlike that of dogs and other experimental animals,[2,3] is normally sterile,[2,4,5] as is normal portal blood.[2] When portal bacterial showers occur,[6] however, the liver is able to eliminate bacteria from the bloodstream. Berg et al[7] showed that animals with normal but contaminated liver parenchyma have sterile bile. Beeson et al[1] demonstrated that patients with subacute bacterial endocarditis had a lower concentration of organisms in the hepatic vein blood than in the peripheral blood. In spite of the filtering function of the liver, bacterial infections are rare and usually occur in the form of abscesses. In most instances, the morphologic changes observed during septicemia are caused by toxic damage to the hepatocytes. Only a few cases of true bacterial hepatitis, mostly streptococcal, have been reported,[8] and it appears to be rare today.[8] Histologically, one can see the invasion of parenchyma by streptococci and scattered focal areas of hepatocellular necrosis. In contrast to toxic damage of the liver by viruses, which is centrilobular, these le-

TABLE 40–1. INFECTIOUS DISEASE WITH HEPATIC INVOLVEMENT

A. Bacterial infections
  1. Gram-positive cocci
    a. Pneumococcus
    b. *Staphylococcus*[a]
    c. *Streptococcus*[a]
  2. Gram-negative cocci
    a. Gonococcus (Fitz-Hugh-Curtis syndrome)
  3. Gram-negative enteric bacteria
    a. *E. coli*[a]
    b. *Salmonella*
    c. *Shigella*
    d. Other enteric bacteria[a]
  4. Other gram-negative bacilli
    a. *Brucellosis*[a]
    b. Tuberculosis[a]
    c. Granuloma inguinale
    d. Tularemia
  5. Spirochaetales
    a. Leptospirosis
    b. Borreliosis
    c. Syphilis
  6. Anaerobic bacteria
    a. *Clostridium*[a]
    b. *Bacteroides*[a]
    c. Other anaerobic bacteria[a]
  7. Rickettsial infections
    a. Q fever
  8. Chlamydiae
    a. Psittacosis
B. Mycotic infections
  1. Actinomycosis[a]
  2. Blastomycosis
  3. Candidiasis[a]
  4. Coccidioidomycosis
  5. Cryptococcosis
  6. Histoplasmosis
  7. Aspergillosis
  8. Mucormycosis
C. Protozoan infections
  1. Malaria
  2. Toxoplasmosis
  3. Amebiasis[a]
D. Viral infections
  1. Adenovirus
  2. Coxsackievirus
  3. Cytomegalovirus
  4. Echovirus
  5. Hepatitis virus A, B, non-A, non-B
  6. Herpes simplex virus
  7. Epstein-Barr virus
  8. "Marburg" virus
  9. Reovirus
  10. Rubella
  11. Varicella zoster HIV

[a] Diseases of surgical significance.
Adapted from Schiff L, Schiff ER (eds): Diseases of the Liver, 7th ed. Philadelphia, Lippincott, 1993.

sions are either periportal or intrazonal. The liver is involved in numerous other infections; only a few bacterial, mycotic, and protozoal infections assume surgical significance (see Table 40–1). Abscesses can develop in granulomas caused by brucellosis, actinomycosis, and candidiasis, which require surgical drainage. Tuberculosis of the liver can develop as large caseating granulomas, which might require resection of the liver. All other diseases that cause diffuse parenchymal damage or miliary abscesses and granulomas are not amenable to surgical therapy. Patients with AIDS can develop opportunistic infections of the liver caused by mycobacteria, viruses, fungi, and protozoa (Table 40–2). In addition, peliosis hepatis, a condition that may have an infectious etiology, has also been observed in eight AIDS patients.[9]

Bacterial Abscess of the Liver

Incidence. Abscess of the liver has always been a rare finding. Two autopsy series conducted before 1900 reported an incidence of liver abscesses between 0.4 and 1.75 percent.[10] Even in 1932, Collins found only 111 cases in 18,300 autopsies (0.606 percent).[11] At the same time, the incidence based on hospital admissions ranged from 0.04 to 0.007 percent.[12] Pyogenic liver abscesses have occurred even less frequently since the advent of antibiotic therapy. Knowles and Rinaldo[13] reported nine cases from the Henry Ford Hospital over the 10 years before 1960 (0.005 percent of all hospital admissions), and Ribaudo and Ochsner[14] found one liver abscess in every 1628 patients in 1973.

Furthermore, the peak incidence of the liver abscesses has shifted from the third and fourth decade to the seventh and eighth decades of life, a

TABLE 40–2. HEPATIC INFECTIONS ASSOCIATED WITH AIDS

Infection	Reported Cases
Mycobacterium avium-intracellulare	92
Other and unknown mycobacterial species	37
Cytomegalovirus	44
Other viral infections	1
Cryptococcus neoformans	15
Coccidioides immitis	9
Histoplasma capsulatum	8
Other fungi	3
Pneumocystis carinii	4
Other protozoa	3

Adapted from Mitchell SC: Am J Gastroenterol 86:1, 1991.

reflection of the previous importance of appendicitis as the main cause of liver abscesses. The current autopsy incidence is not available.

Besides the decline in the incidence of pyogenic liver abscesses, a change in the relative frequency of bacterial and amebic abscesses has been observed. Although Ochsner et al[15] noted that 35 percent of all liver abscesses were amebic in 1938, they now constitute approximately 10 percent.[16]

Etiology. Virtually every bacterium known to medical microbiology has been mentioned as a causative agent of hepatic abscesses; however, reliable data are hard to come by. In the older literature, sterile cultures were found in up to 60 percent of all cases. Even in more recent reviews, the number of sterile abscesses still exceeds 10 percent.[17] Aside from 47 cases observed by Sabbaj et al,[18] only 165 cases of anaerobic liver abscesses have been reported. This low number is probably the result of inadequate anaerobic culture techniques. In a systematic search, Sabbaj and co-workers found that anaerobic bacteria were present in 45 percent of all liver abscesses; the most commonly encountered organisms were anaerobic and microaerophilic streptococci, *Bacteroides fragilis,* and *Fusobacterium.* Of the 47 cases of Sabbaj et al,[18] 19 grew only aerobes, 15 grew only anaerobes, and 6 showed mixed anaerobic and aerobic cultures. In seven instances, either the cultures were sterile or the results were not available. In view of experimental data in which chronic liver abscesses could be reliably reproduced in mice only by the intraperitoneal injection of *Fusobacterium necrophorum,* and the observations of Onderdonk et al[19] that the presence of anaerobic bacteria is necessary to produce intraperitoneal abscesses, it is likely that anaerobic bacteria are involved in a large percentage of hepatic abscesses. Unfortunately, there is little information about the relationship between the pathogenesis of liver abscess and its bacteriology. It seems, however, that anaerobic bacteria are prominent in abscesses, secondary to hepatic tumors, and that the bacteriology of abscesses originating from lesions within the portal circulation closely resembles that of intraperitoneal infections, that is, *E. coli, Enterococcus,* and *Bacteroides.* A summary of the bacteriology of liver abscesses in Table 40–3 excludes the data of Sabbaj et al. Table 40–4 lists the anaerobes in 310 patients with liver abscesses collected by Finegold.[20] Rarely, bacteria that normally elicit granulomatous reactions will cause hepatic abscess as a complication of systemic infection. Brucellosis is commonly complicated by hepatomegaly, splenomegaly, and microscopic hepatic granulomas. Although *Brucella*

TABLE 40–3. BACTERIOLOGY OF HEPATIC ABSCESSES[a]

Organisms	Number (%)	Number (%)
• GRAM-POSITIVE AEROBES		
Staphylococci		34 (18.5)
S. aureus	27 (14.7)	
S. epidermidis	7 (3.8)	
Streptococci		16 (8.7)
Hemolytic streptococci	3 (1.6)	
Nonhemolytic streptococci	13 (7.1)	
Enterococci		20 (10.9)
Others		4 (2.2)
• GRAM-NEGATIVE AEROBES		
Escherichia coli		82 (44.6)
Klebsiella/Enterobacter		61 (33.2)
Proteus		21 (11.4)
Pseudomonas		12 (6.5)
Others		16 (8.7)
• ANAEROBES		
Bacteroides		16 (8.7)
Peptostreptococcus		11 (6.0)
Clostridium		7 (3.8)
Others		5 (2.7)

[a] Represents 305 isolates from 184 patients.[27,29,32,76,78]

abortus is the common human pathogen, abscesses of the liver and spleen have been seen in *B. suis* infections. In these cases, prolonged septic courses with calcific deposits in the liver or the spleen were relieved by drainage.

Most tuberculous lesions of the liver are miliary granulomas. Abscess-like masses (tuberculomas) sometimes form and spread along the walls of the intrahepatic bile ducts (tuberculous cholangitis). Diagnosis may be difficult because both caseation and acid-fast organisms can be absent. Tuberculomas are often, but not always, accompanied by an abdominal focus. Drainage was sometimes curative in the prechemotherapeutic era.

Miliary abscesses have been found in cases of disseminated granuloma inguinale. Hepatic clostridial infections cause gas abscesses, but most of the jaundice in disseminated infections is hemolytic.

Pathogenesis. Table 40–5 lists the pathogenetic factors that are probably involved in the formation of liver abscesses. Primary hepatic causes include trauma, tumor, and ischemia. Direct extension of infections of neighboring organs to the liver has been described, but is rather rare. In a recent survey, trauma caused 5 percent of the liver abscess.[17] According to Robertson et al,[21] 16 percent of all hepatic abscesses observed over a 25-year period orig-

TABLE 40–4. ANAEROBIC ORGANISMS IN PYOGENIC LIVER ABSCESS (310 PATIENTS)

Organisms	Number of Isolates
Anaerobic streptococci	58
Microaerophilic streptococci	38
Anaerobic gram-positive cocci	7
Anaerobic gram-negative cocci	1
Bacteroides species	39
B. fragilis	33
B. oralis	2
B. serpens	3
P. melaninogenicus	7
Bacteroidaceae	6
Fusobacterium species	34
F. girans	3
F. necrophorum	47
Unidentified anaerobic gram-negative rods	16
Clostridium	38
Actinomyces	32
Eubacterium species	2
Lactobacillus species	1
Bifidobacterium	1
Propionibacterium	2
Bacterium halosepticum	1
Unidentified anaerobic gram-positive rods	5
"Anaerobe"	4
Total	379 strains

From Finegold SM, George WL (eds): Anaerobic Bacteria in Human Disease. New York, Harcourt, 1989, p. 342.

inated from secondary infection of neoplastic lesions. Trump et al[22] have stated that of 1262 liver abscesses described in the literature since 1934, only 32 patients had a lesion associated with either primary or metastatic tumor. Jochimsen et al[23] reported several cases of liver abscess that developed after the hepatic artery was ligated for the treatment of neoplasms (hepatic metastases). Although abscesses that are associated with tumors may not be reported in surgical series, the association of infection with metastatic liver disease is probably underreported. Whether infection superimposed on hepatic metastasis is a common undiagnosed problem is speculative.

Because of the liver's dual blood supply, hematogenous spread of infections to the liver can occur by the portal vein or the hepatic artery, although the portal system is the more common pathway. Appendicitis was once the leading course of hepatic abscesses. Today, 20 percent of all liver abscesses are secondary to an infection in the drainage area of the portal vein (see Table 40–5).

Hepatic abscesses that originate from the arterial circulation of the liver constitute 13 to 15 percent of all liver abscesses, a number that has remained rather constant through the years.[15,17] Every infection associated with bacteremia can be the source of this kind of liver abscess. In summary, one-third of all hepatic abscesses are caused by cholangitis and operations or manipulations of the biliary tract.[24]

Even after thorough clinical and pathologic investigation, 20 percent of hepatic abscesses will remain, the source of which cannot be determined (cryptogenic abscesses). Perhaps they develop secondary to bacterial invasion from an unrecognized source within the portal system. Multiple hepatic abscesses due to *Fusobacterium nucleatum* have been described in patients with dental disease.[25] Focal areas of ischemia within the hepatic parenchyma may provide a local site of impaired defense so that bowel bacteria cannot be cleared.[26]

Patients with compromised host defenses have an increased risk of developing pyogenic liver ab-

TABLE 40–5. PATHOGENESIS OF PYOGENIC HEPATIC ABSCESSES

PRIMARY HEPATIC	Trauma Tumor Ischemia Hepatic parasites Foreign bodies
BY DIRECT EXTENSION	Penetrating peptic ulcers Penetrating carcinomas of the UGI tract Cholecystitis Pancreatitis Perihepatic abscess
VIA THE PORTAL CIRCULATION	Inflammatory disease of the small and large bowel Carcinoma of the GI tract with abscess formation Appendicitis Diverticulitis Pancreatitis Splenic infections Peritonitis and intraperitoneal abscesses Omphalitis
VIA THE ARTERIAL CIRCULATION	All infections associated with bacteremia
VIA THE BILIARY SYSTEM	Ascending cholangitis secondary to Stones Strictures Tumor
CRYPTOGENIC	

scesses. Diabetes mellitus was present in 15 percent of the patients of Altemeier et al,[27] and liver abscesses have been found in children with leukemia, chronic granulomatous disease, AIDS, and other immune deficiency disorders. Liver abscesses, usually multiple, occur in recipients of orthotopic liver transplants who suffer thrombosis of the hepatic artery. Ischemia is almost always followed by infective necrosis requiring total hepatic replacement. Enteric organisms are most often found. Liver transplant recipients will develop pyogenic and opportunistic liver abscesses when biliary obstruction, tumor, trauma, or bacteremia occurs.

Pathology. The pathogenesis of liver abscesses is reflected in the gross anatomic picture. If the cause of the abscess is a primary pathologic process of the liver, the abscess is single and corresponds to the primary lesion. Similar observations can be made if the abscess has been created as a direct extension of a perihepatic infection. If the primary lesion is located within the portal circulation, the abscesses are large, single or multiple, and in most cases confined to the right lobe of the liver; the left lobe is rarely affected. Kinney and Ferrebee,[28] in a study based on experiments of Sérégé in 1901,[29] showed that there is a separate flow of blood from the superior mesenteric vein to the right lobe of the liver, and from the splenic vein to the left lobe of the liver. This explains the preferential location of portal hepatic abscesses in the right lobe, which drains the intestines. Hepatic abscesses in both lobes will occur when the portal vein is filled with a septic thrombus.

Bacteria originating from the systemic circulation reach the liver through the hepatic arteries, and usually form many small abscesses—a frequent autopsy finding in debilitated and immunosuppressed hosts. If the hepatic abscesses originated from the biliary system, they are equally distributed over both lobes of the liver, are multiple, and the dilated biliary ducts are filled with pus. Approximately 65 percent of all hepatic abscesses occur in the right lobe; less than 5 percent of the cases involve the left lobe and the remainder involve both lobes. The abscesses are multiple 40 percent of the time.[15,30]

Clinical Manifestations. The symptoms and signs associated with hepatic abscess are either systemic or local. The systemic symptoms are those of sepsis: fever, chills, and profuse sweating. The fever is classically of the septic (picket fence) type, but continuous and intermittent fevers occur. Malaise and anorexia occur early, along with weight loss, weakness, nausea, vomiting, and lethargy. The most prominent local symptom, dull, constant right upper quadrant pain, was present in over 90 percent of the cases reported by Ochsner et al[15]; it appears less frequently in more recent reports.[15,26] Often the patient complains of pain that radiates into the right shoulder.

The salient physical finding in two-thirds of these patients is a large, tender liver. Other findings include localized guarding and thoracic signs of pleural effusion or lower lobe infiltration. Jaundice occurs less commonly; Ochsner et al described it in only 8.3 percent of their patients. This holds true only for those hepatic abscesses that were not caused by an obstruction of the biliary tree.[15] Ascites is rare and is seen only as a terminal event.

COMPLICATIONS OF HEPATIC ABSCESS. Complications from hepatic abscess result from perforation of the abscess into neighboring structures. Pleuropulmonary complications, with a 15 percent occurrence in Ochsner's series,[15] result most often from direct extension of the hepatic abscess through the diaphragm into the parenchyma of the lung or the pleural space. Metastatic abscesses are rare. Even less frequently, a hepatic abscess will rupture into the peritoneal cavity and cause peritonitis or subhepatic abscess. In the preantibiotic era, this complication was observed in 7.2 and 2.5 percent of hepatic abscesses, respectively.[15] Perforations may also occur into the pericardium, the hepatic vein, the thoracic duct, and the abdominal wall. All these complications appear in less than 10 percent in most recent series.[30] Block et al[16] state that 8 of 26 patients with hepatic abscesses had other nonhepatic abscesses that required drainage.

LABORATORY EVALUATION. The laboratory findings in patients with a pyogenic liver abscess reflect systemic infection as well as impairment of the hepatic function. Leukocytosis is common, and occasionally microcytic anemia is present. Hepatic dysfunction is manifested by a moderate elevation of bilirubin, alkaline phosphatase, serum glutamic-oxaloacetic transaminase (SGOT), decreased serum albumin, and prolonged prothrombin time. Usually the alkaline phosphatase is the most constantly and significantly elevated. The abnormalities in the liver function are usually mild and do not correlate with the clinical picture of severe illness with hepatomegaly and systemic sepsis. Although it was once stated that blood cultures are sterile in most cases of hepatic abscesses,[12] Satiani and Davidson[30] recently found positive blood culture results in 58 percent of their patients.

RADIOLOGIC EVALUATION. Certain abnormalities observed by x-ray studies of the chest and plain film of the abdomen may suggest the presence of a hepatic abscess. The x-ray study may show an elevation of the right diaphragm, a right pleural effusion, atalectatic changes in the right lower lobe, or obliteration of the costophrenic angle. Fluoroscopy reveals that the motion of the diaphragm is limited. The plain film of the abdomen may also show signs of hepatic enlargement. Accumulation of gas within the liver indicates the presence of a hepatic abscess. Gas within the unoperated biliary tree suggests septic cholangitis; gas within the portal vein suggests gangrene of the bowel with extension of the infection to the liver. A right lateral view is especially helpful in locating the accumulation of gas and deciding if it is within or outside the liver parenchyma. Large abscesses also show displacement of the stomach or the duodenum, which can be better demonstrated by radiologic examination of the upper gastrointestinal tract.

Ultrasonography and computed tomography (CT) have replaced scans with technetium-99 sulfur colloid as the method of choice for the radiologic proof of hepatic abscesses.[31–33] Abscesses that are large enough to be suitable for diagnostic aspiration or therapeutic drainage can be equally well diagnosed by either imaging technique.[32,34] The multiple abscesses associated with biliary sepsis may be invisible by ultrasonography but can be more readily seen by CT scan. There are some variations in the appearance of hepatic abscesses on ultrasound as well as CT scans. With ultrasonography the lesion can be echogenic as well as nonechogenic. In the case of nonechoic lesions variable amounts of internal echo can be seen. Occasionally, fluid interfaces can also be detected. Most abscesses have only a thin wall that delineates them from the normal parenchyma. However, this wall can be completely absent or very thick. Nearly all abscesses show distal sonic enhancement as long as no gas is present (Fig. 40–1).[35] The appearance of hepatic abscesses on CT scans is also variable. Most abscesses are inhomogeneous, but the density is generally lower than in the surrounding tissue. Intravenous administration of contrast material enhances the ease by which abscesses can be diagnosed, and in a few cases the abscess cannot be detected until the contrast material has been administered (Fig. 40–2). However, rim enhancement is seen only rarely.[36] If there are any doubts about the nature of the hepatic lesion, an aspiration of the abscess under ultrasonographic or CT control should be performed. This not only allows a diagnosis by Gram stain and culture, but also distinguishes a pyogenic abscess from an amebic abscess or a cystic lesion of the liver. Ultrasonographic aspiration should only be performed if the abscess is superficial and fairly large because it is difficult to follow the needle and simultaneously observe the anatomy with ultrasound equipment.

The needle can be inserted after the anatomy has been delineated by ultrasound. Direct visualization of the needle usually can be accomplished by using a regular transducer that is positioned close to an acoustic window, at an angle of 90 degrees from the entrance site. The needle can then be observed on the video screen while it is inserted into the abscess. Because the needle can only be visualized if it is at a right angle to the transducer, special coaxial transducers have been developed that can be placed directly over the entrance site. With modern equipment the angle of the puncture as well as the depth of the puncture can be preselected depending on the ultrasonographic findings. The puncture is performed with a fine needle with a diameter of 0.9 mm or if the abscess content is very viscous of 1.3 mm under local anesthesia with

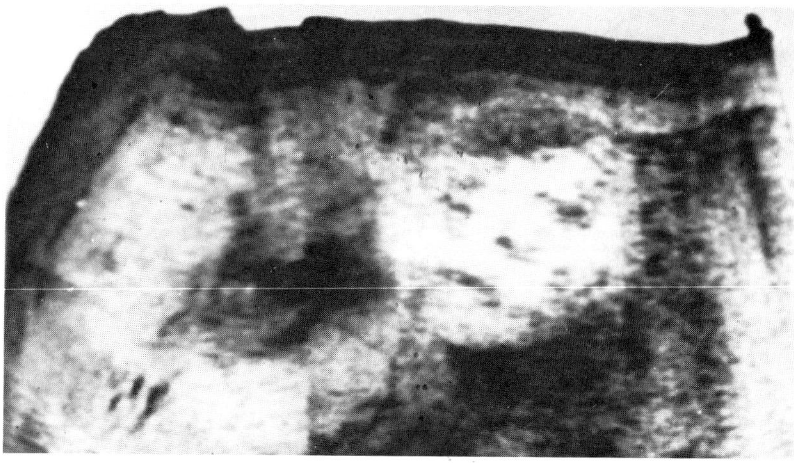

Figure 40–1. Echogram of the liver revealing a large fluid-filled intrahepatic space, which was found to be a hepatic abscess at operation. *(Courtesy of S. B. Feinberg, MD, Department of Radiology, University of Minnesota, Minneapolis.)*

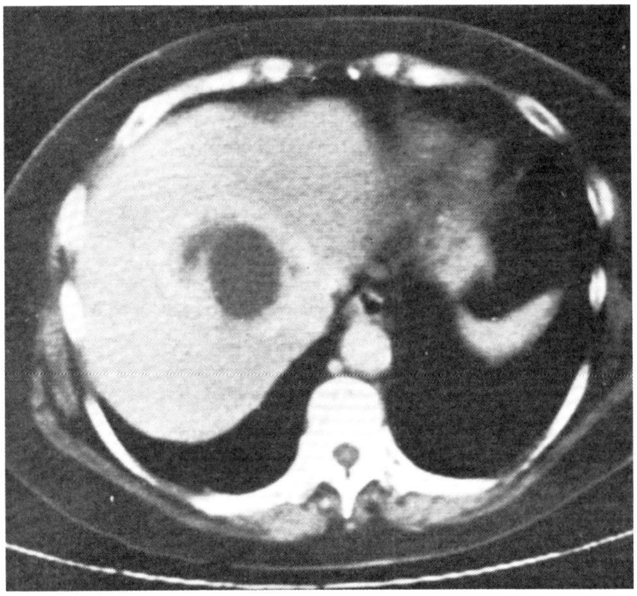

Figure 40–2. Pyogenic abscess of the liver. The density of the well-defined abscess cavity is near that of water. There is a peripheral rim of increased density on the contrast enhanced scan. *(From Stephens DH, Sheedy PF II: The liver. In Haaga JR, Alfidi RJ (eds): Computed Tomography of the Abdomen. St Louis, Mosby, 1985.)*

the patient holding his or her breath. When the needle enters the suspected abscess a "blip" can be seen on the video screen. Today, puncture under sonographic guidance is as safe and successful as under CT guidance.[37–39] After a series of diagnostic scans, a point on the skin surface is chosen that provides the shortest distance to the abscess area. After a metal marker is placed, the distance from the skin to the abscess is measured and a 18-gauge splenoportal plastic-sheathed needle is introduced under CT control. After the needle is introduced 2 cm in the abdominal wall, a repeat scan is performed to adjust the angulation of the needle and assess the depth of the lesion. After these adjustments have been made, the instrument is introduced to the previously measured depth into the abscess cavity. After pus has been withdrawn, the exact location of the needle is verified by CT.[37]

A liver scan with technetium-99 sulfur colloid will show the defect in over 80 percent of all cases,[30,40] but usually takes more time to obtain. The anatomic details are not as clear as with the previously mentioned methods, and these methods do not allow an aspiration. Other radiologic methods, such as scanning with indium-111 labeled leukocytes and gallium-67,[40,41] arteriography, and endoscopic retrograde cholangiography, have been reported in the diagnosis of hepatic abscesses, but are dispensable in view of the modern imaging techniques.

Diagnosis. A combination of systemic sepsis with hepatomegaly, and hepatic tenderness without jaundice, is the characteristic clinical syndrome of hepatic abscesses. The diagnosis can seldom be made on clinical grounds alone. In two older series, only 9 of 24 and 26 of 42 abscesses were diagnosed ante mortem.[21] Lee and Block[26] pointed out that the use of liver scans decreased the incidence of autopsy diagnosis from 26 percent to 8 percent. Although the symptoms seem to be less acute than in the past, they should at least arouse suspicion and lead to the institution of the proper diagnostic procedures. Ultrasonography or CT scan, combined with aspiration of the abscess if necessary, should establish the diagnosis of a hepatic abscess in all cases and make the routine use of other diagnostic measures unnecessary.

An intensive search for the primary source of infection should be conducted, because it has significant prognostic and therapeutic implications. The differentiation from amebic abscesses is discussed later.

Treatment. The treatment of pyogenic abscesses requires both antibiotic therapy and adequate drainage, but no controlled studies have been carried out. The antibiotic treatment is usually started when a hepatic abscess is suspected, because systemic sepsis is obvious in most patients. If this is not the case, antibiotic treatment should be started before operation. The choice of antibiotics can be deduced from the microbiology of hepatic abscesses. As stated earlier, there are three groups of bacteria that may be present singly or in combination: (1) pyogenic gram-positive cocci (staphylococci and streptococci), (2) enterobacteria (eg, *E. coli, Klebsiella, Enterobacter, Proteus*), and (3) anaerobic bacteria (*B. fragilis,* clostridia). Antibiotic treatment is usually started without knowledge of the causative organism or its sensitivity. If the pathogenesis of the hepatic abscess is known, the underlying disease gives some clue to the bacteriology, and with that to the choice of antibiotics. If the abscess is thought to be secondary to an infection in the drainage area of the portal system, one can suspect a similar bacteriology as in intraperitoneal infections, consisting of a mixed flora or gram-negative aerobes, such as *E. coli, Enterobacter, Klebsiella,* and *Proteus* and anaerobic bacteria (mainly *B. fragilis*). The antibiotic therapy, therefore, should consist either of a combination of an aminoglycoside with either clindamycin or metronidazole, or a suitable broad-spectrum beta-lactam antibiotic with satisfactory anaerobic coverage, such as cefoxitin, moxalactam, imipenem, piperacillin, or mezlocillin. If the abscess occurs in the context of systemic sepsis *Staphylococcus aureus* or streptococci are the most likely etiologic agents, and the patient, therefore, should be treated with either a penicillinase-resistant penicillin or a first generation cephalosporin. Hepatic abscesses secondary to biliary infection are most frequently caused by gram-negative Enterobacteriaceae or *Enterococcus faecalis* so that ampicillin or a ureidopenicillin should be combined with an aminoglycoside. These antibiotics also will reach bactericidal concentrations in the bile. If the source of the abscess is not known, a broad spectrum combination therapy is usually necessary, consisting of ampicillin, an aminoglycoside, and clindamycin. The presence of gram-positive facultative or microaerophilic organisms mitigates against the use of ampicillin. The bacteriologic diagnosis should, however, be established as soon as possible through aspiration of the abscess and the antibiotic regimen modified according to the result.[42] There is no evdience that antibiotics instilled into the abscess cavity or infused into the portal system have any advantage over appropriate systemic antibiotic therapy.

Antibiotic treatment alone is not sufficient in the treatment of hepatic abscesses, because bactericidal concentrations of antibiotics may be difficult to achieve within the walled-off abscess cavity. An adequate drainage procedure is, therefore, mandatory. Without drainage, the mortality even today is close to 50 percent. Recently, several reports have been published about treatment of hepatic abscesses with systemic antibiotics and closed-needle aspiration of the abscess cavity.[43,44] The initial results seem to be encouraging. A total of 62 cases with a mortality of 4 percent have been reported, although the aspiration often has to be repeated more than five times,[43] and adequate continuous drainage seems to be preferable.[45] This can be achieved either percutaneously or surgically. The parenchyma of the liver can be reached percutaneously without endangering other intra-abdominal or thoracic organs and without contaminating the pleura or peritoneal cavity. However, if multiple abscesses are present multiple drains may be necessary. If the abscess is secondary to a disease that requires surgical therapy, such as a biliary tract infection or a perforated viscus, a surgical approach is mandatory. In other situations a primary percutaneous approach for the drainage of hepatic abscesses is the procedure of choice. Gerzof et al[31] have recently reviewed 109 continuous percutaneous drainage procedures for liver abscesses with a recurrence rate of 15 percent and a mortality of 3.9 percent. These figures have been confirmed in several recent reports.[45–48] The first step in the percutaneous drainage of hepatic abscesses is the aspiration of the abscesses under ultrasonographic or CT guidance. After pus is aspirated and a positive gram stain has been obtained, an angiographic wire is inserted and the plastic sheath withdrawn. A 7 or 8 French pigtail catheter is then inserted over the guidewire using the standard Seldinger technique. Over the ensuing days the catheter tract can be dilated to accommodate a 14 or 16 French catheter. The final positioning of the catheter is done under fluoroscopic control, and a small amount of contrast material is injected to define the extent of the cavity and compare it with the previously obtained CT scan. It is necessary to make sure that no loculations are overlooked and that the entire abscess cavity is drained. Once the catheter is positioned correctly the entire cavity is evacuated and irrigated with saline until the return is clear. In addition to the usual criteria for removal of a drain, one should be sure to obtain a repeat CT scan to ascertain that the abscess cavity is completely collapsed.[37]

Two operative approaches can be used to drain the liver abscess. Extraserous drainage was once considered mandatory to avoid contamination of the peritoneal cavity.[15] This method is effective only if a solitary abscess is located near the dome of the liver, because the incision permits only a limited exploration of the liver. Smaller abscesses can easily be overlooked, and the limited exposure will not permit any intra-abdominal septic source to be diagnosed. For these reasons, and because of the safety of the transperitoneal approach with appropriate antibiotic coverage and thorough peritoneal toilet, most authors prefer the transperitoneal approach.[27,30,49] Extraperitoneal drainage of an anterior hepatic abscess can be done using a short right subcostal incision. After division of the rectus muscle, the dissection can be carried cephalad between the abdominal wall and the parietal peritoneum until the fluctuant abscess is reached. After needle aspiration confirms its location, the abscess is entered and evacuated. Soft suction drains are left within the cavity and led out through the abdominal wall (Fig. 40–3).

If the abscess is located in the posterior aspect of the dome of the liver, the transpleural approach through the bed of the 10th or 11th rib can be used. After the pleural space has been entered, a chest tube is inserted in the fifth intercostal space. The dome of the liver is palpated, and after the area of

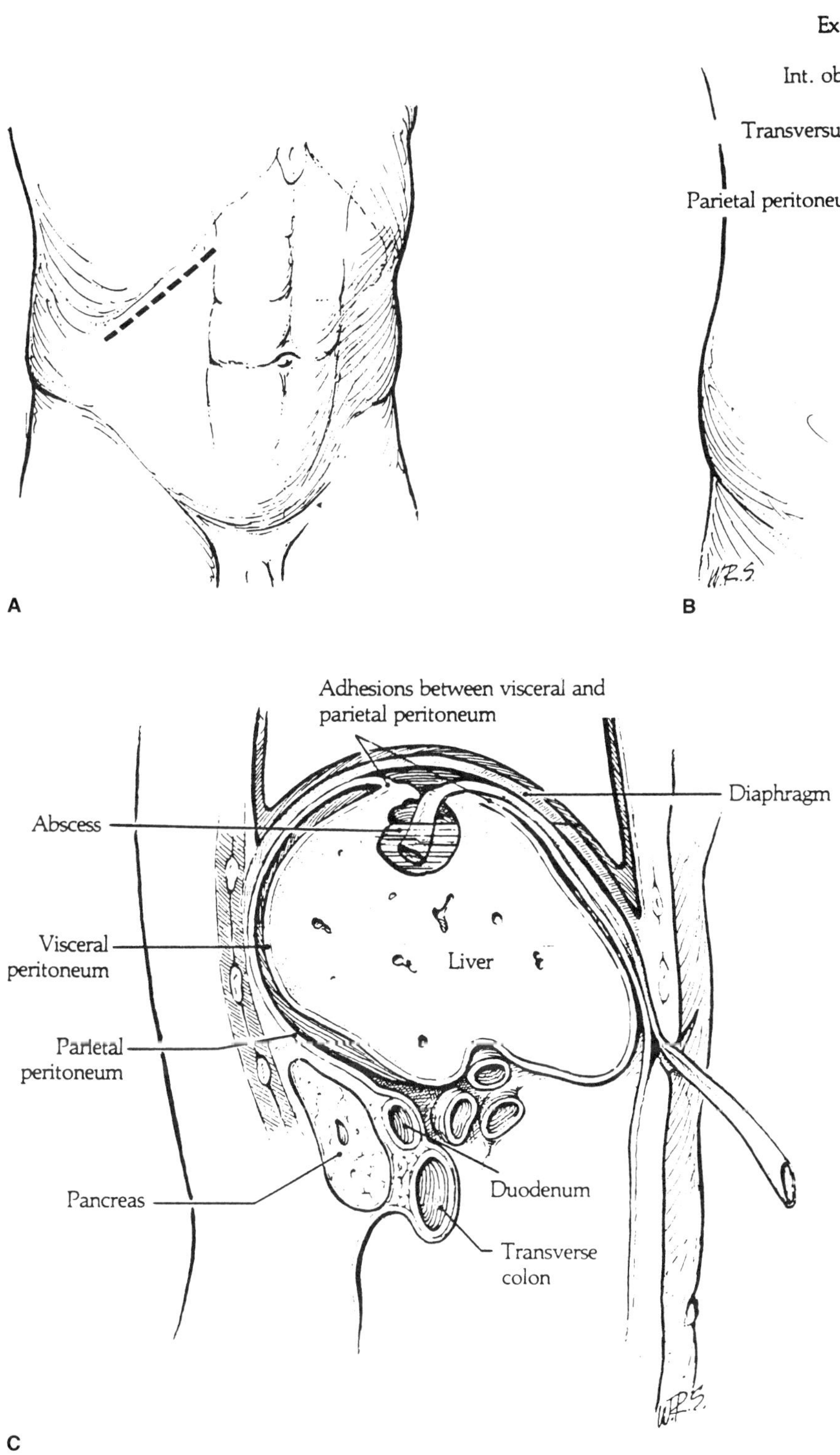

Figure 40–3. A. Drainage of an anterior liver abscess. Skin incision lateral to the rectus abdominus muscle, 2 cm below the costal margin. **B.** Drainage of anterior liver abscess. Division of the abdominal musculature of the parietal peritoneum is not opened. **C.** Drainage of anterior liver abscesses. Position of the drain between the parietal, peritoneum, and diaphragm. *(From Hau T: Drainage, subphrenic and subhepatic abscesses. In Nyhus LM, Baker RJ (eds): Mastery of Surgery. Boston, Little, Brown, 1984.)*

the abscess has been identified, the diaphragmatic pleura is mobilized and sutured to the parietal pleura above the level of the thoracotomy. The diaphragm is then incised, the abscess unroofed, and soft rubber suction drains left in the cavity (Fig. 40–4). Both these methods depend on the preexistence of adhesions between the parietal and visceral peritoneum to prevent contamination of the peritoneal cavity. Transperitoneal drainage of the hepatic abscess can usually be accomplished through a subcostal incision. A midline incision can be used if further exploration of the abdominal cavity is necessary to determine the source of sepsis. If the primary source of infection is not known, a thorough exploration should be carried out to exclude all possible sites. The liver is then palpated, and suspicious areas are aspirated with a needle. After the abscess has been located, its cavity is entered and the entire contents evacuated and irrigated until clear. Loculations should be broken up to create one large cavity. During this procedure, the peritoneal cavity should be protected by a heavy layer of antibiotic-soaked gauze pads. Traditionally, dependent drainage with soft rubber drains is established by appropriate placement of drainage incisions. Soft Silastic suction drains function better without reliance on a dependent position. In addition, the shutter action of the abdominal muscles will not interfere with a suction drain, as it does with Penrose drains brought out through a stab wound. In some cases, marsupialization of an anterior abscess can be used. If the drain tract traverses a long distance across the peritoneal cavity, peritoneal contamination will occur for several days prior to the development of a fibrous tract. For this reason additional drains should be placed in the parahepatic space to permit exit tracts for contaminated spillage (Fig. 40–5).

It is possible to compromise between the transperitoneal and extraserous approaches. For example, after laparotomy and location of the abscess in the liver, a separate retroperitoneal tract can be developed for the actual drainage.[27]

Some patients with suppurative cholangitis will have concurrent or subsequent hepatic abscesses. In addition to drainage of the common duct and evacuation of the hepatic abscesses, they will need irrigation of the common duct to provide through-and-through drainage of hepatic abscess and common duct. This technique can help locate the smaller, less easily detected abscesses within the hepatic parenchyma. Also, hepatic resection for multiple liver abscesses confined to one lobe is possible. Whatever the technique, postoperative management requires prolonged antibiotic treatment and nutritional support. If sepsis continues or recurs, repeated CT scans may be necessary to rule out the reaccumulation of pus within the liver, the appearance of additional abscesses, or the development of a perihepatic abscess.

The postoperative complication rate is still approximately 30 percent. Satiani and Davidson[30] reported a 42 percent rate of recurrent abscesses in the liver, abscess formation within the peritoneal cavity, metastatic abscesses, and wound infections. The reaccumulation of pus, whether within the peritoneal cavity or the cavity of the hepatic abscess, requires reevacuation and drainage. Empyemas must also be drained. Metastatic abscesses in the lung, however, usually respond to antibiotic treatment. Hepatobronchial fistulas result in a spontaneous drainage of the abscess; once it is drained, antibiotic treatment usually leads to closure of the fistula.

Prognosis. In 1938, Ochsner et al[15] reported a mortality of 79.6 percent in a collected series of 432 liver abscesses. This figure did not change significantly, even after introduction of antibiotics, until the introduction of the liver scan in the middle 1960s. Lee and Block[26] found the mortality in the prescan era to be between 70 and 85 percent; in the postscan era it dropped below 30 percent. The improvement in prognosis is mainly the result of earlier and more accurate diagnosis. According to Lee and Block,[26] during the period from 1955 to 1965 the disease was diagnosed antemortem only 20 percent of the time and with an 80 percent mortality.

The mortality in the prescan as well as in the postscan era is influenced by (1) the number of abscesses, (2) the causative bacteria, (3) the mode of treatment, (4) the presence of complications, and (5) the age of the patient. Before the mid-1960s, the differences in prognosis were much more pronounced.

Today, the mortality of hepatic abscesses ranges from 10 to 20 percent.[24,45,46] However, series of patients with a mortality of only 2 percent have been reported.[47] In the past, the number of abscesses, the mode of treatment, the age of the patient, and the bacteriology as well as the origin of the bacteria (portal, arterial, biliary) had a significant impact on the prognosis. These differences are much less marked today, even though the prognosis of multiple abscesses is slightly worse than for single abscesses and the underlying disease has an obvious influence on the overall prognosis especially if the source of the hepatic abscess is a malignant tumor.[24,39,45] Lee and co-workers,[49] using univariant

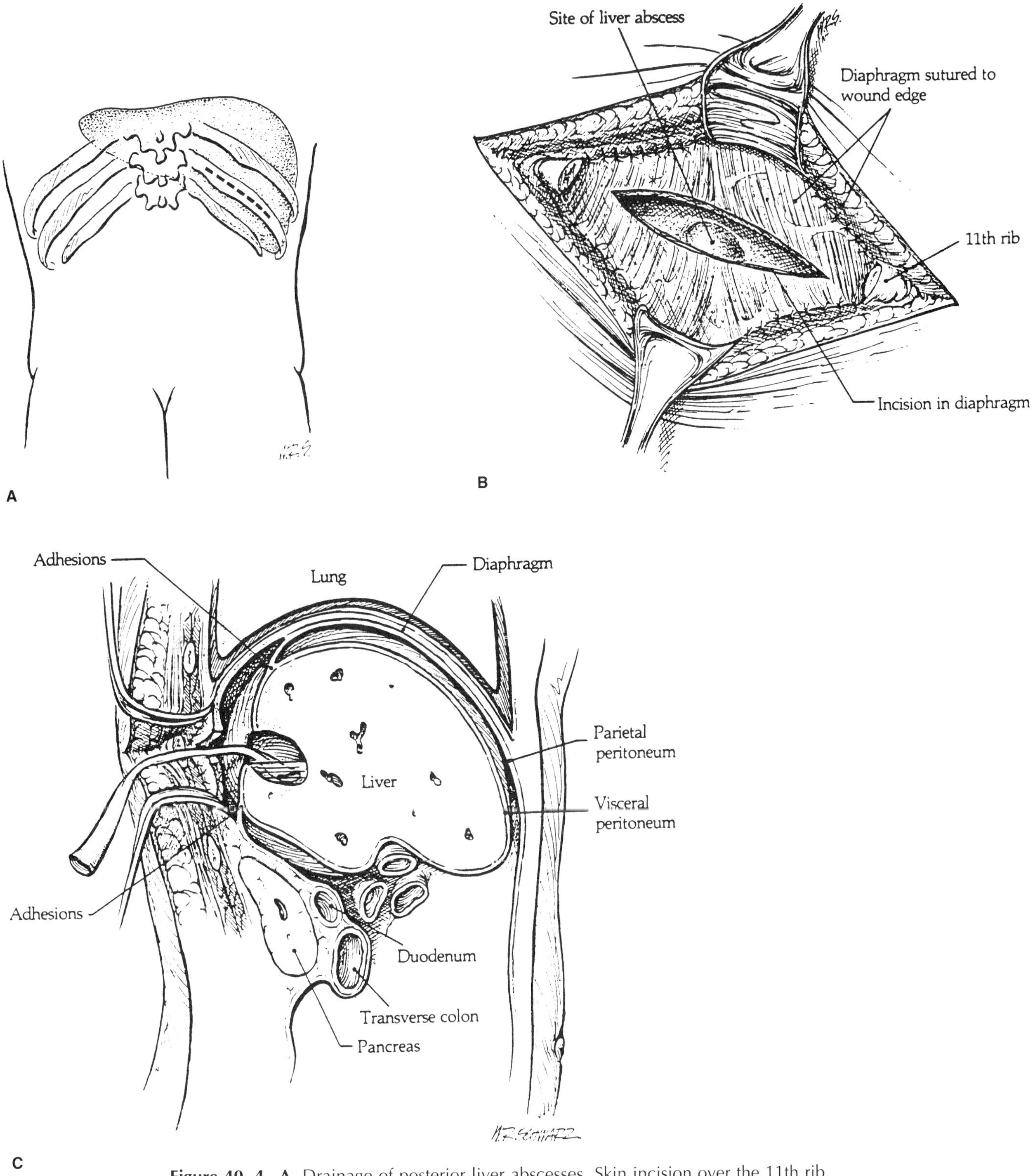

Figure 40–4. **A.** Drainage of posterior liver abscesses. Skin incision over the 11th rib. **B.** Drainage of posterior liver abscesses. The rib has been resected; the diaphragm is then sutured to the parietal pleura surrounding the incision and incised. The liver abscess can be seen as a slight prominence in the liver parenchyma. **C.** Drainage of posterior liver abscesses. Note position of the drain, which violates neither the pleural nor peritoneal cavity. *(From Hau T: Drainage of hepatic, subphrenic and subhepatic abscesses. In Nyhus LM, Baker RJ (eds): Mastery of Surgery. Boston, Little, Brown, 1984.)*

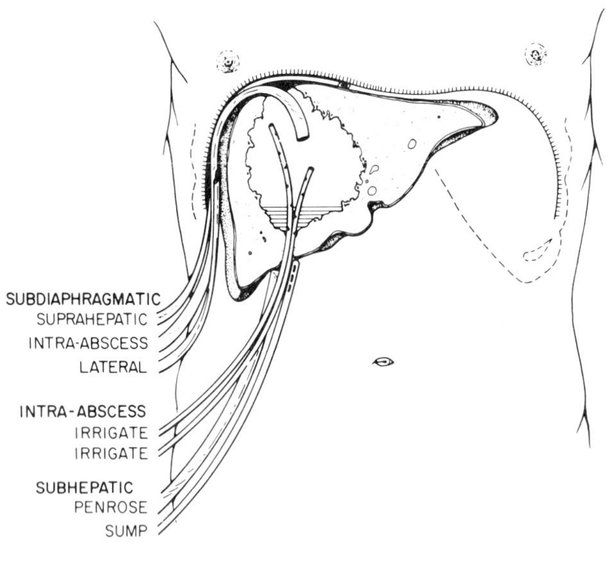

Figure 40–5. Transperitoneal drainage of a hepatic abscess. *(From Goldsmith HS, Chen WF: Surg Clin North Am 53:711, 1973.)*

analysis, have shown that clinical jaundice, pleural effusion, profound hypalbuminemia, hyperbilirubinemia, elevated alkaline phosphatase, and marked leukocytosis were associated with a higher mortality. However, multivariant stepwise logistic regression analysis showed that only three factors—marked leukocytosis (over 20,000) profound hypalbuminemia (under 2.5 g/dl), and presence of a pleural effusion—were independent predictors of mortality.[49]

Amebic Abscess of the Liver

Incidence. Contrary to general opinion, infestation with amebae is relatively common even in temperate zones. Hepatic involvement, though relatively uncommon, is serious. Ochsner and DeBakey[50] found clinical evidence of hepatic involvement in 5 percent of 9696 patients with amebiasis. Of 5211 amebiasis patients who died, however, 36 percent had liver involvement. Contrary to this low incidence, Adams[51] found an incidence of hepatic involvement in 41 percent of over 5000 cases treated in South Africa between 1955 and 1974. Men are more commonly affected by hepatic amebiasis than women; in some series the ratio is 10:1. Although there is no race preference, the native population of endemic regions seems to be less frequently afflicted with hepatic amebiasis.

Etiology. Systemic amebiasis is discussed in Chapter 8.

Pathogenesis and Pathology. It is generally agreed that amebae enter the liver from within the colon by the portal blood. Although it has not been possible to develop an animal model of hepatic amebiasis by creating intestinal amebiasis, experimental observations have shown that intrahepatic portal thrombosis and infarction are key features in the development of the typical lesions.[52] The lesions usually start in the portal triad and extend peripherally toward the capsule. In the early stages, an area of necrotic tissue, which may contain leukocytes, connective tissue cells, and occasional amebae, is surrounded by hyperemia. Later, a more or less well-defined capsule develops in which, unlike the necrotic center, amebae can be found. The contents of the abscess is a viscid, light to dark brown material, that has been classically described as anchovy paste.

The coexistence of amebic hepatitis has been disputed. Regenerative changes, Kupffer cell hyperplasia, increased hyperfuchsin pigment, portal and sinusoidal infiltration, and occasional areas of focal necrosis have been described on light microscopy,[53] and injury to the mitochondria and to endoplasmic reticulum have been seen on electron microscopy. Adams and McLeod[54] and Turrill and Burnham,[55] however, feel that there is no histologic evidence of amebic hepatitis. Aside from the typical abscesses, liver biopsies taken from patients with hepatic amebiasis are normal.

The right lobe of the liver is involved in a single abscess in over 90 percent of the cases. Multiple abscesses are found in only 10 percent. Amebic abscesses are usually bacteriologically sterile. Secondary bacterial infection has been observed in earlier reports in approximately 20 percent,[56] but more recently an incidence of less than 5 percent has been reported.[55,57]

Clinical Manifestations. The symptoms of liver abscesses are similar regardless of etiology. The main symptom is pain located over the right hypochondrium, the chest, or the epigastrium, which radiates occasionally into the right shoulder and is accompanied by cough, fever, weakness, and weight loss. Over 80 percent of the patients have an enlarged, tender liver and tenderness below the right costal margin. An abnormal finding over the right lung base or localized intercostal tenderness can be found in 47 and 38 percent, respectively.[54]

Only one to two-thirds of the patients have either clinical signs of intestinal amebiasis at the time of diagnosis or a history that suggests it.[50,54] If the diarrhea antedates the diagnosis of hepatic amebiasis, the symptom-free interval is less than 2 months in over two-thirds of the patients.

The disease can occur in a chronic or acute form. Ochsner and DeBakey[50] stated that two-thirds of all the cases had a rather chronic course, but more recent reports indicate that over two-thirds of all patients have an acute form, with symptoms lasting approximately 2 weeks before hospital admission.[54,57] In some patients, a rectosigmoidoscopic examination reveals signs of amebic colitis, manifested by mucosal edema, granularity, hyperemia, and increased friability.

RADIOLOGIC EVALUATION. X-ray studies reveal an elevated right diaphragm, the motion of which is decreased on fluoroscopy, pleural effusion or infiltrate at the base of the right lung, and occasionally a bulge in the right diaphragm. According to DeBakey and Ochsner,[56] positive radiologic signs on plain films are present in 80 percent of the patients. If the abscess is situated in the left lobe of the liver, there are usually no findings on x-ray studies of the chest, but an upper gastrointestinal series will show signs of external compression on the stomach. A liver scan will nearly always locate the abscess. It has been generally assumed that the results of gallium-67 scans of amebic abscesses will be normal because of the lack of granulocytes in the abscess, but Geslien et al[58] have found increased uptake in the periphery of amebic abscesses in two patients. As for pyogenic abscesses, however, ultrasonography and CT scan are the most expedient and accurate methods to demonstrate the anatomy of an amebic abscess even though there are no specific features that will distinguish between the two diseases.

COMPLICATIONS. The most common complication of an amebic hepatic abscess involves direct extension into the thorax. Hematogenous and lymphatic spread are rare. Ochsner and DeBakey[12] described a 15.7 percent incidence equally divided between pulmonary consolidation or abscess, bronchopleural fistula, and empyema. More recent reports give an incidence of 4 to 7 percent,[54,57] half of these presenting as bronchopleural fistula, and the rest as empyema or consolidation-pulmonary abscess.[54] Before the actual rupture of the liver abscess into the chest, signs of pleural irritation, such as effusion or atelectasis, can be detected either clinically or by x-ray examination. After rupture, the patients complain of pain located over the right lower thorax that radiates toward the shoulder, a cough (sometimes with hemoptysis or expectoration of large amounts of amebic pus if a bronchopleural fistula is present), and dyspnea. Physical signs are similar to those of pleural effusion or consolidation, usually with an elevated diaphragm.

Rupture of the amebic abscess into the peritoneal cavity may occur in as many as 7 to 11 percent of cases.[50,57] In endemic areas, the incidence may be lower; Adams and McLeod[54] report an incidence of only 1.8 percent in over 2000 cases of hepatic amebiasis. The rupture can result in either a perihepatic abscess or in diffuse peritonitis. Rupture of an amebic abscess into the pericardium has been observed in less than 2 percent of all cases of hepatic amebiasis.[54] The abscess is often located in the left lobe of the liver. The rupture into the pericardial sac can occur suddenly or gradually, and is often preceded by a pericardial effusion or a pericardial friction rub. Three modes of presentation have been observed:

1. About one-third of the patients have typical signs of an hepatic abscess followed by chest pain on the left side and midsternum and signs of pericarditis.
2. Two-thirds of the patients initially have pericardial effusion and congestive heart failure, without any suspicious liver findings; the correct diagnosis is seldom suspected in these patients.
3. Rarely, a patient presents in shock with signs of cardiac tamponade.[51,54]

The diagnosis of amebic pericarditis is based on clinical, electrocardiographic, and radiologic evidence of pericarditis, positive serology, and an elevated diaphragm on the left side. In addition, a defect in the left lobe of the liver can be seen on hepatic imaging.

Secondary bacterial infection, which had been previously quoted to be present in 10 to 20 percent of amebic abscesses,[56] is rarely encountered today.[54] If organisms other than amebae are found, open drainage of the abscess is mandatory. Other rare complications of hepatic amebiasis are the rupture of the abscess into the adjacent gastrointestinal tract, hematobilia and thoracobilia, and metastatic brain abscesses.[50,54,59]

LABORATORY EVALUATION. Patients with hepatic amebiasis usually have moderate leukocytosis (white blood cell count of 16,000 cells/mm^3 with increased band forms), eosinophilia, and mild microcytic anemia. The patients have liver dysfunction, as indicated by moderately elevated bilirubin and liver enzyme levels, decreased albumin, and prolonged prothrombin time. Severe liver dysfunction and jaundice, although rare, can be the initial presentation. DasGupta[60] found that the IgG levels in intestinal amebiasis are significantly higher than in the extraintestinal form. The IgE levels are elevated equally in both forms of the disease, and the IgA and IgM levels do not show any changes. The C3 levels are elevated in invasive amebiasis.

Amebae cannot regularly be found in the stool of patients with hepatic amebiasis, but Ochsner and DeBakey[50] recovered either trophoids or cysts in 36.4 percent. More recent reports show between 7 and 26 percent recovery of amebae from stool.[54,55,61] Healy[62] stressed that in more chronic cases the stool should be examined repeatedly for parasites. The direct wet mount is done to demonstrate trophoids as well as cysts. Polyvinyl alcohol preparations increase the yield in detecting the trophoids, and formalin preparations facilitate the detection of the cystic form (see Chap. 8).

Serologic tests are important in the diagnosis of hepatic amebiasis.[61–63] A summary of the accuracy of serologic tests is presented in Table 40–5.

Other diagnostic measures include the percutaneous aspiration of the abscess, which yields typical anchovy paste abscess fluid in over 80 percent of the cases. The aspirate is lacking in granulocytes and is usually sterile. Bacteria are cultured in only 4 percent, and amebae are rarely found.[55,56]

Diagnosis. Neither the physical findings nor the x-ray studies offer a definite differentiation from bacterial abscesses, either in the liver or under the diaphragm. The clinical symptoms of hepatic amebiasis are usually mild, and toxicity is rarely present. The history of diarrhea is unreliable. Because the treatments of bacterial and amebic abscesses differ considerably, it is important to make the differentiation. If one suspects an amebic abscess on the basis of clinical and radiologic findings, a reliable diagnosis can be made by serologic testing. The most frequently used test is the gel diffusion precipitin test with an accuracy of nearly 100 percent (Table 40–6). The test gradually becomes negative after cure. Diagnostic aspiration should only be necessary in exceptional cases.[64]

The absence of amebae in the stool or in the aspirated abscess material does not exclude the presence of amebiasis. In endemic areas, amebicidal drugs should be tried; the diagnosis of amebiasis can then be confirmed by the response of the patient to this treatment.

Treatment. There is general agreement that amebicidal drugs are the best treatment for hepatic amebiasis.

The essential treatment is both a systemic amebicide (metronidazole, emetine, dehydroemetine, chloroquine) and a luminal amebicide (diiodohydroxyquinoline, diloxanide furoate, tetracycline). Emetine, the classic drug to treat amebiasis, is toxic to skeletal and cardiac muscles. Dehydroemetine is similarly cardiotoxic.[65]

Chloroquine must be combined with either emetine or dehydroemetine for 100 percent cure.[66]

The drug of choice is metronidazole, which produces nearly 100 percent cure in hepatic amebiasis.[67] Side effects, such as nausea, vomiting, drowsiness, headaches, skin rashes, and pruritus, as well as moderate leukopenia are minimal and transient. One effective regimen is metronidazole 750 mg three times a day for 5 to 10 days plus the luminal amebicide didoxanide furoate, 500 mg three times daily for 10 days. Other nitroimidazoles (for example tinidazole) are also highly effective.[68] The doses of these drugs as well as other drugs are noted in Table 8–20.

The effectiveness of metronidazole on intestinal amebiasis is not as constant as on hepatic amebiasis. Approximately 15 to 20 percent of the patients continue to pass cysts and must be treated with a luminal amebicide, such as diiodohydroxyquin.

TABLE 40–6. SEROLOGIC TESTS FOR AMEBIASIS

	Percent Positive Reaction[a]		
Result	*CF*	*IHA*	*GDP*
No amebiasis	0–6	0.6–18	0–18
Noninvasive intestinal amebiasis	11–90	0–90	1–85
Invasive intestinal amebiasis	67–90	33–100	81–95
Hepatic amebiasis	83–100	47–100	80–100

[a] CF, complement fixation test; IHA, indirect hemagglutination test; GDP, gel-diffusion-precipitin test.

Adapted from Juniper K Jr, Worrell CL, Minshew MC, et al: Am J Trop Med Hyg 21:156, 1972.

Although hepatic amebiasis can be cured by the oral administration of metronidazole alone,[61,69] some authors feel that the hepatic abscess should still be aspirated. Powell et al[67] had no treatment failures when they combined metronidazole with aspiration, and Freeman[70] observed a faster clinical recovery and a radiologic resolution of the abscess when he used aspiration in addition to antiamebicides.[70] In our opinion, aspiration should be used selectively. Indications are failure to respond to medical management within 5 days, large left lobe abscesses (greater propensity for intrapericardial rupture), and suspected bacterial superinfection. The only indication for drainage of amebic liver abscess is proven bacterial super-infection.[71] The aspiration must be repeated when more than 150 ml of pus are aspirated the first time.

The thoracic complications of amebiasis are generally treated without operation. The hepatic abscess should be aspirated, and the patient should receive amebicidal drugs. An empyema should also be aspirated. Surgical intervention is rarely necessary for a persistent empyema or a pulmonary abscess that does not respond to conservative therapy. Bronchopleural fistulas always heal under medical treatment.

Laparotomy for drainage purposes, as well as establishment of the diagnosis, is always indicated in suspected intraperitoneal rupture of an amebic abscess and is supplemented by treatment with amebicidal drugs. The treatment of amebic pericarditis consists of antiamebic drugs plus pericardial aspiration.

Prognosis. No patient with uncomplicated hepatic amebic abscesses should die. Ochsner and DeBakey[50] reported no deaths, and Adams and McLeod[54] reported a mortality rate of 0.7 percent in 1959 uncomplicated cases. The presence of complications, however, changes this favorable picture dramatically. Pulmonary complications carry a mortality of 6.2 percent. Amebic peritonitis secondary to hepatic abscess rupture has a mortality of 18.4 percent, which is more favorable than amebic peritonitis secondary to the intestinal perforations, which uniformly involves bacterial superinfection.[54] The most serious complication is the rupture of the abscess into the pericardium, which has a mortality of 30 to 100 percent.[54] Secondary infection converts the amebic abscess to a pyogenic abscess of the liver, with the typical mortality of around 20 percent. Taking all possible complications into account, approximately 2 percent of all patients with hepatic amebiasis will die.

Hydatid Cyst of the Liver

Incidence. Echinococcal disease is rare in the United States. Katz and Pan[72] collected only 556 cases; of those the infestation of only 24 had occurred near the United States. In other countries, however, especially those bordering the Mediterranean Sea, infestation with *Echinococcus* is common. The largest endemic area in North America is Alaska, where an estimated 22 percent of all dogs are infested. In northwestern Canada, approximately 40 percent of the indigenous human population is infested.

Etiology. The details of echinococcal disease are given in Chapter 8. In brief, people can be infested with larvae of two species of *Echinococcus: E. granulosus* and *E. multilocularis.* The tapeworm is only a few millimeters in length and usually has four segments. It lives in the small bowel of canines, mainly dogs, wolves, and foxes. The terminal segment contains eggs, which are discharged into the intestinal contents of the host. The eggs reach the intermediate host by fecal contamination of food, fingers, or water. The capsule of the ova is dissolved in the stomach and the larvae hatch from the ova in the small intestine, penetrate through the intestinal mucosa, and are carried with the portal circulation to the liver where they develop the cyst. The intermediate hosts for *E. granulosus* are sheep, cattle, hogs, and humans. The intermediate hosts for *E. multilocularis* are small silvan rodents. Because small wild canines feed on these animals, this variety of *Echinococcus* is found mainly in foxes.

Pathology. Infestation with *E. granulosus,* which accounts for over 80 percent of all human infestations, results in a large single cyst. The cyst wall has two layers, an outer layer of adventitia that represents the host's reaction to the parasite, and an inner layer, the laminated membrane, which contains the growing organism. The cyst fluid is clear and colorless and is often under considerable pressure. Cysts tend to grow slowly, therefore a person might be infested as a child and be asymptomatic until adulthood.

Infestation with *E. multilocularis* results in the development of multiple small cysts replacing large segments of liver parenchyma. The liver is involved in three-fourths of the cases, and in half of the cases the liver is the only organ affected. Other organs frequently involved are lung (10 percent), spleen (3 percent), and kidney (4 percent), as well as musculature, bone, bladder, pleura, breast, brain, and other structures. As is usually the case in enteric-derived liver disease, the cyst is located in the right lobe in 75 percent of the cases, and can reach a gigantic size.[73]

Clinical Manifestations and Diagnosis. The most common signs and symptoms of hydatic cysts are abdominal fullness, epigastric pain, hepatomegaly, fever, and jaundice.[73-75] X-ray studies reveal typical calcifications in the cyst wall, and the liver scan shows a filling defect (Fig. 40–6). Ultrasonography and CT scan, which are the diagnostic tools of choice, show in most cases a simple cyst with a density of the cyst contents near that of water. However, occasionally sepations within the cyst, or cysts within the cyst, or signs of collapsed germinal center can be demonstrated (see Fig. 40–6). The sensitivity of plain abdominal x-ray studies is 68 percent, of radio nucleate scans 67 percent, of ultrasonography 95 percent, and of CT scan 93 percent.[73] The rarer form of *Echinococcus alveolaris* results in a rather poorly defined lesion with a density lower than normal liver parenchyma but higher than water. Angiographic studies by Rizk et al[76] demonstrated a small rim of increased density surrounding the cyst during the capillary phase. Because the relationship of the biliary system to the cyst is important for the planning of the surgical management,[77] preoperative retrograde cholangiography should be considered.[78] Laboratory results frequently show elevation of liver function test (bilirubin in 20 percent, alkaline phosphatase in 27 percent, transaminases in 41 percent), elevated white blood cell count (37 percent), and eosinophilia (45 percent).[75] Immunologic tests can confirm the diagnosis. The Casoni test consists of an intradermal injection of hydatid cyst fluid, and the development of a large weal surrounding the site of injection is a positive reaction. This test is positive in 60 to 70 percent of the cases and will always be positive even if the cyst has been removed or is inactive. The complement-fixation test is somewhat more specific but less sensitive, and is positive in only 50 to 60 percent of the cases. Recently an IHA test has been developed that shows a sensitivity of 86.7 percent, whereas a simultaneously conducted complement-fixation test has a sensitivity of only 63 percent.[79] The diagnosis is established by combining the results of immunologic, radiologic, and ultrasonographic investigations. A diagnostic puncture of the cyst is not necessary and is dangerous.

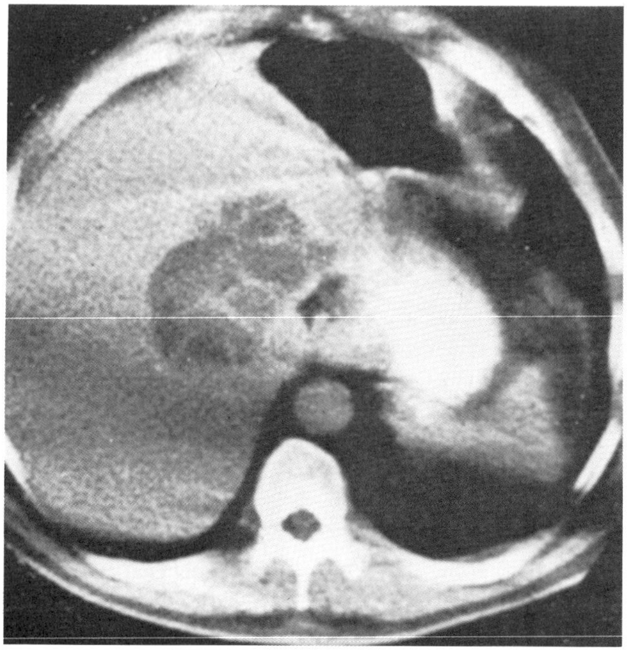

Figure 40–6. Hydatid cyst. Internal septations within the main cyst represent the wall of daughter cysts. *(From Stephens DH, Sheedy PR II: The liver. In Haaga JR, Alfidi RJ (eds): Computed Tomography of the Abdomen. St Louis, Mosby, 1985.)*

COMPLICATIONS. The most common complication of hydatid cysts of the liver is the rupture into the biliary tree. Papadimitriou and Mandrekas[80] described this complication in 6.2 percent of 227 cases, and other authors report even higher incidences. According to Bourgeon and Pietri,[81] a rupture of the cyst into the biliary tree occurs in two phases. In the first phase, minute communications between the cyst and the biliary duct are created by abrupt increased pressure within the cyst during trauma, deep inspiration, or cough. Because the pressure in the echinococcal cyst is higher than in the bile ducts, the contents of the cyst leak into the biliary system. The second phase—the rupture of the cyst into the biliary tree—is caused by weakening of the wall of the bile ducts through areas of recurrent cholangitis caused by the parasite.[81] The classic symptoms of this complication include biliary colic and jaundice, as fragments of the parasite are passed through the biliary tree into the bowel. Other signs and symptoms include spiking fever, enlargement of the liver, allergic reaction manifested by a rash, and high eosinophil count. Rarely, an anaphylactic reaction can occur. If a communication between the hydatid cyst and the biliary tree is suspected, a retrograde cholangiogram can help find the exact location and size of the fistula.[78] The treatment is directed at elimination of the parasitic cyst and internal drainage of the biliary fistula.

The next most common complication (2 percent) is rupture of the cyst through the diaphragm into the pleural space or the bronchial tree. Cysts in the dome of the right lobe of the liver are relatively common,[27,82,83] and the hepatopleural or hepatobronchial fistulas occur slowly with no dramatic symptoms in some of these. Fistulas between cysts and the bronchus result in productive cough, sometimes with bile-stained sputum. Parasites can be found in the sputum. The sudden rupture of the hydatid cyst into the pleural cavity, although uncommon, is accompanied by severe right-sided chest pain that radiates into the shoulder. An x-ray study of the chest will show a pleural effusion on the right, or a consolidation of the right base as well as an elevated and immobile diaphragm.

Rupture of the hydatid cyst into the peritoneal cavity is rather rare. Barros[77] describes only one instance of spontaneous intraperitoneal rupture in 124 cases of hydatid cyst of the liver, and Papadimitriou and Mandrekas[80] describe an incidence of 3.5 percent. Rupture of the cyst and spillage of its contents into the peritoneal cavity, however, is not so rare during operation. Schiller[84] reported 30 cases of spillage of hydatid cyst contents into the abdominal cavity, an incidence of 13.5 percent. In nine of these cases, signs of anaphylaxis were present; two of the patients died of anaphylactic shock and four others died of septic complications.

The last complication is that of superinfection of the cyst which, according to Papadimitriou and Mandrekas,[80] occurs in 7.8 percent of these patients. In those cases, the parasites are frequently destroyed by the bacterial infection, which should be treated like a pyogenic hepatic abscess.

Treatment. Treatment of hydatid disease with abendazole or mebendazole has been reported in patients infected with *Echinococcus granulosus* and multilocularis who were either inoperable or refused surgery. The dose of mebendazole was 50 mg/kg/day for 1 month followed by a period of 2 months without treatment. In most patients the disease process could be arrested. However, progression was noted again in one-third of the patients after therapy was stopped.[85–87] Chemotherapy should therefore be reserved for patients who have either unresectable disease secondary to *E. multilocularis* or spillage of cyst content into the peritoneal cavity during operation or as an adjuvant to surgery in patients with *Echinococcus multilocularis.*[86,88]

The treatment in other cases is purely surgical. Operation should be undertaken as soon as the cyst is diagnosed, because the mortality increases significantly when complications develop. The aim of operation is to remove the entire parasitic cyst (Fig. 40–7). During operation, any spillage of the cyst fluid might infect the entire peritoneal cavity. The operative field is therefore walled off with packs, and the cyst fluid is evacuated by aspiration. A solution designed to kill the parasite is then instilled into the cyst. Two percent formalin has been used in the past, although fatalities with this treatment have been reported.[77] The preferred solutions are 30 percent saline[90,91] or providone-iodine.[89] The adventitia of the cyst is then incised, and the laminated membrane is removed. The laminated membrane containing the parasites must be removed meticulously to prevent relapses. If a fibrous capsule is present, this should be resected to reduce the size of the cyst.[90] A small cyst can usually be closed primarily; however, several methods have been proposed to deal with the resulting space of a large cyst. Harris[91] and Ekrami[90] recommend filling the

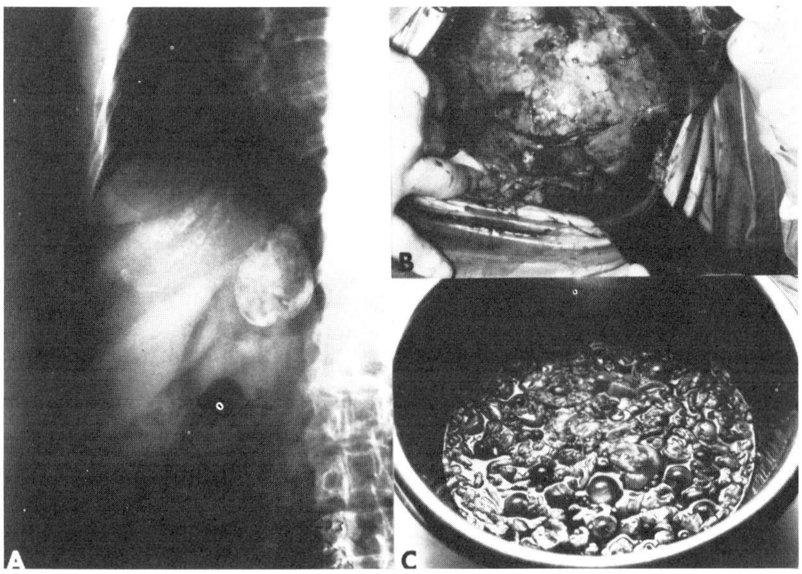

Figure 40–7. Hydatid cyst of liver. **A.** Calcified cyst on plain film of the abdomen. **B.** Gross pathology seen during en bloc excision. **C.** Daughter cysts after en bloc excision of hydatid. *(Courtesy of Basil Golematis, MD, Athens, Greece.)*

entire cyst with water and closing the capsula tightly with a continuous suture. Barros[77] and Papadimitriou and Mandrekas[80] recommend filling the empty space with omentrum. Marsupialization to the outside and drainage have been used, although this technique frequently resulted in persistent biliary fistulas. Papadimitriou and Mandrekas[80] reported bile leaks in 25 percent of marsupialized cases and 61 percent after drainage. With omentoplasty this complication occurred in only 2.5 percent. Recently, low mortality (2.5 percent) and low recurrence rates (9 percent) were reported with high vacuum suction drainage of the residual cyst without the routine use of an omentoplasty.[73] While resecting the laminated membrane, it is important to detect small bile leaks, which must be oversewn. The communication of a large bile duct with the cyst requires internal drainage of the cyst with a Roux-en-Y cyst–jejunostomy to prevent postoperative leakage of bile.[80] The importance of total or subtotal pericystectomy as opposed to less radical procedures (capitonage, partial pericystectomy) is stressed in two recent papers. With more radical surgery, the mortality remained low (2 percent) and the morbidity acceptable (18 percent). The recurrence rate was 6 percent.[92,93] Liver resection is necessary in all cases of *E. multilocularis* and in 15 percent of patients infested with *E. unilocularis.*[93] Orthotopic liver transplantation for otherwise inoperable *E. alveolaris* has been reported in 17 patients with an actuarial survival of 75 percent at 15 months.[94]

Yacoubian[83] and Barros[77] recommend a transthoracic approach for removal of cysts that extend into the thorax, whereas Reventos et al[82] prefer an abdominal approach. If a fistula into the pleural cavity has developed, the pleura has to be cleaned and drained, the diaphragm closed, and the cyst treated as previously described. In case of rupture into the bronchial tree, a segmental resection of the lung may be required.

In treating peritoneal spillage, either spontaneous or operative, thorough cleansing of the peritoneal cavity is mandatory to diminish the number of parasites seeded in the abdomen. Secondary cysts have formed in 50 percent of the patients who were evaluated for prolonged periods after intraperitoneal seeding.[84] Recently, the percutaneous puncture of the cyst under ultrasonographic or CT guidance, aspiration of the content, and installation of hypertonic saline has been used in the treatment of hydatid disease. After the procedure, progressive decrease in the size of the cyst could be observed.[95–97] In a series of 120 patients who were not considered surgical candidates, the procedure was successful in 70 percent of the cases with a recurrence rate of under 5 percent with a follow-up time of up to 36 months.[97] The role of this procedure in the treatment of hydatid disease remains to be determined.

Prognosis. The mortality for removal of an echinococcal cyst is approximately 3.5 percent.[80] When the thorax is involved or intraperitoneal seeding occurs, however, this number increases to 20 percent.[84] Complications of cyst removal include external bile fistulas, which are observed in 2.5 to 3.8 percent, contamination of the peritoneal cavity, intraperitoneal abscesses, and wound infection. The multilocular hydatid disease caused by *E. multilocularis* is a slowly progressive disease and resection can be palliative but is rarely curative.[86]

Infectious Complications of Liver Trauma and Hepatectomy

Infectious complications after liver resection or liver trauma are common. Three recent series report an incidence of septic complications from 15 to 19 percent of patients with liver trauma.[98–100] Although approximately half of the infectious complications in each group were superficial wound infections, severe intraperitoneal infections appear in 10 to 15 percent of all cases.[101–104] Intra-abdominal sepsis in approximately two-thirds of the cases was perihepatic abscess formation. Diffuse peritonitis and intrahepatic abscesses, as well as abscesses remote from the liver, were less common. The likelihood of postoperative infections is, of course, increased with the degree of hepatic injury. Fischer et al[101] noted intraperitoneal sepsis in only 1 percent of the patients with nonbursting liver injuries and 19.6 percent in patients with bursting injuries. In addition to class IV injuries, the use of liver packs and the transfusion requirements seemed to be associated with an increased abscess rate.[102–104] While Bender et al[102] found that other intra-abdominal injuries also resulted in an increased likelihood of abscess formation, Scott et al[104] stated that only transfusion requirements statistically significantly influence the rate of abscess formation.

These septic complications contribute significantly to the mortality of liver injuries. Lim et al[105] describe a series of 681 patients with trauma of the liver, 71 of whom died soon after initial treatment (most commonly of hemorrhage), and 29 patients who died late in the course of their hospitalization (41 percent of septic complications).

Important pathogenic factors for the development of those infections are thought to be presence of blood, bile, and necrotic tissue in the right upper quadrant, all of which are known to be potent adjuvants in the development of intraperitoneal infections.[106,107] The risk of infection is, of course, increased if there is continuous hemorrhage, a bile leak or biliary obstruction. Similar complications have been observed after elective hepatic resections, although their frequency is somewhat lower.

Some guiding principles have emerged with regard to the prophylaxis of these complications. The preoperative administration of antibiotics is effective in reducing the incidence of infectious complications. Stone and Tester[108] have shown that the preoperative administration of a cephalosporin lowers the incidence of infectious complication after laparotomy for trauma, including injuries of the liver. In addition, all researchers have agreed that (1) nonbleeding lacerations should not be sutured; (2) all devitalized tissue should be removed;[105] and (3) hemostatic agents, such as Gelfoam and Surgicell, should not be left in the wound, because they seem to increase the risk of postoperative infection.[99] A major controversy in infection prophylaxis centers around the question of drainage. Prophylactic drainage of the biliary tree was once advocated in order to decompress the biliary system and thereby avoid the development of a biliary fistula. Lucas and Walt[109] have shown that drainage does not lower the incidence of complications but was, instead, detrimental. Nevertheless, endoscopic decompression of the biliary system with a transpapillary catheter or a sphincterotomy has occasionally been useful in the treatment of persistent biliary fistulas.

The recommendation to drain all liver wounds goes back to Madding et al[110] in 1946 and is still advocated by many.[99,105,111] The purpose of these drains is to evacuate blood, bile, and serum, which inevitably escape the cut or damaged surface of the liver. The theoretical disadvantages are the facts that foreign bodies are adjuvants for infection and that exteriorized drains permit the ingress of microbes. Moreover, most drains incompletely evacuate the cavity so that major bile leaks are inadequately drained by any means. More recently, the problem of drainage after surgery for hepatic trauma has been addressed in several prospective and retrospective studies. In a prospective study of 56 patients who were randomly assigned to closed drainage or no drainage after liver injury, Gilmore and co-workers[111] did not find any difference in the rate of intra-abdominal abscesses (closed drain 4.2 percent, no drain 3.1 percent). A study by Fabian and co-workers[103] yielded similar results. The incidence of perihepatic abscesses in 482 with liver injuries who were randomized to no drainage, closed suction drainage, and sump drainage were 6.7 percent, 3.5 percent, and 13 percent, respectively.[103] In summary, it seems that liver injuries should be drained selectively by closed drainage and that sump drainage should be avoided.

Infections After Liver Transplantation

The systemic opportunistic infections that occur in immunodepressed hosts, including recipients of organ transplants, are discussed in Chapters 9 and 47. Orthotopic liver transplantation has, in addition, a number of infectious complications peculiar to the operation. Almost all are related to technical complications. These problems have been described by many authors.[112]

Most life-threatening infections in liver transplant patients are bacterial and fungal infections of the abdomen. The fungal infections usually occur after bacterial infections are treated with antibiotics and in patients who have undergone prolonged or repeated abdominal operations, that is, those who have surgical complications—bile leaks, vascular anastomotic problems, or hemorrhage. Patients with liver failure requiring transplant are nutritionally depleted, immunosuppressed by steroids or their preexisting disease, and have clotting disorders.

Technical problems that predispose to intra-abdominal infections include thrombosis of the hepatic artery or its branches. Characteristically, this results in multiple ischemic areas within the liver, which subsequently become infected; almost all enteric organisms (gram-positive, gram-negative, aerobes, anaerobes) are found. Hepatic artery thrombosis is best treated by retransplantation if infection supervenes. Some liver abscesses can be drained percutaneously or via open techniques.

Cholangitis most often results from technical problems as well. Biliary stricture of the choledochocholedochostomy or the choledochojejunostomy may require dilation or reconstruction (if stricture occurs relatively late in the course), but bile leaks from anastomotic breakdown are a relatively common cause of intra-abdominal sepsis. Cholangitis and indeed all biliary problems associated with decreased liver function are often confused with rejection, cytomegalovirus (CMV) hepatitis, or other infections including adenovirus, herpes simplex virus (HSV) hepatitis, or distant infections. Liver biopsy with careful culture may be necessary to make the distinction. Access to the biliary tract via a T-tube permits significant obstruction to be ruled out by cholangiography. As in cholangitis associated with biliary surgery, a polymicrobial is most common with enteric aerobes and anaerobes.

Peritonitis results from perforation of a viscus—perforated diverticulitis, peptic ulcer, or ischemic necrosis. Bile leaks from around T-tubes or after removal of a T-tube often become infected during the procedures to repair the leak or reconstruct the biliary tree. Additional abscesses without new perforation occur in areas of pancreatitis, fluid, ascites, or hematoma more often than after other intra-abdominal operations.[113,114]

Bacteremia most often arises from intra-abdominal infections, but infected urinary tract, pneumonia, and infected intravenous lines are also sites. In the presence of empiric broad spectrum antibiotics used as prophylaxis in most of these patients, the common aerobic enteric pathogens (*E. coli, Klebsiella, B. fragilis*) are in the minority; enterococci, *Enterobacter, Pseudomonas, S. epidermidis,* and *Candida* predominate.[115,116]

The problems induced by CMV infection in transplant patients have been detailed in Chapters 11 and 51. Primary CMV derived from donor tissue or transfusion is the most important single infection after transplantation of any organ. CMV hepatitis in the donor organ is rare in other organ transplants but common after liver transplantation. CMV duodenitis or colitis can result in perforation or massive hemorrhage.

Recurrent hepatitis after liver transplantation for hepatitis B and C is a common problem. Patients who display HBAg prior to transplant almost inevitably develop clinical recurrence at some time (months to years) after the transplant, despite use of hepatitis B immunoglobulin, IFN-α, or other prophylaxis. Patients with HB$_e$Ag usually develop active hepatitis promptly after the transplant. Hepatitis C also frequently recurs but may take several years to develop.

INFECTIONS OF THE SPLEEN

Many infections can involve the spleen and represent systemic infections that affect the reticuloendothelial system. Few are of special interest to the surgeon. Some of these infections will, on rare occasions, produce sufficient hypersplenism to indicate splenectomy, and others, most notably infectious mononucleosis, will cause such splenic hypertrophy that rupture (either spontaneous or after mild trauma) will occur, requiring operative control.

Splenic Abscess

Incidence and Pathogenesis. Splenic abscesses are rare today. Between 1964 and 1978, Chulay and Lankerani[117] found only 10 cases in 94,460 hospital admissions (0.01 percent), and the incidence in 2840 autopsy reports was 0.22 percent. Up to 1990 less than 250 patients with splenic abscesses have been reported in the literature.[118] Eighty percent of splenic abscesses occur in conjunction with systemic infections[119]: otitis, mastoiditis, peritonsillar, abscess, suppurative parotitis, cutaneous infection, pulmonary abscesses, appendicitis, diverticulitis, cholecystitis, and osteomyelitis. Prior to the antibiotic era, splenic suppuration was found in 10 percent of all cases with bacterial endocarditis, and the incidence of splenic abscess was tripled in patients with typhoid fever compared with the normal population. Today the entity is most commonly seen in immunocompromised patients and drug addicts.[120–123]

The work of Caldarera[124] sheds some light on the pathogenesis of splenic abscesses. Splenic abscesses could not be produced with an injection of *S. aureus* in experimental animals unless a branch of the splenic artery had been previously ligated or the spleen itself traumatized. Thus, it is not surprising that splenic abscesses are more frequent in patients with hemolytic disorders whose spleens undergo repeated infarction. Three-quarters of patients with splenic abscesses in Nigeria suffer from sickle cell disease.[125] The incidence is also increased with thalassemia, malaria, and leukemia.

Fifteen percent of splenic abscesses follow splenic trauma and have also been seen as complications of splenic salvage. With the advent of splenic embolization in the treatment of hypersplenism, cases of development of splenic abscess have been described after this procedure.[126,127]

Etiology. Table 40–7 lists the organisms most often found in splenic abscesses. As expected, staphylococci, streptococci, salmonellae, and other gram-negative bacteria predominate. Recently, a change in flora has been noted with an increase in the enteric and anaerobic bacteria as well as sterile cultures. *Salmonella* species have nearly disappeared, and the incidence of streptococci has declined. If splenic abscesses complicate an infectious endocarditis, however, it is nearly always caused by streptococci or staphylococci.[128] In drug addicts, splenic abscesses are nearly exclusively caused by *S. aureus.*[125] Johnson and Raff[129] have recently col-

TABLE 40–7. BACTERIOLOGY OF SPLENIC ABSCESSES (PERCENT)

Staphylococci	21
Streptococci	16
Salmonellae	15
Escherichia coli	8
Other gram-negative bacilli	17
Anaerobic organisms	5
Others	1
Sterile cultures	24

From Chulay JD, Lankerani MR: Am J Med 61:513, 1976.

lected 19 patients with fungal splenic abscesses, most of whom were immunosuppressed. The most common causative agents were *Candida* species and *Aspergillus*. Tuberculous splenic abscesses in AIDS patients have also been described. They respond rapidly to antituberculous therapy.[130]

Clinical Manifestations. Fever is present in nearly all patients, along with other symptoms of systemic sepsis: chills, malaise, nausea, and vomiting. Two-thirds of the patients have abdominal pain, which is often sharp and radiates into the left shoulder and the left thorax; however, localization to the splenic area is only present in one-half the patients. One-third of the patients have a palpable spleen, and often an abdominal mass can be felt in the epigastrium or left upper quadrant. Laboratory test results reveal a leukocytosis with a shift to the left, and plain x-ray films show a mass in the left upper quadrant, extraluminal gas, and elevated left diaphragm with pleural effusion (Fig. 40–8). Although a liver-spleen scan is helpful in establishing the diagnosis, splenic abscess can be confirmed more quickly and easily with either ultrasonography or CT (Fig. 40–9).[131,132] The lesion usually presents as an irregular area with decreased echogenicity on ultrasound and low density on CT scan, and does not enhance with injection of contrast material.[133]

Treatment and Prognosis. The procedure of choice in splenic abscesses has traditionally been splenectomy accompanied by distal pancreatectomy if the abscess was closely adherent to the tail of the pancreas.[117,119] Lately, however, some new treatment options for splenic abscesses have been considered. A few children have had successful treatment with antibiotics alone,[134,135] but most surgeons feel that those abscesses should either be drained or removed. Successful partial splenectomy[136] and more

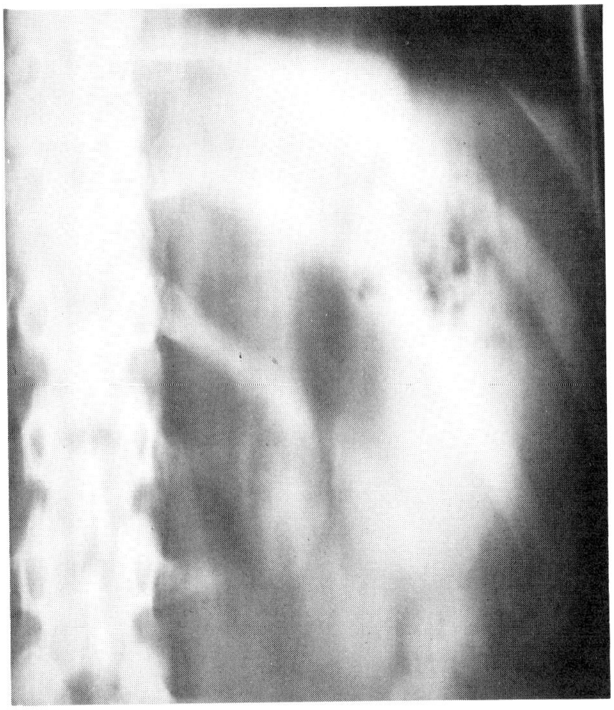

Figure 40–8. Gas formation in the spleen after splenic embolization on tomograms of the RUQ. The patient had a splenic abscess due to Klebsiella. *(Courtesy of D. Spigos, MD, Department of Radiology, University of Illinois Medical Center, Chicago.)*

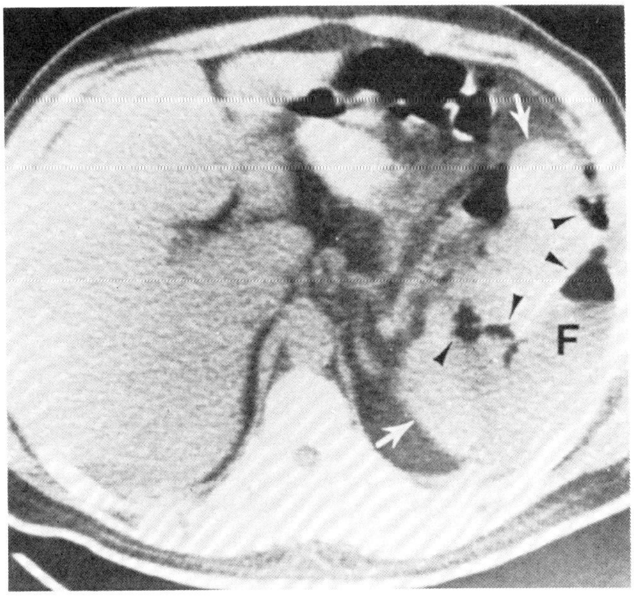

Figure 40–9. Splenic abscess secondary to *Salmonella* infection contains fluid (F), collection of gas (L), and splenic fragments (L). *(From Breiman RS, Korobkin M: The spleen. In Haaga JR, Alfidi RJ (eds): Computed Tomography of the Abdomen. St Louis, Mosby, 1985.)*

often percutaneous drainage have been used. Gleich and co-workers[137] have collected 30 cases of abscess from the literature; percutaneous drainage was successful in 24. They state that while single lesions with a discrete wall and without internal separation lend themselves to percutaneous drainage, multiloculated or complex splenic abscesses should be treated by splenectomy.[137] If serious underlying disease is not present, all patients can be cured.[117] If, however, the diagnosis is not made in time and the splenectomy is delayed, rupture into the peritoneal cavity can occur and nearly always causes death. In ten cases described by Chulay and Lankerani,[117] delay in diagnosis and appropriate therapy was responsible for the death of three of ten patients.

Rupture of the Spleen in Infectious Disease

Rupture of the spleen in association with infectious disease has long been recognized. The most common cause is infectious mononucleosis. However, only 14 percent of the reported cases fit rigid criteria of spontaneous rupture, and most are caused by trauma to an enlarged friable spleen.[135] Other infectious diseases that can cause a spontaneous rupture of the spleen are malaria,[138] endocarditis,[139] viral hepatitis,[140] and actinomycosis.[141] Rupture of the spleen is usually preceded by the development of upper abdominal pain. At the time of actual rupture, an acute abdomen, with shock, develops. Sokolowski and Kent[142] described certain x-ray features that might assist the diagnosis; these include distention of the stomach with a serrated margin of the greater curvature, downward displacement of the gastric cardia, and displacement of the stomach to the right from extrinsic pressure. There is also a downward displacement of the splenic flexure of the colon and elevation and decreased mobility of the left diaphragm.[142] In general, immediate splenectomy is recommended; however, organ-preserving surgery with hemostasis by means of fibrin glue has been described.[143] If a splenic rupture is diagnosed immediately, there should be no deaths caused by the rupture itself. The long-time prognosis is the same as it is for the underlying disease.

Infectious Complications After Splenectomy

The risk of infection after splenectomy is twofold. First, local infections can develop in the postoperative period, and second, splenectomized patients seem to succumb more often to fulminant sepsis with encapsulated bacteria.

Local Infections. Local infectious complications occur in approximately 16 percent of all patients who undergo splenectomy. One-third of those are subphrenic abscesses, the remainder are subcutaneous wound infections.[144] Patients who undergo splenectomy for trauma or for hypersplenism associated with leukemia and other generalized disease have the highest incidence of suppurative infections.[145] Septic complications after splenectomy are especially common when the splenectomy is associated with peritoneal contamination by intestinal contents and in the case of splenectomy for trauma in patients with associated injuries of the pancreas, colon, nervous system, and extremity fractures.[146] Incidental splenectomy during intra-abdominal procedure increases the incidence of an intra-abdominal abscess from 0 to 10.5 percent.[146]

The pathogenesis of subphrenic abscesses after splenectomy is similar to that of the development of perihepatic abscesses after liver trauma and liver resection. Necrotic tissue, blood, and sometimes pancreatic juice from the contused pancreas accumulate in the left upper quadrant and function as adjuvants for a bacterial infection. Good hemostasis, operative evacuation of all fluid, and avoidance of pancreatic trauma will minimize the chances of develoment of septic complications after splenectomy.

The proper use of drains remains controversial. Several authors feel that the drainage of the subphrenic space after splenectomy significantly increases the incidence of the development of postoperative septic complications. Although all available studies are retrospective, clinical observation together with experimental evidence would lead one to avoid drainage of the splenic bed after splenectomy. In a retrospective study, Cohn[119] found intra-abdominal septic complications in 40 percent of the patients in whom drainage of the splenic bed had been carried out; the incidence of septic complications was only 4 percent without drainage. Olson and Beaudoin[147] observed ten subphrenic abscesses and ten infections of the drainage tract in 228 patients who underwent splenectomy with drainage. In 87 patients who did not undergo splenic drainage, only one subphrenic abscess was found.[147] Experimental evidence suggests that bacteria can migrate from the skin surface along the drain tract into the abdominal cavity. Nora et al[148] obtained positive cultures in 34 percent of intra-abdominal drains inserted in a previously sterile area. If drains are to be used, closed suction with soft silastic drains should be employed for as short a period as possible, preferably 24 hours. If drainage after splenectomy is considered necessary it should be done with a closed drainage system, as a closed drainage system is less likely to lead to abscess formation.[149] In general damage to the pancreas that would lead to a pancreatic fistula should be drained, even if the spleen is preserved or repaired after trauma.

Overwhelming Sepsis

Incidence. There is a relatively high incidence of fulminant infections after splenectomy, especially after splenectomy in childhood. Evidence also supports an increased incidence even in otherwise healthy adults.

Singer[150] first reviewed 2795 splenectomy patients and found an incidence of lethal, overwhelming sepsis in 2.5 percent. Similar results have been obtained by Eraklis and Filler,[151] who found an incidence of lethal overwhelming infections in 2.4 percent of patients who underwent splenectomy in childhood. The highest incidence is observed in patients with underlying hematologic or malignant diseases. Splenectomy secondary to trauma or incidental during operative procedures carries a rather low risk of the development of lethal postsplenectomy fulminant sepsis, 0.53 and 0.86 percent, respectively.[152] Though uncommon, the incidence is substantially higher than in similar healthy persons with intact spleens. Indeed, Gopal and Bisno[153] have recently collected 26 patients without underlying disease who developed fulminant pneumococcal sepsis after splenectomy of an injured spleen for an otherwise normal patient. Fifteen of these patients were adults, and none of them was under 7 years of age when the splenectomy was performed. More World War II veterans who had been splenectomized for trauma died from pneumonia and ischemic heart disease than did members of a nonsplenectomized control group.[154] Sekikawa and Shafney[152] found six cases of severe bacterial infection after splenectomy in 242 patients and Malangoni and co-workers[145] found 3 cases in 140 patients; none of these infections resulted in the death of the patient.

Etiology. Approximately half of all cases of overwhelming postsplenectomy infections are caused by pneumococci; mortality is 50 percent. *Neisseria meningitidis, E. coli, Hemophilus influenzae,* and *S. aureus* are found in decreasing frequency.

Pathology. At autopsy, the observations are typical of septicemia but also include adrenal hemorrhage in a high proportion of cases (Waterhouse-Friderichsen syndrome).

Pathogenesis. Several lines of evidence suggest that splenectomized patients have compromised humoral defenses; both immunoglobulin and complement deficiencies have been reported.[155] Numerous defects in immunoglobulins have been reported after splenectomy. Antibody responses to intravenously administered particulate antigens and bacteriophage are reduced. Asplenic individuals have an inability to switch from IgM to IgG antibody.[156] The influence of splenectomy on IgM levels is controversial. Although some authors found a significant decrease of IgM levels after splenectomy for hematologic disease, as well as for trauma,[157] others found this phenomenon only when the spleen was removed for hematologic reasons but not after splenectomy for trauma in an otherwise healthy person.

IgG and IgA immunoglobulins are frequently elevated in healthy and splenectomized patients, and no reliable data on IgD or IgE levels has been gathered.

The IgM deficiency in splenectomized patients does not completely explain the failure to eradicate circulating bacteria. Host defense in most bacteria requires opsonization either by antibody (usually IgG) or by complement. Opsonized bacteria can be cleared by the spleen, and less effectively by the liver. In the absence of opsonins, however, pneumococci are nearly exclusively cleared by the spleen.[158] Pneumococci obviously are best opsonized by specific antibody, but can be opsonized by complement activated by the alternative pathway. In this regard, properdin activity, an alternate complement pathway factor, is reduced in asplenic patients,[157] but this depression is not universal. Several investigators have been unable to show diminished serum opsonic activity after vaccination with a pneumococcal vaccine.[157] Finally, the spleen produces tuftsin, a polypeptide that promotes phagocytosis, and serum levels of this substance are significantly decreased after splenectomy.[159]

Splenectomy also influences the numbers of lymphocytes. Circulating T lymphocytes are somewhat reduced following splenectomy; the lymphocyte mitogen proliferative response is initially decreased, but then returns to normal.[160] Polymorphonuclear leukocyte functions and C3 levels are not changed in asplenic patients. In short, although there are numerous defects of the immune response after splenectomy, none of them totally explains the failure to appropriately eliminate circulating encapsulated organisms. It is probable that the filtering effect of the spleen itself is important in eliminating these organisms and that the liver is far less efficient than the spleen in this regard.

Clinical Manifestations. Overwhelming postsplenectomy infection is characterized by the sudden onset of nausea, vomiting, and confusion, which leads to coma, and often proceeds to death within hours. The case fatality rate ranges from 50 to 75 percent.[157] There is frequently evidence of disseminated intravascular coagulation, severe hypoglycemia, electrolyte imbalance, and shock.

Prevention. Penicillin prophylaxis has effectively reduced the incidence of pneumococcal sepsis after splenectomy. Penicillin should be continually administered for life. Unfortunately, compliance with daily penicillin ingestion is expected to decrease with time, so it is important to educate the patient to the risks after splenectomy.

Pneumococcal vaccination can now be carried out. The present commercially available vaccine contains the capsular polysaccharides of 23 pneumococcal serotypes. These 23 types out of 82 known account for more than 80 percent of the serious pneumococcal infections encountered in people. Because the polysaccharides are highly purified, few side effects of vaccination are seen. The vaccine has an aggregate efficiency of 60 to 70 percent in preventing infection.[134] All asplenic individuals should be vaccinated. The antibody response of splenectomized patients is apparently normal when each antigen is used alone. Giebink (personal communication) has noted that patients splenectomized for trauma respond to fewer of the antigens in the polyvalent vaccines. In addition, the titer of pneumococcal antibody decreases over time and reverts to prevaccination levels in less than 6 months. Whether boosters can be used is unknown. In addition, several patients who were previously vaccinated died of overwhelming pneumococcal sepsis after splenectomy. Even though pneumococcal vaccination cannot be relied upon, it should be used in all patients, in addition to daily penicillin prophylaxis. The realization that splenectomy leads to overwhelming bacterial sepsis has lead to the development of more conservative forms of management of splenic trauma during the last ten years.[161] In children conservative treatment of splenic trauma has been advocated. Clinical surveillance can be carried out in an intensive care setting when vital signs, abdominal findings, and hematocrit are stable and if no greater blood replacement is required.[160,162] Most children and all adults, however, should still undergo exploratory laparotomy. Splenic salvage in these cases is only indicated if there are no associated injuries present, the patient is stable, and the splenorrhaphy can be performed without undue blood loss. In general, this will be possible in approximately one-half of the patients with a range from 8 to 10 percent. When complex procedures, such as partial resection, are required, the complication rate, especially postoperative bleeding and subphrenic abscess, are rather high. Considering the fact that the incidence of overwhelming sepsis after splenectomy for trauma is low, it can be further reduced by either polyvalent pneumococcal vaccine or antibiotic prophylaxis. Clinical and experimental evidence supports the idea that preservation of the spleen by hemostasis, splenorrhaphy, or partial splenectomy can protect the host from pneumococcal sepsis. However, no such evidence exists for autotransplantation of splenic tissue.[163]

REFERENCES

Liver

1. Beeson PB, Brannon ES, Warren JV: Observations on the sites of removal of bacteria from the blood in patients with bacterial endocarditis. J Exp Med 81:9, 1945.
2. Orloff MJ, Peskin GW, Ellis HL: A bacteriologic study of human portal blood: implications regarding hepatic ischemia in man. Ann Surg 148:738, 1958.
3. Schweinburg FB, Sylvester EM: Bacteriology of the healthy experimental animal. Proc Soc Exp Biol Med 82:527, 1953.
4. Romieu C, Brunschwig A: Bacteriologic study of the human liver. Surgery 30:621, 1951.
5. Sborov VH, Morse WC, Giges B, Jahnke EJ: Bacteriology of the human liver. J Clin Invest 31:986, 1952.
6. Klatskin G: Hepatitis associated with systemic infections. In Schiff L (ed): Diseases of the Liver, 4th ed. Philadelphia, Lippincott, 1975.
7. Berg BN, Zau ZD, Jobling JW: Bactericidal function of the liver. Proc Soc Exp Biol Med 24:433, 1926.
8. Weinstein L: Bacterial hepatitis: A case report on an unrecognized cause of fever of unknown origin. N Engl J Med 299:1052, 1978.
9. Mitchell SC: Hepatobiliary manifestations of the acquired immune deficiency syndrome. Am J Gastroenterol 86:1, 1991.

Bacterial Abscess of the Liver

10. Baerensprung C: Der Leberabscess nach Kopfverletzungen. Arch Klin Chir 18:586, 1975.
11. Collins AN: Abscess of the liver. Minn Med 15:756, 1932.
12. Ochsner A, DeBakey M: Pleuropulmonary complications of amebiasis: an analysis of 153 collected and 15 personal cases. J Thorac Surg 5:225, 1936.
13. Knowles R, Rinaldo JA: Pyogenic hepatic abscess secondary to sigmoid diverticulitis. Gastroenterology 38:262, 1960.

14. Ribaudo JM, Ochsner A: Intrahepatic abscess: amebic and pyogenic. Am J Surg 125:570, 1973.
15. Ochsner A, DeBakey M, Murray S: Pyogenic abscess of the liver. II. An analysis of forty-seven cases with review of the literature. Am J Surg 40:292, 1938.
16. Block MA, Schuman BM, Eyler WR, et al: Surgery of liver abscess. Arch Surg 88:602, 1964.
17. Brodine WN, Schwartz SL: Pyogenic hepatic abscess. NY State J Med 73:1657, 1973.
18. Sabbaj J, Sutter VL, Finegold SM: Anaerobic pyogenic liver abscess. Ann Intern Med 77:629, 1972.
19. Onderdonk A, Bartlett J, Louis T, et al: Microbial synergism in experimental intraabdominal abscess. Infect Immun 13:22, 1976.
20. Finegold SM: Anaerobic Bacteria in Human Disease. New York, Harcourt, 1989.
21. Robertson RD, Foster JH, Peterson CG: Pyogenic liver abscess studies by cholangiography: case report and 25-year review. Am Surg 32:521, 1966.
22. Trump DL, Fahnenstock HM, Cloutier CT, Dickman MD: Anaerobic abscess and intrahepatic metastases: a case report and review of the literature. Cancer 41:682, 1978.
23. Jochimsen PR, Zinke WL, Shirazi SS, Pearlman NW: Iatrogenic liver abscess. Arch Surg 113:141, 1978.
24. Matthews JB, Gertsch P, Baer HU, Blumgart LH: Hepatic abscess after biliary tract procedures. Surg Gynecol Obstet 170:469, 1990.
25. Crippin JS, Kenneth KW: An unrecognized etiology for pyogenic hepatic abscesses in normal hosts: dental disease. Am J Gastroenterol 7:1740, 1992.
26. Lee JF, Block GE: The changing clinical pattern of hepatic abscesses. Arch Surg 104:465, 1972.
27. Altemeier WA, Schowengerdt CG, Whitely DH: Abscess of the liver: surgical considerations. Arch Surg 101:258, 1970.
28. Kinney TD, Ferrebee JW: Hepatic abscess: factors determining its localization. Arch Pathol 45:41, 1948.
29. Sérégé H: Contribution á létude de la circulation du sang fort dans le foie et des localisation lobaires hépatiques. J Med Bord 31:208, 217, 291, 312, 1901.
30. Satiani B, Davidson ED: Hepatic abscess: improvement in mortality with early diagnosis and treatment. Am J Surg 135:647, 1978.
31. Gerzof SG, Johnson WC, Robbins AH, Nabseth DC: Intrahepatic pyogenic abscesses: treatment by percutaneous drainage. Am J Surg 149:487, 1985.
32. McDonald MI, Corey GR, Gallis HA, Durack DT: Single and multiple pyogenic liver abscesses. Medicine (Baltimore) 63:291, 1984.
33. Neoptolemos JP, Macpherson DS, Holm J, Fossard DP: Pyogenic liver abscess: a study of forty-four cases in two centres. Acta Chir Scand 148:415, 1982.
34. McFadzcan JS, Chang KPS, Wong CC: Solitary pyogenic abscess of the liver treated by closed aspiration and antibiotics. Br J Surg 41:141, 1953.
35. Kuligowska E, Connors SK, Shapiro JH: Liver abscess. Sonography in diagnosis and treatment. AJR 138:253, 1982.
36. Halvorsen RA, Korobkin M, Foster WL, et al: The variable CT appearance of hepatic abscesses. AJR 142:941, 1984.
37. Hau T, Haaga JR, Aeder MI: Pathophysiology, diagnosis and treatment of abdominal abscesses. Curr Probl Surg 21(7):1, 1984.
38. Schwerk WB, Görg C, Görg K, et al: Perkutane Drainagen von Leber- und Milzabszessen. Z Gastroenterol 29:146, 1991.
39. Gain T, Lorenz R, Classen M: Sonographische Perkutane Drainage von Leberabszessen. Med Klin 85:577, 1990.
40. Thakur ML, Coleman RE, Welch MJ: Indium-111-labeled leukocytes for the localization of abscesses: preparation, analysis, tissue distribution, and comparison with gallium-67 citrate in dogs. J Lab Clin Med 89:217, 1977.
41. Adatepe MH, Welch M, Evens RG, Potchen EJ: Clinical application of the broad-spectrum scanning agent—indium-113m. Am J Roentgenol Radiother Nucl Med 112:701, 1971.
42. Hau T, Nishikawa R, Danziger LH: Antibiotics in surgery. Surg Annu 15:177, 1983.
43. Berger LA, Osborne DR: Treatment of pyogenic liver abscesses by percutaneous needle aspiration. Lancet XX:132, 1982.
44. Herbert DA, Rothman J, Simmons F, et al: Pyogenic liver abscesses: successful nonsurgical therapy. Lancet 1:134, 1982.
45. Donovan AJ, Yellin AE, Ralls PW: Hepatic abscess. World J Surg 15:162, 1991.
46. Robert JH, Mirescu D, Ambrosetti P, et al: Critical review of the treatment of pyogenic hepatic abscess. Surg Gynecol Obstet 174:97, 1992.
47. Stain SC, Yellin AE, Donovan AJ, Brien HW: Pyogenic liver abscess. Arch Surg 126:991, 1991.
48. Wong KP: Percutaneous drainage of pyogenic liver abscesses. World J Surg 14:492, 1990.
49. Lee KT, Sheen PC, Chen JS, Ker CG: Pyogenic liver abscess: multivariate analysis of risk factors. World J Surg 15:372, 1991.

Amebic Abscess of the Liver

50. Ochsner A, DeBakey M: Amebic hepatitis and hepatic abscess: an analysis of 181 cases with review of the literature. Surgery 13:460, 1943.
51. Adams EB: Amoebic pericarditis. Med S Afr 17:1013, 1974.
52. Maegraith GB, Harinasut AC: Experimental amoebic infection of the liver in guinea pigs: infection via the mesenteric vein and via the portal vein. Ann Trop Med 48:421, 1954.
53. Ravi VV, Tandon HD, Tandon BN: Morphological changes in the liver in hepatic amoebiasis. Indian J Med Res 62:1832, 1974.
54. Adams EB, McLeod IN: Invasive amebiasis. II. Amebic liver abscess and its complications. Medicine (Baltimore) 56:325, 1977.

55. Turrill FL, Burnham JR: Hepatic amebiasis. Am J Surg 111:424, 1966.
56. DeBakey ME, Ochsner A: Hepatic amebiasis: a 20-year experience and analysis of 263 cases. Surg Gynecol Obstet 92:209, 1951.
57. Crane PS, Lee YT, Seel DJ: Experience in the treatment of 200 patients with amebic abscess of the liver in Korea. Am J Surg 123:332, 1972.
58. Geslien GE, Thrall JH, Johnson MC: Gallium scanning in acute hepatic amebic abscess. J Nucl Med 15:561, 1974.
59. Amir-Jahed AK, Sadrieh M, Fappour A, et al: Thoracolbilia: a surgical complication of hepatic echinococcosis and amebiasis. Ann Thorac Surg 14:198, 1972.
60. DasGupta A: Immunoglobulin in health and disease. III. Immunoglobulin in the sera of patients with amoebiasis. Clin Exp Immunol 86:163, 1974.
61. Shabot JM, Patterson M: Amebic liver abscess: 1966–1976. Dig Dis 21:110, 1978.
62. Healy GR: The laboratory diagnosis of amebiasis. Am J Gastroenterol 42:191, 1964.
63. Juniper K Jr, Worrell CL, Minshew MC, et al: Serologic diagnosis of amebiasis. Am J Trop Med Hyg 21:156, 1972.
64. Maltz G, Knauer M: Amebic liver abscess: a 15-year experience. Am J Gastroenterol 86:704, 1991.
65. Wilmot AJ, Powell SJ, Adams EB: The comparative value of emetine and chloroquine in amebic liver abscess. Am J Trop Med Hyg 7:197, 1958.
66. Wilmot AJ, Powell SJ, McLeod IN, Elsdon-Dew R: The treatment of amoebic liver abscess with dehydroemetine. In: Proceedings of Third International Congress on Chemotherapy. Stuttgart, Georg Thieme, 1964.
67. Powell SJ, Wilmot AJ, Elsdon-Dew R: Further trials of metronidazole in amoebic dysentery and amoebic liver abscess. Ann Trop Med Parasitol 61:511, 1967.
68. Scragg JN, Proctor EM: Tinidazole in treatment of amebic liver abscess in children. Arch Dis Child 52:408, 1977.
69. Van Allan RJ, Katz MD, Johnson MB, et al: Uncomplicated amebic liver abscess: prospective evaluation of percutaneous therapeutic aspiration. Radiology 183:827, 1992.
70. Freeman O, Akamaguna A, Jarikre LN: Amebic liver abscess: the effect of aspiration on the resolution or healing time. Ann Trop Med Parasitol 84(3):281, 1990.
71. Abuabara S, Barrett J, Hau T, Jonasson O: Amebic liver abscess. Arch Surg. 117:239, 1982.

Hydatid Cyst of the Liver

72. Katz AM, Pan L-T: Echinococcus disease in the United States. Am J Med 25:759, 1958.
73. Karavias DD, Vagianos CE, Bouboulis N, et al: Improved techniques in the surgical treatment of hepatic hydatidosis. Surgery 174:176, 1992.
74. Bilge A, Sözüer EM: Diagnosis and surgical treatment of hepatic hydatid disease. HPB Surg 6:57, 1992.
75. Xynos E, Pechlivanides G, Anastasios T, Papageorgiou A: Hydatid disease of the liver. Diagnosis and surgical treatment. HPB Surg 4:59, 1991.
76. Rizk GK, Tayyarah KH, Ghabdur-Mnaymneh L: The angiographic changes in hydatid cyst of the liver and spleen. Diagn Radiol 99:303, 1971.
77. Barros JL: Hydatid cyst of the liver. Am J Surg 135:597, 1978.
78. Cottone M, Amuso M, Cotton PB: Endoscopic retrograde cholangiography in hepatic hydatid disease. Br J Surg 65:107, 1978.
79. Chematai AK, Bowry TR, Ahman Z: Evaluation of five immunodiagnostic techniques in echinococcosis patients. Bull WHO 59:767, 1982.
80. Papadimitriou J, Mandrekas A: The surgical treatment of hydatid disease of the liver. Br J Surg 57:431, 1970.
81. Bourgeon R, Pietri H: L'ouverture de kystes hydatiques du foie dans les voies biliaires. Sixième Congres International de l'hydatidose. Athènes 16:193, 1956.
82. Reventos J, Nogueras FM, Rius X, Lorenzo T: Hydatid disease of the liver with thoracic involvement. Surg Gynecol Obstet 143:570, 1976.
83. Yacoubian HD: Thoracic problems associated with hydatid cyst of the dome of the liver. Surgery 79:544, 1976.
84. Schiller CR: Complications of *Echinococcus* cyst rupture. JAMA 195:220, 1966.
85. Beard TC, Richard MD, Goodman HT: Medical treatment for hydatids. Med J Aust 1:366, 1978.
86. Ammann RW, Hirsbrunner R, Cotting J, et al: Recurrence rate after discontinuation of long-term mebendazole therapy in alveolar echinococcosis (preliminary results). Am J Trop Med Hyg 43(5):506, 1990.
87. Rippmann K, Dietrich M, Kern P: Langzeittherapie der zystischen Leberechinokokkose mit Mebendazol. Med Klin 87:350, 1992.
88. Morris DL, Dykes PW, Marriner S, et al: Albendazole-objective evidence of response in human hydatid disease. JAMA 253:2053, 1985.
89. Golematis B: Hydatid disease: History, etiology, epidemiology, epizootiology, locations, and prevention. Surg Annu 10:359, 1978.
90. Ekrami Y: Surgical treatment of hydatid disease of the liver. Arch Surg 111:1350, 1976.
91. Harris JD: Rupture of hydatid cysts of the liver into the biliary tracts. Br J Surg 52:210, 1965.
92. González EM, Selas PR, Martinez B, et al: Results of surgical treatment of hepatic hydatidosis: current therapeutic modifications. World J Surg 15:254, 1991.
93. Magistrelli P, Masetti R, Coppola R, et al: Surgical treatment of hydatid disease of the liver. Arch Surg 126:518, 1991.
94. Bresson-Hadni S, Franza A, Miguet JP, et al: Orthotopic liver transplantation for incurable alveolar

echinococcosis of the liver: report of 17 cases. Hepatology 13(6):1061, 1991.
95. Acunas B, Rozanes I, Celik L, et al: Purely cystic hydatid disease of the liver: treatment with percutaneous aspiration and injection of hypertonic saline. Radiology 182:541, 1992.
96. Giorgio A, Tarantino L, Francica G, et al: Unilocular hydatid liver cysts: treatment with US-guided, double percutaneous aspiration and alcohol injection. Radiology 184:705, 1992.
97. Gargouri M, Ben Amor N, Ben Chehida F, et al: Liver cysts and abscesses: percutaneous treatment of hydatid cysts (*Echinococcus granulosus*). Cardiovasc Intervent Radiol 13:169, 1990.

Infectious Complications of Liver Trauma and Hepatectomy

98. Brotman S, Oliver G, Oster-Granite ML, Cowley RA: The treatment of 179 blunt trauma-induced liver injuries in a statewide trauma center. Am Surg 50:603, 1984.
99. McClelland RN, Shires T: Management of liver trauma in 259 consecutive patients. Ann Surg 161:248, 1965.
100. Stone HH, Ansley JD: Management of liver trauma in children. J Pediatr Surg 12:3, 1977.
101. Fischer RP, O'Farrell KO, Perry JF: The value of peritoneal drains in the treatment of liver injuries. J Trauma 18:393, 1978.
102. Bender JS, Geller ER, Wilson RF: Intra-abdominal sepsis following liver trauma. J Trauma 29(8):1140, 1989.
103. Fabian TC, Croce MA, Stanford GG, et al: Factors affecting morbidity following hepatic trauma. Ann Surg 213(6):540, 1991.
104. Scott CM, Grasberger RC, Heeran TF, et al: Intraabdominal sepsis after hepatic trauma. Am J Surg 155:284, 1988.
105. Lim RC, Lau G, Steele M: Prevention of complications after liver trauma. Am J Surg 132:156, 1976.
106. Hau T, Hoffman R, Simmons RL: Mechanisms of the adjuvant effect of hemoglobin in experimental peritonitis. I. In vivo inhibition of peritoneal leukocytosis. Surgery 83:233, 1978.
107. Schneierson SS, Amsterdam D, Perlman E: Enhancement of intraperitoneal staphylococcal virulence for mice with different bile salts. Nature 190:829, 1961.
108. Stone HH, Tester TR Jr: Incisional and peritoneal infections after emergency celiotomy. Ann Surg 117:669, 1973.
109. Lucas CE, Walt AJ: Analysis of randomized biliary drainage in hepatic trauma in 189 patients. J Trauma 12:925, 1972.
110. Madding GF, Lawrence KG, Kennedy PA: War wound of the liver. Tex State J Med 42:267, 1946.
111. Gilmore D, MsSwain NE, Browder IW: Hepatic trauma: to drain or not to drain? J Trauma 27(8):898, 1987.
112. Ho M, Dummer JS, Peterson PK, Simmons RL: Infections in solid organ transplant recipients. In Mandell GL, Douglas RG, Bennett JE (eds): Principles and Practices of Infectious Disease, 3rd ed. New York, Churchill Livingstone, 1990, p 2294.
113. Bilik R, Yellin M, Superina RA: Surgical complications in children after liver transplantation. J Pediatr Surg 27:1371, 1992.
114. George DL, Arnow PM, Fox AS, et al: Bacterial infection as a complication of liver transplantation: epidemiology and risk factors. Rev Infect Dis 13:387, 1991.
115. Kusne S, Dummer JS, Ho M, et al: Infections after liver transplantation. Medicine (Baltimore) 67:132, 1988.
116. Wood RP, Rosenlof LK, Shaw BW Jr, et al: Complications requiring operative intervention after orthotopic liver transplantation. Am J Surg 156:513, 1988.

Splenic Abscess

117. Chulay JD, Lankerani MR: Splenic abscess: report of 10 cases and review of the literature. Am J Med 61:513, 1976.
118. Cohen MAA, Galera MJ, Ruiz M, et al: Splenic abscess. World J Surg 14:513, 1990.
119. Cohn LH: Local infections after splenectomy. Arch Surg 90:320, 1965.
120. Fry DE, Richardson JD, Flint LM: Occult splenic abscess: an unrecognized complication of heroin abuse. Surgery 84:650, 1978.
121. Gaslowitz PL, Labs JD, Fishman EK, Siegelman SS: The changing spectrum of splenic abscess. Clin Imaging 13:201, 1989.
122. Helton WS, Carrico J, Zaveruha PA, Schaller R: Diagnosis and treatment of splenic fungal abscesses in the immune-suppressed patient. Arch Surg 121:580, 1986.
123. Nallathambi MN, Ivatury RR, Lankin DH, Stahl WM: Pyogenic splenic abscess in intravenous drug addiction. Am Surgeon 53(6):342, 1987.
124. Caldarera E: Acute abscess of the spleen. Surg Gynecol Obstet 67 (Suppl):265, 1938.
125. Anand SW, Davey WW: Surgery of the spleen in Nigeria. Br J Surg 52:335, 1965.
126. Spigos DG, Jonasson O, Felix E, Capek V: Transcatheter therapeutic embolization of hypersplenum. Invest Radiol 12:418, 1977.
127. Shah HR, Cué JI, Boyd CM, Cone JB: Solitary splenic abscess: a new complication of splenic salvage treated by percutaneous drainage. J Trauma 27(3):337, 1987.
128. Johnson JD, Raff MJ, Barnwell PA, Chun CH: Splenic abscess complication infections endocarditis. Arch Intern Med 143:906, 1983.
129. Johnson JD, Raff MJ: Fungal splenic abscess. Intern Med 144:1987, 1984.
130. Wolff MJ, Bitran J, Northland RG, Levy IL: Splenic abscesses due to *Mycobacterium tuberculosis* in patients with AIDS. Review Infect Dis 13:373, 1991.

131. Ralls PW, Quinn MF, Colletti P, et al: Sonography of pyogenic splenic abscess. AJR 138:523, 1982.
132. Baruch Y, Levy Y, Brooke JG, et al: Splenic abscess diagnosed with the aid of abdominal computerized tomography: report of two cases. Br J Med 68:137, 1981.
133. Breiman RS, Kokobin M: The spleen. In Haaga JR, Alfidi RJ (eds): Computed Tomography of the Abdomen. St Louis, Mosby, 1985.
134. Fernandes ET, Tavares PB, Garcette CBM: Conservative management of splenic abscesses in children. J Pediatr Surg 27(12):1578, 1992.
135. Bhattacharyya N, Ablin DS, Kosloske AM: Stapled partial splenectomy for splenic abscess in a child. J Pediatr Surg 24(3):316, 1989.
136. Gleich S, Wolin DA, Herbsman H: A review of percutaneous drainage in splenic abscesses. Surg Gynecol Obstet 167:211, 1987.

Rupture of the Spleen in Infectious Disease

137. Rutkow IM: Rupture of the spleen in infectious mononucleosis. Arch Surg 113:718, 1978.
138. Davis R: Spontaneous rupture of the pathalogical spleen in malaria. S Afr Med J 47:1801, 1973.
139. Gonin A, Berthou JD, Roques JC, Dufoix V: Rupture spontanée de la rate: manifestation révèlatrice d'une endocardite infectieuse. Nouv Press Méd 2:1306, 1973.
140. Wood LJ: Pathologic aspects of acute epidemic hepatitis. Arch Pathol 41:345, 1946.
141. Sperling RL, Heredia R, Gillesby WJ, Chomet B: Rupture of the spleen secondary to actinomycosis. Arch Surg 94:344, 1967.
142. Sokolowski JW, Kent DC: Spontaneous rupture of the spleen in infectious mononucleosis: value of roentgenography. NY State J Med 68:1172, 1968.
143. Ormann W, Hopf G: Spontane Milzruptur bei infektiöser Mononucleose—Organerhaltende Operation mittels Fibrinklebung. Langenbecks Arch Chir 373:240, 1988.

Infectious Complications After Splenectomy

144. Hodam RP: The risk of splenectomy: a review of 310 cases. Am J Surg 119:709, 1970.
145. Malangoni MA, Dillon LD, Klamer TW, Condon RE: Factors influencing the risk of early and late serious infection in adults after splenectomy for trauma. Surgery 96:775, 1984.
146. Kassum D, Thomas EJ: Morbidity and mortality of incidental splenectomy. Can J Surg 20:209, 1977.
147. Olson WR, Beaudoin DE: Wound drainage after splenectomy: indications and complications. Am J Surg 117:615, 1969.
148. Nora PF, Vanecuo RM, Bransfield JJ: Prophylactic abdominal drains. Arch Surg 105:173, 1972.
149. Patchen HL, Hofstetter SR, Spencer FC: Evolving concepts of splenic surgery: splenography versus splenectomy and splenectomy drainage. Experience in 105 patients. Ann Surg 105:173, 1972.
150. Singer DB: Postsplenectomy sepsis. In Rosenberg AS, Bolande RP (eds): Perspective in Pediatric Pathology, Vol I. Chicago, Year Book Medical Publishers, 1973.
151. Eraklis AJ, Filler RM: Splenectomy in childhood: a review of 1413 cases. J Pediatr Surg 7:382, 1972.
152. Sekikawa T, Shafney C: Septic sequelae after splenectomy for trauma in adults. Am J Surg 145:667, 1983.
153. Gopal V, Bisno AL: Fulminant pneumococcal infections in "normal" asplenic hosts. Arch Intern Med 137:1526, 1977.
154. Robinette CD, Fraumeni JF: Splenectomy and subsequent mortality in the veterans of the 1939–45 war. Lancet 2:127, 1977.
155. Krivit W, Giebink GS, Leonard A: Overwhelming postsplenectomy infection. Surg Clin North Am 59:223, 1979.
156. Sullivan JL, Ochs HD, Schiffmann G, et al: Immune response after splenectomy. Lancet 1:178, 1978.
157. Krivit W: Overwhelming post-splenectomy infection. Am J Hematol 2:193, 1977.
158. Schulkind ML, Ellis EF, Smith RT: Effect of antibody upon clearance of I-125-labelled pneumococci by the spleen and liver. Pediatr Res 1:178, 1967.
159. Constantopoulus A, Najjar VA, Wish JB, et al: Defective phagocytosis due to tuftsin deficiency in splenectomized subjects. Am J Dis Child 125:663, 1973.
160. Amsbaugh DF, Prescott B, Baker PJ: Effect of splenectomy on the expression of regulatory T cell activity. J Immunol 121:1483, 1978.
161. Morgenstern L: The avoidable complications of splenectomy. Surg Gynecol Obstet 145:525, 1977.
162. Sherman NJ, Asch MD: Conservative surgery for splenic injuries. Pediatrics 61:267, 1978.
163. Perry JF Jr: Injuries of the spleen. Curr Probl Surg 12:753, 1988.

BIBLIOGRAPHY

Adams EB, McLeod IN: Invasive amebiasis. Am J Surg 111:424, 1966.

Branum GD, Tyson GS, Branum MA, Meyers WC: Hepatic abscess. Ann Surg 212(6):655, 1989.

Golematis B: Hydatid disease: history, etiology, epidemiology, epizootiology, locations, and prevention. Surg Annu 10:359, 1978.

Kapoor OP: Amoebic Liver Abscess. Bombay, India, SS Publishers, 1979.

Klatskin G: Hepatitis associated with systemic infections. In Schiff L (ed): Diseases of the Liver, 4th ed. Philadelphia, Lippincott, 1975.

Perry JF Jr: Injuries of the spleen. Curr Probl Surg 12:753, 1988.

Infections of the Pancreas

CHAPTER 41

Ernst Klar, Andrew L. Warshaw

PATHOGENESIS

Infections of the pancreas are of two types. Acute pancreatitis may be an incidental part of systemic infections such as mumps, viral hepatitis, coxsackievirus, and mycoplasma infections. The pancreas develops edema, which most often subsides uneventfully. Similar hematogenous infection of the pancreas by opportunistic infections (mainly cytomegalovirus, *Cryptococcus neoformans,* and mycobacteria) occurs as part of the human immunodeficiency virus (HIV) syndrome and other immunosuppressed states.[1] The second category of pancreatic infections—the focus of this chapter—occurs through secondary infection of established tissue injury after noninfectious pancreatitis. Viable pancreatic tissue is highly resistant to infection, but necrotic tissue is highly susceptible. The chain of events leading to pancreatic necrosis is incompletely understood, but both enzymatic digestion and ischemia seem to be contributing factors. Necrosis of pancreatic and peripancreatic tissues develops in about 15 percent of cases of acute pancreatitis, gallstones, and alcoholism representing the causative factors in 85% of these.[2] Infection occurs in 1 to 9 percent of all patients with pancreatitis.[3,4]

Ectopic intrapancreatic protease activation with resultant autodigestion of the acinar cell is generally believed to be the central pathogenetic mechanism of early acute pancreatitis. Activation of trypsinogen by cleavage to trypsin is probably the key enzymatic event and initiates the autodigestive cascade resulting in activation of other zymogens.[5] Experimental models confirm the appearance of trypsinogen activation peptides (cleavage products of trypsinogen) in plasma, urine, and ascites. The magnitude of these trypsinogen cleavage products correlates with acinar necrosis and other measures of severity, including death.[6]

Experimental models produced by hyperstimulation with the cholecystokinin (CCK)-analog cerulein have also given insights into the earliest origins of the process. An abnormality of processing of intracellular enzymes has been described in which lysosomal enzymes localize with zymogen granules into "autophagic" granules. Such colocalization promotes the intracellular activation of trypsinogen by the lysosomal enzymes, principally cathepsin B.[7] Alternatively, fusion of zymogen granules and abnormal secretion of proteases into the interstitial spaces by basolateral exocytosis have also been described.[8–10] However, it remains unclear why these processes, which have been described in several experimental models, have no correlation with the severity of the pancreatitis,[11] and why in fact the result may be only interstitial or edematous pancreatitis with a predominant picture of single-cell necrosis, which is totally repaired by acinar cell regeneration.[9] Recent evidence suggests that the next critical stage may be the activation of the proteases after discharge into the interstitial space.[10,12] The mechanism of that activation, and why it may or may not occur and thereby convert mild edematous into severe necrotizing pancreatitis, is unknown.

A large body of evidence has accumulated that pancreatic ischemia also plays a critical role in the transition of edematous pancreatitis to necrosis. Quantitation of pancreatic microcirculation by intravital microscopy in the rabbit has shown homogeneous and increased perfusion in edematous pancreatitis as opposed to a progressive reduction of capillary blood flow in necrotizing pancreatitis.[13,14] Parallel changes have been demonstrated in the oxygenation of pancreatic tissues in edematous compared to necrotizing pancreatitis.[15] The severity of cerulein-induced pancreatitis can be increased by reduction of pancreatic capillary perfusion with intravenous vasoconstricting catecholamines.[16,17]

Bacterial infection may occur soon after the necrotizing process. Studies with needle aspiration of pancreatic inflammatory masses show positive bacterial aspirates late in the first week after onset in 20 percent of patients selected for testing.[18] In patients who are operated on within 7 days after the onset of symptoms, bacteria can be cultured in the removed necrotic debris in 24 percent, but the incidence of contamination appears to rise thereafter and may peak in the third week at approximately 71 percent.[2] The amount of necrosis, both of pancreatic parenchyma and extrapancreatic retroperitoneal fatty tissues, correlates with the probability of developing an abscess.[2,19,20] However, infection may appear later in patients whose initial presentation appears to be disarmingly mild.[21–23]

The origin of bacterial contamination is potentially the bile duct in gallstone pancreatitis. Almost 90 percent of patients with common duct stones have positive bile cultures. In acute pancreatitis of other etiology, the source and route taken by the infecting organisms are unsettled. Hematogenous seeding,[24] lymphatic spread,[23] and transmural passage from the colon[25] have been considered. The fact that at least one enteric organism can be detected in more than two-thirds of isolates reflects the likelihood that translocation of bacteria from the gut is most important.[26,27] Shock, bowel ischemia, or inflammation may lead to an increase in permeability of the mucosal barrier.[28–30] Ryan and colleagues[31] have shown that permeability of the bowel to macromolecules is increased in proportion to the severity of experimental pancreatitis. This hypothesis is further supported by the detection of endotoxin in peripheral blood in patients with severe pancreatitis before any sign of local infection.[32,33] Pancreatic infections usually contain multiple organisms rather than a single species.[2,4,18,19,21,23] Coliforms and other enteric species predominate over staphylococci and streptococci (Table 41–1). Despite special efforts to detect them, anaerobes such as *Bacteroides* are found only rarely.[23] *Candida albicans,* found with increasing frequency, is usually recovered from patients who have been exposed to long-term antibiotic therapy and represents a complicating superinfection. There are a few reports of primary *Candida* abscesses[34] and a single report of a primary tuberculous abscess of the pancreas.[35]

In contrast to other forms of intra-abdominal abscesses, pancreatic infections may extend aggressively along tissue planes and by direct destruction of tissues, probably abetted by activated proteolytic and lipolytic enzymes. They may thus extend far beyond the pancreas, reaching up into the mediastinum or down as far as the groin.[25]

TERMINOLOGY

Because of the vast improvement of supportive care during the last two decades, death from acute pancreatitis at its early stages has become uncommon. Most patients now survive the initial phase of cardiopulmonary and circulatory dysfunction, which is due both to fluid loss from the vascular bed and to microcirculatory derangements. They live long enough for the tissue injury to evolve and for septic complications to occur. Sepsis is now the major cause of death from pancreatitis.

The products of infection after acute pancreatitis have long been summarized by the term pancre-

TABLE 41–1. MICROORGANISMS FOUND IN 45 PANCREATIC INFECTIONS

Organism	No.
Escherichia coli	22
Enterococcus	17
Staphylococcus	16
Klebsiella	6
Proteus	4
Candida albicans	3
Pseudomonas	3
Streptococcus	2
Terulopsis glubrata	1
Hemophilus parainfluenzae	1
Diphtheroids	1
Serratia marcescens	1
Negative culture (positive Gram stain for organisms on smear)	5

atic abscess, but there is now emphasis on distinguishing between different forms of pancreatic infection, which may have different clinical presentations, morbidity rates, and treatment needs. These refinements have been facilitated both by clinical observations and by improved imaging, principally through computed tomography (CT).[27,36–39] Originally championed by Beger's studies in Germany, there has been widespread acceptance of new clinical classifications and subdivisions of the postpancreatitis complications that involve infection.[40]

Pancreatic Phlegmon

Pancreatic phlegmon describes an ill-defined pancreatic or peripancreatic tissue swelling representing a combination of edema and inflammatory infiltrate. It is probably sterile initially and usually resolves spontaneously over a period of a few weeks.[25,41–43] A critically important feature of the lesion is that its outcome cannot be predicted.[42] A phlegmon can also evolve to areas of necrosis with a high risk of subsequent infection.[18] Although the use of the term has been debated because of its lack of precise meaning, others find the implied uncertainty a useful concept in that it warns to remain vigilant for deterioration.[44] There is also no other term that encompasses the woody indurated inflammatory masses that may spread to involve wide areas of the extrapancreatic retromesenteric tissues and mesenteries.

Acute Peripancreatic Fluid Collection

An acute peripancreatic fluid collection, also called an acute pseudocyst, is a collection of secretions, exudate, and perhaps blood that has accumulated around the pancreas as a result of the inflammatory process. Ultimately it may be reabsorbed or become encapsulated by granulation tissue.[25] Although relatively uncommon, infection of acute peripancreatic fluid collections is found in approximately 15 percent.[18] This entity must be distinguished from an infected pseudocyst, which has a well-formed capsule[40,45,46] and most commonly becomes infected only after invasive instrumentation such as pancreatography.

Infected Pancreatic Necrosis

This term, promoted by Beger and co-workers, connotes the principal form of postpancreatitis infection.[2,36,47,48] The infection is of the dead pancreatic and peripancreatic tissues with variable proportions of semisolid contents and pus. The clinical presentation of this entity is often fulminant and may blend imperceptibly with the initial attack of acute pancreatitis without a quiescent interval.[36,49] It is frequently lethal.

Pancreatic Abscess

Pancreatic abscess represents a collection of pus with lesser amounts of necrotic tissue within a relatively well-demarcated cavity. It may involve the pancreas and extend into surrounding structures in a multilocular fashion. It is the end result of tissue breakdown, liquefaction, and infection.[21,27] As such, a pancreatic abscess is not truly an entity distinctly different in its pathogenesis from infected necrosis, but rather a later evolution or stage.[44]

CLINICAL PRESENTATION

Fever, abdominal pain, and tenderness, either continuing after an attack of pancreatitis or reappearing after apparent resolution, are the predominant findings[2,19,21,22,27,33] (see Table 41–2). However, the symptoms and signs of pancreatic infection are by no means specific, and even fever is missing in 13 to 35 percent.[21,27] In addition, it has been noted that all the clinical features characterizing pancreatic infections may also be produced by sterile necrosis, including hyperdynamic cardiocirculatory failure.[50–52] While patients with sterile necrosis may stabilize and recover without further complication, those with infected necrosis are often characterized by a progressive deterioration and increasing generalized signs of sepsis. The local inflammatory response may be less impressive than the systemic manifestations in these patients since bacterial toxins can gain ready access to the systemic circulation from the damaged tissues. The average time between the onset of pancreatitis and operative treatment of infected necrosis has been 10 to 18 days,

TABLE 41–2. PRESENTING SYMPTOMS AND SIGNS OF PANCREATIC INFECTIONS IN 45 PATIENTS

Sign or Symptom	N	Percentage
Fever	39	87
Abdominal pain	37	82
Abdominal tenderness	28	62
Palpable mass	22	50
Nausea or vomiting	21	47
Distention	12	27
Jaundice	7	16
Systemic sepsis	3	7
Pulmonary failure	2	4
Gastrointestinal bleeding	1	2

which is 2 weeks less than is typical for pancreatic abscesses.[19–22,27,33]

DIAGNOSIS

A reliable diagnosis of infection must be confirmed by bacterial culture of the tissue in question. Blood cultures are often negative, and, even if positive, other sources of infection such as central venous lines and the urinary tract must be considered.[19,20,23] Percutaneous CT-guided thin-needle aspiration has proved to be a safe technique.[18,53] Gerzof and colleagues found that half of the phlegmons, acute pseudocysts, and solid necrosis were infected, whereas peripancreatic collections showed a much lower incidence of infection (about 15 percent).[18] Their study reported no false-positive or false-negative cultures and no contamination introduced by the needling procedure.

Although others have also reported that infection can be reliably excluded by fine-needle aspiration,[54,55] some studies have found false-negative samples in 10 percent of cases when compared with cultures taken subsequently at operation.[22,52] Needle aspiration studies of symptomatic patients have shown that 22 percent of the infections became apparent and were confirmed within 1 week after the onset of pancreatitis, and the incidence increases to 55 percent within 14 days[18] and to about 70 percent ultimately.[2,52]

The appropriate use of fine-needle aspiration for diagnosis of pancreatic infection is still debated. Because asymptomatic patients, even with necrosis evidenced by contrast-enhanced CT scanning, can often be managed without resort to surgical debridement or drainage, fine-needle aspiration would seem not to have a useful role in decisions regarding therapy in such patients. Conversely, patients who show signs of severe ongoing inflammation, sepsis, or cardiovascular instability probably require surgical intervention whether the necrotic tissues are sterile or infected.[2,51,52] In this latter situation also, needle aspirates do not alter the imperatives of treatment. We therefore reserve guided needle aspiration for those patients whose therapy, operative versus nonoperative, will be determined by the results of the test, that is, those with documented infected necrosis but without severe systemic sepsis.

Contrast-enhanced CT has become the diagnostic gold standard for evaluating the pancreas in acute pancreatitis.[56] The intravenous bolus of contrast dye results in a homogeneous enhancement of the intact normally perfused pancreas. Nonenhanced areas may indicate viable but underperfused tissues, or these may be already necrotic[38,57–59] (Fig. 41–1). Microangiographic studies in resected human specimens confirmed that defects shown by contrast-enhanced CT scan correlate with a microcirculatory injury in necrotizing pancreatitis.[60]

Considerable effort has been directed to the identification of patients at risk of developing an abscess by the use of CT scanning. A CT-scoring system, developed by Vernachia and co-workers,[61] to assess the initial severity of pancreatitis emphasized retroperitoneal spread and extrapancreatic findings, but this system failed to predict infectious complications at a later stage. In contrast, Clavien's group[62] demonstrated that the majority of patients with extensive extrapancreatic extension of the inflammatory process detected within 36 hours of admission eventually developed infection of these tissues. Balthazar and colleagues[63] were able to predict abscess formation in 60 to 80 percent in their patient population with severe pancreatitis by applying a scoring system assessing the inflammatory process and the number of fluid collections in and around the pancreas.

Conventional imaging techniques often yield radiologic abnormalities, but most are nonspecific and do not allow for a differentiation between abscess and other types of pancreatic inflammation.[21] In our previously reported series of 45 patients with pancreatic abscess, upper small bowel dilation (*sentinel loop*) was detected in 46 percent and the classical soap-bubble sign (mottled appearance of the retroperitoneum and necrotic tissues) was noted in

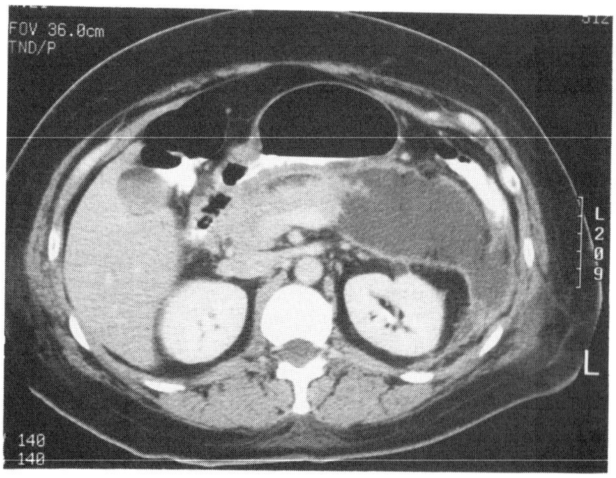

Figure 41–1. Contrast-enhanced CT scan in pancreatic necrosis. The viable, perfused head and body of the pancreas are clearly demarcated from the nonperfused necrotic tail and the fluid that permeates and surrounds it in a well-defined cavity.

only 9 percent of tissues. Gas bubbles in the fluid collection or necrotic tissues (Fig. 41–2) are usually pathognomonic for infection, but this sign is often missing.[62,64] Gas in the tissue most often indicates the presence of insoluble gases from anaerobic bacterial metabolism by either facultative or (less commonly) obligate anaerobic bacteria. On rare occasion, there may be gas detected in the pancreas due to a pancreatic-enteric fistula, rather than from an abscess.[65]

The diagnostic value of ultrasonography in acute pancreatitis is mainly limited to the detection of gallstones. Although pancreatic swelling may be demonstrated, excess bowel gas will impair the visualization of the pancreas in 30 percent of patients.

Routine laboratory tests do not allow for differentiation between infection and acute pancreatitis and a sterile process. The degree of leukocytosis may be similar in both instances and even a very high white blood cell (WBC) count does not necessarily indicate infection. In our series of 45 patients operated on because of pancreatic infection, the leukocyte count was normal in 6 cases and only moderately elevated in over 50 percent of patients, whereas the serum amylase was normal in 26 patients (Table 41–3). The Fedorak et al[27] analysis of 64 patients with secondary pancreatic infections revealed that infected necrosis was associated with a significantly higher WBC count (22,300 cells mm^3) compared to an infected pseudocyst or pancreatic abscess. In 90 percent of patients with infected necrosis, at least one sign of sepsis was recorded as compared to 70 percent with pancreatic abscess and 22 percent with infected pseudocyst. Although some interpret these findings to suggest that infected necrosis is a more virulent form of infection than others, it must still be remembered that the systemic signs of bacterial sepsis are similar to those caused by severe sterile necrosis[50–52] and the latter may be equally lethal.[52]

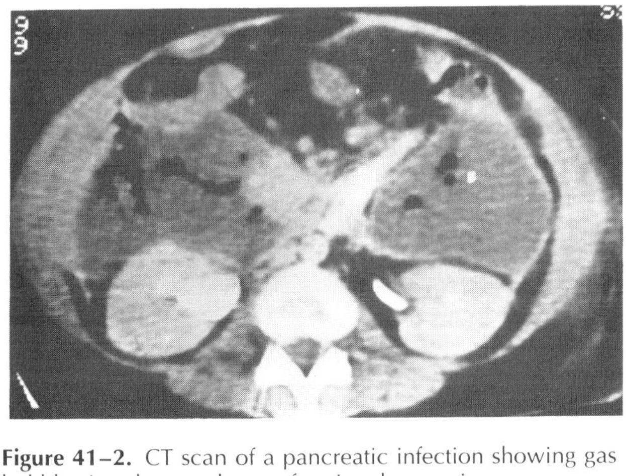

Figure 41–2. CT scan of a pancreatic infection showing gas bubbles in a large volume of regional necrosis.

TABLE 41–3. ROUTINE LABORATORY FINDINGS IN 45 PANCREATIC INFECTIONS

Finding	N
White blood cell count/mm^3	
>20,000	6
15,000–20,000	7
10,000–15,000	26
<10,000	6
Serum amylase value elevated	19
Alkaline phosphatase elevated	18
Transaminase elevated	23
Bilirubin >1.2 mg/dl	17
Calcium <8.5 mg/dl	25
Albumin <3 g/dl	20

Serum levels of C-reactive protein and phospholipase A2 have been shown to correlate well with the severity of pancreatitis and may have up to 95 percent accuracy in predicting the occurrence of pancreatic necrosis.[66–69] Alpha-2-macroglobulin and complement factors C3 and C4 are significantly elevated in only 74 to 85 percent of complicated pancreatitis and are of less diagnostic value. Most recently, trypsinogen activation peptides (TAPs) in plasma have been validated by our group as a predictor of the outcome in different pancreatitis models. There was an excellent correlation of TAP levels with both mortality and acinar necrosis[6] confirming prior clinical reports.[70] Although none of these parameters specifically indicate infection, they may be helpful in pinpointing patients with more severe necrotizing pancreatitis who are at greater risk of developing infection.

TREATMENT

The prevention of parenchymal necrosis, if possible, has to be regarded as a principal therapeutic goal in acute pancreatitis. Pancreatic ischemia has been shown to be important in the transition of edematous to necrotizing pancreatitis.[13,16,71–74] In experimental biliary pancreatitis the expected reduction of functional capillary density can be counteracted by isovolemic hemodilution with dextran 60,[75] with resultant preservation of viable pancreas.[74] The initial clinical application of this experimental concept appears to validate this strategy.[76] Very high molecular weight dextrans (500 kilodaltons) also have been shown to protect the pancreas in acute experimental pancreatitis.[77]

Based on the concept that pancreatic secretion might potentiate the inflammatory process in acute pancreatitis, the attempt to reduce pancreatic secretory activity has traditionally been part of the conservative treatment of pancreatitis. In addition to simple fasting, somatostatin and its long-acting analog octreotide have been evaluated for their action as potent inhibitors of pancreatic secretion. However, three controlled trials have shown no significant effect on the course of patients with mild or severe pancreatitis.[78–80]

It is also believed that inappropriate, uncontrolled, or ectopic activation of proteolytic enzymes within the pancreatic acinar cell or perhaps in the pancreatic interstitium plays an initiating role in the pathogenesis of pancreatitis. Nonetheless, in experimental models, protease inhibition has been effective only when administered prophylactically.[11] In a randomized, double-blind study, gabexate mesilate, a potent inhibitor of proteases and phospholipase A2, which is small enough to enter the acinar cell, was evaluated in 223 patients with severe pancreatitis.[81] No difference between the placebo and treatment group was found with regard to mortality, need for surgical treatment, or the incidence of complications despite the fact that therapy was implemented at a median of only 21 hours after the onset of symptoms. Even with still earlier treatment (about 12 hours after onset) another controlled study of gabexate mesilate also failed to demonstrate a beneficial effect.[82]

An unresolved conundrum in the medical treatment of acute pancreatitis is the use of prophylactic antibiotics. Three earlier prospective controlled trials found that prophylactic antibiotics were ineffective. However, those series comprised almost entirely mild cases of pancreatitis and used antibiotics (principally ampicillin), which are characterized by a low penetration of the pancreas and a narrow spectrum of coverage.[83–85] As noted previously in pancreatitis complicated by pancreatic and peripancreatic necrosis, there is a 40 to 70 percent risk of pancreatic infection, which can become established as early as the first week.[2,18,52,86] Because the spectrum of organisms is that of the colon, an appropriate antibiotic regimen must be broad enough to cover the usual enteric flora. The analysis of tissue samples from perinecrotic areas obtained at the time of surgical debridement revealed that imipenem, ciprofloxacin, and ofloxacin, all of which have an adequate spectrum of coverage, had reached adequate tissue concentration in the pancreas and had good tissue-to-serum ratios.[87] Metronidazole shows similar kinetics and seems to be the drug of first choice against anaerobes.[87] In an Italian multicenter trial, imipenem succeeded in reducing the rate of bacterial infection of necrotic tissues, as determined by surgical debridement and culture, but that apparent benefit did not translate into any reduction in mortality.[88] Thus the clinical impact of prophylactic antibiotic treatment in necrotizing pancreatitis still warrants further studies. No studies have evaluated the use of selective gut decontamination, which, if applied early, might be expected to reduce gut-derived contamination.

Peritoneal lavage extended for a period of 7 days results in a lower incidence of late pancreatic sepsis as compared to the conventional 2-day lavage.[89] The mechanism of action may be through interruption of the transperitoneal pathway by which bacteria reach the pancreas after translocating from the enteric lumen.

General agreement exists that infected necrosis is uniformly lethal unless treated surgically.[52] Controversy persists over the optimal treatment of sterile necrosis.[90] While some patients with sterile necrosis exhibit the same signs of inflammation and systemic instability as those with infected necrosis,[51] a "sepsis syndrome" presumably mediated by similar cytokines, others are remarkably well. The latter can safely be treated conservatively, at least until signs of deterioration press for a change. It is the unstable symptomatic patient who provokes debate. Bradley and Allen[55] treated 11 patients with pancreatic necrosis estimated by dynamic CT planigraphy to involve 38 ± 4 percent of the pancreas. Five of the 11 patients had persisting fever and leukocytosis; 4 developed respiratory failure requiring prolonged mechanical ventilation; and 2 had reversible acute renal failure. Nevertheless, after fine-needle aspiration of the necrotic areas appeared to prove a sterile process, all were treated without operation and all survived.

In contrast, in our own series of 73 patients with pancreatic necrosis, the overall mortality rate was 25 percent. There was no significant difference between the mortality rate of infected or sterile pancreatic necrosis. The only preoperative variables that did correlate with mortality were shock, an APACHE II score greater than 15, and preintervention blood transfusion requirements.[52] Similarly, Karimgani and colleagues[50] report a mortality rate of 38 percent in patients with "severe sterile necrosis" who experienced at least one systemic complication. Secondary organ failure occurred during the first 2 weeks of illness, and in their experience shock was also the best predictor of fatal outcome. Of the 16 patients with sterile necrosis who survived, 7 were surgically debrided, and the remaining 9 patients survived without surgical intervention.

It would appear that sterile necrosis has the capacity to be lethal in much the same manner as infected necrosis. It is therefore our policy to utilize nonoperative treatment as long as there is neither proven sepsis nor compeling signs suggesting sepsis. Percutaneous aspiration is performed in patients who are clearly not sick enough to require operation or so stable as to not need an operation. In these indeterminate cases, the decision for surgical intervention is based on the bacteriologic findings of the aspirate.

The role of percutaneous drainage of pancreatic infection is limited. Despite good results in the cure of intra-abdominal abscesses of other types,[91,92] pancreatic infections do not respond to percutaneous catheter techniques as well.[52,93–99] Whereas late simple abscesses may be successfully drained by catheter, definitive evacuation of infected necrosis through the catheters is hindered by the semisolid debris and solid material. In a series of 30 patients with 59 pancreatic or peripancreatic fluid collections,[94] each patient required an average of three catheter manipulations, seven abdominal CT scans, 5 weeks of catheter drainage, and a mean intensive care unit stay of 31 days. Percutaneous intervention was completely successful only in 1 of 10 central collections and 28 of 49 peripheral collections. Secondary surgical debridement was necessary in 53 percent of all patients due to failure of percutaneous drainage. These results suggest that primary percutaneous interventions of infected necrosis in patients with severe pancreatitis have a poor success rate. Catheter drainage should be limited to plain fluid collections, which develop in distant locations (pararenal space, paracolic gutters) or true abscesses, particularly those following debridement in the attempt to avoid additional operation. In addition, radiologic intervention may be beneficial as a temporary maneuver to decompress and stabilize a critically ill patient.[94]

Surgical debridement and drainage are the cornerstones of therapy for infected pancreatic necrosis and pancreatic abscess. There are basically three different techniques for the management of the patient following debridement: open packing with planned periodic relaparotomy, closed system drainage, and closed system drainage with irrigation of the cavity. Subtotal or total pancreatectomy has been dismissed by most because of the excessive mortality rate.[100,101] Beger et al[48] report an excellent mortality rate of 8.1 percent for necrosectomy and postoperative local lavage in necrotizing pancreatitis. Seventy-four patients with a mean Ranson score of 4.5 points were subjected to debridement and local lavage through two large double lumen tubes at a rate of 4 to 20 liters every 24 hours for 5 to 90 days. The median time in the intensive care unit was 6.5 days. The concept is that high-volume lesser sac lavage promotes a continuous washout and debridement of sloughed material. However, less favorable results were reported by other groups using a similar technique with a mean mortality rate of 22.7 percent.[102,103] Open packing of infected necrosis, which is widely used at present, is particularly well-suited to cases in which the necrotizing process has not yet become finally defined, particularly if the necrotic areas (or areas likely to become necrotic) do not separate easily during manual debridement. This situation is most likely to be found early, perhaps in the first week or two, rather than later in the course of the disease. Programmed reinterventions are performed at 2- to 3-day intervals to change the packs and extend the debridement until the walls of the cavity are clean and granulating.[104] The high rate of enteric (15 to 20 percent) and colonic (13 percent) fistulas may come from aggressive debridement or from pressure by adjacent packs and seems to be a significant disadvantage of the method. Mean mortality rate is 24.5 percent ranging from 11 to 55 percent.[100,104–106]

Our experience has been mainly with a third approach to infected pancreatic necrosis: blunt debridement followed by closed packing with gauze-filled Penrose drains and closed system suction catheters (Fig. 41–3). The areas to be debrided can be reached either through the gastrocolic omentum or through the transverse mesocolon (Fig. 41–4). The latter approach has been of particular advantage in patients with previous upper abdominal surgery. It is frequently a rapid and safe way to the lesion and does not threaten the stomach or transverse colon. The duodenum must be avoided. A blunt digital dissection allows for optimal discrimination between devitalized tissue and major vascular structures. It is essential to clean out the devitalized tissues as completely as possible to leave the least amount of necrotic tissue behind. Inadequate debridement is probably the major determinant of recurrent sepsis.[52] The cavity and its extensions are packed with the drains to discourage oozing of blood from the cavity walls. The multiple soft

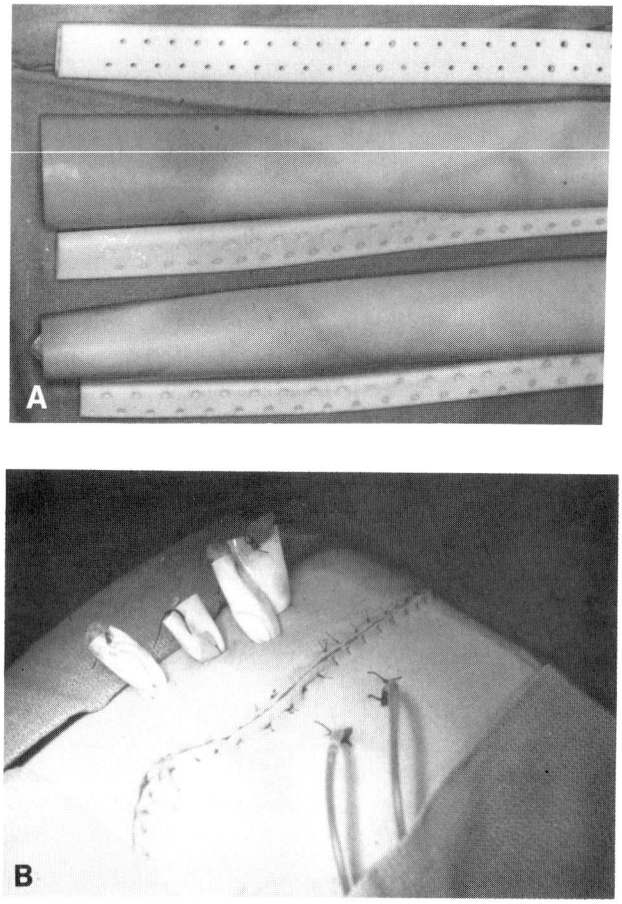

Figure 41–3. Multiple closed-system suction and stuffed drains (A) placed in the cavity left after drainage and debridement of infected pancreatic and peripancreatic necrosis (B).

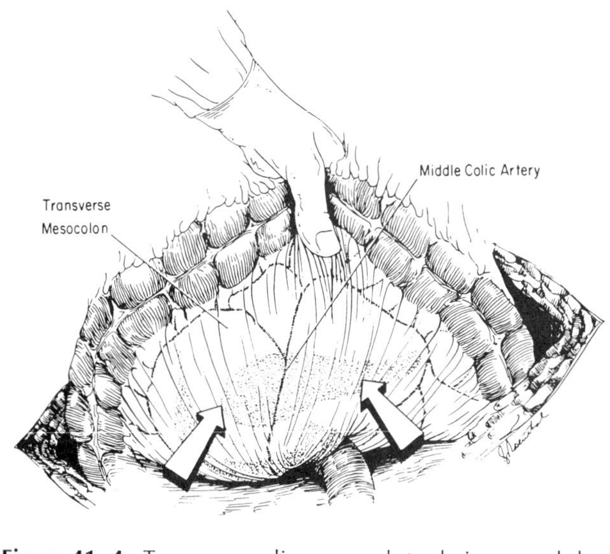

Figure 41–4. Transmesocolic approach to drainage and debridement of the pancreas.

gauze-filled rubber drains provide in aggregate a wide pathway for the egress of solid chunks of debris, and the suction drains prevent pus, pancreatic secretions, and exudate from accumulating. The drains are usually brought through the abdominal wall individually to minimize the risk of wound infections and hernias. No less than a week after the primary intervention the stuffed drains are removed one at a time to facilitate the contraction of the cavity around the remaining suction catheters. When the volume of drainage decreases sufficiently, the suction drains can be extracted. Using this technique we have experienced a mortality rate of 25 percent and a reoperation rate of 27 percent in a group of 73 patients with severe pancreatitis (mean APACHE II score of 11.3).[52]

Separate flank incisions have been proposed for the debridement of retroperitoneal necroses below the transverse colon in order to avoid contamination of the infracolic part of the abdominal cavity. In one series[107] the combination of this approach with closed lavage and programmed reintervention resulted in an extremely low mortality rate of 2.9 percent. Villazon and co-workers[108] report that the mortality rate at their institution decreased from 100 to 22 percent after introducing a similar technique in the treatment of severe necrotizing pancreatitis.

COMPLICATIONS

The sequelae of necrotizing pancreatitis are characterized by local complications of the inflammatory process and multiple organ failure due to uncontrolled sepsis (Table 41–4). The incidences of extension of the infected necrotizing process and recurrent abscesses are high, perhaps 40 percent.[4] The thoroughness of the debridement at the first surgical procedure appears to be the major factor in reducing the recurrence rate to as low as 16 percent.[21,52] While good surgical debridement and drainage remain the mainstay of effective treatment, percutaneous catheter drainage has become a valuable adjunct to evacuate fluid collections and abscess in the postoperative patient, especially when reoperation might carry extra hazards and difficulties.[21,95,109]

Pancreatic fistulas develop in about 30 percent of patients and usually closed spontaneously within weeks.[21,110–113] Loss of continuity between a segment, usually the tail, and the duct may lead to an obligate fistula because the secretions have no exit other than the drainage tract.[111,113]

Enteric fistulas are also common—10 to 31 percent.[19,21,100,104,111,112,114] The most common cause ap-

TABLE 41–4. COMPLICATIONS AFTER DRAINAGE OF 45 CASES OF PANCREATIC ABSCESS AND INFECTED NECROSIS

	Period 1 (1974–1978)		Period 2 (1979–1983)		Periods 1 and 2		Died
Complications	*N*	%	*N*	%	*N*	%	*N*
Hemorrhage	9	35	1	5	10	22	7
Pancreatic fistula	8	31	6	32	14	31	1
Colonic necrosis	1	4	1	5	2	4	1
Colonic fistula	1	4	1	5	2	4	0
Duodenal fistula	1	4	1	5	2	4	1
Gastric fistula	1	4	0	0	1	2	0
Systemic sepsis	1	27	1	5	8	18	8
Recurrent abscess	7	15	3	16	7	16	1
Renal failure	4	12	1	5	4	9	4
Respiratory failure	3	12	0	0	3	7	3
Pulmonary emboli	3	4	0	0	1	2	1
Pneumonia	1	23	3	16	9	20	0
Wound infection	6	19	1	5	6	13	0
Permanent diabetes	5	8	1	5	3	7	0
Splenic vein thrombosis	2	4	0	0	1	2	0
Incisional hernia	0		1	5	1	2	0
Total patients with complications	24	92	14	74	38	84	
Total deaths	10	38	1	5	11	24	26

pears to ischemic necrosis of the enteric wall, whether from thrombosis of the vascular supply or from local enzymatic injury.[114] In addition, iatrogenic damage during surgical debridement or by pressure necrosis from drains occurs. Enteric fistulas may close spontaneously if complete drainage is provided. However, colocutaneous fistulas often require a proximal colostomy and resection of the damaged colonic segment.[115] Similarly, duodenal fistulas may fail to heal and may require a Roux-en-Y jejunal anastomosis or even duodenopancreatectomy to gain control. Gastric fistulas are not common but are particularly troublesome due to their high output, acid content, and proclivity to bleed large amounts from the fistula tract.[114] If a gastric fistula does not heal after 4 weeks of conservative measures, gastric resection has been suggested as definitive treatment.[114]

Progressive sepsis is the most common cause of death, but hemorrhage from the abscess cavity is also commonly fatal. Intraoperative bleeding from major vessels in the pancreatic bed, injured either by the inflammatory process or by the surgeon, may be profuse and difficult to control. If the origin cannot be identified, packing is the therapy of choice.[112] Spontaneous hemorrhage at later stages is often life-threatening due to its magnitude and to difficulties in surgical access and localization of the bleeding source. Angiography with arterial embolization[21,116] or balloon occlusion can control the hemorrhage temporarily to provide time to reexplore, ligate, debride further, and pack the cavity under stable conditions.

REFERENCES

1. Bonacini M: Pancreatic involvement in human immunodeficiency virus infection. J Clin Gastroenterol 13:58, 1991.
2. Beger HG, Bittner R, Block S, Buchler M: Bacterial contamination of pancreatic necrosis. Gastroenterology 91:433, 1986.
3. Donohue PE, Nyhus LM, Baker RJ: Pancreatic abscess after alcoholic pancreatitis. Arch Surg 115:905, 1980.
4. Warshaw AL: Pancreatic abscesses. N Engl J Med 287:1234, 1972.
5. Rinderknecht H: Activation of pancreatic zymogens: normal activation, premature intrapancreatic activation, protective mechanisms against inappropriate activation. Dig Dis Sci 31:314, 1986.
6. Schmidt J, Fernandez-del Castillo C, Rattner DW, et al: Trypsinogen activation peptides in experimental pancreatitis in the rat. Prognostic implications and histopathologic correlates. Gastroenterology 103:1009, 1992.
7. Watanabe O, Baccino FM, Steer ML, Meldolesi J: Supramaximal caerulein stimulation and ultrastructure of rat pancreatic acinar cell: early morphological changes during development of experimental pancreatitis. Am J Physiol 246:G457, 1984.
8. Lampel M, Kern HF: Acute interstitial pancreatitis in the rat induced by excessive doses of a pancreatic secretagogue. Virchows Arch A Pathol Anat Histopathol 373:87, 1977.
9. Adler G, Hupp T, Kern HF: Course and spontaneous regression of acute pancreatitis in the rat. Virchows Arch A Pathol Anat Histopathol 382:31, 1979.
10. Kloppel G, Dreyer T, Willemer S, et al: Human acute pancreatitis: its pathogenesis in the light of immunocytochemical and ultrastructural findings in acinar cells. Virchows Arch A Pathol Anat Histopathol 409:791, 1986.
11. Warshaw AL: Damage prevention versus damage control in acute pancreatitis. Gastroenterology 104:1216, 1993.
12. Fernandez-del Castillo C, Foitzik TH, Schmidt J, et al: A model of fulminant pancreatitis in the rat. Pancreas 7:736(Abstract), 1992.
13. Klar E, Endrich B, Messmer K: Microcirculation of the pancreas. A quantitative study of physiology

and changes in pancreatitis. Int J Microcirc 9:85, 1990.
14. Klar E, Schratt W, Foitzik TH, et al: Different changes in the pancreatic microcirculation in acute edematous and necrotizing pancreatitis—pathophysiological basis for therapy. Langenbecks Arch Chir 377(Suppl):207, 1992.
15. Knoefel WT, Kollias N, Warshaw AL, et al: Altered pancreatic perfusion in pancreatitis of increasing severity. Gastroenterology 100:A280(Abstract), 1991.
16. Klar E, Rattner DW, Compton C, et al: Adverse effect of therapeutic vasoconstrictors in experimental acute pancreatitis. Ann Surg 214:168, 1991.
17. Schratt W, Klar E, Schmidt J, et al: Adverse effect of different catecholamines on pancreatic microcirculation during acute pancreatitis. Eur Surg Res (in press).
18. Gerzof SG, Banks PA, Robbins AH, et al: Early diagnosis of pancreatic infection by computed tomography-guided aspiration. Gastroenterology 93:1315, 1987.
19. Becker JM, Pemberton JH, DiMagno EP, et al: Prognostic factors in pancreatic abscess. Surgery 96:455, 1984.
20. Ranson JHC, Spencer FC: Prevention, diagnosis, and treatment of pancreatic abscess. Surgery 82:99, 1977.
21. Warshaw AL, Jin G: Improved survival in 45 patients with pancreatic abscess. Ann Surg 202:408, 1985.
22. Fink AS, Hiatt JR, Pitt HA, et al: Indolent presentation of pancreatic abscess: experience with 100 cases. Arch Surg 123:1067, 1988.
23. Malangoni MA, Shallcross JC, Seiler JG, et al: Factors contributing to fatal outcome after treatment of pancreatic abscess. Ann Surg 203:605, 1986.
24. Webster WW, Pasculle AW, Myerowitz RL, et al: Postinduction bacteremia in experimental acute pancreatitis. Am J Surg 138:418, 1979.
25. Warshaw AL: Inflammatory masses following acute pancreatitis: phlegmon, pseudocyst, and abscess. Surg Clin North Am 54:621, 1974.
26. Runkel NS, Moody FG, Smith GS, et al: The role of the gut in the development of sepsis in acute pancreatitis. J Surg Res 51:18, 1991.
27. Fedorak IJ, Ko TC, Kjuricin G, et al: Secondary pancreatic infections: are they distinct clinical entities? Surgery 112:824, 1992.
28. O'Dwyer ST, Michie HR, Ziegler TR: A single dose of endotoxin increases intestinal permeability in healthy humans. Arch Surg 123:1459, 1988.
29. Maejima K, Deitch E, Berg RD: Bacterial translocation from the gastrointestinal tracts of rats receiving thermal injury. Infect Immun 43:6, 1984.
30. Baker JW, Deitch EA, Berg RD, Specian RD: Hemorrhagic shock induces bacterial translocation from the gut. J Trauma 28:896, 1988.
31. Ryan CM, Schmidt J, Lewandrowski K, et al: Gut macromolecular permeability in pancreatitis correlates with severity of disease in rats. Gastroenterology 104:890, 1993.
32. Beger HG, Buchler M, Bittner R, et al: Necrosectomy and postoperative local lavage in necrotizing pancreatitis. Br J Surg 75:207, 1988.
33. Block S, Buchler M, Bittner R, Beger HG: Sepsis indicators in acute pancreatitis. Pancreas 2:499, 1987.
34. Richter JM, Jacoby GA, Schapiro RH, Warshaw AL: Pancreatic abscess due to *Candida albicans*. Ann Intern Med 97:221, 1982.
35. Stambler JB, Klibraner MI, Bliss CM, LaMont JT: Tuberculous abscess of the pancreas. Gastroenterology 83:922, 1982.
36. Bittner R, Block S, Buchler M, Beger HG: Pancreatic abscess and infected pancreatic necrosis: different local septic complications in acute pancreatitis. Dig Dis Sci 32:1082, 1987.
37. Freeny PC: Incremental dynamic bolus computed tomography of acute pancreatitis. Int J Pancreatol 12:147, 1993.
38. Bradley EL, Murphy F, Ferguson C: Prediction of pancreatic necrosis by dynamic pancreatography. Ann Surg 210:495, 1989.
39. Ranson JHC, Balthazar E, Caccavale R, Cooper M: Computed tomography and the prediction of pancreatic abscess in acute pancreatitis. Ann Surg 201:656, 1985.
40. Bradley EJ: A clinically based classification system for acute pancreatitis: summary of the International Symposium on Acute Pancreatitis, Atlanta, GA, September 11 through 12, 1992. Arch Surg 128:586, 1993.
41. Kune GA, King R: The late complications of acute pancreatitis: pancreatic swelling, cyst and abscess. Med J Aust N Z 1:1241, 1973.
42. Sostre CF, Flournoy JG, Bova JG, et al: Pancreatic phlegmon: clinical features and course. Dig Dis Sci 30:918, 1985.
43. Fan ST, Choi TK, Chan FL, et al: Pancreatic phlegmon: what is it? Am J Surg 157:544, 1989.
44. Warshaw AL: Lowering the level of uncertainty in late pancreatitis. Gastroenterology 93:1434, 1987.
45. Colhoun E, Murphy JJ, MacEarlean DP: Percutaneous drainage of pancreatic pseudocysts. Br J Surg 71:131, 1984.
46. Glazer G, Dudley HAF: Pancreatic abscess: an incomplete descriptive phrase. Br J Surg 71:131, 1984.
47. Beger HG, Krautzberger W, Bittner R, et al: Results of surgical treatment of necrotizing pancreatitis. World J Surg 9:972, 1985.
48. Beger HG, Buchler M, Bittner R, et al: Necrosectomy and postoperative local lavage in patients with necrotizing pancreatitis: results of a prospective clinical trial. World J Surg 12:255, 1988.
49. Lumsden A, Bradley EL III: Secondary pancreatic infections. Surgery 170:459, 1990.
50. Karimgani I, Porter KA, Langevin RE, Banks PA:

Prognostic factors in sterile pancreatic necrosis. Gastroenterology 103:1636, 1992.
51. Beger HG, Bittner R, Buchler M, et al: Hemodynamic data pattern in patients with acute pancreatitis. Gastroenterology 90:74, 1986.
52. Rattner DW, Legemate DA, Mueller PR, Warshaw AL: Early surgical debridement of pancreatic necrosis is beneficial irrespective of infection. Am J Surg 163:105, 1992.
53. Hiatt JR, Fink AS, King W III, Pitt HA: Percutaneous aspiration of peripancreatic fluid collections: a safe method to detect infection. Surgery 101:523, 1987.
54. Banks PA: Infected necrosis: morbidity and therapeutic consequences. Hepatogastroenterology 38: 116, 1991.
55. Bradley EL, Allen K: A prospective longitudinal study of observation versus surgical intervention in the management of necrotizing pancreatitis. Am J Surg 161:19, 1991.
56. London NJM, Neoptolemos JP, Lavelle J, et al: Contrast-enhanced abdominal computed tomography scanning and prediction of severity of acute pancreatitis: a prospective study. Br J Surg 76:268, 1989.
57. Nuutinen P: Contrast-enhanced computed tomography in acute oedematous pancreatitis. Surg Res Commun 1:251, 1987.
58. Schroder T, Kivisaari L, Standertskjold-Nordenstam CG, et al: The clinical significance of contrast enhanced computed tomography in acute pancreatitis. Ann Chir Gynaecol 73:268, 1984.
59. Kivisaari L, Somer K, Standertskjold-Nordenstam CG, et al: A new method for the diagnosis of acute hemorrhagic-necrotizing pancreatitis using contrast-enhanced CT. Gastrointest Radiol 9:27, 1984.
60. Nuutinen P, Kivisaari L, Schroder T: Contrast-enhanced computed tomography and microangiography of the pancreas in acute human hemorrhagic/necrotizing pancreatitis. Pancreas 3:53, 1988.
61. Vernacchia FS, Jeffrey RB Jr, Federle MP, et al: Pancreatic abscess: predictive value of early abdominal CT. Radiology 162:435, 1987.
62. Clavien PA, Hauser H, Meyer P, Rohner A: Value of contrast-enhanced computerized tomography in the early diagnosis and prognosis of acute pancreatitis. Am J Surg 155:457, 1988.
63. Balthazar E, Ranson JHC, Naidich DP, et al: Acute pancreatitis: prognostic value of CT. Radiology 156:767, 1985.
64. Siegelman SS, Copeland BE, Saba GP, et al: CT of fluid collections associated with pancreatitis. Am J Radiol 134:1121, 1980.
65. White M, Simeone JF, Wittenberg J: Air within a pancreatic inflammatory mass: not necessarily a sign of abscess. J Clin Gastroenterol 5:173, 1983.
66. Wilson C, Heads A, Shenkin A, Imrie CW: C-reactive protein, antiproteases and complement factors as objective markers of severity in acute pancreatitis. Br J Surg 76:177, 1989.
67. Buchler M, Malfertheiner P, Schoetensack C, et al: Sensitivity of antiproteases, complement factors and C-reactive protein in detecting pancreatic necrosis. Results of a prospective clinical study. Int J Pancreatol 1:227, 1986.
68. McMahon MJ, Bowen M, Cooper EH, Mayer AD: C reactive protein: an acid to assessment and monitoring of acute pancreatitis. J Clin Pathol 37:207, 1984.
69. Puolakkainen P, Valtonen V, Paananen A, Schroder T: C-reactive protein (CRP) and serum phospholipase A2 in the assessment of the acute pancreatitis. Gut 28:764, 1987.
70. Gudgeon AM, Heath DI, Hurley P, et al: Trypsinogen activation peptides assay in the early prediction of severity of acute pancreatitis. Lancet 335:4, 1990.
71. Popper HL, Necheles H, Russel K: Transition of pancreatic edema into pancreatic necrosis. Surg Gynecol Obstet 87:79, 1948.
72. Warshaw AL, O'Hara PJ: Susceptibility of the pancreas to ischemic injury in shock. Ann Surg 188:197, 1978.
73. Klar E, Messmer K, Warshaw AL, Herfarth C: Pancreatic ischaemia in experimental acute pancreatitis: mechanism, significance and therapy. Br J Surg 77:1205, 1990.
74. Klar E, Mall G, Messmer K, et al: Improvement of impaired pancreatic microcirculation by isovolemic hemodilution protects pancreatic morphology in acute biliary pancreatitis. Surg Gynecol Obstet 176:144, 1993.
75. Klar E, Herfarth C, Messmer K: Therapeutic effect of isovolemic hemodilution with dextran 60 on the impairment of pancreatic microcirculation in acute biliary pancreatitis. Ann Surg 211:346, 1990.
76. Klar E, Foitzik TH, Buhr H, et al: Isolvolemic hemodilution with dextran 60 as treatment of pancreatic ischemia in acute pancreatitis—clinical practicability of an experimental concept. Ann Surg 217:369, 1993.
77. Schmidt J, Fernandez-del Castillo C, Rattner DW, et al: Hyperoncotic ultrahigh molecular weight dextran solutions reduce trypsinogen activation, prevent acinar necrosis, and lower mortality in rodent pancreatitis. Am J Surg 165:40, 1993.
78. Choi TK, Mok F, Zhan WH, et al: Somatostatin in the treatment of acute pancreatitis: a prospective randomised controlled trial. Gut 30:223, 1989.
79. D'Amico D, Favia G, Biasiato R, et al: The use of somatostatin in acute pancreatitis—results of a multicenter trial. Hepatogastroenterology 37:92, 1990.
80. Glorup I, Roikjaer O, Andersen B, et al: A double blind multicenter trial of somatostatin in the treatment of acute pancreatitis. Surg Gynecol Obstet 175:397, 1992.
81. Buchler M, Malfertheiner P, Uhl W, et al: Gabexate mesilate in human acute pancreatitis. Gastroenterology 104:1165, 1992.
82. Valderrama R, Perez-Mateo M, Navarro S: Multicenter double-blind trial of gabexate mesilate

(FOY) in unselected patients with acute pancreatitis. Digestion 51:65, 1992.
83. Craig RM, Dordal E, Myles L: The use of ampicillin in acute pancreatitis. Ann Surg 183:667, 1976.
84. Finch WT, Sawyers JL, Schenker S: A prospective study to determine the efficacy of antibiotics in acute pancreatitis. Ann Surg 183:667, 1976.
85. Howes R, Zuidema GD, Cameron JL: Evaluation of prophylactic antibiotics in acute pancreatitis. J Surg Res 18:197, 1975.
86. Bassi C, Falconi M, Girelli R, et al: Microbiological findings in severe pancreatitis. Surg Res Commun 4:1, 1989.
87. Buchler M, Malfertheiner P, Friess H, et al: Human pancreatic tissue concentration of bactericidal antibiotics. Gastroenterology 103:1902, 1992.
88. Pederzoli P, Bassi C, Vesentini S, Campedelli A: A randomized multicenter clinical trial of antibiotic prophylaxis of septic complications in acute necrotizing pancreatitis with imipenem. Surg Gynecol Obstet 176:480, 1993.
89. Ranson JHC, Berman RS: Long peritoneal lavage decreases pancreatic sepsis in acute pancreatitis. Ann Surg 211:708, 1990.
90. Reber HA: Surgical intervention in necrotizing pancreatitis. Gastroenterology 91:479, 1986.
91. Gerzof SG, Johnson WC, Robinson AH, Nabseth DC: Expanded criteria for percutaneous abscess drainage. Arch Surg 120:227, 1985.
92. Gerzof SG, Robbins AH, Johnson WC, et al: Percutaneous catheter drainage of abdominal abscesses: a five-year experience. N Engl J Med 305:653, 1981.
93. Adams DB, Harvey TS, Anderson MC: Percutaneous catheter drainage of infected pancreatic and peripancreatic fluid collections. Arch Surg 125:1554, 1990.
94. Lee MJ, Rattner DW, Legemate DA, et al: Acute complicated pancreatitis: redefining the role of interventional radiology. Radiology 183:171, 1992.
95. Pickleman J, Moncada R: The role of percutaneous drainage of pancreatic abscesses. Am Surg 53:451, 1987.
96. Steiner E, Mueller PR, Hahn PF, et al: Complicated pancreatic abscesses: problems in interventional management. Radiology 167:443, 1988.
97. Rotman N, Mathieu D, Anglade MC, Fagniez PL: Failure of percutaneous drainage of pancreatic abscesses complicating severe acute pancreatitis. Surg Gynecol Obstet 174:141, 1992.
98. Traverso LW: Infections complicating severe pancreatitis. Infect Dis Clin North Am 7:601, 1992.
99. Feig BW, Pomerantz RA, Bogelzang R, et al: Treatment of peripancreatic fluid collections in patients with complicated acute pancreatitis. Surg Gynecol Obstet 175:429, 1992.
100. Stone HH, Strom PR, Mullins RJ: Pancreatic abscess management by subtotal resection and packing. World J Surg 8:340, 1984.
101. Alexandre JK, Guerrari MT: Role of total pancreatectomy in the treatment of necrotizing pancreatitis. World J Surg 5:369, 1981.
102. Larvin M, Chalmers AG, Robinson PJ, McMahon MJ: Debridement and closed cavity irrigation for the treatment of pancreatic necrosis. Br J Surg 76:465, 1989.
103. Teerenhovi O, Nordback I, Eskola J: High volume lesser sac lavage in acute necrotizing pancreatitis. Br J Surg 76:370, 1989.
104. Bradley EL III: Management of infected pancreatic necrosis by open drainage. Ann Surg 206:542, 1987.
105. Garcia-Sabrido JL, Tallado JM, Christou NV, et al: Treatment of severe intra-abdominal sepsis and/or necrotic foci by an "open-abdomen" approach: zipper and zipper-mesh techniques. Arch Surg 123:152, 1988.
106. D'Egidio A, Schein M: Surgical strategies in the treatment of pancreatic necrosis and infection. Br J Surg 78:133, 1991.
107. Horn J: Programmed reintervention in necrotizing pancreatitis. In Beger HG, Buchler M, Malfertheiner P (eds): Standards in Pancreatic Surgery. Berlin, Springer-Verlag, 1993, pp 203–212.
108. Villazon A, Villazon O, Terrazas FE, Rana R: Retroperitoneal drainage in the management of the septic phase of severe acute pancreatitis. World J Surg 15:103, 1991.
109. Walters R, Herman CM, Neff R: Percutaneous drainage of abscesses in the postoperative abdomen that is difficult to explore. Am J Surg 149:623, 1985.
110. Aranha GV, Prinz RA, Greenlee HB: Pancreatic abscess: an unresolved surgical problem. Am J Surg 144:534, 1982.
111. Fielding GA, McLatchie GR, Wilson C, et al: Acute pancreatitis and pancreatic fistula formation. Br J Surg 76:1126, 1989.
112. Pemberton JH, Becker JM, Dozois RR, et al: Controlled open lesser sac drainage for pancreatic abscess. Ann Surg 203:600, 1986.
113. Schmidt J, Warshaw AL: Surgical treatment of pancreatic fistulas: rationale, timing and technique. In Bassi C, Vesentini S (eds): Topics on Pancreatic Fistulas. Berlin, Springer-Verlag, 1993, pp 176–194.
114. Warshaw AL, Moncure AC, Rattner DW: Gastrocutaneous fistulas associated with pancreatic abscesses. Ann Surg 210:603, 1989.
115. Russell JC, Welch JP, Clark DG: Colonic complications of acute pancreatitis and pancreatic abscess. Am J Surg 146:558, 1983.
116. Waltman AC, Luers PR, Athanasoulis CA, Warshaw AL: Massive arterial hemorrhage in patients with pancreatitis: complementary roles of surgery and transcatheter occlusive techniques. Arch Surg 121:439, 1986.

Infections of the Upper Gastrointestinal Tract

CHAPTER 42

Alastair C. J. Windsor, Harvey J. Sugerman,
Richard J. Howard

The human gastrointestinal tract contains an enormous variety of aerobic and anaerobic bacteria that interact in a complex ecosystem. The precise number and importance of this complex microflora were underestimated for many years. Recently, however, the development and increasing use of anaerobic bacteriologic techniques have led to a rapid growth of knowledge in this field. It is currently estimated that 95 percent of the bacterial species within the gastrointestinal tract can now be cultured and that between 200 and 500 different bacterial species can exist in the gut of a single individual.[1] Fortunately, despite this large number, consideration of only the most representative microorganisms provides a reasonable outline of this complex microflora.

Of significance to the general public and to underscore the importance of continued investigation of intestinal microflora, it was estimated, more than a decade ago, that gastrointestinal infection causes 200 million work days lost per year in the United States at a cost of 20 billion dollars.[2] In consideration of the problem worldwide, it has been said that there is enough diarrhea in a single day to equal the effluent over Victoria Falls in a minute.[3]

INTESTINAL MICROECOLOGY

The composition of normal microflora is different for different populations and may show individual variation. For example, *Salmonella typhi* may be considered part of the normal flora for a typhoid carrier but not so for an uninfected individual. In contrast, the autochthonous or indigenous flora are regarded as those bacteria that have reached symbiotic status, a process thought to result from a long evolutionary association with the host. Until the mid-1960s, the coliforms were thought to constitute the chief inhabitants of the intestine. However, the advent of anaerobic culturing techniques has clearly established nonsporing anaerobes, including *Bacteroides, Bifidobacterium, Eubacterium,* and many others as the predominant gut species. Bacteria and other pathogens generally enter the gastrointestinal tract through the mouth and leave in the feces. What remains to a large extent conjecture and the subject of ongoing research is what dictates which organisms will become the predominant flora.

The human stomach, unlike that of some other animals, is commonly thought to be sterile, but depending on the time of sampling, it is possible to isolate organisms from gastric juice. Immediately following a test meal, approximately 10^5 bacteria per milliliter of gastric juice can be isolated. As the pH falls, the bacterial content declines and very few organisms are found at a pH of 3 or below. Counts of 10^3 colony forming units per milliliter (CFU/ml) are typically quoted for fasting gastric juice. Organisms such as lactobacilli, aerobic streptococci, and *Candida* are notably more acid tolerant and therefore make up the majority of isolated species. Indeed, some authors would argue that they form part of an indigenous stomach flora.[2] Oral anaerobes, such as *Peptostreptococcus, Bacteroides,* and *Fusobacterium,* may be present in low concentrations but coliforms are distinctly uncommon.

The upper small intestine has a concentration of bacteria approaching that of the stomach, at approximately 10^3 to 10^4 CFU/ml.[4] Aerobic streptococci and lactobacilli predominate. Coliforms and obligate anaerobes, such as *Clostridium* and *Bacteroides* are uncommon, but their isolation becomes progressively more common with sampling further down the small bowel. As in the stomach, the number of bacteria isolated is dependent to a great extent on the time of sampling. For example, Dickman et al[5] found mean colony counts of $10^{1.8}$ CFU/ml in the fasting state and, following a meal, the number increased to 10^4 CFU/ml. The species variation resembled that of oral and gastric flora, though the numbers were much reduced and suggest that large numbers of bacteria are killed by their passage through the stomach.

Most studies of small bowel flora demonstrate increasing bacterial counts with increasing distance down the bowel. Total counts usually reach levels of 10^6 to 10^8 with equal numbers of aerobes and anaerobes. The predominant aerobes are *Escherichia coli* and enterococci, and the predominant anaerobes *Bacteroides* and *Bifidobacterium.* The flora of the terminal ileum resemble that of the colon, with counts increasing to 10^{11} CFU/ml. In the colon, the bacterial content of the feces represents some 70 percent of its dry weight. Qualitatively, in the distal ileum, gram-negative bacteria begin to outnumber gram-positive organisms. Coliforms are consistently present, and *Bacteroides, Bifidobacterium, Fusobacterium,* and *Clostridium* are found in substantial quantities.[6] This subject is covered in greater detail in Chapter 3.

Colonization of the Gut in Newborn Infants

Colonization of the gastrointestinal tract occurs within a few days of birth. Patterns of colonization of anaerobic bacteria depend on factors such as type of delivery, dietary constituents, and gestational age. Long and Swenson[7] found that within 4 to 6 days nearly all full-term, formula-fed, vaginally delivered infants were colonized with anaerobic bacteria. In contrast, only 59 percent of infants delivered by cesarean section were colonized in the same time period. This suggests passage through the birth canal is a key to the subsequent colonization of the gut. The direction of colonization would appear to be from the top down, in that infants with congenital obstructions demonstrate a fecal flora just proximal to, and a sterile bowel distal to the site of obstruction.[8]

Indigenous Flora and Normal Gut Physiology

Far from a one-way existence, the presence of bacteria within the gastrointestinal tract has a number of beneficial effects for the host. The structure and function of the gut are highly dependent on the presence of resident bacterial flora.[9] In the study of germ-free animals, the intestinal wall is considerably thinner and less cellular; villi are thin, fingerlike, and sometimes short. The crypts are shallow and total mucosal surface area is substantially reduced. The lamina propria is poorly developed and infiltrated by few lymphocytes and macrophages. There is little immunologic stimulation and therefore plasma cells are absent and Peyer's patches are small and possess few germinal centers. Labeled thymidine studies demonstrate reduced mucosal cell turnover and slowed mucosal cell migration from crypts to villus tip.[10] Following exposure and colonization of these germ-free animals, the bowel rapidly resumes a normal appearance.[11] Interestingly, the crypt hyperplasia and infiltration of the lamina propria with large numbers of immunologic competent cells suggest that the histologic picture accepted as normal resembles a state of "chronic inflammation."[12] Functional alterations are also present in the bowel of germ-free animals, with a more alkaline pH and a more positive reduction potential, reflecting absent bacterial metabolism, in addition to decreased intestinal motility and gastric emptying.

In some animals, intestinal organisms clearly carry on metabolic and digestive activities, which benefit the host. For example, fibrous food is delayed in the stomach of ruminants for microbial digestion. Similarly, rats derive vitamin B_6 from their indigenous flora. These observations suggest that bacterial metabolism does provide essential nutrients for the benefit of the host. This nutritional role is more difficult to establish in humans, but the microflora are known to metabolize foreign compounds.[13] For example, many drugs are metabolized by enteric bacteria, including lactulose, sulfasalazine, L-dopa, and salicyluric acid. Lindenbaum et al[14] noted that digoxin could also be inactivated by the gut flora in 10 percent of patients and that the use of broad spectrum antibiotics could prevent this metabolic inactivation. The suggestion has been made that intestinal bacteria manufacture secondary bile acids and fecal sterols from bile acids and cholesterol and thereby play a role in carcinogenesis.[15]

The role of indigenous flora as key effectors in the host resistance to pathologic infection is only just becoming clear. Under normal circumstances, an individual's intestinal flora are highly effective at impeding colonization by potentially pathogenic invaders, a phenomenon known as *bacterial interference* or *colonization resistance.* Bacteria basically do this by restricting access of intestinal pathogens to the epithelial surface.[16] Colonization resistance is primarily mediated by endogenous anaerobic bacteria. The human gastrointestinal tract not only contains huge numbers of bacteria (about 10^{14}), the composition is quite stable.[16] Bifidobacteria are thought to be an important stabilizing group.[16] These organisms seem to prosper in saliva and intestinal mucus because they have enzymes that can digest mucus and utilize the glycoproteins for nutrients.[16]

Bacterial competition for nutrients is only one mechanism of colonization resistance. The indigenous flora are capable of secreting antimicrobial substances such as short-chain fatty acids and colicins, which are potentially bactericidal or bacteriostatic. In addition, the resident flora tend to maintain a redox potential and pH that puts invading pathogens at a disadvantage. The efficacy of this bacterial interference was ably illustrated by Bohnhoff et al,[17] who demonstrated a 10,000-fold reduction in the infective dose of *Salmonella typhimurium* in mice whose gut flora had been eradicated by pretreating with streptomycin.

Normal Control of the Enteric Flora

Under optimal growth conditions in the laboratory, coliform organisms divide approximately every 20 minutes. Such rapid growth in the gastrointestinal tract would rapidly overwhelm the host if allowed to proceed unchecked. The same organisms existing in the human gut undergo 1 to 4 divisions per day, a generation time considerably longer than that encountered in vitro. A number of mechanisms serve to limit bacterial growth in the gut and maintain a stable bacterial population under normal conditions.

Anatomical Considerations

Gross Features. The anatomic features most relevant to a discussion regarding control of the gastrointestinal microflora are the sphincters. The pylorus plays a role in regulating the upper gastrointestinal microflora by prolonging the exposure of gastric contents to the bactericidal effects of gastric acid. When the sphincter is bypassed by gastroenterostomy, in conjunction with vagotomy and reduced gastric acid secretion, investigators noted a significant increase in proximal bowel flora. Subtotal gastrectomy almost always results in proximal bacterial overgrowth, but it is questionable as to what extent this is due to the loss of sphincter and to what extent the reduced acid secretion.

The sphincter of Oddi probably serves to prevent colonization of the biliary and pancreatic trees. Under clinical conditions of bacterial overgrowth in the proximal small intestine (10^9 organisms/ml jejunal contents), clinical infection of the normal biliary tract is rare.

The ileocecal valve is probably the most significant of the three sphincters mentioned. It is a physiologically important valve and to some extent isolates the ileum from the fecal flora of the colon. Insofar as it retards the passage of intestinal contents into the colon, the distal ileum becomes the only area of small bowel with any significant stasis. Thus, according to Savage,[1] this is the only area of small bowel with an appreciable colonization by indigenous flora. In this regard the terminal ileum is the segment most often involved in infectious processes.

Microscopic and Fine Structure. The villous configuration of the small intestinal mucosa provides a surface of interstices and niches where bacteria may grow without being washed along by luminal contents. The glycocalyx of the microvillous membrane is a mucous layer on the surface of the epithelium that harbors that portion of the total flora critical for colonization resistance. These organisms not only benefit from the nutrition derived from the interaction, they are firmly attached to it and can not be easily dislodged from this layer even by repeated washings, and remain relatively protected from some of the other control mechanisms at work in the small bowel.

Nonimmunological Defense Mechanisms. In addition to the classic cellular and humoral immune systems, a number of nonimmune mechanisms represent an important and often first-line defense against overgrowth and pathologic infection in the gut. So efficient is this nonimmune system at bacterial control, that infectious bacterial disorders of the gastrointestinal tract are not always observed in patients with humoral and cellular immune deficiency,[18] and it has been suggested that the lymphoid system represents a method of fine tuning the intestinal ecology rather than gross control. The two primary nonimmune mechanisms are intestinal motility and gastric acid secretion. These are backed up by other factors, such as bactericidal effects of bile and pancreatic secretions, bacterial interference, and lysozyme secretion.

Gastric Acid. The importance of gastric acid as a nonimmunologic defense factor has been known for more than 50 years. Sir Arthur Hurst suggested in 1934 that "bacillary and amoebic dysentery occur much more commonly in people with achlorhydria and hypochlorhydria."[19] As discussed previously, patients with normal gastric acid secretion have low bacterial counts in their fasting gastric juice. Swallowed food provides some protection for the bacteria from acid and hence the transient postprandial increase in bacterial counts. The low pH (less than 3.0) of gastric juice is considered to be responsible for its bactericidal properties. Bactericidal substances have been found in the stomachs of suckling rabbits, but similar antibacterial mechanisms are not thought to exist in humans. Indeed, neutralization of gastric acid with 2 g of sodium bicarbonate reduced the infective dose of *Vibrio cholerae* by 10,000 times in healthy volunteers,[20] and the use of H_2 antagonists, such as cimetidine, is associated with increased intragastric bacterial counts.[21] Clinically, the relevance of this increased gastric acid colonization has only recently been fully appreciated and remains somewhat contradictory. The mortality associated with stress ulceration in an intensive care unit (ICU) patient population has prompted the widespread use of ulcer prophylaxis. Increased bacterial colonization of the stomach associated with the use of histamine antagonists (and antacids) raised concern over the possible risk of an increased incidence of subsequent nosocomial pneumonia. Meta-analyses by Tryba et al[22] and Cook et al[23] both indicated an increase in the incidence of pneumonia in H_2-antagonist treated groups when compared to non-acid-reducing treatment such as sucrulfate. The problem with these reports, however, was the confounding effects of antacids, which were often not analyzed as separate groups in some of the trials. Recently, Fabian et al[24] published a prospective evaluation of the effects of stress ulceration prophylaxis in severely injured patients. They concluded that both sucrulfate and cimetidine were effective treatment for preventing stress ulcers and that there was no increase in the incidence of pneumonia associated with the use of cimetidine.

Intestinal Motility. Beyond the pylorus, it is intestinal peristalsis that maintains bacterial control. In particular, it is the "intestinal housekeeper" or the well-defined phase III component of the interdigestive motor complex that occurs every 84 to 112 minutes and sweeps an intense band of contraction down the small bowel at 6 to 8 cm/min, preventing stagnation and bacterial overgrowth.[25] Almost all predispositions to bacterial overgrowth in the small intestine are associated with some sort of interference with this mechanism. A vast increase in microorganisms occurs in intestinal obstruction in both animals and humans. Furthermore, after operative relief of the obstruction, bacterial counts remain high until peristalsis resumes and then fall precipitously.[26] Even though this mechanism is effective under normal conditions, bacterial overgrowth, in particular by organisms that are able to attach firmly to the gut wall, may well induce motility disorders, thus potentiating the condition. The mechanisms behind this effect will be discussed in more detail later.

Pancreatic and Biliary Secretions. Felsenfeld and Gyr[27,28] noted an association between protein-depleted monkeys with exocrine pancreatic insufficiency and a more prolonged and severe episode of diarrhea following cholera challenge. They also noted that the addition of pancreatic extract to the same monkeys modified the course of illness, reducing both duration and severity. Rubinstein et al[29] also showed that canine pancreatic fluid exhibited antibacterial properties in vitro when exposed to a variety of gram-negative organisms. Despite these findings, the precise mechanism behind this antimicrobial effect of pancreatic juice is yet to be fully evaluated. A similar in vitro effect of bacterial inhibition has been seen with bile acids; however, the equivalent observations have not as yet been made in vivo and more work needs to be done to establish the role of bile in enteric bacterial control.

Diet. Dietary factors may be related to resistance to particular pathogens. An interesting example of this phenomenon has come from New Guinea, where enteritis necroticans caused by *Clostridium perfringens* type C is endemic. The organism is 100 percent lethal in guinea pigs when inoculated into the stomachs along with raw sweet potatoes. However, when inoculated alone or with baked sweet potato, the animals are not infected. The raw sweet potato has a trypsin inhibitor that is believed to prevent the inactivation of the B toxin of the microorganism; therefore the consumption of raw sweet potato in New Guinea may be related to the prevalence of the disease.

Bacterial Interference. The presence of a normal, healthy bacterial flora helps prevent bacterial overgrowth and pathologic invasion. Known as bacterial interference or colonization resistance, the precise mechanisms that give rise to the phenomenon are poorly understood. It appears that normal flora metabolize a portion of the available nutrition, tend to adjust their local environment to suit their needs, and may even secrete bactericidal agents into their local environment; in this way, it is difficult for other bacteria to establish a hold and multiply. The use of broad spectrum antibiotics will kill established bowel flora and thus destroy this natural control mechanism, providing access for pathogenic organisms. Recently, it has been suggested that the process of bacterial interference may be used as a therapeutic mechanism. Reid et al[30] reviewed the use of lactobacillus in the prevention of urogenital and intestinal infection. Yogurt lactobacillus (*L. acidophilus*) will not permanently colonize the human gut unless it is fed continuously. A "probiotic" has been defined by Fuller[31] as "a live microbial food supplement which beneficially affects the host . . . by improving its microbial balance." Some bacterial supplements are useful for infantile diarrhea, for example, *Bifidobacterium breve.*[31] Systematic clinical trials have not been done, however.

The Gut Lymphoid System and Immunologic Control. The mucosal immune system within the gastrointestinal tract is conveniently divided into three distinct regions.[32]

Peyer's Patches. The inductive sites, or Peyer's patches, are submucosal collections of lymphoid tissue predominantly composed of B cells with fewer T cells and macrophages. Specialized dome epithelial cells, known as M cells, pinocytose luminal antigens and transport them to other cells within the patch. Once presented to follicular lymphoid cells, local release of cytokines appears to control the growth and differentiation of the B cell lymphocyte population into committed IgA-secreting plasma cells.

Lamina Propria Lymphocytes. A second distinct compartment of the mucosal immune system is represented by lymphocytes found within the lamina propria, the only tissue where large numbers of plasma cells are present under normal conditions. Seventy to 90 percent of these plasma cells secrete IgA and they have an estimated half-life of approximately 5 days.[33] This population must therefore be continually replaced, and prevailing evidence suggests that the committed B cells arise in Peyer's patches and migrate to the lamina propria through mesenteric nodes.

Intraepithelial Lymphocytes. The third compartment is made up of lymphocytes that reside within the epithelium of the intestine itself. The intraepithelial lymphocyte population is possibly the largest lymphoid collection in the body and amounts to approximately 5 to 15 percent of the normal intestinal epithelium. Though the function of this massive cell population is as yet unclear, the predominant cell type is that of T cell lymphocytes. It is therefore currently postulated that they represent the T cell equivalent of the lamina propria plasma cells and are involved in cellular defense of the intestinal mucosa.

Secretory Immunoglobulins. While the predominant plasma immunoglobulin is IgG, the predominant immunoglobulin of intestinal secretions is IgA. In this respect, the secretions of the gut are similar to those of the bronchial epithelium or the salivary glands. The ratio of gut plasma cells making IgA, IgM, and IgG is approximately 10:2:1, respectively. Immunoglobulin A is predominantly a dimer of two 7S molecules made by plasma cells in the lamina propria. The complete secretory molecule has an additional component manufactured and attached by the epithelial cells. The complete secretory IgA molecule is believed to be delivered to the lumen by reverse pinocytosis. The secretory component added by the epithelial cell is probably responsible for the molecule's extraordinary stability in a proteolytic environment. Secretory IgA binds to viruses and bacteria, and a primary function of the molecule may be to bind to those ligands on the microbe that are necessary for bacterial adherence to the mucosa. An additional function of great potential importance may be to prevent the absorption of certain ingested macromolecules or products of bacterial metabolism. Although the surface epithelium does pose a barrier against the absorption of potentially toxic complexes, absorption of some macromolecules can occur. Indeed, there is detectable absorption of endotoxin administered directly into the small intestine. Thus a function of the secretory immunoglobulins may be to combine with certain of these antigens to reduce absorption. In overall function, the barrier is efficient, as few complex molecules from food or bacteria are actually absorbed intact.

Another feature of the secretory IgA defense is that higher levels of immunity are accomplished after local rather than systemic introduction of antigens. Local immunity is illustrated by studies in patients with double-barreled colostomies. An attentuated poliovirus was used to immunize one limb of the colostomy. Subsequently, significant immunization was proved in the test limb of the colostomy when compared to the control, unimmunized limb.[34] Not all bacterial inhabitants of the intestine appear to induce antibodies. Some bacterial inhabitants that were once believed to induce antibodies detectable in serum or secretions turned out on further investigation to be incapable of inducing antibodies on their own. The antibodies appear to be directed against bacteria that share antigens with the surface mucus or mucosa. This factor may select species with antigenic similarities to the host surface. On the other hand, some bacteria clearly evoke immune responses. For example, *Vibrio cholerae* induces antibodies that interfere with its attachment. Antibodies called coproantibodies can be present in high titer in the stool—and totally absent in the serum. These antibodies can be protective against enteric colonization but irrelevant to systemic inoculation.[35]

Paneth Cells. Paneth cells may also be a part of the gastrointestinal host defense system. These cells sit in the deepest reaches of the small intestinal crypts and studies reveal evidence for active phagocytosis and degradation of microorganisms opsonized by IgA within these cells.[36] In addition, immunofluorescence studies show that lysozyme granules are present in Paneth cells and that these granules appear to be discharged into the lumen after stimulation with intravenous pilocarpine. Lysozymes can degrade the cell wall polymer of most bacteria and, in the intestinal lumen, the bactericidal properties of lysozymes may be enhanced by secretory immunoglobulins. In addition to lysosomal enzyme release, recent evidence suggests that Paneth cells are capable of producing defensins, a novel family of antimicrobial peptides. Selsted et al[37] identified five defensins known as *cryptdins* in the intestinal lumen and noted at least three of them are predominantly secreted by Paneth cells.

Microbial Adherence as a Genetic Basis for Resistance. Microbial invasion of intact epithelial surfaces seems to require the presence on the surface of bacteria of specific ligands for receptors on epithelial cells. This property almost certainly represents an important virulence factor for certain bacteria but may also be an important mechanism in colonization resistance, when all the potential sites for pathogen binding are occupied by commensals. Consequently, the unavailability of certain epithelial receptors may render some animals resistant to infection. Genetic resistance to a pathogen may be governed by a similar principle. Thus, in a strain of piglets with receptors for the virulence antigen of a species of *E. coli,* 95 percent of animals die after inoculation. On the other hand, if the piglet strain does not have receptors for the attachment antigen, 95 percent of inoculated animals survive.

Host Pathogenic Factors

In the same way that there are multiple factors that control the gastrointestinal flora, failure of these factors can also contribute to subsequent overgrowth or pathological infection. The clinical syndromes associated with bacterial overgrowth are discussed in a later section. Here we discuss the predisposing conditions.

Intestinal Obstruction. Any disorder that interferes with intestinal motility can result in bacterial overgrowth within the intestine. For example, in scleroderma the peristaltic waves that ordinarily help to clear bacteria from the proximal small bowel may be diminished and bacterial overgrowth may occur as a result of functional obstruction with a patent lumen. Syndromes associated with chronic bacterial overgrowth may ensue. In acute intestinal obstruction, intraluminal bacterial overgrowth also occurs and can be a major source of morbidity and mortality after operative relief. In fact, most deaths after surgery for intestinal obstruction result from sepsis. Studies of the microbial flora in intestinal obstruction are difficult because the intraluminal contents cannot safely be obtained and the laboratory resources for quantitative bacteriology are frequently not available during emergencies. Some studies have negotiated these obstacles. In one, the aerobic bacterial counts in obstructed jejunum were on the order of 10^8/ml.[38] Anaerobes were isolated from 17 of 26 obstructed patients and averaged over 10^2/ml in obstructed jejunum and over 10^4/ml in obstructed ileum. In another study, total bacterial counts in obstructed small intestine were between 10^9 and 10^{11}/ml. The aerobic bacteria were 5 to 6×10^9/ml. More than 90 percent of patients had quantitative anaerobic cultures in the range of 5×10^5/ml with a range of 10^5 to 10^7/ml, although only about 50 percent of unobstructed patients cultured any anaerobic organisms at all.[39] There was a great increase in the frequency of isolation of *Bacteroides* species in obstructed small bowel.

The duration of intestinal obstruction also correlates with the quantitative bacterial counts. In intestinal obstruction of more than 12 hours duration, jejunal aerobic counts rise to 10^{10}/ml and higher. During the recovery phase after intestinal obstruction, the flora return to normal after peristalsis resumes and quantitative counts are back to normal after a few days. In large bowel obstruction, there is also an increase in the number of bacteria in the small intestine. Larger numbers of organisms are isolated at both jejunal and ileal levels, and there is a loss of the normal gradient of bacterial counts. Indeed, 10^{10} to 10^{11} organisms/ml may be cultured from the entire length of the small intestine. In one study, anaerobes were recovered in all of ten specimens, and *Bacteroides* was isolated in all specimens except one. Increases in bacterial numbers in the gut have been strongly correlated with translocation of bacteria out of the otherwise normal gut to mesenteric nodes and to distant sites. This is true not only of all experimental models but in human studies as well. Deitch[40] has shown that almost all mesenteric nodes contained viable *E. coli* in humans undergoing operation for intestinal obstruction. Operations for other acute abdominal illnesses yielded sterile nodes.[40]

Reduced Gastric Acid. Hypochlorhydria and achlorhydria, regardless of the etiology, are associated with bacterial overgrowth in the stomach and sometimes the small intestine. Overgrowth may occur in the course of chronic diseases such as pernicious anemia with reduced gastric acid secretion. Overgrowth also occurs in patients with gastric ulcer benign or malignant. Patients with carcinoma of the stomach are frequently achlorhydric and those with benign gastric ulcer are often relatively hypochlorhydric. Septic complications are far more common after gastric operations for these conditions than for duodenal ulcers. Massive bacterial overgrowth may also occur in the stomach when there is gastric hemorrhage. The blood buffers the gastric acid and provides a broth suited to the exuberant growth of microorganisms. Wound infection and other septic complications after emergency gastric surgery for hemorrhage are correspondingly more common.

The role of stress ulcer prophylaxis in severely ill patients has been discussed. However, it is to be emphasized that there may be a potential danger, in terms of secondary nosocomial pneumonia, following reduction of gastric acidity with H_2 antagonists or antacids. In view of the prevailing evidence that suggests mucosal barrier-enhancing agents such as sucrulfate are as effective as acid reduction for ulcer prophylaxis, but do not carry the potential risks for nosocomial pneumonia, their preferential use may be advisable.

Changes in Local and Systemic Immune Status. Gastrointestinal infection with some microorganisms, such as *Candida,* is virtually unknown except in patients with cancer, diabetes, or immunosuppression. Advanced malnutrition in cancer patients appears to predispose toward serious infection with *Candida.* In experimental animals, T cell-deficient mice have been found to be more susceptible to *Salmonella* enteritis. Patients with acquired immunodeficiency syndrome (AIDS) are more subject to gastroenteritis with a variety of organisms such as *Cryptosporidium* and *Giardia.* Changes in local immune status also appear to predispose toward infections with certain organisms. Infection with *Giardia* is rare except in patients with congenital or acquired deficiencies in IgA. IgA deficiency may be selective or caused by a global immunoglobulin deficiency.

It has been speculated that deficiencies in local antibody production may also result in a breakdown of the mucosal barrier function to macromolecules and lead to the absorption of noxious materials that may be related to hepatic or systemic disease.

Intestinal Ischemia. The mortality of gangrenous small bowel remains high regardless of etiology. The major causes of intestinal gangrene (strangulating obstructions and mesenteric vascular accidents) have remained essentially the same, but little progress has been made in reducing the septic complications of these conditions. The importance of the microflora in intestinal gangrene is easily demonstrable in experimental models. Ischemic injury to bowel has been compared in germ-free versus monocontaminated species. Of the contaminating species studied, *C. perfringens* type A has been found to be extraordinarily toxic and lethal. This organism is capable of virtually dissolving an intestinal segment in animals.[41]

The concept of an intestinal factor in irreversible shock goes back to the 1950s. Fine[42] postulated a role for enteric organisms in contributing to the irreversibility of hemorrhagic shock and showed that denervation of the intestine protected an animal from longer periods of hypotension. Because the arterioles in the intestine undergo spasm during hypotension to redistribute the cardiac output to other organs, the gut becomes progressively ischemic and vulnerable to bacterial invasion and absorption of endotoxins that leak through the epithelial barrier. Denervation allows the arterioles to vasodilate and autoregulate blood flow, resulting in protection of the mucosa.

Even normal gut will permit bacterial translocation into the extraintestinal body. This normally occurs at a slow rate, which accelerates under conditions of shock, sepsis, and bacterial overgrowth. *Bacterial translocation* has attracted massive research interest in recent years and will be the subject of a separate section within this chapter.

Genetic Susceptibility. Almost nothing is known in humans about a genetic basis for the resistance to invasion of the small bowel by microorganisms. Work on piglets has suggested that receptors to certain antigens associated with bacteria enable pathogenic microorganisms to attach to the mucosa. The K-88 antigen of the surface of *E. coli* is a virulence determinant in piglets, as the adhesive properties of the antigen enable the bacteria to attach to the cell surface. Ninety-six percent of animals genetically lacking the K-88 receptor survive inoculation with the organism, whereas 95 percent of animals with the appropriate receptor die after inoculation. Nothing is known in humans about this possible mechanism of resistance to enteric infection.

Underlying Diseases and Metabolic Disorders. Enteric bacterial overgrowth is recognized in a number of systemic diseases. However, most of these associations are explained by the effect of the systemic disease on one of the mechanisms of host defense that has been discussed previously. For example, the bacterial overgrowth associated with diabetes may be related to a motility disturbance related to diabetic neuropathy. Gastric emptying may also be reduced in gastroparesis diabeticorum of diabetes mellitus. Similarly, scleroderma may predispose to bacterial overgrowth from a disturbance in motility. High coliform counts in the proximal bowel are seen in pernicious anemia and this disturbance is probably caused by gastric achlorhydria.

Anatomic Disorders. Several anatomic disorders predispose to bacterial overgrowth in the small intestine. Originally, the pathophysiology of blind loop syndrome was developed experimentally in animals with true antiperistaltic blind loops. Accordingly, the term blind loop syndrome carried over to patients with actual surgical blind loops. These may develop from poorly planned anastomoses or intentionally, as with intestinal bypass operations for obesity popular in the 1960s, which left segments of bowel that did not empty properly by peristalsis and were connected to the large intestine without a sphincter mechanism. Bacterial overgrowth is usually the conspicuous and presenting problem in patients with diverticula of the small intestine. Other anatomic disorders, such as strictures and fistulas that interfere with the peristaltic cleansing of the bowel, predispose to bacterial overgrowth.

Extension from Other Infected Regions. The only ductal system from which bacterial overgrowth spreads to the small bowel is the pancreaticobiliary tree. Bacterial overgrowth has been reported in the small bowel in connection with common duct disease and obstruction of the biliary tract.[43] Once bacterial overgrowth is established in the small intestine, contamination spreads the length of the gastrointestinal tract. Accordingly, bacterial overgrowth originating in the small bowel, for example, in a case of jejunal diverticulosis, tends to traverse the pylorus and contaminate the stomach.

Relationship to Prior Operative Procedures. Infectious complications from operative procedures span a variety of problems that may be broken down into two groups. On the one hand, there are the wound infections and anastomotic leaks that may occur after surgery on the stomach and small bowel; on the other hand, there are the operative procedures that predispose to bacterial overgrowth in the lumen as chronic complications. The former are discussed in other chapters, whereas the latter predispose to blind loop syndrome. Another matter that merits comment here is the problem of bacteremia arising from the small bowel in association with diagnostic procedures. Bacteremias occur after peroral jejunal biopsy or upper gastrointestinal endoscopy; however, these bacteremias rarely induce significant infection elsewhere. Most endocarditis is caused by cocci, which form rigid chains in the bloodstream. However, most enteric organisms are motile rods that do not float in clumps and adhere to the cardiac valves. It is considered advisable, however, to provide prophylactic antibiotic coverage against enterococci before instrumentation of the proximal gastrointestinal tract in patients with rheumatic heart disease or intravascular prostheses.

Surgical procedures that predispose to bacterial overgrowth as a late complication interfere either with peristaltic emptying or gastric acidity.

Anatomic blind loops from side-to-side anastomoses have been mentioned. Perhaps the most common clinical form of this problem is a side-to-side ileotransverse colostomy to bypass Crohn's disease, with the distal ileum terminating in a stricture or inflammatory mass. Although the defunctionalized small intestine after jejunoileal bypass for obesity should empty isoperistaltically, there is evidence that bypass enteropathy may be related to bacterial overgrowth in the excluded segment.

Hypochlorhydria has also been discussed as a predisposition for bacterial overgrowth, regardless of etiology. Bacterial overgrowth has been noted after a variety of gastric procedures for either benign or malignant disease. Manifestations of bacterial overgrowth may occur either as contaminated small bowel syndrome or as a predisposition toward infection with specific organisms such as *Salmonella*. A fecal flora in the small bowel with bacterial counts up to 10^8/ml, predominantly enterobacteria and bifidobacteria,[44,45] have been reported after both Billroth I and Billroth II reconstruction of the stomach. Vitamin B_{12} malabsorption after gastrectomy is probably as likely to occur from bacterial overgrowth as from loss of intrinsic factor and significant changes have also been reported after vagotomy and drainage. Although some have shown major changes after gastroenterostomy,[46] others have claimed that the changes are small. Further studies have included the more contemporary acid-lowering procedures in dogs with a variety of gastric operations.[47] A marked and persistent increase in the flora occurred after subtotal gastrectomy or total vagotomy with antrectomy; the bacterial overgrowth was prominent in the stomach as well as in the jejunum. Only after highly selective vagotomy was there no bacterial overgrowth. All animals were said to have the same degree of acid reduction at 30 and 90 days postoperatively, but acid secretion returned in the animals with highly selective vagotomy at 1 year.

BACTERIAL TRANSLOCATION

The association between critically ill patients and the development of systemic sepsis in the absence of a septic focus has prompted much research into the sources of the bacteremia. The gastrointestinal tract is almost certainly a major reservoir for these bacteria and yet the mechanisms by which they breach the mucosal barrier and initiate the septic process remain to some extent an enigma. The passage of viable bacteria from the gastrointestinal tract through the gut epithelium to sites such as mesenteric lymph nodes, liver, spleen, peritoneal cavity, and bloodstream is termed *bacterial translocation*. The phenomenon is normal in many animals[48] but is augmented in a multitude of experimental situations, notably hemorrhagic shock, thermal injury, malnutrition, sepsis, and jaundice, and may have profound clinical importance.[49–56]

Hemorrhagic Shock

Baker et al[49] demonstrated increasing bacterial translocation and increasing mortality in rats subjected to 30, 60, and 90 minutes of hemorrhage, respectively. Sori et al[50] elegantly demonstrated the source of systemic contamination by prefeeding their rats with isotope-labeled *E. coli* and correlating subsequent postshock mortality with plasma activity. The mechanism of increased bacterial contamination following hemorrhage would appear to be multifactorial. It is established that hypoperfusion leads to direct mucosal injury and loss of the mucosal barrier. However, hemorrhage also leads to complex changes in the host immune system.[51] Therefore the loss of, or impairment of, the gut lymphoid system may also play a role in facilitating bacterial translocation.

Thermal Injury

Although the endogenous contamination of burn wounds is known to occur commonly and the gastrointestinal tract is a primary site of origin, to what extent these organisms arise from translocation and to what extent from the wound is not clear. In the experimental model, however, rats subjected to third degree burns develop bacteremia almost immediately, and viable labeled bacteria were found in lymph nodes within hours, long before the burn wound is colonized.[57]

Nutrition and Sepsis

Although disruption of a normal enteric nutrition can lead to impaired immune systems and an altered gastrointestinal microecology,[52,53] Wells et al[48] and Baker et al[49] demonstrated that malnutrition alone was insufficient to promote bacterial translocation. However, in the presence of endotoxemia, bacterial translocation to mesenteric lymph nodes occurred. The gut, though providing nutrients for host survival, requires certain nutrients of its own in order to function adequately. Glutamine is a specific nutrient used by the gut epithelium and its absence in parenteral nutrition fluids can lead to mucosal atrophy following prolonged feeding. In addition, parenteral feeding can lead to a marked reduction in secretory IgA present in the gut and has been associated, in the absence of enteric stimulation, with increased bacterial translocation.[56] Alverdy et al.[56] demonstrated spontaneous bacterial translocation in 67 percent of rats fed parenterally for 2 weeks. Most evidence suggests that translocation in unfed animals is best explained by bacterial overgrowth secondary to slow gut motility rather than a defect in the mucosa itself.

Mechanisms of Translocation

Bacterial translocation appears to be facilitated by a combination of three clinical settings: (1) physical disruption of the gut mucosa (following hypotension), (2) decreased host immunity (following severe trauma or malnutrition), and (3) an abnormal or overgrown gut flora (following intestinal obstruction, broad spectrum antibiotics, or lack of dietary fiber). The precise mechanism leading to the migration of organisms through the gut wall is poorly understood. It should be emphasized, however, that translocation is a normal phenomenon,[48] the importance of which is increased in sick and immunocompromised patients.

Many pathogens penetrate the intestine and cause no intestinal pathology—listeriosis, brucellosis, salmonellosis, anthrax, toxoplasmosis, Q fever, polio, hepatitis A, and others. Omitted from this list are intestinal pathogens that cause lesions (shigellosis), organisms that cause local disease without systemic translocation (cholera), and organisms that produce exotoxins that are absorbed (botulism). In fact, the intestinal epithelium can be "penetrated" by inert particles like starch granules and latex beads.[48] Yeast has been shown by Alexander et al[58] to enter into small intestinal epithelial cells and pass through to the subepithelial layer; bacteria have been seen passing through intact cells since 1933.[48] When bacteria pass the intestinal barrier, they most often can be cultured from mesenteric lymph nodes.

Wells et al[59] have hypothesized an active uptake of bacteria by gut macrophages, transportation to extraintestinal sites, and then liberation following the death of the macrophages. This argument is based on the evidence that latex particles and fluorinated bacteria in the gut can be found inside macrophages in mesenteric nodes. The bacteria persist alive for some time. It is probably no coincidence that bacteria capable of translocating in normal animals tend to be obligate intracellular pathogens. Bacteria like *E. coli,* which are not obligate intracellular pathogens, also survive inside cells.[59] One can readily see how overgrowth of bacteria in the gut could, via a normal mechanism, induce systemic infection. Simply shifting the endogenous flora by intestinal obstruction or by antibiotics, which deplete the anaerobes responsible for colonization resistance, might permit translocation routinely. Only in those patients with impaired host defenses (eg, hepatic clearance, intracellular killing) would systemic infection ensue.

One cannot argue convincingly that the normal route of translocation is the route taken under conditions of stress in which the intestinal epithelial barrier may be disordered. Since the barrier is composed of normal gastric acid, motility, mucus, IgA, and bacterial receptors (plus many other factors), the mechanism of translocation in stress remains to be worked out. Of the more than 500 strains of bacteria in the normal gut, relatively few have been shown to translocate—*E. coli, K. pneumoniae,* other enterobacteria, *Pseudomonas aeruginosa,* enterococci, other streptococci, lactobacilli, staphylococci—no anaerobes, even though they predominate. The organisms seen are the same as those that invade stressed and immunosuppressed hosts.

Bacterial translocation from the gut is strongly implicated in the pathogenesis of extraintestinal systemic infections in patients with altered flora and compromised host defenses. An equally strong argument can be made for its role in the contamination of sites of inflammation adjacent to the gut, that is, vascular prostheses, sutures, areas of pancreatitis, wounds. Wells et al[60] first demonstrated that normal rats bearing intra-abdominal *Bacteroides*-infected fibrin clots became contaminated with *E. coli;* neither sterile clots in the abdomen nor *Bacteroides* clots in the subcutaneous tissue had a similar fate. Intraluminal latex beads also passed from the gut to peri-intestinal prosthetic biomaterials.[61] Thus translocation into inflammatory foci can occur. Phagocytes appear to engulf bacteria after they pass through the intestinal epithelial cells and transport the bacteria to an inflamed site nearby, thereby contaminating it.

Although bacterial translocation from the gut is important in the dissemination of bacteria and to the pathogenesis of extraintestinal infection, there is little evidence that it is responsible by itself for multiple organ failure in septic patients.

Selective Decontamination of the Digestive Tract

Infection in compromised patients is often derived from the gut, and gut defense against ingested pathogens is well maintained by the endogenous anaerobic flora. For these two reasons, van der Waaij and colleagues[62] devised a prophylactic approach designed to reduce the number of pathogens in the digestive tract while maintaining the anaerobic flora, which resist colonization. Selective decontamination of the digestive tract is designed to serve the purpose of infection prophylaxis in susceptible patients. Nonabsorbable antimicrobials are smeared on the mucosal surfaces of the mouth and nostrils and ingested at doses designed to suppress pathogenic gram-negative bacteria and yeast (*Candida*). The antibiotics are chosen to have no suppressive effect on gram-positive organisms or anaerobes. The narrow spectrum antimicrobials must act rapidly, must be nontoxic, and must be inactivated by intestinal contents.[62] Co-trimoxazole, the quinolones, aminoglycosides, polymyxins, and nystatin pass these criteria and all have been used. Norfloxacin plus nystatin, tobramycin, polymyxin, and nystatin has been used most frequently. The stool generally is freed of cultureable gram-negative enterics within a day. Systemic antibiotics are necessary to eliminate the bacteria in the glycocalyx. On theoretical grounds, van der Waaij et al[62] have reasoned that various groups of high-risk hospitalized patients may be subject to far fewer nosocomial gram-negative infections on such a prophylactic regimen. These include patients with hematologic malignancy, patients receiving chemotherapy for solid tumors, severe trauma patients on ventilatory assistance, burn patients, low birth weight infants, and liver and intestinal transplant patients.[62]

A number of randomized prospective blinded trials have been carried out in high-risk patients, usually critically ill patients in intensive care units.[63–65] Certain results have been consistently noted. Most studies show significant reduction in nosocomial gram-negative infections, especially pneumonia[63]; a few show no such effect.[64] Most show no decrease in the incidence of gram-positive infections, as predicted. Many studies show that surviving patients have shorter stays in the intensive care unit. Only a few studies show a significantly decreased mortality.

The usual protocol involves the short-term use of a broad spectrum systemic antimicrobial, such as intravenous cefotaxime[63] plus a combination of polymyxin, an aminoglycoside, and nystatin applied to the oropharynx and enterally. Some studies have omitted the systemic antibiotics. A few have substituted oral norfloxacin (or polymyxin and aminoglycoside), but these show little effect.[64]

It remains controversial whether these techniques or their slight modifications will significantly affect mortality. All agree that neutropenic patients should have some kind of selective decontamination (see Chap. 51). There is great fear, however, that these patients are so sick and so susceptible to all types of infection that the technique will be ineffective, and multiple resistant nosocomial pathogens will emerge.[64]

INFECTIONS OF THE ESOPHAGUS

The esophagus serves as a conduit through which food passes from the hypopharynx to the stomach. Food and saliva contaminated by mouth organisms pass through the esophagus many times a day. The microbes found in the esophagus, then, are those organisms that have been carried down from the mouth. The esophagus is almost entirely free of infectious problems. The main infection seen is mediastinitis as a result of esophageal perforation or rupture (see Chap. 35). Primary infections of the esophagus tend to occur only in compromised hosts. *Candida,* herpes simplex virus, and cytomegalovirus (CMV) are most commonly seen.[66] They usually do not require surgical treatment but may cause pain, significant bleeding,[67] and perforation, if they occur elsewhere in the gastrointestinal tract.

Perforations of the Esophagus

Perforation of the esophagus is discussed in Chapter 35.[68–72] The major cause of perforation is instrumentation. In one series of 199 perforations, 137 (70 percent) were caused by instrumentation. Endoscopy has a perforation rate of 0.2 to 0.5 percent; the rate is less with the flexible endoscope than with rigid instruments. Dilations are accompanied by a perforation rate of 1.0 to 1.5 percent. Other causes of perforation are postemetic (spontaneous) (12 percent), paraesophageal surgery (10 percent), penetrating trauma (5 percent), foreign body (3 percent), and blunt trauma (2 percent). The site of perforation is cervical esophagus (39 percent), upper thoracic esophagus (12 percent), lower thoracic esophagus (40 percent), and abdominal esophagus (10 percent).

Infection Caused by Perforation. Perforation of the esophagus allows food and saliva contaminated by oral microorganisms to contaminate the neck, mediastinum, or abdomen. Perforation of the esophagus also allows microbes to enter the paravertebral space, which extends from the base of the skull to the diaphragm, and infection of the entire space can occur. Perforation of the anterolateral wall of the esophagus or pyriform sinus allows the infection to extend anteriorly into the pretracheal space. The infection can extend from the pretracheal space into the thorax. If the esophagus is perforated immediately above the diaphragm, the pleural space can be entered, resulting in empyema because the pleurae, especially the left one, are immediately adjacent to the esophagus. Perforation of the abdominal esophagus results in peritonitis. Discussion of infectious problems of these different spaces can be found in Chapters 33, 35, and 38. Of course, leaking anastomoses in these same regions can give rise to similar space infections. Because these infections are caused by mixed anaerobic and aerobic organisms, they can be rapidly necrotizing, leading to gangrene of the esophagus or eroding into the pleura, lung, and even major blood vessels. Infected lacerations of the esophageal mucosa can even result in direct extension of the inflammation without actual perforation. With slower developing perforations, such as those that occur with esophageal carcinomas, fistulas into the trachea, bronchus, and pleural spaces can develop.

Treatment. A thorough discussion of the treatment of esophageal perforations can be found elsewhere.[73] In general, the treatment depends on the size and rapidity of perforation. With large perforations there is immediate and continuous pouring of food, saliva, and bacteria into the mediastinum or abdomen. With postemetic perforations (Boerhaave's syndrome), there is forceful ejection and flooding of the mediastinum with food, bacteria, and irritating gastric juices. On the other hand, with some instrumental or foreign body perforations, the hole in the esophagus may be small and the leak is not continuous. In most esophageal perforations, there is no fibrosis to stop the free dissection of the inflammatory process, but with some perforations the esophageal penetration occurs slowly so that fibrosis and sealing off occur, which prevent free spread of the infection. Perforation of tumors by instruments, however, is usually into the open mediastinum. Strictures occurring after lye ingestion can be accompanied by surrounding fibrosis, which may limit the spread of infection as a result of perforation after dilation.

Most esophageal perforations should be repaired operatively and the surrounding area drained. Perforations of the lower and abdominal esophagus should all be operated on. A trial of nonoperative treatment can be done in selected circumstances *provided the patient is followed closely:* (1) when the perforation occurs high in the neck when there is no continuing leak of air or fluid; (2) when the perforation in the cervical region is due to a sharp foreign body, such as a pin or fishbone, if the object has been removed; (3) when the patient is not seen until several days after the perforation, has no fever, leukocytosis, or radiographic evidence of spreading infection, and has minimal symptoms; (4) when a suspected diagnosis of perforation cannot be proved and the symptoms are minimal; and (5) perforation results from chronic lye stricture. Most patients with esophageal perforation do not meet these requirements and need operation. If symptoms persist, a fever continues or develops, or the white blood cell (WBC) count remains elevated, however, prompt operation should be carried out, to direct the salivary and refluxing gastric fluids and to drain the mediastinum and pleura. Despite operative antibiotic therapy, the mortality rate from esophageal perforation remains high (9 to 49 percent).

Candida *Esophagitis*

Incidence. Candida (monilial) esophagitis usually occurs in patients with compromised host defenses. It is found in patients with malignant neoplasms—especially the lymphoproliferative disorders—who have received radiation therapy or chemotherapy, in persons treated with antibiotics, and in some patients with chronic disorders such as diabetes mellitus, especially after renal transplantation, aplastic anemia, and commonly in congenital and acquired immune deficiency states. Only rarely is it found in otherwise healthy persons who have received antibiotics. *Candida* can occur as a part of the normal flora of the mouth and gastrointestinal tract but overgrowth is prevented by competing bacteria. When this bacterial population is reduced by antibiotic therapy or the balance is altered by malignant neoplasms or chronic diseases, invasive growth of *Candida* can occur.

Pathology. Candida esophagitis is characterized by a pseudomembrane that contains yeasts, hyphae, and necrotic debris. The esophageal mucosa is ulcerated and inflamed and bleeds easily. Microscopically, the esophageal wall is inflamed. Perforation is rare, but stenosis can be a result.

Clinical Features. Esophageal spasm results in dysphagia and retrosternal pain on swallowing. Gastrointestinal bleeding can accompany esophageal ulceration and necrosis in patients receiving cancer chemotherapy.[74] These patients frequently have concurrent oral candidiasis, but oral candidiasis is usually completely painless. Any patient receiving antibiotics, steroids, or chemotherapeutic agents who complains of dysphagia should be suspected of having *Candida* esophagitis. The differential diagnosis involves gastroesophageal reflux with esophagitis, cytomegalovirus, or herpes simplex virus infection.

Diagnosis. A barium study of the esophagus is rarely indicated but will show the typical pseudomembrane with ulcerations and pseudopolypoid changes comparable to that seen in the colon in patients with ulcerative colitis. Esophagoscopy shows a yellow to white pseudomembrane, ulcers, and marked inflammation. A biopsy of the pseudomembrane will show typical mycelia mixed with necrotic debris and bacteria. Viral esophagitis usually presents with vesicular changes. The presence of viral inclusions makes the diagnosis. *Candida* and viral esophagitis can coexist.

Treatment. Topical treatment often suffices. Mycostatin (nystatin) 400,000 to 600,000 units four times a day for 10 days is satisfactory. Clotrimazole and miconazole also work. Improvement is usually prompt, and the dysphagia lessens in 24 to 48 hours. The radiographic appearance returns to normal in about 7 days. Systemic amphotericin B and oral fluconazole are recommended for more severely immunosuppressed patients or for those who do not respond promptly. Only brief courses of systemic therapy are usually required unless systemic candidosis is also present.[75] If the underlying susceptibility persists (eg, the diabetic post-transplant patient), prophylactic long-term mycostatin prophylaxis will be necessary to prevent recurrence.

INFECTIONS OF THE STOMACH

Helicobacter Pylori, *Gastritis, and Peptic Ulceration.*

Methods to reduce gastric acid have dominated the treatment of peptic ulcer disease for decades. Medical methods have generally superceded surgical approaches to peptic ulceration uncomplicated by bleeding, perforation, or obstruction. All medical methods are associated with a high incidence of recurrence. In 1983, Warren and Marshall[76] added another dimension to the peptic ulcer story with their description of a spiral bacterium in the stomach of patients with gastritis. They described spiral-shaped gram-negative rods cultured in a microaerophilic environment on chocolate or blood agar. Initially designated *Campylobacter pylori,* subsequent rRNA sequencing revealed it to be a new genus for which a new name, *Helicobacter pylori* (*H. pylori*), was coined.

Epidemiology. The organism is motile and has flagella at one pole. The organism produces abundant urease catalyzing urea to ammonia, an important characteristic.[77] Most *H. pylori* infections are asymptomatic and a useful rule of thumb is that its prevalence increases 1 percent per year of life in Western societies. Lower socioeconomic status is associated with a higher prevalence so that infection is almost universal in developing countries. The fecal-oral route of transmission is most likely.[78]

Pathology. There seems to be no question that *H. pylori* causes the histologic changes of chronic gastritis. *Helicobacter pylori* is primarily found in the gastric antrum but tends to colonize gastric metaplasia in the duodenum, fundus, and esophagus. The organism lives in the gastric mucus, and the spiral shape of the organism is thought to allow it to corkscrew through the gastric mucus. *Helicobacter pylori* seeks out the intercellular junctions of mucus-secreting cells of the gastric antral epithelium.[79] The precise mechanism by which *H. pylori* causes local injury is not known, but it clearly elicits an acute and chronic inflammatory change in the lamina propria, especially of the gastric antrum. The organism is capable of elaborating extracellular material and cytotoxins plus ammonia, which degrade mucus glycoprotein polymers and are capable of destroying cultured cells in vitro. Because nonprotective antibodies are found in victims, an autoimmune hypothesis has been proposed to explain the pathogenesis of gastritis.

Ingestion causes an acute transient gastritis followed by a year-long period of hypochlorhydria. Gastric secretion remains high. Wherever the organism is found, a chronic, usually asymptomatic gastritis is found as well.

Diagnosis. There are a number of diagnostic techniques available to establish the presence of *H. pylori.* The gold standard is considered to be culture of endoscopically retrieved biopsy material with incubation on blood, chocolate, or Thayer-Martin plates. Histology of multiple biopsies also provides an accurate diagnostic tool, as does the more recent use of brush cytology. The urease-producing activity of *H. pylori* provides alternative methods of diagnosis. Metabolism of urea to ammonia results in a pH change that can be utilized as diagnostic indicator in modified culture plates. In a similar manner, ^{13}C- and ^{14}C-labeled urea administered orally can be used in a breath test to indicate *H. pylori* urease activity. Finally, ELISA kits are currently available to test for specific antibodies. This provides a highly sensitive and specific means of large-scale diagnostic testing.

Clinical Presentation. Type B gastritis is almost universally associated with *H. pylori* infection. Although it was argued that *H. pylori* infection was a marker rather than the cause of gastric inflammation, current evidence would suggest otherwise. When *H. pylori* is present, there is almost always evidence of gastritis; eradication of the organism is followed by resolution of the inflammation, and ingestion of *H. pylori* in a noninfected host led not only to local infection by *H. pylori* but also to evidence of gastritis.[80]

Though a causal link with gastritis is probable, such evidence is not as convincing in the case of peptic ulcer disease or gastric cancer. Much of the evidence is at best circumstantial. The increase in incidence of gastric ulcers with advancing age could be correlated with the increasing incidence of *H. pylori* infection. However, it could equally be associated with increasing use of NSAIDs with advancing age and joint disease. Likewise, the evidence for an association between *H. pylori* and duodenal ulcers relies largely on the important finding in almost all studies that eradication of the infection, in addition to healing the ulcer, reduces the incidence of recurrent ulcer disease. Hentschel et al[81] recently published a randomized, prospective trial that 8 percent of patients receiving H_2 blockade and anti-*H. pylori* antibiotics developed a recurrent ulcer at 1 year follow-up, compared to 42 percent of patients who received just H_2 blockade.

Blaser[77] has summarized several reports of a similar type (Table 42–1). Thus most data suggest that *H. pylori* is important in the pathogenesis of peptic ulcer. There is equally convincing epidemiologic evidence that it is not involved in nonulcer gastric dyspepsia.[77]

Treatment. The organism is sensitive in vitro to penicillin, amoxicillin, quinolone, and aminoglycoside and many other antibiotics. Metronidazole, a first-line treatment drug, leads to the rapid development of resistance if used alone.[77]

For many years, bismuth preparations have been associated with peptic ulcer treatment. Recently, it has been shown that this may be due to its direct anti-*H. pylori* effect. Although bismuth is effective at eradication of *H. pylori* in the short term, it has an almost 100 percent recurrent infection rate on stopping treatment. Chronic control is therefore best achieved with antibiotic administration. Currently, recommended regimens are listed in Table 42–2. Omeprazole, in addition to its antiacid effect, is effective against *H. pylori.*

Safe and effective treatment is available. The question is who should be treated and for how long. Studies are underway to test the efficacy of treatment for nonulcer dyspepsia and patients at high risk for gastric cancer. The only current indications are for patients with refractory peptic ulcer disease; it is not useful for Zollinger-Ellison syndrome.

Suppurative Gastritis. Spontaneous infections of the normal stomach are almost unknown because its acid environment is virtually sterile. Almost all infections arise in achlorhydric stomachs or by extension from contiguous extragastric sources. Indeed, suppurative gastritis is a condition so rare that a worldwide incidence of 2.5 cases/year has been estimated. Obviously, many cases go unreported. The most severe form, emphysematous gastritis, was once considered to be uniformly fatal. Survival is said to have increased from 16 percent in 1938 to 67 percent in 1970.[82]

Etiology. Numerous organisms have been cultured, but 70 percent of patients have alpha-hemolytic

TABLE 42–1. EFFECTS OF ERADICATION OF *H. PYLORI* ON RATES OF RELAPSE OF DUODENAL ULCERS, ON THE BASIS OF PUBLISHED REPORTS

First Author of Study	Follow-up Period (months)	Duodenal Ulcer Relapse: *H. pylori* + N[a]	%[b]	*H. pylori* − N	%[b]
Coghlan (1987)	12	29	76	10	10
Marshall (1988)	12	47	81[c]	23	23[c]
Borody (1989)	9–37	4	75	54	0
Rauws (1990)	12	21	81	17	0
George (1990)	12–48	0	NA	62	0
Graham (1992)	12	36	95	40	0

+, infected; −, uninfected; NA, not applicable.
[a] Number of subjects in whom *H. pylori* organisms were detected 1 month after therapy was discontinued.
[b] Percentage of subjects whose ulcer disease relapsed during the prolonged follow-up period.
[c] Includes patients whose symptoms recurred with no endoscopic confirmation of duodenal ulcer.
From Blaser MJ: Clin Infect Dis 15:386, 1992.

TABLE 42–2. SUMMARY OF SEVERAL REGIMENS USEFUL FOR ERADICATION OF *H. PYLORI* INFECTION

Agents	Oral Dosage for Adults	Eradication Rate Achieved with Regimen
Pepto-Bismol[a]	2 tablets qid for 14 days	
Plus metronidazole	250 mg tid for 14 days	69–96%
Plus amoxicillin	250–500 mg tid for 14 days	
Or tetracycline	500 mg qid for 14 days	
Omeprazole	40 mg bid × 10 days then 20 mg bid for 32 days	58–82%
Plus amoxicillin	1 g bid for 10 days	

[a] Product of Proctor & Gamble, Cincinnati. Active ingredient is bismuth subsalicylate.
Adapted from Blaser MJ: Clin Infect Dis 15:386, 1992.

streptococci in the stomach. Suppurative gastritis due to *Streptococcus pneumoniae* has been associated with pneumonia and endocarditis. Other organisms include *Staphylococcus, E. coli,* and, more rarely, *Proteus vulgaris* and *C. perfringens.*[83] *Clostridium perfringens* is most commonly associated with emphysematous gastritis.

Pathogenesis and Pathology. Predisposing factors include chronic gastritis, hypoacidity, infections elsewhere in the body, and the debilitated, immunosuppressed state. Emphysematous gastritis is most often associated with gastric ischemia such as that which occurs with gastric cancer, corrosive gastritis, and preceding gastric operation. Pathologic findings include a congested edematous gastric wall with gangrene and pockets of pus. Submucosal blebs of gas may be present under the mucosa in emphysematous gastritis.

Clinical Manifestations. Patients usually present with the sudden onset of abdominal pain, nausea, vomiting, and the physical findings of an acute abdomen. Purulent emesis, though rare, is pathognomonic, and in emphysematous gastritis an entire gastric mucosal cast may be vomited. Fever, chills, prostration, and bacteremia are frequent, and peritonitis rapidly ensues. The radiographic findings in the usual case of suppurative gastritis are nonspecific. In emphysematous gastritis, however, bubbles can be seen in the thickened stomach wall. Submucosal gas blebs and intramucosal penetration of contrast medium along intramural sinus tracts can be seen on upper gastrointestinal radiographic series. The differential diagnosis must include pneumatosis cystoides intestinalis and traumatic emphysema of the stomach.

Treatment. The usual treatment has been gastric resection and antibiotics. Near total gastrectomy is required for emphysematous gastritis. There are few survivors who have recovered with antimicrobial treatment alone; most have required gastric resection. One would expect that agents effective against gram-positive cocci or clostridia would be most efficacious. In the absence of careful bacterial studies, however, one must assume that a mixed oral and colonic flora will be found. Therefore a combination of an aminoglycoside, clindamycin, and massive doses of penicillin seem rational. Many other agents have also been used with success.

Prognosis. Death is common, but increasing numbers of survivors are seen. In the rare survivor without gastric resection, cicatricial constriction of the stomach may result.

Gastric Diverticulitis. Gastric diverticulitis is a rare complication of a rare condition. A gastric diverticulum is found in only 0.004 percent of hospital admissions, is most often asymptomatic, is rarely subject to obstruction, and occurs at a site where bacterial contamination is minimal. The complications of hemorrhage and perforation are likely not related to previous obstruction.[84]

Gastric Mycosis. Gastric fungal balls have been reported after gastric surgery.[85] Only one of these patients had a vagotomy. These patients were not taking antibiotics, steroids, or immunosuppressive agents and had no systemic diseases to account for the proliferation of *Candida* in their stomachs. All were achlorhydric, except one who had narrowing of the surgical anastomosis. The fungal ball is not really an infection, but rather a bezoar. There are reports of candidal ulceration, perforation and fistula formation in achlorhydric stomachs of dehydrated hosts.

Granulomas of the Stomach. A variety of infectious and noninfectious granulomas of the stomach can occur. Noninfectious granulomatous diseases of the stomach include sarcoidosis, Crohn's disease, eosinophilic granuloma, and isolated nonspecific granulomas. Infectious granulomas of the stomach can be due to tuberculosis, syphilis, histoplasmosis, and eosinophilic granulomas associated with nematode larvae.[86–90]

Tuberculosis. Gastric tuberculosis occurs in less than 0.6 percent of patients who die of tuberculosis and is rarely, if ever, seen in patients without severe primary or systemic tuberculosis.[81] Like all gastric granulomas, the symptoms are nonspecific and include epigastric pain, vomiting, weight loss, weakness, hematemesis, and gastric outlet obstruction. As with all gastric infections, hypochlorhydria or achlorhydria is common. X-ray studies reveal gastric ulceration, tumor, stenosis of the pylorus and antrum, constricting lesions, concurrent duodenal involvement, and a picture resembling linitis plastica. Gastric cytology can be confusing. In tuberculosis of the stomach, fistula formation and ulceration of the antrum may be confused with Crohn's disease. The diagnosis depends on demonstration of either acid-fast bacilli or caseating granulomas in the stomach by endoscopic or open biopsy. Organisms are rarely cultured from gastric washings in gastric tuberculosis. Antibiotic therapy is effective for gastric tuberculosis and surgery should be used only for the complications of stricture, fistula, stenosis, and ulcers. Gastric tuberculosis can give rise to carcinoma.

Syphilis. Tertiary syphilis rarely affects the stomach. The diagnosis is dependent on biopsy evidence of granulomatous gastritis, a diagnosis of untreated tertiary syphilis, a defect seen on radiographic examination of the stomach, gastric symptoms, and biopsy evidence of a fibrosing obliterative panvasculitis. Most diagnostic radiographic findings include the so-called hour-glass stomach and large shallow ulcerations. Differentiation from extensive involvement of the stomach with cancer may be difficult. Penicillin is the treatment, but the response may be slow so that the suspicion of cancer may grow. If healing is progressing well and a definitive diagnosis of cancer cannot be made, operation should be delayed. Secondary syphilis may be accompanied by syphilitic gastritis—the mucosa is hyperemic, edematous, and friable.

Histoplasmosis. The stomach is rarely involved in disseminated histoplasmosis, though occasionally patients treated with amphotericin B may present with lesions of the fundus and cardia of the stomach, which resemble carcinoma, but biopses reveal noncaseating granulomas. Special stains will demonstrate the organism (see Chap. 9). Although the disease can be cured with amphotericin B, fibrosis and stricture may result in persistent gastric lesions and obstruction.[88]

Differential Diagnosis of Granulomas of Unknown Etiology. Granulomatous disease of the stomach of unknown etiology must always be considered to represent sarcoidosis or Crohn's disease. In the absence of other evidence of these diseases, the diagnosis of isolated sarcoid or isolated Crohn's disease is doubtful. Such patients are frequently considered to have isolated granulomatous gastritis until other systemic involvement appears. Because no case of isolated granulomatous gastritis that evolved into Crohn's disease or sarcoidosis has been described, isolated eosinophilic gastric granulomatosis must be considered a separate entity. In Japan the eating of raw fish permits the larvae of *Anisakis* species (a nematode) to penetrate the human gastric mucosa and establish a symptomatic ulcerating eosinophilic granulomatous reaction. Resection is necessary for the diagnosis, which is made by microscopic examination (see Chap. 8).[87]

Infectious Complications After Gastric Surgery. The wound infections that follow gastric surgery are similar to wound infections following all clean-contaminated operations (see Chap. 22). The more common intraperitoneal infections of subphrenic, subhepatic, and intra-abdominal abscess also follow gastric surgery (see Chap. 38). The incidence is low after elective surgery for duodenal ulcer. Gardner et al[89] reported an overall wound infection rate of only 3.3 percent for elective gastric surgery. However, the incidence increases markedly for emergency surgery, especially that performed for massive bleeding or perforation. Snyder and Stellar[90] reported a wound infection rate of 10 percent in a large series of patients with duodenal ulcers on whom emergency surgery was performed. Rapid overgrowth of oral bacteria within the gastric blood clots and hemorrhagic shock probably account for the increased rate of sepsis in patients undergoing emergency surgery for hemorrhage. A similar increased rate is seen after surgery for chronic pyloric obstruction, which appears to permit bacterial growth secondary to gastric stasis. In patients with gastric ulcer, gastric cancer, or those recovering from operations on achlorhydric or hypochlorhydric stomachs, septic complications can be extremely common because these stomachs are not sterile and may be obstructed or contain necrotic tissue. To minimize infectious complications, the hypochlorhydric or obstructed stomach should be lavaged with either antibiotics or povidone-iodine before operation. In emergencies, gastric lavage with povidone-iodine (1:10 dilution) can be carried out just prior to, or during, the operation. In patients with gastric carcinoma, a colonic bowel prep should be carried out if there is any possibility that a portion of the transverse colon will be resected. Systemic perioperative antibiotic prophylaxis should be used in patients with achlorhydria, gastric carcinoma, or obstruction (see Chap. 25). Since almost all elective gastric operations take place in the presence of previous or concurrent antacid therapy, perioperative prophylaxis should probably be practiced.

Subphrenic and Intra-abdominal Abscess After Gastric Surgery. Sherman and associates[91] reported that subphrenic abscess followed 1.4 percent of 3000 gastric operations. This figure is consistent with other series. Most such abscesses appear because of leakage at the suture lines, especially duodenal stump dehiscence.

Late and Persistent Postgastrectomy Infections. Pulmonary tuberculosis and *Salmonella* enteritis seem to occur with increased frequency after gastric resection.[92] The increased susceptibility of the latter may be caused by the lack of the protective effect of gastric acidity. Prophylactic isoniazid has even been recommended for patients undergoing gastrectomy. Gastric overgrowth syndromes are also common after Billroth II operations with anemia, steatorrhea, diarrhea, and malabsorption syndromes, even though the most common reason for anemia is iron deficiency associated with decreased iron intake, increased gastrointestinal blood loss, and malabsorption of dietary or organic iron in the achlorhydric patient whose duodenum has been bypassed.

Infections of the Upper Small Intestine

Jejunal Diverticulitis

Incidence. Diverticulosis of the jejunum is generally an asymptomatic condition, but it may produce a variety of confusing syndromes, which are surgically correctable. In a group of 62 patients with jejunal diverticulosis seen by Altmeier et al,[93] symptomatic complications occurred in 16, but only two developed inflammation, with one perforation and death. Symptomatic diverticula are rarely seen before age 60.

Pathogenesis and Pathology. Acquired jejunal diverticula appear as thin-walled, round, elliptical, or multilobulated sacs continuous with the walls of the intestine and extending between the leaves of the mesentery. The opening into each diverticulum is usually large but may vary from a few millimeters to 3 cm in diameter. The large ostium and the fluid contents of the duodenum and jejunum make conditions unfavorable for inspissation and prolonged retention of material within the lumen. The wall of the diverticulum consists largely of fibromucosal tissue and consequently lacks the muscular motor power to effectively empty its contents. The most frequent involvement is in the proximal jejunum and the larger diverticula are found near the duodenal-jejunal flexure just proximal or distal to the ligament of Treitz. Multiple diverticula are usually in continuity, although skip areas may occur, and the entire length of the small intestine may occasionally be involved. If partly distended with air and fluid, the sacs are easily seen, but when empty they may be overlooked or their true extent not appreciated. Concomitant duodenal diverticula are present in about 20 percent of patients and ileal diverticula in 10 percent.

Manifestations. Most patients have no symptoms, but six clinical syndromes have been discussed by Altmeier et al[93]: (1) acute inflammation, (2) hemorrhage, (3) intestinal malabsorption, (4) chronic *dyskinesia,* (5) acute high intestinal obstruction, and (6) spontaneous pneumoperitoneum (one patient). The malabsorption syndrome appears to be identical with the bowel overgrowth syndromes discussed elsewhere in this chapter. Neither the acute nor the chronic obstructive symptoms are related to infection. Rare cases of jejunal diverticulitis occur in elderly patients with acute pain and tenderness progressing to peritonitis. It is not known whether obstruction to the diverticulum orifice, vascular compromise, or bowel infection is important.

Treatment. Chronic symptoms are best treated symptomatically, or with resection if severe or if a blind loop syndrome appears. Emergency operation, resection, and treatment of the peritonitis are necessary for acute diverticulitis or hemorrhage. Antibiotics have not been shown to be helpful in the prophylaxis or treatment of the underlying condition. Antibiotics are almost certainly useful for the treatment of acute peritonitis.

Approach to Diarrhea in the Surgical Patient. Diarrhea is a common complication of surgery, but a less common indication for consultation with a surgeon, who is asked to see patients with diarrhea associated with bleeding, perforation, possible obstruction, or toxic colitis. Thus infectious diarrhea is of less interest to surgeons.

Nevertheless, pinpointing the cause of the diarrhea can minimize morbidity. Several tests are of value. (1) Fecal leukocyte examination, preferably using mucus, is important. Presence of many leukocytes indicates inflammation, whereas a negative result indicates a virus, parasite, or toxin. Diarrhea of small bowel origin lacks leukocytes. (2) Parasites can be found if sought. *Giardia, Entamoeba,* and *Cryptosporidium* are the most important in the United States. (3) Stool culture is important even in cases of diarrhea during the postoperative period. *Salmonella, Shigella, Campylobacter, Yersinia,* and *C. difficile* should always be sought. (4) Virus culture is of little import to surgeons even though cytomegalovirus colitis occurs in surgical patients. (5) Proctosigmoidoscopy is important in suspected *C. difficile* colitis and amebiasis.

The homosexual male who practices receptive anal intercourse can present with diarrhea at any time due to *Neisseria gonorrhoeae,* herpes simplex virus, *Chlamydia trachomatis,* or *Treponema pallidum.* AIDS patients present with *Cryptosporidium, Isosporia,* cytomegalovirus, *Salmonella, Mycobacterium,* and herpes simplex virus.

A common cause of diarrhea in postoperative surgical patients is caused by antibiotics that alter the normal flora. *Clostridium difficile* need not be present. Similarly, the use of magnesium antacids, laxatives, and other drugs can lead to similar symptoms.

Diarrhea is best defined as "loose stools," because the surgeon encounters it as a transient symptom, that is, a lesser part of a complex of symptoms and signs, more often than as the predominant problem. Diarrhea is considered mild if three or fewer loose stools are passed per day, and severe if more than 200 g are passed or if cramps or systemic symptoms (fever, dehydration) accompany it.[94]

The historic context for the differential diagnosis is important. Has the patient been traveling? Is the diarrhea associated with drugs? Antibiotic-associated diarrhea is probably the most common diarrhea encountered by the surgeon in postoperative patients, but laxatives, magnesium-containing antacids, and chemotherapeutic drugs are common. Is the patient at risk for AIDS? Is the patient part of a cluster of others exposed to a common source, for example, meats contaminated with enteropathogenic *E. coli*?[94]

The character of the diarrhea is of some diagnostic significance. A few voluminous stools per day generally suggests a small bowel origin consistent with enteropathogenic *E. coli* and cholera. By contrast, multiple small stools are usually of large bowel origin, characteristic of *C. difficile* or infectious colitis (*Shigella, Salmonella, Campylobacter*). Tenesmus suggests colitis. Mucus in large quantities suggests infectious diarrhea; blood suggests invasive disease. Fever tends to accompany infections.

A common dilemma faced by a surgical consultant is the patient with diarrhea and abdominal pain. Most surgeons fail to rule out infectious causes of diarrhea. Several simple tests are sometimes helpful. Many leukocytes in the fecal mucus indicates mucosal inflammation in the colon. Small bowel diarrhea, a virus, or a toxin give a negative result. The stools should be examined for parasites on three or more specimens if this diagnosis is suspected. Stools should be cultured to identify the common pathogen—*Shigella, Salmonella, Campylobacter, Yersinia,* or *C. difficile.* A positive *C. difficile* culture is not diagnostic; the toxin must also be present. Proctosigmoidoscopy in patients with a history of loose stools, with or without systemic toxicity, will hasten the diagnosis of *C. difficile* colitis (see Chap. 43).[94]

Diarrhea requires treatment for dehydration, if present (Table 42–3). Symptomatic treatment is contraindicated in patients with *C. difficile* colitis or other febrile diarrheas, but bismuth subsalicylate and loperamide-like drugs will reduce the volume of stools in most diarrheal disease. Specific antimicrobial treatment is effective for *Shigella, Campylobacter jejuni* enterocolitis, traveler's diarrhea, giardiasis, amebiasis, and *C. difficile.*

Infectious Enteropathies

Bacterial Diarrheas. It has become customary to distinguish the *dysenteric* or inflammatory syndromes from the *choleric* or secretory syndromes. The inflammatory syndromes are characterized by abdominal cramps with blood and pus in the stool, whereas the secretory syndromes are characterized by profuse watery diarrhea.[95] The secretory syndromes are caused by organisms that elaborate an exotoxin (enterotoxin, pharmacotoxin) that stimulates intestinal secretion without actual invasion of the mucosa.[96,97] The classic example, cholera toxin, is heat labile, water soluble, and antigenic. It probably binds to a site on the mucosal side of the cell and stimulates secretion. In addition to *Vibrio cholerae,* enterotoxins that cause secretory diarrheas are also produced by *E. coli, Staphylococcus aureus, C. perfringens,* and *Shigella dysenteriae.* The in-

TABLE 42–3. ANTIMICROBIAL AGENTS AND RECOMMENDED THERAPY IN INFECTIOUS DIARRHEAL DISEASES

Diagnosis	Drug	Dosage
Shigellosis	Trimethoprim-sulfamethoxazole	160 mg TMP/800 mg SMX bid for 3 days
	Norfloxacin	400 mg bid for 3 days
	Ciprofloxacin	500 mg bid for 3 days
Clostridium jejuni enterocolitis	Norfloxacin	400 mg bid for 5 days
	Ciprofloxacin	500 mg bid for 5 days
	Erythromycin	500 mg pid for 5 days
Traveler's diarrhea	As for *Shigella*	
Giardiasis	Quinacrine	100 mg tid for 7 days
	Metronidazole	250 mg tid for 10 days
	Furazolidone	100 mg tid for 7 days
Amebiasis	Metronidazole *plus*	750 mg tid for 5 days
	Diiodohydroxyquin	650 mg tid for 21 days
C. difficile	Vancomycin	500 mg tid for 7–10 days
	Metronidazole	500 mg qid for 7–10 days

Adapted from Bandres JC, Dupont HL: Approach to the patient with diarrhea. In Gorbach SL, Bartlett JG, Blacklow NR (eds): Infectious Diseases. Philadelphia, Saunders, 1992, p 574.

flammatory syndromes, on the other hand, are caused by organisms that invade and destroy the mucosa by means of cytotoxins. Although some species of *Salmonella* work their damage on the gut by invasion alone without enterotoxin production, most organisms that cause dysentery (eg, most species of *Shigella*) produce both cytotoxins and enterotoxins, and the illness produced is both inflammatory and secretory. *Campylobacter fetus* subspecies *jejuni* and *Yersinia* can also cause inflammatory diarrhea.[98,99]

These toxins should not be confused with bacterial endotoxins, which are lipopolysaccharide components of the bacterial cell wall. Intestinal endotoxins have nothing to do with invasion or intestinal secretion, but endotoxin may be absorbed from the gut during invasion by bacteria and contribute to systemic illness. Endotoxemia from the small bowel most commonly occurs when ischemic or gangrenous bowel is invaded by anaerobic species. As this book is devoted to infectious diseases of primary relevance to surgeons, this interesting group of diseases are summarized without elaborate detail (Tables 42–4 and 42–5). The reader may find more comprehensive discussions of these diseases in other sources.[100,101] The only bacterial enteropathies with important, though rare, operative indications are those caused by *Salmonella typhi* and *Clostridium*.

Typhoid Fever. Typhoid fever is an acute febrile disease caused by *S. typhi,* although other *Salmonella* organisms can produce an identical clinical picture with fever, headache, apathy, prostration, cough, splenomegaly, rash, leukopenia, and diarrhea. Several important surgical complications occur.

Etiology. Typhoid fever is spread by food or drink contaminated by human excreta from a patient or an asymptomatic carrier. It is seen principally in areas of the world with poor standards of sanitation, but several hundred cases are reported in the United States yearly. The carrier state is more frequent in women.

Pathogenesis and Pathology. Enteric *S. typhi* organisms pass from the intestinal lumen to the regional lymphoid tissue, where they are phagocytized but not killed. The pathologic hallmark is the proliferation of large mononuclear cells involving the lymphoid tissue of the gastrointestinal tract, particularly the terminal ileum. The bacteria multiply intracellularly, seed the blood, and infect the biliary tract. The organisms are then poured back into the gut and appear in stool during the second week of the illness. Typhoid perforations usually occur in the last 12 inches of the terminal ileum. The perforations are usually 5 to 10 mm in diameter and oriented in the long axis of the gut on its antimesenteric border. The edges of the perforations are edematous, but the margin is usually not so friable that it will not hold sutures. When typhoid perforations of the ileum occur, the abdomen is usually distended with 3 to 4 liters of purulent material or feces.

Clinical Manifestations. Typhoid fever has an incubation period of 1 to 2 weeks and a course of 3 to 4 weeks. Fever and headache are the first signs. The

TABLE 42–4. DISTRIBUTION AND PREVALENCE OF BACTERIAL DIARRHEAS

		In North America		In Developing Countries	
Causative Organism	**General Distribution**	*Age Group Principally Affected*	*Transmission Patterns*	*Age Group Principally Affected*	*Transmission Patterns*
Shigella	Global	Children	Custodial institutions	0–6 years	Direct contact
E. coli	Global	Newborn	Hospital nursery	0–6 years ?Adults	Direct contact ?Direct contact
V. cholerae	Asia and contiguous areas	—	—	0–10 years All ages	Epidemic Water; ?food (epidemic)
V. parahemolyticus	Japan; ?elsewhere	Adults	Raw shellfish	?	?Raw seafood
Salmonella	Global	All	Prepared foods; poultry; egg products	All	Food-borne; direct contact
C. perfringens	?Global	Adults	Cooked meat	Children; nonimmune adults	Pork feasts ("pigbel")
Staphylococci	Industrialized nations	All	Prepared foods	—	(Rare)

From Grady GF, Keusch GT: N Engl J Med 285:831, 1971.

rash of typhoid is described as rose-colored spots on the upper abdomen. Splenomegaly and leukopenia are typical. Diarrhea is not a prominent symptom early in the course of the disease—in fact, constipation is a common complaint, though mild diarrhea occurs. During the second week of fever, diarrhea is more common and may be bloody, but vomiting and abdominal pain are more typical. Tenderness with guarding in the right lower quadrant and increasing distention suggest impending or perforated disease. Severe hemorrhage occurs in about 2 percent of patients and perforation in 1 percent. Perforation is the most serious complication and is frequently preceded by minor or major episodes of bleeding. Pain, tenderness, and local guarding precede signs of generalized peritonitis. In areas where typhoid is endemic, the diagnosis is rarely problematic. For example, at a hospital in Haiti where the disease is

TABLE 42–5. CLINICAL CORRELATIONS OF ENTEROPATHOGENICITY

Organism	Diarrhea/ Dysentery	Abdominal Pain	Vomiting	Incubation Period (hr)	Mucosal Penetration	Enterotoxin	Extraintestinal Manifestations
Shigella	+/+	+	±	24–72	+	+[a]	Seizures: meningismus
E. coli	+/0	±	0	24–72	0	+	Minimal
	0/+	+	0	24–72	+	0(?)	Variable
V. cholerae	+/0	0	±	24–72	0	+	Hypokalemic nephropathy
Salmonella	+/±	±	±	12–36	+	0(?)	Fever: bacteremia
C. perfringens	+/0	++	±	8–15	0	+[b]	Minimal
	+/+[c]	++	+	18–48	±	0(?)	Shock
Staphylococci	+/0[b]	±	++	4–8	0	+[b]	Minimal
	+/+[d]	+	±	Indeterminate	±	+(?)	Shock

[a] ? only *S. dysenteriae* 1.
[b] Preformed toxin ingestion.
[c] Necrotizing jejunitis (enteritis necroticans) may be clinically similar to dysentery.
[d] May occur when enterocolitis is produced by proliferating enterotoxin-producing organisms.
From Grady GF, Keusch GT: N Engl J Med 285:831, 1971.

endemic, patients presenting with a clinical syndrome resembling appendicitis were presumed to have typhoid until proved otherwise. The diagnosis may be established by blood culture during the first week or stool culture during the second or third weeks. A fourfold or greater increase in agglutinin titer against the O antigen confirms the diagnosis.

Treatment. Abdominal exploration must be performed for intestinal perforation with peritonitis. However, some patients in underdeveloped countries are seen so late that they are moribund. Multiple perforations should be sutured in two layers, including areas of apparent incipient perforation. Even for multiple perforations, small bowel resection is inadvisable, since resection seems to increase the mortality rate. Patients treated with end-to-side ileotransverse colostomy in addition to closure of the perforations have fewer complications (Table 42–6). If perforation is seen late, particularly with peritonitis for more than 48 hours, some authorities recommend drainage of the peritoneal cavity through a flank incision. This may be accomplished with local anesthesia, and it has even been carried out as a bedside procedure with local anesthesia, with some survivors. This appears to be a stopgap procedure in underdeveloped areas, however, and cannot be recommended for routine therapy. Typhoid fever should be treated with chloramphenicol but treatment of the perforation requires those antibiotics for polymicrobial flora. Chloramphenicol would not be ideal by itself (see Chap. 38). Early treatment may reduce the incidence of ileal perforation, but perforation and hemorrhage can still occur despite treatment. Ampicillin, amoxacillin, and trimethoprim-sulfamethoxazole are appropriate second choices for resistant strains.

TABLE 42–6. POSTOPERATIVE COMPLICATIONS OF TYPHOID PERFORATIONS OF THE BOWEL

Complication	No Bypass (49)	Bypass (29)
None	8	7
Major wound infection or dehiscence	12	2
Fecal fistula	7	2
Chest infection	16	8
Septicemia	4	5
Intra-abdominal abscess	5	0
Encephalopathy	5	1
Minor wound infection	5	10
Miscellaneous	12	9

From Eggleston FC, Santoshi B, Singh CM: Ann Surg 190:31, 1979.

Prognosis. The two most important factors affecting outcome after typhoid perforations are duration of illness or perforation and adequacy of fluid replacement. In one large series, the patients who lived had been ill for less than 6 days prior to admission, whereas those who died had been ill for 11 days or more. Similarly, duration of the interval between perforation and operation is a highly significant factor. Those who underwent surgery within 24 hours of perforation had a 14 percent mortality, whereas those who had been perforated for more than 72 hours had an 80 to 100 percent mortality.[102,103]

It is noteworthy that the mortality for typhoid perforation is still approximately 33 percent, which is said not to be appreciably lower than the mortality in the presurgical era when nonoperative management was the rule.[104] Also, the antibiotic era has not made much impact on mortality from perforation, although the overall mortality for typhoid fever is lower. Nevertheless, in most series nonoperative management is associated with 100 percent mortality.

Chronic Carrier State. One to 3 percent of patients with typhoid fever become chronic carriers. The chronic carrier state after nontyphoidal *Salmonella* infections is unusual. The gallbladder is the site of infection and chronic carriers of *S. typhi* excrete 10^6 to 10^9 bacteria/ml bile. Antibiotic therapy (ampicillin, 4 to 6 g/day combined with probenicid, 2 g/day, divided into four doses for 6 weeks) can be tried in carriers with normally functioning gallbladders, but it fails in 75 percent of carriers with gallbladder disease. Cholecystectomy should be carried out if antibiotic therapy is not successful.

Clostridial Enterocolitis. Species of *Clostridium* are associated with three noteworthy problems: food poisoning, intestinal gangrene, and antibiotic-associated diarrhea.

Food Poisoning. Clostridium perfringens, usually found in meat products but also in other foods, is a major cause of food-borne diarrhea, overshadowing its importance as a cause of dramatic infections like gas gangrene. It causes a secretory syndrome of cramps and diarrhea, with an onset of 10 to 24 hours and a duration of 24 hours or less (see Table 42–5). The enterotoxin is produced by the type A organism that forms heat-resistant spores, which may not be killed by cooking. These spores may germinate and grow at room temperature. Because the organisms are anaerobic, it is important that anaerobic cultures be performed on suspected foods in search of enterotoxin-producing organisms.[105]

Pseudomembranous Enterocolitis. Clostridium difficile is usually the cause of pseudomembranous enterocolitis.[106] It is likely that many previously reported cases of antibiotic-associated colitis, often attributed to staphylococci, were actually due to overgrowth of this organism. The clue came from a study suggesting that nine of ten patients with pseudomembranous colitis had a bacterial toxin in the feces, which was neutralized by a clostridial antitoxin. These matters are discussed in more detail in Chapter 39.

Necrotizing Enteritis. Certain *Clostridium* species are associated with enteritis necroticans, a rapidly progressive form of gas gangrene of the bowel with diarrhea and shock.[107] *Clostridium perfringens* and *C. septicum* can invade the intestinal wall in the absence of vascular compromise or obstruction. The best studied example is necrotizing enteritis (pigbel), found in New Guinea in association with traditional pig feasting where large amounts of contaminated pork are consumed. *Clostridium perfringens* type C (beta-toxin) appears to be the cause. Because this organism is frequently isolated from resected bowel, beta-antitoxin levels are high, and mortality is reduced by beta-antitoxin. Darmbrand is a form of necrotizing enteritis in Germany, which appears after excessive consumption of rich food associated with type C (formerly thought to be type F) *C. perfringens.* Numerous other case reports have documented the association of *C. perfringens* infections of various serotypes. Finegold summarized the literature through 1976.[105]

The need for overeating in the development of this condition may be related to the need for partial intestinal obstruction or stasis to permit the organisms time to proliferate within the intestine. In the cases scattered throughout the literature, other causes of gangrene of the bowel, such as strangulation, volvulus, intussusception, and mesenteric arterial or venous occlusion, have been excluded. It is possible that transient ischemic disease may also permit invasion by clostridia. Unfortunately, the extensive invasion of the bowel wall with gangrene and the tendency for clostridial overgrowth in the postmortem period do not permit clarification of the pathogenesis. It is possible that similar pathophysiologic events take place in toxic megacolon or necrotizing enterocolitis of the newborn (see Chap. 43). Nausea, vomiting, and crampy abdominal pain rapidly progress to steady pain with distention and peritonitis leading to shock. In general, the clinical picture resembles enteric vascular occlusion with intestinal gangrene, except that the onset is less sudden than that due to vascular compromise. Because food poisoning and intestinal obstruction lie within the differential diagnosis, the diagnosis may be difficult. When necrotizing enteritis is present, resection of the involved bowel segment is required in combination with antibiotics designed to eliminate intestinal organisms from the peritoneal cavity. A Gram stain of the peritoneal contents should show a predominance of clostridia. If the etiologic agent is recognized, high doses of penicillin are required. Even in the absence of the diagnosis, the combination of an aminoglycoside, clindamycin, and ampicillin is recommended for the treatment of polymicrobial peritonitis.

Uncommon Infectious Agents

Although the common bacterial infectious agents affecting the stomach and small bowel rarely produce complications that require surgery, some of the less common infectious and parasitic agents may lead to perforation and obstruction. The helminthic parasites and other unusual intestinal infections are discussed briefly (see Chap. 8).

Roundworms (Nematodes). Ascariasis is common worldwide and is seen with some frequency in the southern United States. It is the largest roundworm found in humans, and the adults live in the small intestine. The eggs laid in the small bowel must reach the soil to develop into an infective stage. After ingestion, the eggs hatch and the larvae begin a migration from the gut via the circulation to the lungs. Then they migrate by the airways and pharynx back to the gut, where they establish residence. Surgical complications arise when a bolus of worms obstructs the ileocecal valve. The mass of worms may also initiate a volvulus or intussusception. If the administration of an antihelminthic, like piperazine, through a long intestinal tube does not relieve the obstruction, laparotomy is required. The mass of worms can usually be milked down into the colon without the necessity for an enterotomy.[108]

Strongyloidiasis is also seen in the southern United States. It has the most complex reproductive cycle of the nematodes and can sometimes cause massive intestinal infestation with bloody diarrhea. Steroids should be avoided in patients with strongyloidiasis because systemic dissemination has been reported.

Four additional nematodes account for most of the other human infestations. Hookworms (*Ancylostoma* and *Necator*) inhabit the small bowel after the larvae enter the skin on contact with contaminated soil. Gastrointestinal complaints are unusual, and patients usually present with anemia. Pinworms and whipworms more commonly inhabit the colon, especially in children. Pinworms (enterobiasis) migrate at night and cause perianal pruritis. They are treated effectively by several antihelminthics. One piperizine tablet is all that is required. However, the child's sheets and clothes need to be thoroughly washed to prevent cyclic self-reinfestation. In addition, it may be necessary to treat the other family members.

Tapeworms. The tapeworms *Taenia saginata* and *Diphyllobothrium latum* may grow to extraordinary size in the gut, sometimes reaching 10 m in length. They cause few symptoms other than anemia. The most dangerous tapeworm for humans is *T. solium* (the pork tapeworm), because humans may harbor a larval stage that migrates and encysts (eg, cysticercosis).

Protozoans. Amebiasis is primarily a colonic infestation and is discussed in Chapters 8, 40, and 43. Giardiasis, on the other hand, is ingested as cysts, and the trophozoites inhabit the duodenum and jejunum attached to the mucosa by sucking disks. Infestation is usually asymptomatic, but in patients with immune deficiencies (hypo- or agammaglobulinemia), *Giardia* may cause diarrhea. Radiographic studies are nonspecific, and duodenal biopsy may resemble sprue. The most rewarding diagnostic step is to search duodenal aspirates for the cysts. There is evidence that *Giardia* can be invasive. In a series of 31 patients with trophozoites in their stool, 12 had invasion of the lamina propria in jejunal biopsy specimens.

Other Agents. Complications of *Candida* overgrowth usually occur either in diabetes mellitus, immunodeficient patients, or terminally ill patients with carcinoma. *Candida* has been reported to be responsible for multiple jejunal perforations.[109] When perforation occurs, yeasts have been seen deep in the intestinal mucosa and also cultured from the perforation site and the peritoneal fluid, supporting the possibility that the primary infection was an invasive process.

Tuberculosis of the small bowel is usually ulcerative and associated with pulmonary disease. Perforation is rare (approximately 2 percent) because of the fibrous adhesions to the bowel and the thick base of a tuberculous ulcer.[110] From a hospital with over 240 cases of abdominal tuberculosis, only three perforations were reported.[111] Tuberculosis of the bowel may also obstruct with strictures and adhesions.

AIDS Associated Gastrointestinal Infections

It is estimated that gastrointestinal symptoms, particularly diarrhea, occur in 30 to 50 percent of North American and European patients with AIDS and in nearly 90 percent of patients from developing countries. Initially, diarrhea may be associated with the general malaise at the time of seroconversion. Later, diarrhea may be the presenting complaint of full-blown AIDS, accompanied by a wide variety of other intestinal symptoms.[112] A useful review is provided by Bartlett.[113] A list of common infections in AIDS patients is shown in Table 42–7.

Diagnostic Evaluation. A three-stage diagnostic work-up is recommended for AIDS patients with diarrhea[112]:

- Step 1. Stool specimens should be cultured for *Salmonella, Shigella, Campylobacter,* and *Clostridium* species. In addition, stool samples are examined microscopically for parasitic infestation.
- Step 2. Upper gastrointestinal endoscopy and colonoscopy then follow to obtain biopsy material. This material is cultured for cytomegalovirus, herpesvirus, and mycobacterium and is histologically examined for protozoa, viral inclusion bodies, fungi, and mycobacterium. Finally, duodenal fluid samples should be examined for the presence of parasites.
- Step 3. Duodenal and colonic tissue may then be subjected to electron microscopy, in an attempt to identify microsporidia and adenovirus, respectively.

Using this protocol, one or more pathogenic processes can be identified in 85 percent of patients.

Gut Immune Consequences of HIV Infection. HIV infection of the lamina propria leads to a marked reduction in the CD4+ T cell population. This reduction is subsequently accompanied by an increase in the CD8+ T cell population, a manifestation of more advanced clinical disease.[114] These T cell changes are also associated with reduced numbers of IgA-secreting B cells (plasma cells) in 75 percent of patients with or without gastrointestinal manifestations.[115] This decrease in immunocompetent B cells is probably responsible for the abundant and opportunistic colonization of the AIDS gut. As HIV disease progresses, CD4+ T cell depletion becomes critical, leading to impaired cytotoxic T cell function and impaired macrophage and monocyte activation and subsequent cytotoxicity. This opens the patient to viral and intracellular pathogenic invasion.

Clinical Manifestations

ESOPHAGUS. Dysphagia, odynophagia, and retrosternal pain are common presenting complaints in AIDS patients. By far the commonest association, particularly with dysphagia, is *Candida* infections. Pain is a more common symptom of cytomegalovirus (CMV) or herpes simplex virus (HSV) infection, both of which can lead to extensive ulceration.

STOMACH. Virtually the whole gastrointestinal tract is susceptible to CMV infection, which is a significant risk factor in AIDS and immunocompromised transplant patients, and the stomach is no exception. Severe ulcerative gastritis is typically diagnosed by the characteristic histopathologic findings of intranuclear inclusion bodies, or an "owls eye" halo.

SMALL INTESTINE. Cramping periumbilical pain, weight loss, and large volume diarrhea are common in patients with AIDS. Mimicking many intra-abdominal pathologies, the majority of these patients will have an intestinal infection as their primary cause. The common bacterial pathogens such as *Salmonella, Shigella,* and *Campylobacter* should initially be ruled out. Atypical and routine parasitic infections, including *Giardia, Entamoeba histolytica, Cryptosporidium,* and *Isospora belli* should be ruled out by examination of stool samples. Microsporidiasis cannot be detected in stool samples and requires electron microscopy of small bowel biopsies.[113] One-third of the remaining patients in whom no other pathogen is isolated or cultured have CMV or *Mycobacterium avium-intracellulare* as the cause of their diarrhea. The clinical spectrum in these cases is highly variable. Many patients remain minimally symptomatic; whereas others have profound dehydrating diarrhea, malabsorption, severe pain, and weight loss. Small bowel vasculitis and ulceration caused by CMV infection may freely perforate into the peritoneum.

AIDS-ASSOCIATED ENTEROPATHY. Changes in the morphology of the small bowel mucosa can develop in the absence of pathogenic infection. These morphologic changes, which include subtotal villous atrophy and decreased crypt mitosis, may contribute to the functional intestinal impairment seen in these patients. Ullrich and colleagues[116] suggested that, because they occurred in patients whose lamina propria contained HIV virus, this enteropathy may well be the result of HIV intestinal infection.

PERITONEUM. AIDS patients occasionally present with the sudden onset of ascites and, although the majority are due to underlying hepatic disease, exudative ascites can sometimes occur. Careful evaluation of the ascitic fluid should rule out malignancy and acid-fast stains may demonstrate disseminated tuberculous infection.

Bacterial Overgrowth Syndromes

Blind Loop Syndrome. The syndrome of bacterial overgrowth in the small intestine that results in anemia, steatorrhea, and malabsorption is usually known as the blind loop syndrome. Because several causes of blind loop syndrome do not involve an anatomic blind loop, the British prefer the term stagnant loop syndrome. Because any cause of bacterial overgrowth within the small intestine may produce the syndrome, the terms *blind loop* and *contaminated small bowel* may be used interchangeably.

Etiology and Pathogenesis. The two factors that keep the proximal small bowel relatively clear of fecal organisms are gastric acid and peristalsis. Thus disturbances of either of these functions may result in bacterial overgrowth. Defects in effective peristalsis arise from certain congenital or acquired anatomic defects (small intestinal diverticula, strictures, fistulas), surgical procedures (gastrectomy, vagotomy, pyloroplasty, afferent loops), or disorders of small bowel function and motility (scleroderma, diabetic autonomic neuropathy, radiation enteritis). Achlorhydria from any cause leads to increased bacterial levels in the jejunum. Most of the abnormalities cause neither symptoms nor malabsorption, as the bacterial overgrowth is composed of coliforms, streptococci, and lactobacilli. Symptoms appear when stasis of small bowel contents is accompanied by overgrowth with anaerobes, especially *Bacteroides, Veillonella, Clostridium,* and anaerobic cocci.

Jejunal diverticulosis is one of the more common predisposing factors in the elderly; it may take many years for the symptoms to develop. An interesting cause of blind loop syndrome is the gastrojejunocolic fistula as a complication of gastrectomy. The diarrhea that results from this fistula is not due to direct passage of ingested nutrients to the colon but rather to the contamination of the small

TABLE 42–7. MOST COMMON GASTROINTESTINAL INFECTIONS IN HOMOSEXUAL MEN AND PATIENTS WITH HIV INFECTION

Site	Infective Agent	
	Patients with HIV Infection	*Homosexual Men*
Mouth	*Candida albicans* Herpes simplex virus	*Neisseria gonorrhoeae* *Chlamydia trachomatis* Herpes simplex virus
Esophagus	*C. albicans* Herpes simplex virus Cytomegalovirus	
Small intestine	Cryptosporidia Microsporidia *Isospora* *Mycobacterium avium* *Salmonella* Cytomegalovirus	*Giardia lamblia*
Colon	*Salmonella* Cytomegalovirus *Clostridium difficile*	*Campylobacter cinaedi* *C. trachomatis* *N. gonorrhoeae* *Treponema pallidum*
Anus or rectum	Herpes simplex virus Cytomegalovirus	Herpes simplex virus

Adapted from Bartlett JG: Gastrointestinal complications of HIV infection. In Gorbach SL, Bartlett JG, Blacklow NR (eds): Infectious Diseases. Philadelphia, Saunders, 1992, p 944.

intestine with colonic organisms that work their pathophysiologic effects by mechanisms to be described. Although bacterial overgrowth within the small intestinal lumen is the common pathogenetic factor, each of the components of the syndrome—anemia, steatorrhea, and malabsorption—is explained by different mechanisms.

ANEMIA. The first case of this syndrome was described in the 19th century in a patient with an intestinal stricture and anemia. Similar cases were described with a macrocytic, hyperchromic anemia, glossitis, and neurologic symptoms. Although the illness mimics pernicious anemia, these patients produce both acid and intrinsic factor. As it appears that some intestinal microorganisms compete directly with the host for vitamin B_{12}, either antibiotics or parenteral vitamin B_{12} will correct the anemia. Binding of vitamin B_{12} to intrinsic factor normally protects the vitamin somewhat from bacterial uptake, but some bacteria can ingest the whole complex. The megaloblastic anemia is not related to malabsorption of folic acid, since serum folate may actually be increased above normal due to bacterial synthesis of folic acid.

STEATORRHEA. Steatorrhea as a result of the blind loop syndrome is principally caused by malabsorbed dietary fat. In addition, bacteria may synthesize hydroxylated fatty acids, which are poorly absorbed. Free fatty acids have a cathartic effect on the colon, which may further aggravate the diarrhea by mechanisms similar to the action of linoleic acid in castor oil. The major cause of fat malabsorption is a short-circuiting of the enterohepatic circulation of bile salts.[117] The enterohepatic circulation temporarily provides bile salts to the proximal small intestine to solubilize dietary fat and recovers the bile salts in the ileum after fat absorption is complete. To solubilize fat for absorption, there must be a critical micellar concentration of at least 2 to 3 millimoles/liter of conjugated bile salts, which is normally 5 to 10 millimoles/liter.

Bile salt conjugation performs two functions essential for normal fat absorption. First, conjugation enables bile salts to form micelles and solubilize dietary fat. Second, conjugation protects bile salts from premature passive reabsorption in the jejunum. If the bile salts become deconjugated in the jejunum, a jejunohepatic circulation occurs rather than the normal ileohepatic circulation, and the bile salts are not retained within the intestinal lumen to solubilize and to facilitate dietary fat absorption.

Bacteroides, Clostridium, and a few other anaerobes have enzymes, such as taurocholate amidase, which can cleave the glycine or taurine conjugate from the bile salt. Most coliforms do not have the enzyme to perform this cleavage. Indeed, *E. coli* may proliferate widely in the proximal small intestine, competing with the host for vitamin B_{12} and causing anemia but not producing steatorrhea. Thus, although most microorganisms can compete with the host for essential nutrients, only particular species with the appropriate amidases can deconjugate the bile salts and disrupt the enterohepatic circulation.

Other hypotheses to explain the pathogenesis of steatorrhea have been proposed over the years:

1. Some have suggested that unconjugated bile salts interfere with lipolysis by pancreatic lipase, but this claim has not been widely accepted.
2. In vitro studies have suggested that conjugated bile salts are essential for intracellular reesterification of lipids.
3. A direct toxic effect of unconjugated bile acids on the epithelium has been proposed and has gained some support from demonstrations of metabolic and morphologic abnormalities in intestinal mucosa exposed to unconjugated bile salts in vivo.[118]

Most evidence still seems to favor decreased micelle formation by normal conjugated bile salts as the primary pathophysiologic mechanism. For example, unconjugated deoxycholic acid has been administered both orally and as a continuous intraduodenal infusion, without any evidence of producing steatorrhea or mucosal damage. In addition, patients may experience symptomatic relief on a regimen that includes feeding conjugated bile salts, even though the amount of unconjugated bile salts in the jejunum increases. Finally, the presence of free bile acid has been demonstrated in patients who do not have steatorrhea, unless the level of unconjugated bile acid is also below the critical micellar concentration.

PANMALABSORPTION. Although the bile salt story seems to be a sufficient explanation for the steatorrhea of blind loop syndrome, other features of the illness are presently not well explained. Some patients with bacterial overgrowth have hypoproteinemia, edema, alopecia, depigmented hair, low essential amino acids in serum, and low-voltage electrocardiograms. These changes reflecting panmalabsorption of carbohydrate and protein are not easily explained by the micelle theory. Some laboratories have also found steatorrhea and bacterial overgrowth in the jejunum of patients after gastrectomy with no evidence of free bile acids in the lumen. Thus there has been an impetus to search for other possible explanations.

Goldstein[119] has developed the concept of bacterial competition for essential nutrients to explain some of these problems. He has calculated that a liter of intestinal fluid in bacterial overgrowth syndromes may contain approximately 10 g of bacteria. At known rates of bacterial multiplication, the nutritional requirements for this mass of organisms can easily run over 100 g of sugar per day. Thus the nutritional requirements of the mass of bacteria alone may pose a significant competitive burden for the host.

Low serum levels of essential amino acids have also been noted in some blind loop patients, but protein-losing enteropathy is rare. It is possible that the bacteria also compete with the host for amino acids.

Carbohydrate malabsorption is also well established in experimental blind loop syndrome. Decreased urinary excretion of D-xylose may also be a result of bacterial competition for sugars. Although xylose is not metabolized by humans, a number of bacterial species that include a variety of aerobic organisms do metabolize xylose. Thus it is not established whether xylose malabsorption in blind loop syndrome is due to uptake and competition by the bacteria or to a possible toxic factor as previously outlined.

Deficiencies of fat-soluble vitamins are common in the steatorrheas, but vitamin K deficiency almost never occurs in blind loop syndrome. Vitamin K is synthesized by intestinal microorganisms, so in this one instance the bacterial mass contributes a molecule that is useful to the host.

Pathology. The mucosa is usually normal by light microscopy in syndromes of bacterial overgrowth except for infiltrates in the submucosa and lamina propria. The significance of these infiltrates is not clear, but they probably represent a development of the gut lymphoid system in defense against the bacterial flora. An increased concentration of Paneth cells has been noted in bypassed intestine and this may also reflect a defense mechanism against the bacteria.

Clinical Manifestations. Anemia and steatorrhea are the hallmarks of blind loop syndrome, but symptoms of abdominal discomfort and cramps (depending on the underlying cause of bacterial overgrowth) may precede the development of the typical metabolic findings for years. In addition to the typical megaloblastic anemia, some patients with chronic hemorrhage also have iron deficiency. Weight loss and neurologic manifestations of vitamin B_{12} deficiency may occur, along with hypoproteinemia and edema. Watery diarrhea may result from the cathartic effects of bacterial synthesis of hydroxyfatty acids.

Laboratory Findings. The steatorrhea should be documented and quantified by stool collection for fat analysis. A routine hematologic work-up should be done, including red blood cell indices and vitamin B_{12} levels. A three-stage Shilling test will usually be abnormal in the first two steps, when vitamin B_{12} is given alone and then with intrinsic factor. However, in the third stage, when vitamin B_{12} is given after a course of oral antibiotics as described below, normal absorption of vitamin B_{12} should be restored.

Jejunal biopsy should be performed to rule out other causes of malabsorption, such as sprue. The small bowel should also be intubated for quantitative bacteriologic studies. If the combined anaerobic and aerobic count is greater than 10^7/ml, the bacterial overgrowth syndrome should be suspected. The quantitative cultures should be repeated after a 5- to 7-day course of tetracycline along with follow-up stool fat determination and the three-stage Shilling test. If these studies show improvement in vitamin B_{12} absorption and reduced stool fat excretion along with a reduction in bacterial count, the diagnosis is considered confirmed. Additional niceties such as serum free bile acids and jejunal levels of free and conjugated bile acids are interesting, but not essential for the diagnosis.

The breath analyzer test for bile salt deconjugation remains an accurate diagnostic tool for overgrowth. Recent studies indicate that when a critical level of bacterial overgrowth is defined as greater than 10^3 anaerobes/ml or greater than 5×10^4 aerobes/ml in the jejunum, the test as presently performed has a sensitivity of 70 percent and a specificity of 90 percent.[120]

Diagnosis. Clues to bacterial overgrowth in blind loops are often present in the history of the patient. Previous gastric or small bowel surgery or a history of an intestinal disorder such as Crohn's disease with a tendency to stricture should arouse suspicion of bacterial overgrowth when noted in patients with steatorrhea or megaloblastic anemia. A history of Raynaud phenomenon or dysphagia may suggest scleroderma. An upper gastrointestinal radiographic series with small bowel follow-through is usually definitive in establishing any predisposing malfunction that can be surgically corrected. Suspicion of the diagnosis should be sustained by the laboratory studies outlined previously.

Treatment. Operative therapy is advisable for those patients with lesions that are correctable without massive resection of the intestine (eg, solitary jejunal diverticulum, mechanical obstruction, gastrojejunocolic fistula). Patients with multiple jejunal diverticula or motility disorders should be treated medically. If medical management is selected, tetracycline, 250 mg daily, is a satisfactory initial antibiotic, with further modifications based on jejunal culture results. Alternate regimens have been discussed by Joiner and Gorbach.[121]

Bypass Enteropathy

Incidence. Within a few years of the introduction and popularization of jejunoileal (JI) bypass for morbid obesity, the complication of bypass enteropathy was recognized.[122] Estimates of the incidence of this complication vary considerably, from a low of approximately 3 percent to as much as 60 percent.[123,124] This variation no doubt relates to different criteria for diagnosis and the recognition of patients in some series with subtle rather than fulminant signs of enteropathy.

Etiology and Pathogenesis. The available evidence strongly suggests that this complication is related to bacterial overgrowth in the bypassed intestine.[124] Although peristaltic activity in bypassed small bowel has not been studied in detail, it seems likely that the bypassed intestine develops a motility disturbance that predisposes toward bacterial overgrowth in the segment. In patients with an end-to-end JI bypass, the bypassed small bowel is connected to the colon without a valve mechanism; this may permit the colonic bacterial flora to enter the small bowel limb, increasing the bacterial overgrowth. In addition, there may be acquired deficiencies in the gut immune system within the bypassed bowel segment, but studies in experimental animals have actually shown Paneth cell hyperplasia, which may reflect a reaction by the gut immune system to the overgrowth of bacteria. Evidence for bacterial overgrowth in the bypassed loop in association with the enteropathic syndrome was found in three patients who had not been on systemic antibiotics. Aspirations of the secretions in the bypass revealed a flora with 10^6 to 10^7 aerobes/ml and 10^7 to 10^9 anaerobes/ml. This evidence of bacterial overgrowth, along with the observation that some patients improve on antibiotic therapy, strongly suggests that bacteria do play a pathogenetic role. On the other hand, an increase in flora may not be specific for the patients with signs of the disease. For example, Corrodi et al[125] have reported a colonic flora in the bypassed loops of patients who are asymptomatic.

Bacterial overgrowth in the small bowel has also been considered a possible cause of liver failure after jejunoileal bypass. Germ-free dogs with jejunoileal bypass do not develop liver failure, but antibiotics given to conventional dogs do not appear to protect them.[126] Absorption of bacterial products has also been implicated in the rheumatoid-like arthropathy seen in JI bypass patients. Endotoxin has been detected in the joint fluid of these patients. They also develop interstitial nephritis, pyoderma nodosum, and pyoderma gangrenosum, which suggests that these too may be manifestations of bacterial translocation. It is also suggested that these phenomena seen in patients with inflammatory bowel diseases may also be secondary to bacterial translocation.

Pathology. There is usually inflamed, hyperemic mucosa in the bypassed intestine. Inflammation may also be apparent on the serosal surface, either of the whole bypassed loop or the ileum adjacent to the colonic anastomosis. There may also be evidence of pneumatosis cystoidis intestinalis. On microscopic examination, the mucosa shows evidence of nonspecific inflammatory changes with blunted villi and infiltrates of lymphocytes and plasma cells in the lamina propria.

Clinical Manifestations. Virtually all patients have diarrhea, Hemocult-positive stools, and abdominal distention with air-fluid levels apparent on radiographic examination. The severity and duration of symptoms are inconstant, however. Symptoms may begin early in the postoperative course or may be delayed for several years. Once bypass enteropathy has developed, the subsequent course is variable. Exacerbations and remissions are common even without antibiotic therapy, although remission is often induced by antibiotics.

Signs and symptoms of an acute abdomen may develop in as many as 25 percent of all patients with enteropathy. These patients have abdominal pain, tenderness, nausea, fever, and leukocytosis. The clinical course may also be complicated by systemic symptoms—skin lesions resembling erythema nodosum, arthralgias and arthritis, and recurrent fevers. Hyperoxaluria and kidney stones do not seem to be more common in patients with enteropathy than in patients without intestinal complications. The systemic symptoms are relieved in some patients by courses of antibiotic therapy or by dismantling the bypass.

Diagnosis. The diagnosis should be suspected in patients with the typical clinical findings of diarrhea and distension. Abdominal films may show distended bowel with air-fluid levels. Liver biopsy should be performed if there is any evidence of liver failure, and a significant percentage of patients with bypass enteropathy have hepatic steatosis and fibrosis. Although steatosis is often seen in patients with jejunoileal bypass who do not have enteropathy, fibrosis is unusual without some degree of enteropathy.

Treatment. The place of antibiotics in the initial management of these patients is well established. In a double-blind antibiotic-crossover study, five jejunoileal bypass patients with colonic pseudo-obstruction had only 9 of 34 pain-free days on placebo, whereas they had 31 out of 33 pain-free days on metronidazole. Metronidazole also resulted in a precipitous decrease from 10^9 to 10^1 in the anaerobic counts per milliliter from the vicinity of the bypassed loop. Kanamycin was relatively ineffective and did not decrease the abdominal girth or bacterial cell counts in the patients studied.[127]

Operation is required under two circumstances: (1) if the symptoms cannot be controlled with antibiotics, an elective dismantling of the bypass should be performed; and (2) emergency exploration should be carried out in the less common patient with an acute abdomen. If serosal inflammation is not intense, restoration of continuity may suffice. However, if there is severe inflammation of a portion of the bypassed bowel, it may be safest to resect the most inflamed portion of bowel.

Prognosis. Because the severity and duration are quite variable, and since exacerbations are common followed by remissions, it is difficult to be dogmatic about the prognosis in this condition. In patients with severe enteropathy with a poor response to antibiotics, dismantling of the bypass is advisable. The late sequelae of bypass enteropathy with long-term antibiotic control are as yet unknown.

Ileoanal Pouch and Continent Ileostomy. The pathophysiology of bacterial overgrowth in ileostomy reservoirs and ileoanal pouch is identical to that described for blind loop syndrome.

The flora of a conventional ileostomy are unique, occupying an intermediate portion of the spectrum between normal ileal flora and the flora of a transverse colostomy. Anaerobic flora are less prevalent than in transverse colostomy effluent, and counts are approximately 10^5 lower than typical feces. On the other hand, the counts are approximately 10^2 higher than the counts in normal ileal contents.[128] Because the purpose of the continent ileostomy is to induce stasis, the microbial ecology would be expected to come to resemble the colonic flora. Bacterial counts are 10^3 higher than effluents of conventional ileostomies.

Two studies have investigated the possible consequences of this increase in flora with respect to the pathophysiology of blind loop syndrome. Schjonsby and co-workers[129] compared steatorrhea in patients with a continent ileostomy versus a conventional ileostomy. Abnormal fat excretion was found in 57 percent of the reservoir patients versus 14 percent of the conventional patients. Similarly, abnormal vitamin B_{12} absorption was found in 71 percent of the reservoir patients versus 29 percent of the conventional patients. The reservoir patients had increased total anaerobic counts and also counts of *Bacteroides;* 29 percent had abnormal breath tests for bile salt deconjugation. Oral lincomycin increased vitamin B_{12} absorption, reduced fecal fat excretion, and reduced microbial counts of *Bacteroides* in four patients. Similarly, four of seven continent ileostomy patients evaluated by Halvorsen and co-workers[130] for blind loop syndrome had malabsorption of fat and vitamin B_{12}. Others have reported enteritis as a complication of continent ileostomy with an incidence of over 50 percent.[131] Pouchitis, or inflammation of the ileoanal pouch, has also been noted in 10 to 30 percent of patients following total abdominal proctocolectomy for ulcerative colitis and familial polyposis.[132–134] The diagnosis is confirmed by endoscopy of the pouch, which reveals an inflamed, friable, bloody mucosa. Aphthous ulcers may be present leading to the incorrect diagnosis of Crohn's enteritis of the pouch. However, the prompt response to antibiotics confirms the diagnosis of pouchitis.

Symptoms typically include bloody diarrhea. Some patients develop new onset extraintestinal manifestations of inflammatory bowel disease such as arthritis and pyoderma nodosa or gangrenosum.[135] The pouchitis is thought to result from the overgrowth of anaerobic bacteria and responds in over 90 percent of patients to oral metronidazole. Once a patient has developed pouchitis he/she remains at risk for recurrent attacks, which can lead to long-term antibiotic therapy. Patients in whom metronidazole does not work almost always respond to bactrim, tetracycline, or cyprofloxacin.

Wound Infection After Small Bowel Operations

Bowel preps for small bowel operations have been studied, with inconclusive results. In one series of 155 jejunoileal bypasses for morbid obesity,[136] positive jejunal and ileal cultures were obtained in 62 and 87 percent of cases, respectively. The jejunal flora were predominantly streptococci, lactobacilli, and staphylococci, while the ileal flora contained these organisms with other coliforms and anaerobes. A mechanical preparation alone lowered the incidence of positive jejunal and ileal cultures to 57 and 56 percent, respectively, with the reduction in positive ileal cultures being statistically significant. The wound infection rate with mechanical preparation alone was 43 percent, in comparison with the infection rate of 11 percent in patients with mechanical and antibiotic preparations. However, the wound infection rate was zero in patients who had no preparation at all, which renders the results of the entire study questionable.

It is known that the oral administration of doxycycline (200 mg, 4 hours before operation) results in tissue levels in the ileum that are approximately twice the serum level.[137] Whether oral doxycycline decreases the incidence of wound infections, however, is unknown. Studies of the wound infection rates after parenteral antibiotics in small bowel surgery are not available. Most evidence suggests that perioperative antibiotic prophylaxis decreases wound infections after clean-contaminated operations (see Chap. 25). Because asymptomatic bacteremias do occur during small intestinal operations, it seems advisable to cover patients with prosthetic vascular grafts or other implants with prophylactic preoperative systemic antibiotics.

REFERENCES

1. Savage DC: Microbial ecology of the gastrointestinal tract. Annu Rev Microbiol 31:107, 1977.
2. Luckey TD: Bicentennial overview of intestinal microecology. Am J Clin Nutr 30:1753, 1977.
3. Brandborg LL: Other infectious inflammatory and miscellaneous diseases. In MH Sleisenger, JS Fordtran (eds): Gastrointestinal Disease. Philadelphia, Saunders, 1973, p 909.
4. Simon GL, Gorbach SL: Intestinal flora in health and disease. Gastroenterology 86:174, 1984.
5. Dickman MD, Chapelka AR, Schaedler RW: The microbial ecology of the upper small bowel. Am J Gastroenterol 65:57, 1976.
6. Gorbach SL, Plaut AG, Nahas L, Weinstein L: Studies of the intestinal microflora: II. Microorganisms

of the small intestine and their relationship to oral and fecal flora. Gastroenterology 53:856, 1967.
7. Long SS, Swenson RM: Development of anaerobic fecal flora in healthy newborn infants. J Pediatr 91:298, 1977.
8. Bishop RF, Anderson CM: The bacterial flora of the stomach and small intestine in children with intestinal obstruction. Arch Dis Child 35:487, 1960.
9. Abrams GD: Microbial effects on mucosal structure and function. Am J Clin Nutr 30:1880, 1977.
10. Lesher S, Walburg HE, Sacher GA: Generation cycle in the duodenal crypt cells of germ free and conventional mice. Nature 202:884, 1964.
11. Kenworthy R: Observations on the reaction of the intestinal mucosa to bacterial challenge. J Clin Pathol 24:138, 1971.
12. Simon GL, Gorbach SL: The human intestinal microflora. Dig Dis Sci 31(Suppl):147s, 1986.
13. Scheline PR: Metabolism of foreign compounds by gastrointestinal microorganisms. Pharmacol Rev 25:451, 1973.
14. Lindenbaum J, Rund DG, Butler VP, et al: Inactivation of digoxin by gut flora: reversal by antibiotic therapy. N Engl J Med 305:789, 1981.
15. Lamont JT, O'Gorman TA: Experimental colon cancer. Gastroenterology 75:1157, 1978.
16. van der Waaij D: The microflora of the gut: recent findings and implications. Dig Dis 9:36, 1991.
17. Bohnhoff M, Miller CP, Martin WR: Resistance of the mouse intestinal tract to experimental *Salmonella* infarction. J Exp Med 120:805, 1964.
18. Sheretz RJ: Aquired immunodeficiency syndrome. Med Clin North Am 69:637, 1985.
19. Hurst AF: The clinical importance of achlorhydria. BMJ 2:665, 1934.
20. Hornick RB, Music SI, Wenzet R, et al: The Broad street pump revisited: response of volunteers to ingested cholera vibrios. Bull NY Acad Med 47:1181, 1971.
21. Ruddel WSJ, Axon ATR, Findlay JM, et al: Effects of cimetidine on gastric bacterial flora. Lancet 1:672, 1980.
22. Tryba M: Sucrulfate versus antacids or H2-antagonists for stress ulcer prophylaxsis: a meta analysis on efficacy and pneumonia rate. Crit Care Med 19:942, 1991.
23. Cook DJ, Laine LA, Guyatt GH, Raffin TA: Nosocomial pneumonia and the role of gastric pH: a meta analysis. Chest 100:7, 1991.
24. Fabian TC, Bradley AB, Croce MA, et al: Pneumonia and stress ulceration in severely injured patients. Arch Surg 128:185, 1993.
25. Sarker SA, Gyr K: Non-immune defence mechanisms of the gut. Gut 33:987, 1992.
26. Sykes PA, Boulter KH, Schoffield PF: Alterations in small bowel microflora in acute intestinal obstruction. J Med Microbiol 9:13, 1976.
27. Felsenfeld O, Gyr K: Action of some pancreatic enzymes on *Vibrio cholerae*. Med Microbiol Immunol 163:53, 1977.
28. Gyr K, Felsenfeld O: The effect of oral pancreatic extract on jejunal bactericidal activity in protein deficient vervet monkeys challenged with *Vibrio cholerae*. Acta Trop 36:147, 1979.
29. Rubinstein E, Mark Z, Haspel J, et al: Antibacterial activity of pancreatic fluid. Gastroenterology 88:926, 1985.
30. Reid G, Bruce AW, McGroaty JA, et al: Is there a role for lactobacilli in prevention of urogenital and intestinal infection? Clin Microbiol Rev 3:335, 1990.
31. Fuller R: Probiotics in human medicine. Gut 32:439, 1991.
32. Beagley KW, Elson CC: Cell and cytokines in mucosal immunity and inflammation. Gastroenterol Clin North Am 21:347, 1992.
33. Brandtzaeg P, Vallaes K, Scott H, et al: The human gastrointestinal secretory immune system in health and disease. Scand J Gastroenterol 114:17, 1985.
34. Ogra PL, Karson DT: Distribution of poliovirus antibody in serum, nasopharynx and alimentary tract following segmental immunization of the lower alimentary tract with polio-vaccine. J Immunol 102:1423, 1969.
35. Fubara ES, Freter R: Protection against enteric bacterial infection by secretory IgA antibodies. J Immunol 111:395, 1973.
36. Rodning CB, Wilson SD, Erlandson SL: Immunoglobulins with human small intestinal Paneth cells. Lancet 1:984, 1976.
37. Selsted ME, Miller SI, Henschen AH, Oullette AJ: Enteric defensins: antibiotic peptide components of intestinal host defense. J Cell Biol 118:929, 1992.
38. Sykes P: Small bowel microflora in intestinal obstruction and Crohn's disease. Proc R Soc Med 69:325, 1976.
39. Sykes PA, Boulter KH, Schofield PF: The microflora of the obstructed bowel. Br J Surg 63:721, 1976.
40. Deitch EA: The role of intestinal barrier failure and bacterial translocation in the development of systemic infection and multiple organ failure. Arch Surg 125:403, 1990.
41. Yale CE, Balish E: The importance of clostridia in experimental intestinal strangulation. Gastroenterology 71:793, 1976.
42. Fine J: The intestinal circulation in shock. Gastroenterology 52:454, 1967.
43. Scott AJ, Khan GA: Partial biliary obstruction with cholangitis producing a blind loop syndrome. Gut 9:187, 1968.
44. Dellipiani AW, Girwood RH: Bacterial changes in the small intestine in malabsorptive states and in pernicious anemia. Clin Sci 26:359, 1964.
45. Gorbach SL, Tabaquali S: Bacteria, bile and the small bowel. Gut 10:963, 1969.
46. Mortimer DC, Reed PI, Vidinli M, Finlay JM: The role of the upper gastrointestinal flora in malabsorption syndrome. Can Med Assoc J 90:559, 1964.
47. Greenlee HB, Gelbart SM, DeOrio AJ, et al: The influence of gastric surgery on the intestinal flora. Am J Clin Nutr 30:1826, 1977.

48. Wells CL, Maddaus MA, Simmons RL: Proposed mechanism for the translocation of intestinal bacteria. Rev Infect Dis 10:958, 1988.
49. Baker JW, Deitch EA, Li M, et al: Hemorrhagic shock induces bacterial translocation from the gut. J Trauma 28:896, 1988.
50. Sori AJ, Rush BF, Lysz TW, et al: The gut as a source of sepsis after hemorrhagic shock. Am J Surg 155:187, 1988.
51. Abraham E, Chang YH: Effects of hemorrhage on inflammatory response. Arch Surg 119:1154, 1987.
52. Chandra RK: Nutrition, infection and immunity: present knowledge and future directions: Lancet 1:688, 1983.
53. Tannock GW, Savage DC: Influences of dietary and environmental stress on microbiological population in the murine gastrointestinal tract. Infect Immun 9:591, 1974.
54. Deitch EA, Winterton J, Ll M, Berg R: The gut as a portal of entry for bacteremia. Role of protein malnutrition. Ann Surg 205:681, 1987.
55. Deitch EA, Winterton J, Specian R: Endotoxin promotes the translocation of bacteria from the gut. Arch Surg 122:185, 1987.
56. Alverdy JC, Aoys E, Moss GS: Total parenteral nutrition promotes bacterial translocation from the gut. Surgery 104:185, 1988.
57. Maejima K, Deitch EA, Berg DB: Bacterial translocation from the gastrointestinal tract of rats receiving thermal injury. Infect Immun 43:6, 1984.
58. Alexander JW, Boyce ST, Babcock GF, et al: The process of microbial translocation. Ann Surg 212:496, 1990.
59. Wells CL, Maddaus MA, Simmons RL: Role of the macrophage in the translocation of intestinal bacteria. Arch Surg 122:48, 1987.
60. Wells CL, Rotstein OD, Pruett TL, Simmons RL: Intestinal bacteria translocate into experimental intra-abdominal abscesses. Arch Surg 121:102, 1986.
61. Mora EM, Cardona MA, Simmons RL: Enteric bacteria and ingested inert particles translocate to intraperitoneal prosthetic materials. Arch Surg 126:157, 1991.
62. van der Waaij D, Manson WL, Arends JP, de Vries-Hospers HG: Clinical use of selective decontamination: the concept. Intensive Care Med 16:S212, 1990.
63. Cockerill FR, Muller SR, Anhalt JP, et al: Prevention of infection in critically ill patients by selective decontamination of the digestive tract. Ann Intern Med 117:545, 1992.
64. Craven DE: Editorial: use of selective decontamination of the digestive tract. Is the light at the end of the tunnel red or green? Ann Intern Med 117:609, 1992.
65. Gastinne H, Wolff M, Delatour F, et al: A controlled trial in intensive care units of selective decontamination of the digestive tract with nonabsorbable antibiotics. N Engl J Med 326:594, 1992.
66. McDonald GB, Sharma P, Hackman RC, et al: Esophageal infections in immunosuppressed patients after marrow transplantation. Gastroenterology 88:1111, 1985.
67. Rattner HM, Cooper DJ, Zaman MB: Severe bleeding from herpes esophagitis. Am J Gastroenterol 80:523, 1985.
68. Schackelford RT: Perforations and ruptures of the esophagus. In Schackelford RT (ed): Surgery of the Alimentary Tract, 2nd ed. Philadelphia, Saunders, 1978, pp 51–87.
69. Wichern WA Jr: Perforation of the esophagus. Am J Surg 19:534, 1970.
70. Borgeskov S, Brynitz S, Siemenssen O: Perforation of the esophagus. Scand J Thorac Cardiovasc Surg 18:93, 1984.
71. Ajalat GM, Mulder DG: Esophageal perforations: the need for an individualized approach. Arch Surg 119:1318, 1984.
72. Shaffer HA, Valenzuela G, Mittal RK: Esophageal perforation: a reassessment of the criteria for choosing medical or surgical therapy. Arch Intern Med 152:757, 1992.
73. Skinner DB, Little AG, DeMeester TR: Management of esophageal perforation. Am J Surg 139:760, 1980.
74. Jones JM: Necrotizing *Candida* esophagitis: failure of symptoms and roentgenographic findings to reflect severity. JAMA 244:2190, 1980.
75. Odds FC: *Candida* and Candidosis. Baltimore, University Park Press, 1979.
76. Warren JR, Marshall B: Unidentified curved bacilli on gastric epithelium in active chronic gastritis. Lancet 1:1273, 1983.
77. Blaser MJ: *Helicobacter pylori:* its role in disease. Clin Infect Dis 15:386, 1992.
78. Dooley CP, Cohen H, Fitzgibbons PL, et al: Prevalence of *Helicobacter pylori* infections and histologic gastritis in asymptomatic persons. N Engl J Med 321:1562, 1989.
79. Hazel SL, Lee A, Brady L, et al: *Campylobacter pylori* and gastritis: association of intercellular spaces and adaption to an environment of mucus as important factors in colonization of the gastric epithelium. J Infect Dis 153:2053, 1986.
80. Marshall BJ, Armstrong JA, McGechie DB, et al: Attempt to fulfill Koch's postulates for pyloric *Campylobacter.* Med J Aust 142:436, 1985.
81. Hentschel E, Brandstatter G, Dragosics B, et al: Effect of ranitidine and amoxicillin plus metronidazole on the eradication of *H. pylori* and the recurrence of duodenal ulcer. N Engl J Med 328:308, 1993.
82. Stephenson SE Jr, Yasrehi H, Rhatigan R, Woodward ER: Acute phlegmasia of the stomach. Am Surg 36:225, 1970.
83. Nevin NC, Eakins D, Clarke SD, Carson DJL: Acute phlegmonous gastritis. Br J Surg 56:268, 1969.
84. Locolio SA, Stahl W: Diverticular disease of the alimentary tract: the esophagus, stomach, and duode-

num and small intestine. Curr Probl Surg 51:3, 1968.
85. Konok G, Haddad H, Strom B: Postoperative gastric mycosis. Surg Gynecol Obstet 150:337, 1980.
86. Chazan BI, Aitchison JD: Gastric tuberculosis. Br Med J 2:1288, 1960.
87. Raffin S: Granulomatous infectious disease of the stomach. In Sleisenger MH, Fordtran JS (eds): Gastrointestinal Disease: Pathophysiology, Diagnosis, Management. Philadelphia, Saunders, 1973, p 573.
88. Nudelman HL, Rakatansky H: Gastric histoplasmosis: a case report. JAMA 195:44, 1966.
89. Gardner B, Butler ED, Goldman L: Early complications of gastrectomy with particular reference to delayed gastric emptying. Arch Surg 89:475, 1964.
90. Snyder EN Jr, Stellar CA: Results from emergency surgery for massively bleeding duodenal ulcer. Am J Surg 116:170, 1968.
91. Sherman JN, Davis JR, Jesseph JE: Subphrenic abscess: a continuing hazard. Am J Surg 117:117, 1969.
92. Brummer DL: Prophylaxis of tuberculosis after gastrectomy (editorial). Am J Dig Dis 14:753, 1969.
93. Altmeier WA, Bryant LR, Wulsin JH: The surgical significance of jejunal diverticulosis. Arch Surg 86:732, 1963.
94. Bandres JC, Dupont HL: Approach to the patient with diarrhea. In Gorbach SL, Bartlett JG, Blacklow NR (eds): Infectious Diseases. Philadelphia, Saunders, 1992, p 572.
95. Grady GF, Keusch GT: Pathogenesis of bacterial diarrheas. N Engl J Med 285:831, 891, 1971.
96. Editorial. Mechanisms in enteropathogenic *Escherichia coli* diarrhea. Lancet 1:1254, 1983.
97. Moss J, Burns DL, Hsia JA, et al: Cyclic nucleotides: mediators of bacterial toxin action in disease. Ann Intern Med 101:653, 1984.
98. Drake AA, Gilchrist MJR, Washington JA II, et al: Diarrhea due to *Campylobacter fetus* subspecies *jeju:* a clinical review of 63 cases. Mayo Clin Proc 56:414, 1981.
99. Blaser MJ, Reller LB: *Campylobacter* enteritis. N Engl J Med 305:1444, 1981.
100. Sleisenger MH, Fordtran JS (eds): Gastrointestinal Disease: Pathophysiology, Diagnosis, Management. Philadelphia, Saunders, 1973.
101. Thoren A, Wolde-Mariam T, Stintzing G, et al: Antibiotics in the treatment of gastroenteritis caused by enteropathogenic *Escherichia coli.* J Infect Dis 141:27, 1980.
102. Archampong EQ: Typhoid ileal perforations: why such mortalities? Br J Surg 63:317, 1976.
103. Singh J, Singh B: Enteric perforation in typhoid fever: a study of 15 cases. Aust N Z J Surg 45:279, 1975.
104. Eggleston FC, Santoshi B, Singh CM: Typhoid perforation of the bowel: experience in 78 cases. Ann Surg 190:31, 1979.
105. Finegold SM: Anaerobic Bacteria in Human Disease. New York, Academic, 1977.
106. Larsen HE, Price AB, Honour P, Borriello SP: *Clostridium difficile* and the aetiology of pseudomembranous colitis. Lancet 1:1063, 1978.
107. Hitchcock CR, Bubrick MP: Gas gangrene infections of the small intestine, colon and rectum. Dis Colon Rectum 19:112, 1976.
108. Asao OG, Solanke TF: Surgical aspects of ascariasis. J Natl Med Assoc 69:149, 1977.
109. Schlossberg D, Devig PM, Travers H, et al: Bowel perforation with candidiasis. JAMA 238:2520, 1977.
110. Aston NO, DeCosta AM: Tuberculous perforation of the small bowel. Postgrad Med J 61:251, 1985.
111. Asraf SM, Mital RN, Prakash A: Tuberculous bowel perforations. Am J Proctol 26:47, 1975.
112. NIH Conference: Moderator Smith PD: Gastrointestinal Infections in AIDS. Ann Intern Med 116:63, 1992.
113. Bartlett JG: Gastrointestinal complications of HIV infection. In Gorbach SL, Bartlett JG, Blacklow NR (eds): Infectious Diseases. Philadelphia, Saunders, 1992, p 944.
114. Ellakany S, Whiteside TL, Schade RR, van Theil DH: Analysis of intestinal lymphocyte subpopulations in patients with AIDS and AIDS related complex. J Clin Pathol 87:356, 1987.
115. Kotler DP, Scoles JV, Tierney AR: Intestinal plasma cell alteration in acquired immune deficiency syndrome. Dig Dis Sci 32:129, 1987.
116. Ullrich R, Zeitz M, Heise W, et al: Small intestinal structure and function in patients infected with HIV. Evidence for HIV induced enteropathy. Ann Intern Med 111:15, 1989.
117. Rosenberg IH: Influence of intestinal bacteria on bile acid metabolism and fat absorption: contributions from studies of blind-loop syndrome. Am J Nutr 22:284, 1969.
118. Gracey M, Burke V, Oshin A, et al: Bacteria, bile salts, and intestinal monosaccharide malabsorption. Gut 12:683, 1971.
119. Goldstein F: Mechanisms of malabsorption and malnutrition in the blind loop syndrome. Gastroenterology 61:780, 1971.
120. Lauterburg BH, Newcomer AD, Hofmann AF: Clinical value of the bile acid breath test. Mayo Clin Proc 53:227, 1978.
121. Joiner KA, Gorbach SL: Antimicrobial therapy of digestive diseases. Clin Gastroenterol 8:3, 1979.
122. Drenick EJ, Ament M, Finegold SM, et al: Bypass enteropathy: intestinal and systemic manifestations following small bowel bypass. JAMA 236:269, 1976.
123. Francis WW, Eunnuccilli E: Acute fulminating transmural ileocolitis after small bowel bypass for morbid obesity. Am J Surg 135:524, 1978.
124. Drenick EJ, Ament M, Finegold SM, Passaro E: Bypass enteropathy: an inflammatory process in the excluded segment with systemic complications. Am J Clin Nutr 30:76, 1977.
125. Corrodi P, Wideman PA, Sutter VL, et al: Bacterial flora of the small bowel before and after bypass procedure for morbid obesity. J Infect Dis 137:1, 1978.

126. Nelson JL, Rees R, Bonneval MM, et al: Jejunoileal bypass, liver morphology and intestinal microflora in conventional and germ-free dogs. Surg Forum 27:73, 1976.
127. Barry RE, Chow AW, Billesdon J, et al: Colonic pseudo-obstruction complicating jejuno-ileal bypass: the role of intestinal flora. Gut 16:825, 1975.
128. Brandberg A, Kock NH, Philipson B: Bacterial flora in intraabdominal ileostomy reservoir. Gastroenterology 63:413, 1972.
129. Schjonsby H, Halvorsen IF, Hofstad T, Hordenak N: Stagnant loop syndrome in patients with continent ileostomy (intraabdominal ileal reservoir). Gut 18:795, 1977.
130. Halvorsen IF, Heimann P, Hoel R: The continent reservoir ileostomy review of a collective series of 36 patients from 3 surgical departments. Surgery 83:252, 1978.
131. King SA: Enteritis and the continent ileostomy. Conn Med 41:477, 1977.
132. O'Connell PR, Rankin DR, Weiland LH, Kelly KA: Enteric bacteriology, absorption, morphology and emptying after ileal pouch–anal anastomosis. Br J Surg 73:909, 1986.
133. Sugerman HJ, Newsome HH, Decosta G, Zfass AM: Stapled ileoanal anastomosis for ulcerative colitis and familial polyposis without a temporary diverting colostomy. Ann Surg 213:606, 1991.
134. Gemlo BT, Wong WD, Rothenberger DA, Goldberg SM: Ileal pouch–anal anastomosis, patterns of failure. Arch Surg 127:784, 1992.
135. Lohmuller RJ, Pemberton JH, Dozois RR, et al: Pouchitis and extra-intestinal manifestations of inflammatory bowel disease after ileal pouch–anal anastomosis. Ann Surg 211:623, 1990.
136. Parker TH, O'Leary IP: Effect of preparation of the small bowel on microflora postoperative wound infection. Surg Gynecol Obstet 146:379, 1978.
137. Hojer H, Wetherfors J: Concentration of doxycycline in bowel tissue and postoperative infections. Scand J Infect Dis Suppl 9:100, 1976.

Infections of the Colon

CHAPTER 43

Alonzo P. Walker, Robert E. Condon

PATHOGENIC FEATURES OF INFECTIONS ARISING IN THE COLON

Anatomic Features

At some point in its course, the colon is situated adjacent to every intra-abdominal organ. Loss of bowel wall integrity can therefore lead to any of the intra-abdominal infections discussed in Chapter 38. Disease of the cecum or the sigmoid colon may remain localized in the right or left lower quadrant, or extend into the pelvis. Disease of the ascending or descending colon can be confined to the paracolic gutters. Hepatic or splenic flexure disease can cause subphrenic or subhepatic abscesses. Disease originating in the intraperitoneal rectosigmoid colon may involve the pelvis and may spread superiorly into the main abdominal cavity.

Only the transverse and sigmoid colon are supported by a mesentery. Disease may extend directly into the mesentery, remaining confined there. Or, it may burst free, resulting in an abscess of the lesser sac originating from the transverse colon, or a pelvic or midabdominal (interloop) abscess originating from the sigmoid colon.

The posterior surfaces of the ascending and descending colon are retroperitoneal. Perforation here can cause a retroperitoneal abscess with subsequent extension to the perineum, thigh, groin, abdominal wall, or chest (posterior mediastinum, pericardium, pleural cavities). Retroperitoneal infection arising from the rectosigmoid or rectum can spread cephalad into the main retroperitoneal spaces; remain localized in the pelvis in the presacral, pararectal, rectovesical, and prevesical spaces; or extend through the levator diaphragm into the ischiorectal space and the perineum.

Physiologic Features

The large bowel conducts the ileal effluent to the rectum, where it is stored until defecation is convenient. Propulsive activity differs in the right and left colon. On the right side, much of the motor activity consists of short runs of circular muscle contraction, involving only a portion of the bowel circumference; bidirectional flow results. Periodically, the cecum contracts, the ascending colon shortens, and a sequential wave of circular muscle contractions strips some of the luminal content into the transverse colon. On the left side, propulsion is predominantly caused by mass contraction of both circular and longitudinal muscle, which occurs most consistently after meals. The mass contractions begin in the left transverse and progress slowly to the proximal sigmoid colon. The colon ahead of the mass contraction relaxes; as a result, the left colon forms a tube through which a large bolus of the fecal mass is moved by the mass contraction.

Segmental contractions also occur throughout the colon, especially between meals, and particularly in the transverse, descending, and sigmoid colon. These localized, almost occlusive contractions temporarily separate the colon into a series of small compartments, producing a kneading action on the feces. There is also some evidence for antiperistaltic activity in the left colon. Barium sulfate instilled into the rectum can be found in the ascending and transverse colon within several hours.

Absorption of water, sodium, and chloride occurs during fecal passage through the large bowel. Whereas 1500 to 2500 ml of ileal content, containing about 185 mEq of sodium, enters the cecum each day, the daily fecal volume of 100 to 150 ml contains only 2 to 5 mEq of sodium.

Colon Flora

The microbial ecology of the alimentary tract is discussed in Chapter 3. The gut is sterile at birth but rapidly becomes populated by both aerobic and anaerobic organisms. Although *Escherichia coli* and *Klebsiella* species appear early in infant feces, aerobic lactobacilli predominate while milk or formula is the primary food. Anaerobes also are present in infant feces within 1 week of birth. *Bacteroides* species predominate in formula-fed babies, whereas *Bifidobacterium* species are more frequent in breast-fed infants.

The concentration of bacteria in the colon approaches 10^{11} to 10^{12} CFU/ml, nearly equaling the theoretical maximum number of bacteria (10^{12}) that can be packed into such a volume. This ecosystem is extremely dense, heterogeneous, and complex. More than 400 distinct bacterial species have been isolated from the feces of a single individual.[1] Most of the organisms in feces are saprophytes and commensals, do not act as pathogens, and have not been recovered in human infections. The fecal flora are remarkably stable in composition and are only slightly affected by environmental or dietary change. Bacteria represent about one-third of the dry weight of human fecal matter.[1]

The colon flora are a mixture of aerobic and anaerobic bacteria (Fig. 43–1). The principal aerobic pathogen is *E. coli* (10^8 per gram of dry fecal matter). Other aerobic coliforms (*Klebsiella, Proteus, Enterobacter*) and the enterococci are present in lower concentrations. The aerobic coliforms are 100 to 1000 times less numerous in feces than are anaerobes,[2] primarily because of the low oxidation-reduction potential of the colon lumen that favors the growth of anaerobic organisms.

The most common anaerobic genera of fecal isolates are *Bacteroides, Fusobacterium, Eubacterium, Bifidobacterium, Clostridium,* and anaerobic cocci (*Peptostreptococcus*).[1,3] *Bacteroides* species are predominant and account for approximately 3 percent of the fecal bacterial mass.[4] The most numerous *Bacteroides* species in human feces are *B. vulgatus, B. distasonis,* and *B. thetaiotamicron* (10^{10} per gram dry weight feces). Although less numerous, *B. fragilis* (10^9 per gram dry fecal weight) is still present in high concentration and is the most common anaerobe isolated from clinical infections associated with colorectal operations.[1,4,5] Other numerically predominant fecal isolates are *Eubacterium aerofaciens, Peptostreptococcus productus, Fusobacterium prausnitzii, Bifidobacterium adolescentis, Clostridium leptum* (10^9 per gram dry feces), and *Peptostreptococcus magnus.*[4,6] Staphylococci and fungi also inhabit the colon in small numbers, their concentration being inversely related to the concentration of *E. coli.* Antimicrobial agents, which act selectively against *E. coli,* will permit staphylococcal and fungal overgrowth. *Salmonella typhosa* and *Vibrio cholerae* are other potential pathogens but they cannot easily colonize the colon unless the inoculum is very high or protein malnutrition is present.

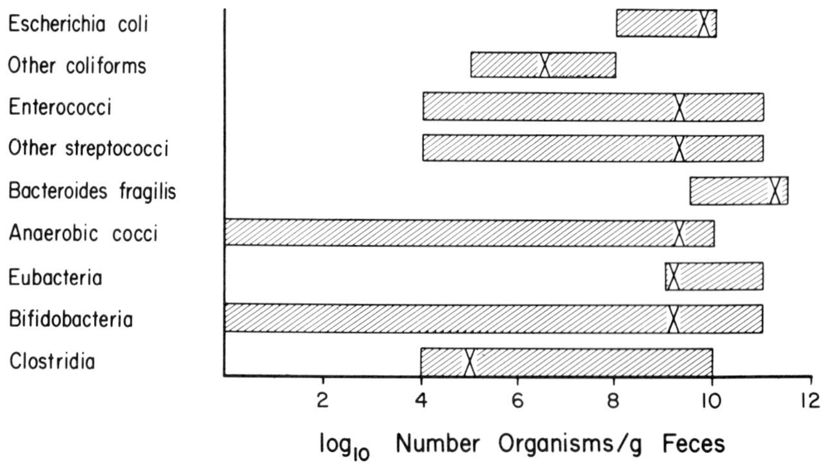

Figure 43–1. Concentrations of fecal bacteria. (X, median; bars, range.)

PERFORATION OF LARGE BOWEL

General Aspects

Epidemiology and Incidence. The causes of large bowel perforation are listed in Table 43–1. In the United States, most perforations are caused by trauma, carcinoma, and diverticulitis. In less developed areas of the world, parasitic disease also is an important cause of colon perforation.

Etiology and Pathogenesis. It is the bacterial component of feces that causes problems after perforation. Sterilized feces injected into the peritoneal cavity of experimental animals have no major adverse consequences. However, feces containing live bacteria produce peritonitis.[7]

Fecal organisms are isolated most frequently from patients with abdominal sepsis (see Chap. 38).[2,8] *Escherichia coli* is recovered in nine of ten cases of infection due to colon perforation and *Klebsiella, Enterobacter, Proteus,* and enterococci are frequent aerobic isolates. *Pseudomonas, Staphylococcus,* and *Candida* are found infrequently. The most common anaerobic pathogen is *B. fragilis,* isolated in 80 to 95 percent of patients with colorectal perforation. Also found are other *Bacteroides* species, *Clostridium, Fusobacterium,* peptostreptococci, *Eubacterium,* and *Bifidobacterium.* The number of anaerobic species recovered varies with the skill of the laboratory.

The importance of synergistic infections caused by multiple organisms has been stressed (see Chaps. 7 and 38). Although most enteric aerobes are relatively noninvasive pathogens, anaerobic organisms may be quite tissue-invasive when necrotic tissue, decreased tissue oxidation-reduction potential, and iron derived from hemoglobin or myoglobin are present. The chief contribution of aerobic organisms in mixed infections may be the use of available tissue oxygen.

There are a number of factors that influence the clinical outcome of peritonitis. The extent of contamination, the underlying cause (trauma, perforation, obstruction), the general condition of the patient, the site of perforation, and the promptness of medical and surgical therapy are some of the major factors that influence the development, progress, and resolution of peritonitis.[9]

TABLE 43–1. CAUSES OF PERFORATION

- Trauma
  - Penetrating injury
  - Blunt injury
  - Iatrogenic
    - Operative injury
    - Drain erosion
    - Enema
    - Endoscopic and diagnostic
    - Thermometer
  - Colostomy irrigation
  - Ingested foreign body
  - Pneumatic rupture
  - Rectal foreign body
- Diverticular disease
  - Sigmoid diverticula
  - Cecal diverticula
- Inflammatory bowel disease
  - Ulcerative colitis
  - Granulomatous colitis
- Carcinoma of large bowel
- Large bowel obstruction
  - Extrinsic tumor
  - Fecal impaction
  - Volvulus
  - Hirschsprung's disease
  - Atresia of colon or anus
  - Meconium ileus
  - Meconium plug syndrome
  - Neonatal small left colon syndrome
- Strangulation of colon
  - Intussusception
  - Hernia
  - Volvulus
  - Strangulated hernia
  - Pseudo-obstruction of colon
- Ischemic colitis
  - Necrotizing colitis
  - Colitis of obstruction
  - Colitis of vascular surgery
  - Radiation colitis
  - Stercoral ulcer and perforation
  - Spontaneous ulcer and perforation
- Bacterial infections
  - Shigellosis
  - Salmonellosis, including typhoid
  - Yersiniosis
- Antibiotic-associated colitis
- Tuberculosis
- Actinomycosis
- Cytomegalovirus disease
- Amebiasis
- Schistosomiasis
- Diseases of infancy and childhood
  - Neonatal necrotizing enterocolitis
  - Idiopathic perforation
  - Obstructive lesions

Clinical Manifestations. Leaking large bowel contents most often cause local peritonitis (see Chap. 38). Abdominal pain is constant, aching, and aggravated by sudden change in position or by coughing or retching. Initially, the pain is localized; however, as the process expands, the pain spreads, first across the lower abdomen and then upward over the entire abdomen. If the diaphragm is involved, unilateral or bilateral shoulder pain may develop. If the process is confined to the pelvis, little or no anterior abdominal pain may be present.

Peritonitis results in disordered secretory and absorptive function of the bowel. Initially, those bowel segments adjacent to the perforation become inflamed, leading to diarrhea. Later, as ileus develops, obstipation results. Fever, most often low grade but sometimes spiking with shaking chills, is present in nearly all patients. With septicemia, the temperature may be subnormal. Usually, malaise and anorexia are present even if pain is absent. If generalized ileus results, nausea and vomiting may occur.

Clinical findings of both hypovolemia and sepsis usually are present. At first, pain may induce tachycardia and mild hypertension. With progression of peritonitis, diarrhea, ileus, and vomiting, the extracellular fluid volume becomes depleted, the heart rate increases, blood pressure declines, and shock eventually ensues. The patient is thirsty, lethargic, and weak and becomes disoriented. Skin turgor may be decreased, and urine output is low. The patient may be flushed owing to septicemia, or pale owing to poor capillary filling if hypovolemia predominates. Blood loss may contribute to pallor.

Inspection of the abdomen may show limited respiratory motion because of local guarding. If generalized peritonitis is present, the abdominal component of respiration may be entirely absent. Distension eventually occurs. Palpation demonstrates localized or generalized guarding. If guarding is not severe, a mass may be palpated. Bowel sounds are hypoactive. The abdomen is distended, tympanitic to percussion, and normal dullness over the liver may be absent. Tenderness can be elicited by percussion and may be localized to the area of involvement, be referred from the local area to elsewhere in the abdominal wall, or be generalized.

Rectal and pelvic examinations may demonstrate exquisite tenderness in the presence of pelvic sepsis or generalized peritonitis. Gross or occult blood may be present in the stool. With a pelvic abscess, a fluctuant mass may bulge into the anterior rectum. With a retroperitoneal abscess, abdominal symptoms and signs may be totally absent.

Septicemia caused by anaerobic organisms is often characterized by jaundice and disorientation as well as high-spiking fever. Occasionally, perforation of the colon and rectum into the retroperitoneal spaces will be detected first as a perianal or perineal abscess, sometimes even as gangrene of the scrotum and perineum or as a psoas abscess even extending into the thigh. Motion at the hip joint may be limited because of muscle spasm or joint involvement. Thus a patient complaining of buttock, perineal, groin, or thigh pain, associated with erythematous or dusky skin, perhaps with bullae or tissue emphysema, may have an occult colon perforation. More bizarre clinical presentations of colon perforation, such as mediastinitis with emphysema or pneumopericardium, have been recorded.

Laboratory Findings. In most cases, the leukocyte count is elevated between 10,000 and 20,000 cells/mm^3. *Bacteroides* septicemia may elicit leukocyte counts as high as 50,000. The differential count usually shows increased numbers of immature neutrophils. A normal urinalysis indicates that the urinary tract is not the source of the problem. However, an infection contiguous to any portion of the urinary system may induce minimal pyuria or hematuria. A fistula between the colon and the urinary tract directly contaminates the urine.

In cases suspected of early peritonitis, abdominal x-rays should be taken in the recumbent, upright, and left and right lateral decubitus positions. Free air may be noted under the diaphragm on upright films (Fig. 43–2A) or in the flank on the lateral decubitus films (see Fig. 43–2B). Loss of the flank preperitoneal fat stripe or the psoas shadow indicates local inflammation in these areas. The kidney outline may be obscured as a result of a perinephric infection. Inflammation in the perirenal and pararenal tissues may impair the movement of the kidneys when the patient moves from a recumbent to an erect position. The presence of free intraperitoneal fluid may be suggested by widening between loops of bowel. Examination of the bowel gas pattern can indicate ileus, obstruction, or volvulus. *Thumbprinting* suggests ischemic or inflamed colon. Displaced loops of bowel indicate an extrinsic mass, and extraluminal gas bubbles point to an abscess. If an intra-abdominal abscess is suspected, computed tomography (CT) scan of the abdomen is the most efficient investigation. Barium should not be used.

In most clinical situations, contrast studies are unnecessary. Intravenous pyelography may help document the location of the ureters. In doubtful cases, water-soluble contrast studies of the colon can confirm the presence of a leak. Barium contrast studies should be avoided. Endoscopy may be considered if the patient is stable and the diagnosis is unclear. The perforation itself, another lesion, or ischemic mucosa may be noted.

In cases of multiple trauma and in obtunded patients or children, the diagnosis may be more difficult. Peritoneal lavage with a liter of crystalloid solution may yield helpful information; finding bacteria, vegetable fibers or other fecal matter, or a white blood cell (WBC) concentration greater than 500 cells/mm^3 of lavage fluid may help establish a diagnosis of perforation. In patients with an obscure clinical picture, compatible with but not diagnostic of intra-abdominal or retroperitoneal sepsis, a variety of techniques to detect and localize septic processes have been proposed (see Chap. 38), none of which appear to be either specific or efficient. Although there is a place for such examinations, the information derived in individual patients must be interpreted in light of the total clinical picture.

Diagnosis. To provide optimum antimicrobial therapy, it is desirable to identify each organism involved in the infection. Chapter 38 lists those bacte-

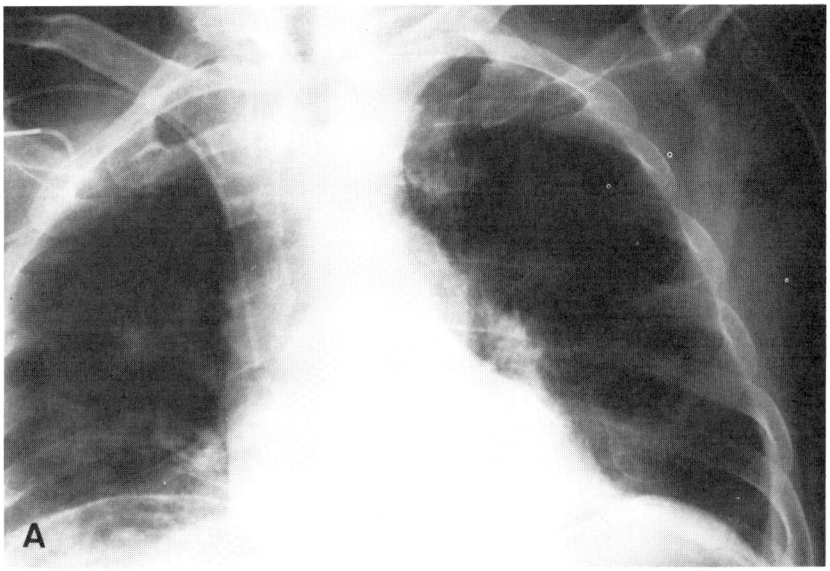

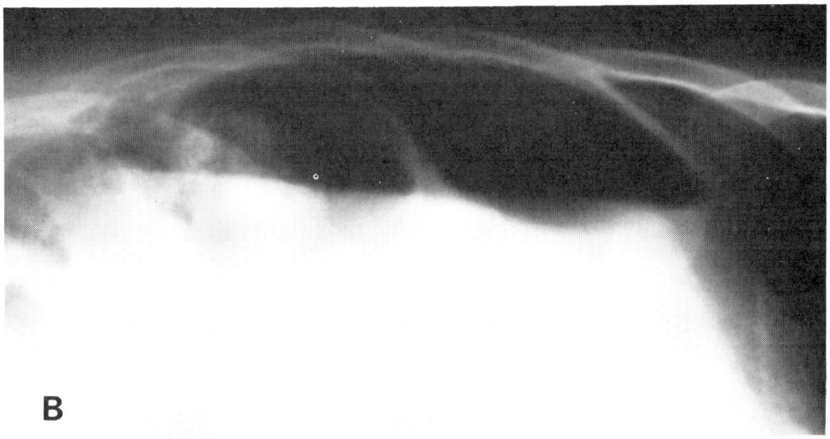

Figure 43–2. A. Colon perforation. Free air is seen under the diaphragm on an upright chest film. **B.** Colon perforation. Free air is seen under the right rib cage on a left lateral decubitus abdominal film.

ria commonly found in feculent peritonitis and the rationale for empiric choice of antibiotics. A Gram stain of the infected material is sometimes helpful in tentative morphologic identification of anaerobes. Even when anaerobes cannot be cultured, they must be assumed to be present in all fresh colon perforations. The best procedures for anaerobic culture are described in Chapter 2.

Treatment and Prognosis. Treatment of a suspected large bowel perforation should be vigorous. The blood volume should be replenished rapidly with intravenous crystalloid solution or blood. A gastric tube should be placed to empty the stomach and reduce the risk of aspiration of vomitus. Intravenous antibiotics should be administered immediately. Because fecal organisms are present, broad spectrum antibiotics effective against both aerobes and anaerobes are recommended. Alternative choices of antibiotics are discussed in Chapter 38.

After the patient is prepared, surgical control of the perforation is obtained. The basic task to be accomplished at operation is control of the perforation and removal of necrotic tissue and pus. On occasion, this may be accomplished by simple suture closure if (1) there is no fecal contamination, (2) the colon wound is small, and (3) the colon wall is otherwise structurally normal. More frequently, the diseased bowel should be resected. There are few circumstances in which large bowel perforation is treated only by drainage.

The reason for thorough peritoneal toilet in the treatment of peritonitis is discussed in Chapter 38. As much necrotic tissue as possible should be debrided. Collections of pus must be drained completely. Abscesses are drained externally, using large closed suction drains. The drains should be brought out through separate stab incisions placed so that the drainage track is as short, direct, and dependent as possible. The peritoneal cavity should be irrigated copiously with large volumes of saline solution to remove as much fecal material and loose debris as possible.

The fascia is closed using a running monofilament suture. The skin is not approximated. The entire dressing is changed postoperatively as often as needed. If the wound is clean and contains no necrotic tissue, delayed closure is accomplished by loose approximation of the wound edges with adhesive strips after the fifth postoperative day.

If there is extensive peritoneal contamination, primary fascia closure should be delayed. The abdominal wall may be approximated temporarily with an artificial device to allow for planned reexplorations. The purpose of these planned reexplorations is to remove residual or reaccumulated pus, debride nonviable tissue, and inspect the bowel and anastomoses if any were performed.[10]

Although the risk of death following perforation of the colon and rectum is still high, the mortality rate of patients with untreated intra-abdominal sepsis approaches 100 percent.[11] Thus expeditious and thorough surgical therapy combined with aggressive postoperative care are essential.

Perforation of the Colon in Infancy

The true incidence of isolated colon perforation secondary to trauma and other diseases is not well documented in the pediatric population because colon perforation, as seen in this population, generally is grouped in the category of *gastrointestinal tract perforation.* In infancy, the leading cause of both gastrointestinal tract and colon perforation is necrotizing enterocolitis.[12,13] Obstructive lesions, that is, Hirschsprung's disease and small left colon syndrome, are no longer frequent causes of colon perforation because of earlier diagnosis and treatment of these lesions. Trauma is probably the most common cause in older children.

Neonatal Necrotizing Enterocolitis. This disease causes more than 50 percent of all gastrointestinal tract perforations seen in neonates.[14] Although the problem became increasingly apparent during the 1970s,[15] the need for operation has decreased as understanding of the pathogenesis of this disease has increased.[16]

Pathology and Pathogenesis. Variable amounts of small and large intestine are affected in neonatal necrotizing enterocolitis. The ileocecal area and ascending colon are involved most often; the entire gut from stomach to rectum is affected in 5 to 15 percent of cases. Skip areas of necrotic and normal bowel are often found. The gut proximal to areas of involvement and the involved bowel are both dilated, the bowel wall being thin and friable. Affected bowel may demonstrate a spectrum of necrosis from areas of apparent subserosal ecchymosis to obvious full-thickness gangrene. Multiple perforations surrounded by deposits of fibrin and exudate are frequent; perforations may be sealed by adherent surrounding loops of bowel. The mucosa is edematous, hemorrhagic, or ulcerated. Frequently, pockets of gas are noted under the mucosa and, less frequently, subserosally. Gas bubbles may be detected in mesenteric veins. Bacteria may be present in the bowel wall. Intramural blood vessels are engorged, but thrombosis is rare except in autopsy specimens.

Certain predisposing factors appear to be critical to the pathogenesis of this condition. The Apgar score is often below 7, and most affected infants (up to 90 percent) are premature or have a low birth weight. Respiratory distress syndrome or apneic episodes occur in 50 to 60 percent, an umbilical artery catheter has been used in 25 to 60 percent, and exchange transfusion has been necessary in another 15 to 45 percent. Congenital heart disease and patent ductus arteriosus are present in 20 to 45 percent. The common factor seems to be bowel ischemia. Thromboembolic phenomena may be involved, but vasospasm in response to hypoxia and stress seems to be more important. Barlow and Santulli[14] have been able to reproduce a similar condition in newborn rats subjected to hypoxia or to cold stress. After the mucosal barrier is injured, gut bacteria invade and cause further damage.

Whether infection is ever a primary (rather than a contributory) cause of neonatal necrotizing enterocolitis is debated. Clustering of cases of enterocolitis suggesting an infectious epidemic has been reported. Book et al[17] were unable to identify any specific responsible organisms, but using infection control procedures, they reduced their incidence of necrotizing enterocolitis from 3.6 to 0.7 percent. In contrast, Bell et al[18] found no unusual organisms in patients with enterocolitis, even though *E. coli* and *K. pneumoniae* were more prevalent in the feces of enterocolitis patients than control patients. On the other hand, Howard et al[19] were able to isolate *C. butyricum* from the blood of nine of ten patients.

Many patients with necrotizing enterocolitis have been fed formula or glucose solution rather than breast milk, which has a protective effect presumably due to its content of IgA and leukocytes.[16]

Formula and glucose solutions are, in addition, hyperosmolar and may further injure ischemic mucosa.

Clinical Manifestations. Although the syndrome usually starts during the first 10 days of life, necrotizing enterocolitis can be delayed in appearance to age 3 or 4 weeks. Initial changes may be subtle: lethargy, acrocyanosis, increased gastric retention between feedings, and vomiting or regurgitation of bile-stained gastric contents. Abdominal distention is almost always present, initially soft and nontender; later, tenderness, erythema, and induration of the abdominal wall supervene. The presence of a pneumoscrotum or an inflammatory mass in the scrotum indicates bowel perforation.[17] In a thin neonate, intramural intestinal air blebs may be detectable by abdominal palpation, a sensation akin to that of palpating Rice Krispies.

Affected infants have usually passed meconium, and the anus is patent. Diarrhea sometimes appears, and one-fourth pass stools of mucus and visible blood. Hypothermia or thermal instability is frequent. As dehydration progresses, tachycardia and hypotension become apparent. Petechiae and oropharyngeal bleeding appear late in the course.

Diagnosis. Laboratory examination at first reveals only a mild anemia, leukocytosis or leukopenia, and thrombocytopenia (50,000 to 75,000). In later stages of illness, diffuse intravascular coagulation, hypoxia, and acidosis will be evident. Stool analysis may reveal the presence of occult blood and of reducing substances (carbohydrate). Stool examinations may be used to screen infants at risk for enterocolitis, but a positive result in the absence of other clinical signs does not establish a diagnosis.

All infants with findings suggestive of sepsis should have cultures of sputum, urine, feces, cerebrospinal fluid, and blood made before institution of antibiotic treatment. Positive blood culture findings are obtained in 20 to 70 percent of patients with necrotizing enterocolitis. In the majority of cases, *E. coli, Klebsiella, Enterobacter,* and *Proteus* are recovered. Positive anaerobic blood culture results are rare, although Howard et al[19] describe a group of patients from whom *C. butyricum* was isolated. Repeated plain abdominal x-ray studies in the recumbent, upright, or lateral decubitus positions at 4- to 6-hour intervals are the most useful tests for diagnosing and following necrotizing enterocolitis. The early images are of generalized ileus, with dilation of the stomach and small and large bowel. As the disease progresses, there is evidence of thickened bowel walls. Intramural collections of gas, pneumatosis cystoides intestinalis, are noted in 75 to 80 percent of patients. In addition, gas may be noted in the mesenteric and portal venous systems. Intra-abdominal fluid is found in later stages of the disease. Free intraperitoneal gas indicates bowel perforation. Fixed loops of bowel may indicate areas of sealed perforation. Early in the disease, one should resist the temptation to perform a contrast enema, because the risk of perforation is great while the diagnostic aid is small.

Treatment. Early enterocolitis can most often be cured by nonoperative treatment. Oral feedings should be stopped, gastric suction instituted, and intravenous antibiotics begun. On the basis of the organisms usually cultured, an aminoglycoside, clindamycin, and ampicillin have been chosen in the past as initial therapy. Substitution of other, less potentially toxic, regimens awaits documentation by clinical trials. On the basis of the work of Cohn et al,[20] which indicates that topical antibiotics can help to heal ischemic bowel, Bell et al[21] also administer aminoglycosides by gastric tube; since oral aminoglycosides are absorbed poorly, potential toxicity is limited.

Intravenous fluids and electrolytes help maintain vital signs, urine output, and normal electrolyte balance. Blood is replaced as necessary. Fresh whole blood or fresh frozen plasma is given if coagulation abnormalities develop. It may be necessary to transfuse platelets. Maintenance of nutrition with intravenous alimentation is essential. Nonoperative therapy is continued as long as improvement is noted.

The indication for operation in acute necrotizing enterocolitis is development of gangrene of the bowel, with or without actual perforation. The clinical task is to detect this state without performing unnecessary operations that only lead to high mortality.[14,21] Kosloske et al[22] recently reviewed 61 infants with this disease. A total of ten proposed clinical, x-ray, and laboratory criteria for operation were considered. Each operative criterion was correlated with the documented presence or absence of intestinal gangrene. Indications for operation verified by this study were (1) pneumoperitoneum, (2) paracentesis findings positive for gangrenous intestine, (3) erythema of the abdominal wall, (4) a fixed abdominal mass, and (5) a persistently dilated loop of intestine on serial abdominal x-ray studies. The first two signs occurred frequently; the latter three were rare. Operative indications that proved to be invalid in this study were (1) clinical deterioration, (2) persistent abdominal tenderness, (3) profuse lower gastrointestinal hemorrhage, (4) x-ray finding of a gasless abdomen with ascites, and (5) severe thrombocytopenia.

Surgical management involves resection of perforated and gangrenous segments of bowel. All free ends of bowel should be brought out as enterostomies rather than performing primary anastomoses. If any doubt exists as to whether bowel is viable it may be assessed intraoperatively by intravenous fluorescein injection. Normal bowel fluoresces quickly while ischemic or dead bowel does not fluoresce. If the bowel is slow to fluoresce a second-look operation in 24 to 48 hours is recommended.

Prognosis. Neonatal necrotizing enterocolitis used to be uniformly fatal. With earlier diagnosis and more aggressive treatment, the present overall survival is greater than 80 percent in most centers.[23] Mortality is related directly to a number of factors, low birth weight being the most important. The mortality of infants greater than 1500 g at birth was 29 percent compared to 47 percent for infants of low birth weight. Additionally, patients without perforation had a 20 to 30 percent mortality compared to a 60 to 65 percent mortality for patients with perforation.[23] Late complications of necrotizing enterocolitis include malabsorption if large lengths of bowel were excised, and obstruction of the small intestine resulting from stricture as the ischemic bowel heals.

Obstructive Lesions Leading to Colonic Perforation in Infants and Children. Hirschsprung's disease,[24–26] atresia of the colon or anus, meconium ileus, meconium plug syndrome, and neonatal small left colon syndrome will result in perforation of the colon if left unattended. Patients with Hirschsprung's disease frequently develop an enterocolitis proximal to the obstructed segment. This condition is distinct from necrotizing enterocolitis in that necrosis of the bowel wall with perforation is unusual even though septicemia can occur; the mucosa demonstrates only a nonspecific colitis.[3]

Hirschsprung's Disease. The clinical picture may vary, but in all instances problems with defecation begin in the first few days of life. There may be no spontaneous passage of meconium, or only small amounts may be passed. Vigorous rectal examination or enemas may result in passage of a large quantity of normal meconium and stool. Typically, abdominal distention develops over weeks or months and peristaltic waves are sometimes visible on the abdominal wall. Feeding is less vigorous, bilious vomiting may occur, and food may be retained only intermittently. The infant is unusually listless and fails to gain weight. Cecal perforation or acute appendicitis in the newborn is commonly caused by Hirschsprung's disease.[26]

Enterocolitis occurs in about one-fourth of patients with Hirschsprung's disease and is responsible for most of the deaths.[27] Explosive diarrhea is associated with abdominal distention, fever, and prostration. Usually, the enterocolitis can be managed for several days with frequent saline enemas. Careful observation by a physician or a parent is necessary to prevent dehydration in severe cases.

Some children with untreated Hirschsprung's disease survive infancy. These patients have problems with chronic constipation, abdominal distention, and flatulence, but encopresis does not occur. Both development and weight gain lag. Although mild, intermittent eposides of diarrhea are more prevalent, enterocolitis continues to be a risk.

Hirschsprung's disease is suspected when a dilated colon filled with feces proximal to the involved narrow segment is seen on barium enema. Usually, there is a rather definite demarcation between segments. To be certain of the diagnosis, a rectal biopsy demonstrating lack of intermuscular ganglion cells is required.

Often the obstruction of Hirschsprung's disease can be initially managed by enemas, but once the diagnosis has been proved by rectal biopsy, a colostomy proximal to the affected segment should be established. When the child has grown sufficiently, and the proximal bowel has returned to normal size, the abnormal bowel is resected and a coloanal or colorectal anastomosis is made in the manner of Swenson, Duhamel, or Soave.

Patients with Hirschsprung's disease rarely survive to adulthood without operation. Death occurs in 2 to 4 percent of patients who undergo elective resection.[26,28] Patients with enterocolitis, especially infants, have a worse prognosis because of the complications of dehydration, perforation, and septicemia. The mortality rate in enterocolitis is 30 percent.[24] The significance of enterocolitis in Hirschsprung's disease is indicated by the mortality rate of diverting colostomy performed in infants before or after the onset of enterocolitis: 4 percent versus 33 percent, respectively. The incidence of postoperative enterocolitis is 5 to 25 percent and is more likely to occur if it had been present preoperatively.

Perforation due to Other Obstructive Colonic Lesions in Infancy. *Strangulation* may occur as a result of an obstructing lesion, such as malrotation of the bowel or incarcerated hernia. In obstructed infants, hernia must be sought not only in the inguinal and umbilical regions, but also in unusual sites such as the diaphragm, perineum, and lumbar areas. Treatment involves resection, usually with primary anastomosis. The *meconium plug syndrome, atresia,* and the *small left colon syndrome* are unusual causes of perforation proximal to the obstruction and rarely are associated with enterocolitis of the obstructed bowel. The diagnosis is usually apparent on barium enema. The meconium plug syndrome and small left colon syndrome do not require operative treatment unless perforation has taken place. Irrigation of the colon with Gastrografin usually suffices to clear obstructing meconium from the bowel. As the child matures and as the distal colon is used, the bowel attains normal caliber. Atresia requires operative correction of the obstruction.

Perforation due to Trauma in Infancy. Children often swallow foreign objects, which may perforate the colon. Iatrogenic perforation with a thermometer or an enema also occurs. Patients with trauma to the colon usually present clinical features similar to those of adults. When the history of the accident is vague, the possibility of child abuse must be considered.

Idiopathic Perforation of the Colon in Infants and Children. Although affected patients do not present the usual picture of necrotizing enterocolitis, ischemia of the gut also may account for these lesions. Idiopathic perforation of the colon can be difficult to detect. The predominant sign is abdominal distention. Obstipation, bilious vomiting, and unstable vital signs usually develop but may be absent. The diagnosis is made by the presence of free air within the peritoneal cavity in the absence of any obstructive or traumatic lesion. The treatment is the same as any secondary bacterial peritonitis (see Chap. 38), plus resection of the diseased bowel.

Traumatic Perforation of Colon and Rectum

Pathogenesis. Trauma to the colon and rectum usually leads to uncontrolled peritoneal contamination that, if left untreated for long, will produce infectious peritonitis.[29-31] Most (92 percent) injuries of colon and rectum are the result of *penetrating trauma.* Gunshot wounds predominate, 3:1. The transverse colon is involved most frequently (36 percent), followed by the left colon (32 percent), right colon (24 percent), and rectum (8 percent). Isolated large bowel injuries are present only about 20 percent of the time. Rectal injuries are frequently accompanied by injuries to the pelvic skeleton and genitourinary system. The severity of the resulting infection and the prognosis are usually determined by the gravity of the overall injury.

The velocity and mass of the penetrating projectile determine the amount of energy delivered to the tissues (see Chap. 24). Stab wounds usually cause little injury beyond the wound track. Multiple fragments obviously may cause more damage than a single missile. The amount of foreign matter (bone, dirt, clothing) carried into the wound is an important infection-potentiating factor, and some missile materials, such as phosphorus, are injurious in themselves. The time between injury and definitive treatment is also important. The longer uncontrolled infection or impaired vascularity is present, the more severe the necrosis. An object, such as a toothpick or bone splinter, that perforates the colon or rectum becomes contaminated with feces so that invasive infection may develop anywhere along the path of injury.[32]

Blunt trauma constitutes 4 to 5 percent of colon and rectal injuries.[11] Most (50 to 70 percent) are the result of vehicular trauma.[29,31] There are four mechanisms of blunt injury to the intra-abdominal colon: (1) rapid deceleration avulses bowel segments that are fixed only at their ends to the retroperitoneum (eg, the transverse or sigmoid colon); intramural hematoma, mesenteric tear producing bowel ischemia, or laceration of the bowel wall all can result; (2) acute increase in intraluminal pressure, typically from compression, can cause blow-out lesions; (3) direct impact; and (4) injury resulting from blunt compressive forces causing injury to the bowel wall, as in crush and explosion. Compression trauma often produces primarily retroperitoneal injury because the increased pressure is distributed evenly to all intraperitoneal structures but unevenly only to the surface of the retroperitoneal portions of the bowel.

Rectal injuries associated with blunt trauma usually accompany comminuted fractures of the pelvis or sacrum or are associated with perineal injury.[33] The rectum may be lacerated by bone fragments. Avulsion injuries of the rectum most often occur at the level of attachment of the levator sling to the rectum. Avulsion of the rectum from the anal sphincter apparatus also may occur.

Iatrogenic trauma is frequent but is reported infrequently. Colon injuries during operation are usually recognized quickly, and fecal spillage is minimal or absent. Erosion of the colon by an adjacent stiff drain usually appears postoperatively as a fecal fistula. Injuries during enema or colostomy irrigation are caused by the enema tip itself or by excessive hydrostatic pressure. Injection of an irritating enema solution, such as hypertonic phosphate, may result in widespread necrosis of tissue. A common cause of rectal injury in infants is perforation by a thermometer. If the perforation is limited to perirectal tissues, only a perirectal or ischiorectal abscess may develop.

Most iatrogenic injuries occur during diagnostic procedures. The rate of perforation after barium enema is about 0.02 percent.[34] Although the resting pressure developed by a barium enema with the reservoir 4 feet above the table is only 8 to 38 mm Hg, spasms of the colon during the procedure can produce pressures of over 170 mm Hg that are sufficient to rupture normal colon.[35] The risk of perforation is increased when a barium enema is performed through a colostomy stoma. Sterile barium sulfate injected experimentally directly into the peritoneal cavity induces a benign, self-limited, acute inflammatory reaction, granuloma formation, and adhesions.[7] In contrast, injection of feces together with barium uniformly produces death. Water-soluble contrast medium mixed with feces also is more lethal than feces alone in laboratory animals but can be treated more successfully than can barium peritonitis. Injection of barium and feces into the paracolic soft tissues leads to soft tissue infection. Intramesenteric perforation also may occur, usually in patients with diverticular disease. Barium injected into the portal venous system[36] usually results in pylephlebitis and death.

Perforation during *proctoscopy* usually is a consequence of biopsy. Perforation may be caused directly by the proctoscope, usually on the anterior surface of the sigmoid colon near the sacral promontory where sigmoid angulation is most acute. The risk of perforation during diagnostic fiberoptic *colonoscopy* is less than 1 percent. During colonoscopic polypectomy, the perforation rate is about 1.5 percent.[37] Most perforations are caused by inexperience of the endoscopist. Air insufflation carries the danger of overinflation, especially of the normal cecum and transverse colon. Particular care must be taken to avoid insufflation directly into the mouth of a diverticulum. In addition, perforation may occur through seromuscular tears induced during the procedure. Perforation also may occur when trying to pass through a stricture or beyond a tumor. Application of pressure to advance the colonoscope can create great tension of the mesentery of a looped portion of colon, particularly the sigmoid.

Occasional perforations of the rectum may occur during cystoscopy and culdoscopy, often causing minimal damage. Small perforations of the colon may occur during paracentesis of the abdominal cavity.

Another potential infectious complication of diagnostic procedures is septicemia. Blood cultures taken during rectal examination have failed to document bacteremia, but bacteremia has been documented during and for up to 30 minutes after proctoscopy, barium enema, and colonoscopy. Transient bacteremia can be expected to cause no problem in healthy persons. Antibiotic prophylaxis is indicated in immunosuppressed patients and in those subject to development of endocarditis.

Perforation of the colon during colostomy dilation or irrigation is rare.[38] The most common mechanism is forcing an irrigation catheter through the wall of a redundant loop of colon. Such loops are frequently associated with a paracolostomy hernia. Perforation may be intraperitoneal or into the abdominal wall. This type of perforation may be avoided by using a cone irrigation device rather than a catheter.

Colon perforation by an *ingested foreign body* occurs in children, denture wearers, and the mentally incompetent. More than 90 percent of all foreign objects and 80 percent of ingested sharp foreign bodies pass per rectum, without incident, usually within a week. After an object has passed out of the stomach, perforation is most likely to occur in the large bowel, especially the cecum and the sigmoid colon. Perforation may be acute, resulting in peritonitis and abscess formation, or chronic, resulting in an abscess adjacent to the site of the perforation, whereas the perforation itself is found to have healed.

Another type of trauma to the perineum and large bowel is impalement injury, usually a fall onto a rigid rod or stake. If the object is long enough, multiple injuries to the bowel and other organs may occur. A similar injury results from insertion of foreign bodies into the rectum for erotic purposes[39,40] or after a sexual assault. Perforation may occur through the extraperitoneal rectum or through the sigmoid colon.

Clinical Manifestations. The clinical presentation in all varieties of traumatic perforation are similar to the typical picture of nontraumatic large bowel perforation described previously.

When the colon has been injured by a penetrating injury, abdominal pain usually develops within an hour or two. The symptoms of colon injury may be overshadowed by those of other concomitant injuries. Entrance and exit wounds are examined to estimate the track of the missile or the weapon. Omentum, bowel, or stool may be present in the wound. Marked abdominal distention suggests intraperitoneal free blood or, occasionally, air. Usually, the abdomen is quiet on auscultation and tender to palpation; signs of peritonitis are present. Blood may be present in the rectum. On occasion, no findings are present initially, and repeated examinations are necessary to detect signs of colon injury as early as possible.

After blunt trauma, examination yields similar findings; ecchymoses may suggest the mechanism of injury. A fracture of the pelvis should make one suspect rectal injury. A quiet tender abdomen suggests significant injury, as does blood in the rectum.

Iatrogenic injuries of large bowel frequently produce immediate abdominal pain and progressive signs of peritonitis temporally related to the procedure. But perforation by biopsy at proctosigmoidoscopy may not be apparent for hours or days. When injury results from an enema or colostomy irrigation, the patient often reports that there was little or no return of the solution. Blood may be found on the catheter or thermometer. Perforation during endoscopy may be immediately apparent when the examiner sees omentum or small intestine, or free air may be seen in the peritoneal cavity on a postcolonoscopy abdominal x-ray. Barium may be seen either leaking into the peritoneal cavity or in an extraluminal location in the evacuation films of a barium enema.

Diagnosis. Laboratory findings after traumatic perforation of the large bowel are similar to those for nontraumatic perforation. X-ray studies of the chest, abdomen, and pelvis are helpful to determine the path taken by bullets and other missiles. Pelvic fractures are detected or confirmed. Contrast studies of the large bowel are contraindicated when perforation is suspected. All patients with indwelling rectal foreign bodies should have biplanar x-ray studies taken of the pelvis to determine the orientation of the object.

Proctoscopy is indicated any time blood is detected on rectal examination. Proctoscopy should also be considered in any patient in whom a missile has transversed the pelvis or who has a pelvic fracture. In addition, proctoscopy is indicated in those with rectal injury or rectal foreign body both before and after extraction.

If the patient is unable to communicate with the physician, as in cases of head trauma or in young children, or when physical examination is otherwise inconclusive, peritoneal lavage is useful in detecting evidence of intra-abdominal injury. The finding of blood (100,000 RBCs/mm^3), leukocytes (500/mm^3), or fecal particles in the lavage aspirate may indicate perforation of the colon. A Gram stain of the lavage return can offer definitive proof of bacterial contamination in doubtful cases.

Treatment. Improved survival rates are achieved when intervention occurs within 6 hours of injury. Broad spectrum antibiotics effective against aerobes and anaerobes are administered intravenously and blood volume is restored.

The importance of separating injured colon segments from adjacent bone injuries at operation to prevent development of osteomyelitis has been stressed by Christy.[41] Devitalized bone fragments should be debrided whenever feasible. In the past, treatment has taken four forms: (1) repair of the injury and protection of the repair with a proximal diverting colostomy or ileostomy, (2) exteriorization of the injury as colostomy, (3) resection of the injured bowel with anastomosis protected by a proximal diverting enterostomy or colostomy, and (4) resection with an end colostomy and mucous fistula or oversewing of the distal remnant.

Primary repair, or resection with immediate primary anastomosis without a proximal diverting stoma, avoids temporary colostomy and, if successful, shortens convalescence. Primary closure, with or without resection, has been found to be as safe as traditional methods if all the following conditions prevail: (1) minimal injury to colon adjacent to the perforation, (2) repair conducted less than 6 hours after injury, (3) stable patient without preceding shock or severe hemorrhage, (4) good basic health prior to injury, (5) injury to no more than one other organ in addition to the large bowel, and (6) minimal or no fecal spillage or peritonitis.[39] Unfortunately, the necessary conditions are not often fulfilled. In addition, if urinary tract injury coexists, primary anastomosis is inherently dangerous even if all other conditions for the direct approach are fulfilled.

Careful observation of extraperitoneal rectal lacerations, with or without primary repair, is feasible when there is no gross fecal leakage, significant hematoma, or necrosis of surrounding tissue. Otherwise, sigmoid colostomy and primary repair or resection of the damaged segment are recommended. Whether or not colostomy is carried out, washout of all fecal matter from the rectum and dependent drainage of traumatized perirectal tissues through the rectum or through the perineum will reduce the incidence and severity of subsequent pelvic infections.

Prognosis. The median mortality rate for a collected series of nearly 4000 patients with traumatic colorectal perforation was 7.5 percent,[42–50] and the median incidence of infectious complications was 28 percent. Traditional management, including treatment by exteriorized primary repair, was employed in 55 percent with a median mortality rate of 10.5 percent and a median infectious morbidity rate of 32.5 percent. Primary repair was performed in 45 percent of patients with a median mortality rate of 6 percent and a median morbidity rate of 24 percent.

Stone and Fabian[51] have reported a prospective, randomized study of traditional colostomy treatment versus primary closure therapy in patients whose wounds fulfilled the six criteria listed in the previous section. The mortality rate (1 percent) was the same in each group. The infectious morbidity rates were greater in the group treated with colostomy (wound sepsis, 57 percent; peritoneal sepsis, 29 percent; anastomotic failure, 10 percent) than in the group treated with primary closure without colostomy (48 percent, 15 percent, and 1 percent, respectively). However, significantly greater complication rates occurred only in patients having intraperitoneal drains.

Right colon injuries could be analyzed specifically in four series.[48–50] This subgroup was composed of 384 patients, 41 percent of whom were treated traditionally and 59 percent by primary repair. The overall mortality rate (4 percent) in patients with right colon trauma was better than for all colon trauma patients and there was no difference in the mortality rate of patients treated traditionally (4 percent) or by primary repair (3 percent). However, the infectious morbidity rate in those treated traditionally (25 percent) was better than that for those treated by primary repair (40 percent). Although primary repair of colon injuries may succeed under favorable circumstances, the available data suggest that traditional measures are indicated in most large bowel injuries.

Spontaneous Colon Perforation Due to Ehlers-Danlos Syndrome. The Ehlers-Danlos syndrome is an uncommon inherited disorder caused by defective collagen synthesis of which there are ten types. One of its most important acute surgical complications is spontaneous colon perforation seen in patients with type IV disorder. In addition to spontaneous colon perforation, it is characterized by joint hyperextensibility, thin skin, easy bruising, and vascular instability. The site of perforation is in the sigmoid colon. There is a high risk of recurrent perforation if bowel continuity is reestablished. Sykes[52] recommends resection of the involved colon with end colostomy and a mucous fistula or Hartman procedure. Repeat colon perforation has been reported following this procedure[53]; total colectomy was required.

DIVERTICULAR DISEASE OF THE COLON

Incidence. The true incidence of diverticulosis of the colon in the general population is unknown because estimates derive either from necropsy or barium enema studies and are, of necessity, biased. Most studies cite an incidence of 6 to 8 percent.[54,55] Diverticulosis is principally a disease of the elderly who reside in Western industrialized nations. Patients less than 40 years of age make up less than 3 percent of the patients with diverticula,[56] and patients older than 70 years of age have an incidence of about 25 percent. Most recent series document a higher incidence of diverticular disease in women, an observation that cannot be explained by the greater longevity of women.

Although colonic diverticular disease is more common in Western countries, it is increasingly common worldwide.[57,58]

Pathogenesis. Typical diverticula are pulsion-type outpouchings of mucosa protruding through the colon circular muscle at sites of apparent weakness, located adjacent to the mesenteric side of each of the antimesenteric taeniae at the point where blood vessels penetrate the colon wall.[59] In addition, smaller vessels penetrate the bowel wall on either side of the mesenteric taeniae. Thus, typically, there are two rows of diverticula on each side of the colon. The mucosa of the diverticulum is covered superficially by a thin layer of muscle and peritoneum. Frequently, diverticula are also invested with the fat of epiploic appendages. Marcus and Watt[60] describe a row of diverticula often found on the antimesenteric, intertaenial aspect of the colon in addition to the more usual locations. Another structural characteristic of diverticular disease is thickness of the bowel wall, primarily caused by prominence of the circular muscle layer but also caused by thickening and apparent shortening of the taeniae. These muscular changes result in an apparent increase in the number of haustra and a narrowed lumen.

The sigmoid colon is affected in 95 percent of diseased patients and is the sole site of disease in

50 to 75 percent; acquired sigmoid diverticula also account for most of the symptoms in this disorder. The descending colon is next most frequently involved, with the transverse and right colon involved in less than 15 percent of patients.[61]

The presence of uncomplicated diverticula is thought to be the result of increased colonic intraluminal pressure. Diseased colonic segments manifest a high rate of muscle contraction and increased pressure responses to administration of prostigmine and morphine.[62] Arfwidsson[63] also noted a high intraluminal pressure. The high pressures are apparently the result of strong segmental contractions of circular muscle. Cineradiographic studies in patients with diverticulosis have shown the formation of small segments of bowel with complete occlusion of the lumen at both ends of the segments; the diverticula in these segments become distended. The muscle alterations are said to be caused by a deficiency of fiber in the diet; and the loss of bulk allows narrowing to occur. If adequate bulk is present, exaggerated segmentation is prevented, narrowing inhibited, and development pressures noted in diverticulosis patients are avoided. This hypothesis is supported by evidence that laboratory animals fed diets low in bulk develop diverticula.[64]

Diverticulitis represents, at the least, an inflammatory response in the vicinity of a diverticulum.[59] Stool and mucus collect in a diverticulum and cause an inflammation in the mucosa. Perforation can then occur, leading to a greater or lesser infection, which may include a phlegmon, abscess, or free perforation. Obstruction may be the result of scar formation, which thickens, narrows, and stiffens the bowel wall. Bleeding is said to be a consequence of the anatomic relationship of arteries to the diverticula; ulceration of the neck of the diverticulum erodes into the colonic artery. Recent clinical experience, however, demonstrates that many episodes of supposed diverticular bleeding are actually hemorrhage from an arteriovenous malformation, often located in the right colon. The so-called giant sigmoid diverticulum develops as the result of a localized perforation, which subsequently develops a mucosal ball valve so that a cyst lined by granulation and fibrous tissue develops.

Solitary diverticula of the cecum seem to have a different pathogenesis. These diverticula are outpouchings from the cecum, within 2 cm of the ileocecal valve, containing all the coats of the bowel. They probably represent congenital lesions, although a pulsion mechanism has been postulated.

Clinical Manifestations

DIVERTICULOSIS. Traditionally, diverticulosis was deemed an asymptomatic condition. Morson's[59] finding that 35 percent of colon specimens removed for *persistent diverticulitis* showed no evidence of inflammation but only abnormally thick musculature raises a question about the accuracy of diagnosis. At least some patients thought to have symptomatic diverticulosis probably have irritable bowel syndrome. Their symptoms cannot be correlated with the number of diverticula or their location.[55] There are no specific physical findings.

DIVERTICULITIS. This is an acute inflammatory process usually involving the sigmoid colon and frequently presenting with pain, which can be intermittent and cramping in nature but more commonly is steady, deep, and aching. Pain is usually located in the left lower quadrant but may be hypogastric or present on the right. Aching in the low back is common. Often, there is a history of altered bowel function, usually constipation, although diarrhea or intermittent constipation and diarrhea also occur. Changes in bowel function are often the result of acute inflammation. This acute process may be complicated or uncomplicated.

Nausea and vomiting may be caused by obstruction but are usually the result of the inflammatory process. The presence of fever is variable, but with the other findings of left lower quadrant pain, tenderness, a palpable mass, and leukocytosis, the diagnosis of acute diverticulitis can be suspected on clinical grounds alone. Blood in the stool is common, but bleeding is rarely profuse (less than 5 percent). Symptoms of suprapubic pain, dysuria, and frequency may indicate inflammation in the region of the urinary tract, or it may indicate the presence of a colovesical fistula. When complicated diverticulitis develops, pain often intensifies and spreads as the inflammatory process progresses. If open perforation occurs, the diffuse pain of generalized peritonitis ensues.

Colovesical fistula is suggested by dysuria, urinary frequency, pneumaturia, and fecaluria. If pneumaturia is present, it is described as a hissing or popping sensation or sound noted at the end of urination. Particles of feces may be seen in the urine. Symptoms of urinary sepsis usually predominate. Other fistulas may be recognized by passage of stool from the vagina or through an abdominal cutaneous fistula site. The development of persisting diarrhea suggests the presence of a fistula to the small bowel.

Diverticulitis in a cecal diverticulum usually produces symptoms similar to those of acute appendicitis. There is less nausea and vomiting than with appendicitis; otherwise, the two conditions cannot be differentiated until operation is performed. Giant sigmoid diverticula rarely produce distinctive symptoms. Sometimes, the patient becomes aware of an intra-abdominal mass.

Physical findings in patients with acute diverticulitis or its complications are like those of a localized or generalized intra-abdominal inflammation. Local tenderness, with guarding and localized rebound, is most frequent. If ileus or obstruction is present, distention will be noted. Frequently, an abdominal mass, most often in the left lower quadrant or pelvis, is noted on abdominal, pelvic, or rectal examination.

Diagnosis. There are no blood tests specific for diverticular disease. The leukocyte count usually is elevated in acute diverticulitis. If there has been bleeding, anemia may be present. Urinalysis may be abnormal when there is impending or actual vesicosigmoid fistula. If only bladder irritation exists, pyuria alone might be noted. With fistulization, bacteria will be detected in the urine on Gram stain or culture. If the fistula is large enough, fecal matter will be noted on gross or microscopic examination.

Endoscopy of the rectum and the colon is performed primarily to rule out other disease, especially carcinoma, and to determine the length of healthy rectum available for an anastomosis. Sigmoidoscopy is of limited value because the involved segments usually cannot be visualized with this instrument because of angulation and fixation of the bowel. Ritchie[65] emphasizes the relationship of mucosal puckering with diverticulosis. Wychulis et al[66] list the following endoscopic observations in patients with diverticular disease: acute angulation at the lower level of the sigmoid, pronounced fixation of the colon, narrowing of the bowel lumen, edema and inflammation of the mucosa, sacculation of the bowel, blood and purulent material in the lumen, and extrarectal mass. Rarely, diverticular ostia may be visualized. Wychulis et al[66] noted one or more of these findings in two-thirds of their patients, but Ochsner and Bargell[54] found abnormalities in only one-fifth. Care must be used in performing proctoscopy on patients with acute diverticulitis. Friable bowel may be injured, and confined areas of sepsis may be disrupted. Colonoscopy offers theoretical advantages, but in the presence of bowel angulation, fixation, and narrowing, it also is difficult to perform. Only one-half of examinations are successful.

The diagnosis of colon carcinoma in patients with suspected diverticulitis requires visualization of abnormal mucosa. Morton and Goldman[67] were able to see only 38 percent of carcinomas in their series of patients with diverticular disease in the era prior to fiberoptic colonoscopy.

X-ray studies are the most productive means of diagnosing diverticular disease. Plain films may demonstrate thickened bowel wall, displaced small bowel, and abnormal collections of air. Barium enema examination demonstrates goblet-like outpouchings from the bowel lumen, sometimes displaced by fecal matter within the diverticula. The lesions may also be obscured by the overlying column of barium. The use of air contrast overcomes this problem but is not advised in patients with acute disease. The postevacuation film demonstrates residual barium-filled diverticula in most instances.

Findings that have been suggested to indicate diverticulitis or abscess include spasticity and hyperactivity of the bowel, prominent sacculations, transverse folds, a sawtooth appearance of the bowel mucosa, stenosis of the bowel, and extraluminal barium in abscess cavities or fistulas (Figs. 43–3 and 43–4). Muscle abnormalities account for most of these findings, whether or not diverticulitis is present. The sawtooth deformity usually corresponds to the presence of diverticula in the antimesenteric intertaenial area.[60] Persistent narrowing suggests scarring in the bowel wall or extrinsic compression by abscess, but most abscesses manifest no x-ray changes. In addition, Parks[68] could demonstrate no significant correlation between x-ray appearance and clinical symptoms and signs of acute diverticulitis. A giant sigmoid diverticulum frequently first becomes apparent on a plain film of the abdomen or on barium enema.[69]

Carcinoma may coexist with diverticular disease. In the presence of narrowing, obstruction, or a mass lesion, one must rule out neoplasm. The following are indicative of diverticular disease rather than cancer: (1) long segments of bowel involvement, (2) gradual tapering of the ends of the segment, (3) preservation of the mucosal pattern, (4) presence of diverticula and other signs of diverticular disease, (5) changing appearance of the lesion in the same examination or in different examinations, and (6) obstruction without demonstrable tumor.[67]

In patients with a clinical diagnosis of acute diverticulitis, the abdominal-pelvic CT scan has emerged as the best initial radiologic diagnostic procedure.[70,71] It is able to identify both uncompli-

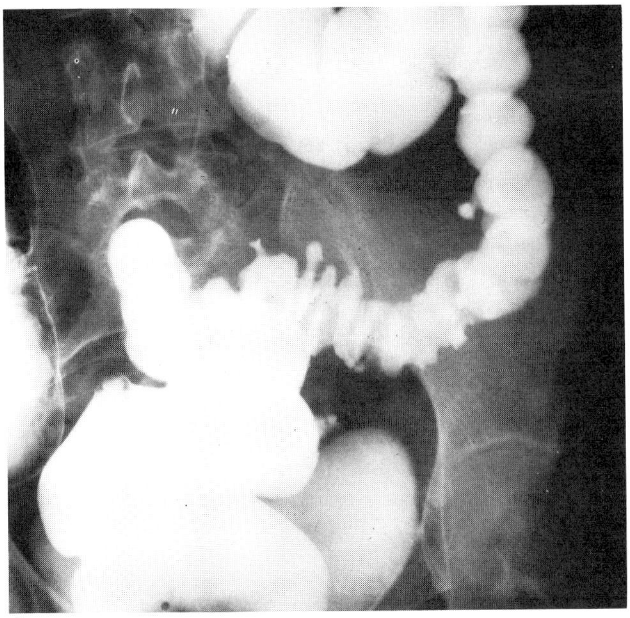

A

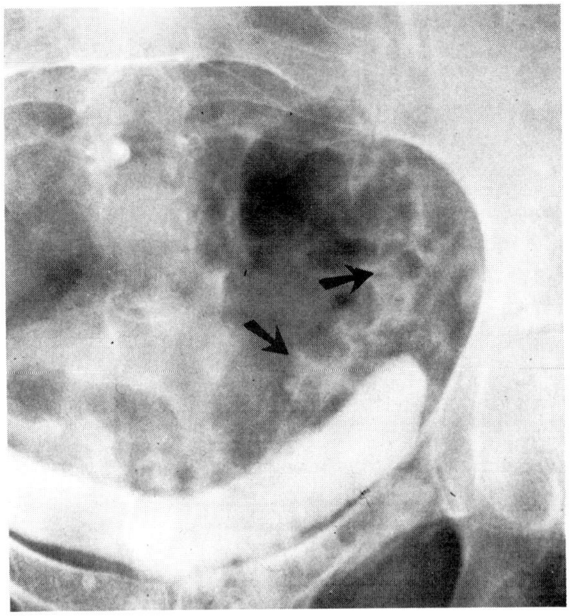

B

Figure 43–3. Diverticulitis. Barium enema demonstrates diverticula, prominent sacculations, and narrowing in the sigmoid colon. The presence of contrast in the bladder proves a colovesical fistula; the patient has received no urinary contrast media. **B.** Colovesical fistula. Cystogram demonstrates contrast leaking into the sigmoid colon (arrows) of a patient with diverticulitis—a rare finding.

cated and complicated disease. The finding associated with uncomplicated disease is effacement of the pericolic fat; localized bowel wall thickening may also be present.[71] In complicated diverticulitis, the CT findings are adjacent or distant abscess, peritonitis, fistula formation, and colonic obstruction. In the report by Hachigian and colleagues[71] of CT changes in 59 patients with a clinical diagnosis of acute diverticulitis, 23 had uncomplicated disease and 19 complicated disease. In the remaining 17 patients, 14 did not have CT findings to support the clinical diagnosis but were treated and responded. Three patients were shown by CT to have other intra-abdominal processes.

Treatment. Nonoperative treatment of patients with diverticular disease is summarized by Eastwood[72] and by Friedman and Janowitz.[73] Adding

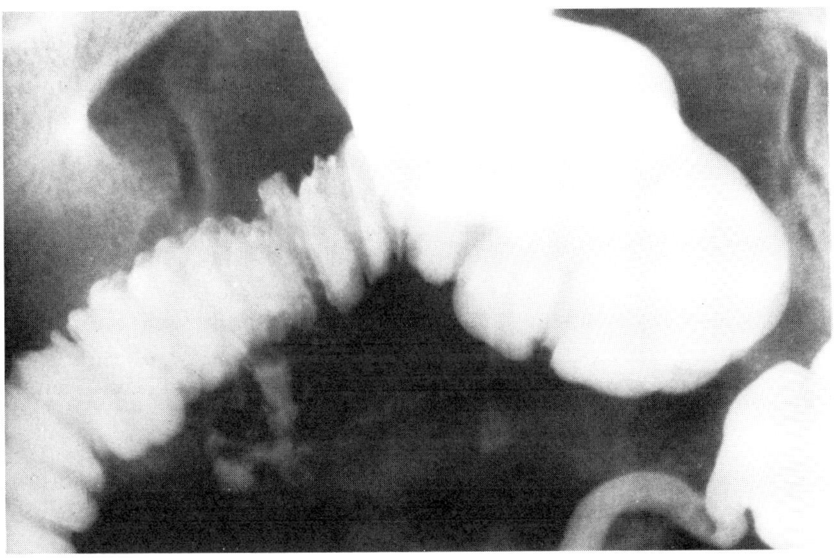

Figure 43–4. Diverticulitis. Barium enema demonstrates extraluminal contrast in a confined paracolic abscess.

bulk to the diet appears to relieve the symptoms of diverticulosis. Although carrots, apples, brussels sprouts, and oranges offer such bulk, emphasis has been placed on bran because it is inexpensive and intake can be quantitated. Alternative but relatively expensive forms of bulk are psyllium colloids (Metamucil) and karaya gum. The estimated bulk requirements are 15 g of brain and 200 g of appropriate fruits and vegetables per day. The goal is to provide enough fecal bulk to prevent excess segmentation and to allow at least one effortless bowel movement per day.

Painter et al[74] offered dietary management with bran to 70 patients. Although 8 patients could not tolerate the diet, 62 experienced relief of their chronic symptoms. Three of the 62 were admitted to the hospital during bran treatment with acute diverticulitis, one with suppuration. All but 7 patients were able to give up chronic use of other laxatives.

Most attacks of acute suppurative diverticulitis can be managed without operation. The patient should be hospitalized, given nothing by mouth, and maintained with intravenous fluids. If obstruction or minimal signs of peritonitis exist, the gastrointestinal tract should be decompressed with a nasogastric tube. Antibiotics efficacious against colon aerobes and anerobes should be administered. As long as the response is prompt, this treatment suffices for the specific episode.

Operative treatment is indicated for repeated attacks of diverticulitis, and for the complications of obstruction, perforation, bleeding, and fistula formation. Inability to rule out the presence of a neoplasm is also an indication for resection. To avoid the increased risks of an operation under urgent conditions, patients with persistent and recurrent symptoms of diverticulitis should be considered for elective resection of the diseased bowel segment. Chronic obstruction (34 percent), abscess (19 percent), acute obstruction (13 percent), perforation (12 percent), fistula (12 percent), and hemorrhage are the most common indications for operation.

OPERATIVE TREATMENT OF COMPLICATIONS. The prime task in surgical treatment is to resect the diseased segment of colon. Proximal *diverting* colostomy has proved to be an unsatisfactory therapy for distal infection. Over 50 years ago, Smithwick[75] documented that colostomy failed to control infection; mortality remained high (8 to 9 percent). Even if temporary control was achieved, exacerbation followed colostomy closure. Drainage of abscesses is equally unsatisfactory, as simple drainage resulted in persistent fecal fistula in 41 to 95 percent of patients, and creation of a proximal colostomy did not result in permanent closure of either cutaneous or colovesical fistulas. Smithwick[75] concluded that a three-stage operative protocol was needed: (1) colostomy and drainage, (2) resection with anastomosis, and (3) closure of colostomy after a 3- to 6-month interval. The mortality was low (4 to 5 percent), and three-fourths of the patients were cured. Although this classic three-stage approach was important in the preantibiotic era, it is no longer recommended as preferred operative therapy.

Most studies have shown that patients do better when diseased bowel is excised at the first operation. A preliminary first-stage proximal colostomy is not effective without resection due to the persistent distal column of feces, or when there is an enterocolic fistula that bypasses the colostomy. Sepsis will continue from an abscess that is not well drained, or if leakage from the perforation persists. In 1961, Madden and Tan[76] reported a 33 percent mortality rate in patients who had diverticular perforation with abscess or peritonitis treated by staged resection. They then successfully treated six patients with resection and primary anastomosis.[77]

However, in the presence of peritonitis, abscess, and partial obstruction, primary anastomosis is still associated with a high rate of leak and other serious morbidity.[78] In a report by Hackford et al,[79] resection with a primary anastomosis was associated with a mortality of 1 percent and morbidity of 18 percent. If the anastomosis was protected by a proximal colostomy, there were no deaths and a 22 percent morbidity rate; with a Hartmann procedure or colostomy and mucous fistula, the mortality rate was 16 percent and the morbidity rate was 23 percent. The three-stage procedure led to a mortality rate of 14 percent and morbidity rate of 24 percent.

Under appropriate conditions, resection with primary anastomosis appears to be a safe initial procedure. The conditions necessary for a successful anastomosis include two healthy ends of bowel with a good blood supply that can be joined without tension. There should be no fecal matter remaining in the bowel. Tissues surrounding the anastomosis must be free of sepsis. Thickened bowel, inflamed bowel, or dilated obstructed bowel that does not return to a normal appearance upon decompression cannot be expected to heal.

Complicated diverticular disease is sometimes encountered in a patient who is operated on, after adequate bowel preparation, for pelvic mass, possible carcinoma, or fistula. In such patients, resection of the diseased bowel and adjacent disease or fistula, with primary anastomosis of the bowel, sometimes can be performed safely if conditions are ideal. Several authors stress the increased risk of anastomotic leak when extraperitoneal bowel is mobilized to make the anastomosis. Therefore they suggest complementary colostomy for low anterior anastomosis in the presence of active disease.

ELECTIVE OPERATION. Elective one-stage colectomy can be performed with a mortality rate of less than 3 percent.[80] Colcock[81] summarized the current indications for elective resection: (1) two or more attacks of acute diverticulitis while on good medical management; the diagnosis of acute diverticulitis should be supported by the presence of acute pain, localized peritoneal signs, palpable mass during the attack, fever, leukocytosis, and x-ray signs of acute diverticulitis; (2) one or more attacks of diverticulitis associated with radiologic evidence of perforation; (3) attacks associated with persistent evidence of obstruction; (4) attacks associated with symptoms of urinary tract irritation; (5) repeated episodes of lower gastrointestinal hemorrhage (in the absence of arteriographic evidence of arteriovenous malformation); (6) inability to rule out the presence of neoplasm; and (7) attacks of diverticulitis in patients less than 50 years of age.

Resection of the diseased segment is successful in preventing recurrence of symptomatic disease in nearly all patients. To achieve the best results, it is necessary to resect all bowel with thickened and hypertrophied muscle, but it is not necessary to remove all diverticula. It is especially important that the distal resection margin be free of both diverticula and hypertrophied muscle.

When the importance of colonic muscular hypertrophy was recognized, longitudinal myotomy of the antimesenteric intertaenial circular muscle was introduced for the treatment of patients with chronic symptoms, but without inflammatory complications.[82] The mortality rate with this procedure has ranged from 0 to 5 percent,[82,83] and successful initial relief of symptoms has been achieved in 85 to 90 percent. When the procedure is used in patients with complications of diverticulitis, however, sepsis and failure occur more frequently. Smith[84] demonstrated that the procedure reduces the high intracolonic pressure seen in diverticular disease. However, 3 to 5 years after myotomy, high pressure has returned. A diet including bran tends to retard return of the high-pressure state.

Others have felt that shortening of the taeniae is more important as a factor contributing to diverticular disease and have performed multiple transverse myotomies in the antimesenteric taeniae. No circular muscle is incised; therefore the risk of mucosal perforation is reduced. This procedure, too, has successfully relieved symptoms and led to reduction of intracolonic pressure. The two procedures have been combined by Kettlewell and Moloney.[85] Myotomy was never widely adopted by surgeons in the United States, and further experience with the myotomy approach has led to its gradual abandonment elsewhere.

CECAL DIVERTICULUM. The diagnosis of cecal diverticulum must be considered in all cases of periappendiceal inflammation. Digital invagination of the cecum may permit palpation of the diverticular os. If an inflamed cecal diverticulum with only minimal surrounding inflammation is detected, excision of the involved tissue is adequate treatment if care is taken to avoid both tension on the repair and obstruction of the ileocecal valve. Generalized cecitis with no apparent diverticulum may be left alone or drained. More advanced inflammation may require ileocecal resection. Perforation with abscess formation requires drainage of the abscess and resection of the cecum. If neoplasm cannot be ruled out, a formal right hemicolectomy should be performed. Primary anastomosis is safe if abscess or peritonitis is not present.

Prognosis. Younger patients with diverticulitis have more complications.[56,61] Eusebio and Eisenberg[56] describe the course of diverticulitis in patients less than 40 years of age. Fifty-eight percent required surgical treatment; 76 percent of the operations were performed for an acute emergency; and, in those treated medically, 53 percent continued to have symptoms when followed up to 4 years. Similar findings were seen in a recent retrospective study reported by Ouriel and Schwartz.[86] Resection of the involved colon at initial presentation should be considered in younger patients with symptomatic disease.

Overall, about 25 percent of patients with diverticulosis will have at least one attack of diverticulitis (range 15 to 82 percent).[55] Factors that affect the incidence of diverticulitis are (1) the number of diverticula, (2) the extent of involved colon, (3) the duration of follow-up, (4) progression of diverticulosis during follow-up, and (5) the criteria used to diagnose diverticulitis. Once a person has a single attack of diverticulitis, the incidence of recurrent disease ranges from 11 to 75 percent (median 30 percent).[61] Three or more episodes of diverticulitis are noted in 6 to 24 percent. Recurrence took place within 1 year in 46 to 83 percent. Symptoms were noted in the interval between attacks in 13 to 92 percent.

Death due to diverticular disease in patients treated nonoperatively occurs in 2 to 6 percent of patients who had diverticulitis; operation was eventually required in 11 to 55 percent (median 25 percent).[61,75] Complications requiring surgical therapy were much more likely to occur in patients who had multiple attacks of diverticulitis. However, of patients requiring operation, 12 to 48 percent (median 37 percent) had never had symptoms before the acute attack that led to operation.[75,87]

Colon resection is effective in preventing recurrent symptoms of diverticulitis. Long-term follow-up in numerous series shows that 69 to 100 percent (median 89 percent) of patients are asymptomatic following resection of the diseased colon.[56,75,87] Wychulis et al[66] and Wolf et al[88] reported recurrence rates of 4 and 11.4 percent, respectively.

INFLAMMATORY BOWEL DISEASE

Most patients with inflammatory bowel disease (ulcerative colitis and granulomatous colitis) can be treated without operation. However, an infectious etiology of these disorders has not been excluded, and significant morbidity and mortality with these diseases result from infectious complications.

Epidemiology. The epidemiologic features of granulomatous and ulcerative colitis are similar. Most cases appear in young adults, although ulcerative colitis is somewhat more likely to appear in children. Both sexes are equally affected. Caucasians are affected more often than members of other races, and these diseases are detected more frequently in industrialized countries.

The incidence of ulcerative colitis has remained stable in recent years, but there has been an increase in the incidence of granulomatous colitis (regional enteritis).[89] The proportion of patients with ulcerative colitis ranges from 32 to 87 percent, with granulomatous colitis from 12 to 58 percent, and with unclassified colitis from 1 to 11 percent. The reported relative incidence varies according to whether the histopathology has been analyzed using modern criteria and whether the subsequent course of the disease has been taken into account. Tompkins et al[90] report that the proportion of their patients with ulcerative colitis decreased from 85 to 39 percent upon histologic review.

Etiology and Pathogenesis. Although theories abound, no specific causative factor for either disease process has been proved. Conditions associated with the onset of ulcerative colitis[91] include pregnancy, severe purgation, a recent surgical procedure, emotional trauma, epidemic diarrhea, and infectious disease in general. Recent work has attempted to identify infectious and immune factors.[92] Current hypotheses include an abnormal immune response to an infectious agent or to a part of the normal flora, and an allergic response to exogenous or endogenous antigens (autoimmune reaction).

Proof of an infectious etiology of inflammatory bowel disease has long been sought. There is no difference in the fecal flora of patients with ulcerative colitis, granulomatous colitis, or a normal bowel. However, microbiologic techniques, especially those necessary to detect fastidious anaerobes, chlamydia, and rare opportunistic agents, continue to be improved and may yet detect a responsible organism. Monteiro et al[92] describe an antibody reacting with fecal anaerobic bacteria in the colonic mucosa of patients with ulcerative colitis.

Evidence supporting a viral agent as the cause of inflammatory bowel disease has been discussed by Brooke[93] and by Kirsner.[89] Simonowitz et al[94] produced histologic changes similar to Crohn's disease in rabbit colon by injecting homogenates of bowel wall from Crohn's disease patients. Hardin and Werder[95] produced a viral cytopathic effect in tissue culture of human amniotic membrane cells by adding sera from ulcerative colitis patients. Antibody to cytomegalovirus has been isolated from the sera of 65 percent of ulcerative colitis patients. In addition, a cytopathic effect similar to that of cytomegalovirus was detected in tissue cultures of the mucosa of three of six patients with ulcerative colitis and one of four with Crohn's disease. Sidi et al[96] discussed 12 ulcerative colitis patients in whom cytomegalovirus inclusions were found in the granulation tissue of mucosal ulcers and in mucosal endothelial cells. Such findings constitute only circumstantial evidence and do not confirm an etiologic relationship between viruses and inflammatory disease of the bowel.

Pathology. Ulcerative colitis nearly always (90 to 96 percent) involves the rectum. The disease extends proximally without skip areas. The rectum alone is involved in 4 to 15 percent, the rectosigmoid and left colon in 6 to 10 percent, and the entire colon in 31 to 43 percent. These figures are based on barium enema examinations and probably underestimate the extent of disease.

Ulcerative colitis is a disease primarily of the mucosa and submucosa of the bowel wall. Grossly there is edema, diffuse granularity, and friability. Extensive mucosal involvement results in denuding the bowel wall and pseudopolyp formation. Discrete ulcers are unusual. Fibrous thickening of the entire bowel wall is not seen, and strictures are uncommon in the absence of neoplasm. Enlargement of mesenteric lymph nodes is unusual. Histologic examination confirms that ulcerative colitis is confined to the mucosa and the superficial submucosa. At first, abscesses are confined to the crypts; later, they also involve the lamina propria. There is a reduction in numbers of goblet cells in the mucosa, and premalignant changes may be seen. Lymphoid aggregates are sometimes found in the mucosa, but granulomas are not. Fissures are absent. Fibrosis is noted only in the mucosa and submucosa. In the absence of toxic megacolon, the muscular and serosal layers are not at all involved.

Granulomatous colitis, on the other hand, is more likely to be distributed segmentally with intervening normal bowel. The rectum is spared in 22 to 81 percent. The small bowel is involved in 27 to 58 percent, and the colon is involved in 35 to 90 percent of all patients with Crohn's disease. Granulomatous colitis is a disease of all bowel wall layers. Early discrete mucosal ulcers later coalesce to form serpiginous longitudinal ulcers with intervening normal mucosa. The development of transverse fissures produces a cobblestone effect. Pseudopolyps may be found. The bowel wall is thickened by fibrosis affecting all layers, and serositis is usually present. The mesentery is edematous with large, succulent lymph nodes. Spontaneous fistula is more likely to occur in this disease. Microscopically, a subacute inflammatory response with thickening and fibrosis involves all layers of the bowel wall. Noncaseating granulomas and deep fistulas are common.

Toxic dilation of the colon is a potentially serious complication of all inflammatory colon disease and leads to many infectious complications. The colon becomes dilated and the wall thins. Serositis is severe, subserosal vessels are engorged, and a fibrinous exudate develops on the serosa. Mucosal ulceration is severe. Histologically, there is transmural inflammation. Muscle cells are separated by exudate. Hyaline degeneration of muscle may be present. Often, inflammation of the ganglia of the intramuscular neural plexus is seen.[97]

Clinical Manifestations. Both ulcerative colitis and granulomatous colitis can have the same symptoms, signs, and complications. The cardinal symptoms are abdominal pain, diarrhea, and hematochezia. Infectious complications that occur in both diseases are perianal sepsis, bowel perforation, fistula, and toxic megacolon. In the following discussion, differences between the two conditions are stressed.

Typically, *ulcerative colitis* is characterized by acute exacerbations with intermittent periods of improvement or remission. Each attack may be mild or severe. Most exacerbations last less than 3 months, but some may remit only after a year. Generally, if the disease has been active for 6 months, it remains so. Instead of undergoing some degree of healing, the colon progressively deteriorates, and the extent of involvement usually increases. There is an increased risk of developing large bowel cancer in the chronic form of the disease. An acute attack may be characterized by rapid, relentless progression of symptoms in 3 to 21 percent of patients. Most deaths and complications occur in this form of the disease, largely the result of bleeding, perforation, or toxic megacolon.

Granulomatous colitis usually develops more slowly and is more relentlessly progressive. Acute fulminant attacks are rare, though symptoms wax and wane. There may be long periods of remission. Infectious complications may develop at any stage. Manifestations of associated small bowel disease may mask those of the colitis.

The most common *symptom* in both diseases is diarrhea. In ulcerative colitis, diarrhea occurs early, often with great frequency, and is associated with urgency. Hematochezia occurs almost universally and, in fulminating attacks, may be exsanguinating. Diarrhea in granulomatous colitis is of lesser frequency and urgency, and serious hemorrhage is rare. Hematochezia is seldom the first symptom of granulomatous colitis (5 percent). Intermittent cramping abdominal pain, in the absence of complications, is usually periumbilical or hypogastric. In ulcerative colitis, cramps tend to occur prior to defecation and are accompanied by tenesmus, whereas in granulomatous colitis, cramps are more continuous and have no regular relationship to defecation.

Physical signs are not diagnostic in either condition unless complications are present. Fever and toxicity are noted in severe or fulminant acute attacks. There may be tenderness overlying the colon. Occasionally, an abdominal mass may be palpated in granulomatous colitis. Rectal examination may reveal blood or pus on the examining finger. There are many noninfectious complications of inflammatory bowel disease (colon carcinoma, growth retardation, arthritis). Malnutrition is a serious accompaniment of acute attacks and can predispose to infectious complications. The most frequent *infectious complication* of inflammatory bowel disease is perianal sepsis in the form of anal fissure, perianal abscess and fistula, or rectovaginal fistula (see Chap. 45). Perianal sepsis is more common in patients with granulomatous colitis (25 to 81 percent)[98] and is the first symptom in 27 percent of patients, especially those with colonic rather than small intestinal involvement.[99]

Colon perforation and fistula occur infrequently in ulcerative colitis. Although the signs and symptoms of perforation may be masked in patients treated with steroids,[98,100] these drugs have not resulted in an increase in the incidence of perforation (11 to 12 percent). Most perforations occur during fulminant acute attacks, especially if toxic dilation of the colon develops. One-half to two-thirds of acute perforations are free; the rest are sealed or confined by abscess formation.[101] In older series, perforations and abscesses progressed so that external fistulas were seen in 1 to 2 percent of patients; such fistulas are rare today.

Free perforation is unusual in granulomatous colitis (2 to 6 percent), because most perforations occur slowly, resulting in an abscess or a fistula. The reported incidence of internal and external fistulas in patients with granulomatous colitis ranges from 3 to 59 percent (median 21 percent).[102] Even when perforation or fistula occurs, it more often originates in the small bowel than in the colon.

Toxic dilation is a common complication of acute fulminating attacks of colitis (2 to 14 percent of patients hospitalized with ulcerative colitis),[98,100,101,103] but it occurs in only 1 percent of patients with granulomatous colitis. Typically, patients show signs of toxicity (fever and tachycardia) and peritonitis (abdominal distention and tenderness). Sirinek et al[103] stress that these signs may be absent, particularly if the patient is very ill. The diagnosis may be missed unless abdominal x-ray studies are done on all patients with acute attacks of colitis. If perforation occurs (24 percent), the mortality is high.

Diagnosis. The diagnosis of inflammatory bowel disease and the differentiation between ulcerative colitis and granulomatous colitis are determined by the clinical picture, endoscopic examination, and histologic appearance. Proctoscopy is abnormal in about 95 percent of patients with ulcerative colitis[98] but reveals changes in only 5 to 25 percent of patients with granulomatous colitis. Colonoscopy increases the diagnostic yield to about 87 percent in ulcerative colitis,[104] and the addition of biopsy increases the yield to nearly 100 percent.

Endoscopic findings in ulcerative colitis are edematous mucosa with petechiae, pits, pinpoint ulcerations, friability, and pseudopolyps. In granulomatous colitis, edematous, friable mucosa with aphthous ulcers and mucosal nodules is seen. Biopsy of perianal lesions may confirm the presence of granulomatous disease. A key distinguishing feature is that ulcerative colitis is a general, diffuse process, whereas granulomatous colitis is characterized by discontinuous involvement with relatively normal mucosa between lesions.

X-ray studies are more important than endoscopy in the diagnosis of infectious complications. Serial plain films of the abdomen are taken in acute attacks to detect unsuspected toxic dilation of the colon (Fig. 43–5). In addition, there may be evidence of perforation or intra-abdominal sepsis. Barium enema should not be used during acute exacerbations for fear of precipitating toxic megacolon.

In the early stages of *ulcerative colitis* (Fig. 43–6), the bowel may be irritable, haustra are thickened and irregular in width, and their mucosal margins may be fuzzy or stippled due to tiny ulcers and exudate or may take on a shaggy appearance as ulcers become large. Postevacuation films may show coarse longitudinal folds instead of the normal transverse folds. As the disease becomes more chronic, there is often progression to continuous involvement, the mucosa is granular, haustra disappear, the lumen becomes narrowed, and the bowel is shortened. Pseudopolyps may become apparent. The presence of a stricture raises the possibility of carcinoma. Typically, there is no involvement of the terminal ileum.

The barium enema findings of *granulomatous colitis* (Fig. 43–7) include an abnormal haustral pattern and ulcerations that eventually progress to typical longitudinal ulcers with transverse fissures. These produce a cobblestone pattern; pseudopolyps also are seen. Involvement is often eccentric, and skip areas are apparent. As the disease progresses, strictures and internal fistulas are seen frequently. The terminal ileum is often involved.[93]

Treatment. In most instances, acute attacks of inflammatory bowel disease are treated without operation. Nutritional and fluid deficits should be replaced. Antidiarrheal agents (diphenoxylate, loperamide, codeine) may help control the diarrhea of mild disease but should never be used during a severe attack because they can precipitate toxic megacolon.

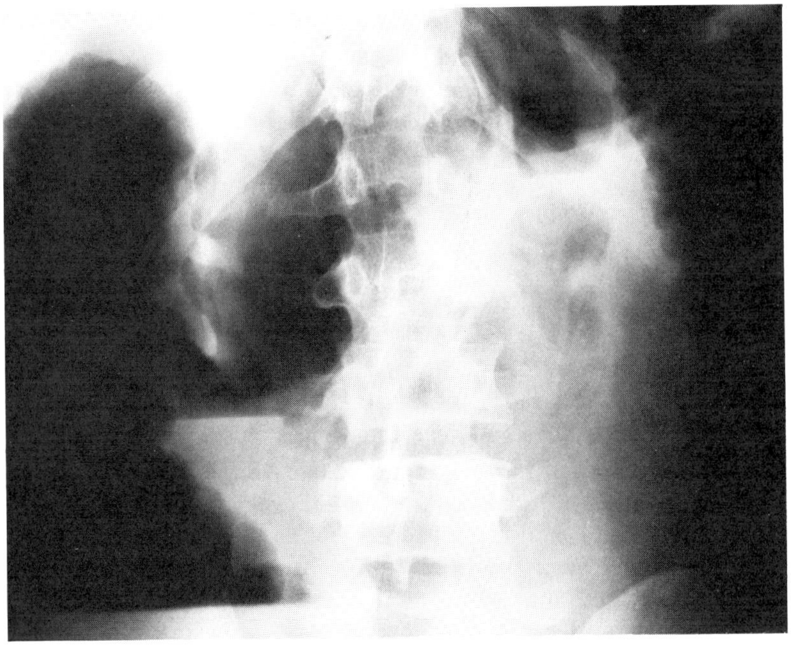

Figure 43–5. Ulcerative colitis. Plain abdominal film demonstrates toxic dilation of the colon.

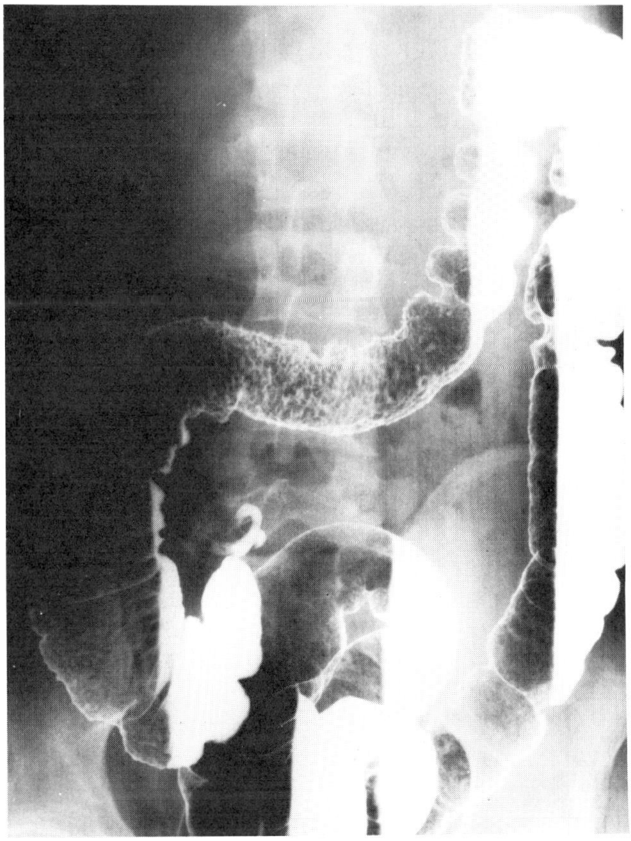

Figure 43–6. Ulcerative colitis. Air contrast barium enema (lateral decubitus position) demonstrates a shaggy mucosal pattern with ulcerated margins. Haustra are sparse in number and thickened. Shortening of the right colon has occurred.

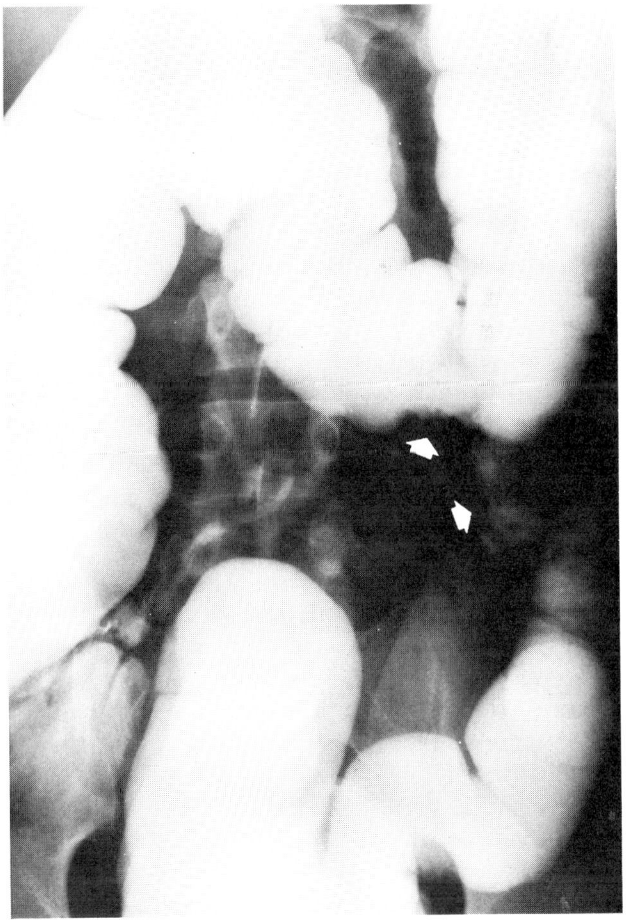

Figure 43–7. Granulomatous colitis. Barium enema demonstrates segmental involvement of transverse and descending colon; intervening colon is normal. Descending colon segment (arrow) is narrowed with ulcers and fissures apparent. Transverse colon involvement (arrow) is eccentric.

The most useful drugs for inflammatory bowel disease are corticosteroids and sulfasalazine.[105,106] Steroids do not increase the complication rate; neither do they prevent relapse of either ulcerative colitis or granulomatous colitis.[107] Steroids may be administered either orally or intravenously; ulcerative proctitis may be treated by steroid suppositories or retention enemas. Sulfasalazine is a less effective anti-inflammatory agent. It must be broken down by gut flora, mainly in the colon, to its metabolites, sulfapyridine and 5-aminosalicylic acid. It does not prevent relapse of Crohn's disease,[107] but it does reduce the early relapse rate in ulcerative colitis. Its antimicrobial effect is incidental. Antibiotics have no proven effect on either disease.

TREATMENT OF COMPLICATIONS. Indications for surgical treatment in ulcerative colitis include fulminating acute disease unresponsive to nonoperative treatment, perforation, fistula (rare), hemorrhage, occurrence of systemic complications, growth failure in children, and persistent rectal disease. The risk of carcinoma in patients with chronic persistent disease also warrants operation. Although severe hemorrhage and cancer occur rarely in granulomatous colitis, the indications for surgical treatment otherwise are the same as in ulcerative colitis.

The surgical treatment of ulcerative colitis requires, as a minimum, removal of the entire abdominal colon. Before 1960, ileostomy alone yielded an immediate postoperative mortality rate of about 25 percent, an eventual mortality rate of 46 to 84 percent (largely within the first postoperative year), and persistent disease requiring eventual colectomy in 41 to 45 percent.[108] If the ileostomy was subsequently closed, only 13 percent had a good result, and 50 percent required a new ileostomy.

The overall mortality rate of total abdominal colectomy with or without proctectomy is 3 to 14 percent (median 8 percent)[100,101] but is higher after emergency colectomy (14 to 54 percent; median 23 percent).[101] Infectious morbidity (incisional and intra-abdominal sepsis) of emergency procedures is 36 to 57 percent.

No single operation is best for the treatment of granulomatous colitis. The disease is segmental, and cure cannot be assured by excision of the involved segment of bowel. The basic choices in treatment of granulomatous colitis are diversion of the fecal stream from the diseased segment by a proximal stoma or bypass, excision of the segment with subsequent anastomosis, abdominal colectomy and ileoproctostomy, or total coloproctectomy and ileostomy. In general, such operations are associated with a mortality rate of about 5 percent,[109] a wound infection rate of 18 percent, and an intra-abdominal sepsis rate of 3 percent. Five percent of anastomoses leak. The recurrence rate ranges from 16 to 94 percent (median 31 percent); recurrences are less common when gross disease is restricted to the colon.

When infectious complications (abscess, perforation) are present, diversion (proximal stoma or bypass) is safer than resection (mortality range 0 to 24 percent).[110] Morbidity, including anastomotic leak, is almost inevitable (94 percent).[109,111] Because of the frequent need for reoperation, Homan and Dineen[110] recommend that diversionary procedures be performed only when an important normal structure (such as a ureter) would be endangered, or entry into an otherwise confined abscess would be needed, to resect diseased bowel.

Resection of only the grossly involved bowel segment with primary anastomosis is appealing because functioning colon is conserved and the need for ileostomy is avoided. The operative mortality rate is low (0 to 2 percent) and morbidity is acceptable (6 percent).[110] After such resections, recurrence ranges from 39 to 85 percent (median 75 percent),[110,112] and the reoperation rate ranges from 11 to 59 percent (median 22 percent).[111,112]

Total colectomy with ileostomy succeeds in removing almost all diseased bowel with low operative mortality (0 to 8 percent)[111,113] and acceptable recurrence (7 to 43 percent)[112,113] and reoperation (2 to 20 percent) rates.[111] In an effort to achieve the benefits of total colectomy and avoid ileostomy, many surgeons perform total abdominal colectomy and ileoproctostomy. The following situations are contraindications to this procedure: (1) emergency operations, (2) active disease in the rectum, and (3) stricture and fibrosis of the anorectum due to chronic anorectal or perianal sepsis. Although it has been claimed that rectal disease in ulcerative colitis often resolves after total abdominal colectomy, subsequent ileorectal anastomosis is almost never possible in any ulcerative colitis patient whose rectum is retained. In patients with granulomatous colitis, the retained rectum frequently develops active disease (50 to 73 percent), and proctectomy is required in 24 to 50 percent (median 30 percent).[113]

If ileoproctostomy is performed, the incidence of anastomotic leak (2 to 25 percent)[113,114] can be reduced by proximal diverting ileostomy. The patient must be warned that the recurrence rate in the rectum is high,[114] and conversion to ileostomy may be necessary.[113,114]

ACUTE TOXIC MEGACOLON. This complication occurs in both granulomatous colitis and ulcerative colitis, more frequently in the latter. In no case is timing more important than in the management of this life-threatening complication. Although medical management may be employed successfully in an initial episode of acute toxic megacolon, nearly 60 percent of patients have unsatisfactory long-term results. Approximately 29 percent may have a second episode of acute toxic colitis.[115] Prolonged medical management in deteriorating patients leads to progression of the inflammatory process involving the bowel wall and ultimate colon perforation. In these cases, the resulting surgical mortality approaches 50 percent compared with 95 percent survival when brief medical management consisting primarily of resuscitation and preparation for operation[115] is employed.

Many colon perforations found at operation for toxic dilation are found to have sealed. But, in the process of performing total colectomy, they are frequently opened again with subsequent fecal spillage. Turnbull et al[97] proposed the temporizing procedure of ileostomy, transverse colostomy, and sigmoid colostomy to avoid extensive dissection. This procedure resulted in a low mortality rate (2 percent); however, 10 percent of the patients did not improve, and 31 percent reactivated their colitis (19 percent with recrudescence of toxic megacolon) before elective colectomy could be performed.

Fry and Atkinson[116] noted that when patients were operated on within 4 days of the onset of toxic dilation, no perforations occurred and total colectomy was performed with no deaths. This experience has been confirmed by others.[103,117] Therefore operative treatment of acute fulminating disease, including toxic dilation of the colon, is indicated when nonoperative measures have failed to produce improvement within 48 to 72 hours. Total abdominal colectomy is the procedure of choice. Proctectomy is indicated in emergent cases only when severe rectal hemorrhage complicates the acute process.[117]

INFECTIOUS COMPLICATIONS OF CARCINOMA OF THE LARGE BOWEL

The acute mortality of large bowel cancer is largely due to infectious complications. In addition to direct complications from the tumor and its surgical treatment, infections of other body systems (eg, urinary and respiratory tracts) are common. There may be impaired immune resistance because of poor nutrition, and adjuvant treatments may impair body resistance. Two infectious complications of large bowel cancer are of pressing concern to the surgeon: (1) acute tumor perforation that necessitates an emergency operation and (2) occurrence of certain opportunistic infections that suggest the diagnosis.

Acute Perforation of Colon Cancer

Epidemiology and Pathogenesis. Perforation most often occurs as a consequence of direct penetration by the tumor (3 to 8 percent).[118,119] The combination of obstruction and proximal perforation occurs in only about 1 percent of patients with large bowel cancer. Both obstruction and perforation occur more frequently in elderly women. Most invasive perforations (about two-thirds) occur in the left colon; those in the right colon are more frequently the result of neglected obstruction. Perforation of nonobstructed colon is more likely to result in abscess or fistula formation, whereas peritonitis results from obstruction-perforation. The frequency of fistula formation ranges from 15 to 28 percent.[118] In contradistinction to fistulas resulting from diverticular disease, the structures most likely to be involved by a carcinomatous fistula are adjacent loops of small bowel and colon; stomach and duodenum are involved in 5 to 10 percent, bladder and female reproductive organs in about 20 percent, and colocutaneous fistula develops in less than 10 percent.

Clinical Manifestations. The picture of acute perforated large bowel cancer, with or without obstruction, does not differ from perforation as discussed previously. Most patients have abdominal pain, local or general signs of peritonitis, fever, and a palpable abdominal or rectal mass. Welch[120] stresses that abscesses may be found in unusual locations. A patient with a fistula, on the other hand, rarely presents as an acute emergency.

It is desirable to be aware preoperatively that carcinoma is present. A prior history of change in bowel habits, weight loss, and gross rectal bleeding suggests the presence of cancer. Other observations that suggest carcinoma include anemia or a stool test positive for occult blood. Generally, the duration of symptoms prior to perforation is less than 5 months, often less than 2 months. Perforating tumors seem to be more aggressive, at least locally, than nonperforating tumors.

A mass may be palpable on abdominal or rectal examination. Hepatomegaly is sometimes found.[118,119] Proctoscopy demonstrates the tumor in 44 to 67 percent of patients; contrast enema (water-soluble) shows the lesion in 95 percent of patients.

Treatment and Prognosis. The treatment of perforation of large bowel cancer has two goals: control of acute sepsis and cure of the tumor. Although it is reported that cancer cure rates for such patients are lower than for unperforated large bowel cancer, cure is certainly possible. Peloquin[119] found no difference in the proportion of patients with either positive nodes or distant metastases in his patients with perforation compared with all large bowel cancer patients.

Proximal diversion or bypass of a tumor perforation is an inadequate procedure. The shortcomings of this approach are that the leaking bowel and an obstructed column of stool remain in situ, and definitive treatment for the tumor is delayed. Primary resection removes the involved bowel segment and provides definitive treatment for the cancer. Drawbacks of this approach are the added stress of the procedure and the risk that the tumor may be unresectable. If the tumor is adherent to adjacent structures, it may be impossible to tell whether these structures are involved by tumor or not. Thus an attempt at curative resection often demands removal of adjacent organs and tissues, maneuvers that may be unwise in a patient with peritonitis. Resection, at least for palliation, is feasible in about 80 percent of patients.[117] Tumor must be assumed to be present in the walls of abscesses and along any fistula track.

Our approach to patients with malignant perforation of the colon stresses aggressive resuscitation. Patients with small, localized abscesses, fistulas, or incomplete obstruction can be treated with fluids, electrolytes, intestinal decompression, parenteral nutrients, and antibiotics; a planned primary operation is then possible. For most patients, however, an emergency operation is needed to control the source of infection. At operation, the technical feasibility of curative resection, including necessity to resect adjacent tissues and organs, and the presence of distant metastasis are ascertained. We prefer to resect both primarily perforated tumors and obstructing tumors with proximal perforation, and to turn out the bowel ends. We do not do primary anastomoses in the presence of peritonitis or obstruction. Although Hartmann's resection for a rectal tumor might be necessary, emergency abdominoperineal resection is not performed. After the intra-abdominal infection is eradicated, staging of the lesion must be completed to rule out second primaries and to interdict further operative procedures in patients whose life expectancy is limited.

Large series report overall mortality rates of 30 to 44 percent for patients with perforated colon cancer. Perforation with diffuse peritonitis is roughly twice as lethal as perforation with abscess. Likewise, the mortality rate of patients with obstruction-perforation is about twice that of penetration. Patients with fistula have mortality rates from 5 to 11 percent.[118] For primary resection, the mortality rate is 8 to 25 percent (median 19 percent).[118,121] Primary resection has half the mortality risk of diversionary procedures for perforated tumor. When the perforation occurs proximal to an obstructing tumor, however, Welch and Donaldson[122] report that preliminary decompression of the perforated bowel followed by staged resection yields a mortality half that of primary resection. Anastomotic leak rates of up to 40 percent have been noted in patients whose perforated cancer is treated by resection and primary anastomosis; others report no leaks.[121]

A crude calculation indicates that the 5-year survival of patients with perforating carcinoma is less than half (8 to 25 percent) that for all colon cancer patients (32 to 50 percent). These results primarily reflect the immediate sepsis-related mortality of patients with perforated tumors. In patients with perforated colon cancer who survive the acute emergency, survival ranges from 36 to 50 percent and is only slightly less than among all colon cancer patients.[118,119] In contrast, patients with both obstruction and perforation remain at a disadvantage. Survival after curative operations ranges from 11 to 25 percent.[122]

Opportunistic Infections in Colon Cancer

Patients with early large bowel cancer are not overly susceptible to systemic opportunistic infections (see Chap. 51). Instead, tumor ulceration allows fecal bacterial access to the bloodstream so that systemic infections caused by *Bacteroides* and *Clostridium* (especially *C. septicum*) occur more frequently in patients with colon cancer.

Colon cancer fosters gut colonization by certain uncommon organisms. *Streptococcus bovis* is recovered from the feces of 56 percent of patients with large bowel cancer versus 10 percent of control patients and has the capacity to cause endocarditis as well as septicemia.[123] *Streptococcus bovis* can be differentiated from other viridans streptococci only by special microbiologic techniques. One may suspect *S. bovis* if a nonenterococcal, group D *streptococcus,* unusually *susceptible* to penicillin, cephalosporins, and clindamycin, is isolated. The special importance of these infections is that their presence may be the only early indication of large bowel cancer. Any patient with such infections without an obvious source should undergo evaluation for colon cancer.

Cancer chemotherapy may induce marked neutropenia that, in turn, may cause typhlitis or other forms of enterocolitis.[124]

INFECTIOUS MANIFESTATIONS OF LARGE BOWEL OBSTRUCTION

Obstruction of the large bowel can be complicated by perforation, strangulation, and colitis proximal to the point of obstruction. The infections that ensue account for much of the morbidity and mortality associated with large bowel obstruction. The conditions that cause bowel obstruction are discussed elsewhere in this chapter and will not be treated in detail here. Ischemia contributes importantly to the colitis of obstruction; this entity is discussed with ischemic and nonspecific colitis. Because they are not included elsewhere, volvulus, hernia, intussusception in adults, and pseudo-obstruction are discussed here.

Epidemiology and Pathogenesis. Large bowel obstruction occurs primarily in the elderly, with nearly equal distribution between the sexes.[125,126] Perforation occurs in 8 to 9 percent, and, of these, 22 to 50 percent occur at the site of obstruction.

The degree of colon distention depends on the duration and completeness of the obstruction and the competence of the ileocecal valve. If the ileocecal valve is competent, decompression into the proximal bowel cannot occur (closed-loop obstruction). Michel et al[127] estimate that the ileocecal valve is competent in about 50 percent of patients. With the development of a closed loop, intestinal contents and gas (mostly swallowed air) flow into the colon, thereby increasing intraluminal pressure. Increased amounts of fluid are secreted, and absorption is inhibited.

Distention of the bowel may result in perforation in two ways. The first is mechanical rupture by increased pressure. The cecum is the usual segment to perforate proximal to an obstruction because it has a thinner wall and distends to a greater diameter at a given pressure (La Place's law: tension = pressure $\times$ π $\times$ radius). The second mechanism of perforation is development of ischemic injury as intraluminal pressure increases. A role for fecal bacteria, promoting necrosis of the bowel wall in obstructed ischemic colon that leads to perforation, is assumed but has not been documented. Strangulation of the colon usually is a result of volvulus or an incarcerated hernia. As the bowel wall loses viability, bacteria and their toxins gain access to the peritoneal cavity, even in the absence of actual perforation.

The more common lesions accounting for large bowel obstruction are listed in Table 43–2. Large bowel obstruction is seldom caused by adhesions. Obstruction caused by extrinsic cancer usually results from gynecologic tumors, although neoplasms of prostate, genitourinary tract, and presacral tumors also may cause obstruction. Massive fecal impaction may occur in patients with motility disorders and occurs frequently in elderly, senile, and institutionalized patients. Massive fecal impaction may occur in opiate drug abusers and in patients taking large quantities of narcotic analgesics. Antacids containing aluminum and calcium may produce fecal impaction.

Most cases of intussusception occur in young children; less than 10 percent are colonic in origin. Intussusception in adults originates in the ileocecal segment in 46 percent, the sigmoid in 18 percent, and the intervening colon in 36 percent.[128] The intussusceptum is usually a benign tumor.

Pseudo-obstruction of the colon occurs in adults of all ages. Although no organic obstruction is present, the danger of colon perforation is as great as if one were, and cecal perforation occurs in about one-fourth of reported cases. Causes of pseudo-obstruction include pregnancy, intra-abdominal inflammation, sepsis, cardiac failure, retroperitoneal disease, pelvic surgery, trauma, and cesarean section; 23 percent of cases are idiopathic.

Clinical Manifestations. Patients with large bowel obstruction usually give a history of cramping hypo-

TABLE 43–2. CAUSES OF LARGE BOWEL OBSTRUCTION[125–131]

Lesion	Range (%)	Median (%)
Large bowel cancer	34–64	53
Volvulus	7–28	13
Congenital	9–16	13
Diverticulitis	3–12	7
Extrinsic cancer	2–13	3
Ileus	3–5	4
Hernia	0–3	2
Adhesions	1–4	3
Fecal impaction	1–6	4
Intussusception	—	1

gastric abdominal pain, associated with obstipation and abdominal distention.[127] There may have been preexisting diarrhea or constipation. Nausea and vomiting can occur but frequently are absent, even in patients with advanced obstruction. If perforation or strangulation occurs, pain becomes localized and more constant as peritonitis develops. Typically, large bowel obstruction develops over days or even weeks.

Abdominal distention, active bowel sounds, tympany, tenderness, and signs of peritonitis may be present, even in the absence of true peritonitis, owing to stretching of the peritoneum. There are no typical signs of gangrenous bowel, although tenderness (86 percent), decreased bowel sounds (46 percent), rebound tenderness (45 percent), and fever (43 percent) are supposed to be classic.[126–129]

In cases of volvulus, there sometimes is a history of prior episodes of abdominal pain, distention, and constipation. The diagnosis of incarcerated hernia usually is obvious. When a diaphragmatic hernia is present, peristaltic sounds or a succussion splash may be heard in the chest. Intussusception in adults may have no distinctive findings although a mass may be palpable. Pseudo-obstruction is associated with abdominal distention and obstipation, but pain is minimal or absent. Pain and signs of peritonitis develop only when perforation is imminent or has occurred.

Diagnosis. Plain abdominal films demonstrate a distended colon, possibly with a cut-off at the site of obstruction. Frequently, small bowel distention causes confusion about the exact site of obstruction. The risk of perforation is increased if cecal distention is greater than 9 cm in diameter. Although frequently omitted, proctoscopy should be done in most obstructed patients.[126] The obstructing lesion may be visualized, and the diagnosis confirmed by biopsy. All stable patients with bowel obstruction without evidence of perforation or strangulation should have a contrast enema to demonstrate the obstructing lesion.

Sigmoid volvulus is suggested by a greatly distended sigmoid colon bent upon itself, a loop extending as far as the diaphragm, and a pattern of mucosal spiraling or a bird's beak cut-off on contrast enema. Classic signs of cecal volvulus are a distended cecum located in the left upper quadrant, midabdomen, or right upper quadrant; a large extragastric air-fluid level in the left upper quadrant; an ileocecal valve seen on the right side of the cecum; beaking and mucosal folds; small bowel in the right lower quadrant in place of the cecum; and small bowel distention.

Intussusception mainly produces findings of small bowel obstruction. A contrast enema may outline the intussuscepted bowel.[128] Absence of an obstructing lesion on contrast enema indicates pseudo-obstruction.

Treatment. Nonoperative treatment is directed toward the prevention of perforation by nasogastric decompression and fluid resuscitation. Uncomplicated fecal impaction is managed by manual disimpaction and saline or Gastrografin enemas. Complete large bowel obstruction, perforation, and strangulation are indications for immediate operation. Distention of the cecum to greater than 12 cm in diameter is also an indication for operation if the cecum does not decompress promptly when intubated.

The two alternative surgical approaches to mechanical large bowel obstruction are proximal decompression of the obstructed segment and primary resection of the obstructing lesion. Proximal decompression by left transverse colostomy or cecostomy[127,129] relieves the obstruction with minimal trauma. The danger of performing rapid decompression alone is that gangrenous bowel or a perforation can be missed. Furthermore, a second major procedure is necessary to provide definitive treatment. Payne and McAlpine[130] suggest making a stoma as close as possible to the obstruction so that the colostomy closure can be performed coincident with removal of the lesion.

We agree with those who prefer to resect the obstructing lesion at the first operation. We do not believe, however, that primary anastomosis in obstructed colon is ever indicated. Perforated segments should be resected; proximal cecal perforation is also managed with a resection. Proximal decompression is performed if the lesion is unresectable or if an abdominal-perineal resection is necessary for its removal.

Contrast enemas and endoscopy are successful in reducing sigmoid volvulus in 50 to 85 percent of patients.[131] Even so, the risk of recurrence makes elective resection of the involved loop of sigmoid colon desirable. Emergency resection is required if nonoperative reduction fails or strangulation occurs; primary anastomosis should be avoided. Cecal volvulus requires emergency reduction with cecopexy or cecostomy. There is an increased incidence of postoperative sepsis when cecostomy is added. If gangrenous bowel is present, right colectomy is indicated. Volvulus of the transverse colon requires emergency resection.

If possible, an incarcerated inguinal hernia should be reduced by gentle manipulation aided by mild sedation. If reduction is unsuccessful or if strangulation is believed present, operation should be performed promptly to reduce the hernia, resect strangulated bowel, and repair the defect.

Because of the high incidence of malignancy as the precipitating cause, attempts to reduce adult colonic intussusception by any means usually are not indicated. The involved bowel should be resected. Only when rectosigmoid intussusception is present should manual reduction be performed to avoid the need for abdominal-perineal resection.

When signs of perforation are absent, pseudo-obstruction of the colon is treated with nasogastric decompression. If the cecal diameter exceeds 12 cm, or if distention persists for more than 48 hours, decompression of the colon by colonoscopy is necessary.

Prognosis. The mortality rate for patients with large bowel obstruction ranges from 6 to 37 percent (median 32 percent).[124,126,129] This rate reflects the advanced age of the typical patient and the associated illnesses in addition to the cause of the obstruction and its complications. Perforation and peritonitis increase the mortality to almost 50 percent for perforated sigmoid or cecal volvulus and pseudo-obstruction.

ISCHEMIC DISEASES OF THE COLON

Ischemic colitis frequently is unrecognized because it is actually a spectrum of conditions ranging from acute focal ulcers of the colon to gangrenous necrotizing colitis. Ischemia alone does not account for the entire clinical picture. Although their role is unproved, the fecal flora probably account for additional tissue necrosis, as well as toxemia and septicemia. This concept is supported by the ability of local antibiotic instillation to protect ischemic bowel anastomoses.[20] In this discussion, the following disorders are considered: ischemic colitis, necrotizing enterocolitis, colitis complicating large bowel obstruction, ischemic colitis complicating vascular surgery, radiation colitis, stercoraceous ulcer and perforation, and spontaneous ulcer with perforation of the colon.

Epidemiology and Pathogenesis. Most ischemic diseases of the colon occur in the elderly with atherosclerotic disease and carcinoma of the colon. Institutionalized patients, many of them elderly, with poor bowel habits, younger patients with radiation damage to the colon after treatment for gynecologic cancer, and those with autoimmune disorders are also susceptible. An obvious although uncommon cause of ischemia of the colon is spontaneous, traumatic, or operative occlusion of the visceral arteries.

Decreased perfusion due to heart disease, shock, sepsis, and the drugs used to treat such disorders (digitalis, vasopressors) also may divert blood from the splanchnic circulation. Enterocolitis, apparently ischemic in nature, has been described in a child with pheochromocytoma. The effects of distention and increased intraluminal pressure on blood flow were discussed in the section above on colon obstruction.

Proliferative intimal changes in small arterioles and medial hypertrophy of small arteries have been seen in ischemic colitis. Thrombosis of submucosal vessels is associated with primary thrombotic disorders such as the hemolytic-uremic syndrome. Use of estrogen compounds is described in patients with ischemic colitis, and discrete colonic ulcers have been noted after use of oral contraceptives.[132] Autoimmune disease may induce vasculitis of the small vessels to the colon.[133] Although early radiation injury of the bowel involves mucosal cells, the late changes include vasculitis characterized by subendothelial proliferation and medial thickening.

Although any fecal organism might be expected to increase the damage to ischemic bowel wall, the anaerobic environment particularly encourages growth of anaerobic organisms such as clostridia. Stasis of stool behind a colon obstruction promotes increased concentrations of anaerobic organisms. Invasion of the colon by clostridia has been implicated in necrotizing enterocolitis of infancy and antibiotic-associated colitis. Likewise, clostridia have been identified in patients reported to have ischemic colitis[134] and necrotizing colitis. Bacteria may play an important role in the development of ischemic colitis,[135] necrotizing colitis, and cecal perforation in leukemia patients receiving chemotherapy. Similar mechanisms may account for some of the problems seen in transplant patients. The occurrence of some acute ulcerative lesions in patients with uremia may be the result of the action of urease-producing gut bacteria resulting in large local concentrations of ammonia.[136]

Early changes of colon ischemia are mucosal and submucosal edema and hemorrhage. Mucosal necrosis follows. With more severe involvement, transmural infarction develops with acute inflammatory changes and bacterial penetration. During the healing phase, mucosal ulcers with granulating bases are present.[137] The surrounding mucosa regenerates over the ulcer. When only the mucosa and the submucosa are involved, complete healing is expected. When the muscularis propria is involved and is replaced with scar tissue, stricture results.

Clinical Manifestations. The clinical features of classic ischemic colitis have been reviewed extensively.[137] Usually, the patient complains of lower abdominal pain, vomiting, and diarrhea. Minimal to moderate amounts of blood are passed per rectum. Frequently, the patient gives no past history of significant bowel disease or other illness. Many patients are already hospitalized for treatment of shock, heart disease, sepsis, or other predisposing illness. Typical physical findings include a normal blood pressure, no more than mild fever, and minimal, if any, abdominal tenderness. Peristaltic sounds are active to hyperactive.

Boley et al[137] observed one group of patients with ischemic colitis who had transient disease that rapidly healed and caused no further trouble (45 percent). A second group recovered within a week, but returned 1 to 12 months later with a large bowel obstruction due to a segmental ischemic stricture (13 percent). A third group developed transmural gangrenous colitis (19 percent), with severe abdominal pain, generalized abdominal distention, and peritoneal signs. A fourth group of patients (19 percent) had symptoms that continued for 1 to 4 months and culminated in perforation, stricture, or a protein-losing enteropathy. The clinical features of necrotizing colitis are similar to those of gangrenous or transmural ischemic colitis, and most surgeons now consider these entities identical.[138,139]

Patients with colitis proximal to a bowel obstruction usually present with the findings of carcinomatous large bowel obstruction. The presence of local abdominal tenderness, diarrhea, and toxicity may suggest colitis, but the diagnosis cannot be made with certainty. Obstructive colitis may not be suspected until a leak occurs after resection and anastomosis for a colon tumor.[140]

The findings of colon ischemia complicating aortic surgery are similar to those of typical colonic ischemia. Unfortunately, postoperative pain obscures the clinical picture. The diagnosis is first considered when diarrhea, often progressing to bloody diarrhea, appears within the first postoperative week. Although this complication is said to occur in 1 to 2 percent of patients undergoing aortic surgery, Ernst et al[141] report that 6 percent of their patients examined routinely in the postoperative period have endoscopic evidence of colon ischemia. Preoperative antibiotic and mechanical bowel preparation decreases the incidence of this complication.

Although colon ischemia rarely occurs after elective abdominal aortic surgery, there is a markedly increased incidence after repair of ruptured abdominal aortic aneurysm. Clinically, this is seen in 7 to 27 percent of patients but up to 60 percent when colonoscopy is routinely performed postoperatively.[142]

Early proctocolitis is a routine sequel to pelvic irradiation; symptoms are cramping pain, diarrhea, and the passage of mucus and blood. This condition is self-limited and disappears soon after the completion of treatment. Late radiation colitis does not become apparent for months or years. Radiation enteritis complicates abdominopelvic radiation therapy in 5 percent of patients. Most damage is done to the rectum and the small bowel. Sigmoid colon damage accompanies 17 percent of small bowel injuries and most frequently follows pelvic operation and irradiation for carcinoma of the cervix. Approximately one-half of radiation colitis patients develop a partial large bowel obstruction caused by stricture. Nearly another one-half have cramping, pain, and diarrhea containing mucus and blood. In occasional patients, ulceration progresses to fistula formation or perforation.

Stercoraceous ulceration with perforation affects the sigmoid (rarely, the cecum) in patients with chronic constipation who are institutionalized, chronically ill, or taking constipating drugs. Patients with scleroderma are especially susceptible.[143] These patients frequently are acutely ill, comatose, and have signs of peritonitis with a palpable fecal mass within the abdomen or the rectum.[144] Perforation of an idiopathic cecal ulcer accounted for about 8 percent of all cecal perforations prior to 1956.[145] These lesions were found most frequently in patients with cardiovascular or autoimmune disease or sepsis, but young, previously healthy victims have been reported. Cecal ulcer causes rectal bleeding or produces abdominal pain of acute onset often mistaken for acute appendicitis. When perforation occurs, peritonitis and sepsis quickly develop.

Diagnosis. Diagnostic features are similar for many ischemic disorders of the colon. Anemia is proportional to the amount of blood loss. Leukocytosis (10,000 to 20,000) and a moderate left shift in the white blood cell count are usual but may be profound in the presence of gangrenous bowel. Conversely, leukopenia may reflect severe sepsis. Heikkinen et al[139] noted metabolic acidosis in patients with severe necrotizing colitis.

Colonoscopy is the ideal method to diagnose colonic ischemia. Because the rectum is involved in only 6 to 20 percent of patients, and the sigmoid colon in less than half,[137,140] proctosigmoidoscopy alone frequently is inadequate to establish the diagnosis. Mucosal edema and pallor are the earliest signs. A congested, bluish appearance accompanied by submucosal bleeding appears next. Blue nodules, the *thumbprints* seen on abdominal x-ray studies, may be seen. The mucosa then becomes friable and ulceration occurs. The subsequent course of the ischemic process determines subsequent findings. The mucosa may become necrotic and pseudomembranes may develop. The ulcers may coalesce, and one may see only a bed of granulation tissue as resolution occurs. Neither gross appearance nor biopsy permits differentiation of ischemic colitis from inflammatory bowel disease or pseudomembranous colitis.

Radiation colitis produces a rather pale, atrophic, granular mucosa. Radiation ulcers tend to be punched out with a shaggy yellow-gray base. Colon involved by radiation changes is often fixed and narrowed by fibrous stricture so that the endoscope cannot be safely passed. When bowel obstruction is present, a tumor, stercoroma, or other lesion may be seen. Endoscopy should be performed in all patients with possible ischemic colitis unless they are unstable from sepsis or shock, or unless they have an acute abdomen. After an ischemic area is found and the diagnosis made, undue effort to pass the instrument further should not be made because of the risk of perforating the bowel.

Contrast enema is the most useful study for diagnosing and following uncomplicated ischemic colitis; in the absence of signs of sepsis or peritonitis, barium enema should be performed within 48 hours of admission.[106] Usually, ischemic colitis is a segmental process. The splenic flexure and descending colon are most frequently involved (57 to 65 percent). The transverse colon is involved in 9 to 21 percent of patients, and the cecum and ascending colon in 4 to 8 percent. Involvement of more than one segment is seen in 12 to 39 percent.[137,138]

Thumbprinting (Fig. 43–8A) is the classic, but transient, sign as ulceration soon occurs over the

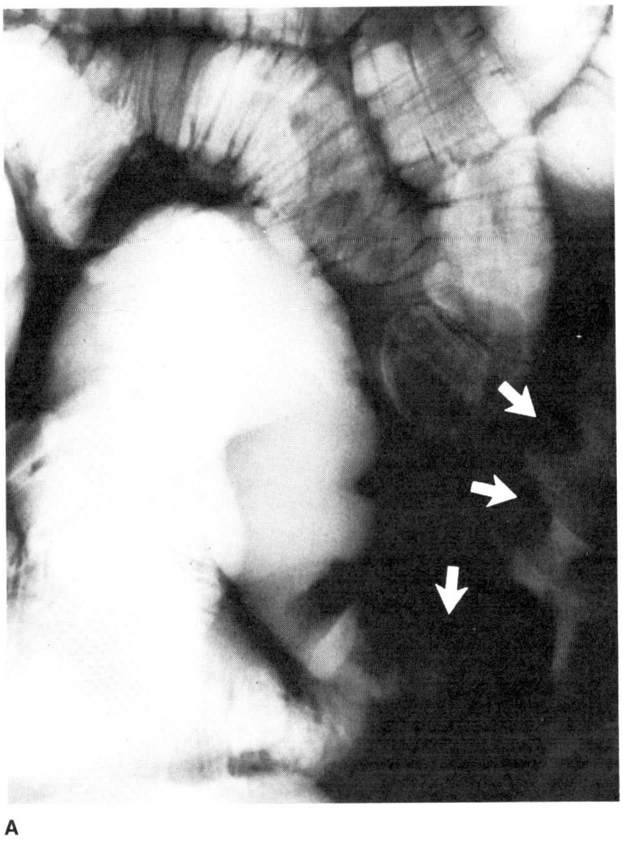

A

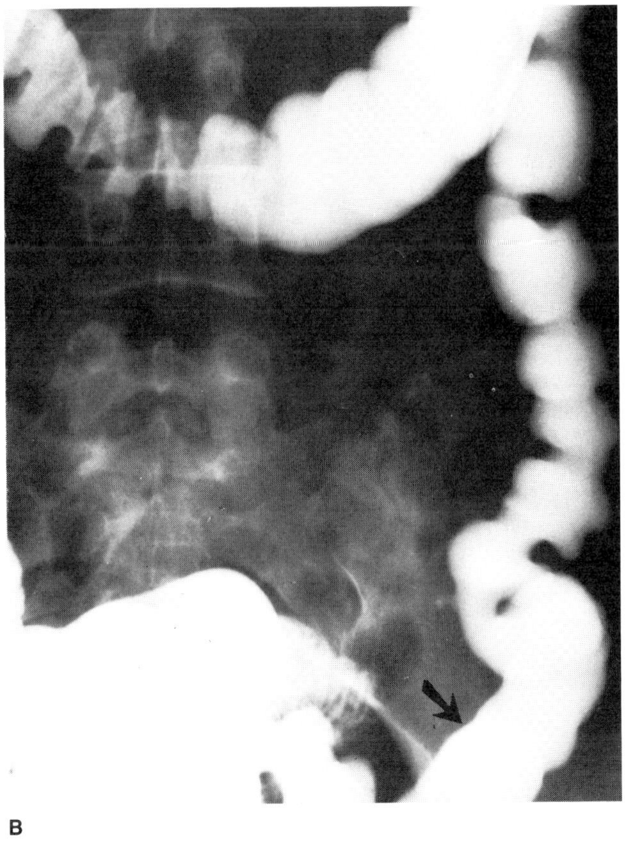

B

Figure 43–8. A. Ischemic colitis. Barium enema demonstrates narrowing of a sigmoid colon segment with "thumbprinting" (arrows). **B.** Ischemic colitis. Repeat barium enema performed 2 weeks later demonstrates resolution of the ischemic changes (arrow).

nodules of submucosal edema and hemorrhage. Subsequent changes include segmental spasm, ulceration, and other changes noted in inflammatory as well as ischemic colitis. Evolution from the early findings to complete resolution within 2 weeks is essential to the diagnosis; barium enema must be repeated (Fig. 43–8B). Persistent findings signify the presence of another disease. The late changes of segmental stricture must be differentiated from other causes of stricture.

Barium enema should not be done when peritoneal signs are present. Findings on plain films may include free intraperitoneal air, intraperitoneal fluid, and distended small or large bowel. When the colon is distended, thumbprinting, thickening of the bowel wall, and ulceration may be apparent on plain films (Fig. 43–9). The presence of a distended colon or colonic segment on a plain film may be of great diagnostic significance. When distention occurs secondary to obstruction, the dilated bowel retains haustral markings and appears otherwise normal. Distended ischemic colon is characterized by haustra that are thickened, blunted, or absent. Spontaneous distention of a segment of ischemic bowel indicates transmural involvement with impending or actual perforation.[134,139] Toxic dilation of the colon may be seen in ischemic colitis.

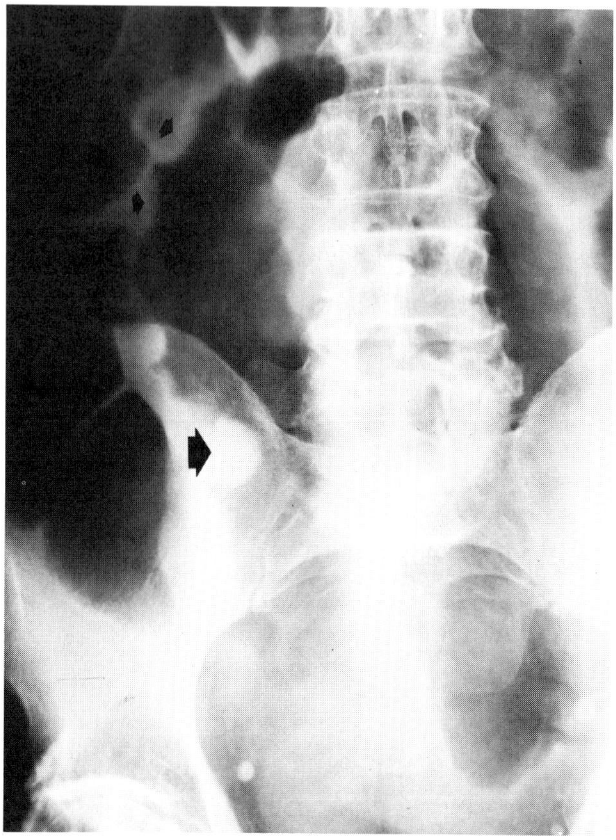

Figure 43–9. Transmural ischemic colitis. Plain abdominal film demonstrates dilation of the sigmoid colon with loss of haustra. Thickening of the bowel wall and "thumbprinting" (arrows) are apparent.

Arteriography is relatively unproductive in ischemic bowel disease because occlusion of large vessels (eg, inferior mesenteric artery) occurs in only 5 percent of patients.[138] The study may be performed in selected patients; vascular reconstruction may be beneficial on occasion.

Treatment. Uncomplicated ischemic colitis does not require operation. Intravenous fluids, avoidance of oral intake, and nasogastric suction should reduce distention. There are no reliable data on the effects of systemic or oral antibiotics in this disease. Operation is indicated when the findings or clinical course suggest transmural involvement. Acute ischemic colitis persisting for more than 2 weeks results in irreversible bowel damage, for which resection of the segment of involved colon is recommended.

Because the serosal surface of involved bowel may appear entirely normal, the extent of resection is determined by examining the margins of the excised bowel segment. Primary colocolonic anastomosis is unwise when peritonitis is present, when bowel preparation has not been performed, and when resection is necessary during the acute phase of the disease. If colitis is found proximal to an acutely obstructing lesion, the entire involved segment should be resected and colostomy performed. If a simple diverting colostomy is performed for distal obstruction, the patient must be observed closely for progression of the colitis.

When colon ischemia complicates an aortic operation, the management is the same. Ernst et al[141] stress several technical factors to prevent this complication: ligation of the inferior mesenteric artery flush with the aorta, restoration of hypogastric artery flow, avoidance of hypotension and trauma to the colon, preservation of a meandering mesenteric artery, and reimplantation of a patent inferior mesenteric artery if the collateral circulation appears inadequate.

Radiation colitis should be treated by a low-residue diet, stool softeners, local or systemic steroids, and sulfasalazine. Operation is necessary for hemorrhage, complete obstruction, perforation, or fistula formation. The entire involved segment should be resected. End colostomy may be necessary, but anastomosis can be attempted if healthy bowel is present distally. If anastomosis is made to the rectum, a diverting colostomy may be necessary. Rarely, colitis is severe enough to require a permanent diverting colostomy; such a stoma must be made far enough proximally to avoid irradiated bowel.

Fecal impaction causing stercoraceous ulceration must be removed rapidly but gently. Once the stool is evacuated, a nonperforated ulcer should heal as long as constipation is prevented. If perforation has occurred, the defect must be exteriorized, resected, or closed and protected by a proximal stoma.

Spontaneous ulcers usually become apparent by perforation. They should be managed by resection or exteriorization. Even though many of these ulcers occur in the cecum, primary colon anastomosis or closure is not recommended if peritonitis is present. Nonperforated cecal ulcers usually are detected during operations for suspected acute appendicitis. For these, excision with primary closure or imbrication is suggested.

LARGE BOWEL FISTULA

Although fistulas between the colon and many organs have been reported, most types of colon fistula are relatively rare. The review of Webster and Carey[146] includes a comprehensive discussion of large bowel fistula. A discussion of intra-abdominal abscesses and fistulas is given in Chapter 38.

Epidemiology and Pathogenesis. A listing of the anatomic types of large bowel fistula and the possible etiologic conditions for each type are presented in Table 43–3. Rectal fistulas are discussed in Chapter 45. Fistulas develop when a diseased organ comes into contact with other organs or when the space between organs is occupied by a mass, a focus of infection, or a foreign body. Pressure, nonspecific inflammation, and digestion by enzymes or other products of infection result in communication between the visceral lumina, or the fistula opens to the skin.

Clinical Manifestations. Colocutaneous fistulas constitute 29 to 44 percent of all external gastrointestinal fistulas. Most colocutaneous fistulas (52 to 94 percent) occur as sequelae of surgical procedures, either as complications (eg, anastomotic leak) or as a persistent drainage track. Diverticular disease, carcinoma, and inflammatory bowel disease account for most spontaneous fistulas. Spontaneous and complicating fistulas initially appear as a fluctuant, localized area of inflammation that subsequently breaks down and drains pus or feces. After the removal of drains, feces continue to drain through the persistent track. Under the best of circumstances, a colocutaneous fistula functions as a colostomy. Possible complications of fistula include intra-abdominal sepsis, fluid-electrolyte and acid-base imbalance, malnutrition, hemorrhage, bowel obstruction, and skin breakdown.

Most *gastrocolic* fistulas result from carcinoma of the colon or the stomach. Gastrojejunocolic fistulas formerly were an occasional complication of retrocolic gastrojejunostomy performed for peptic ulcer disease.[146] Gastrocolic fistula produces upper abdominal pain, diarrhea, and weight loss. Vomiting, occasionally feculent, frequently occurs. A tumor mass may be palpated. Malabsorption is frequent; colonization of the stomach and the upper intestine by large numbers of fecal organisms alters digestion and absorption; undigested food and fluid may pass directly from the stomach to the colon bypassing the small bowel.

Duodenocolic fistula is also usually caused by malignancy, especially carcinoma of the right or transverse colon. Benign duodenocolic fistulas result from peptic ulcer or inflammatory bowel disease. The symptoms are similar to that of gastrocolic fistula with pain, diarrhea, weight loss, malabsorption, and abdominal mass. Vomiting occurs less frequently than with gastrocolic fistula.

Intestinocolic and *colocolic* fistula frequently result from septic complications of diverticular disease or inflammatory bowel disease. Systemic signs of infection are more prevalent than in gastric or duodenal fistula. Otherwise, the symptoms are similar abdominal pain, diarrhea, and weight loss. Symptoms may be minimal if the intestinal communication is located in the distal small bowel. When cancer or abscess is present, an abdominal or pelvic mass may be detected.

Biliary-enteric fistula occurs in 0.4 to 2 percent of patients with biliary tract diseases[146–148]; 8 to 24 percent are cholecystocolonic, and another 2 to 8 percent are cholecystoduodenocolic fistulas. Because 80 to 90 percent of these fistulas are sequelae of chronic cholecystitis and cholelithiasis, many patients give a past history of right upper quadrant pain. The disappearance of right upper quadrant pain, particularly during an acute exacerbation, may herald the development of a fistula.

Elderly patients with cholecystitis, diabetes mellitus, and atherosclerotic vascular disease are especially prone to fistula formation. Patients with a biliary-enteric fistula may develop gallstone ileus.

TABLE 43–3. LARGE BOWEL FISTULA: CLASSIFICATION AND ETIOLOGY

Anatomic Type	Etiology
Colocutaneous fistula	Iatrogenic (anastomotic leak, persistent cecostomy, postabscess drainage, intestinal injury), diverticulitis, carcinoma of large bowel, inflammatory bowel disease, trauma, ingested foreign body, tuberculosis, amebiasis, actinomycosis, strangulated hernia, appendicitis, ischemic perforation
Coloenteric fistula	
Gastrocolic and gastrojejunocolic fistula	Carcinoma of colon, carcinoma of stomach, peptic ulcer disease, gastric ulcer, inflammatory bowel disease, diverticulitis, carcinoma of pancreas or gallbladder, tuberculosis, syphilis, trauma, lymphoma, sarcoma, carcinoid, typhoid, pancreatic abscess, ingested foreign body, subphrenic abscess, iatrogenic (anastomotic leak, gastrostomy tube erosion, inadvertent gastrocolostomy, radiation therapy)
Duodenocolic fistula	Carcinoma of colon, carcinoma of gallbladder, carcinoma of duodenum, carcinoma of pancreas, lymphoma, peptic ulcer disease, duodenal diverticulitis, inflammatory bowel disease, biliary disease, pancreatitis, abdominal and subhepatic abscess, tuberculosis, typhoid, trauma, ingested foreign body, amebiasis
Intestinocolic fistula	Diverticulitis, inflammatory bowel disease, carcinoma of colon, ingested foreign body
Colocolic fistula	Sigmoid volvulus, diverticulitis
Appendicocolic fistula	Appendicitis
Cholecystocolic and colecystoduodenocolic fistula	Chronic cholecystitis and cholelithiasis, carcinoma of colon, carcinoma of gallbladder, peptic ulcer disease, inflammatory bowel disease, diverticulitis coli, duodenal diverticulitis, lymphoma, trauma
Pancreaticocolic and pseudocystocolic fistula	Pancreatic abscess, pancreatic pseudocyst
Genitourinary-colon fistula	
Renocolic fistula	Renal disease—pyelonephritis, tuberculosis, echinococcosis, bilharziasis, renal calculus, renal tumor
Ureterocolic fistula	Renal disease—pyelonephritis, tuberculosis, renal and ureteral calculus, ureteral stricture, pregnancy, pelvic kidney, urinary tumor; bowel disease—carcinoma of colon, diverticulitis, blunt and penetrating trauma, postileal conduit surgery
Vesicocolic fistula	Diverticulitis, carcinoma of colon, carcinoma of cervix, carcinoma of bladder, postradiation treatment, trauma, tuberculosis, amebiasis, syphilis, inflammatory bowel disease, other pelvic tumors
Colovaginal, colouterine, colocervical, tubocolic fistula	Diverticulitis, carcinoma of colon, pelvic cancer, operative trauma, radiation, tuberculosis, pelvic inflammatory disease, endometriosis
Intestinorespiratory fistula	Subphrenic abscess, rupture of the diaphragm, empyema, pyonephrosis
Vascular fistulas	
Aortocolic fistula	Ruptured aortic aneurysm, penetrating trauma
Inferior mesenteric artery-colic fistula	Arteriovenous malformation, arteriovenous fistula after bowel resection
Iliac artery-colic fistula	Foreign body perforation, iliac artery aneurysm, postvascular surgery

The point of obstruction may be located in the terminal ileum if there is a cholecystoduodenal fistula or in the sigmoid colon with cholecystocolonic fistula.[148]

Hematochezia of moderate to severe degree occurs if the cystic artery is involved in the fistula. Diarrhea and malabsorption occur if the duodenum is involved or if there is common bile duct obstruction with diversion of all bile into the colon. Jaundice and cholangitis are more likely to occur when the duct is obstructed. Although a cholecystocolonic fistula is the most likely biliary-enteric fistula to cause cholangitis, the reported incidence ranges widely from 0 to 60 percent. Biliary-colonic fistula may be asymptomatic, with only the x-ray finding of pneumobilia.

Complications involving the colon occur in about 1 percent of patients who are admitted with acute *pancreatitis*, and as many as one-half of these involve fistula formation. Pancreatocolonic fistulas occur spontaneously or as a sequel to operation in 10 to 18 percent of patients with pancreatic abscess,[149] and in 0.6 to 6 percent of patients with pseudocyst.[150] Most pancreatitis patients who develop colonic fistulas have a clinical course characterized by the presence of an abdominal mass, pain, and, in the case of abscess, sepsis. Communication with the colon is heralded by the sudden passage of a brown or yellow watery diarrheal stool; pain and sepsis may be relieved. More than half of affected patients subsequently develop severe hemorrhage. Passage of stool from a pancreatic drain track indicates the presence of a postoperative fistula (see Chap. 41).

Colourinary fistula may originate from disease in either system. Fistulas that communicate with the upper urinary tract are more likely related to primary urinary tract disease,[146] whereas lower urinary tract fistula usually arises from primary bowel disease.[69] Colovesical fistula is rare in women unless a hysterectomy has been performed. Approximately 70 percent of colovesical fistulas are due to diverticular disease and 15 to 20 percent are caused by colon or bladder tumor.[151] Nearly all patients with urinary fistula have urinary sepsis and its symptoms: frequency, dysuria, and hematuria. Pneumaturia and fecaluria are noted in some patients. If present, primary bowel disease may produce such symptoms as rectal bleeding, change in bowel habit, and lower abdominal pain. Other findings may include flank tenderness and pain, upper abdominal mass, presence of a psoas sign with upper urinary tract disease, and a lower abdominal or pelvic mass with bladder fistula. Urine may drain into the colon, causing watery diarrhea.

Colovaginal and *colocervical* fistula occur in women who have had a hysterectomy. These fistulas, along with colouterine fistula, are secondary to diverticulitis or pelvic cancer. In women who have been treated for pelvic cancer, the development of a fistula frequently indicates tumor recurrence. Fistulas between the colon and the female reproductive organs usually are associated with the passage of pus, feces, and flatus per vagina.

Colorespiratory fistulas are rare. The most common cause is extension of a subphrenic abscess into both the colon and the thorax. The presence of the fistula is indicated by mediastinitis, empyema, or recurrent pneumonitis.

Colovascular fistulas are uncommon, even relative to other forms of vascular enteric fistula. Aortocolic fistulas can result from a ruptured aortic aneurysm or penetrating tumor but are more likely to occur at the distal suture line of an aortoiliac graft. Vascular fistula presents with rectal hemorrhage. The initial bleeding is usually minimal and of short duration; however, bleeding continues to occur and eventually reaches exsanguinating proportions.

Diagnosis. Fistulas can be accompanied by sepsis, malnutrition, and fluid-electrolyte and acid-base imbalances. Therefore a complete blood count and electrolyte, arterial blood pH, calcium, magnesium, and vitamin B_{12} determinations are indicated in many patients. A complete nutritional assessment is frequently necessary. Cultures of blood and drainage should be done when sepsis exists. The cause of the fistula should be determined.

The evaluation of a colocutaneous fistula must answer several questions: (1) What is the origin of the fistula? (2) Is there continuity of the bowel? (3) Is there distal obstruction of the bowel? (4) What is the nature of adjacent bowel? (5) Is there an undrained abscess? Plain abdominal x-ray studies, abdominal ultrasonography, and computed tomography may be used to investigate abdominal sepsis. However, the key studies are proctoscopy, barium enema, and injection of the fistula with contrast medium. An upper gastrointestinal series with small bowel follow-through and an intravenous pyelogram are sometimes helpful.

Gastrocolic, gastrojejunocolic, and other coloenteric fistulas are all best demonstrated by barium enema examination.[146] Upper gastrointestinal series and upper gastrointestinal endoscopy are less often successful, although both studies are indicated.[146,152,153] Neither proctoscopy nor colonoscopy demonstrates the fistula, but these studies may establish a diagnosis of the specific colonic disease causing the fistula.

Plain abdominal x-ray studies showing air in the biliary tree (Fig. 43–10A) or a change in the location of previously demonstrated biliary calculi may allow a diagnosis of biliary-colonic fistula. Communication with the colon is often detected by barium enema (Fig. 43–10B). An upper gastrointestinal series may demonstrate the presence of a cholecystoduodenocolic fistula.

Likewise, a pancreatocolonic fistula is usually visualized with barium enema examination. Concurrent gastric or duodenal involvement may be apparent on upper gastrointestinal series. Upper gastrointestinal x-ray studies, ultrasonography, and computed tomography are indicated to determine the extent of the pancreatic disease process.

A urinary-colic fistula is more difficult to demonstrate than a coloenteric fistula. Plain abdominal films may be of some help, because many patients harbor radiopaque calculi in the involved collecting system or in the bladder. When a renocolic or ureterocolic fistula is present, pneumonephrosis or air surrounding the renal shadow or outlining the renal pelvis may be seen. Rarely, in upper or lower urinary tract fistula, an air-fluid level may be seen in the bladder.

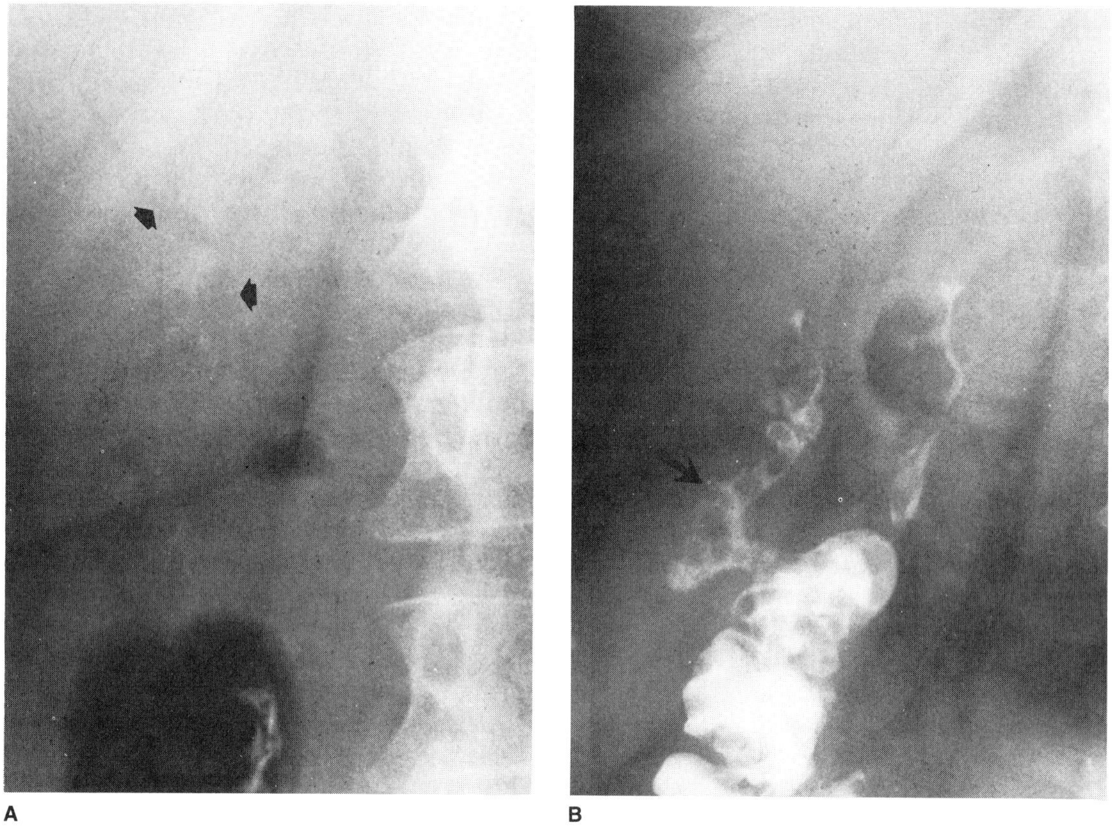

Figure 43–10. A. Cholecystocolonic fistula. Plain abdominal film demonstrates air in the biliary and hepatic ducts (arrows). **B.** Cholecystocolonic fistula. Barium enema demonstrates the fistula and the gallbladder containing calculi (arrow). Contrast from an intravenous pyelogram is seen in the pelvis of the right kidney.

In contrast to coloenteric fistula, it is usually difficult to demonstrate a colourinary fistula by studying the bowel. In most instances, both endoscopy and barium enema demonstrate only the nature of the bowel disease (see Fig. 43–3A). With renocolic or ureterocolic fistula, the colon may be narrowed or inflamed at the site of the fistula. Methylene blue or indigo carmine injected intravenously or directly into the urinary tract only rarely will be seen empyting into the colon.

Urinalysis and urine culture nearly always prove the presence of urinary infection with enteric organisms. Intravenous pyelography and cystography almost never demonstrate the fistula (see Fig. 43–3B). In the event of upper tract fistula, however, the kidney may not be visualized on the involved side. Otherwise, hydronephrosis and hydroureter are seen. Likewise, although the fistula is not seen on the cystogram, a mass effect may be seen at areas of inflammation or tumor involvement. Retrograde ureterography is the examination most likely to demonstrate upper tract fistulas, whereas cystoscopy is the most useful examination in the evaluation of colovesical fistula. Cystitis, either diffuse or localized to the area of the fistula, is found in most patients. Tumor involvement of the bladder may be proved by biopsy. Fecal matter, pus, or air may be seen passing through the fistula or, in the case of upper tract fistula, from the ureteral orifice.

Fistula between the colon and the vagina, cervix, uterus, or fallopian tubes also is not frequently demonstrated on barium enema or large bowel endoscopy. Colon disease may be defined, however. Pelvic examination may demonstrate feces passing into the vagina or through the cervical os, but this is unusual. Hysterography and salpingography may demonstrate uterine and tubal fistulas.

Colorespiratory fistulas are usually demonstrated by barium enema. Vascular fistulas from the colon usually are not diagnosed by arteriography, barium enema, or large bowel endoscopy. However, arteriography may visualize a contributing vascular malformation.

In some patients, the presence of an otherwise obscure fistula originating from the colon can be confirmed by having the patient ingest 2 ounces of powdered charcoal and examining the spun sediment of the urine or other drainage for the presence of the distinctive charcoal particles. Sometimes sufficient charcoal is passed through the fistula to color the urine or drainage gray or black.

Treatment and Prognosis. Before definitive treatment of any fistula is undertaken, metabolic complications must be corrected. Fluid and electrolyte deficits must be replaced and excessive losses controlled. Institution of complete bowel rest with nasogastric drainage and restriction of all oral intake may be necessary to control such losses. Nutritional requirements must be met to correct malnutrition and promote healing. For an external colon fistula, oral alimentation with low-residue nutritional supplements or an elemental diet is usually adequate. However, if the volume of fistula output is high (greater than 200 ml/day), if residue or digestive enzymes prevent healing, or if malnutrition is a sequela of an internal fistula, parenteral hyperalimentation should be used.

Failure to control sepsis is an ominous sign in patients with gastrointestinal fistula. The mortality rate with uncontrolled sepsis is 85 percent. Appropriate antibiotics must be administered, and drainage of any abscess along the fistula track must be performed. Diversion of enteric contents may be necessary to minimize drainage. Spontaneous closure of a colocutaneous fistula is expected in 30 to 70 percent of patients,[146] and recurrence is unusual after closure. When spontaneous closure is to occur, it does so within 1 month of the control of sepsis in 91 percent of patients. Spontaneous closure is rare after more than 8 weeks of supportive care.[146]

Persistence of a fistula is the result of one or a combination of these factors: large size, large volume of output, a rigid wall of the fistula track, presence of carcinoma, persistent foreign body, epithelialization of the track, obstruction distal to the fistula, and separation of the ends of the bowel. Persistent sepsis or infections such as tuberculosis, actinomycosis, and amebiasis also prevent spontaneous healing. Closure is relatively unlikely to occur when the fistula is secondary to diverticulitis, granulomatous colitis, and radiation colitis. Patients receiving steroids or chemotherapy heal poorly.

Unless drainage is minimal, or the patient is a poor operative risk, external fistulas that persist for more than 8 weeks should be treated by operation. The most efficient treatment is excision of the fistula and the involved colon segment with end-to-end anastomosis. Simple turn-in repair leads to frequent recurrence. It may be necessary to achieve fistula closure in stages.[146]

Unless pressed by sepsis or hemorrhage, an internal fistula can be treated by supportive measures until the patient is in optimum condition. Although operation may be necessary to treat sepsis, definitive repair of an internal fistula should not be attempted in the presence of uncontrolled infection.

Gastrocolic or gastrojejunocolic fistula is tolerated poorly if untreated. Resection of the fistula and the involved stomach and bowel with primary anastomoses is recommended. When the fistula is due to recurrent peptic ulcer disease, the cause of recurrence also must be treated.

Duodenocolic fistula is lethal if not closed. The diseased colon, the fistula, and the involved portion of duodenum should be excised.[146,153] Duodenal closure may be a problem. Management options include primary transverse closure, reinforcement of the closure with an omental patch or a jejunal serosal patch, anastomosis of the duodenal opening to either a loop or a Roux-en-Y limb of jejunum, or pancreaticoduodenectomy. Korelitz[152] suggests that duodenocolic fistula caused by Crohn's disease may be managed with a bypassing ileocolostomy or a diverting ileostomy with success equal to that of resection. It has been suggested that surgical correction of duodenocolic fistula secondary to Crohn's disease be dictated by the severity of the disease; the mere presence of the fistula should not be a primary indication for operation.[154–158] The implication is that the symptoms are more related to the activity of the Crohn's disease than to the fistula.

When the lesion is resectable for cure, malignant duodenocolic fistula usually requires an extensive en bloc resection, often a colectomy and pancreatoduodenectomy. If the patient is not curable, a double bypass (gastrojejunostomy and ileocolostomy) provides the best palliation.[146,159]

Colointestinal and colocolic fistulas are treated by en bloc resection of the involved bowel and any focus of sepsis. The 5-year survival of colon cancer patients with a fistula to small bowel is 43 percent.[146]

Elective operative treatment of cholecystocolonic fistula consists of cholecystectomy and closure or resection of the colon. Common duct exploration is performed if indicated. When the procedure is performed in an acute situation, the colon opening may be exteriorized as a colostomy to be closed secondarily. If gallstone ileus has occurred, one should try to milk the stone into the rectum for removal by proctoscopy. If this is unsuccessful, the stone may be removed through a colotomy that is closed primarily, and protected by a proximal colostomy. Opinion is divided as to whether cholecystectomy should be performed at the same operation.[146,147] Patients who are poor operative risks, who have no complications, and who have no bile duct obstruction may be managed nonoperatively if carcinoma can be excluded.

Pancreatic fistula to the colon requires individualized management. The overall mortality is 33 percent, mostly due to sepsis and hemorrhage. When the fistula is secondary to a pancreatic abscess, radical debridement of the pancreas and wide drainage of the pancreatic bed and retrocolic area are necessary procedures. In addition, the splenic flexure and left colon should be mobilized to ensure complete drainage. Repair of the opening in the colon and proximal colostomy may suffice; however, resection of the involved colon segment with colostomy and mucous fistula are necessary in many cases[146,149] (see Chap. 41).

When a pseudocyst ruptures into the colon, spontaneous closure of the cysts and fistula is common; therefore proximal colostomy alone is recommended in most instances. If the fistula persists after 3 to 6 months of decompression, colon resection is necessary. Hemorrhage from such a fistula carries a mortality risk of 50 percent.

Renocolic and ureterocolic fistulas usually require nephrectomy and ureterectomy with resection of the colon. Occasionally, the involved segment of the ureter may be excised and the remainder repaired. Nephrostomy drainage of the kidney may permit preservation of that kidney if any function persists.[146]

Definitive treatment of vesicocolic fistula requires resection of the diseased colon segment and the fistula. If the fistula opening through the bladder wall is tiny or inapparent, it may be closed by suture and the bladder drained via a Foley catheter for 2 weeks. If the fistula is larger, or the bladder wall is scarred, then at least a small segment of involved bladder should be resected and the defect closed by suture, providing Foley catheter drainage.

The complete procedure may require one or more stages, depending on the presence of pelvic sepsis, bowel obstruction, inflamed bowel, and apposition of suture lines. When malignancy is the underlying problem, curative resection should be performed whenever possible. The 5-year survival is dependent on lymph node, rather than local, extension. In cases with massive tumor or involvement of the trigone, this may require pelvic exenteration with end colostomy and ileal conduit urinary diversion. If the disease is unresectable, diverting colostomy is indicated.[69]

Treatment of fistula to the female reproductive organs involves resection of the involved colon segment and the cervix, uterus, or tube, as required. If recurrent carcinoma of the cervix is the cause of the fistula, pelvic exenteration is indicated if technically feasible and if there is no distant spread of tumor.[146]

After abscesses and other septic foci have been drained and controlled, respiratory fistulas are treated by resection of involved colon and irreversibly damaged pulmonary tissue. Vascular fistulas require resection of aneurysms and involved grafts with closure of the colon. Extra-anatomic vascular reconstruction is the best method to avoid subsequent graft sepsis (see Chap. 37).

BACTERIAL ENTEROCOLITIS WITH SURGICAL MANIFESTATIONS

Many bacterial diarrheas are caused by the effects of enterotoxins; diarrhea and dehydration are the usual complications of bacterial enterocolitis (see Chap. 42). When the causative organism is capable of invading the bowel wall, however, surgical complications such as hemorrhage or perforation may occur. Such complications have been documented with *Shigella,*[160] *Salmonella,*[161] and *Yersinia*[162] infections. When perforation occurs, the resulting infection is caused by mixed fecal flora, in addition to the enteric invader. All three diseases are caused by ingestion of contaminated human fecal matter. Yersinosis has been documented in humans only in the past 20 years. Most cases have been reported in Western Europe and in North America, in colder rather than warmer climates. Cases appear in clusters.[162] Many animals and birds probably serve as reservoirs for the organism. The etiologic agents of these diseases are discussed in Chapters 4, 5, and 42.

Etiology and Pathogenesis. Shigella species causing human disease include *S. dysenteriae, S. flexneri, S. boydii,* and *S. sonnei.* All these organisms cause infection by penetrating the mucosa of the terminal ileum and colon. Their endotoxins and exotoxins result in superficial inflammation, coagulation necrosis, pseudomembrane formation, and ulceration. The ulcers may be deep, producing severe hemorrhage or perforation. Healing may be complete or may occur with stricture formation. Gram-negative bacilli are usually present on microscopic examination of affected bowel.

Salmonella gastroenteritis results from infection with *S. typhimurium, S. enteritidis,* and *S. choleraesuis.* Typhoid fever is caused by *S. typhi* and *S. paratyphi* A, B, and C. These organisms infect by penetrating the mucosa of the small bowel and invading lymphoid tissues. They gain access to the bloodstream by way of the lymphatics and are taken up by reticuloendothelial cells where they proliferate. A second period of bacteremia occurs, and the bowel may be reinfected by the bloodstream or by infected bile.

Reinfection in typhoid infections occurs in the bowel lymphoid tissues, especially the Peyer's patches of the distal ileum. Hyperemia, hyperplasia, and mononuclear cell proliferation occur. As the lymphoid aggregates undergo necrosis, ulcers develop in the distal small bowel and ascending colon, which may bleed or perforate. In the fourth week of infection, healing occurs with little or no scar formation. Bacteremia also produces metastatic infection resulting in lymphadenitis, splenomegaly, cholecystitis, pneumonitis, pyelonephritis, meningitis, osteomyelitis, thrombophlebitis, and soft tissue abscess.

Yersinia enterocolitica is responsible for yersinosis. The pathogenesis of yersinosis is similar to that of typhoid, with an initial enteritis and subsequent involvement of bowel and mesenteric lymphoid tissues. Bacteremia has occasionally been lethal. In addition, erythema nodosum and arthritis, apparently secondary to immune complex deposition, may occur.

Clinical Manifestations. The typical incubation period of shigellosis is 2 or 3 days (range, 12 hours to 7 days). In severe acute diseases, the onset of fever (38C to 40C), headache, and malaise is abrupt. Abdominal cramps, vomiting, diarrhea, and severe tenesmus occur, and stool is converted to bloody mucus. Physical examination reveals abdominal guarding and tenderness, especially overlying the colon; peristalsis is hyperactive. Toxemia, dehydration, perforation, or bleeding may cause death. The disease lasts several days. Chronic disease with occasional episodes of diarrhea, flatulence, or rectal bleeding may occur. Asymptomatic patients may be carriers.

The incubation period of *Salmonella* gastroenteritis is short, usually less than 24 hours. Fever, nausea, vomiting, and diarrhea develop suddenly. The temperature usually ranges from 37.5C to 38.5C. The watery stools may contain blood or mucus. Colicky abdominal pain is common. The duration and severity of the disease vary, but surgical complications almost never occur.

The onset of typhoid fever is insidious. The patient may give a history of a mild, nonspecific respiratory infection or enteritis. Typhoid begins with malaise, headache, and myalgia, and arthralgia, bronchitis, epistaxis, lethargy, anorexia, flatulence, and constipation often follow. During the first week, the temperature rises gradually. Fever is high and continuous during the second and third weeks and falls by lysis in the fourth week. Apathy, toxemia delirium, and the typhoid rash (rose spots) accompany the high fever. Most surgical complications occur after the second week. Toxic dilation of the colon in a typhoid patient has been reported. Death may result from septicemia, dehydration, or perforation and peritonitis (see Chap. 42).

Yersinosis presents several clinical pictures. *Yersinia* gastroenteritis produces fever, headache, vomiting, diarrhea, and abdominal pain. Stools are usually watery and bilious. As many as one-third of patients have an exudative pharyngitis.[163] In terminal ileocolitis and mesenteric adenitis, pain is localized to the right lower quadrant. A tender mass may be palpable, and it may be impossible to exclude the presence of acute appendicitis. Polyarthritis and erythema nodosum may be the only signs of disease. Rarely, especially in immunocompromised hosts, hepatosplenic abscess and septicemia occur. In addition to pseudoappendicitis, surgical complications include hemorrhage from ileo-ascending colon ulcer,[162] bowel obstruction secondary to adhesions to inflamed lymph nodes, and pseudocholecystitis. The duration of yersinosis is variable but is in the range of weeks.

Diagnosis. In bacterial enterocolitis, radiologic examinations demonstrate nonspecific changes and are of no help in establishing a diagnosis. If a question of perforation exists, abdominal films are helpful. The rare toxic dilation of the colon also is demonstrated on plain films. If blood is lost, hematologic analysis reveals anemia in all these diseases; on the contrary, dehydration produces an apparent erythrocytosis. The leukocyte count may or may not be elevated; regardless, a left shift in the differential count is typical.

Serologic tests may be useful in the diagnosis of *Salmonella* and, to a lesser extent, *Yersinia* infections. For the tests to be meaningful, high titers of agglutinating antibody must be observed in repeated samples, and comparison with antibody levels in convalescent serum is worthwhile. In yersinosis, the numbers of serotypes and false positives and negatives are a problem.

With shigellosis, proctoscopy may show red, edematous mucosa that subsequently develops dirty gray ulcers. Patches of granulation tissue may be present in patients with chronic disease. Proctoscopy is unlikely to reveal changes in salmonellosis and yersinosis because right colon involvement is most common.

Microscopic analysis of stool may be helpful. Leukocytes are present in the stained specimen in 69 percent of shigellosis patients. A positive stool analysis correlates with positive stool cultures and invasive disease. Only one-third of patients with salmonellosis have fecal leukocytosis; yersinosis may produce similar findings.

Isolation of the organism on culture of a stool specimen is the surest way to establish the diagnosis. Blood cultures are useful in yersinosis and in typhoid and paratyphoid fever. When a normal appendix is found at appendectomy, culture of mesenteric nodes may be productive if the patient has yersinosis. The microbiology laboratory must be alerted if *Yersinia* is suspected, because special culture methods are necessary to isolate these organisms.

Treatment. Because all three diseases are self-limiting, the essential task in treating bacterial enteritis is appropriate fluid and electrolyte support to prevent anemia, dehydration, and their complications.

It is often difficult to detect any effect of antibiotic treatment on the course of the disease. Presently, specific antibiotic treatment is indicated in the following situations: (1) severe disease, (2) septicemia, (3) disease in children and the elderly, (4) disease in an immunocompromised patient, and (5) surgical complications, in which case antibiotics active against the broad spectrum of fecal organisms should be selected.

If antibiotics are to be used, the choice should be dictated by in vitro sensitivity determinations, because drug resistance is a growing problem. Shigellosis usually responds to ampicillin, the sulfas, and tetracycline; trimethoprim-sulfamethoxazole is highly successful against organisms resistant to ampicillin.[163] Although bacteriologic cure usually is achieved in 7 days, antibiotic treatment may prolong the carrier state.

Antibiotic treatment does not alter the duration of diarrhea or the carrier state in *Salmonella* enteritis. Treatment does decrease the degree of toxemia and prostration in septicemia and typhoid fever. Several weeks of treatment are required. Ampicillin, chloramphenicol, and the tetracyclines are the first-line drugs. Trimethoprim-sulfamethoxazole is effective against resistant *Salmonella* as well.

Except for septicemia, the course of yersinosis is not altered by antibiotic therapy. The antibiotics showing most effect against *Yersinia* are tetracycline, chloramphenicol, and the aminoglycosides; ampicillin, trimethoprim-sulfamethoxazole, and cephalosporins are less effective.

Hemorrhage is treated as is lower gastrointestinal bleeding from any other cause. Intra-arterial vasopressor infusion and resection of the involved ileum and colon have been successful. Kim et al[161] reported their experience in treating typhoid perforations of the ileum. Most patients were treated successfully by simple closure of the perforation; resection with anastomosis and bypass with ileostomy or ileotransverse colostomy also gave good results. Drainage alone is less successful, with a mortality rate of 10 to 32 percent. Most patients with toxic dilation of the colon respond well to nonoperative therapy.

Prognosis. Most patients who are supported adequately recover from *Shigella, Salmonella,* and *Yersinia* infections. Prompt treatment of complications also yields successful results. Repeated stool cultures are necessary until two to four successive test results, over a 3-week period, are negative. To prevent spread of the disease, fecal isolation precautions must be followed until the carrier state is cleared. Food handlers, especially, must not return to work until their stool results are negative.

PSEUDOMEMBRANOUS AND ANTIBIOTIC-ASSOCIATED COLITIS

Antibiotic-associated colitis is an inflammatory disease of the colon that usually occurs secondary to antibiotic use. Anatomically, the mucosal changes may range from mild inflammation to severe pseudomembranous colitis. The enteric pathogen, *Clostridium difficile,* is now recognized as the most important cause of antibiotic-associated colitis with or without pseudomembrane formation.[164,165] Other bacteria, such as *Staphylococcus aureus,* which are capable of secreting an epidermolytic exotoxin, also may cause antibiotic-associated colitis.

Epidemiology. With the recognition of *C. difficile* as the putative agent in the majority of cases of antibiotic-associated colitis, attention is usually directed toward the identification of this pathogen in patients who develop diarrhea in association with antibiotic use. Though antibiotic-associated colitis may occur with any antibiotic agent,[164] the most commonly implicated drugs are clindamycin and the beta-lactam antibiotics. On the basis of relative use, the risk of developing antibiotic-associated colitis appears to be higher with clindamycin and cephalosporins than with ampicillin.[166] The incidence of antibiotic-associated colitis does not always appear to be related to the dose or the duration of therapy. The inflammatory process develops secondary to changes in the microecologic system of the colon induced by antibiotic suppression of the normal flora, thereby facilitating growth of toxin-producing *C. difficile.* The major virulent factors produced by *C. difficile* are toxins A and B. Toxin A is an entotoxin and cytotoxin and toxin B is a potent cytotoxin. Toxin B seems not to cause disease by itself but in synergy with toxin A.[167] Superinfection due to organisms resistant to the responsible antibiotic is not considered a part of the pathogenic process.[164,165,168]

In patients with antibiotic-associated diarrhea without colitis, only about 20 percent will have a positive stool culture for *C. difficile;* in those with colitis, about 60 percent will have positive cultures and in patients with antibiotic-associated pseudomembranous colitis, about 95 percent will have positive stool cultures.[164,169] Asymptomatic carriers of *C. difficile* have been identified. In healthy infants and children up to only 1 year of age, up to 40 percent may have positive stool cultures for the organism itself.[164,165,170,171] Additionally, approximately 3 percent of healthy adults have positive stool cultures.[164,169]

Although *C. difficile* infections occur primarily endogenously in association with antibiotic use, there are reports that indicate occurrence of colitis as a result of environmental contamination.[172,173] Finally, Aronsson et al[166] reported that considering the population at risk for *C. difficile* colitis, the observed incidence is highest in patients over 60 years of age. It is now recognized as the major cause of nosocomial diarrhea causing 95 to 97 percent of cases of infectious nosocomial diarrhea in hospitalized patients.[174]

Pathogenesis. Clostridium difficile, a gram-positive anaerobic bacillus, is the pathogen currently primarily responsible for almost all cases of antibiotic-associated pseudomembranous colitis and most cases of antibiotic-associated colitis.[164] Though this relationship is now well established, pseudomembranous colitis was described long before antibiotics were available. The cases reported usually were complications of intestinal surgery, colon carcinoma, intestinal obstruction, heavy metal poisoning, and the hemolytic-uremic syndrome.[164,175]

During the early antibiotic era (1950s and 1960s), antibiotic-associated colitis and pseudomembranous colitis were seen after the use of the broad spectrum antimicrobials, chloramphenicol, and tetracycline.[164] Laboratory and clinical investigations at that time, consisting of stool cultures and Gram stain, suggested *S. aureus* as the pathogen.[164,176] However, review of the early data and recent investigations[175,177,178] of antibiotic-associated colitis fail to support a current role for *S. aureus* in the etiology of this disease process.

During the 1970s, there were numerous reports of pseudomembranous colitis associated with use of clindamycin and lincomycin. The report by Tedesco et al[179] was the most provocative; the authors documented an overall incidence of clindamycin-associated pseudomembranous colitis of 10 percent in treated patients who developed diarrhea. Laboratory studies conducted by Bartlett et al[180,181] and by Fekety's group[173] led to identification of *C. difficile* and its toxin, and clinical studies of stool cultures from patients[182] confirmed the role of *C. difficile.*

Clinical Manifestations. The clinical findings in patients with antibiotic-associated pseudomembranous colitis are variable.[164,168] Diarrhea is the cardinal symptom and is found in most patients. Onset may occur soon after initiation of antibiotic therapy, usually within 5 to 7 days, or may be delayed, occurring up to 4 weeks after discontinuation of antibiotic therapy. Stools may be of large volume and may number up to 30 per day. They may be watery or mucoid; gross blood is unusual but occasionally may be seen. Commonly associated findings[164] are crampy abdominal pain, which may be an initial symptom; abdominal tenderness; fever, with an average peak of 101F; and leukocytosis averaging 15,000/ml. In severe cases, patients may develop dehydration and electrolyte imbalance, hypoalbuminemia, toxic megacolon, or colon perforation. Because of the wide spectrum of symptoms with this disease, ranging from nuisance diarrhea to acute fulminant disease suggesting an intra-abdominal catastrophe, patients should be carefully evaluated to avoid an unnecessary operation.

Diagnosis. The most useful diagnostic measures are sigmoidoscopy or colonoscopy and tissue culture cytotoxicity assays.[183] The endoscopic changes vary from mild mucosal erythema and edema to the classic lesions of pseudomembrane formation. These are yellow-white plaques adherent to the mucosa. If a large amount of mucus is present, it must be removed carefully. Biopsies may be taken if there is a question about the diagnosis. Though usually not necessary to establish the diagnosis, barium enema, preferably a double-contrast study, may be performed. Tissue culture assay for *C. difficile* toxin done on a stool specimen is the preferred method for diagnosis of *C. difficile*-induced colitis. Diagnosis is also made by direct detection of toxin B by the cell culture assay. Overall sensitivity is 67 to 78 percent and specificity is 95 to 99 percent.

Treatment. The treatment of a patient with antibiotic-associated colitis depends on the severity of disease. Discontinuation of the implicated antibiotic is the most important therapeutic maneuver. In case of a source of infection requiring continuing treatment, the antibiotic should be changed. An agent with a lower risk for antibiotic-associated colitis should be preferred. Most patients will respond to discontinuation of the antibiotic with resolution of colitis over a few days. Patients with diarrhea causing moderate to severe dehydration, electrolyte imbalance, or hypoalbuminemia require supportive fluid and electrolyte replacement. Such patients may not have noticeable diarrhea when they are most sick, the diarrhea having been transient or masked by other illness. Immunosuppressed transplant patients or patients in intensive care units are most at risk for progressive fulminant disease without diarrhea. Total parenteral nutrition may be necessary in patients who respond poorly to simpler therapy or who have other debilitating diseases. Diphenoxylate or other antiperistaltic agents should not be used.

Specific agents for antibiotic-induced colitis caused by *C. difficile* are vancomycin, metronidazole, bacitracin, or cholestyramine, all given orally. Vancomycin is most widely used and has the best track record. Bartlett[164] reviewed his experience with 189 patients, reporting a 97 percent favorable response rate. The drug is preferably given orally, 125 to 500 mg, four times daily for 7 to 14 days. Oral vancomycin is poorly absorbed but attains concentrations in the colon lumen to which *C. difficile* is highly susceptible.[164,184] Systemic toxicity has not been reported after oral administration of vancomycin. In spite of good results with vancomycin, relapses after discontinuation of therapy have been reported.[164,185] Metronidazole is a satisfactory alternative to vancomycin. Comparable results were obtained in a prospective, randomized trial of the two drugs.[186] The suggested regimen is 250 mg orally, three times daily for 7 to 14 days. Overall, there is a 10 to 20 percent relapse rate with either agent. Experience with bacitracin is limited, though published reports indicate results comparable to vancomycin.[164] Response rates with cholestyramine are inferior compared to those achieved with specific antibiotics.[164]

Prognosis. In the past, the mortality rate in patients with pseudomembranous colitis was high (50 to 75 percent); even reports from the 1970s document mortality rates up to 25 percent. Tedesco[168] has shown that mortality should approach zero with early diagnosis and cessation of antibiotic treatment. The disease may persist for as long as 4 to 8 weeks, but once it has subsided, the colon returns to normal. There may be an increased tendency to redevelop colitis after subsequent antibiotic treatment.

Patients with fulminant disease are now observed primarily among those who have severe underlying conditions, that is, those whose nosocomial disease was acquired in intensive care units. Such patients respond slowly to oral medications. Parenteral metronidazole has been used with some success. Subtotal colectomy has been found to be successful in toxic, unresponsive patients.[187]

PNEUMATOSIS COLI

Pneumatosis coli is a manifestation of many diseases rather than a disease itself. Table 43–4 lists conditions in which it has been described. Although pneumatosis may be associated with severe disease, it is more often a benign condition requiring no surgical treatment.

The gross appearance is that of multiple spherical and oblong cysts visible in the subserosa or submucosa of the small intestine or the colon. The overlying mucosa may be normal or hemorrhagic. Histologically, the cysts are located in the subserosa, the submucosa, and occasionally the muscularis. There is no active inflammatory response, but multinucleated giant cells are often seen around the cysts. Bacteria are not seen.

In 85 percent of patients, pneumatosis intestinalis is associated with other pathologic conditions. Pneumatosis of the distal colon is more likely to occur in patients with no apparent underlying condition, whereas pneumatosis of the right colon usually is associated with small intestinal disease.

Presently, two hypotheses attempt to explain pneumatosis coli. Most widely accepted is the *mechanical* theory, which suggests that gas reaches the subserosa and submucosa in one of two ways: (1) intraluminal gas enters via a mucosal defect or (2) air from ruptured pulmonary alveoli dissects down the mediastinum into the retroperitoneum and mesentery and along mesenteric vessels. A large number of patients with chronic lung disease have asymptomatic pneumatosis; the blebs contain mostly nitrogen and oxygen.

TABLE 43–4. CONDITIONS ASSOCIATED WITH PNEUMATOSIS COLI INTESTINALIS

Bowel ischemia
  1. Circulatory
    a. Hypoperfusion
    b. Mesenteric vascular occlusion
  2. Simple bowel obstruction (any cause)
  3. Mechanical strangulation
    a. Volvulus
    b. Internal hernia
    c. Intussusception

Inflammatory
  1. Neonatal necrotizing enterocolitis
  2. Septic enterocolitis
  3. Pseudomembranous enterocolitis
  4. Toxic megacolon
  5. Crohn's disease
  6. Inflammatory diarrhea of childhood

Pulmonary
  1. Obstructive lung disease
  2. Pneumothorax
  3. Interstitial emphysema
  4. Pneumomediastinum

Iatrogenic
  1. Endoscopy
  2. Umbilical vein catheter
  3. Hydrogen peroxide enemas

Miscellaneous
  1. Autoimmune diseases (especially scleroderma)
  2. Whipple disease
  3. Leukemia
  4. Sprue
  5. Peptic ulcer
  6. Diverticulitis
  7. Caustic injury
  8. Trauma
  9. Intestinal parasites

The other prevalent theory is that *gas-producing bacteria* gain access to the submucosa and cause cyst formation. This theory has not been accepted widely because, in adults, bacteria are neither seen around nor cultured from the cysts. However, cyst cultures are positive in infants with necrotizing enterocolitis. Moreover, Yale and Balish[188] have reproduced pneumatosis in germ-free laboratory animals after monocontamination of the gut with *C. perfringens* and *C. tertium*.

The clinical features of the underlying disease predominate[189]; patients with associated bowel disease usually are seriously ill. In asymptomatic patients, the discovery of pneumatosis on chest or abdominal x-rays is fortuitous. Pneumoperitoneum occurring in a patient without symptoms of abdominal disease suggests pneumatosis. Most asymptomatic patients have underlying respiratory disorders.

Usually, the diagnosis may be made on plain abdominal films. The cysts are apparent as collections of air along the bowel (Fig. 43–11). Air may be located within the mesentery and may become confined under the diaphragm, regardless of the patient's position. Gastrointestinal contrast studies usually make visualization of the cysts easier. The appearance is that of polypoid or tumor-like radiolucent masses on the margin of the contrast column (Fig. 43–12).

Treatment of underlying disease usually suffices to control secondary pneumatosis coli. It is unnecessary to treat asymptomatic pneumatosis; if symptoms are present, oxygen therapy has been successful.

TUBERCULOSIS OF THE LARGE BOWEL

Primary tuberculous enteritis is rare in countries in which pasteurization of milk is practiced, but recent reports continue to document sporadic cases of secondary infection confined to the abdomen.[190] In the prechemotherapy era, such secondary bowel involvement was common, especially in patients with advanced pulmonary disease. Tuberculous enterocolitis is a disease of young adults (third decade) and is more frequent in women.[191]

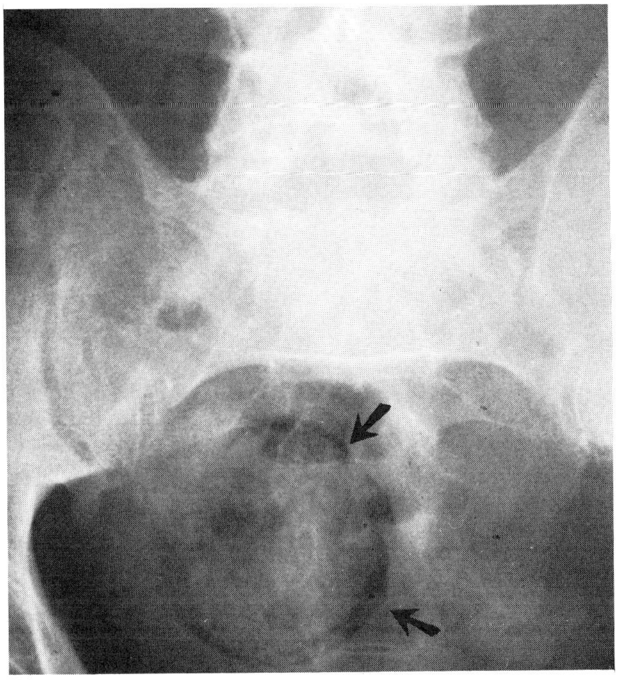

Figure 43–11. Pneumatosis coli indicative of infection. Plain abdominal film of a patient with peritonitis following a cardiac bypass procedure demonstrates intramural collections of air in an infarcted cecum (arrows).

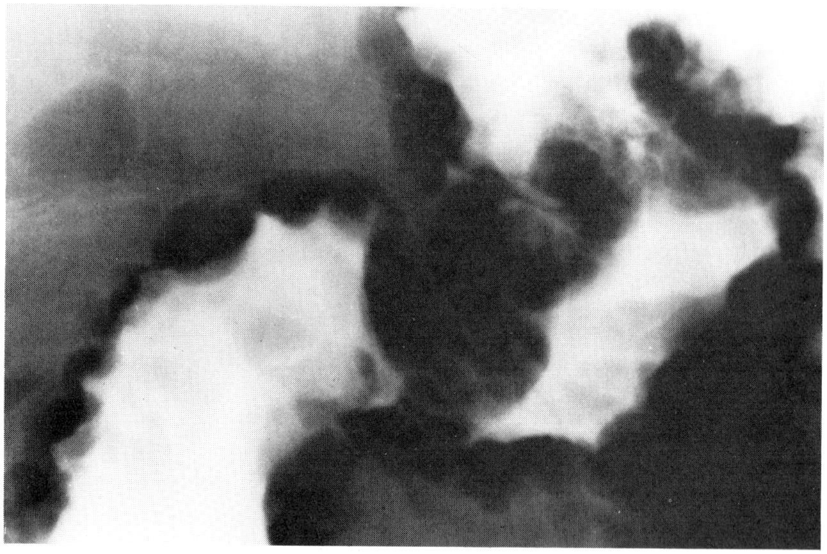

Figure 43–12. Pneumatosis coli—benign form. Barium enema of an asymptomatic patient demonstrates lucent masses surrounding the barium column.

Pathogenesis. Intestinal tuberculosis can be caused by drinking milk contaminated with the bovine strain, but most recent cases have been caused by human strains. The organisms are swallowed in infected sputum. Intestinal involvement may also result from hematogenous spread and, perhaps, direct spread from contiguous involved organs.[191] The most frequently involved segments of bowel are the ileocecal region, the ileum, and the colon, in that order,[192] although Paustian and Monto[191] indicate that disease of the ileum is now being reported more frequently. Anorectal disease, especially fistula, occurs and is discussed in Chapter 45. The frequency of ileocecal involvement seems to be accounted for by the relative stasis of feces in this region, the abundance of lymphoid tissue, and the more digested state of the bowel content (Fig. 43–13).

Infection begins in the depths of the mucosal crypts. After invasion, phagocytes ingest and transport the bacteria to the submucosa, where lymphoid tissues become infected. Marked submucosal thickening occurs with edema, cellular infiltration, lymphoid hyperplasia, and tubercle formation. If the mucosal blood supply is impaired, ulceration occurs. As the process continues, mesenteric lymph nodes become involved. Eventually, the process becomes transmural. Free perforation is unusual because surrounding tissues adhere to the bowel before perforation occurs. Healing of ulcers may be complicated by stricture formation.

Gross examination reveals inflamed bowel and edema of the mesentery and involved lymph nodes. Tubercles are often visible on the serosal surface. Ulcers are oriented in the transverse axis of the bowel and may become circumferential; the resulting strictures occupy only short segments of bowel. Histologic analysis reveals a submucosal chronic inflammatory process with tubercles featuring epitheloid cells, giant cells, and central caseation necrosis. Fibrosis and hyalinization frequently surround the inflamed areas. Myobacteria may be seen with an acid-fast stain.

Clinical Manifestations. The clinical features of tuberculous enteritis, especially when involving the ileocecal region and the colon, have been discussed in several articles.[190,191,193] Currently, the most common surgical complications are obstruction and the presence of a mass that cannot be differentiated from carcinoma; bleeding, fistula formation, and perforation occur infrequently.

The symptoms and signs are those of chronic partial small bowel obstruction: colicky pain, distention, increased peristaltic activity, and right lower quadrant tenderness. Abdominal physical findings are those of small bowel obstruction. A palpable mass is present in up to two-thirds of patients.

Diagnosis. A positive skin test in a patient with abdominal symptoms is supportive, but not diagnostic, evidence of enteric tuberculosis; conversely, a negative result, especially in a chronically or critically ill patient, does not rule out the possibility.

X-ray signs on barium enema and small bowel follow-through examinations provide strong presumptive evidence of tuberculosis enterocolitis, especially if the findings regress on appropriate antitubercular treatment. The following findings suggest tuberculous bowel disease: (1) motility disturbances such as reduced transit time, hypersegmentation, stiffening, and thickening of mucosal folds; (2) lack of barium retention in the involved segment; (3) a short, persistently narrowed stream of barium in a small bowel segment; (4) delay of transit and dilation of short segments of small bowel; and (5) cecal and colonic filling defects, with shortening of the ascending colon, cecal distortion, and gaping of the ileocecal valve.[191]

The only way to establish a definite diagnosis is by culture and histologic analysis of resected tissue. Preoperative chemotherapy may cause difficulty in confirming the diagnosis of tuberculosis enterocolitis. The recovery of acid-fast bacilli from sputum or other sources is diagnostic of tuberculosis but is only strongly suggestive of bowel disease. After bacilli are swallowed, they may be recovered from feces and fistula drainage in the absence of enteric infection.

Treatment. In active disease, antibiotic treatment is initiated with two or three drugs to which the organisms are sensitive (see Chap. 28). The drugs presently used most frequently are isoniazid, pyrazinamide, and rifampin. Treatment is continued for at least 2 years. Antibiotic therapy of intestinal disease usually is effective within 1 or 2 weeks in relieving symptoms. Jordan and DeBakey[192] report perforation occurring in three patients with abnormal bowel involvement after antibiotic therapy.

Operation is indicated to treat complications (obstruction, perforation with abscess or peritonitis, fistula, hemorrhage), to rule out carcinoma of the colon, and to remove disease that does not respond to systemic antimicrobial treatment. Because the diagnosis frequently is unclear, right hemicolectomy and resection of involved ileum are usually indicated.[193] Patients with tuberculosis and coexisting cecal carcinoma have been reported.

Free perforation usually occurs in the terminal ileum. Formerly, simple closure with drainage was performed; the mortality rate with this procedure

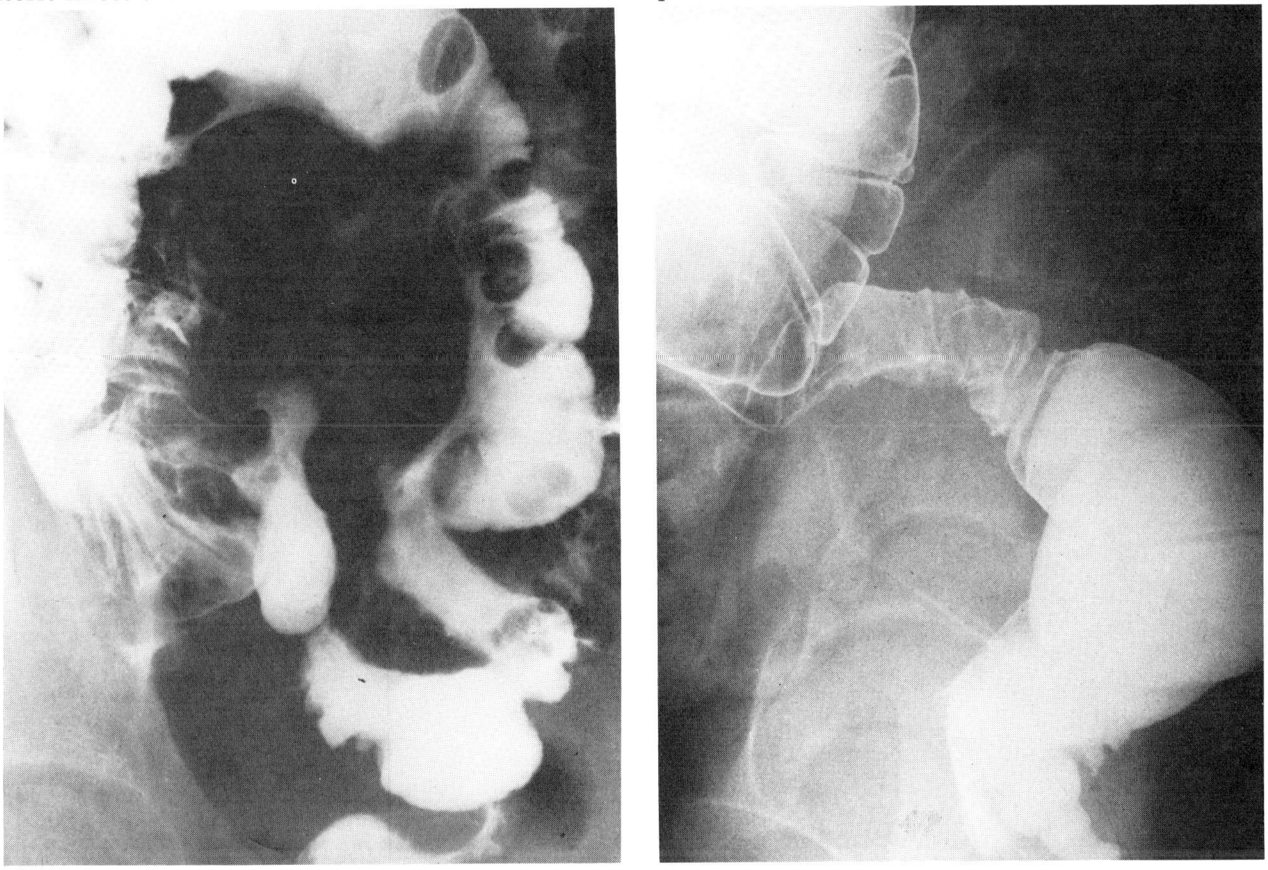

A B

Figure 43–13. A. Tuberculosis. Barium enema with reflux into the terminal ileum demonstrates cecal distortion and filling defects, ileal narrowing with intervening dilated segments, and ileal inflammatory masses. **B.** Lateral rectal film demonstrates involvement of the first sacral vertebra and persistent narrowing of adjacent rectum.

was 50 percent. Resection of the perforated segment is now recommended by most surgeons. However, Porter et al[194] report a patient treated by drainage alone; a second stage became unnecessary when resulting fistula healed with chemotherapy and nutritional support. Katariya et al[195] suggest that resection of all small bowel containing strictures is not necessary. They prefer to incise the bowel longitudinally through short strictures, closing the incision transversely. They reserve resection for segments with numerous strictures.

Adams and Miller[193] stressed the danger of operating on patients with uncontrolled pulmonary disease. Two principles of surgical treatment of enteric tuberculosis continue to apply. First, administer antibiotics for at least 2 weeks before performing elective surgery in patients with known disease in the lung or the bowel. Second, it is unwise to attempt primary anastomosis in diseased bowel because of the dangers of anastomotic leak and fistula formation.

ACTINOMYCOSIS OF THE LARGE BOWEL

Abdominal actinomycosis is an uncommon disease and the diagnosis is usually delayed. Because medical treatment is curative in the early stages of the disease, surgeons should beware. The etiology and pathogenesis of abdominal actinomycosis are discussed in Chapters 6 and 38. Most cases of abdominal actinomycosis occur in young adults, although patients at all ages are affected. There is no predilection for either sex.[196,197]

Actinomyces israelii is the species most often isolated from all forms of human disease. Most, if not all, infections occur after a break in the gut mucosa. Of 192 cases of abdominal actinomycosis,[197] 61 percent resulted from appendiceal perforation; large bowel perforation was associated in 14 percent. Infection due to perforating foreign bodies is frequent. The organism itself does not seem to be invasive. Actinomycotic infection in the abdomen never occurs without involvement of other enteric bacteria. Microscopically, an actinomycotic abscess consists of an outer zone of granulation tissue surrounding a central purulent loculation containing *sulfur granules* made up of numerous gram-positive bacilli. Necrosis in the abscess is unusual. The early actinomycotic abscess in the bowel wall spreads by direct extension and rarely disseminates. Eventually, multiple fistulas characterized by discharge of pus and sulfur granules develop.

Clinical Manifestations. Abdominal actinomycosis develops gradually; occasionally, the precipitating event goes unrecognized.[196] The initial symptoms are nonspecific: malaise, night sweats, and fever. Abdominal pain suggests the source, and a mass may be noted. Frequently, one or more fistula tracks discharge onto the abdominal wall or the perineum. Physical findings include abdominal tenderness, a palpable mass, and the fistulas. The diagnosis is rarely suspected so there usually is a history of multiple failed previous treatments. Rarely, proctoscopy, barium enema, or intravenous pyelography may show evidence of a mass lesion. The differential diagnosis includes carcinoma, Crohn's disease, and other granulomatous infections such as tuberculosis and nocardiosis.

Diagnosis. Cultures from the fistula may yield only enteric organisms. Special attention must be paid to collection of material from deep within the fistula and to proper anaerobic methodology to successfully grow *Actinomyces.* The finding of sulfur granules may lead to the diagnosis. Histologic confirmation of actinomycotic granulomas in resected tissue also is diagnostic.

Treatment. Successful treatment of the later stages of actinomycosis requires an appropriate combination of surgical and antibiotic therapy. Surgical measures may include only incision and drainage of abscesses and fistulas or resection of all affected tissues. Penicillin G is administered in large doses for weeks to months. Alternative antibiotics include erythromycin, the tetracyclines, and clindamycin.[196] With antibiotics, the cure rate exceeds 90 percent,[196] and major operations are rarely indicated.

VIRAL INFECTIONS OF THE COLON

The only viral infections presently known to be of surgical significance cause ulcers that bleed or perforate.[198] Although viruses have been implicated in the development of regional enteritis and ulcerative colitis, an etiologic association has not been established.

Epidemiology. Viral ulcers of the colon rarely are clinically apparent. The most prevalent viral lesion is sexually transmitted herpes simplex B infection of the anus and the rectum (see Chap. 45). Of greater surgical significance are colonic ulcers due to cytomegalovirus (CMV). Many people have had subclinical infections with these viruses and carry latent viral genetic material within body cells. Infections become apparent under conditions of stress or impaired host resistance when latent virus is reactivated. Immunosuppression in transplant patients is a frequent setting.

Etiology and Pathogenesis. The etiology of the herpesvirus infections, including CMV, is discussed in Chapter 11. Most evidence suggests that these viruses infect mucosal and endothelial cells and produce an ischemic vasculitis as part of the infection. Why the viruses become reactivated and produce clinical disease during stress, hyperthermia, neoplasm, and exposure to immunosuppressive and antineoplastic drugs is unknown. Why the colon and especially the cecum preferentially become infected is also unclear but may be related to local blood supply, colonic motility, or intraluminal bacteria. The viral ulcers become a surgical problem when perforation or hemorrhage occurs.[198]

Clinical Manifestations. The clinical features of CMV infection have been discussed in Chapters 9 and 51. Gastrointestinal bleeding from colon ulcers occurs and may be profuse. The diagnosis sometimes can be made by colonoscopy; angiography may be necessary if bleeding is profuse. Also, CMV infection may cause perforation of the colon requiring surgical intervention.

Diagnosis. The diagnosis depends on evidence of a fourfold rise in anti-CMV titer or cultural isolation of the virus from blood. Histologic study of the ulcer reveals inclusion bodies at the base of the ulcer.

Treatment. Both successful and unsuccessful outcomes have followed resection, which is associated with significant morbidity and mortality in the immunocompromised patient. There was no specific agent available to treat CMV infections. Ganciclovir has shown some efficacy.[199]

SURGICAL MANIFESTATIONS OF INFESTATION BY INTESTINAL PARASITES

Infestation with intestinal parasites is a problem of global significance because of population mobility. Colonic infestations of major significance include amebiasis and schistosomiasis. Selected aspects are discussed in Chapters 8 and 40.

Amebiasis

Epidemiology. The pathogenesis and epidemiology of amebiasis are discussed in Chapter 8. The disease is endemic in the Mississippi Valley and adjacent Gulf Coast. The infestation rate in the United States may be as high as 5 percent.[200,201]

Pathogenesis. Invasion by *Entamoeba histolytica* trophozoites occurs by release of lytic enzymes in contact with the intestinal mucosa. Survival of the trophozoite requires the anaerobic environment provided by the fecal flora. Trophozoites appear in the stool of patients with dysentery. Ingestion of trophozoites does not result in infestation because they are killed by gastric acid. Cysts, on the other hand, are found in the formed stool of asymptomatic carriers. Thus spread of disease is by the asymptomatic carrier rather than from the patient with dysentery.

Invasion results initially in formation of minute ulcers located in the center of a tiny nodule of edematous mucosa surrounded by an aggregation of chronic inflammatory cells. The process extends by undermining the mucosa, forming a flask-shaped abscess. If sufficient blood supply is compromised, ulcers enlarge. Occasionally, a proliferative granulomatous reaction occurs, forming an ameboma. The trophozoites are found at the junction of viable and necrotic tissue. Eventually, invasion of blood vessels allows dissemination of the trophozoites to other organs, particularly the liver.

Clinical Manifestations. Nondysenteric colitis is the most frequent manifestation of amebiasis. Symptoms include anorexia, malaise, weight loss, cramping abdominal pain, mild diarrhea, and constipation. Dysenteric colitis may occur at any time after infestation. Dysentery is more likely to occur if host defenses are impaired by concurrent disease or use of immunosuppressive drugs, including chronic use of alcohol. Onset of dysentery may be gradual or rapid. The predominant symptom is diarrhea associated with abdominal cramps and lower abdominal pain.

As many as 12 to 18 stools may be passed daily. The bowel movements are foul smelling, mushy or watery, and contain blood-streaked mucus. Dehydration is relatively uncommon, but severe weight loss, weakness, nausea, vomiting, and fever occur. Abdominal examination reveals hyperperistalsis and tenderness; the liver may be slightly enlarged and tender. Acute dysentery may last 1 to 4 weeks and often regresses without treatment. Recurrent episodes are typical.

Occasionally, localized amebiasis may occur in the rectum or the cecum. Rectal ulcers may be associated with passage of formed stools, but several discharges of bloody exudate are more typical. Cecal ulcers produce right lower quadrant pain and massive hemorrhage, but little or no diarrhea. An ameboma may produce symptoms, usually pain without diarrhea. A tumor mass may be noted, usually in the cecum or the rectosigmoid. Obstruction, intussusception, and volvulus may occur; carcinoma may be suggested. Extraintestinal manifestations often are noted. Foremost among these is amebic liver abscess, which may exist along with fulminant colitis.

Amebiasis becomes a surgical disease with the rare occurrence of fulminating necrotizing amebic colitis, frequently complicated by perforation and peritonitis. Toxic dilation of the colon may stimulate ulcerative colitis. Endoscopy reveals punctate ulcers and tiny nodules, with normal intervening mucosa. More advanced changes are indistinguishable from those of ulcerative colitis. A tumor mass representing an ameboma may be seen. Rectal biopsy usually reveals trophozoites. Barium enema is usually unable to distinguish amebiasis from ulcerative colitis. With localized disease, however, one may see a tumor mass or luminal narrowing; the cecum may fill incompletely (cone-shaped cecum). These changes disappear more or less completely after successful therapy.

Diagnosis. The diagnosis of colitis requires the finding of trophozoites on microscopic examination of fresh stool or colonic biopsy specimens, bloody mucus obtained at endoscopy, or, best of all, scrapings taken from the ulcers themselves. It is most important to realize that feces are rendered unsatisfactory for diagnostic purposes for as long as 2 weeks after a number of otherwise routine maneuvers, including administration of antidiarrheals containing bismuth or kaolin, nonabsorbable antacids, antimicrobials, barium, mineral oil, magnesium hydroxide, and enemas of tapwater, soap or hypertonic solutions. Thus examination of feces for trophozoites must be performed before any other therapeutic or diagnostic maneuver; initial endoscopy must be performed without preparation.

Even when other diagnostic maneuvers fail to demonstrate evidence of amebiasis, serologic tests are indicated to rule out the disease (see Table 8–1). The indirect hemagglutination test (IHA) is positive in 82 to 98 percent of patients with symptomatic amebiasis. Repeated assay, if initially negative, may increase the diagnostic yield. Serologic tests should be performed whenever amebiasis is considered, even if fecal biopsy findings are negative.

Treatment. The treatment of amebiasis is discussed extensively in Chapter 8. Metronidazole is the current drug of choice in the United States for extraintestinal amebiasis. Diiodohydroxyquin and diloxanide furoate are effective in asymptomatic patients, whereas diiodohydroxyquin and paromomycin used sequentially are effective in the dysenteric form of disease. Many investigators also administer broad spectrum antibiotics, especially tetracycline, in addition to amebicides. When antiamebic therapy must be administered parenterally to a postoperative patient, parenteral metronidazole is preferred.

A colon operation in a patient with unrecognized amebiasis often results in septic complications and the mortality risk is high. However, in acute fulminating colitis with perforation, toxic dilation, or in some cases of ameboma, timely surgical treatment is necessary to avoid mortality rates approaching 100 percent. Latimer[201] lists the following indications for operation in acute fulminating amebic colitis: (1) impending or free intraperitoneal perforation, or perforation while receiving antiamebic chemotherapy; (2) failure of a localized perforation to respond to antiamebic therapy; (3) persistence or development of abdominal distention and tenderness while receiving treatment; (4) persistence of severe diarrhea after 5 days of chemotherapy; and (5) severe postamebic colitis symptoms with unremitting anemia and hypoproteinemia.

Indications for operation for ameboma include (1) failure of the ameboma to regress after appropriate chemotherapy, (2) persistent ulceration, (3) intestinal obstruction, (4) stricture formation, (5) intussusception, (6) hemorrhage, (7) internal fistula formation, and (8) perforation. Most surgeons believe the procedure of choice is resection of all involved intra-abdominal colon; proctectomy is rarely necessary. Eggleston et al,[202] however, report better success with diversion and drainage procedures. Primary anastomosis should not be attempted in the presence of active amebiasis. Whenever possible, operative intervention should be postponed until antiamebic therapy has been administered for at least 24 hours.

Schistosomiasis

Schistosomiasis is the subject of several reviews[203,204] and the etiology, epidemiology, and pathogenesis are discussed in Chapter 8. The human phase of this infection is initiated when the individual is exposed to cercariae, the second-stage larvae of this infection, which are released by the snail host into stagnant and slow-moving water. The cercariae penetrate skin or mucous membranes and become schistosomulae, which migrate to the lungs and liver, where maturation to the adult worm occurs. The adult females lay their eggs in the venules of the colon, from which they may be carried back to the liver or deposited in intestinal tissues. Some of the eggs erode into the bowel lumen and are passed in the feces. Eggs reaching maturity provoke a granulomatous reaction within intestinal serosa, mesenteric and retroperitoneal tissues, and lymphatics. In the acute phase, involved rectum and colon become edematous and hyperemic, and many fine granulations, pinpoint hemorrhages, and small ulcerations result. In the chronic phase, granuloma formation predominates.

In severe bowel disease, pseudoneoplastic tumors develop and may extend into the abdominal cavity or the bowel lumen. Polypoid lesions are found, especially in the rectosigmoid. Eventually, these lesions lose their blood supply and slough, leaving behind an ulcer that may bleed. Rarely, stricture occurs.

Clinical Manifestations. The systemic clinical manifestations are discussed in Chapter 8. In the acute phase, diarrhea is seen. Chronic colonic disease is associated with sporadic diarrhea, productive of bloody mucus, and constipation. Bowel polyps bleed, pseudoneoplastic tumors may compress or obstruct bowel, and abdominal masses may be palpable.[204] Perforation through the ulcers may occur. Segmental ischemia of the colon due to vascular occlusion of small vessels has been reported.[205] Endoscopy may reveal discrete or clustered hemorrhages and erosions. Surrounding inflammation is absent. The mucous membrane usually is pale and edematous. Small excrescences and polypoid lesions may be noted. The intestinal manifestations are important, but hepatic fibrosis, subsequent portal hypertension, and pulmonary hypertension are the more troublesome complications of this disease.

Diagnosis and Treatment. Diagnosis of schistosomiasis depends on visualization of eggs in feces or in a rectal biopsy taken from an upper rectal valve. Serologic studies are sometimes helpful (see Chap. 8). Effective drug therapy is outlined in Table 8–4. Surgical therapy is indicated to treat obstructive complications and to rule out neoplasm.

INFECTIOUS COMPLICATIONS OF COLONIC OPERATIONS

Anastomotic Leak

Anastomotic leak and its consequences constitute the major potentially preventable technical complication of operations on the large bowel. The incidence of anastomotic leak in specific diseases and after specific procedures is noted in the other sections of this chapter. Clinically significant leaks have been noted in 3 to 23 percent of patients having colon resection.[206–210] One-third to one-half of patients with an anastomotic leak die; anastomotic leak accounts for one-quarter to one-half of all the operative mortality risk of colon surgery.

Anastomotic Healing

Laboratory studies of anastomotic healing have focused on collagen metabolism at the anastomosis and in the adjacent colon. The amount, concentration, and structure of the collagen determine anastomotic strength, at least in part. Collagen lysis occurs at an increased rate at the anastomosis, and for several centimeters to each side, nearly immediately after operation. As a counterbalance to this, collagen synthesis increases in the same sites within 2 days. The balance of these factors is such that the total collagen content in the anastomosis and surrounding colon is decreased by about one-half in the third postoperative week; the anastomosis is stronger than surrounding normal colon. Any factor that increases the rate of collagen lysis or retards its synthesis may contribute to anastomotic leak. Factors contributing to anastomotic leak are discussed by Schrock et al,[208] Morgenstern et al,[209] and Irvin and Goligher.[211]

The prime factor contributing to anastomotic leak is the presence at operation of peritonitis, abscess, or fistula. Sepsis causes both an increase of collagen lysis and a decrease in collagen synthesis. Any colonic anastomosis is subject to this effect—ileocolic as well as colocolic or colorectal anastomoses. Debas and Thomson[210] found that because of leaks, right hemicolectomy in the presence of peritonitis was associated with a mortality rate of 23 percent versus 3 percent for elective procedures.

Any extraperitoneal anastomosis is more likely to leak. Leak rates of 58 percent have been documented when routine contrast enemas have been used to detect early minor postoperative leaks.[206] The incidence of clinically significant anastomotic leak is about 5 percent.[212] The main reasons seem to be the presence of dead space around the anastomosis, the separation of the anastomosis from intraperitoneal defense and healing mechanisms, and the absence of serosa that appears to reduce suture-holding integrity. The dead space collects blood and serum, which easily become infected.[213] Otherwise, the segment of resected colon has no influence on leak rate.

Anything that decreases blood flow to the anastomosis results in a potential increase in leak rate. Hypoxia retards collagen synthesis so that increased risk of leak is associated with a preoperative hematocrit of less than 35 percent, transfusion intraoperatively of more than two units of blood, or intraoperative hypotension. Colonic blood flow is particularly sensitive to hypovolemia. Blood flow to the colon decreased markedly when greater than 10 percent of the blood volume was lost and was only partially reversed by blood replacement. Other facts that increase leak rate, such as emergency operation, duration of operation of greater than 5 hours, or fixation of tumor to the pelvis, probably also relate to the degree of blood loss. Both trauma and hypovolemia have been shown to result in decreased collagen synthesis as well as decreased blood flow. Radiation injury of bowel leads to decreased protein synthesis, although no decrease in anastomotic strength results when the anastomosis is made between 8 and 23 days after radiotherapy.[214] Clinically, a history of prior radiotherapy is associated with an increased risk of leak. Chronic radiation damage is associated with decreased vascularity of tissue.

Nutritional factors should be important in anastomotic healing. Starvation (specifically protein depletion) is associated with decreased collagen synthesis and a weaker anastomosis. Morgenstern et al[209] and Irvin and Goligher[211] identified malnutrition and hypoalbuminemia as factors associated with leak. In the article of Schrock et al,[208] nutritional factors just missed being of statistical significance. Ascorbic acid, iron, and zinc, among other nutrients, are necessary for proper wound healing.

Drugs that impair collagen synthesis include dicumarol, chloramphenicol, and the cancer chemotherapeutic agents actinomycin D, nitrogen mustard, cyclophosphamide, 5-fluorouracil, and methotrexate. Steroids produce lysis of collagen as well as decreased synthesis. Morgenstern et al[209] recognized an increase of leaks in patients dependent on steroids, but Schrock et al[208] could demonstrate no such effect. Other factors generally agreed on as influencing the leak rate are age greater than 60 years and cancer at the margin of resection. Schrock et al[208] found that neither the colon disease necessitating operation nor the presence of other illnesses was associated with an increased leak rate. Morgenstern et al[209] found a positive correlation with obesity, coagulopathy, uremia, and diabetes mellitus.

The risk of anastomotic leak is reduced in clinical studies by effective preoperative mechanical colon cleansing[209,211] and by administration of oral antibiotics effective against both aerobes and anaerobes.[215] Bowel preparation and use of systemic antibiotics are discussed in subsequent sections of this chapter.

Schrock et al[208] could find no technical factors that increased the safety of colon anastomosis. A number of suture techniques have been tested. No significant difference between single-layer and two-layer anastomosis is demonstrable,[206] but everting anastomoses are inferior to inverting anastomoses.[216] Proximal diversion does not prevent leaks but colostomy (not cecostomy) does reduce the risk of death. The use of neostigmine to reverse muscle relaxants is not associated with an increased leak rate.[217] Goldsmith[218] describes the use of a pedicle flap of omentum placed in the pelvis and wrapped around a low rectal anastomosis to fill the dead space and to use the protective properties of the omentum. This maneuver is helpful in experimental animals.[219]

Insertion of a rectal tube through the anastomosis to allow colon decompression and instillation of antibiotic solution has been associated with good results, but no prospective controlled studies have been reported.[220] Many surgeons place drains in the vicinity of the anastomosis (particularly with low anastomosis), supposedly to establish a track through which feces will drain if a leak occurs. Such drains increase the incidence of anastomotic leak.[221] Drainage was rarely used by Schrock's group[208]; therefore its effect was not analyzed. Fazio[213] reports good results using sump suction catheters with continuous irrigation to prevent the collection of a hematoma around an extraperitoneal rectal anastomosis. This practice has not been compared with alternative methods in a randomized trial.

In summary, the primary technical requirements for a safe colon anastomosis are healthy bowel, good blood supply, absence of tension, and a watertight seal. A primary unprotected anastomosis should not be constructed in any segment of colon in the presence of localized or generalized abdominal sepsis. A conservative attitude (ie, constructing a colostomy rather than performing a primary anastomosis) is especially indicated in any emergency operation.

Diagnosis. Debas and Thomson[210] stressed that the second most difficult problem with anastomotic leak is delay in diagnosis and management. They classified anastomotic leaks into three types: minor separation, major separation, and gross necrosis of the bowel. Minor separations occurred in 34 percent of patients with anastomotic leak. Patients with minor separation usually developed a fecal fistula through the wound on the seventh to tenth postoperative day. Fever and leukocytosis were minimal; sepsis was absent. These fistulas usually healed spontaneously with nonoperative management.

Major separations occurred in 56 percent of all leaks. In these patients, fever and toxicity appeared in the early postoperative period. One-third presented findings of generalized peritonitis. Half the patients were treated conservatively for fecal fistula, and 31 percent died. The other half were treated by reoperation, with an 11 percent mortality rate.

Gross necrosis of at least one segment of a colon anastomosis occurred in 10 percent of patients. These patients demonstrated fever, disorientation, and signs of peritonitis; septic shock appeared within 36 hours. All patients passed blood per rectum or through a drain. All of these patients died.

Early diagnosis and treatment of a major anastomotic leak are imperative. Postoperative examination of the anastomosis with water-soluble contrast medium should be done in any patient who has unexplained signs of postoperative infection.

Treatment. The treatment of uncomplicated colocutaneous fistulas is described in a preceding section of this chapter. Simple proximal diversion is sufficient treatment for some patients. The anastomosis should be explored (1) when the proximal segment is ileum, (2) when a fecal fistula is associated with findings of peritonitis, and (3) when the patient deteriorates in the early postoperative period. With major leak, proximal diversion plus adequate drainage is preferred; with a small leak, an attempt may be made to repair the anastomosis as well. When stool is present in the proximal bowel, the anastomotic defect is large, or necrosis has occurred, the anastomosis should be taken down and the ends exteriorized or a Hartmann's procedure done. Resection and reanastomosis with proximal diversion are rarely indicated.

PREVENTION OF INFECTIOUS COMPLICATIONS OF COLON OPERATIONS

Preoperative Preparation of the Bowel

Preoperative bowel preparation has been the subject of considerable discussion for three decades. The goals of bowel preparation are to empty the bowel of all bulk fecal matter (mechanical preparation) and to render the remaining bowel contents less infective (antimicrobial preparation). By accomplishing these goals, postoperative wound infection, anastomotic leak, intra-abdominal sepsis, and death are reduced.

There is little argument that adequate mechanical bowel preparation is important for successful colon surgery. The standard method of bowel cleansing used to involve restriction of diet to low-residue and liquid foods, and purgation with laxatives and enemas for 3 to 5 days before operation. Preoperative administration of an oral elemental diet (1800 to 2500 calories/day) plus laxatives has been tried[222] and is successful in producing good mechanical preparation; but hospital time is not saved, and currently available elemental diets have a poor taste.

Whole-gut lavage techniques have been adopted that have the advantages of more effective mechanical cleansing, shortened hospital stay, and better patient acceptance.[223-225] Our current regimens are listed in Table 43–5. Patients given whole-gut irrigation preparation must be alert and able to help themselves. An intelligent patient can control the rate of infusion to permit comfort. Patients with obstructive bowel lesions, or with fluid retention states associated with heart, kidney, and liver disease, are not candidates for whole-gut irrigation.

Mechanical preparation of the bowel removes bulk fecal matter. In so doing, the absolute numbers of gut bacteria are reduced, and the chances of gross fecal spillage during operation are decreased. The concentration of bacteria residual in the colon is unchanged, however, and the concentration of bacteria is the most important factor determining the incidence of septic complications. In a prospective study,[226] none of three methods of bowel preparation showed any significant differences from untreated controls or each other in residual bacterial concentration following preparation. Use of oral an-

TABLE 43–5. MECHANICAL BOWEL PREPARATION (COLON CLEANSING REGIMENS)

LAVAGE METHOD (PREFERRED)	
Preop Day 1	Insert nasogastric tube; weigh patient. Start polyethylene glycol cleansing solution via nasogastric tube at 9 a.m. at an initial rate of 1000 ml/20 min; adjust (or have patient adjust) rate to minimize cramps and distention. Place patient on commode. Continue lavage until a minimum volume of 4 liters has been administered and the anal effluent is clear; up to 10 liters may be needed in chronically constipated patients. After lavage has been completed, weigh patient and determine serum potassium; order diuretics or potassium supplements, as needed.
Operation Day	Patient evacuates rectum at 6 a.m.; no enemas. Schedule operation for 8 a.m.
CATHARSIS METHOD	
Preop Day 3	Order low-residue or clear liquid diet; administer bisacodyl 1 capsule orally, at 6 p.m.
Preop Day 2	Continue low-residue or clear liquid diet; administer magnesium sulfate, 30 ml of 50 percent solution (15 g) orally at 10 a.m., 2 p.m., and 6 p.m.; order saline enemas in the evening (three-position technique) to be repeated until the returns are clear.
Preop Day 1	Clear liquid diet; administer magnesium sulfate (in dose above) at 10 a.m. and 2 p.m.; administer supplemental IV fluids as needed; do *not* administer enemas on this day. Administer antibiotic prophylaxis.
Operation Day	Patient evacuates rectum at 6 a.m.; no enemas. Schedule operation for 8 a.m.

tibiotic agents is necessary to produce a significant reduction in the bacterial concentration of large bowel content.

Poth[227] enumerated the ideal characteristics of a colonic antiseptic: (1) broad spectrum of effect, (2) low host toxicity, (3) chemical stability with the gastrointestinal tract, (4) low rate of stimulating bacterial resistance, (5) rapidity of action, (6) limited absorption from the gastrointestinal tract, (7) activity in presence of food, (8) capacity to aid bowel cleansing without causing dehydration, (9) lack of irritation of gastrointestinal mucosa, (10) no interference with anastomotic healing, (11) low dosage requirement, (12) water solubility, (13) palatability, (14) inhibition of excessive fungal growth, and (15) limited clinical use. An additional important characteristic has been stressed in subsequent discussions: efficacy against pathogenic organisms. For over 30 years, investigators have been trying to find agents and regimens to fulfill all these criteria.

Until the 1970s, the prominent role of anaerobic organisms in the septic complications of large bowel operations was not recognized. The target organisms were *E. coli,* other Enterobacteriaceae, and aerobic streptococci. Special effort was made to avoid the pseudomembranous enterocolitis thought to be associated with staphylococcal overgrowth. The drugs and combinations used most widely were neomycin, neomycin and phthalylsulfathiazole, neomycin and tetracycline, neomycin and bacitracin, and kanamycin. Nystatin was sometimes added to prevent overgrowth of *Candida.* In 1971, Nichols and Condon[228] reviewed the status of antibacterial bowel preparation and reached several important conclusions. First, in light of the frequency of *B. fragilis* in postoperative infections, the then current regimens were inadequate. Second, nearly all prior clinical studies of the efficacy of antibacterial bowel preparation were retrospective and poorly controlled. The effects of several commonly used regimens were evaluated for their effects on bowel flora,[229] using modern techniques of anaerobic microbiology. Kanamycin, neomycin, and neomycin-phthalylsulfathiazole preparations were effective against aerobic and facultative organisms. Kanamycin showed no effect on anaerobes. Neomycin alone or with phthalylsulfathiazole produced no effect on anaerobes in half the patients.

In the selection of agents to use for bowel preparation, it is reasonable to aim specifically against fecal organisms that most often cause postoperative sepsis. The most important aerobe is *E. coli,* and the most important anaerobe is *B. fragilis.* Drugs effective against these organisms are listed in Table 43–6. Nichols et al[229,230] chose to test the combination of neomycin and erythromycin, drugs that best fit Poth's criteria. Neomycin and erythromycin produced nearly complete suppression of both aerobic and anaerobic organisms. Arabi et al[231] were able to produce equally remarkable reductions in colon bacterial counts using neomycin and metronidazole.

A number of prospective randomized trials of preoperative oral antibacterial bowel preparation have been conducted. These trials used drugs expected to have effect against anaerobes as well as aerobes. The results of these trials are tabulated in Table 43–7. All studies but two showed a statisti-

TABLE 43–6. ANTIBIOTICS EFFECTIVE AGAINST FECAL BACTERIA

Aerobes (*E. coli*)	Anaerobes (*B. fragilis*)
Cephalosporins (all generations)	Metronidazole
Trimethoprim-sulfamethoxazole	Clindamycin
Ampicillin, amoxicillin	Imipenem
Anti-pseudomonal penicillins (carbenicillin, etc)	Cefoxitin
Aminoglycosides (gentamicin, etc)	Moxalactam
Imipenem	Chloramphenicol
Aztreonam	Tetracyclines
Tetracyclines	Erythromycin

cally significant reduction in infection rate. Regimens combining an aminoglycoside with a drug active against anaerobes provided superior results. In most studies the combination of neomycin and erythromycin produced wound infection rates of under 10 percent. Studies that included microbiologic analysis uniformly demonstrated suppression of aerobic and anaerobic organisms. There was no overgrowth of organisms resistant to aminoglycosides. Thus recent prospective, randomized studies demonstrate a reduction in bacterial counts (aerobic and anaerobic) and a decrease in incidence of septic complications when appropriate oral antibiotic regimens are used. There were no instances of worse infection rates, overgrowth by resistant organisms, and no cases of pseudomembranous colitis. No impairment of anastomotic healing has been noted.

Prophylactic administration of parenteral antibiotics to patients undergoing elective colon surgery and to patients undergoing emergency operations for possible perforation of the colon (see Chap. 25) is another controversial practice. Laboratory experiments have shown that antimicrobial agents must be present in tissues before bacterial inoculation if maximum inhibition of infection is to be achieved.[232–234]

To determine how long prior to operation antibiotics should be administered and by what route, antibiotic concentrations in tissues have been measured in several reports. Maximum tissue antibiotic levels are achieved within 1 to 2 hours when drugs are given intramuscularly; tissue levels are achieved faster by intravenous administration.[235] In the absence of tissue infection, there is no advantage to prophylactic administration prior to the time required to achieve bactericidal tissue levels during operation.

Another question relating to the prophylactic use of parenteral antibiotics concerns the postoperative duration of administration. In most prospective studies, these agents have been administered for 24 hours or less. Studies examining this question specifically have shown no significant differ-

TABLE 43–7. CLINICAL TRIALS OF EFFICACIOUS ORAL ANTIMICROBIAL BOWEL PREPARATION REGIMENS

Author	Antibiotic(s) Studied	Infection Rate: Placebo Number	Placebo %	Treated Number	Treated %	Significant ($p < 0.05$?)
St. John 1973	neo-tetra	76/317	24	127/509	25	NS
Washington 1974	neo-tetra	43/63	68	5/65	8	Yes
Goldring 1975	kana-metro	11/25	44	2/25	8	Yes
Clarke 1977	neo-erythro	26/60	43	5/56	9	Yes
Pollock 1978	neo-tetra-phthalyl	29/44	66	8/27	30	Yes
Gillespie 1978	kana-metro	17/37	46	4/34	12	Yes
Fiddian 1978	genta-metro	11/19	58	0/27	0	Yes
Matheson 1978	neo-metro	25/59	42	9/51	18	Yes
Proud 1979	kana-metro	11/24	46	3/24	13	Yes
Montariol 1979	neo-tetra	27/41	66	17/46	37	Yes
Molin 1979	neo-oxytetra	41/66	62	9/75	12	Yes
Proud 1979	metro	11/24	46	5/19	26	NS
Hunt 1979	tinidazole	11/42	35	3/43	8	Yes
Hares 1982	genta-metro	14/27	52	8/30	27	Yes

neo, neomycin; tetra, tetracycline; kana, kanamycin; metro, metronidazole; erythro, erythromycin; phthalyl, phthalylsulfathiazole; genta, gentamicin; oxytetra, oxytetracycline; tobra, tobramycin; linco, lincomycin; cefurox, cefuroxime; clinda, clindamycin; mezlo, mezlocillin; pen, penicillin.

ence between groups who received antibiotics only during the perioperative period compared with treatment for 5 to 7 days postoperatively.[236–240]

Systemic antibiotics are useful in patients undergoing elective colectomy and in patients with possible perforation of the large bowel. Administration of parenteral antibiotics for periods longer than 24 hours postoperatively does not seem to improve results, although treatment of known intraperitoneal sepsis should certainly be more prolonged. Preoperative mechanical preparation with administration of oral antibiotics, such as neomycin and erythromycin base, seems to be more important in elective procedures than the use of systemic antibiotics.[241,242] The combination of oral antibiotics with systemic antibiotics offers only a marginal advantage over oral drugs alone but is the practice of the majority of surgeons.

The results of prospective, randomized trials of prophylaxis with parenteral antibiotics in colon surgery are listed in Table 43–8. Only those studies in which antibiotics were administered before or during operation are included. Parenteral antibiotic prophylaxis is probably effective, although the results of controlled trials are less consistent than studies with oral prophylaxis. Studies comparing various oral to parenteral antibiotic regimens are recorded in Table 43–9; oral antibiotics appear to be more effective than parenteral antibiotics in reducing infections. Studies comparing oral antibiotic preparation alone to oral plus parenteral ("belt and suspenders") antibiotics are summarized in Table 43–10.

Drainage

Routine drainage after operations on the large bowel is not the usual practice of many surgeons and continues to be the subject of debate. No one argues against draining localized collections of infected body fluids (pus, blood, feces). The debate concerns prophylactic drainage. The rationale for prophylactic drainage includes (1) prevention of generalized peritonitis, (2) prevention of fluid collections, and (3) obliteration of cavities.

TABLE 43–8. CLINICAL TRIALS OF EFFICACIOUS PARENTERAL ANTIBIOTICS IN COLORECTAL OPERATIONS

Author	Antibiotic(s) Studied	Infection Rate				Significant ($p < 0.05$?)
		Placebo		Treated		
		Number	*%*	*Number*	*%*	
Polk 1969	cephaloridine	15/50	30	4/54	7	Yes
Evans 1973	cephaloridine	20/46	44	14/41	34	NS
Burton 1975	gentamicin	12/41	29	14/39	36	NS
Griffiths 1976	tobra-linco	3/6	50	2/6	33	NS
Brote 1976	cephalothin	8/30	27	9/37	24	NS
Wetterfors 1976	doxycycline	16/43	37	3/39	8	Yes
Burdon 1977	cephalothin	16/36	44	14/39	36	NS
Kjellgren 1977	cephalothin	24/41	59	7/45	16	Yes
Feathers 1977	genta-linco/metro	12/25	48	2/28	4	Yes
Galland 1977	tobra-linco	16/38	42	3/37	8	Yes
Hojer 1978	doxycycline	25/60	42	5/58	9	Yes
Keighley 1978	tobra-linco	7/31	23	6/31	19	NS
Hughes 1979	cephaloridine	31/81	38	12/78	27	Yes
Mitchell 1980	cefurox-metro	5/7	71	0/6	6	NS
Mitchell 1980	cefuroxime	5/7	71	3/8	38	NS
Nygaard 1980	doxycycline	8/49	16	6/55	11	NS
Hoffmann 1981	cefoxitin	9/33	27	1/32	3	Yes
Mehigan 1981	cefamandol	1/38	3	2/36	6	Yes
Brown 1982	ticarcillin	12/45	27	0/29	0	Yes
Wenzel 1982	mezlocillin	22/48	46	5/52	10	Yes
Wittmann 1982	cefamandol	8/26	31	3/24	13	Yes
Coppa 1983	cefoxitin	22/120	18	8/121	7	Yes
Winker 1983	cefoxitin	11/27	47	2/30	7	Yes
Gomez-Alonso 1984	genta-metro	15/31	48	6/37	17	NS

For abbreviation key see Table 43–7.

TABLE 43–9. STUDIES COMPARING ORAL AND PARENTERAL ANTIBIOTICS IN COLORECTAL OPERATIONS

Author	Oral Antibiotic(s) Studied	Number Infected/Total	Infected (%)	Parenteral Antibiotic(s) Studied	Number Infected/Total	Infected (%)	Significant ($p < 0.05$?)
Lewis 1978	neo-erythro	5/41	12	cephaloridine	5/38	13	NS
Aeberhard 1979	kano-metro	4/25	16	kana-metro	3/27	11	NS
Condon 1979	neo-erythro	7/126	6	cephalothin	26/67	39	Yes
Keighley 1979	kana-metro	17/47	36	kana-metro	3/46	7	Yes
Fluckiger 1980	kana-metro	6/35	17	kana-metro	6/37	16	NS
Dion 1980	neo-metro	1/39	3	metro	3/39	8	NS
Eisenberg 1981	neo-erythro	10/141	7	cefamandol	4/112	4	NS
Hares 1981	genta-metro	11/35	31	cefoxitin	12/52	23	NS
Lewis 1981	metro-erythro	6/60	10	cephradine	25/70	36	Yes
Edmondson 1982	neo-erythro	1/58	2	cephaloridine	8/60	13	Yes
Beggs 1982	neo-metro	6/46	13	neo-metro	5/51	10	NS
Lazorthes 1982	kana-metro	9/30	30	cephradine-metro	7/30	23	NS
Gahos 1982	neo-metro	3/43	7	neo-clinda	0/38	0	NS
McDonald 1983	genta-metro	12/48	25	cefoxitin	12/52	23	NS
Marti 1983	genta-metro	4/55	7	genta-clinda	5/52	10	NS
Figueras 1984	neo-erythro	4/45	9	genta-metro	13/48	35	Yes
McCulloch 1986	genta-metro	6/45	13	moxalactam	5/41	12	NS
Hanke 1986	neo-metro	0/50	0	mezlo-metro	1/50	2	NS
Lau 1988	neo-erythro	14/62	23	genta-metro	5/67	7	Yes
Raahave 1988	neo-erythro	6/50	12	cefotaxime	2/50	4	NS
Stellato 1990	neo-erythro	5/44	11	cefoxitin	6/51	11	NS
Kling 1989	neo-erythro	1/27	4	ceftri-metro	2/27	7	NS

For abbreviation key see Table 43–7.

Yates[243] demonstrated that drains placed within the abdominal cavity are sealed off from the cavity in less than 24 hours. This observation has been confirmed by Agrama et al.[244] It is impossible to drain the peritoneal cavity. Even if a large amount of fluid is present within the abdominal cavity, the bowel or omentum usually adheres around the drain and isolates it from the peritoneal cavity in a matter of hours.

Although few suggest that it is beneficial to drain intraperitoneal anastomoses, many surgeons routinely drain a low rectal extraperitoneal anastomosis. It is reasoned that bloody fluid frequently collects in the sacral hollow, preventing apposition of the rectum to presacral tissues and serving as a growth medium for bacteria. Drainage is supposed to prevent these events. The efficacy of such drainage has not been demonstrated. Another reason given for prophylactic pelvic drainage is to provide a conduit through which pus will drain if an abscess develops. Stone et al[245] found that intraperitoneal abscesses, in patients whose wounds had already been drained, ultimately presented through the wound three times more frequently than they did by the drain track.

Drains are not innocuous. Yates[243] demonstrated that peritoneal resistance to infection was impaired by the presence of drains. Stone et al[245,246] documented in controlled clinical studies that, after intraperitoneal contamination, prophylactic drainage increased the incidence of intraperitoneal sepsis and wound infections. Berliner et al[247] found that the presence of drains in the vicinity of an anastomosis resulted in impaired anastomotic healing and a higher leak rate. Drains are two-way conduits; surface bacteria quickly colonize the drain track.[243] Even sump drains with bacterial filters allow drain track infection. In clean cases, infections occurring in drained patients are more often caused by hospital pathogens.[245]

When drainage is used, the type of drain must be carefully selected. Active suction drains are superior to passive Penrose drains in almost all ways: (1) Penrose drainage by gravity is inefficient; (2) passive drains are open to the environment, facilitating secondary infection; (3) suction drains, as long as they remain patient, actively remove any liquid with which they come in contact; (4) the force of suction assists obliteration of dead spaces; and (5) if low suction (15 cm H_2O) is used, sump drains

TABLE 43–10. STUDIES COMPARING EFFECTIVE ORAL ANTIBIOTICS USED ALONE VERSUS COMBINED ORAL PLUS PARENTERAL ANTIBIOTICS IN COLORECTAL OPERATIONS

Author	Oral Antibiotic(s) Studied	Number Infected/Total	Infected (%)	Oral plus Parenteral Antibiotic(s) Studied	Number Infected/Total	Infected (%)	Significant ($p < 0.05$?)
Stone 1976	neo-erythro	7/43	16	neo-erythro + cefazolin	6/101	6	Yes
Barber 1979	neo-erythro	3/28	11	neo-erythro + genta-clinda	2/31	7	NS
Eisenberg 1981	neo-erythro	10/141	7	neo-erythro + cephalothin	9/111	8	NS
	neo-erythro	7/80	9	neo-erythro + cefamandole	3/85	4	NS
Mehigan 1981	neo-erythro	1/38	3	neo-erythro + cefamandole	2/36	6	NS
				neo-erythro + pen-genta-clinda	1/39	3	NS
Brown 1982	neo-erythro	3/14	21	neo-erythro + ticarcillin	0/29	0	NS
				neo-erythro + cephalothin	1/19	5	NS
Lazorthes 1982	kana-metro	9/30	30	kana-metro + cephradine-genta	1/30	3	Yes
Coppa 1983	neo-erythro	22/120	18	neo-erythro + cefoxitin	8/121	7	Yes
Condon 1983	neo-erythro	42/540	8	neo-erythro + cephalothin	31/542	6	NS
Portnoy 1983	neo-erythro	6/17	35	neo-erythro + cefazolin	3/43	7	Yes
				neo-erythro + ticarcillin	2/44	5	Yes
Petrelli 1988	neo-erythro	1/36	3	neo-erythro + cefamandole	0/34	0	NS
Stellato 1990	neo-erythro	5/44	11	neo-erythro + cefoxitin	4/51	8	NS
Schoetz 1990	neo-erythro	14/96	15	neo-erythro + cefoxitin	5/101	5	Yes

For abbreviation key see Table 43–7.

allow more limited access of bacteria to the drain track than does a passive drain. Suction drainage of low rectal anastomoses results in a lower incidence of complications than does drainage using Penrose drains. Stone et al[245] suggest that if Penrose drains are used, they be dressed with a sterile stoma appliance to reduce contamination from external sources.

REFERENCES

Pathogenesis

1. Moore WEC, Holdeman LV: Human fecal flora: the normal flora of 20 Japanese-Hawaiians. Appl Microbiol 27:961, 1974.
2. Finegold SM: Anaerobic Bacteria in Human Disease. New York, Academic, 1977.
3. Simon GL, Gorback SL: Intestinal flora in health and disease. Gastroenterology 86:174, 1984.
4. Salyers AA: *Bacteroides* of the human lower intestinal tract. Annu Rev Microbiol 38:293, 1984.
5. Wilson AJ, Strachan CJL: Perioperative prevention of infection in abdominal surgery. Antibiot Chemother 33:30, 1985.
6. Holdeman LV, Cood IJ, Moore WEC: Human fecal flora: variation in bacterial composition within individuals and a possible effect on emotional stress. Appl Environ Microbiol 31:359, 1976.

Colonic Perforations

7. Cochran DQ, Almond CH, Shucart WA: An experimental study of the effects of barium and intestinal

contents on the peritoneal cavity. Am Roentgenol 89:883, 1963.
8. Stone HH, Kolb LD, Geheber CE: Incidence and significance of intraperitoneal anaerobic bacteria. Ann Surg 181:705, 1975.
9. Anderson CB, Marr JJ, Ballinger WF: Anaerobic infections in surgery: clinical review. Surgery 79:313, 1976.
10. Wittmann DH, Aprahamian C, Bergstein JM: Etappenlavage: advanced diffuse peritonitis managed by planned multiple laparotomies utilizing zippers, slide fastener, and velcro analogue for temporary abdominal closure. World J Surg 14:218, 1990.
11. Altemeier WA, Culbertson, WR, Fullen WD, Shook CD: Intra-abdominal abcesses. Am J Surg 125:70, 1973.
12. Emanuel B, Zlotnik P, Raffensperger JC: Perforation of the gastrointestinal tract in infancy and childhood. Surg Gynecol Obstet 146:926, 1978.
13. Bell MJ: Perforation of the gastrointestinal tract and peritonitis in the neonate. Surg Gynecol Obstet 160:20, 1985.
14. Barlow B, Santulli TV: Importance of multiple episodes of hypoxia or cold stress on the development of enterocolitis in animal model. Surgery 77:687, 1975.
15. O'Neill JA, Holcomb GW: Surgical experience with neonatal necrotizing enterocolitis. Ann Surg 189:612, 1979.
16. Kleinhaus S, Weinberg G, Gregor MD: Necrotizing enterocolitis in infancy. Surg Clin North Am 72:261, 1992.
17. Book LS, Overall JC, Herbst JJ, et al: Clustering of necrotizing enterocolitis: interruption by infection-control measures. N Engl J Med 287:984, 1977.
18. Bell MJ, Feigin RD, Ternberg JL, Brotherton T: Evaluation of gastrointestinal microflora in necrotizing enterocolitis. J Pediatr 92:589, 1978.
19. Howard FM, Flynn DM, Bradley JM, et al: Outbreak of necrotizing enterocolitis caused by *Clostridium butyricum*. Lancet 2:1099, 1977.
20. Cohn I, Langford D, Rives JD: Antibiotic support of colon anastomoses. Surg Gynecol Obstet 104:1, 1957.
21. Bell MJ, Ternberg JL, Feigin RD, et al: Neonatal necrotizing enterocolitis: therapeutic decisions based upon clinical staging. Ann Surg 187:1, 1978.
22. Kosloske AM, Papile L, Burstein J: Indications for operation in acute necrotizing enterocolitis of the neonate. Surgery 87:502, 1980.
23. Kanto WP, Wilson R, Ricketts PR: Management and outcome of necrotizing enterocolitis. Clin Pediatr 24:79, 1985.
24. Kleinhaus SJ, Boley MS, Sieber NK: Hirschsprung's disease: a survey of the members of the surgical section of the American Academy of Pediatrics. J Pediatr Surg 14:588, 1979.
25. Corkery JJ: Hirschsprung's disease. Clin Gastroenterol 4:531, 1975.
26. Sieber WK, Soave F: Hirschsprung's disease, with a note on the Soave operation. Curr Probl Surg 15:1, 1978.
27. Bill AH, Chapman ND: The enterocolitis of Hirschsprung's disease: its natural history and treatment. Am J Surg 103:70, 1962.
28. Rescorla FJ, Morrison AM, Engles D, et al: Hirschsprung's disease. Evaluation of mortality and long-term function in 260 cases. Arch Surg 127:934, 1992.
29. Howell HS, Baritzal JF, Freeark RJ: Blunt trauma involving the colon and rectum. J Trauma 16:624, 1976.
30. Haas PA, Fox TA: Civilian injurics of the rectum and anus. Dis Colon Rectum 22:17, 1979.
31. Davis JJ, Cohn I, Nance FC: Diagnosis and management of blunt abdominal trauma. Ann Surg 183:672, 1976.
32. Flint LM, Voyles CR, Richardson JD, Fry DE: Missile tract infections after transcolonic gunshot wounds. Arch Surg 113:727, 1978.
33. Strate RG, Grieco JG: Blunt injury to the colon and rectum. J Trauma 23:384, 1983.
34. Lorinc P, Brahme F: Perforation of the colon during examination by the double contrast method. Gastroenterology 37:770, 1959.
35. Burt CAV: Pneumatic rupture of the intestinal canal with experimental data showing the mechanism of perforation and the pressure required. Arch Surg 22:875, 1931.
36. Salvo AF, Leigh KE: Barium intravasation into portal venous system during barium enema examination. JAMA 235:749, 1976.
37. Schwesinger WH, Levine BA, Ramos R: Complications in colonoscopy. Surg Gynecol Obstet 148:270, 1979.
38. Terranova O, Sandei F, Rebuffat C, et al: Irrigation vs. natural evacuation of left colostomy: a comparative study of 340 patients. Dis Colon Rectum 22:31, 1979.
39. Sohn N, Weinstein MA, Gonchar J: Social injuries of the rectum. Am J Surg 134:611, 1977.
40. Crass RA, Tranbaugh RF, Kudak DA, Trunkey DD: Colorectal foreign bodies and perforation. Am J Surg 142:85, 1981.
41. Christy JP: Complications of combat casualities with combined injuries of bone and bowel: personal experience with nineteen patients. Surgery 71:270, 1972.
42. Roof WR, Morris GC, DeBakey ME: Management of perforating injuries to the colon in civilian practice. Am J Surg 99:641, 1960.
43. Vannix RS, Carter R, Hinshaw DB, Joergenson EJ: Surgical management of colon—trauma in civilian practice. Am J Surg 106:364, 1963.
44. Beall AC, Bricker DL, Alessi FJ, et al: Surgical considerations in the management of civilian colon injuries. Ann Surg 173:971, 1971.
45. McGown C, Khan MO, Rousufuddin M: Colon injuries in civilian practice. Am Surg 38:218, 1972.
46. Garfinkle SE, Cohen SE, Matolo NM, et al: Civilian

colonic injuries: changing concepts of management. Arch Surg 109:402, 1974.
47. LoCicero J, Tajima T, Drapanas T: A half-century of experience in the management of colon injuries: changing concepts. J Trauma 15:575, 1975.
48. Chilimindris C, Boyd DR, Carlson LE, et al: A critical review of management of right colon injuries. J Trauma 11:651, 1971.
49. Quarantillo EP, Nemhauser GM: Survey of cecal and ascending colon injuries among Vietnam casualties in Japan (1967–1970). Am J Surg 125:607, 1973.
50. Bartizal JF, Boyd DR, Folk FA, et al: A critical review of management of 392 colonic and rectal injuries. Dis Colon Rectum 17:313, 1974.
51. Stone HH, Fabian TC: Management of perforating colon trauma. Ann Surg 190:430, 1979.
52. Sykes EM: Colon perforation in Ehlers-Danlos syndrome. Am J Surg 147:410, 1984.
53. Sherry RM, Fisch A, Grey DP, Lubbock CA: Embolization of a hepatoportal fistula in a patient with Ehlers-Danlos syndrome and colon perforation. Surgery 111(4):475, 1992.

Diverticular Disease

54. Ochsner HC, Bargell JA: Diverticulosis of the large intestine and evaluation of historical and personal observations. Ann Intern Med 9:282, 1935.
55. Willard JH, Bockus HL: Clinical and therapeutic status of cases of colonic diverticulosis seen in office practice. Am J Dig Dis Nutr 3:580, 1936.
56. Eusebio EB, Eisenberg MM: Natural history of diverticular disease of the colon in young patients. Am J Surg 125:308, 1973.
57. Fatayer WT, A-Khalaf MM, Shalan KA, et al: Diverticular disease of the colon in Jordan. Dis Colon Rectum 26:247, 1983.
58. Sugihara K, Muto T, Moriuka Y, et al: Diverticular disease of the colon in Japan: a review of 615 cases. Dis Colon Rectum 27:531, 1984.
59. Morson CB: Pathology of diverticular disease of the colon. Clin Gastroenterol 4:37, 1975.
60. Marcus R, Watt J: The radiological appearances of diverticula in the antimesenteric intertaenia area of the pelvic colon. Clin Radiol 16:87, 1965.
61. Parks TG: Natural history of diverticular disease of the colon: a review of 521 cases. Br Med J 4:639, 1969.
62. Painter NS, Truelove SC: Potential dangers of morphine in acute diverticulitis of the colon. Br Med J 2:33, 1963.
63. Arfwidsson S: Pathogenesis of multiple diverticula of the sigmoid colon in diverticular disease. Acta Chir Scand Suppl 342:47, 1964.
64. Painter NS, Burkitt DP: Diverticular disease of the colon, a 20th century problem. Clin Gastroenterol 4:3, 1975.
65. Ritchie JA: Rectosigmoidal mucosal puckering and diverticulosis. Dis Colon Rectum 18:221, 1975.
66. Wychulis AR, Beahrs OH, Judd ES: Surgical management of diverticulitis of the colon. Surg Clin North Am 47:961, 1967.
67. Morton DL, Goldman L: Differential diagnosis of diverticulitis and carcinoma of the sigmoid colon. Am J Surg 103:55, 1962.
68. Parks TG: Reappraisal of clinical features of diverticular disease of the colon. Br Med J 4:642, 1969.
69. Wetstein L, Camera A, Trillo RA, Zamora BO: Giant sigmoidal diverticulum: report of a case and review of the literature. Dis Colon Rectum 21:110, 1978.
70. Labs JD, Sarr MG, Fishman EK, et al: Complications of acute diverticulitis of the colon: improved early diagnosis and computed tomography. Am J Surg 155:331, 1988.
71. Hachigian MP, Honickman S, Eisenstat TE, et al: Computed tomography in the initial management of acute left-sided diverticulitis. Dis Colon Rectum 35:1123, 1992.
72. Eastwood MA: Medical and dietary management. Clin Gastroenterol 4:85, 1975.
73. Friedman G, Janowitz HD: Diverticular disease: the medical aspects. Contemp Surg 11:29, 1977.
74. Painter NS, Almeida AZ, Colebone KW: Unprocessed bran in treatment of diverticular disease of the colon. Br Med J 2:137, 1972.
75. Smithwick RH: Experiences with the surgical management of diverticulitis of the sigmoid. Ann Surg 115:969, 1942.
76. Madden JL, Tan PY: Primary resection and anastomosis in the treatment of perforated lesions of the colon, with abscess of diffusing peritonitis. Surg Gynecol Obstet 113:646, 1961.
77. Madden JL: Treatment of perforated lesions of the colon by primary resection and anastomosis. Dis Colon Rectum 9:413, 1966.
78. McSherry CK, Grafe WR Jr, Perry HS, Glenn F: Surgery of the large bowel for emergent conditions: staged vs. primary resection. Arch Surg 98:749, 1969.
79. Hackford AW, Schoetz DJ, Coller JA, Veidenheimer MC: Surgical management of complicated diverticulitis. Dis Colon Rectum 28:317, 1985.
80. Rodkey GV, Welch CE: Colonic diverticular disease with surgical treatment: a study of 338 cases. Surg Clin North Am 54:655, 1974.
81. Colcock BP: Diverticular disease: proven surgical management. Clin Gastroenterol 4:99, 1975.
82. Reilly M: Sigmoid myotomy. Part I: Development of the operation; its application and results. Clin Gastroenterol 4:121, 1975.
83. Taylor SA, Good CS, Porter NH: Sigmoid myotomy: a retrospective study of 28 patients. Br J Clin Pract 28:153, 1974.
84. Smith AN: Sigmoid myotomy. Part II: Manometric and clinical results; comparison with resection and the effect of bran; transverse myotomy. Clin Gastroenterol 4:135, 1975.
85. Kettlewell W, Moloney GE: Combined horizontal and longitudinal colomyotomy for diverticular dis-

ease: preliminary report. Dis Colon Rectum 20:24, 1977.

86. Ouriel K, Schwartz SL: Diverticular disease in the young patient. Surg Gynecol Obstet 156:1, 1983.
87. Charnock ML, Rennie JR, Wellwood JM, Todd IP: Results of colectomy for diverticular disease of the colon. Br J Surg 64:417, 1977.
88. Wolf BG, Ready RR, MacCarty RL, et al: Influence of sigmoid resection on progression of diverticular disease of the colon. Dis Colon Rectum 84:645, 1984.

Inflammatory Bowel Disease

89. Kirsner JB: Inflammatory bowel disease: consideration of etiology and pathogenesis. Am J Gastroenterol 69:253, 1978.
90. Tompkins RK, Weinstein MH, Foroozan P, et al: Reappraisal of rectum-retaining operations for ulcerative and granulomatous colitis. Am J Surg 125:159, 1973.
91. Sloan WP, Bargen JA, Gage RP: Life histories of patients with chronic ulcerative colitis: a review of 2,000 cases. Gastroenterology 16:25, 1950.
92. Monteiro E, Fossey J, Shiner M, et al: Antibacterial antibodies in rectal and colonic mucosa in ulcerative colitis. Lancet 1:249, 1971.
93. Brooke BN: The pathogenesis of ulcerative and granulomatous colitis: surgical implications. Surg Clin North Am 52:971, 1972.
94. Simonowitz D, Block GE, Riddell RH, et al: The production of an unusual tissue reaction in rabbit bowel injected with Crohn's disease homogenates. Surgery 82:221, 1977.
95. Hardin CA, Werder AA: Tissue culture of sera in human ulcerative colitis. Am J Surg 130:20, 1975.
96. Sidi S, Graham JH, Razvi SA, Banks PA: Cytomegalovirus infection of the colon associated with ulcerative colitis. Arch Surg 114:857, 1979.
97. Turnbull RB, Hawk WA, Weakley FL: Surgical treatment of toxic megacolon: ileostomy and colostomy to prepare patients for colectomy. Am J Surg 122:325, 1971.
98. Korelitz BI, Gribetz D, Kopel FB: Granulomatous colitis in children: a study of 25 cases and comparison with ulcerative colitis. Pediatrics 42:446, 1968.
99. Homan WP, Tang C, Thorbjarnarson B: Anal lesions complicating Crohn disease. Arch Surg 111:1333, 1976.
100. Binder SC, Miller HH, Deterling RA: Emergency and urgent operations for ulcerative colitis: the procedure of choice. Arch Surg 110:284, 1975.
101. Ritchie JK: Ulcerative colitis treated by ileostomy and excisional surgery: fifteen years experience at St. Mark's Hospital. Br J Surg 59:345, 1972.
102. Lindner AE, Marshak RH, Wolf BS, Janowitz HD: Granulomatous colitis: a clinical study. N Engl J Med 269:379, 1963.
103. Sirinek KR, Tetirick CE, Thomford NR, Pace WG: Total proctocolectomy and ileostomy: procedure of choice for acute toxic megacolon. Arch Surg 112:518, 1977.
104. Meuwissen SGM, Pape KSSB, Agenant D, et al: Crohn's disease of the colon: analysis of the diagnostic value of radiology, endoscopy, and histology. Am J Dig Dis 21:81, 1976.
105. Lennard-Jones JE, Powell-Tuck J: During treatment of inflammatory bowel disease. Clin Gastroenterol 8:187, 1979.
106. Summers RW, Switz DM, Sessions JT Jr, et al: National Cooperative Crohn's Disease Study: results of drug treatment. Gastroenterology 77:847, 1979.
107. Singleton JW: National Cooperative Crohn's Disease Study (NCCDS): results of drug treatment. Gastroenterology 72:A110, 1977.
108. Michener WM, Gage RP, Sauer WG, Stickler CB: The prognosis of chronic ulcerative colitis in children. N Engl J Med 265:1075, 1961.
109. DeDombal FT: Results of surgery for Crohn's disease. Clin Gastroenterol 2:493, 1972.
110. Homan WP, Dineen P: Comparison of the results of resection bypass, and bypass with exclusion for ileocecal Crohn's disease. Ann Surg 198:530, 1978.
111. Jones JH, Lennard-Jones JE, Lockhart-Mummery HE: Experience in the treatment of Crohn's disease of the large intestine. Gut 7:448, 1966.
112. Fawaz KA, Glotzer DJ, Goldman H, et al: Ulcerative colitis and Crohn's disease of the colon—a comparison of the long-term postoperative courses. Gastroenterology 71:372, 1976.
113. Goligher JC: The outcome of excisional operation for primary and recurrent Crohn's disease of the large intestine. Surg Gynecol Obstet 148:1, 1979.
114. Khubchandani IT, Trimpi HD, Sheets JA, et al: Ileorectal anastomosis for ulcerative and Crohn's colitis. Am J Surg 135:751, 1978.
115. Grant CS, Dozois RR: Toxic megacolon: ultimate fate of patients after successful medical management. Am J Surg 1417:106, 1984.
116. Fry PD, Atkinson KG: Current surgical approach to toxic megacolon. Surg Gynecol Obstet 143:26, 1976.
117. Block GE, Moossa AR, Simonowitz D, Hassan SZ: Emergency colectomy for inflammatory bowel disease. Surgery 82:531, 1977.

Infectious Complications of Cancer

118. Welch JP, Donaldson GA: Perforative carcinoma of colon and rectum. Ann Surg 180:734, 1974.
119. Peloquin AB: Factors influencing survival with complete obstruction and free perforation of colorectal cancers. Dis Colon Rectum 18:11, 1975.
120. Welch JP: Unusual abscesses in perforation colorectal cancer. Am J Surg 131:270, 1976.
121. Valerio D, Jones PF: Immediate resection in the treatment of large bowel emergencies. Br J Surg 65:712, 1978.
122. Welch JP, Donaldson GA: Management of severe obstruction of the large bowel due to malignant disease. Am J Surg 127:492, 1974.
123. Klein RS, Recco RA, Catalano MT, et al: Association

of *Streptococcus bovis* with carcinoma of the colon. N Engl J Med 297:800, 1977.
124. Wade DS, Nova HR, Douglas HO Jr: Neutropenic enterocolitis, clinical diagnosis and treatment. Cancer 69:17, 1992.

Infection Related to Large Bowel Obstruction

125. Greene WW: Bowel obstruction in the aged patient: a review of 300 cases. Am J Surg 118:541, 1969.
126. Greenlee HB, Pienkos EJ, Vanderbilt PC, et al: Acute large bowel obstruction: comparison of county, Veterans Administration, and community hospital populations. Arch Surg 108:470, 1974.
127. Michel ML, Tanner GR, Rohr ME: Obstructions of the colon. In Ballinger WF, Drapanas T (eds): Practice of Surgery—Current Review, Vol II. St Louis, Mosby, 1975, p 90.
128. Weillbaecher D, Bolin JA, Hearn D, Ogden W: Intussusception in adults: review of 160 cases. Am J Surg 121:531, 1971.
129. Smith GA, Perry JF, Yonehiro EG: Mechanical intestinal obstructions: a study of 1,252 cases. Surg Gynecol Obstet 100:651, 1955.
130. Payne RL, McApline RE: Obstruction of the colon: resection in two stages. Ann Surg 153:871, 1961.
131. Starling JR: Initial treatment of sigmoid volvulus by colonoscopy. Ann Surg 190:36, 1979.

Colonic Ischemia

132. Bernardino ME, Lawson TL: Discrete colonic ulcers associated with oral contraceptives. Am J Dig Dis 21:503, 1976.
133. Kistin MG, Kaplan MM, Harrington JT: Diffuse ischemic colitis associated with systemic lupus erythematosus—response to subtotal colectomy. Gastroenterology 75:1147, 1978.
134. Hagihara PF, Parker JC, Griffen WO: Spontaneous ischemic colitis. Dis Colon Rectum 20:23, 1977.
135. O'Connell TX, Kadell B, Tompkins RK: Ischemia of the colon. Surg Gynecol Obstet 142:332, 1976.
136. LeVeen EG, Falk G, Ip M, et al: Urease as a contributing factor in ulcerative lesions of the colon. Am J Surg 135:53, 1978.
137. Boley SJ, Brandt LJ, Veith FJ: Ischemic disorders of the intestines. Curr Probl Surg 15:1, 1978.
138. Williams LF, Wittenberg J: Ischemic colitis: a useful clinical diagnosis, but is it ischemic? Ann Surg 182:430, 1975.
139. Heikkinen E, Larmi TKI, Huttunen R: Necrotizing colitis. Am J Surg 128:362, 1974.
140. Feldman PS: Ulcerative disease of the colon proximal to partially obstructive lesions. Report of two cases and review of the literature. Dis Colon Rectum 18:601, 1975.
141. Ernst CB, Hagihara PF, Daugherty ME, et al: Ischemic colitis incidence following abdominal aortic reconstruction: a prospective study. Surgery 80:417, 1976.
142. Meissner MH, Johanson KH: Colon infarction after ruptured abdominal aortic aneurysm. Arch Surg 127:979, 1992.
143. Robinson JC, Teitelbaum SL: Stercoral ulceration and perforation of the sclerodermatous colon: report of two cases and review of the literature. Dis Colon Rectum 17:622, 1974.
144. Russell WL: Stercoraceous ulcer. Am Surg 42:416, 1976.
145. Albers JH, Smith LL, Carter R: Perforation of the cecum. Ann Surg 143:251, 1956.

Large Bowel Fistula

146. Webster MW, Carey LC: Fistulae of the intestinal tract. Curr Probl Surg 13:1, 1976.
147. Haff RC, Wise L, Ballinger WF: Biliary-enteric fistulas. Surg Gynecol Obstet 133:84, 1971.
148. ReMine WH: Biliary-enteric fistulas: natural history and management. In Hardy JD, Zollinger RM (eds): Advances in Surgery, Vol 7. Chicago, Year Book Medical Publishers, 1973, p 69.
149. Holden JL, Berne TV, Rosoff L: Pancreatic abscess following acute pancreatitis. Arch Surg 111:858, 1976.
150. Grace RR, Jordan PH: Unresolved problems of pancreatic pseudocysts. Ann Surg 184:16, 1976.
151. Holmes SAV, Christmas TJ, Kirby RS, Hendry WF: Management of colovesical fistulae associated with pelvic malignancy. Br J Surg 79:432, 1992.
152. Korelitz BI: Colonic duodenal fistula in Crohn's disease. Am J Dig Dis 22:1040, 1977.
153. Howat JMT, Schofield PF: Benign duodenocolic fistula. Br J Surg 65:513, 1978.
154. Murray JJ, Schoetz DJ, Nugent FW, et al: Surgical management of Crohn's disease involving the duodenum. Am J Surg 147:58, 1984.
155. Glass RE, Ritchie JK, Lennard-Jones JE, et al: Internal fistulas in Crohn's disease. Dis Colon Rectum 28:557, 1985.
156. Jacobson IM, Schapiro RH, Warshaw AL: Gastric and duodenal fistulas in Crohn's disease. Gastroenterology 89:1347, 1985.
157. Klein S, Greenstein AJ, Sachar DB: Duodenal fistulas in Crohn's disease. J Clin Gastroenterol 9:46, 1987.
158. Pichney LS, Fanty GT, Graham SM: Gastrocolic and duodenocolic fistulas in Crohn's disease. J Clin Gastroenterol 15:205, 1992.
159. Ergin MA, Alfonso A, Auda SP, Waxman M: Primary carcinoma of the duodenum producing a malignant duodenocolic fistula. Dis Colon Rectum 21:408, 1978.

Bacterial Enterocolitis

160. Viranuvatti V: Infectious diarrheas, Part II. Cholera, salmonellosis and shigellosis. In Bockus H (ed): Gastroenterology. Philadelphia, Saunders, 1976, p 959.

161. Kim HJ, Oh S, Jarrett F: Management of ileal perforation due to typhoid fever. Ann Surg 181:88, 1975.
162. Gutman LT, Ottesen EA, Quan TJ, et al: An interfamilial outbreak of *Yersinia enterocolitica* enteritis. N Engl J Med 288:1372, 1973.
163. Nelson JD, Kusmiesz H, Jackson LH, Woodman E: Trimethoprim-sulfamethoxazole therapy for shigellosis. JAMA 235:1239, 1976.
164. Bartlett JG: Antibiotic-associated colitis. Dis Mon 30:1, 1984.
165. Trnak YM, Lamont JT: *Clostridium difficile* colitis. Adv Intern Med 29:85, 1984.
166. Aronsson B, Mollby R, Nord CE: Diagnosis and etiology of *Clostridium difficile* enterocolitis in Sweden. J Antimicrob Chemother I 14(Suppl D):85, 1984.
167. Wilkins TD, Lyerly DM: Toxins of *Clostridium difficile* and *Clostridium sordelli.* In Rambaud JC, Ducluzean R (eds): *Clostridium difficile* Intestinal Diseases. Paris, Springer-Verlag 1990, pp 45–53.
168. Tedesco FJ: Clindamycin-associated colitis: review of the clinical spectrum of 47 cases. Am J Dig Dis 21:26, 1976.
169. Viscidi R, Wiley S, Bartlett JG: Isolation rates and toxigenic potential of *Clostridium difficile* isolates from various patient populations. Gastroenterology 81:5, 1981.
170. Holst E, Helin I, Mardh PA: Recovery of *Clostridium difficile* from children. Scand J Infect Dis 13:41, 1981.
171. Hall IC, O'Toole E: Intestinal flora in new born infants with a description of a new pathogenic anaerobe *Bacillus difficilis.* Am J Dis Child 49:390, 1935.
172. Mulligan ME, Rolfe RD, Finegold SM, et al: Contamination of a hospital environment by *Clostridium difficile.* Curr Microbiol 3:173, 1979.
173. Fekety R, Kim K-H, Brown D, et al: Epidemiology of antibiotic-associated colitis: isolation of *Clostridium difficile* from the hospital environment. Am J Med 70:906, 1981.
174. Dupont HL, Ribner BS: Infectious gastroenteritis. In Bennett JV, Brachman PS, Sanford JP (eds): Hospital Infections, 3rd ed. Boston, Little, Brown, 1992, pp 641–658.
175. Bartlett JG, Gorbach SL: Pseudomembranous enterocolitis (antibiotic-related colitis). Adv Intern Med 22:455, 1977.
176. George WL: Antimicrobial agent-associated colitis and diarrhea: historical background and clinical aspects. Rev Infect Dis 6(Suppl 1):S208, 1984.
177. George WL: Post operative pseudomembranous enterocolitis, staphylococcal colitis and *Clostridium difficile* (antimicrobial associated) diarrhea. In Wilson SE, Finegold SM, Williams RA (eds): Intra-abdominal Infections. New York, McGraw-Hill, 1982, p 286.
178. Tedesco FJ: Pseudomembranous colitis, pathogenesis and therapy. Med Clin North Am 66:655, 1982.
179. Tedesco FJ, Barton RW, Alpers HD: Clindamycin-associated colitis. Ann Intern Med 81:429, 1974.
180. Bartlett JG, Chang TW, Gurwith M, et al: Antibiotic-associated pseudomembranous colitis due to toxin-producing *Clostridia.* N Engl J Med 298:531, 1978.
181. Bartlett JG, Onderdonk AB, Cisneros AB, et al: Clindamycin-associated colitis due to toxin producing species of *Clostridium* in hamsters. J Infect Dis 136:701, 1977.
182. Bartlett JG: *Clostridium difficile:* clinical considerations. Rev Infect Dis 12:S243, 1990.
183. Doern GV, Coughlin RT, Wu L: Laboratory diagnosis of *Clostridium difficile*–associated gastrointestinal diseases: comparison of a monoclonal antibody enzyme immunoassay for toxin A and toxin B with a monoclonal antibody enzyme immunoassay for toxin A only and two cytotoxicity assays. J Clin Microbiol 30:2042, 1992.
184. George WL, Sutter VL, Finegold SM: Toxigenicity and antimicrobial susceptibility of *Clostridium difficile,* a cause of antimicrobial agent-associated colitis. Curr Microbiol 1:55, 1978.
185. Miller SD, Blake M, Miliotis M, et al: Antibiotic-associated diarrhea and pseudomembranous colitis caused by *Clostridium difficile.* A review of 40 cases. S Afr Med J 63:936, 1983.
186. Teasley DG, Gerding DN, Olson MM, et al: Prospective randomized trial of metronidazole versus vancomycin for *Clostridium difficile* associated diarrhea and colitis. Lancet 1:1843, 1983.
187. Medich DS, Lee KKW, Simmons RL, et al: Laparotomy for fulminant pseudomembranous colitis. Arch Surg 127:847, 1992.
188. Yale CE, Balish E: Pneumatosis cystoides intestinalis. Dis Colon Rectum 19:107, 1976.
189. Gruenberg JC, Grodsinsky C, Ponka JL: Pneumatosis intestinalis: a clinical classification. Dis Colon Rectum 22:5, 1979.

Granulomatous Infections

190. Shukla HS, Hughes LE: Abdominal tuberculosis in the 1970's: a continuing problem. Br J Surg 65:403, 1978.
191. Paustian FF, Monto GL: Tuberculosis of the intestines. In Bockus HL (ed): Gastroenterology. Philadelphia, Saunders, 1976, p 750.
192. Jordan GL, DeBakey ME: Complications of tuberculous enteritis occurring during antimicrobial therapy. Arch Surg 69:688, 1954.
193. Adams R, Miller WH: Surgical treatment of intestinal tuberculosis. Surg Clin North Am 26:656, 1946.
194. Porter JM, Snowe RJ, Silver D: Tuberculous enteritis with perforation and abscess formation in childhood. Surgery 71:254, 1972.
195. Katariya RN, Sood S, Rao PG, Rao PLNG: Stricture-plasty for tubercular strictures of the gastrointestinal tract. Br J Surg 64:496, 1977.

196. Berardi RS: Abdominal actinomycosis. Surg Gynecol Obstet 149:257, 1979.
197. Cowgill R, Quan SH: Colonic actinomycosis mimicking carcinoma. Dis Colon Rectum 22:45, 1979.
198. Howard RJ, Balfour HH, Simmons RL: The surgical significance of viruses. Curr Probl Surg 14:1, 1977.
199. Dieterich DT, Kotler DP, Busch DF, et al: Ganciclovir treatment of cytomegalovirus colitis in AIDS: a randomized double-blind, placebo-controlled multicenter study. J Infect Dis 167:278, 1993.
200. Krogstad DJ, Spencer HC Jr, Healy GR: Amebiasis. N Engl J Med 298:262, 1978.
201. Latimer RG: Surgical intervention in intestinal amebiasis. Am Surg 41:385, 1975.
202. Eggleston FC, Verghese M, Handa AK: Amoebic perforation of the bowel: experiences with 26 cases. Br J Surg 65:748, 1978.
203. Warren KS: Schistosomiasis japonicum. Clin Gastroenterol 7:77, 1978.
204. Prata A: Schistosomiasis mansoni. Clin Gastroenterol 7:49, 1978.
205. Boley SJ, Schwartz S, Lash J, Sternhill V: Reversible vascular occlusion of the colon. Surg Gynecol Obstet 116:53, 1963.
206. Goligher JC, Lee PWG, Simpkins KC, Lintott DJ: A controlled comparison of one- and two-layer techniques of suture for high and low colorectal anastomoses. Br J Surg 64:609, 1977.
207. Jonsell G, Edelmann G: Single-layer anastomosis of the colon: a review of 165 cases. Am J Surg 135:630, 1978.
208. Schrock TR, Deveney CW, Dunphy JE: Factors contributing to leakage of colonic anastomoses. Ann Surg 177:513, 1973.
209. Morgenstern L, Yamakawa T, Ben-Shoshan M, Lippman H: Anastomotic leakage after low colonic anastomosis: clinical and experimental aspects. Am J Surg 123:104, 1972.
210. Debas HT, Thomson FB: A critical review of colectomy with anastomosis. Surg Gynecol Obstet 135:747, 1972.
211. Irvin TT, Goligher JC: Aetiology of disruption of intestinal anastomoses. Br J Surg 60:461, 1973.
212. Dunphy JE: The cut gut. Am J Surg 119:1, 1970.
213. Fazio VW: Sump suction and irrigation of the presacral space. Dis Colon Rectum 21:401, 1978.
214. Crowley LG, Anders CJ, Nelsen T, Bagshaw M: Effect of radiation on canine intestinal anastomoses. Arch Surg 96:423, 1968.
215. Condon RE, Wittmann DH: The use of antibiotics in general surgery. Curr Probl Surg 28:893, 1991.
216. Goligher JC, Morris C, McAdam WAF, et al: A controlled trial of inverting versus everting intestinal suture in clinical large-bowel surgery. Br J Surg 57:817, 1970.
217. Cofer TW, Ray JE, Gathright JB Jr: Does neostigmine cause disruption of large intestinal anastomoses? A negative answer. Dis Colon Rectum 17:235, 1974.
218. Goldsmith HS: Protection of low rectal anastomosis with intact omentum. Surg Gynecol Obstet 144:584, 1977.
219. McLachlin AD, Denton DW: Omental protection of intestinal anastomoses. Am J Surg 125:134, 1973.
220. Balz J, Samson RB, Stewart WRC: Rectal-tube decompression in left colectomy. Dis Colon Rectum 21:94, 1978.
221. Crowson WN, Wilson CS: An experimental study of the effects of drains on colon anastomoses. Am Surg 39:597, 1973.
222. Cooney DR, Wassner JD, Grossfeld JL, Jesseph JE: Are elemental diets useful in bowel preparation? Arch Surg 109:206, 1974.
223. Hewitt J, Rigby J, Reeve J, Cox AG: Whole-gut irrigation in preparation for large-bowel surgery. Lancet 2:337, 1973.
224. Crapp AR, Powis SJA, Tillotson P, et al: Preparation of the bowel by whole gut irrigation. Lancet 2:1239, 1975.
225. Davis GR, Santa Ana CA, Morawski SG, Fordtran JS: Development of a lavage solution associated with minimal water and electrolyte absorption or secretion. Gastroenterology 78:991, 1980.
226. Dickman MD, Chappelka AR, Schaedler RW: Evaluation of gut microflora during administration of an elemental diet in a patient with an ileoproctostomy. Am J Dig Dis 20:377, 1975.
227. Poth EJ: Intestinal antisepsis in surgery. JAMA 153:1516, 1953.
228. Nichols RL, Condon RE: Preoperative preparation of the colon. Surg Gynecol Obstet 132:323, 1971.
229. Nichols RL, Condon RE, Gorbach SL, Nyhus LM: Efficacy of preoperative antimicrobial preparation of the bowel. Ann Surg 176:227, 1972.
230. Nichols RL, Broido P, Condon RE, et al: Effect of preoperative neomycin-erythromycin intestinal preparation on the incidence of infectious complications following colon surgery. Ann Surg 178:453, 1973.
231. Arabi Y, Dimock F, Burdon DW, et al: Influence of bowel preparation and antimicrobials on colonic microflora. Br J Surg 65:555, 1978.
232. Miles AA, Miles EM, Burke J: The value and duration of defence reactions of the skin to the primary lodgement of bacteria. Br J Exp Pathol 38:79, 1957.
233. Burke JF: The effective period of preventive antibiotic action in experimental incisions and dermal lesions. Surgery 50:161, 1961.
234. Polk HC, Miles AA: The decisive period in the primary infection of muscle by *Escherichia coli*. Br J Exp Pathol 54:99, 1973.
235. Stone HH, Hooper CA, Kolb LD, et al: Antibiotic prophylaxis in gastric biliary and colonic surgery. Ann Surg 184:443, 1976.
236. Griffiths DA, Shorey BA, Simpson RA, et al: Single-dose preoperative antibiotic prophylaxis in gastrointestinal surgery. Lancet 2:325, 1976.
237. Downing R, McLeish AR, Burdon DW, et al: Duration of systemic prophylactic antibiotic cover

against anaerobic sepsis in intestinal surgery. Dis Colon Rectum 20:401, 1977.
238. Stone HH, Haney BB, Kolb LK, et al: Prophylactic and preventive antibiotic therapy: timing, duration and economics. Ann Surg 189:691, 1979.
239. Goransson G, Nilsson-Ehle I, Olson S-A, et al: Single versus multiple dose doxycycline prophylaxis in elective colorectal surgery. Acta Chir Scand I 50:245, 1984.
240. Roland M, Bergan T, Bjerkset T, et al: Prophylactic regimens in colorectal surgery: comparisons between metronidazole used alone or with ampicillin for one or three days. World J Surg 9:626, 1985.
241. Condon RE, Bartlett JG, Nichols RL, et al: Preoperative prophylactic cephalothin fails to control septic complications of colorectal operations: results of controlled clinical trial. Am J Surg 137:68, 1979.
242. Figueras-Felip J, Basilio-Bonet E, Lara-Eisman F, et al: Oral is superior to systemic antibiotic prophylaxis in operations upon the colon and rectum. Surg Gynecol Obstet 158:359, 1984.
243. Yates JL: An experimental study of the local effects of peritoneal drainage. Am Surg 21:1048, 1955.
244. Agrama HM, Blackwood JM, Brown CS, et al: Functional longevity of intraperitoneal drains: an experimental evaluation. Am J Surg 132:418, 1976.
245. Stone HH, Hooper CA, Millikan WJ: Abdominal drainage following appendectomy and cholecystectomy. Ann Surg 187:606, 1978.
246. Stonc HH, Hester TR: Incisional and peritoneal infection after emergency celiotomy. Ann Surg 177:669, 1973.
247. Berliner SD, Burson LC, Lear PE: Use and abuse of intraperitoneal drains in colon surgery. Arch Surg 89:686, 1964.

Appendicitis

CHAPTER 44

Russell A. Williams, Samuel E. Wilson

The appendix ranks as knave among the abdominal organs, having no important function, yet attracting surgical attention most commonly of them all.

The first reported appendectomy was done in 1735, by Claudius Amyand at St. George's Hospital, London.[1,2] In addition to being the founder of St. George's Hospital, he was Sergeant Surgeon to Queen Ann, George I, and George II, and his description of this case was published in *Philosophical Transactions of the Royal Society*. The patient, a 12-year-old boy, had a long-standing scrotal hernia and fecal fistula of the thigh. The appendix was surrounded by omentum and perforated by a pin, forming the fecal fistula.

In 1886, Reginald Ritz, Professor of Pathological Anatomy at Harvard University, presented his classical contribution on appendicitis entitled "Perforating Inflammation of the Vermiform Appendix; with Special Reference to Its Early Diagnosis and Treatment."[3] He made the point that most inflammatory disease of the right lower quadrant begins in the appendix, and substantiated his belief, opposed to contemporary thinking, that early typhlitis and paratyphlitic abscess were the same disease. He suggested that the more precise term appendicitis should be used to describe them. The mortality for appendicitis at the time of his presentation was 26 percent.

Charles McBurney of New York and Frederick Treves of London fathered the method we use today for treatment of appendicitis. In 1889, each recommended independently that removal of the diseased appendix was comparatively safe and preferable for treating appendicitis.[4,5] An editorial in *Annals of Surgery* that year cautioned against widespread adoption of this practice, yet hailed it as a significant advance in the treatment of appendicitis[6]: "A very grave responsibility, therefore, must be attached to the surgeon in any given case in deciding upon laparotomy and excision of the appendix. It is evident it could only be proper for one who was a perfect master of aseptic abdominal technique to offer such a procedure as less dangerous than the policy of delay and palliation." By the early part of this century numerous cases of appendicitis had been described.

The average hospital mortality rate for appendicitis when reviewed by Murphy, in the 1920s, was 10 percent. At present, the mortality rate for appendicitis is 0.8 percent, with most deaths occurring in patients older than 50 years of age and some in young patients.

Anatomy. The appendix is a 5- to 10-cm finger-like outpouching from the cecum with its base attached to the cecum at the confluence of the taenia coli as they continue onto it, forming a complete longitudinal outer muscle layer. Its lumenal diameter is small, averaging about 7 mm.

The appendix arises at a fairly constant site on the cecum, but its position in the abdomen varies with that of the cecum; the body of the appendix may be located behind the cecum (retrocecal), in the iliac fossa or pelvis, or in a paracecal or paraileal position.

The appendix artery courses near the free edge of the mesoappendix to reach the appendix tip; the veins drain into the portal venous system, and its epithelium is similar to that of the colon, containing tubular glands and crypts of Lieberkühn. Lymphoid tissue is prominent in the submucosal and mucosal layers of the appendix, accounting for more than half of the cross-sectional area in the younger patient. With age this diminishes, and it is barely seen in the later stages of life. At birth there are only meager quantities of lymphoid tissue present, but these increase and are most well developed during the early teens.

Pathogenesis. The appendix is an attenuation of the cecum and, like it and the remainder of the colon, has an abundant bacterial flora within its lumen. Modestly sized aggregates of fecal material or hypertrophy of the lymphoid tissue in its wall will encroach significantly on the small lumen, producing occlusion and distal stasis. Bacterial multiplication continues and, coupled with continued mucosal secretion, results in a rapid rise of intralumenal pressure. Progressive venous obstruction follows, leading to thrombosis of the appendix artery, an end artery, and ischemia and gangrene of the appendix.

Mechanical obstruction is most often produced by a fecalith impacting at the appendix base. Fecaliths are concretions of fecal material found in about 40 percent of patients with simple acute appendicitis, whereas in patients with rupture of a gangrenous appendix this increases to about 90 percent. Appendiceal obstruction may also be produced by hypertrophy of the abundant intramural lymphoid aggregates, possibly stimulated to hypertrophy by an intercurrent viral infection. This gives credence to the often repeated but anecdotal observation that there is a *seasonal incidence* or *epidemics* of appendicitis, in addition to the association between an attack of rubella followed by appendicitis. Each may be the clinical symptom resulting from passage of a particular virus through the community at the time.[7] Less frequently, obstruction results from vegetable material, intestinal worms, or ingested foreign bodies. In other cases it may be a tumor, with appendicitis bringing to light an adenocarcinoma of the cecum or carcinoid of the appendix that has encroached on the lumen.

In the stagnant environment of early appendicitis, organism numbers increase, greatly enhancing their virulence, with invasion of the partly ischemic appendix wall; thus, infective appendicitis develops. The inflammation spreads through the appendix wall to the serosa, and histologic examination will show submucosal edema and congestion of the vessels, with bacteria in the wall of the appendix, an infiltration of white blood cells, and ulceration of the appendix mucosa, termed acute catarrhal or focal appendicitis.

The inflammatory exudate developing with appendicitis accumulates in the peritoneal cavity adjacent to the appendix. In the same area local peritonitis develops; however, the fluid cultured from this region is usually sterile in the early stages of appendicitis.

While the foregoing evolves, the omentum is stimulated to envelop the inflamed appendix, tending to mechanically localize the inflammatory process and any abscess that may develop. One of the earliest operative findings may be amassing of omentum around the appendix.

With unremitting appendiceal obstruction the intralumenal pressure continues to rise, and the appendix itself enlarges from the inflammatory swelling of its walls and the accumulation of pus. On microscopic examination, pus is seen in its walls and lumen; this is termed acute suppurative appendicitis. Acute gangrenous appendicitis develops when infarction occurs. The infarcted areas allow relatively unimpeded passage of the infected material into the adjacent peritoneal cavity, finally detaching or rupturing; this stage of the disease is termed perforated or ruptured appendicitis. The appendix tip (part most remote from the blood supply) and the wall overlying the fecalith (due to pressure necrosis) are the sites most likely to become gangrenous and rupture.

Obstructive appendicitis is a form of closed loop bowel obstruction; untreated, there is perforation with periappendiceal abscess formation. In otherwise healthy patients, the process is usually localized by developing inflammatory adhesions and by the omentum. In those who are malnourished or elderly, or in very young children with a poorly formed omentum, however, the inflammation is not so well contained and infected colonic contents may disseminate widely throughout the peritoneal cavity, establishing generalized fecal peritonitis. Uncommonly, in some patients without any of the previous conditions, obstructive appendicitis may progress so rapidly that early perforation occurs before localization by these potential mechanisms.

Some patients, particularly those with more

advanced appendicitis and generalized peritonitis, develop abscesses at other sites within the abdomen, commonly in the pelvic or right subphrenic spaces. Prior to treatment of appendicitis by early operation, a not uncommon complication was portal pylephlebitis when the venous spread of the infection to the liver resulted in liver abscesses. Although rare today, this was once the commonest cause of liver abscesses.

Spontaneous resolution of appendicitis, rather than unrelenting progression to gangrenous rupture, does occur, presumably through relief of the intralumenal pressure as it dislodges the fecalith or overcomes only partial obstruction of the lumen, discharging the infected appendix contents into the cecum before ischemia and gangrene develop. In these patients the appendix may later appear partly fibrotic, kinked, or involved in adhesions. Fitz[3] concluded that resolution of appendicitis occurs in about one-third of the patients with perforated appendicitis, but he cautioned that it is imprudent to delay operation in expectation of this. He also noted that 11 percent of patients had recurrent symptoms of appendicitis, and suggested that appendectomy would have been better done during an earlier episode of milder appendicitis. A review of 1000 cases of appendicitis treated in the last decade found that 9 percent of patients had experienced a previous similar clinical illness and 4 percent had this illness on more than one occasion.[8]

Epidemiology. Appendicitis is the most common acute surgical condition of the abdomen, and is estimated to afflict 1 in 700 of the population each year.[9] It occurs at any age, but is rare in patients under 3 or over 50 years of age. Men are affected in the ratio of 3 to 2 women; and 70 percent of patients are under 30 years of age.

There has been a fall in the incidence of appendicitis during the last four decades, mostly during the first of these decades. In part, it may be due to the more accurate preoperative diagnosis, as one study showed appendicitis was confirmed microscopically in 73 percent of cases reviewed in 1951 compared with 52 percent in 1941.[10] Another explanation is a change in composition of the Western diet in which more roughage is being consumed. Burkitt[11] believes that the high fiber contained in the diets of native Africans accounts for the very low incidence of acute appendicitis in these people.

Bacteriology. The flora of an inflamed appendix is polymicrobial, consisting mostly of anaerobic organisms particularly of the bacteroides species. *Escherichia coli* and *Streptococcus* are the most common aerobic flora. The peritoneal fluid around an inflamed appendix grows bacteria in about half the patients. *Bacteroides* is found in 78 percent of these cultures, and organisms are most likely to be isolated in perforated appendicitis (80 percent of cases).[12]

Sepsis in sites remote from the inflamed appendix is more likely to develop with the more severe types of appendicitis (ie, more often with perforated than with simple acute appendicitis). The organisms cultured from these abscesses are similar to those cultured from fluid and pus in the inflamed appendix.

Aschoff, the 19th century pathologist, maintained that appendicitis was a specific bacterial disease resulting from infection by the enterococcus type B of Gundel. *Yersinia enterocolitica* and *S. milleri* have more recently been suggested to be specific organisms causing acute appendicitis in an occasional patient.

Clinical Manifestations. Pain, nausea or vomiting, abdominal sensitivity, and fever (usually appearing in that order) are a sound basis for the diagnosis of appendicitis.[4] Pain is present in about 99 percent of the patients. It is commonly of sudden onset, located in the periumbilical or epigastric areas, and colicky, especially in patients with obstructive appendicitis. Early in the disease the pain is only moderately severe. After 6 hours or so it moves to the right lower abdominal quadrant and becomes constant rather than colicky, at the same time increasing in severity. The initial, diffuse, milder, colicky pain in the midline is visceral in origin, being transmitted by visceral afferent nerves stimulated by inflammation and distention of the appendix. As the inflammation spreads from the mucosa through the appendix wall, the adjacent somatically innervated peritoneum is inflamed and stimulated, and the poorly localized visceral character of pain changes, now felt in the area adjacent to the inflamed appendix, and becoming more constant and severe.

Anorexia is reported by most patients, and nausea and vomiting by about three-quarters of them. Vomiting is usually not marked and does not appear before the pain. Many patients relate these early symptoms to a recent dietary indiscretion, describing them as a *liverish attack* or *stomach flu*.

Constipation is usual, but diarrhea does occur in some cases, particularly in children, and also when the inflamed appendix lies in contact with the ileum, where it can cause a local enteritis. Later in the disease, mucous diarrhea usually heralds formation of a pelvic abscess, which irritates the overlying rectal mucosa, stimulating secretion of large amounts of mucus. Diarrhea may confuse the physician, who wrongly diagnoses gastroenteritis in a patient who has appendicitis. It nearly always indicates extension of the inflammation beyond the appendix.

The abdomen is usually not tender in early appendicitis. Tenderness is found with periappendiceal peritonitis, at about the same time as the colicky, visceral pain changes into the constant, severe pain in the right lower quadrant of the abdomen. Usually the tenderness is located at McBurney's point, which "when one examines with the fingertips is in adults one and one-half to two inches inside the right anterior spinous process on a line drawn to the umbilicus."[4]

Other clinical findings on examination of the patient relate to differences in location of the inflamed appendix. In the retrocecal position, the appendix is cushioned from the examiner's finger by the gas-filled cecum and ascending colon, reducing the expected degree of tenderness. In these patients there may be more tenderness in the right flank extending posteriorly. If the inflamed appendix lies on the ileopsoas or obturator muscles, manipulation of the leg by passively stretching these muscles produces pain (the psoas or obturator sign). Rectal or vaginal examination elicits tenderness when the inflamed appendix lies in contact with these organs, usually on their right side. Palpation and compression of the sigmoid colon in the left lower quadrant of the abdomen may cause the complaint of concomitant pain in the right lower quadrant as the column of gas in the colon is compressed, distending the cecum and inflamed base of the appendix (Rovsing's sign). In some patients the foregoing signs may have no accompanying anterior abdominal tenderness.

At times, a phlegmonous appendix mass is felt in the right lower quadrant, formed by appendiceal and periappendiceal inflammatory swelling, amassing of the omentum in response to the inflammation, and, in some patients, a collection of purulent material. The mass is usually tender and may not be appreciated when the patient is first examined because of protective muscle guarding, only becoming evident under anesthesia. Although the mass may contain pus, its size is not related to the amount of pus present. With large abscesses, fluctuation or even crepitus may be found in the overlying abdominal tissues late in the course of the disease. Should an abscess form, it is usually in the right iliac fossa, and it may point onto the skin of the loin, flank, or abdomen, or enlarge downward into the pelvis. With the latter, rectal examination confirms its presence through a bulging of the anterior wall of the rectum by the tender, often fluctuant mass, in addition to mucous diarrhea.

With free perforation of the appendix and fecal peritonitis, the tenderness relates to the extent of involvement of the peritoneal cavity, therefore in advanced cases there may be guarding or even board-like rigidity over the entire anterior abdominal wall. With careful examination, however, it may be possible to detect that the tenderness is most severe in the right lower quadrant.

Bowel sounds are usually present in the earlier stages of the disease, but with extension of the peritonitis these disappear and paralytic ileus distends the abdomen.

With early appendicitis, the patient's temperature is only slightly above normal, but as peritonitis or an abscess develops, it usually rises to about 38C to 38.5C and may take on a *spiking* pattern. A high body temperature early in the course of suspected appendicitis is unusual, and other diagnoses should be considered.

As with any acute inflammatory abdominal condition, a neutrophil leukocytosis is seen, usually with a mean count of 15,000 white blood cells/mm^3, with no reliable differences in level or pattern that correlate with the severity of the appendicitis. A sudden large increase in the white blood cell count, accompanied by other symptoms, however, usually indicates the onset of extensive peritonitis.

The urine may contain white cells and some red cells, but not a significant number of organisms, when the inflamed appendix is in contact with part of the urinary tract, particularly the right ureter or dome of the bladder. Large numbers of bacteria in the urine indicate a probable urinary tract infection.

Appendicitis is a clinical diagnosis, and is not usually made radiologically. *Abdominal radiographs* can be useful in excluding other diseases, such as renal colic or a perforated peptic ulcer, where the clinical findings may be similar to acute appendicitis. On plain film, in patients with appendicitis, air-fluid levels may be seen in loops of the small bowel in the right lower quadrant (the sentinel loop), and there may be an increase in soft tissue density in the iliac area, a blurred distal psoas shadow, or with bacterial invasion, gas in the appendix or adjacent tissues.[13,14] An appendolith or gas-filled appendix with the proper history and physical findings usually indicates gangrenous appendicitis.

Barium enema or *barium swallow* have been useful in diagnosing appendicitis, particularly in equivocal cases in adults and children or when the patient has another serious illness, such as leukemia.[15,16] With the latter, every effort is made to avoid the much higher risks associated with an unnecessary operation. The corollary, however, is that not making the diagnosis of appendicitis is a very serious error in these patients. The study is done without preparation of the colon, by instilling barium with no external manipulation or pressure. Findings that indicate appendicitis include no filling of the appendix (Fig. 44–1), which may also be seen in 20 to 30 percent of healthy persons, or partial filling of the root of the appendix only, persistent extrinsic deformity of the cecal wall, or displacement of the terminal ileum by an extrinsic inflammatory mass (Fig. 44–2) or the outlining of an abscess cavity. Complete filling of the appendix with no abnormalities of the mucosa or the appendix contour makes the diagnosis of appendicitis unlikely. About 5 percent of patients with this picture do have appendicitis, however, and ultimately, the decision to operate is based on the patient's clinical condition.

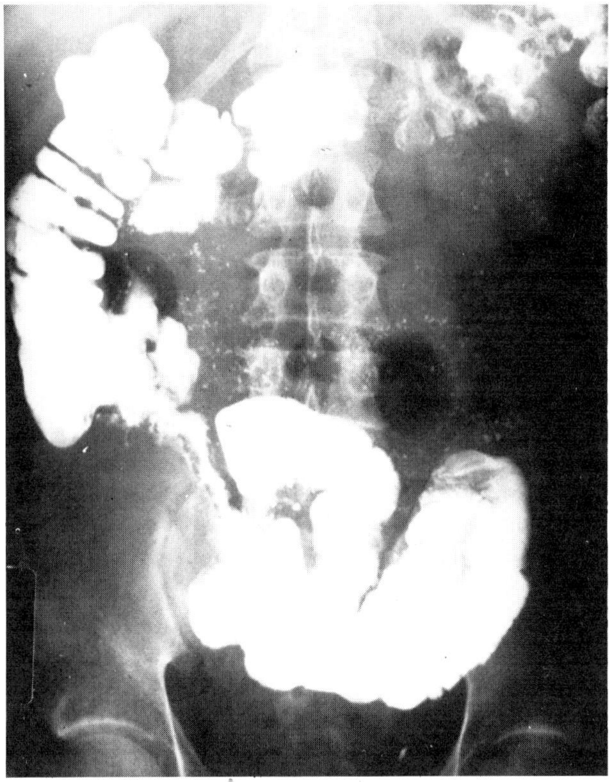

Figure 44–2. An appendix abscess deforming the terminal ileum, with barium outlining the abscess cavity adjacent to ileocecal angle.

ULTRASONOGRAPHY

Ultrasonography in experienced hands can improve the diagnostic accuracy of acute appendicitis and aid in determining the etiology of right lower quadrant abdominal pain due to causes other than appendicitis. The ultrasound scan appearance of acute appendicitis is characterized by visualization of a noncompressible aperistaltic appendix presenting with a "target-like" cross-sectional view due to the different echogenicity of inflammatory thickened wall layers and a tubular appearance with a blind tip on longitudinal scan. There is a widespread spectrum of echomorphologic appearances of abscesses associated with ruptured appendicitis.

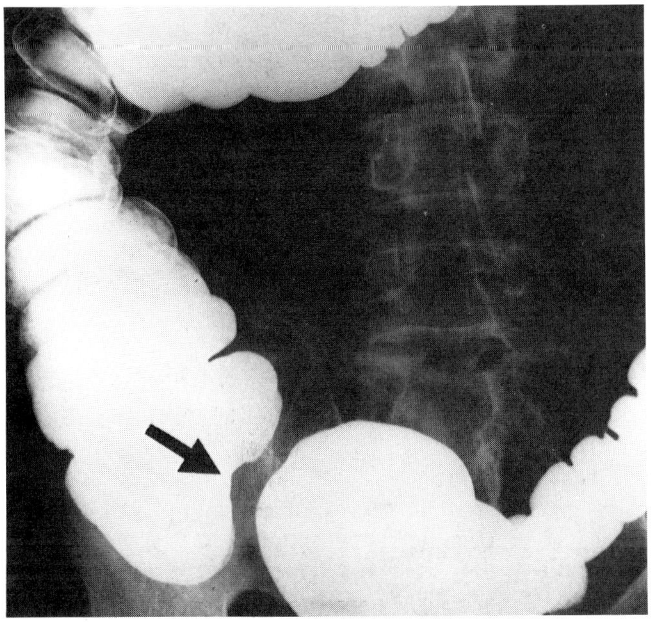

Figure 44–1. The appendix is not seen, and there is a persistent cecal deformity in a patient with a 4-day history of lower abdominal pain. He had very little tenderness and was found to have an appendix phlegmon at operation.

Ultrasound scan may be of assistance in patients where the diagnosis is unclear and is most useful in patients admitted with a diagnosis of "rule-out appendicitis." This may be a problem, particularly in women where other diagnoses such as a gynecologic disease may present with symptoms and signs suggestive of appendicitis. Ultrasonography should not be used as a screening test to rule out appendicitis as there are a significant number of false-negative studies. The diagnosis of appendicitis still remains clinical, supplemented in some cases with laboratory and radiologic studies.

Laparoscopy may also be useful in patients suspected of having appendicitis but in whom the clinical history or examination is equivocal and insufficient to establish the diagnosis.[17] This may constitute 10 to 15 percent of patients, who have features such as prolonged history and other intercurrent diseases, or who have been treated with antibiotics or other drugs such as steroids. With this technique the negative appendectomy rate was decreased from 10 to 1 percent. Laparoscopy, unlike barium enema, may reveal other conditions outside the bowel, such as leukemic infiltrates, mittelschmerz, tumor implants, torsion or rupture of an ovarian cyst, or salpingitis. The appendix must be seen through the laparoscope, otherwise laparotomy is required; hence operation is needed for all retrocecal inflamed or normal appendices. It is suggested that laparoscopy with this group of patients is cost effective and safer than a laparotomy.

Radionuclide studies using gallium-67 or indium-111 labeled autologous leukocytes may aid in localizing an abscess in difficult clinical situations. These are most likely to be helpful in the patient who has not had an operation, as these nucleotides accumulate in sites of recent injury, such as the surgical wound and the appendix bed after recent appendectomy. Thus the technique may be useful to detect an abscess in a patient who initially presents with a fever of undetermined origin.

COMPUTED TOMOGRAPHY

In some patients with lower abdominal pain and tenderness but no nausea, vomiting, fever, or leukocytosis, computed tomography (CT) has been useful in determining the underlying cause of the symptoms. The number of patients that fall into this category varies but in one study it was approximately 20 percent of patients operated on for acute appendicitis during the study. The diagnosis of acute appendicitis is made with CT scan if the appendix is visualized with cross and longitudinal axis as a small tubular structure 4 to 20 mm (outer diameter) and usually fluid filled. Other abnormalities seen on CT scan may be a combination of localized inflammatory changes and a phlegmon or abscess in a pericecal or retrocolic location, which is often accompanied by a calcified appendicolith.

VARIATIONS IN THE ELDERLY, THE YOUNG, AND THE PREGNANT PATIENT

In the elderly and the young, a surgeon is far more likely to find a ruptured appendix at operation. In collected series of hospital patients, the rate of perforation of the appendix varies from 10 to 37 percent. In two United States series, each with about 1000 patients, the perforation rate was 27 percent at a large public hospital (San Francisco General)[8] and 19 percent for patients in a health maintenance organization (Kaiser Foundation Hospital, Los Angeles).[18] At San Francisco General, patients under 10 years of age and over 50 years of age had perforation rates of 39 and 65 percent respectively. In the Kaiser study, 77 percent of perforated appendices occurred in patients younger than 15 or older than 35.

The reasons for this higher rate of perforation are not clear. Less than 10 percent of operations for acute appendicitis are done on patients over 60 years of age; however, the majority of deaths due to appendicitis occur in this group. The mortality rate in older patients, derived from seven large series, was 6 percent, with a perforation rate that varied from 32 to 74 percent.[19] In the elderly, the appendix is often narrowed or even partly obliterated with atrophy of its lymphoid tissue, accompanied by atherosclerosis of the blood vessels, but these characteristics do not adequately explain their different clinical course. Older patients with intra-abdominal sepsis usually manifest fewer symptoms and a lower white cell count with a less marked febrile response. Pain and tenderness are no less frequent, however, and an awareness that perforation is more likely to occur in the older patient should lead to operation without delay once appendicitis is thought to be present. Unfortunately, there is often a delay averaging 58 hours before medical treatment is sought, which correlates with the higher incidence of rupture. In addition, over half of the elderly patients have taken cathartics, and about 40 percent have other coexistent serious illnesses.[20]

In children there is a 30 to 50 percent incidence of appendix perforation, which rises to 85 percent in infants. After perforation, the infection rapidly contaminates the peritoneal cavity, probably because the poorly developed omentum in infants is unable to contain it.[21] In children with ruptured appendices, the mortality is not necessarily high, overall being less than 1 percent, with the majority occurring in patients less than 6 years of age. Of this group, most of the deaths occur in infants under 2 years of age.[22]

In children, the physician is often hindered in making the diagnosis of appendicitis because of the child's inability to complain or give a coherent history, particularly the very young child. Crying and straining, in addition, make interpretation of physical signs difficult. Often it is the mother who notes that something is wrong because the infant refuses feedings, vomits, or clutches the abdomen. If the child is older, he or she may complain of abdominal pain. In any case, most mothers will have a suspicion that their child has a sore abdomen. The most common presenting complaints in children under 2 years of age are fever, vomiting, diarrhea, and distention, whereas in children over 2 years of age, the complaints are pain, nausea, vomiting, and anorexia.

Once the physician has gained the confidence of the sick child, an unhurried, gentle examination of the abdomen may reveal tenderness and muscle guarding localized in the right lower quadrant. It is important that the physician look for disease elsewhere, especially in the lungs, throat, and ears, and for the signs of meningitis. These infections may all present with abdominal manifestations similar to those of appendicitis.

As with adults, there are no distinct radiographic signs of appendicitis; however, ileus or a fecalith suggests that the disease process is in the abdomen and not one of the other organ systems. Barium enema is often quite nondiagnostic, and the burden of proof of the diagnosis rests on the clinical examination and the patient's history.

Appendicitis is the most frequent extrauterine surgical complication in the pregnant woman. Understandably, the symptoms of appendicitis will very likely be attributed to changes that occur with the pregnancy, and hence treatment will be delayed. Abdominal pain, particularly in the right lower quadrant, is considered the most reliable symptom of appendicitis during pregnancy.[23] The most constant complaint in the pregnant patient with appendicitis is of a vague pain in the right side of the abdomen. In the latter part of the pregnancy, when the appendix has risen above the iliac crest level, pain and tenderness are more likely to be in the right upper quadrant or the flank, rather than in the iliac fossa. Anorexia is usually not the pathognomonic symptom, as it is in other patients.

Urinary tract infections develop commonly in pregnancy, and the finding of fever and bacteruria, with accompanying vague abdominal or flank pain, may result in appendicitis being overlooked. A urinary infection is confirmed by urinalysis and culture. The leukocytosis of pregnancy, where normal white blood cell counts may be as high as 15,000, can confuse the clinician.

In the early part of this century, maternal and fetal mortality were 24 and 40 percent, respectively; with peritonitis the fetal mortality increased to about 80 percent. At present, maternal death is rare (less than 1 percent) and fetal loss is about 9 percent with simple appendicitis, rising to 36 percent in those with peritonitis.[24]

APPENDICITIS IN PATIENTS WITH HUMAN IMMUNODEFICIENCY VIRUS (HIV) INFECTION

The presentation of acute appendicitis in patients with AIDS/HIV infection is not different from that in nonimmunocompromised patients except there may be a lack of the usual increase in white blood cell (WBC) count.[25] Some AIDS patients with bacterial appendicitis may have an apparently normal WBC count when first seen, but in reality this WBC count is much elevated over their baseline relative leukopenia. Drug prophylaxis may result in the WBC count elevation, showing a relative neutropenia. A relative leukocytosis is an important finding and in some patients an increase in the WBC count from that found at a previous recent examination may be a significant observation even though both counts are within normal limits.[26]

The etiology of right lower quadrant pain in AIDS patients is sometimes difficult to determine, particularly to know if it is a complication of the AIDS itself or in fact is appendicitis. Most AIDS patients are young men who are also the group most likely to develop bacterial peritonitis unrelated to their HIV infection.[27–29]

Some patients with AIDS may develop a specific AIDS-related appendicitis, different from the usual suppurative bacterial peritonitis. In these patients cytomegalovirus (CMV) is typically the inciting infective agent, or, alternatively, the appendix has been involved with Kaposi's sarcoma. Because CMV colitis primarily affects the right colon, CMV appendicitis is not an unexpected development and is possibly more frequent than the absence of published reports suggests. There are no preoperative signs or symptoms that are statistically useful in differentiating AIDS-related appendicitis from routine suppurative appendicitis.

Typically, a non-HIV-infected patient with symptoms and signs suggesting appendicitis is operated on within 6 hours of admission, whereas a patient who has AIDS or HIV infection with similar symptoms and signs, again suggesting appendicitis, often incurs considerable delay before operation. In these patients there is concern that the acute disease is related to AIDS, possibly due to an opportunistic infection for which treatment is antimicrobial therapy, not operation. This delay may result in patients with AIDS/HIV having a more advanced stage of acute appendicitis with a higher incidence of perforation and subsequently an increased rate of complications.

Earlier, accurate diagnosis of appendicitis in patients with AIDS/HIV may be facilitated by using diagnostic laparoscopy.

Diagnosis. Laparoscopy is an effective means for diagnosing acute appendicitis in patients with borderline or early symptoms and furthermore can be used to perform appendectomy. A prospective randomized trial comparing the open and laparoscopic techniques for appendectomy found the in-hospital stay for laparoscopy was 2 days versus 3 days for the open technique ($p < 0.1$), the median operating time was 61 minutes for laparoscopic and 51 minutes for open appendectomy (not significant). In addition, there were no episodes of wound infection, acute urinary retention, or paralytic ileus in patients undergoing laparoscopy. There was one wound infection, two episodes of acute urinary retention, and one episode of paralytic ileus in patients undergoing an open appendectomy.

Because laparoscopy can be used for both diagnosis and treatment, it offers several advantages compared with the traditional approach to diagnosis and the treatment of appendicitis. Those with minimal physical findings can undergo direct visualization of the appendix with early appendectomy, bringing the progression of inflammation to an early termination and preventing perforation. Furthermore, patients with ambiguous signs are spared the additional delay and expense required for a further diagnostic work-up. Laparoscopy in these patients provides an early diagnosis of appendicitis or another condition. If open operation is required, the patient can then be explored through an incision made appropriately over the underlying disease.

Treatment. Acute appendicitis is treated by removal of the inflamed appendix. If this is done before perforation and peritoneal contamination occur, the patient will very likely have a short hospital stay of 3.5 days.[8] The average hospital stay for all patients with appendicitis is 5.4, rising to 10.2 in those with a ruptured or perforated appendix.[30]

Delay before removing the appendix, particularly in elderly and very young patients, results in perforation, which in many cases leads to other septic complications, particularly of the wound, or to localized and generalized peritonitis and abscesses.

Antimicrobial agents should not be administered in a mistaken attempt to cure the disease. These agents will only obscure the clinical features by dampening the inflammatory reaction and, in fact, result in further delay. Antimicrobials, however, are used to limit the extension of cellulitis surrounding the inflamed appendix and to control development of peritonitis and septicemia. In addition, they have been shown to lower wound infection rates. Antimicrobial agents to be considered for treatment of appendicitis should be effective against anaerobes and aerobes, particularly *Bacteroides* and *E. coli.* A popular regimen has been the use of an aminoglycoside, such as gentamicin, together with an antianaerobic agent. There are other antimicrobials that cover these bacterial flora, however, including the second- and third-generation cephalosporins and the extended spectrum penicillins. Metronidazole or clindamycin are alternative choices for an anaerobic antimicrobial agent.[31]

In patients diagnosed as having appendicitis, perioperative antibiotics are generally used, the first dose given immediately before operation to ensure that effective blood and tissue levels are present at the time of potential contamination during the operation. Two further doses are usually given if unruptured appendicitis is found. If the appendix is ruptured and abscesses are present, the agents are continued until there is clinical evidence that the sepsis has been eradicated, usually when the patient is afebrile and has a WBC count that has returned to less than 12,000 cells/mm^3.

A *periappendiceal abscess* is usually treated by surgical drainage, and develops in about 2 percent of patients with acute appendicitis, compared with 21 percent of patients 40 years ago.[32] In some of these patients, abscess drainage alone may be the only initial surgical treatment, particularly if the appendix cannot be easily removed because it is situated in the midst of dense inflammatory adhesions that would require forceful dissection to liberate it. This dissection could contaminate the remainder of the peritoneal cavity or result in large amounts of bleeding, and has a high likelihood of producing traumatic perforation of the bowel, particularly the cecum or terminal ileum, leading to a fecal fistula formation.

A 3 to 5 percent mortality rate is associated with appendix abscess if reports combined over the last 50 years are considered. These figures are biased by older results, however, and in the last decade,[32–34] the mortality for operative treatment has been reduced to about 1 percent.

An abscess may be associated with a palpable appendix mass; features suggesting to the surgeon that pus is present include symptoms for longer than 48 hours, a temperature higher than 39C, and no signs of generalized peritonitis.

In some patients, appendix abscesses have been drained percutaneously, using computed tomography or ultrasonography to guide placement of the catheter.[35] This technique precludes removal of the appendix and avoids an operation, although the catheter may penetrate the bowel and produce an enteric fistula, which may require prolonged catheter drainage but usually spontaneously closes. Criteria for effective treatment are that the patient feels well and has a decrease in temperature within 12 hours after treatment. If this does not occur, a repeat scan is done to reassess the disease, particularly to identify a previously undefined abscess. Antibiotics are administered concurrently.[36]

If the appendix is not removed, the patient may develop recurrent appendicitis in 10 to 20 percent of cases.[37] In addition, those few cases of appendicitis associated with an obstructing carcinoma or carcinoid are inadequately treated by simple abscess drainage. To avoid these problems, *interval* or *à froid* appendectomy some months later, when the inflammation has resolved, is usually advised. At that time, operation is usually easier and safer than when the patient is first treated. If interval appendectomy is not undertaken, patients over 40 years of age who have had an abscess drained are studied by barium enema or colonoscopy.

Generalized peritonitis is the most serious complication of appendicitis, and not uncommonly leads to septicemia and intraperitoneal abscess formation. Patients with generalized peritonitis are initially treated with intravenous fluids and antimicrobial agents. If septic shock has developed, this treatment resuscitates the patient and is continued until hemodynamic abnormalities are corrected, or at least stabilized. At this stage, the perforated appendix, being the source of sepsis and focus for its continuation, is removed by operation.

Wound infection is the most frequent cause of morbidity in appendicitis. It occurs in over 50 percent of patients with perforated appendicitis, and in about 5 to 15 percent of patients with acute or gangrenous appendicitis, respectively. Removal of the normal appendix is associated with a wound infection rate of 1.4 to 4.5 percent, which is higher than that for clean operations (1 to 3 percent).[31,38]

Wound infections are rarely lethal, but prolong the patient's hospital stay. Occasionally, synergistic gangrene develops in the confines of the closed infected appendectomy wound and is life threatening; it requires wide excision of the adjacent abdominal wall tissues to control its spread. In addition, high doses of penicillin are administered to eradicate the anaerobic streptococci, which is usually one of the causative organisms in this synergistic process.

To decrease the likelihood of an infection after appendectomy for perforated appendicitis, the wound may be managed by delayed primary closure, or may be deliberately left open to heal by secondary intention. With delayed primary closure, wound infection rates are reduced to less than 15 percent. If the wound heals by secondary intention and it is of the usual muscle splitting type with the skin incision in Langer's lines, it heals within 3 to 4 weeks with minimal scarring. Healing by secondary intention practically eliminates the likelihood of a closed wound abscess. Many antimicrobials, given systemically or topically, have been shown to significantly reduce the wound infection rate in patients with appendicitis.

Appendicitis presents with a palpable *appendix mass* in 11 to 13 percent of patients.[37] This mass, usually in the right iliac fossa, is composed of an aggregation of the omentum and edematous inflammatory tissue, and very effectively incarcerates the inflammation and any perforation from the adjacent peritoneal cavity, aiding the patient's own immunologic defenses to eradicate the sepsis. Upon finding an appendix mass in the right iliac fossa, if the patient is not septic, a trial of nonoperative treatment is worthwhile. During the 24 to 48 hours after discovery of the mass the patient is observed, especially for a rise in temperature or pulse, or for an increase in the size or tenderness of the mass. Any of these changes would suggest that the mass is in fact an evolving abscess and not a well-contained perforation or phlegmon. To avoid confusing the clinical picture, antimicrobial agents are not administered during this observation period. If the patient's physical signs and symptoms resolve, however, the treatment is continued, and 6 to 8 weeks after recovery an interval appendectomy is generally recommended.

Again, the argument against immediate appendectomy for the patient presenting with an appendiceal mass is that the infection may be disseminated and the edematous, friable bowel damaged, leading to fecal fistula formation. In some of these cases operated on early, a right hemicolectomy may have been performed on the mistaken notion that the mass was a malignant tumor; the converse situation is removal of only the appendix when a tumor is actually present. The risk for recurrent appendicitis in patients with an appendix mass is similar to that of patients with an appendix abscess that has been drained only.

When Reginald Fitz[3] published his paper, "Perforating Inflammation of the Vermiform Appendix;

with Special Reference to Its Early Diagnosis and Treatment," all patients with appendicitis had an abscess. Today, in patients with appendicitis there is still a correlation between the diagnostic accuracy and perforation so that among 14,000 patients a high diagnostic accuracy of 89 percent was found among those with the highest perforation rate of 29 percent, whereas the lowest diagnostic rate of 67 percent was found among patients with a 14 percent perforation rate. Thus the clinical picture becomes clearer as complications of appendicitis develop.

Quality of Care and Outcome Committees have the notion that an acceptable negative appendectomy rate may be as low as 10 and 15 percent for men and women, respectively. A more realistic level, however, has been suggested as 23 percent.[39]

The diagnostic accuracy for appendicitis in 444 patients among surgical trainees who had performed more than 25 appendectomies each increased with experience from 54 to 95 percent. The diagnosis was wrong twice as often in women compared with men and appendicitis was found in 70 percent of women and in 85 percent of men.[40]

The quest by surgeons for a high level of accuracy in the clinical diagnosis of acute appendicitis has resulted in the development of many predictive scoring systems such as the Alvarado Score, in which the clinical symptoms and signs are summed and weighed to give a number that suggests a high or low probability of the patient having appendicitis.[41] Along similar lines the "appendix index" was developed using logistic regression analysis. These indices, which have included computer-aided diagnostic systems, formalize the analytic process every clinician uses in deciding the likelihood of a patient having appendicitis and are of little practical value.[42] Utilization of conventional radiographic examinations such as the plain x-ray and barium enema, computed tomography, WBC scanning techniques, ultrasonography, and laparoscopy can each be helpful in increasing diagnostic accuracy in selected clinical situations.

The incidence of finding a *normal appendix on exploration for appendicitis,* or *the negative appendectomy rate,* varies from 5 to 20 percent. It is thought that a percentage of negative findings with appendectomy must be accepted, otherwise, the rate of perforation, with consequent complications, will be considerably increased and attempts to further lower the negative appendectomy rates will fail to diagnose appendicitis in some cases.[43,44]

For this practice to be acceptable, the mortality rate associated with a negative laparotomy has to be practically nonexistent, as it is. This is weighed against the much higher morbidity and mortality rates that attend the train of complications set in motion by missed appendicitis.

Alternative conditions that can mimic appendicitis, giving rise to a negative appendectomy, include pelvic inflammatory diseases, torsion or rupture of ovarian cysts, ectopic pregnancy, and other gynecologic abnormalities. In addition, other diseases include mesenteric adenitis, gastroenteritis, or diseases of the renal and biliary tracts. It is evident that a normal appendix is found more often in women suspected of having appendicitis because of the possibility of gynecologic disease; the negative appendectomy rate in women is accepted at about three times the rate in men.

Patients with normal appendices and without a diagnosis to account for symptoms are followed regularly for up to 12 months. Diagnoses in these patients after surgery have included pancreatitis, gallstones, and some gastrointestinal infections.

REFERENCES

1. Meade RH: The evolution of surgery for appendicitis. Surgery 55:741, 1964.
2. Williams GR: A history of appendicitis. Ann Surg 197:495, 1983.
3. Fitz RH: Perforating inflammation of the vermiform appendix; with special reference to its early diagnosis and treatment. Am J Med Sci 92:321, 1886.
4. McBurney C: Experience with early operative interference in cases of disease of the vermiform appendix. NY Med J 50:676, 1889.
5. Treves F, Swallow JD: A case of relapsing typhlitis treated by removal of the vermiform appendix. Lancet 1:267, 1889.
6. Pilcher LC: The treatment of appendicitis by early laparotomy. Am Surg 10:434, 1889.
7. Jackson RH, Kennedy J, Gardner PS, McQuillan J: Viruses in the aetiology of acute appendicitis. Lancet 2:711, 1966.
8. Lewis FR, Holcroft JW, Boey J, Demphy JE: Appendicitis: a critical review of diagnosis and treatment in 1000 cases. Arch Surg 110:677, 1975.
9. Maloney GE, Russell WT, Wilson DC: Appendicitis: a report on its social pathology and recent surgical experience. Br J Surg 38:52, 1950.
10. Castleman KB, Puestow CB, Sauer D: Is appendicitis decreasing in frequency? Arch Surg 78:794, 1959.
11. Burkitt DP: The aetiology of appendicitis. Br J Surg 58:695, 1971.
12. Leigh DA, Simmons K, Norman E: Bacterial flora of the appendix fossa in appendicitis and postoperative wound infection. J Clin Pathol 27:997, 1974.
13. Shimkin PM: Radiology of acute appendicitis. Am J Roentgenol 130:1001, 1978.

14. Fee HJ, Jones PC, Kadell B, O'Connell TX: Radiological diagnosis of appendicitis. Arch Surg 112:742, 1977.
15. Schisgall RM: Use of the barium swallow in the diagnosis of acute appendicitis. Am J Surg 146:663, 1983.
16. Rajagpalan AE, Mason JH, Kennedy M, Rawlikowski J: The value of barium enema in the diagnosis of acute appendicitis. Arch Surg 112:531, 1977.
17. Leape L, Ramenofsky ML: Laparoscopy for questionable appendicitis. Am Surg 191:410, 1980.
18. Silberman VA: Appendectomy in a large metropolitan hospital. Am J Surg 142:615, 1981.
19. Anderson A, Bergdahl L: Acute appendicitis in patients over sixty. Am Surg 44:445, 1978.
20. Owen BJ, Hamit HF: Appendicitis in the elderly. Am Surg 187:392, 1978.
21. Marchildon MB, Dudgeon DL: Perforated appendicitis: current experience in a children's hospital. Ann Surg 185:84, 1977.
22. McFee AS: Diagnosing appendicitis in the pediatric patient. Infect Surg 1:42, 1982.
23. Masters K, Levine BA, Gaskill HV, Sirinek KR: Diagnosing appendicitis during pregnancy. Am J Surg 148:768, 1984.
24. Gomez A, MacDonald W: Acute appendicitis during pregnancy. Am J Surg 137:180, 1979.
25. Binderow SR, Shaked AA: Acute appendicitis in patients with AIDS-HIV infection. Am J Surg 162:9, 1991.
26. Whitney TM, Macho JR, Russell TR, et al: Appendicitis in acquired immunodeficiency syndrome. Am J Surg 164:467, 1992.
27. Deziel DJ, Hyser MJ, Doolas A, et al: Major abdominal operations in acquired immunodeficiency syndrome. Am Surg 56:445, 1990.
28. LaRaja RD, Rothenberg RE, Odom JW, Mueller SC: The incidence of intra-abdominal surgery in acquired immunodeficiency syndrome: a statistical review of 904 patients. Surgery 105:175, 1989.
29. Davidson T, Allen-Mersh TG, Miles AJ: Emergency laparotomy in patients with AIDS. Br J Surg 78:924, 1991.
30. Detmer DE, Nevers LE, Sikes ED: Regional results of acute appendicitis care. JAMA 246:1318, 1981.
31. Condon RE: Selective antibiotic therapy in surgery. Part 2: Appendicitis and antibiotics. Surg Pract News, p 8, Jan 1983.
32. Bradley EL, Isaacs J: Appendiceal abscess revisited. Arch Surg 113:130, 1978.
33. Barnes BA, Behringer GE, Wheelock FC, et al: Treatment of appendicitis at the Massachusetts General Hospital (1937–1959). JAMA 180:122, 1962.
34. Paull DL, Bloom GP: Appendiceal abscess. Arch Surg 117:1017, 1982.
35. Gerzof SG, Robbins AH, Johnson WC, et al: Percutaneous catheter drainage of abdominal abscesses: a 5-year experience. N Engl J Med 305:653, 1981.
36. Johnson WC, Gerzof SG: Appendiceal abscess: operative drainage or percutaneous drainage? Infect Surg 4:367, 1985.
37. Hoffmann J, Lindhaud A, Jensen HE: Appendix mass: conservative management without interval appendectomy. Am J Surg 148:379, 1984.
38. Cruse PJE, Foord R: The epidemiology of wound infection: a 20-year prospective study of 62,939 wounds. Surg Clin North Am 60:27, 1980.
39. Malt RA: The perforated appendix. N Engl J Med 315:1546, 1986.
40. Gilmore OJA, Browett JT, Griffin PH, et al: Appendicitis and mimicking conditions. Lancet 421, 1975.
41. Alvarado A: A practical score for the early diagnosis of acute appendicitis. Ann Emerg Med 15:557, 1986.
42. Nordestgaard AG, Butler JA, Marcus CJ, et al: Value of clinical factors in predicting acute appendicitis in young women: a logistic regression analysis. Surg Forum 38:456, 1987.
43. Bell MJ, Bower RJ, Ternberg JL: Appendectomy in childhood: analyses of 105 negative explorations. Am J Surg 144:335, 1982.
44. Lau WY, Fau ST, Yin TF, et al: Negative findings at appendectomy. Am J Surg 148:375, 1984.

Anal and Perianal Infections

CHAPTER 45

Julio Garcia-Aguilar, David A. Rothenberger

Although infections of the anorectal region and their consequences have been recognized for hundreds of years, they still represent a significant diagnostic and therapeutic challenge to the medical profession. The accurate diagnosis and effective treatment of anal and perianal infections require an understanding of their etiology and pathogenesis and a thorough three-dimensional knowledge of the regional anatomy and potential routes of spread of infection. Surgical adventures without a precise diagnosis and understanding of the relationship of the infectious process to the sphincter mechanism may lead to incomplete eradication of the infection and/or permanent impairment of anorectal function. The increased number of immunocompromised patients secondary to cancer chemotherapy, transplant immunosuppression, leukemia, and acquired immunodeficiency syndrome (AIDS) has introduced a new dimension to this old problem.

SURGICAL ANATOMY OF THE ANORECTUM

The rectum is the portion of the large bowel extending from the level of the sacral promontory where the taenia coli spread out to form a continuous layer of longitudinal muscle to the level of the levator ani muscles. The anorectal ring represents the point at which the puborectalis wraps around the upper limit of the surgical anal canal, which extends distally for 3 to 4 cm to the anal verge.

An important anatomic landmark in the anal canal is a row of crypts situated approximately 2 cm from the anal verge known as the dentate line (Fig. 45–1). Embryologically, this line represents the junction of the hindgut and the proctodeum. The ducts of the anal glands empty at the bottom of the anal crypts. Proximal to the dentate line, the mucosa protrudes into the lumen producing eight to ten folds, known as columns of Morgagni, that extend distally to the spaces in-between the anal crypts at the level of the dentate line (see Fig. 45–1).

The upper portion of the anal canal is covered by columnar epithelium. For approximately 1 cm above the dentate line, the anal canal is lined by a transitional or cloacogenic epithelium. The anal canal distal to the dentate line is covered by modified squamous epithelium, devoid of skin appendages. The mucosa of the anal canal overlies a highly vascularized submucosa that at the level of the columns of Morgagni contains the internal hemorrhoidal plexus (see Fig. 45–1).

The inner muscular layer of the anal canal, known as the *internal sphincter,* represents the thickened distal continuation of the circular muscular layer of the rectum (see Fig. 45–1). As is true of the rest of the musculature of the gut, the internal

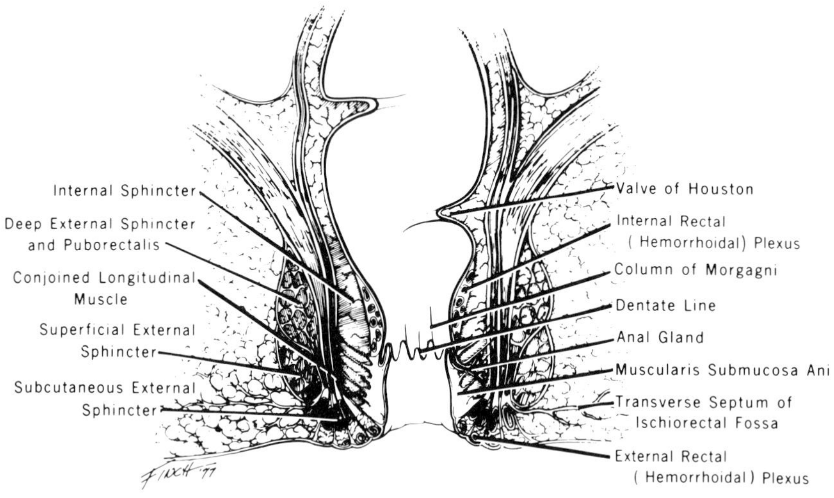

Figure 45–1. Coronal section of the rectum and anal canal, showing sphincter muscles and the lining of the anal canal. *(From Storer EH, Goldberg SM, Nivatvongs S: Colon, rectum, and anus. In Schwartz SI, Shires GT, Spencer FC, Storer ED (eds): Principles of Surgery, 4th ed. New York, McGraw-Hill, 1984.)*

sphincter is innervated by the autonomic nervous system.

Outside the internal sphincter, the longitudinal muscular coat of the rectum is joined by muscular fibers of the levator ani and puborectalis muscle to form the *conjoined longitudinal muscle* (see Fig. 45–1). The distal fibers traverse the superficial portion of the external sphincter to insert in the perianal skin. This portion of the muscle causes wrinkling of the anal verge and is referred to as the *corrugator cutis ani.*

The internal sphincter and conjoined longitudinal muscle are surrounded by a tube of skeletal muscle with somatic innervation. The distal portion, called the *external sphincter,* is an elliptical cylinder of muscle attached posteriorly to the perianal skin and the anococcygeal ligament and anteriorly to the perineal body and transverse perineal muscle (see Fig. 45–1). Anatomically, the external sphincter is described as consisting of subcutaneous, superficial, and deep components; but electromyographically, it behaves as a single functional unit. The lowest portion of the external sphincter lies underneath the skin, slightly distal and lateral to the inferior edge of the internal sphincter. A depression palpable between these two muscles is known as the intersphincteric groove.

The proximal portion of the external sphincter is fused superiorly with the puborectalis and the levator ani muscle (see Fig. 45–1). The puborectalis originates from the back of the symphysis pubis and the superior fascia of the urogenital diaphragm and runs posteriorly forming a U-shaped loop around the rectum. The impression of this muscle in the rectal wall, along with the upper borders of the internal and external sphincters, was called the *anorectal ring* by Milligan and Morgan.[1] This anatomic landmark is critically important during the treatment of abscesses and fistula, because its division will usually result in anal incontinence.

The *levator ani muscle* is a broad plate of muscle that consists of the iliococcygeus and pubococcygeus, which forms the greater part of the pelvic floor. The *pubococcygeus muscle* originates in the back of the pubis and anterior portion of the obturator fascia. Its fibers are directed posteriorly, inferiorly, and medially, fusing in the midline with the fibers from the opposite side to form the anococcygeal raphe. Some of the most posterior fibers insert directly into the coccyx and distal segments of the sacrum. The *iliococcygeus muscle* arises from the iliac spine and the posterior part of the obturator fascia and, after a posterior, inferior, and medial course, inserts on the last two segments of the sacrum and the anococcygeal raphe. The medial fibers of the pubococcygeus form an elliptical space called the *levator hiatus* through which pass the distal rectum, urethra, and dorsal vein of the penis in a man or vagina in a woman. The pelvic diaphragm is completed by part of the pelvic fascia that is more condensed at the level of the anorectal junction and has been called the *hiatal ligament* and binds together the intrahiatal viscera. In a more superficial plane and anterior to the superficial and deep transverse perineus muscles, the levator hiatus is partially covered by the structures of the urogenital diaphragm.

The anatomic structures of the pelvis and anorectal region demarcate several potential spaces that are normally filled with fat or areolar tissue (Fig. 45–2). Perianal infections can spread to these spaces producing well-defined abscesses.

The intersphincteric space lies between the internal and external sphincters. It contains the conjoined longitudinal muscle that theoretically facilitates spreading of infection to the perianal and supralevator spaces. The perianal space is the potential space surrounding the anal verge that communicates with the intersphincteric plane and is continuous with the fat of the buttocks. The ischiorectal space is limited superiorly by the levator ani; medially by the anal sphincter; laterally by the obturator internus, obturator fascia, and ischium; and inferiorly by the skin of the perineum. Both ischiorectal spaces communicate with each other posteriorly behind the anal canal via the so-called postanal space. The anococcygeal ligament divides the postanal space into superficial and deep components. The supralevator space is situated around the rectum, above the levator ani, and is bounded superiorly by the pelvic peritoneum and laterally by the pelvic wall. Both sides are connected posteriorly around the rectum.

Normal anorectal continence is a complex process that requires integrity of the internal and external sphincters and puborectalis muscle. The internal sphincter provides most of the resting tone of the anal canal,[2] while the squeeze pressure is generated by the combined action of the external sphincter and the puborectalis.[3]

ANORECTAL ABSCESS

Etiology and Pathogenesis. The cryptoglandular theory suggests that anorectal abscesses and fistulas-in-ano represent the acute and chronic stages of the same pathologic condition: an infection that originates in the glands of the anal canal. It is generally thought that obstructions of the glandular ducts by fecal material, foreign bodies, or trauma will result in stasis and secondary infection. After the abscess is drained, either spontaneously or surgically, the abnormal communication that often

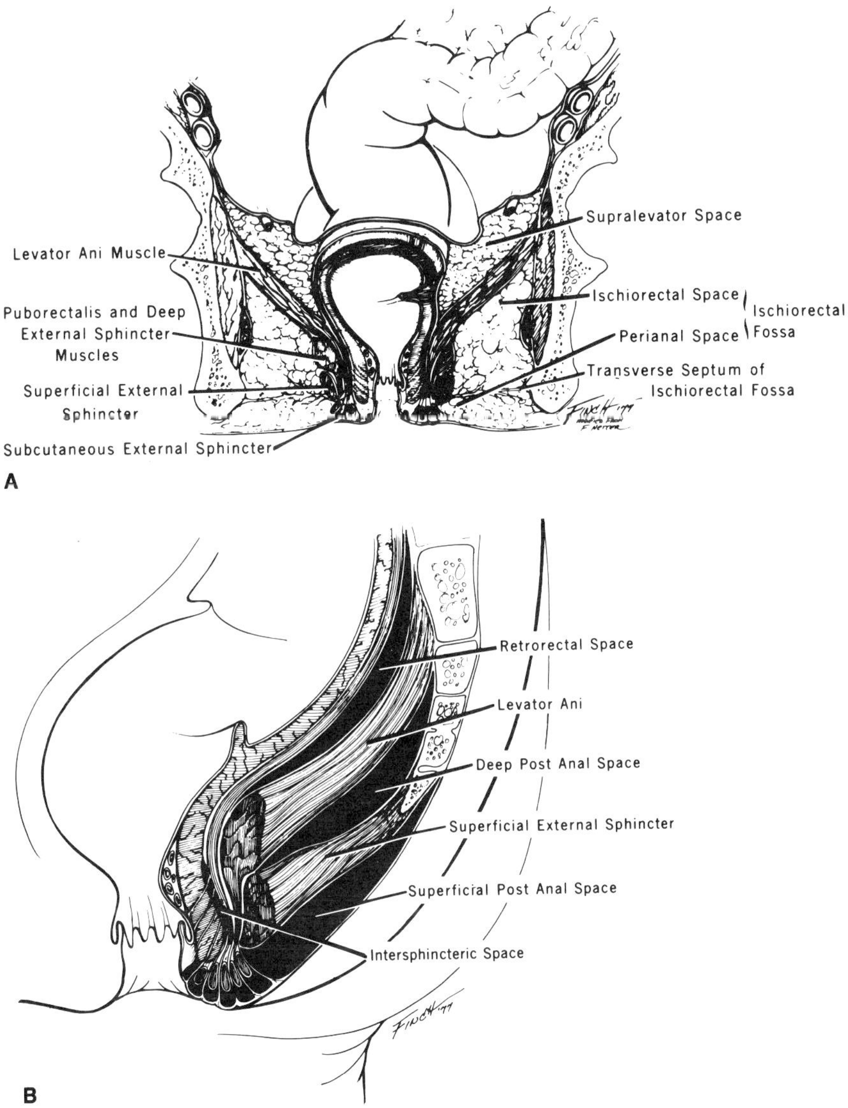

Figure 45–2. A. Coronal section of the perianal and perirectal spaces. **B.** Sagittal section of the perianal and perirectal spaces. *(From Storer EH, Goldberg SM, Nivatvongs S: Colon, rectum, and anus. In Schwartz SI, Shires GT, Spencer FC, Storer ED (eds): Principles of Surgery, 4th ed. New York, McGraw-Hill, 1984.)*

persists between the anal canal and the perianal skin is called a fistula-in-ano.

The anal glands, originally described by Chiari in 1887,[4] have been the subject of multiple studies. They are tubular glands lined by stratified squamous epithelium with a direct opening into the base of an anal crypt. Parks[5] found that two-thirds of the anal glands send branches to the internal sphincter, and one-half crossed the internal sphincter completely to end in the longitudinal muscle. No branch was observed to penetrate the external sphincter.

The glandular origin of anorectal abscesses was suggested in 1880 by Herrmann and Desfosses,[6] but it was Eisenhammer[7,8] who ascribed most anorectal abscesses and fistulas-in-ano to a glandular infection in the intersphincteric space (Fig. 45–3). From this location, the infectious process may extend distally along the fibers of the conjoined longitudinal muscle to emerge subcutaneously as a perianal abscess. The infection may spread laterally through the longitudinal muscle and external sphincter, producing an ischiorectal abscess. Upward extension in the intersphincteric space gives rise to a high intersphincteric abscess. It may then break through the longitudinal muscle into the supralevator space, causing a supralevator abscess.

In addition to tracking upward, downward, and laterally, the suppurative process may spread circumferentially around the anus. This type of spreading can occur at three tissue planes: the ischiorectal fossa, the intersphincteric space, and the supralevator space. This circumferential spread is known as horseshoeing.

The cryptoglandular theory of anorectal abscess and fistula-in-ano is not universally accepted. Goligher et al[9] found only 8 intersphincteric abscesses in 28 patients with anorectal sepsis. However, the cryptoglandular theory is supported by the constant location of the internal fistulous opening at the level of the dentate line.

Anorectal abscesses usually contain bowel derived organisms, particularly *Escherichia coli* and *Bacteroides fragilis,* but up to 21 percent contain skin-derived organisms.[10–12] Grace et al[11] and Whitehead et al[12] have demonstrated a strong correlation between gut-derived flora, but not skin-derived flora, and the presence of a fistula. They suggest that perirectal abscesses with and without fistulas may have a different etiology and that anorectal sepsis may sometimes result from secondary infection of blocked apocrine glands. They believe that appropriate bacteriologic investigations will differentiate both types of abscesses and thus guide treatment.

Anal and perianal infections can also be secondary to other anorectal pathologic conditions such as inflammatory bowel disease, tuberculosis, actinomycosis, lymphogranuloma venereum, carcinoma, lymphoma, infectious complications of AIDS, trauma, surgery, and radiation.

Clinical Manifestations. Patients with anorectal sepsis usually complain of perianal pain. Depending on the location of the abscess, the pain can be described as throbbing or as a dull ache and is usually aggravated by sitting, walking, and sudden increases of abdominal pressure produced by coughing and sneezing. General symptoms include malaise and fever. Minor anal bleeding or purulent discharge is usually secondary to pus draining through the crypt of origin into the anal canal. A larger amount of discharge, often followed by symptomatic improvement, suggests spontaneous drainage of the abscess through the skin.

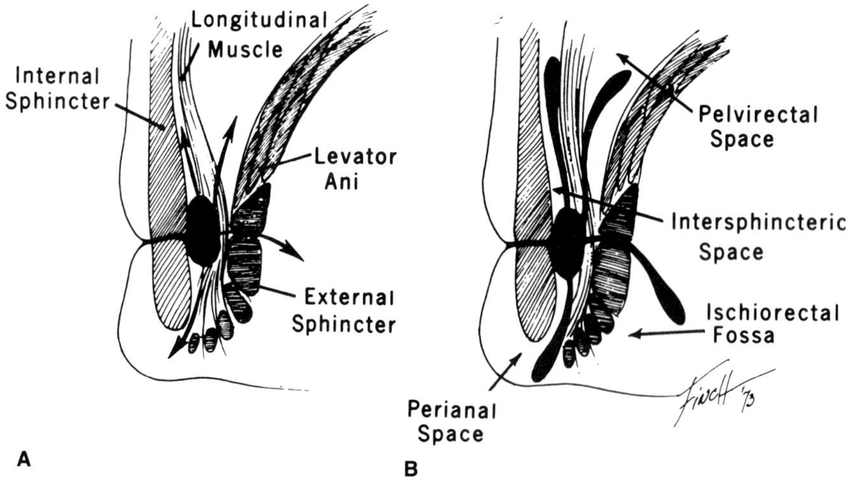

Figure 45–3. A. Pathways of infection from the intersphincteric space at the base of the anal duct. **B.** The intersphincteric abscess then spreads to form perianal, ischiorectal, or pelvirectal abscesses. *(From Storer EH, Goldberg SM, Nivatvongs S: Colon, rectum, and anus. In Schwartz SI, Shires GT, Spencer FC, Storer ED (eds): Principles of Surgery, 4th ed. New York, McGraw-Hill, 1984.)*

Physical examination usually reveals the classic signs of inflammation: swelling, redness, tenderness, and a local increase in temperature. Fluctuation tends to be a late finding and may be difficult to elicit because of local tenderness. Its absence should not delay the diagnosis or treatment.

With intersphincteric and supralevator abscesses, there may be no visible swelling or induration in the perianal region. Anal and rectal examination is usually extremely painful and thus generally ill-advised; but in a few cases, an anal mass or sensation of fullness may be palpable. A tender pelvic mass diagnosed by rectal or vaginal examination, along with lower abdominal pain and tenderness, is characteristic of a supralevator abscess. Though usually not needed, anal ultrasonography can be helpful in the diagnosis of intersphincteric abscesses,[13] while pelvic computed tomography (CT) scanning can assist in the diagnosis of supralevator abscesses.[14]

The differential diagnosis of perianal abscess includes hidradenitis suppurativa, pilonidal abscess, thrombosed hemorrhoid, anal fissure, Bartholin gland abscess, and folliculitis of the perianal skin. Patients with significant anal pain, but without abnormal perianal findings, should be examined under anesthesia. Most such patients are found to have a condition amenable to surgical treatment, usually an abscess or a fissure. If a patient with a classic history suggestive of an intersphincteric abscess is examined under anesthesia and found to have no obvious abnormalities, one should strongly consider needling or creating a small internal sphincterotomy in the posterior midline. This maneuver is often rewarded by drainage of an intersphincteric abscess. Neglect of an abscess will only allow its extension into adjacent spaces and can result in life-threatening sepsis.

Treatment. At the time of diagnosis, most anal and perianal infections are in the suppurative phase and therefore unlikely to respond to antibiotic therapy alone. As for abscesses in other parts of the body, the treatment of anorectal abscess is immediate, adequate drainage. Antibiotics are used as a supplement in the occasional patient who is immunosuppressed or who has significant soft tissue cellulitis.

PERIANAL ABSCESSES. Perianal abscesses almost always can be drained under local anesthesia in the office or outpatient department. Preparation of the skin with an antiseptic solution is probably not necessary but easy to do. A 2-cm area of skin over the point of maximal tenderness is infiltrated with 1 percent lidocaine with 1:200,000 epinephrine. A cruciate incision in the anesthetized area allows immediate drainage of the pus. The skin edges are excised to prevent early sealing of the incision and recurrence of the abscess. Except when temporarily required for hemostasis, wounds are not packed. Tight packing occludes the incision, impeding the drainage of pus, and is unnecessarily painful.

ISCHIORECTAL ABSCESSES. Simple ischiorectal abscesses can also be treated under local anesthesia in an identical manner. However, larger abscesses and those with horseshoe extensions are usually best drained in the operating room with the patient under regional or general anesthesia. The same principles outlined for the treatment of perianal abscesses can be applied for ischiorectal abscesses: cruciate incision, excision of skin edges, and no packing. In general, when draining perianal and ischiorectal abscesses, the skin incision should be made as close as possible to the anus, thereby minimizing the amount of tissue to be incised in case a fistula develops after resolution of the abscess. Care is taken to avoid cutting the sphincter muscle.

Alternatively, ischiorectal abscesses can be treated by catheter drainage.[15] With this technique, the abscess is drained through a small stab incision using a number 11 scalpel blade. A 10F to 16F mushroom catheter is inserted into the abscess cavity and the external portion is shortened to leave 2 or 3 cm outside the skin. The catheter is left in place and covered with a bandage until the drainage has ceased and the cavity has closed around the catheter. At the time of removal of the catheter, the patient undergoes a careful examination to exclude an associated fistula. If present, a fistulotomy should be performed once the inflammation has subsided.

The treatment of anorectal abscess by incision, curettage, and primary closure under antibiotic coverage was introduced by Ellis more than 40 years ago.[16–18] Although the fistula rate after this form of treatment was reported in one study to be lower than after conventional incision and drainage,[19] it has never gained significant acceptance, perhaps because the initial stage is painful, requiring regional or general anesthesia.

Horseshoe ischiorectal abscesses usually start as a posterior intersphincteric abscess that extends to the deep postanal space and from there to both ischiorectal fossae. The deep postanal abscess is inferior to the levator, posterior to the deep external sphincter, and superior to the superficial external sphincter. This type of abscess should be treated by drainage and primary fistulotomy.[20] The crypt of origin is almost always located in the posterior midline. The operation is usually started by inserting a crypt hook through the primary opening in the direction of the coccyx. Using the probe as a guide, the postanal space is entered by dividing the distal portion of the internal sphincter and subcutaneous external sphincter and splitting the fibers of the coccygeal attachment of the superficial external sphincter. The anterior ischiorectal extensions of the abscess are drained through separate para-anal incisions.

INTERSPHINCTERIC ABSCESSES. Adequate exposure and treatment of intersphincteric abscesses require regional or general anesthesia. This type of abscess is drained by internal sphincterotomy over the area of fullness. The internal sphincter should be divided from its lower edge to the dentate line or higher if the abscess has a high extension.

SUPRALEVATOR ABSCESSES. The appropriate treatment of a supralevator abscess requires understanding of its etiology. Supralevator abscesses secondary to pelvic pathology, such as perforated diverticulitis, Crohn's disease, or appendicitis, can be drained through the rectum through the ischiorectal fossa or percutaneously with the help of CT scan. Permanent eradication of the abscess may require treatment of the abdominal process. Supralevator abscesses secondary to upward extension of a high intersphincteric abscess should be drained through the rectum, because drainage through the ischiorectal fossa will result in a suprasphincteric fistula (Fig. 45–4). On the other hand, supralevator abscesses secondary to upward extension of ischiorectal abscess should be drained through the ischiorectal fossa, because drainage through the rectum will result in an extrasphincteric fistula. It is fortunate that supralevator abscesses are rare, because their origin is not always clear and their treatment is somewhat empirical.

A point of controversy in the management of perianal and ischiorectal abscesses is whether a fistulotomy should be done at the time of the initial incision and drainage. Proponents of primary fistulotomy believe that the abscess treated by incision and drainage alone will inevitably recur or result in a fistula, and that by performing a primary fistulotomy at the time of drainage of the abscess, the source of infection and the risk of recurrence and fistula are eliminated. They feel that the originating crypt can easily be identified during the acute phase.[21] Opponents to primary fistulotomy argue that a majority of anorectal abscesses treated with incision and drainage alone will heal without any further problem.[22,23] They believe that subjecting all patients to fistulotomy is, at best, unnecessary in the majority of cases; and, at worst, dangerous because overzealous attempts to find the fistulous tract in friable tissue may result in the creation of a false passage, thus increasing the risks of persistent sepsis and anal incontinence. In a prospective randomized study, the combined recurrence or persistence rate was 2.9 percent in the group treated with primary fistulotomy and 40.6 percent in the group treated by incision and drainage alone.[23] More patients with primary fistulotomy had deterioration of anal continence after their treatment (39.4 percent versus 21.4 percent), but the difference was not statistically significant. Combining primary fistulotomy with incision and drainage complicates the procedure to the point that most patients require treatment in the operating room, whereas simple incision and drainage under local anesthesia are readily accomplished quickly and effectively in the clinic in the vast majority of cases. The authors thus recommend outpatient clinic drainage under local anesthesia for most anorectal and ischiorectal abscesses, reserving fistulotomy for those who demonstrate a persistent fistula or a recurrent abscess.

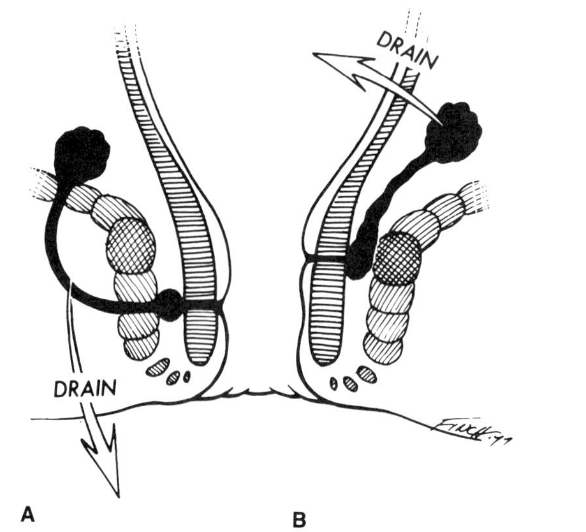

Figure 45–4. Two routes of drainage of supralevator abscesses. **A.** Supralevator abscess secondary to upward extension of an ischiorectal abscess should be drained through the ischiorectal fossa. **B.** A supralevator abscess secondary to upward extension of an intersphincteric abscess should be drained through the rectum. *(From Storer EH, Goldberg SM, Nivatvongs S: Colon, rectum, and anus. In Schwartz SI, Shires GT, Spencer FC, Storer ED (eds): Principles of Surgery, 4th ed. New York, McGraw-Hill, 1984.)*

The use of antibiotics is another controversial point in the management of anorectal abscesses.

There are no data to support their use in uncomplicated abscesses, but antibiotic coverage may be useful in patients with diabetes, an immunocompromised state, or an intravascular prosthesis. Patients with extensive soft tissue cellulitis or necrotizing synergistic infections must be treated aggressively with broad spectrum systemic antibiotics and operative debridement of nonviable tissue.

Neglected perianal infections, particularly in patients with associated debilitating diseases, can spread along fascial planes causing synergistic necrotizing perineal infections.[24,25] Spread along Colles' fascia produces a severe necrotizing infection of the perineum and scrotum known as Fournier's gangrene.[26] Treatment requires broad spectrum antibiotics initially based on Gram stain, wide debridement of all nonviable tissue, tetanus prophylaxis, and nutritional support. Suprapubic cystostomy may be necessary in patients with urethral disruption, while colostomy may be required in patients with infections secondary to rectal trauma or with destruction of the anal sphincters.[27–29]

ANORECTAL ABSCESSES IN HEMATOLOGIC DISEASE. Anorectal infections in patients with hematologic disease represent a special diagnostic and therapeutic challenge. Up to 3.5 percent of patients with acute leukemia develop anorectal abscess, and the incidence is usually related to the degree of the granulocytopenia.[30,31] Infection usually starts following a course of chemotherapy at the time of maximal granulocytopenia, and therefore symptoms of systemic involvement predominate. Later, after the white blood cell (WBC) count increases, suppuration starts and local tenderness, swelling, and erythema develop. Fluctuation is a late and uncommon finding. Concerns about the development of septicemia secondary to digital rectal examination or instrumentation are not supported by recent publications.[32] The more commonly isolated microorganisms are *Bacteroides, Escherichia coli, Klebsiella, Proteus,* and *Streptococcus faecalis.*[33] *Pseudomonas aeruginosa* seems to be more common in children.[34]

The difficulty in distinguishing anorectal abscess from perianal leukemic infiltrates and the concern that surgical instrumentation of the anorectal region may result in spread of the infection and impaired wound healing are responsible for the controversy regarding the surgical management of these lesions. Most of these patients can be treated with precautionary measures such as sitz baths, stool softeners, analgesics, antibiotics, and granulocyte stimulating factor, while avoiding digital rectal examinations, suppositories, or enemas. As the WBC count returns to normal levels, most areas of inflammation and infection resolve. Others develop an abscess that drains spontaneously or requires surgical drainage. Each case should be treated individually depending on the underlying malignant disease, the patient's general condition, and the degree of immunosuppression. Appropriate surgical intervention can relieve pain, prevent local spread of infection, and avoid development of septicemia. Antibiotics, either a third-generation cephalosporin plus an antianaerobic agent or the combination of an extended spectrum penicillin, an aminoglycoside, and an antianaerobic agent, should be used in these patients. If a necrotizing infection is suspected, immediate examination under anesthesia and aggressive debridement will be necessary. Patients with associated thrombocytopenia may require platelet transfusion prior to such debridement.

FISTULA-IN-ANO

A fistula is an unnatural connection between two epithelium-lined surfaces, and a fistula-in-ano is a connection between the epithelium of the anal canal and the epidermis of the perianal skin.

Pathogenesis. The cryptoglandular hypothesis postulates that fistula-in-ano represents the late sequela of a drained anorectal abscess. Fifty percent of the anorectal abscesses will heal after surgical or spontaneous drainage.[35,36] In the other half, a chronic inflammatory process will persist in the tract connecting the anal gland with the perianal skin. Spreading of the intersphincteric abscess to the different anorectal spaces results in different types of abscesses. Drainage of each one of these abscesses may lead to the development of different types of fistula.

Classification. The surgical treatment of fistula-in-ano requires understanding of the relationship of the fistulous tract and the anal sphincters. Therefore anatomic criteria have been used over the years for the development of a classification that would facilitate the understanding of fistula-in-ano and the comparison of therapeutic options.

Many classifications have been used in the past but most of them are complex and impractical. The most helpful and commonly used classification of fistula-in-ano was proposed by Parks et al[37] in 1976 (Fig. 45–5). They based their classification on the presumed cryptoglandular pathogenesis of anal fistula and on the anatomic relationship of the fistulous tract with the anal musculature. They classified anal fistulas in four major groups.

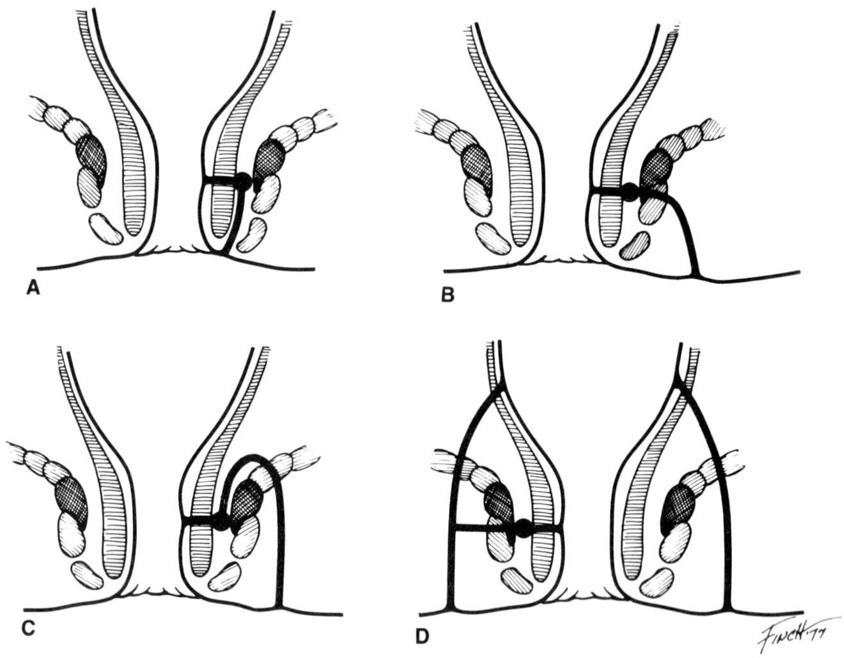

Figure 45–5. The four main anatomic types of fistula. **A.** Intersphincteric (most common). **B.** Transsphincteric (frequent). **C.** Suprasphincteric (uncommon). **D.** Extrasphincteric (rare). *(From Storer EH, Goldberg SM, Nivatvongs S: Colon, rectum, and anus. In Schwartz SI, Shires GT, Spencer FC, Storer ED (eds): Principles of Surgery, 4th ed. New York, McGraw-Hill, 1984.)*

INTERSPHINCTERIC. The fistulous tract remains in the intersphincteric plane. This is the most common type and, in its simplest variety, represents the sequela of a drained perianal abscess. In this case, the track passes from the primary abscess in the intersphincteric plane straight downward to the anal verge (see Fig. 45–5A). The intersphincteric fistula may have an upward extension between the internal sphincter and the conjoined longitudinal muscle that is called a *high blind track.* Occasionally, the high track may have a secondary opening in the rectal wall that may be confused with the internal opening of an extrasphincteric fistula. A high tract may extend all the way up to the supralevator space. Not infrequently, an intersphincteric abscess that drains back to the anal canal through the primary opening originates a fistulous tract in the intersphincteric plane without an external opening.

TRANSSPHINCTERIC. This type of fistula results from an ischiorectal abscess and is the second most common variety. The fistulous tract passes from the intersphincteric plane, through the external sphincter, into the ischiorectal fossa, and then to the skin (see Fig. 45–5B). The level at which the tract passes across the external sphincter varies, and a transsphincteric fistula may involve almost the entire external sphincter or only its most superficial portion. Transsphincteric fistulas can also have a high blind tract that may reach the apex of the ischiorectal fossa or even pass through the levator ani muscle into the pelvis. In a significant number of transsphincteric fistulas, the primary fistulous opening is located in the posterior midline; and the fistulous tract, after crossing the external sphincter, opens into the postanal space. From there, the fistula extends laterally, in a horseshoe fashion, to one or both ischiorectal fossa.

SUPRASPHINCTERIC. This uncommon type of fistula results from a supralevator abscess that has drained downward through the levator ani muscle into the ischiorectal fossa and finally through the skin (see Fig. 45–5C). The fistula tracks upward in the intersphincteric plane to a point above the puborectalis muscle, then laterally over this muscle, and finally downward through the levator ani muscle into the ischiorectal fossa. A high blind tract and horseshoe extension in the supralevator plane are possible in this type of fistula.

EXTRASPHINCTERIC. This is the rarest type of fistula-in-ano. The tract passes from the perineal skin, to the ischiorectal fossa, through the levator ani muscles, and finally into the rectum (see Fig. 45–5D). The tract lies completely outside the sphincter mechanism. When this type of fistula has a cryptoglandular origin, it usually starts as a transsphincteric fistula that iatrogenically opens into the rectum by vigorous probing while attempting to find the internal fistulous opening. Extrasphincteric fistulas may also be secondary to penetrating perineal injuries, inflammatory bowel disease, cancer, or pelvic abscesses drained through the perineum.

The terms *high anal fistula* and *complex fistula* are frequently used in the medical literature to describe those fistulas whose surgical treatment carries significant risk of recurrence or incontinence. They include extrasphincteric, suprasphincteric, and those transsphincteric fistulas that encircle a significant portion of the external sphincter.

Diagnosis. Most patients have a previous history of anorectal abscesses that drained spontaneously or have been drained surgically. The cutaneous opening persists and becomes the external opening of the fistula-in-ano. Patients complain of purulent or seropurulent drainage that is usually intermittent but may be constant. The presence of drainage produces a sensation of wetness and pruritus ani.

A systematic physical examination should be carried out. Inspection of the perianal area, anal digital examination, anoscopy, and sigmoidoscopy are mandatory in every patient with a history suggestive of fistula-in-ano. The examiner should try to determine the external opening, the course of the fistulous tract and its relationship to the sphincter mechanism, the internal opening, and the presence of associated pathology.

The external opening or openings may be found at the bottom of a depressed area or surrounded by granulation tissue. Occasionally, it may heal temporarily, leaving only an area of scarring and induration corresponding to the site of previous drainage. An indurated cord extending from the external opening toward the anal canal can sometimes be palpated, particularly in patients with intersphincteric fistulas. Simultaneous digital palpation of the anal canal and the external fistulous opening in the unanesthetized patient can provide valuable information about the direction and depth of the fistulous tract. The internal opening can be felt as an area of induration or visualized as a dimple at the level of the dentate line. Probing of the fistula in the unanesthetized patient, even when performed gently, is uncomfortable for the patient and carries the risk of creating a false passage. Except in very superficial fistulas, the chances of probing the entire tract and finding the internal opening are very small.

As originally described by Goodsall and Miles,[38] the position of the external fistulous opening may help to predict the direction of the tract and the location of the internal opening (Fig. 45–6). In fistulas secondary to ischiorectal abscesses, when the external opening is posterior to the transverse anal line, the course of the tract is curved and the internal opening is located in the posterior midline. When anterior to that line, the course is straight and the internal opening is in the same radial line as the external one. Fistulas superficial to the ischiorectal fossa take a straight course to the anal canal from the external opening.

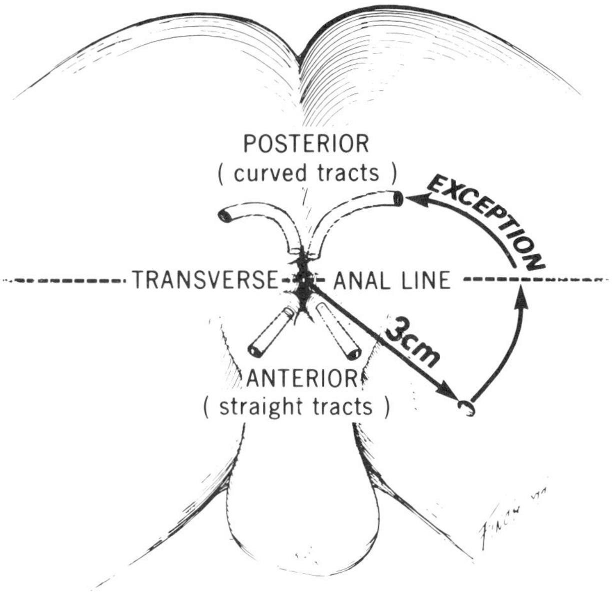

Figure 45–6. Goodsall's rule. *(From Storer EH, Goldberg SM, Nivatvongs S: Colon, rectum, and anus. In Schwartz SI, Shires GT, Spencer FC, Storer ED (eds): Principles of Surgery, 4th ed. New York, McGraw-Hill, 1984.)*

The accurate delineation of the fistulous opening and tract and its relationship to the sphincter mechanism is essential for correct anatomic classification and planning of proper surgical treatment. Given the limitations of preoperative clinical assessment, several diagnostic procedures have been recommended. Fistulography, which involves the injection of contrast material under minimal pressure through the external fistulous opening, has been found to be inaccurate and unreliable.[39] However, a recent retrospective review indicated that fistulography had significant impact in the surgical management of 48 percent of the patients.[40]

Anal endosonography is being used with increasing frequency in the evaluation of patients with anorectal abscess and fistula.[13,41] Endosonography seems to accurately identify the fistulous tract but not the internal opening. When a water-filled balloon is used to cover the ultrasonic transducer, anal endosonography is very sensitive at localizing anorectal abscesses and identifying unsuspected purulent loculations. A prospective study demonstrated that preoperative clinical evaluation was superior to endoanal ultrasonography in defining the anatomy of anal fistulas when compared with the surgical findings.[42]

Preoperative documentation of the status of continence is important in all patients undergoing surgery for fistula-in-ano, particularly in those who had undergone previous fistula surgery or in whom continence can be expected to be compromised (eg, history of traumatic vaginal delivery). Pescatori et al[43] have suggested that preoperative manometric evaluation of the anal sphincter helps to select the appropriate surgical treatment and improves the functional outcome of surgery for fistula-in-ano. However, the systematic use of preoperative anal manometry has not gained widespread acceptance. In our opinion, preoperative anorectal physiology testing is indicated in patients with questionable sphincter function on physical examination, because a significant functional defect in the sphincter mechanism may influence the selection of the surgical procedure.

The anatomy of some fistulas and the relationship of their tracts to the sphincter muscles are impossible to delineate preoperatively, even with the assistance of auxiliary diagnostic procedures. Adequate diagnosis of these patients requires examination under anesthesia.

Treatment. The goal of the surgical treatment of fistula-in-ano is the definitive eradication of the suppurative process without compromising anal continence.

FISTULOTOMY. Fistula operations are performed at our institution under general or regional anesthesia with the patient in the prone jackknife position. The buttocks are spread apart with adhesive tape. The need for good illumination, ideally with a headlight, cannot be overemphasized. The perianal skin is prepared and if local anesthesia is used, a perianal block with 0.25 percent bupivacaine and epinephrine 1:200,000 is established. If local anesthesia is not used, the fistulotomy is performed and early postoperative analgesia is provided by injecting bupivacaine at the sites of the surgical wounds. Occasionally, injecting such solutions before the fistulotomy can make the tissues edematous and difficult to examine, thus making it harder to find all fistula tracts.

The operation begins with a careful inspection of the perianal area and a digital anorectal examination. After localizing the external opening, the anal canal is visually inspected with the help of a Pratt bivalve anoscope. The internal opening may be marked by an area of induration or visualized as an ulcer or a dimple at the level of the dentate line. Occasionally, by pressing in the perianal skin over the suspected fistulous tract, it is possible to express a drop of pus which exudes out of the crypt in which the internal opening is located. The fistulous tract is gently probed starting from the external opening and advancing the probe along the fistulous tract until the internal opening is reached or until the probe cannot be advanced easily. If the probe cannot be passed to the internal opening, a dilute solution of hydrogen peroxide may gently be injected through the external opening. Small bubbles at the level of the dentate line may help localize the internal opening. Alternatively, if after a gentle attempt the internal opening cannot be identified with the fistula probe, the external portion of the track is unroofed starting at the external opening. By "following the granulation tissue," it is usually possible to identify the changes in direction of the fistulous tract and to demonstrate the internal opening. The use of electrocautery during fistula surgery facilitates hemostasis and allows better identification of the granulation tissue in the fistulous track. Sometimes, despite these maneuvers, no internal opening is identified. One should not force the probe through the anal canal but should accept the fact that the internal opening was not apparent and that there may be a persistence of the fistula. Forcing the probe through the anal sphincter risks creation of iatrogenic incontinence and will not resolve the underlying infection.

Once the entire tract has been probed and the internal opening identified, an attempt is made to determine the relationship of the primary fistula tract with the external sphincter and the puborectalis and to evaluate the amount of muscle encircled by the fistula. Occasionally, this maneuver is facilitated by the passage of a seton because a rigid probe distorts the anatomy more than a thread or an elastic ligature.

Most anal fistulas are intersphincteric or low transsphincteric and they are effectively treated by fistulotomy and marsupialization (Fig. 45–7). Once the probe is passed into the internal sphincter, the tissue over the tract is divided over a grooved probe director. After laying open any secondary tract, the granulation tissue is curetted and hemostasis is obtained with the electrocautery. To prevent immediate postoperative bleeding and to shorten the healing time by minimizing the wound, the skin edges are marsupialized to the edge of the tract with a running absorbable suture. A loose cotton dressing may be applied over the area.

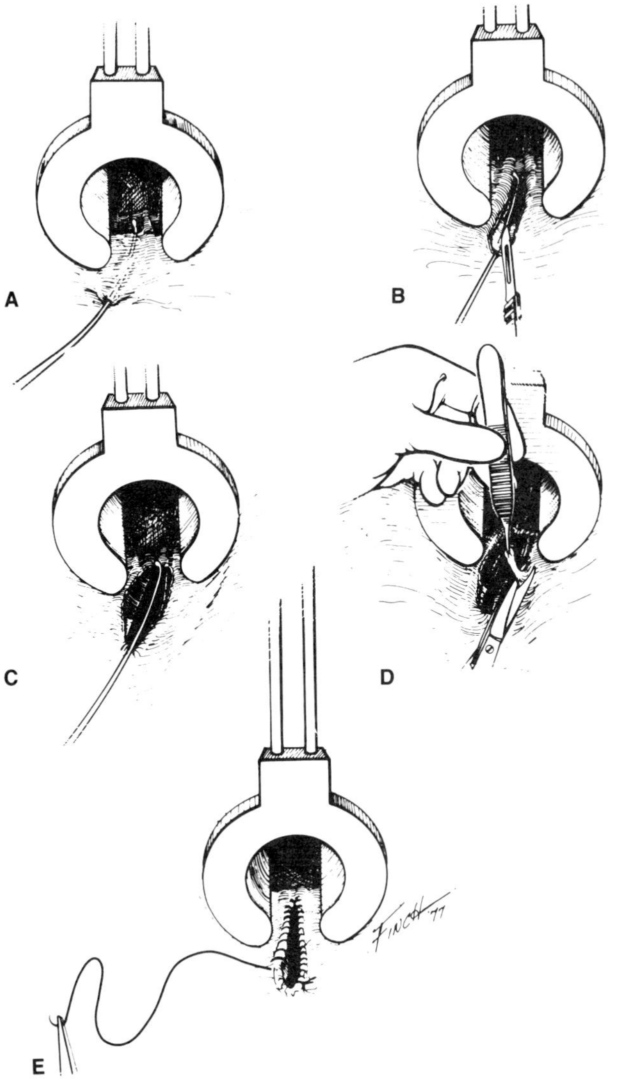

Figure 45–7. Fistulotomy. **A.** The probe is in the fistulous tract. **B,C.** Unroofing of the fistulous tract over the probe. **D.** Redundant skin is excised. **E.** The wound is marsupialized. *(From Storer EH, Goldberg SM, Nivatvongs S: Colon, rectum, and anus. In Schwartz SI, Shires GT, Spencer FC, Storer ED (eds): Principles of Surgery, 4th ed. New York, McGraw-Hill, 1984.)*

ALTERNATIVES TO FISTULOTOMY. The treatment of high anal fistulas (high transsphincteric, suprasphincteric, and extrasphincteric) remains controversial and none of the surgical procedures developed to date has gained widespread acceptance. The idea that the internal and external sphincters can be divided without significant functional loss, provided the puborectalis is preserved, has been challenged.[44] Procedures that divide the muscle encircled by the fistulous tract carry a risk of incontinence, which is proportional to the amount of muscle divided. On the other hand, procedures that attempt to close the internal fistulous opening are penalized by a significant rate of fistula recurrence. The dilemma is how to adequately treat the fistula without causing incontinence.

Fistulotomy and marsupialization are not indicated in those patients in whom it is suspected that the portion of the sphincter complex left after dividing the muscle encircled by the fistulous tract would be insufficient to preserve continence. In general, primary fistulotomy should be avoided when the fistulous tract encircles more than 30 percent of the external sphincter. However, the evaluation of the amount of muscle encircled by a fistula is a difficult judgment; and in most cases, decisions are made based on experience, careful clinical evaluation, and knowledge of the patient's preoperative sphincter competence and bowel function.

The location of the fistula is of paramount importance at the time of evaluating the amount of sphincter involved by the fistula. The external sphincter is reinforced posteriorly and laterally by the sling of the puborectalis muscle. Anteriorly, the sphincter mechanism is devoid of this important muscular element. Therefore, when laid open, fistulas encircling the same amount of external sphincter are more likely to result in incontinence if they are located anteriorly rather than posteriorly.

Setons have been used in the management of anal fistula ever since surgeons recognized the disastrous consequences of dividing the anal sphincter. The rationale behind their use in the management of fistula-in-ano lies in the fibrotic reaction that they induce in the tissue surrounding the fistulous tract. Theoretically, the fibrous tissue fixes the sphincter and prevents its retraction once the portion of the muscle encircled by the seton is divided.

When a seton is used, the portion of the tract outside the sphincter mechanism is laid open and the granulation tissue is removed with a curette. The anoderm and perianal skin overlying the portion of the sphincter complex to be divided by the seton are incised, and the intersphincteric space is drained by division of the internal sphincter. A high blind tract, when present, is managed by cephalad extension of the internal sphincterotomy. The edges of the anoderm and skin are marsupialized with a running absorbable suture. At this point, the seton is passed through the remaining muscular portion of the fistulous tract (Fig. 45–8).

If the seton is to be used as a two-stage procedure, a soft material such as number 0 silk is tied loosely around the sphincter mechanism. The seton is left in place for approximately 8 weeks, at which time fistulotomy is completed by division of the muscle encircled by the seton, either in the office

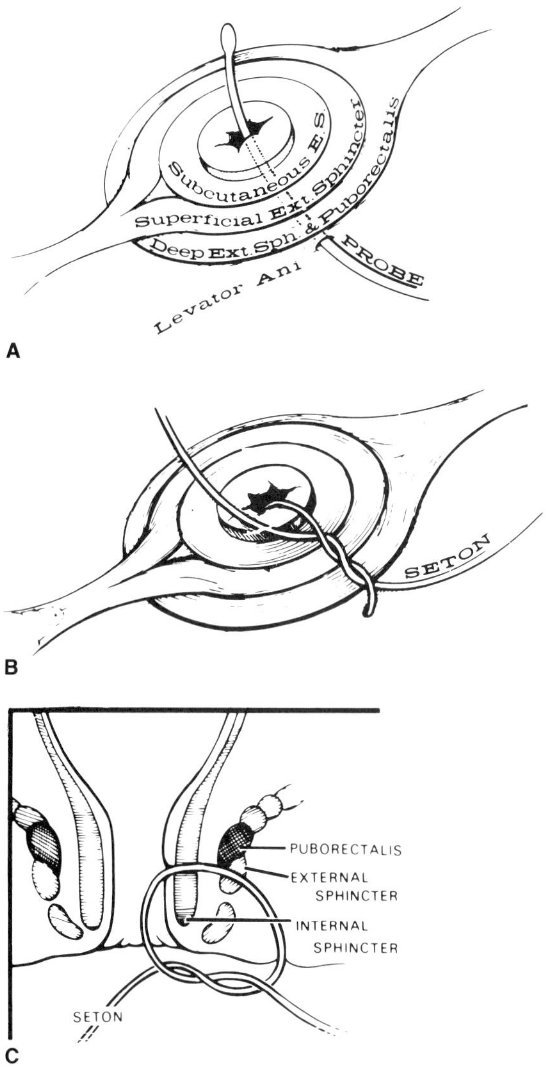

Figure 45–8. Use of seton in high fistula. **A.** The probe is in the fistulous tract. **B.** A seton or suture is inserted into the fistulous tract and tied loosely (**C**) over the sphincter to create fibrosis. The fistulous tract will be laid open in the second stage 6 to 8 weeks later. *(From Storer EH, Goldberg SM, Nivatvongs S: Colon, rectum, and anus. In Schwartz SI, Shires GT, Spencer FC, Storer ED (eds): Principles of Surgery, 4th ed. New York, McGraw-Hill, 1984.)*

under local anesthesia or in the operating room under regional or general anesthesia.

In the cutting seton technique, a rubber band is used that is periodically tightened until it gradually cuts its way through the involved muscle. The tightening of the rubber band seton is not started until the suppurative process has resolved and the fistulotomy wound is starting to heal, usually 3 weeks after the operation. The seton can be tightened by applying a silk tie or a "Barron" ligature to the stretched rubber band. After the first visit, the tightening is repeated every 2 weeks until the seton cuts through the muscle. The entire process takes an average of 16 weeks. Tightening the rubber band at shorter intervals may defeat the purpose of the cutting seton by not allowing adequate fibrosis to develop before sphincter division. Alternatively, the patient can simply "wiggle" the silk seton daily. It gradually cuts through the sphincter fiber by fiber, working its way distally until it is completely through the sphincter, which has healed by fibrosis during this slow cutting process.

The results of the two-stage seton fistulotomy[45–49] and the cutting seton[49–53] are very similar in terms of fistula recurrence and incontinence. The recurrence rate is low, but continence problems, usually in the form of minor soiling and flatus control, are common. The rate of major incontinence ranges from 0 to 39 percent (Table 45–1).

Thomson and Ross[54] and Kennedy and Zegarra[55] used the seton as a drain in the treatment of high anal fistula. They placed a nonelastic seton as described above and removed it when adequate wound healing around the fistulous tract had occurred. The external sphincter is divided only if the fistula fails to heal after seton removal or if sepsis persists around the seton. In their series, the percentages of fistulas healed without the need to divide the external sphincter was 44 and 78 percent, respectively (see Table 45–1).

Anorectal advancement flap, combined with closure of the internal opening and excision of the external portion of the fistulous tract, is another surgical alternative in the management of high anal fistulas. The anatomy of the fistula should be defined precisely and the internal opening identified, excised, and closed with absorbable suture. A flap that consists of mucosa, submucosa, and circular muscle should be raised, advanced beyond the original internal opening, and sutured to the anal canal distal to the internal opening.[56] Aguilar et al[57] have reported an impressive 1.5 percent recurrence rate and 10 percent minor incontinence in 189 patients operated with this technique. Their results are even more remarkable if one considers that 11 percent of their operations were performed at the time of drainage of an abscess. However, the procedure was used in all types of fistulas and the percentage of patients with high anal fistulas was not specified. Similar results have been reported by Wedell et al[58] in 27 patients with high transsphincteric and suprasphincteric fistulas. Our limited experience with this technique is similar to that of Oh[59] and Shemesh et al,[60] who reported no incontinence but a significant recurrence rate in a small series (see Table 45–1).

Closure of the internal fistulous opening and excision[48] or drainage[61] of the tract are technically

TABLE 45–1. COMPARATIVE RESULTS OF SURGICAL TREATMENT OF HIGH ANAL FISTULAS WITH AND WITHOUT DIVISION OF THE EXTERNAL SPHINCTER

Author	Method	Number of Patients	Recurrence (%)	Incontinence	
				Minor (%)	*Major (%)*
• NONDIVISION OF THE SPHINCTER					
Parks and Stitz[48]	Fistulectomy/closure	15	33	NS	NS
Reznick and Bailey[61]	Drainage/closure	7	28.5	0	0
Mann and Clifton[62]	Rerouting	5	0	0	0
Oh[59]	Fistulectomy/flap	15	13	NS	NS
Aguilar et al[57]	Fistulectomy/flap	189	1.5	10	0
Wedell et al[58]	Flap	27	0	30	0
Shemesh et al[60]	Flap	8	12.5	0	0
Thomson and Ross[54]	Draining seton	34	56	0	6
Kennedy and Zegarra[55]	Draining seton	32	22	58	4
• DIVISION OF THE SPHINCTER					
Parks and Stitz[48]	Seton/fistulotomy	30	3	39	0
Kuijpers[45]	Seton/fistulotomy	10	0	60	10
Ramanujam et al[46]	Seton/fistulotomy	45	2	2	0
Thomson and Ross[54]	Seton/fistulotomy	19	0	56	12
Williams et al[49]	Seton/fistulotomy	24	8	54	4
Pearl et al[47]	Seton/fistulotomy	116	3.3	NS	5.4
Culp[50]	Cutting seton	20	0	15	0
Christensen et al[51]	Cutting seton	21	0	29	39
Ustynosky et al[52]	Cutting seton	11	18	NS	NS
Williams et al[49]	Cutting seton	13	0	54	7

NS, non specified.

difficult alternatives that are followed by a high recurrence rate. Mann and Clifton[62] proposed rerouting the tract of a high anal fistula into an intersphincteric position. The external sphincter is immediately repaired and the newly created intersphincteric fistula is treated by a delayed procedure. Their small experience with five patients has not been duplicated (see Table 45–1).

The key to the treatment of horseshoe fistula is the identification of the internal opening, which is usually located in the posterior midline. The principles of treatment of any fistula-in-ano apply to the primary tract of a horseshoe fistula.[20,51,63] After the internal opening is identified, the postanal space is opened in the posterior midline and the primary fistulous tract is treated according to its relationship to the sphincter mechanism. The secondary lateral limbs of the horseshoe tract can be laid open and marsupialized or curetted through the previously enlarged external openings.

One of the main difficulties encountered when comparing the results of different treatment modalities in high anal fistulas is the small number of cases in most reported series. Differences in diagnostic criteria, patient selection, and length of follow-up make it extremely difficult to reliably compare different treatment modalities. Based on the available data and our own experience, we generally use a two-stage seton fistulotomy for transsphincteric fistulas encircling more than 30 percent of the sphincter mechanisms and consider an anorectal advancement flap for suprasphincteric fistulas.

The treatment of an extrasphincteric fistula depends on its etiology. When the fistula has a cryptoglandular origin, the supralevator extension is usually iatrogenic, in most cases secondary to vigorous probing during drainage of an ischiorectal abscess or treatment of a transsphincteric fistula. In this case, the transsphincteric fistula should be treated by a simple fistulotomy or a seton, depending on the level at which the fistulous tract crosses the external sphincter, and the rectal opening is closed primarily. A temporary diverting colostomy, advocated in the past, is being replaced by preoperative mechanical bowel preparation and postoperative elemental diet. Extrasphincteric fistulas secondary to intra-abdominal pathology or trauma are managed according to the causative process.[64]

Most fistula operations are done as an outpatient procedure. The few patients admitted into the hospital are usually discharged to home within 24 hours after the operation. Postoperative orders include sitz baths, oral or parenteral analgesics, and a bulk agent to maintain regular and soft bowel movements.

PERINEAL ABSCESS AND FISTULA IN PATIENTS WITH CROHN'S DISEASE

The reported incidence of perianal involvement in patients with Crohn's disease ranges from 22 to 80 percent, reflecting the investigator definition of what constitutes anorectal Crohn's disease and referral patterns.[65] The National Cooperative Crohn's Disease Study found that 36 percent of patients with Crohn's disease had a history of perianal disease and that anorectal involvement is more common in patients with Crohn's colitis than in patients with ileitis or ileocolitis.[66] Anal involvement is the rule in patients with Crohn's disease of the rectum. In a small number of patients, the anal lesions develop before the intestinal disease is recognized.

Anorectal suppurative complications are among the most common perianal complications in patients with Crohn's disease. Although some authors believe that these complications are secondary to an ulcerated lesion in the anal canal, others believe that they have a cryptoglandular origin as in patients without Crohn's disease.

A Crohn's anus usually has a characteristic appearance with edema, cyanosis, and maceration of the skin. Deep, eccentrically located fissures or ulcers, which are surprisingly nonpainful, and skin tags are common. Anorectal abscesses are manifested by pain in a previously asymptomatic area. Most fistulas are superficial and simple, but some are very complex with multiple external openings and tracts, sometimes extending a long distance from the anus. Horseshoe extension, both anterior and posterior, is particularly common. Such fistulas tend to have a chronic, painless course, punctuated by symptomatic episodes secondary to inadequate drainage. If neglected, a "watering-pot perineum" develops characterized by excessive drainage of pus through multiple external openings on the perianal skin.

The diagnosis is relatively simple in patients with these types of lesions and gastrointestinal manifestations of Crohn's disease. However, in patients without previous history of Crohn's disease, the diagnosis should be contemplated if the anorectal process displays unusual features such as wide-based, eccentrically located, painless fissures; multiple fistulous tracts; or nonhealing perineal wounds. Any of these findings warrants endoscopic and radiologic investigation of the small and large bowel to exclude Crohn's disease. A biopsy of a rectal mucosal lesion may be diagnostic but histologic examination of the perianal lesions is unreliable.

The potentially complex nature of the perianal suppurative lesions in Crohn's patients has promoted the use of imaging techniques that would help to define their extension, location, and relationship to the sphincter mechanism. Fistulogram,[40] ultrasonography,[40] CT scan,[14,67] and magnetic resonance imaging (MRI)[68] can be useful in selected circumstances to identify unsuspected abscesses and fistulas or to delineate the anatomy of a complex fistulous tract.

Simple abscesses in patients with anorectal Crohn's disease should be treated by incision and drainage under local anesthesia. Patients with recurrent, complex, or horseshoe abscesses or patients with questionable adequate drainage should be examined under regional or general anesthesia. The healing time after abscess drainage tends to be long, and Fry et al[69] and Pritchard et al[70] recommend the use of a mushroom catheter to ensure drainage and prevent recurrence.

Several anecdotal reports suggest a beneficial effect of metronidazole in patients with perianal Crohn's disease.[71,72] However, metronidazole should not delay incision and drainage of a perirectal abscess. Its use after abscess drainage has not decreased the incidence of abscess recurrence or the development of a fistula. A prospective study has demonstrated that 6-mercaptopurine can improve or close perianal fistulas; however, the fistulas tend to exacerbate after discontinuation of the medication.[73]

Most perianal fistulas in Crohn's disease have a benign course and some heal spontaneously. Surgical treatment should be reserved for symptomatic anal fistulas.[74] In the past, aggressive surgical therapy in the management of perianal fistulas in Crohn's disease was followed by significant morbidity, particularly in the form of incontinence, anal stenosis, and nonhealing perineal wounds; and therefore a conservative approach has been recommended.[75] However, recent evidence suggests that simple fistulas, particularly intersphincteric fistulas with an internal opening at the level of the dentate line, can be safely treated by conventional fistulotomy.[76,77] Although, in one report, wound healing was not influenced by the presence of rectal Crohn's disease or granulomatous inflammation of the fistulous tract,[78] others stated that the success of the operation correlated with the absence of rectal Crohn's and quiescent disease elsewhere in the gastrointestinal tract.[79]

It should be emphasized that fistulotomy is appropriate to unroof the subcutaneous portion of multiple tracts. The patient with a "watering-pot perineum" often has extensive, interconnecting subcutaneous tracts that eventually communicate with one or, at most, two deep submuscular tracts. Unroofing these multiple subcutaneous tracts quickly improves the patient's situation without risking incontinence. The deep portion of the fistula is managed with a draining seton or advancement flap. High and complex anal fistulas are best treated by opening and marsupialization of the external fistulous tracts and adequate drainage of the primary tract by insertion of a draining seton.[80] The goal of treatment for these patients is to preserve function and prevent recurrent suppuration; therefore the seton should be loosely tied to avoid cutting through the tissue and left in place for a prolonged period of time. A silicone elastomer tube is an ideal seton under these circumstances.

Anorectal advancement flap has been used in selected patients with Crohn's fistulas. Jones et al[81] have reported a success rate of 33 percent in the outcomes of six patients with an anorectal fistula and Crohn's disease, while Lewis and Bartolo[82] had only one recurrence in six patients. Although their experience is small, both groups agree that the anorectal advancement flap should not be attempted in patients with active Crohn's proctitis.

Proctectomy is a reasonable surgical option for patients with a long history of extensive anorectal Crohn's disease, particularly after the development of incontinence and severe stenosis. In order to avoid the high incidence of an unhealed perineal wound, a low Hartmann's procedure has been proposed as an alternative for these patients.[83] We generally use an intersphincteric proctectomy for such cases and find that the resulting small perineal wound heals well.

PILONIDAL DISEASE

The inclusion of pilonidal disease in a chapter dedicated to anal and perianal infections is due to the anatomic proximity of this process to the anorectal region rather than to a shared etiology. The term pilonidal disease was introduced by Hodges[84] to describe a chronic sinus containing hair found between the buttocks.

The process affects young adults after puberty and is rare after age 40 years. In routine physical examinations performed on Minnesota college students, pilonidal disease was identified in 1.1 percent of males and 0.11 percent of females.[85] However, more females undergo treatment, and therefore the sex ratio reported in most surgical series is closer to 4:1. The incidence of pilonidal disease is higher in hirsute, obese, Caucasian patients.[86]

The congenital theory of pilonidal disease ascribed its origin to remnants of the medullary canal, epidermal inclusions due to abnormal fusion of the median raphe, or a vestigial sex gland. Although the congenital theory was supported by the familial tendency to pilonidal disease, it was challenged by the high rate of recurrence after removal of all epithelial tracts, the more cranial location of congenital neural canal sinuses, and the absence of histologic evidence of intermediate conditions such as vestigial sex glands or epidermal inclusions.

The acquired theory proposed in 1946 by Patey and Scarff[87] suggests that pilonidal disease is caused by a foreign body reaction to hair embedded in the skin. The movement between the surface of the buttocks at the natal cleft results in twisting of the hair into a bundle that might drill its way into the skin. The hair penetrates the skin and subcutaneous tissue and eventually becomes detached from the skin surrounding the opening. The finding of pilonidal disease caused by hair in the interdigital clefts and periareolar skin of barbers supports this theory.

A recent alternative to this theory proposed by Bascom[88] ascribes the origin of pilonidal disease to the normal follicles located in the midline of the natal cleft. He proposes that the follicle, enlarged by the accumulation of keratin, becomes infected; and the edema, secondary to the infection, shuts its mouth, blocking the escape of follicular content. Eventually, the bottom of the follicle bursts into the fat, resulting in a pilonidal abscess. As the abscess is drained and the edema subsides, the mouth of the follicle opens, leaving a follicular remnant open at both ends. Change from sitting to standing creates a vacuum effect in the chronic abscess cavity that sucks the natal cleft hair through the follicular remnant into the cavity. Epithelium from the edges of the broken follicle advances along the tract to cover the walls of the chronic abscess cavity.

Pilonidal disease can be classified into three clinical categories: (1) acute pilonidal abscess, (2) chronic pilonidal disease, and (3) complex or recurrent pilonidal disease. Approximately half of all cases of pilonidal disease present as acute abscesses, usually located proximal to the follicular pit. Acute pilonidal abscesses are treated in the clinic by incision and drainage using local anesthesia. With the patient in the prone position, the skin of the natal cleft is prepared with an antiseptic solution and the area of inflammation is anesthetized using 1 percent lidocaine with 1:200,000 epinephrine. The hair surrounding the natal cleft is shaved to facilitate hygiene and healing. A cruciate incision is made over the most fluctuant or tender area. The skin edges of the cruciate incision are excised to allow adequate drainage and prevent premature closure of the skin over the abscess cavity. Wound packing is not used except for hemostatic reasons. Cultures of the abscess contents are usually unnecessary because in most cases antibiotics are generally not required. Postoperatively, the wound is irrigated twice a day with warm tapwater using either sitz baths or a shower attachment followed by careful drying to prevent skin maceration. The skin of the natal cleft surrounding the area of inflammation should be shaved at the time of the clinic visit every 2 weeks. Incision and drainage relieve the symptoms of acute pilonidal abscesses in all patients and result in complete healing in 58 percent of the patients within 10 weeks. However, 40 percent of patients with pilonidal abscesses treated by incision and drainage will develop chronic pilonidal sinuses.

In order to reduce the rate of recurrence after incision and drainage of acute pilonidal abscess, Bascom has introduced the concept of follicle removal after lateral drainage of the abscess.[88,89] During the first operation, the abscess is drained in the clinic under local anesthesia using a longitudinal incision parallel to the natal cleft and one finger's breadth laterally. One week later, once the acute inflammation and edema have subsided, the enlarged midline follicles are individually excised, leaving several wounds 2 to 4 mm in diameter. These small wounds are sutured and neither packs nor antibiotics are used. When epithelized tubes are present, they are removed through the lateral incision. Treatment was completed as an outpatient; the average healing time was 3 weeks and mean disability, defined as missing school or work, was only 1 day. After a mean follow-up of 3.5 years, the 5-year cumulative incidence of new pilonidal trouble after complete healing of the primary surgery was 17 percent.[89]

Chronic pilonidal disease, also called pilonidal sinus, occurs when the chronic abscess cavity remains open as an area of granulation onto the skin, usually lateral to the midline. One or more follicular openings can be identified in the natal cleft 4 to 8 cm cephalad to the anus. The sinus can be palpated as an area of induration under the sacral skin running cephalad from the follicular opening to the laterally situated granulation-lined opening. Patients usually complain of intermittent pain and discharge associated with recurrent bouts of infection.

There are many methods for treatment of chronic pilonidal disease but none has gained widespread acceptance. The ideal treatment of chronic pilonidal disease should (1) eradicate the disease with minimal recurrence rate, (2) avoid hospital admission, (3) produce minimal wound morbidity, and (4) enable the patient to return to daily activities as soon as possible. Many operative procedures claim to meet these criteria, but comparisons of results among different series are difficult because of differences in patient selection, length of follow-up, and lack of consideration of patient inconvenience and financial costs.

Treatment by wide and deep excision is based on the assumption that pilonidal disease is a congenital process and that its eradication requires removal of all epithelial cell rests extending both laterally and down to the presacral fascia. The average healing time is 73 days when the wound is left open to granulate, but it is reduced to 27 days when the skin edges are marsupialized to the presacral fascia.[86] This form of treatment has no practical advantage. It usually requires general anesthesia and hospitalization with aggressive wound management by the patient and the doctor. The recurrence rate at 1 year is similar to that after lay open and marsupialization, and therefore we do not use this technique.

Excision of the follicular opening with tract curettage by brushing[90] or phenol injection[91,92] produces similar early results but higher recurrence rates after 1 year than after lay open techniques. We have had minimal experience with this technique.

Excision of the involved tissue and primary closure have the potential advantage of early wound healing and greater convenience for the patient since prolonged care of an open wound is avoided. However, the procedure usually requires general anesthesia, a longer hospital stay, and restricted physical activity. In 10 percent of the patients, the wound fails to heal primarily, usually secondary to infection, requiring opening of the wound and subsequent treatment by the open technique. The proportion of patients with open wounds at 2 months after primary closure is similar to the proportion of unhealed wounds after the lay open technique.[86] The recurrence rate after primary closure is higher than after open methods of treatment. Displacement of the scar from the midline after primary closure, either by asymmetric skin incision or skin flaps, is associated with lower rates of recurrence.[93–96] However, these procedures are technically more demanding and, if they fail, cause loss of all or part of the skin flap.

Lay open of the fistulous tract with marsupialization of the wound edges is a compromise between wide and deep excision and primary closure.[97] This approach results in a small wound that is reduced even further by marsupializing the skin edges to the floor of the sinus tract over the exposed subcutaneous fat. The average healing time is 43 days. Recurrence rate after lay open and marsupialization is lower than after primary closure, probably because suturing the skin edges to the firm base of the tract changes the contour of the natal cleft, modifying some of the factors that contribute to the development of pilonidal disease.

Lay open of a chronic pilonidal sinus can be performed as an outpatient under local anesthesia with light sedation. With the patient in the prone jackknife position, a field block is achieved around the sinus tracts and skin openings by injecting 1 percent lidocaine with 1:200,000 epinephrine using a fine needle. The sinus is probed and the tissue overlying the tract is incised, unroofing the fistulous tract. The granulation tissue from the sinus tract, side fistulas, and walls of the chronic cystic cavity is curetted, but the firm granular base of the tract is preserved. Devitalized tissue and overhanging skin are excised and the skin edges are marsupialized to the firm base of the tract using a running, absorbable suture. Wounds are kept clean with the aid of daily sitz baths or showers. Patients are examined in the clinic initially every week and later biweekly to inspect the wound and instruct the patient about self-care until the wounds are completely healed. At each visit, necrotic tissue is debrided, excess granulation tissue is removed, and premature skin bridges are divided. The skin around the wound is carefully shaved. After complete healing, patients are instructed to maintain the natal cleft free of hair for at least 6 months.

While late recurrences after treatment for pilonidal disease can be secondary to new follicular infection, most cases of early recurrences represent incompletely healed surgical wounds. Skin debris and hair maintain a chronic infection and foreign body reaction that results in a granulation-lined sinus tract. With time, these tracts can even develop a squamous epithelial lining. This type of complex pilonidal disease is usually the result of a wide excision of a chronic pilonidal sinus, and therefore wider excision to attack the source of the disease and recurrence rarely achieves good results. A number of more aggressive surgical procedures such as wide excision and skin graft,[98] excision and Z-plasty,[99] rotation myocutaneous flaps,[100] and reverse bandaging[101] have been used. Although the healing rate with these techniques has been satisfactory, most of them are technically complex, require prolonged hospitalization, and are sometimes associated with loss of skin sensation or skin necrosis.

Bascom has developed a rotation flap technique that changes the deep and draining cleft into a shallow groove covered with normal skin.[102] Cleft closure is performed by elevating skin flaps, removing skin from the damaged side, and covering the defect with skin from the less damaged side. Raising the flaps exposes the chronic cavity, which is wiped free of granulation tissue and debris. The fat and muscle are not mobilized. After leaving a suction drain, the skin is approximated with subcuticular absorbable suture. Bascom reports 100 percent healing in 30 patients with minimal disability and infrequent and correctable complications.

HIDRADENITIS SUPPURATIVA

Hidradenitis suppurativa is a chronic suppurative and cicatricial disease of the apocrine gland-bearing areas of the skin, particularly the axilla and anogenital region.[103] The disease is unusual before puberty and a postmenopausal onset is rare. Hidradenitis suppurativa affects both sexes, but perianal involvement is more frequent in men. Although the exact sequence of events is unclear, hidradenitis suppurativa appears to be an occlusive disease of the pores of the apocrine glands combined with an element of bacterial infection. Gland rupture leads to local extension with tissue destruction, fibrosis, and sinus tract formation. Assessment of the bacterial role and response to antibiotics in hidradenitis suppurativa is complicated by the chronic relapsing course of the disease, the frequent isolation of mixed cultures, and the fact that most isolated bacteria are human skin flora. The most commonly isolated organisms are *Staphylococcus, Streptococcus, Bacteroides, Proteus,* coliform bacteria, and *Pseudomonas.*[104] Hidradenitis suppurativa has been associated with physiologic hormonal events, overt endocrine disorders, reduced cutaneous levels of zinc and ascorbate, and other skin diseases.[105]

In the early stages of the disease, subcutaneous nodules coalesce to form elevated cords or plaques, which enlarge gradually in size to form large areas of induration. Small abscesses open periodically, draining small amounts of pus and leaving ulcerations and small tracks in the perianal skin. The process involves the perianal region outside the anal canal and, unlike fistula-in-ano, the tracks of hidradenitis suppurativa do not connect with the anal canal or rectum. Severe pain is unusual and most complaints are related to the persistent purulent drainage.

The first step in the treatment of hidradenitis suppurativa is a correct diagnosis because it is frequently misdiagnosed as fistula-in-ano, pilonidal disease, or anorectal abscess. In the early stages, the disease is treated conservatively with sitz baths, warm compresses, antiseptics, and oral antibiotics, particularly erythromycin with or without metronidazole. Antiandrogens[106] and synthetic vitamin A derivatives[107] have been used with variable success.

Incision and drainage of individual lesions may produce temporary relief of symptoms, but lesions inevitably recur.[103] Definitive treatment after control of the acute infection includes radical excision of the involved skin and subcutaneous tissue to the level of healthy fat or fascia.[108] Care should be taken to avoid injury to the sphincter mechanism. The wound may be left to granulate by secondary intention, marsupialized, or covered by a split-thickness or rotational skin graft. Diverting colostomy has been advocated for patients with involvement of the entire perianal area,[109] but other authors treat these patients with staged wide local excisions and reserve colostomy for patients with complex reconstructive procedures or wounds so large that fecal diversion is necessary for adequate hygiene.[108] Patients with extensive perianal disease have been treated with relative success by a "deroofing procedure," a technique that we favor.[110] With this technique, all the abscesses are drained, the sinus tracts unroofed, and the overhanging skin excised. Local recurrences are common and should be treated by local excision of the diseased area with healing by secondary intention.[111]

SEXUALLY TRANSMITTED DISEASES OF THE ANUS

The increase of anal-based erotic practices in recent years has been responsible for the explosive growth in the incidence and variety of sexually transmitted diseases of the anorectal region among homosexual and bisexual men and among women that practice anal receptive intercourse.[112] Promiscuity plays a significant role in the transmission of the majority of these diseases. Some of these patients have more than one disease. Most sexually transmitted diseases are treated by nonsurgical means but are in the differential diagnosis of surgical anorectal problems; therefore colorectal surgeons should have working familiarity with each one of these disorders.

Anorectal Syphilis. Primary anal syphilis is a disease of homosexual men. The causative organism, *Treponema pallidum,* penetrates the anoderm or anal mucosa during anal intercourse. The incubation period ranges from 10 to 90 days, with an average of 21 days.

The primary lesions are usually raised, circular, and indurated. Later, the skin breaks and the lesions ulcerate, producing the typical chancre: an indurated, clean-based ulcer, 1 to 2 cm in diameter, located in the anal margin or anal canal.[113] The chancre is sometimes extremely painful and can therefore be mistaken for an anal fissure. Syphilitic lesions can be eccentrically located, irregular, and multiple, sometimes opposite each other in a "mirror image" or "kissing" configuration. Soon after the development of the primary lesion, inguinal adenopathy develops. The enlarged inguinal lymph nodes have a rubbery consistency and are typically nontender, although secondary bacterial infection of the primary lesion may make them quite tender.

Rectal syphilis appears as localized, thickened, edematous, granular lesions that bleed easily when traumatized. The affected area may be small or extensive and circumferential extension may occur as a result of intramural lymphatic spread. When ulcerated rectal lesions have raised margins, they can be mistaken for adenocarcinoma of the rectum.[114] Rectal syphilis has also been mistaken for lymphoma because both diseases present with submucosal rectal lesions and inguinal lymphadenopathy. Rectal syphilis can be asymptomatic but is often accompanied by tenesmus, mucous discharge, and rectal pain. Primary lesions usually heal spontaneously in 3 to 6 weeks but the patient may develop the secondary stage of syphilis.

Secondary syphilis appears 6 weeks to 6 months after the onset of the primary disease. The manifestations include localized or diffuse mucocutaneous lesions and generalized, nontender lymphadenopathy. The perianal manifestations of secondary syphilis are raised, verrucous, moist, pink or white-gray, highly infectious lesions known as condyloma latum. Superficial mucosal erosions of the anal canal, known as mucous patches, are also common. The secondary lesions and the primary chancre may coexist. Condyloma latum is easily differentiated from condyloma acuminatum. In the latter, the lesions are more desiccated, pedunculated, and keratinized than in condyloma latum.

Syphilis should be in the differential diagnosis of any anal ulcer in homosexual or bisexual men or women with history of anal-receptive intercourse. The diagnosis should be confirmed by dark-field examination of scrapings from the chancre of primary syphilis or condyloma latum of secondary syphilis or by serology. For dark-field examination, the suspected ulcerated lesion should be cleaned with saline and gauze. Any initial exudate should be discarded. Then the serous fluid that flows spontaneously or is squeezed out is mounted on a glass slide, mixed with a drop of saline if necessary, covered with a coverslip, and examined immediately with a dark-field or a phase-contrast microscope. A single negative examination does not exclude syphilis, and the dark-field examination should be repeated on three consecutive days before being considered negative. Gonorrhea frequently coexists with syphilis, and cultures for *Neisseria gonorrhoeae* should be obtained in all cases of anorectal syphilis.

The most commonly used serologic tests for syphilis are the VDRL and RPR, which are nonspecific reagin antibody tests, and the FTA-ABS, which is a specific treponemal antibody test. The nontreponemal tests are inexpensive, easy to perform, and sensitive, making them useful screening tests for syphilis. Individuals with reactive nontreponemal tests should have the diagnosis confirmed by a treponemal serologic test. Treponemal tests usually become reactive before reaginic tests, and, in primary syphilis, the VDRL is negative in almost one-third of the cases, while FTA-ABS is positive in 91 percent. Therefore in patients with suspected primary syphilis, serologic diagnosis can be maximized by performing an FTA-ABS test or by repeating a VDRL after 1 to 2 weeks if the initial VDRL was negative. Both tests are always positive during secondary syphilis.[115]

Patients with primary, secondary, or latent syphilis of less than 1-year duration should be treated with a single intramuscular dose of 2.4 million units of benzathine penicillin. Patients with syphilis of more than 1-year duration require this dose to be repeated at weekly intervals for three successive weeks (7.2 million units total).[116] For patients who are allergic to penicillin, doxycycline, 100 mg orally twice a day, or tetracyline, 500 mg orally four times a day for 14 days, can be used. Erythromycin is an alternative for those patients who cannot tolerate tetracycline. In addition to antibiotic therapy, management of syphilis patients should include HIV counseling. Sexual contacts of patients with syphilis in the preceding 12 months should be prophylactically treated, but before treatment is given, every effort should be made to establish a diagnosis by examination and serologic testing. Patients and sexual partners must abstain from all sexual contacts until proved noninfective by low titers. Follow-up serologic testing should be undertaken at 3-month intervals for 1 year. Appropriate response to therapy is generally defined as a sustained fourfold or greater decline in titer.

Gonococcal Proctitis. Gonorrhea is a common sexually transmitted disease caused by *Neisseria gonorrhoeae,* a gram-negative intracellular diplococcus. Gonococcal proctitis is common in homosexual men. Transmission in men is by anal intercourse, while in women the vast majority of cases are caused by direct extension of vaginal secretions flowing over the anus. While the rectum is the only site of infection in 40 to 50 percent of homosexual men, proctitis is only reported in 6 percent of women without cervical or urethral involvement.[112]

The large number of asymptomatic patients with gonococcal proctitis facilitates the spread of the disease. Symptomatic patients complain of pruritus ani, tenesmus, or mucopurulent or bloody rectal discharge. In advanced cases, dissemination via the bloodstream can occur. The most common manifestations of disseminated disease are arthritis, dermatitis, endocarditis, and meningitis.

Because stratified squamous epithelium is remarkably resistant to invasion by the gonococcus, the anal canal is typically uninvolved. On proctoscopic examination, the rectal mucosa appears erythematous, friable, ulcerated, and covered by a light brown or purulent exudate. Mucopurulent drainage from the anal crypts is characteristic of the disease.

Diagnosis of anorectal gonococcal infections requires a culture on selective media. Ideally, the sample should be obtained by swabbing the mucopurulent exudate during anoscopic examination. Lubricants other than water should be avoided because most of them contain antimicrobial agents. Except in the presence of frank pus, the Gram stain is usually negative. However, the identification of gram-negative intracellular diplococci allows earlier diagnosis and treatment. Samples should be placed immediately on Thayer-Martin or Stuart's medium, which selectively inhibits most other organisms. Because of the changing pattern of antimicrobial resistance, testing for antimicrobial sensitivity is required. Appropriate studies to rule out concomitant syphilis and chlamydial infection should also be performed.

The traditional treatment of gonococcal proctitis is 4.8 million units of aqueous procaine penicillin G administered intramuscularly (2.4 million in each buttock), accompanied by 1 g of probenecid by mouth. However, recent surveillance data indicate that more than 2.2 percent of all gonococci in the United States have plasmid-mediated penicillin resistance, 1.0 percent have plasmid-mediated tetracycline resistance, and 16.8 percent have clinically significant chromosomally mediated resistance.[117] Ceftriaxone is active against all types of resistant strains of *Neisseria gonorrhoeae,* and therefore a single 250-mg intramuscular dose has become the treatment of choice for uncomplicated urethral, endocervical, anorectal, and pharyngeal infection. Because a high proportion of patients with gonorrhea have chlamydial infection, it is recommended that all patients should also be treated with doxycycline, 100 mg orally, twice a day. However, homosexual men are less likely to have chlamydial infections than heterosexual men and women; therefore routine addition of doxycycline has been questioned in this group of patients. Alternatives for treatment of gonorrhea include the use of fluorinated quinolones (ciprofloxacin, norfloxcin, ofloxacin) or a single dose of spectinomycin, 2 g intramuscularly.[118]

Sexual partners exposed to gonorrhea should be examined, cultured, and treated for gonorrhea. Follow-up cultures should be obtained 3 to 7 days after completion of treatment. Cultures should be obtained from the rectum of all women treated for gonorrhea, regardless of whether gonococcal proctitis was documented prior to therapy.

Granuloma Inguinale. Granuloma inguinale is a lesion of tropical regions, caused by *Calymmatobacterium granulomatis,* a gram-negative bacillus transmitted by sexual contact. The initial lesion is a papule at the site of inoculation that develops into a painless, shallow ulcer with a bright red granulation tissue in the base and a raised inflammatory border. Satellite papules and ulcers are common and the perianal lesions are usually extensions of the genital ulcers. Although the lymph nodes are usually spared, the keloid-like scarring that develops after healing of the ulcers may eventually produce lymphatic obstruction and elephantiasis of the external genitalia. The diagnosis of granuloma inguinale should be suspected in any perianal ulcer associated with a genital ulcer without inguinal adenopathy that lasts more than several weeks. The organism cannot be successfully cultured and diagnosis depends on visualization of phagocytized organisms, termed Donovan bodies, within biopsy specimens stained with Giemsa or Wright stain. No serology is available. Treatment is 500 mg of tetracycline given orally four times a day for 7 days.[119]

Chancroid. Chancroid is an acute process characterized by a necrotic ulcer at the site of inoculation and a suppurative inflammation of the regional lymph nodes caused by *Hemophilus ducreyi,* a small gram-negative bacillus. The typical lesion is a painless, nonindurated ulcer known as a soft chancre. Perianal involvement is usually secondary to genital lesions. Two weeks after the appearance of the ulcer, half of the patients develop tender inguinal adenopathy that may become fluctuant and even drain to the skin. Gram stain is unreliable because of limited sensitivity and specificity, and isolation of *H. ducreyi* from ulcers and/or lymph nodes is difficult. Even in experienced laboratories, *H. ducreyi* is recovered from no more than 80 percent of clinically suspected cases. Therefore, in many cases, diagnosis is based on clinical grounds. The susceptibility of this organism to antimicrobial agents varies; and if clinical improvement does not occur after the initial course of therapy, a different antibiotic should be tried. Recommended antibiotic regimens are erythromycin, 500 mg orally four times a day for 7 days; trimethoprim-sulfamethoxazole, one double-strength tablet (160/800 mg) orally twice a day for 7 days; ceftriaxone, 250 mg intramuscular in a single dose; ciprofloxacin, 500 mg orally twice a day for 3 days; or amoxicillin plus clavulinic acid, 500 mg and 125 mg, respectively, three times a day for 7 days. Clinical improvement of ulcerated lesions is expected within a week after institution of therapy, but resolution of adenopathy is slower. Fluctuant lymph nodes should be aspirated to prevent rupture but not surgically drained.[120]

Lymphogranuloma Venereum. Chlamydial infections are the most common sexually transmitted disease in the United States and a frequent cause of proctitis in the homosexual population. Lymphogranuloma venereum is a sexually transmitted disease caused by *Chlamydia trachomatis.* The acute lesion in men is characterized by a transient primary genital lesion followed by regional lymphadenopathy, but women and homosexual men may develop hemorrhagic proctitis with regional lymphadenitis.

Chlamydia trachomatis organisms are obligate intracellular bacteria that, on the basis of outer membrane protein antigenic differences, are divided into 17 different immunotypes. The vast majority of sexually transmitted infections are caused by immunotypes D through K. The L1, L2, and L3 serotypes responsible for the lymphogranuloma venereum syndrome are easier to grow in tissue culture than other immunotypes.[121]

Primary anorectal infection usually occurs after sexual intercourse; but in women, this may also occur by direct spread from a genital infection along the perineum. After an incubation period of an unknown length, multiplication of the chlamydia in the epithelial intestinal cells leads to symptoms that include mucopurulent or bloody discharge, diarrhea, tenesmus, and rectal pain. Complications of anorectal infection include perirectal abscesses, ulcers, perianal fistulas, rectal stenosis, and rectovaginal fistulas. Anal infection can lead to inguinal and femoral lymphadenopathy, but rectal infection produces hypogastric and deep iliac lymphadenitis. Constitutional symptoms are common and include fever, chills, headache, anorexia, myalgias, and arthralgias.[122]

Sigmoidoscopic examination reveals a hemorrhagic, friable, granular mucosa that may resemble ulcerative colitis. In long-standing proctitis, stricture or stenosis that starts within 3 cm of the anal verge and may reach the splenic flexure has been described. In women, the area of stenosis may be adherent to the posterior vaginal wall, occasionally associated with a rectovaginal fistula. In these chronic cases, the rectal mucosa appears pale, atrophic, and friable. Other causes of stricture such as inflammatory bowel disease, ischemia, and malignancy should be excluded.

Because *C. trachomatis* is an intracellular pathogen, confirmatory diagnosis requires culture in mammalian cell lines. McCoy cells are most commonly used. Culture of rectal secretions are usually unrewarding; and in most cases, isolation of the microorganism requires culture of a biopsy of the inflamed rectal mucosa obtained under direct visualization. Nonculture diagnostic tests include direct immunofluorescence with chlamydia-specific monoclonal antibodies and enzyme immunoassay.

The standard therapy for chlamydial infections is tetracycline, 500 mg orally four times a day for 7 days. Alternative regimens include erythromycin, 500 mg orally four times a day; doxycycline, 100 mg orally twice a day; or sulfamethoxazole, 1 g orally twice a day. In cases of anorectal lymphogranuloma venereum, therapy should be maintained for at least 3 weeks.[116]

Efficacy of treatment is reflected in resolution of systemic manifestations and local disease. Antibiotics are usually not helpful in improving late complications such as rectal stricture, but a 3-week course should be attempted in patients with symptomatic stricture. In a soft stricture, gentle dilation should be attempted but hard fibrotic strictures do not respond to dilations. Overzealous attempts at dilation may result in rectal perforation. In some patients, sphincter-saving, excisional surgery may be the only curative alternative.[123]

Herpes Simplex Infection of the Anal and Perianal Area. Genital herpes is a common ulcerative sexually transmitted disease caused by the herpes simplex virus types 1 and 2. Most cases of herpetic proctitis are caused by herpes simplex virus 2. Perianal herpes simplex infection is acquired by anal intercourse and is common in homosexual men.[124] In one study, herpes simplex virus was isolated from 36 percent of homosexual men with proctitis.

The lesions frequently develop 4 to 21 days after anal intercourse. Patients usually present with mild anal irritation followed by severe pain that is exacerbated by bowel movements, enemas, and anal intercourse. Pruritus, tenesmus, reflex constipation, and constitutional symptoms of viremia are also common. Some patients develop a lumbosacral radiculopathy characterized by pain in the pelvis, thighs, or buttocks; paresthesias; urinary dysfunction; and impotence.

During the acute phase of the disease, the anorectum is very tender and physical examination may be impossible without topical anesthesia. Small vesicles, solitary or in clusters, surrounded by a red areola are the first lesions in the perianal area. The vesicles soon rupture leaving aphthous-like ulcerations that coalesce to become larger ulcers. In the anal canal and lower rectum, eroded areas have a grayish floor bordered by edematous, erythematous, and friable mucosa. Many patients have bilateral, tender inguinal lymphadenopathy. These changes are almost always limited to the distal 10 cm of the rectum. The lesions are usually self-limited, with complete healing in approximately 2 to 3 weeks. A chronic relapsing course is common with recurrence rates of 40 percent.

Herpes simplex infection should be considered in the differential diagnosis of any patient with genital or anorectal vesicles, pustules or ulcers, particularly if they are recurrent. Viral culture is the most sensitive and specific way to confirm the diagnosis. Cytologic, immunologic, electron microscopic, and DNA hybridization methods are available for rapid diagnosis of herpes simplex virus infection. Direct immunofluorescence, immunoperoxidase staining, and ELISA are useful for rapid diagnosis. Serotyping of viruses can be achieved with monoclonal antibodies or using restriction endonuclease mapping. The polymerase chain reaction has been applied to the detection of herpes simplex virus infection in patients who are asymptomatically shedding the virus.[125] Serologic response to herpes simplex infection is useful for screening and to document seroconversion in primary genital herpes infection but has no role in the diagnosis of recurrent infection. Concurrent venereal diseases should be ruled out.

In the past, treatment of anal and perianal herpes infections was limited to comfort measures such as sitz baths, cold compresses, local anesthetic ointment, and oral analgesics. At the present time, there is no way to eradicate an established infection; but treatment with oral and topical acyclovir shortens the course, decreases the severity, and suppresses episodes of herpes infections in normal and immunocompromised patients. Most patients with perianal herpes simplex infection should be treated with 400 mg of acyclovir given orally four times a day for 10 days.[126] In addition, topical acyclovir should be used five times a day. Patients with severe perianal involvement or herpes proctitis require intravenous acyclovir, 5 mg/kg over 1 hour every 8 hours for 5 to 7 days followed by oral acyclovir to complete a 10-day course. Chronic suppressive acyclovir therapy, 400 mg twice a day, has been used in patients with frequent recurrences, particularly in AIDS patients. Foscarnet and vidarabine have been used for the treatment of acyclovir-resistant herpes simplex infections. Currently, promotion of safe sex is the only available approach for prevention of transmission.

Condyloma Acuminatum. Condyloma acuminatum is probably the most common sexually transmitted disease treated by colorectal surgeons. Condylomas are small, pink or white, wart-like lesions, usually multiple, with a size ranging from a pinhead to projecting cauliflower-like masses. Condyloma acuminatum lesions are located in the urogenital and anorectal regions up to the dentate line. Extension cephalad to the dentate line is unusual except in immunocompromised patients. They may grow as large clusters completely covering the anal aperture, forming the so-called Buschke-Lowenstein tumor or giant condyloma. Microscopically, condylomas show marked parakeratosis and extreme acanthosis of the epidermis with vacuolization of the cells of the upper prickle layer. Occasionally, condyloma acuminatum is associated with carcinoma in situ.

The causative agent is the human papillomavirus.[127] Of the more than 40 subtypes of papillomavirus described, subtypes 6, 11, 16, and 18 are the most commonly isolated from perianal condylomas. There is strong epidemiologic and clinical evidence suggesting causative relationship between papillomavirus, particularly serotypes 16 and 18, and the development of anal and genital intraepithelial and invasive squamous cell carcinoma.[128]

The prevalence and location of condyloma acuminatum points toward a sexual mode of transmission. Although the lesions can be seen in women and heterosexual men, they are most common among active homosexual and bisexual men. Although autoinoculation from genital warts may occur, anal-receptive intercourse is the usual mode of transmission. In one study, almost half of the male patients with condyloma acuminatum lesions were homosexual. Ninety percent of 70 patients reported by Abcarian and Sharon[129] practiced anal-receptive intercourse. Carr and William[130] reported a 40 to 70 percent prevalence of anal condyloma in a population of homosexual men. More than 50 percent of asymptomatic homosexual men harbor anal condyloma.

Patients with condyloma acuminatum present with relatively minor complaints. Almost all notice visible perianal warts, two-thirds experience pruritus, half describe bleeding with defecation, a few complain of anal wetness, and a minority experience discomfort or pain. Because of the moisture and warmth in the anal region, they may produce a foul-smelling, irritant discharge.

In most cases, the clinical appearance of the lesions makes the diagnosis obvious. Successful therapy requires eradication of all lesions, and therefore localization of intra-anal lesions is extremely important. Sohn and Robilotti[131] found that in only 6 percent of the patients harboring anal condylomas were these confined to the perianal region, while in 84 percent, both perianal and intra-anal lesions were present. Therefore all patients should undergo anoscopy, proctosigmoidoscopy, and genital examination. Condyloma latum is the main differential diagnosis. The lesions of secondary syphilis are smoother, flatter, and more moist than condyloma acuminatum, and they contain spirochetes on dark-field examination. Because of the common association of more than one sexually transmitted disease, condyloma acuminatum and condyloma latum may occur concomitantly. The presence of induration suggests the development of squamous cell carcinoma. A biopsy will establish the diagnosis.

Numerous therapeutic modalities have been used in the treatment of condyloma acuminatum. The inability to destroy small lesions invisible to the naked eye, the potentially long incubating period, and the resumption of sexual contacts before therapy is completed complicate the distinction between true recurrences or reinfection and comparisons between different treatments. Regardless of the method of treatment, patients should be warned about the high recurrence rate of anal condyloma.

The goal of treatment is to eliminate the condylomas while avoiding damage to the surrounding normal skin. Each method has its own advantages and limitations. Local destruction of anal condylomas can be achieved in the office with caustic agents such as podophyllin and bichloracetic acid. Podophyllin is applied as a 25 percent suspension in a vehicle such as liquid paraffin or tincture of benzoin. The warts are accurately painted and patients are instructed to wash the treated area approximately 6 hours after each application. The treatment is repeated at weekly intervals as required. Podophyllin is irritating to skin and local reactions may be severe. It cannot be used in the anal canal, and the application of large amounts may result in systemic toxic effects.[132] Furthermore, chronic use of podophyllin induces skin changes difficult to distinguish from carcinoma in situ.[133] In a prospective, randomized study on the treatment of first-episode anal condylomas, podophyllin application was followed by a higher recurrence rate than after surgical excision.[134]

Bichloracetic acid is a caustic agent that should be applied carefully to condyloma after drying the skin. The treated lesions change from a pink to a frosty white color. Bichloracetic acid is a skin irritant; excess acid should be wiped off, the area washed with water, and sodium bicarbonate used as an antidote. It can be used for anal canal lesions, but the treated lesions should be dabbed gently with a cotton ball before the walls of the anal canal are allowed to fall back together. Bichloracetic acid does not cause systemic toxicity or produce histologic changes that mimic carcinoma in situ. The number of treatments, repeated at weekly intervals, varies according to the size and number of anal condylomas. Recurrence rates as high as 25 percent have been reported,[135] but they can be treated with further short courses of therapy.

Excision and fulguration under local or regional anesthesia are the treatments of choice for extensive perianal involvement. Excision of large lesions allows complete histologic examination while electrocoagulation is used in controlling bleeding points and destroying small lesions. Patients are given two disposable phosphate enemas 30 to 60 minutes before the procedure. The operation is performed with the patient in the prone-jackknife position and the buttocks taped apart. Subcutaneous and submucosal injection of a 1 percent solution of lidocaine with 1:200,000 epinephrine achieves a field block and separates the warts, allowing more precise excision of the individual lesions. Condylomas are removed using a pair of fine-toothed forceps and fine-pointed scissors. Washing the perianal skin with a dilute acetic acid solution and using loops or an operating microscope allow the surgeon to see tiny warts that might otherwise go untreated. Bleeding points and small lesions are electrocoagulated. The aim of electrocoagulation is to produce a white coagulum, which is the equivalent of a superficial, second-degree burn. The white coagulum is wiped away with a gauze. Care should be taken to avoid third-degree burns. Anal stenosis is a potential complication of excision and fulguration and is best avoided by preserving normal skin and mucosa between condylomas. The recurrence rate is approximately 10 to 25 percent.

Cryotherapy has been used in the treatment of condyloma acuminatum, but its main limitation is the inability to control the depth of tissue destruction. Because of the need to store liquid nitrogen or the use of special equipment, cryotherapy is rarely used. The claim that laser therapy produces less pain and fewer recurrences than other forms of therapy has not been corroborated by randomized studies. Furthermore, laser equipment is more expensive and requires special training by the physician and the ancillary staff. The presence of aerosolized, active particles in the laser smoke represents an additional risk to the health care personnel that requires the use of special filter masks and devices to evacuate the smoke.[136] For these reasons, the use of lasers has not gained widespread acceptance.

Intralesional and intramuscular interferon alpha-2 has been used in the treatment of condyloma acuminatum, but clinical results were not better than with excision and fulguration.[137–139] Immunotherapy was originally introduced by Biberstein in 1944.[140] Abcarian and Sharon,[129,141] using six weekly intramuscular injections of an autologous vaccine, reported disappearance of the warts in 84 percent of the patients and partial reduction in an additional 11 percent. These results have been confirmed in later reports.[142] The authors conclude that immunotherapy may be the treatment of choice in extensive, persistent, or recurrent condyloma acuminatum.

Regardless of the type of treatment, condyloma acuminatum has a high rate of recurrence. Patients should be followed in the clinic at monthly intervals for at least 3 months after disappearance of all warts. Unprotected sexual activity may probably be resumed after 3 months free of disease. Limited recurrences can be treated in the clinic with bichloracetic acid or podophyllin.

ANORECTAL SURGERY IN PATIENTS WITH HIV DISEASE AND AIDS

Surgery in patients with AIDS is treated in detail in Chapter 53. It is emphasized that anorectal infections are common in HIV-positive patients.[143] Miles et al[144] found a 5.6 percent incidence of anorectal disease among 1090 HIV-positive patients attending one inner-city hospital. The incidence appears to be much higher in male homosexual patients. In the above-mentioned study, anorectal disease was the most common reason for surgical referral. The list of anorectal conditions in HIV-positive patients includes the entire spectrum of anorectal pathology, but the most common presenting problems are condyloma acuminatum, proctitis, and perianal sepsis. In one study, 63 percent of the patients had more than one anorectal condition.[145]

There is a significant body of evidence suggesting that asymptomatic HIV-positive patients tolerate anorectal surgery better than originally suspected and therefore deserve aggressive surgical treatment of their anorectal ailments.[146] Symptomatic HIV-positive patients demonstrate impaired wound healing and significant rates of morbidity and 6-month mortality.[147–150] The treatment of these patients should be individualized. Before submitting these patients to major anorectal surgery, a careful evaluation of their risk factors and the potential benefits of surgical therapy versus nonoperative treatment is essential.

REFERENCES

1. Milligan ETC, Morgan CN: Surgical anatomy of anal canal with special reference to anorectal fistulae. Lancet 2:1150, 1934.
2. Speakman CTM, Kamm MA: The internal anal sphincter—new insights into faecal incontinence. Gut 32:345, 1991.
3. Gabriel WB, Lloyd-Davies OV: Surgical anatomy of the rectum and anal canal. In: The Principles and Practice of Rectal Surgery, 5th ed. London, HK Lewis and Company, 1963, pp 1–33.
4. Chiari H: Uber die nalen divertikel der rectumschleimhaut und ihre beziehung zu den anal fisteln. Med Jahrbucher Wien 8:418, 1887.
5. Parks AG: Pathogenesis and treatment of fistula-in-ano. Br Med J 5224:463, 1961.
6. Herrmann G, Desfosses L: Sur la muqueuse de la région cloacale du rectum. C R Acad Sci [III] 90:1301, 1880.
7. Eisenhammer S: The internal anal sphincter and the anorectal abscess. Surg Gynecol Obstet 103:501, 1956.
8. Eisenhammer S: A new approach to the anorectal fistulous abscess based on the high intermuscular lesion. Surg Gynecol Obstet 106:595, 1958.
9. Goligher JC, Ellis M, Pissidis AG: A critique of anal glandular infection in the aetiology and treatment of idiopathic anorectal abscesses and fistulas. Br J Surg 54:977, 1967.
10. Eykyn SJ, Grace RH: The relevance of microbiology in the management of anorectal sepsis. Ann R Coll Surg Engl 68:237, 1986.
11. Grace RH, Harper IA, Thompson RG: Anorectal sepsis: microbiology in relation to fistula-in-ano. Br J Surg 69:401, 1982.
12. Whitehead SM, Leach RD, Eykyn SJ, et al: The aetiology of perirectal sepsis. Br J Surg 69:166, 1982.
13. Law PJ, Talbot RW, Bartram CI, et al: Anal endosonography in the evaluation of perianal sepsis and fistula in ano. Br J Surg 76:752, 1989.
14. Guillaumin E, Jeffrey RB Jr, Shea WJ, et al: Perirectal inflammatory disease: CT findings. Radiology 161:153, 1986.
15. Beck DE, Fazio VW, Lavery IC, et al: Catheter drainage of ischiorectal abscesses. South Med J 81:444, 1988.
16. Ellis M: Use of penicillin and sulphonamides in treatment of suppuration. Lancet 1:774, 1951.
17. Wilson DH: The late results of anorectal abscess treated by incision, curettage, and primary suture under antibiotic cover. Br J Surg 51:828, 1964.
18. Leaper DJ, Page RE, Rosenberg IL, et al: A controlled study comparing the conventional treatment of idiopathic anorectal abscess with that of incision, curettage and primary suture under systemic antibiotic cover. Dis Colon Rectum 19:46, 1976.
19. Kronborg O, Olsen H: Incision and drainage v. incision, curettage and suture under antibiotic cover in anorectal abscess. A randomized study with 3-year follow-up. Acta Chir Scand 150:689, 1984.
20. Hanley PH, Ray JE, Pennington EE, et al: Fistula-in-ano: a ten-year follow-up study of horseshoe-abscess fistula-in-ano. Dis Colon Rectum 19:507, 1976.
21. Fucini C: One-stage treatment of anal abscesses and fistulas. A clinical appraisal on the basis of two different classifications. Int J Colorectal Dis 6:12, 1991.
22. Hebjorn M, Olsen O, Haakansson T, et al: A randomized trial of fistulotomy in perianal abscess. Scand J Gastroenterol 22:174, 1987.
23. Schouten WR, van Vroonhoven TJ: Treatment of anorectal abscess with or without primary fistulec-

tomy. Results of a prospective randomized trial. Dis Colon Rectum 34:60, 1991.
24. Bubrick MP, Hitchcock CR: Necrotizing anorectal and perineal infections. Surgery 86:655, 1979.
25. Clayton MD, Fowler JE Jr, Sharifi R, et al: Causes, presentation and survival of fifty-seven patients with necrotizing fasciitis of the male genitalia. Surg Gynecol Obstet 170:49, 1990.
26. Fournier AJ: Gangrene foudrayante de la verge. Semin Med 3:345, 1883.
27. Barkel DC, Villalba MR: A reappraisal of surgical management in necrotizing perineal infections. Am Surg 52:395, 1986.
28. Di Falco G, Guccione C, D'Annibale A: Fournier's gangrene following a perianal abscess. Dis Colon Rectum 29:582, 1986.
29. Enriquez JM, Moreno S, Devesa M, et al: Fournier's syndrome of urogenital and anorectal origin. A retrospective, comparative study. Dis Colon Rectum 30:33, 1987.
30. Blank WA: Anorectal complications in leukemia. Am J Surg 90:738, 1955.
31. Sickles EA, Greene WH, Wiernik PH: Clinical presentation of infection in granulocytopenic patients. Arch Intern Med 135:715, 1975.
32. Boddie AW Jr, Bines SD: Management of acute rectal problems in leukemic patients. J Surg Oncol 33:53, 1986.
33. Corfitsen MT, Hansen CP, Christensen TH, et al: Anorectal abscesses in immunosuppressed patients. Eur J Surg 158:51, 1992.
34. Angel C, Patrick CC, Lobe T, et al: Management of anorectal/perineal infections caused by *Pseudomonas aeruginosa* in children with malignant diseases. J Pediatr Surg 26:487, 1991.
35. Vasilevsky CA, Gordon PH: The incidence of recurrent abscesses or fistula-in-ano following anorectal suppuration. Dis Colon Rectum 27:126, 1984.
36. Scoma JA, Salvati EP, Rubin RJ: Incidence of fistulas subsequent to anal abscesses. Dis Colon Rectum 17:357, 1974.
37. Parks AG, Gordon PH, Hardcastle JD: A classification of fistula-in-ano. Br J Surg 63:1, 1976.
38. Goodsall DH, Miles WE: Ano-rectal fistula. Dis Colon Rectum 25:262, 1982.
39. Kuijpers HC, Schulpen T: Fistulography for fistula-in-ano. Is it useful? Dis Colon Rectum 28:103, 1985.
40. Weisman RI, Orsay CP, Pearl RK, et al: The role of fistulography in fistula-in-ano. Report of five cases. Dis Colon Rectum 34:181, 1991.
41. Cataldo PA, Senagore AJ, Luchtefeld MA: Intrarectal ultrasound in the evaluation of perirectal abscesses. Dis Colon Rectum 36:554, 1993.
42. Choen S, Burnett S, Bartram CI, et al: Comparison between anal endosonography and digital examination in the evaluation of anal fistulae. Br J Surg 78:445, 1991.
43. Pescatori M, Maria G, Anastasio G, et al: Anal manometry improves the outcome of surgery for fistula-in-ano. Dis Colon Rectum 32:588, 1989.
44. Belliveau P, Thomson JP, Parks AG. Fistula-in-ano. A manometric study. Dis Colon Rectum 26:152, 1983.
45. Kuijpers HC: Use of the seton in the treatment of extrasphincteric anal fistula. Dis Colon Rectum 27:109, 1984.
46. Ramanujam PS, Prasad ML, Abcarian H: The role of seton in fistulotomy of the anus. Surg Gynecol Obstet 157:419, 1983.
47. Pearl RK, Andrews JR, Orsay CP, et al: Role of the seton in the management of anorectal fistulas. Dis Colon Rectum 36:573, 1993.
48. Parks AG, Stitz RW: The treatment of high fistula-in-ano. Dis Colon Rectum 19:487, 1976.
49. Williams JG, MacLeod CA, Rothenberger DA, et al: Seton treatment of high anal fistulae. Br J Surg 78:1159, 1991.
50. Culp CE: Use of Penrose drains to treat certain anal fistulas: a primary operative seton. Mayo Clin Proc 59:613, 1984.
51. Christensen A, Nilas L, Christiansen J: Treatment of transsphincteric anal fistulas by the seton technique. Dis Colon Rectum 29:454, 1986.
52. Ustynosky K, Rosen L, Stasik J, et al: Horseshoe abscess fistula. Seton treatment. Dis Colon Rectum 33:602, 1990.
53. Hanley PH: Rubber band seton in the management of abscess-anal fistula. Ann Surg 187:435, 1978.
54. Thomson JP, Ross AH: Can the external anal sphincter be preserved in the treatment of transsphincteric fistula-in-ano? Int J Colorectal Dis 4:247, 1989.
55. Kennedy HL, Zegarra JP: Fistulotomy without external sphincter division for high anal fistulae. Br J Surg 77:898, 1990.
56. Stone JM, Goldberg SM: The endorectal advancement flap procedure. Int J Colorectal Dis 5:232, 1990.
57. Aguilar PS, Plasencia G, Hardy TG Jr, et al: Mucosal advancement in the treatment of anal fistula. Dis Colon Rectum 28:496, 1985.
58. Wedell J, Meier zu Eissen P, Banzhaf G, et al: Sliding flap advancement for the treatment of high level fistulae. Br J Surg 74:390, 1987.
59. Oh C: Management of high recurrent anal fistula. Surgery 93:330, 1983.
60. Shemesh EI, Kodner IJ, Fry RD, et al: Endorectal sliding flap repair of complicated anterior anoperineal fistulas. Dis Colon Rectum 31:22, 1988.
61. Reznick RK, Bailey HR: Closure of the internal opening for treatment of complex fistula-in-ano. Dis Colon Rectum 31:116, 1988.
62. Mann CV, Clifton MA: Re-routing of the track for the treatment of high anal and anorectal fistulae. Br J Surg 72:134, 1985.
63. Held D, Khubchandani I, Sheets J, et al: Management of anorectal horseshoe abscess and fistula. Dis Colon Rectum 29:793, 1986.
64. Parks AG, Gordon PH: Fistula-in-ano: perineal fistula of intra-abdominal or intrapelvic origin simu-

lating fistula-in-ano—report of seven cases. Dis Colon Rectum 19:500, 1976.
65. Nogueras JJ, Rothenberger DA: Surgical management of anorectal Crohn's disease. Prob Gen Surg 10:169, 1993.
66. Rankin GB, Watts HD, Melnyk CS, et al: National Cooperative Crohn's Disease Study: extraintestinal manifestations and perianal complications. Gastroenterology 77:914, 1979.
67. van Outryve MJV, Pelckmans PA, Michielsen PP, et al: Value of transrectal ultrasonography in Crohn's disease. Gastroenterology 101:1171, 1991.
68. Koelbel G, Schmiedl U, Majer MC, et al: Diagnosis of fistulae and sinus tracts in patients with Crohn's disease: value of MR imaging. Am J Roentgenol 152:999, 1989.
69. Fry RD, Shemesh EI, Kodner IJ, et al: Techniques and results in the management of anal and perianal Crohn's disease. Surg Gynecol Obstet 168:42, 1989.
70. Pritchard TJ, Schoetz DJ Jr, Roberts PL, et al: Perirectal abscess in Crohn's disease: drainage and outcome. Dis Colon Rectum 33:933, 1990.
71. Bernstein LH, Frank MS, Brandt LJ, et al: Healing of perineal Crohn's disease with metronidazole. Gastroenterology 79:357, 1980.
72. Brandt LJ, Bernstein LH, Boley SJ, et al: Metronidazole therapy for perineal Crohn's disease: a follow-up study. Gastroenterology 83:383, 1982.
73. Korelitz BI, Present DH: Favorable effect of 6-mercaptopurine on fistula of Crohn's disease. Dig Dis Sci 30:58, 1985.
74. Alexander-Williams J: Fistula-in-ano: management of Crohn's fistula. Dis Colon Rectum 19:518, 1976.
75. Keighley MR, Allan RN: Current status and influence of operation on perineal Crohn's disease. Int J Colorectal Dis 1:104, 1986.
76. Fuhrman GM, Larach SW: Experience with perirectal fistulas in patients with Crohn's disease. Dis Colon Rectum 32:847, 1989.
77. Levien DH, Surrell J, Mazier WP: Surgical treatment of anorectal fistula in patients with Crohn's disease. Surg Gynecol Obstet 169:133, 1989.
78. Williams JG, Rothenberger DA, Nemer FD, et al: Fistula-in-ano in Crohn's disease. Results of aggressive surgical treatment. Dis Colon Rectum 34:378, 1991.
79. Morrison JG, Gathright JB Jr, Ray JE, et al: Surgical management of anorectal fistulas in Crohn's disease. Dis Colon Rectum 32:492, 1989.
80. White RA, Eisenstat TE, Rubin RJ, et al: Seton management of complex anorectal fistulas in patients with Crohn's disease. Dis Colon Rectum 33:587, 1990.
81. Jones IT, Fazio VW, Jagelman DG: The use of transanal advancement flaps in the management of fistulas involving the anorectum. Dis Colon Rectum 30:919, 1987.
82. Lewis P, Bartolo DCC: Treatment of trans-sphincteric fistulae by full thickness anorectal advancement flaps. Br J Surg 77:1187, 1990.
83. Sher ME, Bauer JJ, Gorphine S, et al: Low Hartmann's procedure for severe anorectal Crohn's disease. Dis Colon Rectum 35:975, 1992.
84. Hodges RM: Pilonidal sinus. Boston Med Surg J 103:485, 1880.
85. Dwight RW, Maloy JK: Pilonidal sinus: experience with 449 cases. N Engl J Med 249:926, 1953.
86. Allen-Mersh TG: Pilonidal sinus: finding the right track for treatment. Br J Surg 77:123, 1990.
87. Patey DH, Scarff RW: Pathology of postnatal pilonidal sinus: its bearing on treatment. Lancet 2:484, 1946.
88. Bascom J: Pilonidal disease: origin from follicles of hairs and results of follicle removal as treatment. Surgery 87:567, 1980.
89. Bascom J: Pilonidal disease: long-term results of follicle removal. Dis Colon Rectum 26:800, 1983.
90. Lord PH, Millar DM: Pilonidal sinus: a simple treatment. Br J Surg 52:298, 1965.
91. Maurice BA, Greenwood RK: A conservative treatment of pilonidal sinus. Br J Surg 51:510, 1964.
92. Hegge HG, Vos GA, Patka P, et al: Treatment of complicated or infected pilonidal sinus by local application of phenol. Surgery 102:52, 1987.
93. Farringer JL Jr, Pickens DR Jr: Pilonidal cyst: an operative approach. Am J Surg 135:262, 1978.
94. Fishbein RH, Handelsman JC: A method for primary reconstruction following radical excision of sacrococcygeal pilonidal disease. Ann Surg 190:231, 1979.
95. Manterola C, Barroso M, Araya JC, et al: Pilonidal disease: 25 cases treated by the Dufourmentel technique. Dis Colon Rectum 34:649, 1991.
96. Karydakis GE: Easy and successful treatment of pilonidal sinus after explanation of its causative process. Aust N Z J Surg 62:385, 1992.
97. Solla JA, Rothenberger DA: Chronic pilonidal disease. An assessment of 150 cases. Dis Colon Rectum 33:758, 1990.
98. Guyuron B, Dinner MI, Dowden RV: Excision and grafting in treatment of recurrent pilonidal sinus disease. Surg Gynecol Obstet 156:201, 1983.
99. McDermott FT: Pilonidal sinus treated by Z-plasty. Aust N Z J Surg 37:64, 1967.
100. Perez-Gurri JA, Temple WJ, Ketcham AS: Gluteus maximus myocutaneous flap for the treatment of recalcitrant pilonidal disease. Dis Colon Rectum 27:262, 1984.
101. Rosenberg I: The dilemma of pilonidal disease: reverse bandaging for cure of the reluctant pilonidal wound. Dis Colon Rectum 20:290, 1977.
102. Bascom JU: Repeat pilonidal operations. Am J Surg 154:118, 1987.
103. Banerjee AK: Surgical treatment of hidradenitis suppurativa. Br J Surg 79:863, 1992.
104. Highet AS, Warren RE, Weekes AJ: Bacteriology and antibiotic treatment of perineal suppurative hidradenitis. Arch Dermatol 124:1047, 1988.
105. Harrison BJ, Read GF, Hughes LE: Endocrine basis

for the clinical presentation of hidradenitis suppurativa. Br J Surg 75:972, 1988.
106. Sawers RS, Randall VA, Ebling FJ: Control of hidradenitis suppurativa in women using antiandrogen (cyproterone acetate) and oestrogen therapy. Br J Dermatol 115:269, 1985.
107. Brown CF, Gallup DG, Brown VM: Hidradenitis suppurativa of the anogenital region: response to isotretinoin. Am J Obstet Gynecol 158:12, 1988.
108. Wiltz O, Schoetz DJ Jr, Murray JJ, et al: Perianal hidradenitis suppurativa. The Lahey Clinic experience. Dis Colon Rectum 33:731, 1990.
109. Ching CC, Stahlgren LH: Clinical review of hidradenitis suppurativa: management of cases with severe perianal involvement. Dis Colon Rectum 8:349, 1965.
110. Brown SC, Kazzazi N, Lord PH: Surgical treatment of perineal hidradenitis suppurativa with special reference to recognition of the perianal form. Br J Surg 73:978, 1986.
111. Harrison BJ, Mudge M, Hughes LE: Recurrence after surgical treatment of hidradenitis suppurativa. Br Med J Clin Res 294:487, 1987.
112. Wexner SD: Sexually transmitted diseases of the colon, rectum, and anus: the challenge of the nineties. Dis Colon Rectum 33:1048, 1990.
113. Akdamar K, Martin RJ, Ichinose H: Syphilitic proctitis. Am J Dig Dis 22:701, 1977.
114. Drusin LM, Singer C, Valenti AJ, et al: Infectious syphilis mimicking neoplastic disease. Arch Intern Med 137:156, 1977.
115. Miller JN: Value and limitations of nontreponemal and treponemal tests in the laboratory diagnosis of syphilis. Clin Obstet Gynecol 18:191, 1975.
116. Sexually transmitted diseases treatment guidelines. MMWR Morb Mortal Wkly Rep 38:S-8, 1989.
117. Schwarcz SK, Zenilman JM, Schnell D, et al: National surveillance of antimicrobial resistance in *Neisseria gonorrhoeae*. The gonococcal isolate surveillance project. JAMA 264:1413, 1990.
118. Judson FN: Gonorrhea. Med Clin North Am 74:1353, 1990.
119. Richens J: Donovanosis—a review. Papua New Guinea Med J 28:67, 1985.
120. Morse SA: Chancroid and *Haemophilus ducreyi*. Clin Microbiol Rev 2:137, 1989.
121. Wang SP, Grayston JT: Immunologic relationship between genital TRIC, lymphogranuloma venereum, and related organisms in the new microtiter indirect immunofluorescence test. Am J Ophthalmol 70:367, 1970.
122. Grace AW: Anorectal lymphogranuloma venereum. JAMA 122:74, 1943.
123. Goligher JC: Sexually transmitted diseases. In: Surgery of the Anus, Rectum, and Colon, 5th ed. London, Balliere-Tindall, 1984, pp 1033–1046.
124. Goodell SE, Quinn TC, Mkrtichian E, et al: Herpes simplex virus proctitis in homosexual men. Clinical, sigmoidoscopic, and histopathological features. N Engl J Med 308:868, 1983.
125. Hardy DA, Arvin AM, Yasukawa LL, et al: Use of polymerase chain reaction for successful identification of asymptomatic genital infection with herpes simplex viius in pregnant woman at delivery. J Infect Dis 162:1031, 1990.
126. Rompalo AM, Mertz GJ, Davis LG, et al: Oral acyclovir for treatment of first-episode herpes simplex virus proctitis. JAMA 259:2879, 1988.
127. Oriel JD, Almeida JD: Demonstration of virus particles in human genital warts. Br J Venereal Dis 46:37, 1970.
128. Palmer JG, Scholefield JH, Coates PJ, et al: Anal cancer and human papillomaviruses. Dis Colon Rectum 32:1016, 1989.
129. Abcarian H, Sharon N: The effectiveness of immunotherapy in the treatment of anal condyloma acuminatum. J Surg Res 22:231, 1977.
130. Carr G, William DC: Anal warts in a population of gay men in New York City. Sex Transm Dis 4:56, 1977.
131. Sohn N, Robilotti JG: The gay bowel syndrome. A review of colonic and rectal conditions in 200 male homosexuals. Am J Gastroenterol 67:478, 1977.
132. Montaldi DH, Giambrone JP, Courey NG, et al: Podophyllin poisoning associated with the treatment of condyloma acuminatum: a case report. Am J Obstet Gynecol 119:1130, 1974.
133. Connors RC, Ackerman AB: Histologic pseudomalignancies of the skin. Arch Dermatol 112:1767, 1976.
134. Jensen SL: Comparison of podophyllin application with simple surgical excision in clearance and recurrence of perianal condylomata acuminata. Lancet 2:1146, 1985.
135. Swerdlow DB, Salvati EP: Condyloma acuminatum. Dis Colon Rectum 14:226, 1971.
136. Garden JM, O'Banion MK, Shelnitz LS, et al: Papillomavirus in the vapor of carbon dioxide laser-treated verrucae. JAMA 259:1199, 1988.
137. Schonfeld A, Nitke S, Schattner A, et al: Intramuscular human interferon-beta injections in treatment of condylomata acuminata. Lancet 1:1038, 1984.
138. Eron LJ, Judson F, Tucker S, et al: Interferon therapy for condylomata acuminata. N Engl J Med 315:1059, 1986.
139. Friedman-Kien AE, Eron LJ, Conant M, et al: Natural interferon alpha for treatment of condylomata acuminata. JAMA 259:533, 1988.
140. Biberstein H: Immunization therapy of warts. Arch Dermatol Syph 50:12, 1944.
141. Abcarian H, Sharon N: Long-term effectiveness of the immunotherapy of anal condyloma acuminatum. Dis Colon Rectum 25:648, 1982.
142. Eftaiha MS, Amshel AL, Shonberg IL, et al: Giant and recurrent condyloma acuminatum: appraisal of immunotherapy. Dis Colon Rectum 25:136, 1982.
143. Scholefield JH, Northover JM, Carr ND: Male homosexuality, HIV infection and colorectal surgery. Br J Surg 77:493, 1990.
144. Miles AJ, Mellor CH, Gazzard B, et al: Surgical

management of anorectal disease in HIV-positive homosexuals. Br J Surg 77:869, 1990.
145. Orkin BA, Smith LE: Perineal manifestations of HIV infection. Dis Colon Rectum 35:310, 1992.
146. Wexner SD, Smithy WB, Milson JW, et al: The surgical management of anorectal diseases in AIDS and pre-AIDS patients. Dis Colon Rectum 29:719, 1986.
147. Beck DE, Jaso RG, Zajac RA: Proctologic management of the HIV-positive patient. South Med J 83:900, 1990.
148. Wolkomir AF, Barone JE, Hardy HW III, et al: Abdominal and anorectal surgery and the acquired immune deficiency syndrome in heterosexual intravenous drug users. Dis Colon Rectum 33:267, 1990.
149. Safavi A, Gottesman L, Dailey TH: Anorectal surgery in the HIV+ patient: update. Dis Colon Rectum 34:299, 1991.
150. Burke EC, Orloff SL, Freise CE, et al: Wound healing after anorectal surgery in human immunodeficiency virus–infected patients. Arch Surg 126:1267, 1991.

Infections of the Skeletal System

CHAPTER 46

Robert H. Fitzgerald, Jr., Patrick J. Kelly

> When a Cartilage therefore is inflamed, and soaked in purulent Matter, the transverse or connecting Fibres will the soonest give way, and the Cartilage becomes more or less red and soft. If the Disorder goes on a little longer, and Cartilage does not throw off a Slough, but separates from the Bone, where the Force of Cohesion is least, and where the Disease soon arrives, by reason of the Thinness of the Cartilage. . . . But if, unfortunately, the Patient labours under a bad Habit of Body, the Malignancy, having got Root in the Bone, will daily gain ground, the *Caries* will spread, and at last the unhappy Person must submit to Extirpation, a doubtful Remedy, or wear out a painful, though probably a short Life.
>
> William Hunter, 1743[1]

The introduction of antimicrobial drugs dramatically improved the treatment of a spectrum of serious infectious diseases. Although the results of treatment of acute hematogenous osteomyelitis have been improved by the introduction of newer and more potent agents over that described by William Hunter, chronic osteomyelitis and established septic arthritis remain recalcitrant.

Even though an extensive vascular network exists in osseous tissue, sequestration of devascularized areas of bone creates an environment that permits continued bacterial growth without interference by host defense mechanisms or antimicrobial agents. This basic response of infected osseous tissue isolated from the systemic circulation is fundamental in the development of chronic osseous infections.

Sepsis of the skeletal system can be divided into osteomyelitis, septic arthritis, and postoperative wound sepsis. The microbiologic findings and the medical and surgical treatment of septic arthritis and osteomyelitis differ with various causes, that is, hematogenous, post-traumatic, and postoperative.

OSTEOMYELITIS

Wilensky credits Nelaton with introducing the term *osteomyelitis* in 1834.[2] Nelaton distinguished inflammation of cortical bone, *osteite*, from inflammation of the medulla, *osteomyelitie.* Although osteomyelitis frequently begins in the medullary portion of tubular bones, the term is generally understood to signify an infection of either the cortical or medullary portion of a bone. Pyogenic or bacterial osteomyelitis can be subdivided into hematogenous and secondary forms, which include osteomyelitis from a contiguous focus of infection, as well as post-traumatic and postoperative osteomyelitis.

Pathobiology of Bone Infections

Osteomyelitis is usually initiated by bacteremia lodging in a receptive bony site, usually the metaphysis in children and infants, and in the middle of the shaft of the long bone, pelvic bone, or body of a vertebra in adults.

The vascular supply of the metaphysis in a child older than 1 year seems to be critical for the localization of infection. In growing long bones, the blood supply to the metaphysis is separate from that of the epiphysis. The metaphyseal nutrient artery terminates in acutely looped capillaries beneath the cartilaginous growth plate that flow into venous sinusoids in which blood flow is sluggish. Furthermore, the circulating polymorphonuclear leukocytes can be found in this area. Although there is an abundance of chondroblasts, there is a paucity of tissue-based phagocytes. Septic emboli apparently lodge here and thrombose the terminal capillaries of the nutrient artery, which fosters spread of infection from the venous lakes. The lack of circulating and tissue-based phagocytes permits bacterial growth. In the child, the cartilaginous growth plate is an effective barrier to communication between the blood supply of the shaft and that of the epiphysis. Thus, in a child older than 1 year, bacteremia that leads to metaphyseal osteomyelitis rarely involves the epiphysis. Septic arthritis is an unusual complication of metaphyseal or diaphyseal osteomyelitis in children.

In infancy, blood vessels from the metaphysis perforate the cartilaginous growth plates of the long bones and penetrate the epiphysis, forming venous lakes similar to those in the metaphysis. Because of these vascular communications through the growth plate, infection of the shaft and metaphysis by the nutrient artery can invade the epiphysis and extend secondarily into the joint to produce septic arthritis.

In adulthood, the growth plate has fused, and the old cartilage growth plate has been penetrated by metaphyseal vessels. Vascular communications are then reestablished between the metaphyseal and epiphyseal circulations so that osteomyelitis can once again extend beneath the articular cartilage and into the involved joint. For these reasons, infants have severe, often permanent epiphyseal damage and joint infection, a large involucrum, but only transient damage to the shaft and metaphysis. Children have extensive cortical damage with involucrum and, rarely, damage to the growth cartilage and to joints. Adults have cortical atrophy, chronic infection of the marrow cavity, and chronic discharging sinuses, often with extraperiosteal abscesses and joint involvement.

Infecting agents of low virulence may be inhibited and eradicated by host defense mechanisms. Alternately, host tissue may isolate and wall off the nidus of infection, forming a Brodie abscess (Fig. 46–1). When a Brodie abscess is formed, the remaining microorganisms are usually destroyed, resulting in serous fluid or fibrous tissues filling the cavity. When classic osteomyelitis occurs, necrosis and increased pressure result in the spread of the infection through paths of least resistance—the haversian and Volkmann canals—as well as the intramedullary space. A subperiosteal abscess occurs if the process continues unabated. When the endosteal and the periosteal blood supplies are occluded, sequestration or separation of the entire cortex can occur. Frequently, only a portion of the cortex is involved. The host attempts to isolate the infectious process with new periosteal and endosteal bone forming an involucrum about the necrotic bone (the sequestrum). An inflammatory reaction occurs in adjacent areas, which is the basis for the reactive synovitis so frequently seen in adjacent joints.

This sequence can be altered at any stage by host defense mechanisms or by the administration of antimicrobial agents. If significant necrosis has occurred, operative intervention is usually required to halt the progression of the disease.

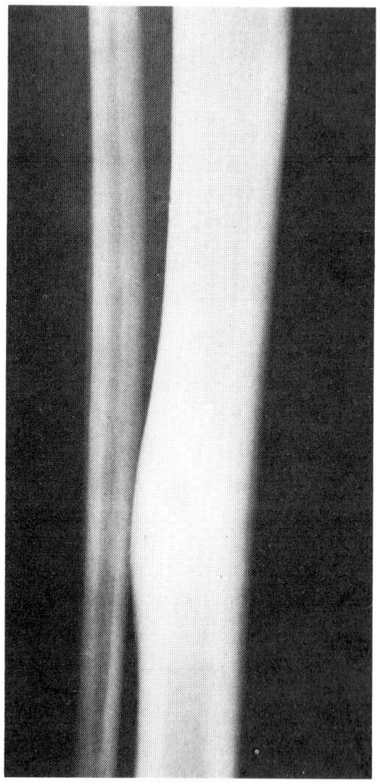

Figure 46–1. Brodie's abscess of tibial diaphysis. Lytic zone is surrounded by zone of sclerosis in middle third of tibia.

Hematogenous Osteomyelitis in Infants and Children

Incidence. Acute hematogenous osteomyelitis is primarily a disease of children between the ages of 3 and 15 years[3] but has been noted in neonates. A predilection for the metaphyseal region of a long tubular bone is seen, so that the most frequent sites of involvement include the proximal tibial and distal femoral metaphysis. The humerus, fibula, radius, and ulna are involved less frequently. Spinal involvement in the pediatric patient is usually limited to the intervertebral disc (Table 46–1).

Most of the patients in whom the proximal femoral metaphysis is involved are infants, and most of these are associated with septic arthritis of the hip. In older children, the distal femur and proximal tibia are frequent sites of involvement. All three sites account for a large percentage of the growth of the extremity and can easily be damaged by uncontrolled infection.

Etiology. Staphylococcus aureus can be isolated from material obtained by aspiration or open biopsy in 80 to 90 percent of the patients. Most of the staphylococcal isolates will be resistant to penicillin. Streptococcal osteomyelitis is less frequent and is usually limited to patients who are 3 years of age or younger. In contrast to the adult patient with osteomyelitis, gram-negative bacilli are rarely isolated from infections in the pediatric patient (Table 46–2).

TABLE 46–1. SITES OF INVOLVEMENT, BY AGE, IN CHILDREN WITH HEMATOGENOUS OSTEOMYELITIS[a]

Site	Age: *2*	*3–8*	*9–16*	Total
Femur (*N* = 50)				
Proximal	8	12	9	29
Middle	0	2	3	5
Distal	3	4	9	16
Tibia (*N* = 42)				
Proximal	3	3	12	18
Middle	1	1	2	4
Distal	2	7	11	20
Humerus	3	4	5	12
Fibula	1	3	4	8
Radius	1	1	1	3
Ulna	0	1	1	2
Pelvis	0	5	5	10
Total	22	43	62	127[b]

[a] Three patients had multiple sites of involvement.
[b] Total does not reflect patients with involvement of cranium (2), talus (1), clavicle (2), calcaneus (3), tarsal navicular (1), scapula (1), and rib (1).
Adapted from Morrey BF, Peterson HA: Orthop Clin North Am 6:935, 1975.

TABLE 46–2. CULTURE RESULTS, BY AGE, IN CHILDREN WITH HEMATOGENOUS OSTEOMYELITIS

Culture	Age: *2*	*3–8*	*9–16*	Total
Staphylococci				
Penicillin-resistant	5	10	23	38
Penicillin-sensitive	0	6	5	11
Unclassified	2	7	11	20
Coagulase-negative	1	1	4	6
Streptococci	7	0	3	10
Gram-negative rods	1	1	0	2
Anaerobic	0	2	0	2
Culture negative	6	12	14	32
Not done	1	4	9	14
Total	23	43	69	135

Adapted from Morrey BF, Peterson HA: Orthop Clin North Am 6:935, 1975.

Clinical Manifestations

IN CHILDREN. Clinically, acute hematogenous osteomyelitis is characterized by an abrupt onset of pain of increasing severity and pyrexia.[4] The patient may be lethargic, dehydrated, and irritable. Early in the infection, the lack of local signs of inflammation may be misleading. A limp or limited use of an involved extremity may be the only clinical finding. In the younger child, pseudoparalysis can be the earliest sign. Close scrutiny reveals that the adjacent joints are flexed and the regional muscles are in spasm. If examination is performed gently, passive motion can be demonstrated in adjacent joints, an important sign in differentiating osteomyelitis from septic arthritis. If an abscess has ruptured through the periosteum, a fluctuant mass can be palpated in the soft tissues. Leukocytosis with a definite shift to the left and an elevation of the erythrocyte sedimentation rate are characteristically present.

It is important to emphasize that x-ray studies initially will reveal only soft tissue changes. A technetium-99 scan can be helpful in making an early diagnosis and localizing the site of involvement. Not until 10 to 14 days after the onset of the infection will a localized destruction surrounded by a zone of decalcification in the metaphysis be visualized by x-ray. Lacy periosteal new bone formation can be observed 2 to 4 weeks after onset. A moth-eaten appearance in the metaphysis appears if the infection continues without treatment (Fig. 46–2).

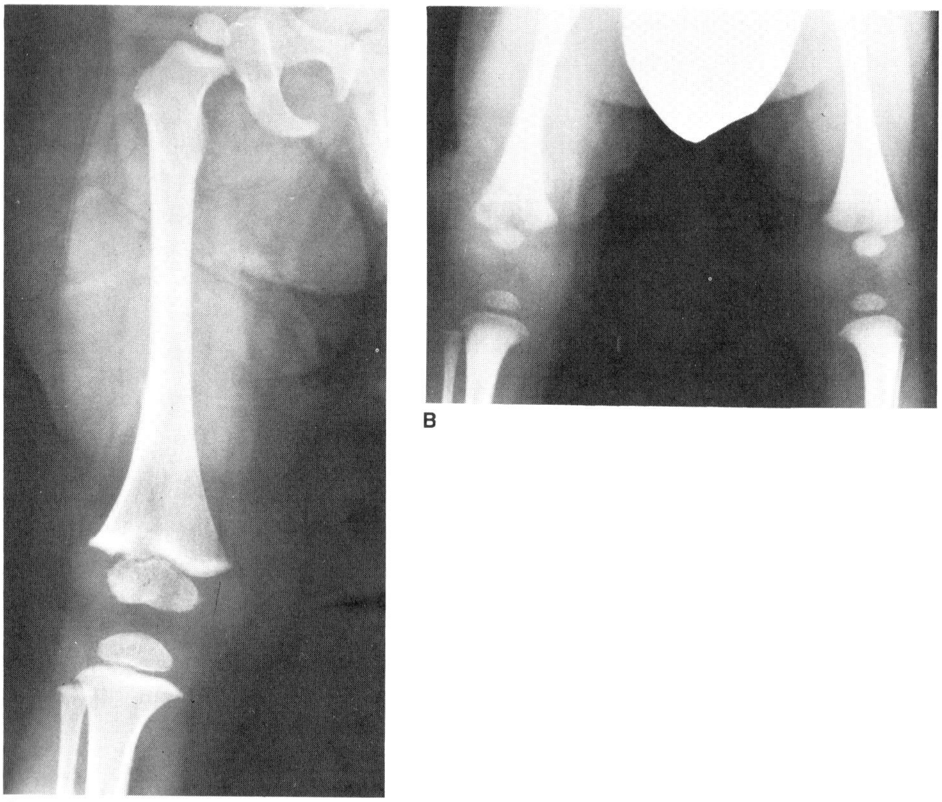

A B

Figure 46–2. A. Newborn child with soft-tissue swelling and early lytic involvement of distal femoral epiphyseal plate. **B.** Three weeks later, further destruction of distal femoral epiphyseal plate and metaphysis has occurred despite parenteral antibiotic therapy. Surgical debridement was required to eradicate infection.

Inadequate administration of antimicrobial agents results in a subacute form of the disease characterized by persistence of regional physical findings and a lack of systemic symptoms. The erythrocyte sedimentation rate remains elevated in spite of a normal leukocyte count. Alteration of the osseous structures can be identified by x-ray studies.

Diagnosis. It is important to obtain clinical material culture to identify the specific organism(s) and determine antibiotic sensitivities in all cases of osteomyelitis. Subperiosteal or intraosseous needle aspiration and aspiration of a contiguous joint are useful procedures when x-ray studies are unrevealing. If there is evidence, however, of a lytic lesion in a metaphysis, the area can be drained through a cortical window and tissue obtained for culture.

Osteomyelitis can be difficult to distinguish from Ewing sarcoma when x-ray changes have occurred in the subacute form. Urgent operative exploration, biopsy, and culture are mandatory.[4]

Treatment. When acute hematogenous osteomyelitis is diagnosed early, parenteral administration of an antimicrobial agent and splinting of the involved extremity will arrest the infection.[4] If, however, the infection has become established, debridement will be required. Usually, removal of a cortical window for the metaphyseal area permits decompression of intramedullary abscesses and excision of sequestrated osseous tissue. Closure can be accomplished over suction drainage a few days later.

Acute Osteomyelitis in Adults. Acute hematogenous osteomyelitis in adults is uncommon in diaphyseal long bones and usually is limited to the axial skeleton in debilitated patients who are in their fifth or sixth decade. The thoracolumbar segments of the spinal column are most frequently involved. *Staphylococcus aureus* is the usual etiologic agent. Residual *S. aureus* infections from childhood osteomyelitis are sometimes seen in the long bones. When retrograde seeding of the vertebral body through the interconnecting plexus of valveless veins occurs from an antecedent infection of the pelvic organs or after instrumentation of the urogenital tract, gram-negative bacillary organisms (most commonly *Pseudomonas aeruginosa*, *Proteus mirabilis*, *Enterobacter*, and *Escherichia coli*) are found.[5] Osteomyelitis caused by *Salmonella* is becoming more common, especially in immunocompromised patients and in the long tubular bones of patients with hemoglobinopathies. An increasing number of young adults, particularly drug addicts, have hematogenous vertebral or clavicular osteomyelitis.[6] Submission of tissue specimens to the microbiology laboratory before initiating antimicrobial therapy is important because unusual causative organisms, such as *P. aeruginosa* and *Candida albicans*, are frequently isolated.

Most adults with hematogenous osteomyelitis of the axial skeleton have fever symptoms and an elevated leukocyte count and sedimentation rate, and most can be treated with bed rest and specific antimicrobial therapy. After the initial symptoms subside, the spinal column should be protected with either a cast or a brace.

Contiguous Osteomyelitis. Osteomyelitis after incomplete antimicrobial therapy for exogenous contamination or an antecedent contiguous soft tissue infection in children has been noted more frequently in recent years. Many of the children with this type of osteomyelitis have sustained puncture wounds of the foot. Their clinical course is altered by oral antimicrobial therapy prescribed in emergency rooms. A progressive limp necessitates further medical consultation. The patient is usually afebrile. Examination reveals an exquisitely tender site with or without an inflammatory response near the previous plantar puncture wound. The erythrocyte sedimentation rate is elevated.

Previous antimicrobial therapy can make identification of the causal organism(s) difficult. Gram-negative bacillary rods predominate in patients with secondary forms of osteomyelitis.

Pseudomonas aeruginosa has been isolated from tissue specimens in more than 90 percent of the patients who have sustained puncture wounds of the foot. Interestingly, *P. aeruginosa* has been isolated from used sneakers and from sneakers worn at the time of the puncture.[7] Surgical debridement is invariably required for eradication of the infection. A retained foreign body can occasionally be identified at operation. When a foreign body is not located during debridement, the central nidus of the infection involves a cartilaginous surface—articular, epiphyseal, or apophyseal.

Chronic Osteomyelitis

Incidence. In the adult, chronic osteomyelitis of the femur and tibia can be categorized into four clinical subsets: fracture with nonunion (FN), fracture with union (FU), postoperative/posttraumatic (PO) in which osteomyelitis occurs after surgery or a penetrating wound, and hematogenous (H). In a series of 401 patients, the following incidences of the various categories were observed: FN, 42.6 percent; FU, 30.2 percent; H, 18.2 percent; and PO, 9 percent. There has been a dramatic increase in FN and a similar dramatic decrease in H. A more recent experience over the last decade and a half reveals little change: FN, 42 percent; FU, 31 percent; H, 19 percent; and PO, 8 percent.[8]

Chronic osteomyelitis after elective musculoskeletal surgery accounts for an increasing number of the patients with chronic osteomyelitis. The prognosis depends on the area involved. In patients with spinal involvement, eradication of the septic process without sacrificing osseous stability or creating neural deficit can create formidable problems. If other areas are involved, a reasonably successful outcome can be anticipated, with removal of foreign bodies, saucerization, and sequestrectomy.

West and associates[9] report that the most frequent sites of involvement in chronic osteomyelitis include the tibia and the femur. The upper extremity is less often involved. However, when osteomyelitis occurs in the arm, the humerus, radius, and ulna are the most frequent sites. Osteomyelitis of the small bones of the hand is usually secondary to penetrating wounds. Involvement of the foot is frequently associated with occlusive vascular disease or diabetes mellitus. The prognosis obviously reflects the severity of the underlying problem, and when the appropriate vascular procedure is successful, a localized amputation will rectify the problem.

Etiology. Chronic osteomyelitis appearing as a late complication of the acute disease in childhood is most often caused by a penicillin-sensitive *S. aureus*. Chronic posttraumatic osteomyelitis is usually caused by polymicrobic, gram-negative organisms, especially *P. aeruginosa* and *P. mirabilis*, with or without *S. aureus*.

Anaerobes have been isolated infrequently from surgical specimens in patients with osteomyelitis. We have isolated anaerobes from 22 percent of 182 patients with osteomyelitis treated over a 28-month period.[10] Actinomycosis of the mandible and other head and neck sites is an obvious exception. More recently, improved transportation vials and increased physician awareness have led to the isolation of increasing numbers of anaerobic organisms from tissue cultures in patients with osteomyelitis, especially after trauma. In a study of *Bacteroides* infections of the musculoskeletal system by Nettles and co-workers,[11] 4 of the 11 patients had chronic osteomyelitis. In a recent study of 182 patients, anaerobic organisms were isolated from 40 (22 percent).[12] A wide variety of gram-positive and gram-negative anaerobic isolates were recovered. In all but one patient, the anaerobes were isolated from a mixed culture consisting of both aerobic and anaerobic organisms.

In a series reported by Finegold,[13] 22 of 58 patients with osteomyelitis had anaerobes recovered. Only 3 of the 22 had only anaerobes. In the group of 22 patients, there were 92 aerobic or facultative isolates (14 *S. aureus*, 32 Enterobacteriaceae, 9 *P. aeruginosa*, 22 streptococci) and 98 anaerobic isolates (33 *Bacteroides*, 4 *Fusobacterium*, 29 *Peptococcus*, 8 *Peptostreptococcus*, 6 *Actinomyces*). In brief, the flora resembled that of long-standing soft tissue infections.

When anaerobic organisms are recovered from tissue specimens harboring mixed aerobic-anaerobic organisms, the incidence of recurrent sepsis is 62 percent. In contrast, pure anaerobic infections have proved to be highly responsive to the combination of surgery and specific antimicrobial therapy.[10]

Diagnosis. The clinical and radiographic findings, including tomography results, should outline the diseased areas. Sinograms may be helpful in demonstrating the degree of soft tissue involvement. The microbiologic diagnosis is more complicated. Because various causal organisms are isolated from the different types of osteomyelitis, separate deep tissue specimens should be obtained from bone, muscle, and fascia. Swab cultures of sinus tract drainage are notoriously misleading. Most organisms isolated from sinus tract drainage will not be recovered from cultures of deep tissue. If *S. aureus* is isolated from the drainage, however, it will invariably be isolated from deep tissue cultures. Furthermore, as treatment progresses the saucerized cavity should be recultured and susceptibility studies performed. An irrigation-suction system, formerly employed in the treatment of osteomyelitis, should not be used, as gram-negative bacterial contamination and superinfection of the irrigation-suction system are common.

Treatment. The treatment of chronic osteomyelitis is prolonged, requiring at least 4 weeks of parenteral antimicrobial therapy and two operations. Surgical treatment of chronic osteomyelitis is based on four principles: (1) excision of dead bone, (2) removal of infected granulation tissue, (3) obliteration of dead space, and (4) obtaining union when nonunion exists.[14] Achieving union in a nonunited and infected fracture may seem difficult, but many fractures unite without further operation after the infection has resolved. The recent introduction of external fixation devices has been invaluable in the management of the infected nonunion, especially if fixed in two planes. In these authors' experience, union was achieved in 85 percent of the 71 patients with a tibial nonunion in whom bone grafts were used and 86 percent of the patients in whom bone grafts were not utilized. In 60 patients with femoral nonunion, 31 patients received bone grafting procedures and 90 percent achieved union. In contrast, only 79 percent of the 29 patients treated without a bone graft experienced union of the femur.

CHRONIC HEMATOGENOUS OSTEOMYELITIS. Tomograms and bone scans are valuable in planning the operations. Exposure of cavities invaded by infected granulation tissue with unroofing procedures is essential. Because patients with chronic hematogenous osteomyelitis have bony stability, external splinting is unnecessary unless excessive bone has been excised, but pathologic fracture can occur when extensive debridement and saucerization have been performed (Fig. 46–3).

Delayed closure over an irrigation-suction system has been abandoned in favor of closure over drains if soft tissues are suitable. In point of fact, closure now is more likely to be obtained by local muscle transfer or by free flap techniques.

POST-TRAUMATIC CHRONIC OSTEOMYELITIS WITH NONUNION. Opinions differ on the management of chronic osteomyelitis and nonunited fractures.[15] Traditionally, primary emphasis has been placed on controlling the infection. Once the infection is eradicated, those patients with a persistent nonunion are treated with autogenous bone grafts and stabilization. The alternate approach is based on the rationale that once union has been achieved, an adequate blood supply exists, permitting the host defense mechanisms to eradicate the infection. We believe that the latter approach, in which internal fixation devices are placed concurrently with wound debridement, has been followed too often by persistent sepsis. Thus, we continue to favor the traditional approach of controlling the infection first. Even in the femur biplane, external fixation is feasible and removes the fixation device from the area of infection.

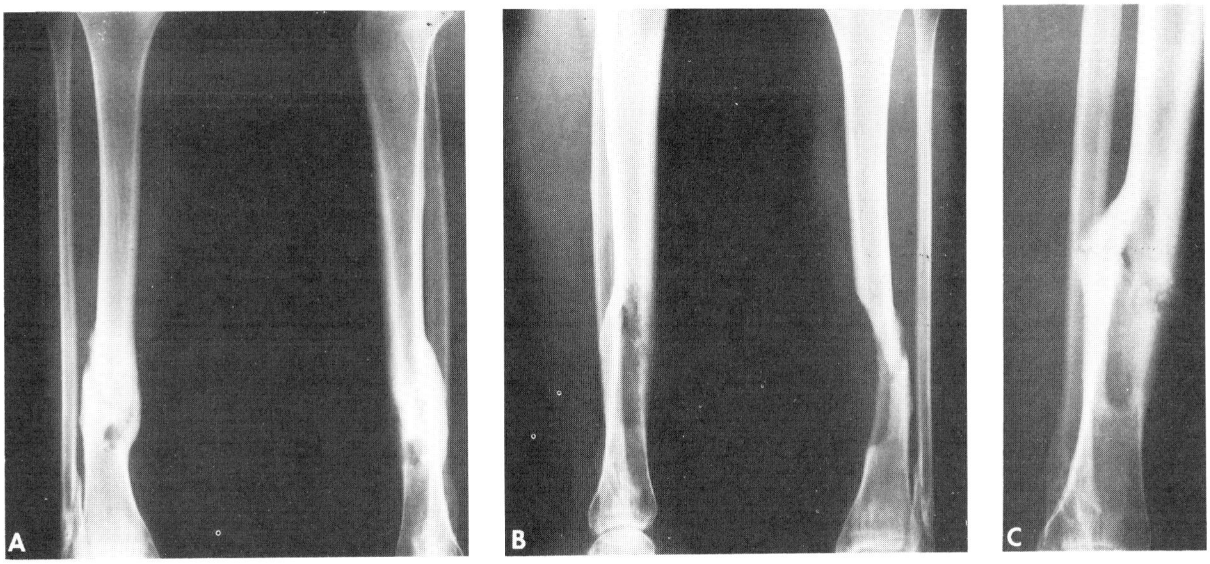

Figure 46–3. Pathologic fracture after saucerization of post-traumatic osteomyelitis of tibia. **A.** Post-traumatic osteomyelitis of tibia with a draining sinus 1 year after removal of foreign bodies (screws) used to achieve stabilization. Lytic destruction of proximal fracture fragment on anteroposterior view is noted. **B.** Tibia was saucerized, and local muscle flap placed in cavity. The degree of infected bone was greater than that appreciated on preoperative x-ray studies. Extensive unroofing procedure was required, leaving only posterior cortex intact. **C.** Healing fracture through saucerized cavity 6 months after surgical treatment.

In our experience, 50 percent of patients with infected nonunions of the femur and tibia will obtain union of their fracture if the infection is eradicated, stability maintained, and early ambulation encouraged, especially if functional casts are used.

For the patient with an infected tibial nonunion, preservation of an intact fibula is important because removal of infected and dead bone may lead to diaphyseal discontinuities. After arrest of the infection, autogenous iliac grafts can be inserted posteriorly, above and below the nonunion, if the fibula is intact. Autogenous iliac crest bone is the material of choice.

In treating an infected nonunion of the femur, debridement and soft tissue healing should be the first objective. After 6 to 12 weeks of freedom from clinical evidence of infection, long strips of autologous iliac bone are placed medially and posteriorly, preferably with an external fixation device for stabilization (Fig. 46–4).

For nonunion of the humerus, radius, or ulna, an iliac graft can be fashioned to fill in defects and maintain length. In these anatomic areas, plates or external fixators are preferable for achieving stability.

If primary stabilization is elected in the treatment of the infected nonunion, the newer devices that provide rigid internal fixation are probably necessary. Burri[15] proposed that rigid internal fixation and cancellous autogenous iliac bone grafts be used to achieve union of the fracture after thorough debridement. If soft tissue closure is not possible, the wound is allowed to heal by granulation tissue and epithelialization. Using these techniques in the treatment of 200 patients with posttraumatic osteomyelitis (102 patients had a united fracture), Burri arrested the osteomyelitic process in 180. Nine patients required amputation for persistent infection, and 11 patients developed recurrent sepsis.

The advent of rigid external fixation has made the preceding debate academic because it permits concurrent stabilization and control of the infection without implanted foreign material traversing the nonunion. Currently, a complete debridement and saucerization can be done at the initial operation. When the secondary debridement is performed 2 to 3 days later, the application of a two-plane fixation device for infected nonunion of the tibia, humerus, radius, or ulna as well as for infected nonunions of the femur (Fig. 46–5) will provide rigid external fixation.

CHRONIC POST-TRAUMATIC OSTEOMYELITIS WITH UNION. The treatment of post-traumatic osteomyelitis with a united fracture can be difficult. Repeated surgical procedures in an area of chronic infection cause extensive scars that make the anatomy ob-

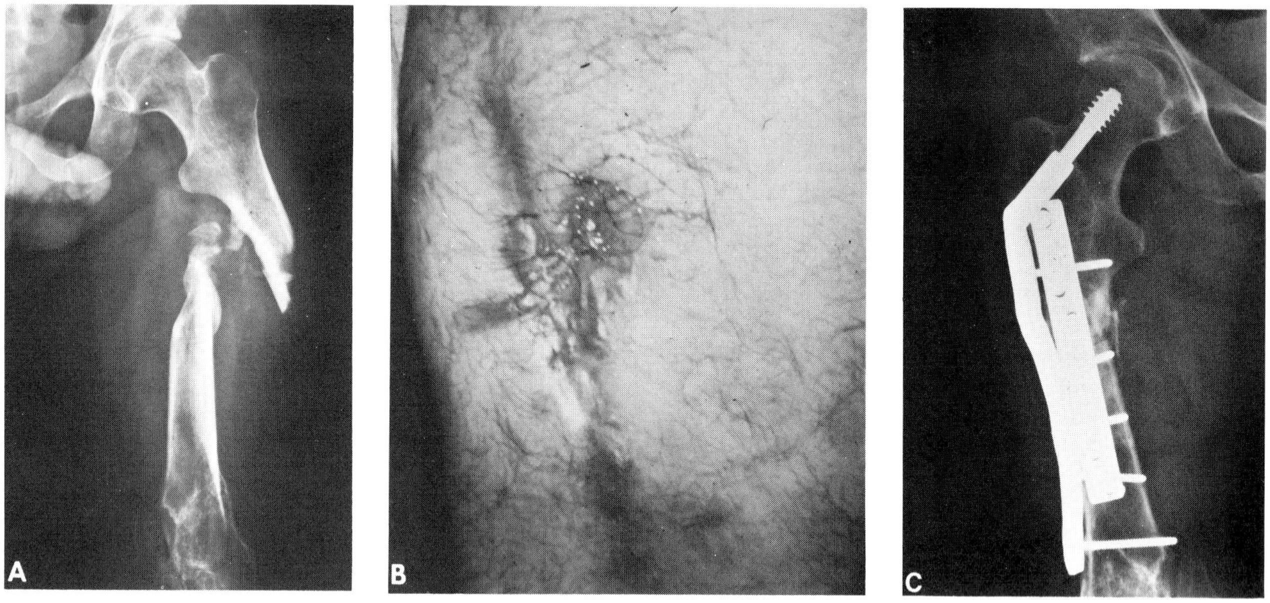

Figure 46–4. Infected nonunion of femur. **A.** Anteroposterior x-ray of femur demonstrating osteomyelitic changes with concomitant nonunion. **B.** Sinus tract located on lateral thigh. **C.** Anteroposterior x-ray 1 year after debridement and soft tissue closure. Internal fixation and autogenous bone grafting were performed 6 months after debridement. Early union of femoral fracture is evident on x-ray.

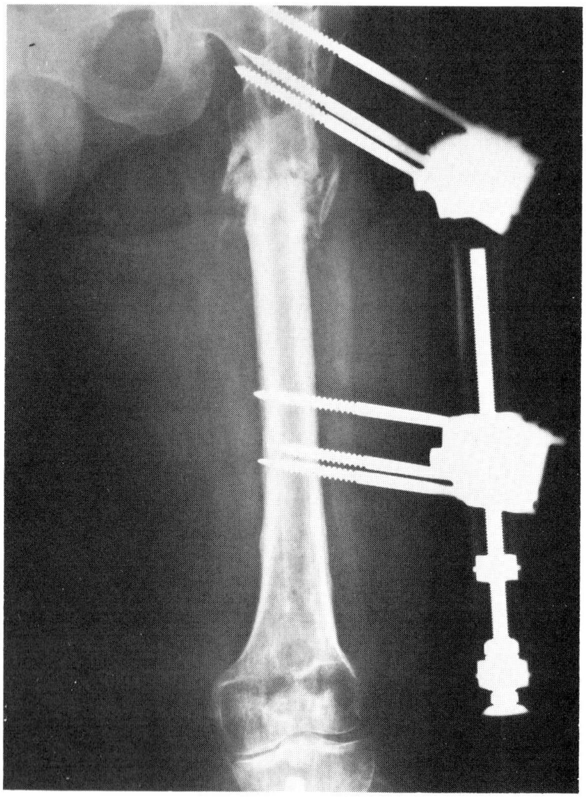

Figure 46–5. Infected nonunion of femur after insertion of intramedullary nail. Intramedullary device was removed, wound debrided, and Wagner apparatus applied. Three months later, there was evidence of early union.

scure, dissection difficult, and healing poor. Excision of bone must be judicious if pathologic fracture is to be avoided, yet saucerization must be sufficient to permit the eradication of the infected granulation tissue and sequestra. Methylene blue can be used to identify avascular tissue and to follow the sinus tracts. If the dye is injected into the sinus tract with a soft catheter 12 hours before operation, all avascular tissues will be stained at the time of debridement.

Because bone is rigid and will not collapse and obliterate the dead space after saucerization, a variety of techniques are employed to close the dead space. The time-honored techniques include open packing of the wound with healing from within, or, alternately, marsupialization of the osseous cavity with subsequent application of a split-thickness skin graft directly to the granulating osseous cavity. The placement of cancellous bone grafts directly into the osseous bed was common 2 to 3 decades ago. In 1944, Mowlem[16] placed cancellous bone into mandibular defects, some of which communicated with the oral cavity. About the same time, Knight and Wood[17] and Robertson and Barron[18] initially applied a split-thickness skin graft to the saucerized cavity. When the infectious process was controlled, the skin graft was replaced by autogenous iliac bone graft. Coleman and co-workers[19] advocated a one-stage procedure consisting of saucerization, bone grafting, and closure. They noted that, although skin necrosis might occur, exposure of the bone grafts had no adverse effect. The exposed grafts were gradually covered by granulation tissue, which could be covered with a second split-thickness skin graft. Bickel and co-workers[20] reported a failure rate of 22 percent with this technique. Recently, this technique has been repopularized by Papineau,[21] who placed the cancellous grafts directly into the saucerized cavity. The grafts are slowly covered with granulation tissue. Secondary epithelialization or placement of split-thickness skin grafts can be used to achieve skin coverage.

In many anatomic locations, especially the tibia, a muscle flap can obliterate the dead space and provide a new blood supply to the saucerized osseous cavity.[22] Muscle tissue has excellent reconstructive properties,[23] rapidly attaches itself to the walls of the cavity, and introduces a new blood supply, which allows host defense mechanisms and parenterally administered antimicrobial agents to reach the wound. The muscle flap can be a pedicle graft or a local flap. Cross-leg pedicle grafts, used in the past, subject the opposite normal extremity to surgical trauma and expose it to infection.

Local flaps have been advocated by Ger[22] for the treatment of osteomyelitis. Although Uyama[24] and Popkirov[25] have each reported replacement of muscle fibers with fibrous tissue, modern techniques take both the blood supply and the innervation of the flap into consideration so that the muscle will remain viable and contractile. We have had gratifying results with this technique in those tibial and femoral lesions in which extensive scar tissue has replaced the soft tissue envelope. In a review of our experience with the use of a local muscle flap in the treatment of osteomyelitis in 42 patients, we were able to successfully eradicate the infectious process in 93 percent of the patients.[26] Even in infected nonunions of the tibia, a local muscle flap and an external fixation device provide a new blood supply and rigid stabilization—prerequisites for healing (Fig. 46–6).

Specific parenteral antimicrobial therapy is as important as good surgical technique. Either modality alone results in a high incidence of recurrent sepsis. We have learned to give parenteral antimicrobial therapy for at least 4 weeks. Data on whether a shorter or longer course of parenteral antimicrobial therapy is better are not available. Nelson and co-workers[27] reported the successful management of pediatric osteomyelitis with oral agents if serum and tissue fluid levels were monitored frequently. The agent used must be selected on the basis of results of susceptibility studies, and some organisms, for example, *P. aeruginosa*, will still require synergistic parenteral treatment with an aminoglycoside and carbenicillin or ticarcillin. Because microorganisms can alter their susceptibility patterns, additional clinical specimens for culture and susceptibility studies should be obtained at subsequent debridements. When the microbes are susceptible to an oral agent, we administer an oral agent for 4 to 6 weeks after parenteral therapy.

Using the techniques described, we arrested the infectious process in 80 percent of the patients treated between 1971 and 1983. Our criteria for resolution of the osteomyelitic process included freedom from clinical signs and symptoms of the infection, a normal erythrocyte sedimentation rate, and resolution of the associated x-ray changes a minimum of 2 years after treatment.

BACTERIAL ARTHRITIS

About 18 of the 250,000 adult patients seen yearly in the authors' experience have septic arthritis. Almost any joint of the upper or lower extremity can be involved, but there is a predilection for the knee, hip, and glenohumeral joints (Table 46–3).

Etiology. Although a variety of bacteria have been isolated from synovial fluid, *S. aureus* is by far the most frequent. Table 46–4 lists those organisms found in patients with septic arthritis treated by the authors. Goldenberg et al[28] have noted a similar distribution. Gram-negative bacilli were isolated from 20 percent of patients with septic arthritis. In recent years, many medial centers have noted a dis-

TABLE 46–3. BACTERIAL ARTHRITIS IN 260 PATIENTS

Joint Affected	Monarticular (Patients)	Polyarticular		Total Joints
		Patients	*Joints*	
Knee	97	10	16	113
Glenohumeral	46	3	4	50
Hip	49	5	6	55
Ankle	13	2	5	18
Elbow	9	4	7	16
Wrist	13	2	5	18
Sternoclavicular	7	2	2	9
Sacroiliac	4	0	0	4
Tarsal	2	0	0	2
Subtalar	1	0	0	1
Acromioclavicular	1	0	0	1
Total	242	18[a]	45	287

[a] Two or more joints were involved in 18 patients.

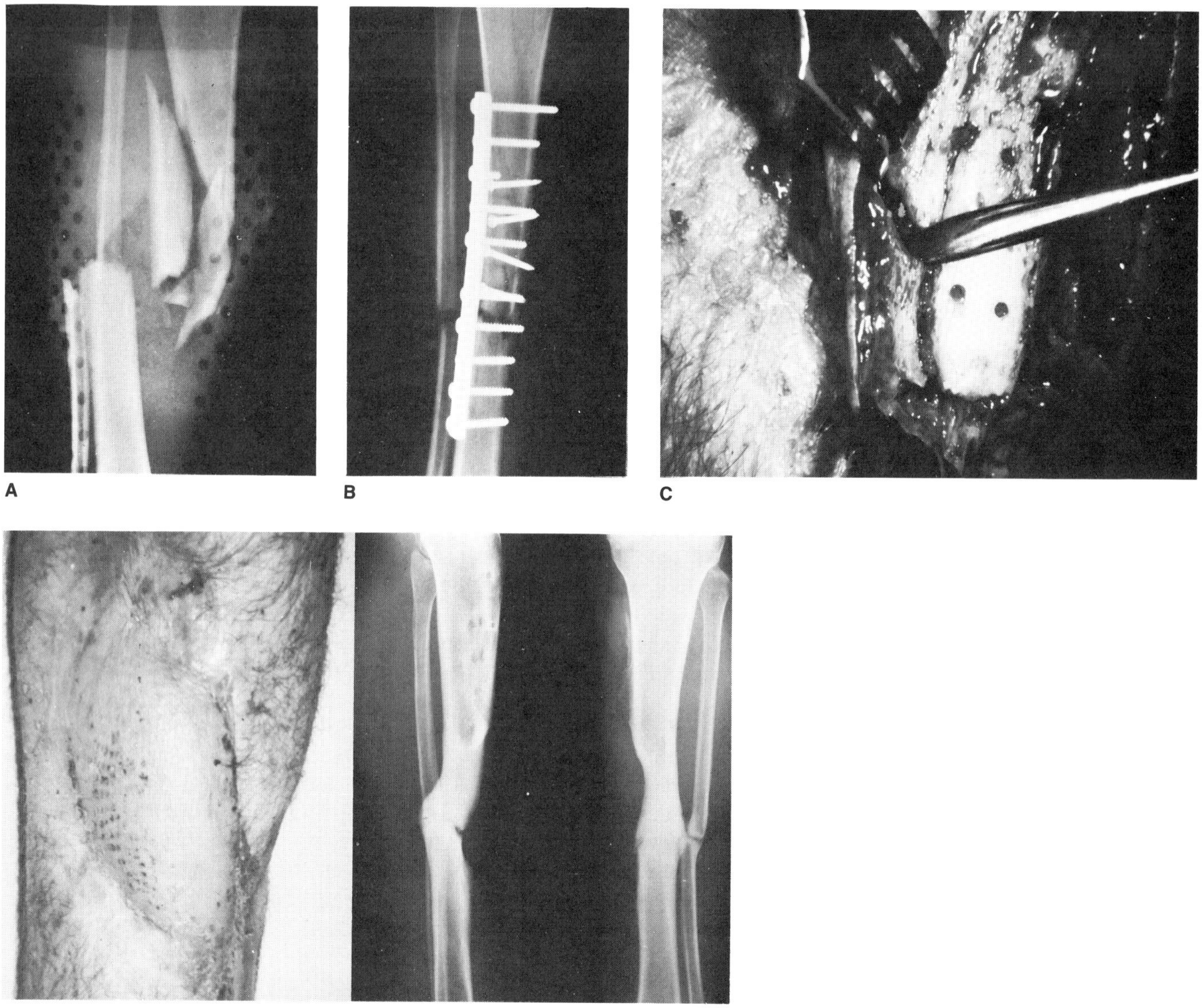

A B C D E

Figure 46–6. Post-traumatic osteomyelitis of tibia with nonunion. A. Anteroposterior x-ray of compound fracture in tibia and fibula of 17-year-old boy. B. Drainage and resorption of osseous tissue at fracture line 4 months after open reduction and internal fixation. C. Multiple sequestra were excised at time of surgical debridement. Modified Vidal-Hoffmann external fixation device was used to stabilize nonunion. D. Localized gastrocnemius-soleus muscle flap was rotated into resulting saucerized cavity. Muscle flap was covered with split-thickness skin graft. Well-healed wound 10 months later. E. Ten months after surgical and antimicrobial treatment, union has occurred. Fracture line is almost obliterated on anteroposterior and lateral x-rays.

tinct increase in the incidence of gonococcal arthritis. Cultures of blood, skin lesions, endocervix, rectum, oropharynx, and urethra are frequently necessary for the isolation of the causative agent.

Hematogenous anaerobic septic arthritis is distinctly uncommon. Anaerobic septic arthritis in association with joint implants, associated with 15 to 20 percent of infected total joint arthroplasties following the introduction of this procedure in North America, is being recognized less frequently. The gram-negative anaerobic bacilli predominate in patients with hematogenous anaerobic septic arthritis. These patients usually have a serious, debilitating, medical illness with gastrointestinal involvement. *Bacteroides fragilis* is the most frequently isolated organism.

TABLE 46–4. BACTERIOLOGIC DATA FROM 260 PATIENTS WITH BACTERIAL ARTHRITIS

Organism	Number
• GRAM-POSITIVE BACILLI	
Staphylococcus aureus	166
S. epidermidis	13
S. aureus and gram-negative bacilli	9
Gram-negative bacilli	41
Streptococci	21
Neisseria	10
Total	260
• GRAM-NEGATIVE BACILLI	
Escherichia coli	13
Pseudomonas	8
E. coli and beta-hemolytic streptococci	3
Bacteroides species	4
Proteus species	1
Enterobacter and *Pseudomonas* species	1
Bacteroides species and *Streptococcus veridans*	1
Pseudomonas species and *Proteus*	1
Citrobacter diversus	3
E. coli and *Pseudomonas* species	1
Klebsiella species	1
Enterobacter and *E. coli*	2
Enterobacter	1
Total	41
• *NEISSERIA*	
Neisseria gonorrhoeae	6
N. meningitis	3
N. catarrhalis	1
Total	10

Salmonella septic arthritis is rarely seen in adult patients. Goldenberg and associates[28] reported the isolation of *Salmonella choleraesuis* and *S. typhimurium* from 2 of 13 patients with gram-negative septic arthritis. This type of septic arthritis often occurs in patients with sickle cell anemia and other types of hemoglobinopathies.

Although pneumococcal and streptococcal organisms were at one time frequently isolated from patients with septic arthritis, they are rare in the modern antibiotic era.

Predisposing Factors. The frequent association of bacterial arthritis with a systemic disease that alters host defenses is more than coincidental. Among the diseases most frequently associated with bacterial arthritis are diabetes mellitus, malignancy, and rheumatoid arthritis. The hypocomplementemic subgroup of patients with rheumatoid arthritis, described by Hunder and McDuffie,[29] appears to be predisposed to various infections, including bacterial arthritis. This group has peripheral manifestations of the rheumatoid process (increased IgM and decreased IgG levels) and depressed serum complement levels.

Preexisting infection elsewhere in the body is frequently seen in patients with bacterial arthritis.

Many patients will report a history of corticosteroid use. Frequently, those who have received oral corticosteroids have rheumatoid arthritis or systemic lupus erythematosus. The frequent local injection of steroid preparations for tendinitis and bursitis has been associated with a precipitous increase in the incidence of septic arthritis, especially septic arthritis of the glenohumeral joint. Prior to 1957, only one patient with septic arthritis of the glenohumeral joint had been seen at the Mayo Clinic. Since then it is as common as hip infection (see Table 46–3).

In children, soft tissue trauma has been implicated in the development of septic arthritis. Bacterial arthritis is a frequent complication of osteomyelitis—classically in infants and adults but also in children. In children, joints in which the metaphysis is located within synovial lining (hip, shoulder, ankle, radiohumeral joints) are typically involved.

Pathophysiology. In 1924, Phemister's investigation[30] of the destructive processes associated with septic arthritis demonstrated that articular cartilage does not have a purely passive role. Phemister incubated articular cartilage with a staphylococcal suspension, a purulent exudate, and saline at 55C. Because the bacterial action of staphylococci was inhibited at this temperature, he concluded that the resulting destruction of articular cartilage occurred through the action of proteolytic ferments present in the purulent exudate. He theorized that the ferments were released by polymorphonuclear leukocytes.

Curtiss and Klein[31] repeated these experiments in 1963. They noted that incubation of articular cartilage and a purulent exudate, with or without staphylococci, at 37C had no visible effect on the articular cartilage. However, incubation of articular cartilage and a purulent exudate at 55C resulted in destruction of the articular cartilage. By measuring the hydroxyproline content, these authors demonstrated that the dissolution of visible cartilage was directly related to the destruction of collagen. Thus, they concluded that Phemister's[30] observations were based on the action of proteolytic enzymes on the collagen of denatured cartilage. At the more physiologic temperature of 37C, they noted that various proteolytic enzymes, such as papain, trypsin, plasmin, streptococcal kinase, and leukocytic proteinase, had no deleterious effect on the collagen content of articular cartilage. In fact, at this temperature, only clostridial collagenase dissolved hyaline cartilage. Curtiss and Klein[32] demonstrated that the proteolytic enzymes had an adverse effect on the cartilage matrix, with a loss of chondroitin sulfate by articular cartilage.

The catabolic activity of stimulated chondrocytes has been an area of intense research activity over the past decade as an explanation for the continued erosion of the glycosaminoglycan resorption following sterilization of the joint in patients with septic arthritis. Fell and Jubb[33] introduced the term *catabolin* in the work demonstrating the importance of viable chondrocytes in this process. This theory suggests the microorganism or its by-product stimulates the synoviocytes, which elaborate catabolins that in turn stimulate the chondrocyte to degrade its matrix. It is thought that the catabolin is IL-1. To date, only cortisone has been found to be effective in reversing this phenomenon.[34]

Clinical Manifestations. In the past, bacterial arthritis was considered to be a disease of children. Although still prevalent in children and young adults, it is not exclusively a pediatric disease. In fact, at the Mayo Clinic, twice as many adult patients as children have been treated for bacterial arthritis during the past 25 years. Adult patients at greatest risk are those with remote infections, urinary tract or bowel disease, the elderly, the chronically ill, those with rheumatoid arthritis, and patients being treated for malignant disease with cytotoxic drugs or radiation. Bacterial arthritis begins as a painful, swollen joint, and the erythrocyte sedimentation rate and peripheral leukocyte count can be helpful in the diagnosis. An elevation of the sedimentation rate in a patient with hip joint or sacroiliac pain should alert the physician to the possibility of septic arthritis. Although x-ray changes are later findings, technetium or gallium scans can provide valuable information early in the disease.

Two clinical forms of gonococcal arthritis are seen. Patients with monarticular involvement, or less often polyarticular involvement, have asymptomatic bacteremia without fever and chills. The characteristic cutaneous manifestation of gonococcemia, that is, erythematous papules surmounted by a hemorrhagic vesiculopustular lesion, is uncommon. Usually, gonococci will be isolated from synovial specimens. The second group of patients with gonococcal arthritis have a septic course. A history of fever and chills, characteristic skin lesions, and polyarticular involvement are characteristic. Although blood and skin lesion cultures are frequently positive, the synovial fluid is usually sterile. In contrast to previous experience, gonococcal arthritis occurs more frequently in female patients.

Fever, chills, and a rash, found in patients with polyarticular involvement, can make differentiation from Reiter's syndrome difficult. Patients with Reiter's syndrome have histories of previous arthritis, persistent low-back pain, or previous urethritis. Patients with gonococcal arthritis experience a rapid clinical response to parenterally administered penicillin, whereas those with Reiter's syndrome respond more slowly to nonsteroidal anti-inflammatory agents. Reiter's syndrome tends to be associated with lower extremity involvement, as well as plantar fasciitis and tendinitis, whereas gonococcal arthritis occurs initially in the upper extremity and is associated with a fever and a positive culture from an orifice or synovial fluid.

More characteristic symptoms and physical findings occur in the pediatric patient with septic arthritis. Rheumatic fever and juvenile rheumatoid arthritis must be included in the differential diagnosis. A more difficult distinction to make is that between transient synovitis of the hip and septic arthritis. In bacterial infections of the hip, the patient tends to be febrile and younger. The erythrocyte sedimentation rate is elevated, and the synovial leukocyte counts are higher. Only the isolation of microorganisms from synovial fluid or blood can prove the final diagnosis.

Diagnosis. Salvage of a functional joint in septic arthritis requires early diagnosis, and tissue culture of synovial fluid obtained by aspiration or of synovial membrane obtained at arthrotomy should be done. Table 46–5 lists the differential diagnostic characteristics of joint fluid. The isolation and subsequent susceptibility studies of the infective agent are essential.

Treatment. Antimicrobial drugs cross the synovial membrane readily in health and disease.[35] If the diagnosis of septic arthritis is made promptly, antimicrobial therapy alone may result in eradication of the infection. The duration of parenteral antimicrobial therapy remains empiric. Four weeks of therapy can be considered a helpful, albeit arbitrary, guide.

The management of the infected synovial fluid precipitates considerable controversy. Animal ex-

TABLE 46–5. SYNOVIAL FLUID CHARACTERISTICS IN MAJOR JOINT DISEASES

Diagnosis	Appearance	Fibrin Clot	Mucin Clot[a]	WBC/mm³	PMN[b] (%)	Sugar (% of blood level)
Normal	Straw-colored, clear	None	Good	<200	<25	~100
Degenerative joint disease	Slightly turbid	Small	Good	<2,000	<25	~100
Traumatic arthritis	Straw-colored, bloody, or xanthochromic	Small	Good	2,000	<25	~100
Rheumatoid arthritis	Turbid	Large	Fair to poor	5,000–50,000	>65	75[c]
Other types of inflammatory arthritis[d]	Turbid	Large	Fair to poor	5,000–50,000	>50	75
Acute gout or pseudo-gout	Turbid	Large	Fair to poor	5,000–50,000	>75	90
Septic arthritis	Very turbid or purulent	Large	Poor	50,000–200,000	>80	<50
Tuberculous arthritis	Turbid	Large	Poor	~25,000	Variable	<50

[a] Correlates with viscosity.
[b] PMN, polymorphonuclear cells.
[c] May be less than 50 percent.
[d] Includes Reiter's syndrome, psoriatic arthritis, ankylosing spondylitis (peripheral joints), and arthritis associated with intestinal diseases.
From Gilliland BC, Mannik M: Approach to disorders of the joints. In Thorn GW, Adams RD, Braunwald E, et al (eds): Harrison's Principles of Internal Medicine. New York, McGraw-Hill, 1977, p 2048.

perimentation suggests that infected synovial fluid interferes with hyaline cartilage metabolism. Daniel and co-workers[36] demonstrated that removal of the infected synovial fluid improved cartilage metabolism, with preservation of collagen content. Thus, most orthopedic surgeons favor removal of the synovial fluid. Arthrocentesis can be readily accomplished in superficially located joints (ie, knee, ankle, shoulder). However, if thick purulent joint fluid is present or if the joint is not readily accessible, such as the hip or sacroiliac joints, open debridement and drainage are indicated. The use of an irrigation-suction system in joint debridement, which was once common,[37] is no longer utilized, as this may provide a route for colonization of the tissues with secondary invaders (usually gram-negative bacilli) and may precipitate superinfection. As mentioned in the treatment of osteomyelitis, such systems are not proper for the delivery of antimicrobial agents. If debridement has been thorough, the remaining tissue has an adequate blood supply that will allow bactericidal concentrations of parenterally administered antimicrobial agents within the tissues of the joint.

The treatment becomes far more complex when the diagnosis of septic arthritis has been delayed. Frequently, delay in diagnosis and treatment precludes salvage of a functional joint. As William Hunter[1] pointed out two centuries ago, "an ulcerated Cartilage is universally allowed to be a very troublesome Disease; . . . it admits of a Cure with more Difficulty than a curious Bone; and, . . . when destroyed, it is never recovered."

Even though it may be irregular and pitted, an attempt should be made to salvage a functional joint if some articular cartilage remains after debridement. Early functional rehabilitation after debridement may provide the patient with a stable and minimally painful joint. If, however, significant destruction of the articular surfaces with exposure or erosion (or both) of subchondral bone has occurred, a more definitive procedure is indicated. When the knee, ankle, elbow, wrist, interphalangeal, or subtalar joints are involved, compression arthrodesis is indicated. Destruction of the articular surfaces of the hip can be treated by either arthrodesis or joint resection, depending on the degree of involvement and the patient's occupation and level of activity. The acromioclavicular and sternoclavicular joints can be treated by joint resection, with remarkably good results. The glenohumeral joint is amenable to treatment with debridement and protected motion or arthrodesis.

Septic arthritis of the hip in children is best treated by early debridement and drainage. Delay in diagnosis and treatment of septic arthritis in the hip in the child is catastrophic. Every effort should be made to salvage the involved joint. The child has an infinitely greater ability to attain a functional joint than does the adult patient. The presence of an open epiphyseal plate makes the salvage operation used in adult patients (which destroys the epiphyseal plate) far more difficult to use in children.

Prognosis. Death attributable to septic arthritis, even in this era of sophisticated antimicrobial therapy, has been noted in as many as 15 percent of afflicted patients. Joint instability and subluxation, when the capsule and associated ligaments are involved, necessitate external support, for example, cane, crutch, or braces. Prolonged immobilization can create stiff, immobile joints. If immobilization is inadequate, flexion contractures are common. Delay in diagnosis in children can result in functional impairment from discrepancy in leg length, persistent pain, limitation of motion, or soft tissue contracture. Because the epiphysis is intra-articular in the glenohumeral and hip joints, septic arthritis can compromise the blood supply and result in osteonecrosis.

UNCOMMON SKELETAL INFECTIONS

Mycobacterial Infections

The various mycobacteria are discussed briefly in Chapter 9 and in many other chapters on regional infection. Although the incidence of tuberculosis has declined, tuberculosis of the spinal column and major joints is still seen. With the advent of total joint arthroplasty, many patients with joints destroyed by tuberculosis years before are now seeking reconstructive surgery. New cases can occur in patients of any age, but adults are more often affected. Because classic tuberculosis of bone appears to arise from a hematogenous source, primary tuberculosis, usually pulmonary, is said to be commonly present. In our experience, however, skeletal involvement with tuberculosis has seldom been associated with pulmonary tuberculosis, but disseminated disease can afflict both multiple bones and soft tissues simultaneously. The tubercle bacilli lodge in the metaphyseal regions of long bones or in the anterior portions of vertebral bodies (Pott's disease). Tuberculous arthritis is probably secondary to tuberculous osteomyelitis.

The spinal column is the most frequent site of involvement with *Mycobacterium tuberculosis* and classically can lead to paraplegia. However, any bone or joint may be afflicted—the hip, the knee, and the tendons of the hand are the most frequent nonspinal sites. The usual clinical findings are insidious, with fever, malaise, and bone or joint pain. Rheumatoid arthritis is a common clinical impression in nonspinal disease.

Unfortunately, x-ray studies are not diagnostic. A range of radiographic alterations from soft tissue swelling to joint destruction can be seen. Initially, soft tissue swelling and distention of a joint capsule may be seen. Cartilage destruction occurs. If bone destruction occurs, the lucent area is surrounded by sclerotic bone, and there may be subperiosteal new bone formation. When infection of the spinal column occurs, destruction of several contiguous vertebral bodies, narrowing of interpectoral spaces, and paraspinal abscess as indicated by anterior vertebral scalloping may be present. Kyphosis or scoliosis, or both, may be observed.

A positive skin test is helpful, but the diagnosis depends on histopathologic demonstration of granulomas with caseous necrosis and Langerhans giant cells, acid-fast stain, and culture. Drug treatment for tuberculosis is essential regardless of the surgical treatment. Nondestructive bony lesions respond to prolonged chemotherapy and immobilization. Moderate joint involvement should probably be treated with synovectomy plus chemotherapy. Extensive joint disease responds best to debridement and arthrodesis. Spondylitis may be best treated with anterior spinal fusion and early drainage of any paraspinal abscess. Paraplegia demands operative decompression and responds remarkably well.[38]

Nontuberculous mycobacterial infections are discussed in Chapter 9. Such infections of the musculoskeletal system are common. In fact, the authors have encountered such infections more frequently than typical tuberculous infections of the musculoskeletal system. It is convenient to separate the nontuberculous mycobacterial infections into the four groups originally described by Runyon[39] based on morphologic characteristics well documented over the past three decades. These four groups include:

- **I.** Photochromogens (*M. kansasii, M. marinum, M. simlae*). These organisms form a yellow carotene pigment on exposure to light.
- **II.** Scotochromogens (*M. flavescens, M. gordonae, M. scrofulaceum*). The colonies of these organisms are pigmented when grown in the dark or the light.
- **III.** Nonphotochromogens (*M. avium, M. gastri, M. terrae, M. triviale, M. xenopi, M. intracellulare*). The buff of the colonies of these organisms does not change with exposure to light.
- **IV.** Rapid growers (*M. chelonei, M. fortuitum*). Mature colonies of these organisms arise in 4 to 6 days of incubation.

Inoculation of the hand and the fingers after minor trauma probably accounts for the frequent involvement of the tendon sheaths of the hand and the wrist. Bone infections are rare, but synovial and bursal infections may be related to injections of anesthetics or steroids into these locations. Because these organisms do not respond to the standard antituberculosis drugs, bacteriologic culture, identification, and susceptibility studies are invaluable. Synovial biopsy is useful for culture. Surgical debridement of all of the involved synovial tissue is frequently required. Further discussion of laboratory diagnosis and treatment of mycobacterial infections appears in Chapters 10 and 28.

Fungal Infections

The more common but still rare fungal infections of bone include blastomycosis, cryptococcosis, coccidioidomycosis, and sporotrichosis.[40] The systemic character of these infections is discussed in Chapter 8. *Actinomyces* is an anaerobic bacterium that can grow like a fungus.

Blastomycosis. Blastomycosis (*Blastomyces dermatitidis*) is acquired by inhalation of the spores from soil, and bone lesions occur only with disseminated disease, frequently in conjunction with cutaneous ulcers and subcutanoeus sinuses.[41] Multicentric osseous lesions are common when the spinal column is infected, the most frequent sites being tubular bones (especially the tibia) and ribs.

Pathology and Pathogenesis. The metaphyses or epiphyses and subarticular regions are commonly involved. Joints become secondarily infected, and the synovium, ligaments, and surrounding soft tissues are destroyed with subluxation of the joints. Draining sinuses are common. Paravertebral dissection occurs after vertebral infection, and even skip areas occur as the infection dissects along the anterior longitudinal ligament.

Clinical Manifestations. Recent respiratory symptoms will have occurred in about half the patients who have skin involvement. The patient is acutely and chronically ill with fever, weight loss, night sweats, and cough. Skin ulcers and draining sinus tracts occur in association with bony involvement. The radiologic genographic appearance of blastomycosis has been described by Gehweiler et al.[40] In spinal disease, several vertebral bodies are infected along with the adjacent ribs—an important differential point. Three forms of disease may be seen: a cystic or focal form: a diffuse form; and, in long bones, a circumscribed, soft, saucer-shape erosion of cortical bone. The differential diagnosis includes neoplasms, sarcoidosis, other fungal diseases, gout, and rheumatoid arthritis.

Diagnosis. Histopathologic examination with special stains may reveal the yeasts in tissue. Culture, however, is necessary for definitive diagnosis. Amphotericin B is the best treatment and is described in Chapter 10. Operative debridement of the extensive sinus tracts, drainage of the abscesses, sequestrectomy, or even amputation may be necessary.

Sporotrichosis. Sporotrichosis (*Sporothrix schenckii*) arthritis should be included in the differential diagnosis of chronic monarticular or polyarticular arthritis.[42] Bone and joint disease is most often the result of hematogenous spread in the rare systemic form of the disease, although direct extension from a local lesion or spread by lymphatic extension may occur. The unifocal form, in which joint infection is the sole manifestation of the disease, predominates. X-ray studies are nonspecific, and the diagnosis depends on cultures of synovial tissue. Patients with destructive changes tend to have had symptoms for a longer time. Debridement with systemically administered amphotericin B is the treatment of choice. Treatment with potassium iodide will not suffice in this form of the disease.

Cryptococcosis. Osseous lesions in cryptococcosis (*Cryptococcus neoformans*) are rare and usually result from direct extension. For this reason, the cranium is the most commonly affected site, secondary to cryptococcal meningitis. The other osseous lesions are usually multiple because of hematogenous spread. Because cryptococcosis can be widespread without systemic or local signs of host response, sinuses and ulcers are unusual. Bone pain may be present. Radiolucent lesions without new periosteal bone formation are the characteristic radiographic alterations. The organisms can be demonstrated on clinical tissue specimens with the periodic acid-Schiff stain, and can be grown on Sabouraud's medium. Cryptococcosis is rarely seen except in patients with debilitating disease. The patient frequently seeks medical attention for evaluation of a fever of unknown origin or dysfunction of the central nervous system. Amphotericin B and 5-fluorocytosine combinations are the treatments of choice. Surgical debridement is frequently necessary.[38]

Coccidioidomycosis. As noted in Chapter 10, primary infection with *Coccidioides immitis* can be accompanied by arthritis (desert rheumatism). Pain, tenderness, and swelling of a joint occur, but the condition is transient, as are most manifestations of the primary infection.

Some patients do not recover from the primary infection, and bone and joint complaints may be the initial signs of the chronic disease.[38] Pain, swelling, and draining abscesses may be the first findings.

Disseminated coccidioidomycosis will occasionally infect one or more joints or the vertebral column. The large joints—hip, knee, and shoulder—are most often afflicted. Coccidioidomycosis tends to involve the metaphysis of large tubular bones and bony prominences. When the vertebral bodies are infected, the disc is spared. The lesions are usually radiolucent and well demarcated without sclerosis or sequestra. As with the other fungal infections, diagnosis depends on the identification of spherules on histologic examination of biopsy material, or on the isolation of the fungus on solid medium (the serologic and skin tests interpretations are discussed in Chapter 10). Systemic involvement requires parenteral administration of amphotericin B. Osseous lesions and septic arthritis have not uniformly responded to ketakonazole. Immobilization of joints and relief from weight bearing may be helpful. Synovectomy of extensively involved joints or saucerization of osseous lesions is occasionally necessary.[38]

Unusual Bacterial Infections

Actinomycosis. Actinomycosis of bone occurs with the cervicofascial form and frequently invades the mandible after tooth extraction. Osseous infection at other sites is distinctly uncommon. Involvement of the second rib has been noted in the thoracic form of the disease. A mixed lytic and sclerotic appearance is seen radiographically, and the picture of cervicofascial actinomycosis (see Chap. 33) is easily recognized. This diagnosis depends on finding sulfur granules in the sinus drainage, gram-positive organisms in smear, and culture. Penicillin G in large doses of 10 to 20 million units per day should be given for an extended period. Tetracycline has also been administered successfully if given for a sufficient duration. Surgical debridement can be helpful.[38]

Brucellosis. Brucellosis (*Brucella abortus*) in the United States is limited to farmers, veterinarians, and others working with infected cattle (see Chap. 9). There are two forms of the disease: an acute form with systemic complaints, and a chronic form with intermittent recurrent (undulant) fever. *B. abortus* is isolated most frequently in the systemic form, and *B. suis* in the localized form.

The spinal column, knees, and hip can be affected. However, invasion of phalanges, pelvis, and diaphyses has been reported. Brucellar spondylitis and prepatellar bursitis are the two most frequent types of skeletal involvement. An insidious onset of nonspecific symptoms is characteristic. Backache and joint pain are characteristic. Agglutination titers are elevated in the spondylitic form and may be normal in the localized form. Treatment of the patient with brucellosis includes debridement and the administration of tetracycline for 3 weeks. In patients with severe disease, streptomycin can also be administered for 10 days.

POSTOPERATIVE WOUND SEPSIS

Even though postoperative skeletal sepsis is not associated with a high mortality rate, the increased morbidity and loss of function of the infected limb make it one of the most formidable complications of orthopedic surgery. The resultant loss of function and the reliance on crutches or canes frequently preclude the patient's return to his or her premorbid occupation. Although newer reconstructive procedures can restore function to a destroyed joint, they are contraindicated in the presence of sepsis. Even with eradication of the infection, the rate of failure of a total joint arthroplasty implanted into a previously infected joint is significantly increased. Thus, prevention of skeletal sepsis and early eradication when infection occurs are the primary goals of orthopedic surgeons.

Incidence and Etiology. The incidence of nosocomial wound infections of the skeletal system is unknown. In a prospective study of postoperative wound sepsis by the National Academy of Sciences,[43] only 692 orthopedic procedures were included among the 15,613 operations studied. Septic complications occurred in 54 (7.8 percent) of the orthopedic procedures.

As expected, the regional anatomy and type of skeletal operation influence the incidence of deep sepsis. The rich vascular supply of the hand helps make postoperative infection uncommon. In contrast, Boyd et al[44] and Tengve and Kjellander[45] have noted wound sepsis in 4.8 and 16.9 percent, respectively, after internal fixation of fractured hips. Thus, in any evaluation of postoperative wound sepsis of the skeletal system, elective and traumatic operations should be considered separately. The variations in anatomy, dissection, and residual dead space necessitate subdivision of elective operations into adult, pediatric, and oncologic procedures. Traumatic procedures are subdivided into open and closed injuries.

In a prospective study, Miller and Counts[46] noted 22 (5.8 percent) wound infections after clean, elective skeletal procedures in 378 patients. In 12 (3.2 percent), the tissues deep to the fascia were infected. Patients treated for closed hip fractures had the highest incidence of deep infections (6 of 65 patients, 9.2 percent), whereas elective reconstructive hip procedures were associated with the lowest incidence (2 of 59 patients, 3.4 percent).

Postoperative sepsis is defined as an inflamed wound that drains purulent material. Even wounds from which microorganisms cannot be isolated are included if many polymorphonuclear leukocytes can be seen.[45] When purulent material extends beneath the fascia, the infection is classified as deep.

ELECTIVE RECONSTRUCTION. Deep sepsis after elective reconstructive procedures in adult patients occurs in 0.4 to 0.5 percent of our patients. The incidence has remained fairly constant.[47] Gram-positive isolates, staphylococci in particular, predominate. Gram-negative bacilli are isolated from 20 to 35 percent of the infected wounds. The anaerobic cocci, *Peptococcus* and *Peptostreptococcus*, have been recovered.

The prophylactic administration of antimicrobial therapy to patients having a total hip arthroplasty has been documented to be efficacious by prospective studies.[48] During the initial experience with total hip and knee arthroplasty in the United States, the incidence of postoperative infections was extraordinarily high. Subsequent experience has led to a dramatic reduction. The incidence for primary total hip arthroplasty for patients with osteoarthritis has been reduced to 0.06 percent. Following total knee arthroplasty for a patient with osteoarthritis, the incidence of deep postoperative sepsis has been decreased to 0.5 percent (see Prevention section that follows).

A new pattern of enzymatic microbial resistance (beta-lactamase production) has emerged from infections about total joint implants (Table 46–6). Eighty percent of the staphylococci produce beta-lactamase, which renders them resistant to commonly administered antibiotics. The general distribution of the causal microorganisms recovered from surgical tissue specimens of 104 patients—47 infected THA, 35 infected TKA, 14 infected Girdlestone resection arthroplasties, and 8 infected resection arthroplasties of the knee—with an infection treated between 1989 and 1992 has not changed: 77 percent of the isolates were gram-positive cocci; 21 percent were gram-negative bacilli; and 2 percent were other microorganisms. There has, however, been a major shift in the type and the susceptibility studies of the gram-positive cocci: 54 percent of gram-positive isolates are *S. epidermidis*, while 25 percent are *S. aureus* and 21 percent are streptococci. Only three of the *S. epidermidis* isolates were methicillin-resistant. However, 93 percent of *S. epidermidis* isolates produced beta-lactamase. Methicillin resistance (MRSA) was encountered in 45 percent of the *S. aureus* isolates. Beta-lactamase was produced by another 50 percent of the *S. aureus* isolates. Three of the streptococci isolates were multidrug resistant *Enterococcus faecalis*. Thus 75 percent of the gram-positive isolates exhibited one form or another of resistance. The most common form of resistance was the elaboration of beta-lactamase, which renders the organism resistant to the antibiotics with a beta-lactam ring—the cephalosporins, penicillin, oxacillin, and nafcillin—even though the microbiology report indicates that they may be susceptible. This change

TABLE 46–6. INFECTED TOTAL JOINT ARTHROPLASTY

Microorganism	Number of Isolates
Staphylococcus epidermidis	29
S. aureus	14
Streptococcus agalactiae	3
Group D Streptococci, enterococcus	4
Peptostreptococcus species	3
Micrococcus varians	2
Staphylococcus species	1
Streptococcus species	1
Streptococcus viridans group	1
Beta-hemolytic streptococci	1
Enterococcus faecalis	1
Pseudomonas aeruginosa	4
Enterobacter cloacae	4
Acinetobacter calcoaceticus	3
Proteus mirabilis	2
Morganella morganii	2
Enterobacter agglomerans	1
Xanthomanas maltophilia	1
Serratia marcescens	1
Corynebacterium species	3
Proprionibacterium acnes	2
Mycobacterium tuberculosis	1
Clostridium sporogenes	1
Sporothrix schenckii	1

in the susceptibility pattern frequently necessitates the administration of potentially toxic antimicrobial agents. While the microbiology laboratory reports beta-lactamase organisms to be susceptible to cephalosporins, oxacillin, or nafcillin, they are usually resistant and treatment with these agents can result in recurrent infection.

ONCOLOGIC PROCEDURES. The incidence of deep sepsis after orthopedic oncologic procedures is low (range 0.7 to 1.4 percent) in spite of acquired immunologic defects in cancer patients and the magnitude of tissue dissection required to treat these diseases. Although gram-positive isolates predominate, gram-negative bacilli are noted after inguinal lymphadenectomies and hemipelvectomies.

PEDIATRIC ORTHOPEDICS. Deep sepsis after elective orthopedic procedures in children tends to be associated with chronic urinary tract infections (patients with myelomeningoceles) and long operations requiring foreign body implantation (eg, scoliosis fusions with implantation of spinal instrumentation). Penicillin- and methicillin-resistant staphylococci are common isolates, and gram-negative bacilli are seen occasionally.

TRAUMA. In trauma surgery, the overall incidence of deep sepsis is low. However, when open fractures and dislocations are separated from closed injuries, a fourfold increase in the incidence of sepsis is seen. This difference reflects the contamination of devitalized tissue by soil and water organisms. The etiology of infections after operative treatment of closed fractures is similar to that of infections seen after elective reconstruction if internal fixation devices are implanted for stabilization of the fracture. In contrast, after operations for open fractures and dislocations, gram-negative bacilli alone or in mixed cultures are found in most infections.

In a study of compound fractures, Gustilo and Anderson[49] noted deep sepsis in 2.5 to 9 percent of patients, proportional to the degree of soft tissue injury. The surgical treatment of open fractures was accompanied by an infection rate of 13.9 percent in patients receiving no antimicrobial therapy.[47] A reduction of the incidence of deep sepsis to 2.3 percent occurred with the administration of cephalosporins. In that prospective study, *S. aureus* was the predominant organism in patients who received either no antimicrobial therapy or penicillin and streptomycin. Gram-negative bacilli were isolated in 11 of 14 infections occurring in patients who received cephalosporins.

Prevention. Prevention of septic complications following musculoskeletal surgery includes careful preoperative evaluation of the patient, especially focused to identify remote sites of sepsis; the selection and appropriate administration of prophylactic antimicrobial agents; the establishment of discipline within the operating room; and possibly the use of the ultraclean operating room.

PREOPERATIVE ASSESSMENT OF THE PATIENT. Many patients requiring musculoskeletal surgery are malnourished; 10 to 15 percent of patients scheduled for total hip arthroplasty are severely malnourished and have evidence of immunosuppression. The incidence of similar clinical findings are even more common in the elderly patient with an intracapsular or inter-trochanteric fracture. Since protein depletion can adversely influence wound healing and impair humoral and cell-mediated immunity, such patients need to be identified preoperatively to permit nutritional therapy prior to elective surgery and to institute it postoperatively in patients requiring emergent surgical intervention.

Identification of such patients can be accomplished by a number of ways. Anthropometric measurements, biochemical testing, and skin antigen testing provide data that permit assessment of patients' nutritional status. Anthropometric studies found to be useful in the preoperative assessment for nutritional depletion include measurement of the triceps skinfold and arm circumference in addition to the height and weight of the patient. A newer technique, bioelectrical impedance, provides more accurate assessment than the measurement of the triceps skinfold. This technique involves measurement of the impedance of electrical impulses by the soft tissues of the extremity. Measurement of the serum albumin, transferrin, and creatinine concentrations constitute the biochemical testing. When combined with the total peripheral lymphocyte count and nitrogen balance, the presence or absence of nutritional depletion can be ascertained. A total lymphocyte count less than 1500 cell/mm^3 is associated with impaired cellular defense mechanisms and malnutrition. Similarly, a serum transferrin level below 200 mg/dl is associated with visceral protein depletion. Levels below 150 mg/dl would be considered to be associated with severe depletion. Patients with evidence of nutritional depletion and scheduled for elective surgical treatment of a condition of the musculoskeletal system should be treated with nutritional therapy prior to surgical intervention.

Preoperatively, each patient should be examined carefully for remote infections, which could lead to hematogenous seeding of the postoperative wound. The surgeon must inspect such sites as infected hair follicles or sebaceous glands of the skin, necessitating examination of skin of a disrobed patient. Infected toenails are often overlooked during the preoperative evaluation of patients unless the patient is examined after removal of clothes, including shoes and socks. Such infections should be treated before musculoskeletal surgery is performed. Asymptomatic urinary tract infections can usually be identified by the presence of bacteria on a routine preoperative urinalysis. They can then be confirmed with a Gram stain and urine culture. Surgical intervention should be delayed until the infection has been treated and a sterile urine culture has been obtained with the patient off antibiotic therapy.

Occasionally, patients live symbiotically with chronic urinary infections that are recalcitrant to treatment. The infection can be suppressed during the perioperative period, but the patient has an increased risk of developing postoperative sepsis. This is especially true if the contemplated reconstructive procedure includes the implantation of a foreign body such as an artificial knee or hip prosthesis. Under such circumstances the patient and surgeon must carefully individualize the risk-benefit ratios.

Another area of concern is the prostate in men over the age of 55 years. Such patients should be queried concerning nocturia and urinary frequency. Should the prostate gland feel enlarged to palpation, urologic consultation is necessary. When transurethral prostate resection is necessary, it is more desirable to have such surgery performed prior to the surgical placement of orthopedic implants than to request it postoperatively as urinary catheters are necessary following prostatic resection. Such circumstances certainly place the patient in a compromised position and increase the risk of hematogenous infection. If a transurethral prostatic resection is required, elective musculoskeletal surgery involving the implantation of foreign bodies should be delayed for 12 weeks to allow the resected portion of the prostate gland to reepithelialize.

Orthopedic surgeons should not overlook the oral cavity during the preoperative evaluation of patients. Although it can be difficult to identify carious teeth, poor oral hygiene is usually apparent. When present, the patient should have appropriate dental examinations and treatment prior to musculoskeletal surgery.

Although such an extensive search for remote infections or potential causes of infection during the preoperative evaluation may seem excessive, it is surprising how often remote infections are responsible for septic complications of total joint arthroplasty. These are simple techniques requiring minimal time and provide both the surgeon and the patient with additional insurance against postoperative infections.

PREVENTION OF SEPSIS IN THE OPERATING ROOM. Considerable effort has been extended to define those factors active in the operating room that increase the incidence of postoperative infection. The traffic in and out of the conventional operating room, as well as the total number of personnel in the operating room during the procedure being performed, influences the airborne bacterial counts. Elevated rates of airborne bacterial counts are associated with higher rates of deep postoperative infection. Thus older operating rooms with lower rates of room air exchanges per hour have statistically higher rates of deep postoperative infections following total hip arthroplasty. Sir John Charnley introduced the concept of a unidirectional airflow operating room to eliminate this source of wound contamination and reduce his overall infection rate. His personal experience was associated with a dramatic reduction of septic complications. Other surgeons also reported the incidence of deep sepsis to be reduced: 0.5 to 0.8 percent. However, the concept remained controversial, particularly in North America, as none of these reports were prospective or randomized. The Medical Research Council of Great Britain initiated a prospective study of the ultraclean operating room in 1974. Lidwell and co-workers[56] reported in 1982 the results of this randomized, prospective study of 8056 patients having total hip or knee arthroplasty who were followed for 2 years or more in 1982. These investigators found the incidence of deep infection to be 1.5 percent in a conventional operating room (63 infections among 4133 arthroplasties). In contrast, only 23 of 3922 arthroplasties performed in an ultraclean operating room with unidirectional airflow developed deep wound infections (0.6 percent; $p < 0.001$). Unfortunately, Lidwell and co-workers[56] did not control the prophylactic administration of antibiotics. They did, however, observe a lower incidence of septic complications in those patients receiving prophylactic antibiotics: 34 of 6831 (0.6 percent). In contrast 52 of 2221 (2.3 percent) of those patients not receiving prophylactic antibiotics developed a deep wound infection. More importantly, the investigators noted a reduction in the incidence of deep sepsis from 3.4 percent (39 of 1161 arthroplasties) to 0.8 percent

(24 of 2968 arthroplasties) with the administration of prophylactic antibiotics to those patients having their procedure in a conventional operating room. In the ultraclean operating room, the incidence of deep sepsis was reduced from 1.2 percent (13 of 1060 arthroplasties) to 0.3 percent (10 of 2863 arthroplasties). The differences between the incidence of deep infection in a conventional operating room and an ultraclean operating room with the prophylactic administration of antibiotics were no longer statistically significant! Failure to include randomization of the administration of prophylactic antibiotics has unfortunately raised doubts about the overall impact of this otherwise elegant study.

In 1981 the senior author initiated a randomized, prospective, and blinded study comparing the incidence of deep sepsis following total hip and knee arthroplasty in a conventional operating room with a horizontal (laminar flow) clean room (Table 46–7). All procedures were performed by one group of surgeons who followed a standardized protocol. All patients received prophylactic antimicrobial therapy for 48 to 72 hours postoperatively. Antibiotic impregnated polymethyl methacrylate was not utilized and personnel isolator systems were not worn during the surgical procedures. Each of the ten operating rooms functioned as a standard conventional operating room with turbulent airflow or an operating room with horizontal clean air in a randomized, blinded fashion. The discipline within the operating room and traffic flow were controlled as if the unidirectional flow system were functioning during each and every procedure (eg, placement of the operating table and surgical personnel).

Since the study has only recently been completed, long-term (minimum 2-year) follow-up examination has as yet to be performed. A preliminary analysis is possible on the 7306 arthroplasties performed between 1981 and 1990. During this period of time, 4456 total hip arthroplasties and 2749 total knee arthroplasties were performed. Air sampling revealed a statistically significant reduction in the mean number of viable particles per cubic foot of air with the unidirectional airflow system functioning: 0.2445 versus 2.1776 ($p < 0.01$).

Overall, 19 deep wound infections have been identified to date among 3762 procedures with the room functioning as a conventional operating room. Twenty deep wound infections have been identified among 3543 procedures performed with unidirectional air system functioning. During total hip arthroplasty, 6 deep infections were noted among 2324 procedures with the room functioning as a conventional operating room and 11 deep infections were identified among 2232 procedures with the room functioning as a unidirectional airflow system. During total knee arthroplasty, 13 deep infections were noted among 1438 procedures with the room functioning as a conventional operating room and 9 deep infections were identified among 1311 procedures performed with the room functioning as a horizontal clean room. These differences are not statistically significant ($p > 0.05$). Primary total hip or knee arthroplasties were performed in 5868 patients. Ten deep infections were noted among 3202 arthroplasties performed with the operating room functioning as a conventional operating room. Eight deep infections were identified among 2848 procedures performed while the horizontal unidirectional airflow system was functioning. Among the primary total hip arthroplasties, there were 4 deep infections among 1739 procedures (0.23 percent) while the operating room was functioning as a conventional operating room. With the unidirec-

TABLE 46–7. INCIDENCE OF DEEP SEPSIS AFTER TOTAL HIP ARTHROPLASTY

	No Previous Surgery			Previous Surgery			Total		
		With Sepsis			With Sepsis			With Sepsis	
Environment	*Total*	*Number*	*%*	*Total*	*Number*	*%*	*Number*	*Number*	*%*
Vertical unidirectional airflow	321	1	0.3	197	2	1.0	518	3	0.6
Horizontal unidirectional airflow	511	9	1.8	200	7	3.5	711	16	2.3
Vertical unidirectional airflow	1187	5	0.4	234	2	0.9	1500	7	0.5
Conventional operating room	2224	19	0.9	991	23	2.3	3215	42	1.3
Total	4243	34	0.8	1662	34	2.1	5944	68	1.1

Adapted from Fitzgerald RH, Bechtol CO, Eftekhar N, Nelson JP: Arch Surg 114:803, 1979.

tional airflow system functioning, 1 deep infection was noted among 1682 primary total hip arthroplasties (0.06 percent). With primary total knee arthroplasty, there were 4 deep infections noted among 1281 procedures performed with the room functioning as a conventional operating room (0.31 percent). This contrasted with 8 deep infections among 1166 procedures performed with the horizontal unidirectional airflow system functioning (0.69 percent). There was no statistical significant difference among these observations ($p > 0.5$).

There were 9 deep infections among 742 (1.2 percent) revision procedures performed with the room functioning as a conventional operating room. While the horizontal unidirectional airflow system was functioning, 13 deep infections were noted among 695 revision procedures (1.9 percent). Among 585 revision total hip arthroplasties performed while the operating room was functioning as a conventional operating room, 2 deep infections were identified (0.34 percent). However, 10 deep infections were identified among 550 revision total hip arthroplasties performed with unidirectional airflow system functioning (1.82 percent). This contrasted with 7 deep infections among 157 revision total knee arthroplasties performed with the room functioning as a conventional operating room (4.4 percent). In contrast, only 3 deep infections were noted among 145 revision total knee arthroplasties performed with the horizontally unidirectional airflow system functioning (2.07 percent). Again, no statistically significant difference was noted between these observations ($p > 0.05$).

Since the period of follow-up examination was quite variable, ranging from 8 years to less than 1 year, among this group of 7305 arthroplasties, the data were analyzed with Kaplan-Meier probability analysis. The accumulative probability of deep sepsis following total hip arthroplasty with the unidirectional airflow off was 0.3 percent and with the unidirectional airflow system functioning it was 0.7 percent ($p > 0.05$). The accumulative probability of deep sepsis following total knee arthroplasty with the airflow system off was 1.3 percent and with the unidirectional airflow system functioning it was 0.8 percent ($p > 0.05$). Thus the preliminary analysis of these data does not identify any statistically significant difference. However, there are some suggestions that a horizontal unidirectional airflow system may reduce the deep infection rate during primary total hip arthroplasty, but the current database is not significantly large to statistically support this difference. The data also suggest that the array of equipment and traffic during revision total hip arthroplasty need to be carefully directed and if possible curtailed. The data also suggest that performing total knee arthroplasty in a horizontal unidirectional airflow system without the use of a personnel isolator system can be safely done without an increase in the incidence of deep postoperative sepsis. Finally, the data support the concept that prophylactic antimicrobial agents may be the single most important aspect in the reduction of deep sepsis following total hip or total knee arthroplasty.

PROPHYLACTIC ANTIMICROBIAL AGENTS. The prophylactic administration of antimicrobial agents has become a well-established principle for the reduction of postoperative sepsis. There is, however, some confusion over the application of this principle by surgeons. Should all patients having musculoskeletal surgery receive prophylactic antimicrobials? If not, which patient should and which patient should not? Which antimicrobial agent should be administered and when should it be administered?

Preoperative and intraoperative prophylactic antimicrobial agents are effective in high-risk orthopedic procedures. Antimicrobial agents administered within 3 hours after an operation enter the hematoma and adjacent tissues in sufficient concentrations to lower the incidence of experimental infections.[58] Fogelberg and co-workers[58] noted a statistically significant reduction in the incidence of deep sepsis with the prophylactic administration of penicillin in a prospective randomized series of patients undergoing either mold arthroplasty of the hip or spinal fusion. Boyd and co-workers[44] also noted a significant reduction of wound sepsis in a randomized, prospective study with the prophylactic administration of nafcillin in patients undergoing operations for fracture of the hip. In a study with the randomized administration of cephaloridine to 1591 patients undergoing elective orthopedic procedures, Pavel et al[59] noted a reduction in the incidence of deep sepsis from 5 percent in the placebo group to 2.8 percent in the treatment group ($p = 0.025$). A similar reduction in the incidence of deep sepsis was reported by Patzakis et al[60] with the use of cephalothin in adult patients who had open fractures. Thus, the prophylactic administration of antimicrobial agents reduces the incidence of deep sepsis in patients with open fractures, in those with extensive reconstructive procedures with the implantation of foreign bodies, and in those having procedures in which a large dead space remains. The choice of agent should be based not only on the expected contaminating flora, but also on the distribution and excretion characteristics of the various drugs.[61] Chapter 28 contains a comprehensive review on this subject.

Hill and co-workers[48] documented in a multicenter, randomized, prospective study that cefazolin administered prophylactically was associated with a reduced incidence of deep wound infection following total hip arthroplasty. Unfortunately, these investigators failed to control for the type of operating room in their study. While those patients having total hip arthroplasty in a conventional operating room had a statistically significant reduction ($p < 0.05$) in the incidence of deep sepsis with the prophylactic administration of cefazolin, there was not a statistically significant difference ($p > 0.05$) for those patients receiving the prophylactic administration of cefazolin who had their arthroplasty performed in a unidirectional airflow operating room. Interestingly, the incidence of postoperative wound infection was statistically equivalent among patients receiving the prophylactic administration of cefazolin who had total hip arthroplasty performed in a conventional operating room and patients who did and did not receive the prophylactic administration of cefazolin but had their arthroplasties performed in a unidirectional operating room. This study again points to the importance of the prophylactic administration of antimicrobial therapy in patients who will receive an orthopedic implant.

All surgeons would agree that those procedures involving the implantation of large foreign bodies necessitate the prophylactic administration of antimicrobial agents (see Chap. 25). The indications for the prophylactic administration of antimicrobial agents during operations involving the application of one or two screws or Steinmann pins are less clear. Certainly, any operation where a dead space permits the formation of a hematoma should be associated with the administration of prophylactic antimicrobials. Operations requiring 2 hours or more would also justify the prophylactic administration of antimicrobial agents. In general, soft tissue operations, procedures implanting minimal metal devices, and those of short duration are not usually considered for the prophylactic administration of antimicrobial agents. However, Henley and coworkers[57] recently reported a statistically significant reduction in the incidence of postoperative sepsis in soft tissue and other musculoskeletal procedures not requiring a prosthetic device lasting 2 hours or more with the prophylactic administration of antimicrobials. Procedures requiring less than 2 hours did not have an associated reduction in the incidence of sepsis. The application of these principles to musculoskeletal procedures must be left to the discretion of the individual surgeon, who is capable of making the wisest decision for each patient. The principle, derived from experimental and clinical studies over 30 years, is clear. The infection rate can be reduced if contamination is normally sufficient to induce an infection rate of 2 to 3 percent. Since most evidence suggests that a single perioperative dose of antibiotics is as good as multiple preoperative and postoperative doses, the cost is small.

When the prophylactic administration of antimicrobial agents is thought to be indicated, the surgeon must select an agent that is bactericidal against the microorganisms associated with postoperative musculoskeletal sepsis in his or her hospital. Furthermore, the agent selected should be safe and inexpensive. In North America, *Staphylococcus aureus* and *S. epidermidis* remain the most common causal organisms isolated from postoperative infections of the musculoskeletal system. Streptococci are the third commonest isolates recovered. Gram-negative bacillary organisms are less common isolates. Recently, a prospective multicenter clinical study comparing a first- and second-generation cephalosporin revealed equivalent efficacy with a 25 to 30 percent reduction in cost with the administration of the second-generation cephalosporin. The second-generation cephalosporin—cefuroxime—had a long half-life, permitting 12-hour dosing as compared to cefazolin, which has a shorter half-life that requires dosing every 8 hours. Thus 1 day of cefuroxime was as efficacious as 3 days of cefazolin and less expensive. The obvious remaining question arising from this study is: would 1 day of cefazolin be as effective as 1 day of cefuroxime? At this time, there appears to be a cost savings with 1 day of cefuroxime administered prophylactically for patients having total joint arthroplasty.

The timing of the administration and the duration of prophylactic antimicrobials remain controversial. Although most surgeons initiate the administration of prophylactic antibiotics during surgery, the duration of administration varies widely. It would appear that most surgeons discontinue antimicrobials 48 to 72 hours after surgery. There is certainly no need to continue the administration of antibiotics for 5 to 7 days. In fact, such prolonged administration of antimicrobials appears to permit the development of remote infections. More recently, some authorities have suggested that the antimicrobials may be discontinued after one to two doses administered during surgery and in the recovery room. Though such a brief period of administration may prove to be efficacious and cost effective in general surgery, it has as yet to be studied in depth in orthopedic surgery.

Clinical Manifestations and Diagnosis

ELECTIVE RECONSTRUCTIVE SURGERY. The clinical features of sepsis after skeletal operations vary with the procedure performed. Most infections occur within the first 2 weeks after elective reconstruction in adults if neither foreign body nor prophylactic antibiotics are used. Spiking temperatures (39C to 40C), increasing pain, progressive swelling, and an enlarging area of erythema are first seen. Frequently, there is either serous drainage or a draining hematoma. Because the leukocyte count and erythrocyte sedimentation rate are elevated after most major operations, they are of little value in the differential diagnosis. Similarly, routine x-ray studies and technetium-99 scans will reflect only postoperative changes. Gallium and technetium differential imaging have been supplemented by autologous indium white blood cell scintigraphy. Recent experience has demonstrated accurate evaluation in 94 percent of low grade infections about implants. Similarly, this technique was found to be efficacious in the diagnosis of osteomyelitis.[50,51,53,54] Most acute infections are diagnosed on clinical examination alone. At the time of debridement, fluid and tissue specimens should be submitted for aerobic and anaerobic cultures (see Chap. 3). Susceptibility studies should be performed on all isolates to permit the selection of specific antimicrobial agent(s) for parenteral therapy.

INTERVERTEBRAL DISC OPERATIONS. The clinical and laboratory expressions of postoperative wound infection after intervertebral diskectomy do not conform to the pattern described. The onset of symptoms varies from 1 to 10 weeks after operation. Excruciating pain, unrelieved by narcotics, is the most characteristic symptom. It is described as severe back spasms and extends into both flanks, the lower abdomen, and groin. Sciatic radiation is uncommon. Little fever is noted. Paraspinal spasm and resistance to all spinal motion are noted on physical examination. The erythrocyte sedimentation rate remains elevated for longer than the 6 to 8 weeks that are normally associated with this procedure. X-ray studies during the first few weeks reveal only postoperative changes. Loss of the distinct margins of the usually sclerotic end plate of the cephalad and caudal vertebrae in the lateral projection is the first change. Subsequently, the disc space narrows. Eventually, the adjacent vertebrae fuse with new bone formation. The sedimentation rate remains elevated until bony fusion occurs.

Infected granulation tissue rather than gross purulence is noted if debridement is performed. Tissue specimens from the involved disc space obtained either by needle biopsy or at operation should be submitted for aerobic and anaerobic culture and susceptibility studies. Because *S. aureus* is generally cultured, intravenous antimicrobial therapy with a semisynthetic penicillinase-resistant penicillin or a cephalosporin should be administered until the results of the culture and susceptibility studies are available. The patient should be immobilized in a plaster jacket to control pain.

ELECTIVE RECONSTRUCTIVE SURGERY WITH FOREIGN BODY IMPLANT. The use of prophylactic antimicrobial therapy during operations that require the implantation of plates, screws, or nails has altered the clinical manifestations of postoperative wound sepsis. The infection discloses itself late, 3 months or more after operation. Low-grade infection with commensal organisms, previously considered to be nonpathogenic, is partly responsible for this altered clinical course. The patient usually complains of pain but has little clinical evidence of sepsis. Fever is absent, and the wound appears normal but may be tender. Laboratory evaluation can reveal an elevated leukocyte count with a shift to the left, a moderate anemia, and, usually, an elevated erythrocyte sedimentation rate. X-ray studies reveal various changes, but they are usually subtle—lacy, periosteal new bone formation and cystic erosion around the screws or intramedullary nail.

INTRA-ARTICULAR SURGERY. Septic arthritis after arthrotomy and intra-articular procedures can be difficult to differentiate from intra-articular hematoma. A swollen, painful joint occurs with both conditions. The febrile response associated with septic arthritis varies with the virulence of the bacteria. The peripheral leukocyte count and the erythrocyte sedimentation rate are elevated because of the operation itself. Needle aspiration of the involved joint can provide diagnostic information. If the infection seems superficial to the capsule, the subcutaneous or subfascial space (depending upon the joint) is aspirated without entering the joint. All material obtained is submitted for cell count, Gram stain, and culture. If few leukocytes are seen and no organisms are noted on Gram stain (or if the process is definitely intra-articular), the intra-articular space can then be aspirated. If an infection is present, the aspirate will vary from turbid to purulent, and the viscosity will be decreased. Mucin clot, as measured by acid preparation, will be poor. An elevated total leukocyte count ranging from 15,000 to 20,000/mm^3, with 90 percent polymorphonuclear leukocytes, is common. The synovial glucose level will be decreased, averaging 50 mg/dl less than the serum glucose level. Gram stain of the aspirate will identify microorganisms, allowing the physician to begin administering antimicrobial therapy. A portion of the specimen should be submitted for aerobic and anaerobic cultures. If a postoperative hematoma is present, the aspirate will be bloody with small clots. The viscosity and mucin clot test results are decreased and poor. The leukocyte count may be only slightly elevated, and the percentage of polymorphonuclear leukocytes is not elevated. No organisms will be seen on Gram stain.

INTERNAL FIXATION OF FEMORAL NECK FRACTURES. When low-grade sepsis occurs after open reduction and internal fixation of femoral neck fractures, the patient experiences continuous pain. The erythrocyte sedimentation rate and total leukocyte count remain elevated. X-ray studies reveal a series of characteristic changes, the first of which is the loss of height of the normal joint space. Subsequently, subluxation of the hip joint occurs. With further progression of the infection, cystic erosion of the acetabulum and femoral head usually occurs.

TOTAL JOINT ARTHROPLASTY. Deep sepsis after total joint arthroplasty can be subdivided into three stages based on the time of presentation and the clinical course: stage 1, an acute fulminating infection, which usually develops within the first weeks after surgery; stage 2, delayed deep sepsis, which develops as creeping infection within the first 2 postoperative years; and stage 3, hematogenous infection, which develops in a previously asymptomatic patient, usually occurring 2 to 5 years after operation.

Because most patients who have an elective procedure in which a large foreign body is implanted receive prophylactic antimicrobial therapy, acute fulminating infections (stage 1) are uncommon. Most of these stage 1 infections are infected hematomas that drain postoperatively and can be diagnosed on examination (Fig. 46–7).

Stage 2 infections (delayed deep sepsis) can be difficult to diagnose because the usual clinical signs of wound infection—fever, drainage, and so forth—are rarely seen. The patient complains of pain

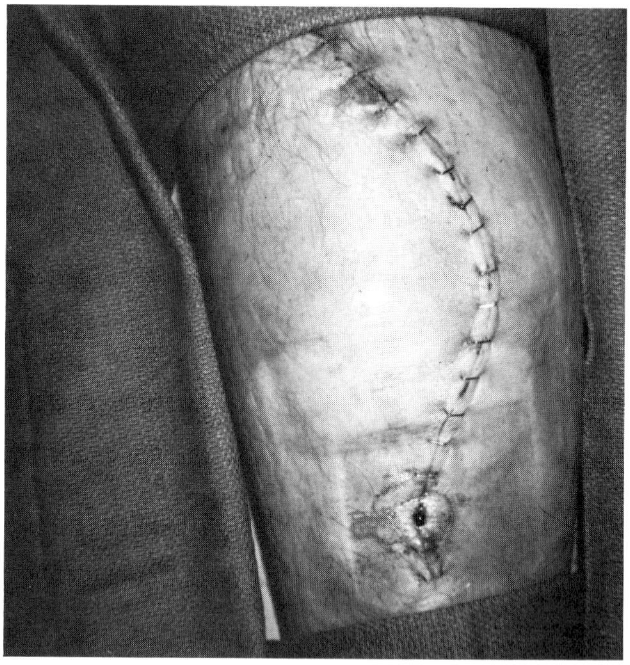

Figure 46–7. Draining hematoma from distal aspect of knee 12 days after total knee arthroplasty.

about the joint, especially when using the extremity. The differential diagnosis includes mechanical loosening at the bone-cement interface and loosening secondary to low-grade infection. Although the leukocyte count is not generally abnormal, the erythrocyte sedimentation rate is frequently elevated—greater than 60 mm in 1 hour (Westergren) in women and greater than 40 mm in men. X-ray studies reveal a lucent zone at the bone-cement interface about one or both components of the total joint arthroplasty. If cystic erosion or periosteal new bone formation is seen, an injection may be present (Fig. 46–8). An arthrogram of the joint frequently is helpful. Before the dye is injected, an aspirate should be sent for culture and susceptibility studies. Penetration of the dye into the bone-cement interface suggests loosening. Murray and Rodrigo,[52] however, have seen such penetration in the bone-cement interface of some asymptomatic patients who have had total hip arthroplasty. If lateral pocketing of the dye beyond the pseudocapsule is noted, an infectious cause is more likely (Fig. 46–9). A technetium-99 scan frequently reveals increased uptake with either mechanical or infectious loosening. Although a gallium-67 scan usually reveals increased uptake only if the cause is infectious, false-positive scan results have been encountered. Indium-111 autologous white blood cell images have proved to be more reliable.[53,54]

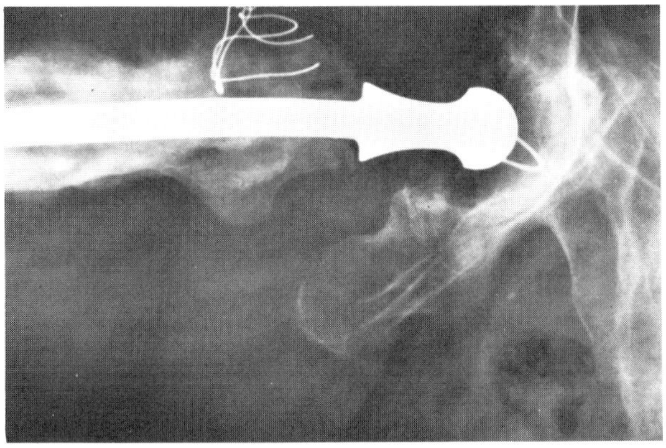

Figure 46–8. Lateral view of Charnley total hip arthroplasty. Periosteal new bone formation of anterior and posterior femoral cortices is well demonstrated. Erosion of bone-cement interface about femoral compartment. Lucent zone is present at bone–cement interface of entire circumference of acetabular component.

Frequently, the clinical and laboratory evaluations will not be diagnostic in the patient with low-grade *S. epidermidis* or anaerobic infections. Frozen-section histologic examination of tissue specimens obtained at operation has been diagnostic. If many polymorphonuclear leukocytes are seen in each high-power field, low-grade sepsis is present, and a complete debridement with removal of the prosthesis should be performed. However, if lymphocytes and histiocytes without polymorphonuclear leukocytes are seen on frozen-section study,

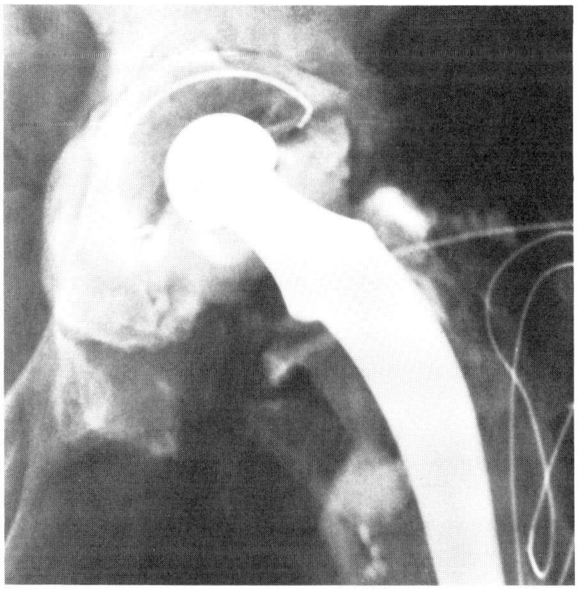

Figure 46–9. Arthrogram of hip reveals penetration of bone-cement interface of femoral components, pocketing of dye inferomedially and superolaterally, and small pocket of dye indicating erosion of greater trochanter.

mechanical loosening is the diagnosis, and revision arthroplasty is indicated.

In stage 3 infections (late hematogenous infections), the patient describes a previously asymptomatic arthroplasty with the acute onset of fever, chills, and pain around the involved joint. Unlike patients with stage 2 infections, who are never completely free of pain after operation, patients with stage 3 infections are asymptomatic until the acute episode. Frequently, the patient has a history of an antecedent infection at a remote site (eg, urinary tract infection, infected toenail). The leukocyte count is elevated, with a shift to the left, and the erythrocyte sedimentation rate is elevated. X-ray studies of the arthroplasty are normal. The acute nature of the infection usually precludes the use of nuclear imaging. When debridement is performed early in the disease, purulent material is found rather than infected granulation tissue permeating the bone-cement interface, so characteristic of delayed deep sepsis (stage 2).

AFTER OPERATION FOR INJURY. Septic complications in the traumatized patient vary with the surgical techniques used in the initial management of the wound. Sepsis after debridement and open packing of the wound is usually associated with purulence within the depths of the wound. A progressive necrosis frequently can be the predominant clinical feature. Clostridial cellulitis or myonecrosis may occur when debridement, followed by primary closure, is the initial operative treatment. In fact, Brown and Kinman,[55] in a study of gas gangrene in 27 patients, stressed the association of clostridial myonecrosis and the premature closure of traumatic wounds.

Virulent microorganisms are associated with wound sepsis after the primary closure of traumatized wounds. Thus, most patients will have systemic signs and symptoms of sepsis. In addition to a spiking temperature, dehydration, and delirium, the patient will experience progressive localized pain. Occasionally, the organism will be one of the less virulent types, for example, *S. epidermidis*. In this group of patients, only local symptoms herald the presence of sepsis. Wound drainage is usually minimal. X-ray studies reveal resorption of bone around internal fixation devices, resulting in their loosening.

Treatment. The management of septic complications after skeletal operations usually requires aggressive intervention. To ignore a draining hematoma during the first few postoperative weeks in a patient with local or systemic signs of sepsis is an invitation to disaster. When there are no implanted foreign bodies in the wound, early debridement and specific parenteral antimicrobial therapy can frequently control, if not eradicate, the infection.

Although the factors influencing the incidence of postoperative sepsis are protean, careful evaluation of operative wound sepsis can identify changing trends in the microbiology of nosocomial infections and alterations in the susceptibility patterns. The information obtained can be invaluable to the physician in determining empiric therapeutic regimens for the patient with a postoperative septic complication while awaiting microbiologic identification and susceptibility studies.[5]

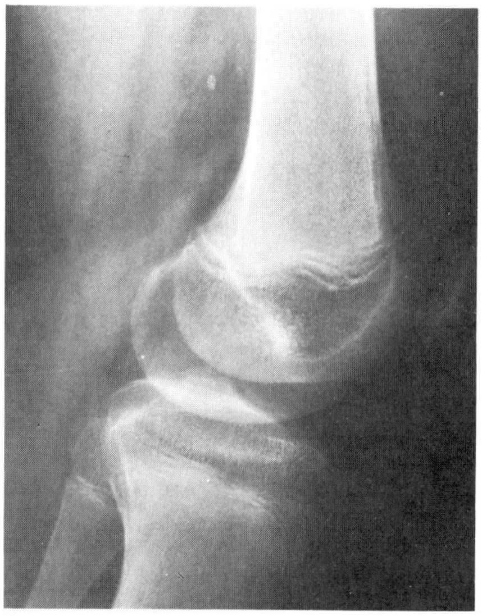

A

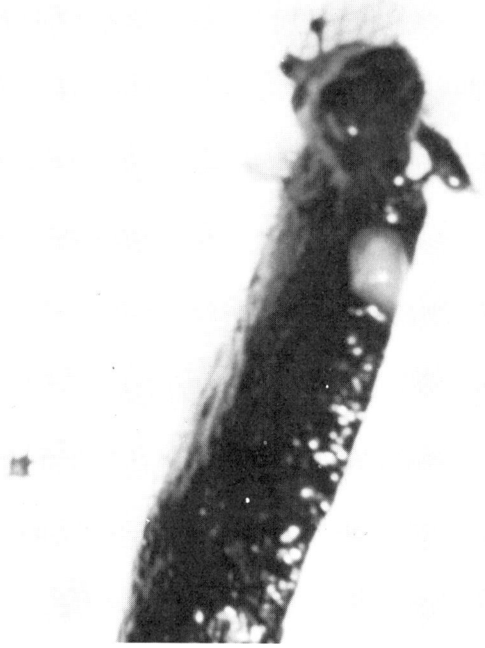

B

Figure 46–10. Persistent drainage about medial aspect of distal thigh, after two subsequent debridements, of 15-year-old boy 1 year after falling on tree branch. **A.** Lateral x-ray of knee. Soft tissue swelling and effusion of knee are seen. **B.** Large (3 by 0.5 cm) twig found. Foreign body had eroded into suprapatellar pouch. Infection cleared after operation and specific antimicrobial therapy.

Debridement provides not only for excision of dead and infected tissue, but also an opportunity to obtain deep tissue specimens for aerobic and anaerobic cultures and susceptibility studies. While the results of the microbiologic studies are being awaited, empiric antimicrobial therapy should be initiated on the basis of the type of infection, the local anatomy, and Gram stain of the clinical material submitted to the laboratory. If necessary, the therapeutic agents can be altered after the organism is identified and the results of susceptibility studies become available.

Early aseptic debridement of hematomas that are about to drain or of those that begin to drain after suture removal can prevent deep sepsis. Foreign bodies that are providing stability to osseous structures (compression plates and intramedullary nails) should not be removed. Frequently, a thorough debridement followed by fascial closure and secondary closure of the subcutaneous tissues and skin will control the infection until first-stage osseous healing has occurred. When early bony union has been achieved, the internal fixation devices can be removed and cast-immobilization used until healing is complete.

In wounds without bone grafts or foreign bodies, debridement followed by open packing will control the sepsis. The wound can be closed in a delayed primary or secondary fashion. Alternately, the fascia alone can be closed, closure allowing the superficial tissues to heal by secondary intention.

Persistent sepsis after soft tissue trauma is often associated with the presence of retained foreign bodies that are frequently radiolucent. Thus x-ray studies are of little value in identifying their location (Fig. 46–10). Removal of the foreign body and debridement of infected and necrotic tissue, combined with specific antimicrobial therapy, usually will eradicate the infection.

The treatment of deep sepsis around an artificial joint varies with the stage of the infection. Stage 1 infected hematomas usually are amenable to debridement with retention of the artificial joint. In contrast, stage 1 fulminative infections require removal of the foreign bodies. Most stage 2 delayed deep infections require removal of the implant. Early operative debridement and parenteral antimicrobial therapy may permit retention of the arthroplasty in stage 3 hematogenous infections.

Quantitative microbiologic techniques have been useful in the management of open fractures and dislocations[62] (R H Fitzgerald, Jr., W P Cooney, and J H Dobyns, unpublished data). A 1 ml tissue specimen is weighed, homogenized, serially diluted, and stained, and bacteria are counted so that the result can be available to the surgeon within 30 minutes. Our experience suggests a high (98 percent) correlation between a positive quantitative Gram stain and a colony count of 10^5 per gram or greater. In our prospective study of open fractures and dislocation in 82 patients, a similar correlation was found between the results of quantitative microbiology techniques and the development of wound sepsis. For these reasons, positive quantitative Gram stains at the conclusion of the debridement are used as an indication for open packing of the wound and the parenteral administration of antibiotic drugs. A negative quantitative Gram stain allows the surgeon greater latitude in the management of the wound.

Joint Reconstruction After Operative Wound Sepsis. Limited function and a painful joint occur frequently after alteration of the articular cartilage by the infection. In certain conditions, the residual pain can be alleviated by extra-articular reconstructive procedures. Pain after incomplete destruction of either the medial or the lateral compartment of knees can be relieved by transferring the weight-bearing focus to the asymptomatic compartment with an upper tibial osteotomy. More commonly, the partially destroyed joint will require that the articular surfaces be replaced by a total joint arthroplasty.

It is desirable to perform a second total joint arthroplasty after removal of the first and eradication of the infection. Few objective criteria are available, however, to determine whether the infection has been completely eliminated and whether a second implant will not be complicated by recurrent infection. Experience with reimplantation includes both total hip and total knee arthroplasties.[63–65] Favorable results have been reported by Wilson et al[66] in the treatment of subacute sepsis of the hip with immediate total joint arthroplasty combined with large doses of parenteral antimicrobial drugs. Because many patients do not wish immediate reoperation, we believe that reimplantation generally should be delayed for 1 year after the treatment of the infection around the hip implant if the causal organism is a virulent isolate.[65] Patients who have continued pain and difficulty in walking with a resection (Girdlestone) arthroplasty and have no evidence of sepsis are candidates for reimplantation. Recurrent deep sepsis is more common in patients with previous gram-negative bacterial infections and those with early reimplantation (less than 6 months). In our experience, if organisms of low pathogenicity are isolated during the initial infection, reimplantation of a total joint is associated with a better prognosis.

Preliminary experience is promising with a similar technique in the treatment of the infected total knee arthroplasty. Reimplantation of the prosthetic components can be performed if, after three debridements, the bony and soft tissues are sterile.

Buchholz and Gartmann[67] used gentamicin-impregnated bone-cement in a single-stage treatment of the infected total hip arthroplasty. In contrast to the delayed reconstruction with total hip arthroplasty performed by the author, their technique involved removal of the infected components, complete debridement of the bone and soft tissues, and immediate reimplantation of a new total hip with gentamicin-impregnated cement. Sixty-nine percent of their early results with this technique were successful. Subsequent experience has demonstrated that in their hands this technique has been successful in three-quarters of their patients. However, the failure rate appears to have a direct relationship to the toxicity of the causal organism (Table 46–8).[68] Recent experience with this technique in North America reported by Garvin and colleagues[64] has been favorable.

Complications of Chronic Skeletal Sepsis. Malignant degeneration and amyloidosis are occasionally seen in patients who have chronic infections of bones and joints.[12,15] Both carcinomas and sarcomas probably result from a long-standing reparative process. Squamous cell carcinoma appears in association with a draining sinus of long duration. Increased pain, drainage, hemorrhage, an enlarging mass, or a pathologic fracture suggests neoplastic degeneration. The sedimentation rate and leukocyte count are frequently normal. X-ray studies usually demonstrate lytic and sclerotic changes indistinguishable from those of chronic osteomyelitis.

TABLE 46–8. ONE-STAGE EXCHANGE ARTHROPLASTY ANTIBIOTIC-IMPREGNATED BONE CEMENT

Microorganism	Failure (%)
Gram-negative bacilli (*Pseudomonas aeruginosa, Escherichia coli, Klebsiella* species)	≥50
Staphylococcus aureus	28
Peptococcus species	24
Corynebacterium species	16
Sterile	11

Adapted from Buchholtz HW, Elson RA, Engelbrecht E, et al: J Bone Joint Surg [Br] 63:342, 1981.

However, a severely destructive lesion clearly different from the usual osteomyelitic process can be seen. Biopsy of the sinus tract usually reveals bone invasion. Cure usually can be achieved with amputation.

Sarcomatous change in chronic osteomyelitis is usually associated with a pathologic fracture or an enlarging mass. Biopsy delineates the histologic diagnosis.

The association of amyloidosis with long-standing osteomyelitis and tuberculosis of the skeletal system was recognized years ago. Although secondary amyloidosis complicating chronic osteomyelitis has been seen occasionally in the patient who fails to receive treatment, modern drug therapy has significantly reduced this complication. Secondary amyloidosis is seen with equal frequency in patients who have chronic hematogenous and posttraumatic osteomyelitis. In general, chronic or recurring osteomyelitis will have been present for 20 years or more. Hepatosplenomegaly, a common finding in primary amyloidosis, is seldom noted. Laboratory evaluation of renal function reveals an elevation of the serum creatinine and blood urea nitrogen levels. Proteinuria is noted on routine urinalysis. Renal or rectal biopsies are necessary to confirm the diagnosis. A technetium-99 scan and a gallium-67 scan of the area reveal increased activity. An invasive type of subacute and chronic inflammatory granulation tissue is noted on tissue study.

REFERENCES

Osteomyelitis

1. Hunter W: Of the structure and diseases of articulating cartilages. Philos Trans R Soc Lond 42:514, 1743.
2. Wilensky AO: Osteomyelitis: Its Pathogenesis, Symptomatology and Treatment. New York, Macmillan, 1934.
3. Dich VQ, Nelson JD, Haltalin KC: Osteomyelitis in infants and children: a review of 163 cases. Am J Dis Child 129:1273, 1975.
4. Morrey BF, Peterson HA: Hematogenous pyogenic osteomyelitis in children. Orthop Clin North Am 6:935, 1975.
5. Waldvogel FA, Medoff G, Swartz MN: Osteomyelitis: a review of clinical features, therapeutic considerations and unusual aspects. N Engl J Med 282:198, 260, 317, 1970.
6. Lewis R, Gorbach S, Altner P: Spinal pseudomonas chondrosteomyelitis in heroin users. N Engl J Med 286:1303, 1972.
7. Wold ER: Risk factors for osteomyelitis. Am J Med 78:206, 1985.

8. Kelly PJ, Fitzgerald RH Jr, Cabanela ME, et al: Results of treatment of tibial and femoral osteomyelitis in adults. Clin Orthop Relat Res 259:295, 1990.
9. West WF, Kelly PJ, Martin WJ: Chronic osteomyelitis. I. Factors affecting the results of treatment in 186 patients. JAMA 213:1837, 1970.
10. Hall BB, Fitzgerald RH Jr, Rosenblatt JE: Anaerobic osteomyelitis. J Bone Joint Surg 65A:30, 1983.
11. Nettles JL, Kelly PJ, Martin WJ, Washington JA II: Musculoskeletal infections due to bacteroides: a study of eleven cases. J Bone Joint Surg [Am] 51:230, 1969.
12. Hall BB, Rosenblatt JE, Fitzgerald RH Jr: Anaerobic septic arthritis and osteomyelitis. Orthop Clin North Am 15:505, 1984.
13. Finegold SM: Anaerobic Bacteria in Human Disease. New York, Academic Press, 1977.
14. Kelly PJ: Infections of bones and joints in adult patients. Instructional Course Lectures. Am Acad Orthop Surg 26:3, 1977.
15. Burri C: Post-traumatic Osteomyelitis. Bern, Huber, 1975.
16. Mowlem R: Cancellous chip bone-grafts: report on 75 cases. Lancet 2:746, 1944.
17. Knight MP, Wood GO: Surgical obliteration of bone cavities following traumatic osteomyelitis. J Bone Joint Surg 27:547, 1945.
18. Robertson IM, Barron JN: A method of treatment of chronic infective osteitis. J Bone Joint Surg 28:19, 1946.
19. Coleman HM, Bateman JE, Dale GM, Starr DE: Cancellous bone grafts for infected bone defects: a single stage procedure. Surg Gynecol Obstet 83:392, 1946.
20. Bickel WH, Bateman JG, Johnson WE: Treatment of chronic hematogenous osteomyelitis by means of saucerization and bone grafting. Surg Gynecol Obstet 96:265, 1953.
21. Papineau LJ: L'excision-gréffe avec fermeture retardée délibérée dans l'osteomyelite chronique. Nouv Presse Med 2:2753, 1973.
22. Ger R: Muscle transposition for treatment and prevention of chronic posttraumatic osteomyelitis of the tibia. J Bone Joint Surg [Am] 59:784, 1977.
23. Prigge EK: The treatment of chronic osteomyelitis by the use of muscle transplant or iliac graft. J Bone Joint Surg 28:576, 1946.
24. Uyama S: Die Plombierung, von Knochenhöhlen durch Muskeltransplantation. Bruns Beitr Klin Chir 104:707, 1917.
25. Popkirov SG: Die Behandlung der hämatogenen und der traumatischen Osteomyelitis. Berlin, Volk und Gesundheit, 1971.
26. Fitzgerald RH Jr, Ruttle PE, Arnold PG, et al: Local muscle flaps in treatment of chronic osteomyelitis. J Bone Joint Surg 67A:175, 1985.
27. Nelson JD, Howard JB, Shelton S: Oral antibiotic therapy for skeletal infections in children. I. Antibiotic concentrations in suppurative synovial fluid. J Pediatr 92:131, 1978.

Septic Arthritis

28. Goldenberg DL, Brandt KD, Cathcart ES, Cohen AS: Acute arthritis caused by gram-negative bacilli: a clinical characterization. Medicine (Baltimore) 53:197, 1974.
29. Hunder GG, McDuffie FC: Hypocomplementemia in rheumatoid arthritis. Am J Med 54:461, 1973.
30. Phemister DB: The effect of pressure on articular surfaces in pyogenic and tuberculous arthritides and its bearing on treatment. Ann Surg 80:481, 1924.
31. Curtiss PH Jr, Klein L: Destruction of articular cartilage in septic arthritis. I. In vitro studies. J Bone Joint Surg [Am] 45:797, 1963.
32. Curtiss PH Jr, Klein L: Destruction of articular cartilage in septic arthritis. II. In vivo studies. J Bone Joint Surg [Am] 47:1595, 1965.
33. Fell HB, Jubb RW: The effect of synovial tissue on breakdown of articular cartilage in organ culture. Arthritis Rheum 20:1359, 1977.
34. Steinberg JJ, Sledge CB: Synovial factors and chondrocyte-mediated breakdown of cartilage: inhibition by hydrocortisone. J Orthop Res 1:13, 1983.
35. Marsh DC Jr, Matthew EB, Persellin RH: Transport of gentamicin into synovial fluid. JAMA 228:607, 1974.
36. Daniel D, Akeson W, Amiel D: The effect of joint lavage in preventing cartilage destruction in an experimentally produced *Staphylococcus aureus* joint infection (abstract). J Bone Joint Surg [Am] 57:583, 1975.
37. Anderson LD, Horn LG: Irrigation-suction technic in the treatment of acute hematogenous osteomyelitis, chronic osteomyelitis, and acute and chronic joint infections. South Med J 63:745, 1970.

Granulomatous Infections of Bones and Joints

38. Pritchard DJ: Granulomatous infections of bones and joints. Orthop Clin North Am 6:1029, 1975.
39. Runyon EH: Anonymous *Mycobacterium* in pulmonary disease. Med Clin North Am 43:273, 1959.
40. Gehweiler JA, Capp MP, Chick EW: Observations on the roentgen patterns and blastomycosis of bone. Am J Roentgenol Radium Ther Nucl Med 108:497, 1970.
41. Bassett FH III, Tindall JP: Blastomycosis of bone. South Med J 65:547, 1972.
42. Crout JE, Brewer NS, Tompkins RB: Sporotrichosis arthritis: clinical features in seven patients. Ann Intern Med 86:294, 1977.

Postoperative Infections

43. Ad Hoc Committee of the Committee on Trauma: Postoperative wound infections: the influence of ultraviolet irradiation of the operating room and of various other factors. Ann Surg 160[Suppl]:1, 1964.
44. Boyd RJ, Burke JF, Colton T: A double-blind clinical trial of prophylactic antibiotics in hip fractures. J Bone Joint Surg [Am] 55:1251, 1973.
45. Tengve B, Kjellander J: Antibiotic prophylaxis in op-

erations on trochanteric femoral fractures. J Bone Joint Surg [Am] 60:97, 1978.
46. Miller WE, Counts GW: Orthopedic infections: a prospective study of 378 clean procedures. South Med J 68:386, 1975.
47. Fitzgerald RH Jr: The epidemiology of nosocomial infections of the musculoskeletal system. In Gröschel D (ed): Handbook on Hospital-Associated Infections, Vol 3. New York, Dekker, 1979, pp 25–35.
48. Hill C, Mazas F, Flamont R, Eorard J: Prophylactic cefazolin versus placebo in total hip replacement. Lancet 11:795, 1981.
49. Gustilo RB, Anderson JT: Prevention of infection in the treatment of 1025 open fractures of long bones: Retrospective and prospective analyses. J Bone Joint Surg [Am] 58:453, 1976.
50. Merkel KD, Brown ML, Dewangee MK, Fitzgerald RH Jr: Comparison of indium-labeled leukocyte imaging with sequential technetium–gallium scanning in the diagnosis of low-grade musculoskeletal sepsis: a prospective study. J Bone Joint Surg [Am] 67:465, 1985.
51. Merkel KD, Fitzgerald RH Jr, Brown ML: Scintigraphic examination of total hip arthroplasty: comparison of indium with technetium–gallium in loose and infected canine arthroplasty. In Welch R (ed): The Hip. St Louis, Mosby, 1984, pp 163–192.
52. Murray WR, Rodrigo JJ: Arthrography for the assessment of pain after total hip replacement: a comparison of arthrographic findings in patients with and without pain. J Bone Joint Surg [Am] 57:1060, 1975.
53. Merkel KD, Brown ML, Fitzgerald RH Jr: Scintigraphic evaluation in musculoskeletal sepsis. Orthop Clin North Am 15:401, 1984.
54. Merkel KD, Brown ML, Dewanjee MK, Fitzgerald RH Jr: Comparison of indium-labeled-leukocyte imaging with sequential technetium-gallium scanning in the diagnosis of low-grade musculoskeletal sepsis. J. Bone Joint Surg [Am] 67:465, 1985.
55. Brown PW, Kinman PB: Gas gangrene in a metropolitan community. J Bone Joint Surg [Am] 56:1445, 1974.
56. Lidwell OM, Lowbury EJ, Whyte W, et al: Effect of ultraclean air in operating rooms on deep sepsis in the joint after total hip or knee replacement: a randomised study. Br Med J 285:10, 1982.
57. Henley MB, Jones RE, Wyatt RWB, et al: Prophylaxis with cefamandole nafate in elective orthopaedic surgery. Clin Orthop 209:249, 1986.
58. Fogelberg EV, Zitzmann EK, Stinchfield FE: Prophylatic penicillin in orthopaedic surgery. J Bone Joint Surg [Am] 52:95, 1970.
59. Pavel A, Smith RL, Ballard A, Larson IJ: Prophylactic antibiotics in elective orthopedic surgery: a prospective study of 1,591 cases. South Med J 70[Suppl 1]:50, 1977.
60. Patzakis MJ, Harvey JP Jr, Ivler D: The role of antibiotics in the management of open fractures. J Bone Joint Surg [Am] 56:532, 1974.
61. Hill C, Flamant R, Mazas F, Evrard J: Prophylactic cefazoline versus placebo in total hip replacement. Lancet 1:795, 1981.
62. Robson MC, Lea CE, Dalton JB, Heggers JP: Quantitative bacteriology and delayed wound closure. Surg Forum 19:501, 1968.
63. Fremont-Smith P: Sepsis and total hip arthroplasty. Part I. Antibiotic management of septic total hip replacement: a therapeutic trial. Proc Sci Meet Hip Soc 2:301, 1974.
64. Garvin K, Fitzgerald RH Jr, Salvati E: Reconstruction of the infected total hip and knee arthroplasty with gentamicin-impregnated palacos bone cement. Instructional Course Lectures. Am Acad Orthop Surg 42:293, 1993.
65. McDonald DJ, Fitzgerald RH Jr, Ilstrup DM: Two-stage reconstruction of a total hip arthroplasty because of infection. J Bone Joint Surg [Am] 71:828, 1989.
66. Wilson PD Jr, Aglietti P, Salvati EA: Subacute sepsis of the hip treated by antibiotics and cemented prosthesis. J Bone Joint Surg [Am] 56:879, 1974.
67. Buchholz WH, Gartmann HD: Infektionsprophylaxe und operative Behandlung der schleichenden tiefen Infektion bei der totalen Endoprosthese. Chirurgie 43:446, 1972.
68. Buchholtz HW, Elson RA, Engelbrecht E, et al: Management of deep infection of total hip replacement. J Bone Joint Surg [Br] 63:342, 1981.

BIBLIOGRAPHY

Esterhai JL Jr. Orthopedic infections. Orthop Clin North Am 22:363, 1991.

Fitzgerald RH Jr: The epidemiology of nosocomial infections of the musculoskeletal system. In Gröschel D (ed): Handbook on Hospital-Associated Infections. Vol 3. New York, Dekker, 1979, p 25.

Fitzgerald RH Jr, Kelly PJ: Musculoskeletal sepsis. Orthop Clin North Am 15:399, 1984.

Infections of the Hand

CHAPTER 47

William Lineaweaver

The treatment of hand infections is a contest between the infecting agents and the physician played out on the intricate terrain of the hand's anatomy. Early in this century, Kanavel synthesized the fundamental principles of bacteriologic identification and anatomically based surgical intervention that remain the foundations of modern treatment of hand infections.[1,2] The introduction of antibiotics was an important addition to the maneuvers available to the physician, and antibiotics have changed the entity of hand infections from one with a measurable mortality and great morbidity[3,4] to one in which a successful resolution can be anticipated following appropriate treatment. Modern techniques of surgical reconstruction also allow the surgeon to pursue more ambitious approaches of ablation and restoration.

Diagnosis. The specific diagnosis of a hand infection must be based on a careful history, an anatomically based physical examination, and, in most cases, an x-ray study of the hand.

The history should include onset of pain and swelling, details of injury, and details of previous hand infections, hand injuries, and hand operations (a source of foreign bodies). Systemic diseases should be noted, and circumstances associated with specific anatomic and bacteriologic infections (eg, human bites) considered.

Physical examination should begin with a search for fluctuance around the nailbed, within the finger pulp, and within the web spaces. Palmar swelling and erythema can indicate deep space infection and should be evaluated carefully. Passive and active range of motion of all joints should be performed to elicit signs of joint and tendon inflammation, fracture, dislocation, or impinging foreign bodies. Skin lesions and draining wounds should be noted, as should cellulitis and lymphadenopathy. Painful, firm veins can represent suppurative phlebitis, and any network of symptomatic veins in a febrile patient must be explored surgically.

An x-ray study is an invaluable adjunct to the physical examination. Abscesses may be related to occult foreign bodies, pyogenic arthritis complicated by fracture, and draining wounds continuous with chronic osteomyelitis. Treatment of a hand infection must include proper management of skeletal lesion and foreign bodies, and these complicating factors must be defined by x-ray studies.

The findings should allow the examining physician to decide whether or not a hand infection should be treated with antibiotics alone or surgically. Any acute suppurative lesion should be explored and drained, and any findings that suggest skeletal or joint infection, deep space infection, or infection spreading along anatomic planes or involving fascia or muscle must also lead promptly to surgery. Delay can result in dangerous spread of the infection as well as significant damage to skin, joints, and tendons. If an infection is judged to be nonsurgical, treatment with antibiotics alone must be accompanied by frequent reexamination of the patient to determine whether or not a surgical lesion develops or becomes apparent. As stated by Watson, "the prescription of antibiotics as the sole treatment of a hand infection must . . . be undertaken with great circumspection. The penalty for error is great."[5]

Microbiology. Whether or not a hand infection is initially judged to be surgical, antibiotic administration is begun either as primary therapy or as a preoperative adjunct. Antibiotic treatment must initially be based on a general knowledge of the microbiology of hand infection and modified according to response to treatment and availability of culture results when microbiologic specimens are analyzed. Any etiologic agent capable of infecting soft tissue or bone (discussed in Chap. 27) can infect the hand. Most primary hand infections in otherwise healthy individuals have a mixed but broadly predictable bacterial population. Group A *Streptococcus pyogenes* and *Staphylococcus aureus* are the organisms most commonly found in primary hand infections, but single-agent infections are reported less frequently than in the days of Kanavel. Polymicrobial infections now comprise between 30 and 60 percent of the current hand infection population,[6,7] and the presence of gram-negative organisms and anaerobic bacteria can be documented in up to 50 and 29 percent of cases, respectively.[4,7] Initial antibiotic therapy should therefore be directed at common gram-positive organisms, gram-negative organisms, and anaerobes. Although this bacterial population may give the impression of requiring complicated antibiotic coverage, empirically the sensitivities of the organisms found in hand infections permit relatively simple antibiotic coverage. Spiegel and Szabo[7] initially treated 67 cases of hand infections with penicillin and cefazolin. Gentamicin was added when the patient gave a history of injected drug use. This coverage adequately treated 342 of the 346 bacterial isolates cultured from these patients[7] (Table 47–1). Other authors have reasonably proposed second- and third-generation cephalosporins as initial antibiotic therapy.[4,8,9]

Certain subsets of patients merit wider initial antibiotic coverage because of a predisposition to more complicated and virulent infections. Chronic users of injectible drugs, as suggested above, develop hand infections often containing gram-negative and gram-positive organisms in a setting of advanced, complicated lesions.[9,10] Initial antibiotic therapy in these cases can reasonably be broadened to include aminoglycosides as suggested by Spiegel and Szabo.[7] Hand infections in diabetics also include a large percentage of mixed organism infections (63 percent of cases in a recent report[11]). Aminoglycosides can play a significant role in the initial management of these cases. Renal transplant patients with functioning arteriovenous fistulas on rare occasions develop severe, gangrenous hand infections that may require broad antibiotic coverage, aggressive debridement, and takedown of the fistula with arterial reconstruction for hand salvage.[11] A single report of hand infections in patients with acquired immune deficiency syndrome (AIDS) suggested that these patients might have a more frequent progression of soft tissue infection to os-

TABLE 47–1. BACTERIAL ISOLATES (346) CULTURED FROM HAND INFECTIONS IN 67 PATIENTS

Bacterium	Number
Gram-positive aerobes	
Streptococcus	111
Staphylococcus aureus	70
Staphylococcus epidermidis	29
Streptococcus faecalis	3
Bacillus species	1
Gram-negative aerobes	
Hemophilus parainfluenzae	25
Hemophilus influenzae	4
Hemophilus species	1
Branhamella catarrhalis	7
Neisseria sicca	2
Gram-positive anaerobes	
Corynebacterium species	5
Lactobacillus	3
Peptococcus	7
Peptostreptococcus	11
Clostridium perfringens	1
Gram-negative anaerobes	
Eikenella corrodens	16
Bacteroides melaninogenicus	13
Bacteroides species	8
Veillonella species	3
Fusobacterium nucleatum	3
Acinetobacter lwoffi	1
Acinetobacter anitratus	3
Pasteurella multocida	5
Gram-negative enteric bacteria	
Enterobacter cloacae	5
Enterobacter agglomerans	1
Klebsiella oxytoca	2
Klebsiella pneumonia	1
Escherichia coli	2
Hafnia alvei	1
Proteus mirabilis	1
Pseudomonas aeruginosa	1
Total	346

From Spiegel JD, Szabo R: J Hand Surg 13A:254, 1988.

teomyelitis but no evidence was presented that distinguished these infections from those lesions seen in injectible drug users (who in fact formed a subset of the reported population).[12]

Specific circumstances can produce hand infections that may harbor unusual bacteria and justify wide presumptive antibiotic coverage. Large traumatic wounds of the hand and upper extremity may be contaminated by environmental elements such as soil, grass, grease, and oil. This sort of contamination creates the possibility of mixed organism infection in a large area containing compromised and devitalized tissue. Although debridement is of paramount importance in the management of these wounds, antibiotic coverage should initially include penicillin and a third-generation cephalosporin or penicillin, a second-generation cephalosporin, and an aminoglycoside.[13,14] Coverage can subsequently be narrowed when culture results become available. As the definition of acute complex hand injuries becomes more certain and acute reconstruction more ambitious,[15] quantitative cultures may play a role in the timing of surgical repairs and the duration of antibiotic treatment.[14]

Wounds contaminated by salt and fresh water (eg, wounds resulting from boating accidents) can harbor organisms unique to the contaminant. Salt water contamination can produce wound infections by marine *Vibrio* species.[16,17] These infections can be extensive and lethal and should be anticipated by administration of tetracycline or an aminoglycoside. Fresh water contamination can result in infection by *Aeromonas hydrophila,* an organism capable of producing cellulitis, abscess, myonecrosis, and sepsis.[18–21] Antibiotic coverage of *Aeromonas hydrophila* includes third-generation cephalosporins, cefoxitin, and aminoglycosides, and an effective agent should be included in initial antibiotic coverage of these wounds.[22] *Aeromonas hydrophila* is a normal resident of the gut of medicinal leeches, and such infections can be caused when leeches are used to treat venous congestion in replanted fingers. Patients undergoing leech application to traumatized tissue should receive antibiotics effective against *Aeromonas* prior to leech application.[22,23] The organism is sensitive to ciprofloxacin if oral treatment is in order.

Bite wounds are frequently complicated by injection of contaminated material into deep tissues or joints, foreign body introduction (tooth fragments and plaque), and fractures. These wounds should all be examined by x-ray, and all but the most superficial of them merit debridement and careful operative exploration. *Streptococcus viridans* is the most common organism cultured from bite wounds, and additional agents usually include staphylococci and a wide variety of gram-negative and anaerobic organisms. *Eikenilla corrodens* is an organism specifically found in human bites, and *Pasteurella multocida* is a specific complication of domestic animal bites. Initial antibiotic coverage should include penicillin for oral anaerobes (as well as *Eikenella* and *Pasteurella* organisms) and a cephalosporin for staphylococcus coverage.[9,24] Animal bites or exposure to contaminated animal tissues can also lead to infection by such organisms as *Bacillus anthracis, Erysipelothrix rhusiopathiae, Francisella tularensis,* and *Brucella* species.[9,25] Chronic or unusual wounds should be debrided and carefully cultured to identify these organisms.

Chronic wounds may be caused by unusual organisms that require meticulous cultures and stains from resected involved tissue for proper identification. Mycobacterial infection, including lesions caused by *M. tuberculosis, M. marinum, M. kansasii,* and other species, can manifest themselves as skin lesions, proliferative synovitis, arthritis, and osteomyelitis. Extensive and sequestered sites of diseased tissue will need to be ablated surgically (eg, synovectomy, sequestrectomy), but careful identification of the organism is necessary to plan both definitive (and frequently prolonged) antibiotic therapy as well as proper surgical treatment.[25,26] Chronic draining wounds can also be caused by *Actinomyces israelii,* an anaerobic gram-positive organism that is difficult to grow in culture. The presence of this organism must be sought in sections of resected tissue where distinct basophilic bacterial colonies (traditionally called "sulfur granules") can be identified.[25]

Chronic fungal infections can produce cutaneous, subcutaneous, or deep infections. Superficial lesions (including infection caused by *Treponema rubrum, Treponema mentagrophytes,* and *Candida* species) can usually be treated with topical antifungal agents once the fungi are identified. Lesions involving the nails may require plate removal, tangential excision of involved skin, topical agents, and oral administration of griseofulvin. Subcutaneous or deep infection (ie, infection of synovium, bone, joint) requires debridement of involved tissue and careful use of the surgical specimen to identify the causative organism, which could be a *Candida* species, *Sporothrix schenckii,* or a local manifestation of a systemic fungal disease such as histoplasmosis, coccidioidomycosis, or blastomycosis. The plans for surgical debridement must take into account the expected results of systemic antifungal administration. Careful follow-up is necessary to determine the effects of drug therapies and the possible need for further surgical debridement.[27] A recent interest in acute fungal wound infections, initially described in burn patients,[28] has extended to complicated wounds of the hand. In such cases, a clear distinction between fungal contamination and invasive fungal infection must be made. Fungal contamination merely requires debridement of devitalized tissue, and the administration of potentially toxic systemic antifungal agents may not be indicated. True invasive fungal infections are defined as cases manifesting fungemia or microvascular fungal invasion demonstrated in a wound biopsy. These rare infections can be lethal and do require systemic antifungal medications.

Viral infections of the hand are generally caused by one of the herpesviruses. These lesions begin with pain and the appearance of vesicles that progress to an ulcerating lesion that generally resolves in 2 to 3 weeks. Diagnosis is generally made from the course of the disease and can be confirmed by staining and viral culture of vesicular fluid. Treatment should be symptomatic, although antibiotic treatment of staphylococcal superinfection may be necessary. Acyclovir can be considered in severe or recurrent cases. Incision, drainage, and debridement do not favorably change the course of the disease and may cause increased local tissue damage and viremia.[29]

Operative Treatment: General Consideration. Based on their reported clinical experience, Spiegel and Szabo[7] concluded that treatment of suppurative hand infections in the operating room with proper lighting, anesthesia, and equipment resulted in more thorough ablation of the infection and faster recovery time. I share their bias for formal operative treatment; only the most obviously limited lesions should be drained in emergency rooms or clinics. Even simple lesions should be followed closely to detect inadequate initial treatment.

Regional or axillary block anesthesia can be considered if short operative and tourniquet times are securely anticipated. Intravenous lidocaine anesthesia (Bier block technique) has no place in an infected upper extremity. If an extensive, unpredictable, or lengthy procedure is anticipated, general anesthesia should be considered.

Tourniquet use is a valuable asset in these cases, but exsanguination prior to tourniquet inflation should avoid the use of pressure devices like elastic bandages, which can rupture infected loculations and spread purulent material along tissue planes. Therefore only extremity elevation should be employed to empty the vessels prior to inflation of the tourniquet.

Incisions must include the area of infection, but extensions should be made according to the general principles of hand surgery (Fig. 47–1).[30]

Careful collection of surgical microbiology specimens is of great importance in determining correct antibiotic therapy. Swab cultures are generally misleading. Pus and involved tissue from the deep and wide margins of the wound, as well as bone if osteomyelitis is suspected, should be sent to the laboratory for proper diagnosis of the involved infectious agents.[14,31,32]

Operative Treatment: Specific Entities

ABSCESS. Loculated purulence anywhere in the hand deserves prompt and thorough drainage. Pre-

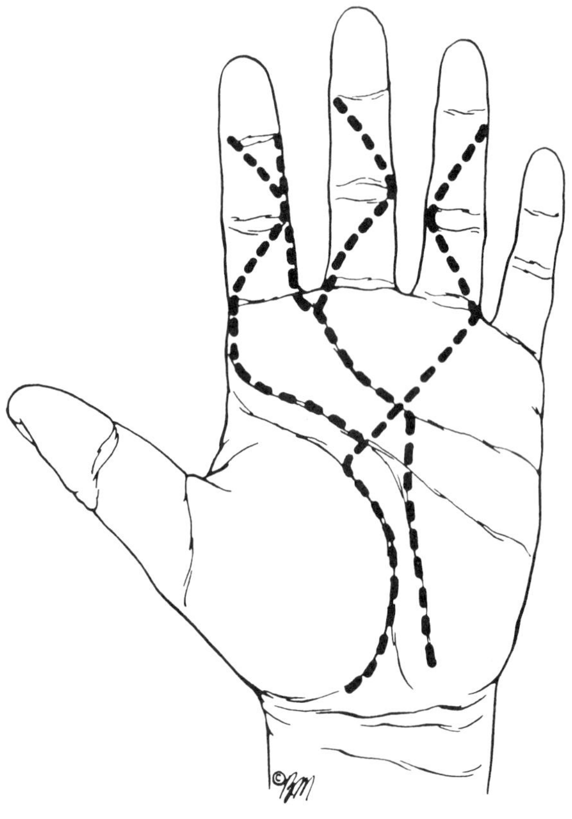

Figure 47–1. Extension of hand incisions for drainage of infection should be extended according to the principles of elective hand incision. Generally, palmar incisions of the finger traverse each phalanx diagonally, coming to points at the joint creases. These incisions provide wide exposure and avoid contracting scars across the joint creases. Palmar incisions generally follow creases and can be extended through the carpal tunnel and into the forearm in a zigzag manner. *(From Adamson JE, Fleury F: Incisions in the hand and wrist. In Green DP (ed): Operative Hand Surgery, 3rd ed. New York, Churchill Livingstone, 1988, p 1799.)*

operative x-ray studies should routinely be obtained to detect foreign bodies or skeletal lesions. The abscess cavity should be explored carefully to determine if the loculation is limited to subcutaneous tissue or if the infection involves communicating structures or anatomic compartments. Many of the specific hand infections discussed below can be considered abscesses requiring detailed knowledge of hand anatomy. Abscess cavities, once evacuated and explored, should be left open to drain until a secondary healing or later reconstruction closes the wound.

PARONYCHIA. Acute infections around the nail are called paronychia. Early, nonfluctuant infections may resolve with antibiotics effective against *Staphylococcus aureus,* but infections that have progressed to fluctuance should be treated by incising the margin of the involved nail fold and lifting it away from the nail plate (Fig. 47–2). If the infection extends beneath the nail plate, the nail should be removed.

Chronic paronychia, characterized by maceration and progressive scarring around the nail, is usually a fungal disease with bacterial superinfection. If the lesion does not resolve with topical antifungal therapy, an excision of the involved skin down to the germinal matrix can effectively drain the infection. The area of excision is allowed to heal secondarily. Extensive involvement may require removal of the nail plate.[33,34]

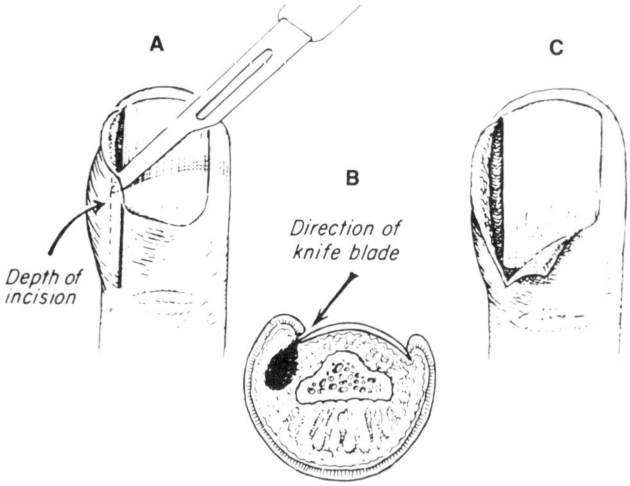

Figure 47–2. A paronychia involving a single side of a nail fold (**A**) is incised to its depth (**B**) and left open to drain and heal. (**C**) Infections including the fold at the base of the nail are drained by two parallel incisions extending proximally from each lateral nail fold and elevation of the involved fold. *(From Flynn JE: Hand Surgery. Baltimore, Williams & Wilkins, 1975.)*

FELON. The skin of the finger pulp is stabilized by multiple fibrous trabeculae that connect the dermis to the distal phalanx. These trabeculae divide the subcutaneous tissue into compartments, and established infection in these spaces is called a felon. Untreated, these infections can cause infarction of the pulp skin. Incision and drainage of these wounds must include careful inspection of the pulp to detect and drain multiple loculations. *Staphylococcus aureus* is the most common causative organism.[33]

TENOSYNOVITIS. Acute flexor tenosynovitis was characterized by Kanavel as presenting with fusiform swelling of the finger, semiflexed finger posture, tenderness to palpation along the flexor sheath, and pain with passive extension.[2] These findings indicate the presence of pus in the flexor tendon sheath. *Staphylococcus aureus* is the most common organism found. Early treatment consisting of elevation and antibiotics may resolve the infection, but persistence of physical findings for 48 hours or any local or systemic evidence of progression requires surgical drainage.[34,35] If untreated, these infections can result in severe damage to tendons and joints, skin infarction, and sepsis. The infection can be reliably drained by incising the tendon sheath in the finger at the distal interphalangeal joint and in the palm proximal to the first annular pulley (Fig. 47–3). An irrigation catheter can be passed through the sheath by way of these incisions and used to irrigate the sheath with antibiotics for 24 to 48 hours. This intervention, followed by physical therapy, can usually result in a functioning finger.

Chronic tenosynovitis can involve the flexor sheaths, the flexor synovium in the carpal tunnel, or the extensor synovium. The flexor sheaths are the most common sites of infection. The disease is characterized by slow, progressive swelling of the involved synovium. These lesions are usually caused by mycobacterial organisms (especially *M. marinum* and *M. kansasii*),[35] and diagnosis is obtained from cultured biopsies. Treatment consists of excision of involved tissue and systemic antibiotic therapy.

WEB SPACE ABSCESSES. Abscesses of the web spaces can involve volar and dorsal subcutaneous spaces. A volar web space abscess, for example, can extend into the dorsal subcutaneous space dermally or into spaces in the palmar fascia in the region of the superficial transverse metacarpal ligaments. Drainage of these "collar button" abscesses requires incision of both the volar and dorsal components

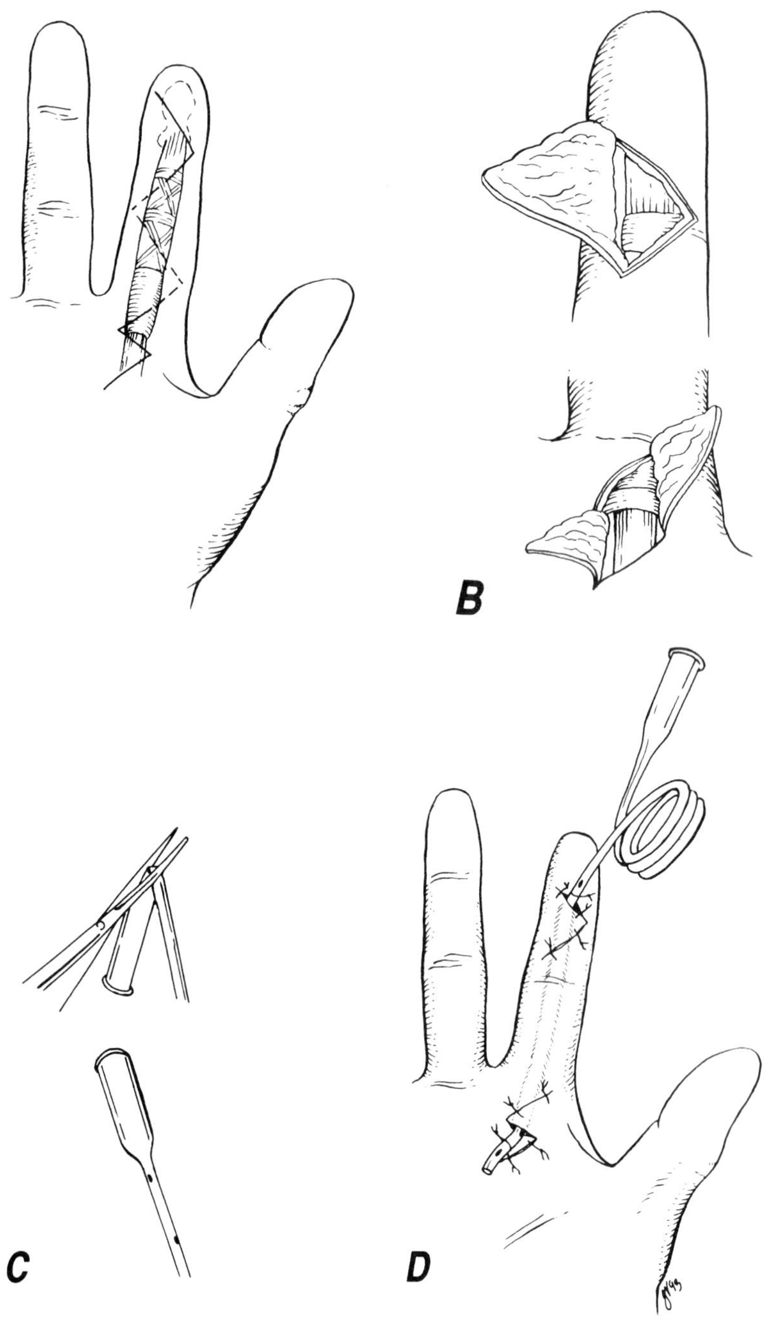

Figure 47–3. Acute flexor tenosynovitis. **A.** Exposure of the flexor sheath should be obtained over the distal interphalangeal joint and proximal to the first annular pulley (solid lines). These incisions can be extended (dotted lines) if further exposure is required. **B.** Reflection of local flaps permits clear visualization of the flexor sheath. **C.** An irrigation catheter can be fashioned from a pediatric feeding tube by fenestrating the tube with fine scissors. **D.** The irrigation catheter is passed through the sheath, distal to proximal. Holes are left outside the loose skin closure to prevent pressure buildup within the finger. Antibiotic infusion can most safely be done with an infusion pump. *(From Lineaweaver W: Surgical treatment of hand infection. In Cohen M (ed): Mastery of Plastic Surgery. Boston, Little, Brown, 1993.)*

through incisions designed to avoid web space contracture (Fig. 47–4).[34]

DEEP SPACE INFECTION. These anatomically defined spaces in the hand can become the sites of loculated infections (Fig. 47–5). Infection can be initiated by penetrating wounds or extension of infection from communicating sites (eg, a flexor tendon sheath).[34,36] The midpalmar space is bounded by the flexor tendons superficially and deep by the fascia over the second and third interosseous muscles and the third and fourth metacarpals. The radial border of the midpalmar space is the vertical septum between the middle finger metacarpal and the sheath of the profundus tendon of the middle finger, and its ulnar border is the fascia of the hypothenar muscle. The space extends from the vertical septa of the palmar fascia near the web space to the distal carpal tunnel. The thenar space is on the radial side of the radial septum of the midpalmar spaces and extends to the lateral edge of the adductor pol-

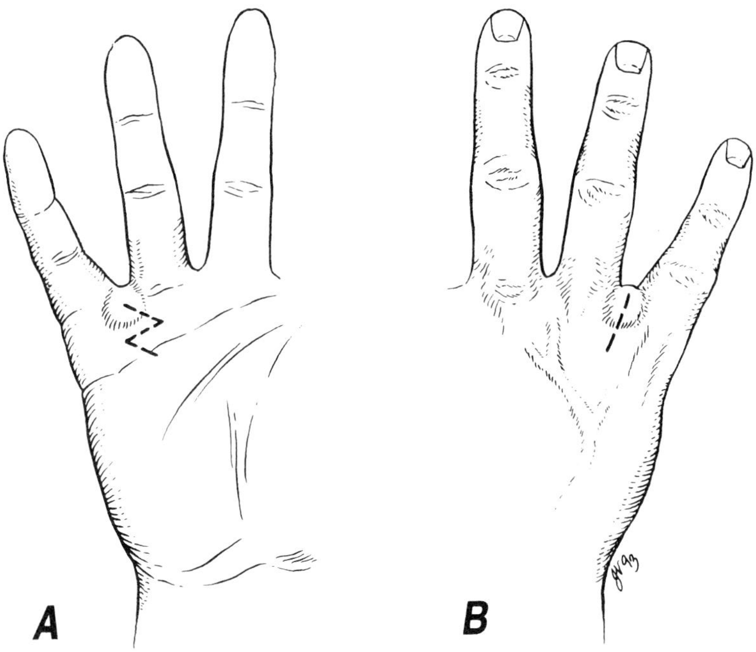

Figure 47–4. Drainage of web space abscesses. **A.** A volar zigzag incision permits drainage and visualization of the neurovascular bundles. **B.** The linear dorsal incision adequately drains the abscess and avoids web space contractures associated with transverse incisions. *(From Lineaweaver W: Surgical treatment of hand infection. In Cohen M (ed): Mastery of Plastic Surgery. Boston, Little, Brown, 1993.)*

licis. The hypothenar space contains the hypothenar muscles and is defined by their inverting fascia.

Infections in these spaces produce pain in the palm and loss of normal palmar concavity. The dorsum of the hand may swell from edema, but actual spread of purulence to the dorsal hand is unusual. Incision and drainage should be performed through palmar and first web space exposures, which can be extended into the carpal tunnel as necessary.[30,34]

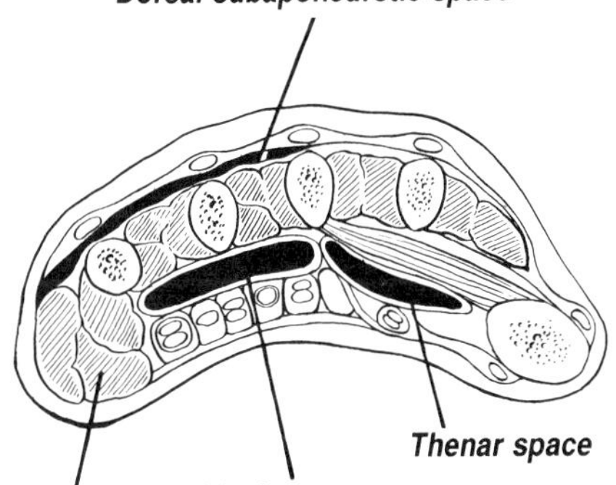

Figure 47–5. Shown at the level of the midpalm, four deep spaces can become infected. Midpalmar and thenar space infections may become confluent. Hypothenar space infections are rare but may progress to significant myonecrosis. Dorsal subaponeurotic space infections are rare, and most dorsal swelling is only reactive edema. *(From Lineaweaver W: Surgical treatment of hand infection. In Cohen M (ed): Mastery of Plastic Surgery. Boston, Little, Brown, 1993.)*

BURSAL INFECTIONS. The so-called radial and ulnar bursae are the palmar portion of, respectively, the synovia of the flexor pollicis longus and the flexor digitorum profundus of the little finger. Infection of these synovia can result from distal tenosynovitis, and infection of one bursa can spread to the other and to the wrist through Parona's space, the anatomic compartment defined by the flexor pollicis longus, the profundus tendon, and the pronator quadratus.[36] Drainage of either bursa can be accomplished through palmar incision. The wrist should also be opened through the carpal tunnel and the proximal margins of the bursae drained from this exposure. Distal tenosynovitis, if present, must also be drained, and catheters can be passed from either finger or palmar wound to the wrist for through-and-through irrigation (Fig. 47–6).

JOINT INFECTIONS. Infections of the metacarpophalangeal or interphalangeal joints are usually the result of bites, impact injuries, other penetrating injuries, or extension of other infections. Pain and swelling characterize these infections, and x-ray studies should be taken to look for skeletal damage and foreign bodies. The joints must be drained promptly, and exposure is obtained through dorsal incisions and entry lateral to the extensor hood. Catheter irrigation for 24 to 48 hours is frequently employed, and motion is begun after removal of the catheter (Fig. 47–7).

Joint infections unrelated to trauma may be the result of bacterial seeding from remote sites of

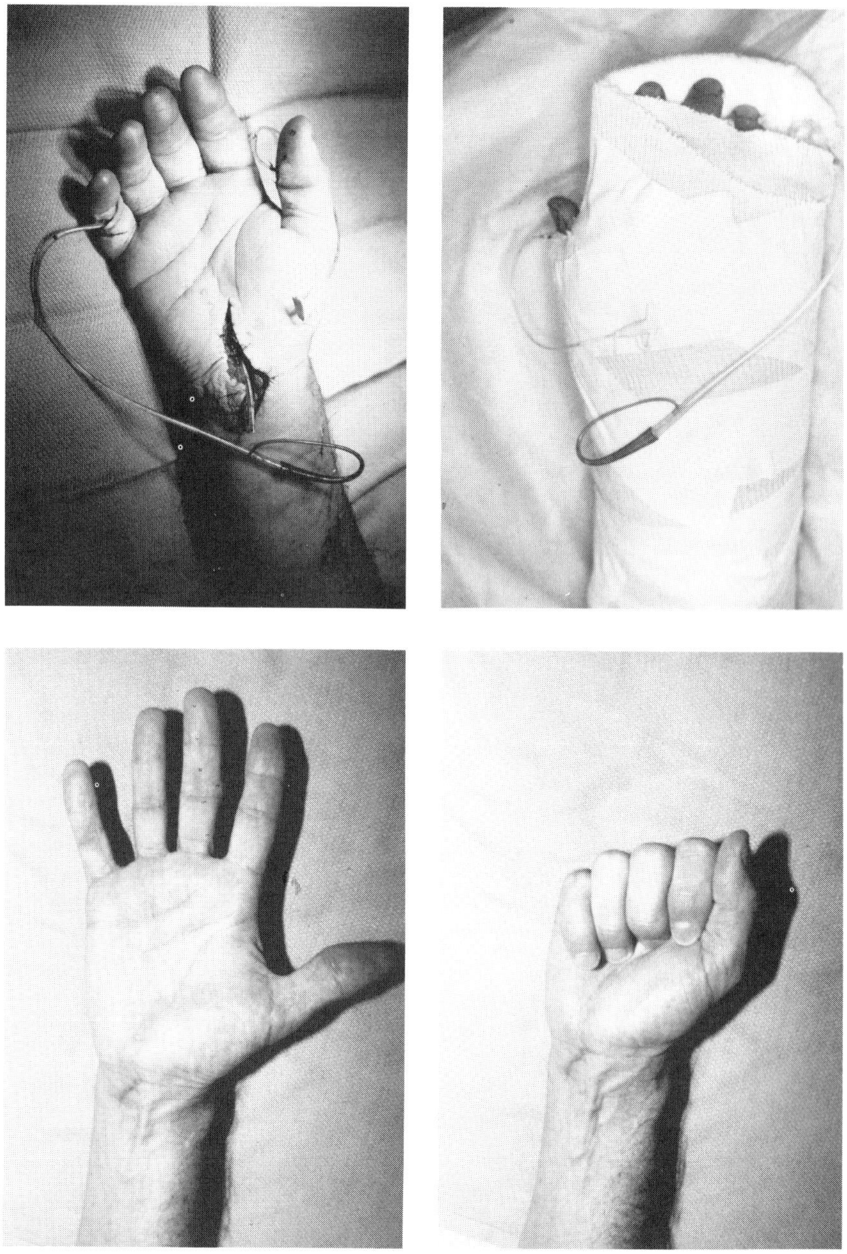

A B C D

Figure 47–6. A. This patient developed tenosynovitis of the thumb, which spread along the radial bursa to the wrist, ulna bursa, and flexor sheath of the little finger. The flexor sheaths were drained, as were the bursae through the carpal tunnel. Irrigation catheters were passed from the thumb and little finger to the wrist. **B.** The hand was elevated in a bulky, splinted dressing and irrigated for 48 hours. **C** and **D.** Following secondary closure, the patient regained excellent function.

infection. *Neisseria gonorrheae* should be considered in such cases.[9,37] Incision and drainage of the joint are still necessary, and evaluation and treatment of the primary infection are also required.

OSTEOMYELITIS. In the hand, osteomyelitis most frequently occurs following open injuries, although hematogenous spread may be encountered. Acute wounds with bone involvement are usually successfully managed with debridement, irrigation, fixation, and closure,[14,15] but established osteomyelitis requires resection of the involved bone, careful culturing, and 4 to 6 weeks of antibiotic therapy.[38] These infections often present with local swelling and chronic drainage. X-ray studies usually clearly demonstrate the established bone lesion. Extensive involvement of phalanges can result in amputation but large skeletal defects in significant areas (eg, thumb or midpalm) can be salvaged with bone grafting and flap coverage.

NECROTIZING FASCIITIS. Although much abused, the term necrotizing fasciitis specifically refers to infection of superficial fascia resulting in necrosis

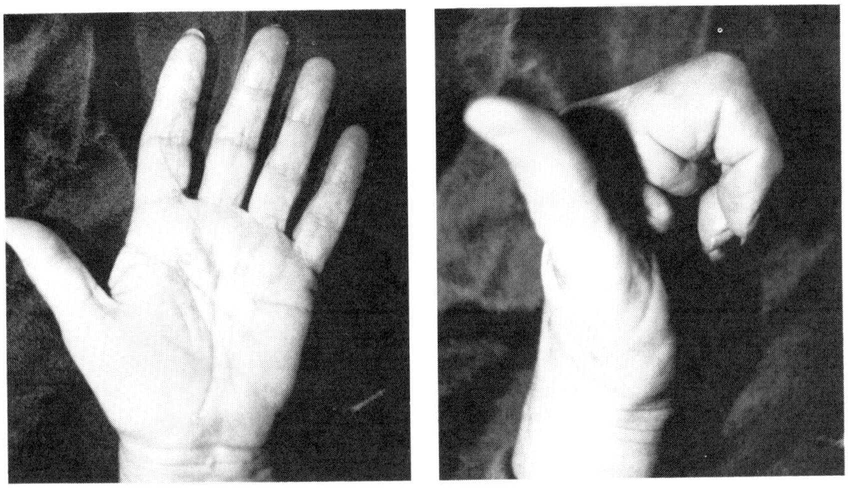

Figure 47–7. Functional result after prompt drainage of proximal interphalangeal joint infection and contiguous flexor tenosynovitis in a 63-year-old woman.

of the fascia, eventual infarction of overlying subcutaneous tissue and skin, rapid spread, and sepsis.[39,40] In the hand, unlike the trunk, the infection is commonly caused by group A *Streptococcus pyogenes* after trivial penetrating wounds, but many organisms can create this anatomic infection and necrotizing fasciitis should be considered a "clinical entity and not a specific bacterial infection."[40] In the hand, the palmar fascia is the most clearly defined structure that can become involved. Treatment consists of wide exposure and resection of all involved fascia, debridement of devitalized overlying tissue, and antibiotics. Definitive surgical resection of involved tissue may require multiple procedures, and closure and reconstruction should begin only after complete resolution of the infection.

MIXED INFECTIONS. Mixed infections following complicated injuries require aggressive debridement. Acutely, complex wounds are populated by contaminating organisms, and thorough removal of involved tissue can permit early closure and reconstruction.[14] Established infection in damaged tissue must be treated with wide drainage and meticulous resection of all involved structures. Clostridial infections can occur in these circumstances.

POSTOPERATIVE INFECTIONS. Infections occurring after elective hand surgery are rare but potentially destructive. Incisional cellulitis can resolve with antibiotics, but evidence of deep infection requires prompt opening of the incision. Deep postoperative infections most often occur within hematomas in the field of dissection, and all this material must be removed. Established postoperative infection usually also requires removal of any foreign bodies such as tendon rods and joint prostheses.

REFERENCES

1. Kanavel AB: An anatomical, experimental, and clinical study of acute phlegmons of the hand. Surg Gynecol Obstet 1:221, 1905.
2. Kanavel AB: Infections of the Hand, 5th ed. Philadelphia, Lea & Febiger, 1925.
3. Flynn JE: Severe infections of the hand: a historical perspective. In Jupiter JB (ed): Flynn's Hand Surgery, 4th ed. Baltimore, Williams & Wilkins, 1991, p 689.
4. Krizek TJ, Perry AW: Infections of the hand. In Jurkiewicz MJ, Mathes SL, Ariyan S (eds): Plastic Surgery, Principles and Practice. St Louis, Mosby, 1990, p 803.
5. Watson N: Antibiotics in hand infections. Br Med J 290.491, 1985.
6. Stromberg BV: Changing bacteriologic flora of hand infections. J Trauma 25:530, 1985.
7. Spiegel JD, Szabo R: A protocol for the treatment of severe infections of the hand. J Hand Surg 13A:254, 1988.
8. Robson MC, Schmidt D, Heggars JP: Cefamandole therapy in hand infection. J Hand Surg 8:560, 1983.
9. McGrath M: Infections of the hand. In McCarthy JG (ed): Plastic Surgery. Philadelphia, Saunders, 1990, p 5529.
10. Reyes F: Infections secondary to intravenous drug use. Hand Clin 5:629, 1989.
11. Francel T, Marshall KA, Savage RC: Hand infections in the diabetic and the diabetic renal transplant patient. Ann Plast Surg 24:304, 1990.
12. Glickel S: Hand infections in patients with acquired immunodeficiency syndrome. J Hand Surg 13A:770, 1988.
13. Brown PW: Open wounds of the hand. In Green DP (ed): Operative Hand Surgery, 3rd ed. New York, Churchill Livingstone, 1993, p 1533.
14. Breidenbach WC: Emergency free tissue transfer for reconstruction of acute upper extremity wounds. Clin Plast Surg 16:505, 1989.

15. Buchler U, Hastings H: Combined injuries. In Green DP (ed): Operative Hand Surgery, 3rd ed. New York, Churchill Livingstone, 1993, p 1563.
16. Howard R, Pessa MF, Brennaman BH, Ramphal R: Necrotizing soft tissue infections caused by marine vibrios. Surgery 98:126, 1985.
17. Howard RJ, Lieb S: Soft tissue infections caused by halophilic marine vibrios. Arch Surg 123:245, 1988.
18. Lineaweaver W, Follansbee S, Hing D: Cefatoxime-sensitive *Aeromonas hydrophila* in a revascularized foot. Ann Plast Surg 20:322, 1988.
19. Semel JD, Trenholme G: *Aeromonas hydrophila* water associated traumatic wounds: a review. J Trauma 30:324, 1990.
20. Lowen RM, Rodgers CN, Ketch LL, Phelps DB: *Aeromonas hydrophila* infection complicating digital replantation and revascularization. J Hand Surg 14A:714, 1989.
21. Sanger JR, Yousif NJ, Matloub HS: *Aeromonas hydrophila* upper extremity infection. J Hand Surg 14A:719, 1989.
22. Lineaweaver W, Hill MK, Buncke GM, et al: *Aeromonas hydrophila* infections following use of medicinal leeches in replantation and flap surgery. Ann Plast Surg 29:238, 1992.
23. Lineaweaver W, Furnas H, Follansbee S, et al: Post prandial *Aeromonas hydrophila* cultures and antibiotic levels of enteric aspirates from medicinal leeches applied to patients receiving antibiotics. Ann Plast Surg 29:245, 1992.
24. Faciszewski T, Coleman DA: Human bite wounds. Hand Clin 5:561, 1989.
25. Pruitt B, McManus AT, McManus WF, Graves TA: Infections: bacteriology, antibiotics, and chemotherapy. In Jupiter JB (ed): Flynn's Hand Surgery, 4th ed. Baltimore, Williams & Wilkins, 1991, p 704.
26. Gunther SF, Levy C: Mycobacterial infections. Hand Clin 5:591, 1989.
27. Hitchcock T, Amadio PC: Fungal infections. Hand Clin 5:599, 1989.
28. Becker WK, Cioffi WG, McManus AT, et al: Fungal burn wound infection. Arch Surg 126:44, 1991.
29. Fowler JR: Viral infections. Hand Clin 5:613, 1989.
30. Adamson JE, Fleury AF: Incisions in the hand and wrist. In Green DP (ed): Operative Hand Surgery, 2nd ed. New York, Churchill Livingstone, 1988, p 1985.
31. Sharp CS, Bessman A, Wagner FW, et al: Microbiology of superficial and deep tissues in infected diabetic gangrene. Surg Gynecol Obstet 149:217, 1979.
32. Brook I, Frazier EH: Aerobic and anaerobic bacteriology of wounds and cutaneous abscesses. Arch Surg 125:1445, 1990.
33. Canales F, Newmeyer WL, Kilgore ES: The treatment of felons and paronychia. Hand Clin 5:515, 1989.
34. Neviaser RJ: Infections. In Green DP (ed): Operative Hand Surgery, 3rd ed. New York, Churchill Livingstone, 1993, p 1021.
35. Neviaser RJ: Tenosynovitis. Hand Clin 5:525, 1989.
36. Brenman SA: Hand infections and related injuries. In Georgiade NG, Riefkohl R, Barwick WJ (eds): Textbook of Plastic, Maxillofacial and Reconstructive Surgery, 2nd ed. Baltimore, Williams & Wilkins, 1992, p 1211.
37. Cahill JM: Special infections of the hand. In Jupiter JB (ed): Flynn's Hand Surgery, 4th ed. Baltimore, Williams & Wilkins, 1991, p 773.
38. Freeland AE, Senter BS: Septic arthritis and osteomyelitis. Hand Clin 5:533, 1989.
39. Meleney F: Hemolytic streptococcus gangrene. Arch Surg 9:317, 1924.
40. Rea WJ, Wyrick WJ: Necrotizing fasciitis. Ann Surg 172:957, 1970.

Infections of the Female Genital Tract

CHAPTER 48

Daniel V. Landers, Richard L. Sweet

Infection of the genital tract is among the most common clinical problems encountered in women's health care. Among office gynecology patients, lower genital tract infections, such as vaginitis and cervicitis, are the most frequent diagnoses. In addition, it is estimated that nearly 1 million women are treated for acute pelvic inflammatory disease annually in the United States alone.[1] Genital tract infections following obstetric and gynecologic surgery are also very prevalent. In fact, the rate of postoperative infection after cesarean section has been reported to be as high as 85 percent in some populations prior to the widespread introduction of prophylactic antibiotics.[2,3] Similarly, the rate of postoperative infection after vaginal hysterectomy has been reported to be as high as 64 percent in some populations.[4]

The polymicrobial (mixed aerobic and anaerobic) nature of pelvic infections has led to intensive investigation into the etiology, prevention, and treatment of female genital tract infections over the past decade. The pathogenic role of exogenous and endogenous genital tract microorganisms and their interactions with local host defenses have been the focus of extensive study.

The clarification of the pathogenesis of genital tract infections, combined with current diagnostic technology and the ever expanding antimicrobial armamentarium available to the clinician, have vastly improved our ability to recognize and effectively treat a variety of genital tract infections.

NORMAL MICROBIAL FLORA OF THE FEMALE GENITAL TRACT

The normally sterile upper genital tract is separated at the level of the endocervix from the lower genital tract, which contains a rich endogenous microflora made up of a multitude of microorganisms. The microflora of the vagina and the endocervix have received considerable attention because of the significant association with genital tract infections. The vagina normally contains in the range of 10^9 bacterial colony forming units of bacteria per gram of secretions. This includes a variety of facultative and anaerobic organisms (see Chap. 3).

Studies on the normal flora of the lower genital tract have shown that most women have some species of facultative and anaerobic organisms present. The most common gram-positive aerobic organisms isolated from asymptomatic, premenopausal women are *Lactobacillus, Corynebacterium* (diphtheroids), *Staphylococcus epidermidis,* and *Strepto-*

coccus.[5] Lactobacilli have been the most prevalent and are usually present in the highest concentration. Of particular importance are the hydrogen peroxide-producing lactobacilli that play a major role in controlling the microbial milieu in the normal healthy vagina. The gram-negative aerobes have been less frequently isolated, with *Escherichia coli* being the species most commonly found. Recently, the presence of *Gardnerella vaginalis* as part of the normal flora in up to 60 percent of healthy women has been demonstrated. Yeasts (usually *Candida albicans*) can be found in up to 30 percent of asymptomatic women. Mycoplasmas, especially *Ureaplasma urealyticum* and *Mycoplasma hominis,* have been isolated from the lower genital tract of healthy, asymptomatic women as well.[6]

Obligate anaerobes have been isolated from the lower genital tract in about 70 to 90 percent of asymptomatic, premenopausal women.[5] The most common gram-positive anaerobes have been *Peptococcus asaccharolyticus, P. magnus, P. prevotii* (now all reclassified as *Peptostreptococcus*), and even more common was *Peptostreptococcus anaerobius,* which has been found in up to one-third of women.[7] The gram-negative anaerobes most frequently isolated from the lower genital tract of asymptomatic, premenopausal women include *Prevotella* (formerly *Bacteroides*) *bivius, P. disiens,* black-pigmented *Bacteroides,* and *Fusobacterium.*[5,8,9] Although *B. fragilis* has been referred to as endogenous flora of the vagina and the endocervix, it is an infrequent isolate from these sites.[5,7,8]

In reviewing the most common isolates from the lower genital tract, one must keep in mind the dynamic nature of the vaginal microflora, characterized by frequent variation with respect to both species and concentration of organisms at various times in the menstrual cycle.[10] These variations in microflora may be further influenced by other factors such as pregnancy, hormonal therapy, menopause, and pelvic surgery. Furthermore, the factors influencing vaginal pH and the role of pH in altering vaginal microflora remain poorly understood aspects of the vaginal ecosystem.[11] The organisms commonly isolated from the site of the upper genital tract infections are listed in Table 48–1. With the exception of sexually transmitted organisms, such as *Neisseria gonorrhoeae* and *Chlamydia trachomatis,* the organisms are much the same as those isolated from the lower genital tract of asymptomatic, premenopausal women. In addition, beta-hemolytic *Streptococcus* is another exogenous microorganism that can produce severe upper genital tract sepsis.

TABLE 48–1. ORGANISMS COMMONLY ISOLATED FROM UPPER GENITAL TRACT INFECTIONS

• ANAEROBES	• FACULTATIVE (AEROBES)
Peptostreptococci (including bacteria formerly classified as peptococci or *Gaffkya*)	Streptococci
Prevotella species	Staphylococci
P. bivius	*Escherichia coli*
P. disiens	*Gardnerella vaginalis*
P. asaccharolyticus	Lactobacilli
P. melaninogenicus	• SEXUALLY TRANSMITTED ORGANISMS
Fusobacterium	*Neisseria gonorrhoeae*
Bacteroides fragilis group	*Chlamydia trachomatis*
	Mycoplasma hominis
	Ureaplasma urealyticum

Local Host Defense

The mucosal surface of the vagina and the endocervix serves as the portal of entry for most genital tract pathogens. The local host defense system of the lower genital tract must afford protection against the attack of exogenous pathogens, iatrogenic alterations in endogenous microflora, and the trauma of sexual intercourse. The normal vaginal flora are thought to play a protective role, to some degree, from exogenous and endogenous lower genital tract pathogens. Some vaginal species, such as lactobacilli, may inhibit the growth of *N. gonorrhoeae,* anaerobic bacteria, and *C. albicans.* Conversely, some forms of vaginitis are associated with markedly reduced concentrations of lactobacilli, especially species that produce hydrogen peroxide, and gram-positive rods.[12] A failure in mucosal host defenses may lead to alterations in the vaginal flora that permit one or more pathogenic organisms to proliferate.

In considering the local host defenses in the female lower genital tract, both nonspecific factors and those factors that occur in direct response to invading pathogens must be taken into account. The nonspecific responses include the protective barrier of mucus overlying the epithelium, particularly at the level of the endocervix, and a number of substances contained in mucosal secretions that may afford nonspecific protection, including lysozyme, lactoferrin, zinc, fibronectin, and complement.[13] The more specific host defenses of the lower genital tract include the increased concentrations of secretory IgA that is released in response to specific pathogens and the migration of neutrophils in response to microbial invasion.[13] The combined efforts of these generalized and specific host defenses serve to limit the type and the severity of infections in the female genital tract.

Unfortunately, our knowledge in regard to the mucosal immune system of the female reproductive tract is very limited. Factors that determine whether microorganisms remain limited to the lower genital tract or ascend to colonize and infect the upper genital tract are poorly understood. The role played by the mucosal immune system in this key aspect of pathogenesis has not been elucidated.

INFECTIONS OF THE LOWER FEMALE GENITAL TRACT

A wide spectrum of clinical complaints involving the lower female genital tract have an infectious cause. These patients may present with complaints of abnormal vaginal discharge, irritation, itching, lumps, ulcers, and other bothersome conditions. Although these symptoms may have noninfectious causes, such as genital neoplasms, atrophic vaginitis, and allergic vulvitis, infectious causes are the most common. The conditions most commonly attributed to lower genital tract infections are vaginitis, cervicitis, and vulvitis. The most common causative agents are the sexually transmitted organisms, such as *N. gonorrhoeae, C. trachomatis,* herpes simplex, and *Trichomonas vaginalis* (Table 48–2). However, endogenous facultative and anaerobic flora also play a role in the pathogenesis of these infections, especially bacterial vaginosis (nonspecific vaginitis).

TABLE 48–2. LOWER GENITAL TRACT INFECTIONS

Clinical Diagnosis	Etiologic Agents
Vaginitis	*Trichomonas vaginalis* *Candida albicans* *Gardnerella vaginalis* and anaerobes (bacterial vaginosis)
Vulvitis	*Candida albicans* Herpes simplex virus
Cervicitis	*Neisseria gonorrhoeae* *Chlamydia trachomatis* Herpes simplex virus
Bartholinitis/Skenitis	*N. gonorrhoeae* Mixed anaerobes *C. trachomatis*
Genital tract ulcers	
Herpes	Herpes simplex virus
Syphilis	*Treponema pallidum*
Lymphogranuloma venereum	*C. trachomatis*
Granuloma inguinale	*C. granulomatis*
Chancroid	*Hemophilis ducreyi*
Papules	
Condylomata acuminata	Human papilloma virus
Syphilis	*Treponema pallidum*
Molluscum	Molluscum contagiosum virus
Scabies	*Sarcoptes scabiei*

Vaginitis

Vaginitis is one of the most frequent reasons for office gynecology visits and probably the most common infectious disease encountered by the practicing gynecologist. The cause can be identified and treated simply in the majority of cases; however, some women are plagued with persistent or recurrent symptoms of vaginitis in spite of repeated treatment.

Vaginitis is usually associated with abnormal vaginal discharge or pruritis, or both. The most common types are trichomoniasis, monilial vaginitis, and bacterial vaginosis.

Trichomoniasis. *Trichomonas vaginalis* is a motile parasite that can be identified by wet mount vaginal preparations in 90 percent of infected women. Culture media, such as Diamond's media, will detect 100 percent of *T. vaginalis,* but its cost usually does not provide enough increased benefit to justify its routine use over wet mounts in symptomatic women.

Trichomoniasis is often associated with copious, malodorous, bubbly, frothy, nonhomogeneous vaginal discharge with a pH above 4.5. The color of the discharge is usually gray or yellow-green. Examination of the cervix may reveal small, punctate, mucosal hemorrhages (sometimes referred to as *strawberry cervix*) but this finding is infrequent.

Trichomoniasis is most effectively treated with metronidazole or related 5-nitroimidazole derivatives. Metronidazole is given orally in a 2-g dose taken all at once for best compliance; or as 250 mg, three times daily for 7 days. Abstinence from alcohol should be recommended for 24 hours after completion of therapy. Sexual partners should be treated simultaneously to prevent reinfection. Concern with the use of metronidazole during pregnancy and a possible teratogenic effect are unfounded. No documentation has been provided demonstrating that metronidazole, despite widespread use in pregnancy, is a teratogen. However, the use of metronidazole during pregnancy is generally withheld until after 14 weeks gestation when major organogenesis is complete. There are no other currently available agents that offer equivalent efficacy in the treatment of trichomoniasis. Failure to eradicate the infection with the above regimens may be related to reinfection, inactivation of metronidazole by vaginal bacteria, or resistance to metronidazole. Several resistant strains of *T. vaginalis* have been identified, but fortunately this has thus far been an infrequent problem and has generally been relative rather than absolute resistance. If *T. vaginalis* persists, patients should be treated with either larger doses of metronidazole orally or intravenously (ie, 2 to 3 g/day for 5 to 7 days) or a metronidazole combination with 1 g bid orally plus 0.5 g intravaginally bid for 5 to 7 days. With continued persistence, antimicrobial susceptibility studies should be considered. These can be obtained from the Centers for Disease Control and Prevention.

Recent investigations have demonstrated that *T. vaginalis* is associated with an increased risk of adverse pregnancy outcomes including preterm labor and delivery, preterm rupture of the membranes, and low birth weight.[14] If future studies confirm these findings and placebo-controlled treatment trials demonstrate that eradication of *T. vaginalis* improves pregnancy outcome, routine screening and treatment for *T. vaginalis* in pregnancy will be recommended.

Candida Vulvovaginitis. Yeast vaginitis is most commonly caused by *C. albicans,* which can be identified by the presence of pseudohyphae on a 10 percent KOH preparation or by methylene blue staining. Culture is available, but generally not necessary.

Symptomatic patients most often complain of pruritis with or without discharge. Certain conditions, such as glycosuria, diabetes mellitus, pregnancy, obesity, recent broad spectrum antibiotics, steroids, or immunosuppressants, may predispose to the growth of yeast in the vagina. Findings consistent with yeast infection include reddened vulvar or vaginal areas with vulvar scaling, edema, or excoriation. The vagina may contain raised white or yellow adherent plaques.

Recurrent and/or persistent *Candida vulvovaginitis* is one of the more common clinical findings among human immunodeficiency virus (HIV)-infected women. However, the presence of recurrent *Candida vulvovaginitis* is not considered an indication for HIV counseling and/or HIV testing. In general, local application of antifungal therapy is effective. The imidazole derivatives are more effective than nystatin and thus are the preferred topical treatment for vulvovaginal candidiasis.[15] The available imidazole antifungal treatment regimens are listed in Table 48–3. All these regimens have similar therapeutic effectiveness. Ketoconazole, an imidazole antifungal agent, has been used orally to treat vaginal candidiasis. The efficacy of a 200-mg bid dose for 5 days is approximately 90 percent.[15] However, it has not been shown to be superior to miconazole therapy. In addition, hepatotoxicity is a concern with ketoconazole use. Other oral azole agents such as fluconazole and itraconazole may be as effective as topical agents. Boric acid (600 mg in a size 0 gelatin capsule) has also been used, and excellent results have been reported with a 14-day course.[16] Care must be taken to keep boric acid out of the reach of infants.

TABLE 48–3. TOPICAL INTRAVAGINAL PREPARATIONS FOR THE TREATMENT OF VULVOVAGINAL CANDIDIASIS

Butoconazole 2% cream, 5 g × 3 days
Clotrimazole[a] 1% cream, 5 g × 7–14 days
Clotrimazole[a] 100 mg tablet × 7 days
Clotrimazole 100 mg tablet, 2 tablets × 3 days
Clotrimazole 500 mg tablet, 1 tablet single application
Miconazole[a] 2% cream, 5 g × 7 days
Miconazole 200 mg suppository, 1 suppository × 3 days
Miconazole 100 mg suppository, 1 suppository × 7 days
Terconazole 6.5% ointment, 5 g single application
Terconazole 0.4% cream, 5 g × 7 days
Terconazole 0.8% cream, 5 g × 3 days
Terconazole 80 mg suppository, 1 suppository × 3 days

[a] Available over the counter.

The problem of recurrent disease or failure of therapy is not uncommon when dealing with yeast vaginitis. Despite the removal of predisposing factors, and the advent of multiple treatment courses and treatment of partners, there is a subgroup of patients who have persistent symptoms of yeast vaginitis. It remains unclear whether this condition is a result of altered local host defenses, or simply of persistence or recolonization from a rectal reservoir. Alternatively, it has been proposed that rather than eradicating *C. albicans* from the vagina, treatment only suppresses growth so patients become asymptomatic. Then with stimulation of *C. albicans* by estrogen and progesterone over the next several menstrual cycles, clinical symptoms again appear. Based on this premise, several long-term approaches to the treatment of recurrent *Candida vulvovaginitis* have been suggested. Topical imidazole therapy for 5 to 7 days premenses each cycle for 6 months or systemic therapy with ketoconazole (200 mg daily for 5 days) or fluconazole (single dose premenses) has been shown to result in good response rates during therapy. However, after therapy is stopped, recurrent disease occurs in many of these patients. Another approach has been a 6-month course of daily ketoconazole (200 mg). Once again, after treatment is halted, symptoms tend to recur.

Bacterial Vaginosis (Nonspecific Vaginitis). Bacterial vaginosis is the most common vaginal infection seen in sexually active women.[15] In the past, this condition has been referred to as nonspecific vaginitis and has been attributed to *Hemophilus vaginalis, Corynebacterium vaginalis,* and, more recently, *Gardnerella vaginalis.* These names have been used to identify the same organism, a gram-variable coccobacillus; however, it has become clear that this organism is not, in and of itself, a cause of vaginitis. The clinical entity of nonspecific vaginitis has most recently been termed *bacterial vaginosis* in an effort to indicate that it is characterized by an outgrowth of bacteria (bacterial) and a foul odor due to amine production (vaginosis).

Several investigators[12,17–19] have documented a 90 to 100 percent prevalence of *G. vaginalis* among women with bacterial vaginosis, whereas others[20,21] have isolated the organism in only 55 to 65 percent. However, *G. vaginalis* can be isolated from the vagina in up to 60 percent of asymptomatic, healthy women. Thus a culture positive for *G. vaginalis* is not diagnostic of vaginosis and should not be used clinically in such a way. Bacterial vaginosis is characterized by a significantly increased concentration of *G. vaginalis* and reduced levels of lactobacilli, particularly those strains that produce hydrogen peroxide. In general, this reduction in lactobacilli is accompanied by an increase in the concentration of anaerobes, particularly *Prevotella* (formerly *Bacteroides*) species such as *P. bivius* and *P. disiens,* and peptostreptococci. In addition, a curved motile aerobic gram-negative rod, recently assigned to the genus *Mobiluncus,* has also been associated with bacterial vaginosis.[18,21,22] Lastly, increased concentrations of the genital tract mycoplasmas, *Mycoplasma hominis* and *Ureaplasma urealyticum,* also are noted.

It is likely that bacterial vaginosis is caused by, or at least accompanied by, an alteration in the microenvironment of the lower genital tract that supports the proliferation of the more pathogenic anaerobic flora at the expense of lactobacillus. *Gardnerella vaginalis* may, in fact, turn out to be primarily a marker for high concentrations of pathogenic anaerobic organisms.

The traditional diagnostic approach to bacterial vaginosis is not microbiologic. A diagnosis of bacterial vaginosis requires three of the following four findings: (1) homogeneous vaginal discharge; (2) a pH of 4.7 or higher; (3) positive "sniff" test when addition of 10 percent potassium hydroxide to the vaginal discharge produces a fishy, foul odor; and (4) presence of "clue" cells. Recently, Nugent et al[23] have demonstrated that a Gram stain of the lateral vaginal wall is equivalent to the use of clinical criteria and thus can be utilized for the diagnosis of bacterial vaginosis. With this approach three major groups of morphotypes are evaluated (*Lactobacillus,* gram-negative rods, and *Mobiluncus* species) and semiquantitated with a composite score being given as follows: normal, 0 to 3; intermediate, 4 to 6; bacterial vaginosis, 7 to 10.

The treatment of bacterial vaginosis has evolved considerably with the recognition that topical sulfa creams applied intravaginally were largely ineffective. Oral metronidazole was the first antimicrobial agent with demonstrated effectiveness and 85 percent cure rates at 28 days post-treatment. Originally, the recommended therapy for bacterial vaginosis was metronidazole 500 mg bid for 7 days.[12] More recently, it has been suggested that a single 2-g loading dose of metronidazole may be as effective as the multiple day dosing.[24] In addition, intravaginal topical therapy for bacterial vaginosis has become available. Clindamycin cream instilled intravaginally once a day for 7 days[25] and metronidazole gel used bid for 5 days[26] have been demonstrated to have clinical cure rates equivalent to those seen with oral metronidazole.

Bacterial vaginosis has been demonstrated to be associated with a variety of complications and adverse pregnancy events. These recent studies are summarized in Table 48–4.

TABLE 48–4. COMPLICATIONS ASSOCIATED WITH BACTERIAL VAGINOSIS

Complication	Relative Risk	*P* Value	Author
Pelvic inflammatory disease (PID)	9.2	0.4	Eschenbach et al,[27] 1988
		0.023	Paavonen et al,[28] 1987
Postabortion PID	3.0	<0.05	Larsson et al,[29] 1992
Posthysterectomy infection	4.3	<0.1	Larsson et al,[30] 1991
	3.2	0.0005	Soper et al,[31] 1991
Preterm delivery	1.4	<0.1	Hillier et al,[32] 1991
	2.6	0.03	McGregor et al,[33] 1990
	3.8	0.02	Gravett et al,[34] 1986
	2.3	<0.5	Martius et al,[35] 1988
Premature ruptured membranes	2.4	<0.1	Gravett et al,[36] 1986
Amniotic fluid infection	1.5	0.03	Silver et al,[37] 1989
	2.7	<0.5	Gravett et al,[36] 1986
Chorioamnionitis	2.6	0.05	Hillier et al,[38] 1988
Postpartum endometritis	5.8	<0.001	Watts et al,[39] 1990
	2.2	<0.001	Newton et al,[40] 1990

The diagnosis of vaginitis can be simplified by a systematic approach to patients presenting with lower genital tract complaints. Some useful clinical features are listed in Table 48–5, which describes the characteristics of each condition, including suggested treatment regimens. Although this approach is usually successful, persistent or recurrent infections remain a problem for health providers. Recurrent vaginal candidiasis, persistent bacterial vaginosis, and trichomoniasis that is resistant to high doses of metronidazole are among the most difficult problems faced in outpatient gynecology clinics.

Cervicitis

Cervicitis or inflammation of the endocervix is most commonly caused by *C. trachomatis* or *N. gonorrhoeae*. The clinical diagnosis is made by visual inspection of the cervix and identification of mucopurulent discharge, edema, and friability.[8] The diagnosis is confirmed by isolation of one or more of the causative agents. *Neisseria gonorrhoeae* can be isolated by a single endocervical swab plated onto specific media (ie, modified Thayer-Martin) in 90 percent of infected patients. Two consecutive endocervical swabs or an endocervical and an anal swab will recover over 99 percent of *N. gonorrhoeae.*

The most common site of female genital tract infection with *C. trachomatis* is the cervix. *Chlamydia trachomatis* infections are best confirmed by tissue culture isolation from epithelial cells obtained with an endocervical swabbing or scraping. An alternate method is the recently marketed fluorescent-labeled monoclonal antibody to *C. trachomatis.* The sensitivity of this method compared with tissue culture may vary from 70 to 98 percent, depending on the prevalence of *C. trachomatis* in the population studied and the tissue culture method used for comparison.[41,42]

Neisseria gonorrhoeae and *C. trachomatis* can cause both symptomatic and asymptomatic endocervitis; however, they usually do not cause vagini-

TABLE 48–5. CLINICAL FEATURES OF VAGINITIS/CERVICITIS

Clinical Features	Trichomoniasis	Candidiasis	Bacterial Vaginitis (Nonspecific Vaginitis)	Cervicitis
Chief symptom	Malodorous discharge	Pruritis	Discharge	Discharge, history of STD exposure
Character of discharge	Copious, nonhomogeneous	Adherent, floccular (or discharge may be scant)	Homogeneous, odorous	Purulent
Color of discharge	Yellow-green, gray	White	Gray	Yellow, white
pH	>4.5	<4.5	>4.5	Variable
Most prominent features	Motile trichomonads on wet mount	Mycelia and/or pseudohyphae on KOH mount	Amine odor after KOH contact; clue cells; pH 4.5	WBCs on wet mount or Gram stain
Amine (sniff) test	Variable	Negative	Positive	Variable
White blood cells	Present	Absent	Usually absent	Present
Lactobacilli	Absent	Often present	Absent	Variable
Key to diagnosis	Identification of trichomonads	Identification of yeast forms	Clinical features	Visual inspection of cervix and identification of etiologic agent
Etiologic agents	*Trichomonas vaginalis*	*Candida albicans* *Torulopsis glubrata* Other *Candida* species	*Gardnerella vaginalis,* anaerobic bacteria, including *Mobiluncus* species	*Neisseria gonorrhoeae* *Chlamydia trachomatis* Herpes simplex
Treatment	Metronidazole 2 g orally or 250 mg tid × 7–10 days	Many regimens effective: —2% miconazole cream, 1 applicator per vagina daily × 7 days —clotrimazole suppositories 200 mg daily × 3 days or 100 mg daily × 7 days	Metronidazole 500 mg bid × 7 days	Direct treatment against specific etiologic agent

tis. Tissue culture has been considered the gold standard for identification of *C. trachomatis*. However, even in the most experienced laboratories the sensitivity of culture is 80 to 90 percent (ie, 10 to 20 percent false negatives) and is decreased further in most laboratories. Moreover, culture requires cold storage, cold transport, and 5 to 7 days to obtain results. Currently, antigen detection methods are the most commonly used methodology for identification of *C. trachomatis*. Two major antigen detection techniques are available. These are fluorescent-labeled monoclonal antibody smear (Microtrac) and immunoassay (Chlamydiazyme). These tests are more widely available, easier to perform, and quicker than culture. While their sensitivity and specificity are excellent, in a low prevalence population their positive predictive value decreases to 50 to 70 percent (ie, increased false positives). Recently, DNA probes and polymerase chain reaction (PCR) have been introduced into clinical practice for identifying the presence of *C. trachomatis*.

Because *C. trachomatis* coexists in 30 to 50 percent of women with gonococcal cervicitis,[43] both organisms should be treated unless specific cultures have been done. The Centers for Disease Control and Prevention (CDC) recommendations for the treatment of uncomplicated gonorrhea and chlamydia cervicitis are listed in Table 48–6.

Herpes simplex virus (HSV) is a third pathogen capable of producing cervicitis. This organism causes both ectocervicitis and endocervicitis. HSV may cause vesicles, pustules, ulcers, or nonspecific inflammation of the endocervix or the ectocervix. The organism is best identified by isolation of the virus in cell culture. Demonstration of multinucleate giant cells on Papanicolau smears from the cervix may be diagnostic, but negative smears do not rule out HSV infection.

TABLE 48–6. CDC GUIDELINES FOR TREATMENT OF UNCOMPLICATED GONOCOCCAL[a] AND CHLAMYDIAL INFECTIONS

• NEISSERIA GONORRHOEAE
Recommended regimens for uncomplicated infections
Ceftriaxone 125 mg IM once
Ciprofloxacin 500 mg PO once
Cefixime 400 mg PO once
Ofloxacin 400 mg PO once
Alternative regimens
Ceftizoxime 500 mg IM once
Cefotaxime 500 mg IM once
Cefotetan 1 g IM once
Cefoxitin 1 g IM once
Cefuroxime axetil 1 g PO once
Cefpodoxime 200 mg PO once
Enoxacin 400 mg PO once
Lomefloxacin 400 mg PO once
Norfloxacin 800 mg PO once
Spectinomycin 2 g IM once
• CHLAMYDIA TRACHOMATIS
Recommended regimens
Doxycycline 100 mg bid orally × 7 days
Azithromycin 1 g orally
Alternative regimens
Ofloxacin 300 mg bid orally × 7 days
Erythromycin base 500 mg qid orally × 7 days
Erythromycin ethylsuccinate 800 mg qid orally × 7 days
Sulfisoxazole 500 mg qid orally × 7 days

[a] CDC guidelines recommend concurrent treatment for *Chlamydia* whenever gonorrhea is treated, because of the high incidence of coexistence of these organisms.

Adapted from 1993 STD Treatment Guidelines: Morb Mortal Wkly Rep (in press).

Vulvar Infections

The vulva is composed of the labia majora, labia minora, mons pubis, vestibule, vestibular bulb, vestibular glands, and vaginal orifice. The vulva may be involved in a wide variety of infections, including genital herpes, condylomata acuminata, syphilis, bartholinitis, skenitis, chancroid, lymphogranuloma venereum, granuloma inguinale, molluscum contagiosum, candidiasis, furunculosis, scabies, and lice. The correct identification and treatment of the specific causative agents are fundamental to successful management of these lesions.

Genital Herpes Simplex. Genital herpes is a sexually transmitted disease caused by herpes simplex virus types 1 and 2 (HSV-1 and HSV-2). Primary genital herpes infections are about 85 percent HSV-2 and 15 percent HSV-1. Recurrent genital lesions are virtually all HSV-2 in origin.[44] Recent investigations utilizing antibody to HSV-2 glycoprotein have revealed that up to 35 percent of individuals in the United States have had previous HSV-2 infection. Genital herpes commonly involves the cervix but is far more painful when it infects the vagina and the vulva. The majority of patients presenting with genital herpes have recurrent or reactivated disease from a previous primary infection. Patients with primary herpes may present with pain, fever, malaise, nausea, myalgias, multiple lesions, diffuse vulvovaginitis, urinary incontinence, and inguinal adenopathy, whereas patients with recurrent disease tend to have more localized disease of shorter duration. The mean duration of pain in women with recurrent disease is 6 days, compared with 12 days for primary disease.[44] The mean duration of viral shedding from genital lesions is 4 days in recurrent disease and 12 days for primary disease.[44] The most common presenting lesions are a small cluster of painful vesicles or shallow ulcers with pain out of proportion to their size and location. The diagnosis is best confirmed by viral culture. A third clinical presentation for HSV infection is nonprimary first clinical episode of HSV. While clinical findings may help distinguish between primary and recurrent disease, definitive differentiation relies on serologic studies. With primary infection the initial serum contains no anti-HSV-2 antibody while the convalescent specimen does. With either recurrent genital HSV or nonprimary first clinical episode of HSV, the initial specimen demonstrates anti-HSV antibody.

Treatment with oral acyclovir (200 mg, five times daily) reduces the duration of viral shedding, accelerates healing time, and reduces the duration and severity of symptoms in primary episodes of herpes.[45] In severely ill patients, acyclovir may be administered intravenously. Oral acyclovir also suppresses genital herpes in patients with frequently recurrent HSV disease but has no influence on the natural history of the disease.[46,47] The long-term safety and risk of inducing drug resistance with suppressive therapy are unknown. To date continuous suppression of recurrent genital HSV with acyclovir for up to 5 years has been reported to be effective and safe.[48]

Condyloma Acuminata. Condylomata acuminata are benign epithelial tumors of the genitalia and the perineal area caused by the human papillomavirus. Often referred to as genital or venereal warts because of their wart-like appearance, this sexually transmitted infection is appearing in epidemic proportions in the United States according to CDC reports.[49] The lesions are typically multiple, discrete, well-differentiated papillary growths, that may coalesce to form cauliflower-like masses in the vulvar area, vagina, inner thighs, perineum, and perianal area. These lesions may also occur on the cervix, where they tend to be flat and endophytic. These lesions often require colposcopy for recognition and have frequently been classified as mild dysplasia of the cervix.

The diagnosis is usually made on clinical grounds alone; however, atypical lesions should be biopsied to exclude malignancy.

The usual treatment for condylomata acuminata is podophyllin 10 to 25 percent in tincture of benzoin carefully applied to lesions, avoiding normal tissue. The solution should be washed off within 4 hours of the application. Podophyllin must be used with great care in the vagina, and its use is discouraged in the treatment of cervical or anorectal condyloma where cryotherapy, laser therapy, or surgical excision (anorectal) are more appropriate. Podophyllin may be teratogenic and should not be used in pregnancy. Studies are currently under way to evaluate the usefulness of local and systemic use of immune-enhancing agents, such as interferon, as well as the role of antiviral chemotherapy in the treatment of genital warts. Recently, patient-applied podofilox has been shown to be a safe and effective therapy for genital condylomata in women.[49–51]

Primary Syphilis

Treponema pallidum, the causative agent of syphilis, is a strictly anaerobic sexually transmitted spirochete. Syphilis can present in any one of its stages and with almost any variety of symptoms. Syphilitic lesions of the female genital tract are most often the primary chancres that arise at the spirochete point of entry. This painless, ulcerated lesion with raised borders and an indurated base may go unnoticed, particularly if it occurs on the cervix or in the vagina. Even without treatment the chancre will heal and patients enter the secondary stage of syphilis (bacteremia systemic form) in which multiple organs and systems are involved. Characteristically, patients develop a papillosquamous symmetrical rash that typically involves the palms and soles. Other manifestations include mucous patches, condyloma latum, lymphadenopathy, and alopecia. Once again, even without treatment, the clinical manifestations of syphilis resolve and the patient enters the latent state of syphilis.

Most cases of syphilis are diagnosed in the latent phase by positive serologic tests. There are nonspecific nontreponemal tests available, including the VDRL and the rapid plasma reagin test (RPR). If these screening tests are positive, they are followed by treponema-specific tests, such as the *T. pallidum* immobilization (TPI) test, the fluorescent treponemal antibody absorption (FTA-ABS) test, or the microhemagglutination assay (MHA-TP) test, to confirm the diagnosis.

The most specific method for diagnosis of syphilis is the demonstration of *T. pallidum* on dark-field examination of fresh specimens for the lesions of infected patients. It should be remembered that when the syphilitic chancre first appears, both the nonspecific (VDRL, RPR) and specific (FTA-ABS, MHA-TP) serologic tests may be nonreactive.

Penicillin is the drug of choice for the treatment of syphilis. The CDC recommends benzathine penicillin G, 2.4 million units intramuscularly once for early syphilis (ie, duration less than 1 year) and once a week for 3 successive weeks (7.2 million units total) for syphilis of more than 1 year's duration. Alternative drugs include tetracycline (contraindicated in pregnancy) or erythromycin (500 mg qid for 15 days). Most authorities now recommend that patients allergic to penicillin be desensitized and treated. Treatment should be monitored with serial quantitative VDRL titers every 3 months for at least 1 year.

Bartholinitis

Bartholin's glands lie on either side of the vagina at the base of the labia minora. Blockage of the drainage duct may lead to cyst or abscess formation. Patients may present with a unilateral, tender, swollen, cystic mass (abscess) or an asymptomatic, cystic mass (cyst) at the vaginal introitus. Bartholin's abscesses may be accompanied by local cellulitis and edema. As the abscess enlarges and approaches the surface, it may spontaneously rupture or require incision and drainage for symptomatic relief.

Bartholin's abscesses, once thought to be caused exclusively by the gonococcus, have been shown to contain a variety of organisms, including mixed facultative and anaerobic organisms, such as aerobic streptococci, *E. coli, Proteus mirabilis,* and *Bacteroides* species, as well as *C. trachomatis* and *N. gonorrhoeae.*[52,53]

Treatment of a Bartholin's abscess includes hot soaks or sitz baths. As the abscess begins to point, local incision just inside the hymenal ring may provide adequate drainage. Following drainage, the insertion of a drainage catheter may prevent early recurrence. Antibiotics, such as ampicillin or tetracycline, should provide broad spectrum coverage when necessary, and the isolation of any sexually transmitted pathogens, such as *C. trachomatis* or *N. gonorrhoeae,* should be treated with the appropriate regimen.

Bartholin's abscesses are frequently associated with recurrences, which should be treated by marsupialization of the gland to provide permanent drainage of secretions. The bleeding complications associated with the rich vascular bed underlying Bartholin's gland have led to the use of marsupialization rather than complete gland excision for the treatment of recurrent Bartholin abscesses whenever feasible.

The Skene's glands, which lie on either side of the urethra, can become infected, causing dysuria and local pain and swelling. The causative organisms are likely to be the same as seen in bartholinitis; however, this has not been systematically studied. Treatment is with hot soaks and antibiotics as necessary. Abscesses may require incision and drainage; however, abscess formation at this site is far less common than with Bartholin's glands.

INFECTIONS OF THE UPPER FEMALE GENITAL TRACT

Infections of the upper female genital tract may be community acquired (acute salpingitis), postpartum (endomyometritis), or occur after gynecologic procedures (postoperative hysterectomy cuff cellulitis). It is preferable to refer to these infections by the nature and site of infection, for example, acute salpingitis or postpartum endometritis.

Pelvic Inflammatory Disease

History. Pelvic inflammatory disease (PID) is a very imprecise term, but it has become rather ingrained into the medical literature. This entity most often refers to acute infection of the fallopian tubes or acute salpingitis. Because these are presumed to be ascending infections, it is most likely that there is a concurrent endometritis and frequently an oophoritis as well.

The epidemic of sexually transmitted diseases (STDs) combined with the widespread use of the intrauterine contraceptive device (IUD) has led to a rising incidence of acute salpingitis.[54,55] It has been estimated that as many as 1 million women are treated for acute salpingitis in the United States annually, at a cost of 4 billion dollars.[1,56] Even more important are the significant medical sequelae of PID. One-fourth of all women who have had acute PID will experience one or more long-term sequelae, the most important of which is involuntary infertility in 20 percent of patients.[55] The incidence of ectopic pregnancy is increased six- to tenfold after an episode of acute salpingitis.[55] Chronic pelvic pain, dyspareunia, pelvic adhesions, chronic pyosalpinges, hydrosalpinges, and tubo-ovarian abscess may also occur as a result of PID.

Etiology. The classification of salpingitis into gonococcal and nongonococcal disease has proved to be grossly inadequate. Fallopian tube and peritoneal fluid cultures from acute salpingitis patients have demonstrated the true polymicrobial nature of the disease.[57,58] Isolation of *N. gonorrhoeae* from the endocervix in no way confirms that this organism is the predominant organism present in the fallopian tubes. Studies in which cultures were taken directly from the fallopian tubes demonstrated that correlation between endocervical and fallopian tubes isolates is quite variable.[57] Studies using culdocentesis and laparoscopy to obtain culture specimens from the peritoneal fluid or fallopian tube exudate, in combination with good anaerobic culture techniques, have provided valuable information on the causative agents of acute salpingitis PID.[57–60] The organisms most frequently recovered in these studies were *N. gonorrhoeae* and anaerobic bacteria, including peptostreptococci, peptococci, and *Bacteroides* species. In one of these studies using cultures from the fallopian tubes only, it was found that *N. gonorrhoeae,* which was isolated from nearly 50 percent of all endocervical cultures, was recovered from the fallopian tubes in only 23 percent of patients and 42 percent of those with endocervical gonorrhea.[59] Anaerobic bacteria were the most frequent fallopian tube isolates from these women with acute salpingitis, being recovered from 29 percent of patients.

Although *N. gonorrhoeae* is an important organism contributing to the etiology of acute PID, its presence in the cervix does not guarantee its presence in the fallopian tubes, nor does it indicate what other organisms may be present and playing a pathogenic role.

Chlamydia trachomatis, an even more common sexually transmitted organism, has also been implicated in the pathogenesis of acute PID.[61–66] Approximately half of the cases of acute PID occurring in Scandinavia are due to *C. trachomatis.* Sweet et al[67] reported the recovery of *C. trachomatis* from the upper genital tract in 23 percent of patients hospitalized in San Francisco with acute PID and demonstrated that *C. trachomatis* persisted in the upper genital tract of women treated with antimicrobial agents that were not active against *C. trachomatis.* Similarly, Kiviat et al[68] and Wasserheit et al[69] have reported the presence of *Chlamydia* in up to 40 percent of patients with acute PID. Most dramatic have been the numerous investigations that have demonstrated that women with tubal factor infertility or ruptured ectopic pregnancy are significantly more likely to have had previous chlamydial infection than women with other types of infertility or pregnant controls.

Mycoplasma hominis and *Ureaplasma urealyticum* have also been implicated as potential pathogens in acute PID; however, their exact roles in the etiology and pathogenesis have yet to be determined.[59,63,65]

The organisms most frequently isolated from endometrial or fallopian tube cultures are summarized in Table 48–7. *Neisseria gonorrhoeae* was recovered from 45 percent and *C. trachomatis* from 18 percent. The most frequently recovered organisms were nongonococcal, nonchlamydial bacteria. Anaerobic bacteria predominated, being present in 92 percent of patients with nongonococcal, nonchlamydial organisms. The most common of the nongonococcal, nonchlamydial organisms found included *Prevotella* species, *P. bivius,* anaerobic cocci, *G. vaginalis,* group B streptococci, and *E. coli.* Thus acute PID is usually a polymicrobial infection involving combinations of sexually transmitted organisms and endogenous facultative and anaerobic bacteria. In summary, STD organisms (*C. trachomatis* and/or *N. gonorrhoeae*) are involved in approximately two-thirds of cases of acute PID. In

TABLE 48–7. MICROBIOLOGY OF ACUTE PID FROM HOSPITALIZED PATIENTS AT SAN FRANCISCO GENERAL HOSPITAL

Organism	Number Positive/ Number Cultured	Percent Positive
Sexually transmitted organisms		
Neisseria gonorrhoeae	172/380	45
Chlamydia trachomatis	68/380	18
Nongonococcal nonchlamydial bacteria	267/380	67
Anaerobic bacteria		
Prevotella species	88/188	47
Other *Prevotella*	99/188	53
P. bivius	72/188	38
P. disiens	25/188	13
Peptostreptococcus asaccharolyticus	93/188	49
P. anaerobius	71/188	38
Facultative bacteria		
Gardnerella vaginalis	121/188	64
Escherichia coli	25/188	13
Nonhemolytic streptococci	49/188	26
Group B streptococci	29/188	15
Coagulase-negative staphylococci	72/188	38

one-third of acute PID cases only anaerobic and/or facultative organisms (mostly those organisms associated with bacterial vaginosis) are present. Roughly 50 percent of the PID associated with STD organisms also have anaerobic and/or facultative bacteria recovered.

Diagnosis. There is considerable evidence demonstrating the inaccuracy of diagnosing acute PID by clinical criteria. Jacobson and Westrom[70] reported results on 814 women with a clinical diagnosis of acute salpingitis who underwent diagnostic laparoscopy, of whom only 65 percent had the diagnosis confirmed. Furthermore, analysis of their data failed to identify clinical features that could reliably differentiate between patients with and without acute PID. Because it is not logistically or economically practical to subject all patients suspected to have acute PID to laparoscopy, an attempt has been made to standardize the criteria used in the diagnosis of acute PID.[71] Those criteria, listed in Table 48–8, are intended only to provide guidelines for the diagnosis of acute PID based on clinical findings alone, and are not expected to provide a highly sensitive method of detecting patients with acute PID. Whenever there is serious doubt about the diagnosis, the clinician must consider laparoscopy, particularly if a potentially life-threatening disorder, such as appendicitis or ectopic pregnancy, is a likely alternative diagnosis.

Treatment. To provide the optimal therapy for patients with acute PID, the clinician must institute early therapy with antimicrobial agents effective against the known pathogenic organisms. Although a prompt response is the first goal of therapy, equally important is the prevention of subsequent infertility, recurrent infection, and the chronic residual sequelae of the infection. Combination antimicrobial regimens are currently employed, aimed at broad spectrum coverage that includes mixed aerobic and anaerobic bacteria, as well as sexually transmitted organisms such as *N. gonorrhoeae* and *C. trachomatis*. The CDC, recognizing the need for broad spectrum coverage, have recommended two different antibiotic regimens for the treatment of acute PID.[72] These treatment regimens are listed in Table 48–9. These treatment regimens for both inpatient and outpatient therapy will continue to undergo revision as more information on the etiology and pathogenesis of acute PID and newer, improved antimicrobials become available.

There are no studies to date that provide good data comparing the efficacy of inpatient versus outpatient treatment of acute PID. The major weakness of the outpatient regimens, as recommended by the CDC in the past, was the difficulty in effectively treating mixed infections that include penicillin-resistant gram-negative anaerobes. Theoretically, the current recommendations for outpatient therapy with ofloxacin plus clindamycin or metronidazole would avert this problem.

Patients should definitely be treated as inpatients if they have significant fever, the diagnosis is in question, there is evidence of a pelvic abscess, or

TABLE 48–8. DIAGNOSTIC CRITERIA FOR ACUTE PID

Patients must have:
- A. Lower abdominal pain and tenderness
- B. Cervical motion tenderness
- C. Adnexal tenderness

Patients must also have one or more of the following:
- A. Temperature > 38C
- B. Elevated white blood cell count (>10,500/ml[3])
- C. Elevated erythrocyte sedimentation rate
- D. Presence of an inflammatory mass on examination or ultrasonography
- E. WBCs and bacteria on culdocentesis if this procedure is done prior to treatment
- F. Evidence of endocervical gram-negative intracellular diplococci suggesting *Neisseria gonorrhoeae* or a positive monoclonal antibody suggesting *Chlamydia trachomatis*

Adapted from Hager WE, Eschenbach DA, Spence MR, Sweet RL: Obstet Gynecol 61:113, 1983.

TABLE 48–9. CDC TREATMENT RECOMMENDATIONS FOR ACUTE PID 1993

Inpatients	A. Doxycycline 100 mg IV, twice daily plus Cefoxitin 2g, IV, four times daily Continue drugs IV for at least 4 days and 48 hours after improvement of symptoms. Then continue doxycycline 100 mg, PO, twice daily to complete 10 to 14 days of therapy B. Clindamycin 600 mg, IV, four times daily plus Gentamicin 2.0 mg/kg, IV, followed by 1.5 mg/kg, three times daily in patients with normal renal function Continue drugs IV for at least 4 days and 48 hours after improvement of symptoms. Then continue clindamycin 450 mg, PO, four times daily to complete 10 to 14 days of therapy
Outpatients	Ofloxucin 400 mg bid, orally plus clindamycin 450 mg qid orally or metronidazole 500 mg bid orally for 14 days or Cefoxitin 2 g IM single dose plus doxycycline 100 mg bid orally for 14 days

1993 STD Treatment Guidelines: Morb Mortal Wkly Rep (in press).

they cannot tolerate or fail to respond to oral medications. Adolescents and patients with IUD-related infections should also be considered for inpatient therapy. Most patients with acute PID respond to one of the above mentioned treatment regimens, although surgical intervention may be necessary to effect a cure in some patients. Most patients requiring surgery have deep-seated infections because of multiple recurrences or because treatment was begun late in the course of the disease. Tubo-ovarian abscess, pyosalpinx, and inflammatory complexes all increase the likelihood that antibiotics alone will fail to cure the infection.

Tubo-ovarian Abscess. The incidence of tubo-ovarian abscesses in patients hospitalized with acute PID is about 10 to 15 percent, but has been reported to be as high as 34 percent.[73] The presence of an inflammatory mass, such as a tubo-ovarian abscess, a pyosalpinx, or an inflammatory complex involving the fallopian tube and any surrounding contiguous structures, may complicate the course of acute PID. These deep-seated infections may be difficult to control, and early recognition and proper selection of antimicrobial regimens may improve the outcome. Ultrasonography is a useful tool with which to supplement the physical examination, particularly if the diagnosis is in question. Studies have shown that ultrasonography is remarkably accurate in confirming the presence and complexity of pelvic masses.[74,75]

The treatment of patients with acute PID complicated with tubo-ovarian abscesses, pyosalpinges, or other inflammatory masses is quite similar to that for uncomplicated acute PID. The principle of therapy is to use parenteral antimicrobial agents that are effective against the suspected pathogens, penetrate abscesses, and remain stable and active to some degree within the abscess environment. Studies using animal models have shown that a number of antibiotics penetrate abscesses and maintain activity within the abscesses' environment.[76,77] Most notable were clindamycin, metronidazole, cefoxitin, and moxalactam, although not all of the newer antimicrobial agents have been tested in this model.

Current data indicate that 60 to 70 percent of patients with an unruptured tubo-ovarian abscess will have an initial response to antibiotics alone.[73,75,78,79] Furthermore, this response rate may be considerably higher if the antimicrobial agents chosen are active against the resistant anaerobes and can penetrate into the abscess cavity.[73,75] Sweet and co-workers[80] compared the efficacy of the CDC inpatient regimens clindamycin plus gentamicin and cefoxitin plus doxycycline in the treatment of tubo-ovarian abscess. In 125 tubo-ovarian abscesses, both regimens were equally effective with an overall clinical success rate of 70 percent.

Indications for surgical intervention in patients with acute PID include the suspicion of a ruptured abscess, uncertainty of the diagnosis when an alternative surgical disease may be present (ie, appendicitis, ectopic pregnancy), or failure to respond after 48 to 72 hours of antibiotic therapy. Once surgery is undertaken, a conservative approach with unilateral adnexectomy for one-sided abscesses is appropriate if future fertility or hormone production is desired.[73] The surgery may be difficult because of the loss of the normal architecture of the pelvic viscera. Postoperative intraperitoneal closed drainage, use of permanent fascial sutures, and delayed primary closure may all serve to reduce postoperative infectious complications.

Fitz-Hugh-Curtis Syndrome. The Fitz-Hugh-Curtis syndrome is an acute perihepatitis characterized by a localized fibrinous inflammation affecting the anterior surface of the liver and adjacent parietal peritoneum. This infection frequently results in fibrous adhesion formation between the liver and the diaphragm or anterior peritoneal surface. The Fitz-Hugh-Curtis syndrome is usually associated with acute PID.

In the past, the Fitz-Hugh-Curtis syndrome was believed to be a complication of gonococcal infection. More recent evidence suggests that *C. trachomatis* may have an etiologic role in this syndrome.[81,82] It is likely that other organisms involved in acute PID contribute to this syndrome as well.

INFECTIONS AFTER GYNECOLOGIC PROCEDURES

Postoperative infections may be seen after most gynecologic procedures. The close proximity of vaginal and endocervical microflora provides a potential source of infection to the operative site. The most common gynecologic procedures currently being done include dilatation and curettage, suction curettage for incomplete or therapeutic abortion, vaginal and abdominal hysterectomy, extended or radical gynecologic procedures for malignancy, and a variety of adnexal procedures such as ovarian cystectomy, removal of ectopic pregnancies, and tubal procedures for infertility. The risk of infection after these procedures is directly related to the amount of contamination with genital flora that occurs during the surgery. It is not surprising that without the use of prophylactic antibiotics the highest postoperative infection rates are associated with hysterectomy, radical surgery, and to a lesser extent, uterine curettage procedures.

Infections After Uterine Curettage

Postabortal Endometritis and Septic Abortion. Uterine curettage is one of the most common gynecologic procedures performed. It is done with a suction curette for retained products of conception after incomplete abortion and for early pregnancy termination. Sharp uterine curettage is a frequently used method to evaluate abnormal uterine bleeding, particularly in older women at risk for endometrial carcinoma. Infection after curettage may be caused by sexually transmitted organisms, such as *C. trachomatis* and *N. gonorrhoeae,* or by the endogenous microflora of the lower genital tract. Infection after diagnostic curettage is an uncommon occurrence. There are several factors that contribute to the likelihood of infection after curettage performed for pregnancy termination. Infections after suction abortion range from mild to severe. Several factors may contribute to the severity of the infection, including the presence of sexually transmitted pathogens, uterine perforation during the procedure, and retained products of conception after the procedure. Additionally, the length of gestation may influence the postoperative infection rate because later gestation may require instrumentation beyond a simple suction cannula and the procedure may take significantly more time.

The routine use of prophylactic antibiotics for patients undergoing early pregnancy termination has been controversial, as the infection rate in most centers remains well below 10 percent. While many centers utilize routine prophylaxis (usually tetracycline or doxycycline), we reserve the use of prophylactic antibiotics for suction curettage, usually tetracycline, for patients with a history of PID, gonorrhea, or chlamydia, or patients with an IUD.

Patients with endometritis after curettage usually present with fever, lower abdominal pain, and pelvic tenderness indistinguishable from acute PID. They may also complain of cramping and vaginal bleeding secondary to retained products of conception.

The term *septic abortion* usually refers to sepsis associated with an abortion performed in the community by intrauterine mechanical or chemical manipulation. The incidence and morbidity of septic abortion dropped dramatically with the widespread availability of legal, medically approved abortions. When patients do present with septic abortion, they may have any combination of aerobic or anaerobic sepsis, shock, and infected, necrotic, retained products of conception. They may have hypotension, fever, chills, lower abdominal pain, and bloody, purulent vaginal discharge.

The organisms involved in postabortal endometritis and septic abortion are similar to those described for acute PID. There is usually a mixed infection involving any combination of the sexually transmitted organisms and the endogenous aerobic and anaerobic flora of the lower genital tract.

The treatment of pelvic infections after abortion or dilatation and curettage is much the same as that for acute PID. Patients should be treated with broad spectrum antibiotic regimens, such as those listed in Table 48–9 for acute PID. In addition to antibiotic treatment, these patients may need evacuation of the uterus if there is suspicion of retained products of conception. This procedure should be performed as soon as satisfactory tissue levels of antibiotics have been achieved. Occasionally a patient may have widespread pelvic infection that does not respond to antibiotics; evacuation of the uterus and more extensive surgical intervention may be necessary to either drain or remove a pelvic abscess or remove a uterus with multiple microabscesses unresponsive to parenteral antimicrobial agents.

Postoperative Infection After Hysterectomy

Pelvic infection after hysterectomy has been a common occurrence on most gynecologic services, particularly before the widespread use of prophylactic antibiotics. The most common type of soft tissue infection after hysterectomy is the vaginal cuff infection. The cuff, created when the uterus is removed from the vaginal vault, is virtually always contaminated with vaginal microflora and, therefore, highly susceptible to postoperative infection. Vaginal cuff infections are especially common after vaginal hysterectomy but can also occur after abdominal hysterectomy. These cuff infections may be complicated by pelvic cellulitis and abscess formation. Cuff infections, like other wound infections, tend to present with fever. Pelvic examination may reveal a tender, indurated vaginal cuff. Purulent material may be seen draining from the cuff. If postoperative abscess formation has occurred, drainage is usually necessary.

The microbiology of posthysterectomy pelvic infections involves, not surprisingly, the endogenous aerobic and anaerobic microflora of the lower genital tract, especially anaerobic bacteria such as *P. bivius, Prevotella* species, and peptostreptococci. Treatment of these infections begins with the initiation of broad spectrum antimicrobial agents. Because of the paucity of sexually transmitted pathogens associated with posthysterectomy infections, these patients frequently respond to single agent therapy directed at the mixed aerobic and anaerobic organisms involved in these infections. This would include a myriad of second- and third-generation cephalosporins and extended spectrum penicillins with activity against mixed aerobic and anaerobic bacteria including the resistant gram-negative anaerobes such as *P. bivius.* Examples of reasonable single agents or combination agents for the treatment of mixed aerobic and anaerobic soft tissue infections of the female pelvis are listed in Table 48–10.

Wound Infections

Abdominal wound infections may be seen after cesarean section or routine gynecologic procedures. Most cesarean sections and hysterectomies done in the absence of gross infection, such as chorioamnionitis, PID, or tubo-ovarian abscess, are classified as clean-contaminated wounds. The infection rate after these procedures may, however, be slightly higher than expected for clean-contaminated cases, depending on a number of risk factors for postoperative infection. In addition to the usual risk factors for wound infection, such as operating time, age, obesity, and underlying medical diseases, postcesarean section wound infections may be more influenced by temperature on admission, number of vaginal examinations, duration of ruptured membranes, duration of labor, and duration of internal monitoring.[83–85] The rate of wound infection after abdominal hysterectomy is estimated to range between 3 and 6 percent, whereas for cesarean section it ranges between 4 and 8 percent.[86] Abdominal wound infections generally fall into two categories: (1) the early onset wound infections and (2) the late onset wound infections. The sources of wound contamination may include both skin and lower genital tract, as well as exogenous contamination from surgical personnel. Early onset wound infections in obstetrics and gynecology are most commonly associated with group A streptococci or, less commonly, group B streptococci and *Clostridium perfringens.* These infections occur within the first 48 hours postoperatively and, frequently, in the initial 12 to 24 hours, presenting with fever and a spreading wound cellulitis or discoloration. Progression of this process can be seen over a period of hours. A Gram stain of material aspirated from the active margin of infection may help differentiate *Streptococcus* (gram-positive cocci) from *Clostridium* (gram-positive rods). A bronze appearance of the skin and nearby crepitance may also raise suspicion of clostridial infection.

These early onset wound infections should be treated promptly with penicillin if possible, or ampicillin, cephalosporins, or erythromycin if penicillin is unacceptable. Excision of necrotic tissue is equally important to prevent necrotizing fasciitis, bacteremia, and disseminated intravascular coagulation. Recently, toxic shock syndrome associated with early onset wound infection caused by toxin producing strains of *S. aureus* has been reported.[87] These patients present with the classic signs and symptoms of toxic shock syndrome in addition to the findings of a rather mild appearing wound infection. However, patients with toxic shock syndrome secondary to wound infection do not require extensive debridement after opening the wound. Rather, antibiotics plus supportive therapy directed at maintaining intravascular volume and perfusion of tissue is the keystone.

Late onset wound infections are the type more commonly seen and occur at about 4 to 8 days postoperatively. These infections are usually associated with mixed facultative and anaerobic bacteria arising from the endogenous flora of the vagina and the cervix. The symptoms of late onset wound infection usually include fever with an erythematous, swollen, or draining wound. The crucial part of treatment is incision and drainage, which usually effects a response within 12 hours. Antibiotic therapy is usually not necessary unless there is associated cellulitis. If an infected wound does not respond to drainage within about 12 hours, antibiotics directed at mixed aerobic and anaerobic bacteria should be

TABLE 48–10. ANTIMICROBIAL REGIMENS FOR SOFT TISSUE PELVIC INFECTIONS

Combination therapy	
Clindamycin + aminoglycoside	
Metronidazole + aminoglycoside	
Clindamycin + aztreonam	
Single agent	
Cephalosporins	Cephamycin
Ceftizoxime	Cefoxitin
Moxalactam	Cefotetan
Cefotaxime	
Extended spectrum penicillins	Beta-lactam plus enzyme blocker
Mezlocillin	Amoxicillin plus clavulanic acid
Piperacillin	Tirarcillin plus clavulanic acid
Carbapenems	Ampicillin plus sulbactam
Imipenem	

instituted, and a more extensive infectious process should be ruled out.

The possibility of necrotizing fasciitis should always be considered in patients who do not respond to simple incision and drainage of uncomplicated wound infections. Necrotizing fasciitis is a polymicrobial infection that usually involves aerobic and anaerobic organisms. It requires early diagnosis, extensive surgical debridement, and potent broad spectrum antimicrobial therapy.

The use of prophylactic antibiotics to prevent postoperative pelvic infections after hysterectomy and cesarean section has also served to reduce the risk of postoperative wound infection. In addition, the incidence of wound infections will likely be reduced with good surgical and sterile technique. If there is an anticipated increased risk of wound infection, as with surgery for a ruptured pelvic abscess, then a delayed primary closure may reduce the risk of wound infection.[88]

Infections Associated with Pregnancy

Chorioamnionitis. Intrauterine infection may occur during late pregnancy, and has been referred to as chorioamnionitis, amnionitis, or intra-amnionitic infection. The infection may involve the uterus, the membranes (amnion and chorion), the placenta, the umbilical cord, and the fetus. Approximately 10 percent of pregnancies show histologic evidence of chorioamnionitis, but the correlation with clinical symptoms is poor. Clinical evidence of chorioamnionitis is seen in only about 1 percent of pregnancies, and is associated with an increase in perinatal morbidity and mortality, as well as maternal morbidity. However, recent studies using sophisticated microbiologic studies have demonstrated that subclinical amnionitis is present in 4.6 to 10.8 percent of laboring parturients.

The placental membranes and cervical mucus normally protect the amniotic cavity from bacterial colonization. Chorioamnionitis usually occurs in patients with ruptured membranes, and after the onset of labor. The most common mode of transmission of organisms to the amniotic cavity is ascending infection from the lower genital tract.[89] There are, however, reported cases of documented chorioamnionitis in patients without labor or rupture of membranes, presumedly infected via transplacental or hematogenous spread. In particular, *Listeria monocytogenes* has been noted to cause chorioamnionitis and fetal demise in patients without labor or rupture of membranes.[90] Another organism associated with chorioamnionitis that is especially worrisome is the group B streptococcus. This organism has been associated with a severe form of neonatal sepsis having a mortality rate near 50 percent, as well as postpartum endomyometritis in the mother.[91] Most clinicians will treat patients with premature ruptured membranes and who have lower genital tract colonization with group B streptococcus in hopes of preventing the transmission of the organism to the fetus and the upper genital tract. These patients can be treated with intravenous ampicillin, which will achieve reasonable levels in the mother and her fetus.

A number of diagnostic and therapeutic procedures, such as amniocentesis, cervical cerclage, and intrauterine transfusion, have been reported to increase the risk of intra-amniotic infection. The benefits of these procedures are thought to outweigh the risks, but these patients should be watched closely for signs of amnionitis.

The microorganisms most frequently isolated from the amniotic cavity of patients with chorioamnionitis include *Prevotella* species, *P. bivius,* group B streptococci, other aerobic streptococci, *E. coli, Clostridium* species, peptostreptococci, and *Fusobacterium.*[92,93] *Mycoplasma hominis* has also been isolated from as many as 35 percent of patients with intra-amniotic infections, but usually in conjunction with other organisms thought to be of high virulence in the genital tract.[94]

Gibbs and co-workers[95] have reported that the recovery of *E. coli* and/or group B streptococci from the amniotic fluid of patients with amnionitis is associated with a significantly increased risk of severe neonatal sepsis and/or mortality.[96,97]

The diagnosis of chorioamnionitis is difficult to make early in the course of the infection. As a result, the infection is usually well established before any clinical signs are evident. The earliest signs are maternal fever, leukocytosis, and maternal or fetal tachycardia. Uterine tenderness and foul smelling amniotic fluid tend to be later findings. Analysis of Gram stain and culture of amniotic fluid, although useful in ruling out infection in asymptomatic patients with premature rupture of membranes, have limited value in laboring patients with clinical evidence of chorioamnionitis. These specimens are difficult to collect without contamination and may not always reveal the true polymicrobial nature of the infection.

The treatment of chorioamnionitis generally includes the administration of broad spectrum antimicrobial agents and delivery of the fetus to effect drainage of the infected amniotic cavity. The antimicrobial agents chosen should provide broad spectrum coverage directed toward the organisms most frequently isolated from patients with these infections, ie, group B streptococci and other aerobic gram-positive and gram-negative organisms, as well as the anaerobes, including the penicillin-resistant gram-negative anaerobes such as *P. bivius.* The regimen most often used at our institution is a combination of ampicillin and cefoxitin. Other regimens that have been used successfully include combinations of penicillin with an aminoglycoside, with the addition of clindamycin, particularly if the patients are delivered by cesarean section. Some of the newer agents recently developed that cover group B streptococci and the mixed aerobic and anaerobic microflora of the genital tract may also prove to be effective in the treatment of chorioamnionitis.

Most authors recommend that the uterus be emptied to effect drainage of the infected amniotic cavity. This does not need to be done by immediate cesarean section but, rather, within a reasonable amount of time, ie, 12 to 24 hours. With electronic fetal monitoring and intravenous antibiotics, patients can continue labor, or labor can be induced or augmented, without undue risk to the mother or her fetus. Recent studies have shown that cesarean section can be reserved for those with obstetric indications and, in fact, the maternal outcome was significantly better in those patients delivered vaginally.[89] There is some evidence, however, that cesarean section may be necessary more often in patients with chorioamnionitis because of dysfunction of the infected uterus.[98] If cesarean section is required, recent data suggest that there is no advantage to an extraperitoneal approach compared with transperitoneal when broad spectrum antibiotics are used in patients with chorioamnionitis.[99] With grossly infected amniotic fluid noted at cesarean section, a delayed primary wound closure should be considered. The risk of chorioamnionitis in patients with prolonged rupture of membranes has led clinicians to consider delivery of these patients regardless of gestational age. In recent years, many clinicians have favored expectant management of patients with premature ruptured membranes if the fetus was between 26 and 34 or 35 weeks gestational age. Studies are currently under way to evaluate the use of prophylactic antibiotics in these patients to reduce the risk of chorioamnionitis. If chorioamnionitis does occur at any gestational age, it is generally felt that expeditious delivery should be part of the management plan.

Postpartum Infections. The overall estimated rate of postpartum infection ranges from about 1 to 8 percent.[100] The most common type of postpartum infection is infection of the uterus. These infections are commonly referred to as postpartum endometritis, endomyometritis, or endoparametritis. A number of risk factors have been identified that may predispose women to developing postpartum endometritis. Delivery by cesarean section is far and away the major predisposing factor. The rate of endometritis rarely exceeds 3 percent after vaginal delivery, whereas the rate after cesarean section has been reported to range from 12 to 85 percent.[100] Infection rates after cesarean section are further determined by additional risk factors. Duration of labor was the most significant factor affecting postpartum morbidity after cesarean section when other confounding variables were controlled.[101] Other factors that have been reported to influence the risk of postpartum infection include duration of ruptured membranes, number of vaginal or rectal examinations, internal fetal monitoring, duration of surgery, estimated blood loss, and obesity.[102–105]

Much like other genital tract infections, the pathogenic organisms that normally inhabit the lower genital tract are thought to play an etiologic role in patients with endometritis. These infections tend to be mixed aerobic and anaerobic bacterial infections. It is reported that anaerobic organisms can be found in 80 percent of postpartum infections.[100] Gram-negative anaerobes, such as *P. bivius,* are of particular concern because of their penicillin resistance. Genital mycoplasmas have also been associated with postpartum infection, although patients with puerperal infections respond well to antimicrobial regimens that do not cover the genital mycoplasmas. In addition, *C. trachomatis* has been associated with a late onset, mild endometritis in a small number of cases.[106] Postpartum endometritis should be suspected in patients with fever during the postpartum period. Additional findings that may secure the diagnosis include chills, uterine tenderness, and foul smelling lochia.

The vast majority of patients with simple postpartum endometritis respond to antimicrobial therapy within 48 to 72 hours. Although patients with postpartum endometritis will respond to a wide variety of antimicrobial regimens, it is important to provide adequate coverage against the major pathogens involved in these infections, particularly the resistant gram-negative anaerobes. DiZerega and co-workers,[107] in a study of 200 patients with post-cesarean section endometritis, found that patients treated with clindamycin and gentamicin had a significantly higher cure rate than those treated with penicillin and gentamicin. Furthermore, an abscess, two cases of septic pelvic thrombophlebitis, and a wound evisceration all occurred in the penicillin-gentamicin group. The improved outcome with clindamycin-gentamicin probably reflects the effectiveness of this regimen against *B. fragilis, P. bivius,* and other anaerobes. Thus therapy for postpartum endometritis should be directed against these resistant anaerobes as well as gram-positive and gram-negative anaerobes. Presently, the combination regimen of clindamycin and gentamicin is considered the standard for comparison. These two drugs, however, are not the least toxic agents available, nor the most effective. Based on small comparative clinical trials, many single agents have been recommended for the treatment of postpartum endometritis. Unfortunately, the low incidence of complications, such as pelvic abscess and septic pelvic thrombophlebitis, makes it difficult to assess efficacy of these regimens in preventing these complications. In obstetric infections, the newer extended spectrum penicillins and the second- and third-generation cephalosporins may have a role in the treatment of mild to moderate postpartum endometritis. Those shown to be effective include mezlocillin, piperacillin, cefoxitin, moxalactam, cefotaxime, cefotetan, ceftizoxime, ticarcillin/clavulanic acid, and ampicillin/sulbactam. None of these single agents, however, has ever been shown to be superior to the others in prospective, randomized clinical trials.

Failure to respond to antimicrobial therapy beyond 72 hours should alert the clinician to the possibility of pelvic abscess formation, septic pelvic thrombophlebitis, or wound abscess. The presence of one of these complications, rather than failure of antibiotics to cure a simple endometritis, should be suspected. Recent studies have demonstrated the emergence of enterococcal infections as an important cause of infectious morbidity in postcesarean endometritis patients, especially where broad spectrum cephalosporins have been used for prophylaxis. In patients who have not responded to initial therapy, a complete exam including the pelvis should be performed. If exam does not reveal an infected mass requiring drainage, antimicrobial therapy is adjusted to provide coverage against potential pathogens that may not be covered by the initial empiric regimen. Ultrasonography may be useful in identifying the presence of a pelvic abscess or an infected hematoma. A trial of heparin therapy may be necessary to confirm suspected septic pelvic thrombophlebitis. These patients will usually show a dramatic response 12 to 24 hours after heparin therapy is begun if the cause of their resistance to antibiotics alone is septic pelvic thrombophlebitis. The wound should be inspected daily to ensure that patients unresponsive to antibiotics do not have deep-seated wound infections. Finally, some patients, in rare circumstances, will have extensive myonecrosis or microabscess formation within the uterine walls that will be unresponsive to antibiotic therapy alone. Although surgical intervention is seldom necessary in patients with postpartum endometritis, it can be a necessary adjunct to therapy in some patients. Retained necrotic placental tissue may require curettage before response is evident. Colpotomy or laparotomy may be necessary in patients with pelvic abscess formation. Rarely, hysterectomy may be necessary in patients with infections unresponsive to antimicrobial therapy, particularly if they have necrotizing endometritis associated with clostridial infection, or in patients with septic shock unresponsive to antibiotics and supportive therapy.

PROPHYLACTIC ANTIBIOTICS IN OBSTETRICS AND GYNECOLOGY

The short-term administration of perioperative antibiotics has been shown to dramatically reduce the risk of postoperative infection in a large number of procedures associated with bacterial contamination at the time of surgery. Because infections occur commonly after cesarean section and hysterectomy, there has been a great deal of interest in antibiotic prophylaxis in obstetrics and gynecology (see Chap. 25).

The incidence of postoperative infection after cesarean section has been reported to be as high as 85 percent in some populations.[2,3] Not all cesarean deliveries carry such a risk; in fact, elective repeat cesarean deliveries in some populations carry a postoperative infection rate well below 10 percent and therefore do not warrant prophylactic antibiotics. The patients that benefit the most from the use of prophylactic antibiotics are those undergoing cesarean section after labor with ruptured membranes and multiple examinations. In randomized trials of prophylactic antibiotics for primary cesarean sections, there is a marked reduction in the infection rate in the prophylaxis groups.[108] Furthermore, short courses of antibiotic prophylaxis have been found to be just as effective as the longer courses.[109] Studies evaluating single-dose prophylaxis in cesarean sections immediately after cord clamping have documented excellent results. Because withholding the antibiotics until after the umbilical cord is clamped will allow full evaluation of the infant for sepsis, it remains the current recommendation of most authors to administer the prophylactic agents after cord clamping. Although a number of different antibiotics have been shown to be effective prophylactic agents for cesarean section, there are no good prospective randomized trials that demonstrate any benefit of using the more expensive second- and third-generation cephalosporins or extended spectrum penicillins over the first generation cephalosporins or ampicillin. Some investigators have evaluated the efficacy of antibiotic prophylaxis given as intraoperative local irrigation of the uterus and peritoneal cavity instead of systemic administration.[110] They found that this was an effective means of prophylaxis. However, others[111] have found that appreciable systemic absorption of antibiotics administered by this route may permit blood levels to reach concentrations well beyond the minimal inhibitory concentration for many genital tract pathogens, and the levels are not as consistent as when antibiotics are administered by the intravenous route.

The use of prophylactic antibiotics in gynecology has been primarily directed toward preventing posthysterectomy infections. The majority of studies have shown that the use of prophylactic antibiotics significantly reduces the rate of postoperative infection after vaginal hysterectomy.[112] There were no statistically significant differences between single dose and multiple dose prophylaxis if the single dose was administered 30 to 60 minutes prior to surgery.[112–114] Furthermore, there have been no prospective randomized studies in which any of the newer broad spectrum antimicrobial agents have been shown to be more effective than the inexpensive first generation cephalosporins, such as cefazolin or cephalothin.[85,87,88,112,114,115]

The use of prophylactic antibiotics to prevent infection after abdominal hysterectomy has not been as widely recommended as for vaginal hysterectomy. The infection rate after abdominal hysterectomy tends to be significantly lower at most institutions. In 16 studies evaluating prophylactic antibiotics for abdominal hysterectomy, only seven showed statistically significant differences in pelvic cellulitis or wound infections.[115] The postoperative infection rate after abdominal hysterectomy may vary depending on risk factors and patient population. Clinicians should evaluate their own postoperative infection rates and the individual patient's risk factors in determining whether or not to use prophylactic antibiotics for abdominal hysterectomy. In a study of patients undergoing radical hysterectomy, Marsden and co-workers[116] found that, although there was a trend, there was no statistically significant difference in surgical site infections in the antibiotic group versus the placebo group. They did find that several factors, including operative time, patient weight, blood loss, and blood replacement, were related to the incidence of infectious morbidity. It is clear from this and other studies that certain groups of patients are at higher risk for postoperative infections after abdominal hysterectomy and may benefit from the selective use of prophylactic antibiotics.

Elective abortions in the absence of risk factors, such as a history of sexually transmitted diseases or the presence of an IUD, have been associated with a low infection rate ranging from 0.5 to 10 percent depending on the population.[115] We generally reserve prophylactic antibiotics for those patients with a history of PID, a current sexually transmitted disease, an IUD, or valvular heart disease.

Prophylactic antibiotics have been used in infertility surgery. Although there are no good studies demonstrating the efficacy of prophylaxis for these procedures, the devastating consequences of operative site infection for these patients has been cited as a reasonable concern.[115]

When prophylactic antibiotics are used to prevent postoperative infections after gynecologic surgery, the agent chosen should be short-term, efficacious, and cost effective. Ampicillin or cefazolin for hysterectomy and tetracycline or ampicillin for high-risk elective abortions would be appropriate choices. Tetracycline is our choice for patients undergoing infertility surgery where chlamydial infection is of paramount concern.

The American Heart Association[117] noted that bacterial endocarditis after vaginal delivery is extremely rare. We continue to use prophylactic antibiotics for vaginal delivery in patients with underlying heart disease to prevent this rare complication. The indication for prophylactic antibiotics is more firmly established for complicated deliveries such as cesarean section. Antibiotic prophylaxis has also been recommended for patients with underlying heart disease undergoing gynecologic surgery, such as hysterectomy, and for patients with prosthetic valves undergoing dilatation and curettage or IUD insertion or removal. The recommended prophylaxis regimen to prevent bacterial endocarditis in obstetric and gynecologic procedures is ampicillin (2.0 g intramuscularly or intravenously) plus gentamicin (1.5 mg/kg intramuscularly or intravenously) given 30 minutes to 1 hour before the procedure. A follow-up dose may be given 8 hours after the initial dose.[118,119] Vancomycin (1.0 g intravenously over 1 hour) may be substituted for ampicillin in penicillin-allergic patients. Drug dosages may need to be reduced for patients with compromised renal function.

REFERENCES

1. Curran JW: Economic consequences of pelvic inflammatory disease in the United States. Am J Obstet Gynecol 138:848, 1980.
2. Gibbs RS: Clinical risk factors for puerperal infections. Obstet Gynecol 55:178(s), 1980.
3. Gilstrap LC, Cunningham FG: The bacterial pathogenesis of infection following cesarean section. Obstet Gynecol 53:545, 1979.
4. Mendelson J, Portnoy J, DeSaint V, et al: Effect of single and multidose cephradine prophylaxis on infectious morbidity of vaginal hysterectomy. Obstet Gynecol 53:31, 1979.
5. Hill GB, Eschenbach DA, Holmes KK: Bacteriology of the vagina. In Mardh P-A, Taylor-Robinson D (eds): Bacterial Vaginosis. Stockholm, Sweden, Almqvist and Wiksell International, 1984, pp 23–39.
6. Tashjian JH, Coulam CB, Washington JA: Vaginal flora in asymptomatic women. Mayo Clin Proc 51:557, 1976.
7. Ohm MJ, Galask RP: Bacterial flora of the cervix in prehysterectomy patients. Am J Obstet Gynecol 122:683, 1975.
8. Hill GB: Anaerobic flora of the female genital tract. In Lambe DW, Gencot RJ, Mayberry-Carson KJ (eds): Anaerobic Bacteria: Selected Topics. New York, Plenum, 1980, pp 39–50.
9. Hammann R: A reassessment of the microbial flora of the female genital tract, with special reference to the occurrence of *Bacteroides* species. J Med Microbiol 15:293, 1982.
10. Bartlett JG, Onderdonk AB, Drude E, et al: Quantitative bacteriology of the vaginal flora. J Infect Dis 136:271, 1977.
11. Mardh PA, Soltesz LV: Interactions between lactobacilli and other organisms occurring in the vaginal flora. Scand J Infect Dis Suppl 40:47, 1983.
12. Pheifer TA, Forsythe PS, Durfee MA, et al: Nonspecific vaginitis. N Engl J Med 98:1429, 1978.
13. Cohen MS, Black JR, Procter RA, Sparling PF: Host defences and the vaginal mucosa. In Mardh PA, Taylor-Robinson D (eds): Bacterial Vaginosis. Stockholm, Sweden, Almqvist and Wiksell International, 1984, p 13.
14. McGregor JA, French JI, Jones W, et al: Association of cervicovaginal infections with increased vaginal fluid phospholipase A2 activity. Am J Obstet Gynecol 167:1588, 1992.
15. Sweet RL, Gibbs RS: Infectious vulvovaginitis. In Sweet RL, Gibbs RS (eds): Infectious Diseases of the Female Genital Tract. Baltimore, Williams & Wilkins, 1990.
16. VanSlyke KK, Michel VP, Rein MF: Treatment of vulvovaginal candidiasis with boric acid powder. Am J Obstet Gynecol 141:145, 1981.
17. Spiegel CA, Amsel R, Eschenbach D, et al: Anaerobic bacteria in nonspecific vaginitis. N Engl J Med 303:601, 1980.
18. Blackwell AL, Fox AR, Phillips I, Barlow D: Anaerobic vaginosis: clinical, microbiological and therapeutic findings. Lancet 2:1379, 1983.
19. Tabaqchali S, Wilks M, Thin RN: *Gardnerella vaginalis* and anaerobic bacteria in genital disease. Br J Vener Dis 59:111, 1983.
20. Taylor E, Blackwell AL, Barlow D, Phillips I: *Gardnerella vaginalis* anaerobes and vaginal discharge. Lancet 1:1376, 1982.
21. Skarin A, Mardh PA: Comma-shaped bacteria associated with vaginitis. Lancet 1:342, 1982.
22. Speigel CA, Eschenbach DA, Amsel R, Holmes KK: Curved anaerobic bacteria in bacterial (nonspecific) vaginosis and their response to antimicrobial therapy. J Infect Dis 148:817, 1983.
23. Nugent RP, Krohn MJ, Hillier SL: Reliability of diagnosing bacterial vaginosis is improved by a standardized method of Gram stain interpretation. J Clin Microbiol 29:297, 1991.
24. Lugo-Miro VI, Green M, Mazur L: Comparison of different metronidazole therapeutic regimens for bacterial vaginosis: a meta-analysis. JAMA 268:92, 1992.
25. Livengood CH, Thomasen JL, Hill GB: Bacterial vaginosis: treatment with topical intravaginal clindamycin phosphate. Obstet Gynecol 76:118, 1990.
26. Hillier S, Lipinski C, Briseldon AM, Eschenbach DA: Efficacy of intravaginal 0.75% metronidazole gel for treatment of bacterial vaginosis. Obstet Gynecol 81:963, 1993.
27. Eschenbach DA, Hillier S, Crithlow C, et al: Diagnosis and clinical manifestations of bacterial vaginosis. Am J Obstet Gynecol 158:819, 1988.
28. Paavonen J, Teisala K, Heinonen PK, et al: Microbiological and histopathological findings in acute pelvic inflammatory disease. Br J Obstet Gynaecol 94:454, 1987.
29. Larsson P-G, Platz-Christensen J-J, Thejis H, et al: Incidence of pelvic inflammatory disease after first-trimester legal abortion in women with bacterial vaginosis after treatment with metronidazole: a double-blind, randomized study. Am J Obstet Gynecol 166:100, 1992.
30. Larsson P-G, Platz-Christensen JJ, Forsum U, Pahlson C: Clue cells in predicting infections after abdominal hysterectomy. Obstet Gynecol 77:450, 1991.
31. Soper DE, Bump RC, Hurt WG: Bacterial vaginosis and *Trichomonas vaginitis* are risk factors for cuff cellulitis after abdominal hysterectomy. Am J Obstet Gynecol 163:1016, 1990.
32. Hillier SL, Nugent RP, Krohn MA, et al: The association of bacterial vaginosis with adverse pregnancy outcome. 1991 Presentation at ICAAC, October 1991.
33. McGregor JA, French JI, Richter R, et al: Antenatal microbiologic and maternal risk factors associated with prematurity. Am J Obstet Gynecol 163:1465, 1990.
34. Gravett MG, Nelson HP, DeRoven T, et al: Indepen-

dent associations of bacterial vaginosis and *Chlamydia trachomatis* infection with adverse pregnancy outcome. JAMA 256:1899, 1986.

35. Martius J, Krohn MA, Hillier SL, et al: Relationship of vaginal *Lactobacillus* species, cervical *Chlamydia trachomatis* and bacterial vaginosis to preterm birth. Obstet Gynecol 71:89, 1988.
36. Gravett MG, Hummel D, Eschenbach DA, et al: Preterm labor associated with subclinical amniotic fluid infection and with bacterial vaginosis. Obstet Gynecol 67:229, 1986.
37. Silver HM, Sperling RS, St Clair PJ, Gibbs RS: Evidence relating bacterial vaginosis to intraamniotic infection. Am J Obstet Gynecol 161:808, 1989.
38. Hillier SL, Martius J, Krohn MA, et al: A case-controlled study of chorioamnionic infection and histologic chorioamnionitis in prematurity. N Engl J Med 319:972, 1988.
39. Watts DH, Krohn MA, Hillier SL, Eschenbach DA: Bacterial vaginosis as a risk factor for post-cesarean endometritis. Obstet Gynecol 75:52, 1990.
40. Newton ER, Prihoda TJ, Gibbs RS: A clinical and microbiologic analysis of risk factors for puerperal endometritis. Obstet Gynecol 74:402, 1990.
41. Tam MR, Stamm WE, Handsfield HH, et al: Culture dependent diagnosis of *Chlamydia trachomatis* using monoclonal antibodies. N Engl J Med 310:1146, 1984.
42. Lipkin E, Moncada J, Schachter J: Comparison of monoclonal antibody staining and culture in diagnosis of chlamydial infection. Abstract #377, American Society for Microbiology, 85th Annual Meeting, March, 1985, Las Vegas, Nevada.
43. Sweet RL, Schachter J, Landers DV: Chlamydial infections in obstetrics and gynecology. Clin Obstet Gynecol 26(s):143, 1983.
44. Corey L, Adams HG, Brown ZA, Holmes KK: Genital herpes simplex virus infections: clinical manifestations, course and complications. Ann Intern Med 98:958, 1983.
45. Bryson YJ, Dillon M, Lovett M, et al: Treatment of first episodes of genital herpes simplex virus infections with oral acyclovir. N Engl J Med 308:916, 1983.
46. Straus SE, Takiff HE, Seidlin M, et al: Suppression of frequently recurring genital herpes: a placebo-controlled double-blind study of oral acyclovir. N Engl J Med 310:1545, 1984.
47. Douglas JM, Critchlow C, Benedetti J, et al: A double-blind study of orally acyclovir for suppression of recurrences of genital herpes simplex virus infection. N Engl J Med 310:1551, 1984.
48. Straus SE, Croen KD, Sawyer MH, et al: Aryclovir suppression of frequently recurring genital herpes: Efficacy and diminishing need during successive years of treatment. JAMA 2227–2230, 1988.
49. Centers for Disease Control: *Condyloma acuminatum*—United States 1966–1981. Morb Mortal Wkly Rep 32:306, 1983.
50. Greenberg MD, Rutledge LH, Reid R, et al: A double-blind, randomized trial of 0.5% podofilox and placebo for the treatment of genital warts in women. Obstet Gynecol 77:735, 1991.
51. Baker DA, Douglas JM, Buntin DM, et al: Topical podofilox for the treatment of condylomata acuminatum in women. Obstet Gynecol 76:656, 1990.
52. Lee YH, Rankin JS, Alport S, et al: Microbiological investigation of Bartholin's gland abscesses and cysts. Am J Obstet Gynecol 129:150, 1977.
53. Davies JA, Rees E, Hobson D, Karayiannis P: Isolation of *Chlamydia trachomatis* from Bartholin's ducts. Br J Vener Dis 54:409, 1978.
54. Eschenbach DA, Harnisch JP, Holmes KK: Pathogenesis of acute pelvic inflammatory disease: role of contraception and other risk factors. Am J Obstet Gynecol 128:880, 1980.
55. Westrom L: Incidence, prevalence and trends of acute pelvic inflammatory disease and its consequences in industrialized countries. Am J Obstet Gynecol 138:880, 1980.
56. Jones OG, Saida AA, St John RK: Frequency and distribution of salpingitis and pelvic inflammatory disease in short stay hospitals in the United States. Am J Obstet Gynecol 1338:905, 1980.
57. Eschenbach DA, Buchanan T, Pollack HM, et al: Polymicrobial etiology of acute pelvic inflammatory disease. N Engl J Med 293:166, 1975.
58. Sweet RL, Mills J, Hadley WK, et al: Use of laparoscopy to determine the microbiologic etiology of acute salpingitis. Am J Obstet Gynecol 134:68, 1979.
59. Sweet RL, Draper DL, Schachter J, et al: Microbiology and pathogenesis of acute salpingitis as determined by laparoscopy: what is the appropriate site to sample? Am J Obstet Gynecol 138:985, 1980.
60. Cunningham FG, Hauth JC, Gilstrap LC, et al: The bacterial pathogenesis of acute pelvic inflammatory disease. Obstet Gynecol 52:161, 1978.
61. Mardh P-A, Ripa T, Svensson L, Westrom L: *Chlamydia trachomatis* infection in patients with acute salpingitis. N Engl J Med 298:1377, 1977.
62. Osser S, Persson K: Epidemiology and serodiagnostic aspects of chlamydia salpingitis. Obstet Gynecol 59:206, 1982.
63. Moller BR, Mardh P-A, Ahrons S, Nussler E: Infections with *Chlamydia trachomatis, Mycoplasma hominis,* and *Neisseria gonorrhoeae* in patients with acute pelvic inflammatory disease. Sex Transm Dis 8:198,1981.
64. Gjonnaess H, Dalaker K, Anestad G, et al: Pelvic inflammatory disease: etiologic studies with emphasis on chlamydial infection. Obstet Gynecol 59:550, 1982.
65. Mardh P-A, Lund I, Svensson L, et al: Antibodies to *Chlamydia trachomatis, Mycoplasma hominis,* and *Neisseria gonorrhoeae* in sera from patients with acute salpingitis. Br J Vener Dis 57:125, 1981.
66. Ripa KT, Svensson L, Treharne JD, et al: *Chlamydia trachomatis* infections in patients with laparoscopically verified salpingitis: results of isolation

and antibody determinations. Am J Obstet Gynecol 138:960, 1980.

67. Sweet RL, Schachter J, Robbie MO: Failure of betalactam antibiotics to eradicate *Chlamydia trachomatis* in the endometrium despite apparent clinical cure of acute salpingitis. JAMA 250:2641, 1983.
68. Kiviat NB, Wolner-Hanssen P, Peterson M, et al: Localization of *Chlamydia trachomatis* infection by direct immunofluorescence and culture in pelvic inflammatory disease. Am J Obstet Gynecol 154:865, 1986.
69. Wasserheit JN, Bell TA, Kiviat NB, et al: Microbial causes of proven pelvic inflammatory disease and efficiency of clindamycin and tobramycin. Ann Intern Med 104:187, 1986.
70. Jacobson L, Westrom L: Objective diagnosis of acute pelvic inflammatory disease. Am J Obstet Gynecol 105:1088, 1969.
71. Hager WE, Eschenbach DA, Spence MR, Sweet RL: Criteria for diagnosis and grading of salpingitis. Obstet Gynecol 61:113, 1983.
72. Centers for Disease Control and Prevention: 1993 STD Treatment Guidelines: Morb Mortal Wkly Rep 42(RR-14):1, 1993.
73. Landers DV, Sweet RL: Current trends in the diagnosis and treatment of tuboovarian abscess. Am J Obstet Gynecol 151:1098, 1985.
74. Taylor KJK, Degraaft MCI, Wasson JF, et al: Accuracy of grey-scale ultrasound diagnosis of abdominal and pelvic abscesses in 220 patients. Lancet 1:83, 1978.
75. Landers DV, Sweet RL: Tubo-ovarian abscess: contemporary approach to management. Rev Infect Dis 5:876, 1983.
76. Joiner KA, Lowe BR, Dzink JL, Bartlett JG: Antibiotic levels in infected and sterile subcutaneous abscesses in mice. J Infect Dis 143:487, 1981.
77. Joiner KA, Lowe BR, Dzink JL, Bartlett JG: Comparative efficacy of 10 antimicrobial agents in experimental *Bacteroides fragilis* infections. J Infect Dis 145:561, 1982.
78. Ginsberg DS, Stern JL, Hamod KA, et al: Tuboovarian abscess: a retrospective review. Am J Obstet Gynecol 138:541, 1980.
79. Franklin EW, Hevron JE, Thompson JD: Management of the pelvic abscess. Clin Obstet Gynecol 24:1187, 1981.
80. Reed SD, Lauders DV, Sweet RL: Antibiotic treatment of tubo-ovarian abscess: Comparison of broad spectrum betalactam agents versus clindamycin-containing regimens. Am J Obstet Gynecol 164: 1556–1562, 1991.
81. Paavonen J, Saikuu P, vonKnorring J, et al: Association of infection with *Chlamydia trachomatis* with Fitz-Hugh-Curtis syndrome. J Infect Dis 144:176, 1981.
82. Wang SP, Eschenbach DA, Holmes KK, et al: *Chlamydia trachomatis* infection in Fitz-Hugh-Curtis syndrome. Am J Obstet Gynecol 138:1034, 1980.
83. Stage AH, Long H, Silberman R, et al: Wound infection following cesarean section. Surg Gynecol Obstet 145:882, 1977.
84. Gibbs RS, Listwa HM, Read JA: The effect of internal fetal monitoring on maternal infection following cesarean section. Obstet Gynecol 48:653, 1976.
85. Sweet RL, Gibbs RS: Wound and episiotomy infections. In Sweet RL, Gibbs RS (eds): Infectious Disease of the Female Genital Tract. Baltimore, Williams & Wilkins, 1985, p 155.
86. Daly JW: Wound Infections. In Monif G (ed): Infectious Diseases in Obstetrics and Gynecology, 2nd ed. Philadelphia, Harper & Row, 1982, p 611.
87. Bartlett P, Reingold AL, Graham DR, et al: Toxic shock syndrome associated with surgical wound infections. JAMA 247:1448, 1982.
88. Brown SE, Allen HH, Robin RN: The use of delayed primary wound closure. Am J Obstet Gynecol 127:713, 1977.
89. Gibbs RS, Castillo MS, Rodgers PJ: Management of acute chorioamnionitis. Am J Obstet Gynecol 136:209, 1980.
90. Halliday HL, Hirata T: Perinatal listeriosis: a review of twelve patients. Am J Obstet Gynecol 133:404, 1979.
91. Sweet RL, Gibbs RS: Intraamniotic infections. In Sweet RL, Gibbs RS (eds): Infectious Diseases of the Female Genital Tract. Baltimore, Williams & Wilkins, 1981, p 263.
92. Gibbs RS, Blanco JD, St Clari PJ, et al: Quantitative bacteriology of amniotic fluid from patients with clinical intra-amniotic infection at term. J Infect Dis 145:1, 1982.
93. Gravett MG, Eschenbach DA, Speigel-Brown CA, Holmes KK: Rapid diagnosis of amniotic fluid infection by gas–liquid chromatography. N Engl J Med 306:725, 1982.
94. Blanco JD, Gibbs RS, Malherbe H, et al: A controlled study of genital mycoplasmas in amniotic fluid from patients with intraamniotic infection. J Infect Dis 147:650, 1983.
95. Gibbs RS, Dinsmoor MJ, Newton E, Ramamurthy RS: A randomized trial of intrapartum vs. immediate postpartum treatment of women with IAI. Obstet Gynecol 72:823, 1988.
96. Sperling RS, Ramamurthy RS, Gibbs RS: A comparison of intrapartum vs. immediate postpartum treatment of intra-amniotic infection. Obstet Gynecol 70:861, 1987.
97. Gilstrap LC, Leven KS: Intrapartum treatment of acute chorioamnionitis impact on neonatal sepsis. Am J Obstet Gynecol 159:579, 1988.
98. Duff P, Sanders R, Gibbs RS: The course of labor in term patients with chorioamnionitis. Am J Obstet Gynecol, 147:391, 1983.
99. Yonekura ML, Wallace R, Eglinton GL: Amnionitis—optimal operative management: extraperitoneal cesarean section vs. low cervical transperitoneal cesarean section. Third Annual Meeting,

Society of Perinatal Obstetricians, Abst. 24A, San Antonio, TX, 1983.
100. Sweet RL, Gibbs RS: Postpartum infections. In Sweet RL, Gibbs RS (eds): Infectious Diseases of the Female Genital Tract. Baltimore, Williams & Wilkins, 1985, p 277.
101. D'angelo LJ, Sokol RJ: Time-related peripartum determinants of postpartum morbidity. Obstet Gynecol 55:319, 1980.
102. Rehu M, Nilsson CG: Risk factors for febrile morbidity associated with cesarean section. Obstet Gynecol 56:269, 1980.
103. Hager D: Maternal febrile morbidity associated with fetal monitoring and cesarean section. Obstet Gynecol 46:260, 1975.
104. Hagglund L, Christensen KK, Christensen P, et al: Risk factors in cesarean section infection. Obstet Gynecol 46:145, 1983.
105. Nielsen TK, Hokegard KH: Postoperative cesarean section morbidity: a prospective study. Am J Obstet Gynecol 146:911, 1983.
106. Wager GP, Martin DH, Koutsky L, et al: Puerperal infectious morbidity: relationship to route of delivery and to antepartum *Chlamydia trachomatis* infection. Am J Obstet Gynecol 138:1028, 1980.
107. diZerega G, Yonekura L, Roy S, et al: A comparison of clindamycin–gentamicin and penicillin–gentamicin in the treatment of post cesarean section and myometritis. Am J Obstet Gynecol 52:31, 1979.
108. Polk BF: Antimicrobial prophylaxis to prevent mixed bacterial infections. J Antimicrob Chemother 8[Suppl]:115, 1981.
109. Swartz WH, Grolle K: The use of prophylactic antibiotics in cesarean section: a review of the literature. J Reprod Med 26:595, 1981.
110. Long WH, Rudd EG,Dillon MB: Intrauterine irrigation with cefamandole naflate solution at cesarean section: a preliminary report. Am J Obstet Gynecol 138:755, 1980.
111. Duff P, Gibbs RS, Jorgenson JH, et al: The pharmacokinetics of prophylactic antibiotics administered by intraoperative irrigation at the time of cesarean section. Obstet Gynecol 60:409, 1982.
112. Hamod KA, Spence MR, King TM: Prophylactic antibiotics in vaginal hysterectomy. Obstet Gynecol Surv 37:207, 1982.
113. Lett WJ, Ansbacher R, Davison BL, Otterson WN: Prophylactic antibiotics for women undergoing vaginal hysterectomy. J Reprod Med 19:51, 1977.
114. Hamod KA, Spence MA, Rosenshein NB, Dillon MB: Single and multidose prophylaxis in vaginal hysterectomy: a comparison of sodium cephalothin and metronidazole. Am J Gynecol 136:976, 1980.
115. Cartwright PS, Pittaway DE, Jones HW, Entman SS: The use of prophylactic antibiotics in obstetrics and gynecology. A review. Obstet Gynecol Surv 39:537, 1984.
116. Marsden DE, Cavanaugh D, Wisniewski RN, et al: Factors affecting the incidence of infectious morbidity after radical hysterectomy. Am J Obstet Gynecol 132:817, 1985.
117. Kaplan EL, Anthony BF, Bisno A, et al: Prevention of bacterial endocarditis. AHA News 139A, 1977.
118. Shulman ST, Amren DP, Bisno AL, et al: Prevention of bacterial endocarditis. Circulation 70:1123, 1984.
119. Prevention of Bacterial Endocarditis. Med Lett 26:2, 1984.

Infections of the Genitourinary Tract

CHAPTER 49

James A. Roberts

Urinary tract infections (UTIs) are the second most common infection (after upper respiratory infection) in females.[1] They are also a frequent cause of infection in neonatal males and postadolescent and aged men. They are the most common cause of nosocomial infection, even more common than wound infections.[2] These iatrogenic or hospital-acquired infections are often due to less virulent bacteria and most often follow catheterization. However, if the organisms are hospital-acquired, the infection is often more difficult to clear because they are resistant to more antibacterials.

A normal urinary tract is one without bacteria, stone, tumor, obstruction, vesicoureteral reflux, or neurologic disorder. It will not have been affected by drugs such as analgesics or lead. The patient will have no systemic abnormality such as diabetes mellitus or immunosuppression, which can predispose to infection. Within these restrictions, the pathogenesis of UTI can more readily be explored. The mechanisms by which bacteria enter the normal urinary tract involve bacterial adhesion and colonization. This is most frequently due to bacterial fimbriae adhering to specific receptors, but other proposed virulence factors may be necessary for invasive disease. The majority of what will be discussed is concerned with nonobstructive infections and thus deals more with bacterial than host factors. However, host factors must be considered. For instance, acute pyelonephritis is often associated with sepsis, especially in the presence of obstruction. Thus obstructing ureteral stone with infection, as an example, becomes a surgical emergency.

PATHOGENESIS OF URINARY TRACT INFECTIONS

Physicians, as contrasted with urologists, have conveniently divided UTIs into three groups: (1) acute uncomplicated cystitis in women, (2) uncomplicated pyelonephritis in women, and (3) complicated UTI in men and women. Urologists principally deal with the latter group.

Etiology. Table 49–1 lists the microbes found in the three groups.[3] *Escherichia coli* causes more than 95 percent of UTIs, but other organisms are found in upper tract, recurrent, or complicated infections. *Staphylococcus saprophyticus,* a coagulase-negative organism resistant to novobiocin, is increasingly prominent. Other fecal organisms contaminating the perineum are usually contaminants causing UTIs, as in *Gardnerella vaginalis. Mycoplasma* and *Chlamydia* probably also cause urethritis.

TABLE 49–1. MICROBIAL SPECIES MOST OFTEN ASSOCIATED WITH SPECIFIC TYPES OF UTI

Microbe	Acute Uncomplicated Cystitis[a] (%)	Acute Uncomplicated Pyelonephritis[a] (%)	Complicated UTI[b] (%)	Catheter-Associated UTI[b] (%)
E. coli	79	89	32	24
S. saprophyticus	11	0	1	0
Proteus	2	4	4	6
Klebsiella	3	4	5	8
Enterococcus	2	0	22	7
Pseudomonas	0	0	20	9
Mixed	3	5	10	11
Other	0	2	5	10
Yeast	0	0	1	28
S. epidermidis	0	0	15	8

[a] Data are from 607 episodes of cystitis and 84 episodes of pyelonephritis in Seattle.
[b] Data are from *Platt R, Polk BF, Murdock B, et al: Am J Epidemiol 124:977, 1986; and Gasser TC, Graverson PH, Madsen PO: Am J Med 82(Suppl 4):278, 1987.*
From Stamm WE: Approach to the patient with urinary tract infection. In Gorbach WL, Bartlett JG, Blacklow NR (eds): Infectious Diseases. Philadelphia, Saunders, 1992, p 789.

Stamm[3] devised Table 49–2 as an overview of the epidemiology of UTI, by sex and age. Infections in boys are associated with an intact foreskin and congenital abnormalities. Proteus infections that colonize the prepuce are common in uncircumcised boys. UTI predominates in females aged 1 to 35, associated with a short urethra directly entering the contaminated perineum, sexual intercourse, and diaphragm/spermicide use. Not until obstructions and incomplete voiding occur does the incidence in men and women approximate one another.

PATHOGENESIS OF NOSOCOMIAL URINARY TRACT INFECTION

The highest rate for nosocomial infection occurs on surgical services. Of these nosocomial infections, 67 percent occur because of catheterization, instrumentation of the bladder, or surgery on the lower urinary tract.[2] Such instrumentation breaks down the normal body defenses against infection. Indeed, bacteriuria occurs in 1 to 5 percent of patients after a single catheterization.[4] With an indwelling catheter, the risk of acquiring an infection increases with time, being 5 to 10 percent for each day of catheterization. Despite this high rate, patients with a normal lower urinary tract will often spontaneously rid themselves of the infection once the catheter is removed. It was shown in one late follow-up that only 8 to 10 percent of patients (after catheter drainage for up to a week) had bacteriuria and less than 1 percent developed a clinical infection.[5]

Because an estimated 15 percent of all hospitalized patients develop nosocomial bacteriuria, serious attempts at prevention must be made. Bacteriuria is associated with increased mortality,

TABLE 49–2. OVERVIEW OF THE EPIDEMIOLOGY OF UTI BY AGE GROUP

Age Group (yr)	Females: *Prevalence* (%)	Females: *Risk Factors*	Males: *Prevalence* (%)	Males: *Risk Factors*
<1	1	Anatomic or functional urologic abnormalities	1	Anatomic or functional urologic abnormalities
1–5	4–5	Congenital abnormalities, vesicoureteral reflex	0.5	Congenital abnormalities, uncircumcised penis
6–15	4–5	Vesicoureteral reflux	0.5	None
16–35	20	Sexual intercourse, diaphragm use	0.5	Homosexuality
36–65	35	Gynecologic surgery, bladder prolapse	20	Prostatic hypertrophy, obstruction, catheterization, surgery
Over 65	40	As above, plus incontinence, chronic catheterization	35	As above, plus incontinence, long-term catheterization

From Stamm WE: Approach to the patient with urinary tract infection. In Gorbach WL, Bartlett JG, Blacklow NR (eds): Infectious Diseases. Philadelphia, Saunders, 1992, p 789.

although the direct cause for the mortality could not be proved to be urinary tract infection or sepsis. First, an attempt should be made to decrease the number of patients catheterized. The catheter cannot be avoided completely, however, because urethral catheterization is mandatory treatment for a variety of conditions. If, however, a catheter is needed for postoperative urinary retention in young adults, single catheterization rather than an indwelling catheter is suggested. Even multiple single catheterizations lead to fewer symptomatic febrile infections, as has been shown in the treatment of neurogenic bladders.[6] An indwelling catheter should be used only in surgical procedures where continuous monitoring of urine output is mandatory. In the case of abdominal surgery, if the full bladder interferes with the procedure, it can temporarily be emptied by needle puncture and aspiration.

When the indwelling catheter cannot be avoided, proper care will reduce the infection rate. The use of a closed drainage system has greatly decreased the incidence of bacteriuria.[7] If the system is broken, a new catheter and closed system should be used. Cleansing around the meatus should not be done, as this may increase the chance of ascending infection.[8] If bacteriuria occurs, treatment should be delayed either until the catheter is removed or until a febrile infection occurs. Most often, simply removing the foreign body may permit the normal bladder defense mechanisms to clear the infection. In the case of the incontinent male, an external condom catheter should be tried. If successful, it should be changed and the penis cleaned daily to prevent damage to the penis. Suprapubic catheter drainage should also be considered when it is obvious that long-term catheterization will be needed.

BACTERIAL FACTORS IN THE PATHOGENESIS OF URINARY TRACT INFECTION

It is generally accepted that contamination of the urinary tract ascends along the lower tract. Although some hospital-acquired infections associated with catheters or instrumentation may be transferred directly by personnel, most infections originate from gut bacteria that colonize the perineum.[9]

Bacterial Adherence

Bacteria attach to host tissues in a highly selective manner. If they do not attach, colonization is impeded.[10] Most bacteria that cause UTI possess adhesins, or chemical ligands, which endow the bacteria with the ability to attach to specific receptors on either uromucoid or uroepithelial cells. Such attachments permit the bacteria to resist cleansing activities of these surfaces, such as the urinary flow.

The proteinaceous adhesions of most urinary pathogens lie along the bacterial fimbriae, which are rigid, filamentous appendages of proteinaceous material found on most gram-negative organisms.[11] The adhesion-receptor complex acts to oppose the usual repulsive forces between microbial and epithelial surfaces, both of which are hydrophobic and negatively charged.[12] Various types of bacterial fimbriae and their complementary receptors have been found. The receptors recognized by fimbriae may be host glycoproteins and/or glycolipids (such as the P blood group antigen-related glycosphingolipids in the case of P fimbriae).[13] The essential receptor of type 1 fimbriae of uropathogenic *E. coli* strains contains mannosyl residues and such adherence is blocked by the addition of D-mannose.[14] The type 1 fimbriae have been found to be important in colonization of the bladder, while the type P fimbriae which bind to αGal-(1$\rightarrow$4)βGal are involved in colonization of the upper urinary tract.[10] Adherence to uromucoid cells (such as Tamm-Horsfall protein) by type 1 fimbriae may provide a mechanism by which bacteria can be shed, since this glycoprotein only coats uroepithelial cells and may aid in clearing the infection as the coating is shed.[15] Excess mucus production, as may occur in response to a foreign body such as a catheter, may, however, be the means by which infection ascends to the bladder around the catheter.

Other Virulence Factors

Although bacterial adherence is an important initiating factor, it is not the only suspected virulence factor. The O serotype does not appear to differentiate which strains are pathogenic in the urinary tract. Plasmid-mediated pathogenicity has been shown for some *E. coli,* such as plasmid coding for enterotoxins of enterotoxigenic *E. coli* in humans,[16] and the K88 fimbriae responsible for adhesion relevant to porcine epidemic diarrhea.[17] Whether plasmids are responsible for pathogenicity in the urinary tract has not been proved. Colicin V plasmids have been said to be common and may well code for virulence for some markers common to uropathogenic species such as serum bactericidal resistance, production of hemolysins, K antigen, and mannose-resistant bacterial adhesion.[18] There is no evidence, however, that colicin V itself is responsible for the increased virulence of the bacteria producing it.[19] Using the mouse assay (a measure of mortality from intravenous infection), it has been shown that *E. coli* isolated from patients with pyelonephritis would cause death more often than those with either cystitis or asymptomatic bacteriuria.[20] Strains with particular O serotypes were not more common, but rather certain combinations of virulence factors seemed more important. Strains of O type O1, O4, O6, O8, and O75 are the five most frequent serotypes in symptomatic UTIs. These are most often both hemolytic and show mannose-resistant hemagglutination patterns. The same association was not found for K antigen as some K antigens were associated with hemolysins and others were not. Hemolysin activity was found to be present in bacteria that were negative for colicin V.[18]

Colicin V has been found in some cases of UTI pathogens, but it and some others such as K1 and R factors are probably all plasmid-mediated, which would be a decisive factor in only individual strains.[21] Both hemolysin production and the fimbrial determinants of UTI pathogenic bacteria appear to be carried on the chromosome.[22] Virulent strains carry both hemolysin and mannose-resistant fimbriae, and sometimes type 1 fimbriae, and these strains may represent descendants from a small number of clones that are nephropathogenic as well as some more frequently causing cystitis.[18]

Other *E. coli* not containing these virulence factors often cause cystitis and asymptomatic bacteriuria (ABU). They will, however, probably have the common type 1 fimbriae as the means of colonization of the perineum and the bladder. Colonization of the bladder does not always cause a symptomatic infection, probably because of the lack of other virulence factors.

HOST FACTORS IN URINARY TRACT INFECTION

Host Defense Mechanisms

The flushing, diluting effect of voiding urine is probably the most important host defense mechanism. In addition, the acidity, high urea concentration, and osmolarity impede the growth of many but not all bacteria.[10] The sloughing of the uroepithelium acts as a natural debridement of adherent bacteria, but excessive epithelial sloughing causes damage.

Residual Urine

Urologists generally hold that abnormalities that cause residual urine predispose to infection. Proof is difficult to find in either the clinical or experimental literature. Partial ureteral obstruction in the rabbit leads to hydronephrosis. The hydronephrotic kidney, however, is barely more susceptible to infection.[23] If the ureter of a rat is totally obstructed and ascending pyelonephritis produced in the opposite kidney, the obstructed kidney does not become infected.[24] A clinical study of benign prostatic hyperplasia showed that only 8.6 percent of those men (who had not been instrumented) with a residual of over 50 ml were infected.[25] Thus the impression that infection is common in these patients may be due to iatrogenic infection from the instrument used to determine residual urine. Women with residual urine also do not seem harmed by it. When women with persistent bacteriuria after infection during pregnancy were compared to those with sterile urine, the residual urine was the same.[26] Small amounts of residual urine have been found in both children[27] and older adults[28] with bacteriuria as opposed to those without bacteriuria. Thus bacteria may affect bladder function to the point of residual urine. The long-term results in these patients, found by screening studies, however, were no different from the controls.

Anatomic Abnormalities

There is no doubt that urologic abnormalities cause persistent recurrent infections. Thus abnormalities such as struvite infection stones, urethral diverticula, fistulas, and chronic atrophic pyelonephritis should be sought when recurrent symptomatic infections are caused by the same (or persistent) organism.[29]

Vesicoureteral Reflux

Many believe that bacteria only reach the kidney by vesicoureteral reflux. While 20 to 30 percent of all children with recurrent urinary tract infection have reflux,[30,31] of those infants and children investigated after their first episode of acute pyelonephritis, less than half had reflux.[32] Studies in both adult and infant monkeys have shown that infection causes reflux only if the ureterovesical junction has been made marginally competent by surgical means.[33] These studies agree with the theories of Hutch and Amar,[34] as well as the studies done in children by Gross and Lebowitz,[35] which show that infection does not cause reflux if the ureterovesical junction is normal.

Reflux does not predispose to infection,[36] but the presence of vesicoureteral reflux does appear to allow relatively avirulent bacteria to cause pyelonephritis.[37] Thus in the growing child with recurrent infections, whose reflux should disappear with maturation, prophylactic antibiotics should be continued until the reflux disappears. It has now been shown that even high-grade reflux may be treated medically as renal damage does not occur when either medical or surgical therapy is used.[38]

Pregnancy

Pregnancy is associated with a high incidence of acute pyelonephritis once bacteria colonize the urinary tract.[39] This is probably because hydronephrosis of pregnancy is due to ureteral obstruction by the gravid uterus.[40] Any bacteria reaching the ureter would then easily enter the kidney by intrarenal reflux as obstruction changes the shape of the renal papilla to allow free intrarenal reflux at low pressures.

Diabetes Mellitus

The incidence of bacteriuria in diabetic women is twice as high as in other women.[41] This may be due to the frequency of catheterization needed during management of episodes of diabetic coma, or the increased incidence of neurogenic bladder in these patients. Although there are no hard data to show an increase in renal damage from infection, indirect studies suggest that renal infection is common. Both renal papillary necrosis and renal abscess are more common in diabetics than others.[42]

Infection Stone

Infection stone follows urinary tract infection with urease-producing bacteria, most frequently *Proteus* species, although *Providencia*, *Pseudomonas*, *Klebsiella, Morganella, Serratia,* and some *E. coli* may also produce urease and cause such stones. Urease produces a highly alkaline pH by splitting urea and producing ammonia. This is a pH at which magnesium salts are insoluble, and with the increase in ammonia concentration magnesium ammonium phosphate stones are formed. Recurrent *Proteus* urinary tract infections should lead one to request radiographic studies to look for silent struvite stones. Staghorn calculi may occur in patients even in the absence of a febrile episode as they do not commonly cause acute pyelonephritis until a stone obstructs the ureter. Treatment consists of a combination of complete stone removal, while at the same time treating with culture-specific antibiotics. This most frequently now is done by percutaneous nephrolithotomy with additional extracorporeal shock wave lithotripsy of residual fragments. Following removal of stones percutaneously, the nephrostomy tube is irrigated with Suby's G solution, maintaining a sterile urine with antibacterials until plain film tomogram shows no residual fragments. If irrigation is required for more than several days, the addition of extracorporeal shock wave lithotripsy would be indicated. When the kidney is clear of stone, the urine should be kept sterile by continuous antibiotic therapy for 1 month, during which time the urine should also be acidified by treatment with ammonium chloride, adjusting the dose from 2 to 8 g depending on urinary pH to maintain the urine pH at 5 to 6. Despite all these therapies, the recurrence rate for infection stones is approximately 15 percent.[43,44]

Receptors for Pathogenic Bacteria

The specific urothelial receptor for nephropathogenic P-fimbriated *E. coli* is now known to be a glycolipid. The minimally active factor is a disaccharide α-D-Gal*p*-1-4-β-D-Gal*p*.[45] Over 99 percent of all females have this glycolipid receptor for P-fimbriated *E. coli.* Adhesion of these bacteria has been shown to be important in over 95 percent of children or adults with uncomplicated acute pyelonephritis.[46] Indeed, adhesion by these P fimbriae can cause ascending acute pyelonephritis even in the absence of vesicoureteral reflux as we have shown in the monkey.[47]

Why, then, do only 20 percent of all women develop a urinary tract infection? It appears that this is due in part to a more or less random colonization of the gut by P-fimbriated *E. coli.* In addition, there may be only a few clones of *E. coli* that are P-fimbriated but also carry other virulence factors necessary for invasive disease.[48] In addition, we have found that more P-fimbriated *E. coli* adhere to the urothelial cells of patients who have had acute pyelonephritis than to age-matched controls.[49] Thus receptor density availability is increased in infection-prone women.

Diagnosis. The diagnosis of uncomplicated UTI is best accomplished by midstream quantitative urine culture. Although a measurement of 10^5 organisms/ml of fresh urine has been considered diagnostic, even lower numbers (10^2 to 10^3) are diagnostic in symptomatic patients, especially if pyuria is present. Pyuria should not be determined on spun sediment; it should be quantitated by a hemocytometer technique. Pyuria is not a sensitive determination in complicated or upper tract infections. Cystitis is frequently accompanied by microscopic hematuria. Culture and sensitivities are essential for all complicated infections and for pyelonephritis in women, but it is not always indicated in uncomplicated lower tract infections in women. Pyuria, bacteria, and dysuria suffice for empiric treatment.[3]

SPECIFIC INFECTIONS AND THEIR TREATMENT

Principles of Treatment

Uncomplicated symptomatic UTIs in women should be treated with antimicrobial drugs. The urinary concentration of drug, not the tissue level, is critical. The cheapest drug that achieves good urine levels should be prescribed, for example, trimethoprim-sulfamethoxazole, norfloxacin, ciprofloxacin, or nitrofuradantin, for uncomplicated cystitis or pyelonephritis in women. If sepsis is suspected, treatment should be begun in the hospital with parenteral drugs. Recurrence should prompt a search for complicating factors and treatment should be governed by careful culture and sensitivities. Adjunctive measures include large fluid intake to prompt a normal diuresis, but excessive fluids dilute the antimicrobial concentrations in the urine. It is probably not necessary to treat asymptomatic bacteriuria. Women with more than three episodes of cystitis per year should be treated with low-dose or intermittent doses of prophylactic antibiotics.[3]

Acute Urethral Syndrome. This disease of females is characterized by frequency and dysuria without many bacteria. Indeed in over 70 percent of the cases a colony count of less than 10^5 bacteria/ml is found.[50] If pyuria is found (more than 10 WBC/ml^3) the infection is considered significant[51] and should be treated. These patients are most frequently infected with *E. coli.* Treatment with trimethoprim-sulfamethoxazole or nitrofurantoin is usually effective. *Chlamydia trachomatis* or *Neisseria gonorrheae,*[52] *Gardnerella vaginalis,*[53] and *Ureaplasma urealyticum* can also be causative.[54]

Nongonococcal (Nonspecific) Urethritis. The most common sexually transmitted disease is not gonococcal urethritis.[55] Thirty to 50 percent of the cases are caused by *C. trachomatis.*[56] Two genital mycoplasma organisms, *Ureaplasma urealyticum* and *Mycoplasma hominis,* may also cause nonspecific urethritis,[57,58] although their real importance as etiologic agents has been debated for years. Nongonococcal urethritis occurs in the same age group as gonorrhea. Men with the disease are more likely to be caucasian, in a higher socioeconomic group, and better educated and to have fewer sexual partners than men with gonorrhea.[59]

The urethral discharge in nongonococcal urethritis is clear and watery, and the disease frequently causes only minor symptoms of mild dysuria, perineal ache, urinary frequency, premature ejaculation, and pain on ejaculation. Urethral stricture does not occur.

The most serious sequela is Reiter's syndrome, which consists of nongonococcal urethritis associated with ocular, arthritic, and dermatologic findings.[60] The incubation period is approximately 14 days. The ocular manifestations vary from the usual mild transient conjunctivitis to anterior uveitis that may lead to blindness. The arthritis characteristically affects the large joints of the legs, Achilles tendons, plantar fascia, and sacroiliac joints. The arthritis usually remits after several months, although permanent disability can occur. Recurrences are common. The skin lesions are distinctive; balanitis circinata, well-demarcated erythematous erosions surrounded by a light border, occur on the glans penis in up to 80 percent of cases. Hyperkeratotic lesions occur on the soles of the feet and occasionally on the hands. Small superficial ulcers may also occur on the palate, oral mucosa, and tongue.

Nongonococcal urethritis is important because of its frequency and the need to distinguish it from gonorrhea, prostatitis, and cystitis. The diagnosis is usually made by clinical features characteristic of the urethral discharge and failure to demonstrate gonococci by Gram stain or culture. *Chlamydia trachomatis* can be cultured if special techniques are used.[61]

Tetracycline, 500 mg four times daily, or doxycycline, 100 mg twice daily, for 14 to 21 days, should be used for nongonococcal urethritis caused by *C. trachomatis.* Relapses are common: 17 percent of *Chlamydia*-positive and 47 percent of *Chlamydia*-negative patients have recurrences.[62] For patients who recur after tetracycline therapy, trimethoprim-sulfamethoxazole is the second-choice antimicrobial agent. Erythromycin, 500 mg four times daily for 7 days, is also active against *C. trachomatis* and is moderately active against *U. urealyticum.*

Gonorrhea. In 1983, 900,435 cases of gonorrhea were reported. This is a continued decrease in incidence since the peak in 1975.[63] The number of cases was probably a good deal greater, since many cases are not reported. The incidence of gonorrhea has increased markedly in the past 20 years. This increase is believed to be due to changing sexual mores and a decrease in the use of the condom, brought about in part by the widespread use of oral contraceptives. The incidence of gonorrhea in the United States is estimated to be three to ten times higher than in England because of the failure to trace and treat infected contacts. The highest incidence of gonorrhea occurs in people between 20 and 24 years of age.

Asymptomatic female carriers have long been known to be potential sources of spread. Handsfield et al[64] have now shown that men too can be asymptomatic carriers. The carrier rate is low, however, and more than 95 percent of men who become infected develop symptoms. Nevertheless, the men who remain asymptomatic or who ignore their symptoms become a reservoir of gonorrhea and can spread the infection to women. Handsfield et al[64] found that two-thirds of the men with asymptomatic gonorrhea remained asymptomatic carriers for as long as 165 days if treatment was withheld.

The gonococcus first adheres to the urethral epithelial cells by the fimbriae on the bacterial cells. The bacteria then penetrate the interepithelial spaces to reach the subepithelial connective tissue. An intense inflammatory reaction develops, with extensive exudate and abundant polymorphonuclear leukocytes. The overlying epithelium may be destroyed. The inflammatory reaction gives rise to the characteristic purulent discharge.[65,66]

The bacteria and neutrophils accumulate in the mucosal infoldings and in the periurethral glands of Littré. Infection in these mucous glands results in microabscesses. The infection may then extend to the corpus spongiosum. Lymphangitis and thrombophlebitis can result in extensive edema of the penis.

Gonococci can be demonstrated in prostatic secretions,[67] but infection of the prostate and seminal vesicles is rare. The infection can spread into the epididymis, however, through the vas deferens. Most infections are unilateral, but if both glands are involved the rate of infertility is high. The epididymis is involved in approximately 2 percent of cases of gonorrhea.[68]

The incubation period is 3 to 4 days, though it can be as long as 14 days. The patient usually has a purulent urethral discharge and symptoms of dysuria, urinary frequency, and meatal erythema. Because most symptomatic men seek prompt medical attention, the disease is usually promptly arrested. Men who do not develop symptoms and those who ignore their symptoms are at risk for developing complications. With the advent of effective chemotherapy, epididymitis, prostatitis, edema of the penis from dorsal lymphangitis or thrombophlebitis, inflammation of the corpus spongiosum, paraurethral abscess or fistula, infection of Cowper glands, and seminal vesiculitis are much less common.

Anorectal gonococcal infection causes rectal pain, tenesmus, mucopurulent rectal discharge, and rectal bleeding. Systemic gonococcal infection produces fever; arthralgia; petechial, pustular, and hemorrhagic skin lesions; and tenosynovitis. The infection may cause endocarditis, meningitis, myocarditis, and hepatitis.

The preferred drugs for treatment of gonococcal infection are penicillin G, ampicillin or amoxicillin, tetracycline, and spectinomycin. Because gonorrhea and syphilis often are contracted at the same time, the preferred treatment is aqueous procaine penicillin G, 4.8 million units given in two equal portions intramuscularly in two sites at one visit. Probenecid, 1 g orally, is also given as a single dose. This therapy is also adequate treatment for incubating syphilis. Spectinomycin, 2 g intramuscularly as a single dose, and tetracycline, 30 mg/kg/day orally four times a day for 4 days, are alternate regimens if the patient is allergic to penicillin. Recently, it has been shown that gonorrhea may be cured by a single 400-mg dose of ofloxacin. Follow-up serologic tests for syphilis should be done 6 weeks to 3 months later.

One-fourth to two-thirds of men develop a mild form of urethritis, termed postgonococcal urethritis,[69] 1 to 3 weeks after treatment for gonorrhea. In about half the cases, *C. trachomatis* is responsible. The cause in the other half is unknown. Probably the gonorrhea and *Chlamydia* infection were obtained together, but the incubation period for the *Chlamydia* is longer or antibiotic therapy may have eradicated the gonorrhea but only suppressed the *Chlamydia*.

Urethritis Associated with Indwelling Catheters. A urethral catheter or urethral foreign body not only perpetuates infection by its irritative effect but may also obstruct periurethral glands leading to periurethral infection. A thick yellow discharge from around the long-term indwelling urethral catheter is indicative of severe urethral infection. All urethral catheters left for more than a few days will have some associated mild urethritis unless antibiotics are given at the same time, as has been suggested in women who will only be catheterized for several days.[70]

The patient with bacterial urethritis usually complains of urethral pain around the catheter. If the infection is not cleared quickly, the patient will likely develop a urethral stricture some time after the catheter is removed. Proper treatment is removal of the catheter to facilitate urethral drainage. Most often, bladder drainage will still be necessary, so a suprapubic catheter should be placed by either operative or percutaneous techniques. The urethral infections caused by catheters are usually mixed, with gram-negative organisms predominating, so that a broad spectrum antibiotic should be given. Complications of urethral infections are stricture and periurethral abscess.

Catheter-induced urethritis can be reduced in incidence and severity by proper catheter care.[71] The choice of size and material of the urethral catheter will also bear on the frequency and severity of urethral infections. Large-bore catheters obstruct free urethral drainage of secretions and should be avoided in routine use. There are advocates of cutting side holes in the urethral catheters to allow urethral secretion drainage.[72] Teflon-coated, Silastic, or catheters with a hydrophilic coating cause less foreign body reaction than latex catheters.

Urethral Stricture and Its Complications. Urethral strictures can be a complication of gonococcal urethral infection as well as of trauma from indwelling catheters or urethral instrumentation. Dysuria, urgency, frequency, persistent urinary tract infections, alteration of the force, diameter, and appearance of the stream, and a split, narrowed, or dribbled flow of urine can all be due to urethral stricture. Strictures are occasionally discovered in asymptomatic patients when passage of a catheter is attempted. The diagnosis of stricture is established by cystoscopy, urethrography,[73] and calibration by bougie à boule.

Treatment depends on location, severity, age, and health of the patient. Strictures in nursing home patients, for instance, who require intermittent or continuous catheter drainage, are best managed by suprapubic cystostomy. In other patients, the initial treatment of strictures is dilatation. The stricture should be dilated without causing urethral tears, which in turn can lead to more scar formation and further narrowing. Dilatation may then be performed weekly or biweekly until a No. 28 or 30 French sound may be passed easily. Dilatation may be required for life. If the stricture recurs or becomes resistant to dilatation, a number of surgical procedures can be performed: internal or external urethrotomy,[74,75] stricture excision with urethral reapproximation, patch-graft urethroplasty, and marsupialization with or without later reconstruction.[75–78] If a stricture recurs quickly after dilatation, biopsy should be performed to rule out carcinoma. Chronic inflammation associated with urethral strictures can also lead to malignant degeneration and squamous cell carcinoma.

Urethral Diverticulum and Periurethral Abscess. Urethral diverticulum and periurethral abscess in men are complications of strictures and their treatment or may follow urethroplasty for hypospadias. Diverticula may be formed by infection behind the stricture or by traumatic urethral dilatations. Spinal cord injury patients develop diverticula and strictures as a result of applying condom catheters too tightly around the penis and causing compression and erosion of the penis and urethra. Urethral diverticula usually drain poorly and often become infected. Diagnosis is made by urethrography and cystoscopy. They should be resected and the associated urethral stricture repaired.[79]

Infected diverticula or infected periurethral glands may form periurethral abscesses in men or women. Infected urethral carcinoma may present as a periurethral abscess and should be looked for in any patient with the recent onset of stricture.

Periurethral abscesses present with fever and a fluctuant mass. They may rupture spontaneously or require incision and drainage. A urethrocutaneous fistula often forms after incision and drainage or spontaneous rupture. Adequate drainage and debridement are essential. Left undrained, the abscess may spread to involve the scrotum and lower abdominal wall. Frequently, suprapubic cystostomy will aid in local care by diverting urine from the wound. Extensive periurethral abscesses and urethrocutaneous fistulas in the bulbous urethra lead to the "watering pot perineum." Surgical repair of the causative stricture should be delayed until healing of the acute abscess has occurred.

Acute Cystitis. The patient with acute cystitis often presents with gross hematuria, thus another name is acute hemorrhagic cystitis. Within hours following this, however, the patient develops urgency, frequency, and dysuria. Treatment is indicated if pyuria is found and more than 100 colony forming units of any Enterobacteriaceae, *Staphylococcus saprophyticus,* or *Enterobacter* are found. While *E. coli* is still responsible for most of the cases, in young sexually active females, *S. saprophyticus* now causes up to 22 percent of all cases.[80] While previous therapy was 10 days of antibacterial agents, it has been found that single-dose therapy may be as effective.[81] A better response has been found with 3-day therapy. In those patients with over two recurrences per year either self-administered single-dose therapy with trimethoprim-sulfamethoxazole (four regular strength tablets) or continuous prophylaxis with either daily single-dose trimethoprim or nitrofurantoin has been shown to be both effective and economical treatment.[82]

Nonobstructive Pyelonephritis. The urinary tract proximal to the urethra is normally sterile. Thus colonization with bacteria that are pathogenic to the host must occur to cause an infection. Bacterial adhesion has been found to be a necessary event for colonization of any mucous membrane, be it the respiratory, gastrointestinal, or urinary tract. In some instances, this appears to be protective to the host. As an example, colonization of the perineum and vagina by lactobacilli may protect against colonization with pathogenic *E. coli* as suggested by in vitro studies of urothelial cells.[83] To begin, however, the gut must first be colonized with the bacteria in question. As to the urinary tract, these bacteria are Enterobacteriaceae, which most frequently adhere by means of fimbriae. The ubiquitous type 1 fimbriae, which adhere to mannose receptors on glycoproteins, are probably responsible for gut adherence to mucous membranes though this has not been proved. The *E. coli* organisms, which are the most frequent cause of urinary tract infection, are not pathogenic in the gut. They are not the enterotoxigenic *E. coli* that cause diarrheal disease by release of an exotoxin after adherence by means of fimbriae.[16]

Escherichia coli organisms must colonize the perineum prior to causing an ascending infection as has been shown in both women[84] and children.[85] After colonization for varying periods of time, ascent and colonization of the bladder will occur. The bacterial adhesion allows the bacteria to remain for a sufficient time to reach the critical concentration necessary to cause invasive disease. The host response to eradicate the infection would include sloughing of uromucoid cells to which bacteria are attached. In addition, the inflammatory response occurs, with chemotactic events leading to migration of polymorphonuclear cells into the bladder.[86] Cystitis is not thought to frequently involve bacterial invasion below the mucosa. While it was suggested by an in vitro study that granulocytes do not function well in the high osmolality of urine, in vivo they appear to phagocytose well.[87]

It is only when the host response is not sufficient or the bacterial virulence overcomes this response that further disease will occur. P-fimbriation of *E. coli* appears to be at least a marker of this virulence. Thus, while only 10 to 15 percent of all *E. coli* that cause urinary tract infections are P-fimbriated, 70 to 100 percent of all cases of nonobstructive pyelonephritis are caused by P-fimbriated *E. coli.*[88,89] P-fimbriation is not the only important factor, as hemolysin production and resistance to serum bactericidal activity also are commonly found with these organisms.[90] P-fimbriated *E. coli* organisms, as opposed to those without fimbriae or those with type 1 fimbriae, thus appear to be nephropathogenic.

Once colonization of the ureter occurs, the usual flow through a tube promotes adhesion of bacteria. This is because although flow through a tube is laminar in the center, at its outer edges, because of friction, turbulent flow is seen. This is essentially no flow.[91] Bacteria in the center would thus be washed out, while those at the wall would not be affected by flow. In addition, if the bacteria are P-fimbriated, they can adhere to the specific urothelial glycolipid receptor. This would allow bacterial growth and ascent, with new attachment of the bacterial progency. Growth will cover the urothelium within 48 hours of ureteral inoculation of the monkey with P-fimbriated *E. coli.*[92]

The close association between urothelium and bacteria that then ensues may well allow the effect of endotoxin, hemolysin, and other as yet unknown factors to affect surrounding cells. Indeed, it appears that colonization allows the effect of endotoxin to paralyze the ureter, as peristalsis ceases after infection.[93] When it does, the ureter becomes dilated and both resting and perfusion pressures increase. While the conical renal papillae ordinarily prevent intrarenal reflux until pressures are very high, this ureteral obstruction flattens the papillae, allowing intrarenal reflux of infected urine.[94] Intrarenal reflux of bacteria in studies of both pigs[95] and monkeys[96] always leads to pyelonephritis. This may well be because both monkeys[97] and pigs,[95] as well as humans, have receptors for P-fimbriated *E. coli* and adhesion to renal tubular cells occurs. Its importance in initiation of the disease has been shown by the fact that immunization with purified P fimbriae prevents both acute and chronic pyelonephritis in monkeys.[98]

At this point a very rapid sequence of events occurs—a host response to eradicate the bacteria, which may also lead to damage to the host. Complement activation occurs even in the first infection; thus activation may occur by the alternate pathway. Cytokine activation with production of interleukin 1 rapidly follows.[99] This is an important event as it leads to leukocyte adhesiveness and migration to the site of the bacterial antigen. This chemotactic event occurs rapidly, within 1 minute of bacterial inoculation of the renal tubule in our recent studies.[100] Damage may follow this event, however, as agglutination of leukocytes and platelets follows and capillary obstruction with ischemia and hemorrhage ensues. This is most significant 10 minutes after inoculation, the ischemia being obvious because of elevation of renal vein renin.[101] A more indirect method of showing the importance of complement in these events is to decomplement with cobra venom factor. This prevents acute pyelonephritis in both the rat[101] and monkey.[102]

Although phagocytosis of bacteria is an important event in clearing a bacterial infection, it appears to be harmful to the host as well. It has been shown in the rat that ablation of the granulocytic response by pretreatment with nitrogen mustard prevents renal tissue destruction.[103] Activation of phagocytes by bacterial antigen leads to both the degranulation and lysosome release and the respiratory burst. This appears to occur within 24 to 48 hours after infection.[92] On contact with bacteria, endocytosis occurs to form a phagocytic vacuole within which bacteria are killed. Later, contact of lysosomes with the vacuole allows release of enzymes into the vacuole. Since these enzymes also are released to the exterior, they may damage the tubular cells. However, at the time of initial phagocytic respiratory burst, the cell begins to release superoxide into the vacuole and at the same time from its cell surface.[104] The free radical superoxide and/or its metabolites, hydrogen peroxide, hydroxyl radical, or singlet oxygen (radical oxygen intermediates, ROI), may all be toxic not only to the bacteria but also to host tissues.[105] To test this hypothesis superoxide dismutase was administered to monkeys with pyelonephritis.[106] While the peripheral leukocytic response was the same in treated and control animals, the renal inflammatory response was decreased in the monkeys treated with superoxide dismutase and protection of the renal tubular cells was shown ultrastructurally. Thus the studies gave support to the idea that the initial renal events after infection are inflammatory and that phagocytosis may be harmful to the host as well as the parasite.

The foregoing suggest that prevention and early treatment of infection are critical to prevent renal damage. Since bacterial adherence appears to be the initial event in pyelonephritis, immunization against P fimbriae holds the most promise for the future as a preventive method. Treatment of an established renal infection must be rapid and rigorous. The initial therapy of acute pyelonephritis should be by a parenteral fluoroquinolone or cephalosporin until the results of culture and sensitivity are at hand when specific antibacterials may be used. Either a renal scan or intravenous pyelogram should be done within 24 hours to rule out obstruction. Obstruction must be relieved, either by percutaneous nephrostomy, surgical therapy, or cytoscopic insertion of indwelling ureteral catheter. If no obstruction is found, parenteral therapy is continued until the patient is afebrile for 48 hours. At this time, oral treatment with antibacterials is continued for a 2-week period. Later evaluation with a cystogram is suggested, at least in children, to rule out vesicoureteral reflux.

Emphysematous Pyelonephritis. Acute pyelonephritis associated with formation of gas in the collecting system may occur in both diabetics and nondiabetics. However, the finding of gas within renal tissue itself has been found only in patients with diabetes. Quite commonly, the infection is also associated with ureteral obstruction. Because gas within renal tissue in diabetics is associated with a mortality of 75 percent if treated medically, surgery is indicated and lowers the mortality rate to 25 percent. Nephrectomy within hours of the diagnosis is the treatment of choice.

Renal Abscess. A variety of abscesses can be found within the renal parenchyma: renal cortical abscesses, renal corticomedullary abscesses, and perinephric abscesses.

Renal cortical abscess (renal carbuncle) is most commonly the result of *S. aureus* septicemia, usually from skin infections of diabetics, drug abusers, and patients on dialysis. Most are unilateral solitary right kidney lesions, and the rest of the urinary system is normal. The patient presents with chills, fever, and costovertebral tenderness; laboratory values show a normal urinalysis and leukocytosis. The imaging study of greatest value is ultrasonography, but intravenous pyelograms are generally nondiagnostic and even the ultrasound can look like a neoplasm. Aspiration under guidance makes the diagnosis and initiates therapeutic percutaneous drainage. Open surgical drainage remains an option. Antibiotic treatment with oxacillin, nafcillin, and vancomycin have been successful even without drainage.

A renal corticomedullary abscess occurs secondary to an underlying lower tract disorder so that the usual gram-negative enteric pathogens (see Table 49–1) are etiologic.[3] Acute focal bacterial nephritis may precede the areas of liquefaction. Most of the predisposing abnormalities include renal calculi, obstructive uropathy, vesicoureteral reflux, and diabetes. The urinalysis and urine culture assist the diagnosis, which is best confirmed by ultrasonography and computed tomography (CT). Percutaneous drainage plus antibiotics (ampicillin plus an aminoglycoside is a good empiric choice) should be curative.

Perinephric Abscess. A perinephric abscess arises by direct extension from an infected kidney or by hematogenous spread, usually from sites of skin infection. While in the past *S. aureus* was the usual cause, now the bacteria most frequently cultured are gram-negative enteric bacteria such as *E. coli, Proteus, Pseudomonas,* and *Klebsiella,* especially in the presence of stone or obstruction.

Clinical manifestations include chills and fever, dysuria, unilateral flank pain, tenderness, abdominal pain and tenderness, abdominal mass, and flank mass. Tenderness to compression of the eleventh rib is often found. Ultrasonography is helpful in confirming the presence of a fluid-filled mass; however, CT scanning is now considered to be the best diagnostic study.

The treatment of perinephric abscess has in the past always been surgical drainage through the flank. However, it has been found possible to drain the abscess by percutaneously introduced catheters through which antibiotics may also be given. Relief of any concomitant ureteral obstruction by ureteral catheterization of nephrostomy tube is necessary, with later definitive surgical therapy.

Initial antibiotic therapy should be broad spectrum, because a variety of organisms can cause perinephric abscess. The antibacterial regimen can be more specific once a specimen has been obtained and can be further altered by culture results.

Infections of the Prostate

Acute Prostatitis. Prostatic infections may be caused by almost any bacterial agent. The gram-negative organisms *E. coli, Proteus, Klebsiella, Enterobacter,* and *Pseudomonas* predominate in acute and chronic bacterial prostatic infection. The gram-positive organisms *S. epidermidis,* alpha-hemolytic *Streptococcus, Enterococcus,* and diphtheroids are often thought of as normal flora in the distal urethra but have been reported to cause chronic prostatitis.[107] This is the only such report. It may well be that the previously reported *S. epidermidis* is actually *S. saprophyticus,* a common cause of acute cystitis in females as well.[108,109] Colonization of the urethra by Enterobacteriaceae is common, but ascending infection infrequently occurs probably because of the bactericidal activity of normal prostatic fluid.[110] The bacteria colonizing the normal man are the same ones colonizing the vagina of his sexual partner.[111] Therefore this is the probable source of catheter- or instrument-induced UTI in men. It has been suggested, but not universally agreed to, that all urethral instrumentation of men should be followed by antibacterial therapy. When the man's sexual partner gives a history of UTI, there is even more reason to do so. Parasite infections of the prostate do occur, but only *Trichomonas vaginalis* is a significant problem in the United States and Canada, and it more commonly causes urethritis. Tuberculosis of the prostate occurs when mycobacteria invade the prostate from upper urinary tract infection. Rarely, tuberculous prostatitis may occur as a sexually transmitted ascending infection.

Infections of the prostate are caused either by (1) infectious agents ascending the urethra, entering the prostatic ducts, and proliferating within the prostatic acini, causing marked inflammation in part or all of the prostate gland; or (2) infection in the urine entering the prostatic ducts during voiding, particularly if there is urethral obstruction distal to the prostate causing high voiding pressures within the prostatic urethra. Prostatic calculi may also act as foreign bodies to perpetuate infections.

Histologically, acute bacterial prostatitis shows polymorphonuclear leukocytes within and around prostatic acini and diffuse edema and hyperemia of the stroma. Small abscesses are common, therefore acute bacterial prostatitis presents with sudden onset of moderate to high fever and chills. Other symptoms are often nonspecific with general malaise and myalgia being prominent. Urinary symptoms may be absent or include frequency, urgency, dysuria, decreased urinary flow rate, intermittency and spraying, a sensation of incomplete bladder emptying, and occasionally total urinary retention.

The expressed prostatic secretions contain numerous leukocytes, but the prostate examination should not be vigorous, as bacteremia may occur. Manipulation or instrumentation can also cause retrograde movement of bacteria into the vasa deferentia, leading to epididymitis. Thus if urinary retention occurs, either a very small urethral catheter or suprapubic catheter should be used to relieve the retention.

The laboratory assessment of acute bacterial prostatitis should include a white blood cell count, which is usually elevated. Urine should be cultured, as bacteria are found in the urine even though the primary infection is in the prostate. Patients with acute bacterial prostatitis usually have ascending bacterial cystitis. Indeed, cystitis should not occur in the absence of prostatitis in men.[111]

Treatment of acute bacterial prostatitis consists of bed rest and antimicrobial therapy specific to the culture's sensitivity. Parenteral therapy with a cephalosporin or fluoroquinolone is often begun while awaiting the culture results. Because of the high concentration of fluoroquinolones in prostatic fluid, parenteral therapy with ciprofloxacin, norfloxacin, or ofloxacin is now used.[112]

Chronic prostatic infection is difficult to treat because most antibiotics do not diffuse into the prostate from the blood. The acute inflammatory reaction of the acute disease allows therapeutic levels of most antibiotics to reach the gland. In an attempt to prevent progression of the disease to the chronic state, it is recommended that an orally administered antibacterial be continued for at least 1 month after the patient has recovered from the acute disease and until the prostatic fluid has returned to normal.

Chronic Prostatitis. The clinical manifestations of chronic prostatitis vary widely. Although chronic prostatitis may follow acute prostatitis, most patients have no history of acute prostatitis.

Most patients have irritative voiding symptoms such as dysuria, urinary frequency and urgency, and nocturia. Low back pain, perineal discomfort, and painful ejaculation can also be found. Physical examination is frequently normal unless benign prostatic hyperplasia or calculi are also present. The differential diagnosis includes prostatosis, when more than 10 leukocytes per high-power field are found but culture is negative, and prostatodynia, when no leukocytes or bacteria are found.[113]

Meares' technique of urine and prostate fluid should be used for diagnosis.[114] A saline mount of the prostatic fluid should be examined for *T. vaginalis.*

The irritative voiding symptoms caused by prostatic infection can be mimicked by in situ carcinoma of the bladder, a serious disease that can be cured if detected early. Patients should have urine cytologies performed for irritative voiding symptoms if infection is not present, and then undergo cystoscopy. Infections in the prostate, including tuberculosis, can lead to formation of a palpable nodule. Biopsy of these nodules is mandatory to rule out carcinoma of the prostate in patients over 40 years old.

Chronic bacterial prostatitis is difficult to cure with most antimicrobial agents, probably because they do not diffuse from the plasma to the prostatic tissue and fluid. Thus the therapy of prostatic infections depends more on physiology than on the infectious agents. Prostatic fluid has a pH of 7.3, and this fluid becomes more alkaline (pH 8.3) with infections.[114,115] This would suggest that only a few antibiotics like trimethoprim-sulfamethoxazole and a fluoroquinolone would be effective in prostatic fluid. Recent studies have shown that the newer tetracyclines, such as doxycycline and minocycline, as well as carbenicillin, may also be effective. Long-term therapy for at least 6 weeks is suggested to increase this cure rate.[116] The bladder symptoms of prostatitis can be kept under control with long-term suppressive antibacterial therapy with nitrofurantoin. With this regimen, most patients remain relatively asymptomatic. Discontinuing the antibacterial therapy, even after months or years, may cause reinfection of the bladder urine and recurrence of symptoms.

Total prostatectomy offers the most definitive cure for patients with debilitating symptoms. Transurethral resection of the prostate can be curative if all infected tissue is removed. In a small series, Meares[117] cured only one-third of the patients. None of the patients who were not cured were made worse, although transurethral resection of the prostate can make the patient's irritative voiding symptoms worse.

Prostatic Abscess. Occasionally, acute prostatitis may lead to prostatic abscess. This occurs most often in patients with diabetes mellitus or immunosuppression. Transrectal needle biopsy of the prostate can also lead to abscess formation; thus prophylactic antibiotics such as a fluoroquinlone should be given prior to biopsy. Symptoms include acute urinary retention, frequency, dysuria, fever, and rectal discomfort. Since perirectal abscess may cause all these symptoms, it must be kept in mind in the differential diagnosis. The gland is enlarged, tender, and fluctuant. The abscess may spontaneously rupture and drain intraurethrally, or it may require endoscopic transurethral incision or perineal incision for drainage. Appropriate antimicrobial therapy should also be given. Abscesses usually leave no sequelae and usually do not recur.

Epididymitis. Epidydymitis rarely affects the prepubertal child in the absence of urethral manipulation. An indwelling urethral catheter is often the cause for urethritis and subsequent epididymitis.[118] It is thought therefore that retrograde ascent of bacteria from the prostatic urethra up to vas deferens is the cause. In young men, *C. trachomatis* is the most common organism,[119] but in older men, enteric bacteria, staphylococci, and occasionally streptococci predominate. In patients with long-term indwelling urethral catheters, unusual bacteria, such as *Serratia marcescens,* may cause epididymitis.

The epididymis is enlarged and tender. Some patients present with fever and systemic symptoms of toxicity. With rapid progression, suppuration, abscess formation, and extension into the testicle may occur but are unusual. In these cases, fluctuance is found with abscess formation. A reactive hydrocele often occurs, making differentiation of the epididymis and testis difficult. Aspiration of the hydrocele may thus be necessary. Infiltration of the spermatic cord with 1 percent xylocaine will often produce a reduction of pain that is lasting. In chronic epididymitis, tenderness may be mild, and the epididymis may only be indurated and slightly enlarged.

Urine culture should be obtained before treatment and the antibacterials used should be those indicated in acute prostatitis. If there is doubt about the diagnosis or if epididymitis does not promptly resolve, inguinal exploration of the testis should be performed to rule out testicular cancer. Because torsion of the testis occurs in young men as well, the distinction between epididymitis and torsion must be made. Early surgical exploration may be necessary to resolve any diagnostic questions and save the testis. In addition to antibiotic therapy, bed rest and scrotal elevation are very important in the treatment of acute epididymitis. Folded bath towels may be placed under the scrotum or alternatively, a wide band of tape can be placed across the upper thigh to provide scrotal elevation. Walking while wearing a scrotal supporter is permissible after the pain and swelling have subsided, but lifting and manual labor should be avoided for 2 to 6 weeks. If an abscess forms, surgical drainage is required.

Chronic epididymitis is an annoying and painful condition. Patients with chronic epididymitis are liable to recurrent acute attacks, especially if there is infection of the prostate and seminal vesicles that cannot be eradicated. Epididymectomy may be necessary for cure.

Orchitis. Infections of the testicle are rare and are usually caused by systemic viral infections, most notably mumps. Mumps orchitis is rare before puberty and occurs 4 to 6 days after mumps parotitis. Approximately 5 to 10 percent of adult men with mumps parotitis develop orchitis. The orchitis is unilateral in about 70 percent of cases and results in some degree of testicular atrophy.[120] The epididymis may also be involved, and sterility can result. The rich blood and lymphatic supplies of the testis give it a high degree of resistance to bacteria.

Although infection may occur by direct extension from severe epididymitis to involve the testis, producing epididymo-orchitis, this is rare. In this form of orchitis, the testicle is swollen and tense and has many punctate hemorrhages on its surface. Multiple foci of necrosis may be found. Suppuration may progress to involve the entire gland.

Acute pyogenic infection usually begins with chills and fever and sudden pain in the involved testicle. The pain radiates to the inguinal canal and is usually accompanied by nausea and vomiting. The involved testicle is swollen, tense, and extremely tender with a reactive hydrocele. If suppuration involves the entire gland, it becomes fluctuant. Testicular pain will often cause cremasteric contraction, drawing the testis high up into the scrotum where it is difficult to examine. The spermatic cord can be infiltrated with 1 percent xylocaine as in epididymitis, which will reduce the pain and permit better examination of the testis.

The patient is treated with bed rest, scrotal elevation, and antibacterial therapy. Bed rest, scrotal elevation, and warm or cold compresses provide symptomatic relief. Broad spectrum antibiotic therapy should be initiated until the specific causative agent can be identified by Gram stain or culture of urine or aspirated material. With prompt institution of antibacterial therapy, there is less suppuration, but orchiectomy is usually required.

Specific immunoglobulin or plasma can reduce the incidence of mumps orchitis by 75 percent if given early after the onset of parotitis.[121,122] Steroids or ACTH were thought to reduce testicular pain and swelling in men with mumps orchitis and reduce the incidence of orchitis if given prophylactically, but their efficacy has not been proved in controlled trials.[122]

Balanitis and Balanoposthitis. Bacterial infections of the glans penis usually occur in uncircumcised men with poor hygiene. Initially, an acute viral infection may cause open sores, and superinfection with mixed organisms, often anaerobes, quickly follows in the warm, moist environment. In other cases, especially diabetics, the infection is caused by yeast such as *Candida albicans.* Bacterial balanitis can be the initial presentation of other, more serious diseases or can be confused with these diseases (such as Kaposi's sarcoma, squamous cell carcinoma) and premalignant conditions (such as erythroplasia of Queyrat). Other skin disorders can also present on the penis, such as drug eruptions, leukoplakia, lichen planus, psoriasis, neurodermatitis, and eczematous eruptions. Biopsy may be required to differentiate them from infections or neoplastic lesions.

Without treatment, the infection may progress to cause gangrene and necrosis of the foreskin and glans penis. The organisms causing gangrenous balanitis are frequently oral anaerobes, the salivary contact occurring by fellatio. The first sign of gangrene is erythema, which progresses to ulceration, induration, and swelling of the prepuce, which then turns black. Gangrene of the prepuce can be accompanied by necrosis of the glans and in some instances entire penile shaft. The inguinal nodes are enlarged, and the patient will have systemic manifestations of infection such as malaise, chills, and fever.

Treatment of balanoposthitis consists in retraction of the foreskin, cleansing of the glans penis, application of topical antibiotics, and broad spectrum systemic antibiotics. Exposure of the glans penis to the air is helpful in treating the infection, and often a dorsal slit of the foreskin under local anesthesia is required. Gangrene, of course, requires appropriate surgical therapy.

Fulminating Gangrene of the Penis. Primary spontaneous fulminating gangrene of the penis is an entity distinct from the slowly progressive gangrenous conditions that may involve the penis secondary to other infections such as balanitis. Fulminating gangrene is commonly associated with gangrene of the scrotum (Fournier's gangrene)[123] and other types of perineal necrotizing infections.

Alpha-hemolytic streptococci and staphylococci are commonly listed as the causal organisms, but *E. coli, Clostridium perfringens,* and diphtheroids have also been implicated. Careful aerobic and anaerobic culture techniques will usually yield aerobic and anaerobic fecal flora. Thrombosed vessels are seen histologically at the periphery of the lesion.

The onset is sudden, with rapid progression to the gangrenous state. The infection may be confined to the penis. Within 24 hours, exudation and desquamation of the skin begin. Gangrene ensues and spreads rapidly to involve the entire penis. A line of demarcation spontaneously occurs, and the gangrenous portion sloughs down to the primary fascial planes. The corpora and testicles are not involved. At times, the gangrene also involves the scrotum and even the entire pubic region. The sloughed region may bleed and soon begins to granulate and heal. Systemic symptoms occur such as chills, fever, and pain. The mortality rate has been estimated to be 17 to 27 percent.

Treatment consists of debridement of necrotic tissue, irrigation with antiseptic solutions, and systemic antibiotic therapy. Antibiotic therapy should initially be based on Gram stains of the tissue specimens and modified depending on the culture results. Penicillin should be instituted if clostridial species are suspected. An aminoglycoside and clindamycin are a good initial combination for polymicrobial perineal infections.

Gangrene of the Scrotum (Fournier's Gangrene) Gangrene of the scrotum is a rapidly progressive, frequently mixed infection, usually caused by microaerophilic streptococci, enteric organisms, and gas-forming anaerobes. It is probably similar to necrotizing, synergistic gangrene found in other sites. Even *Entamoeba histolytica* and Rocky Mountain spotted fever (caused by *Rickettsia rickettsii*) have been associated with scrotal gangrene. Histologically, subcutaneous and dermal necrosis are seen together with an obliterative endarteritis.

The source of the infection is usually gastrointestinal organisms from such sources as an ischiorectal abscess or anal fissure,[124–126] but it can also occur with urethral stricture after extravasation of urine. In the otherwise normal diabetic, the organisms may enter the scrotum through tiny defects in the skin caused by abrasions or scratching.

The onset is sudden in the patient who does not have a stricture. This otherwise healthy individual is suddenly stricken with pain. Scrotal edema and swelling soon appear. The scrotum becomes tense, red, glossy, and moist. The gangrene is usually limited to the scrotum, but it may involve the penis or extend onto the abdominal wall. Systemic manifestations of fever, chills, nausea, vomiting, and prostration occur. Left untreated, the infection progresses to rapid death from sepsis.

Treatment is aimed at the scrotal gangrene, as well as any underlying pathology. The necrotic tissue should be debrided aggressively and widely until uninfected tissues are exposed. Culture of tissue and wound fluid should be incubated aerobically and anaerobically. Proper debridement will usually necessitate removal of most of the scrotum.

The testicles are not involved and can be left intact uncovered by skin or placed subcutaneously in the thigh. If clostridia are present, therapeutic hyperbaric oxygen should be considered.[126] If the penis or abdominal wall is involved or if urine extravasation had a role in the etiology of the gangrene, a suprapubic catheter should be placed. Upon resolution of the acute infection, split-thickness skin grafts can be placed on healthy granulation tissue when it appears over the exposed testicles. Ultimately, these grafts will assume the corrugated appearance of the normal scrotum.

Combination broad spectrum antibiotics should be given because of the likelihood of a mixed infection. If crepitation is present, penicillin in high doses should also be administered. The antibiotic regimen should be adjusted on the basis of Gram stains of debrided tissue and the results of the cultures, but antibiotic therapy should never replace debridement and drainage. An underlying infection such as ischiorectal abscess, epididymitis, or prostatitis should also be sought and treated.

Genitourinary Tuberculosis. Genitourinary tuberculosis rarely, if ever, occurs as an isolated infection. Rather, it is a local manifestation of a generalized infection that is disseminated via the bloodstream to any part of the body. Death from tuberculosis had been declining in the United States for the past 60 years, and the incidence of new cases of pulmonary and genitourinary tuberculosis was decreasing until recently. Pulmonary tuberculosis remains a major problem in developing countries, but in Europe the incidence has increased by approximately one-third and in the United States by approximately 15 percent. *Mycobacterium tuberculosis* remains the most frequent cause but in immunosuppressed individuals *M. bovis, M. avium-intracellulare,* and *M. kansasii* have also been reported. It is believed that the increase in the incidence of tuberculosis is due to several factors, one being the human immunodeficiency virus (HIV) epidemic with its immunosuppression as well as immigration of persons with tuberculous infection from other parts of the world. A contributing factor, however, is nonadherence in prescribing the recommended treatment regimens by the physician or patient nonadherence in following recommended treatment regimens, particularly in drug users who are at risk as well.

Because tubercle bacilli reach the kidneys via the bloodstream, both kidneys should be assumed to be involved in patients with renal tuberculosis. From the kidney, the tubercle bacilli may migrate down the urinary tract to involve the ureter, bladder, prostate, seminal vesicle, and epididymis. The kidneys in patients with renal tuberculosis can be destroyed by parenchymal involvement and destruction by *M. tuberculosis* or as a result of hydronephrosis due to ureteral stricture from tuberculous involvement of these sites. Most frequently, however, these strictures occur during the healing state after treatment.

The symptoms and signs of genitourinary tuberculosis vary markedly from one patient to another. In male patients, the earliest indication may be epididymitis.[127] Most patients, however, present with signs and symptoms of cystitis: urinary frequency, burning, and dysuria even though the site of infection is the kidney. Albuminuria and pyuria are found, but routine urine culture is sterile.

The physical examination in women is usually normal as it is in men who only have renal involvement. In men, the prostate may be shrunken and irregularly nodular from involvement of that organ. Epididymal involvement presents as nontender spermatic cord masses (the beaded vas) or it may be a solitary mass explored because of the suspicion of neoplasm. Rupture of an epididymal tuberculoma can lead to chronic draining scrotal sinus tract.

The diagnosis is most commonly made by finding tubercle bacilli in the urine. Patients with pulmonary tuberculosis should have periodic urine cultures to rule out renal involvement. In patients suspected to have prostatic or epididymal involvement, the semen should be cultured as well. Culture for tuberculosis and biopsy should also be performed on all nonhealing scrotal sinus tracts. The preferred therapy remains triple drug for 1 year, with the usual combination being isoniazide, rifampin, and ethambutal.[128]

REFERENCES

1. Gottschalk CW, Lassiter WE: Research Needs in Nephrology and Urology, Vol 1, DHEW Publ. No. (NIH) 78-1481. Bethesda, Department of Health, Education, and Welfare, 1978, pp 48–59.
2. Mulholland SG, Bruun JA: A study of urinary tract infections. J Urol 110:245, 1973.
3. Stamm WE: Approach to the patient with urinary tract infection. In Gorbach WL, Bartlett JG, Blacklow NR (eds): Infectious Diseases. Philadelphia, Saunders, 1992, p 788.
4. Stamm WE: Guidelines for prevention of catheter-associated urinary tract infections. Ann Intern Med 82:386, 1975.
5. Guinan PD, Bayley BC, Metzger WI, et al: The case against "The case against the catheter": initial report. J Urol 101:909, 1969.
6. McGuire EJ, Savastano JA: Long-term follow-up of spinal cord injury patients managed by intermittent catheterization. J Urol 129:775, 1983.
7. Kunin CM, McCormack RC: Prevention of catheter-induced urinary tract infections by sterile closed drainage. N Engl J Med 274:1155, 1966.

8. Burke JP, Garibaldi RA, Britt MR, et al: Prevention of catheter-associated urinary tract infections. Efficacy of daily meatal care regimes. Am J Med 70:655, 1981.
9. Bollgren I, Winberg J: The periurethral aerobic flora in girls highly susceptible to urinary infections. Acta Paediatr Scand 65:74, 1976.
10. Gibbons RJ: Bacterial attachment to host tissues. In: Gorbach WL, Bartlett JG, Blacklow NR, eds. Infectious Diseases. Philadelphia: Saunders, 1992, p 7.
11. Duguid JP, Clegg S, Wilson MI: The fimbrial and non-fimbrial hemagglutinins of *Escherichia coli.* J Med Microbiol 12:213, 1978.
12. Jones GW, Isaacson RE: Proteinaceous bacterial adhesions and their receptors. CRC Crit Rev Microbiol 10:229, 1983.
13. Källenius G, Möllby R, Hultberg H, et al: Structure of carbohydrate part of receptor on human uroepithelial cells for pyelonephritogenic *Escherichia coli.* Lancet 2:604, 1981.
14. Aronson M, Medalia O, Schori L, et al: Prevention of colonization of the urinary tract of mice with *Escherichia coli* by blocking of bacterial adherence with methyl α-D-mannopyranoside. J Infect Dis 139:329, 1979.
15. Balish MJ, Jensen J, Uehling DT: Bladder mucin: a scanning electron microscopy study in experimental cystitis. J Urol 128:1060, 1982.
16. Evans DG, Evans DJ Jr: New surface-associated heat-labile colonization factor antigen (CFA/II) produced by enterotoxigenic *Escherichia coli* of serographs O6 and O8. Infect Immun 21:638, 1978.
17. Rutter JM, Burrows RM, Sellwood R, Gibbons RA: Genetic basis for resistance to enteric disease caused by *E. coli.* Nature 257:135, 1975.
18. Hughes C, Hacker J, Roberts A, Goebel W: Hemolysin production as a virulence marker in symptomatic and asymptomatic urinary tract infections caused by *Escherichia coli.* Infect Immun 39:546, 1983.
19. Quackenbush RL, Falkow S: Relationship between colicin V activity and virulence in *Escherichia coli.* Infect Immun 24:562, 1979.
20. van den Bosch JF, Oe PL, Postma P, et al: Virulence of *Escherichia coli* in acute pyelonephritis, acute cystitis and asymptomatic bacteriuria. Antonie Van Leeuwenhoek 46:321, 1980.
21. Hughes C, Phillips R, Roberts AR: Serum resistance among *Escherichia coli* strains causing urinary tract infection in relation to O type and the carriage of hemolysin, colicin, and antibiotic resistance determinants. Infect Immun 35:270, 1982.
22. Swaney LM, Liu YP, Ippen-Ihler K, Brinton CC Jr: Genetic complementation analysis of *Escherichia coli* type 1 somatic pilus mutants. J Bacteriol 130:506, 1977.
23. Guze LB, Beeson PB: Experimental pyelonephritis. II. Effect of partial ureteral obstruction on the course of bacterial infection in the kidney of the rat and the rabbit. Yale J Biol Med 30:315, 1958.
24. Vivaldi E, Cotran R, Zangewill DP, Kass EH: Ascending infection as a mechanism in pathogenesis of experimental nonobstructive pyelonephritis. Proc Soc Exp Biol Med 102:242, 1959.
25. Hasner E: Prostatic urinary infection. Acta Chir Scand 285[Suppl]:1, 1962.
26. Williams GL, Davies DKL, Evans KT, Williams JE: Vesicoureteric reflux in patients with bacteriuria in pregnancy. Lancet 2:1202, 1968.
27. Lindberg U, Bjure J, Haugstvedt S, Jodal U: Asymptomatic bacteriuria in schoolgirls. III. Relation between residual urine volume and recurrence. Acta Paediatr Scand 64:437, 1975.
28. Shand DG, Nimmon CC, O'Grady F, Cattell WR: Relation between residual urine volume and response to treatment of urinary infection. Lancet 1:1305, 1970.
29. Stamey TA: Urinary tract infections in males. In Stamey TA (ed): Pathogenesis and Treatment of Urinary Tract Infections. Baltimore, Williams & Wilkins, 1980, pp 342–429.
30. Filly R, Friedland GW, Govan ED, Fair WR: Development and progression of clubbing and scarring in children with recurrent urinary tract infections. Radiology 113:145, 1974.
31. Rolleston GL, Maling TMJ, Hodson CJ: Intrarenal reflux and the scarred kidney. Arch Dis Child 49:531, 1974.
32. Winberg J, Bergstrom T, Jacobsson B: Morbidity, age and sex distribution, recurrences and renal scarring in symptomatic urinary tract infection in childhood. Kidney Int 4(Suppl):S101, 1975.
33. Roberts JA: Vesicoureteral reflux in the monkey: a review. Urol Radiol 5:211, 1983.
34. Hutch JA, Amar AD: In Hutch JA, Amar AD (eds): Vesicoureteral Reflux and Pyelonephritis. New York, Appleton-Century-Crofts, 1972, pp 145–189.
35. Gross GW, Lebowitz RL: Infection does not cause reflux. Am J Roentgenol 137:929, 1981.
36. Shopfner CE: Vesicoureteral influx. Five-year reevaluation. Radiology 95:637, 1970.
37. Lomberg H, Hanson LÅ, Jacobsson B, Jodal U: Correlation of P blood group, vesicoureteral reflux, and bacterial attachment in patients with recurrent pyelonephritis. N Engl J Med 308:1189, 1983.
38. Allen TD, Arant BS Jr, Roberts JA: Commentary: vesico-ureteral reflux—1992. J Urol 148:1758, 1992.
39. Savage WE, Hajj SN, Kass EH: Demographic and prognostic characteristics of bacteriuria in pregnancy. Medicine (Baltimore) 456:385, 1967.
40. Roberts JA: Hydronephrosis of pregnancy. Urology 8:1, 1976.
41. Vejlsgaard R: Studies on urinary infections in diabetes. IV. Significant bacteriuria in pregnancy in relation to age of onset, duration of diabetes, angiopathy and urological symptoms. Acta Med Scand 193:343, 1973.

42. Forland M, Thomas V, Shelokov A: Urinary tract infections in patients with diabetes mellitus. Studies on antibody coating of bacteria. JAMA 238:1924, 1977.
43. Griffith DP: Stuvite stones. Kidney Int 13:372, 1978.
44. Nemoy NJ, Stamey TA: Surgical, bacteriological, and biochemical management of "infection stones." JAMA 215:1470, 1971.
45. Källenius G, Svenson SB, Möllby R, et al: Carbohydrate receptor structures recognized by uropathogenic *E. coli.* Scand J Infect Dis 33(Suppl):52, 1982.
46. Källenius G, Möllby R, Svenson SB, et al: Occurrence of P-fimbriated *Escherichia coli* in urinary tract infections. Lancet 2:1369, 1981.
47. Roberts JA, Suarez GM, Kaack B, et al: Experimental pyelonephritis in the monkey: VII. Ascending pyelonephritis in the absence of vesicoureteral reflux. J Urol 133:1068, 1985.
48. Achtman M, Mercer A, Kusecek B, et al: Six widespread bacterial clones among *Escherichia coli* K1 isolates. Infect Immun 39:315, 1983.
49. Roberts JA, Suarez GM, Kaack B, et al: Host–parasite relationships in acute pyelonephritis. Am J Kidney Dis 8:139, 1986.
50. Stamm WE, Wagner KF, Amset R, et al: Causes of the acute urethral syndrome in women. N Engl J Med 303:409, 1980.
51. Stamm WE, Counts GW, Running KR, et al: Diagnosis of coliform infection in acutely dysuric women. N Engl J Med 307:463, 1982.
52. Curran JW: Gonorrhea and the urethral syndrome. Sex Transm Dis 4:119, 1978.
53. Fairley KF, Birch DF: Unconventional bacteria in urinary tract disease: *Gardnerella vaginalis.* Kidney Int 23:862, 1983.
54. McDonald MI, Lam MH, Birch DF, et al: *Ureaplasma urealyticum* in patients with acute symptoms of urinary tract infection. J Urol 128:517, 1982.
55. Dunlop EMC, Jones BR, Darougar S, et al: Chlamydia and non-specific urethritis. Br Med J 2:575, 1972.
56. Schachter J: Chlamydial infections (3 parts). N Engl J Med 298:428, 1978.
57. Bowie WR, Wang SP, Alexander ER, Holmes KK: Etiology of nongonococcal urethritis. In Hobson D, Holmes KK (eds): Non-gonococcal Urethritis and Related Infections. Washington, DC, American Society of Microbiology, 1977, pp 19–29.
58. McCormack WM, Braun P, Lee YH, et al: The genital mycoplasmas. N Engl J Med 288:78, 1973.
59. Weisner PJ: Selected aspects of the epidemiology of nongonococcal urethritis. In Hobson D, Holmes KK (eds): Non-gonococcal Urethritis and Related Infections. Washington, DC, American Society of Microbiology, 1977, pp 9–14.
60. Farber GA, Forshner JG, O'Quinn SE: Reiter's syndrome. Treatment with methotrexate. JAMA 200: 171, 1967.
61. Levy NJ, Munoz A, McCormack WM: Enzyme-linked immunosorbent assay for the detection of antibody *Chlamydia trachomatis* and *Chlamydia psittaci.* J Lab Clin Med 102:918, 1983.
62. Handsfield HH, Alexander ER, Wang SP, et al: Differences in the therapeutic response of chlamydia-positive and chlamydia-negative forms of nongonococcal urethritis. J Am Vener Dis Assoc 2:5, 1976.
63. Centers for Disease Control: Gonorrhea—United States, 1983. Morb Mortal Wkly Rep 33:361, 1984.
64. Handsfield HH, Lipman TO, Harnish JP, et al: Asymptomatic gonorrhea in men. Diagnosis, natural course, prevalence and significance. N Engl J Med 290:117, 1974.
65. King GJ, Swanson J: Studies on gonococcus infection. XV. Identification of surface portions of *Neisseria gonorrhoeae* correlated with leukocyte association. Infect Immun 21:575, 1978.
66. Swanson J, Sparks E, Young D, King G: Studies on gonococcus infection. X. Pili and leukocyte association factor as mediators of interactions between gonococci and eukaryotic cells in vitro. Infect Immun 11:1352, 1975.
67. Danielsson D, Mulin L: Demonstration of *Neisseria gonorrhoeae* in prostatic fluid after treatment of uncomplicated gonorrheal urethritis. Acta Derm Venereol (Stockh) 51:73, 1971.
68. Kraus SJ: Complications of gonococcal infections. Med Clin North Am 56:1115, 1972.
69. Holmes KK, Johnson DW, Floyd TM, Kuale PA: Studies of veneral disease. II. Observations on the incidence, etiology and treatment of postgonococcal urethritis syndrome. JAMA 202:467, 1967.
70. van der Wall E, Verkooyen RP, Mintjes-DeGroot J, et al: Prophylactic cipro-floxacin for catheter-associated urinary-tract infection. Lancet 339:946, 1992.
71. Uehling DT: The normal caliber of the adult female urethra. J Urol 120:176, 1978.
72. Turner-Warwick R: Complex traumatic posterior urethral strictures. J Urol 118:564, 1977.
73. Bissada NK, Cole AT, Fried FA, et al: Urethrography in the investigation of proximal urethral strictures. J Urol 110:299, 1973.
74. Kirchheim D, Tremann JA, Ansell JS: Transurethral urethrotomy under vision. J Urol 119:496, 1978.
75. Carlton FE, Scardino PL, Quattlebaum RB: Treatment of urethral strictures with internal urethrotomy and 6 weeks of Silastic catheter drainage. J Urol 111:191, 1974.
76. Olsson CA, Krane RJ: The controversy of single versus multi-staged urethroplasty. J Urol 120:414, 1978.
77. Devine PC, Fallon B, Devine CJ Jr: Free full thickness skin graft urethroplasty. J Urol 116:444, 1976.
78. Wein AJ, Leoni JV, Sansone TC, et al: Two-stage urethroplasty for urethral stricture disease. J Urol 118:392, 1977.
79. Devine CJ Jr, Horton CE: Urethral diverticula. In Horton CE (ed): Plastic and Reconstructive Surgery

of the Genital Area. Boston, Little, Brown, 1973, pp 405–406.
80. Wallmark G, Arremark I, Telander B: *Staphylococcus saprophyticus:* a frequent cause of acute urinary tract infection among female outpatients. J Infect Dis 138:791, 1978.
81. Wong ES, McKevitt M, Running K, et al: Management of recurrent urinary tract infections with patient-administered single-dose therapy. Ann Intern Med 102:302, 1985.
82. Stamm WE, Counts GW, Wagner KF, et al: Antimicrobial prophylaxis of recurrent urinary tract infections. A double-blind, placebo-controlled trial. Ann Intern Med 92:770, 1980.
83. Chan RCY, Reid G, Irvin RT, et al: Competitive exclusion of uropathogens from human uroepithelial cells by *Lactobacillus* whole cells and cell wall fragments. Infect Immun 47:84, 1985.
84. Stamey TA, Timothy M, Millar M, Mihara G: Recurrent urinary infection in adult women: the role of introital Enterobacteriaceae. Calif Med 155:1, 1971.
85. Bollgren I, Winberg J: The periurethral aerobic flora in girls highly susceptible to urinary infections. Acta Paediatr Scand 65:81, 1976.
86. Fukushi Y, Orikasa S: The role of intravesical polymorphonuclear leukocytes in experimental cystitis. Invest Urol 18:471, 1981.
87. Bryant RE, Sutcliffe MC, McGee ZA: Human polymorphonuclear leukocyte function in urine. Yale J Biol Med 46:113, 1973.
88. Väisänen V, Elo J, Tallgren LG, et al: Mannose-resistant haemagglutination and P antigen recognition are characteristic of *Escherichia coli* causing primary pyelonephritis. Lancet 2:1366, 1981.
89. Domingue GJ, Roberts JA, Laucirica R, et al: Pathogenic significance of P-fimbriated *Escherichia coli* in urinary tract infections. J Urol 133:983, 1985.
90. Caugant DA, Levin BR, Liden-Janson G, et al: Genetic diversity and relationships among strains of *Escherichia coli* in the intestine and those causing urinary tract infections. Prog Allergy 33:203,1983.
91. Weinberg SL, Jaffrin MY, Shapiro AH: Hydrodynamic model of ureteral function. In Boyarsky S, Tanagho EA, Gottschalk CW, Zimskind PD (eds): Urodynamics: Hydrodynamics of the Ureter and Renal Pelvis, Sec 3. New York, Academic Press, 1971, pp 217–231.
92. Fussell EN, Roberts JA: The ultrastructure of acute pyelonephritis in the monkey. J Urol 132:179, 1984.
93. Roberts JA: Experimental pyelonephritis in the monkey. III. Pathophysiology of ureteral malfunction induced by bacteria. Invest Urol 13:117, 1975.
94. Roberts JA, Angel JR, Roth JK Jr: The hydrodynamics of pyelorenal reflux. II. The effect of chronic obstructive changes on papillary shape. Invest Urol 18:296, 1981.
95. Ransley PG, Risdon RA: Reflux and renal scarring. Br J Radiol 14(Suppl):1, 1978.
96. Janson KL, Roberts JA: Experimental pyelonephritis. V. Functional characteristics of pyelonephritis. Invest Urol 15:397, 1978.
97. Roberts JA, Kaack B, Källenius G, et al: Receptors for pyelonephritogenic *Escherichia coli* in primates. J Urol 131:163, 1984.
98. Roberts JA, Hardaway K, Kaack B, et al: Prevention of pyelonephritis by immunization with P-fimbriae. J Urol 131:602, 1984.
99. Dinarello CA: Role of interleukin-1 in infectious diseases. Immunol Res 127:119, 1992.
100. Kaack MB, Dowling KJ, Patterson GM, Roberts JA: Immunology of pyelonephritis. VIII. *E. coli* causes granulocytic aggregation and renal ischemia. J Urol 136:1117, 1986.
101. Sullivan MJ, Harvey RA, Shimamura T: The effects of cobra venom factor, an inhibitor of the complement system, on the sequence of morphological events in the rat kidney in experimental pyelonephritis. Yale J Biol Med 50:267, 1977.
102. Roberts JA, Roth JK Jr, Domingue G, et al: Immunology of pyelonephritis in the primate model. VI. Effect of complement depletion. J Urol 129:193, 1983.
103. Shimamura T: Mechanisms of renal tissue destruction in an experimental acute pyelonephritis. Exp Mol Pathol 34:34, 1981.
104. Johnston RB Jr, Lehmeyer JE: Neutrophil and monocyte oxidative metabolism in inflammation: stimulation by surface contact and suppression by anti-inflammation agents. In Rossi F, Patriarca P, Romeo D (eds): Movement Metabolism and Bactericidal Mechanisms of Phagocytes. Padua, Italy, Piccin Medical Books, 1977, pp 243–256.
105. McCord JM, Wong K: Phagocyte-produced free radicals: roles in cytotoxicity and inflammation. In Fitzsimmons, DW (ed): Oxygen-free Radicals and Tissue Damage. Amsterdam, Elsevier/North-Holland, 1979, pp 343–360.
106. Roberts JA, Roth JK Jr, Domingue G, et al: Immunology of pyelonephritis in the primate model. V. Effect of superoxide dismutase. J Urol 128:1394, 1982.
107. Drach GW: Prostatitis: man's hidden infection. Urol Clin North Am 2:499, 1975.
108. Hovelius B, Mardh PA: On the diagnosis of coagulase-negative staphylococci with emphasis on *Staphylococcus saprophyticus.* Acta Pathol Microbiol Scand 85B:427, 1977.
109. Mardh PA, Hovelius B: *Staphylococcus saprophyticus* infections. Lancet 2:875, 1977.
110. Stamey TA, Fair WR, Timonthy MM, Chung HD: Antibacterial nature of prostatic fluid. Nature 218:444, 1968.
111. Stamey TA, Govan DE, Palmer JM: The localization and treatment of urinary tract infections: the role of bactericidal urine levels as opposed to serum levels. Medicine (Baltimore) 44:1, 1965.
112. Naber KG: Use of quinolones in urinary tract infec-

tions and prostatitis. Rev Infect Dis 11(Suppl 5):S1321, 1989.
113. Orland SM, Hanno PM, Wein AJ: Prostatitis, prostatosis, and prostatodynia. Urology 25:439, 1985.
114. Meares EM, Stamey TA: Bacteriologic localization patterns in bacterial prostatitis and urethritis. Invest Urol 5:492, 1968.
115. Fair WR, Couch J, Wehner N: Prostatic antibacterial factor: identity and significance. Urology 7:169, 1976.
116. Meares EM Jr: Serum antibody titers in urethritis and chronic bacterial prostatitis. Urology 10:305, 1977.
117. Meares EM Jr: Urinary tract infections in men. In Harrison JH, Gittes RF, Perlmutter AD, et al (eds): Campbell's Urology, Vol 1. Philadelphia, Saunders, 1978, pp 509–537.
118. Jacobs SC, Kaufmann JM: Complications of permanent bladder cathether drainage in spinal cord injury patients. J Urol 119:740, 1978.
119. Berger RE, Alexander ER, Monda GD, et al: *Chlamydia trachomatis* as a cause of "idiopathic" epididymitis. N Engl J Med 298:301, 1978.
120. Gall EA: The histopathology of acute mumps orchitis. Am J Pathol 23:647, 1947.
121. Smith RG: Plasma treatment of mumps orchitis. US Naval Med Bull 44:159, 1945.
122. Mongan ES: Treatment of mumps orchitis with prednisone. Am J Med Sci 237:749, 1959.
123. Jones RB, Hirschmann JV, Brown GS, Tremann JA: Fournier's syndrome: necrotizing subcutaneous infection of male genitalia. J Urol 122:279, 1979.
124. Burpee JF, Edwards P: Fournier's gangrene. J Urol 107:812, 1972.
125. Flanigan RC, Kursh ED, McDougal WS, Persky L: Synergistic gangrene of the scrotum and penis secondary to colorectal disease. J Urol 119:369, 1978.
126. Riegels-Nielsen P, Hesselfeldt-Nielsen J, Bang-Jensen E, Jacobsen E: Fournier's gangrene: 5 patients treated with hyperbaric oxygen. J Urol 132:918, 1984.
127. Wechsler H, Westfall M, Lattimer JK: The earliest signs and symptoms in 127 male patients with genitourinary tuberculosis. J Urol 83:801,1960.
128. Cos LR, Cockett ATK: Genitourinary tuberculosis revisited. Urology 20:111, 1982.

SPECIAL PROBLEMS IN SURGICAL INFECTIONS

PART VII

Tetanus

CHAPTER 50

Wesley Furste, Augusto Aguirre

Tetanus (lockjaw) is a dreaded infectious complication of wounds, caused by the neurotoxin, tetanospasmin, which is produced by *Clostridium tetani.*

This disease is characterized by tonic spasms of the voluntary muscles and by a tendency to episodes of respiratory arrest. Total prevention by immunization with tetanus toxoid is possible.

Tetanus has been recognized as a terrifying disease for 2300 years. Hippocrates referred to a patient, the master of a large ship, who smashed the index finger of his right hand with the anchor: "Seven days later a somewhat foul discharge appeared; then trouble with his tongue . . . on the third day opisthotonos occurred with sweating . . . 6 days later he died."[1] In the second century, Aretaeus, the Cappadocian, called the disease an inhuman calamity, an unseemly sight, a spectacle painful even to the beholder.[2] He wrote, "The wish of the physician that the patient should expire, otherwise irreverent and objectionable, is, in this case well taken" (Fig. 50–1).

In spite of the many advances in medicine and surgery, tetanus, although completely preventable, still occurs and appears as it was described centuries ago.[3] For example, in 1991, an 80-year-old woman in Ohio died of tetanus due to a wood splinter in her left lower leg. In 1992, a 31-year-old woman in Vermont developed tetanus from a puncture wound at the base of her right great toe sustained while walking in her yard. She recovered.

The results of the therapy of tetanus are not yet ideal. Tetanus can become a disease of only historic significance if physicians constantly consider and implement four basic principles: (1) administration of tetanus toxoid when indicated; (2) immediate, meticulous surgical care of all wounds; (3) administration of tetanus immune globulin when indicated; and (4) use of emergency medical identification devices for all individuals (Fig. 50–2).

Incidence and Epidemiology. The clinical introduction of tetanus toxoid a half a century ago was followed in many parts of the world by immunization of entire populations and contributed greatly to the control of tetanus.

In developed countries, like the United States, the incidence of tetanus is less frequent (Fig. 50–3). Certain populations have a higher incidence; it is greatest in the South. Noncaucasians have a fivefold greater incidence, men are more frequently affected than women, and older adults who have not been immunized have the highest incidence (Fig. 50–4). Most cases appear in the spring, summer, and early fall, when outdoor activity and exposure to the organism in the soil are the greatest. Heroin addicts are particularly susceptible, especially when quinine is injected, because this agent appears to produce locally anaerobic conditions.

At the Eighth International Conference in Leningrad, Russia, in 1987, the Conference partici-

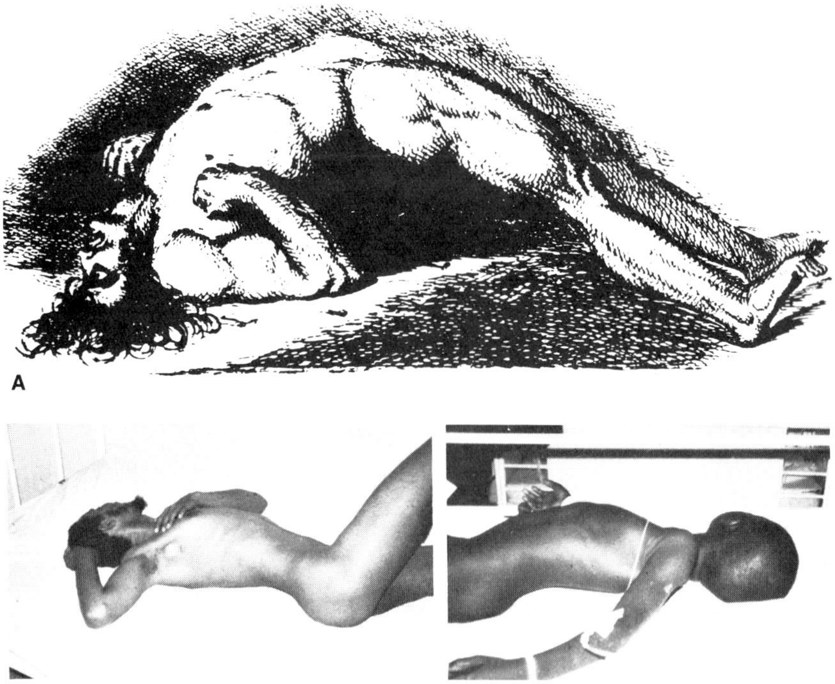

A B C

Figure 50–1. **A.** Tetanus as depicted by Sir Charles Bell during the 19th century. **B.** In a man. **C.** In a boy. *(Courtesy of United States National Library of Medicine.)*

to put E.M.I. to work for you...

fill in both sides of this card. **For example,** under

Immunizations

The date is important. If you note immunization over three years old, ask your doctor about a booster immunization. For tetanus toxoid, note the date of your first immunization as well as your last.

Present Medical Problems

Epilepsy	Tracheotomy (neck breather)
Diabetes	Pneumothorax
Glaucoma	Pneumoperitoneum
Hemophilia	Colostomy
Chorea	

Dangerous Allergies

Drug allergies	Feathers (pillows)
Horse serum (as in tetanus antitoxin)	Common foods
	Penicillin sensitivity

Medicines Taken Regularly

Anticoagulants	When noting drugs, ask your doctor for the name to use that will be easy to identify in an emergency.
Cortisone or ACTH	
Heart drugs such as digitalis or nitrites	
Thyroid preparation	

Other Information

Scuba diver	Speak no English (note the language you speak)
Recurring unconsciousness	Wearing contact lenses
Hard of hearing	

Additional copies may be purchased from:
Order Department OP-2
American Medical Association
535 N. Dearborn St.
Chicago, Illinois 60611

YA:5025:907-N:25M:10/77

Medical Information

Last Immunization Date

diphtheria ______ **mumps** ______ **tetanus toxoid** ______

German measles ______ **polio Sabin** ______

measles ______ **small pox** ______ **typhoid** ______

Present Medical Problems ______

Medicine Taken Regularly ______

Dangerous Allergies ______

Other Information ______

Copyright 1970, 1977 American Medical Association

EMERGENCY MEDICAL IDENTIFICATION

American Medical Association
535 North Dearborn Street
Chicago, Illinois 60610

Why You Should Carry Emergency Medical Identification

An emergency medical identification card is your protection in an emergency. If you are not able to tell your medical story after an accident or sudden illness, the information entered on this card can save your life.

You may have health problems which can affect your recovery from an emergency. You may have a problem which is no emergency but often is treated as one, such as epilepsy. Even if you do not have a health problem, the information on this card can be of valuable assistance to the first aid attendant.

Why You Should Wear an Emergency Medical Signal Device

In an emergency, you may be separated from your pocket card. Possibly you are one who has a medical problem so critical that it must be immediately known to those who help you. If so, a signal device of durable material should be worn around your neck or wrist so that it can be present at all times, even while swimming.

The device should be fastened to the person wearing it with a strong nonelastic cord or chain so designed that it does not become an accident hazard in itself.

On this device there should be:

- The symbol of emergency medical identification
- The name of your major health problem
- For children and the aging, the name and address of a responsible relative and a telephone number, including area code.

Carry Your Card and Wear Your Signal Device at All Times!

Emergency Medical Identification

My name is ______

Please call ______

My Doctor is ______

Figure 50–2. Front and back sides of an effective emergency medical identification device. *(Courtesy of American Medical Association.)*

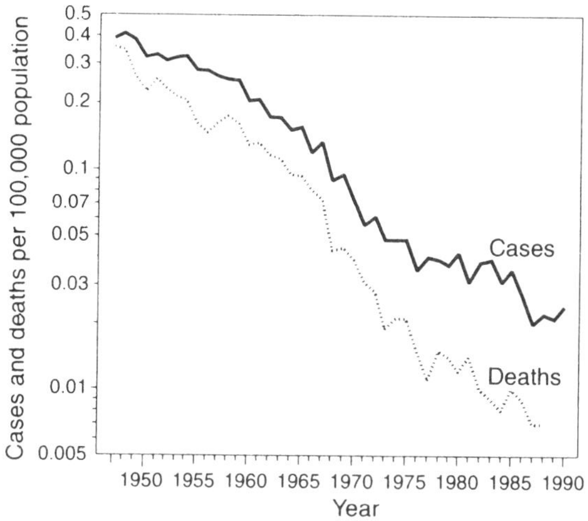

Figure 50–3. Reported incidence of tetanus and tetanus-related deaths—United States, 1947 to 1990. After substantial declines in occurrence following widespread vaccination of children, the annual number of reported tetanus cases has been stable since 1986. The lack of further decline probably reflects continued inadequate vaccination coverage of the older portion of the population. *(From Centers for Disease Control and Prevention: Morb Mortal Wkly Rep 41(SS-8):3, 1992.)*

pants estimated a yearly incidence in developing and underdeveloped countries of possibly 1,700,000 cases and of a worldwide mortality rate ranging from 25 to 85 percent. Most of these are neonatal with a mortality rate of 85 percent.[4] Such figures are only estimates, because accurate data are very difficult to obtain.

Etiology

MICROBIOLOGY. *Clostridium tetani* is a large, gram-positive, actively motile bacillus, which in its spore-bearing form has a characteristic drumstick appearance. Spores may develop at either end of the bacillus, giving a dumbbell appearance. It is strictly anaerobic; spores will not germinate in the presence of even the smallest amount of oxygen. The spores of *C. tetani* are found worldwide in soils, dust, and the feces of humans and animals. The spores resist killing by phenol and boiling, although autoclaving destroys them.

After germination, *C. tetani* produces two exotoxins, tetanospasmin and tetanolysin. Of these, tetanospasmin is the neurotoxin that produces the typical muscle spasms of tetanus. The organism itself apparently has almost no properties that permit it to invade tissue or elicit inflammatory responses.

Pathogenesis and Pathology. Clostridium tetani is almost always acquired by implantation of the organism into tissues via breaks in mucosal or skin barriers.[5–8] The routes of infection for a large number of cases of tetanus in India are listed in Table 50–1. Of particular interest is the absence of any apparent wounds in 14.2 percent, the high incidence of puerperal and umbilical tetanus (neonatal tetanus), and the high incidence associated with otorrhea.[5]

Table 50–2 lists the injuries associated with 285 cases of tetanus in the United States.[8] The majority appeared after punctures, lacerations, and abrasions. Only a small number appeared in wounds classically associated with large amounts of anaerobic devitalized tissue. Many wounds appear to be healed (cryptogenic tetanus). No injury seems categorically unsuited for spore germination, especially if infection with facultatively anaerobic organisms further reduces redox potential. Spores

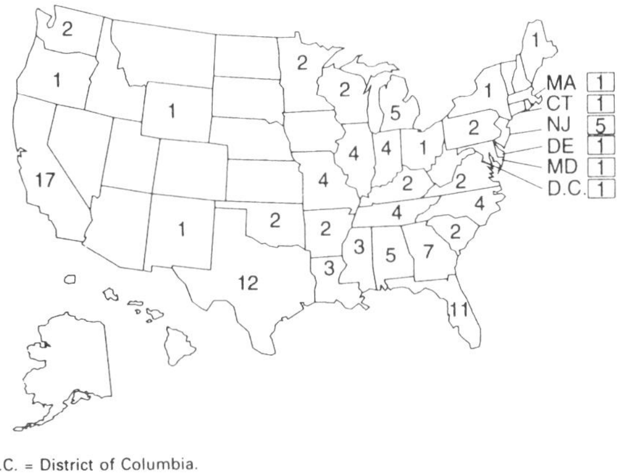

*D.C. = District of Columbia.

Figure 50–4. Number of reported tetanus cases by state—United States, 1989 to 1990. *(From Centers for Disease Control and Prevention: Morb Mortal Wkly Rep 41(SS-8):4, 1992.)*

TABLE 50–1. ROUTE OF INFECTION OF *C. TETANI* IN A LARGE SERIES OF TETANUS CASES AT THE KING EDWARD MEMORIAL HOSPITAL, BOMBAY, INDIA

Route	Total	Percentage
Injury	892	44.5
Otorrhea	406	20.2
Umbilicus	292	14.5
Unknown	283	14.2
Puerperal	67	3.3
Injection	32	1.6
Vaccination	20	1.0
Operation	15	0.7

Adapted from Patel JD, Mehta BC: Indian J Med Sci 17:791, 1963.

TABLE 50–2. TETANUS CASES BY TYPE OF ASSOCIATION INJURY IN THE UNITED STATES

Type of Wound	Number of Cases	Proportion Total Cases (%)	Case/Fatality Ratio (%)
Puncture	105	36.8	51.5
Laceration	101	35.4	45.6
Abrasion	22	7.7	60.0
Crush	10	3.5	50.0
Surgical	9	3.2	62.5
Injection	2	0.7	100
Multiple injury	31	10.9	46.7
No injury	5	1.8	25.0
Total	285	100	49.4

From Smith A: Tetanus. In Beeson PB, McDermott W (eds): Cecil-Loeb Textbook of Medicine, 13th ed. Philadelphia, Saunders, 1971, p 566.

may persist in healed wounds for years and will occasionally germinate later after reinjury or operation. Postoperative tetanus, however, usually results from breaks in sterile technique or wound contamination with intestinal contents.

During 1989 to 1990 in the United States, 86 cases of tetanus occurred after an identified acute injury.[7] Most (52 percent) occurred following puncture wounds, 23 percent after lacerations, and 17 percent after abrasions. Most of the wounds were due to a sharp object (splinter, nail) penetrating the lower extremity, but all wounds in all sites are susceptible. The injury most often occurred during farming, gardening, or other outdoor activities. Only one case occurred following operation (mammoplasty).

Table 50–3 presents the vaccination status of persons with reported tetanus in the United States during 1989 to 1990. The cases with more than two doses always raise the possibility that the history of previous doses is incorrect.

TABLE 50–3. VACCINATION STATUS OF PERSONS WITH REPORTED TETANUS—UNITED STATES, 1989 to 1990

Vaccination Status	Number	Percentage
0 doses	34	31.2
1 dose	9	8.3
2 doses	2	1.8
3 doses	2	1.8
≥4 doses	10	9.2
Unknown	53	48.2
Total	110	100.0

From Centers for Disease Control and Prevention: Morb Mortal Wkly Rep 41(SS-8):6, 1992.

The mere presence of *C. tetani* in a wound does not necessarily mean that the patient has or will develop tetanus. The organisms proliferate only in the presence of an oxidation-reduction potential far lower than that existing in normal living tissue. As soon as *C. tetani* begins to multiply, it produces tetanospasmin, which is transported to the central nervous system, where it becomes fixed and is responsible for the development of tetanus. Tetanospasmin is a protein with a molecular weight of 67,000 with a potency equivalent to botulinus toxin; a dose of approximately 130 μg of purified tetanospasmin is lethal. There have been differences of opinion concerning the site of action of tetanospasmin and the route by which it spreads.[8] Apparently, wound toxin spreads centrally along the motor nerve trunks to the spinal cord and brain stem.[9] Tetanus will develop after an intravenous injection of toxin into animals.

The route by which toxin clears the blood-brain barrier and enters the central nervous system is not clear. Toxin injected intramuscularly apparently spreads both by passing centrally in nerves and by absorption into the blood.

The toxin, which can be neutralized by antitoxin at the site of production in a wound or en route to the nervous system, becomes bound to central nervous system gangliosides. Early involvement of the lower cranial nerves is most frequent, but widespread central nervous system involvement is common when tetanus is fatal. The action of tetanospasmin mimics that of strychnine in suppressing the central inhibitory influences on motor neuron activity, leading to intensified, reflex responses to afferent stimuli. Convulsions and spasticity result. The sympathetic, neurocirculatory, and neuroendocrine systems are also involved so that hypertension, tachycardia, peripheral vasoconstriction, and cardiac arrhythmias may be seen.

The causes of death in treated tetanus are complex. Pulmonary complications appear to be important in patients who survive more than 1 week. Degenerative changes in the respiratory muscles may play an important role, because such changes become more severe with increased survival time.[10] If the patient survives, the toxin is metabolized, and no permanent neurologic injury is evident.

Clinical Picture. The incubation period between wounding and the onset of symptoms is variable. The median incubation period is approximately 7 days (range, 0 to 123 days); 70 percent of disease appears between 4 and 14 days. The incubation period does not correlate with mortality.

Tetanus almost always appears in a general form, but occasionally it may appear as local tetanus with increased muscle tone and spasms confined to muscles near a wound, without systemic signs. Neonatal tetanus is first recognized as a difficulty in sucking, beginning at 3 to 10 days of age, progressing to generalized tetanus. Cephalic tetanus may follow injury to the head or otitis. The incubation period is short and the mortality extremely high. In this form, cranial motor nerve palsies are common, but if the patient survives, total recovery ensues.

In general tetanus, some patients have prodromal symptoms of restlessness and headaches. In others, the first symptoms are those stemming from the developing muscle rigidity, with vague discomfort in the jaws, neck, or lumbar region. In an early stage, spasm of the muscles of mastication causes trismus and difficulty with chewing, ie, lockjaw. Sustained contraction of the facial muscles produces a distorted grin (risus sardonicus). Spasm of the pharyngeal muscles makes swallowing difficult; a stiff neck is among the early signs. Progressively, other muscle groups become involved. Tightness of the chest and rigidity of the abdominal wall, the back, and the limbs become evident. Orthotonos, opisthotonos, or emprosthotonos may develop.[11] Generalized tonic convulsions are frequent, exhausting, and unpredictable. Any external stimulus (a breeze, sudden movement, noise, light) and many internal stimuli (cough, swallow, distended bladder) may trigger such generalized convulsions. In association with these convulsions, spasms may occur of the laryngeal and respiratory muscles, possibly with occasional fatal, acute asphyxia.

The patient is mentally alert throughout the course of the disease and suffers great pain from the muscle spasms. The pulse rate is elevated, and there is profuse perspiration. Fever may or may not be present. Neurologic examination discloses hyperactive tendon reflexes, often with sustained clonus. There are no sensory changes.

Cases have been classified as mild, moderate, and severe corresponding to the length of incubation, severity of paroxysms, and degree of autonomic dysfunction. In severe cases, patients may experience sudden changes in hemodynamic vital signs, either spontaneously or in response to external stimuli. Patients who survive more than 1 week gradually improve over 2 to 6 weeks, but total recovery may take months.

The diagnosis of tetanus must be based on the clinical picture, associated with no prior history of immunization, because laboratory examinations are not available for routine use. The demonstration of *C. tetani* in a wound does not diagnose tetanus; the failure to demonstrate the bacillus in a wound does not eliminate the diagnosis. Fever is initially mild, leukocytosis moderate, and cerebrospinal fluid normal.

Rarely has the surgical literature included notes on the progress of these patients. After giving the clinician's account of successful treatment of tetanus in a 20-year-old analytical chemist, Cole et al[12] included their patient's personal account of his illness.

> The first symptoms started approximately a week after I had cut my finger. They consisted in a sudden tightening around my throat causing extreme difficulty in breathing and making swallowing virtually impossible. During this spasm, coughing or expectoration added to the difficulty in obtaining air as my throat seemed to collapse when I tried to inspire.
>
> Spasms of the throat usually appeared at rest and lasted about ten minutes in the early stages. Later on, they were more prolonged. Two days after admission they seemed continuous, and about this time my voice became reduced to a whisper and my jaw felt stiff. The symptoms from then on are only snatches of memory. I felt like snarling, my upper lip involuntarily drawing back over the teeth, and a peculiar twitch was vaguely present in my limbs. . . .
>
> After several days I lost the fear of never being able to breathe when off the respirator, as it was always restored quickly. I only had one really scary time, when the tube fell out after replacement. I know it felt more secure when the tube from the ventilator was *screwed* into the tracheostomy socket and not just pushed in. Also, when the tube was taken off before the suction apparatus was made ready, the time taken was terrifyingly long. . . .

Diagnosis. The differential diagnosis may be difficult to make in early tetanus, but severe tetanus can be confused with a few other diseases, such as the following.

Heterologous serum sickness may be confused with early tetanus in patients who have received heterologous antisera in an effort to prevent the disease. In the United States, heterologous tetanus antitoxin should no longer be given.

Hypocalcemic tetany is less severe than tetanus and may follow operations on the thyroid or parathyroid glands when the latter are injured or removed. The upper extremities are primarily affected, the serum calcium is low, and calcium infusions provide easy control.

Meningitis and encephalitis usually provide enough signs to enable a physician to differentiate them from tetanus. In addition, the cerebrospinal fluid examination is an aid to diagnosis.

Rabies is indicated early by an inability to swallow, drooling of saliva, and spasms of the muscles of deglutition. Trismus is rare, and spinal fluid pleocytosis is frequent. Animal bites may precede both tetanus and rabies, but the incubation period is much longer for rabies.

Strychnine poisoning may mimic tetanus closely, except that the muscles are relaxed between seizures in strychnine intoxication, whereas spasms tend to persist in tetanus.

Central nervous system cancer metastases can mimic the symptoms of tetanus.

Drug toxicity to penicillin, to haloperidol, to lead, or to phenothiazine tranquilizer drugs may be differentiated from tetanus by an adequately taken history.

Acute hysteria and *acute psychoses* may be quite difficult to differentiate from early or mild tetanus until the patient has been evaluated for several days.

Spasms of a localized group of voluntary muscles that result from soft tissue or bone injuries may simulate local tetanus.

Trismus not caused by tetanus may occur with peritonsillar abscess, dental infections, and other local infections of the mouth and cervical regions, and with dentomandibular problems.

Meningitis, sepsis, hypocalcemic tetany, hypomagnesemia, metabolic alkalosis, and *intracranial hemorrhage* can be confused with neonatal tetanus. Newborns of drug-addicted mothers can have temporary tetanus-like symptoms.

Stiff-man syndrome, said to be associated with occult breast cancer, can at first be confused with subacute tetanus, but the slow progression, for months or years, eventually differentiates it from tetanus.[13]

Malingering, mimicking the signs of mild tetanus, may be used for monetary or other reasons. One unusual patient did so to remain near a ward nurse (OH Wangensteen, personal communication).

The failure to demonstrate a wound does not eliminate a diagnosis of tetanus, for many cases have occurred without a demonstrable wound.

Prognosis. Even when treatment is adequate, the mortality rate may exceed 50 percent.[4,6] Patients who survive 10 days or more have a good chance of total recovery.[10] Many combinations of nonfatal complications may be responsible for death. Pulmonary atelectasis and aspiration can be followed by pneumonia. Traumatic glossitis is often seen. Compression fractures of the vertebrae may result from the convulsive seizures. Decubitus ulcers may occur. Constipation, fecal impaction, and urinary retention are often encountered. Cystitis and pyelonephritis may develop in patients who require catheterization. Foot drop and muscle contractures may follow prolonged unconsciousness. Asphyxia from respiratory or laryngeal muscle spasm or from aspiration of secretions, vomitus, or food can be the immediate cause of death. Coagulopathy can develop, as can fatal pulmonary emboli.

In long-term follow-up studies, irritability, insomnia, fits, myoclonus, decreased libido, postural hypotension, and electroencephalographic abnormalities have been recorded.

The professional liability law suit is an annoying complication for the physician, which can occur months or years after a case of tetanus, and for which well-documented records are most important.[10]

Prevention. Tetanus is almost of historic significance in the United States because of the implementation of the effective and inexpensive methods of tetanus prophylaxis that are available. Such methods are outlined in Tables 50–3 to 50–6, which represent the combined thinking and recommendations of many. If the elderly were properly immunized with tetanus toxoid, there would be fewer cases in the United States (Fig. 50–5).[14–26]

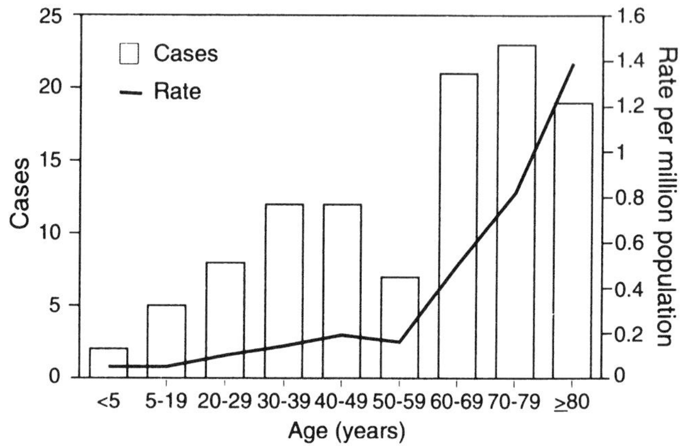

Figure 50–5. Reported tetanus cases and incidence rates by age group—United States, 1989 and 1990. The largest number of cases occurred among persons 60 years of age and older. This is consistent with serosurveys that show that 31 to 71 percent of older adults lack protective levels of tetanus antibodies. Health care providers who treat the elderly should take every opportunity to ensure that their patients are protected against tetanus and diphtheria in accordance with Immunization Practices Advisory Committee (ACIP) recommendations. *(From Centers for Disease Control and Prevention: Morb Mortal Wkly Rep 41(SS-8):5, 1992.)*

TABLE 50–4. ROUTINE DIPHTHERIA, TETANUS, AND PERTUSSIS VACCINATION SCHEDULE SUMMARY FOR CHILDREN UNDER 7 YEARS OF AGE—UNITED STATES, 1992

Dose	Age	Customary Age/Interval	Product
Primary 1	2 months	>6 weeks of age	DTP[a]
Primary 2	4 months	4–8 weeks after first dose[b]	DTP[a]
Primary 3	6 months	4–8 weeks after second dose[b]	DTP[a]
Primary 4	15 months	6–12 months after third dose[b]	DTaP or DTP[a,c]
Booster	Age 4–6 years, before entering kindergarten or elementary school (not necessary if fourth primary vaccinating dose administered after fourth birthday)		DTaP or DTP[a,c]
Additional boosters	Every 10 years after last dose		Td[d]

[a] Use DT if pertussis vaccine is contraindicated. If the child is age 1 year or older at the time that primary dose 3 is due, a third dose 6 to 12 months after the second dose is administered completes primary vaccination with DT.
[b] Prolonging the interval does not require restarting series.
[c] Either DTaP or whole-cell DTP can be used for the fourth and fifth doses; DTaP is generally preferred, if available.
[d] Tetanus-diphtheria toxoids adsorbed (Td) (for adult use).
From Centers for Disease Control and Prevention: Morb Mortal Wkly Rep 41(RR-2):6, 1992.

Tetanus Toxoid. Active immunization with adsorbed tetanus toxoid is the best way to prevent tetanus. Unfortunately, many individuals, even in developed countries, are not adequately immunized,[22,27] and primary immunization after wounding, though essential, will not provide protection from tetanus arising from this wound (see Tables 50–4 to 50–6). In healthy individuals, two injections of adsorbed toxoid 8 weeks apart provide the *initial series* and a third injection (the *reinforcing injection*) 6 to 12 months later completes the primary *basic immunization.* Antibody (circulating antitoxin) develops soon after the second dose. Adsorbed toxoid should be used for primary immunization and for booster doses after injury, or routinely about every 10 years. In the previously immunized, booster injections will elicit protective levels of antitoxin in 4 to 7 days. Local reactions are unusual except in those who have received frequent booster injections. Most reactions are confined to local erythema and swelling. A few cases of tetanus have occurred with alleged prior tetanus toxoid immunization (complete or incomplete).[28–32] Cases have been reported with a circulating serum tetanus antitoxin titer greater than 0.01 units of anti-

TABLE 50–5. ROUTINE DIPHTHERIA, TETANUS, AND PERTUSSIS VACCINATION SCHEDULE SUMMARY FOR PERSONS 7 YEARS OF AGE AND OLDER—UNITED STATES, 1991

Dose	Age/Interval	Product
Primary 1	First dose	Td
Primary 2	4–8 weeks after first dose[a]	Td
Primary 3	6–12 months after second dose[a]	Td
Booster	Every 10 years after last dose	Td

[a] Prolonging the interval does not require restarting series.
From Centers for Disease Control and Prevention: Morb Mortal Wkly Rep 40(RR-10):6, 1991.

TABLE 50–6. SUMMARY OF RECOMMENDATIONS OF ADVISORY COMMITTEE ON IMMUNIZATION PRACTICES FOR TETANUS PROPHYLAXIS IN ROUTINE WOUND MANAGEMENT—UNITED STATES, 1991

History of Adsorbed Tetanus Toxoid (Doses)	Clean, Minor Wounds		All Other Wounds[a]	
	Td[b]	*TIG*	*Td*[b]	*TIG*
Unknown or <3	Yes	No	Yes	Yes
≥3[c]	No[d]	No	No[e]	No

[a] Such as, but not limited to, wounds contaminated with dirt, feces, soil, saliva; puncture wounds; avulsions; and wounds resulting from missiles, crushing, burns, and frostbite.
[b] For children less than 7 years old, DTP (DT, if pertussis vaccine is contraindicated) is preferred to tetanus toxoid alone. For persons 7 years of age or older, Td is preferred to tetanus toxoid alone. Diphtheria and tetanus toxoids and acellular pertussis vaccine (DTaP) may be used instead of DTP for the fourth and fifth doses.
[c] If only three doses of *fluid* toxoid have been received, then a fourth dose of toxoid, preferably an adsorbed toxoid, should be given.
[d] Yes, if more than 10 years since last dose.
[e] Yes, if more than 5 years since last dose. (More frequent boosters are not needed and can accentuate side effects.)
From Centers for Disease Control and Prevention: Morb Mortal Wkly Rep 41(SS-8):7, 1992.

toxin per milliliter of serum, which has been considered a protective level.[23,33]

For those 7 years or older, tetanus and diphtheria toxoids (adult type) (Td) are recommended for routine or wound boosters; but if there is any reason to suspect hypersensitivity to the diphtheria component, tetanus toxoid (T) should be substituted for Td.

Failure of toxoid can be due to (1) agammaglobulinemia, (2) exposure to acute doses of radiation, (3) immunosuppressive drugs, (4) carcinoma of the breast, (5) poor toxoid, or (6) an inaccurate toxoid history.[10] Individuals with acquired immune deficiency syndrome (AIDS) might not respond to an initial injection of toxoid so they might not have an anamnestic response to booster injections of toxoid. Bernstein et al[15] assessed specific antibody production in five young children with AIDS. No antibody was found in serum obtained before tetanus toxoid booster immunization. Three patients had no demonstrable antibody after immunization; the other two patients had a diminished response that was less than the lowest titer measured in age-matched controls.

It seems reasonable (1) to administer tetanus toxoid (active immunization) to injured patients with AIDS in accordance with the guidelines for tetanus toxoid injections in individuals without this syndrome and, in addition, (2) to give tetanus immune globulin (passive immunization) to injured patients with the syndrome.

Surgical Wound Care. Operative prophylaxis consists of the removal of *C. tetani* and nonviable tissue from wounds and of the best possible reconstruction of aerobic wounds. Optimal prophylaxis includes the following steps.[10,34]

1. The wounds are treated at the earliest possible moment.
2. Aseptic technique must be observed, including the use of gloves, gowns, masks, sterile instruments, and proper antiseptic skin preparation.
3. During preparation of the skin, the wounds should be covered with gauze to prevent further contamination from surrounding contaminated tissue.
4. Proper lighting is needed to help identify and protect fine structures such as nerves and vessels.
5. Adequate instruments and assistance are needed for optimal exposure.
6. Hemostasis should be achieved with delicate instruments and with fine suture material to minimize the amount of necrotic tissue left in wounds.
7. Tissues should be handled gently to prevent additional tissue necrosis.
8. Complete debridement with excision of necrotic tissue must be carried out so that no pabulum is left on which residual *C. tetani* can propagate. If reevaluation of wounds indicates the development of more necrotic tissue, debridements must be repeated.
9. All foreign bodies must be excised.
10. Wounds should be irrigated copiously with large amounts of physiologic saline solution.
11. If they might provide the anaerobic conditions for growth of the tetanus bacillus and production of its lethal toxin, wounds should be left open and drainage instituted when necessary.

Antitoxin. Since 1966, the recommended prophylactic dose of tetanus immune globulin (TIG) in the United States has been 250 units. An increase to 500 units is recommended for severe, neglected, or old (more than 24 hours) tetanus-prone wounds.[23] During 1970 and 1971, only five of 207 (2.4 percent) of the patients with tetanus in the United States, with information on prophylaxis, had received prophylactic antitoxin before the onset of tetanus; two of these received more than eight doses of tetanus immune globulin (more than 1000 units). The two cases may represent therapy after the onset of tetanus that was incorrectly reported as prophylaxis.[35] Nevertheless, higher dosage of TIG may be indicated for major burns, septic abortions, retained foreign bodies, open fractures, inadequate debridement, or wounds contaminated with herbivore feces.[25,36] TIG must not be given intravenously. Passive immunization with TIG is no substitute for active immunization or adequate surgical care of a local wound. Different needles, syringes, and sites of injection should be used when both tetanus toxoid and TIG are given.

Emergency Medical Identification Devices. In the United States, where more and more individuals are actively immunized for tetanus, emergency medical identification devices are becoming more important. Clinicians constantly ask these questions during the management of the wounded: (1) Has the patient been actively immunized for tetanus? (2) If actively immunized for tetanus, when? (3) Have there been severe—and hence significant—reactions to tetanus toxoid? (4) Should TIG be given? Such questions can be answered immedi-

TABLE 50–7. USE OF EMERGENCY MEDICAL IDENTIFICATION DEVICE (EMID) IN THE UNITED STATES IN AUGUST AND SEPTEMBER 1991[a]

Persons Surveyed	Number of Individuals	Number with EMID	Number with Tetanus Data on EMID
Nonmedical students	137	19 (13.9%)	11 (8.0%)
Medical students	43	3 (7.0%)	2 (4.7%)
Total	180	22 (12.2%)	13 (7.2%)

[a] Data were obtained by a survey of patients and their friends encountered in the practice of one of the authors (WF) and by a survey of medical students.

ately if every citizen carries an up-to-date emergency medical identification device (see Fig. 50–2). Memory alone can be inadequate. Many who have thought they had received tetanus toxoid injections in the past are discovered to have received tetanus antitoxin, diphtheria toxoid, or perhaps typhoid vaccine instead. The possession of some type of emergency medical identification device could simplify and expedite history taking after injury before treatment is begun. Tetanus toxoid immunization could be performed accurately, and overdoses and unnecessary injections of tetanus toxoid could be avoided in the rare individual who is sensitive to toxoid. Unfortunately, only a few individuals have with them emergency medical identification devices (Table 50–7).

Antibiotics. The consensus reached at the Second International Conference on Tetanus in 1966 was that antibiotics, such as penicillin, are effective against vegetative tetanus bacilli, both in vitro and in experimental animals. Antibiotics have no effect against toxin and must not be relied on to the exclusion of active and passive immunization procedures. The effectiveness of antibiotics for prophylaxis remains unproved; if used, they should be given for at least 5 days.[37] Therefore antibiotics should be used as a deterrent to the growth of tetanus organisms that cannot be surgically removed from wounds. Huge doses are generally recommended to penetrate into partially devitalized areas.

Of 86 patients who developed tetanus in 1989 to 1990 after a wound, only 32 percent sought medical treatment. Approximately half received tetanus toxoid but half did not.[7] In 1989 to 1990, 14 patients developed tetanus from chronic wounds such as skin ulcers, abscesses, or gangrene. Some of these patients were diabetics and others were drug addicts. Ten patients with tetanus in these years had no known injury, chronic wound, or other preexisting medical condition.[7]

TREATMENT: MANAGEMENT OF THE VICTIM OF TETANUS

The therapeutic recommendations that follow have been discussed in detail at the eighth International Conference on Tetanus, most recently in Leningrad, Russia, August 1987.[4,25,35–43]

1. Establishment of a diagnosis of tetanus. Be as certain as possible of the diagnosis. Other diseases mimic tetanus.
2. Complete history and physical examination. This information forms a baseline for the recognition of complications.
3. Antitoxin: *Intramuscular Injection.* As soon as the diagnosis of tetanus is made, give intramuscular injections of 500 to 10,000 units of TIG.[7] Intravenous administration of aggregated gammaglobulin may produce hypertension and is contraindicated. The exact, effective dosage of TIG has not been established. A dose of only 500 units may be as effective as 3,000 to 10,000 units.[40] Patel and his associates[41] in Bombay, India, found no significant difference in mortality for doses ranging from 5,000 units (the lowest dose) to 60,000 units, and interpreted larger doses as being probably detrimental. In countries where there are adequate supplies of tetanus immune globulin, there are no indications for the administration of heterologous equine antitoxin. In countries in which it is not available, heterologous antitoxins are still being used.
   Intrathecal Injection. At the International Tetanus Conference, many tetanologists have been enthusiastic about—in addition to the intramuscular injection of TIG—a simultaneous single injection of TIG and prednisolone intrathecally.[4,25] For neonatal tetanus, 250 units of TIG and 12.5 mg of prednisolone are administered intrathe-

cally, and 250 units of TIG are given intramuscularly. For adults, the dose of TIG for the intrathecal route is increased to 1,000 units and—for the intramuscular route—500 to 10,000 units. Complications of intrathecal administration are believed to be due to the preservatives rather than to the antitoxin itself.[25,42,43]

4. Laboratory tests. Our protocol for laboratory tests in the hospital is shown in Table 50–8.

5. Nursing care. Nursing care must be provided constantly in an intensive care unit. A respirator, oxygen, suction, and tracheostomy equipment must be immediately at hand.

6. Analgesics. The use of appropriate doses of codeine, meperidine (Demerol), and morphine will relieve the pain associated with the tonic contractions of tetanus, without causing excess respiratory depression.

7. Sedatives and muscle relaxants. The purpose of sedatives is to reduce the patient's threshold to external stimuli, with the hope of reducing the number and severity of seizures. The mildest cases of tetanus can be sedated adequately with phenobarbital or paraldehyde, but the more severe cases require thiopental sodium (Pentothal). Some physicians have been enthusiastic about the use of muscle relaxant drugs to control convulsive seizures. These drugs are difficult to administer because of the problems of overdosage or underdosage. Drugs more commonly suggested for use are diazepam (Valium), D-tubocurarine, succinylcholine (Anectine), pancuronium (Pavilon), atracurium (Tracrium), vecuronium (Norcuron), and midazolam (Versed).

TABLE 50–8. PROTOCOL FOR ADMISSION LABORATORY TESTS

Order the following:
1. Complete blood cell count with differential white blood cell count
2. Urinalysis
3. Prothrombin time and partial thromboplastin time
4. Blood chemistry tests: urea nitrogen, creatinine, electrolytes, bilirubin, calcium, glucose
5. Arterial blood gases
6. Chest roentgenogram
7. Electrocardiogram
8. Electroencephalogram if it can be obtained so that—if necessary for later brain evaluation—serial electroencephalograms may be available from the time of initial care
9. Wound and—if the patient is febrile—both aerobic and anaerobic blood cultures and sensitivity tests
10. If necessary for diagnosis, cerebrospinal fluid for culture, Gram smear, cells, and chemistry tests
11. Diazepam levels of serum

TABLE 50–9. ANTIBIOTICS THAT MAY HAVE A POSSIBLE DETERRENT ACTION ON ANY *C. TETANI* THAT HAVE NOT BEEN OR CANNOT BE REMOVED SURGICALLY FROM A WOUND

Ampicillin
Cephalosporins
Chloramphenicol
Clindamycin
Erythromycin
Metronidazole
Penicillin[a]
Tetracyclines

[a] Penicillin is the most effective.

8. Surgical wound care. Meticulous surgical care of wounds must be used, with removal of all necrotic tissue and foreign bodies, as outlined in the previous section on prevention.

9. Antibiotics. In vitro, penicillin and other antibiotics (Table 50–9) are effective against the tetanus bacillus.[10] However, antibiotic therapy will be disappointing insofar as it is directed against the tetanus itself, because tetanus is a toxemia, not a bacteremia. In addition, the organism's lethal antibiotic concentrations within the wound may not be attained, because avascular conditions are frequently present. Nevertheless, penicillin may be a useful adjunct to surgical wound care.

On the other hand, antibiotics are part of the therapy plan. They are irreplaceable in the care of infectious complications of tetanus, especially in combating pneumonia or secondary invasive wound infections. Of course, the choice of most effective antibiotics for the infectious complications should be determined by prior experience and by culture and sensitivity tests.

10. Tracheostomy. If personnel and facilities, including adequate tracheostomy tubes and mechanical respiration units, are available to care adequately for the patient, perform a tracheostomy. Tracheostomy and controlled ventilation are not necessary for every patient, but patients with short incubation periods or those who manifest periods of respiratory arrest will require long-term respiratory control.

11. Iatrogenic problems. Be constantly on the alert to avoid iatrogenic problems. For example, rectal probes left in place for the constant recording of temperature must be checked to prevent trauma to the rectal mucosa and anorectal veins during convulsions.
12. Private, dark, quiet room. It is traditional to place the patient in a private, dark, quiet room, but with adequate sedation and muscle relaxation, this may no longer be necessary.
13. Proper environment for infants. Infants with tetanus must have a proper environment in which the oxygen partial pressure, temperature, and humidity can be monitored and maintained. An infant radiant warmer will maintain body temperature and allow for availability of nursing care.
14. X-ray studies. X-ray studies are useful for fractures associated with the initial injury, or with tonic muscle contractions, or for pulmonary complications.
15. Padded tongue depressor. A padded tongue depressor should be inserted to protect the tongue from being bitten during tonic contractions.
16. Oral hygiene. The lips, teeth, tongue, and oral cavity must be cleaned daily to lessen the possibility of growth of pathologic bacteria and viruses.
17. Nutrition. Central intravenous hyperalimentation is best during the convulsive phase of tetanus. Enteral alimentation via mouth, gastrostomy, or nasogastric feeding tube is best deferred until convalescence so that the risk of aspiration is minimized. It is extremely difficult to maintain adequate nutrition. Adults may require up to 7000 calories daily. Only the mildest cases would be able to tolerate oral nutrition. Nasogastric tube feedings can be used, but they increase the risk of aspiration and gastrointestinal bleeding. Parenteral hyperalimentation appears to be the method of choice for providing nutrition.
18. Alimentary tract elimination. Provide for adequate gastrointestinal elimination by saline laxatives prophylactically and enemas as required.
19. Urine elimination. When necessary, a Foley catheter can provide for elimination of urine. Remove the catheter as soon as possible to prevent urinary tract infections.
20. Intake and output records. Record the fluid and electrolyte balance. If facilities permit, weigh the patient daily.
21. Protection of the eyes. To prevent desiccation, an ophthalmic ointment and moist gauze sponges should be used.
22. Prevention of decubitus ulcers. Decubitus ulcers can be prevented by appropriate cushions, pads, skin hygiene, and frequent turning of the patient.
23. Blood dyscrasias and bleeding problems. If there is a possibility of blood dyscrasias or bleeding problems, order frequent complete blood cell counts and promptly investigate the clotting mechanisms.
24. Prevention of pulmonary emboli. Some patients may require heparin to prevent or treat thromboembolic disease.
25. Prevention of cardiac exhaustion and circulatory disruption resulting from sympathetic overstimulation. Use propranolol to treat cardiac dysrhythmias, and add bethanidine for persistent hypertension.[44] When possible, if indicated, continuously monitor the heart rate and the arterial and central venous blood pressures. Cardiac arrhythmias are a major cause of death, but there is no general agreement about the methods to prevent fatal arrhythmias. Both alpha- and beta-adrenergic blockers have been advocated.
26. Consideration of temporary endocardial pacemaker in cases with severe bradycardiac episodes. A temporary endocardial pacemaker may be indicated when severe, medically refractory bradycardia of unknown cause occurs.[45]
27. Prevention of muscle contractures. Prevent muscle contractures with resulting deformities, such as foot drop, by temporary splints. Physiotherapy should be started as soon as recovery permits.
28. Control of body temperature. Carry out necessary procedures to lower excessively high body temperatures.
29. Tetanus toxoid. One month after the diagnosis of tetanus is made, give 0.5 ml of adsorbed tetanus toxoid intramuscularly for active immunization, and instruct the patient to complete basic immunization. Exposure to tetanospasmin does not provide immunity because the amount of tetano-

spasmin that causes tetanus is so very, very small. A complete course of active immunization is necessary.[10]

30. **30.** Emergency medical identification device. At the time of discharge from the hospital, give the cured patient a completed emergency medical identification device (see Fig. 50–2).
31. **31.** Hyperbaric oxygen. Hyperbaric oxygen is not recommended because it is ineffective and dangerous. Oyxgen has no effect on the toxemia.
32. **32.** Recording of data. The possibility of professional liability problems require that complete and accurate records of the course of treatment of tetanus cases be kept.

Results of Treatment

The Centers for Disease Control and Prevention Tetanus Surveillance for 1989 to 1990 revealed therapeutic TIG administration to 99 patients.[7] The median TIG dosage used was 3,000 IU (range, 250 to 19,000 IU). Of the patients who received TIG, 22 percent died; one (25 percent) of four patients who did not receive TIG died. Dosage did not correlate with outcome. The median duration of hospitalization was 17 days (range, 2 to 131 days). Fifty-eight percent required assisted ventilation. Only 15 percent of those who did not require ventilation died; 27 percent of those who required ventilation died.[7]

Professional Liability Problems

Unfortunately, in the United States professional liability problems are greatly overemphasized (Table 50–10). In addition to the impressive dollar values involved, such problems encircle the physician with a girdle from which he or she cannot escape. Lawyers have frequently been consulted for professional liability problems involving tetanus prophylaxis or treatment.

A factor that may influence the availability as well as the use of the very effective tetanus toxoid is the liability of the producers of the toxoid. At the end of 1984 and the beginning of 1985, only Lederle Laboratories continued the production and distribution of the multivalent DTP vaccine because of monetary awards that had been given and that were currently being litigated. Fortunately, by April 1985, Connaught Laboratories and Wyeth Laboratories were again distributing DTP.[46]

The producers of immunization agents have been favorably influenced by a 1992 decision, which found no evidence that a DTP vaccine caused a 7-year-old patient to have a stroke.[47]

TABLE 50–10. PROFESSIONAL LIABILITY ASPECTS OF A POSSIBLE CASE OF TETANUS

Tetanus (?); No Trial: 1978[a]	
Responsible individual	$100,000
First care providers	231,000
Third care providers	100,000
Local government	19,800
SUBTOTAL	$450,800
Lawyers	?

[a] Estimate of $750,000 if trial.
Pretrial settlements, as indicated, were made because a much higher total settlement (possibly $750,000) might have resulted if the case had been evaluated by a judge and/or jury in court. The responsible individual (the defendant) was involved in an automobile accident with the plaintiff *(RK Quinn, personal communication).*

Progress in the United States

The tetanus prophylaxis record of the United States has steadily improved (see Figs. 50–3 to 50–5). In 1992, only 40 cases of tetanus were reported to the Centers for Disease Control and Prevention, considerably less than one case per million population per year.[48]

The U.S. armed forces have had an outstanding record of tetanus prophylaxis for many years. Among the several million people who have served in the Navy and Marine Corps from 1946 to 1977, none had an injury while on active duty that was responsible for tetanus (WP Arentzen, personal communication). The only case of tetanus in the Navy during this period was seen in a man who had never received a tetanus inoculation and was circumcised several days before enlisting in the Navy; he developed tetanus several days after his induction.

In a continuing study of the Army's Individual Patient Data System, located in San Antonio, Texas, through October 10, 1991, Lieutenant General Frank F. Ledford, Jr., Surgeon General of the United States Army, found only one case of tetanus occurred in an active duty Army soldier since 1971. This individual was diagnosed in April 1989 following a puncture wound. His last tetanus immunization had been approximately 11 years previously (F Ledford, Jr., personal communication).

REFERENCES

1. Hippocrates (with an English translation by WHS Jones), Vol 1. Cambridge, Harvard University Press, 1923, p 165.

2. Aretaeus, the Cappadocian: On tetanus. In Adams F (ed): The Extant Works, London, 1856, pp 246–249, 400–404.
3. Centers for Disease Control and Prevention: Tetanus fatality—Ohio, 1991. Morb Mortal Wkly Rep 42:148, 1993.
4. Furste W: Editorial: The Eighth International Conference on Tetanus, Leningrad, Union of Soviet Socialist Republics, 24–28 August 1987. J Trauma 29:268, 1989.
5. Patel J, Mehta B: Tetanus: a study of 2007 cases. Indian J Med Sci 17:791, 1963.
6. Centers for Disease Control and Prevention: Tetanus—United States, 1982–1984. Morb Mortal Wkly Rep 39:602, 1985.
7. Centers for Disease Control and Prevention: Tetanus surveillance—United States 1989–1990. Morb Mortal Wkly Rep 41(SS-8):1, 1992.
8. Smith A: Tetanus. In Beeson PB, McDermott W (eds): Cecil-Loeb Textbook of Medicine, 13th ed. Philadelphia, Saunders, 1971, p 566.
9. Kryzhanovsky G: Tetanus: A polysystemic disease. In: Comptes rendus de la quatriéme conférence internationale sur le tétanos (Proceedings of the fourth international conference on tetanus). Lyon, France, Lips, 1975, p 189.
10. Furste W, Wheeler W: Tetanus: a team disease. Curr Probl Surg October, 1972.
11. Glenn F: Tetanus—a preventable disease: including an experience with civilian casualties in the battle for Manila (1945). Ann Surg 124:1030, 1946.
12. Cole L, Youngman H, Gandy A: An attack of tetanus. Lancet 2:567, 1968.
13. Foll F, Solimena M, Cofiell R, et al: Autoantibodies to a 128-kd synaptic protein in three women with the stiff-man syndrome and breast cancer. N Engl J Med 328:546, 1993.
14. American Academy of Pediatrics: Report of the Committee on the Control of Infectious Diseases. Evanston, IL, The Academy, 1977, p 11.
15. Bernstein LJ, Ochs HD, Wedgwood RJ, et al: Defective humoral immunity in pediatric acquired immune deficiency syndrome. J Pediatr 107:352, 1985.
16. Centers for Disease Control, Public Health Service, US Department of Health, Education, and Welfare: Recommendation of the Public Health Service Advisory Committee on Immunization Practices. Morb Mortal Wkly Rep 30:420, 1981; 32:4, 1983.
17. Committee on Control of Surgical Infections, American College of Surgeons: Manual on Control of Infection in Surgical Patients. Philadelphia, Lippincott, 1976, pp 180, 189.
18. Committee on Trauma, American College of Surgeons Poster: Prophylaxis against tetanus in wound management. Am Coll Surg April, 1984.
19. Department of the Army, the Navy, the Air Force, and Transportation: Immunization. AR 40–562, BUMEDINST 6230.1H, AFR 161–13, CG COMDINST 6230.4C. Washington, DC, June 7, 1977.
20. Dull H: Active immunization for infectious diseases. In Conn H (ed): Current Therapy, 1978. Philadelphia, Saunders, 1978, p 86.
21. Furste W, Aguirre A: Preventing tetanus. Am J Nurs 78:834, 1978.
22. Krugman S, Katz S: Childhood immunization procedures. JAMA 237:2228, 1977.
23. McComb J: The combined use of homologous tetanus immune globulin and toxoid in man. In Eckmann L (ed): Principles on Tetanus. Bern, Hans Huber, 1967, p 359.
24. Peebles T, Levine L, Eldred M, Edsall G: Tetanus toxoid emergency boosters. A reappraisal. N Engl J Med 280:575, 1969.
25. Proceedings of the Seventh International Conference on Tetanus. Copanello, Italy, 1984.
26. Sandusky W: Tetanus. In Conn H (ed): Current Therapy, 1978. Philadelphia, Saunders, 1978, p 71.
27. Chase A: Immunization. Med Trib 19:11, 1978.
28. Long A: The Army Immunization Program. Vol III. Preventive Medicine in World War II, Medical Department. United States Army, Washington, DC, United States GPO, 1955, p 287.
29. Long A, Sartwell P: Tetanus in the U.S. Army in World War II. Bull US Army Med Dept 7:371, 1947.
30. Murphy K: Fatal tetanus with brainstem involvement and myocarditis in an ex-serviceman. Med J Aust 2:542, 1970.
31. Sakurai N, Hashizume S, Fujishiro K: Tetanus infection after immunization with tetanus toxoid. Part I. Human incidence. Presentation at Fifth International Conference on Tetanus, 1978.
32. Sakurai N, Ogonuki M, Niro M, et al: Tetanus infection after immunization with tetanus toxoid. II. Cases in guinea-pigs in experiments and calves in the farms. Presentation at Fifth International Conference on Tetanus, 1978.
33. Crone E, Reder A: Severe tetanus in immunized patients with high anti-tetanus titers. Neurology 42:761, 1992.
34. Furste W: The role of surgical prophylaxis. In Eckmann L (ed): Principles on Tetanus. Bern, Hans Huber, 1967, p 369.
35. Centers for Disease Control, Public Health Service, US Department of Health, Education, and Welfare: Tetanus Surveillance. Report No 4, March 31, 1974, p 9.
36. Santangelo Y, Moreira I: Tetanus prophylaxis of wounds. Rev Bras Med 33:257, 1976.
37. Eckmann L (ed): Principles on Tetanus. Bern, Hans Huber, 1967.
38. Furste W: The Second International Conference on Tetanus. Int Med Dig 82:469, 1966.
39. Furste W, Editorial: The Sixth International Conference on Tetanus. J Trauma 22:1032, 1982.
40. Blake P, Feldman R, Buchanan T, et al: Serologic therapy of tetanus in the United States, 1965–1971. JAMA 235:42, 1976.
41. Patel J, Mehta B, Nanavati B, et al: Role of serum therapy in tetanus. Lancet 1:740, 1963.

42. Ildirim I: Intrathecal treatment of tetanus with antitetanus serum and prednisolone mixture. Report at Third International Conference on Tetanus, Sao Paulo, Brazil, 1970.
43. Tetanus immune globulin: the intrathecal route: Editorial. Lancet 2:464, 1980.
44. Prys-Roberts C, Corbett J, Kerr J, et al: Treatment of sympathetic over-activity in tetanus. Lancet 1:542, 1969.
45. Pikelj F, Lazar M, Vidmar L: Treatment of asystole and bradycardia in tetanus with endocardial demand pacemaker. Presentation at Fifth International Conference on Tetanus, 1978.
46. Centers for Disease Control, Public Health Service, US Department of Health, Education and Welfare: Morb Mortal Wkly Rep 33:695, 1984; 34:231, 1985.
47. Toon v. Lederle Laboratories, 603. So.2d 245 (La. Ct. of App., June 24, 1992). The Citation 64:2, 1993.
48. Centers for Disease Control and Prevention: Summary-cases of specified notifiable diseases, United States. Morb Mortal Wkly Rep 41:974, 1993.

BIBLIOGRAPHY

Bartlett JG: *Clostridium tetani.* In Gorbach SL, Bartlett JG, Blacklow NR (eds): Infectious Diseases. Philadelphia, Saunders, 1992, p 1580.

Cate TR: *Clostridium tetani* (tetanus). In Mandell GL, Douglas RG Jr, Bennett JE (eds): Principles and Practice of Infectious Diseases, 3rd ed. New York, Churchill Livingstone, 1990, p 1842.

Furste W, Wheeler W: Tetanus: a team disease. Curr Probl Surg October, 1972.

Infections in the Immunocompromised Host

CHAPTER 51

Robert H. Rubin, A. Benedict Cosimi

The past two decades have witnessed a major increase in the numbers of individuals who might be characterized as immunocompromised hosts, highly susceptible to life-threatening infection. Major advances in immunosuppressive therapy have greatly extended the productive years of people who would formerly have succumbed quickly to uremia, end-stage liver and heart disease, and a variety of malignant and auto-immune diseases. Such potential, however, may only be realized if life-threatening infections, which arise from the major host defense defects present in these patients, can be prevented or treated. Infection, not the primary illness, has become a major cause of both morbidity and mortality for many of these individuals.

In addition, the unprecedented epidemic of opportunistic infection and viral-associated malignancies seen in previously well individuals, the acquired immune deficiency syndrome (AIDS), has placed an even greater emphasis on the problems of infection in the immunocompromised host. Physicians at every level of specialization must now become familiar with both the unusual infectious diseases that occur in these patients and also the way in which the underlying disease and its therapy can modify the clinical presentation and management of common conditions.

SPECIFIC AND NONSPECIFIC HOST DEFENSE DEFECTS AND THEIR INFECTIOUS COMPLICATIONS

The Mucocutaneous Barriers to Infection

The mucocutaneous surfaces of the body serve as the primary barrier between the individual and the surrounding microbial world. The importance of this primary barrier becomes even greater in individuals whose secondary host defenses—humoral immunity, cell-mediated immunity, phagocytic function, and so on—are impaired. Damage to the primary barrier in such patients provides a common portal of entry for invasive infection. The gastrointestinal mucosa, particularly at the mouth and the anorectal areas, requires protection from trauma, and aggressive management of even trivial infection at these sites.

Likewise, the skin and subcutaneous tissues play an important role in the care and evaluation of the immunocompromised patient. In this population, disseminated infection caused by both bacteria and opportunistic fungi, such as *Aspergillus, Candida,* and *Rhizopus* species, has occurred all too frequently after iatrogenic trauma, such as maceration of the skin caused by occlusive dressings and adhesive tape. The rich blood supply of the skin provides an opportunity for metastatic spread of infection both *from* the skin as the initial portal of entry and *to* the skin from other bodily sites. Because the impaired inflammatory response of many of these patients will modify the appearance of invasive infection of the skin, the physician must be prepared to protect the skin and to biopsy even *minor* unexplained skin lesions in patients with significant host defense defects.[1]

Neutrophil, B Lymphocyte, T Lymphocyte, and Complement Function

Host defenses are discussed in detail in Chapters 12–16. Both primary (inborn) and secondary (acquired) disorders of neutrophil, B lymphocyte, T lymphocyte, and complement function have been described, and these disorders increase the susceptibility of the host to infection. Each disorder gives rise to certain types of infection (Table 51–1).[2] Thus the discovery of depressed neutrophil function and number is associated with an increased frequency of bacterial, candidal, and *Aspergillus* infection. Patients with impaired neutrophil function, such as those with chronic granulomatous disease, are especially susceptible to recurrent abscesses of the skin, lymph nodes, and visceral organs caused by *Staphylococcus aureus* and various gram-negative bacilli. Particularly common is a decrease in the number of circulating neutrophils, either because of leukemia or aplastic anemia or as a consequence of radiation and cytotoxic chemotherapy used in the treatment of malignancy. Once the circulating neutrophil count falls below 1000/mm^3, the risk of infection begins to rise and becomes particularly common at levels below 100/mm^3. In patients receiving chemotherapy, the rate of decline in the neutrophil count is as important as the degree of neutropenia. In such instances, breaks in the integrity of the primary mucocutaneous barriers to infection can result in invasive infection: bacteremia due to the Enterobacteriaceae and *Pseudomonas aeruginosa* from the gastrointestinal tract (due to the effects of chemotherapy on the gut mucosa), gram-positive bacteremia particularly from indwelling venous access devices, and gram-negative pneumonia that can be a result of oral mucositis, gram-negative colonization, and then aspiration. In addition, the patient with sustained, severe neutropenia is at high risk from invasive disease due to *Candida* species and *Aspergillus* species.[3–5]

B lymphocyte disorders, whether congenital or due to such acquired conditions as multiple myeloma or chronic lymphocytic leukemia, result in the inadequate production of opsonizing and bactericidal antibody. This is clinically expressed by an increased susceptibility to bacteremia, pneumonia, sinusitis, and otitis due to the encapsulated bacteria—*Streptococcus pneumoniae, Hemophilus influenzae* type B, and *Neisseria meningitidis.* In addition to these bacterial infections that are most commonly observed in children with congenital disorders of antibody synthesis, patients with hypogammaglobulinemia appear to have an increased incidence of infection with the gastrointestinal pathogens *Giardia lamblia,* nontyphoidal salmonel-

TABLE 51–1. RELATIONSHIP BETWEEN INFECTION WITH PARTICULAR MICROORGANISMS AND SPECIFIC HOST DEFENSE DEFECTS

Host Defense Defect	Microorganisms Commonly Causing Significant Infection	Commonly Associated Conditions
Impaired antibody function	*Streptococcus pneumoniae, Hemophilus influenzae* type B, *Neisseria meningitidis,* Enteroviruses	Congenital and acquired hypoglobulinemia, B cell malignancies, AIDS
Defects in complement	*Streptococcus pneumoniae, Hemophilus influenzae* type B, *Neisseria* species	Congenital and acquired hypocomplementemic states, hypocomplementemic vasculitis
Depressed cell-mediated immunity	Typical and atypical *Mycobacteria, Listeria monocytogenes, Nocardia asteroides,* fungi (including *Pneumocystis carinii*), *Toxoplasma gondii, Strongyloides stercoralis,* herpes group viruses, measles	AIDS, transplant recipients, lymphoma, prolonged corticosteroid therapy, congenital defects
Decrease in the number of fully functional granulocytes	Enterobacteriaceae, *Pseudomonas aeruginosa, Staphylococcus aureus,* oral bacterial flora, *Aspergillus* species, *Candida* species	Myeloproliferative disorders, cytotoxic chemotherapy, congenital disorders

From Rubin RH, Ferraro MJ. Hematol Oncol Clin North Am 7:795, 1993.

lae, and *Campylobacter jejuni.* These individuals do not appear to have an unusual susceptibility to fungi (with the possible exception of *Pneumocystis carinii*) or to most viruses. Patients with hypogammaglobulinemia do appear to be quite susceptible to severe infection with the enteroviruses and rotavirus—chronic, progressive meningoencephalitis due to enteroviruses (including the attenuated, live Oral polio vaccine) and protracted diarrhea due to rotavirus infection.[6]

Patients with depressed cell-mediated immunity (whether due to defects in T lymphocyte or monocyte-macrophage function) have an increased susceptibility to a variety of viruses (particularly the herpes group viruses—cytomegalovirus, Epstein-Barr virus, varicella-zoster virus, and herpes simplex virus); such fungal infections as those due to *Pneumocystis carinii, Candida* species, the geographically restricted systemic mycoses (blastomycosis, coccidioidomycosis, histoplasmosis) and *Aspergillus* species; bacteria that can survive intracellularly (*Mycobacteria* species, *Salmonella, Nocardia asteroides,* and *Listeria monocytogenes*); and certain protozoans (most notably *Strongyloides stercoralis,* and *Toxoplasma gondii*).[5,6]

Patients with defects in the terminal components of complement are at risk for disseminated infection with both *Neisseria meningitidis* and *N. gonorrhoeae.* The rare patient with a combined deficiency in the alternative pathway and the second component of complement is at major risk of life-threatening infection with the same encapsulated bacteria that cause difficulty in patients with hypogammaglobulinemia.[5,6]

Adverse Effects of Splenectomy

It has become apparent that the spleen is important to people who develop bacteremia with an organism to which they have little or no preexisting antibody. Although well-opsonized bacteria are removed primarily by the liver, the spleen is responsible for removing unopsonized bacteria from the bloodstream. The spleen plays an important role in the humoral response, as the primary immunoglobulin response takes place in the spleen, and low levels of IgM have been observed after splenectomy in children. In addition, a reduced level of the complement factor *properdin* has been demonstrated after splenectomy. The spleen also serves as a major site of synthesis of *tuftsin,* a basic tetrapeptide that coats polymorphonuclear leukocytes to promote phagocytosis. The unique microcirculation of the spleen appears to be crucial to the survival of the nonimmune patient with pneumococcal or type B *H. influenzae* bacteremia. Even healthy adults who are splenectomized after trauma exhibit an increased risk of catastrophic, overwhelming infection with these organisms. This phenomenon is particularly important in individuals who are asplenic after sickle cell anemia or as part of the management of hematologic malignancy. Children are clearly more susceptible than adults, especially during the first 6 to 12 months after splenectomy, although there have been several instances of late pneumococcal sepsis.[6] Every effort should be made to protect the spleen from needless removal. Patients who have been splenectomized should receive pneumococcal vaccine, and young children should receive the newly available *H. influenzae* type B vaccine. Although these vaccines are useful, infection may still occur—particularly in small children and in individuals with malignant disease who are receiving combined radiation and chemotherapy. Therefore, all patients with functional or anatomic asplenia should be assumed to be susceptible to the development of overwhelming sepsis with the encapsulated organisms, and because the syndrome may follow otherwise trivial upper respiratory infections, the onset of a frank rigor in such an individual, even if he or she has received the vaccine, should be regarded with great concern. Antibiotic therapy aimed at the encapsulated organisms should be promptly initiated in such individuals, immunized or not.

Malnutrition

The interaction of inadequate nutrition and infectious agents is complex. The host defense defects produced by malnutrition predispose to infection, and the infection increases nutritional requirements. Increased nutrition is needed to avoid infection during malignant disease, major thermal injury, conditions associated with major losses of protein of the body, such as the nephrotic syndrome, advanced cirrhosis, malabsorption, and gastrointestinal fistulas, and chronic peritoneal dialysis. Protein-calorie-vitamin malnutrition causes (1) atrophy of lymphoid tissue, particularly thymus and thymic-dependent areas of peripheral lymphoid tissues; (2) an associated decrease and function of circulating T lymphocytes; (3) normal or increased numbers of circulatory B lymphocytes, with depressed primary antibody responses; (4) impaired intracellular killing of organisms by neutrophils; (5) a decrease in both classic and alternate complement pathway components. It is little wonder that a major effort is now devoted to correcting and preventing nutritional abnormalities in all surgical patients, but most particularly in those with other defects in host defense.[7–9]

Uremia

The host defense defects observed in the uremic patient can be divided into two general categories: those caused directly by the metabolic abnormalities of uremia and those caused by therapeutic interventions. The net result is an increased susceptibility to pneumonia, bacteremia, peritonitis, and chronic viral infection. When one is considering the pathogenesis of these infections in uremic individuals, the following factors have been identified: the direct immunosuppressing effects of uremic toxins; the indirect effects of metabolic abnormalities such as protein, trace metal, or vitamin deficiency that are induced by the life-sustaining therapies these patients undergo; the effects of the hemodialysis membrane on such blood constituents as complement factors and white blood cells; and the necessity for vascular access for hemodialysis and peritoneal access for peritoneal dialysis—both of these bypassing the critical cutaneous barrier to infection.[10]

The most clearly demonstrable defect in host defense of the uremic patient is in cell-mediated immunity. Enhanced survival of skin, renal, and cardic allografts, suppression of cutaneous delayed-type hypersensitivity reactions, defective lymphocyte blastogenesis in response to transplantation antigens and a variety of mitogenic agents, and, in some instances, lymphopenia and thymic atrophy have all been demonstrated in uremic patients and animals. An additional function of T lymphocytes, the production of interferon in response to viral infection, likewise seems to be significantly depressed in uremia.[6,10]

The other component of cell-mediated immunity, namely, monocyte and macrophage function, likewise appears to be affected by the uremic state. Thus depressed phagocytic function and impaired antigen processing have been noted, with this depressed function of alveolar macrophages probably playing an important role in the increased rate of pneumonia in these patients. Impaired clearance of immunoglobulin-coated particles by splenic macrophages, probably involving the Fc_rRI receptor, has been demonstrated in vivo in uremic patients. Particularly noteworthy has been the correlation with this observation and the risk of infection: the greater the extent of this defect in splenic function, the higher the risk of invasive infection.[11] It has been hypothesized that these defects in cell-mediated immunity and interferon production play an important role in the uremic patient's frequent inability to eliminate hepatitis virus after acute exposure and the development of the prolonged carrier state.[6,10]

Less is known about the function of the B lymphocyte system in uremia. Available data suggest that the nature of the inciting antigen is important in predicting the antibody response. Although uremic patients appear to respond normally to such potent antigens as tetanus and diphtheria toxoids, other vaccines, most notably hepatitis B, typhoid, influenza, and pneumococcal vaccines, are far less effective. Granulocyte function in uremia similarly may be impaired. Studies performed more than two decades ago show that the injection of noxious agents, such as sodium urate or bacteria, into the skin of uremic animals causes a diminished inflammatory response. Thus signs of peritonitis and other acute infections may be attenuated in uremic individuals.[6,10,12,13]

Uremic patients are susceptible to host defense abnormalities induced by such correctable nutritional deficiencies as protein malnutrition and zinc and pyridoxine deficiencies.[10] Mobilization of iron stores by means of deferoxamine therapy has been correlated with a markedly increased risk of mucormycosis and perhaps other infections.[14] Finally, contact of blood during hemodialysis with the standard Cuprophane membrane results in complement activation, transient leukopenia and hypoxemia due to pulmonary leukosequestration, and leukocyte activation. The repetitive occurrence of these events with each hemodialysis session may have significant impact on the individual's risk of infection—although the quantitative aspects of this relationship remain to be determined.[10]

Diabetes

Diabetes mellitus is associated with increased risk of infection, particularly mucocutaneous infections caused by *S. aureus* and urinary tract infections. It is still unclear how much of the vulnerability is related to the patient's general debility, increased exposure to the hospital environment, and vascular and neuropathic complications of the disease as opposed to direct inhibitory effects of the molecular consequences of diabetes on host defenses. At present, it would appear that diabetics have an increased susceptibility only to (1) urinary tract infections in women, particularly a form of pyelonephritis complicated by renal papillary necrosis; (2) pulmonary tuberculosis; (3) vaginal candidiasis; (4) rhinocerebral mucormycosis, especially in association with ketoacidosis; and (5) malignant otitis externa, caused by *Pseudomonas aeruginosa*. Other serious infections, for example, staphylococcal, gram-negative bacteremias, and viral influenza, may have a greater impact in the diabetic because of his or her general debility and metabolic complications. Individuals with impaired circulation secondary to diabetic vascular disease often develop osteomyelitis and chronic skin ulcerations of the feet, but the primary lesion is neuropathic and vascular. The increased propensity to urinary tract infections in certain patients may be primarily due to abnormalities in bladder emptying caused by a diabetic neuropathy. Hyperglycemia may be a risk factor in predisposing organ transplant patients to infection. Defects in neutrophil chemotactic responsiveness, adherence, and phagocytic function can be demonstrated in patients with hyperglycemia, although the significance of these findings is at present unclear.[6,15]

Hemolysis

Blockade of the reticuloendothelial system renders the patient more susceptible to infection with intracellular parasites (*Salmonella, Listeria, Babesia*). Chronic hemolysis, malaria, relapsing fever, bartonellosis, and certain neoplastic conditions result in decreased monocyte-macrophage function.[16]

EFFECTS OF TREATMENT REGIMENS ON HOST DEFENSE

There are many therapeutic programs that adversely affect the patient's ability to resist infection, particularly when more than one therapeutic agent is being used at a time—antimicrobial agents, hyperalimentation, radiation therapy, corticosteroids, and cytotoxic chemotherapeutic agents. Antimicrobial agents create selection pressures for colonization with antibiotic-resistant organisms. This is accomplished by both suppression of normal flora and increased availability of nutrients caused by this suppression. All too often, the result is a treatment-resistant primary infection or superinfection, both of which are common in this patient population. In addition, there is increasing evidence that many of the antimicrobial agents can have a suppressing effect on certain parts of the host defense. Thus antibiotic therapy should be as specific as possible and should not be used needlessly.[17]

Intravenous hyperalimentation can be life saving in the repair of nutritional defects, but organisms can be infused in this manner. Thus, staphylococcal and gram-negative bacteremias and, most importantly, *Candida* fungemias may occur. In the patient with underlying granulocytopenia or a defect in T lymphocyte function, *Candida* introduced by this route is associated with at least a 50 percent rate of dissemination throughout the body.[18] Radiation therapy can cause a variety of dose-related systemic and local side effects that will impair the ability of the patient to resist infection. Factors influencing this impairment include the volume of irradiated marrow-bearing tissue, whether the bowel is included, and the extent of anatomic derangement caused by postirradiation fibrosis. The serious side effects caused by radiation therapy include (1) granulocytopenias and lymphopenia (especially T cells); (2) decreased bactericidal function of monocytes and macrophages; (3) damage to mucocutaneous surfaces, providing a portal of entry for resident microbes; and (4) impaired circulation, providing a fertile soil for anaerobic infection.[19]

Corticosteroids have the most global immunosuppressive effects. They impair the mobilization, adherence, phagocytosis, and bactericidal activity of neutrophils, monocytes, and macrophages. They depress B and T lymphocyte activity, diminish production of interferon, and alter the gastrointestinal flora and local tissue integrity, resulting in easier invasion by endogenous flora. These effects are related to both the dose and the duration of therapy. Thus, high-dose steroids are usually well tolerated for up to 3 weeks, but after that the incidence of life-threatening infection is increased. Alternate-day steroids have less suppressing effects on host defense and are associated with significantly fewer serious clinical infections than is daily therapy.[6,20–22] When prolonged daily use is required to achieve the desired anti-inflammatory or immunosuppressive effect, the dosage of prednisone should remain under 20 mg/day, even if this requires the addition of a second drug, such as azathioprine or cyclophosphamide. Experience has demonstrated that using prednisone with a second agent at low doses or moderate doses of both is associated with fewer side effects than the use of one of these agents at much higher dosage.

Cytotoxic drugs also have broad-ranging immunosuppressive properties. The most common adverse effect is granulocytopenia. Patients myelosuppressed by cytotoxic drugs usually have both neutropenia and monocytopenia and, thus, may be at greater risk for infection than patients with chronic granulocytopenia of other etiologies. Other adverse effects include ablation or suppression of both antibody synthesis and cell-mediated immunity, suppression of the reticuloendothelial system, and damage to mucocutaneous surfaces. Because mucosal damage to the gut may predispose to gram-negative bacteremia, the simultaneous reticuloendothelial depression may contribute to the high mortality rate from gram-negative sepsis observed in patients receiving cytotoxic therapy. Other defects of importance produced by some of these agents include decreased white blood cell mobilization, chemotaxis, phagocytosis, and bactericidal function (particularly by the *Vinca* alkaloids) and diminished opsonic activity by the cytotoxic agents, such as cyclophosphamide and nitrogen mustard compounds.[6]

The cumulative effects of individual immunosuppressive agents may far exceed the effects of each alone. For example, splenectomized adult lymphoma patients are not at greater risk for overwhelming sepsis than are healthy individuals undergoing posttraumatic splenectomies. However, if one adds granulocytopenia and age less than 12 years, or, most particularly, a history of combined radiation and chemotherapy, the risk is significantly increased. Patients with Hodgkin's disease subjected to this most intensive therapeutic regimen have lower circulating IgM levels and lower titers of antibody to *H. influenzae* type B and respond poorly to pneumococcal vaccine. Thus, the net effect of successful therapy for a T lymphocyte disorder (Hodgkin's disease) has been the creation of a B lymphocyte disorder.[23]

In the past decade, as part of the continuing effort to make immunosuppression more specific, a number of additional immunosuppressive agents have come into clinical use, particularly in transplantation. Thus both cyclosporine and FK-506 (cyclosporine is currently the cornerstone of immunosuppression for the transplant patient, while FK-506 is currently under intensive study) inhibit helper-inducer and cytotoxic T cell activities, while leaving B lymphocyte, neutrophil, and monocyte function relatively intact. The end result is a decreased risk of bacterial infection, although such other problems as cytomegalovirus (CMV) infection and Epstein-Barr virus (EBV) related lymphoproliferative disease may be exacerbated by these potent drugs.[24]

Both clinical observations and careful study in animal models have shown that different immunosuppressive drugs, even when administered in dosage schedules that are equal in terms of such immunosuppressing effects as the treatment of allograft rejection, can have very different effects on the course of important infections. Thus, in the case of CMV and EBV, perhaps the most important causes of infectious disease morbidity and mortality in the transplant patient, the following statements can be made[24]:

1. Cyclosporine, corticosteroids, and FK-506 have no ability to reactivate latent infection due to these viruses; in contrast, such anti-lymphocyte antibody preparations as OKT3 (a monoclonal anti-T cell antibody), antithymocyte globulin, and anti-lymphocyte serum are extremely potent in their ability to reactivate these and other herpes group viruses. Cytotoxic agents, such as azathioprine and cyclophosphamide, are moderately active in terms of their ability to reactivate these viruses.
2. Once replicating virus is present, cyclosporine and FK-506 are extremely potent in terms of blocking the patient's response to these viruses, thus amplifying the extent and impact of these infections (indeed, we have called these immunosuppressive agents "an in vivo PCR" in terms of their ability to promote the growth and clinical impact of these viruses). The anti-lymphocyte antibodies and the cytotoxic agents, in the dosages that are currently used, are only moderately active in terms of their abilities to promote these infections.
3. From these observations, it is clear that the temporal sequence in which immunosuppressive agents are deployed can have an effect in determining clinical impact. Anti-lymphocyte antibody therapy followed by cyclosporine or FK-506 will be the most potent regimen in terms of the promotion of these infections. Recent studies have shown that the administration of the antiviral agent during the anti-lymphocyte antibody therapy (so-called preemptive therapy, vide infra) can provide significant protection against these infections that would otherwise result from this particular sequence of immunosuppressive therapy.[25]

APPROACH TO PATIENTS WITH POSSIBLE HOST DEFENSE DEFECT

The major clue to the presence of a significant host defense defect is an increased susceptibility to infection. This is usually manifested by increased frequency, severity, or duration of infection; the development of an unusual complication or manifestation of the primary infection; or the demonstration of invasive infection with organisms that are normally relatively avirulent. In children, the clinical clues suggesting a primary immunodeficiency syndrome are as listed in Table 51–2.

The ideal test to screen for a possible immunodeficiency should be inexpensive, noninvasive, easy to perform, and reliable. Table 51–3 delineates the

TABLE 51–2. PEDIATRIC PRIMARY IMMUNODEFICIENCY SYNDROME

Usually Present	Frequently Present	Occasionally Present
Recurrent respiratory infections	Draining ears	Mucocutaneous candidal infection
Severe infections Pneumonia Bacteremia Meningitis	Irritability	Vaccinia gangrenosum
	Anemia	*Pneumocystis carinii* pneumonia
	Chronic pneumonia	Skin rashes and alopecia
Recurrent diarrhea	Bronchiectasis	Severe viral disease
Overall failure to thrive	Pyoderma	Arthritis
	Chronic conjunctivitis	Hepatosplenomegaly or lymphadenopathy
	Malabsorption A paucity of lymph nodes and tonsils	Hematologic abnormalities

TABLE 51–3. LABORATORY EVALUATION OF POSSIBLE IMMUNODEFICIENCY

Type of Deficiency	Screening Test	Definitive Tests
Antibody deficiency	Immunoelectrophoresis Schick test Isoagglutinin titers	Quantitative immunoglobulin determination Enumeration of B lymphocytes Secretory immunglobulins and antibodies Rectal or lymph node biopsy Lateral pharyngeal x-ray study Preexistent antibodies to polio, tetanus, and so on Antibody response to injected antigens Immunoglobulin kinetics IgG subclass determination
Cell-mediated immunity deficiency	Lymphocyte count and morphology Thymic x-ray study Skin tests with battery of skin test antigens (*Candida*, mumps, *Trichophyton*)	Enumeration of T lymphocytes Dinitrochlorobenzene challenge Assay of lymphokine and blastogenic response in vitro Lymph node biopsy Skin homograft
Phagocytic deficiency	White blood cell count, differential, and morphology	Nitrobluetetrazolium assay Assays of chemotactic responsiveness, random migration, phagocytosis, bactericidal activity Antileukocyte antibodies Rebuck skin window Splenic scan
Complement and opsonic deficiency	Total hemolytic complement (CH_{50}) C3 level	Assay of specific complement components Generation of chemotactic factors Opsonic assay

Adapted from Stiehm ER: Immunodeficiency disorders: general considerations. In Stiehm ER, Fulginiti VA (eds): Immunologic Disorders in Infants and Children. Philadelphia, Saunders, 1980, p 183.

approach developed by Stiehm—initial screening test followed by more specific evaluation of abnormalities.

Risk of Infection in the Compromised Host

The risk of infection in the compromised host, particularly opportunistic infection, is detemined largely by the interaction between two factors: the patient's *net state of immunosuppression* and the *epidemiologic exposures* the patient encounters. The relationship between these two factors is at least semiquantitative. Thus if the exposure is great enough, even an immunologically normal individual will develop life-threatening infection; conversely, if the net state of immunosuppression is great enough, even trivial exposures to normally innocuous organisms can likewise cause life-threatening disease.[24,26]

The net state of immunosuppression is a complex function determined by the interaction of a number of factors: the host defense defects engendered by the underlying disease; the dose, duration, and temporal sequence of immunosuppressive regimens; the presence or absence of neutropenia, defects to the mucocutaneous surfaces, or an indwelling foreign body that bypasses the protection usually provided by these surfaces; such metabolic factors as protein-calorie malnutrition, uremia, and hyperglycemia; and the presence of infection that is immunomodulating, particularly such viruses as cytomegalovirus, Epstein-Barr virus, hepatitis B and C viruses, and the human immunodeficiency virus. The contribution of these viral infections to the net state of immunosuppression is illustrated by the following statistic: at the Massachusetts General Hospital over a 10-year period, more than 90 percent of the opportunistic infections occurred in the setting of infection with one or more of these viruses. Indeed, the exceptions turned out to be instances in which excessive epidemiologic hazards were subsequently identified.[24,26]

The epidemiologic exposures of importance to the compromised host can be divided into two general categories: those encountered in the community and those encountered within the hospital. Within the community the major concerns are exposures to the geographically restricted systemic mycoses (*Blastomyces dermatitidis, Coccidioides immitis, Histoplasma capsulatum*), *Mycobacterium tuberculosis, Strongyloides stercoralis,* and such respiratory viruses as influenza. As far as the systemic mycoses and *M. tuberculosis* are concerned, three patterns of infection are observed: progressive primary infection, with systemic dissemination, when the exposure to the organisms (usually via the respiratory route) first occurs after the immunosuppressed state has developed; reactivation infection, with secondary dissemination, when a long dormant focus breaks down and is not contained due to the immunocompromised condition of the patient; and superinfection, again with the potential for systemic dissemination, when immunity gained by previous exposures is attenuated by the patient's immunosuppressed state and reinfection, with the potential for systemic spread, occurs when the organism is once again encountered. The emphasis is thus on life-threatening infection of the lung and/or metastatic sites. Thus the clinical syndromes that should lead to a consideration of these possibilities include the following: fever of unknown origin; miliary lung disease; metastatic infections of the skin, skeletal system, and central nervous system; and a chronic wasting illness resembling malignancy. The clinician needs to keep in mind that both recent and remote epidemiologic histories are pertinent in evaluating compromised patients with one or more of these clinical presentations.[5,24,26]

Strongyloides stercoralis is unique among helminthic infections of humans in being maintained in the gastrointestinal tract of individuals for decades after the individual was infected due to an autoinoculation cycle. The onset of impaired cell-mediated immunity, particularly that engendered by exogenous immunosuppressive therapy, can result in the transformation of a hitherto asymptomatic infestation into a life-threatening infection. Two forms of strongyloidiasis can occur when this happens: a hyperinfection syndrome, which is an exaggerated form of the clinical events that occur in the normal host—in this case resulting in hemorrhagic enterocolitis and/or hemorrhagic pneumonia; and a disseminated infection, in which these parasites actually disseminate to other tissues, often accompanied by gut flora so that the clinical presentation is often that of antibiotic unresponsive gram-negative bacteremia or meningitis. Because of the gravity of these clinical syndromes, great emphasis is placed on evaluating patients for this infestation and treating it with thiobendazole or ivormectin prior to the initiation of immunosuppressive therapy. Thus candidates for organ transplantation with a history of residence in Southeast Asia, Latin America, and other endemic sites should be evaluated as to the need for pretransplant therapy. Routine examination of stool specimens for ova and parasites has a sensitivity of less than 30 percent, so that in an individual with an appropriate epidemiologic history one of two approaches is possible: examine purged stools and specimens obtained at duodenal intubation; or, alternatively, treat patients on the basis of their epidemiologic history alone.[5,24]

As more and more immunocompromised patients are surviving within the community for longer periods of time, common viral infections that circulate within the community periodically are being reported as having an increased impact on these individuals. Thus influenza, parainfluenza, respiratory syncytial virus, and other respiratory viruses appear to cause more severe and prolonged disease in these individuals, with a higher rate of pneumonia and of bacterial superinfection than is observed in immunologically normal individuals. Similarly, prolonged rotavirus and enterovirus infection and overwhelming adenovirus infection have likewise been observed in many immunocompromised patients, including both organ and bone marrow transplant recipients. Unfortunately, vaccines are relatively ineffective, and specific antiviral therapy with such drugs as amantadine and ribavirin has not been adequately evaluated in these patients. At present, the emphasis must be on the avoidance of exposures.[24]

An even more important group of epidemiologic problems occurs within the hospital environment, where both epidemic and endemic problems can occur. Epidemics occuring within the hospital are of two types: *domiciliary,* in which patients are exposed to contaminated air or water where they are housed within the hospital (such events are usually discovered quite expeditiously because of clustering of cases in time and space); and *nondomiciliary,* in which the epidemiologic exposure occurs at a central location, such as the operating room or radiology suite, to which large numbers of patients from throughout the hospital are taken for essential procedures (these outbreaks may be more difficult to recognize because of the lack of clustering of cases on one unit or floor of the hospital). The organisms commonly involved with both types of outbreak are similar—*Pseudomonas aeruginosa* and other gram-negative bacilli, *Aspergillus* species, and *Legionella* species. The common denominator is often hospital construction, which can liberate aerosols of organisms, particularly *Aspergillus.* A major clue to the presence of a potential excessive nosocomial hazard is the occurrence of infection with one of these organisms at a time when the net state of immunosuppression is not normally great enough for such an infection to occur.[27,28] Table 51–4 outlines the general approach to preventing nosocomial infection.

Among hospitalized cancer and leukemia patients, careful studies have shown that although 86 percent of infections arise from the patient's endogenous flora, approximately half of these organisms were first acquired from the hospital environment. The incidence of nosocomial infections among cancer patients is approximately four times that of the general population. Such infections are most frequently caused by Enterobacteriaceae, especially *Klebsiella* and *Enterobacter* species, *P. aeruginosa,* and *Candida* species. Of particular importance is the fact that once colonization with *P. aeruginosa* occurs, 40 to 68 percent of patients will develop septicemia during periods of drug-induced severe neutropenia.[29] Goldschmidt and Body[30] have made the interesting observation that many of the cytotoxic agents employed for cancer chemotherapy have antibacterial activity for much of the intestinal flora, with the exception of *P. aeruginosa,* thus creating another selection pressure for the emergence of such difficult to treat infections.

TABLE 51–4. PRINCIPLES OF INFECTION PREVENTION IN THE COMPROMISED HOST

- Reduce acquisition of ambient organisms from hospital environment
  - Avoid hospitalization
  - Segregate patients with potentially communicable diseases
  - Avoid overcrowding in wards and intensive care units
  - Enforce strict hygiene, particularly handwashing, among physicians, nurses, and aides
- Avoid invasive procedures whenever possible
  - Employ indwelling intravenous and urinary catheters only if absolutely necessary
  - Change scalp vein needles, tubing, and intravenous bottles daily
  - Use respiratory assistance devices, particularly those requiring intubation, with great care and with close monitoring to ensure that they are adequately decontaminated
- Reduce number of colonizing organisms
  - Remove or reduce sites of prior infection
  - Consider the use of isoniazid prophylaxis in patients with histories, positive skin tests, or chest x-ray findings of old tuberculosis
  - Closely monitor serologic tests and clinical course in patients with evidence of old coccidioidomycosis or histoplasmosis who have now become immunosuppressed
- Bolster host defense mechanisms
  - Successfully treat the underlying disease
  - Prescribe adequate nutrition and exercise
  - Improve respiratory toilet
  - Control diabetes mellitus, congestive heart failure, or respiratory insufficiency
  - Reduce local obstruction caused by tumor
  - Protect the integrity of oral and anorectal mucosae
  - When appropriate, prescribe immunotherapy with vaccines and/or immunoglobulin preparation

Adapted from Levine AS, Schimpff SC, Graw RG Jr, et al: Semin Hematol 11:141, 1974.

Antimicrobial Strategies in the Immunocompromised Host

There are three modes in which antimicrobial agents can be utilized: a therapeutic mode, a prophylactic mode, and a preemptive mode. The term therapeutic describes the use of antimicrobial therapy to treat established clinical disease—the standard use of antimicrobial drugs. In general, in the immunocompromised host, clinical bacterial infection is treated for 5 to 7 days beyond the point when the patient becomes afebrile, and bactericidal regimens are preferred. In the case of fungal and nocardial infections, where markers of clinical activity may be less available and more prolonged therapies are required, our general rule is to treat for 2 to 4 weeks beyond the point when clinical evidence of active infection is present. The major factor determining the success of therapeutic programs in the compromised patient is early diagnosis followed by the immediate institution of effective therapy.[31]

Because of the potentially grave consequences of infection in the compromised host, there is a particular emphasis on prevention of infection by means of either prophylactic or preemptive therapy. Several important hypotheses underline the preventive aspects of antimicrobial therapy. Observations in animals with and without tumors have shown that if the animals are rendered germ free, there is an increased tolerance of chemotherapy, and larger doses may be given with enhanced tumoricidal effect and a greater chance for induction of remission from the neoplastic condition. Germ-free animals can tolerate a greater degree and duration of myelosuppression without added risk. Similarly, in transplantation, the greater the freedom from infection, the more intensively can rejection be treated or prevented, and the greater the rate of transplant success.[31,32] Thus an important precept in the care of patients requiring immunosuppressing therapy is the following: the therapeutic prescription has two components—an immunosuppressive component to control the disease process and an antimicrobial strategy to make it safe.[31]

The prophylactic use of antimicrobial therapy describes the administration of these drugs to an entire population of individuals prior to an event in order to prevent infection from developing. For prophylaxis to be worthwhile, two requirements must be fulfilled: the infection that is to be prevented is important enough and prevalent enough to justify prophylaxing a large group of individuals; and an effective prophylactic regimen is available that is nontoxic. In addition to surgical prophylaxis, perhaps the most successful examples of prophylaxis are the following: anti-*Pneumocystis* prophylaxis with trimethoprim-sulfamethoxazole or other strategies in the AIDS patient, the transplant recipient, the child with acute lymphocytic leukemia undergoing cycles of chemotherapy, and perhaps other patient groups; and the prevention of urosepsis, *Pneumocystis,* nocardiosis, and listeriosis in transplant patients with trimethoprim-sulfamethoxazole prophylaxis.[31]

What is less clear is the optimal approach for preventing bacterial and candidal infection in the cancer patient undergoing intensive chemotherapy that will result in prolonged neutropenia. Programs with protected environments (such as laminar airflow rooms with high-efficiency air filters), topical antiseptic and antimicrobial agents, sterile water and diets, and bowel decontamination with nonabsorbable antimicrobial agents have been tested in an effort to reduce infectious disease morbidity and mortality. Such programs markedly increase cost and are disliked by the patients because of the psychologic effects of the isolation and the abdominal discomfort and diarrhea caused by the antimicrobial agents. They do decrease the infectious disease events and mortality, but there is no difference in long-term patient survival, and these programs have largely fallen out of favor. More recently, simpler programs in which fluoroquinolones, such as ciprofloxacin, norfloxacin, or ofloxacin, are administered prophylactically have received attention. These agents are active against the normal aerobic flora of the gut, while leaving the anaerobes intact, thus preserving the *colonization resistance* activity that the anaerobic flora provide against the engraftment of potential pathogens. Such programs have become widely used not only in oncology patients but also in the liver transplant patient, with a number of promising reports of apparent efficacy.[32–37]

Less well established is the optimal approach to antifungal prophylaxis. Oral nystatin, clotrimazole, and amphotericin have been useful in the prevention and treatment of oral and esophageal candidiasis but appear to be ineffective in the prevention of invasive fungal infection. Fluconazole, particularly in dosages greater than 100 mg/day, may offer some protection, although the clinician needs to be alert for the appearance of candidal strains resistant to this drug, that is, *C. krusei, C. glabrata,* and other of the unusual strains. Fluconazole does appear to be active in preventing and treating invasive infection due to the most common and virulent of candidal species—*C. albicans* and *C. tropicalis.*[38]

Nonantimicrobial strategies that are beginning to be deployed prophylactically with some success in the immunocompromised host include the following: intravenous immunoglobulin replacement in patients with antibody deficiency and problems with recurrent infection (usually sinopulmonary or gastrointestinal) due to chronic lymphocytic leukemia or primary hypogammaglobulinemia; granulocyte colony-stimulating factor in neutropenic patients; interferon alpha (IFN-α) in patients with hairy cell leukemia; and interferon gamma (IFN-α) in patients with chronic granulomatous disease. As more and more of these cytokines, growth factors, and immunoglobulin preparations become available, the challenge will be not just to show clinical efficacy but to develop programs that are cost effective with these agents, which are both potent and quite expensive.[38]

Preemptive therapy is a new preventive concept applicable to the immunocompromised patient, in which intensive antimicrobial therapy is administered before the onset of clinical disease to a subgroup of individuals at especially high risk of clinical disease (rather than to everyone). The criteria for initiating preemptive therapy are either a clinical epidemiologic characteristic or a laboratory marker that delineates a patient as being at particularly high risk of life-threatening infection.[39] A number of examples of successful preemptive therapy have now been defined. In the organ transplant patient, the administration of anti-lymphocyte antibody therapy to treat allograft rejection to someone at risk of cytomegalovirus (CMV) infection (as defined by seropositivity prior to transplant) is associated with a two- to fourfold increase in the incidence of clinical CMV disease.[25] The administration of small doses of ganciclovir just during the course of anti-lymphocyte antibody therapy effectively eliminates this excessive incidence of clinical disease. In the bone marrow transplant recipient, the demonstration of CMV replication while the individual is still asymptomatic is highly associated with the subsequent development of pneumonia (a highly lethal condition in this patient population). If full-dose ganciclovir therapy is initiated on the basis of virologic data, while the patient is still asymptomatic, CMV pneumonia can be effectively preempted.[40,41] Similarly, preemptive fluconazole therapy in the renal transplant patient with asymptomatic candiduria will effectively prevent the development of obstructive fungal balls and candidal pyelonephritis; and fluconazole therapy following surgical excision of fungal nodules effectively eliminates the 5 to 10 percent incidence of dissemination previously observed following such a procedure, when it is unaccompanied by effective preemptive treatment.[24] Whether or not such a strategy offers similar protection to the critically ill surgical patient, who is colonized at multiple sites with candidal species and is at high risk for invasive disease, requires careful study—although the concept is quite appealing.

Timetable of Infection

An important clue to the etiology of an infectious disease syndrome in an immunocompromised patient is the duration of the immunosuppressed state prior to the onset of the fever, pneumonia, or other symptoms suggesting infection; that is, each immunocompromised state has a typical timetable that delineates what infections are apt to occur at particular points of time. Thus although pneumonia may occur at any point in a leukemia patient's course, the etiology is very different in the first few days (bacterial, often gram-positive), after 7 to 10 days of chemotherapy (predominantly gram-negative bacterial), or after 2 to 3 weeks of neutropenia (an increasing incidence of opportunistic infection, particularly that due to *Aspergillus* species). Perhaps the most carefully studied timetable is that for the organ transplant patient (Fig. 51–1), which is worth reviewing in detail, because of the lessons it contains. The post-transplant course can be divided into three time periods: the first month post-transplant; the period 1 to 6 months post-transplant; and the late period, more than 6 months post-transplant.[24,26]

In the first month post transplant the infectious disease problems can be divided into three general categories[24,26]:

1. Infection present in the recipient prior to transplant, which is exacerbated by the transplant operation and post-transplant immunosuppressive therapy. This is a particular problem in liver and cardiac transplant recipients whose precarious status prior to transplant can lead to pneumonia or intravenous line-related sepsis. Performing a transplant in such individuals is doomed to failure due to progressive infection in the case of pneumonia, and a high risk of seeding of the vascular suture lines if bacteria or fungal species are present in the bloodstream at the time of transplant. The cardinal rule is that all treatable infections must be eradicated prior to transplant.
2. Active infection conveyed with the allograft. Fortunately, this is an uncommon event, as

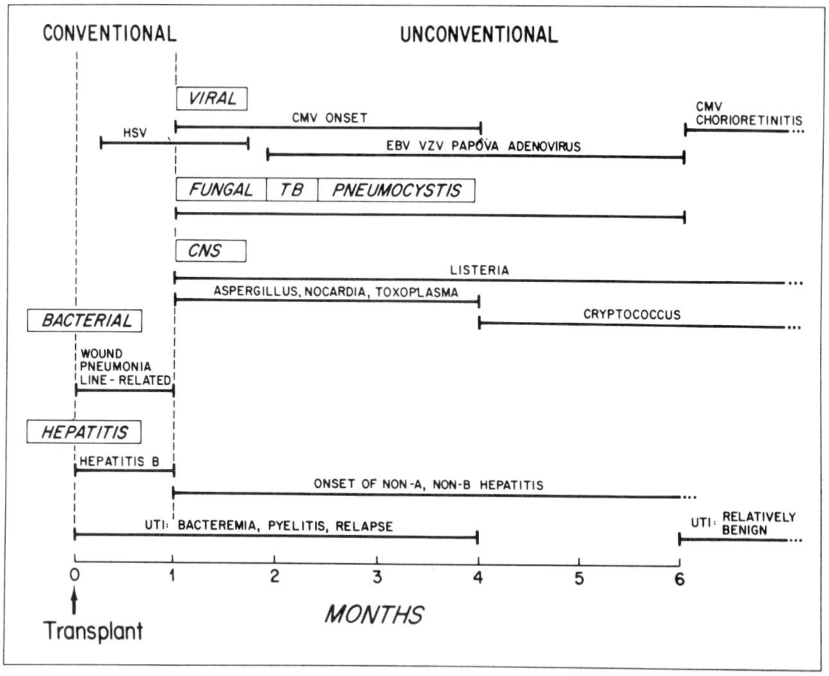

Figure 51–1. Timetable for the occurrence of infection in the renal transplant patient. Exceptions to the timetable should initiate a search for unusual epidemiology exposure (usually an excessive nosocomial hazard). CMV, cytomegalovirus; HSV, herpes simplex virus; EBV, Epstein-Barr virus; VZV, varicella-zoster virus; CNS, central nervous system; UTI, urinary tract infection. *(From Rubin RH, Wolfon JS, Cosimi AB, Tolkoff-Rubin NE: Am J Med 70:405, 1981.)*

transplantation of a contaminated organ will result in either systemic sepsis or infection of suture lines, with catastrophic rupture—particularly of vascular anastomoses.

3. More than 95 percent of the infections occurring in this time period are the same bacterial and candidal infections of the lungs, surgical wound, bladder, intravenous lines, or drainage catheters that occur in nonimmunosuppressed patients undergoing comparable amounts of surgery. The consequences may be greater, although the etiologies are the same, and the incidence in both populations is largely related to the technical skill with which the patient has been managed. This emphasis on technical excellence applies not only to the surgery but also to the management of the endotracheal tube, the vascular lines, and the drainage catheter and tubes. Surgery in the immunocompromised patient is the most technically demanding form of surgery possible, as a technical error invariably results in potentially life-threatening infection.

Notable by their absence in this first month post-transplant are opportunistic infections due to such organisms as *Pneumocystis carinii, Aspergillus* species, *Legionella* species, and *Listeria monocytogenes.* Exceptions to this rule should be regarded as strong evidence that an excessive epidemiologic exposure has occurred. This absence of opportunistic infection at a time when the daily dose of immunosuppressive drugs is at its highest underlines an important point: the net state of immunosuppression is predominantly determined by the intensity of therapy over a prolonged period, the area under the curve, rather than what is occurring on a single day or even several days.

In the period 1 to 6 months post-transplant, very different causes of infection occur. The most important of these are the viral infections—CMV, EBV, HIV, and hepatitis B and C. Not only do these cause clinical syndromes by themselves, but they also contribute significantly to the net state of immunosuppression, combining with the immunosuppressive therapy (the duration of which is now great enough to have a significant effect) to render the individual vulnerable to opportunistic infection with a wide variety of pathogens—even after very minor exposures.

Patients continuing on immunosuppression with functioning allografts more than 6 months post-transplant can be divided into three categories on the basis of their infectious disease problems:

1. Approximately 75 percent of patients who are on baseline immunosuppression with good allograft function and are at minimal risk of opportunistic infection. Their infections resemble those of the general community—pneumococcal pneumonia, influenza, urinary tract infection, and so on.

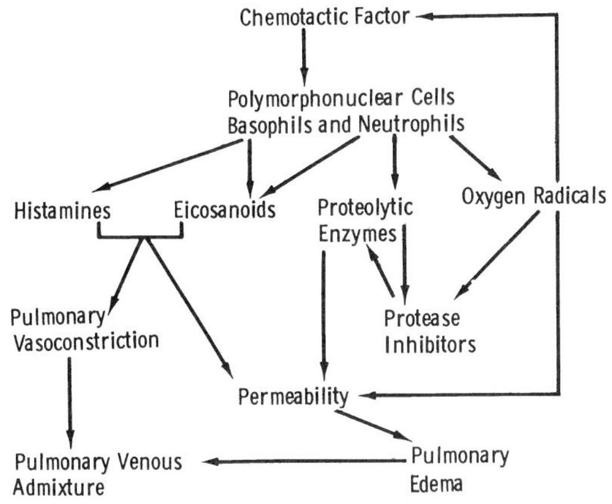

Figure 51–2. Timetable for infectious causes of fever in the bone marrow transplant patient. *(From Hibberd PL, Rubin RH: Fever in the immunocompromised host. In Mackowiak PA (ed): Fever, Basic Mechanisms and Management. New York, Raven Press, 1991.)*

2. Approximately 15 percent of patients who have had significant acute and chronic rejection, and thus have received excessive amounts of immunosuppression, are at high risk of infection with such opportunistic pathogens as *Cryptococcus neoformans, Pneumocystis carinii,* and *Listeria monocytogenes.*
3. Approximately 10 percent of patients with chronic viral infection will have inexorable progression of their infection, with destruction of the involved organ (progressive liver disease due to hepatitis B or C viruses, or chorioretinitis due to CMV) or the development of virus-associated malignancy (hepatocellular carcinoma due to the hepatitis viruses, lymphoproliferative disease due to EBV, or squamous cell carcinoma due to papillomaviruses).

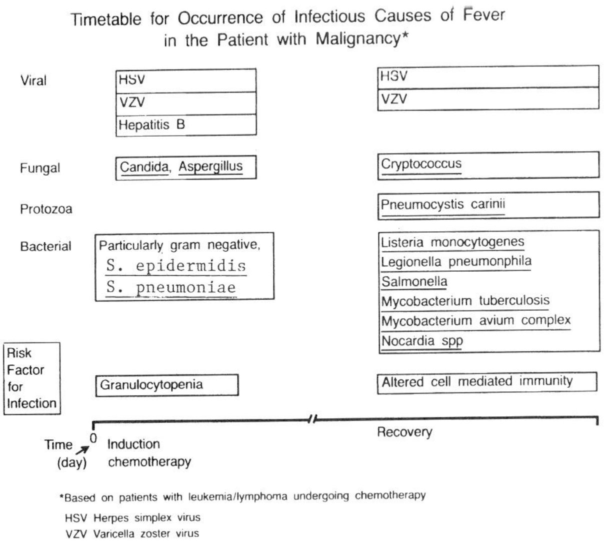

Figure 51–3. Timetable for infectious causes of fever in the patient with malignancy. *(From Hibberd PL, Rubin RH: Fever in the immunocompromised host. In Mackowiak PA (ed): Fever, Basic Mechanisms and Management. New York, Raven Press, 1991.)*

Figures 51–2, 51–3, and 51–4 outline the expected timetables of infection for other immunocompromised populations. Experience has shown that such timetables can be useful in two ways: in the evaluation of an individual patient with a clinical syndrome due to invasive infection and as an epidemiological tool, since exceptions to the timetable usually connote an unusual epidemiologic hazard.[24,26,42]

SPECIAL CLINICAL PROBLEMS IN THE IMMUNOSUPPRESSED PATIENT

Fever Without Evident Cause

Perhaps the most common clinical infectious disease problem in the compromised host is fever without evidence of a localized infection. The evaluation of such fevers in this patient population is often greatly complicated by the diminished inflammatory response that is frequently seen. For example, meningeal signs may be absent from patients with meningitis, or cough and sputum production may be impaired in patients with pneumonia.

The differential diagnosis of fever in these patients is extensive. Figure 51–5 illustrates the evaluation procedures used at one transplant center when a kidney recipient develops a fever of unknown origin. Fever may be due to noninfectious causes such as allograft rejection, malignancy, graft-versus-host disease, thromboembolic disease, allergic reactions to anti-lymphocyte serum, antimicrobial agents, anticonvulsants, and blood product transfusion reactions. Overall, more than 50 percent of the fevers, however, are caused by infections.[38,43]

Neutropenic patients, especially, can have life-threatening infection with few localizing findings. Gram-negative bacilli of gastrointestinal origin are particuarly common and usually enter through minor defects in the gastrointestinal mucosa, particularly in the mouth, the oropharynx, and the anorectum. In addition to minimal lesions leading to serious bacteremias, large areas of cellulitis, phlegmon, and frank abscess formation may develop. Another major site of entry is the lungs,

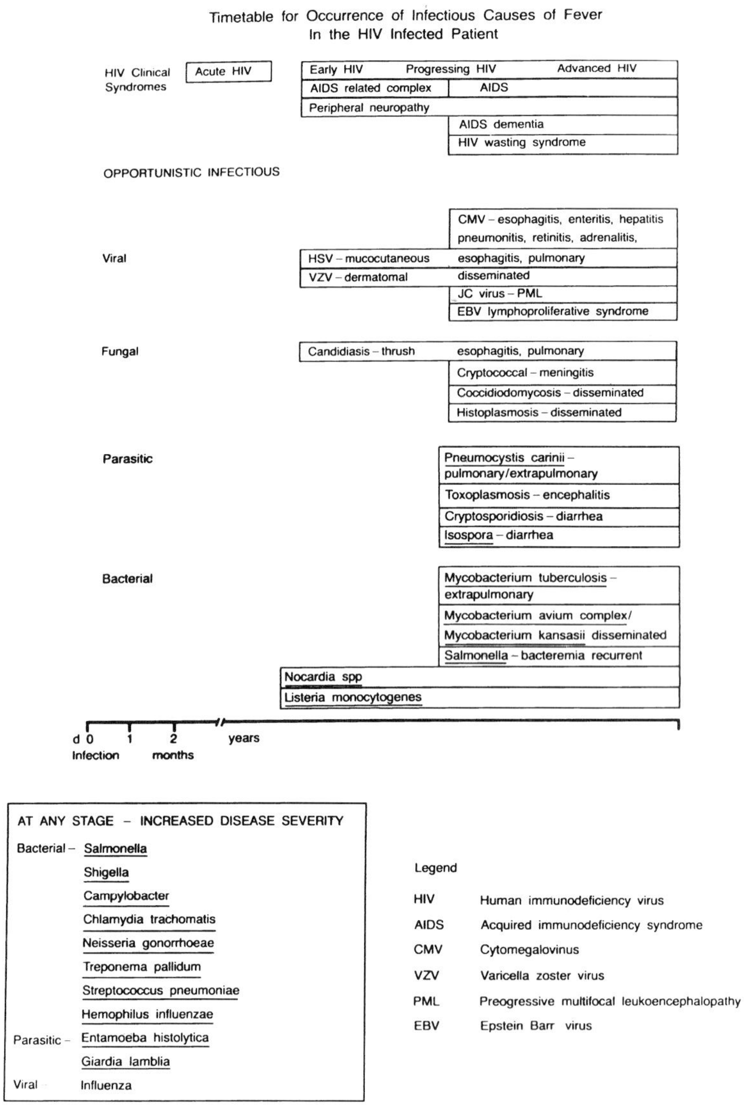

Figure 51–4. Timetable for infectious causes of fever in the HIV-infected patient. *(From Hibberd PL, Rubin RH: Fever in the immunocompromised host. In Mackowiak PA (ed): Fever, Basic Mechanisms and Management. New York, Raven Press, 1991.)*

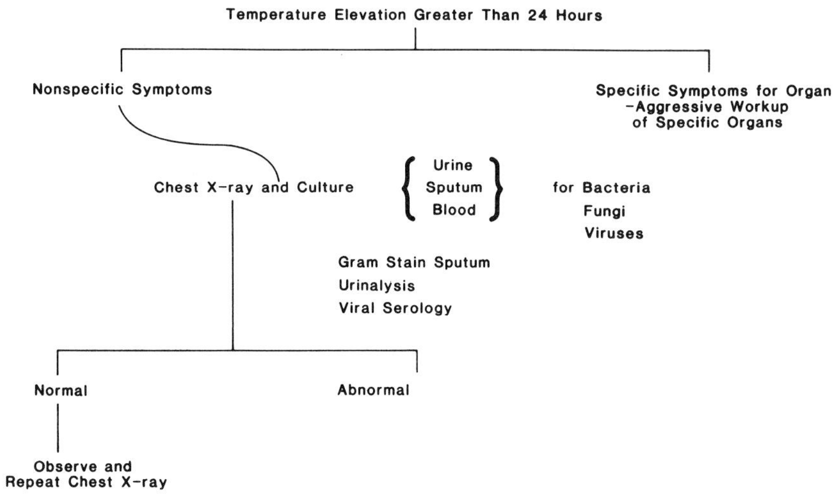

Figure 51–5. Flow diagram illustrating the evaluation of a transplant recipient with fever and nonlocalizing symptoms. *(From Matas AS, Simmons RL, Najarian JS: In Hardy JD (ed): Critical Surgical Illness. Philadelphia, Saunders, 1980.)*

where even a minimal infiltrate can cause overwhelming bacteremia. Perhaps the best example of this phenomenon comes from the studies of children with leukemia who develop pneumonia. The incidence of bacteremia is directly related to the neutrophil count. Patients with neutrophil counts greater than 1000/mm^3 had no positive blood cultures, compared with an incidence of 64 percent in those with counts less than 1000/mm^3.[44]

In recent years, mainly because of the common use of Hickman-Broviac catheters for venous access in the care of neutropenic patients (and also in part because of the selective pressures of quinolone prophylaxis), gram-positive organisms of cutaneous origin, such as *S. epidermidis, S. aureus, Corynebacterium* species (particularly group JK), and *Clostridium* species, have become the most common proved causes of bacteremia. Although gram-negative infections are rapidly lethal in the neutropenic patient, thus necessitating the immediate institution of therapy when such infections are thought to be present, such is not true for the majority of gram-positive infections. Thus the addition of vancomycin to the antimicrobial regimen can be delayed in most instances until either positive blood cultures are obtained or the patient has shown evidence of not responding to an initial program aimed primarily at gram-negative organisms. Approximately 85 percent of catheter-related infections can be cleared without removing the catheter. Venous access catheters must be removed to control the infection in the following circumstances: when significant infection of the catheter exit site or the subcutaneous tunnel is present; and when the infections are caused by *Candida* species, *Bacillus* species, and *Corynebacterium* group JK. Finally, when the decision is made to treat infections with the venous access catheter left in place, care should be taken to deliver the antimicrobial therapy in rotation to each of the lumen ports of these multiport catheters.[37,38]

Life-threatening sepsis may be present, even though there is no fever. More subtle signs of serious infection include unexplained tachypnea, hypotension, continuous volume requirement, and acidosis. Whatever the manifestation of infection, the critical consideration is speed, because these patients rapidly succumb unless antimicrobial therapy is instituted. When the initial physical examination, chest x-ray studies, Gram stain of the urine, and other immediate bedside evaluations are unrevealing, and cultures have been done, empiric therapy with broad spectrum antibiotics directed against a given hospital's most common infecting gram-negative bacteria in these populations of patients should be instituted immediately. The choice of antibiotics in these circumstances has become somewhat controversial. Traditionally, a two- or three-drug combination of an aminoglycoside, an antipseudomonal penicillin, and/or a cephalosporin has been employed for initial therapy to achieve broad spectrum antibacterial coverage and to increase the potential for synergistic therapy against the most common infecting bacteria. With the advent of the third- and fourth-generation cephalosporins, as well as some of the newer antipseudomonal penicillins and monobactams and thienamycins, the possibility of an alternative approach is increasingly being explored. With the use of these new agents, there is the potential for achieving broad spectrum coverage without the risk of aminoglycoside toxicity. The issue then becomes the importance of antimicrobial synergy. Preliminary studies have suggested that approaches using two of the newer agents together without an aminoglycoside and potentially only one of these agents, such as imipenem, can be quite successful with a decreased risk of toxicity.[45–47] One caution, however, remains in that many of these newer agents will induce the production of beta-lactamases by some of the gram-negative bacilli that infect these patients, resulting in ineffective therapy. Therefore more information is needed to choose between these two approaches. Although some groups prefer to use vancomycin as part of the initial therapy, as previously stated, our usual preference is to add vancomycin after evidence of gram-positive infection has developed. The major exception to this approach is the patient who is critically ill and deteriorating rapidly. In this instance, vancomycin is added to the gram-negative regimen immediately. Whatever antibacterial therapy is used, it is recommended that oral antifungal prophylaxis with either mycostatin or chlortrimazole troches be given simultaneously to retard fungal overgrowth of the gastrointestinal tract.

Several series show that the early use of empiric antibiotics in the febrile neutropenic patient lowers mortality, despite the fact that microbiologic proof of infection never emerges.[48,49] How, then, can therapy be terminated, particularly because the risk of superinfection apparently goes up after 7 days of broad spectrum antimicrobial therapy? Empiric antibiotic treatment and clinical evaluation should be continued for 5 to 7 days after antibiotics are initiated. If clinical infection has been documented, or if a clinical response to therapy has been demonstrated, treatment should be continued until the patient has been afebrile for a minimum of 7 days or there is clear evidence that the infection has disappeared. A more difficult decision has to be made in the patient who has manifested no clinical response to the antibacterial therapy and in whom no microbiologic diagnosis has been made. These individuals must be continuously reevaluated, looking first for overlooked clues to the presence of infection. The most frequently missed infection in these patients includes peridontal sepsis, perirectal abscess, occult pneumonia, and infections with fungi, protozoa, or viruses (particularly CMV). Once these possibilities have been eliminated, the question that then arises is whether or not an empiric trial of parenteral amphotericin therapy should be instituted. Clearly, in patients with esophagitis, prolonged diarrhea, history of exposure to broad spectrum antibiotics for greater than 10 days, or positive surveillance cultures for fungi, and continuing unexplained fever, an empiric trial of antifungal therapy is indicated. What remains controversial is whether or not, in patients with continuing fever without these clues to the possible presence of fungal infection, empiric amphotericin therapy should be added to the regimen.[50]

The same pressure for immediate empiric antimicrobial therapy is not present in patients with host defense defects who have normal levels of functioning neutrophils and who have fever but no other local findings. Therefore, in the renal transplant patient or the lymphoma patient with a normal white blood cell count, a more leisurely diagnostic work-up can usually be undertaken. In such patients with fever but no other localized findings, the major indication for initiating broad spectrum antimicrobial therapy without definite evidence of infection is the presence of rigors. The presence of frank rigors in a febrile transplant or lymphoma patient is highly associated with the presence of treatable bacterial infection. In our experience, more than 50 percent of such patients will have treatable infection.

Fever and Pneumonitis

The differential diagnosis of fever and pneumonitis in an immunocompromised patient includes both noninfectious and infectious causes. The noninfectious causes include radiation pneumonitis, drug-induced pneumonitis (bleomycin, busulfan, methotrexate, cyclophosphamide, procarbazine, nitrosurea compounds, chlorambucil, and rarely azathioprine, cytarabine, and cyclophosphamide); parenchymal invasion of the lung by tumor (particularly lymphoma); leukoagglutinin reaction; pulmonary emboli; pulmonary hemorrhage; and atypical congestive heart failure.[51]

Overall, infection is the cause of approximately 75 percent of the episodes of fever and pneumonitis in the immunocompromised patient, although in the patient with severe neutropenia, infection is the primary problem in more than 90 percent of such episodes.[52] Despite the emphasis that unusual opportunistic pathogens have received in many reports of pneumonitis in the immunocompromised host, it must be emphasized that common bacterial pathogens still predominate. Primary bacterial pneumonias occurring in outpatients are usually caused by *S. pneumoniae* and *H. influenzae.* Those that are nosocomially acquired are predominantly caused by enteric gram-negative bacilli. Bacterial pneumonia in the immunosuppressed population is similar to that in the general population. The onset is acute (within hours), the x-ray patterns are characteristic, and the response to therapy is prompt. The major difference lies in the risk of superinfection with antibiotic-resistant bacteria or fungi. In fact, superinfection is the major cause of death in the immunosuppressed patient. At autopsy, it is often impossible to find the original infecting pathogen, although several other agents are usually present (eg, herpes simplex virus, *Candida*). These organisms rarely cause primary pulmonary infection but are frequently part of a fatal polymicrobial superinfection.[51,52]

A major factor that can predispose to superinfection is cytomegalovirus infection, which exerts its major effect 1 to 4 months postorgan transplantation or 1 to 2 months after transfusion of leukocyte-containing blood products in patients with lymphoproliferative disorders. This agent not only can produce pneumonia by itself, but also damages the lung and the alveolar macrophages, which are an important local host defense against infection, and also has a major effect on other host defenses. The net effect is a higher level of immunosuppression and an injured lung that is very vulnerable to superinfection with a wide variety of opportunistic pathogens.[24,51]

Whatever the underlying factors, speed in establishing a diagnosis and initiating therapy is the most important factor in determining the outcome. Important clues may be gained by using information concerning the pace of the illness, the history of the underlying disease, the therapy used to manage it, and the pattern of pulmonary infiltrate observed on chest x-ray studies. As outlined in Table 51–5, a grid can be constructed that suggests the differential diagnosis based on the chest x-ray study and the pace at which the process is proceeding. Thus an illness that develops over a relatively few hours suggests acute bacterial infection, pulmonary embolus, acute pulmonary edema, or pulmonary hemorrhage. A subacute onset (over a few

TABLE 51–5. DIFFERENTIAL DIAGNOSIS OF FEVER AND PULMONARY INFILTRATES IN THE COMPROMISED HOST ACCORDING TO X-RAY ABNORMALITY AND THE RATE OF PROGRESSION OF THE SYMPTOMS[a]

	Etiology According to the Rate of Progression of the Illness	
Chest X-Ray Abnormality	*Acute*	*Subacute-Chronic*
Consolidation	Conventional bacterial *Legionella* Thromboembolic Hemorrhage (pulmonary edema)	Fungal Nocardial Tuberculous Tumor (viral, *Pneumocystis, Mycoplasma,* radiation, drug-induced)
Peribronchovascular ("interstitial") infiltrate	Pulmonary edema Leukoagglutinin reaction (bacterial)	Viral *Pneumocystis* Radiation Drug-induced (fungal, nocardial, tuberculous, tumor)
Nodular infiltrate	(bacterial, pulmonary edema)	Tumor Fungal Nocardial Tuberculous *(Pneumocystis)*

[a] An acute illness is one developing and requiring medical attention in a matter of a relatively few hours (less than 24 hours). A subacute-chronic process develops over several days to weeks. Note that unusual causes of a process are placed in parentheses.
Adapted from Ramsey PG, Rubin RH, Tolkoff-Rubin NE, et al: Medicine (Baltimore) 59:206, 1980.

days) suggests viral infection, *Pneumocystis, Aspergillus,* or *Nocardia.* A more chronic course (over several days to weeks) suggests fungal, nocardial, or tuberculous infection, or tumor-, drug-, or radiation-induced pneumonitis.[51] The exemplary review by Williams and colleagues[53] points out that no radiologic pattern is specific for one particular pathogen, although certain patterns are more characteristic of some infectious agents than of others. Consolidation seen on air bronchograms suggests pneumococcal or *Klebsiella* infection, pulmonary hemorrhage, or other processes primarily infecting the distal air spaces. In contrast, an interstitial pattern suggests *Pneumocystis,* viral, leukoagglutinin, or drug-related disease. Cavitary lesions suggest fungal, nocardial, or tuberculous infection. Thus a series of clues will considerably narrow the diagnostic possibilities.

Even with these clues, an exact diagnosis must be aggressively sought so that specific therapy can be instituted quickly. Figure 51–6 shows the steps used at one center for evaluating a kidney transplant patient who has a fever and symptoms of pulmonary involvement. The classic approach to pneumonia has centered on the microscopic and cultural examination of expectorated sputum, and indeed this should be the first test employed in the evaluation in all patients. However, several factors make this approach unreliable in many immunocompromised patients. (1) These patients often fail to produce sputum, even after the most aggressive induction methods. (2) These patients have a high incidence of pharyngeal colonization by a variety of potentially invasive pathogens, particularly gram-negative bacilli, *S. aureus,* and fungi, that may have nothing to do with the process going on in the lung. Therefore the distinction between colonizers and invaders is difficult. (3) Several of the pathogens that invade this population are not shed into the sputum (*Aspergillus, Pneumocystis, Legionella*); therefore false-negative results are to be expected. (4) The noninfectious causes of the febrile pneumonitis syndrome in this population cannot be diagnosed in this fashion.[51] Therefore invasive techniques have been designed to obtain more accurate information—induced sputum, bronchoscopy with bronchoalveolar lavage and/or transbronchial biopsy, transthoracic biopsy via the thoracoscope, and open lung biopsy. Indeed, the critical decision-making involved in an immunocompromised host with fever and pneumonia is the proper deployment of these diagnostic techniques. The key issue that must be addressed before any invasive procedure in this patient population is the likelihood that information will be gained that will result in a major change in therapy and meaningful prolongation of the patient's life. Thus invasive procedures (beyond an induced sputum examination) are rarely indicated in

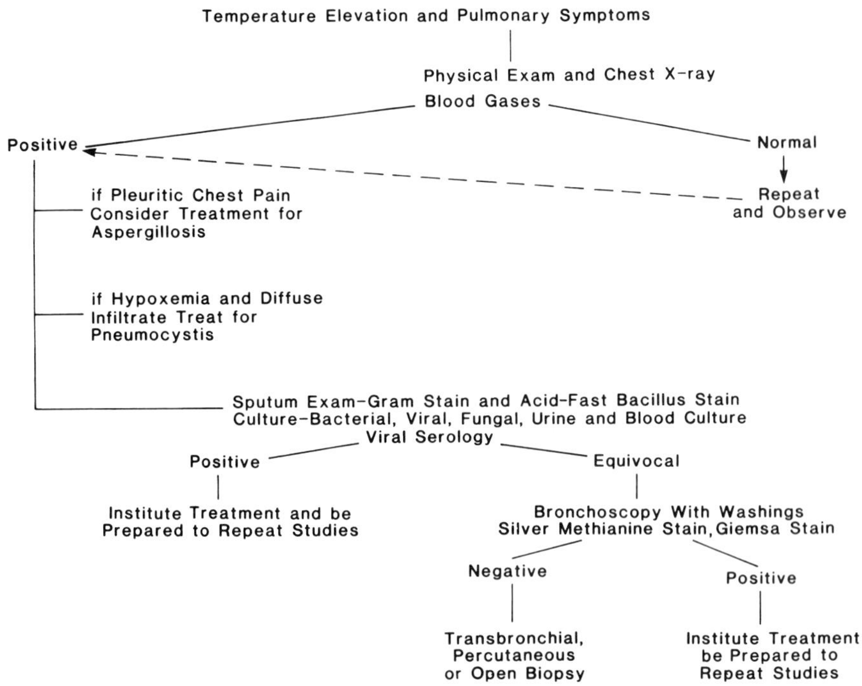

Figure 51–6. Flow diagram illustrating the evaluation of a transplant recipient with fever and pulmonary symptoms. *(From Matas AS, Simmons RL, Najarian JS: In Hardy JD (ed): Critical Surgical Illness. Philadelphia, Saunders, 1980.)*

patients with advanced leukemia, AIDS, or metastatic cancer. In contrast, they usually are indicated in transplant patients, patients with treatable lymphoma, and patients being treated with immunosuppression for collagen vascular or inflammatory bowel disease.[51]

The AIDS epidemic, with its high incidence of *Pneumocystis* pneumonia, has been the driving force behind the widespread deployment of the induced sputum technique. Indeed, when the specimen obtained by sputum induction techniques is subjected to immunofluorescent staining with a monoclonal antibody specific for *P. carinii,* a sensitivity and specificity of more than 90 percent can be obtained in AIDS patients.[54] One caution must be underlined, however: since non-AIDS patients with *Pneumocystis* have a significantly lower organism burden, the diagnostic yield of an induced sputum is considerably less (at least 25 percent less in our experience with organ transplant patients). Although precise data are currently lacking as to the usefulness of this approach, many groups have been utilizing the induced sputum examination to diagnose bacterial and fungal pneumonias. Indeed, this approach has largely replaced transtracheal aspiration in the initial evaluation of patients with pneumonia of unclear cause.[51]

If the diagnosis is not clear after examination of the induced sputum, then the next diagnostic step assumes great importance, with the appropriate choice being made on the basis of several factors: the degree of patient illness, the rate of progression of the process, the type of infiltrate present on x-ray study, and the expertise and experience of personnel at a given institution. If the pneumonitis and the degree of hypoxia are progressing rapidly, the definitive diagnostic procedure—the open lung biopsy—should be carried out immediately. This is particularly true when the pattern of infiltrate is diffuse or multifocal. If the pulmonary process is progressing at a more desultory pace, progressive hypoxia is not an immediate problem, and the clinical problem is more of a diagnostic dilemma than a therapeutic emergency, then less invasive techniques can be attempted, with the open lung biopsy being available if these other techniques fail.[51–53]

The choice among these moderately invasive techniques, assuming that adequate expertise is available, is then guided by the pattern of infiltrate present. Fiberoptic bronchoscopy, with the accompanying procedures it makes possible, is the approach of choice in the immunocompromised patient with diffuse lung disease. In the patient with *Pneumocystis,* bronchoalveolar lavage is so sensitive—if the resulting samples are handled properly—that transbronchial biopsy and bronchial brushing add little to the diagnostic yield, while adding considerably to the complication rate.[51,55] Transbronchial biopsy is particularly useful in the diagnosis of allograft rejection in lung transplant recipients, leukemic infiltrates, radiation- and drug-induced pneumonitis, in various forms of interstitial pneumonitis, and some viral infections.[51–53,56] In recent years, because of the desire for larger tissue samples for diagnosis, many centers, including our own, have turned to transpleural biopsy through the thoracoscope in patients with diffuse interstitial or pleural based focal disease.[51,57]

The initial procedure of choice for diagnosing focal pulmonary processes in the compromised host, particularly when infection is the primary consideration, is percutaneous, aspiration needle biopsy. A sensitivity greater than 80 percent has been noted for infection, and greater than 90 percent for malignancy. When 22- or 23-gauge Chiba needles are employed, the incidence of even moderate hemoptysis postprocedure is less than 1 percent.[51,58,59] The major complication of percutaneous needle aspiration of the lung is pneumothorax, with an average reported incidence of 20 to 25 percent. However, when appropriate precautions are taken (a single pleural puncture at biopsy; the patients being placed with the puncture site down for a period of at least 1 hour or until air leakage has ceased; and restriction of coughing, talking, and activity for this time period), the requirement for chest tube placement is approximately 1 percent.[51,60]

The final consideration is when empirical antimicrobial therapy should be initiated without attempts at specific diagnosis. In our experience, the following are the most common situations in which such an approach appears warranted: (1) patients with far-advanced AIDS, relapsing acute myelogenous leukemia, and other advanced malignancies where life expectancy is limited because of the severity of the underlying illness; (2) patients with leukemia prior to therapy, as there is an exceedingly low probability of opportunistic infection, and antibacterial therapy has a high probability of success; (3) a patient with either an uncorrectable bleeding disorder or respiratory function that would not permit an invasive study; and (4) patients who refuse invasive diagnostic studies. In such clinical situations, the precise nature of the empirical therapy is decided on the basis of the epidemiologic and clinical setting, the host defense defects present, the pace of the pulmonary process, and the radiographic pattern.[51]

SPECIFIC INFECTIONS IN THE COMPROMISED HOST

Acquired Immune Deficiency Syndrome

The acquired immune deficiency syndrome (AIDS) is defined as the occurrence of life-threatening opportunistic infection, Kaposi's sarcoma, or both in patients who have not received immunosuppressive therapy and who have no apparent immunosuppressing disease. In addition, as of 1993, the Centers for Disease Control and Prevention (CDC) has broadened the definition to include individuals infected with the human immunodeficiency virus (HIV, the causative agent of AIDS) who have CD4+ T cell counts of less than 200/mm. Currently available evidence suggests that 80 percent of this last group of individuals will develop an AIDS-related opportunistic infection or malignancy over a 3-year period. Table 51–6 summarizes the current criteria for making the diagnosis of AIDS.[61–63]

Epidemiology. AIDS is initiated by infection with the human retrovirus, HIV. At present, more than one million individuals in the United States are believed to harbor the virus, with an estimated 40,000 adults and 2,000 newborns being newly infected each year. Approximately 300,000 cases of AIDS have occurred in the United States since the first reports in 1981, with approximately two-thirds of these individuals having died. Worldwide, AIDS has been estimated to have occurred in more than one million adults and 500,000 children, with expectations that this number will increase more than tenfold, particularly in Africa and Southeast Asia. Current estimates suggest that 54 percent of individuals will develop overt AIDS within 10 years of being infected with HIV, with virtually all the rest eventually developing AIDS if they live long enough.[61]

HIV is a transmissible, blood-borne infection that can also be spread by intimate contact. Thus transmission occurs primarily through sexual contact, pregnancy, delivery, or breast-feeding; transfusion of blood products; or communal intravenous drug abuse.[64] Four population groups have accounted for the vast majority of AIDS cases in the United States: 59 percent have been homosexual or bisexual men (8 percent of whom also have a history of intravenous drug use); 21 percent have been heterosexual intravenous drug users; 2 percent acquired their infections from transfusions, virtually all before testing of blood became possible in 1985 (although, because of the long latent period between HIV infection and the development of AIDS, new cases of post-transfusion AIDS are still being identified); and 1 percent were hemophiliacs who likewise were infected by contaminated blood products. With currently available techniques for testing of blood for HIV (vide infra), the risk of transmitting this virus by blood transfusion is approximately 1 in 153,000 per unit of blood. Thus far in the United States, less than 10 percent of cases have occurred as a result of heterosexual contact,

TABLE 51–6. CDC SURVEILLANCE CASE DEFINITION FOR AIDS

I. *HIV Status of Patient Is Unknown or Inconclusive*

If laboratory tests for HIV infection were not performed or gave inconclusive results and the patient had no other cause of immunodeficiency listed in I*A* (see below), a definitive diagnosis of any disease listed in I*B* (see below) indicates AIDS.

A. Causes of immunodeficiency that disqualify a disease as an indication of AIDS in the absence of laboratory evidence of HIV infection

1. The use of high-dose or long-term systemic corticosteroid therapy or other immunosuppressive/cytotoxic therapy within 3 months before the onset of the indicator disease.
2. A diagnosis of any of the following diseases within 3 months after diagnosis of the indicator disease: Hodgkin's disease, non-Hodgkin's lymphoma (other than primary brain lymphoma), lymphocytic leukemia, multiple myeloma, any other cancer of lymphoreticular or histiocytic tissue, or angioimmunoblastic lymphadenopathy.
3. A genetic (congenital) immunodeficiency syndrome or an acquired immunodeficiency syndrome that is atypical of HIV infection, such as one involving hypogammaglobulinemia.

B. Diseases that indicate AIDS (*requires definitive diagnosis*)

1. Candidiasis of the esophagus, trachea, bronchi, or lungs.
2. Cryptococcosis, extrapulmonary.
3. Cryptosporidiosis with diarrhea persisting for more than 1 month.
4. Cytomegalovirus disease of an organ other than the liver, spleen, or lymph nodes in a patient older than 1 month.
5. Herpes simplex virus infection causing a mucocutaneous ulcer that persists longer than 1 month; or herpes simplex virus infection causing bronchitis, pneumonitis, or esophagitis for any duration in a patient older than 1 month.
6. Kaposi's sarcoma in a patient younger than 60 years.
7. Lymphoid interstitial pneumonia or pulmonary lymphoid hyperplasia (LIP/PLH complex) in a patient younger than 13 years.
8. Lymphoma of the brain (primary) affecting a patient younger than 60 years.
9. *Mycobacterium avium* complex or *M. kansasii* disease, disseminated (at a site other than or in addition to the lungs, skin, or cervical or hilar lymph nodes).
10. *Pneumocystis carinii* pneumonia.
11. Progressive multifocal leukoencephalopathy.
12. Toxoplasmosis of the brain in a patient older than 1 month.

II. *Patient Is HIV Positive*

Regardless of the presence of other causes of immunodeficiency (see I*A*, above), in the presence of laboratory evidence of HIV infection, any disease listed in I*B* (see above) or in II*A* or II*B* (see below) indicates a diagnosis of AIDS. In addition, beginning in 1993, all HIV-positive adults and adolescents with CD4+ T cell counts less than 200/mm^3 or with pulmonary tuberculosis, recurrent pneumonia, or invasive cervical carcinoma should also be included in the AIDS case definition.

A. Diseases that indicate AIDS (*requires definitive diagnosis*)

1. Bacterial infections, multiple or recurrent (any combination of at least two within a 2- to 4-year period), of the following types in a patient younger than 13 years: septicemia, pneumonia, meningitis, bone or joint infection, or abscess of an internal organ or body cavity (excluding otitis media or superficial skin or mucosal abscesses) caused by *Hemophilus, Streptococcus* (including pneumococcus), or other pyogenic bacteria.
2. Coccidioidomycosis, disseminated (at a site other than or in addition to the lungs or cervical or hilar lymph nodes).
3. Histoplasmosis, disseminated (at a site other than or in addition to the lungs or cervical or hilar lymph nodes).
4. HIV encephalopathy.
5. HIV wasting syndrome.
6. Isosporiasis with diarrhea persisting for more than 1 month.
7. Kaposi's sarcoma at any age.
8. Lymphoma of the brain (primary) at any age.
9. *M. tuberculosis* disease, extrapulmonary (involving at least one site outside the lungs, regardless of whether there is concurrent pulmonary involvement).
10. Mycobacterial disease caused by mycobacteria other than *M. tuberculosis,* disseminated (at a site other than or in addition to the lungs, skin, or cervical or hilar lymph nodes).
11. Non-Hodgkin's lymphoma of B cell or unknown immunologic phenotype and the following histologic types: small noncleaved lymphoma (Burkitt's or non-Burkitt's) or immunoblastic sarcoma.
12. *Salmonella* (nontyphoidal) septicemia, recurrent.

B. Diseases that indicate AIDS (*presumptive diagnosis*)

1. Candidiasis of the esophagus.
2. Cytomegalovirus retinitis, with loss of vision.
3. Kaposi's sarcoma.
4. Lymphoid interstitial pneumonia or pulmonary lymphoid hyperplasia (LIP/PLH complex) in a patient younger than 13 years.
5. Mycobacterial disease (acid-fast bacilli with species not identified by culture), disseminated (involving at least one site other than or in addition to the lungs, skin, or cervical or hilar lymph nodes).
6. *P. carinii* pneumonia.
7. Toxoplasmosis of the brain in a patient older than 1 month.

III. *Patient Is HIV Negative*

With laboratory test results negative for HIV infection, a diagnosis of AIDS for surveillance purposes is ruled out *unless*

A. All the other causes of immunodeficiency listed in 1*A* (see above) are excluded; and

B. The patient has had either of the following:

1. *P. carinii* pneumonia diagnosed by a definitive method.
2. A definitive diagnosis of any of the other diseases indicative of AIDS listed in I*B* (see above) and a CD4+ helper-inducer T cell count of less than 400/mm^3.

but this number is increasing. In the developing countries of the world that are particularly afflicted with this plague, heterosexual transmission is the predominant mode of spread. In the 1990s, it is likely that an increasing proportion of AIDS cases will be in women, as a result of heterosexual transmission, in intravenous drug users, and in young children infected perinatally. It is already clear that HIV infection has and will continue to have a particularly great impact on minority populations who live in the inner cities.[61,64–67]

Pathogenesis. AIDS is initiated by infection with the human immunodeficiency virus, a member of the cytopathic lentivirus family of retroviruses, which as a group produce fatal illnesses characterized by immunosuppression and/or neurodegenerative disease. HIV-1, the prototype virus, is responsible for virtually all cases of AIDS outside Africa; HIV-2, a retrovirus that more closely resembles the simian immunodeficiency virus, has been isolated from patients in West Africa and from individuals with some type of epidemiologic link to West Africa.[61,67–70]

HIV binds to cells bearing the CD4 surface molecule, which serves as the high-affinity cell surface receptor for the virus. Thus CD4+ T cells, which have the highest density of this molecule on their surfaces, are most affected by the virus. Certain populations of monocytes and macrophages, as well as certain neurons and brain glial cells, are also easily infected by this virus. Different isolates of the virus appear to exhibit particular tropisms for one or another cell type. Virtually all the immunodeficiency engendered by HIV infection (Table 51–7) is explained by its depletion of the CD4+ T cell function, as this cell, with its helper/inducer function, has a major effect on virtually every limb of host defense. HIV infection of CD4+ T cells can take one of two forms: active viral replication and latent infection. As HIV infection progresses from the asymptomatic stage to overt AIDS, the number of cells with actively replicating virus increases. In addition, lymphocyte activation will upregulate HIV replication, with a variety of processes commonly present in HIV-infected individuals causing such activation: antigenic or mitogenic stimulation, allogeneic reactions, certain cytokines, and the gene products of such viruses as CMV, EBV, other herpesviruses, and hepatitis B virus.[61,68–73]

The second cell population that becomes infected with HIV is the CD4-bearing subset of monocytes and macrophages. It has been hypothesized that these infected cells serve as important reservoirs of persistent infection within the host and as vehicles for transporting HIV to the central nervous system. In addition, it is likely that disordered macrophage function induced by HIV infection has more direct clinical consequences. Thus alveolar macrophage dysfunction induced by HIV probably plays a significant role in the pathogenesis of *Pneumocystis* pneumonia in these patients. Interleukin 1 (IL-1) and tumor necrosis factor (TNF) release by HIV-infected monocytes and macrophages probably is responsible for the chronic fevers and cachexia that may otherwise be unexplained in an AIDS patient.[68–71,74]

An indirect effect of HIV infection in many AIDS patients is profound B cell dysfunction, as manifested by one or more of the following: polyclonal B cell activation, hypergammaglobulinemia, circulating immune complexes, autoantibodies, and

TABLE 51–7. IMMUNOLOGIC ABNORMALITIES NOTED IN PATIENTS WITH AIDS

Prevalence	Specific Abnormality
Almost always present	Lymphopenia
	Selective T cell deficiency based on a quantitative reduction of the helper-inducer subset (T4-positive)
	Decreased or absent delayed cutaneous hypersensitivity to both recall and new antigens
	Elevated serum immunoglobulins, predominantly IgG and IgA in adults and including IgM in children
	Increased spontaneous immunoglobulin secretion by individual B-lymphocytes
Constantly observed	Decreased in vitro lymphocyte proliferative responses
	Decreased cytotoxic responses
	Decreased ability to mount a de novo antibody response to a new antigen
	Altered monocyte function
	Elevated serum levels of immune complexes
Occasionally present	Increased levels of acid-labile interferon alpha
	Antilymphocyte syndrome
	Suppressor factors
	Increased levels of β_2 microglobulins and thymosin alpha-1; decreased serum thymulin levels

Adapted from Seligman M, Chess L, Fahey JL, et al: N Engl J Med 311:1286, 1984.

a deficient antibody (particularly IgM) response to primary immunizations. Clinically, this has been correlated with an increased risk of bloodstream invasion and dissemination with the encapsulated bacteria, *Streptococcus pneumoniae,* and *Hemophilus influenzae* type B. This B cell dysfunction is due to the fact that the virus itself and certain subunits of the virus, most notably the gp120 envelope glycoprotein, are polyclonal activators of B cells.[61,68–71,74]

HIV shares the ability of other retroviruses of this class to produce progressive neurodegenerative disease. In addition to the fact that glial cells and certain neurons bear the CD4 molecule on their surfaces, evidence has also been put forth that galactosylceramide found in neuronal surface membrane can also serve as an alternative receptor for the virus in the brain. In addition to the direct consequences of viral infection to the brain, cytolytic T cells aimed at viral determinants presumably also contribute to the pathogenesis of neuronal injury.[61,68–71,74,75]

Clinical Manifestations It is convenient to divide the clinical manifestations of AIDS into four general categories: those due to the direct effects of HIV, those due to the opportunistic infections stemming from the immunosuppression initiated by this virus, those due to Kaposi's sarcoma, and those due to the other malignant diseases that are caused by the combined effects of HIV-induced immunosuppression and the malignancy-promoting effects of the other viruses commonly found in this patient population.

A variety of clinical syndromes have now been correlated with infection with HIV. It is now clear that acute infection of seronegative individuals with the virus can cause a mononucleosis-like syndrome that has been characterized by sudden onset, duration of 7 to 21 days, and complaints of fever, sweats, malaise, easy fatiguability, myalgias, arthralgias, headaches, sore throat, diarrhea, generalized lymphadenopathy, macular erythematous truncal eruption, and thrombocytopenia.[76,77] Even more commonly recognized than this acute mononucleosis-like syndrome is a chronic version of this. Approximately 10 to 30 percent of homosexual men who eventually developed AIDS have a persistent version of this syndrome that may go on for months. Of these patients with the chronic lymphadenopathy syndrome, approximately 15 to 20 percent will develop full-blown AIDS over the next year. Because the individuals with this persistent mononucleosis or chronic lymphadenopathy syndrome have similar epidemiologic features as patients with AIDS, have antibody to HIV, and have similar immunologic abnormalities, it is believed by most that this syndrome is a prodromal form of AIDS and has been termed the AIDS-related complex, or pre-AIDS.[77,78]

A number of organs may be particular sites of attack for the virus. Most notable is the central nervous system, where unexplained dementia or encephalopathy has been described in patients with AIDS, with direct infection of the brain with HIV being responsible for these central nervous system symptoms.[75,79] In addition, an enteropathy characterized by malabsorption and mucosal abnormalities of the small intestine has been associated with this virus[80]; renal dysfunction due to glomerular disease has been observed,[81] as well as autoimmune thrombocytopenia, a variety of endocrine-metabolic disorders, including hypercalcemia and adrenal insufficiency,[82] a recrudescence of atopy, and a marked increase in the incidence and severity of allergic reactions to a drug that is important in the therapy of many of these patients, namely trimethoprim-sulfamethoxazole.[61]

Much more common in AIDS patients than these direct effects of the virus are the clinical syndromes caused by invasion with opportunistic infection. By far, the most common clinical presentation of AIDS is with *P. carinii* pneumonia (approximately 50 percent of cases).[61,78,83] Typically, the patients present with a subacute onset of a nonproductive cough and progressive dyspnea over days to weeks. Interstitial pneumonitis is evident on chest x-ray studies, and arterial blood gas studies reveal hypoxia and hypocarbia. However, a significant minority of AIDS patients with cough and dyspnea have biopsy-provable *P. carinii* infection, despite a negative chest x-ray, presumably due to the impaired inflammatory response to the presence of this organism in these individuals. In such patients, abnormal pulmonary function tests or a positive gallium scan can provide an early clue to the presence of *Pneumocystis* infection.

Probably the most important secondary infection besides *Pneumocystis* in AIDS patients is that due to *Mycobacterium tuberculosis,* which is having a major effect both on HIV-infected individuals and on their communities and medical facilities. On the one hand, the profound defect in cell-mediated immunity present in AIDS patients permits the rapid proliferation and dissemination of the tubercle bacilli throughout the individual; on the other hand, the impaired inflammatory response will obscure the clinical and radiologic manifestations of the disease until very late in the course. This has two consequences: far advanced tuberculosis in the AIDS patient is exceedingly difficult to treat; and the public health consequences of individuals with a large burden of organisms who are not under treatment can be catastrophic. All these unfortunate events are exacerbated by the spread of HIV infection in the inner city populations with a high incidence of multidrug-resistant tuberculosis, thus amplifying the public health consequences of tuberculosis in these communities. The end result has been the occurrence of epidemics of tuberculosis, especially multidrug-resistant tuberculosis, in urban health facilities and correctional institutions. Patients, staff, family members, and other contacts are all affected.[61,84–87]

Table 51–8 outlines the other opportunistic infections that are seen in these patients, obviously manifestations of the seriously depressed cell-mediated immunity that are observed. In addition, it must be emphasized that multiple infections may be present simultaneously in the individual patient, as well as sequential infections.

Approximately 30 percent of AIDS patients present with Kaposi's sarcoma, with an additional 7 percent presenting with both *Pneumocystis* pneumonia and Kaposi's sarcoma.[61,78] Not only do these patients have Kaposi's sarcoma, but this is clearly a different clinical entity from that observed with patients with classic Kaposi's sarcoma, which usually has a cutaneous presentation and indolent course. In contrast, patients with AIDS typically have a multicentric process involving lymph nodes and visceral organs, particularly the gastrointestinal tract, as well as the skin. In addition, Kaposi's sarcoma can cause both pulmonary infiltrates and respiratory failure in AIDS patients.[61,78]

A variety of malignancies other than Kaposi's sarcoma occur at an increased rate in AIDS patients, presumably due to the interaction between certain potentially oncogenic viruses and the altered immune system. The most notable examples are EBV-associated B cell lymphoproliferative disease and Burkitt's lymphoma. Other malignancies and their possible viral associations include the following: Hodgkin's disease (EBV), carcinoma of the cervix uteri (papillomavirus), certain carcinomas of the anus and rectum (herpes simplex type 2), and carcinoma of the tongue (herpes simplex type 1).[61]

Diagnosis. There are three separate diagnostic issues that must be addressed when dealing with patients with possible HIV-related disease: the diagnosis of HIV infection; the diagnosis of overt AIDS; and the diagnosis of any secondary opportunistic infection or malignancy that might be present.[88,89] The cornerstone of HIV diagnosis is measuring the

TABLE 51–8. INFECTIOUS COMPLICATIONS OF AIDS

Infecting Organism	Type of Infection
VIRUSES	
Cytomegalovirus	Pneumonia, disseminated infection, retinitis, encephalitis, gastroinestinal ulcerations
Epstein-Barr virus	Important pathogenic factor in B cell lymphoproliferative disorders and Burkitt's lymphoma, oral hairy leukoplakia
Herpes simplex virus	Recurrent severe localized infection
Papovavirus	Progressive multifocal leukoencephalopathy
Varicella-zoster virus	Localized or disseminated infection
FUNGI	
Aspergillus	Invasive pulmonary infection with potential for dissemination
Candida albicans	Mucocutaneous infection, esophagitis, disseminated infection
Coccidioides immitis	Disseminated infection
Cryptococcus neoformans	Meningitis, disseminated infection
Histoplasma capsulatum	Disseminated infection
Petriellidium boydii	Pneumonia
Pneumocystis carinii	Pneumonia, retinal infection
PROTOZOA	
Cryptosporidium	Enteritis
Isospora belli	Enteritis
Toxoplasma gondii	Encephalitis
MYCOBACTERIA	
Mycobacterium avium-intracellulare	Pulmonary, extrapulmonary, or disseminated infection
M. tuberculosis	Pulmonary, extrapulmonary, or disseminated infection
Atypical mycobacteria (eg, *M. kansasii, M. haemophilum)*	Pulmonary, extrapulmonary, or disseminated infection
BACTERIA	
Hemophilus influenzae type b	Pneumonia, disseminated infection
Legionella	Pneumonia
Listeria monocytogenes	Bacteremia, meningitis, meningoencephalitis
Nocardia	Pneumonia, disseminated infection
Pseudomonas aeruginosa	Bacteremia, pneumonia
Salmonella	Gastroenteritis, disseminated infection
Streptococcus pneumoniae	Pneumonia, disseminated infection

From Rubin RH: Acquired immunodeficiency syndrome. In Rubenstein E, Federman DD (eds): The Scientific American Textbook of Medicine. New York, Scientific American, 1993.

presence of antibody to the virus; two levels of testing are commonly used. The current generation of ELISA assays, which serve as the usual screening test, measures antibody to HIV envelope proteins and has a false-positive rate of less than 1 percent and a false-negative rate of less than 3 percent.[88,89] Serum samples that are positive by ELISA on two consecutive assays are then subjected to a confirmatory test, usually the Western blot assay, which detects the presence of antibodies to multiple HIV antigens, thus increasing the specificity of the test. The great majority of individuals seroconvert 1 to 3 months after being infected with the virus, often coincident with the acute mononucleosis syndrome caused by HIV. Uncommonly, patients can be infected for prolonged periods without ever seroconverting: this appears to be a rare event except, perhaps, in individuals who acquire their HIV infection in the setting of another immunosuppressing condition (eg, post-transplantation).

Particularly at this point in time, when our antiretroviral therapies are just being developed, early recognition, diagnosis, and treatment of complicating infections and malignancies remain a critically important part of the approach to the HIV-infected individual. Thus the same aggressive approach outlined in other immunosuppressed patients is essential with AIDS patients: prompt diagnosis of pulmonary disease, if not by induced sputum then by bronchoalveolar lavage; central nervous system symptoms merit a computed tomography (CT) scan and lumbar puncture; prolonged fevers require a full work-up; and abnormal lymph nodes indicate a biopsy.

Management. Therapy for patients with AIDS can be divided into three categories: therapy aimed at HIV itself, therapy aimed at the complicating illnesses, and social and psychological support to protect the dignity and comfort of individuals through the course of this catastrophic illness.

Zidovudine (AZT), one of a group of dideoxynucleosides that block HIV replication by inhibiting HIV reverse transcriptase, remains the cornerstone of HIV therapy. AZT has been shown to improve survival, improve neurologic and immunologic function, and reduce the severity of opportunistic infections in patients with AIDS or AIDS-related complex. At the presently recommended doses of 500 to 600 mg/day, bone marrow toxicity and other toxicities have been less frequent. Unfortunately, drug resistance develops probably because of viral mutation, so that the value of therapy decreases with prolonged use. The merits of instituting early AZT therapy, at a time when the patient is asymptomatic but with a CD4+ T cell count of less than 500/mm^3, have consequently come into question. Currently available data suggest that early institution of therapy will delay the onset of symptomatic disease, but time to death is unchanged. Sequential therapy with AZT, followed by another drug, didanosine, after 4 months, may help alleviate this problem. Indeed, there is considerable interest in terms of sequential or combination therapy with these drugs and/or dideoxycytidine, in order to delay or prevent the emergence of resistance—a strategy that is the basis for the standard approach to tuberculosis.[61,90–95]

Few AIDS patients die directly from HIV-related events: most succumb to the secondary infections or malignancies. Three aspects of the therapy of these components of the illness bear emphasis here: (1) whenever possible, infection must be prevented, with the best example of effective prevention being anti-*Pneumocystis* strategies, which are indicated in every AIDS patient with a CD4+ T cell count under 200/mm^3 or a history of previous *Pneumocystis* infection; (2) prompt diagnosis and early therapy are essential; and (3) prolonged or indefinite therapy is usually required, particularly for those infections that are amplified by an impaired cell-mediated immune system (eg, fungal, mycobacterial, and *Salmonella* infection).[61]

Effects of the AIDS Epidemic on Surgical Practice. Of increasing importance to the surgeon, as it is for the entire medical profession, is the issue of transmission of the human immunodeficiency virus (HIV) within the medical setting. This subject is also discussed in Chapter 23. Recent events emphasize that there are two aspects of this problem that are of special importance to the surgeon: the possibility that a surgeon will acquire HIV infection due to percutaneous or mucosal inoculation with infected blood; and the possibility that an HIV-positive surgeon could transmit the virus to a patient during the course of an invasive procedure.[61,64,96]

Currently available data suggest that the risk of HIV acquisition through percutaneous inoculation is low. The risk of HIV acquisition from needle sticks or in the operating room appears to be on the order of 0.3 to 0.5 percent per percutaneous exposure to HIV-infected blood. There may be a somewhat greater risk associated with the inoculation of concentrated viral specimens in the research laboratory. There are three recorded instances in which HIV infection apparently followed the exposure of skin lesions or mucous membranes to infected blood, although the efficiency of transmission via this route appears to be significantly less than with needle sticks. Of particular importance is the observation that two health care workers who became infected within the hospital setting acquired their infection due to accidental inoculation by co-workers during the course of a resuscitation effort on an HIV-infected individual. This observation and reports of a slowly rising incidence of undiagnosed HIV infection among patients presenting to urban hospitals for emergency care underline the need for great care on the part of health care workers. Such care should include the implementation of universal blood and body fluid precautions within the health care setting to protect against transmissions of this type (Table 51–9). In the operating room, increased attention to effective barrier precautions such as face shields and fluid-resistant gowns, the development of puncture-resistant glove materials, and improved surgical techniques to minimize percutaneous needle sticks will decrease the risk of HIV transmission even more. Even with presently available gloves, data suggest that there is significant reduction in the volume of blood (and presumably the amount of virus) transmitted via needle stick when the needles pass through glove material before entering the skin.[61,64,96–100]

Recent studies of the epidemiology of health care worker exposure to HIV are extremely relevant to this discussion. Needle stick and other sharp injuries account for more than 80 percent of occupationally acquired cases of HIV infection among health care workers. Whereas outside the operating room the majority of needle stick injuries involve nursing personnel, in the operating room more than 90 percent of such injuries involve surgeons or residents. Percutaneous sharp injury occurs in approximately 7 percent of operative procedures, with an observed rate of injury among surgeons of about 2.5 injuries per 100 procedures. Most of these injuries involve solid suture needle sticks, usually occurring on the palmar surface of the fingers of the nondominant hand. These occur predominantly during the unsafe practice of manipulating the needle tip by blind palpation rather than by instrument control. Not surprisingly, certain operations, such as vaginal hysterectomy and other gynecologic procedures, carry a higher risk of percutaneous injury than others—the explanation being that deep pelvic surgery where visibility is poor is more frequently associated with the blind palpation of suture needles.[99,100]

Once a recognized exposure to HIV-infected blood has occurred, a series of steps should be initiated. The patient and the health care worker in question should be evaluated clinically, epidemiologically, and by laboratory testing for HIV (as well as hepatitis B and C viruses). In the case of HIV, this presently requires the informed consent of the individuals involved, although the emotionally charged issue of HIV testing of both patients and health care workers is undergoing continuing discussion and evolution. Although no data are currently available to document the efficacy of such procedures (indeed, there is a report of HIV acquisition by a health care worker who had rinsed a site of injury with bleach), it would seem reasonable to copiously rinse and decontaminate the local wound. The exposure should be reported to the responsible office within the hospital. The CDC currently recommends follow-up HIV testing, if the exposure indeed involved HIV-infected material, 6 weeks, 3 months, and 6 months postexposure. If unexplained fever, lymphadenopathy, rash, pharyngitis, aseptic meningitis, and lymphopenia—features of acute retroviral illness—develop, then the worker should return immediately for thorough clinical and laboratory evaluation. Counseling of the worker and/or the worker's family may be needed during the follow-up period and should be made easily available.[61,64,96]

The big unanswered question is whether chemoprophylaxis with zidovudine should be initiated following occupational exposure to HIV. The theory supporting this approach is that although zidovudine does not prevent the initial entry of HIV into cells, it might prevent the establishment of latent infection, or prevent or limit dissemination. Animal studies, utilizing nonhuman primates and the related simian immunodeficiency virus, as well as HIV in the SCID-hu mouse model, suggest the following[96,101]: efficacy of zidovudine prophylaxis is at best incomplete, very time dependent, and may be overcome by large infecting inocula. In humans there are at least six anecdotal reports of zidovudine prophylaxis failure, but these represented relatively massive exposures and/or significant delay in initiating therapy. Significant but not life-threatening bone marrow and gastrointestinal toxicity was frequently observed in individuals receiving such prophylaxis. Thus the issue is at present unsettled, and many centers have taken the position that the decision to initiate zidovudine prophylaxis should be made by the health care worker himself/herself after complete disclosure of the available information. One group of individuals for whom chemoprophylaxis is currently not recommended is women who are pregnant or who might become pregnant in the near future.[61,96]

The second issue regarding HIV infection and surgical practice is the possibility that the virus

TABLE 51–9. UNIVERSAL PRECAUTIONS TO PREVENT TRANSMISSION OF HIV

Universal Precautions

Because a medical history and physical examination cannot reliably identify all patients infected with HIV or other blood-borne pathogens, blood and body-fluid precautions should be consistently used for all patients, especially those in emergency care settings in which the risk of blood exposure is increased and the infection status of the patient is usually not known.

1. Use appropriate barrier precautions to prevent skin and mucous membrane exposure when exposure to blood, body fluids containing blood, or other body fluids to which universal precautions apply (see below) is anticipated. Wear gloves when touching blood or body fluids, mucous membranes, or nonintact skin of all patients; when handling items or surfaces soiled with blood or body fluids; and when performing venipuncture and other vascular access procedures. Change gloves after contact with each patient; do not wash or disinfect gloves for reuse. Wear masks and protective eye wear or face shields during procedures that are likely to generate droplets of blood or other body fluids to prevent exposure of mucous membranes of the mouth, nose, and eyes. Wear gowns or aprons during procedures that are likely to generate splashes of blood or other body fluids.
2. Wash hands and other skin surfaces immediately and thoroughly after contaminations with blood, body fluids containing blood, or other body fluids to which universal precautions apply. Wash hands immediately after gloves are removed.
3. Take care to prevent injuries when using needles, scalpels, and other sharp instruments or devices; when handling sharp instruments after procedures; when cleaning used instruments; and when disposing of used needles. Do not recap used needles by hand; do not remove used needles from disposable syringes by hand; and do not bend, break, or otherwise manipulate used needles by hand. Place used disposable syringes and needles, scalpel blades, and other sharp items in puncture-resistant disposal containers, which should be located as close to the use area as is practical.
4. Although saliva has not been implicated in HIV transmission, the need for emergency mouth-to-mouth resuscitation should be minimized by making mouthpieces, resuscitation bags, or other ventilation devices available for use in areas in which the need for resuscitation is predictable.
5. Health care workers with exudative lesions or weeping dermatitis should refrain from all direct patient care and from handling patient-care equipment until the condition resolves.

Universal precautions are intended to supplement rather than replace recommendations for routine infection control, such as hand washing and use of gloves to prevent gross microbial contamination of hands. In addition, implementation of universal precautions does not eliminate the need for other category- or disease-specific isolation precautions, such as enteric precautions for infectious diarrhea or isolation for pulmonary tuberculosis. Universal precautions are not intended to change waste management programs undertaken in accordance with state and local regulations.

Body Fluids to Which Universal Precautions Apply

Universal precautions apply to blood and other body fluids containing visible blood. Blood is the single most important source of HIV, hepatitis B virus, and other blood-borne pathogens in the occupational setting. Universal precautions also apply to tissues, semen, vaginal secretions, and the following fluids: cerebrospinal, synovial, pleural, peritoneal, pericardial, and amniotic.

Universal precautions do not apply to feces, nasal secretions, sputum, sweat, tears, urine, and vomitus unless they contain visible blood. Universal precautions also do not apply to human breast milk, although gloves may be worn by health care workers in situations in which exposure to breast milk might be frequent. In addition, universal precautions do not apply to saliva. Gloves need not be worn

could be transmitted from an infected surgeon to a patient undergoing an invasive procedure. This theoretical possibility was brought to the public's attention when a well-publicized group of five individuals receiving dental care from a dentist with AIDS acquired HIV infection. Since then extensive evaluation of more than 15,000 individuals who had received surgical, medical, or dental care from HIV-infected individuals have failed to identify a single instance of HIV positivity when other risk factors for HIV acquisition were not also present. Therefore, although the risk of transmission of HIV from a health care worker to a patient may not be zero, it appears to be vanishingly small. Therefore routine screening of health care workers for HIV positivity is not currently recommended. Rather, the following recommendations have been made by the CDC for health care providers[61,96]:

1. All health care workers should adhere to universal precautions (see Table 51–9), including the appropriate use of hand washing, protective barriers, and care in the use and disposal of needles and other sharp instruments. Health care workers who have exudative lesions or weeping dermatitis should refrain from all direct patient care and from handling patient care equipment and devices used in performing invasive procedures until the condition resolves. Health care workers should also comply with current guidelines for disinfection and sterilization of reusable devices used in invasive procedures.
2. Currently available data provide no basis for recommendations to restrict the practice of health care workers infected with HIV or

TABLE 51–9. *Continued*

when feeding patients or wiping saliva from skin, although special precautions are recommended for dentistry, in which contamination of saliva with blood is predictable. The risk of transmission of HIV, as well as hepatitis B virus, from these fluids and materials is extremely low or nonexistent.

Use of Gloves for Phlebotomy

Gloves should be effective in reducing the incidence of blood contamination of hands during phlebotomy (drawing of blood samples), but they cannot prevent penetrating injuries caused by needles or other sharp instruments. In universal precautions, all blood is assumed to be potentially infectious for blood-borne pathogens. Some institutions have relaxed recommendations for the use of gloves for phlebotomy by skilled health care workers in settings in which the prevalence of blood-borne pathogens is known to be very low (eg, volunteer blood-donation centers). Institutions that judge that routine use of gloves for all phlebotomies is not necessary should periodically reevaluate their policy. Gloves should always be available for those who wish to use them for phlebotomy. In addition, the following general guidelines apply:

1. Use gloves for performing phlebotomy if cuts, scratches, or other breaks in the skin are present.
2. Use gloves in situations in which contamination with blood may occur—for example, when performing phlebotomy on an uncooperative patient.
3. Use gloves for performing finger or heel sticks on infants and children.
4. Use gloves when training persons to do phlebotomies.

Precautions for Laboratories

Blood and other body fluids from all patients should be considered infective. To supplement the universal precautions listed above, the following precautions are recommended for workers in clinical laboratories:

1. Put all specimens of blood and body fluids in a well-constructed container with a secure lid to prevent leakage during transport. Take care when collecting each specimen to avoid contaminating the outside of the container or the laboratory form accompanying the specimen.
2. Wear gloves when processing blood and body-fluid specimens (eg, when removing tops from vacuum tubes). Wear masks and protective eye wear if it is anticipated that mucous membranes will come in contact with blood or body fluids. Change gloves and wash hands after completion of specimen processing.
3. For routine procedures, such as histologic and pathological studies or microbiological culturing, a biologic safety cabinet is not necessary. However, use a biologic safety cabinet (class I or II) when procedures are conducted that have a high potential for generating droplets, such as blending, sonicating, and vigorous mixing.
4. Use a mechanical pipetting device for manipulating all liquids in the laboratory. Do not pipette by mouth.
5. Limit use of needles and syringes to situations in which there is no alternative.
6. Decontaminate laboratory work surfaces with an appropriate chemical germicide after a spill of blood or other body fluids and after work is completed.
7. Decontaminate materials contaminated during laboratory tests before reprocessing them. Place contaminated materials for disposal in bags and discard in accordance with institutional policies for disposal of infective waste.
8. Decontaminate and clean scientific equipment that has been contaminated by blood or body fluids if repair in the laboratory or transport to the manufacturer is necessary.
9. Wash hands after completing laboratory work and remove protective clothing before leaving the laboratory.

Implementation of universal precautions eliminates the need for warning labels on specimens because blood and body fluids from all patients should be considered infective.

---

hepatitis B virus who perform invasive procedures not identified as exposure-prone, provided the infected health care workers practice recommended surgical or dental technique and comply with universal precautions and current recommendations for sterilization/disinfection.

3. Exposure-prone procedures should be identified by medical/surgical/dental organizations and institutions at which the procedures are performed.
4. Health care workers who perform exposure-prone procedures should know their HIV antibody status.
5. Health care workers who are infected with HIV should not perform exposure-prone procedures unless they have sought counsel from an expert review panel and been advised under what circumstances, if any, they may continue to perform these procedures. Such circumstances would include notifying prospective patients of the health care worker's seropositivity before they undergo exposure-prone invasive procedures.

Bacterial Infections

Although unusual pathogens are important in the immunocompromised host, common bacteria are still the most frequent cause of serious infection. There are two groups of infections caused by aerobic gram-negative bacilli: those caused by common endogenous organisms, *Escherichia coli*, *Klebsiella*, *Proteus*, and *Enterobacter*; and those acquired in the hospital environment, antibiotic-resistant *E. coli* and *Klebsiella*, *Pseudomonas*, *Serratia*, and *Acinetobacter*. In addition, in the past few years, there has been an increasing incidence of staphylococcal infection, both *S. aureus* and *S. epidermidis*, usually associated with intravenous line-related sepsis. The increasing use of indwelling central lines, such as Hickman catheters for blood drawing and chemotherapy purposes, has been particularly associated with the occurrence of such staphylococcal infections.[38] Anaerobic infection, especially that with *Bacteroides* and *Clostridium*, is rare, except in patients with solid tumors, or leukemia, but particularly tumors involving the gastrointestinal or genitourinary tracts. In fact, unexplained bacteremias with one of these organisms can be a clue to the presence of such neoplasms.[102] Similarly, *S. bovis* bacteremia is highly associated with the presence of colonic malignancy. The principle here is that significant breaks in mucosal integrity are necessary for bacteremia to occur with these organisms. Among the less common bacterial species, infections caused by *Salmonella*, *Listeria*, *Bacillus*, and *Nocardia*, deserve comment.

Salmonella. Nontyphoidal *Salmonella* infections are more common and more severe in immunocompromised patients. Nosocomial transmission of the intracellular organism appears to be an important factor. The risk of bacteremia, metastatic infection, prolonged clinical illness, and a sustained carrier state are significantly increased in patients with AIDS, renal transplant recipients, patients with lymphoproliferative disorders, those with defects in intracellular killing of bacteria, patients with immunoglobulin disturbances, and patients with solid tumors that may actually become infected with these organisms. In each of these instances, prolonged therapy with bacteriocidal antibiotics is required to control the infection.[16]

Listeria Monocytogenes. *Listeria monocytogenes* is discussed in Chapter 9. Although listeriosis may occur among healthy individuals, 50 to 75 percent of children above the age of 12 years and adults in whom listerial infection develops have a significant predisposing disease. Underlying conditions associated with *Listeria* infection include lymphoproliferative disorders, prolonged corticosteroid or cytotoxic drug therapy, organ transplantation, AIDS, and other diseases associated with impaired cell-mediated immunity, such as sarcoidosis and cirrhosis of the liver. The most common form of listerial infection observed in the immunocompromised patient is meningitis, which occurs in 60 to 70 percent of these patients. In most instances, listerial meningitis is clinically indistinguishable from other forms of acute pyogenic meningitis. Occasionally, however, in immunosuppressed patients, the manifestations of listerial meningitis may be less acute, without clear-cut evidence of meningeal irritation.

The other major form of listerial infection observed in the immunocompromised patient is that of bacteremia without evident central nervous system seeding, which occurs in as many as 30 percent of immunocompromised individuals with listerial infections. No specific clinical features distinguish this disorder from other bacteremic illnesses. When bacteremia does occur, metastatic spread to other sites, particularly the heart valves and the skeletal system, may occur.

The treatment of listeriosis is discussed in Chapter 9. We use ampicillin (12 g daily, intravenously in adults) or penicillin G (2 million units intravenously every 2 hours in adults) with or without accompanying aminoglycoside therapy, which may provide synergistic killing of the organism. The issue of how to treat life-threatening *Listeria* infection in individuals who are penicillin allergic is not completely settled. Traditionally, high-dose intravenous tetracycline (1 to 2 g/day in four divided doses) or erythromycin (4 g/day in four divided doses) has been employed. Because treatment failures have occurred with this regimen, our own preference is to desensitize the penicillin allergic patients with penicillin so that the optimal regimen can be employed in immunocompromised patients. Central nervous system infection with *Listeria* has a distinct tendency to relapse, therefore therapy should be continued for a minimum of 10 to 14 days after the patient has become afebrile.[103]

Bacillus. The saprophytic species of *Bacillus*, *B. subtilis* and *B. cereus*, particularly the latter, are capable of producing invasive pulmonary and disseminated blood-borne infections in the immunologically compromised host, comparable with that produced by *B. anthracis* in the normal host (see Chap. 9). Although *B. subtilis*, like *B. anthracis*, is sensitive to penicillin, *B. cereus* requires therapy with gentamicin.

Nocardia. The major focus of infection with *Nocardia* is the lungs, but there is a relatively high rate of disseminated disease, particularly to the brain, skeletal system, skin, and kidneys, sometimes without obvious preceding pulmonary disease (see Chap. 9). Patients with chronic deficits of host defense (eg, lymphoma, organ transplant recipients, AIDS) are most susceptible.

Diagnosis of nocardial infection depends on the awareness of the clinical setting in which it occurs and the prompt and liberal use of biopsy wherever the lesion appears. Positive blood or sputum culture results are unusual, although nocardial colonization of the respiratory tract without disease has been noted. Treatment of nocardial infection in the immunosuppressed patient requires at least 4 to 6 months of therapy with high-dose sulfonamide or trimethoprim-sulfamethoxazole. Minocycline is an alternative agent.

Fungal Infection

Fungal infections are the greatest concern in the compromised host. Aspergillosis, candidiasis, cryptococcosis, blastomycosis, coccidiomycosis, histoplasmosis, and mucormycosis all occur in this population. These agents have been extensively discussed in Chapter 10. *Aspergillus* and *Candida* species require reemphasis here.

Invasive Aspergillosis. Two species, *A. fumigatus* and *A. flavus*, account for more than 90 percent of the invasive aspergillosis in compromised patients. The air supply in hospital environments may serve as a source of epidemic infection in this patient population. *Aspergillus* infection in the compromised host is invasive aspergillosis, a necrotizing bronchopneumonia and bronchitis featuring blood vessel invasion with hemorrhage, infarction, and dissemination to every conceivable organ. Brain abscesses are common and usually fatal.

The pneumonic form causes dyspnea, tachypnea, nonproductive cough, pleurisy, hemoptysis, fever, and chills. Twenty to 30 percent of these patients have these symptoms before the appearance of clear x-ray abnormalities, in which case lung scans can be useful in demonstrating perfusion defects and can suggest a diagnosis. The x-ray studies can be varied, with the most characteristic image showing single or multiple nodular lesions that progress rapidly to cavitation and frequently cross lung fissures. Less commonly, interstitial pneumonia, lobar consolidation, and miliary disease may be observed. Dual infections are common, with *Aspergillus* complicating primary cytomegaloviral or bacterial pneumonia or simultaneously presenting with *Nocardia* and *M. tuberculosis. Aspergillus* is by far the most lethal of the common superinfections afflicting this patient population.[51–53]

Invasive biopsy techniques are still the cornerstone of early diagnosis and therapy. The importance of early diagnosis is underscored by the results obtained in the treatment of this disease. For example, Aisner et al[104] studied patients with acute nonlymphocytic leukemia. Of six patients diagnosed and treated within 4 days of onset, three were cured, and three showed a partial response. In contrast, all 11 patients in whom diagnosis was delayed for at least 2 weeks died with disseminated disease.

The best treatment for invasive aspergillosis is amphotericin B, with a minimum of 2 to 2.5 g used as the total dose. The new azole agent itraconazole has activity against *Aspergillus*, but its role as more than "wrap-up" therapy in an immunocompromised host remains to be demonstrated.

Candidiasis. Infection caused by *Candida* in the immunocompromised host can range from the trivial to the life threatening (see Chap. 10). The most virulent of the *Candida* species are *C. albicans* and *C. tropicalis*.

In the immunosuppressed patient population, the patient who is receiving concomitant steroid and antibiotic therapy is the best candidate for candidal overgrowth. In addition, mucocutaneous candidal infection in individuals without any of these risk factors can be an early sign of AIDS. Even with such overgrowth, however, candidal infection remains trivial unless the colonized mucocutaneous surfaces are penetrated. Tumor, trauma, operation, and immunosuppression encourage penetration into the bloodstream, with possible visceral dissemination. The most frequent means of penetration is provided by intravenous therapy, particularly hyperalimentation.[18]

In the healthy human, even when *Candida* organisms penetrate beyond the primary mucocutaneous barriers into the bloodstream, infection is usually easily controlled by natural defense mechanisms. The host defenses that appear to be the most important are adequate numbers of normally functioning neutrophils and normal T lymphocyte-monocyte interactions. Patients with hematologic malignancy and those receiving corticosteroids are, therefore, particularly at risk for invasive candidal infection. A practical example of the difference in the nature of candidal infection in the healthy person and compromised patient is what happens after transient fungemia related to contaminated intravenous infusions. In the nonimmunosuppressed patient, transient fungemia results in serious disease in less than 5 percent of patients, as long as the source of the infection is removed promptly. In contrast, in the patient with leukemia or lymphoma or the patient on steroids, transient fungemia is associated with at least a 50 percent risk of visceral invasion, and antifungal therapy is indicated at the first sign of transient fungemia.[18,53]

In the compromised patient, overgrowth of *Candida* on mucosal surfaces may result in local discomfort and a risk of dissemination. In the oropharynx, raised, discrete, white patches on an erythematous base may appear. Such lesions are frequently painful but may be asymptomatic and, more important, may be associated with candidal overgrowth in the rest of the gastrointestinal tract. In the esophagus, the usual symptom complex is severe retrosternal pain and dysphagia, usually beginning in close association with a course of broad spectrum antibiotic therapy. Although in the appropriate clinical setting a presumptive diagnosis can usually be made, diagnosis may be confirmed by esophagoscopy (the most sensitive technique) or barium swallow.

In the compromised host, *Candida* are by far the most commonly cultured fungal organisms recovered from sputum, bronchial secretions, or postmortem lung biopsies, although its clinical significance is often questionable. Most commonly, *Candida* are present as colonizers of the tracheobronchial tree but are not actually invading the pulmonary parenchyma. Even if the patient has concomitant pneumonia, the odds are overwhelming that the candidal isolates have more to do with the pathogenesis of an accompanying stomatitis or esophagitis than with the pneumonia. Although primary candidal pneumonia exists in the immunosuppressed host, it is rare, it cannot be reliably diagnosed by the examination of sputum or serologic testing, and it should be accepted as a diagnosis only when proved by lung biopsy. In contrast, *Candida* are frequently part of a multimicrobial superinfection. *Candida* may also invade the lung, producing miliary microabscesses as part of a generalized hematogenous dissemination of the organism.[51–53]

Disseminated candidal infection, with metastatic spread to one or more visceral organs, is common in the following circumstances: (1) intravenous catheter-related infections, (2) operative manipulations of sites of candidal overgrowth (particularly the gastrointestinal tract), and (3) spontaneous bloodstream invasion from gastrointestinal disease or its therapy in patients with major defects in lymphocyte-monocyte interaction and function. All these factors are exacerbated if concomitant steroid therapy is being given.[18]

The consequences of candidal dissemination are many. Perhaps the major site of metastatic seeding is to the kidneys. In fact, in a patient at risk for candidal invasion, the demonstration of candiduria in the absence of an indwelling catheter indicates the presence of disseminated candidiasis and the need for systemic anticandidal therapy. The other easily diagnosed metastatic site of candidal infection is the eye—candidal endophthalmitis is a frequent complication of sustained candidemia. Repeated examination of the optic fundi should be carried out in any patient with suspected disseminated candidiasis or in any compromised patient who is on prolonged hyperalimentation. The classic funduscopic finding is one or more white, cottonball-like areas of chorio-retinitis extending out into the vitreous. Another site of metastatic infection that may be of diagnostic help is the skin. Hematogenous spread of *Candida* to the skin is usually associated with erythematous, macronodular, occasionally hemorrhagic skin lesions that are 0.5 to 1.0 cm in size. Such lesions should be biopsied soon after they appear.[1] Less common sites of metastatic infection include the myocardium, the skeletal system, and the meninges.[18]

As with invasive aspergillosis, invasive candidiasis is difficult to diagnose. Routine blood cultures are usually negative (50 to 75 percent of the time), and even when positive, they may not be recognized for a long time. Serologic studies are useless in immunosuppressed patients. It is little wonder that a premortem diagnosis of disseminated candidiasis is made in only 15 to 40 percent of patients. Even though newer techniques for demonstrating candidal antigen appear promising, aggressive biopsy techniques and empiric anticandidal therapy will have to be employed if mortality is to be reduced.[18]

There are two aspects to the therapy of candidal infection in the immunosuppressed host: (1) correction of the circumstances that lead to candidal overgrowth and invasion in the first place and (2) specific antifungal chemotherapy. The first step, then, is to remove urinary and intravenous catheters, discontinue broad spectrum antibacterial therapy, control diabetes, and decrease, if possible, corticosteroid and other immunosuppressive therapy.

The antifungal therapy used depends, in part, on the type of candidal invasion observed. Even in immunosuppressed patients, mucocutaneous infection will often respond to correction of predisposing factors and topical therapy. Cutaneous and vaginal candidiasis are effectively treated with creams and lotions containing nystatin, clotrimazole, or miconazole. Frequent gargling and swallowing of suspensions of nystatin or amphotericin B will usually clear oropharyngeal and esophageal infection. Such therapy is more effective prophylactically, and, therefore, we place susceptible patients on prophylactic nystatin whenever antibacterial therapy is initiated.

In patients with severe mucosal disease, not responsive to topical therapies, systemic antifungal therapy is indicated. The advent of fluconazole, administered at doses of 200 to 400 mg/day, has been a major advance in this situation, since the drug can be administered once a day either orally or intravenously. Alternatively, low-dose amphotericin (approximately 10 mg/day for 10 to 14 days) can achieve the same objective. The big controversy at present is the question of when to use fluconazole and when to use amphotericin in the treatment of systemic candidiasis. Randomized trials that are currently in progress will help to answer this question, but until these data are available, we find the following guidelines to be useful when dealing with both invasive candidal and cryptococcal infection[24]:

1. The first question to be asked is whether the patient is a therapeutic emergency or is more subacutely ill. That is, is immediate control of the disease essential, or do you have several days to accomplish this? If the patient is a therapeutic emergency, then amphotericin (with or without flucytosine) is the initial therapy of choice, as it will gain control of the process more quickly than will fluconazole. If the patient is more subacutely ill, then both drugs appear to have comparable long-term efficacies (provided infection is not with one of the fluconazole-resistant species, most notably *Candida krusei* and *C. glabrata*). Hepatosplenic candidiasis and candidal urinary tract infection appear to be particularly responsive to fluconazole therapy.
2. Even if therapy is initiated with amphotericin B, this does not require that the entire course of antifungal treatment be accomplished with this drug. Once control of the disease has been achieved, fluconazole can be substituted, thus permitting oral therapy with less of a risk of toxicity.
3. Patients, such as transplant recipients, who are receiving cyclosporine represent a particular challenge: idiopathic, synergistic nephrotoxicity occurs in a significant number of patients when amphotericin B is added to the cyclosporine-based regimen. We have observed oliguric renal failure occur following the administration of as little as 10 mg of amphotericin B to a transplant patient with previously normal renal function. Because of this, we utilize fluconazole as the treatment of choice in virtually all transplant patients with invasive infection due to *C. albicans*, *C. tropicalis*, and *Cryptococcus neoformans*.

Cryptococcal Infection

Cryptococcus neoformans is discussed in Chapter 10. Only a few points will be emphasized here. More than half of the patients in whom cryptococcal infection develops have an easily recognizable defect in host defenses, usually caused by lymphoma, corticosteroid administration, AIDS, or sarcoidosis. In fact, the diagnosis of cryptococcal infection indicates the possibility of a disease state associated with defects in cell-mediated immunity. The major clinical impact of *C. neoformans* infection is on the lungs and central nervous system, although miliary disease occurs in patients with the most profound defects in host defense.[51,103]

Infection of the lung with *C. neoformans* produces a subacute to chronic illness. Despite the presence of rather extensive pulmonary infiltrates, the symptoms are often minimal, and at least one-third of patients are asymptomatic. The most common symptoms are low-grade fever and nonproductive cough. The typical x-ray finding is a mass or a segmental consolidation, occasionally with some cavitation. Rarely, multiple nodules or diffuse disease, either in an interstitial or a miliary pattern, may also be seen. Hilar adenopathy is present in 10 percent of patients and pleural effusions occur in less than 5 percent.[51–53,105]

It is important to emphasize that the isolation of *C. neoformans* on sputum culture does not prove that a lesion seen radiographically is caused by this organism, because *Cryptococcus* may only be colonizing the tracheobronchial tree. There appears to be a particular association between cryptococcal colonization and lung cancer. For example, the Mayo Clinic[106] noted that 25 percent of their sputum isolates of *C. neoformans* were from patients with lung cancer without fungal pulmonary invasion. Relying on sputum cultures alone, particularly in patients with coin lesions, to rule out the presence of tumor and the need for thoracotomy could have disastrous consequences. Mixed infections with *Nocardia*, tuberculosis, and *Aspergillus* may be present. In the patient with depressed cell-mediated immunity, the diagnosis of pulmonary cryptococcal infection should lead to a search for disseminated disease, particularly of the meninges.

Cryptococcal meningitis is a chronic meningitis that follows a waxing and waning course over months to years before death inevitably occurs. The clinical onset is usually insidious, and asymptomatic intervals may occur. The most common symptoms are fever and persistent headache, or headache alone, although headaches can be absent in 5 to 20 percent of patients. It is important to reemphasize that because of the benignity of the symptoms frequently associated with the onset of cryptococcal and listerial meningitis, the indications for a lumbar puncture in a compromised host include both unexplained fever and unexplained headache (Fig. 51–7). Nausea, dizziness, impaired mentation, irritability, and ataxia are common. Seizures rarely occur early, but they occasionally develop as the disease progresses, as may decreased visual acuity, diplopia, and facial numbness and weakness. Papilledema is present in about one-third of patients and cranial nerve palsies are present in about one-fifth. Although patients commonly complain of neck stiffness, fully developed meningismus is rare. Focal neurologic lesions, except those caused by the effects of the basilar meningitis on the cranial nerves, are rare. In patients who are severely immunosuppressed, meningitis can be associated with multiple sites of extraneural infection, particularly the skin, lungs, skeletal system, and urinary tract.[103]

Although cryptococci may be disseminated by the bloodstream to any organ in the body, the most commonly affected extraneural sites are the skin, skeletal system, and urinary tract. Any unexplained skin eruption in an immunosuppressed host merits biopsy to make an early diagnosis of disseminated opportunistic infection, whatever the cause. Cryptococcal skin lesions most commonly appear as erythematous papules or acneiform lesions at body sites atypical of acne. Cellulitis closely mimicking bacterial cellulitis and vesicular lesions resembling herpetic vesicles may also occur. Whatever the initial lesion, ulceration usually develops subsequently. Approximately 10 to 30 percent of patients with cryptococcal infection will have cutaneous involvement.[1]

Cryptococcal osteomyelitis and arthritis occur in approximately 10 percent of patients with cryptococcal infection and develop as slowly progressive osteolytic lesions without accompanying periosteal proliferation. In patients with long-standing bony infection, direct extension to the skin may occur. Particularly in patients with underlying malignancies, solitary bony lesions caused by *C. neoformans* may be mistaken, histologically, for Hodgkin's disease or osteogenic sarcoma unless special fungal stains are used.

The diagnosis of cryptococcal infection depends on the isolation of the organism or the demonstration of cryptococcal antigen in a body fluid. These issues are discussed in Chapter 10, as is the appropriate therapy.

One final consideration is the need for antifungal therapy in patients who undergo operation for the removal of cryptococcal lesions. Campbell[105] has reported that 7 of 62 patients undergoing pulmonary resection for cryptococcal infection developed postoperative meningitis. Although amphotericin B is too toxic to justify its use as antifungal prophy-

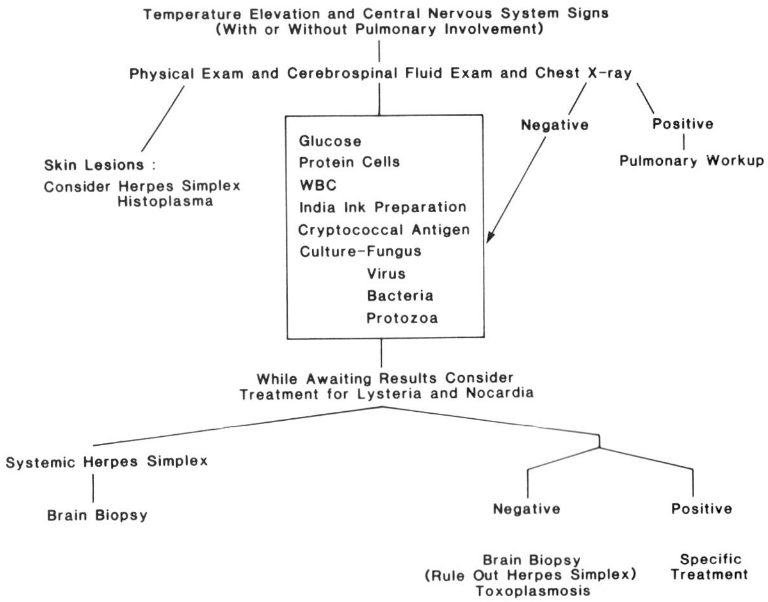

Figure 51–7. Flow diagram illustrating the evaluation of a transplant recipient with fever and neurologic symptoms. *(From Matas AS, Simmons RL, Najarian JS: In Hardy JD (ed): Critical Surgical Illness. Philadelphia, Saunders, 1980.)*

laxis in this situation, we believe that the availability of the less toxic and more easily administered fluconazole has obviated this problem and that a perioperative course of fluconazole may safely prevent postoperative meningitis.

Pneumocystis carinii *Infection*

Pathogenesis. *Pneumocystis carinii* causes a diffuse interstitial plasma cell pneumonia in patients who are immunosuppressed by a variety of diseases. Two epidemiologic patterns of disease have been noted. The first is an endemic infantile pattern found among the malnourished (war refugees). The second pattern of *Pneumocystis* infection is an acute to subacute interstitial pneumonia in patients immunosuppressed by AIDS, malignancy, or chemotherapy.

Pneumocystis is probably acquired by air-borne human-to-human transmission, although there is considerable evidence that immunosuppression can reactivate a latent or asymptomatic infection. The practical implications of such observations are that patients with active *Pneumocystis* pneumonia should be kept isolated from other immunosuppressed patients, and strict respirator precautions should be used in their care.[53,107]

Whatever the means by which *Pneumocystis* infection is acquired, clinical disease only occurs in combination with significant immunosuppression. As previously noted, *Pneumocystis* (including repeated episodes) is the most common infectious problem in patients with AIDS. *Pneumocystis* infection develops in organ transplant recipients and cancer patients only after exposure to corticosteroids and chemotherapy. Patients with hematologic malignancies that are themselves immunosuppressive, such as Hodgkin's disease, rarely develop *Pneumocystis* pneumonia unless immunosuppressive therapy has been initiated. As far as steroids are concerned, the interesting observation has been made that, in many patients, *Pneumocystis* disease becomes clinically manifest only after the steroid dosage has been tapered. Nutritional status is clearly important, as shown by studies in which serum albumin levels and body weights were significantly lower in children with cancer who developed *Pneumocystis* infection than in children with cancer who did not. Likewise, normal B lymphocyte function must be important in protecting against *Pneumocystis*, as shown by the many reports of *Pneumocystis* infection in patients with hypogammaglobulinemia, intact cellular immunity, and no history of steroid or cyclophosphamide exposure.[107,108]

Pathology. *Pneumocystis* pulmonary infection is characterized by an interstitial pneumonia with thickening of the alveolar septae and the alveoli, hyperplasia of alveolar lining cells, and large numbers of infiltrating plasma cells in the septae. Foamy eosinophilic material fills the alveolar spaces. When the Gomori methenamine silver stain or Giemsa stain is used, this material is shown to be filled with organisms (Fig. 51–8B). The diagnostic finding is a 4- to 6-μm cyst containing six to eight oval bodies, the merozoites. Rarely, *Pneumocystis* organisms have been found in draining hilar and thoracic lymph nodes, and a few instances of systemic dissemination have been reported.[107,108]

Clinical Manifestations. *Pneumocystis* pneumonia presents with fever, a hacking nonproductive cough, tachypnea, and progressive dyspnea without pleurisy over a few days to weeks. The patient is tachypneic and may be cyanotic but has normal breath sounds. A surprising degree of hypoxia is demonstrable on arterial blood gas determination. The differential diagnosis must include cytomegaloviral infection, which may coexist or predispose to *Pneumocystis* infection.[51–53,108]

The classic radiologic appearance of *P. carinii* pneumonia is a diffuse, bilateral, symmetric, interstitial, and alveolar pattern with a predominantly perihilar distribution (Fig. 51–8A). Unilateral consolidations and nodular densities, however, have also been reported with this organism, but about 80 percent of our patients have had the classic pattern. Pleural effusions, cavitation, and lymphadenopathy on x-ray studies are quite unusual and, when present, should suggest the possibility of a concomitant process. There have been a number of reports of simultaneous infection by *Pneumocystis* and other opportunistic pathogens, such as *Nocardia* and *Aspergillus*, and an atypical chest x-ray examination or an atypical clinical course, or both, should alert the clinician to that possibility. In addition, particularly in the AIDS patient, *Pneumocystis* infection may be causing significant pulmonary dysfunction in the face of a negative chest x-ray study. In such individuals, a positive gallium scan or otherwise unexplained abnormalities in pulmonary function testing can lead to the appropriate diagnosis.[51–53,107,108]

Treatment. The first treatment demonstrated to be effective against *Pneumocystis carinii* pneumonia was pentamidine isethionate. In a dose of 4 mg/kg/day intramuscularly or intravenously for 2 to 3 weeks, this drug has reduced mortality from 100 to 25 percent. Because of such toxicities as hypoten-

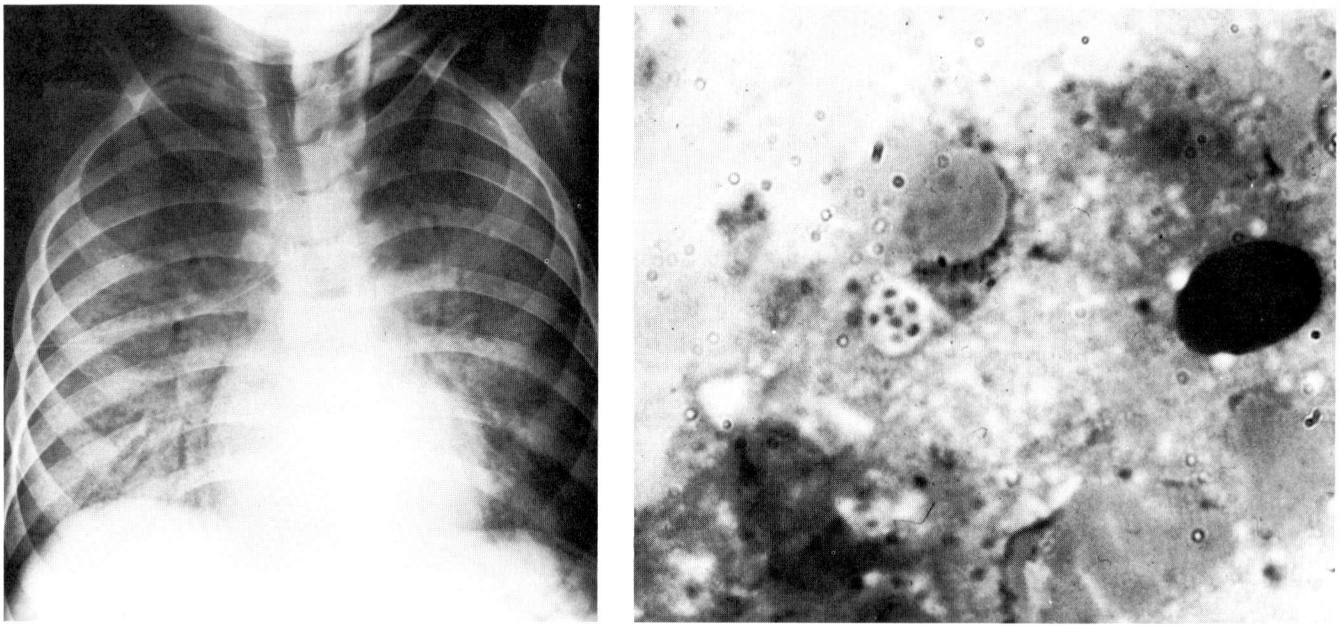

A B

Figure 51–8. **A.** The alveolar infiltrate that extends to the periphery of both lungs with an air bronchogram is characteristic of *Pneumocystis carinii.* This patient, an 8-year-old boy, died 3 weeks after the disease was confirmed by open lung biopsy. **B.** Lung biopsy showing *P. carinii* with cysts (Giemsa stain). *(From Simmons RL, Kjellstrand CM, Najarian JS: In Hardy JD (ed): Critical Surgical Illness. Philadelphia, Saunders, 1971.)*

sion, tachycardia, nausea, vomiting, facial flushing, pleuritis, local irritation, hypoglycemia, azotemia, bone marrow suppression, and sterile abscess formation at injection sites, pentamidine is now usually reserved for patients who do not tolerate trimethoprim-sulfamethoxazole. These drugs, administered for 14 to 21 days either orally or intravenously at a dose of 20 mg of trimethoprim and 100 mg of sulfamethoxazole/kg/day in three or four divided doses, are as effective as pentamidine and in non-AIDS patients are better tolerated[38,107,108]; in AIDS patients, significant allergic reactions to trimethoprim-sulfamethoxazole often intervene, and pentamidine, or such other regimens as dapsone plus trimethoprim, or atovaquone may be needed.[109]

As previously noted, in such populations as HIV-infected individuals with CD4+ T cell counts under 200/mm^3, transplant recipients, and certain patients with lymphoproliferative disease on therapy, *Pneumocystis* infection is common enough to justify prophylaxis. Low-dose trimethoprim-sulfamethoxazole is the drug of choice, with monthly aerosolized pentamidine being an alternative. This latter regimen, in AIDS patients, has been associated with both extrapulmonary infection and unusual forms of *Pneumocystis* pneumonia such as infection restricted to the upper lobes.[61]

The biggest change in the therapy of *Pneumocystis* pneumonia has been the addition of corticosteroids to the treatment regimen. When combined with effective anti-*Pneumocystis* therapy, steroids (a sample regimen being prednisone 40 mg twice per day for 5 days, then 40 mg/day for 5 days, followed by 20 mg/day for 11 days, together with a 21-day course of trimethoprim-sulfamethoxazole or pentamidine) decrease mortality, the incidence of respiratory failure, and the extent of hypoxia that develops in patients with moderate or severe *Pneumocystis* infection. Although the studies documenting this were only performed in AIDS patients, it would seem reasonable to apply this information to any patient with *Pneumocystis* pneumonia.[108,110,111]

Toxoplasmosis

Toxoplasmosis, a systemic protozoan infection caused by *T. gondii*, is endemic worldwide. It has a particular impact on the immunosuppressed patient, because life-threatening disease can develop after the acquisition of primary infection or the reactivation of previously acquired latent infection.[108,112]

Pathogenesis and Pathology. The most common sites of tissue invasion and the subsequent formation of cysts are the brain and the skeletal and cardiac muscle, although all organs may be affected by this obligate intracellular parasite. Because intact cell-mediated immunity is most important in limiting the extent of toxoplasmosis, patients with AIDS, Hodgkin's disease, and those receiving immunosuppressive therapy are most commonly affected.[108,112]

Clinical Manifestations. In healthy individuals, toxoplasmosis is often asymptomatic or is associated with silent lymphadenopathy. It is most frequently diagnosed when a full-blown infectious mononucleosis-like syndrome occurs, with fever, myalgias, sore throat, headache, diffuse lymphadenopathy, hepatosplenomegaly, maculopapular rash, and atypical lymphocytosis. Rarely, acute acquired toxoplasmosis may develop, with carditis, hepatitis, encephalitis, polymyositis, pneumonitis, or chorioretinitis.

In the compromised host, the clinical manifestations are more serious—50 percent involve the central nervous system, with diffuse encephalopathy, meningoencephalitis, or a cerebral mass lesion. The heart and lungs are also affected in the compromised host. In patients with lymphoma, it is easy to misdiagnose a recurrence of lymphadenopathy as being caused by the malignancy rather than by toxoplasmosis. Simultaneous infections with herpes group viruses, particularly cytomegalovirus, and *T. gondii* are quite common. In the AIDS patient, toxoplasma encephalitis has been the most common cause of central nervous system disease. A very typical CAT scan finding is focal contrast-enhancing ring lesions. It should be emphasized, however, that this picture is not unique to toxoplasmosis, and a tissue diagnosis is still needed.[103,108,112,113]

Although rare cases of disseminated toxoplasmosis have been reported in renal transplant recipients, the major transplant population at risk consists of patients receiving cardiac transplants. When the allograft donor is seropositive for toxoplasmosis and the recipient is seronegative, there is a greater than 50 percent chance that the recipient will develop myocarditis with or without disseminated infection that primarily will impact on the central nervous system. The myocarditis that occurs can be diagnosed as rejection on biopsy, with increases in immunosuppression then exacerbating the problem. Because of these events, cardiac donors and recipients are routinely screened serologically for this infection, and any individual receiving a cardiac allograft who is at risk for primary infection (donor seropositive, recipient seronegative) is placed on prophylaxis for 3 to 6 months, usually with pyrimethamine and a sulfonamide. Since this regimen also provides effective prophylaxis against *Pneumocystis*, trimethoprim-sulfamethoxazole prophylaxis is not necessary in these individuals.[24,114–117]

Diagnosis. Ruskin and Remington[112] pointed out the difficulties in making a diagnosis of toxoplasmosis in this population by demonstrating the trophozoites themselves. Brain biopsy results appear to be most useful, particularly when electron microscopic examination is performed. Of greater use is the fact that the lymph nodes exhibit pathognomonic changes in the absence of the parasite—reactive follicular hyperplasia associated with irregular groupings of epithelioid histiocytes in cortical and paracortical zones, as well as focal distention of subcapsular and trabecular sinuses by monocytoid cells. Immunofluorescent studies for *Toxoplasma* antigen and lymphangiograms are also useful.[108,112]

Serologic testing can be helpful. Greater than fourfold rises in titer by any serologic method and very high titers without a documented rise are diagnostic in a patient with a typical illness. Because some immunocompromised patients will not mount a characteristic serologic response, biopsy is required in a patient with a clinically compatible syndrome, particularly if this syndrome includes undiagnosed central nervous system disease. Unfortunately, in AIDS patients, serologic methods are not useful, and brain biopsy is necessary for diagnosis.[108,112,113]

Pyrimethamine plus sulfadiazine is the treatment of choice. Pyrimethamine is given in an initial dose of 100 to 200 mg and 25 mg/day thereafter. The usual dose of sulfadiazine is 75 to 100 mg/kg/day in four divided doses after an initial loading dose of 50 to 75 mg/kg. Therapy should probably be continued for at least 4 to 6 weeks, and indefinitely in the AIDS patient. To prevent pyrimethamine-induced bone marrow toxicity, folinic acid (leucovorin calcium) should be administered in dosages of 2 to 10 mg/day.

Viral Infection

The most important viral infections other than HIV to affect the compromised host are those caused by the four members of the human herpes group—herpes simplex virus, varicella-zoster virus, Epstein-Barr virus, and cytomegalovirus. Although the clinical impact of each of these may be different, they share a number of characteristics (see Chap. 11).[24]

Herpesviruses are enveloped DNA viruses that range in size from 180 to 200 nm and characteristically produce intranuclear inclusion bodies in infected cells. Like other enveloped viruses, herpesviruses are relatively unstable at room temperature, and direct contact between susceptible cells and infected cell secretions is usually necessary for disease transmission. As soon as primary infection has occurred, latent infection develops, with the virus remaining dormant in one or more different cell types for months to decades, with poorly understood perturbations in host defenses resulting in viral reactivation and even dissemination. Although clearly recognized disease syndromes caused by these agents are commonly observed in the healthy individual, the extent and impact of the illnesses are enhanced by immunosuppression. Antibody responses to each of these agents can be easily defined and are often useful for diagnosis. The role of antibody in preventing and limiting the extent of such infections remains undefined, with cell-mediated immunity apparently of greater importance. This is best shown by the clinical impact of these agents in patients with defects in cell-mediated immune function.

Herpes Simplex Virus Infection. Herpes simplex virus (HSV) is of two antigenic types. HSV-1, primarily transmitted by infected oral secretions, is the major cause of oral, encephalitic, and ocular infections in the adult. HSV-2 is venerally transmitted and is the major cause of genital and neonatal infection. Both primary and recurrent infections occur and are common in the community.[118]

Pathogenesis. The pathogenesis of both primary and reactivation HSV infection requires the viral invasion of skin epithelium and mucous membranes. Viral replication kills the cell and elicits an inflammatory response, producing the typical vesicle on an erythematous base. Regional adenopathy may then occur, and systemic symptoms of viral infection, such as fever, myalgias, malaise, or anorexia, are common. After a primary infection, the virus travels centripetally via neuronal axons to reside in the sensory ganglia that correspond to the site of primary infection. The virus remains latent within these ganglia until reactivated by such factors as immunosuppression, fever, sunlight, trauma, operative manipulation of the nerve root, or a variety of circumstances, including menstruation. After reactivation, the virus travels centrifugally down the axon to reinfect the appropriate epithelial cells. This process may be repeated many times in the lifetime of a patient. In general, unless an acquired immunosuppressed state has developed, primary infection is more severe than recurrent infection, which is manifested by smaller lesions, fewer vesicles, less viral shedding, less adenopathy, fewer systemic symptoms, and a shorter time required for healing. Viremia has been documented in both healthy and immunosuppressed individuals, but its importance is unclear, except in the few patients with disseminated visceral disease.[118]

Humoral antibodies to HSV are not protective. Recurrent and even fatal disease can occur with high titers. Humoral immunity may play a role in attenuating the severity of recurrent illness, making it less severe than primary infection. Such antibodies may act as blocking antibodies and contribute to the development of viral latency. An antibody-dependent, cell-mediated cytotoxicity system appears to be important in controlling HSV infection.[118]

Cell-mediated immunity appears to be more important than humoral immunity in protection. Prospective studies of organ transplant patients have correlated decreased lymphocyte transformation and interferon production in response to HSV antigen in the early posttransplant period with the peak incidence of both symptomatic and asymptomatic HSV excretion. The appearance of intravesicle interferon, in particular, appears to correlate with healing of the individual lesions.[118,119]

People at risk for severe HSV infection include all those with defects either in cellular immunity or in the mucocutaneous surfaces that are the primary sites of attachment, including organ transplant recipients, burn patients, and the debilitated, the malnourished, and the elderly. As with mucocutaneous candidiasis, recurrent or particularly severe mucocutaneous HSV infection can be an important manifestation of AIDS.[118,119]

Clinical Manifestations. Chronic, large, ulcerated lesions (herpes phagedena) may persist at either oral or genital sites for weeks to months. Eczema herpeticum (Kaposi varicelliform eruption) is a diffuse vesicular eruption caused by cutaneous dissemination of HSV at sites of previous skin damage (ie, burns, eczema). In addition to the cosmetic and physical discomfort associated with this condition, visceral dissemination may occur, with mortality rates of 10 to 50 percent. More commonly, secondary bacteremias may ensue because of viral-induced mucocutaneous damage at sites (mouth, anogenital area) heavily contaminated with potentially invasive bacteria.[118]

The prolonged presence of an endotracheal tube or a nasogastric tube can result in a superficial necrotizing mucositis, characterized grossly by multiple punched-out lesions. Coexistent candidal infection is often present. Primary infection of the lungs in the absence of endotracheal intubation or generalized visceral dissemination is rare.[118]

Widespread visceral dissemination of HSV may occur in the compromised host. This is often associated with disseminated intravascular coagulation. Previously, treatment of this condition was ineffective, and mortality rates approached 100 percent. The advent of acyclovir therapy is beginning to change this outcome.

Treatment. Effective chemotherapy for HSV infection began with the success of vidarabine (adenine arabinoside) in the treatment of HSV encephalitis. Acyclovir has now superseded vidarabine for this purpose. In addition, acyclovir has been a major advance in the treatment of severe mucocutaneous infections seen in patients with morbidly impaired cell-mediated immunity. Unfortunately, acyclovir does not appear to influence recurrence rates or the course of postherpetic neuralgia. In the AIDS patient, recurrent, severe mucocutaneous infection with a heavy viral burden and requiring extended courses of acyclovir to control the infection is the rule, particularly as the CD4+ T cell count falls. Because of these characteristics, it is not surprising that acyclovir-resistant HSV infection has become a common feature in advanced AIDS. In these circumstances, foscarnet can be quite useful in controlling the infection, although the toxicity of this therapy can be quite marked, particularly the nephrotoxicity.[120,121]

Varicella-Zoster Viral Infection. A single virus causes both varicella (chickenpox) and zoster (shingles). Varicella-zoster virus (VZV) is presumably acquired through the respiratory tract with subsequent dissemination to skin and visceral organs, resulting in clinical varicella. It remains dormant within sensory ganglia until activated, then travels down the nerve root to the skin to produce zoster (see Chap. 11).

Pathogenesis. As with HSV infection, antibodies to VZV can be demonstrated during both varicella and zoster, with the pattern in zoster suggesting an anamnestic response. In transplant patients, serial antibody titers fluctuate, suggesting to Luby et al[122] that subclinical viral release and antigenic stimulation may be occurring. Humoral antibody must play some role in protection against this infection, as witnessed by the successful prophylactic use of zoster immune globulin or plasma when given early after exposure to immunosuppressed children at high risk for varicella, those with leukemia, lymphoma, and primary immunodeficiency syndromes. In contrast, administration of antibody after the incubation period is ineffective. Apparently, after this strongly cell-bound virus reaches cellular sites, circulating antibody has little effect on it, and cell-mediated immunity and the production of interferon become more important in limiting the extent of these infections. Patients with particular susceptibility to VZV, bone marrow transplant recipients, lymphoma patients, and those receiving corticosteroid therapy have diminished lymphocyte responsiveness to this agent and delayed local interferon production, even with adequate antibody responsiveness.[118,123]

Disseminated visceral infection following varicella occurs in 20 to 35 percent of children with malignant disease who are receiving chemotherapy, with an associated morbidity of 7 to 30 percent from varicella pneumonia or encephalitis. Among adults, the risk of developing zoster is 13 to 15 percent for those with Hodgkin's disease, 7 to 9 percent for non-Hodgkin's lymphoma patients, and 1 to 3 percent for patients with solid tumors. Of the Hodgkin's patients, approximately 15 to 30 percent with zoster will develop disseminated disease.[118] As expected, patients with AIDS have a high incidence of zoster, with the first episode often signaling the beginning of AIDS. Recurrent episodes are not uncommon, and disseminated disease occurs occasionally in patients with advanced AIDS.[61]

Clinical Manifestations. Zoster appears to develop more frequently at areas of regionalized tumor and localized radiation therapy. Its severity is proportional to the stage of cancer and the intensity of radiation and chemotherapy.[118]

Localized zoster will develop in 10 to 20 percent of organ transplant patients. Rarely, pain due to VZV without rash will be present. Although clinical zoster is usually well tolerated, primary varicella is often severe, with a high rate of visceral dissemination. Pediatric transplant recipients, in particular, should be carefully protected from exposure to VZV.[118,119] In 50 percent of bone marrow transplant recipients who survive longer than 6 months, either varicella or zoster will develop, with an exceedingly high mortality rate. Similarly, children with primary immunodeficiency syndromes associated with impaired cell-mediated immunity have a high rate of disseminated VZV infection.[118]

Treatment. An attenuated live virus vaccine is being developed so that active prophylaxis of high-risk children may be possible. In immunocompromised patients with zoster, trials of vidarabine, exogenous interferon derived from human leukocytes, and acyclovir have been quite encouraging in controlling dissemination (see Chap. 28). At the present time, high-dose acyclovir therapy should be considered the treatment of choice for this purpose.[118] As with the other herpesviruses, acyclovir-resistant VZV has been observed in patients with AIDS, which requires therapy.[118,124]

Epstein-Barr Viral Infection. Epstein-Barr virus (EBV) causes classic heterophil antibody-positive infectious mononucleosis (and some cases of heterophil-negative mononucleosis) and probably causes African Burkitt's lymphoma and certain forms of nasopharyngeal carcinoma. Here, too, cell-mediated immunity plays an important role in limiting the extent of the infection.[118]

The first evidence that EBV infection would have a significant impact on immunocompromised patients came from the recognition of the X-linked recessive immunodeficiency syndrome. In these young men, EBV infection causes both a B cell lymphoproliferative syndrome (eg, Burkitt's lymphoma, immunoblastic sarcoma) and/or an aproliferative syndrome characterized by agammaglobulinemia, agranulocytosis, and aplastic anemia.[118]

Although EBV can cause a typical mononucleosis syndrome in other immunocompromised hosts in association with primary infection, its major impact is its role in the pathogenesis of the EBV-associated lymphoproliferative disease—an increasingly common event in AIDS patients and organ transplant recipients. At present, it appears that the incidence of lymphoproliferative disease is related to the interaction between the amount of EBV replication that is present and the level of functioning of the key host defense against EBV—the MHC-restricted, EBV-specific cytotoxic T cells (which are greatly inhibited both in AIDS patients and in transplant patients treated with high doses of cyclosporine). Since more than 90 percent of adults are seropositive for EBV, and hence harbor latent virus, most of the EBV events observed in immunocompromised patients are the result of reactivation infection. It should be noted, however, that studies in transplant patients suggest that patients with primary infection have a higher level of EBV replication (as assayed in the oropharynx) and a higher risk of lymphoproliferative disease than those with reactivation disease.[24,125–127]

Unlike CMV (vide infra), the latency of EBV is relatively unstable, with spontaneous reactivation occurring commonly. Thus 20 percent of seropositive normal individuals have replicating virus demonstrable in their oropharyngeal secretions at any one point in time. In organ transplant recipients, this figure goes up to 30 percent for those on maintenance immunosuppression and rises to 80 percent in association with anti-lymphocyte antibody therapy (which also increases the level of virus replication). Cyclosporine and, to a lesser extent, the other parts of the immunosuppressive program, in a dose-related fashion, block the cytotoxic T cell response to the virus, permitting the survival and amplification of the EBV-transformed, immortalized B cells that initiate the lymphoproliferative syndrome.[24,126]

The clinical presentation of EBV-associated lymphoproliferative disease can be quite variable and includes one or more of the following[24,125,127]: unexplained fever (an FUO); a mononucleosis-type syndrome with fever, malaise, and lymphadenopathy, with or without pharyngitis or tonsillitis; a gastrointestinal (GI) presentation, which can include GI bleeding, abdominal pain, and perforation or obstruction; hepatocellular dysfunction; and central nervous system dysfunction such as seizures, change in mental status, and focal neurologic disease. In transplant patients, the allograft is not uncommonly involved, not surprisingly given the MHC restriction of the key host defense against these events, the virus-specific, cytotoxic T cell surveillance mechanism.[24,125–127] Involvement of the bone marrow, lungs, and virtually every other organ has been described. Pathologically, the EBV-related lymphoproliferative disease represents a continuum, both in terms of histology (nonspecific reactive hyperplasia, polymorphic B cell hyperplasia, polymorphic B cell lymphoma, immunoblastic sarcoma) and clonality (polyclonal, oligoclonal, monoclonal), from the reactive to the frankly malignant. Optimal management of this entity, other than decreasing the level of immunosuppression, is currently an area of some debate, with the options including no additional therapy (which does work in 20 percent or more of transplant patients), cytotoxic chemotherapy, an anti-B cell monoclonal antibody, the combination of interferon alpha with intravenous IgG, or some combination of these. The hope is that with aggressive antiviral therapy in conjunction with periods of increased immunosuppression, the pathogenetic events involved in this process can be interrupted, as this disease is clearly one that is better prevented than treated.[24,125–127]

Cytomegalovirus Infection. The viral infection with the greatest clinical impact on the compromised host is caused by CMV. In the AIDS patient, its primary effect is in the causation of a progressive chorioretinitis, but it may also cause enterocolitis, adrenalitis, pneumonia, and encephalitis. In addition, CMV may play a role in modulating HIV replication.[61] In the transplant patient, it is the most important single microbial pathogen. In the bone marrow transplant recipient, the most important effect is the causation of CMV pneumonia, which has had a 15 to 20 percent incidence among allogeneic bone marrow transplant recipients and, until recently, a mortality rate of more than 85 percent. In organ transplant patients, CMV's effects can be placed into three separate categories: it directly produces a variety of clinical infectious disease syndromes such as fever, leukopenia, thrombocytopenia, hepatitis, gastrointestinal ulcerations, pneumonia, and chorioretinitis; it contributes significantly to the net state of immunosuppression; and it may play a role in the pathogenesis of acute and chronic allograft injury. In other immunocompromised patients, the most common effect of CMV infection is the production of a post-transfusion mononucleosis syndrome.[24,128,129]

There are three major modes, and one minor one, by which immunocompromised individuals may acquire active CMV infection: from viable leukocyte-containing blood products that harbor latent virus from seropositive donors (a particular issue in bone marrow and liver transplant patients and other individuals receiving large amounts of blood); from latently infected allografts from seropositive donors; from immunosuppression-induced reactivation of endogenous virus in seropositive individuals; and, finally, due to acquisition of the virus in the general community following intimate contact with an actively infected individual.[24]

There are thus three major epidemiologic patterns of CMV infection in transplant recipients, each with its own rate of clinical illness (as delineated in the following statistics from organ transplant patients)[24,129]:

1. *Primary* CMV infection occurs when the individual has had no pretransplant experience with this virus (and is seronegative for CMV before the transplant) and is infected with virus carried latently in cells from a seropositive, latently infected donor. Among organ transplant patients, approximately 60 percent of individuals at risk for primary CMV infection develop symptomatic disease.
2. *Reactivation* infection occurs when endogenous, latent virus is reactivated, usually due to the effects of immunosuppression, in seropositive individuals. Among organ transplant patients 10 to 20 percent of these individuals become ill.
3. *Superinfection* occurs when a CMV-seropositive individual receives latently infected cells from a seropositive donor (this has been defined primarily in organ transplant patients, when the allograft is the source of the virus), and the virus that is reactivated is of donor rather than recipient origin. It has been suggested that a greater percentage of these individuals become ill (possibly 20 to 40 percent) than those with reactivation infection.

Intravenous ganciclovir at a dose of 5 mg/kg twice a day (with appropriate corrections for renal dysfunction) represents a major advance in the treatment of symptomatic CMV infection. The addition of CMV hyperimmune globulin to the ganciclovir has markedly increased the effectiveness of the antiviral in bone marrow transplant patients with CMV pneumonia and in a murine model of CMV infection. Whether or not this is true in other immunosuppressed patients with symptomatic CMV infection is unclear, although many experts would utilize such a combined regimen in those patients with life-threatening CMV disease. Prevention of CMV infection is still being developed, with high-dose acyclovir and hyperimmune globulin offering some protection. As previously described, preemptive therapy coordinated with antirejection therapy or based on early markers of infection has become an increasingly important component of preventative strategies against this infection. In addition, the use of CMV-seronegative blood products or an effective leukocyte filter during transfusion of red blood cells or platelets can have an important impact on the occurrence of CMV disease in transplant patients and in selected other immunosuppressed populations.[24,31]

SURGICAL CONSIDERATIONS IN IMMUNOCOMPROMISED PATIENTS

With increasing frequency, surgical evaluation and therapy are required for patients with altered host defenses (malnutrition or advanced malignancy, steroid therapy, uremia, or diabetes, or patients who are immunosuppressed). Signs and symptoms of inflammation are frequently masked in immunologically compromised patients. Thus peritonitis may be present in a patient receiving steroids, despite only modest abdominal pain, low-grade fever, and leukocytosis. Within hours, this same patient may be moribund with gram-negative sepsis. For example, in several reports of colonic perforation in steroid-treated patients, the paucity of symptoms, signs, and laboratory evidence of visceral perforation led to frequent delays in treatment and to incorrect preoperative diagnosis in almost all cases.[9,130]

Diagnostic Approach

An aggressive diagnostic approach, therefore, must be undertaken. In patients with only mild abdominal pain, paracentesis and peritoneal lavage have been particularly helpful in diagnosis, often providing purulent fluid despite the absence of free air on plain x-ray studies. If the diagnosis remains in doubt, contrast x-ray studies of the gastrointestinal tract should not be delayed for fear of peritoneal soilage. In general, a water-soluble contrast agent is preferred.

In patients with occult fever but without evidence of peritonitis, the search for an intraperitoneal infection often requires the use of ultrasonography, computed tomography, and radioactive isotope scanning. Negative results with any of these methods do not rule out active infection. Diagnostic laparotomy is probably indicated in any patient with steady, undiagnosed abdominal pain.

Previous, apparently healed incisions should also be regarded with suspicion in these patients with occult fever. Hidden infections may be demonstrated even years after apparent healing. Needle aspiration of any area of tenderness, erythema, or questionable fluctuance is frequently helpful.[9]

Preoperative Preparation

The degree to which preoperative preparation can be extended in an immunoincompetent patient is determined primarily by the nature and urgency of the operation. The usual preoperative resuscitative measures, including volume replacement, institution of antibiotic therapy, and correction of electrolyte imbalances, should be followed. Certain conditions unique to these patients, however, must also be considered. For example, acute adrenal insufficiency must be avoided in patients receiving steroids. Adrenal crisis can be avoided by administering hydrocortisone, 300 mg the day of operation, 150 mg the following day, and 75 mg the third day. By this time, resumption of the preoperative maintenance dosage should be adequate, providing there is no continuing stress.

Uremia may necessitate preoperative dialysis or, at least, correction of hyperkalemia and fluid overload. Ketoacidosis should be corrected in diabetic patients. Given time, there may be some benefit in reducing immunosuppression or improving nutrition.

Intraoperative Considerations

Specific operative procedures often must be modified in these patients. In urgent gastrointestinal tract operations, for example, stomas should be used in preference to anastomoses. Local drainage and proximal colonic diversion are inadequate therapy for sigmoid perforation. Despite the diversion of fecal stream, the inflammatory response is inadequate to provide local containment. Primary resection of the involved bowel and construction of a descending colostomy and distal mucous fistula must, therefore, be undertaken.

The technique of intraperitoneal toilet described in Chapter 38 should be followed in these patients.

After abdominal surgery in the immunocompromised host, prolonged periods of bowel dysfunction will result. Some surgeons advocate gastric drainage by gastrostomy to avoid pulmonary and esophageal complications of nasogastric suction. Others object to unnecessary enterotomies that may leak. At the same time, consideration should be given to using the small bowel for resumption of nutritional support as soon as possible. In fact, it has been observed that most patients with a reasonable length of healthy small intestine can be given full nutrition by jejunostomy in the early postoperative period. Motility and absorption of the small intestine usually return within hours of abdominal exploration. Moreover, because the elemental diet is absorbed in the proximal intestine without the need for digestion, an early return to anabolism is achieved without the risks associated with prolonged hyperalimentation by central venous lines. Placement of a needle or tube catheter jejunostomy at the time of surgery for instillation of elemental diet postoperatively should be a regular consideration in these patients.[9]

Wound complications and delayed healing should be expected. In transplant recipients, the incidence of wound infection may be as high as 39 percent, but usually it is far less than 5 percent if the techniques described in Chapters 22 and 24 are used.[9,24]

Specific Surgical Conditions

Certain surgical conditions are seen so regularly in the immunocompromised host that they deserve special emphasis. One of these is acute perforation of the colon in patients who are receiving steroids. Some authors suggest a direct adverse effect of steroids on the normal colon. Certainly, inhibition of the normal inflammatory response, antifibroblastic activity, and atrophy of lymphoid elements of the bowel wall could interfere with normal barriers to invasive infection by intraluminal bacteria. Perforation could occur whether the colon wall was previously diseased or not and, indeed, has been documented in apparently healthy areas of the bowel.[9,130]

Interestingly, appendicitis rarely occurs in most immunosuppressed hosts, except perhaps in children receiving chemotherapy for leukemia. In this group, abdominal pain and fever are often considered sufficient findings to justify immediate appendectomy. In renal transplant patients, on the other hand, appendicitis is seldom reported. Perhaps the lymphoid atrophy in the bowel wall makes obstruction and inflammation of the appendix unlikely.[9]

Acute pancreatitis in immunosuppressed patients occurs with considerable frequency, even in the absence of alcoholism or biliary tract disease. In one autopsy study of 54 patients who had received steroids, acute focal pancreatitis was found in 28.5 percent of the subjects, as compared with 3.7 percent of 54 matched but nonsteroid-treated autopsy subjects.[131] The mechanism whereby steroids could produce pancreatitis may be ductal ectasia and epithelial metaplasia, resulting in obstruction. Azathioprine is also suspect. Perhaps more important is the fact that many of these patients have a coincident, severe, often viral infection. Cytomegaloviral inclusions have been found in the pancreas of many immunosuppressed patients. This condition in transplant patients carries a mortality rate as high as 70 percent.[132] The factors responsible for this high rate were considerable in establishing the diagnosis and the unusually high incidence of postpancreatic complications (pseudocyst and abscess).[9]

REFERENCES

1. Wolfson JS, Sober AJ, Rubin RH: Dermatologic manifestations of infection in immunocompromised patients. Medicine (Baltimore) 64:115, 1985.
2. Howard RJ: Host defense against infection. Curr Probl Surg 17:1, 1980.
3. Bodey GP, Buckley M, Sathe YS, et al: Quantitative relationships between circulating leucocytes and infection in patients with acute leukemia. Ann Intern Med 64:328, 1966.
4. Wiernik PH: The management of infection in the cancer patient. JAMA 244:185, 1980.
5. Rubin RH, Ferraro MJ: Understanding and diagnosing infectious complications in the immunocompromised host; current issues and trends. Hematol Oncol Clin North Am 7:795, 1993.
6. Van der Meer JWM: Defects in host defense mechanisms. In Rubin RH, Young LS (eds): Clinical Approach to Infection in the Compromised Host, 2nd ed. New York, Plenum Press, 1986.
7. Chandra RK: Nutrition, immunity and infection: present knowledge and future directions. Lancet 1:688, 1983.
8. Keusch GT: Host defense mechanisms in protein energy malnutrition. Adv Exp Med Biol 135:183, 1981.
9. Cosimi AB: Surgical aspects of infection in the compromised host. In Rubin RH, Young LS (eds): Clinical Approach to Infection in the Compromised Host, 2nd ed. New York, Plenum Press, 1986.
10. Tolkoff-Rubin NE, Rubin RH: Uremia and host defenses. N Engl J Med 322:770, 1990.
11. Ruiz P, Gomez F, Schreiber AD: Impaired function of macrophage Fc_r receptors in end-stage renal disease. N Engl J Med 322:717, 1990.
12. Montgomerie JZ, Kalmanson GM, Guze LB: Renal failure and infection. Medicine (Baltimore) 47:1, 1968.
13. Goldbaum SE, Reed WP: Host defenses and immunologic alterations associated with chronic hemodialysis. Ann Intern Med 93:597, 1980.
14. Windus DW, Stokes TJ, Julian BA, Fenves AZ: Fatal *Rhizopus* infections in hemodialysis patients receiving deferoxamine. Ann Intern Med 107:678, 1987.
15. Allen JC: The diabetic as a compromised host. In Allen JC (ed): Infection and the Compromised Host. Clinical Correlations and Therapeutic Approaches, 2nd ed. Baltimore, Williams & Wilkins, 1981, p 229.
16. Rubin RH, Weinstein L: Salmonellosis: Microbiologic, Pathologic and Clinical Features. New York, Stratton Intercontinental Medical Book, 1977, p 66.
17. Hauser WE Jr, Remington JS: Effect of antibiotics on the immune response. Am J Med 72:711, 1982.
18. Edwards JE Jr, Lehrer RI, Stiehm ER, et al: Severe candidal infections: clinical perspective, immune defense mechanism, and current concepts of therapy. Ann Intern Med 89:91, 1978.
19. Campbell AC, Hersey P, MacLennan ICM, et al, and Medical Research Council's Working Party on Leukaemia in Childhood: Immunosuppressive consequences of radiotherapy and chemotherapy in patients with acute lymphoblastic leukemia. Br Med J 2:385, 1973.
20. Fauci AS, Dale DC, Balow JE: Glucocorticosteroid therapy. Mechanisms of action and clinical considerations. Ann Intern Med 84:304, 1976.
21. Dale DC, Fauci AS, Wolff SM: Alternate-day prednisone: leukocyte kinetics and susceptibility to infections. N Engl J Med 291:1154, 1974.
22. Cupps TR, Fauci AS: Corticosteroid-mediated immunoregulation in man. Immunol Rev 65:134, 1982.
23. Weitzman SA, Aisenberg AC, Siber GR, Smith DH: Impaired humoral immunity in treated Hodgkin's disease. N Engl J Med 297:245, 1977.
24. Rubin RH: Infection in the organ transplant recipi-

ent. In Rubin RH, Young LS (eds): Clinical Approach to Infections in the Compromised Host, 3rd ed. New York, Plenum Press 1994, pp 629–706.
25. Hibberd PL, Tolkoff-Rubin NE, Cosimi AB, et al: Symptomatic cytomegalovirus disease in the cytomegalovirus antibody seropositive renal transplant recipient treated with muromonab-CD3 (OKT3). Transplantation 53:68, 1992.
26. Rubin RH, Wolfson JS, Cosimi AB, et al: Infection in the renal transplant recipient. Am J Med 70:405, 1981.
27. Hopkins CC, Weber DJ, Rubin RH: Invasive *Aspergillus* infection: possible non-ward common source within the hospital environment. J Hosp Infect 12:19, 1989.
28. Rubin RH: The compromised host as sentinel chicken. N Engl J Med 317:1151, 1987.
29. Schimpff SC, Greene WH, Young VM, Wiernik PH: Significance of *Pseudomonas aeruginosa* in the patient with leukemia or lymphoma. J Infect Dis Suppl 130:S24, 1974.
30. Goldschmidt MC, Bodey GP: Effects of chemotherapeutic agents upon microorganisms isolated from cancer patients. Antimicrob Agents Chemother 1:348, 1972.
31. Rubin RH, Tolkoff-Rubin NE: Antimicrobial strategies in the care of organ transplant recipients. Antimicrob Agents Chemother 37:619, 1993.
32. Levine AS, Schimpff SC, Grew RG Jr, et al: Hematologic malignancies and other marrow failure states: progress in the management of complicating infections. Semin Hematol 11:141, 1974.
33. Wade JC: Epidemiology and prevention of infection in the compromised host. In Rubin RH, Young LS (eds): Clinical Approach to Infection in the Compromised Host, 3rd ed. New York, Plenum Press 1994, pp 5–32.
34. Prevention of bacterial infection in neutropenic patients with hematologic malignancies: a randomized, multicenter trial comparing norfloxacin with ciprofloxacin. The GIMEMA Infection Program. Ann Intern Med 115:7, 1991.
35. Hughes WT, Armstrong D, Bodey GP, et al: Guidelines for the use of antimicrobial agents in neutropenic patients with unexplained fever. J Infect Dis 161:381, 1990.
36. Verhoef J, Rozenberg-Arska M, Dekker A: Prevention of infection in the neutropenic patient. Rev Infect Dis 11(Suppl 7):S1545, 1989.
37. Pizzo PA: Considerations for the prevention of infectious complications in patients with cancer. Rev Infect Dis 11(Suppl 7):S1551, 1989.
38. Rubin RH: Infection in the immunosuppressed host. In Rubenstein E, Federman DD (eds): The Scientific American Textbook of Medicine. New York, Scientific American, 1993.
39. Rubin RH: Preemptive therapy in immunocompromised hosts. N Engl J Med 324:1057, 1991.
40. Schmidt GM, Horak DA, Niland JC, et al: A randomized, controlled trial of prophylactic ganciclovir for cytomegalovirus pulmonary infection in recipients of allogeneic bone marrow transplant. N Engl J Med 32:1005, 1991.
41. Goodrich JM, Mori M, Gleaves CA, et al: Early treatment with ganciclovir to prevent cytomegalovirus disease after allogeneic bone marrow transplantation. N Engl J Med 235:1601, 1991.
42. Hibberd PL, Rubin RH: Fever in the immunocompromised host. In Mackowiak PA (ed): Fever, Basic Mechanisms and Management. New York, Raven Press, 1991.
43. Peterson PK, Balfour HH, Fryd DS, et al: Fever in renal transplant recipients: causes, prognostic significance and changing patterns at the University of Minnesota Hospital. Am J Med 71:345, 1981.
44. Bodey GP: Microbiologic aspects in patients with leukemia. Hum Pathol 5:687, 1974.
45. De Jongh CA, Joshi JH, Thompson BW, et al: A double beta-lactam combination versus an aminoglycoside-containing regimen as empiric antibiotic therapy for febrile granulocytopenic cancer patients. Am J Med 80:101, 1986.
46. Wade JC, Standiford HC, Drusano GL, et al: Potential of imipenem as a single-agent empiric antibiotic therapy of febrile neutropenic patients with cancer. Am J Med 78(Suppl 6A):62, 1985.
47. Wade JC: Antibiotic therapy for the febrile granulocytopenic cancer patient: combination therapy vs. monotherapy. Rev Infect Dis 11(Suppl 7):S1572, 1989.
48. Lau WK, Young LS, Black RE, et al: Comparative efficacy and toxicity of amikocin-carbenecillin versus gentamicin/carbenecillin in leukopenic patients. A randomized prospective trial. Am J Med 62:959, 1977.
49. Bloomfield CD, Kennedy BJ: Cephalothin, carbenecillin and gentamicin therapy for febrile patients with acute non-lymphocytic leukemia. Cancer 34:431, 1974.
50. Pizzo, PA, Commers J, Cotton D, et al: Approaching the controversies in antibacterial management of cancer patients. Am J Med 76:436, 1984.
51. Rubin RH, Green R: Clinical approach to the compromised host with fever and pulmonary infiltrates. In Rubin RH, Young LS (eds): Clinical Approach to Infection in the Compromised Host, 3rd ed. New York, Plenum Press 1994, pp 121–162.
52. Rosenow EC III, Wilson WR, Cockerill FR III: Pulmonary disease in the immunocompromised host. Mayo Clin Proc 60:473, 610, 1985.
53. Williams DM, Krick JA, Remington JS: Pulmonary infection in the compromised host. Am Rev Respir Dis 114:359, 593, 1976.
54. Kovacs JA, Ng JL, Masur H, et al: Diagnosis of *Pneumocystis carinii* pneumonia: improved detection in sputum with use of monoclonal antibodies. N Engl J Med 318:589, 1988.
55. Weldon-Linne CM, Rhone DP, Bourassa R: Bronchoscopy specimens in adults with AIDS; comparative yields of cytology, histology, and culture for diagnosis of infectious agents. Chest 98:24, 1990.

56. Ettinger NA, Trulock EP: Pulmonary considerations of organ transplantation: Parts I–III. Am Rev Respir Dis 143:1386, 1991; 144:213, 433, 1991.
57. Ferson PF, Landreneau RJ, Dowling RD, et al: Comparison of open versus thoracoscopic lung biopsy for diffuse infiltrative pulmonary disease. J Thorac Cardiovasc Surg 106:194, 1993.
58. Dijkman JH, van der Meer JWM, Bakker W, et al: Transpleural lung biopsy by the thoroscopic route in patients with diffuse interstitial pulmonary disease. Chest 82:76, 1982.
59. Perlmutt LM, Johnston WW, Dunnick NR: Percutaneous transthoracic needle aspiration: a review. AJR 152:451, 1989.
60. Moore EH, Shepard JO, McCloud TC, et al: Positional precautions in needle aspiration lung biopsy. Radiology 175:733, 1990.
61. Rubin RH: Acquired immunodeficiency syndrome. In Rubenstein E, Federman DD (eds): The Scientific American Textbook of Medicine. New York, Scientific American, 1993.
62. Revision of the CDC surveillance case definition for acquired immunodeficiency syndrome. Council of State and Territorial Epidemiologists; AIDS Program, Center for Infectious Disease. Morb Mortal Wkly Rep 36(Suppl 1):15, 1987.
63. 1993 Revised classification system for HIV infection and expanded surveillance case definition for AIDS among adolescents and adults. Morb Mortal Wkly Rep 41:961, 1992.
64. Curran JW, Jaffe HW, Hardy AM, et al: Epidemiology of HIV infection and AIDS in the United States. Science 239:610, 1988.
65. Centers for Disease Control and Prevention: The second 100,000 cases of acquired immunodeficiency syndrome—United States, June 1981–December 1991. Morb Mortal Wkly Rep 41:28, 1992.
66. Mann JM: AIDS—the second decade: a global perspective. J Infect Dis 165:245, 1992.
67. O'Brien TR, Shaffer N, Jaffe HW: Acquisition and transmission of HIV. In Sande MA, Volberding PA (eds): The Medical Management of AIDS, 3rd ed. Philadelphia, Saunders, 1992, p 3.
68. Ho DD, Pomerantz RJ, Kaplan JC: Pathogenesis of infection with human immunodeficiency virus. N Engl J Med 317:278, 1987.
69. Fauci AS: The human immunodeficiency virus: infectivity and mechanisms of pathogenesis. Science 239:617, 1988.
70. Levy JA: Viral and immunological factors in HIV infection. In Sande MA, Volberding PA (eds): The Medical Management of AIDS, 3rd ed. Philadelphia, Saunders, 1992, p 18.
71. Greene WC: The molecular biology of human immunodeficiency virus type 1. N Engl J Med 324:308, 1991.
72. Bukrinsky MI, Stanwick TL, Dempsey MP, et al: Quiescent T lymphocytes as an inducible virus reservoir in HIV-I infection. Science 254:423, 1991.
73. Saag MS, Crain MJ, Decker WD, et al: High level viremia in adults and children infected with human immunodeficiency virus: relation to disease stage and CD4+ lymphocyte level. J Infect Dis 164:72, 1991.
74. Fauci AS, Schnittman SM, Poli G, et al: Immunopathogenic mechanisms in human immunodeficiency virus (HIV) infection. Ann Intern Med 114:678, 1991.
75. Worley JM, Price RW: Management of neurologic complications of HIV-I infection and AIDS. In Sande MA, Volberding PA (eds): The Medical Management of AIDS, 3rd ed. Philadelphia, Saunders, 1992, p 193.
76. Cooper DA, Gold J, MacLean P, et al: Acute AIDS retrovirus infection: definition of a clinical illness associated with seroconversion. Lancet 1:537, 1985.
77. Valle SL, Saxinger C, Ranki A, et al: Diversity of clinical spectrum of HTLV-III infection. Lancet 1:301, 1985.
78. Fauci AS, Masur H, Gelmann EP, et al: The acquired immunodeficiency syndrome: an update. Ann Intern Med 102:800, 1985.
79. Shaw GM, Harper ME, Hahn BH, et al: HTLV-III infection in brains of children and adults with AIDS encephalopathy. Science 227:177, 1985.
80. Greenson JK, Belitsos PC, Yardley JH, et al: AIDS enteropathy: occult enteric infection and duodenal mucosal alterations in chronic diarrhea. Ann Intern Med 114:366, 1991.
81. Glassock RJ, Cohen AH, Danovitch G, et al: Human immunodeficiency virus (HIV) infection and the kidney. Ann Intern Med 112:35, 1990.
82. Grunfeld C, Feingold KR: Metabolic disturbances and wasting in the acquired immunodeficiency syndrome. N Engl J Med 327:329, 1992.
83. Hopewell PC: *Pneumocystis carinii* pneumonia: current concepts. In Sande MA, Volberding PA (eds): The Medical Management of AIDS, 3rd ed. Philadelphia, Saunders, 1992, p 261.
84. Fischl MA, Uttamchandani RB, Daikos GL, et al: An outbreak of tuberculosis caused by multiple-drug-resistant tubercle bacilli among patients with HIV infection. Ann Intern Med 117:177, 1992.
85. Pearson ML, Jereb JA, Frieden TR, et al: Nosocomial transmission of multidrug-resistant *Mycobacterium tuberculosis:* a risk for patients and health care workers. Ann Intern Med 117:191, 1992.
86. Onorato IM, McCray E: Prevalence of human immunodeficiency virus infection among patients attending tuberculosis clinics in the United States. J Infect Dis 165:87, 1992.
87. Fischl MA, Daikos GL, Uttamchandani RB, et al: Clinical presentation and outcome of patients with HIV infection and tuberculosis caused by multiple-drug-resistant bacilli. Ann Intern Med 117:184, 1992.
88. Davey RT Jr, Lane HC: Laboratory methods in the diagnostic and prognostic staging of infection with human immunodeficiency virus type 1. Rev Infect Dis 12:912, 1990.
89. Sloand EM, Pitt E, Chiarello RJ, et al: HIV testing: state of the art. JAMA 266:2861, 1991.

90. Broder S, Mitsuya H, Yarchoan R, et al: NIH conference: antiretroviral therapy in AIDS. Ann Intern Med 113:604, 1990.
91. Hirsch MS: Chemotherapy of human immunodeficiency virus infections: current practice and future prospects. J Infect Dis 161:845, 1990.
92. Corey L, Fleming TR: Treatment of HIV infections: progress in perspective. N Engl J Med 326:484, 1992.
93. Hamilton JD, Hartregan PM, Simberkoff MS, et al: A controlled trial of early versus late treatment with zidovudine in symptomatic human immunodeficiency virus infection: results of the Veterans Affairs Cooperative Study. N Engl J Med 326:437, 1992.
94. Kahn JD, Lagakos SW, Richman DD, et al: A controlled trial comparing continual zidovudine with didanosine in human immunodeficiency virus infection: the NIAID AIDS Clinical Trial Group. N Engl J Med 327:581, 1992.
95. Fauci AS: Combination therapy for HIV infection: getting closer. Ann Intern Med 116:85, 1992.
96. Gerberding JL: HIV transmission to providers and their patients. In Sande MA, Volberding PA (eds): The Medical Management of AIDS, 3rd ed. Philadelphia, Saunders, 1992, p 54.
97. Becker CE, Cone JE, Gerberding J: Occupational infection with human immunodeficiency virus (HIV): risks and risk reduction. Ann Intern Med 110:653, 1989.
98. Kelen GD, DiGiovanna T, Bisson L, et al: Human immunodeficiency virus infection in emergency department patients: epidemiology, clinical presentations, and risk to health care workers: the Johns Hopkins experience. JAMA 262:516, 1989.
99. Panlilo AL, Foy DR, Edwards JR, et al: Blood contacts during surgical procedures. JAMA 265:1533, 1991.
100. Gerberding JL, Schecter WP: Surgery and AIDS: reducing the risk. JAMA 265:1572, 1991.
101. Shih CC, Kaneshima H, Rabin L, et al: Postexposure prophylaxis with zidovudine suppresses human immunodeficiency virus type I infection in SCID-hu mice in a time-dependent manner. J Infect Dis 163:625, 1991.
102. Koransky JR, Stargel MD, Dowell VR Jr: *Clostridium septicum* bacteremia: its clinical significance. Am J Med 66:63, 1979.
103. Rubin RH, Hooper DC: Central nervous system infection in the compromised host. Med Clin North Am 69:281, 1985.
104. Aisner J, Schimpff SC, Wiernik PH: Treatment of invasive aspergillosis: relation of early diagnosis and treatment to response. Ann Intern Med 86:539, 1977.
105. Campbell GD: Primary pulmonary *Cryptococcus.* Am Rev Respir Dis 94:236, 1966.
106. Duperval R, Hermans PE, Brewer NS, Roberts GD: Cryptococcosis, with emphasis on the significance of isolation of *Cryptococcus neoformans* from the respiratory tract. Chest 72:13, 1977.
107. Hughes WT: Current concepts: *Pneumocystis carinii* pneumonia. N Engl J Med 297:1381, 1977.
108. Fishman JA: *Pneumocystis carinii* and parasitic infections in the unimmunocompromised host. In Rubin RH, Young LS (eds): Clinical Approach to Infection in the Compromised Host, 3rd ed. New York, Plenum Press 1994, pp 275–334.
109. Gordin FM, Simon GL, Wofsy CB, et al: Adverse reaction to trimethoprim–sulfamethoxazole in patients with the acquired immunodeficiency syndrome. Ann Intern Med 100:495, 1984.
110. Gagnon S, Boota AM, Fischl MA, et al: Corticosteroids as adjunctive therapy for severe *Pneumocystis carinii* pneumonia in the acquired immunodeficiency syndrome: a double-blind, placebo controlled trial. N Engl J Med 323:1444, 1990.
111. Montaner JGS, Lawson LM, Levitt N, et al: Corticosteroids prevent early deterioration in patients with moderately severe *Pneumocystis carinii* pneumonia and the acquired immunodeficiency syndrome (AIDS). Ann Intern Med 113:14, 1990.
112. Ruskin J, Remington JS: Toxoplasmosis in the compromised host. Ann Intern Med 84:193, 1976.
113. Luft BJ, Brooks RG, Conley FK, et al: Toxoplasmic encephalitis in patients with acquired immune deficiency syndrome. JAMA 252:913, 1984.
114. Hall WA, Martinez AJ, Dummer JS, et al: Central nervous system infections in heart and heart–lung transplant recipients. Arch Neurol 46:173, 1987.
115. Luft BJ, Billingham M, Remington JS: Endomyocardial biopsy in the diagnosis of toxoplasmic myocarditis. Transplant Proc 18:1871, 1986.
116. Michaels MG, Wald ER, Fricker FJ, et al: Toxoplasmosis in pediatric recipients of heart transplants. Clin Infect Dis 14:847, 1992.
117. Wreghett TG, Gray JJ, Pavel P, et al: Efficacy of pyrimethamine for the prevention of donor-acquired *Toxoplasma gondii* infection in heart and heart–lung transplant patients. Transplant Int 5:197, 1992.
118. Hirsch MS: Herpes group virus infections in the compromised host. In Rubin RH, Young LS (eds): Clinical Approach to Infection in the Compromised Host, 3rd ed. New York, Plenum 1994, pp 379–396.
119. Rand KH, Rasmussen LE, Pollard RB, et al: Cellular immunity and herpesvirus in cardiac transplant patients. N Engl J Med 296:1372, 1977.
120. Chatis PA, Miller CH, Schrager LE, et al: Successful treatment with foscarnet of an acyclovir-resistant mucocutaneous infection with herpes simplex virus in a patient with acquired immunodeficiency syndrome. N Engl J Med 320:297, 1989.
121. Erlich KS, Jacobson MA, Kochler JE, et al: Foscarnet therapy for severe acyclovir-resistant herpes simplex virus type-2 infection in patients with the acquired immunodeficiency syndrome (AIDS): an uncontrolled trial. Ann Intern Med 110:710, 1989.
122. Luby JP, Ramirez-Ronda C, Rinner S, et al: A longitudinal study of varicella-zoster infections in renal transplant recipients. J Infect Dis 135:659, 1977.

123. Arvin AM, Pollard RB, Rasmussen LE, Merigan TC: Selective impairment of lymphocyte reactivity to varicella-zoster virus antigen among untreated patients with lymphoma. J Infect Dis 137:531, 1978.
124. Jacobson MA, Berger TG, Fikrig S, et al: Acyclovir-resistant varicella-zoster virus infection after chronic oral acyclovir therapy in patients with the acquired immunodeficiency syndrome (AIDS). Ann Intern Med 112:187, 1990.
125. Stephaman E, Gruber SA, Dunn DL, et al: Posttransplant lymphoproliferative disorders. Transplant Rev 5:120, 1991.
126. Preiksaitis JK, Diaz-Mitoma F, Mirzayans F, et al: Quantitative oropharyngeal Epstein-Barr virus shedding in renal and cardiac transplant recipients: relationship to immunosuppressive therapy, serologic responses, and the risk of posttransplant lymphoproliferative disorder. J Infect Dis 166:986, 1992.
127. Straus SE, Cohen JI, Tosato G, et al: Epstein-Barr virus infections: biology, pathogenesis, and management. Ann Intern Med 118:45, 1993.
128. Ho M: Cytomegalovirus, Biology and Infection. New York, Plenum Press, 1982.
129. Rubin RH: Impact of cytomegalovirus infection on organ transplant recipients. Rev Infect Dis 12(Suppl 7):S754, 1990.
130. Warshaw AL, Welch JP, Ottinger LW: Acute perforation of the colon associated with chronic corticosteroid therapy. Am J Surg 131:442, 1976.
131. Carone FA, Liebow AA: Acute pancreatic lesions in patients treated with ACTH and adrenal corticoids. N Engl J Med 257:690, 1957.
132. Fernandez JA, Rosenberg JC: Post-transplantation pancreatitis. Surg Gynecol Obstet 143:795, 1976.

Infections in Burned Patients

CHAPTER 52

Randi L. Rutan, Thuan T. Nguyen, David N. Herndon

Although the survival of burned patients has significantly improved over the past few decades, infection remains one of the major causes of morbidity and mortality in this population.[1-4] The use of effective topical and antimicrobial agents to control microbiologic proliferation within the burn wound itself and early surgical removal of necrotic tissue prior to microbial invasion have significantly reduced the relative contribution of burn wound sepsis to infective morbidity.[5-7] In fact, pneumonias have supplanted burn wound sepsis as the most common cause of death in the burned patient.[8,9] Fungal infections have also become increasingly common.[7,10,11] The potential for infection, sepsis, and altered organ function still directly correlates with increased burn size[12] and the presence of concomitant smoke inhalation injury, but these correlations simply reflect the combined effects of impaired host resistance and microbiologic virulence.[13]

The first line of microbial host defense is the mechanical barrier of the epithelium. The initial injury from thermal trauma directly disrupts the skin and lung and indirectly impairs the gut epithelial barrier. The induced alterations create a pathway for the migration of bacteria, fungi, and viruses into viable tissue and the systemic circulation. These three portals of entry represent the three major sources of microbial contamination in the burned patient.

SKIN

The host defenses provided to the skin and its normal microbial flora are described in Chapters 3 and 12. Alteration of this environment allows for bacterial overgrowth of both commensals and exogenous bacterial contaminants derived from contact with the environment and attending personnel. Both the quantity of microorganisms present on the burn wound and the depth of their penetration into the necrotic tissue increase progressively with time after injury. Within 2 weeks of injury, the predominantly gram-positive normal skin flora are replaced with gram-negative bacteria.[14]

Local factors influence the susceptibility of the wound to support bacterial growth and promote infection. The blood supply is cut off by thermal coagulation; devitalized tissue is an excellent microbial culture medium; leukocytes cannot penetrate the necrotic tissue; phagocytosis and intracellular killing are inhibited; and the low local oxygen tension creates an anaerobic environment, which further impedes the efficacy of leukocytes.[15] Local blood supply is further impaired by the development of edema secondary to the inflammatory reaction, hypovolemia, and the local release of vasoconstrictive substances.[16] Jackson[17] long ago hypothesized that the burn wound could be represented by three concentric zones of injury. The central zone of coagulation is completely destroyed by the injury. This area was surrounded, in all three concentric dimensions, by the zones of stasis and hyperemia, respectively. Jackson hypothesized that the zone of hyperemia would completely recover from the injury, whereas the zone of stasis has the ability to recover only if given appropriate treatment.

Unfortunately, the problem is far more complex. The wound detritus impels an ongoing inflammatory process,[18–20] which has important systemic components. Whereas inflammation is an essential step in wound repair and the local control and containment of infection, persistent inflammation impairs the subsequent tissue reparative processes. In small injuries, this response is confined to the area of injury. Major thermal injuries, however, stimulate a systemic response, with inflammatory changes occurring in areas distant from the actual wounds. The inflammatory response liberates large quantities of inflammatory mediators (see Chap. 16) in the wound.[21,22] Normally, these agents are short-lived and locally contained by inhibitory enzymes.[22,23] However, with such a massive release, local inhibitory mechanisms are overwhelmed and local acute phase responses become systemic. Once activated, these mediators initiate systemic cascades, which have profound pathophysiologic responses and depress the body's immune system.[22–25] Surgical manipulation, wound contamination, and infection episodically stimulate the inflammatory process, not only impeding wound closure but having adverse systemic consequences.

GUT

A significant portion of the cardiac output is normally directed to the splanchnic vascular bed. Hypovolemic shock, as seen in patients with large burns, is associated with an increase in total peripheral resistance and an even more profound effect on the mesenteric circulation. Increased angiotensin II and vasopressin may have roles in the selective splanchnic vasoconstriction observed following trauma.[26] Splanchnic vasoconstriction results in a disproportionate decrease in blood flow in the mucosa and submucosa and a major reduction in capillary surface area. The level of tissue oxygenation is a function of prevailing oxygen consumption and oxygen delivery. Normally, the mucosal villus partial pressure of oxygen exhibits a large oxygen gradient and there is higher resting oxygen consumption in the tip of the villus compared to the base. When the blood flow is drastically reduced and compensatory mechanisms are overwhelmed, mucosal damage ensues. The villus tips slough as a direct result of ischemia plus the added insults of reperfusion injury and edema. Bacteria more readily cross the mucosal barrier into the systemic blood or lymphatic circulation, increasing the risk of systemic sepsis. In a retrospective review, Desai et al[27] determined that more than half of burned patients were noted to have ischemic intestinal pathology at autopsy. However, only rarely were these changes reflected by the clinical picture. A high mortality (over 60 percent) accompanies bleeding or perforation of the gastrointestinal tract in burn patients.[27]

There is known to be a strong correlation between the microflora of the feces and the bacteria colonizing the burn wound.[14,28] Nearly 30 years ago, Hildebrand and Wolochow[29] described bacterial translocation across the intestinal wall of rats (see Chap. 38). Studies have confirmed microbial translocation from gut mesenteric lymph nodes and blood in various disease states including burns, hemorrhagic shock, malnutrition, bacterial overgrowth, immunosuppression, skeletal trauma, radiation, and cancer.[30–39]

Decreased mesenteric blood flow has been associated with bacterial translocation in experimental animals.[40] Fifty-six percent of hypotensive trauma patients develop bacteremias within 3 hours of injury.[41] Following major thermal injury, despite appropriate resuscitation, a decrease in mesenteric blood flow has been demonstrated during the first 8 hours postburn with concomitant bacterial translocation.[42,43] Conversely, maintenance of normal mesenteric blood flow using selective vasodilatory agents effectively prevents gut bacterial translocation.[44]

There is indirect evidence that mesenteric ischemia may damage the intestinal mucosa. Ornithine decarboxylase (ODC) is the rate-limiting step in the formation of putrescine, which is one of the many polyamines identified in rapidly dividing cells. Following thermal injury, there is an increase in intestinal ODC and DNA activity, suggesting an ongoing reparative process.[45] Furthermore, translocation can be effectively reduced by the administration of mucosal growth factors.[46]

Although the precise role of gastrointestinal bacterial and endotoxin translocation in the development of systemic sepsis remains to be clarified in humans, animal studies suggest that the migration of bacteria and their products through the intestinal wall occurs soon after thermal injury.[47,48] Sittig and Deitch[49] estimated that approximately 80 percent of all lethal bacteremias arise from wound or pulmonary sources; however, the multiple and recurrent episodes of hypovolemia, endotoxemia, hypotension, malnutrition, hypothermia, and overall immunosuppression experienced by a burned patient during recovery may result in numerous opportunities for bacterial translocation from the gastrointestinal tract to occur, which seed the wound and lungs.

LUNGS

Prior to the routine use of topical chemotherapeutic agents to control bacterial proliferation of the burn wound, the majority of pulmonary infections were thought to be caused by hematogenous dissemination of bacteria from wound to lung.[50] Pneumonias arising from systemic wound sepsis are now uncommon. Bronchopneumonias are most often caused by exogenous airborne organisms or those contained in aspirated gastric or nasopharyngeal secretions. These secretions tend to become colonized with antibiotic-resistant pathogens, each one peculiar to a particular burn treatment center. The common epidemiologic features are the frequent use of parenteral antibiotics and the use of gastric antacids.[51,52]

The caustic constituents of smoke produce a local inflammatory reaction and a diffuse chemical tracheobronchitis. Almost immediately following inhalation injury, a marked hyperemia results from the changes in the local blood supply.[53,54] The inhalation of organic acids, aldehydes, or noxious gases reduces the ability of the lung to clear bacteria and interferes with mucociliary transport.[55–57] The local inflammatory response stimulates leukocyte infiltration and exudate formation. The ciliated epithelial lining of the airways becomes necrotic and sloughs shortly before the appearance of exudate. A pseudomembrane forms from the collection of fibrin, mucus, leukocytes, and shed epithelium. The resultant casts may be sufficiently small to be expectorated or may be so extensive as to cause partial or complete obstruction of the bronchi (Fig. 52–1). The casts may act as ball valves within the smaller airways, creating areas of hyperinflation and atelectasis. In addition, generalized bronchoconstriction is stimulated by mediators of the cyclooxygenase cascade.[58,59] Changes in surfactant activity have been documented.[60–62] Gas exchange may be further compromised by the inhibition of thoracic excursion due to cutaneous burn scar.

Pulmonary parenchymal injury is unrelated to direct thermal injury but is rather the result of cellular and humoral reaction to inhaled toxic gases (Fig. 52–2). Edema formation is thought to be mediated by the release of oxygen radicals from leukocytes,[58,59] because fluid accumulation following experimental smoke inhalation is reduced when leukocytes are depleted[63] or when oxygen radicals are scavenged[65] or proteolytic enzymes are inhibited.[64] Smoke inhalation injury stimulates the release of chemotactic substances resulting in the recruitment of leukocytes into the parenchyma,[63] and their activation is mediated through the complement system.[66]

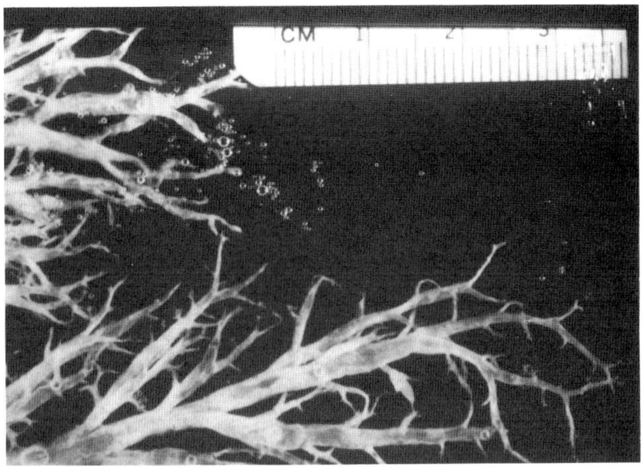

Figure 52–1. A well defined bronchoalveolar cast removed from postmortem sheep lung 2 days postinhalation injury.

Inhalation injury itself causes some systemic effects. An isolated smoke inhalation injury has been noted to decrease mesenteric blood flow by 20 percent, and in combination with a cutaneous burn injury by 36 percent.[46] A concomitant increase in the quantity of bacterial translocation was noted with the combined experimental burn and inhalation injury models over that seen with either isolated injury.

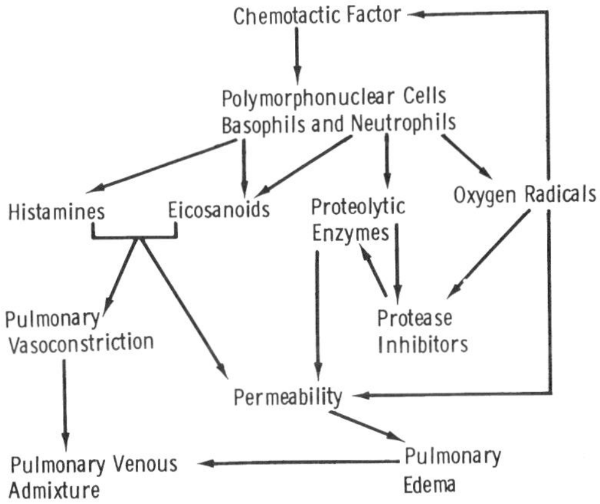

Figure 52–2. Cascade of pulmonary pathophysiology of inhalation injury.

Pulmonary edema and mucous plug formation, bronchoconstriction, and changes in surfactant activity, in combination with bed rest and generalized immunosuppression, leads to the high incidence of pneumonia, infection, and death in the burn-injured patient. These effects are compounded if control of wound colonization is lost so that large amounts of aerosolized bacteria are released during wound manipulation.

TYPES OF CONTAMINANTS

The normal bacterial flora of the human skin consist almost entirely of gram-positive bacteria. Moist areas, such as the groin, web spaces, and axillae, support the growth of gram-negative species as well as some yeasts (see Chap. 3). Figure 52–3 indicates the frequency of recovery of microbes from burn wounds at a single large burn center.[67]

Bacteria

In the 1940s, *Streptococcus pyogenes* was the most frequently isolated contaminant of the burn wound.[68] Following the introduction of penicillin and topical sulfonamides, *S. aureus* became the prevalent bacterial invader of the burn wound, replaced by gram-negative bacteria in the 1960s when topical antibiotic treatment of burn wounds became standard practice.[69] Both staphylococcal and streptococcal infections now occur most commonly on the freshly burned wound, donor sites, new skin grafts, or recently epithelialized partial-thickness burn wounds. *Staphylococcus epidermidis* is frequently the causative organism of local infections of percutaneous and "cut down" intravenous infusion sites. Recently, methicillin-resistant *S. aureus* (MRSA) has emerged as the predominant contaminant of burn wounds, grafts, and injured lungs. The virulence of this strain is felt to be less than the methicillin-sensitive types, but its resistant nature has led to considerable morbidity, particularly skin graft loss.

The most commonly isolated gram-negative bacteria are *Pseudomonas aeruginosa, Enterobacter cloacae, Providencia stuartii, Serratia marcescens,* and *Klebsiella. Pseudomonas* organisms occasionally invade viable tissue and lymphatic and blood vessels, disseminating the bacteria to uninjured subcutaneous tissue, producing a syndrome called *ecthyma gangrenosum* (Fig. 52–4). Of particular importance are the endotoxins released by gram-negative organisms. Endotoxin may possess direct cytotoxic properties, inhibit the function of various

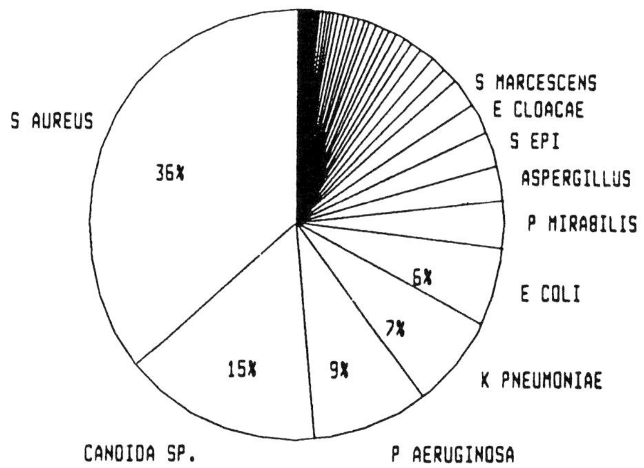

Figure 52–3. Frequency of recovery of microorganisms from infections in burn patients treated at the United States Army Burn Center from 1984 to 1988. Unlabeled segments represent organisms causing less than 4 percent of infections. *(From Pruitt BA Jr, McManus AT, Kim SH: Burns. In Gorbach SL, Bartlett JG, Blacklow NR (eds): Infectious Diseases. Philadelphia, Saunders, 1992, p 784.)*

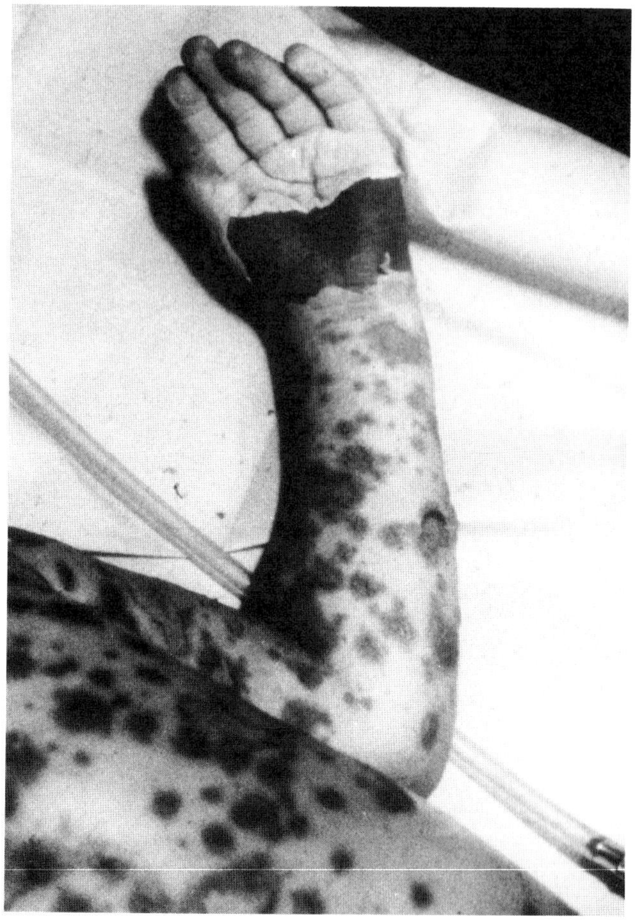

Figure 52–4. Blood-borne invasion of skin tissue classically known as ecthyma gangrenosum is depicted. Clinical course is the sudden appearance of circumscribed brown or black lesions often visible through eschar.

components of the immune system, or produce the classic clinical symptoms of shock.

Anaerobic infections in burned patients are usually associated with avascular muscle found in electrical injuries, frost bite, or cutaneous flame burns with concomitant crush type injuries.[70–74] The high risk of developing tetanus (*Clostridium tetani*), even with small burns, has led to the accepted practice of tetanus prophylaxis (tetanus toxoid 0.5 ml) as a routine part of the admission protocol for most burn centers.[75,76] In addition, if prior immunization is absent or unclear, or the last booster was more than 10 years ago, 250 units of tetanus antitoxin is also given (see Chap. 50).

Fungi

Until the advent of topical antimicrobial agents, fungal infections were not common in burned patients. However, the incidence of mycotic invasion has doubled since the implementation of topical antimicrobial agents to control bacterial colonization.[10,77] The burn wound is the most commonly infected site,[10] although local or disseminated fungal infections of the respiratory tract, urinary tract, gastrointestinal tract, and vagina are increasingly common.[11,78,79] *Candida* species are the most common nonbacterial colonizers of the burn wound, although true fungi such as *Aspergillus, Rhizopus, Mucor,* and *Fusarium* are not uncommon and have a much greater invasive potential than the yeasts[80–83] (Table 52–1).

Early diagnosis of fungal infection is difficult because clinical symptoms frequently mimic low-grade bacterial infections. Standard culture techniques may require up to 7 days to identify fungal contaminants, delaying the initiation of treatment.[77,84] Because of their relatively large size, *Candida* organisms are usually filtered out of blood at the capillary level. Therefore venous blood cultures may not reflect the causative organism.[83] Arterial blood cultures and retinal examination for characteristic candidal lesions can be useful. Organisms are usually found in the urine when sepsis from a distant site occurs. The isolation of *Candida* species from three organ sites is usually required for the definitive diagnosis of candidal sepsis.[78] *Candida* antibody titers in the serum have recently been advocated to assist in early diagnosis.[85] Premortem diagnosis, confirmed with sufficient time to implement appropriate treatment, occurs in less than 40 percent of infected patients.[86]

TABLE 52–1. INVASIVENESS OF ORGANISMS

Measurement	*Candida*	Filamentous Fungi
Incidence		
Colonization	30–40%	2–4.4%
Infection	5–7%	1–2%
Dissemination	2–4%	1–2%
Time of occurrence	Late	Early
Mortality		
With invasive infection	80–100%	90–100%

Candida is omnipresent in the burned patient, appearing in stools, nasopharynx swabs, urine samples, and cultures of intact integument; however, fewer than 20 percent of patients with candidal wound colonization develop widespread candidiasis.[82,87] Only when the controlling bacterial populations are eradicated by systemic antibiotics or the host becomes immunosuppressed does candidal infection occur,[88] frequently following a bacterial sepsis. There is a 3 to 5 percent incidence of candidemia in the burned population[78,80,87,89] and a comparable rate of burn wound invasion.[80] Candidal infections occur most commonly in patients with large burn injuries who are hospitalized for long periods of time and have received multiple courses of antibiotics. Prophylactic treatment with oropharyngeal and topical nystatin has therefore been recommended.[78]

Unlike candidal infections, true fungal infections occur early in the hospital course of patients with specific predisposing characteristics. Most frequently, burned patients infected with fungi have been exposed to spores in the environment by either rolling on the ground or jumping into surface water at the time of injury. Nosocomial sources have also been implicated in fungal infection, especially mucormycosis and aspergillosis. These include bandaging supplies left open to air, heating and air conditioning ducts, and floor drains.[90–92]

Infection with *Aspergillus* or *Mucor* species (see Chap. 10) is truly invasive. Broad nonbranching hyphae extend into subcutaneous tissue, stimulating an inflammatory response. Vascular invasion is common with accompanied thrombosis and avascular necrosis, clinically observed as rapidly advancing dark discolorations of the wound margins or well-described lesions.[76,80] Wound biopsy with appropriate stains yields the diagnosis rapidly. Local treatment must be vigorous if systemic dissemination of the infection via the vasculature is to be avoided.

Viruses

Viral infections are now more frequently recognized in burned patients than in the past. Prospective and retrospective assays of sera have documented a large incidence of subclinical viral infection. Linneman and MacMillan[93] assayed stored sera of burned children and found a fourfold increase in antibodies to cytomegalovirus (CMV) in 22 percent of patients, to herpes simplex virus (HSV) titers in 8 percent, and to varicella-zoster virus (VZV), in 5 percent. In a prospective study, 33 percent of children developed CMV infection, 25 percent herpetic infections, and 17 percent adenovirus infection.[93]

CMV infection typically occurs approximately 1 month postburn and clinically presents with lymphocytosis.[94] Rarely are patients with less than 50 percent total body surface area burn infected. CMV infection frequently occurs concurrently with bacterial and fungal infections but rarely alters the patient's clinical course. CMV inclusions may be identified in the cells of multiple organs but have not been reported in the burn wound.[95] The burned patients who most commonly contract the infection are known to have received multiple blood transfusions, which is the probable infective source.

Herpetic lesions most commonly appear in healing partial-thickness burns or split-thickness donor sites, although other epithelial surfaces such as the oral or intestinal mucosa can be involved. In the latter case, herpetic lesions may lead to erosion and perforation. The cutaneous manifestations may be preceded by unexplained fever unresponsive to empiric antibiotic coverage.[96] Partial-thickness burns and donor sites infected with HSV may "convert" to full-thickness injuries, requiring skin grafting for ultimate closure. Necrotizing hepatic and adrenal involvement may lead to multisystem organ failure. Mortality in patients with disseminated HSV infection is about twice that expected for patients of similar age and burn size.

Chickenpox is a highly contagious disease in school-aged children, and mini-epidemics have occurred within pediatric burn units,[97] where it is life-threatening. The characteristic fluid-filled lesions appear in both normal skin and in healing partial-thickness burn. Due to the fragility of the newly healed or healing skin, the vesicles are much more destructive in the injured than the uninjured skin and may present as hemorrhagic, oozing pockmarks that are prone to secondary infection and subsequent scarring. New, neovascularized skin grafts may be lost and further grafting procedures should be delayed until the lesions are quiescent. In burn patients, HSV and VZV require intravenous acyclovir, because absorption of the oral drug is poor.

SYSTEMIC IMMUNOSUPPRESSION

The complex multifaceted host defense system is reviewed in Chapters 12 to 16. In general, thermal injury results in a generalized downregulation of all immunologic activities: reduced macrophage and neutrophil phagocytic killing ability; decreased levels of opsonins, immunoglobulins, protease inhibitors, and chemotactic factors; and reduced numbers of various lymphocyte function.[24,98,99] There is also the suggestion that the expression of neutrophil receptors[100–102] and the binding properties of intracellular adhesion molecules (ICAMs) are altered to stimulate neutrophil migration.[103,104]

Warden et al[105,106] demonstrated that leukocyte chemotaxis was inversely correlated with clinical status and is predictive of ultimate survival. Similar changes have been noted in monocytes.[107] In addition, commonly used topical[106,108] and systemic[109] antimicrobial agents suppress leukocyte chemotaxis.

Neutrophil bactericidal capacity is also depressed after burn injury. Cole et al[110] have suggested that there are defects in lysosomal enzyme levels (beta-glucuronidase, lysozyme, myeloperoxidease) and Curreri et al[111] have suggested that there are defects in the production of hydrogen peroxide and superoxide. In vitro, oxygen consumption of neutrophils harvested from burned patients is significantly depressed when compared with cells harvested from normal controls.[112]

The primary antibacterial defense mechanisms of the lung are the alveolar macrophages.[113,114] These are thought to be the agents responsible for halting the systemic dissemination of bacteria from the pulmonary vasculature, and an increase in their phagocytic ability has been documented for up to a week following thermal injury.

Delayed allograft rejection, altered rosette forming ability, decreased delayed hypersensitivity, and diminished stimulative and responsive capacity of lymphocytes in mixed lymphocyte culture reactions have been reported in both thermally injured patients and experimentally burned animals.[115–119]

In the course of managing the burned patient, blood replacement frequently becomes necessary. Comparisons of infection rates between patients receiving homologous versus autologous transfusions have demonstrated significantly fewer infectious complications among patients receiving their own blood.[120,121] Most studies have concluded that blood transfusion induces a generalized systemic immunosuppression with decreased helper/suppressor ratios, inhibition of natural killer (NK) cell activity, and decreased nacrophage activity[122–124] while not impairing local responses.[125]

INFECTIONS AND SEPTIC COMPLICATIONS

Burned patients are predisposed to many infections that are commonly seen in other critically ill patients; however, there are also infections that are specific to burn patients. Infection is the most common and most serious complication of a major burn injury and is directly related to size of the burn area. Sepsis account for 50 to 60 percent of deaths in burn patients today despite improvements in antimicrobial therapies. Sepsis in burns is commonly due to bronchopneumonia, pyelonephritis, thrombophlebitis, or invasive wound infection. However, other less common causes of sepsis are sinusitis, endocarditis, chondritis, and candidiasis. Infection is promoted by loss of the epithelial barrier, by malnutrition induced by the hypermetabolic response to burn injury, and by a generalized postburn immunosuppression due to immunoactive agents released from the burn wound into the circulation.

Cellulitis

Prophylactic penicillin was formerly used to treat burn wound cellulitis, because streptococcal septicemia was a primary killer of burn patients in the 1920s and 1930s. Recent studies have shown that the incidence of cellulitis in burned patients was similar whether or not penicillin was given. Burn centers should reassess practice in this regard, because penicillin-resistant organisms have become predominant.

The most common complication of small burn wounds is rubor, dolor, and calor. These changes are typically seen 24 hours to 5 days postburn. The most common organisms cultured are *Staphylococcus* and *Streptococcus*. Surface cultures should be taken, but presumptive therapy must be instituted as soon as recognized. In outpatients, many physicians still use penicillin; in hospitalized patients, the therapy chosen should be based on the major nosocomial organism in that center and its sensitivity. We consider nafcillin to be sufficient for uncomplicated cases while for patients who are diabetic and immunocompromised, a combination of nafcillin and gentamicin is the therapy of choice. For some burn units, the incidence of MRSA as a colonizing organism can be as high as 80 percent, presenting a strong argument for using systemic vancomycin. It should be noted that this agent is potentially ototoxic and the dosage should be titrated by measuring drug levels. Cellulitis usually responds within 2 to 5 days of systemic treatment.

Controversy exists as to whether to excise the wound in an area of cellulitis infection. The decision to do this or not is dependent primarily on the depth of the wound. We have routinely excised these areas, after establishing antibiotic drug levels, if the involved wounds were of sufficient depth to require excision at some time. It is our impression that there is a decrease in the duration of cellulitis if this is done and no increase in graft loss, as was earlier feared. There have, however, been no randomized studies to validate this approach.

Pneumonia

Pulmonary pathology remains one of the most common causes of death in the burned patient. When a patient develops a fever of unknown origin and a sputum Gram stain from an endotracheal source demonstrates leukocytes and uniform bacterial morphology (ie, not contaminated with oropharyngeal secretions), a presumptive diagnosis of pulmonary infection is made. The presence of a positive chest x-ray study or other suspicious physical findings would require immediate institution of intravenous antibiotics and supportive therapies. The routine use of agents that maintain a high gastric pH plus the high risk of aspiration now that enteral feeding is routinely employed through nasogastric tube may have increased the frequency of this complication.

Supportive therapies include avoidance of bed rest, ambulation, and aggressive pulmonary toilet. If not contraindicated, fluids should be administered. Various mucolytic and bronchodilator agents can be nebulized into the bronchial tree. Nebulized epinenefrin, with or without mucomyst, has proved to be clinically beneficial. In addition, recent institution of nebulized heparin has helped "soften" mucous plugs and facilitate suction.

Oro- and nasopharyngeal intubation should be avoided if possible, as it simply opens another pathway for bacterial contamination. Although prolonged endotracheal intubation is associated with decreased survival rate,[126] if intubation is necessary, mechanical ventilation should be instituted immediately if only to provide for positive end expiratory pressure (PEEP). The epiglottis is unable to close when a tube is in place, and normal intrathoracic pressures cannot be preserved without a closed circuit ventilator.

Urinary Tract Infections

One of the major clinical indicators of adequate fluid resuscitation is urine output. In small burns, this can be monitored effectively through voluntary voiding; however, in larger injuries where replacement is titrated to the hourly output, an indwelling catheter is necessary. Particular attention should be paid to those patients who have perineal or penile burns as their risk for intra- or extraluminal ascending bacterial contamination is greater.[127] Periurethral and prostatic abscesses have been observed.

Careful aseptic technique should be used for the placement of the catheter to avoid bladder contamination and the gravity drainage system should be maintained to prevent reflux of urine into the bladder. Catheter care should be performed on a routine basis and the catheter changed on a weekly basis. Urine should be frequently examined for the presence of both red and white blood cells and urine cultures should be routinely collected on all catheterized patients. Bladder catheterization should be maintained only as long as necessary.

Sepsis

Every patient with a major burn has to be examined daily for signs of sepsis. The primary cause of death is sepsis arising from the wound, lung, or urine. Burn wound sepsis may be defined as more than 10^5 bacteria per gram of tissue with invasion of viable tissue on histologic section. Most wounds are normally colonized without any apparent sign of impaired wound healing. Indeed, there is some evidence to suggest that the presence of bacteria in a wound can aid healing by locally stimulating the host's immune system.

Burned patients develop a hypermetabolic state in which they exhibit an elevated basal metabolic rate with a true temperature reset such that their core temperature is 38.5C. Under these circumstances, the clinical diagnosis of wound infection can be difficult. Surveillance schemes using blood cultures, regular skin swabs, and clinical measurements are of limited value when used alone. However, in 1973, Pruitt et al[128] described the use of wound biopsy for diagnosing burn wound infection. With this now standardized technique, biopsied wound tissue is sent for microbiologic culture and histologic examination. A classification system consisting of both histologic and microbiologic features was established.

The clinical diagnosis of sepsis can be made when clinical symptoms appear and a septic source can be identified (Table 52–2). A septic source can be documented as (1) burn wound biopsy with greater than 10^5 organisms/g tissue and/or histologic evidence of viable tissue invasion, (2) positive blood culture, (3) urinary tract infection with greater than 10^5 organisms/ml urine, or (4) pulmonary infection with bacteria and white blood cells present in a class III or better sputum specimen. In addition to the identification of a septic source, at least three of the following criteria should be met: tachypnea (more than 40 breaths/min in adults), prolonged paralytic ileus, hyperthermia (less than 36.5C) or hypothermia (greater than 38.5C), altered mental status, thrombocytopenia (less than 50,000 platelets/mm^3), leukopenia (less than 3,000 cells/mm^3) or leukocytosis (greater than 20,000 cells/mm^3), unexplained acidosis, or hyperglycemia. Local evidence of invasive wound infection includes black or brown patches of wound discoloration, rapid eschar separation, conversion of wounds to full-thickness, spreading periwound erythema, punctate hemorrhagic subeschar lesions, and violaceous or black lesions in unburned tissue (ecthyma gangrenosum). When a patient exhibits signs and symptoms of sepsis, immediate institution of antibiotics is obligatory. A delay of 3 to 4 days in a patient with a major burn would result in an inordinately high morbidity. Specific treatment is only administered if routine surveillance has identified a predominant organism.

TABLE 52–2. DIAGNOSIS OF BURN SEPSIS

The presence of three of the criteria listed below establishes the diagnosis of sepsis, and appropriate interventions should be performed, despite the absence of bacterial culture confirmation.

- Burn wound infection (>10^5 organisms/g tissue) and histologic or clinical evidence of invasion
- Thrombocytopenia (<50,000/mm^3)
- Leukocytosis or leukopenia (>20,000 or <3000 cells/mm^3)
- Unexplained hypoxia, acidosis, or glucose shifts
- Prolonged paralytic ileus
- Hyperthermia (>39C) or hypothermia (<36.5C)
- Positive blood cultures
- Documented catheter or pulmonary infection
- Altered mental status
- Progressive renal or pulmonary dysfunction

Bacterial Endocarditis

Transient bacteremia is associated with burn wound manipulations[129–131] and many other procedures required by burn patients (eg, endotracheal intubation). The generalized immunosuppression associated with burns in previously healthy people plus the procedures they undergo increase the risk for endocarditis. Bacterial endocarditis occurs more commonly in burn patients as we become more capable of supporting the sequelae of major injuries. However, its development is usually occult and, like suppurative thrombophlebitis, may not be noted until there are persistent positive blood cultures.

The patients with the highest risk for the development of bacterial endocarditis are those with repetitive bacteremias. These patients should be monitored closely for the development of heart murmurs and, if found, should undergo echocardiography to determine the presence of vegetations. Serial blood cultures should be obtained over a 24 hour interval, then appropriate broad spectrum antibiotics initiated and continued for the next 6 weeks.

Suppurative Thrombophlebitis and Cannula Infections

Infectious complications associated with intravenous and intra-arterial catheters represent a major problem despite strict attention to aseptic technique for insertion and appropriate maintenance.[132] Burned patients appear to be particularly susceptible to this complication, with catheter infection rates reported ranging from 8 to 57 percent.[133,134] Suppurative thrombophlebitis may be confirmed in up to 5 percent of hospitalized patients with burns over 20 percent total body surface area (TBSA).[134]

A recent prospective study documented that contamination of indwelling catheter tips and hubs correlates with proximity of the insertion site to the burn wound.[135] Bacteria cultured from infected catheters can be traced to the skin in 96 percent of the cases.[136] Much data thus support the hypothesis that catheter infections primarily arise from burn wound contaminants migrating down the catheter to the tip. Strict aseptic technique for insertion of intravascular catheters, the use of Teflon catheters, and rotation of the catheter site, tubing, and apparatus every 72 hours have been associated with a decrease in the rate of catheter infections.[121,137–139]

Suppurative thrombophlebitis should be suspected in patients with persistently positive blood cultures in the absence of local infection. Suppuration may occur long after catheter removal so that cultures at the time of removal may be an unreliable predictor of infection. Gross clinical signs of suppurative thrombophlebitis are most often absent.[140] Careful records of previously cannulated sites may allow for sequential venotomy and examination for intraluminal pus and histologic examination for intimal colonization. Upon confirmation of the diagnosis, immediate operative excision is essential to prevent progressive sepsis. Excision of a vein in its entirety to the point of entry into the central circulation may be required because of the tendency of phlebitis to skip to vein valves, leaving apparently normal vein between infected foci. The subcutaneous tissue and skin should be packed open after a grossly purulent vein is removed and allowed to heal by secondary intention.

Suppurative Chondritis

Burns to the ear are a challenge to clinical management. Full-thickness injuries can injure the cartilage of the ear, resulting in autoamputation of a part or the entire external auricle. Because cartilage has no intrinsic blood supply, chondritis is common following partial- to full-thickness injury. Chondritis is usually seen 3 to 5 weeks following the injury but may be seen earlier and may occur following partial- and full-thickness injuries. Since the introduction of mafenide acetate for burn wound chemprophylaxis, it has become the topical agent of choice for burned cartilagenous surfaces and its use has significantly decreased the incidence of suppurative chondritis.

Characteristically, the patient will complain of dull pain in the ear. The ear becomes warm, red, edematous, and tender (Fig. 52–5). Appropriate antibiotics should be initiated immediately. Any overlying fluid collection should be incised and drained and culture and sensitivity measurements obtained. Should tenderness and induration persist, a more extensive debridement is necessary. Most commonly, the helix is bivalved at the posterior helical margin and all necrotic cartilage debrided with a curette. Difficulty may arise in differentiating between viable and necrotic cartilage and frequently normal cartilage is removed to ensure adequate debridement. However, infected cartilage is usually soft while normal cartilage will feel gritty on curettage. If all necrotic tissue is not removed and the infection controlled, suppurative chondritis can proceed to invade the mastoid bone and there is the potential for intracranial abscess formation.

Suppurative Sinusitis

Both long-term nasotracheal intubation and the use of nasogastric or nasoduodenal tubes for enteral feeding have increased the incidence of this problem. The diagnosis is frequently delayed because there are few local symptoms or signs to accompany the fever. The diagnosis can be confirmed by aspiration once radiologic studies are performed. Therapy is initiated with broad spectrum antibiotics, but surgical drainage of the involved sinuses may be necessary if the infection is unresponsive to antibiotic and decongestive therapy. Oral intubation and orogastric feeding may be necessary as temporary measures until the sinusitis resolves. Tracheostomy

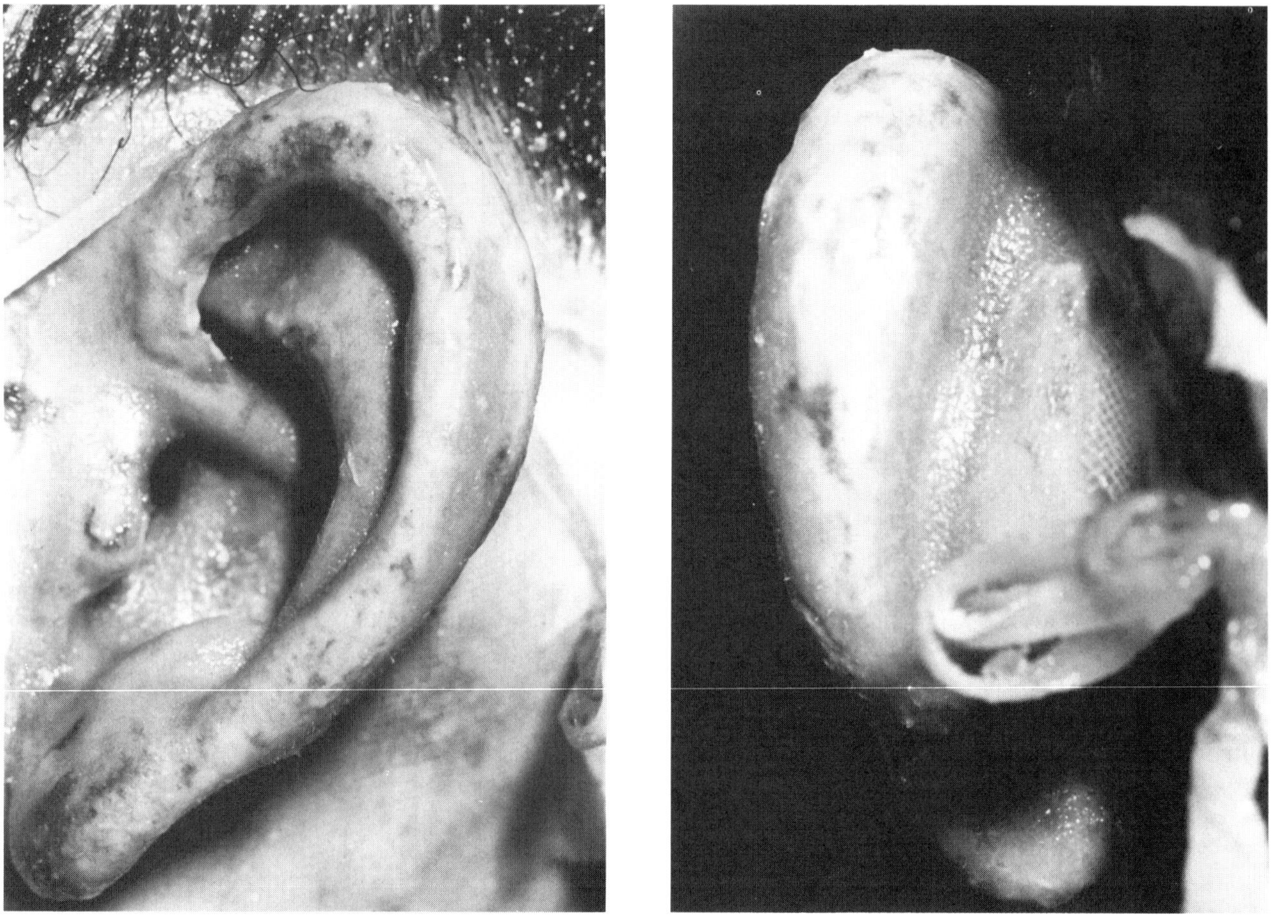

Figure 52–5. Despite the small burn area, the helix of the ear is susceptible to the development of chondritis due to the limited vascularity of cartilage. In addition, the progressive edema further decreases blood flow. The combined effects result in bacterial proliferation and a decreased effectiveness of systemic therapies.

and/or gastrostomy may be necessary if the sinusitis requires prolonged treatment.

PREVENTION AND TREATMENT OF BURN WOUND SEPSIS

Infection Control Practices

Control of burn wound infection is the cornerstone of infection control in any burn unit. Wound colonization progresses to infection only when the surface bacterial counts exceed some threshold value. Accurate quantification of the burned patient's bacterial load is therefore the cornerstone of infection surveillance. This is accomplished through routine cultures of sputum, urine, and wound. Quantitative cultures obtained on a routine basis allow the progress of bacterial colonization to be monitored, provides guidance should empiric antibiotic therapy become necessary, and encourages prompt surgical intervention for bacterial invasion. Cultures of sputum, urine, and the wound should be obtained three times weekly. We routinely biopsy any adherent eschar and use swab cultures for other open wounds.

Maintaining wounds at low contamination levels reduces the number and duration of septic episodes caused by wound flora. The wound should be cleansed two to three times per day by either shower or "tubbing." Some authorities immerse patients in a tub to remove debris and exudate that accumulates between dressing changes, but most no longer advocate tubbing because it may spread surface bacteria to all areas of the burn. We have chosen the shower technique to remove the debris. It is important to note that wound cleansing can be quite painful, and the associated blood loss with each cleansing may cumulatively be significant. The technique of early excision may obviate these disadvantages. An alternative for treatment of small second degree burn is biologic dressing. Biologic dressings have no direct toxins or antimicrobial properties. However, they create a wound environment that prevents desiccation; diminishes bacterial proliferation; reduces loss of heat, water, protein, and red blood cells; and promotes more rapid wound healing. Biologic dressings also reduce burn wound pain. Examples of synthetic covers include Biobrane, Op-site, and Omiderm.

Daily inspection of the wound is essential. Burn wound biopsies should be taken from any area of the wound that has changed in appearance. Bacterial invasion is often signaled by changes in the color, odor, or amount of excudate from the wound; fungal invasion is marked by the appearance or expansion of dark discolorations. Few histologically demonstrated fungal infections are confirmed by culture; therefore treatment should be initiated when invasive hyphae are seen on biopsy specimens.

There is a controversy over the best method to determine infections, with some burn centers using surface qualitative and quantitative cultures and others using contact plates. The area of greatest concern is the identification of the organism. We have found quantitative biopsies to be quite useful. Robson and Krizek[140] found that graft takes were greater than 90 percent when colony counts were less than 10^2/g, but were only 60 percent when colony counts were greater than 10^5/g. We have routinely altered our topical antimicrobial prophylaxis, alternating between silver sulfadiazine and mafenide acetate when colony counts are greater than 10^5. Mafenide is more successful at penetrating necrotic detritis than is silver sulfadiazine. This technique has been demonstrated to be successful in decreasing wound colony counts.

Quantitative wound biopsies are a better determinant of bacterial loads than qualitative swab or smear cultures. However, quantitative cultures showing high bacterial counts correlate with histologic evidence of burn wound infection in less than 50 percent of cases. Quantitative cultures should be accompanied by histologic examination. If quantitative biopsies reveal greater than 10^3 organisms/g of tissue, a change in topical therapy is indicated. If bacterial counts exceed 10^5 organisms/g of tissue, wound infection should be suspected and a histologic examination performed. If histologic evidence of invasion is present, systemic antibiotics should be instituted and the wound should be excised.

Additional measures can be taken to decrease burn wound colonization. The microorganisms populating the wounds of burned patients represent a mixture of endogenous resident flora and exogenous contaminants seeded by contact with the environment and attending personnel. Immunosuppressed burned patients should be protected from exposure to environmental contaminants. Even the most elaborate methods of isolation, however, have failed to effectively reduce the incidence of infection, although significantly reducing the incidence of cross-contamination.[141–144] The most effective means of reducing exposure of burned patients to exogenous bacteria is universal closely enforced handwashing by the care providers before and after every wound contact. Waterproof cover gowns and gloves should be worn whenever direct contact with body fluids and wound exudates are expected, protecting both the patient and the care provider from inadvertent contamination. Dressing materials should be maintained as patient specific. Intravenous pumps and poles, sphygmomanometers, monitoring equipment, bedside tables, and beds should be cleaned daily with bactericidal solutions. Terminal cleaning of the patient's room following discharge should include the walls, ceiling, baseboards, and floors. Mattresses should be covered with vinyl and frequently inspected for cracks in their surfaces. Air filters should be monitored frequently for bacterial and fungal growth.

Most burn units now house patients within individual, self-contained isolation rooms. However, common bathing or showering facilities exist even within these units. These areas should be scrupulously cleaned before and after every use with effective bactericidal agents, which must be chosen to be effective against those organisms most prominant in each individual unit. Disposable or single-use sterilizable instruments should be used for blunt debridements and the use of attendant-owned instruments discouraged.

Topical Antimicrobial Agents

Prophylactic topical agents provide control of colonizing organisms. Maintaining wounds at low contamination levels reduces the number and duration of septic episodes caused by wound flora,[145] which, in turn, reduces the caloric and fluid demands placed on the patient with each septic episode. The introduction of topical antimicrobial agents produced a significant reduction in burn mortality.[146] However, no single agent is totally effective against all organisms and each possesses its own advantages and disadvantages. Almost all currently used topical agents retard wound healing and their application increases the metabolic rate. Their effectiveness must be measured by their ability to inhibit bacterial growth in vitro and reduce wound colony counts in vivo. Studies have demonstrated that agents used in the past may not be effective in inhibiting bacterial growth in vitro.[147] Wounds in which the quantitative culture counts remain less than 10^2 organisms/g of tissue may remain dressed in the topical agent of choice. However, should colony counts increase beyond that point, a change in topical agent is indicated.

Silver Sulfadiazine. Silver sulfadiazine (Silvadene, Flamazine, SSD) is the most commonly used topical agent in burn treatment. It possesses a broad antimicrobial spectrum including gram-positive and gram-negative bacteria and some yeasts.[148] Its activity is related to its silver and sulfa moieties. Recently, some gram-negative organisms have developed a plasmid-related resistance. Silver sulfadiazine is painless and easy to apply. It can be used with or without cover dressings, although when exposed to sunlight it will take on a gray discoloration. SSD does not appear to inhibit epithelialization but does hamper fibroblast contraction. True allergic sensitivities are rare, although patients may develop a transient leukopenia secondary to margination of white blood cells.[149,150] Whether silver sulfadiazine is withheld or not, white blood cell counts usually return to normal within several days. Those few patients with true allergies will experience no return of white blood cell counts and the agent should be permanently discontinued. Silver sulfadiazine does not penetrate eschar well.

Mafenide Acetate. Mafenide acetate (Sulfamylon) is one of the oldest effective topical agents. Mafenide possesses a broad spectrum of antibacterial activity, including resistant *Pseudomonas* species, but limited antifungal properties. Mafenide acetate cream (11.2 percent) is toxic to fibroblasts and epithelial cells. Unlike other topical agents, it is able to penetrate full-thickness eschar and provide some protection to the underlying tissue. For this reason, mafenide is commonly used on heavily colonized or infected full-thickness wounds, electrical injuries, and burns to cartilagenous tissues such as ears. It is painful upon application to viable tissue, although the discomfort subsides in about 30 minutes. Mafenide has been noted to cause allergic skin reactions. Although bicarbonate washing can occur through carbonic anhydrase inhibition, severe metabolic acidosis typically occurs only in those patients with insufficient pulmonary reserve for respiratory compensation. Those patients with extensive burn injuries and a concomitant inhalation injury should be monitored closely for pulmonary compromise if mafenide acetate is to be used.

Mupirocin. Bactroban is derived from *Pseudomonas fluorescens* and has been reported to be more effective than silver sulfadiazine or mafenide acetate in its activity against gram-positive organisms infecting burn wounds.[151] However, it was effective against only 71 percent of gram-negative isolates, comparable to silver sulfadiazine, but significantly inferior to the 89 percent susceptibility to mafenide acetate. Of particular importance is its significantly inferior activity on all species of *P. aeruginosa* compared to both silver sulfadiazine and mafenide acetate. Mupirocin is painless and easy to apply. The data and the expense suggest that mupirocin should be used specifically for the treatment of gram-positive burn wound infections, rather than as a prophylactic topical agent.

Surgical Treatment

Although care of the burn wound is not the initial priority, subsequent survival depends on it. The avascular burn eschar is rapidly colonized within 5 days postburn despite the use of topical antimicrobial agents. If the bacterial density exceeds the immune defenses of the host, then invasive burn sepsis may ensue. When bacterial wound counts are greater than 10^5 microorganisms per gram of tissue, risk of wound infection is great, skin graft survival is poor, and wound closure is delayed.

The goals of local wound management are the prevention of desiccation of viable tissue and the control of bacteria. These are usually achieved by use of topical antimicrobial agents and/or biologic dressings. It is unrealistic to expect to keep a burn wound sterile. Bacterial counts less than 10^3 organisms/g are not usually invasive and allow skin graft survival rates of greater than 90 percent.[140]

Antimicrobial therapy is directed by bacterial surveillance through routine triweekly sputum, urine, and wound cultures. Quantitative wound biopsy is a better determinant of significant pathogens than qualitative surface swabs. Organism identification and in vivo sensitivities to antibiotics are obtained within 48 hours. Agar diffusion assays can also be performed to test susceptibilities to topical antimicrobials. The available topical agents maintain the bacterial density in the burn wound of most patients below the level of 10^5 organisms/g of tissue but do not sterilize the wound. Consequently, the bacteria in the burn wounds of any patient may escape control and invade the underlying tissue. If bacterial counts are greater than 10^5

organisms/g of tissue, wound infection should be suspected, and rapid histologic analysis and Gram stain should be performed to confirm this. Wound infection is confirmed by histologic evidence of tissue invasion or clinical sepsis.

The concept of burn wound sepsis was initially established by Teplitz and colleagues[145] based on autopsy material. The definition evolved so that burn wound sepsis is now considered to be present when the wound is the site of bacteria that are actively invading subjacent unburned tissue. The importance of burn wound sepsis as a complication of burn injury is exemplified in a series of 100 autopsies performed at one burn unit wherein sepsis was confirmed in 76 percent of the patients and the source of the sepsis was the burn wound in 74 percent.[152] To treat burn wound sepsis, systemic antibiotics must be instituted and the wound excised. Parks et al[153] found that tangential or fascial excision of sites of burn wound sepsis in 22 burned children resulted in only a 14 percent mortality rate. Children surviving the septic episodes showed a marked improvement in the clinical course shortly after undergoing therapeutic surgical excision. Since initiation of surgical intervention in burn wound sepsis, the overall mortality in pediatric burn patients has decreased from 11.2 to 2.8 percent.[153]

Early excision as proposed by Burke et al[154] and Alexander et al[155] is extremely attractive in that early elimination of the burn eschar may decrease toxin production and reduce septic episodes, with an improved patient prognosis. In experimental models, complete excision of the wound with 24 hours of injury prevented hypermetabolism and immune suppression in the postburn period.[156] In children with greater than 60 percent BSA burns, excisional therapy has resulted in improved survival.[157]

First described by Janzekovic[158] 20 years ago, tangential excision involves sequential removal of eschar in layers with a dermatome or guarded knife (Goulian or Weck) until viable dermis or subcutaneous fat is reached. An acceptable wound bed is identified by active punctate bleeding. By using this technique, a maximum of viable tissue is preserved and optimal functional and cosmetic results are achieved. By contrast, fascial excision removes all layers of eschar plus the underlying tissue to the level of fascia. Excision to this plane minimizes bleeding and provides a reliable, clean, vascular bed. Fascial excision is recommended if the subcutaneous fat is burned and in selected patients with greater than 60 percent BSA full-thickness who are at high risk for infection, blood loss, or skin graft slough. Fascial excision results in considerable cosmetic deformity and therefore is not used except in the worst burns.

It is also important to examine the graft site daily after the third postoperative day for ghosting. The term *ghosting* is applied to the disappearance or thinning of graft after it initially appears well taken. This process is due to localized infection at the graft site and will result in the eventual loss of the graft. The usual bacteria responsible are *Staphylococcus, Streptococcus,* and gram-negative organisms like *Proteus* and *Pseudomonas.* If the phenomenon is detected early, the graft may be saved with aggressive topical therapy, alternating silver sulfadiazine with mupirocin two or three times per day.

Nutrition

Not until 20 years ago was the importance of nutrition in burn injury appreciated by burn surgeons. The physiologic response to burn is characterized by a greatly increased metabolic rate, thermogenic futile substrate cycling, catabolism with negative nitrogen balance, and increased lipolysis with central fat redistribution.[159–161] This hypermetabolic response may be quite prolonged.[160] Substantial catabolism results in loss of body weight and lean muscle mass, delayed wound healing, immunologic compromise, and increased morbidity and mortality.[162,163] These effects are mediated, at least in part, by large increases in the counter-regulatory or stress hormones, catecholamines, glucagon, and cortisol,[160,164–166] and the inflammatory cytokines (see Chap. 16). Growth hormone levels are decreased during the same period.[167] Most important, the magnitude of protein loss is closely correlated with clinical outcome.[168] In a prospective, randomized study to determine the effects of increasing the amount of protein in the diet, patients receiving a high-protein diet had significantly higher levels of total serum protein, transferrin, C3, and IgG and also had an improved opsonic index.[169] There was a significant reduction in mortality (0 versus 44 percent) and a significant reduction in infection as reflected by fewer days of bacteremia and antibiotic therapy. Supportive findings, found by other investigators, demonstrated that early enteral feeding successfully prevented the postburn hypermetabolism and catabolism.[170,171]

To counter this catabolic response, human growth hormone and high-caloric nutritional supplementation have been administered to patients with severe burns.[172] The effect of this treatment on massively burned children is dramatic. This regimen not only significantly accelerates skin graft donor site wound healing but also results in attenuation of urinary nitrogen loss, hence sparing protein and lean body mass.[173,174] Jiang et al[175] further demonstrated that human growth hormone blunted protein catabolism following major intra-abdominal operations, as indicated by significantly less loss of body weight and urinary nitrogen in rhGH-treated patients than in placebo-treated patients, despite inadequate nutritional intake.

In burned patients, caloric support is best provided with enteral feedings. We recommend beginning nasogastric or nasoduodenal tube feedings within 6 hours following injury and slowly increase volumes to meet caloric requirements. Gastric residual volumes are checked hourly then returned. Rates of enteral infusion are gradually increased as tolerated and intravenous infusion is reduced to keep total fluid intake rate constant. By 48 hours, most fluid requirements may be delivered enterally. Despite postburn gastric hypomotility, postburn intestinal ileus rarely occurs. Early enteral feeding sustains intestinal mucosa, maintains caloric support in the resuscitation period, and may reduce the degree of the hypermetabolic stress response.[170,171] In addition, continuous or small bolus feedings into the stomach may be sufficient to raise gastric pH and reduce risk for stress ulcers (Curling's ulcer), which were formerly the most frequent life-threatening gastrointestinal complication of burn patients.[176] Many scientists and clinicians interested in the pathophysiology of the multiple system organ failure syndrome seen in critically ill patients, including burned patients, believe that the gut is a source of toxic mediators after a period of ischemia or sepsis. Impaired perfusion, as experienced in trauma and burn, may jeopardize the integrity of the mucosal barrier and increase the incidence of bacterial translocation and endotoxin absorption from the gut.[40–42] The superior mesenteric artery syndrome has been identified in burns as associated with intestinal ischemia and sepsis.[177] The treatment for this syndrome is bowel rest with nasogastric suction and intravenous antibiotics.

The precise energy requirements needed to reach weight and nitrogen balance and energy equilibrium have been calculated by Curreri et al[178] based on linear regression analysis of weight change versus predicted dietary intake. The Curreri formula, which is the most popular estimation method, calculates caloric requirements of 25 kcal/kg/day plus 40 kcal/kg/%BSA burned/day in a burned adult. For children, formulas based on body surface area rather than weight may be more appropriate. Our recommendation for caloric replacement in burned children is 1500 kcal/mBSA (total)/day for maintenance plus 1500 kcal/mBSA burn/day for burn losses.[179]

The composition of the nutritional supplement is also important. Caloric replacement should be based on nonprotein calories only. At least 30 percent of the calories should be supplied as fat. In adults, protein requirements are 100 to 150 g/day, or about 1 to 2 g/kg/day. In general, protein should be provided to achieve a calorie/nitrogen ratio of 100:1, which results in better immune function and survival in experimental and clinical burn trials than a ratio of 150:1.[169] For a balanced daily diet, administration of vitamins C, A, and E, zinc, iron, folate, and trace minerals are essential.

Parenteral nutrition should be avoided in burned patients if possible. Despite delivery of more calories, the use of parenteral nutrition results in greater immune suppression and reduced survival in burn patients during clinical trials.[180] Not only is there the additional complication of placement of a central venous catheter and inherent risk of catheter sepsis, but total parenteral nutrition (TPN) is associated with intestinal mucosal atrophy[181] with more depressed immune function and increased mortality, as well as contributing to a more permeable barrier to the bacterial translocation.[181] Enteral feeding is the preferred route of nutritional support in the burn patient and can be safely used even through the perioperative period.

Antibiotics

There are three major phases of burn care during which the choice of systemic antibiotics is of concern: prophylactic, perioperative, and therapeutic. Prophylactic penicillin is frequently administered soon after burning to circumvent the emergence of *Streptococcus pyogenes* and other beta-hemolytic streptococci responsible for early cellulitis, graft loss, and other sequelae related to such infections. However, some authorities no longer advocate its use because it does not decrease the overall rate of cellulitis resulting from a streptococcal infection.

When burns are over 40 percent TBSA and are to be excised, we suggest they be treated perioperatively with amikacin and vancomycin for 48 hours until quantitative biopsies are available. Alternatively, if quantitative biopsies have already been obtained and the agent of infection and its susceptibility pattern are known, more specific therapy can be chosen. Although antibiotic therapy for a localized granulating wound may be questionable, it is important to prevent systemic spread during wound manipulation. There is no question, however, that antibiotic coverage is essential when large burn wounds over 50 percent TBSA are debrided. Sasaki and his colleagues[129] showed that tangential excision induced bacteremia in approximately 50 percent of patients. A larger initial burn size was associated with a higher incidence of bacteremia. Patients with positive blood cultures had a 46.6 percent TBSA injury versus 25.5 percent TBSA injury for those with negative blood cultures.

Our antibiotic regimens currently vary between vancomycin and amikacin, pipercillin and ticarcillin/clavulanate, amoxicillin/clavulanate, and ticarcillin/clavulanate. Vancomycin is used because 80 percent of our *Staphylococcus* is MRSA. Ticarcillin/clavulanate is a valuable adjunct in that it contains clavulanic acid, which inhibits beta-lactamase, prevents plasmid exchange, and discourages the development of resistance. Routinely administered antibiotic regimens are alternated every 3 months, depending on the changes in predominant organisms. When an agent has developed a degree of resistance, its use is curtailed for approximately 6 months, during which time the original susceptibility patterns usually return. The overall fear is that a multiply resistant organism will appear and predominate. We have, in the past, seen gram-negative bacteria resistant to all known antibiotics on routine sensitivity testing. It is obligatory when such organisms are found that synergy tests be performed. Imipenem, amoxicillin/clavulanate, and ticarcillin/clavulanate in combination have been able to suitably control the microbe. Indiscriminate use of antibiotics will, of course, produce an intolerable situation. We have yet to see MRSA resistant to vancomycin, but it is certainly only a matter of time until this occurs.

Therapeutically, systemic antimicrobial agents are usually reserved for patients with evidence of systemic infection. Administration should be continued for 72 hours following the resolution of systemic signs after a minimum of 10 days. Recent data indicated that there is an increasing frequency of bacterial endocarditis and valvular vegetations diagnosed in burn patients.[182] It appears that the multiple bacteremic episodes are inadequately treated and/or diagnosed in such patients. Frequently, specific data concerning the infecting site are unavailable and systemic antibiotics must be empirically administered. Differentiating between gram-negative and gram-positive infections is difficult despite many attempts (Table 52–3). If differentiation is impossible, the safest approach is to select an initial antibiotic therapy that is effective against all the likely pathogens that could be responsible for the septic state. Broad spectrum antibiotic coverage should be the rule, given in combination to cover gram-positive, gram-negative, and anaerobic organisms. A systematic search should be made to ascertain the source of the infecting organisms including culture and/or Gram stains of blood, urine, sputum, cutaneous wounds, and all indwelling catheters. The antibiotics selected should be administered intravenously to prevent the further spread of the infection and should possess a rapid onset of action. It is critical that drug levels are brought into therapeutic range as quickly as possible. To that end, some agents require a loading dose that compensates for the initially skewed distribution of the drug.

It may be tempting to use one of the newer, broad spectrum antibiotics for the initial treatment of the patient. Most serious infections, however, are polymicrobial and no single agent will adequately address all the likely pathogens. Additionally, many antibiotics work synergistically when given in combination, increasing their efficacy. Combined antibiotic therapy may be advantageous in that by varying the dosing pattern so that the peak of one antibiotic's action occurs in the trough of the other, a more sustained level of antibacterial activity may be achieved. It has also been noted that the hypermetabolism in burn patients is associated with an

TABLE 52–3. DIFFERENTIATION OF INFECTIONS

Sign	Gram-Positive	Gram-Negative
Onset	Insidious, 2–6 days	Sudden, 12–36 hours
Temperature	Persistent hyperthermia	Elevation, then hypothermia
Blood pressure	Gradual hypotension	Precipitous fall
Urine output	Gradual oliguria	Sudden anuria
WBC count	Sudden elevation	Sudden elevation, then leukopenia
Sensorium	Confusion	Clouded, obtunded
GI symptoms	Severe	Severe
Serum glucose	>130 mg/dl	<110 mg/dl
Wound	Macerated, exudate	Focal lesions

Adapted from Polk CH Jr, Stone HH: Pseudomonas and other gram-negative bacteria. In Artz C, Moncrief W, Pruitt BA Jr (eds): Burns: A Team Approach. Saunders, Philadelphia, 1979, p 304.

increase in clearance of the antimicrobial.[183] In most cases, this is relatively insignificant. However, in the case of aminoglycosides, a higher dose is required to maintain a therapeutic drug level in the plasma. This results in the accumulation of drug in the perilymph and vestibular and cochlear tissues, damaging them. Hall et al[184] reported a 13 percent incidence of auditory deficit on long-term follow-up of burned children. One method to reduce this potential ototoxicity of aminoglycosides is to use a three-level technique (instead of peak/trough technique) so that the disappearance curve of the drug can be generated to better monitor the dose.

Antifungal Therapy

Prompt diagnosis and treatment are essential for a successful outcome. Before amphotericin B, untreated invasive *Candida* wound infection and sepsis resulted in very high mortality. With aggressive medical and surgical therapies, this mortality has been modestly reduced.[185] Even though the prophylactic treatment with oral nystatin and the combination of nystatin with topical antimicrobials (polysporin and silver sulfadiazine 1:1) have significantly decreased the frequency of candidal superinfections in our patients, it will continue to appear as long as the widespread use of broad spectrum antibiotics and immunosuppression associated with burns persist.[78] If prophylaxis is ineffective in preventing extension of this usually superficial infection, excision should be carried out and amphotericin B administered systemically. Amphotericin B treatment, when it is indicated, requires a dose of 0.5 mg/kg/day for a total treatment dose of 1 g intravenously.

Treatment of the most aggressive true fungi such as *Aspergillus* and *Phycomycetes* requires both amphotericin B systemic administration and wide surgical excision of the infected tissue. Itraconazole has recently become available for the systemic treatment of *Aspergillus*. When the infection on a limb has traversed the investing fascia and involves significant amount of underlying muscle or blood invasion under histologic examination, amputation may be necessary to control the infectious process.

CONCLUSION

Infection is the most common and most serious complication of a major burn injury. Sepsis accounts for 50 to 60 percent of deaths in burn patients today despite improvements in antimicrobial therapies. Sepsis in burns is commonly due to bronchopneumonia, pyelonephritis, thrombophlebitis, or invasive wound infection. Infection is promoted by loss of the epithelial barrier, by malnutrition induced by the hypermetabolic response to burn injury, and by a generalized postburn immunosuppression due to release of immunoactive agents from the burn wound. Understanding the pathophysiology of infections in burns is essential, not only in the treatment but also in prevention and prompt response when infection occurs. Besides the improved infection control practices, the most important factor introduced in recent years to alter the biologic balance between host resistance and microorganism infection has been the use of topical and systemic antimicrobial agents. The administration of an antimicrobial agent at the proper time and in sufficient quantity to be therapeutically active should, theoretically, be uniformly effective in preventing or treating infections of susceptible organisms. However, the ready availability and wide usage of antibiotics have neither eliminated burn infection as a threat to the patients nor even reduced the incidence of such infection in most cases. In addition, there is evidence that the widespread, and often indiscriminate, use of these agents may be responsible for the changing pattern of bacteria implicated in nosocomial infections and for the emergence of pathogenicity in certain bacterial species. A continual surveillance of the invading microbial population and its susceptibility should provide the advantage necessary to prevent morbidity and mortality from sepsis. With constant monitoring and alternating the prophylactic, perioperative, and therapeutic systemic antibiotic approaches, appropriate topical antimicrobials are essential to a good infection-control program in a burn center.

Augmentation of the patient's local and general ability to resist microbial invasion through appropriate resuscitative therapies, particularly nutritional therapies, and immunologic procedures to enhance host resistance may potentially make a difference in the incidence of burn infections and the outcome of these patients. As advances in growth factors continue, this would appear to make an important impact in reversing the severe protein catabolism and immunosuppression of burns and also in speeding up total body wound healing. Antibiotic regimens, when indicated, should be used with therapeutic precision and a recognition of their limitations. The burn wound, as well as the patient as a whole, must be monitored closely using wound biopsies, blood and other body fluid cultures, and operative intervention to prevent, diagnose, and treat infection in a timely manner. Early burn wound excision and excision of wound infection remain the definitive treatments for the prevention of wound sepsis.

REFERENCES

1. Benheir P, Sagi A, Greber B, et al: An analysis of mortality in patients with burns covering 40 percent BSA or more: a retrospective review covering 24 years (1964–88). Burns 17(5):402, 1991.
2. Curreri PW, Luterman A, Braun D, et al: Burn injury: analysis of survival and hospitalization time for 937 patients. Ann Surg 192(4):472, 1980.
3. Dasco C, Luterman A, Curreri PW: Systemic antibiotic treatment in burned patients. Surg Clin North Am 67(1):47, 1987.
4. Moran K, Munster A: Alterations of the host defense mechanism in burned patients. Surg Clin North Am 67(1):47, 1987.
5. Pruitt BA: Infection: cause or effect of pathophysiologic change in burn and trauma patients. In Paubert-Braquet M (ed): Lipid Mediators in the Immunology of Shock. New York, Plenum Press, 1987, pp 31–42.
6. Heggers JP, McCauley RL, Herndon DN: Antimicrobial therapy in burn patient. Part 1. Surg Rounds 15(7):613, 1992.
7. Burdge JJ, Rea F, Ayers L: Noncandidal fungal infections of the burn wound. J Burn Care Rehabil 9(6):599, 1988.
8. Pruitt BA Jr, McManus AT: The changing epidemiology in burn patients. World J Surg 16(1):57, 1992.
9. Shirani KZ, Pruitt BA Jr, Mason AD Jr: The influence of inhalation injury and pneumonia on burn mortality. Ann Surg 205(1):82, 1987.
10. Becker WK, Cioffi WG Jr, McManus AT, et al: Fungal burn wound infection. A 10 year experience. Arch Surg 126(1):44, 1991.
11. Pensler JM, Herndon DN, Ptak H, et al: Fungal sepsis: an increasing problem in major thermal injuries. J Burn Care Rehabil 7(6):488, 1986.
12. Pruitt BA Jr: The burn patient. I. Initial care. Curr Probl Surg 16:8, 1979.
13. Rabin ER, Graber CD, Vogel EH, et al: Fatal *Pseudomonas* infection in burned patients: a clinical, bacteriologic and anatomic study. N Engl J Med 265(25):1225, 1961.
14. Pruitt BA Jr, Lindberg RB, McManus WF, Mason AD Jr: Current approach to prevention and treatment of *Pseudomonas aeruginosa* infections in burned patients. Rev Infect Dis 5(S5):S889, 1983.

Skin

15. Connolly WB, Hunt TK, Dunphy JE: Management of contaminated surgical wounds. Surg Gynecol Obstet 129(3):593, 1969.
16. Heggers JP, Robson MC, London MC: Prevention of microabscess formation following thermal injury. J Am Technol 22:215, 1982.
17. Jackson D: The diagnosis of the depth of burning. Br J Surg 40:588, 1953.
18. Edlich RF, Rodeheaver GT, Thacker JG, Edgerton NT: Technical factors in wound management. In Dunphy JE, Hunt TK (eds): Fundamentals of Wound Management in Surgery. South Plainfield, NJ, Chirurgeocom, 1977, pp 1–80.
19. Howe CW: Experimental studies on determinants of wound infection. Surg 60(5):1072, 1966.
20. Robson MC: The equilibrium between bacteria and host. In Heggers JP, Robson MC (eds): Quantitative Bacteriology: Its Role in the Armamentarium of the Surgeon. Boca Raton, FL, CRC Press, 1991, pp 1–8.
21. Holder IA, Neely A: Hageman factor dependent kinin activation in burns and its theoretical relationship to postburn immunosuppression syndrome and infection. J Burn Care Rehabil 11:496, 1990.
22. Holder IA, Neely A: The role of proteases in *Pseudomonas* infections in burn patients: a current hypothesis. Antibiot Chemother 4:99, 1991.
23. Fearon DD, Ruddy S, Schur P, McCabe WR: Activation of the properdin pathway of complement in patients with gram negative bacteremia. N Engl J Med 292(18):937, 1975.
24. Barbour A, Alfred C, Solber C, et al: Chemiluminescence by polymorphonuclear leukocytes from patients with active bacterial infection. J Infect Dis 141(1):14, 1980.
25. Phillips LG, Heggers JP, Robson MC: Burn and trauma units as sources of methicillin resistant *Staphylococcus aureus*. J Burn Care Rehabil 2(2):293, 1987.

Gut

26. Hilton JG, Marullo DS: Trauma induced increase in plasma vasopressin and angiotensin II. Life Sci 41:2195, 1987.
27. Desai MH, Herndon DN, Rutan RL, et al: Ischemic intestinal complications in patients with burns. Surg Gynecol Obstet 172:257, 1991.
28. Manson WL, Dijkema H, Klasen HJ: Alteration of wound colonization by selective intestinal decontamination in thermally injured mice. Burns 16(3):166, 1990.
29. Hildebrand GJ, Wolochow H: Translocation of bacteriophage across the intestinal wall of the rat. Proc Soc Exp Biol Med 109:183, 1962.
30. Fuller R, Jayne-Williams DJ: Resistance of the fowl (*Gallus domesticus*) to invasion by its intestinal flora. II. Clearance of translocated intestinal bacteria. Res Vet Sci 11:368, 1970.
31. Berg RD, Garlington AW: Translocation of certain indigenous bacteria from the gastrointestinal tract to the mesenteric lymph nodes and other organs in a gnotobiotic mouse model. Infect Immun 23:403, 1979.
32. Maejima K, Deitch EA, Berg RA: Promotion by burn stress of the translocation of bacteria from the gastrointestinal tracts of mice. Arch Surg 119:166, 1984.

33. Redan JA, Rush BF, McCullough JN, et al: Organ distribution of radio-labelled enteric *Escherichia coli* during and after hemorrhagic shock. Ann Surg 211:663, 1990.
34. Deitch EA, Ma WJ, Ma L, et al: Protein malnutrition predisposes to inflammatory-induced gut origin septic states. Ann Surg 211:560, 1990.
35. Berg RD, Wommack E, Deitch EA: Immunosuppression and intestinal bacterial overgrowth synergistically prompts bacterial translocation. Arch Surg 123:1359, 1988.
36. Steffen EK, Berg RD: Relationship between cecal population levels of indigenous bacteria and translocation to the mesenteric lymph node. Infect Immunol 39(3):1252, 1983.
37. Deitch EA, Bridges RM: Effect of stress and trauma on bacterial translocation from the gut. J Surg Res 42:536, 1987.
38. Guzman-Stein G, Bonsack M, Liberty, J, et al: Abdominal radiation causes bacterial translocation. J Surg Res 46:104, 1989.
39. Tancrede CH, Andremont AO: Bacterial translocation and gram-negative bacteremia in patients with hematological malignancies. J Infect Dis 2:99, 1985.
40. Morris SE, Navaratnam N, Townsend CM, Herndon DN: Decreased mesenteric blood flow independently promotes bacterial translocation in chronically instrumented sheep. Surg Forum 40:88, 1989.
41. Rush BF Jr, Sori AJ, Murphy MS, et al: Endotoxemia and bacteremia during hemorrhagic shock: the link between trauma and sepsis. Ann Surg 207(5):549, 1988.
42. Morris SE, Navaratnam N, Townsend CM, et al: Bacterial translocation and mesenteric blood flow in a large animal model after cutaneous thermal and inhalation injury. Surg Forum 39:189, 1988.
43. Morris SE, Navaratnam N, Herndon DN: A comparison of effects of thermal injury and smoke inhalation on bacterial translocation. J Trauma 30:639, 1990.
44. Navaratnam N, Morris SE, Townsend CM, et al: Bacterial translocation and selective mesenteric artery perfusion in an ovine model. Proc Am Burn Assoc 21:240, 1989.
45. Saydjari R, Herndon DN, Beerthuizen GIMJ, et al: Bacterial translocation and its relationship to visceral blood flow, gut mucosal ornithine decarboxylase activity and DNA in pigs. J Trauma 31(5):639, 1991.
46. Coffey JA, Milhoan RA, Abdullah A, et al: Bombesin inhibits bacterial translocation from the gut in burned rats. Surg Forum 39:109, 1988.
47. O'Brien R, Murdoch J, Kuehn R, Marshall JC: The effect of albumin or crystalloid resuscitation on bacterial translocation and endotoxin absorption following experimental burn injury. J Surg Res 191(2):171, 1992.
48. Tokyay R, Zeigler ST, Heggers JP, et al: Effects of anesthesia, surgery, fluid resuscitation and endotoxin administration on postburn bacterial translocation. J Trauma 31(10):1375, 1991.
49. Sittig K, Deitch EA: Effect of bacteremia on mortality after thermal injury. Arch Surg 123(11):1367, 1988.

Lungs

50. Pruitt BA Jr, DiVincenti FC, Mason AD Jr, et al: The occurrence and significance of pneumonia and other pulmonary complications in burned patients: comparison of conventional and topical treatments. J Trauma 10(7):519, 1970.
51. Hillman KF, Riordan T, O'Farrell SM, et al: Colonization of the gastric contents in critically ill patients. Crit Care Med 10:44, 1982.
52. du Moulin GF, Hedley White J, Paterson DG, et al: Aspiration of bacteria in antacid treated patients: a frequent cause of postoperative colonization of the airway. Lancet 1:242, 1982.
53. Kramer GC, Herndon DN, Linares HA, et al: Effects of inhalation injury on airway bloodflow and edema formation. J Burn Care Rehabil 10(1):45, 1989.
54. Maguire JP, Traber LD, Sugi K, et al: Bronchial blood flow in response to inhalation injury. Am Rev Respir Dis 137(4):194, 1988.
55. Green GM, Jakab GJ, Low RD, et al: Defense mechanisms of the respiratory membrane. Am Rev Respir Dis 115:479, 1977.
56. Wanner A: Clinical aspects of mucociliary transport. Am Rev Respir Dis 116:73, 1977.
57. Zikria BA, Ferrer JM: The chemical factors contributing to the pulmonary damage of "smoke poisoning." Surgery 71:704, 1972.
58. Kimura R, Traber DL, Herndon DN, et al: Ibuprofen reduces the lung lymph flow changes associated with inhalation injury. Circ Shock 24:183, 1988.
59. Shinozawa Y, Hales CA, Jung W, et al: Ibuprofen prevents synthetic smoke induced pulmonary edema. Am Rev Respir Dis 134:1145, 1986.
60. Garzon AA, Seltzer B, Song IC, et al: Respiratory mechanics in patients with inhalation burns. J Trauma 20:57, 1970.
61. Head JM: Inhalation injury in burns. Am J Surg 139:508, 1980.
62. Nieman GF, Clarke WR Jr, Wax SD, et al: The effect of smoke inhalation on pulmonary surfactant. Ann Surg 191(2):171, 1980.
63. Basadre JO, Sugi K, Traber DL, et al: The effect of leukocyte depletion on smoke inhalation injury in sheep. Surgery 104:208, 1988.
64. Weissman G, Smolen JE, Hoffstein S: Polymorphonuclear leukocytes as secretory organs in inflammation. J Invest Dermatol 71:95, 1978.
65. Brown M, Desai MH, Traber LD, et al: Dimethylsulfoxide with heparin in the treatment of smoke inhalation injury. J Burn Care Rehabil 9(1):22, 1988.
66. Till GO, Johnson KJ, Kunkel R, Ward PA: Intravascular activation of complement and acute lung injury. J Clin Invest 69:1126, 1982.

67. Pruitt BA Jr, McManus AT, Kim SH: In Gorbach SL, Barlett JG, Blacklow NR (eds): Infectious Diseases. Philadelphia, Saunders, 1992, p 779.

Bacteria

68. Altemeier WA, MacMillan BG: The dynamics of infection of burns. In Artz CP (ed): Research in Burns. Philadelphia, Davis, 1962, pp 203–211.
69. Stone HH: Control of infection in major burns with special emphasis on *Pseudomonas* infections. J Pediatr Surg 3:3, 1968.
70. McManus WF, Goodwin CW, Mason AD Jr, Pruitt BA Jr: Burn wound infection. J Trauma 21(9):753, 1981.
71. Brook I, Randolph JG: Aerobic and anaerobic bacterial flora of burns in children. J Trauma 21:3133, 1981.
72. Hartford CE, Ziffren SE: Electrical injury. J Trauma 11:331, 1971.
73. Gorbach SL, Thadepalli H: Isolation of *Clostridium* in human infections: evaluation of 114 cases. J Infect Dis 131(Suppl):S81, 1975.
74. Davies DM: Gas gangrene as a complication of burns. Scand J Plast Reconstr Surg 12:73,1979.
75. Sherman RT: The prevention and treatment of tetanus in the burn patient. Surg Clin North Am 50:1277, 1970.
76. Larkin JM, Moylan JA: Tetanus following a minor burn. J Trauma 15:546, 1975.

Fungi

77. Bruck HM, Nash G, Foley FD, et al: Opportunistic fungal infection of the burn wound with *Phycomycetes* and *Aspergillus*. Arch Surg 102:476, 1971.
78. Desai MH, Herndon DN, Abston S: *Candida* infection in massively burned patients. J Trauma 27(10):1186, 1987.
79. Nash G, Foley FD, Goodwin MN Jr, et al: Fungal burn wound infection. JAMA 215:1664, 1971.
80. Spebar MJ, Pruitt BA Jr: Candidiasis in the burned patient. J Trauma 21(3):237, 1981.
81. Spebar MJ, Lindberg RB: Fungal infection of the burn wound. Am J Surg 138:879, 1979.
82. Burdge JJ, Rea F, Ayers L: Noncandidal, fungal infections of the burn wound. J Burn Care Rehabil 9(6):599, 1988.
83. Pruitt BA Jr: Phycomycotic infections. Probl Gen Surg 1:664, 1984.
84. Neame P, Rayner D: Mucormycosis: a report of 22 cases. Arch Pathol 70:261, 1960.
85. Kobayashi K, Mukae N, Matsunaga Y, Motchi M: Diagnostic value of serum antibody to *Candida* in an extensively burned patient. Burns 16(6):414, 1990.
86. Goldstein E, Hoeprich PD: Problems in the diagnosis and treatment of systemic conditions. J Infect Dis 125:190, 1980.
87. Kidson A, Lowbury EJL: *Candida* infection of burns. Burns 6:228, 1980.
88. Solomkin JS, Simmons RL: *Candida* infection in surgical patients. World J Surg 4:381, 1980.
89. Prasad JK, Feller IF, Thomson PD: A ten year review of *Candida* sepsis and mortality in burn patients. Surgery 101:213, 1987.
90. Mead JH, Lupton GP, Dillavou CL, et al: Cutaneous *Rhizopus* infection. JAMA 242:272, 1979.
91. Del Pelacio Hernandez A: Nosocomial infection by *Rhizomucor pusillus* in a clinical haematology unit. J Hosp Infect 4(1):45, 1983.
92. Gartenberg G, Bottone EJ, Keusch FT, et al: Hospital acquired mucormycosis (*Rhizopus rhizopodoformis*) of skin and subcutaneous tissue: epidemiology, mycology and treatment. N Engl J Med 299:1115, 1978.

Viruses

93. Linneman CC Jr, MacMillan BC: Viral infections in pediatric burn patients. Am J Dis Child 135:750, 1983.
94. Deepe GS Jr, MacMillan BC, Linnemann CC Jr: Unexplained fever in burned patients due to cytomegalovirus infection. JAMA 248:2299, 1982.
95. Goodwin CW, McManus WF: Viral infections in burned patients. Immunology 12:3, 8, 1985.
96. Edgar P, Kravitz M, Heggers JP, et al: Herpes simplex in pediatric burn patients. Proc Am Burn Assoc 22:56, 1990.
97. Weintraub WH, Lilly AB, Randolph JG: A chickenpox epidemic in a pediatric burn unit. Surgery 76:490, 1974.

Immunosuppression

98. Burleson DG, Mason AD Jr, Pruitt BA Jr: Lymphoid subpopulation changes after thermal injury and thermal injury with infection in an experimental model. Ann Surg 207(2):208, 1988.
99. Hansbrough JF, Gadd MA: Temporal analysis of murine lymphocyte subpopulations by monoclonal antibodies and dual color flow cytometry after burn and non-burn injury. Surgery 106(1):69, 1989.
100. Bjerknes R, Bindenes H, Laerum OP: Altered neutrophil functions in patients with large burns. Blood Cells 17(5):402, 1990.
101. Hasslen SR, Nelson RD, Kishimoto TK, et al: Down regulation of homing receptors: a mechanism for impaired recruitment of human phagocytes in sepsis. J Trauma 31(5):645, 1991.
102. Ogle JD, Noel JG, Sramkoski RM, et al: Effect of antibiotics on CR1 receptor levels on human neutrophils and on the binding and phagocytosis of opsonized polystyrene microspheres by these leukocytes. Burns 15(3):141, 1989.
103. Dunn SM, Hillam AJ, Stomski F, et al: Leukocyte adhesion molecules involved in inflammation. Transplant Proc 21(1):31, 1989.
104. Mileski W, Borgstrom D, Lightfoot E, et al: Inhibition of leukocyte endothelial adhesion following thermal injury. J Surg Res 52:334, 1992.

105. Warden GD, Mason AD Jr, Pruitt BA Jr: Evaluation of leukocyte chemotaxis in vitro in thermally injured patients. J Clin Invest 54(5):1001, 1974.
106. Warden GD, Mason AD Jr, Pruitt BA Jr: Suppression of leukocyte chemotaxis in vitro by chemotherapeutic agents used in the management of thermal injuries. Ann Surg 181(3):363, 1975.
107. Altman LC, Klebanoff SJ, Curreri PW: Abnormalities of monocyte chemotaxis following thermal injury. J Surg Res 22(6):616, 1977.
108. Fikrig SM, Karl SC, Suntharalingam K: Neutrophil chemotaxis in patients with burns. Ann Surg 186(6):746, 1977.
109. Majeski JA, McClellan MA, Alexander JW: Evaluation of leukocyte chemotactic response in the presence of antibiotics. Surg Forum 26:83, 1975.
110. Cole WQ, Cook JJ, Grogan JB: In vitro neutrophil function and lysosomal enzyme levels in patients with sepsis. Surg Forum 26:79, 1975.
111. Curreri PW, Heck EL, Browne L, Baxter CR: Stimulated nitroblue tetrazolium test to assess neutrophil antibacterial function: prediction of wound sepsis in burned patients. Surgery 74(1):6, 1973.
112. Heck EL, Browne L, Curreri PW, Baxter CR: Evaluation of leukocyte function in burned individuals by in vitro oxygen consumption. J Trauma 15(6):486, 1975.
113. Dressler DP, Skornik WA: Alveolar macrophage in the burned rat. J Trauma 14(12):1036, 1975.
114. Harmon JW, Skornik WA, McDonald J, Dressler DP: Pulmonary bacterial defense: effect of burn wound on transfer of alveolar macrophage activation in rats by parabiosis. Am J Surg 131(4):447, 1976.
115. Howard RJ, Simmons RL: Acquired immunologic deficiencies after trauma and surgical procedures. Surg Gynecol Obstet 39:771, 1974.
116. Casson P, Solowey AC, Converse JM, Rapaport FT: Delayed hypersensitivity status of burned patients. Surg Forum 17:268, 1966.
117. Chambler K, Batchelor JR: Influence of defined incompatibilities and area of burn on skin homograft survival in burned subjects. Lancet 1:16, 1969.
118. Munster AM, Eurenius K, Katz RM, et al: Cell mediated immunity after thermal injury. Ann Surg 177:139, 1973.
119. Neilan BA, Taddeini L, Strate RG: T lymphocyte rosette formation after major burns. JAMA 238:493, 1977.
120. Mezrow CK, Bergstein I, Tartter PI: Postoperative infection following autologous and homologous blood transfusions. Transfusion 32:27, 1992.
121. Murphy P, Heal JM, Blumberg N: Infection or suspected infection after hip replacement surgery with autologous or homologous blood transfusions. Transfusion 31:212, 1991.
122. Gascon P, Zoumbos NC, Young NS: Immunologic abnormalities in patients receiving multiple blood transfusions. Ann Intern Med 100:173, 1984.
123. Waymack JP, Rapien J, Garnett D, et al: Effect of transfusion on immune function in a traumatized animal model. Arch Surg 121:50, 1986.
124. Waymack JP, Galon L, Barcelli U, Alexander JW: Effect of blood transfusions on macrophage function in a burned animal model. Curr Surg 43:305, 1986.
125. Waymack JP, Yurt RW: The effect of blood transfusions on immune function: V. The effect on the inflammatory response to bacterial infections. J Surg Res 48:147, 1990.

Infections

126. Muller MJ, Barrow RE, Mlcak R, et al: Endotracheal intubation increases the incidence of pneumonia in severely burned children with inhalation injury. Proc Am Burn Assoc 25:158, 1993.
127. Kreiger JN, Kaiser DL, Wenzel RP: Nosocomial urinary tract infections: secular trends, treatment and economics in a university hospital. J Urol 130(1):102, 1983.
128. Pruitt BA Jr, Foley F: The use of biopsies in burn patient care. Surgery 73:8878, 1973.
129. Sasaki TM, Welch GW, Herndon DN, et al: Burn wound manipulation induced bacteremia. J Trauma 19(1):46, 1979.
130. Beard CH, Ribeiro CD, Jones DM: The bacteremia associated with burn surgery. Br J Surg 62:638, 1975.
131. Hamory BH: Nosocomial sepsis related to intravascular access. Crit Care Nurs Q 11(4):58, 1989.
132. Samsoondar W, Freeman JB, Coultish I, et al: Colonization of intravascular catheters in the intensive care unit. Am J Surg 149:730, 1985.
133. Maki DG, Jarrett F, Sarafin HW: A semiquantitative culture method for identification of catheter related infection in the burn patient. J Surg Res 22:513, 1977.
134. Stein JM, Pruitt BA Jr: Suppurative thrombophlebitis: a lethal iatrogenic disease. N Engl J Med 282:1452, 1970.
135. Franceschi D, Gerding RL, Phillips G, Fratianne RB: Risk factors associated with intravascular catheter infection in burned patients; a prospective randomized study. J Trauma 29(6):811, 1989.
136. Smallman L, Burdon DW, Alexander-Williams J: The effect of skin preparation and care on the incidence of superficial thrombophlebitis. Br J Surg 67:861, 1980.
137. Sheth NK, Franson TR, Rose HD, et al: Colonization of bacteria on polyvinyl chloride and Teflon intravascular catheters in hospitalized patients. J Clin Microbiol 18:1061, 1983.
138. Maki DG, Botticelli JT, LeRoy ML, et al: Prospective study of replacing administration sets for intravenous therapy at 48 to 72 hour intervals. JAMA 258:1777, 1987.
139. Pruitt BA Jr, Stein JM, Foley FD, et al: Intravenous therapy in burn patients: suppurative thrombophlebitis and other life threatening complications. Arch Surg 100:399, 1970.

Treatment

140. Robson MC, Krizek TS: Predicting skin graft survival. J Trauma 13(3):213, 1973.
141. Robson MC: Burn sepsis. Crit Care Clin 4(2):281, 1988.
142. Levenson SM, Alpert S, DelGuerico L, et al: The use of whole and partial body isolators for the care of severely burned patients. Ann NY Acad Sci 150(3):1009, 1968.
143. Lowbury ESL, Babb SR, Ford PM: Protective isolation in a burn unit: the use of plastic isolators and air curtains. J Hyg 69(4):529, 1971.
144. Nance FC, Lewis V, Bornside GH: Absolute barrier isolation and antibiotics in the treatment of experimental burn wound sepsis. J Surg Res 10:33, 1970.
145. Teplitz C, Davis D, Mason AD Jr, Moncrief JA: *Pseudomonas* burn wound sepsis. I. Pathogenesis of experimental *Pseudomonas* burn wound sepsis. J Surg Res 4:200, 1964.
146. Moncrief JA, Lindberg RB, Switzer WE, Pruitt BA: The use of a topical sulfonamide in the control of burn wound sepsis. J Trauma 6(3):407, 1966.
147. Holder IA, Schwab M, Jackson L: Eighteen months of routine topical antimicrobial susceptibility testing of isolates from burn patients: results and conclusions. J Antimicrob Chemother 5:455, 1979.
148. Fox CL, Rappole WB, Stanford W: Control of *Pseudomonas* infection in burns by silver sulfadiazine. Surg Gynecol Obstet 128:1021, 1969.
149. Jarrett F, Ellerbee S, Demling R: Acute leukopenia during topical burn therapy with silver sulfadiazine. Am J Surg 135:818, 1978.
150. Chan CK, Jarrett F, Moylan JA: Acute leukopenia as an allergic reaction to silver sulfadiazine in burn patients. J Trauma 16(6):395, 1976.
151. Strock LL, Lee MM, Rutan RL, et al: Topical bactroban (mupirocin): efficacy in treating burn wounds infected with methicillin resistant staphylococci. J Burn Care Rehabil 11(5):454, 1990.
152. Linares HA: A report of 115 consecutive autopsies in burned children: 1966–1980. Burns 8:263, 1982.
153. Parks DH, Linares HA, Thompson PH: Surgical management of burn wound sepsis. Surg Gynecol Obstet 153:374, 1981.
154. Burke JF, Quinby WC Jr, Bondoc CC: Primary excision and prompt grafting as routine therapy for treatment of thermal burns in children. Surg Clin North Am 56:477, 1976.
155. Alexander JW, MacMillan BF, Law E, et al: Treatment of burns with widely meshed skin autograft and meshed skin allograft overlay. J Trauma 21:433, 1981.
156. LaLonde C, Demling R: The effect of complete burn wound excision and closure on postburn oxygen consumption. Surgery 102:862, 1987.
157. Herndon DN, Parks DH: Comparison of serial debridement and autografting and early massive excision with cadaver skin overlay in the treatment of large burns in children. J Trauma 26:149, 1986.
158. Janzekovic Z: A new concept in early excision and immediate grafting of burns. J Trauma 10:1103, 1970.

Nutrition

159. Wilmore DW, Long JM, Mason AD Jr, et al: Catecholamines: mediators of the hypermetabolic response to thermal injury. Ann Surg 180(4):653, 1974.
160. Wolfe RR: Nutrition and metabolism in burns. Crit Care Med 7:19, 1986.
161. Herndon DN, Wilmore DW, Mason AD Jr: Development and analysis of a small animal model simulating the human postburn hypermetabolic response. J Surg Res 25(5):394, 1978.
162. Davies JWL, Fell GS: Tissue catabolism in patient with burns. Clin Chim Acta 51:83, 1974.
163. Hiebert JM, McGough M, Radeheaver G, et al: The influence of catabolism on immunocompetence in burned patients. Surgery 86:242, 1979.
164. Volenec FJ: Metabolic profiles of thermal trauma. Ann Surg 190:694, 1979.
165. Herndon DN, Wilmore DW, Mason AD Jr, et al: Humoral mediators of non-temperature dependent hypermetabolism in 50% burned adult rats. Surg Forum 28:37, 1977.
166. Balogh D, Bauer M, Hortnagl H: Effect of surgery and anesthesia on plasma catecholamine level and rate of urea production in severely burned patients. Anesthetist 32(3):105, 1983.
167. Dolecek R, Zavada M, Besha F, Buryskova D: Plasma immunoreactive insulin and growth hormone levels in burned subjects. Acta Chir Plast 14:179, 1972.
168. Gottschlich MM, Jenkins M, Warden GD, et al: Differential effects of 3 enteral dietary regimens on selected outcome variable in burn patients. JPEN 14(3):225, 1990.
169. Alexander JW, MacMillan BG, Stinnett JD, et al: Beneficial effects of aggressive protein feeding in severely burned children. Ann Surg 192:505, 1980.
170. Mochizuki H, Trocki O, Dominioni L, et al: Reduction of postburn hypermetabolism by early enteral feeding. Curr Surg 42(2):121, 1985.
171. Mochizuki H, Trocki O, Dominioni L, et al: Mechanism of prevention of postburn hypermetabolism and catabolism by early enteral feeding. Ann Surg 200:297, 1984.
172. Wilmore DW, Moylan JA Jr, Bristow BF, et al: Anabolic effects of growth hormone and high caloric feedings following thermal injury. Surg Gynecol Obstet 138:875, 1974.
173. Herndon DN, Barrow RE, Broemeling LD, et al: Effect of exogenous growth hormone on the rate of donor site healing in pediatric burn patients. Ann Surg 212:424, 1990.
174. Gore DC, Honeycutt D, Jahoor F, et al: Effect of exogenous growth hormone in whole body and isolated limb protein kinetics in burned patients. Arch Surg 126:38, 1991.

175. Jiang ZM, He GZ, Zhang SY, et al: Low dose growth hormone and hypocaloric nutrition attenuate the protein catabolic response after major operation. Ann Surg 210(4):513, 1989.
176. Seavitt S: Duodenal and gastric ulceration after burns. Br J Surg 54:32, 1967.
177. Lescher TJ, Sirinek KR, Pruitt BA: Superior mesenteric artery syndrome in thermally injured patients. J Trauma 19(8):567, 1979.
178. Curreri PW, Richmond D, Marvin JA, et al: Dietary requirement of patients with major burns. J Am Diet Assoc 65:415, 1974.
179. Hildreth MA, Herndon DN, Desai MH, et al: Current treatment reduces calories required to maintain weight in pediatric patients with burns. J Burn Care Rehabil 11:405, 1990.
180. Herndon DN, Barrow RE, Stein MD, et al: Increased mortality with intravenous supplemental feeding in severely burned patients. Ann Surg 208:484, 1988.
181. Saito H, Trocki O, Alexander JW, et al: The effect of route of nutrient administration on the nutritional state, catabolic hormone secretion and gut mucosal integrity after burn injury. JPEN 11(1):1, 1987.

Antibiotics

182. Baskin TM, Rosenthal A, Pruitt BA Jr: Acute bacterial endocarditis: a silent source of sepsis in the burn patient. Ann Surg 184(5):618, 1976.
183. Sawchuk RJ, Rector TS: Drug kinetics in burned patients. Clin Pharmacokinet 5(6):548, 1980.
184. Hall JW III, Herndon DN, Gary LB, Winkler JB: Auditory brainstem response in young burn wound patients treated with ototoxic drugs. Int J Pediatr Otorhinolaryngol 12(2):187, 1986.
185. Grube BJ, Marvin JA, Heimbach DM: *Candida:* a decreasing problem for the burned patient. Arch Surg 123:194, 1988.

Surgery in Patients with Acquired Immune Deficiency Syndrome

CHAPTER 53

Timothy P. Connall, Samuel E. Wilson, Russell A. Williams

As of January 1993 the World Health Organization (WHO) estimated that 13 million people are infected with the human immunodeficiency virus (HIV), including 1 million children.[1] In the second half of 1992, over 1 million new HIV infections occurred worldwide. There have been over 610,000 cases of the acquired immunodeficiency syndrome (AIDS) reported worldwide and it is estimated that the actual number of people with AIDS is 2.5 million. Over 300,000 people have died from the virus worldwide. The WHO projects that by the year 2000 there will be between 30 and 50 million people infected with HIV, with the majority of the growth of infection rate in Africa and South and Southeast Asia[2] (Fig. 53–1).

In the United States there are over 240,000 reported cases of AIDS. Taking effect January 1993, the Centers for Disease Control and Prevention (CDC) revised the classification system for HIV infection for adolescents and adults to emphasize the clinical importance of CD4+ T lymphocyte counts in the categorization of HIV-related clinical conditions.[3] The new system incorporates the previous clinical criteria (with the addition of invasive lymphoma, pneumonia, and *Mycoplasma tuberculosis* pulmonary infection) with three categories of CD4+ T lymphocyte counts to create nine clinical classifications of HIV infection (Tables 53–1 and 53–2). In the new system, all patients with HIV having CD4+ T lymphocyte counts fewer than 200 cells per microliter are classified with AIDS. The CDC estimate that this expanded classification system will result in a 75 percent increase in reported cases in 1993, which would project a total of 85,000 to 90,000 new cases of AIDS in the United States for 1993.

Since the beginning of the epidemic, surgeons have been operating on HIV-infected patients for AIDS-related and nonrelated diseases. Given the large variety and ubiquitous nature of HIV-associated diseases, remarkably few patients ever require surgery for HIV-related pathology. Of 904 AIDS patients admitted to a New York hospital, only 36 (4.5 percent) underwent abdominal surgery and in our review from eight hospitals (3500 beds) in Southern California over a 4-year period, only 35 patients required abdominal surgery.[4,5] Even with the low incidence of surgical disease, these patients often have

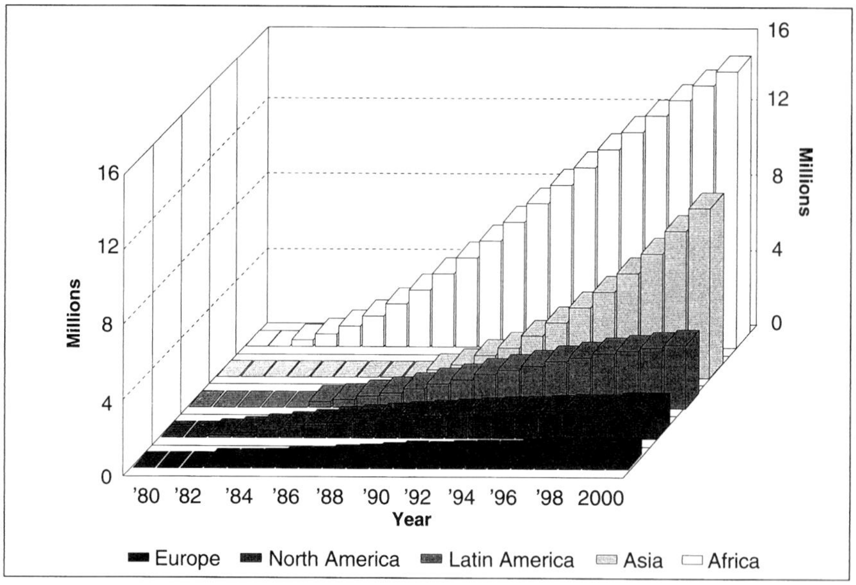

Figure 53–1. Cumulative worldwide incidence of HIV infection in adults, 1980 to 2000. *(From Chaisson RE: Infect Med 9(Suppl F):7, 1992.)*

severe abdominal signs and symptoms and the surgeon is frequently consulted for evaluation of suspected peritonitis. In a review by Barone and colleagues,[6] of 235 patients with AIDS, 29 had abdominal pain, but only 5 required operation. In most cases the abdominal pain is from infectious gastroenteritis, and antimicrobial treatment and close observation are appropriate. However, the surgeon must be aware of surgical HIV-related syndromes to detect and appropriately treat the unusual patient requiring operation.

Several HIV-associated syndromes requiring surgery and surgical procedures for HIV-related diseases have been identified. These include cytomegalovirus enterocolitis, non-Hodgkin's lymphoma of the gastrointestinal tract, Kaposi's sarcoma of the gastrointestinal tract, opportunistic intra-abdominal or retroperitoneal infections, splenectomy, anorectal procedures, and emergency laparotomy. Surgery can be performed with acceptably low morbidity and mortality and can provide significant enhancement of quality and length of life for patients infected with HIV. In the Southern California experience, the 30-day mortality of AIDS patients who underwent elective abdominal surgery was 9 percent, and in a review of 66 major elective general surgery procedures performed on patients with HIV or AIDS the 30-day mortality was 2 percent.[5,7]

CYTOMEGALOVIRUS ENTEROCOLITIS

Cytomegalovirus (CMV), a herpesvirus, is the third most common pathogen in patients with AIDS, superseded only by *Pneumocystis carinii* and *Can-*

TABLE 53–1. 1992 REVISED CLASSIFICATION SYSTEM OF HIV INFECTION AND EXPANDED AIDS SURVEILLANCE CASE DEFINITION FOR ADOLESCENTS AND ADULTS[a]

CD4+ Cell Categories	A Asymptomatic, or Persistent Generalized Lymphadenopathy	B Symptomatic; Not (A) or (C) Conditions	C AIDS-Indicator Conditions
(1) >500/μl	A1	B1	C1
(2) 200–499/μl	A2	B2	C2
(3) <200/μl	A3	B3	C3

[a] Persons with AIDS-indicator conditions (C1, C2, C3) and those with CD4+ T lymphocyte counts less than 200/μl are classified as having AIDS.

From Centers for Disease Control and Prevention. 1993 Revised classification system for HIV infection and expanded surveillance case definition for AIDS among adolescents and adults: Morb Mortal Wkly Rep 41(RR-17):1, 1992.

TABLE 53–2. CASE-DEFINING CLINICAL CATEGORIES

- CATEGORY A
  - Asymptomatic HIV infection
  - Persistent generalized lymphadenopathy
  - Acute HIV infection with accompanying illness or history of acute HIV infection
- CATEGORY B
  - Bacillary angiomatosis
  - Candidiasis; oropharyngeal or vulvovaginal
  - Cervical dysplasia (moderate, severe, or carcinoma in situ)
  - Constitutional symptoms; such as fever or diarrhea lasting more than 1 month
  - Hairy leukoplakia, oral
  - Herpes zoster, involving at least two distinct episodes or more than one dermatome
  - Idiopathic thrombocytopenic purpura
  - Listeriosis
  - Nocardiosis
  - Pelvic inflammatory disease
  - Peripheral neuropathy
- CATEGORY C
  - Candidiasis of bronchi, trachea, or lungs
  - Candidiasis of the esophagus
  - Coccidioidomycosis, disseminated or extrapulmonary
  - Cryptosporidiosis, chronic intestinal (>1 month duration)
  - Cytomegalovirus disease (other than liver, spleen, or nodes)
  - Cytomegalovirus retinitis (with loss of vision)
  - HIV encephalopathy
  - Herpes simplex: chronic ulcer(s) (>1 month duration); or bronchitis, pneumonitis, or esophagitis
  - Histoplasmosis, disseminated or extrapulmonary
  - Isosporiasis, chronic intestinal (>1 month duration)
  - Kaposi's sarcoma
  - Lymphoma, small noncleaved cell (Burkitt's), large cell, and immunoblastic
  - *Mycobacterium avium* complex or *M. Kansasii,* disseminated or extrapulmonary
  - *Mycobacterium tuberculosis,* disseminated or extrapulmonary
  - *Mycobacterium,* other species or unidentified species, disseminated or extrapulmonary
  - *Pneumocystis carinii* pneumonia
  - Progressive multifocal leukoencephalopathy
  - *Salmonella* septicemia, recurrent
  - Toxoplasmosis of brain
  - Wasting syndrome due to HIV
  - Cervical carcinoma, invasive (added in 1992)
  - *Mycobacterium tuberculosis,* pulmonary (added in 1992)
  - Pneumonia, recurrent

dida. Nearly all homosexual men with HIV have serologic evidence of recently acquired or recently activated CMV infection, and over 90 percent of patients with AIDS have evidence of CMV infection at autopsy.[8] The predominant clinical manifestations of CMV in this population are retinitis, gastrointestinal disorders, pneumonitis, and cerebral infection.[9] Jacobson and Mills[8] estimate a prevalence of 2.2 percent of serious CMV gastrointestinal disease in patients with AIDS, second in prevalence after retinitis. Gastrointestinal invasion can involve any organ and is often multifocal.

The diagnosis of CMV invasion of the gastrointestinal tract is made by endoscopy and biopsy of suspicious edematous, erythematous, erosive, or ulcerative lesions.[10] Histology of the specimens may show acute and chronic inflammation, vasculitis, and/or mucosal ulceration, with the diagnosis of CMV made by visualization of nuclear or cytoplasmic viral inclusions with routine or immunocytochemical stains. Epithelial cells, endothelial cells, pericytes, inflammatory cells, and muscle cells may be infected depending on the anatomic location of the biopsy. Francis and colleagues[9] found a predilection for infection of colonic muscularis cells, perhaps owing to the relative predilection for perforation of the colon. CMV cultures may also be performed from biopsy specimens but are less sensitive than histology for confirming the diagnosis.

Severe inflammation and vasculitis caused by CMV may lead to ischemia and transmural necrosis of the bowel, resulting in perforation and peritonitis. These complications are the commonest indication for emergency laparotomy in patients with AIDS.[5,11] Perforation is usually a late complication in these patients, often in those with a history of CMV colitis. It occurs most often in the colon, though several small bowel and a few appendicial perforations have been reported.[5,11,12] At operation, discoloration of the serosa may be seen with the punctate perforations of the bowel. The typically late stage of AIDS in which perforation occurs, together with the peritoneal contamination that follows, portends a poor prognosis for these patients.

To optimize outcome after resection of the perforated segment, a diverting stoma is constructed, retention sutures are used to close the abdomen, and the skin and subcutaneous tissue are allowed to heal by secondary intention. Ganciclovir, an inhibitor of viral DNA polymerase, is administered to suppress CMV, and broad spectrum antibiotics are given to eradicate enteric flora from the contaminated peritoneum (see Chap. 28). In a review of 15 cases of intestinal perforation due to CMV in patients with AIDS, 1-month and 6-month mortality rates were 54 percent and 87 percent, respectively.[11]

CMV is the most common cause of colitis in patients with AIDS.[9,13] Characteristic symptoms of CMV colitis are abdominal pain, diarrhea, fever, weight loss, and, occasionally, bleeding. Other causes of colitis in these patients include shigellosis, salmonellosis, *Campylobacter jejuni* infection, *Mycobacterium avium-intracellulare* disseminated infection, cryptosporidiosis, *Histoplasma capsulatum, Entamoeba histolytica,* and *Clostridium difficile,* and appropriate studies of stool specimens should be performed to exclude these etiologies. If the above are negative, then coloscopy and biopsy should be performed to establish the diagnosis of CMV. Since stool cultures rarely yield virus in patients with CMV colitis and have questionable significance if positive, these studies are not necessary.[8] Therapy consists of a 10- to 14-day induction phase with ganciclovir, followed by lifelong maintenance with ganciclovir to reduce the likelihood of clinical and viral CMV relapse.[8]

Invasive CMV infection can involve the esophagus and stomach and may lead to dysphagia and substernal and epigastric pain. Diagnosis of CMV infection of the upper gastrointestinal tract is also made with biopsy and histologic identification of cytomegaloviral cells. These cells are found in endothelial cells, pericytes, and inflammatory cells of the esophagus and in the glandular epithelial cells of the stomach and small intestine.[9] These infections also require treatment with ganciclovir to avoid progressive symptoms and perforation.[8] CMV has caused sclerosing cholangitis, cholecystitis, and extensive small bowel disease, resulting in diarrhea and marked malabsorption. Mass lesions in the gastrointestinal tract, similar in radiographic and endoscopic appearance to neoplasms, have also been caused by CMV.[14] The pancreas has also been found involved with CMV at autopsy, but there was no associated pancreatitis.

NON-HODGKIN'S LYMPHOMA OF THE GASTROINTESTINAL TRACT

A disproportionately high incidence of non-Hodgkin's lymphoma (NHL) in persons infected with HIV was recognized relatively early in the epidemic and NHL was added to the AIDS case-defining criteria by the CDC. Lymphomas occur in approximately 6 percent of patients with AIDS, 25 to 100 times the prevalence in the normal population.[15] Presently, the CDC recognize three basic subtypes of NHL as criteria for AIDS: small noncleaved cell (Burkitt's) lymphoma, large cell lymphoma, and immunoblastic lymphoma. The criteria include HIV serology and B cell phenotype of lymphoma.[15] These lymphomas are particularly aggressive, often with extranodal distribution at initial presentation, similar to the lymphomas found in immunosuppressed patients with transplants and those with congenital immunodeficiencies.[15]

As in African Burkitt's lymphoma in patients without AIDS, there may be a causative role for Epstein-Barr virus (EBV) in the pathogenesis of NHL in patients with AIDS. The EBV genome has been demonstrated in AIDS-related lymphomas using Southern blot or in situ hybridization techniques in 28 to 78 percent of lymphomas.[16] It has been postulated that the lack of immune surveillance found in AIDS patients provides conditions in which long-lived, EBV-transformed B cells may undergo numerous cell divisions, increasing the probability of critical gene rearrangements that could lead to neoplastic proliferation.[17]

Initial clinical presentation is often with NHL found at extranodal sites including the bone marrow, brain, lung, heart, kidneys, adrenal glands, and the gastrointestinal tract, the later comprising the most common extranodal site and found in 27 to 74 percent of AIDS patients with NHL.[15] Lymphoma may be found at nearly any site in the gastrointestinal tract, commonly developing in the liver, stomach, duodenum, and terminal ileum. Gut involvement is often heralded by the finding of an abdominal mass, intestinal obstruction or perforation, or gastrointestinal bleeding. These symptoms may be the earliest presentation of AIDS, a fact that is revealed only after histologic examination of the resected tumor prompts serologic testing that confirms HIV infection.

Complications resulting from gastrointestinal tract involvement of NHL in these patients may be managed similarly to those of other gastrointestinal tumors. Resection of involved bowel is the first approach. If tumor involvement if too expansive for resection, then the tumor may be bypassed with restoration of intestinal continuity. Surgical treatment usually successfully resolves the acute process, but long-term survival is limited for these patients. Of five AIDS patients who underwent emergency laparotomy for gastrointestinal lymphoma, three died within 3 months of operation.[18]

Most AIDS patients with noncomplicated NHL initially present with a history of fever, weight loss, and night sweats.[15] Many of these patients are managed nonoperatively with combination chemotherapy and/or radiation therapy. Though remission rates exceed 50 percent, high recurrence rates and short disease-free intervals are typical.[15] In a trial at San Francisco General Hospital, 84 patients were treated with either standard chemotherapy regimens, a novel chemotherapy regimen, or radiation therapy alone. No regimen afforded an advantage for survival; rather, survival was predicted by CD4+ T lymphocyte count, presence of extranodal disease, and medical disability performance score.[15]

We have found that if the tumor is resectable, operation is an expedient and worthwhile palliative treatment of the complications of obstruction and bleeding of gastrointestinal lymphomas and may be followed by chemotherapy and radiation regimens. Resection may be necessary during chemotherapy or radiation to treat hollow viscus perforation caused by tumor lysis.

Median survival for AIDS patients with lymphoma (based on any site) is 5 to 10.5 months.[15,16] Approximately 50 percent of deaths are secondary to recurrence of lymphoma; with the others dying from opportunistic infection.[15]

KAPOSI'S SARCOMA

Kaposi's sarcoma (KS) is a multicentric spindle cell neoplasm, likely of lymphatic endothelial cell origin.[15] Prior to 1981, KS was a rare neoplasm, typically manifested as purple, nodular lesions in the skin of the legs of elderly caucasian men and renal allograft recipients. Though early in the epidemic KS was found only in homosexual men with AIDS and is still predominantly found in that group, KS has been found in all risk groups of patients with AIDS.[19] Based on upper and lower endoscopy, 40 to 50 percent of AIDS patients with cutaneous lesions have also been found to have gastrointestinal tract involvement with KS.[19]

The pathogenesis of KS in AIDS patients is unknown. Based on the evidence that several cases of KS have occurred in HIV-negative homosexual men, that KS in Africans from Zaire is not associated with HIV, and that the incidence of KS in the developed world is declining including in homosexual men with AIDS, it has been suggested that KS is caused by a second infectious agent that is an epiphenomenon with HIV infection.[15] Oncogenic viruses have been proposed, but a causative pathogen has not been identified.

KS may occur in any part of the gastrointestinal tract. Best diagnosed by endoscopic examination of the gut, KS appears as violaceous macular or nodular lesions several centimeters in width and length, occasionally with central ulceration or hemorrhage. KS lesions are most often submucosal, accounting for the poor (less than 50 percent) diagnostic yield of endoscopically obtained biopsies. Even though the variant found in patients with AIDS is an aggressive form of KS, the neoplasm is most often asymptomatic and patients with KS most often die from other causes, particularly opportunistic infections. However, with longer survival of patients with AIDS, it may be that KS of the gastrointestinal tract will become a more frequent cause of complications.

Advanced KS of the viscera may cause complications that require surgical management. Hemorrhage is the most common of these, having necessitated local resection of stomach, small and large bowel, and rectum. In such cases, preoperative angiography is often required to localize the bleeding. A group at New York University Hospital has successfully used endoscopic injection sclerotherapy to control hemorrhage from KS of the antrum, fundus, duodenum, and rectum.[20] We have treated by operation patients with diverse manifestations of KS such as a cystic duct obstruction or a rectal tumor that caused tenesmus. KS may also cause abdominal pain, bowel obstruction, perforation, colitis with toxic megacolon, and malabsorption.

KS is responsive to chemotherapy and interferon alpha. The neoplasm is also susceptible to radiation therapy—this modality being best used to ameliorate localized symptomatic lesions that can be treated with one field, such as KS of the rectum. Some argue that since KS does not change the outcome of AIDS and that KS is rarely fatal, only symptomatic lesions should be treated.[15]

MYCOBACTERIA AND OTHER INFECTIONS

Mycobacterium avium-intracellulare (MAI) has been isolated from soil, water, dairy products, and tissue from birds and mammals. Prior to AIDS, diseases attributed to MAI were rare, especially those outside the lungs. In patients with AIDS, MAI is commonly found, often disseminated, and associated at times with invasion of the gastrointestinal tract. Clinical manifestations of gastrointestinal MAI are nonspecific and include diffuse abdominal pain, diarrhea, weight loss, and fever. The diagnosis rests on identifying the acid-fast bacilli in tissue specimens or observing their growth in culture. Blood, bone marrow, and liver biopsies are sources of tissue for study. Blood cultures are less useful because long-term growth is often required and definitive results may not be available for up to 7 weeks.[21]

Endoscopy may be the most expedient method of diagnosing gastrointestinal MAI. Characteristic 2- to 4-mm diameter studded white nodules are seen, often with superficial erosion and surrounding erythema.[21] The second portion of the duodenum is typically involved with sparing of the stomach and duodenal bulb. Other possible sites of abdominal involvement include the terminal ileum, appendix, colon, and periportal and peripancreatic lymph nodes.[21] Histology of affected tissue demonstrates foamy macrophages throughout the mucosa with intracellular and extracellular acid-fast organisms. The inflammation caused by MAI is not transmural, and MAI has not been implicated in intestinal perforation.[22] MAI responds poorly to conventional antituberculosis chemotherapy, but quadruple therapy of ansamycin, clofazimine, isoniazid, and ethambutol produces some improvement in symptoms (see Chap. 9).

Mycobacterium tuberculosis infections of the gastrointestinal tract have signs and symptoms similar to those associated with MAI. In a review of 21 immunocompromised patients (most secondary to HIV) with abdominal mycobacterial infection, diffuse abdominal pain was the most common symptom, although 19 percent had no abdominal pain and 28 percent lacked abdominal findings on physical examination.[23] Only 38 percent of patients had fever; while only three had increased white blood cell counts, and none had a significant abnormal trend in leukocyte differential count.[23] In this series, eight patients had peritoneal infection, seven ileocecal involvement, three hepatic infection, and three psoas abscess. Computed tomography (CT) scan is useful in making the diagnosis and can yield findings that will differentiate between intra-abdominal MAI and *M. tuberculosis* infection[23,24] and suggested abdominal mycobacterial infection in 9 of 14 patients studied.[23] Ten patients were treated with operation, including drainage of psoas abscess, ileocolic resection, appendectomy, and diagnostic laparotomy. *Mycobacterium tuberculosis* was isolated from 15 of these patients and MAI was identified in 4 patients.[23] The mortality of this group 1 year later was 24 percent.[23] Intestinal perforation due to *M. tuberculosis* has been reported but is a rare complication.[22] Multidrug antimicrobial therapy is the first line of treatment of abdominal mycobacterial infections, surgery being used to treat abscess, perforation, or obstruction.

As previously mentioned in reference to CMV colitis, these patients are susceptible to many bacterial, protozoal, viral, fungal, and parasitic infections of the gastrointestinal tract. AIDS patients are predisposed to infection with salmonellae, at times with septicemia. Antimicrobial therapy is effective, but eradication of the organism can be difficult and relapses are common.[25] Esophagitis is most frequently caused by *Candida albicans.* Oral thrush is common, with the diagnosis based on the finding of characteristic white plaques in the mouth. Although the presence of oral thrush and dysphagia is high suggestive of *Candida* esophagitis, the diagnosis is best made with endoscopy. *Candida* esophagitis may lead to a fulminant systemic candidiasis and is also a common cause of gastrointestinal bleeding in these patients.[26,27] A single case of intestinal perforation in a patient with AIDS has been reported.[28]

SPLENECTOMY

Splenectomy is one of the most frequently performed intra-abdominal operations on patients infected with HIV, usually for HIV-associated thrombocytopenia (HAT).[4,5,7] Extrasplenic destruction of platelets due to adsorption of circulating immune complexes, specific anti-platelet antibodies, and defective thrombopoiesis have been implicated in this disease, leaving the spleen normal size and with little associated pathology.[29,30] Medical regimens for HAT include steroids, intravenous immunoglobulin, platelet infusions, and zidovudine (AZT).[30]

Splenectomy is often indicated in symptomatic patients with HAT refractory to medical therapy and those refractory asymptomatic patients with platelet counts less than 20,000/mm^3.[30] In 117 reported splenectomies for HAT, there were no perioperative deaths, the combined complete (sustained platelet count greater than 150,000/mm^3) and partial response (sustained platelet count greater than 50,000/mm^3) rate was 86 percent, and the complication rate was approximately 5 percent.[30,31] The administration of intravenous immunoglobulin in the 48 hours preceding splenectomy may obviate the need for platelet transfusion during surgery on these patients.[30]

Splenomegaly is a common finding in patients with AIDS, reported in up to 72 percent of cases, with splenic enlargement usually 1.5 to 3 times the normal size.[32] Splenomegaly may be associated with an AIDS-related neoplasm, especially non-Hodgkin's lymphoma, and rarely Kaposi's sarcoma. In cases of acute illness with splenomegaly, CT scan should be performed as splenic abscess or infarct may be found, necessitating splenectomy. Mathew and colleagues[32] have reported poor outcomes in AIDS patients with splenomegaly from MAI or CMV and advise against operation in these cases. While operation is not necessary for diagnosis, splenectomy is effective treatment for MAI abscess of the spleen.

Pneumococcal vaccine given to HIV-infected homosexual men has been shown to produce effective antibody titers.[33] All patients with HIV undergoing splenectomy should receive pneumococcal vaccine, preferably at least 1 week prior to surgery.

ANORECTAL SURGERY

Anorectal disease had been reported to occur in up to 34 percent of patients infected with HIV.[34] Pathology commonly encountered includes fistula-in-ano, condylomata acuminata, perianal ulcer, perirectal abscess, fissure-in-ano, hemorrhoids, and neoplasms.[34,35] As in other regions of the gastrointestinal tract, there is a predisposition for infections (herpes simplex virus, CMV, MAI, *Chlamydia, Candida,* condylomata, primary HIV-induced anal ulcer) and neoplasms (non-Hodgkin's lymphoma, Kaposi's sarcoma, anorectal carcinoma) in this region associated with HIV infection.[34] Given the preponderance of these diseases, especially neoplasms, proper treatment requires a diagnosis based on thorough cultures and biopsies of the affected region. Topical and/or systemic antimicrobial therapy is the first line of treatment for many anal fissures, perianal ulcers, and condylomata. Acceptable responses may occur with HSV- and CMV-infected lesions, while the results with condylomata are poor, often necessitating fulguration of the lesion.[34]

There has been concern that these lesions will not respond to or heal adequately after surgery. Safavi and colleagues[34] have demonstrated that surgical management of these disorders will yield symptomatic relief and a high rate of complete or partial wound healing. In 75 procedures, 53 percent completely healed, 30 percent partially healed and yielded symptomatic relief, 4 percent resulted in symptomatic relief but no healing, and 13 percent yielded no relief and no healing.[34] In addition, this group found that while there was a decrease in healing in patients with AIDS compared to HIV-seropositive patients, there was no correlation between CD4+ T lymphocyte count and healing of the surgically treated anorectal lesion.[34]

ACUTE ABDOMEN

The diagnosis of an acute surgical process in the HIV-infected patient is confounded by several factors. The foremost difficulty arises with the large number of nonsurgical diseases that often manifest as abdominal pain. These more common, nonsurgical, infectious etiologies must be balanced with the knowledge that a HIV-related surgical syndrome or a common, non-HIV-related surgical process, such as appendicitis or diverticulitis, may be present—in which case, expedient diagnosis and surgery are critical to minimize the development of fulminant sepsis. A lack of physical signs and absence of leukocytosis also confound the diagnosis. Of 28 AIDS patients undergoing emergency laparotomy, 19 had abdominal tenderness without signs of peritonitis.[18] In a review of patients with HIV or AIDS and acute surgical disease, some had low or normal blood leukocyte counts and 60 percent of patients had normal leukocyte differential counts.[7]

Cognizant of these pitfalls, the diagnostic approach is similar to that for patients without HIV. In patients without clear indications for laparotomy based on physical signs and laboratory studies, the early use of abdominal x-ray studies, ultrasonography, computed tomography, and laparoscopy is essential to expeditiously diagnose perforated viscus, abscess, bowel obstruction, toxic megacolon, and other diseases that require emergent laparotomy.[36] The majority of emergency laparotomies in these patients are for CMV ileocolitis, often with perforation of the bowel.[5,37]

In most cases of bowel perforation, especially secondary to CMV enteritis, an anastomosis is avoided and a diverting stoma is constructed. If drainage is indicated, closed drain systems should be used to facilitate safe collection and disposal of the fluid. Retention sutures should be used liberally, since procedures for diseases associated with intra-abdominal sepsis in these patients have a wound dehiscence rate of 31 percent.[7]

As expected, perioperative mortality in these patients is much higher than those undergoing elective laparotomy.[5,18,37] In Southern California, perioperative mortality for emergency laparotomy was 46 percent,[5] and in a series by Wexner and associates[37] mortality was 71 percent. In a more recent series by Davidson et al[18] of 28 emergency laparotomies in patients with AIDS, mortality at 30 days, 3 months, and 6 months was 11 percent, 64 percent, and 48 percent, respectively. The improved survival reported by Davidson and co-workers may be due to an earlier diagnosis and medical treatment of AIDS.[38]

Appendicitis

Appendicitis in AIDS patients usually displays classic pathology. In about one-third of patients, appendicitis is due to CMV-mediated transmural inflammation and, occasionally, perforation.[12,18,36,39] Appendicitis caused by obstructing Kaposi's sarcoma has also been reported in patients with AIDS.[39]

With the exception of leukocytosis, the classic signs and symptoms of appendicitis are found in AIDS patients with appendicitis, though perhaps with a lower incidence. In a series from the University of San Francisco, of 23 AIDS patients with appendicitis, 83 percent were anorexic preoperatively, 65 percent had fever, 43 percent had right lower quadrant pain, and 38 percent had physical signs of peritonitis.[39] In that series, with the exception of diffuse (more often found in non-AIDS-related appendicitis) versus localized abdominal pain, no preoperative findings were useful in distinguishing between AIDS-related and non-AIDS-related appendicitis.[39] AIDS patients with appendicitis rarely have a leukocytosis, though the leukocyte count may be elevated from the patient's low baseline.[12,36,39]

Error in diagnosis and prolonged preoperative evaluation are common and many perforations and periappendicial abscesses are found at operation.[39] Physicians should maintain a high suspicion for the disease in AIDS patients with abdominal complaints, and appropriate diagnostic tests should be used expeditiously to avoid the late stages of appendicitis. Appendectomy can be performed with low mortality and morbidity in patients with AIDS. In 46 cases of appendectomy for appendicitis in AIDS patients, one perioperative death occurred in a patient with *Pneumocystis carinii* pneumonia on admission to the hospital.[4,5,12,18,36,39] Abdominal wounds heal well either by primary or secondary intention.[39]

Cholecystectomy

In the Southern California experience, cholecystectomy has been used to treat *Candida albicans* acalculous cholecystitis, *Salmonella* and CMV cholecystitis, cholelithiasis, and biliary colic resulting from Kaposi's sarcoma obstruction of the cystic duct. In a series by LaRaja and associates,[4] of 12 patients with AIDS undergoing cholecystectomy, 9 had acalculous cholecystitis. Gallbladder cultures were also remarkable for CMV in two patients and *Candida albicans* in one patient.[4]

Gastrointestinal Bleeding

Frequently encountered causes of AIDS-related gastrointestinal bleeding include *Candida* esophagitis, non-Hodgkin's lymphoma and Kaposi's sarcoma, and enteritis secondary to CMV, MAI, or tuberculosis.[26,27,40] In a series by Cappell and Geller,[26] in-hospital mortality was 39 percent for HIV-seropositive patients with gastrointestinal bleeding, with 91 percent mortality for patients presenting with two or more major concurrent illnesses and 13 percent mortality for patients with no major concurrent illnesses.[26] Effective angiographic diagnosis and transcatheter embolization or endoscopic injection sclerotherapy of lesions with focal bleeding have been reported.[20,40] In the Southern California experience, two patients undergoing gastric resection for bleeding gastric lymphoma survived through 1 month from surgery, and a patient with massive colonic bleeding from lymphoma and CMV died in the perioperative period.[5]

REFERENCES

1. World Health Organization: Acquired immunodeficiency syndrome (AIDS)—data as of 31 December 1992. Wkly Epidemiol Rec 68:9, 1993.
2. World Health Organization: Update on AIDS. Wkly Epidemiol Rec 66:353, 1991.
3. Centers for Disease Control and Prevention: 1993 Revised classification system for HIV infection and expanded surveillance case definition for AIDS among adolescents and adults. MMWR Morb Mortal Wkly Rep 41(RR-17):1, 1992.
4. LaRaja RD, Rothenberg RE, Odom JW, Mueller SC: The incidence of intra-abdominal surgery in acquired immunodeficiency syndrome: a statistical review of 904 patients. Surgery 210:428, 1989.
5. Wilson SE, Robinson G, Williams RA, et al: Acquired immune deficiency syndrome (AIDS). Indications for abdominal surgery, pathology, and outcome. Ann Surg 210:428, 1989.
6. Barone JE, Gingold BS, Nealon TF, Avanites ML: Abdominal pain in patients with acquired immune deficiency syndrome. Ann Surg 204:619, 1986.
7. Diettrich NA, Cacioppo JC, Kaplan G, Cohen SM: A growing spectrum of surgical disease in patients with human immunodeficiency virus/acquired immunodeficiency syndrome. Experience with 120 major cases. Arch Surg 126:860, 1991.
8. Jacobson MA, Mills J: Serious cytomegalovirus disease in the acquired immunodeficiency syndrome (AIDS). Ann Intern Med 108:585, 1988.
9. Francis ND, Boylston AW, Roberts AH, et al: Cytomegalovirus infection in gastrointestinal tracts of pa-

tients infected with HIV-1 or AIDS. J Clin Pathol 42:1055, 1989.
10. Goodgame RW, Genta RM, Estrada R, et al: Frequency of positive tests for cytomegalovirus in AIDS patients: endoscopic lesions compared with normal mucosa. Am J Gastroenterol 88:338, 1993.
11. Kram HB, Shoemaker WC: Intestinal perforation due to cytomegalovirus infection in patients with AIDS. Dis Colon Rectum 33:1037, 1990.
12. Neumayer LA, Makar R, Ampel NM, Zukoski CF: Cytomegalovirus appendicitis in a patient with human immunodeficiency virus infection. Arch Surg 128:467, 1993.
13. Schwarz ED, Greene JB: Diagnostic considerations in the human immunodeficiency virus-infected patient with gastrointestinal or abdominal symptoms. Semin Liver Dis 12:142, 1992.
14. Rich JD, Crawford JM, Kazanjian SN, Kazanjian PH: Discrete gastrointestinal mass lesions caused by cytomegalovirus in patients with AIDS: report of three cases and review. Clin Infect Dis 15:609, 1992.
15. Herndier BG, Friedman SL: Neoplasms of the gastrointestinal tract and hepatobiliary system in acquired immunodeficiency syndrome. Semin Liver Dis 12: 128, 1992.
16. Guarner J, Del RC, Carr D, et al: Non-Hodgkin's lymphomas in patients with human immunodeficiency virus infection. Presence of Epstein-Barr virus by in situ hybridization, clinical presentation, and follow-up. Cancer 68:2460, 1991.
17. Ioachim HL, Dorsett B, Cronin W, et al: Acquired immunodeficiency syndrome-associated lymphomas: clinical, pathologic, immunologic, and viral characteristics of 111 cases. Hum Pathol 22:659, 1991.
18. Davidson T, Allen MT, Miles AJ, et al: Emergency laparotomy in patients with AIDS. Br J Surg 78:924, 1991.
19. Parente F, Cernuschi M, Orlando G, et al: Kaposi's sarcoma and AIDS: frequency of gastrointestinal involvement and its effect on survival. A prospective study in a heterogeneous population. Scand J Gastroenterol 26:1007, 1991.
20. Lew EA, Dieterich DT: Severe hemorrhage caused by gastrointestinal Kaposi's syndrome in patients with the acquired immunodeficiency syndrome: treatment with endoscopic injection sclerotherapy. Am J Gastroenterol 87:1471, 1992.
21. Monsour HJ, Quigley EM, Markin RS, et al: Endoscopy in the diagnosis of gastrointestinal *Mycobacterium avium-intracellulare* infection. J Clin Gastroenterol 13:20, 1991.
22. Friedenberg KA, Draguesku JO, Kiyabu M, Valenzuela JE: Intestinal perforation due to *Mycobacterium tuberculosis* in HIV-infected individuals: report of two cases. Am J Gastroenterology 88(4):604, 1993.
23. Rosengart TK, Coppa GF: Abdominal mycobacterial infections in immunocompromised patients. Am J Surg 159:125, 1990.
24. Radin DR: Intraabdominal *Mycobacterium tuberculosis* vs *Mycobacterium avium-intracellulare* infections in patients with AIDS: distinction based on CT findings. Am J Roentgenol 156:487, 1991.
25. Nelson MR, Shanson DC, Hawkins DA, Gazzard BG: *Salmonella, Campylobacter* and *Shigella* in HIV-seropositive patients. AIDS 6:1495, 1992.
26. Cappell MS, Geller AJ: The high mortality of gastrointestinal bleeding in HIV-seropositive patients: a multivariate analysis of risk factors and warning signs of mortality in 50 consecutive patients. Am J Gastroenterol 87:815, 1992.
27. Cappell MS, Gupta A: Gastrointestinal hemorrhage due to gastrointestinal *Mycobacterium avium-intracellulare* or esophageal candidiasis in patients with the acquired immunodeficiency syndrome. Am J Gastroenterol 87:224, 1992.
28. Heneghan SJ, Li J, Petrossian E, Bizer LS: Intestinal perforation from gastrointestinal histoplasmosis in acquired immunodeficiency syndrome. Arch Surg 128:464, 1993.
29. Blockmans D, Vermylen J: HIV-related thrombocytopenia. Acta Clin Belg 47:117, 1992.
30. Tyler DS, Shaunak S, Bartlett JA, Iglehart JD: HIV-1-associated thrombocytopenia: the role of splenectomy. Ann Surg 211:211, 1989.
31. Alonso M, Gossot D, Bourstyn E, et al: Splenectomy in human immunodeficiency virus-related thrombocytopenia. Br J Surg 80:330, 1993.
32. Mathew A, Raviglione MC, Niranjan U, et al: Splenectomy in patients with AIDS. Am J Hematol 32:184, 1989.
33. Huang KL, Ruben FL, Rinaldo CJ, et al: Antibody responses after influenza and pneumococcal immunization in HIV-infected homosexual men. JAMA 257:2047, 1987.
34. Safavi A, Gottesman L, Dailey TH: Anorectal surgery in the HIV+ patient: update. Dis Colon Rectum 34:299, 1991.
35. Orkin BA, Smith LE: Perineal manifestations of HIV infection. Dis Colon Rectum 35:310, 1992.
36. Binderow SR, Shaked AA: Acute appendicitis in patients with AIDS/HIV infection. Am J Surg 162:9, 1991.
37. Wexner SD, Smithy WB, Trillo C: Emergency colectomy for cytomegalovirus ileocolitis in patients with the acquired immune deficiency syndrome. Dis Colon Rectum 31:755, 1988.
38. Wexner SD: Emergency laparotomy in patients with AIDS. Br J Surg 79:(1), 1992.
39. Whitney TM, Macho JR, Russell TR, et al: Appendicitis in acquired immunodeficiency syndrome. Am J Surg 164:467, 1992.
40. Sharma VS, Valji K, Bookstein JJ: Gastrointestinal hemorrhage in AIDS: arteriographic diagnosis and transcatheter treatment. Radiology 185:447, 1992.

Diabetic Foot Infections

CHAPTER 54

Gary W. Gibbons

Diabetes effects approximately 6 percent of the U.S. population (about 14 million people). Approximately 25 percent of diabetics will seek the assistance of a health care professional because of a foot-related problem and 15 percent of diabetics will develop some type of skin ulceration during their lifetime. Many of these will become nonhealing ulcers, leading to amputation, with both lower extremities at risk. Diabetics are 17 times more likely to develop gangrene (a word to be avoided in front of the patient) than nondiabetics. More in-hospital days are spent treating diabetic foot infections than any other complication of diabetes. Forty-five percent of all lower extremity amputations are performed on people with diabetes (more than 50,000) each year. U.S. health objectives propose a 40 percent reduction in diabetic amputations by the year 2000.[1] Unfortunately, despite all the advances in medical care and technology, amputation rates are increasing. We think many major amputations can be avoided with better patient and physician education and understanding and also by eliminating misconceptions about the treatment of diabetic foot infections. Reduced health care dollars further mandate that any treatment be cost effective.

THE PROBLEM

Although careful control of diabetes may postpone the development of foot problems, it will not prevent them. There are three primary pathologic situations that occur in the diabetic and either singularly or in combination are responsible for the development of foot problems: neuropathy, infection, and arterial insufficiency.

Neuropathy

Somatic and autonomic neuropathies probably represent the greatest risk for ulcer development.[2] The loss of touch and pain sensation results in an anesthetic foot. Although it may look healthy, the diabetic neuropathic foot has altered proprioception (position and vibration) so that the patient is unaware of the position of the foot. Furthermore, peripheral neuropathy affects the intrinsic and skeletal muscles of the foot, causing atrophy and deformity. Neuropathy also affects the autonomic system, resulting in autosympathectomy. There are two results: sweating is reduced, and the dry foot is very susceptible to fissuring and cracking. Furthermore, arteriovenous shunting creates a false sense of security about the blood supply. The foot is therefore highly susceptible to even small amounts of trauma. Trauma can lead to cutaneous ulceration with bacterial invasion and the development of an acute infection that threatens the limb.

Infection

Diabetics tolerate infection poorly. Infection affects diabetic control, and uncontrolled diabetes affects infection. Defects in the host defense mechanism of many diabetics may predispose them to infection and certainly may alter their response to an infectious process. Chemotaxis phagocytosis and bactericidal function of neutrophils are diminished during hyperglycemia and/or ketoacidosis. Lymphocytes are also adversely affected by hyperglycemia. Obesity, diminished renal function, and immunosuppressive therapy after transplantation further compromise an already altered resistance to infection. Defects in wound healing have also been identified.

Not only is resistance to infection reduced, but systemic signs and symptoms of infection often occur late or are even absent. In the diabetic, unexplained and/or uncontrolled hyperglycemia may be the only reliable sign of a potentially serious infection. Any diabetic presenting with uncontrolled blood sugars must be fully and carefully examined in all areas including the feet. No diabetic patient should be discharged from a facility simply because he/she lacks elevation in the white blood count, temperature, or pulse rate. Less than one-third of our diabetic patients with documented pedal osteomyelitis demonstrated systemic signs and symptoms.[3]

Ischemia

Peripheral vascular disease is estimated to be 20 times more common in the diabetic population, with woman being equally affected. Pecoraro and colleagues[4] reported that critical ischemia was associated with 62 percent of cases with nonhealing ulceration and was a causal factor in 56 percent of amputations. Unrecognized and/or inappropriately treated ischemia increases the risk for major amputation. Although the pathology of atherosclerosis is similar to the nondiabetic, it appears at a younger age with a predilection for the more distal vessels (tibial, peroneal) of the lower leg. There is no inherent occlusive microvascular disease affecting the diabetic foot that precludes revascularization.[5] Indeed, many studies have clearly shown that tissue perfusion in the ischemic diabetic foot can be restored by appropriate vascular reconstruction.[6] Unfortunately, the calcification and relative rigidity of atherosclerotic vessels make noninvasive laboratory evaluation unreliable. The ankle/brachial index is often falsely high. The transcutaneous oxygen tension is, however, a reliable measure of skin perfusion. If clinical judgment reveals that vascular insufficiency is complicating a diabetic foot ulcer, then arteriography visualizing the foot vessels is mandatory. A compromised local circulation delays an already altered host response to infection, the delivery of antimicrobial agents, and proper wound healing. One must always be careful, however, to minimize the potential nephrotoxicity of the contrast agent in performing arteriography.

Diabetic Foot Infections

The complications of hyperglycemia, odor, or circulatory collapse often are the symptoms that bring the patient to the hospital with a septic foot. The diabetic is frequently unaware of the severity of tissue destruction and sepsis, because the anesthetic limb is painless and visual acuity is impaired. Overlying callus can hide an undermining infection from an untrained observer. It is imperative to unroof all encrusted areas and inspect the wound to determine the extent of deep tissue destruction and possible bone and joint involvement.[7] Because of neuropathy, this can be done at the bedside using a sterile probe, scissors, and forceps. If a sterile probe penetrates to the bone, joint, or tendon sheath, these areas are involved. The sensitivity and specificity of this examination are equal to any of the currently used radiologic imaging techniques. Prior to debridement, both the patient and family must be informed of the extent of the disease; otherwise, the surgeon may be accused of causing the ulcer, which is, to a casual observer, hidden.

Microbiologic studies of foot infections in the diabetic have emphasized the importance of mixed infections with aerobic gram-positive bacteria, enteric gram-negative bacteria, and obligate anaerobes (Table 54–1).[8,9] Any wound that has crepitance, a foul fetid odor, or gas by x-ray study is harboring an anaerobic infection capable of producing an insoluble gas. Gas formation in this setting rarely reflects infection caused by *Clostridium* species. Even the presence of *Clostridium* species is not diagnostic of gas gangrene and is not synonymous with guillotine amputation. Urgent surgical debridement will be required, however, to excise all diseased tissue. Most gas-forming infections are the product of facultative gram-negative bacilli and anaerobes. Multiple organisms are the rule; single organisms are the exception. Reliable cultures can be attained only by sending tissue and involved bone to the laboratory.

TABLE 54–1. FREQUENCY OF ISOLATION OF BACTERIAL SPECIES

	Non-Limb-Threatening Group I (17 Patients)		Limb-Threatening Group II (41 Patients) No Systemic Toxicity		Limb-Threatening Group III (42 Patients) Systemic Toxicity	
	Number of Patients	*Total Number of Patients*	*Number of Patients*	*Total Number of Patients*	*Number of Patients*	*Total Number of Patients*
• GRAM-POSITIVE AEROBES		15		35		39
Staphylococcus aureus	9		23		22	
S. epidermidis	6		14		12	
Streptococcus	6		10		13	
Enterococcus	4		12		16	
Diphtheroids	5		7		7	
Total number of isolates	30		66		70	
• GRAM-NEGATIVE AEROBES		6		24		21
Escherichia coli	2		3		7	
Proteus	1		10		11	
Klebsiella	1		4		4	
Enterobacter	0		5		3	
Serratia	1		1		0	
Pseudomonas	1		10		3	
Citrobacter	1		1		2	
Acinetobacter					1	
Total number of isolates	17		34		31	
• ANAEROBES		9		14		29
Clostridium perfringens	0		9		2	
Bacteroides	4		3		12	
Anaerobic cocci	9		13		21	
Total number of isolates	13		16		35	
Total number of isolates	50		116		136	
Average number of isolates per patient	3.0		2.8		3.2	

PRINCIPLES OF TREATMENT

The initial treatment of an infected diabetic foot ulcer depends on its extent and severity (Fig. 54–1). We have simplified our algorithm to encompass today's practice and its cost constraints. Basically, we divide foot ulcers into those that do not threaten the limb and require outpatient treatment, and those that are limb-threatening and require immediate admission. Inspection of the wound determines severity, as mentioned previously.

If the ulcer is superficial with minimal cellulitis (less than 2 cm), if there is no significant ischemia, if the patient has no signs or symptoms of systemic toxicity, and if the patient is compliant, reliable, and has an appropriate support system, then outpatient treatment is indicated. First and extremely important is rest of the injured part. All efforts at outpatient treatment will be unsuccessful unless weight-dependant ulcers are put to complete and total rest, a tough task for many patients. Crutches or a walker (not a cane) are needed. Specialized contact casting or felted foam dressings should be left to experts to apply on patients who absolutely cannot stay off their feet. The wound is cultured and an oral antibiotic targeting gram-positive cocci is initiated. The quinolones have a limited gram-positive spectrum when used alone.

Dressings are kept simple. For cracks and fissures, antibiotic ointment or creams are preferred. Open ulcers are best treated with plain gauze wetted with saline or diluted isotonic antiseptic solutions and changed one to two times a day. While the use of growth factors in local care has been advocated by some, their routine use is expensive and has not as yet been shown to be cost effective. Full-strength solutions or astringents such as enzymatic debriding agents should be avoided, as well as heat,

DIABETIC FOOT ULCER

MILD (NON-LIMB-THREATENING)	SEVERE (LIMB-THREATENING)
SUPERFICIAL MINIMAL OR NO CELLULITIS NO BONE INVOLVEMENT NO SYSTEMIC TOXICITY	DEEP ULCER ± BONE INVOLVEMENT > 2 CM CELLULITIS THREATENED LIMB LOSS ± SYSTEMIC TOXICITY
TREATMENT	TREATMENT
REST OF INJURED PART CULTURE & SENSITIVITIES INITIAL BROAD SPECTRUM ANTIBIOTIC BASED ON SENSITIVITIES CAREFUL DEBRIDEMENT LOCAL DRESSINGS PODIATRIC APPLIANCES AND SPECIAL SHOES CAREFUL FOLLOW-UP	IMMEDIATE ADMISSION CONTROL BLOOD SUGAR CULTURE & SENSITIVITIES INITIAL BROAD SPECTRUM INTRAVENOUS ANTIBIOTICS SPECIFIC ANTIBIOTICS BASED ON SENSITIVITIES EARLY SURGICAL DEBRIDEMENT, DEPENDENT DRAINAGE & OPEN AMPUTATION LOCAL DRESSINGS LATER SELECTED REVASCULARIZATION & CONSERVATIVE AMPUTATIONS OR REVISIONS PODIATRIC APPLICANCES & SPECIAL SHOES CAREFUL FOLLOW-UP

Figure 54–1. Approach to the diabetic with a foot ulcer.

soaks, or whirlpools in any form, as they may burn or macerate tissue and spread the bacteria. Hospitalization is advised if there is no significant improvement in 24 to 48 hours. If there is improvement, regular follow-up must be maintained. Patients with questionable vascular impairment should be referred to a vascular specialist for further vascular evaluation and follow-up. Once healing is achieved, full weight-bearing is begun slowly, examining for recurrent breakdown or the develoment of an acute Charcot's foot (neuropathic joint disease of the diabetic). Modification of footwear using podiatric appliances and/or shoeing may be required to protect sensitive high-risk areas.

Limb-Threatening Ulcers

Why seemingly uncomplicated diabetic foot ulcers progress to limb- and life-threatening infections is not completely understood. We know that control of diabetes, severity of vascular disease, continued trauma including any kind of weight-bearing, and local care are important contributions. An altered host defense as discussed earlier and the invasion by specific bacteria are also important. Any patient who has a potentially limb-threatening ulcer (see Fig. 54–1) should be admitted immediately to the hospital on complete bed rest. Again, careful inspection is most important as the lack of systemic signs and symptoms does not exclude a more severe local infection or distant spread. Patients with larger, deeper ulcers with spreading cellulitis (greater than 2 cm) or lymphangitis or with ulcers that probe to bone, joint, or into tendon sheaths should also be admitted. Gangrene, significant ischemia, immunocompromise, unreliability, and/or the lack of a support system also affect our decision. It should always be remembered, especially by managed care providers, that an early aggressive in-hospital approach to patients with potentially limb-threatening infected ulcers is supported by the fact that up to one-third of these extremities are lost to major amputation (below the knee or above the knee).[10] Upon admission, the patient should be stabilized medically and the blood sugar controlled immediately. Medical stabilization must not delay emergent surgical intervention, including delays caused by the pursuit of radiologic imaging studies. Deep cultures are obtained either at the initial bedside evaluation or in the operating room. We obtain blood cultures in patients manifesting systemic signs and symptoms. Broad spectrum, intravenous antibiotics are administered to ensure adequate serum levels. The choice of an initial antibiotic regimen is influenced by several variables: knowing that these are polymicrobial infections (see Table 54–1) or, as indicated by Gram stain of the purulent material, local bacterial resistance patterns; prior antibiotic therapy; preexisting renal or hepatic dysfunction; and the severity of the infection.[11] We avoid the use of aminoglycosides because of their potential nephrotoxicity and the fact that we are doing so many more arteriograms. Changes in antibiotics are made based on sensitivity reports and the response of the wound. Antibiotic coverage appropriate for the infection should be continued through any revascularization surgery, but prolonged courses of intravenous antibiotics have not been required when early aggressive and appropriate surgical debridement is performed.

As important as the need for intravenous antibiotics is the surgical management of the limb-threatening infection. Antibiotics can only work at the infection-host interface. Surgical debridement of all necrotic tissue and dependent drainage of infected fluid are essential to the cure.[12] This is required no matter what the circulatory status of the patient is. Patients with systemic toxicity will not improve until adequate surgical debridement and drainage are performed. Many of these procedures can be carried out with little or no anesthesia. It should always be remembered that diabetics do not tolerate undrained sepsis. Incisions are carefully placed, ensuring adequate debridement yet conserving as much healthy tissue as possible. Small stab wounds and the use of drains are inappropriate. Multiple visits to the operating room may be required for infection control.

The location of the ulcer, the extent of the infection, and the adequacy of circulation will determine what the final result will be. A neuropathic foot with excellent circulation must be managed differently than the same infection in an ischemic foot. Patients with deep serious infection in which much of the foot architecture is destroyed must be emotionally prepared for open guillotine amputation. Definitive amputations should not be done until the infection is controlled by adequate debridement.

Osteomyelitis

Inadequately diagnosed and/or treated contiguous osteomyelitis in a diabetic foot ulcer increases the risk of amputation. Unfortunately, the reports that document the success of any radiologic imaging test have not correlated bone histopathology or microbiology with the particular test. These tests are not only unreliable, they are also costly. We have shown that probing to bone has the same positive and negative predictive value as any of the radiologic imaging studies currently used.[3] Imaging tests should be reserved for occasions when there is confusion about the diagnosis or a question of Charcot's disease.

Reports supporting a long-term course of antibiotic as sole therapy to cure osteomyelitis are highly suspect, because definitive diagnosis by histopathology or microbiology is lacking.[13,14] Such studies report a 30 percent major amputation failure rate and a 20 percent minor amputation failure rate. A 6-week course of outpatient intravenous antibiotic therapy costs at least $12,000, according to published reports.

We believe that all devitalized bone, including the bony cortex, of any protruding metatarsal or phalanx should be debrided carefully during the operative procedure and sent for culture. If the blood supply is adequate, granulation tissue will form over the bone and the wound will heal. Removal of the infected boy prominence does not represent a therapeutic failure, since it probably was responsible for the problem to begin with and its removal will help to prevent local recurrence. The routine use of hyperbaric oxygen is expensive and unsupported by randomized controlled trial.

Dressings help establish an environment conducive to healing after debridement. Dressings are not therapeutic per se. We prefer to keep dressings simple, using plain gauze sponges wetted with saline or diluted isotonic antiseptic solutions. Dressings should be changed two to three times per day, keeping the wound environment moist. Astringents, occlusive dressings, soaks, whirlpools, or heat in any form should be avoided for the reasons mentioned previously. Dressings do not replace debridement and it is important to inspect the wound to be sure infection is controlled.

Nutritional replenishment is important, especially in the chronically ill, geriatric, or immunocompromised patient. Control of edema is also important throughout the course of wound healing.

Once infection is controlled, evaluation and treatment of ischemia are the next most important steps in the treatment algorithm. It should be noted that routine vascular reconstruction of the foot arteries is not successful with patency and limb salvage rates of 88 percent and 92 percent at 3 years.[15] We have appreciated the fact that diabetic patients with extensive tissue loss or gangrene of the foot need the return of a foot pulse whenever possible to achieve the most rapid and effective healing. Since 1984 our team approach to the diabetic foot has demonstrated a significant reduction in every category of amputation at the New England Deaconess Hospital and Joslin Diabetes Center.[16] Again, absolute non-weight-bearing is essential until healing is certain. Progressed weight-bearing with modification of footwear prescribed to protect sensitive high-risk areas is closely monitored by careful follow-up.

SUMMARY

Diabetic patients can live in symbiosis with neuropathy, ischemia, and even an altered host defense. Patient and physician education and understanding correlate directly with not only prevention but also the development and successful treatment of diabetic foot problems. The challenge for all health care systems and practitioners is to cost effectively manage lower extremity problems, thereby reducing major amputation in a climate of continually reduced health care dollars. We have shown that our team approach has reduced amputation rate at all levels since 1984 and we have achieved this while reducing the hospital length of stay and cost of care.[17] Quality of care is the best way to reduce the cost of care.

REFERENCES

1. US Department of Health and Human Services: Healthy People 2000—National Health Promotion and Disease Prevention Objectives (DHHS Publication #91-5023). Washington, DC, US Government Printing Office, 1991, pp 73–117.
2. Bolton AJM: The diabetic foot. Med Clin North Am 72:1513, 1988.
3. Grayson ML, Gibbons GW, Balough K, et al: Probing to bone: a useful clinical sign of osteomyelitis in diabetic fetid feet. Submitted for publication.
4. Pecoraro RE, Reiber GE, Burgess EM: Pathways to diabetic limb amputation: basis of prevention: Diabetes Care 13:513, 1990.
5. LoGerfo FW, Coffman JD: Vascular and microvascular disease of the foot in diabetes: implications for foot care. N Engl J Med 311:1615, 1984.
6. Pomposelli FB Jr, Jepson SJ, Gibbons GW, et al: Efficacy of the dorsal pedal bypass for limb salvage in diabetic patients. Vasc Surg 11:745, 1990.
7. Gibbons GW: Diabetic foot sepsis. Semin Vasc Surg 5:244, 1992.
8. Gibbons GW, Eliopoulos G: Infection of the diabetic foot. In Kozak GP, Hoar CS, Rowbatham JL (eds): Management of Diabetic Foot Problems. Philadelphia, Saunders, 1984, pp 92–96.
9. Lipsky BS, Pecoraro RE, Wheat LJ: The diabetic foot: soft tissue and bone infection. Infect Dis Clin North Am 4(3):409, 1990.
10. Gibbons GW: Toe and foot amputations. In Ernst BS, Stanley JC (eds): Current Therapy in Vascular Surgery II. Toronto, BC Decker, 1991, pp 694–696.
11. Karchmer AW, Gibbons GW: Foot infections in diabetics: evaluation and management. In Remington JS, Swartz MH (eds): Current Clinical Topics in Infectious Diseases, 14th ed. Boston, Blackwell Scientific Publications, 1994, pp 1–22.
12. Gibbons GW: The diabetic foot: amputation and drainage of infection. J Vasc Surg 5:791, 1987.
13. Peterson LR, Lissack LM, Canter K, et al: Therapy of lower extremity infection with ciprofloxacin in patients with diabetes mellitus, peripheral vascular disease or both. Am J Med 87:801, 1989.
14. Bamberger DM, Daus GP, Gerding DN, et al: Osteomyelitis in the feet of the diabetic patients: long term results, prognostic factors and the role of antimicrobial and surgical therapy. Am J Med 83:653, 1987.
15. Pomposelli FB Jr, Jepson SJ, Gibbons GW, et al: A flexible approach to infra-popliteal vein grafts in patients with diabetes mellitus. Arch Surg 126:724, 1993.
16. LoGerfo JW, Gibbons GW, Pomposelli FB, et al: Trends in the care of the diabetic foot; expanded role of arterial reconstruction. Arch Surg 127:617, 1992.
17. Gibbons GW, Marcaccio EJ Jr, Burgess ARN, et al: Improved quality of diabetic foot care, 1984 vs 1990: reduced length of stay and costs, insufficient reimbursement. Arch Surg 128:576–581, 1993.

Index

C

I

O

P

Q

R

S